CURRENT

Pediatric Diagnosis & Treatment

W9-BXZ-793

a LANGE medical book

CURRENT

Pediatric Diagnosis & Treatment

14th Edition

Edited by

William W. Hay, Jr., MD
Professor, Department of Pediatrics
Director, Training Program in Neonatal-Perinatal Medicine
Director, Neonatal Clinical Research Center
Section of Neonatology and the Division of Perinatal Medicine and Research
University of Colorado School of Medicine and The Children's Hospital, Denver

Anthony R. Hayward, MD, PhD
Professor, Departments of Pediatrics and Immunology
Head, Section of Pediatric Allergy and Immunology
University of Colorado School of Medicine and The Children's Hospital, Denver

Myron J. Levin, MD
Professor, Departments of Pediatrics and Medicine
Head, Section of Pediatric Infectious Diseases
University of Colorado School of Medicine and The Children's Hospital, Denver

Judith M. Sondheimer, MD
Professor, Department of Pediatrics
Head, Section of Pediatric Gastroenterology, Hepatology, and Nutrition
University of Colorado School of Medicine and The Children's Hospital, Denver

and Associate Authors

The Department of Pediatrics at the University of Colorado School of Medicine is affiliated with
The Children's Hospital of Denver, Colorado.

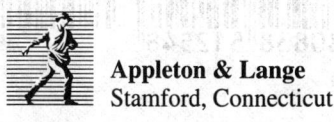
Appleton & Lange
Stamford, Connecticut

Notice: The authors and the publisher of this volume have taken care to make certain that the doses of drugs and schedules of treatment are correct and compatible with the standards generally accepted at the time of publication. Nevertheless, as new information becomes available, changes in treatment and in the use of drugs become necessary. The reader is advised to carefully consult the instruction and information material included in the package insert of each drug or therapeutic agent before administration. This advice is especially important when using, administering, or recommending new or infrequently used drugs. The authors and publisher disclaim all responsibility for any liability, loss, injury, or damage incurred as a consequence, directly or indirectly, of the use and application of any of the contents of this volume.

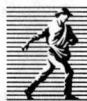

Copyright © 1999 by Appleton & Lange
A Simon & Schuster Company
Copyright © 1997, 1995, 1991, 1987 by Appleton & Lange

All rights reserved. This book, or any parts thereof, may not be used or reproduced in any manner without written permission. For information, address Appleton & Lange, Four Stamford Plaza, PO Box 120041, Stamford, Connecticut 06912-0041.

www.appletonlange.com

99 00 01 02 03 / 10 9 8 7 6 5 4 3 2 1

Prentice Hall International (UK) Limited, *London*
Prentice Hall of Australia Pty. Limited, *Sydney*
Prentice Hall Canada, Inc. *Toronto*
Prentice Hall Hispanoamericana, S.A., *Mexico*
Prentice Hall of India Private Limited, *New Delhi*
Prentice Hall of Japan, Inc., *Tokyo*
Simon & Schuster Asia Pte. Ltd., *Singapore*
Editora Prentice Hall do Brasil Ltda., *Rio de Janeiro*
Prentice Hall, *Upper Saddle River, New Jersey*

ISBN 0-8385-1254-2
ISSN 0093-8556

Acquisitions Editor: Shelley Reinhardt
Senior Development Editor: Cara Lyn Coffey
Development Editor: Isabel Nogueira
Production Editor: Meredith Phillips
Manager of Art Services: Eve Siegel

PRINTED IN THE UNITED STATES OF AMERICA

Table of Contents

Contributors

R. B. Abrams, DDS
Assistant Clinical Professor, Department of Growth and Development, University of Colorado School of Dentistry, Denver; Private Practice Pediatric Dentistry, Longmont, Colorado
Oral Medicine & Dentistry

Frank J. Accurso, MD
Professor, Department of Pediatrics, Section of Pediatric Pulmonary Medicine, University of Colorado School of Medicine and The Children's Hospital, Denver
Internet: accurso.frank@tchden.org
Respiratory Tract & Mediastinum

Edythe A. Albano, MD
Assistant Professor, Department of Pediatrics, Section of Pediatric Hematology and Oncology, University of Colorado School of Medicine; Pediatric Oncologist, The Children's Hospital, Denver
Internet: albano.edie@tchden.org
Neoplastic Disease

Daniel R. Ambruso, MD
Professor, Department of Pediatrics, Section of Pediatric Hematology and Oncology, University of Colorado School of Medicine; Associate Medical Director, Bonfils Blood Center, and The Children's Hospital, Denver
Internet: daniel.ambruso@uchsc.edu
Hematologic Disorders

F. Keith Battan, MD
Assistant Professor, Department of Pediatrics, Sections of Emergency and General Academic Pediatrics, University of Colorado School of Medicine; Associate Director, Emergency Services, The Children's Hospital, Denver
Internet: battan.keith@tchden.org
Emergencies, Injuries, & Poisoning

Donald W. Bechtold, MD
Associate Professor and Co-Director, Child Psychiatry Division; Director, Department of Psychiatry, University of Colorado School of Medicine, Children's Day Psychiatric Hospital, Denver
Internet: dbechtold@crete.uchsc.edu
Psychosocial Aspects of Pediatrics & Child & Adolescent Psychiatric Disorders

Stephen Berman, MD
Professor, Department of Pediatrics, Head, Section of General Academic Pediatrics, University of Colorado School of Medicine and The Children's Hospital; Director of Health Policy, University of Colorado Health Sciences Center, Denver
Ear, Nose, & Throat

Mark Boguniewicz, MD
Associate Professor, Department of Pediatrics, University of Colorado School of Medicine, National Jewish Medical and Research Center, Denver
Internet: boguniewiczm@njc.org
Allergic Disorders

Mark M. Boucek, MD
Professor, Department of Pediatrics, and Head, Section of Pediatric Cardiology, University of Colorado School of Medicine and The Children's Hospital, Denver
Cardiovascular Diseases

Robert M. Brayden, MD
Associate Professor, Department of Pediatrics, Section of General Academic Pediatrics, University of Colorado School of Medicine and The Children's Hospital, Denver
Internet: brayden.robert@tchden.org
Ambulatory Pediatrics

Kenny Chan, MD
Associate Professor, Department of Otolaryngology, University of Colorado School of Medicine; Chairman, Department of Pediatric Otolaryngology, The Children's Hospital, Denver
Internet: chan.kenny@tchden.org
Ear, Nose, & Throat

H. Peter Chase, MD
Professor, Department of Pediatrics, Clinical Director, Barbara Davis Center for Childhood Diabetes, University of Colorado School of Medicine, Denver
Diabetes Mellitus

R. Barkley Clark, MD
Associate Clinical Professor, Department of Psychiatry, Division of Child Psychiatry, University of Colorado School of Medicine, Denver
Psychosocial Aspects of Pediatrics & Child & Adolescent Psychiatric Disorders

Richard C. Dart, MD, PhD
Associate Professor of Surgery, Departments of Medicine and Pharmacy, University of Colorado School of Medicine; Director, Rocky Mountain Poison and Drug Center, Denver
Emergencies, Injuries & Poisoning

Robin R. Deterding, MD
Assistant Professor, Department of Pediatrics, Section of Pediatric Critical Care Medicine, University of Colorado School of Medicine and The Children's Hospital, Denver
Internet: deterding.robin@tchden.org
Respiratory Tract & Mediastinum

Emily L. Dobyns, MD
Assistant Professor, Department of Pediatrics, Section of Pediatric Critical Care Medicine, University of Colorado School of Medicine and The Children's Hospital, Denver
Internet: dobyns.emily@tchden.org
Critical Care

Anthony G. Durmowicz, MD
Assistant Professor, Department of Pediatrics, Section of Pediatric Critical Care Medicine, University of Colorado School of Medicine and The Children's Hospital, Denver
Internet: tony.durmowicz@uchsc.edu
Critical Care

Robert E. Eilert, MD
Professor, Department of Orthopedics, University of Colorado School of Medicine; Chairman, Department of Orthopedic Surgery, The Children's Hospital, Denver
Internet: eilert.robert@tchden.org
Orthopedics

George S. Eisenbarth, MD, PhD
Professor, Departments of Pediatrics, Medicine, and Immunology, University of Colorado School of Medicine; Executive Director, Barbara Davis Center for Childhood Diabetes, Denver
Internet: george.eisenbarth@uchsc.edu
Diabetes Mellitus

Allan M. Eisenbaum, MD
Associate Clinical Professor, Department of Ophthalmology, University of Colorado School of Medicine, Denver
Internet: aeisenoptc@aol.com
Eye

Douglas M. Ford, MD
Associate Professor, Department of Pediatrics, Section of Pediatric Nephrology, University of Colorado School of Medicine and The Children's Hospital, Denver
Internet: ford.douglas@tchden.org
Fluid, Electrolyte, & Acid-Base Disorders & Therapy

Nicholas K. Foreman, MD
Associate Professor, Department of Pediatrics, Section of Pediatric Hematology and Oncology, University of Colorado School of Medicine; Director of Neuro-Oncology, The Children's Hospital, Denver
Neoplastic Disease

Erwin W. Gelfand, MD
Professor, Department of Pediatrics and Microbiology/Immunology, University of Colorado School of Medicine; Chairman, Department of Pediatrics, National Jewish Center for Immunology and Respiratory Medicine, Denver
Internet: gelfande@njc.org
Immunodeficiency

Gaia Georgopoulos, MD
Assistant Professor, Department of Orthopedic Surgery, University of Colorado School of Medicine and The Children's Hospital, Denver
Orthopedics

Edward Goldson, MD
Associate Professor, Department of Pediatrics, Section of Developmental and Behavioral Pediatrics, University of Colorado School of Medicine and The Children's Hospital, Denver
Internet: goldson.edward@tchden.org
Developmental Disorders & Behavioral Problems

Stephen I. Goodman, MD
Professor, Department of Pediatrics, Head, Section of Genetics, Metabolism, and Birth Defects, University of Colorado School of Medicine and The Children's Hospital, Denver
Inborn Errors of Metabolism

Ronald W. Gotlin, MD
Professor, Department of Pediatrics, Section of Pediatric Endocrinology, University of Colorado School of Medicine and The Children's Hospital, Denver
Endocrine Disorders

Carol L. Greene, MD
Associate Professor, Department of Pediatrics, Section of Genetics, Metabolism, and Birth Defects, University of Colorado School of Medicine and The Children's Hospital, Denver
Internet: greene.carol@tchden.org
Inborn Errors of Metabolism

Brian S. Greffe, MD, CM
Assistant Professor, Department of Pediatrics, Section of Pediatric Hematology and Oncology, University of Colorado School of Medicine and The Children's Hospital, Denver
Internet: greffe.brian@tchden.org
Neoplastic Disease

Randi Jenssen Hagerman, MD
Professor, Department of Pediatrics, Head, Section of Developmental and Behavioral Medicine, University of Colorado School of Medicine and The Children's Hospital, Denver
Growth & Development

Ann C. Halbower, MD
Assistant Professor, Department of Pediatrics, Section of Pediatric Pulmonary Medicine, University of Colorado School of Medicine and The Children's Hospital, Denver
Internet: halbower.ann@tchden.org
Respiratory Tract & Mediastinum

K. Michael Hambidge, MD, BChir, ScD
Professor, Department of Pediatrics, University of Colorado School of Medicine and The Children's Hospital, Denver
Internet: michael.hambidge@uchsc.edu
Normal Childhood Nutrition & Its Disorders

Keith B. Hammond, MS, FIMLS
Senior Instructor, Departments of Pediatrics and Pathology, and Director, Pediatric Clinical Research Center Laboratory, University of Colorado School of Medicine and The Children's Hospital, Denver
Internet: keith.hammond@uchsc.edu
Normal Biochemical & Hematologic Values

Anthony R. Hayward, MD, PhD
Professor, Departments of Pediatrics and Immunology, and Head, Section of Pediatric Allergy and Immunology, University of Colorado School of Medicine and The Children's Hospital, Denver
Internet: anthony.hayward@uchsc.edu
Immunodeficiency

Roxann M. Headley, MD
Assistant Professor, Department of Pediatrics, Section of General Academic Pediatrics, University of Colorado School of Medicine; Medical Director, Child Health Clinic, The Children's Hospital, Denver
Ambulatory Pediatrics

Desmond B. Henry, Jr., MD
Assistant Clinical Professor, Department of Anesthesiology and Pediatrics, University of Colorado School of Medicine; Director, Surgical Services, The Children's Hospital, Denver
Internet: henry.desmond@tchden.org
Critical Care

J. Roger Hollister, MD
Professor, Department of Pediatrics, University of Colorado School of Medicine; Head, Section of Pediatric Rheumatology, University of Colorado and The Children's Hospital, Denver
Rheumatic Diseases

David W. Kaplan, MD, MPH
Professor, Department of Pediatrics, and Head, Section of Adolescent Medicine, University of Colorado School of Medicine and The Children's Hospital, Denver
Internet: kaplan.david@tchden.org
Adolescence

Michael S. Kappy, MD, PhD
Professor, Department of Pediatrics, and Head, Section of Pediatric Endocrinology, University of Colorado School of Medicine and The Children's Hospital, Denver
Internet: kappy.michael@tchden.org
Endocrine Disorders

Nancy F. Krebs, MD, MS
Assistant Professor, Department of Pediatrics, and Head, Section of Nutrition, and Associate Director, University of Colorado Center for Human Nutrition, University of Colorado School of Medicine and The Children's Hospital, Denver
Normal Childhood Nutrition & Its Disorders

Richard D. Krugman, MD
Professor, Department of Pediatrics, and Dean, University of Colorado School of Medicine, Denver
Internet: richard.krugman@uchsc.edu
Child Abuse & Neglect

Peter A. Lane, MD
Associate Professor, Department of Pediatrics, Section of Pediatric Hematology and Oncology, and Bone Marrow Transplantation, and Director, Colorado Sickle Cell Treatment and Research Center, University of Colorado School of Medicine and The Children's Hospital, Denver
Hematologic Disorders

Gary L. Larsen, MD
Professor, Department of Pediatrics, and Head, Section of Pediatric Pulmonary Medicine, University of Colorado School of Medicine; Senior Faculty Member, National Jewish Medical and Research Center, Denver
Respiratory Tract & Mediastinum

Donald Y. M. Leung, MD, PhD
Professor, Department of Pediatrics, University of Colorado School of Medicine; Head, Division of Pediatric Allergy-Immunology, National Jewish Medical and Research Center, Denver
Allergic Disorders

Myron J. Levin, MD
Professor, Departments of Pediatrics and Medicine, and Head, Section of Pediatric Infectious Diseases, University of Colorado School of Medicine and The Children's Hospital, Denver
Internet: myron.levin@uchsc.edu
Infections: Viral & Rickettsial
Infections: Parasitic & Mycotic

Stanley L. Loftness, MD
Assistant Clinical Professor, Department of Pediatrics, and Staff Anesthesiologist and Intensivist, University of Colorado School of Medicine and The Children's Hospital, Denver
Critical Care

Gary M. Lum, MD
Professor, Departments of Pediatrics and Medicine, and Head, Section of Pediatric Nephrology, University of Colorado School of Medicine and The Children's Hospital, Denver
Internet: lum.gary@tchden.org
Kidney & Urinary Tract

Kathleen A. Mammel, MD
Clinical Assistant Professor, Wayne State University School of Medicine, Detroit; Chief, Adolescent Pediatrics, William Beaumont Hospital, Royal Oak, Michigan
Adolescence

David K. Manchester, MD
Associate Professor, Departments of Pediatrics and Pharmacology, Section of Genetics, Metabolism, and Birth Defects, University of Colorado School of Medicine; Co-Director, Division of Genetic Services, The Children's Hospital, Denver
Genetics & Dysmorphology

Elizabeth J. McFarland, MD
Assistant Professor, Department of Pediatrics, Section of Pediatric Infectious Diseases, University of Colorado School of Medicine and The Children's Hospital, Denver
Human Immunodeficiency Virus (HIV) Infection

Susan Miller, PharmD
Adjunct Assistant Professor, School of Pharmacy, University of Colorado School of Medicine, Denver
Internet: larkin.susan@tchden.org
Drug Therapy

Paul G. Moe, MD
Professor, Departments of Pediatrics and Neurology, University of Colorado School of Medicine and the Children's Hospital, Denver
Internet:moe.paul@tchden.org
Neurologic & Muscular Disorders

Joseph G. Morelli, MD
Associate Professor, Departments of Dermatology and Pediatrics, University of Colorado School of Medicine, Denver
Internet: joseph.morelli@uchsc.edu
Skin

William A. Mueller, DMD
Chairman, Department of Pediatric Dentistry, The Children's Hospital; Clinical Associate Professor, University of Colorado School of Dentistry, Denver
Internet: mueller.william@tchden.org
Oral Medicine & Dentistry

Michael R. Narkewicz, MD
Associate Professor, Department of Pediatrics, Section of Pediatric Gastroenterology, Hepatology, and Nutrition, and The Pediatric Liver Center, University of Colorado School of Medicine and The Children's Hospital, Denver
Liver & Pancreas

Rachelle Nuss, MD
Associate Professor, Department of Pediatrics, Section of Pediatric Hematology and Oncology, University of Colorado School of Medicine and The Children's Hospital, Denver
Internet: rnuss@msrhc.uhcoloorado.edu
Hematologic Disorders

Lorrie F. Odom, MD
Professor, Department of Pediatrics, Section of Pediatric Hematology and Oncology, University of Colorado School of Medicine; Director, Clinical Oncology, The Children's Hospital, Denver
Internet: odom.lorrie@tchden.org
Neoplastic Disease

John W. Ogle, MD
Professor and Vice Chairman, Department of Pediatrics, University of Colorado School of Medicine, Denver; Director, Department of Pediatrics, Denver General Hospital
Internet:jogle@dhha.org
Antimicrobial Therapy; Infections: Bacterial & Spirochetal

Christopher M. Paap, PharmD, BCPS
Medical Sciences Manager, Bristol-Myers Squibb, Highlands Ranch, Colorado
Internet: paapc@sprynet.com
Drug Therapy

Adam A. Rosenberg, MD
Professor, Department of Pediatrics, Section of Neonatology, University of Colorado School of Medicine and The Children's Hospital; Medical Director, Neonatal High Risk Follow-up Clinic; Medical Director, Newborn Service, University Hospital, Denver
Internet:arosenberg@ewok.uhcolorado.edu
The Newborn Infant

Barry H. Rumack, MD
Clinical Professor, Department of Pediatrics, University of Colorado School of Medicine; President and Chief Executive Officer, Micromedex, Inc., Denver
Emergencies, Injuries, & Poisoning

Michael S. Schaffer, MD
Associate Professor, Department of Pediatrics, Section of Pediatric Cardiology; Director of Electrophysiology; University of Colorado School of Medicine and The Children's Hospital, Denver
Internet:schaffer.michael@tchden.org
Cardiovascular Diseases

Alan R. Seay, MD
Professor, Departments of Pediatrics and Neurology, and Chief, Division of Child Neurology, University of Colorado School of Medicine and The Children's Hospital, Denver
Neurologic & Muscular Disorders

Eric J. Sigel, MD
Assistant Professor, Department of Pediatrics, Section of Adolescent Medicine, and Clinical Director, Adolescent Clinic, University of Colorado School of Medicine and The Children's Hospital, Denver
Internet: sigel.eric@tchden.org
Sexually Transmitted Diseases

Eric A. F. Simoes, MD, DCH
Associate Professor, Department of Pediatrics, Section of Pediatric Infectious Diseases, University of Colorado School of Medicine and The Children's Hospital, Denver
Immunization

Andrew P. Sirotnak, MD
Assistant Professor of Pediatrics, University of Colorado School of Medicine; Director, Kempe Child Protection Team, The Children's Hospital, Denver
Internet: sirotnak.andrew@tchden.org
Child Abuse & Neglect

Robert H. Slover, MD
Associate Professor, Department of Pediatrics, Section of Pediatric Endocrinology and the Barbara Davis Center for Childhood Diabetes, University of Colorado School of Medicine and The Children's Hospital, Denver
Internet: robert.slover@uchsc.edu
Endocrine Disorders

Ronald J. Sokol, MD
Professor, Department of Pediatrics, Section of Pediatric Gastroenterology, Hepatology, and Nutrition; Medical Director, Pediatric Liver Center; Director, Pediatric Clinical Research Center, University of Colorado School of Medicine and The Children's Hospital, Denver
Internet: sokol.ronald@tchden.org
Liver & Pancreas

Judith M. Sondheimer, MD
Professor, Department of Pediatrics, and Head, Section of Pediatric Gastroenterology, Hepatology, and Nutrition, University of Colorado School of Medicine and The Children's Hospital, Denver
Internet: sondheimer.judith@tchden.org
Gastrointestinal Tract

Kurt R. Stenmark, MD
Professor, Department of Pediatrics, and Head, Section of Pediatric Critical Care Medicine, University of Colorado School of Medicine and The Children's Hospital, Denver
Internet: kurt.stenmark@uchsc.edu
Critical Care

Catherine Stevens-Simon, MD
Associate Professor, Department of Pediatrics, Section of Adolescent Medicine, University of Colorado School of Medicine and The Children's Hospital, Denver
Substance Abuse in Pediatrics

Janet M. Stewart, MD
Associate Professor, Department of Pediatrics, Section of Genetics, Metabolism, and Birth Defects, University of Colorado School of Medicine and The Children's Hospital, Denver
Genetics & Dysmorphology

Linda C. Stork, MD
Associate Professor, Department of Pediatrics, Section of Hematology and Oncology, University of Colorado School of Medicine and The Children's Hospital, Denver
Internet: stork.linda@tchden.org
Neoplastic Disease

Eva Sujansky, MD
Associate Professor, Departments of Pediatrics and Biochemistry & Mollecular Genetics, Section of Genetics, Metabolism and Birth Defects, University of Colorado School of Medicine and the Children's Hospital; Co-Director, Division of Genetic Services, The Children's Hospital, Denver
Internet: sujansky.eva@tchden.org
Genetics & Dysmorphology

Elizabeth H. Thilo, MD
Associate Professor, Department of Pediatrics, Section of Neonatology, University of Colorado School of Medicine and The Children's Hospital; Medical Director of Nurseries, Centura-St. Anthony Central Hospital, Denver
Internet: thilo.elizabeth@tchden.org
The Newborn Infant

Adriana Weinberg, MD
Assistant Professor, Departments of Pediatrics and Medicine, and Director, Diagnostic Virology Laboratory, University of Colorado School of Medicine, Denver
Internet: adriana.weinberg@uchsc.edu
Infections: Parasitic & Mycotic

William L. Weston, MD
Professor and Chairman, Department of Dermatology, and Professor, Department of Pediatrics, University of Colorado School of Medicine, Denver.
Skin

Carl W. White, MD
Professor, Department of Pediatrics, Section of Pediatric Pulmonary Medicine, University of Colorado School of Medicine; Senior Faculty Member, National Jewish Medical and Research Center, Denver
Respiratory Tract & Mediastinum

James W. Wiggins, Jr., MD
Clinical Professor, Department of Pediatrics, Section of Pediatric Cardiology, University of Colorado School of Medicine and The Children's Hospital, Denver
Cardiovascular Diseases

Robert R. Wolfe, MD
Professor, Department of Pediatrics, Section of Pediatric Cardiology, University of Colorado School of Medicine and The Children's Hospital, Denver
Internet: wolfe.robert@tchden.org
Cardiovascular Diseases

Philip S. Zeitler, MD, PhD
Assistant Professor of Pediatrics, Section of Pediatric Endocrinology, University of Colorado School of Medicine and The Children's Hospital, Denver
Internet: zeitlerp@jove.uchsc.edu
Endocrine Disorders

Preface

The 14th edition of *Current Pediatric Diagnosis & Treatment* features practical, up-to-date, well-referenced information on the care of children from birth through infancy and adolescence. *CPDT* emphasizes the clinical aspects of pediatric care while also covering the important underlying principles. Its goal is to provide a guide to diagnosis, understanding, and treatment of the medical problems of all pediatric patients in an easy-to-use and readable format.

INTENDED AUDIENCE

Like all Lange medical books, *CPDT* provides a concise yet comprehensive source of current information. Students will find *CPDT* an authoritative introduction to pediatrics and an excellent source for reference and review. Residents in pediatrics (and other specialties) will appreciate the detailed descriptions of diseases and diagnostic and therapeutic procedures. Pediatricians, family practitioners, nurses, and other health-care providers who work with infants and children also will find *CPDT* a useful reference on management aspects of pediatric medicine.

COVERAGE

Forty-one chapters cover a wide range of topics, including normal growth and development, neonatal medicine, emergency and critical care medicine, and diagnosis and treatment of specific disorders according to major problems and organ systems. A wealth of tables and figures summarize such important information as acute and critical care procedures in the delivery room, the office, the emergency room, and the critical care unit; anti-infective agents; drug dosages; immunization schedules; differential diagnosis; and the development screening tests. The final chapter is a handy guide to normal laboratory values.

NEW TO THE EDITION

The 14th edition of *CPDT* remains an up-to-date, comprehensive pediatric treatise, but this edition is *the most comprehensive revision to date* and a significant improvement of this classic book. The editors and contributing authors have continued to substantially revise the book, providing recent medical advances and increasing the book's emphasis on ambulatory care, acute critical care, and the practical approach to pediatric disorders. As editors and practicing pediatricians, we have tried to ensure that each chapter reflects the needs and realities of day-to-day practice.

New Editor: Judith M. Sondheimer, MD, has joined the 14th edition of *CPDT* as editor, replacing Dr. Jessie Groothuis. Dr. Sondheimer is Professor of Pediatrics at the Univeristy of Colorado School of Medicine/The Children's Hospital and Head of the Section of Pediatric Gastroenterology, Hepatology, and Nutrition. Dr. Sondheimer is a nationally acclaimed clinician and scientist and brings to our book a wealth of experience in scholarship and editing.

New Chapters: Four new chapters deal with some of the most important and timely subjects in pediatric medicine today:

   3. Developmental Disorders & Behavioral Problems
   5. Substance Abuse in Pediatrics
 32. Allergic Disorders
 39. Fluid, Electrolyte, and Acid-Base Disorders and Therapy

Chapter Revisions: Six chapters have been extensively revised, with new authors added in several cases, reflecting substantial new information in each of their areas of pediatric medicine. These chapters are as follows:

   2. The Newborn Infant
   6. Psychosocial Aspects of Pediatrics & Child & Adolescent Psychiatric Disorders
   7. Child Abuse & Neglect
   8. Ambulatory Pediatrics
 11. Emergencies, Injuries, & Poisoning
 28. Endocrine Disorders

All other chapters are substantially revised and references have been updated.

ACKNOWLEDGMENTS

The editors want to acknowledge the superb editorial work done over the past four editions of *CPDT* by Dr. Jessie Groothuis. We wish her well in her new position as Director of Vaccine Clinical Research, Ross Products Division, Abbott Laboratories, Columbus, Ohio.

William W. Hay, Jr., MD
Anthony R. Hayward, MD, PhD
Myron J. Levin, MD
Judith M. Sondheimer, MD

Denver
November 1998

Growth & Development

Randi Jenssen Hagerman, MD

The continuous and dynamic process of growth and development in children is the subject of this chapter. The author's intention is to emphasize the interactive aspects of physical, cognitive, social, and emotional development so that the reader can appreciate the impact of each of these domains throughout the span of development.

The chapter is divided into sections according to age so that the interactions of central nervous system maturation; physical, cognitive, and emotional growth; genetic variations; and environmental influences can be discussed at critical age levels. Major theories of development (Freud, Piaget, Erikson) are reviewed, and longitudinal changes are summarized in charts and tables to serve as an organizational framework for study and retention.

THE NEWBORN

Normal newborns are endowed with a set of reflexes—including rooting and sucking reflexes—that serve to facilitate survival as well as remarkable sensory abilities. The newborn is no longer considered a "blank slate" or *tabula rasa* that gradually develops in response to environmental influences. Instead, the newborn is seen as having genetic strengths and weaknesses in neurocognitive organization that are reflected in temperament, adaptability, responsiveness, and interaction with the environment. These responses in turn prompt reciprocal interactions from the parents, which further shape development. The Neonatal Behavioral Assessment Scale by Brazelton was developed to measure many of the newborn's characteristics of temperament, including social behavior, orienting responses to stimuli, ability to deal with disturbing stimuli, state of arousal, and motor skills. When these abilities are described to the mother, this assessment can further sensitize her to the unique aspects of her child's behavior and responsiveness. This knowledge may in turn improve their interactions.

The newborn has significant sensory abilities. Hearing is well developed at birth, and the baby shows a preference for speech sounds over other sounds. The infant becomes alert and oriented to a female voice with high-pitched tones more readily than to a low-pitched male voice. The lower-frequency tones of a male voice are more likely to soothe an infant. High-pitched crying is distressing not only to the newborn but also to adults. Infants can shut out loud or aversive stimuli and simply not respond. Within the first few weeks of life, they learn to recognize the mother's voice and differentiate it from other female voices.

Smell is well-developed at birth and plays a significant role in how infants orient themselves to the environment. Infants turn away from aversive smells and respond positively to pleasant ones. By 1 week of age, breast-fed infants recognize and discriminate the smell of their mother's breast milk. They recognize the odor of their mother, not that of milk alone. The infant has a definite taste preference for sweet at birth. Infants have more taste buds than adults do and avoid bitter or aversive tastes.

At birth, the retina is well developed, but the lens is rather immobile. Fixation and tracking through the visual field are well developed by 2 months of age. Infants prefer to gaze at a human face rather than geometric designs, and they also prefer curved lines, bright colors, and high contrast. The length of time an infant fixates on a paired visual stimulus has been interpreted as visual preference and has been positively correlated with later cognitive development. Visual fixation tasks are the basis of the "infant IQ" tests marketed recently. Although visual acuity is poor at birth (approximately 20/400), it improves rapidly in the first 6 months of life to 20/40.

[Newborn age 0–3]
    http://www.zerotothree.org. (A web site for information and research on physical, cognitive, and social development of infants and toddlers.)

Brazelton TB: *Neonatal Behavioral Assessment Scale,* 3rd ed. MacKeith Press, 1995.

Gemelli R: *Normal Child and Adolescent Development.* American Psychiatric Press, 1996.

THE FIRST YEAR

Crying is common in the first few weeks of life. It gradually increases during the first 6–12 weeks because it is the main modality by which infants respond to stimuli, both aversive and nonaversive. Crying can be a response to a variety of stimuli, including hunger, a wet diaper, fear, fatigue, and overstimulation. Crying gradually diminishes after 12 weeks of age as the infant develops other responses, such as smiling or reaching, or becomes more adept at self-soothing, such as by sucking the fingers or thumb. In the first weeks of life, however, crying can be a distressing problem for the parents. Crying associated with irritability is often called colic. Particularly sensitive infants with a low tolerance for stimuli can be irritable and difficult to deal with at home. It is useful to help parents understand the infant's temperament and to teach them techniques for avoiding excessive stimuli—because parents often respond to excessive crying by creating excessive stimuli. Parents should be taught ways to calm the child, such as offering nonnutritive sucking, rocking or singing to the child, and walking while holding the child. Perhaps most important for the parents is an understanding of the developmental aspects of crying and the emergence of improved coping skills in the baby after 12 weeks of age.

Piaget describes the first 2 years of life as the sensorimotor period, during which infants learn with increasing sophistication how to link sensory input from the environment with a motor response. Infants build on primitive reflex patterns of behavior (termed "schemata"—sucking is an example) and constantly incorporate or assimilate new experiences. The schemata evolve over time as infants accommodate new experiences and as new levels of cognitive ability unfold in an orderly sequence. Enhancement of neural networks through dendritic branching occurs in spurts throughout the sensorimotor period. In the first year of life, the infant's perception of reality revolves around itself and what it can see or touch. It follows the trajectory of an object through the field of vision, but before 6 months the object ceases to exist once it leaves the field of vision. At 9–12 months, the infant gradually develops the concept of object permanence, or the realization that objects exist even when not seen. The development of object permanence correlates with enhanced frontal activity on the EEG. The concept attaches first to the image of the mother because of her emotional importance and is a critical part of attachment behavior (discussed below). In the second year, children extend their ability to manipulate objects by using instruments, first by imitation and later by trial and error (Table 1–1).

Freud describes the first year of life as the oral stage because so many of the infant's needs are fulfilled by oral means. Nutrition is obtained through sucking on the breast or bottle, and self-soothing also occurs through sucking on fingers or a pacifier. This is a stage of symbiosis with the mother during which the boundaries between mother and infant are blurred. The baby's needs are totally met by the mother, and the mother has been described as manifesting "narcissistic possessiveness" of the infant. This is a very positive interaction in the bidirectional attachment process called "bonding." The parents learn to be aware of and interpret the infant's cues, which reflect its needs. A more sensitive emotional interaction process develops that can be seen in the mirroring of facial expressions by mother and infant and in their mutual engagement in cycles of attention and inattention, which further develops into social play. A mother who is depressed or cannot respond to the baby's expressions and cues has a profound adverse effect on its future development. Erikson's terms of basic trust versus mistrust are another way of describing the reciprocal interaction that characterizes this stage (Table 1–1).

Turn-taking games, which occur between 3 and 6 months of age, are a pleasure for both the parents and the infant and are an extension of mirroring behavior. They also represent an early form of imitative behavior, which is important in later social and cognitive development. More sophisticated games, such as "peek-a-boo," occur at approximately 9 months. The infant's thrill at the reappearance of the face that vanished momentarily demonstrates the emerging understanding of object permanence.

Eight to 9 months is also a critical time in the attachment process because this is when separation anxiety and stranger anxiety become marked. The infant at this stage is able to appreciate discrepant events that match previously known schemata only partially. These new events cause uncertainty and subsequently fear and anxiety. The infant must be able to retrieve previous schemata and incorporate new information over an extended time. These abilities are developed by 8 months and give rise to the fears that subsequently develop: stranger anxiety and separation anxiety. In stranger anxiety, the infant analyzes the face of a stranger, detects the mismatch with previous schemata, and may subsequently respond with fear or anxiety, leading to crying. In separation anxiety, the child perceives the difference between the mother's presence and her absence by remembering the schema of her presence. Perceiving the inconsistency, the child first becomes uncertain and then anxious and fearful. This begins at 8 months, reaches a peak at 15 months, and disappears by the end of 2 years in a relatively orderly progression as central nervous system maturation facilitates the development of new skills. A parent can put the child's understanding of object permanence to good use by placing a picture of the mother near the child or by leaving an object (eg, her sweater) where the child can see it during her absence. A visual substitute for her actual presence may comfort the child.

Table 1–1. Perspectives of human behavior.[1]

Age	Theories of Development			Skill Areas		Psychopathology
	Freud	Erikson	Piaget	Language	Motor	
Birth to 18 months	Oral	Basic trust versus mistrust	Sensorimotor	Body actions; crying; naming; pointing	Reflex sitting, reaching, grasping, walking	Autism; anaclitic depression, colic; disorders of attachment; feeding, sleeping problems
18 months–3 years	Anal	Autonomy versus shame, doubt	Symbolic (preoperational)	Sentences; telegraph jargon	Climbing, running	Separation issues; negativism; fearfulness; constipation; shyness, withdrawal
3–6 years	Oedipal	Initiative versus guilt	Intuition (preoperational)	Connective words; can be readily understood	Increased coordination; tricycle; jumping	Enuresis; encopresis; anxiety; aggressive acting out; phobias; nightmares
6–11 years	Latency	Industry versus inferiority	Concrete operational	Subordinate sentences; reading and writing; language reasoning	Increased skills; sports, recreational cooperative games	School phobias; obsessive reactions; conversion reactions; depressive equivalents
12–17 years	Adolescence (genital)	Identity versus role confusion	Formal operational	Reason abstract; using language; abstract manipulation	Refinement of skills	Delinquency; promiscuity; schizophrenia; anorexia nervosa; suicide
17–30 years	Young adulthood	Intimacy versus isolation	Formal operational	Reason abstract; using language; abstract manipulation	Refinement of skills	Schizophrenia; borderline personality; adjustment disorders; development of intimate relationship and difficulties with relationships
30–60 years	Adulthood	Generativity versus stagnation	Formal operational	Reason abstract; using language; abstract manipulation	Refinement of skills	Depression; self-doubts; career development issues; family, social network; neuroses
60 years and over	Old age	Ego integration versus despair	Formal operational		Loss of functions (?)	Involutional depression; anxiety; anger; increased dependency

[1]Adapted and reproduced, with permission, from Dixon S: Setting the stage: Theories and concepts of child development. In: *Encounters With Children*, 2nd ed. Dixon S, Stein M (editors). Year Book, 1992.

Bayley N (editor): *Bayley Scales of Infant Development,* 2nd ed. Psychological Corporation, 1993.

Fischer KW, Rose SP: Dynamic development of coordination of components in brain and behavior. In: *Human Behavior and the Developing Brain.* Dawson G, Fischer KW (editors). Guilford Press, 1994.

Papousek M, Papousek H: Infantile persistent crying, state regulation, and interaction with parents; a systems view. In: *Child Development and Behavioral Pediatrics.* Bornstein MH, Genevro IL (editors). Lawrence Erlbaum Associates, 1996.

GROWTH IN THE FIRST 3 YEARS

Increase in fetal length is most rapid during the fourth to sixth months of gestation. However, adipose tissue begins to develop at 7 months, and weight gain accelerates, causing fetal weight to double during the last 2 months in utero. The rate of growth of males in late fetal development and during the first 6 months postnatally is more rapid than that of females because of the higher level of testosterone. The birth weight of the newborn correlates with the size, nutritional state, and general health of the mother and represents the influence of uterine constraints on ultimate size. Newborns may lose up to 10% of their birth weight in the first few days of life, but with normal nutrition birth weight is regained in about 10 days. The infant subsequently gains approximately 30 g/d for the first several months.

After the first 6 months, genetic factors influencing ultimate height begin to exert their effect. The growth percentile may therefore shift significantly in the first 4–18 months. This shift can be either up or down. An infant who is small for gestational age and has a genetic predisposition to larger stature usually experiences accelerated growth in the first 6 months, and by 18 months a relatively stable new growth percentile is established. The downward shift is seen in large infants who have a genetic predisposition to short stature. A fall-off in growth percentiles may be misconstrued as growth deficiency, or failure to thrive. A stable growth percentile should be achieved by 18 months of age.

By 1 year of age, infants weigh three times as much as they did at birth and are 1½ times as long. By age 2, the growth velocity curve has stabilized into the rate for mid childhood, which is a weight gain of 2–3 kg/y and a height gain of 5–7.5 cm/y (Figures 1–1 to 1–6). At the second birthday, a child has attained approximately 50% of its adult height.

The energy requirement during growth also changes dramatically in the first few years of life. Approximately 110 kcal/kg/d is necessary in early infancy because up to 40% of this total energy requirement is used for growth. The percentage used for growth gradually decreases to 3% at 2 years and remains at this level even during adolescence. After age 2 years, the overall energy requirement gradually decreases from 90 kcal/kg/d to 60 kcal/kg/d during mid childhood, and the majority of the energy expenditure is accounted for by activity and the basal metabolic rate of the tissues. The gradual decrease is secondary to a decline in the relative mass of organs, such as the brain and the liver, that have a high requirement for energy compared with resting muscle. The relative energy expended during activity increases in adolescence, particularly for males. In males, the percentage of body weight that is muscle increases from 22% at 3 months to 35% at 5 years and to 40% at maturity. In contrast, organ weight is 17% of body weight in the infant, with 75% of organ weight accounted for by the brain. By maturity, only 5% of body weight is organ weight. Fat increases during the first year of life from 12% of body weight at birth. After the infant begins to walk and explore, however, the proportion of fat decreases and remains stable throughout childhood. In adolescence, the proportion of body weight that is fat increases with sexual maturation in girls but not in boys. For further information, see Chapter 10.

Falkner F, Tanner JM (editors): *Developmental Biology: Prenatal Growth.* Vol 1 of *Human Growth: A Comprehensive Treatise,* 2nd ed. Plenum, 1986.

Falkner F, Tanner JM (editors): *Postnatal Growth Neurobiology.* Vol 2 of *Human Growth: A Comprehensive Treatise,* 2nd ed. Plenum, 1986.

Buckler IMH: *Growth Disorders in Children.* BMJ Publishing Group, 1994.

Brain Growth

About 100 billion neurons are present in the fully developed brain, and replication of neurons is completed before birth. Most of this growth occurs in the first 3 months of gestation. Cell density subsequently decreases rapidly until birth. After birth, the decrease is slower and ceases at 15 months. At birth, the head is 75% of its adult size and makes up 25% of the baby's length. This ratio changes dramatically in time so that by 25 years of age, the head measures one-eighth of body length. Postnatally, the brain continues to grow rapidly, completing half of its lifetime growth by the end of the first year. Postnatal growth is the result of an increase in white matter and a proliferation of synaptic connections. Environmental stimulation enhances synaptic maturity and dendritic branching. After age 2 years, head circumference increases only 2 cm/y during mid childhood (see Figures 1–5 and 1–6). By 7 years of age, 90% of brain growth is completed, and many 10-year-olds have achieved adult brain weight.

The cerebellum is the area of the gray matter that develops last. It begins its growth at 30 weeks of gestation and ends at approximately 1 year of age. It is thus particularly vulnerable to trauma, which may occur in late gestation or during delivery. The spinal cord extends through the length of the neural canal until the third month of gestation. After this time, the torso of the fetus grows faster than the spinal cord, which is fixed in position superiorly by the brain. The lower end of the spinal cord subsequently rests at a gradually higher vertebral level through later fetal life and, by the time of birth, is located at the third lumbar vertebra. The spinal cord doubles its weight in the first year of life and has increased eightfold by adulthood.

Myelinization begins in the spinal cord by the fourth month of gestation and begins in the brain during the last trimester. At birth, the autonomic system is matured and myelinated. The cranial nerves, except for the optic and olfactory nerves, are also myelinated. The cortex and most of its connection to the thalamus and basal ganglia are incompletely myelinated. It takes at least 2 years for myelinization of these areas and the spinal cord to be complete.

Newborn Reflexes

Reflex movement begins in fetal development as early as 9 weeks of gestation. However, most of the reflexes associated with the newborn develop

GIRLS: BIRTH TO 36 MONTHS
PHYSICAL GROWTH NCHS PERCENTILES*

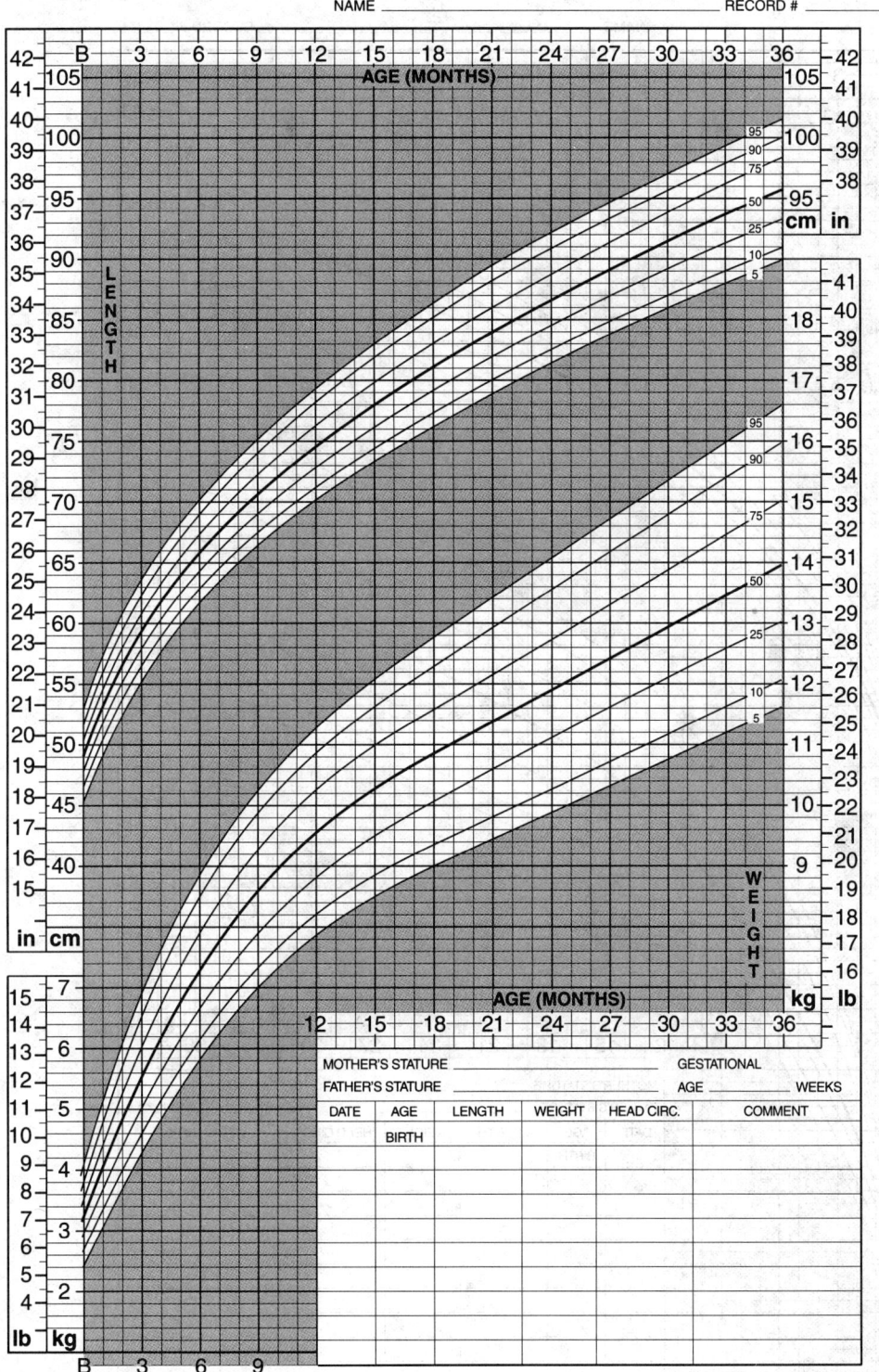

Figure 1–1. Percentile standards for weight and height in girls birth to 3 years. (Reproduced, with permission, from Ross Laboratories, Columbus, OH. © 1982 Ross Laboratories.)

BOYS: BIRTH TO 36 MONTHS
PHYSICAL GROWTH NCHS PERCENTILES*

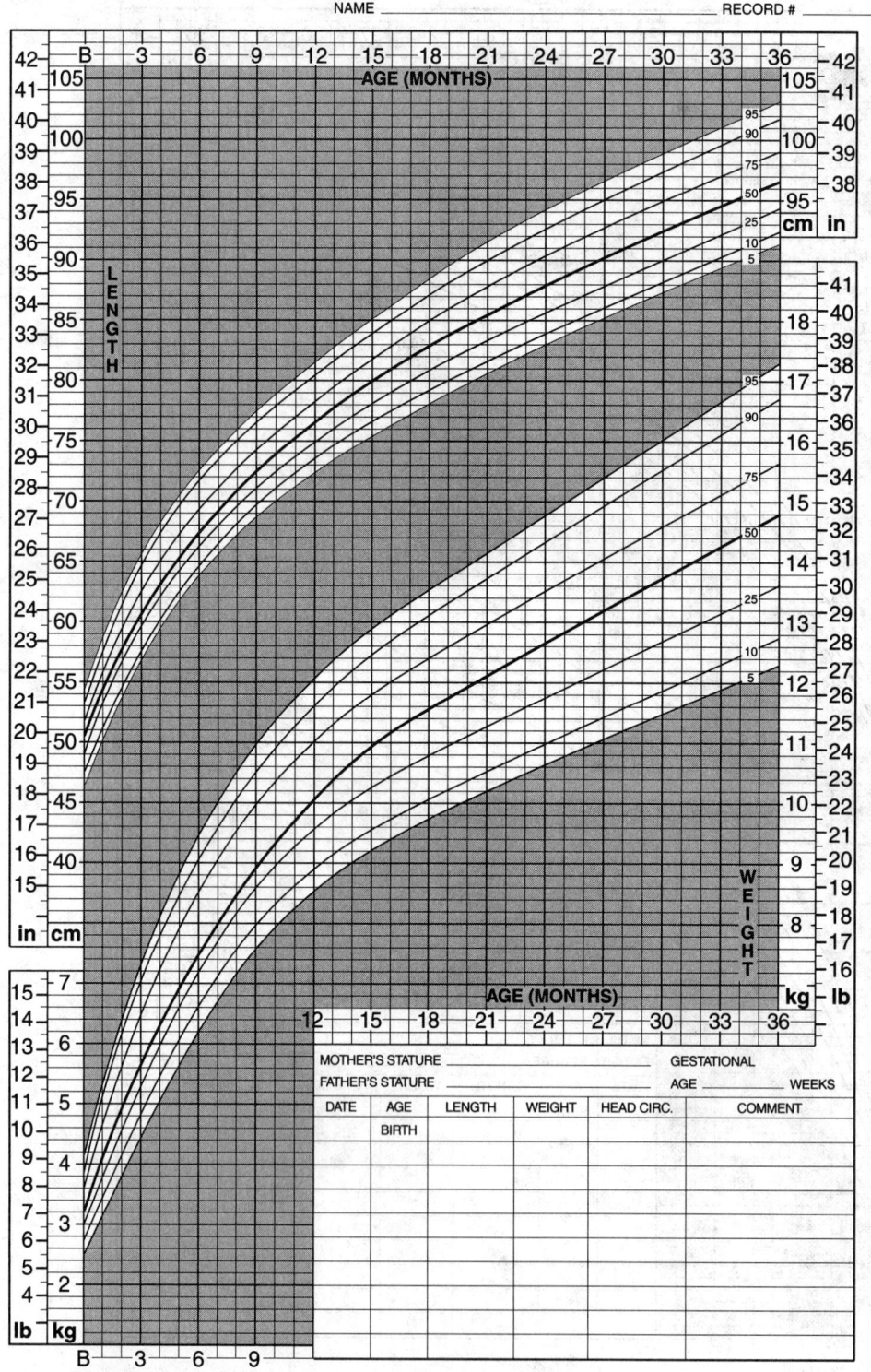

Figure 1–2. Percentile standards for weight and height in boys birth to 3 years. (Reproduced, with permission, from Ross Laboratories, Columbus, OH. © 1982 Ross Laboratories.)

GIRLS: 2 TO 18 YEARS
PHYSICAL GROWTH
NCHS PERCENTILES*

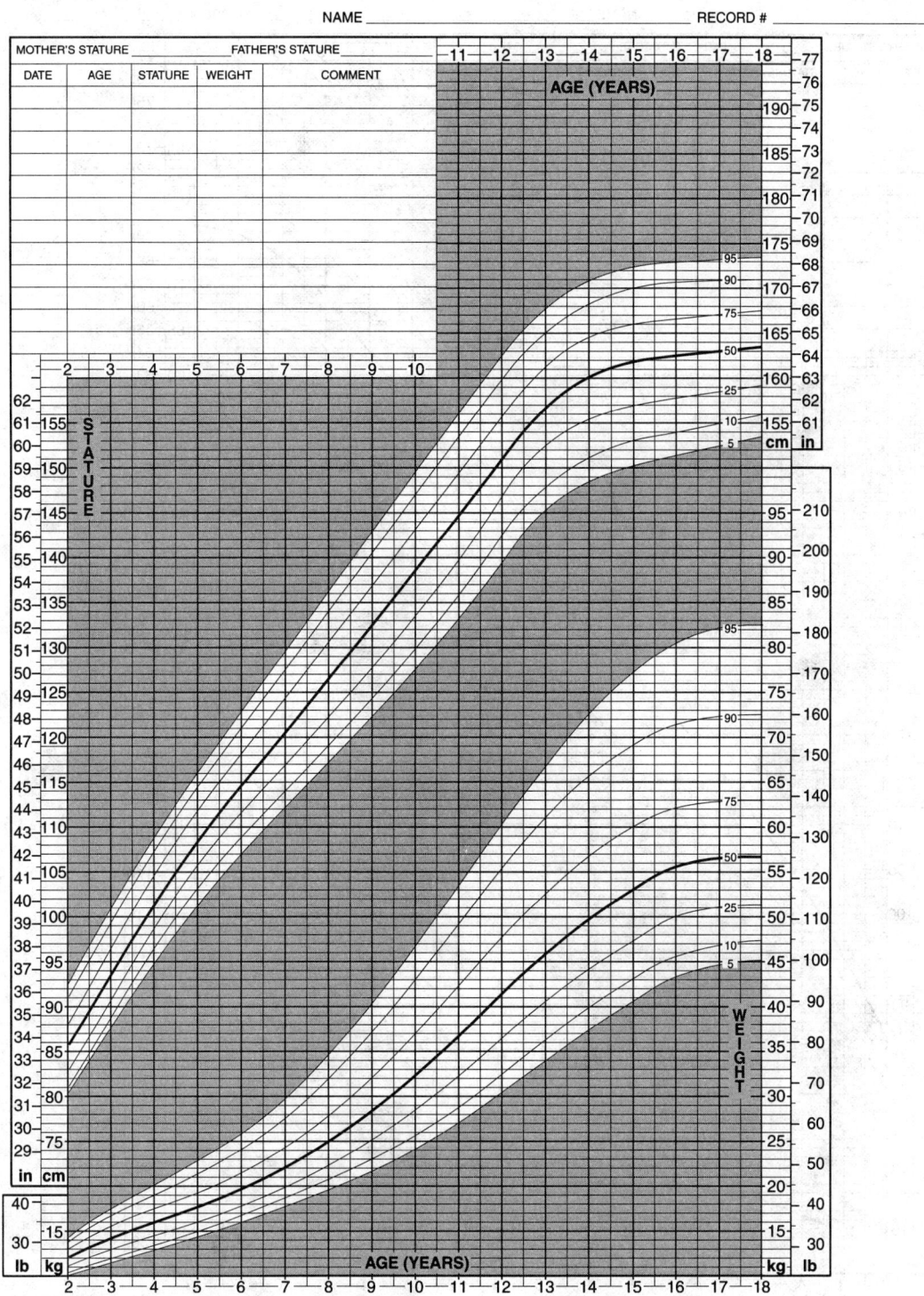

Figure 1–3. Percentile standards for weight and height in girls 2–18 years. (Reproduced, with permission, from Ross Laboratories, Columbus, OH. © 1982 Ross Laboratories.)

BOYS: 2 TO 18 YEARS
PHYSICAL GROWTH
NCHS PERCENTILES*

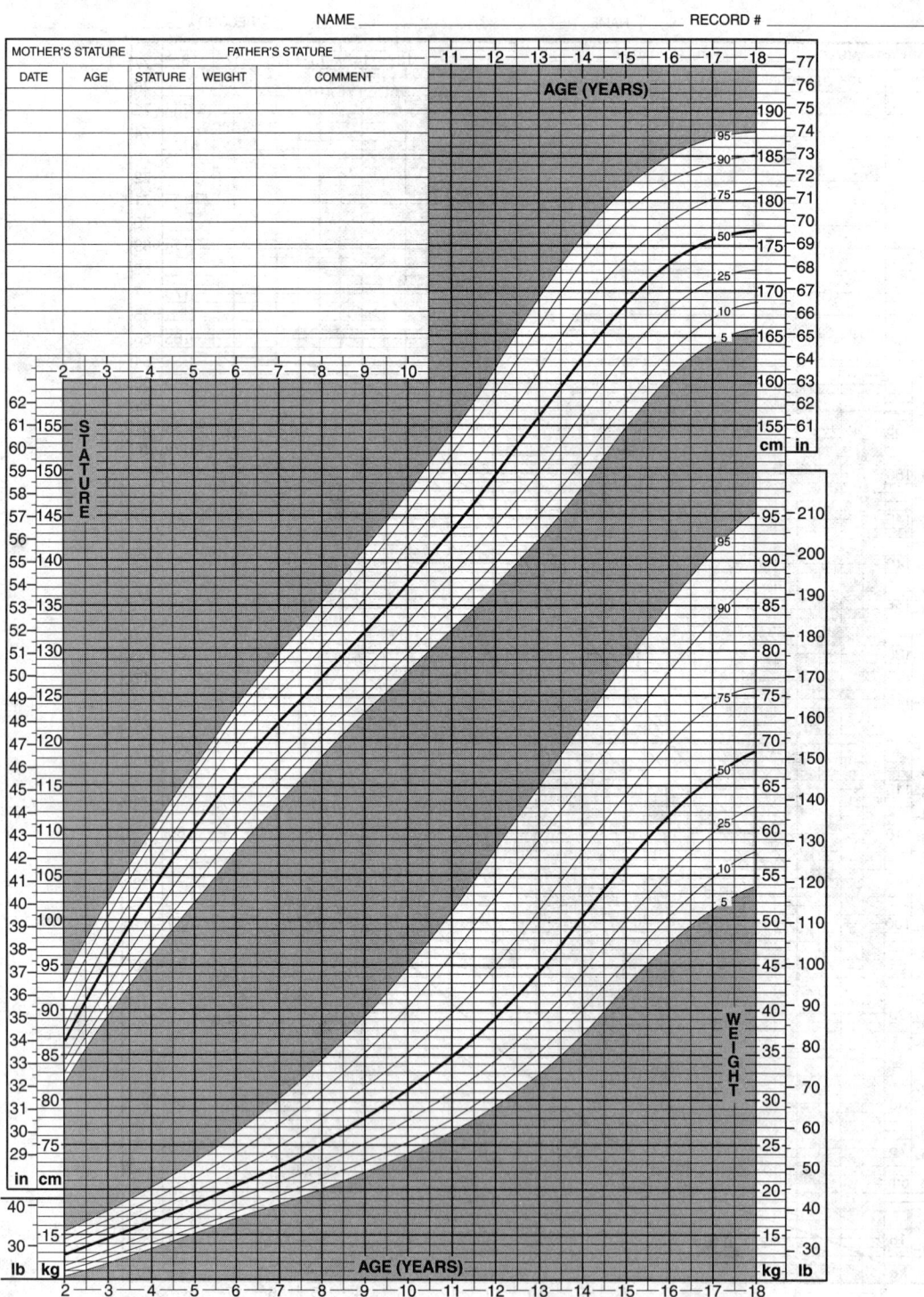

Figure 1–4. Percentile standards for weight and height in boys 2–18 years. (Reproduced, with permission, from Ross Laboratories, Columbus, OH. © 1982 Ross Laboratories.)

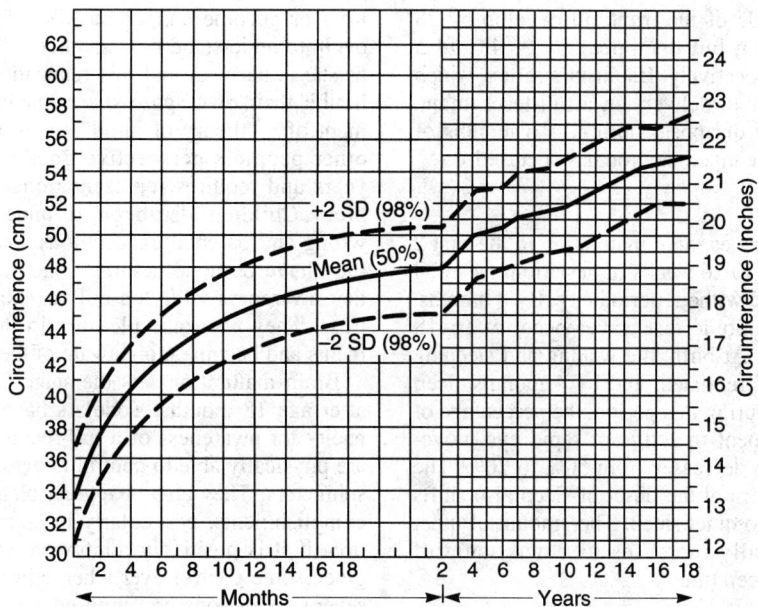

Figure 1–5. Head circumference of girls. (Modified and reproduced, with permission, from Nellhaus G: Pediatrics 1968;41:106.)

between 20 and 38 weeks. Sucking occurs in utero as early as 14 weeks. The rooting reflex, in which the infant turns the head and sucks in response to a touch on the cheek, develops at 28 weeks. The tonic neck reflex is elicited by forcibly turning the infant's head. In response, the infant extends the arm and leg on the side toward which the head is turned and flexes the opposite side ("fencing position"). This reflex disappears by 8 months of age unless myelinization or brain development is defective. The Moro reflex (an embracing movement as a startle response), palmar grasp, and trunk incurving in response to a tactile

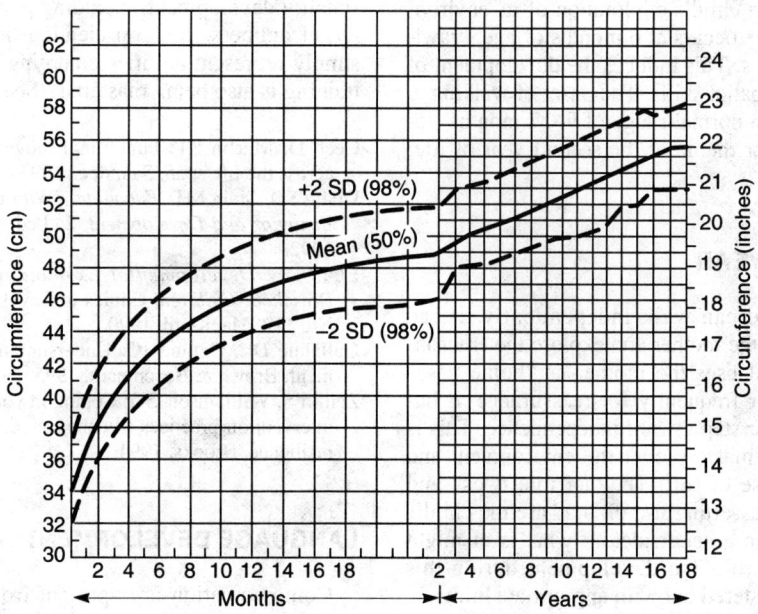

Figure 1–6. Head circumference of boys. (Modified and reproduced, with permission, from Nellhaus G: Pediatrics 1968;41:106.)

stimulus to the side of the trunk all develop by 28 weeks of gestation but disappear by 3, 4, and 5 months of age, respectively. Babinski's reflex, which develops just prior to delivery in a full-term infant, does not normally disappear until 12–16 months of age, when adequate myelinization has occurred.

EEG & Sleep

The brain undergoes rapid maturation in the first 2 years of life. Prior to 26 weeks of gestation, the EEG is disorganized and without periodicity. By 8 months, however, low-amplitude fast waves occur at 16–18 cycles per second. At birth, the waking and sleeping cycles can be differentiated, and by 4 months sleep spindles appear. During this period, the percentage of total sleep time spent in active or rapid eye movement (REM) sleep decreases from 50% to 20%. The infant's sleep pattern at the onset of sleep also shifts from REM sleep to quiet sleep. The amount of quiet sleep also gradually increases to a maximum of 70–80% of total sleep time.

Motor Dexterity

The developmental progression of grasp through the first year illustrates a gradual improvement in motor dexterity. The grasp begins as a raking motion involving mainly the ulnar aspect of the hand at 3–4 months. The thumb is used just before 5 months as the focus shifts to the radial side of the hand. The thumb opposes the finger for picking up a cube just before 7 months, but the neat pincer grasp used for smaller objects, such as a pellet, does not develop until approximately 9 months.

The changes in gross motor skills have a significant impact on the child's exploration of its environment. Sitting alone occurs at 6 months of age, crawling at 7–10 months. This induces the development of a wide range of spatial skills. The onset of walking at 12 months (with a normal range of 9–17 months) introduces the major theme of the second year of life: autonomy.

THE SECOND YEAR

Once the child can walk independently, it can move away from the mother and explore the environment. Although it uses the mother as "home base" and returns to her frequently for reassurance, it has now taken a major step toward independence. This is the beginning of mastery over the environment and an emerging sense of self. The "terrible twos" and the frequent self-asserting use of "no" are the child's attempt to develop a better idea of what is or might be under its control. Ego development during this time should be fostered but with appropriate limits.

As children develop a sense of self, they begin to understand the feelings of others and develop empathy. They hug another child who is in perceived distress or become concerned when one is hurt. They begin to understand how another child feels when he or she is harmed, and this realization helps them to inhibit their own aggressive behavior. The development of a "theory of mind" or an understanding of other people's perspective does not occur until 4 years and requires representational mapping in the brain. Children also begin to understand right and wrong and parental expectations. They realize when they have done something "bad" and may signify that awareness with "uh-oh!" or expressions of distress. They also take pleasure in their accomplishments and become more aware of their bodies.

Brain maturation sets the stage for toilet training after age 18 months. Toddlers have the sensory capacity for awareness of a full rectum or bladder and are physically able to control bowel and urinary tract sphincters. They also take great pleasure in their accomplishments, particularly in appropriate elimination, if it is positively reinforced. Children must be given some control over when elimination occurs. If severe restrictions are imposed, the accomplishment of this developmental milestone can become a battle between parent and child, and long-term struggles of control predisposing to encopresis may develop later. Freud terms this period the anal stage because the developmental issue of bowel control is the major task requiring mastery. It basically represents a more generalized theme of socialized behavior and overall body cleanliness, which is begun to be taught or imposed on the child at this age. The child is encouraged to control impulsive and aggressive behavior by acting in socially appropriate ways. Although Freud describes the by-products of anal regularity on personality development, including punctuality, reliability, cleanliness, and conscientiousness, these themes simply represent abilities emerging at the time toilet training is also being mastered. (See Chapter 6.)

Cech D, Martin ST: Functional movement development across the life span. Saunders, 1995.

Dixon SD, Stein MT: *Encounters With Children: Pediatric Behavior and Development,* 2nd ed. Mosby Year Book, 1992.

Egan DF: *Developmental Examination of Infants and Preschool Children.* Clinics in Developmental Medicine No. 112. MacKeith, 1990.

Gallahue DL, Ozmun JC: Understanding motor development. Brown & Benchmark, 1995.

Zeitlin S, Williamson GG: Coping in young children: Early intervention practices to enhance adaptive behavior and resilience. Brooks, 1994.

LANGUAGE DEVELOPMENT: 1–4 YEARS

Communication is important from birth, particularly the nonverbal reciprocal interactions between the infant and caretaker. By 2 months of age, these interactions begin to include vocalizations that involve cooing and reciprocal vocal play between mother and child. Babbling begins by 6–10 months of age, and the repetition of sounds, such as "da-da-da-da," is facilitated by increasing oral muscular control. Babbling reaches a peak at 12 months. The child then moves into a stage of having needs met by using individual words to represent objects or actions. It is common at this age for children to express wants and needs by pointing to objects and eliciting "joint attention" from the parents. There is significant variability in the number of words acquired by 18 months, with an average of 20–50 words. The failure of parents or siblings to encourage vocalization and overuse of nonverbal communication, such as pointing, slows the development of expressive vocabulary. Recurrent otitis media, which causes a fluctuating conductive hearing loss, may also have an impact on the achievement of early language milestones.

Receptive language usually develops more rapidly than expressive language. Word comprehension be-gins at 9 months; by 13 months, the receptive vocabulary may be as high as 20–100 words. After 18 months, there is a dramatic increase in expressive and receptive vocabulary, and by the end of the second year a quantum leap in language development represents a major change in cognitive development. The child begins to put words and phrases together and begins to use language to represent a new world, the symbolic world. Although the infant begins to use single words to represent objects or people in the latter part of the first year, it is not until the end of the second year that language ability begins to blossom. Children now begin to put verbs into their phrases and focus much of their language on describing their new abilities: "I go out." They incorporate prepositions into speech and ask "why?" and "what?" questions more frequently. They also begin to appreciate time factors and to understand and use this concept in their speech (Table 1–2).

The Early Language Milestone Scale (ELM) is a

Table 1–2. Normal speech and language development.

Age	Speech	Language	Articulation[1]
1 month	Throaty sounds		Vowels: \ah\, \uh\, \ee\
2 months	Vowel sounds ("eh"), coos		
2½ months	Squeals		
3 months	Babbles, initial vowels		
4 months	Guttural sounds ("ah," "go")		Consonants, m, p, b
5 months			Vowels: \o\, \u\
7 months	Imitates speech sounds		
8 months			Syllables: da, ba, ka
10 months		"Dada" or "mama" nonspecifically	Approximates names: baba/bottle
12 months	Jargon begins (own language)	One word other than "mama" or "dada"	Understandable: 2–3 words
13 months		Three words	
16 months		Six words	Consonants: t, d, w, n, h
18–24 months		Two-word phrases	Understandable 2-word phrases
24–30 months		Three-word phrases	Understandable 3-word phrases
2 years	Vowels uttered correctly	Approximately 270 words; uses pronouns	Approximately 270 words; uses phrases
3 years	Some degree of hesitancy and uncertainty common	Approximately 900 words; intelligible 4-word phrases	Approximately 900 words; intelligible 4-word phrases
4 years		Approximately 1540 words; intelligible 5-word phrases or sentences	Approximately 1540 words; intelligible 5-word phrases
6 years		Approximately 2560 words; intelligible 6- or 7-word sentences	Approximately 2560 words; intelligible 6- or 7-word sentences
7–8 years	Adult proficiency		

[1]Data on articulation from Berry MF: *Language Disorders of Children.* Appleton-Century-Crofts, 1969; and from Bzoch K, League R: *Receptive-Expressive Emergent Language Scale.* University Park Press, 1970.

simple tool for assessing early language development in the pediatric office setting (Figure 1–7). It is scored in the same way as the Denver II (Figure 1–8) but tests both receptive and expressive language areas in greater depth.

Piaget characterizes the 2- to 6-year-old stage as "preoperational." This stage begins when language has facilitated the creation of mental images in the symbolic sense. The child begins to manipulate the symbolic world, sorts out reality from fantasy imperfectly, and may be terrified of dreams, wishes, and foolish threats. Most of the child's perception of the world is egocentric or interpreted in reference to wants, needs, or influence. Cause-effect relationships are confused with temporal ones or interpreted egocentrically. Children may focus their understanding of divorce, for example, on themselves. ("My father left because I was bad," or "My father left because he didn't love me.") Illness and the need for medical care are also commonly misinterpreted at this age. The child may make a mental connection between a sibling's illness and a recent argument, a negative comment, or a wish for the sibling to be ill. The child may experience significant guilt unless the parents are aware of these misperceptions and take time to deal with them.

At this age, children also endow inanimate objects with human feelings. They also assume that humans cause or create all natural events. For instance, when asked why the sun sets, they may say that "the sun goes to his house" or "it is pushed down by someone else."

Magical thinking blossoms during ages of 3–5 as symbolic thinking incorporates more elaborate fantasy. Fantasy facilitates development of role playing, sexual identity, and emotional growth. Children test new experiences in fantasy, both in their imagination and in play. In their play, children often create magical stories and novel situations that reflect issues they are dealing with, such as aggression, relationships, fears, and control. Children often invent imaginary friends at this time, and nightmares or fears of monsters are common. At this stage, other children become important in facilitating play, such as in a preschool group. Play gradually becomes more cooperative; shared fantasy leads to game playing. Freud describes the oedipal phase between the ages of 3 and 6, when there is strong attachment to the parent of the opposite sex. The child's fantasies may focus on play-acting the adult role with that parent, though by 6 years of age oedipal issues are usually resolved and attachment is redirected to the parent of the same sex.

Bayley N (editor): *Bayley Scales of Infant Development,* 2nd ed. Psychological Corporation, 1993.

Billeaud FP: *Communication Disorders in Infants and Toddlers.* Andover Medical, 1993.

Bjorklund DF: *Children's Thinking.* Brooks/Cole, 1995.

Coplan J: *Early Language Milestone Scale—2.* Pro Ed, 1993.

Dixon SD, Stein MT: *Encounters With Children: Pediatric Behavior and Development,* 2nd ed. Mosby Year Book, 1992.

Frankenberg WK et al: The Denver II: A major revision and restandardization of the Denver Developmental Screening Test. Pediatrics 1991;89:91.

Glascoe FP, Dvorkin PH: The role of parents in the detection of developmental and behavioral problems. Pediatrics 1995;95:829.

THE EARLY SCHOOL YEARS: 5–7

Attendance at kindergarten at age 5 years marks an acceleration in the separation-individuation theme initiated in the preschool years. The child is ready to relate to peers in a more interactive manner than parallel play. The brain has reached 90% of its adult weight. Sensorimotor coordination abilities are maturing and facilitating pencil-and-paper tasks and sports, both part of the school experience.

Cognitive abilities are still at the preoperational stage, and children focus on one variable in a problem at a time. However, by 5½ years, most children have mastered conservation of length; by 6½ years, conservation of mass and weight; and by 8 years, conservation of volume.

By first grade, there is more pressure on the child to master academic tasks, including the recognition of numbers, letters, and words, and to learn how to write. Piaget describes the "stage of concrete operations" beginning after age 6, when the child is able to perform mental operations concerning concrete objects that involve manipulation of more than one variable. The child is able to order, number, and classify because these activities are related to concrete objects in the environment and because these activities are stressed in early schooling. Magical thinking diminishes greatly at this time, and the reality of cause-effect relationships is better understood. Fantasy and imagination are still strong and are reflected in themes of play. Table 1–3 lists specific developmental abilities through mid childhood and adolescence.

THE MIDDLE CHILDHOOD YEARS: 7–11

Freud characterizes ages 7–11 as the "latency years," during which children are not bothered by significant aggressive or sexual drives but instead devote most of their energies to school and peer group interactions. In reality, throughout this period there is a gradual increase in sex drive, manifested by increasingly aggressive play and interactions with the opposite sex. Fantasy still has an active role in dealing with sexuality before adolescence, and fantasies often focus on movie stars and rock heroes. Orga-

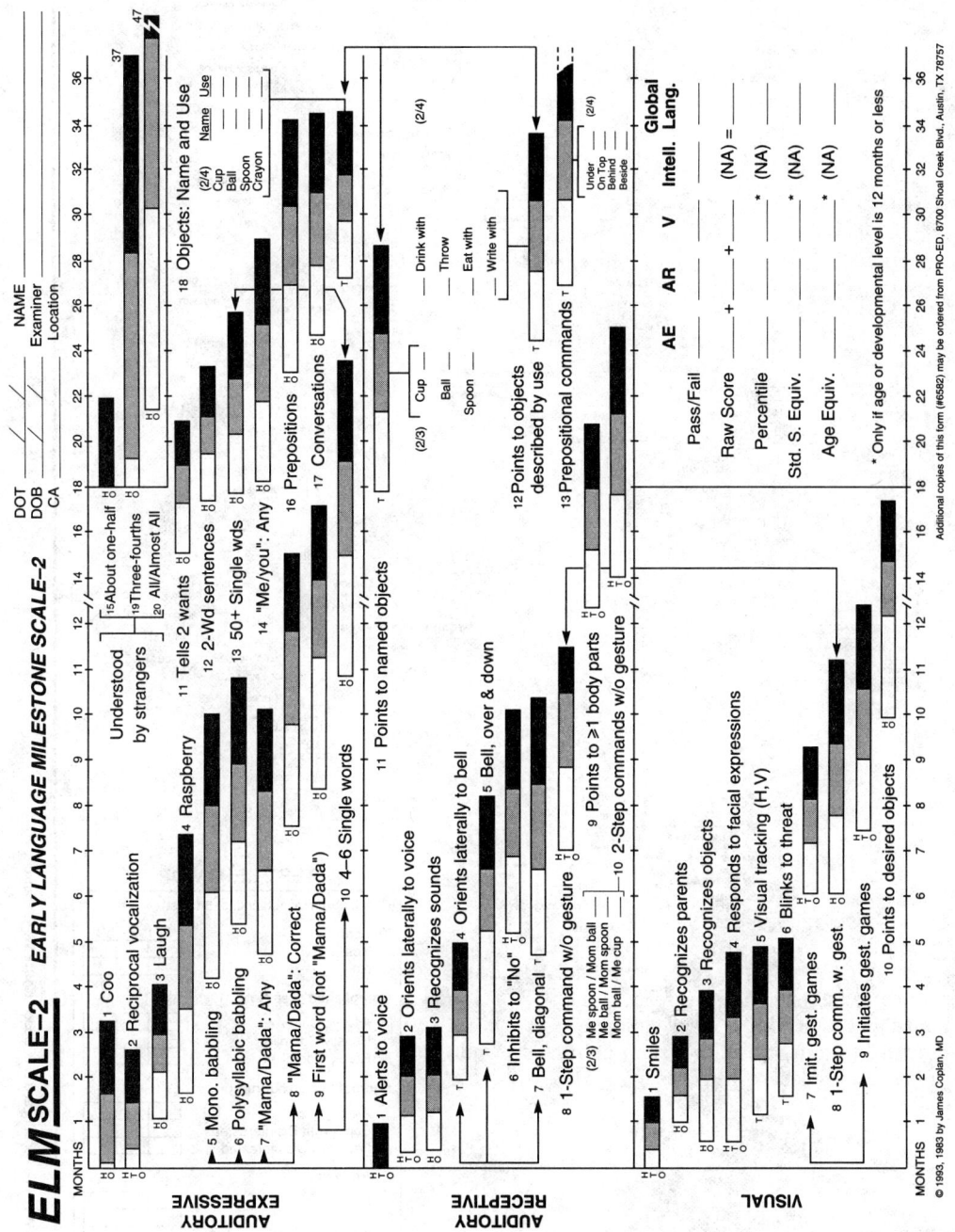

Figure 1–7. Early Language Milestone Scale—2. (Reproduced, with permission, from Coplan J: Early Language Milestone Scale. Pro Ed, 1993.)

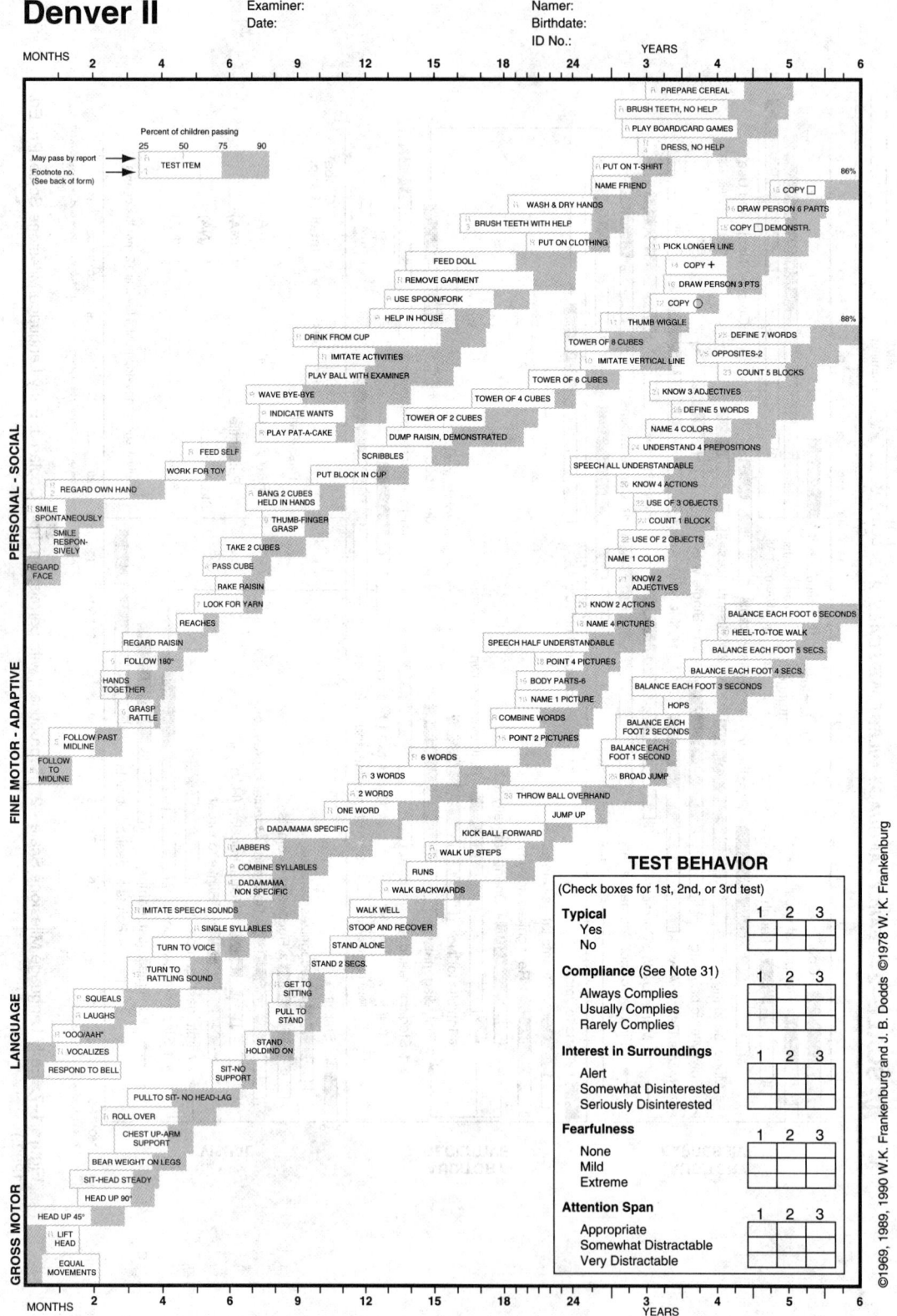

Figure 1–8. Denver II.

Table 1–3. Developmental charts.[1]

1–2 months

Activities to be observed:
Holds head erect and lifts head.
Turns from side to back.
Regards faces and follows objects through visual field.
Drops toys.
Becomes alert in response to voice.

Activities related by parent:
Recognizes parents.
Engages in vocalizations.
Smiles spontaneously.

3–5 months

Activities to be observed:
Grasps cube—first ulnar then later thumb opposition.
Reaches for and brings objects to mouth.
Makes "raspberry" sound.
Sits with support.

Activities related by parent:
Laughs.
Anticipates food on sight.
Turns from back to side.

6–8 months

Activities to be observed:
Sits alone for a short period.
Reaches with one hand.
First scoops up a pellet then grasps it using thumb
    opposition.
Imitates "bye-bye."
Passes object from hand to hand in midline.
Babbles.

Activities related by parent:
Rolls from back to stomach.
Is inhibited by the word *no*.

9–11 months

Activities to be observed:
Stands alone.
Imitates pat-a-cake and peek-a-boo.
Uses thumb and index finger to pick up pellet.

Activities related by parent:
Walks by supporting self on furniture.
Follows one-step verbal commands, eg,
    "Come here," "Give it to me."

1 year

Activities to be observed:
Walks independently.
Says "mama" and "dada" with meaning.
Can use a neat pincer grasp to pick up a pellet.
Releases cube into cup after demonstration.
Gives toys on request.
Tries to build a tower of 2 cubes.

Activities related by parent:
Points to desired objects.
Says 1 or 2 other words.

18 months

Activities to be observed:
Builds tower of 3–4 cubes.
Throws ball.
Scribbles spontaneously.
Seats self in chair.
Dumps pellet from bottle.

Activities related by parent:
Walks up and down stairs with help.
Says 4–20 words.
Understands a 2-step command.
Carries and hugs doll.
Feeds self.

24 months

Activities to be observed:
Speaks short phrases, 2 words or more.
Kicks ball on request.
Builds tower of 6–7 cubes.
Points to named objects or pictures.
Jumps off floor with both feet.
Stands on either foot alone.
Uses pronouns.

Activities related by parent:
Verbalizes toilet needs.
Pulls on simple garment.
Turns pages of book singly.
Plays with domestic mimicry.

30 months

Activities to be observed:
Walks backward.
Begins to hop on one foot.
Uses prepositions.
Copies a crude circle.
Points to objects described by use.
Refers to self as I.
Holds crayon in fist.

Activities related by parent:
Helps put things away.
Carries on a conversation.

3 years

Activities to be observed:
Holds crayon with fingers.
Builds tower of 9–10 cubes.
Imitates 3-cube bridge.
Copies circle.
Gives first and last name.

Activities related by parent:
Rides tricycle using pedals.
Dresses with supervision.

3–4 years

Activities to be observed:
Climbs stairs with alternating feet.
Begins to button and unbutton.
"What do you like to do that's fun?" (Answers using
    plurals, personal pronouns, and verbs.)
Responds to command to place toy *in, on,* or *under* table.
Draws a circle when asked to draw a person.
Knows own sex. ("Are you a boy or a girl?")
Gives full name.
Copies a circle already drawn. ("Can you make one like
    this?")

Activities related by parent:
Feeds self at mealtime.
Takes off shoes and jacket.

4–5 years

Activities to be observed:
Runs and turns without losing balance.
May stand on one leg for at least 10 seconds.

(continued)

Table 1–3. Developmental charts. (continued)

Buttons clothes and laces shoes. (Does not tie.)
Counts to 4 by rote.
"Give me 2 sticks." (Able to do so from pile of 4 tongue depressors.)
Draws a person. (Head, 2 appendages, and possibly 2 eyes. No torso yet.)
Knows the days of the week. ("What day comes after Tuesday?")
Gives appropriate answers to: "What must you do if you are sleepy? Hungry? Cold?"
Copies + in imitation.

Activities related by parent:
Self-care at toilet. (May need help with wiping.)
Plays outside for at least 30 minutes.
Dresses self except for tying.

5–6 years

Activities to be observed:
Can catch ball.
Skips smoothly.
Copies a + already drawn.
Tells age.
Concept of 10 (eg, counts 10 tongue depressors). May recite to higher number by rote.
Knows right and left hand.
Draws recognizable person with at least 8 details.
Can describe favorite television program in some detail.

Activities related by parent:
Does simple chores at home (eg, taking out garbage, drying silverware).
Goes to school unattended or meets school bus.
Good motor ability but little awareness of dangers.

6–7 years

Activities to be observed:
Copies a Δ.
Defines words by use. ("What is an orange?" "To eat.")
Knows if morning or afternoon.
Draws a person with 12 details.
Reads several one-syllable printed words. (My, dog, see, boy.)
Uses pencil for printing name.

7–8 years

Activities to be observed:
Counts by 2s and 5s.
Ties shoes.
Copies a ◊.
Knows what day of the week it is. (Not date or year.)
Reads paragraph #1 Durrell:

Reading:
Muff is a little yellow kitten. She drinks milk. She sleeps on a chair. She does not like to get wet.

Corresponding arithmetic:

$$\begin{array}{cccc} 7 & 6 & 6 & 8 \\ +4 & +7 & -4 & -3 \end{array}$$

No evidence of sound substitution in speech (eg, *fr* for *thr*).
Adds and subtracts one-digit numbers.
Draws a man with 16 details.

8–9 years

Activities to be observed:
Defines words better than by use. ("What is an orange?" "A fruit.")
Can give an appropriate answer to the following:

"What is the thing for you to do if . . .
—you've broken something that belongs to someone else?"
—a playmate hits you without meaning to do so?"
Reads paragraph #2 Durrell:

Reading:
A little black dog ran away from home. He played with two big dogs. They ran away from him. It began to rain. He went under a tree. He wanted to go home, but he did not know the way. He saw a boy he knew. The boy took him home.

Corresponding arithmetic:

$$\begin{array}{cccc} & 45 & & \\ 67 & 16 & 14 & 84 \\ + 4 & +27 & - 8 & -36 \end{array}$$

Is learning borrowing and carrying processes in addition and subtraction.

9–10 years

Activities to be observed:
Knows the month, day, and year.
Names the months in order. (15 seconds, 1 error.)
Makes a sentence with these 3 words in it: (1 or 2. Can use words orally in proper context.)
1. work . . . money . . . men
2. boy . . . river . . . ball
Reads paragraph #3 Durrell:

Reading:
Six boys put up a tent by the side of a river. They took things to eat with them. When the sun went down, they went into the tent to sleep. In the night, a cow came and began to eat grass around the tent. The boys were afraid. They thought it was a bear.

Corresponding arithmetic:

$$\begin{array}{ccc} 5204 & 23 & 837 \\ - 530 & \times 3 & \times 7 \end{array}$$

Should comprehend and answer the question: "What was the cow doing?"
Learning simple multiplication.

10–12 years

Activities to be observed:
Should read and comprehend paragraph #5 Durrell:
Reading:
In 1807, Robert Fulton took the first long trip in a steamboat. He went one hundred and fifty miles up the Hudson River. The boat went five miles an hour. This was faster than a steamboat had ever gone before. Crowds gathered on both banks of the river to see this new kind of boat. They were afraid that its noise and splashing would drive away all the fish.

Corresponding arithmetic:

$$\begin{array}{ccc} 420 & & \\ \times 29 & 9\overline{)72} & 31\overline{)62} \end{array}$$

Answer: "What river was the trip made on?"
Ask to write the sentence: "The fishermen did not like the boat."
Should do multiplication and simple division.

12–15 years

Activities to be observed:
Reads paragraph #7 Durrell:

(continued)

Table 1–3. Developmental charts. (continued)

Reading:	Corresponding arithmetic:

Reading:
  Golf originated in Holland as a game played on ice. The game in its present form first appeared in Scotland. It became unusually popular and kings found it so enjoyable that it was known as "the royal game." James IV, however, thought that people neglected their work to indulge in this fascinating sport so that it was forbidden in 1457. James relented when he found how attractive the game was, and it immediately regained its former popularity. Golf spread gradually to other countries, being introduced in America in 1890. It has grown in favor until there is hardly a town that does not boast of a private or public course.

Corresponding arithmetic:

$$536\overline{)4762} \qquad \tfrac{1}{3} \qquad 7\tfrac{1}{6}$$
$$+\tfrac{1}{3} \qquad -\tfrac{3}{4}$$

Reduce fractions to lowest forms.

Ask to write a sentence: "Golf originated in Holland as a game played on ice."
Answers questions:
  "Why was golf forbidden by James IV?"
  "Why did he change his mind?"
Does long division, adds and subtracts fractions.

[1]Modified from Leavitt SR, Goodman H, Harvin D: Pediatrics 1963;31:499.

nized sports, clubs, and other activities are other modalities that permit preadolescent children to display socially acceptable forms of aggression and sexual interest.

For the 7-year-old, the major developmental tasks are achievement in school and acceptance by peers. Academic expectations have intensified and require the child to concentrate, attend, and process increasingly complex auditory and visual information. Children with significant learning disabilities or problems of attention span may have difficulty in these tasks and subsequently may receive negative reinforcement from teachers and even parents. Such children may develop a poor self-image manifested as behavioral difficulties. The pediatrician must evaluate potential learning disabilities in any child who is not developing adequately at this stage or who presents with emotional or behavioral problems. The developmental status of school-age children is not as easily documented as that of the younger child because of the complexity of the milestones. In the school-age child, the quality of the response, the attentional abilities, and the child's emotional approach to the task can make a dramatic difference in success at school. The clinician must consider all of these aspects in the differential diagnosis of learning disabilities. (See Chapter 3.)

Leffert N, Petersen AC: Biology, challenge and coping in adolescence: Effects on physical and mental health. In: *Child Development and Behavioral Pediatrics.* Bornstein MH, Genevro J (editors). Lawrence Erlbaum Associates, 1996.
Parker S, Zuckerman B (editors): *Behavioral & Developmental Pediatrics: A Handbook for Primary Care.* Little, Brown, 1995.

PREPUBERTAL & PUBERTAL GROWTH

The pubertal growth spurt occurs at about 10 years in girls and 12½ years in boys. The speed of growth increases, reaching a peak of approximately 9 cm/y in girls and 10.3 cm/y in boys. Different areas of the skeleton attain their peak growth at different times. This is seen most dramatically in the feet, which first experience a growth spurt. This is followed by a rapid increase in leg length and subsequently trunk growth. Facial growth occurs after peak height velocity. The mandible changes most remarkably, demonstrating a 25% increase in height between 12 and 20 years of age, compared with only a 6–7% increase in size of the cranial base.

Boys have just over 2 more years of preadolescent growth than girls do; during this time, leg growth increases more dramatically than trunk growth. Girls have a greater spurt in hip width, related to stature, than boys do, though boys exceed girls in most other areas of bone growth.

The Hypothalamic-Pituitary-Gonadal Axis & Puberty

Gonadal development is initiated in the fetus by 10 weeks of gestation and in the male is almost complete by age 3 months. This process occurs without significant input from gonadotropins, though placental human chorionic gonadotropin (hCG) plays a significant role in migration of germ cells and differentiation of Leydig cells. By the 21st week of gestation, the hypothalamus secretes gonadotropin-releasing hormone (GnRH) and the anterior pituitary releases follicle-stimulating hormone (FSH) and luteinizing hormone (LH). These hormone levels reach a peak by the 23rd–24th weeks of gestation, which coincides with oocyte maturation in utero, including the development of primary follicles.

In the newborn period, GnRH is secreted in a pulsatile fashion, causing episodic elevations of both FSH and LH. In females, FSH predominates; in males LH predominates. These hormones stimulate elevations in estrogen and testosterone in the first few months of life. After this period of significant neuroendocrine activity, a quiescent period, with almost undetectable levels of gonadotropins, lasts through childhood. Hypothalamic secretion of GnRH is suppressed until puberty.

The large fetal adrenal gland regresses significantly after birth until adrenarche at 6–9 years of age. Adrenarche refers to the regrowth of the zona reticularis and activation of its enzyme systems to produce adrenal steroids such as dehydroepiandrosterone sulfate and 17-ketosteroids. These steroids are partially responsible for body odor, the development of pubic and axillary hair, and stimulation of linear growth. Adrenarche occurs before gonadarche and is probably under the control of adrenocorticotropic hormone (ACTH).

Gonadarche is initiated by pulsatile secretion of GnRH from the hypothalamus, which in turn stimulates the release of gonadotropins. In early puberty, FSH and LH are secreted during sleep, and there is an increasing amplitude in its pulses as puberty progresses. The efficacy of FSH and LH also changes in that biopotency of these hormones improves as puberty progresses. For additional information on puberty, see Chapter 5.

Gemelli R: *Normal Child and Adolescent Development.* American Psychiatric Press, 1996.

The Newborn Infant

2

Elizabeth H. Thilo, MD, & Adam A. Rosenberg, MD

The first 28 days of life are usually considered the newborn period. In practice, however, neonatal care may extend to many months for sick or very immature infants. Table 2–1 summarizes the levels of nursery care commonly required.

EVALUATION OF THE NEWBORN INFANT

HISTORY

Taking the history in newborn medicine involves three key areas: (1) the medical history of the mother and father, including a relevant genetic history; (2) the history pertaining to the mother's previous pregnancies; and (3) the history of the current pregnancy, including antepartum and intrapartum events.

The mother's medical history should include any chronic medical conditions, medications taken during pregnancy, unusual dietary habits, smoking history, occupational exposures to chemicals or infections of potential risk to the fetus, and pertinent aspects of the social history that may suggest increased risks for parenting problems and child abuse. Family illnesses with genetic implications should be sought. The past pregnancy history should include maternal age, gravidity and parity, blood type, and pregnancy outcomes. The current obstetric history should include documentation and results of procedures such as ultrasound, amniocentesis, screening tests (eg, HBsAg, antibody screen, serum AFP, HIV), and antepartum tests of fetal well-being (eg, biophysical profiles or nonstress tests). Information should be sought regarding pregnancy-related illnesses in the mother such as urinary tract infection, pregnancy-induced hypertension or preeclampsia-eclampsia, vaginal bleeding, and preterm labor. Peripartum events of importance include duration of ruptured membranes, maternal fever, fetal distress or meconium-stained amniotic fluid, type of delivery (vaginal or cesarean section), anesthesia and analgesia used, reason for operative or forceps delivery, and condition of the infant at birth, including any resuscitation needed and Apgar scores.

ASSESSMENT OF GROWTH & GESTATIONAL AGE

It is important to know an infant's gestational age since its behavior and anticipated problems can be predicted on this basis. Accurate recall of the date of the last menstrual period is the best indicator of gestational age. Other obstetric observations, such as fundal height, time of auscultation of fetal heartbeat with a stethoscope, and early ultrasound examination, provide supporting information. A postnatal examination can also be used because fetal physical characteristics and neurologic development progress in predictable fashion. Table 2–2 lists the physical and neurologic criteria to be examined. The upper panel is the neuromuscular examination, assessing primarily muscle tone and strength. The lower panel catalogs a variety of physical characteristics. Adding the scores assigned to each characteristic yields a total score that corresponds to the gestational age.

Disappearance of the anterior vascular capsule of the lens is also helpful in determining gestational age. At 27–28 weeks of gestation, the lens capsule is covered by vessels; by 34 weeks, this vascular plexus is completely atrophied. Foot length, measured carefully from the heel to the tip of the longest toe, also correlates with gestational age in appropriately grown infants. The foot measures 4.5 cm at 25 weeks' gestation and increases by 0.25 cm/wk until term.

By convention, unless the physical examination indicates a gestational age more than 2 weeks different (in either direction) from the obstetric dates, the gestational age is as assigned by the dates. The birth weight and gestational age must be plotted on an appropriate standard to determine if the infant's weight is appropriate for gestational age (AGA infant), small

Table 2–1. Levels of nursery care.

Level 1 nurseries
These nurseries care for infants presumed healthy. In such units, screening and surveillance are primary responsibilities. "Rooming-in" units are encouraged, with emphasis on support of breast feeding and assessment of parenting skills.

Level 2 nurseries
These nurseries care for infants > 30 weeks of gestation and birth weight > 1200 g who require special attention short of the need for circulatory or prolonged ventilator support and major surgical procedures. Because they address the greatest diversity of neonatal disorders, these nurseries present perhaps the greatest challenge to health care providers.

Level 3 nurseries
These nurseries are staffed and equipped to care for all newborn infants who are critically ill, regardless of the level of support required. They are regional institutions serving as referral centers for other nurseries and for this reason are often linked with transport services. These nurseries are in many cases part of a perinatal center.

Perinatal center
A perinatal center provides services both to high-risk mothers and to infants requiring level 3 nursery care. Ample data now clearly demonstrate a higher neonatal survival rate for high-risk pregnancies cared for in such centers. The transport of high-risk mothers to perinatal centers is preferred, therefore, to the transport of a critically ill infant following delivery.

for gestational age (SGA infant) or intrauterine growth restricted (IUGR infant), or large for gestational age (LGA infant) (Figure 2–1). Birth weight and gestational age distributions vary from one population to the next depending on factors such as those listed in Table 2–3. Whenever possible, standards should be prepared from data derived from the local population, but when such information is not available any regional standard may be used. The birth weight-gestational age distribution of an infant is a screening tool that should be supplemented by clinical data confirming a tentative diagnosis of intrauterine growth restriction or excessive fetal growth. These data include not only the clinical features of the infant determined during the physical examination but also factors such as the size of the parents and the birth weight-gestational age distribution of infants previously born to the parents.

Table 2–4 lists causes of variations in neonatal size in relation to gestational age. An important distinction, particularly in SGA infants, is whether the growth disorder is symmetric (weight, length, and occipitofrontal circumference [OFC] all ≤ 10%) or asymmetric (only weight ≤ 10%). Asymmetric growth retardation implies a problem late in the pregnancy, such as pregnancy-induced hypertension or placental insufficiency. Symmetric growth restriction implies an event of early pregnancy: chromosomal abnormality, drug or alcohol use, congenital viral in-

fections. In general, the outlook for normal growth and development is better in the asymmetrically growth-restricted infant whose intrauterine brain growth has been spared.

The fact that SGA infants have fewer problems (such as respiratory distress syndrome) than AGA infants of the same birth weight but a lower gestational age has led to the common misconception that SGA infants have accelerated maturation. SGA infants, when compared to AGA infants of the same gestational age, actually have increased morbidity and mortality rates.

Knowledge of a baby's birth weight in relation to gestational age is also helpful in anticipating neonatal problems. LGA babies are at risk for birth trauma, hypoglycemia, polycythemia, congenital anomalies, cardiomyopathy, hyperbilirubinemia, and hypocalcemia. SGA babies are at risk for fetal distress during labor and delivery, polycythemia, hypoglycemia, and hypocalcemia.

American Academy of Pediatrics: *Guidelines for Perinatal Care,* 4th ed. American Academy of Pediatrics, 1997.
Ballard JL et al: New Ballard score, expanded to include extremely premature infants. J Pediatr 1991;119:417.
McCarton CM et al: Cognitive and neurologic development of the premature, small for gestational age infant through age 6: Comparison by birth weight and gestational age. Pediatrics 1996;98:1167.
Tyson JE et al: The small for gestational age infant: Accelerated or delayed pulmonary maturation? Increased or decreased survival? Pediatrics 1995;95:534.
Wright K et al: New postnatal growth grids for very low birth weight infants. Pediatrics 1993;91:922.

EXAMINATION AT BIRTH

The extent of the newborn physical examination depends on the condition of the infant and the environment in which it is being performed. In the delivery room, the examination consists largely of observation plus auscultation of the chest and inspection for congenital anomalies and birth trauma. Major congenital anomalies are present in 1.5% of live births and account for 20–25% of perinatal and neonatal deaths. Because the infant is recovering from the stress of birth, the examination should not be extensive. The Apgar score (Table 2–5) should be recorded at 1 and 5 minutes of age. In the case of severely depressed infants, a 10-minute score should also be recorded. Although the 1- and 5-minute Apgar scores have almost no predictive value for long-term outcome, serial scores do provide a useful shorthand description of the severity of perinatal depression and the quality of the resuscitative efforts pursued.

The color of the skin is a useful indicator of cardiac output. Because there is normally a high blood flow to the skin, any stress that triggers a cate-

Table 2–2. New Ballard Score for assessment of fetal maturation of newly born infants.[*][1]

Neuromuscular Maturity

Neuromuscular Maturity Sign	Score							Record Score Here
	-1	0	1	2	3	4	5	
Posture								
Square window (wrist)	>90°	90°	60°	45°	30°	0°		
Arm recoil		180°	140° to 180°	110° to 140°	90° to 110°	<90°		
Popliteal angle	180°	160°	140°	120°	100°	90°	<90°	
Scarf sign								
Heel to ear								

Total Neuromuscular Maturity Score [ ]

Physical Maturity

Physical Maturity Sign	Score							Record Score Here
	−1	0	1	2	3	4	5	
Skin	Sticky, friable, transparent	Gelatinous, red, translucent	Smooth, pink, visible veins	Superficial peeling &/or rash; few veins	Cracking pale areas rare veins	Parchment, deep cracking; no vessels	Leathery, cracked, wrinkled	
Lanugo	None	Sparse	Abundant	Thinning	Bald areas	Mostly bald		
Plantar surface	Heel toe 40–50 mm: −1 <40 mm:−2	> 50 mm: no crease	Faint red marks	Anterior transverse crease only	Creases anterior ⅔	Creases over entire sole		
Breast	Imperceptible	Barely perceptible	Flat areola; no bud	Stippled areola; 1- to 2-mm bud	Raised areola; 3- to 4-mm bud	Full areola; 5- to 10-mm bud		
Eye/Ear	Lids fused loosely: −1 tightly: −2	Lids open; pinna flat; stays folded	Slightly curved pinna; soft; slow recoil	Well-curved pinna; soft but ready recoil	Formed & firm instant recoil	Thick cartilage; ear stiff		
Genitals (male)	Scrotum flat, smooth	Scrotum empty; faint rugae	Testes in upper canal; rare rugae	Testes descending; few rugae	Testes down; good rugae	Testes pendulous; deep rugae		
Genitals (female)	Clitoris prominent & labia flat	Prominent clitoris & small labia minora	Prominent clitoris & enlarging minora	Majora & minora equally prominent	Majora large; minora small	Majora cover clitoris & minora		

Total Physical Maturity Score [ ]

Maturity	Score	−10	−5	0	5	10	15	20	25	30	35	40	45	50
Rating	Weeks	20	22	24	26	28	30	32	34	36	38	40	42	44

*Reproduced, with permission, from Ballard JL et al: New Ballard Score, expanded to include extremely premature infants. J Pediatr 1991;119:417.
[1]See text for a description of the clinical gestational age examination.

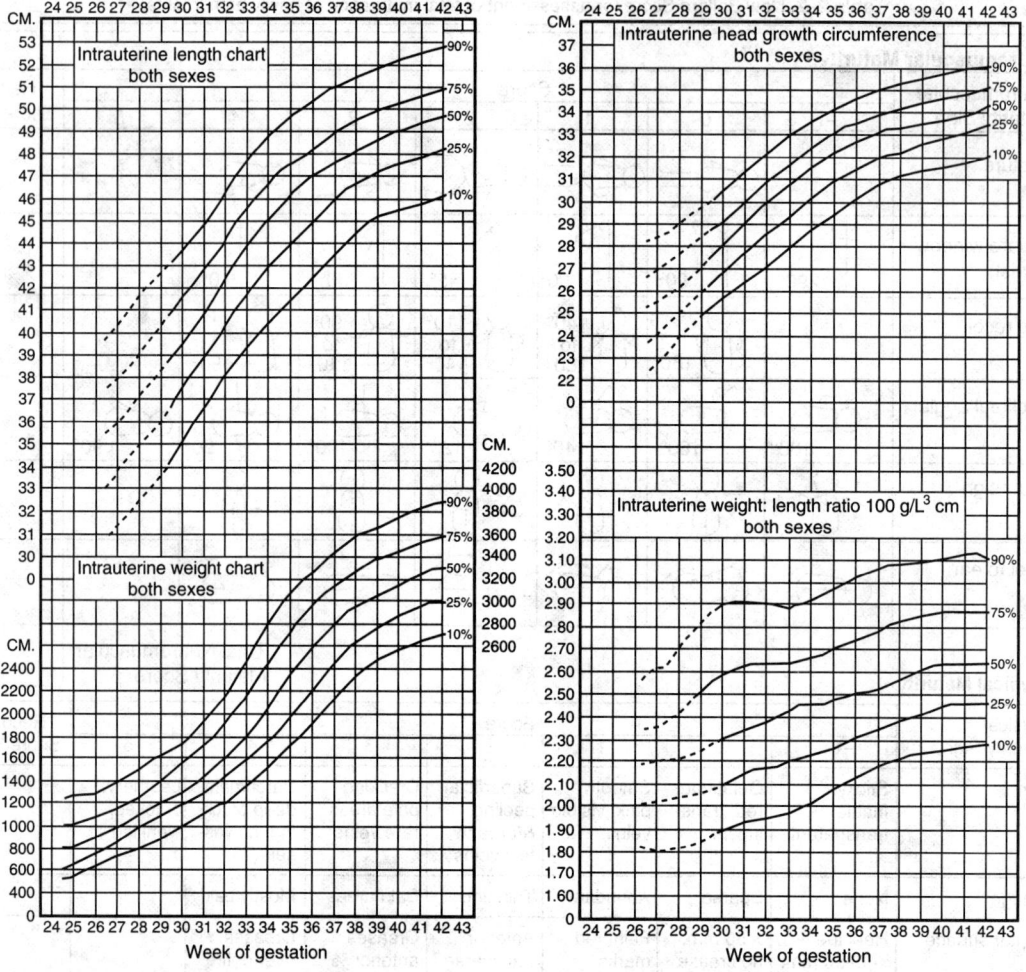

Figure 2–1. Intrauterine growth curves for weight, length, and head circumference for singleton births in Colorado. (Reproduced, with permission, from Lubchenco LO et al: Intrauterine growth in length and head circumference as estimated from live births at gestational ages from 26 to 42 weeks. Pediatrics 1966;37:403.)

cholamine response produces fairly dramatic changes in skin color secondary to changes in the distribution of the cardiac output and perfusion of the skin. Cyanosis and pallor are two signs reflecting inadequate oxygenation and skin blood flow.

The skeletal examination immediately after delivery serves two purposes: (1) to detect any obvious congenital anomalies and (2) to detect signs of birth trauma, particularly in LGA infants or those born after a protracted second stage of labor—in whom a fractured clavicle or humerus might be found.

The umbilical cord should be examined for the number of vessels. Normally, there are two arteries and one vein. In 1% of deliveries (5–6% of twin deliveries), the cord has only two vessels: an artery and a vein. The latter may be considered a minor anomaly and, as with other minor anomalies, carries a slightly increased risk of associated defects. The placenta is usually examined by the physician delivering it. Small placentas are always associated with small infants. The placental examination emphasizes the identification of membranes and vessels—particularly in multiple gestations—as well as the presence

Table 2–3. Factors affecting birth weight–gestational age distributions.

1. Socioeconomic factors that affect nutritional level and access to health care
2. Altitude
3. Environmental factors that affect birth weight (eg, smoking, alcohol, illicit drug use)
4. Race

Table 2–4. Etiology of variations in neonatal size in relation to gestational age.

Infants large for gestational age
Infant of a diabetic mother

Infants small for gestational age
Asymmetric
Placental insufficiency secondary to pregnancy-induced hypertension or other maternal vascular disease
Maternal age > 35 y
Poor weight gain during pregnancy
Multiple gestation
Symmetric
Maternal drug use
Narcotics
Cocaine
Alcohol
Chromosomal abnormalities
Intrauterine viral infection (eg, cytomegalovirus)

Table 2–5. Infant evaluation at birth (Apgar score).[1,2]

	Score		
	0	1	2
Heart rate	Absent	Slow (< 100)	> 100
Respiratory effort	Absent	Slow, irregular	Good, crying
Muscle tone	Limp	Some flexion	Active motion
Response to catheter in nostril[3]	No response	Grimace	Cough or sneeze
Color	Blue or pale	Body pink; extremities blue	Completely pink

[1]Reproduced, with permission, from Apgar V et al: Evaluation of the newborn infant—Second report. JAMA 1958;168:1985. © 1958 American Medical Association.
[2]One minute and 5 minutes after complete birth of the infant (disregarding the cord and the placenta), the following objective signs should be observed and recorded.
[3]Tested after oropharynx is clear.

and severity of placental infarcts or evidence of clot (placental abruption) on the maternal side.

GENERAL EXAMINATION IN THE NURSERY

It is important that the examiner have warm hands and a gentle approach. Start with observation, then auscultation of the chest, and then palpation of the abdomen. Examination of the eyes, ears, throat, and hips should be done last, since these maneuvers are most disturbing to the infant. The heart rate should range from 120 to 160 beats/min and the respiratory rate from 30 to 60/min; blood pressure is affected by perinatal asphyxia and the need for mechanical ventilation more so than by gestational age or birth weight. Systolic blood pressure on day 1 ranges from 50 to 70 mm Hg and increases steadily during the first week of life. *Note:* An irregularly irregular heart rate, usually caused by premature atrial contractions, is not uncommon. This irregularity should resolve in the first days of life and is not of pathologic significance.

Skin

Observe for bruising, petechiae (common over the presenting part), meconium staining, and jaundice. Peripheral cyanosis is commonly present when the extremities are cool or the infant is polycythemic. Generalized cyanosis merits immediate evaluation. Pallor may be caused by acute or chronic blood loss or by acidosis. In dark-skinned infants, pallor and cyanosis should be assessed in the oral region and nail beds. Plethora suggests polycythemia. Note vernix caseosa (a whitish, greasy material covering the body that decreases as term approaches) and lanugo (the fine hair covering the preterm infant's

skin). Dry skin with cracking and peeling of the superficial layers is common in postterm infants. Edema may be generalized (hydrops) or localized (eg, on the dorsum of the feet in Turner's syndrome). Check for birthmarks such as capillary hemangiomas (lower occiput, eyelids, forehead) and mongolian spot (bluish-black pigmentation over the back and buttocks). Milia—small white keratogenous cysts—can be found scattered over the cheeks, forehead, nose, and nasolabial folds. Miliaria (blocked ducts of sweat glands) occurs in intertriginous areas and on the face or scalp. It can occur as small vesicles (crystallina), small erythematous papules (rubra), or pustules. Erythema toxicum is a benign rash characterized by fleeting erythematous papules and pustules which are filled with eosinophils. Pustular melanosis leaves pigmented macules when the pustules rupture. The pustules are noninfectious but contain neutrophils. Jaundice presenting in the first 24 hours is considered abnormal and should be evaluated. (See section on Neonatal Jaundice, below.)

Head

Check for cephalohematoma (a swelling over one or both parietal bones contained within suture lines) and caput succedaneum (edema over the presenting part that crosses suture lines). Subgaleal hemorrhages (beneath the scalp) are uncommon but can lead to extensive blood loss into this large potential space with resultant hypovolemic shock. Skull fractures may be linear or depressed and may be associated with cephalhematoma. Check the size and presence of the fontanelles. The anterior fontanelle varies from 1 to 4 cm in any direction, whereas the posterior fontanelle should be less than 1 cm. A third fontanelle is a bony defect along the sagittal suture in the parietal bones and may be a feature of certain syndromes such as trisomy 21. Sutures should be freely mobile. Craniosynostosis is a prematurely fused suture.

Face

Odd facies may be associated with a specific syndrome. Bruising from birth trauma (especially with face presentation) and forceps marks should be identified. Face presentation may be associated with considerable soft tissue swelling around the nose and mouth, causing considerable distortion. Facial nerve palsy is observed when the infant cries; the unaffected side of the mouth moves normally, giving a distorted grimace.

Eyes

Subconjunctival hemorrhages are seen frequently as a result of the birth process. Less commonly, a corneal tear may occur, presenting as a clouded cornea. Ophthalmologic consultation is indicated in such cases. Extraocular movements should be assessed. Occasional uncoordinated eye movements are common, but persistent irregular movements are abnormal. The iris should be inspected for abnormalities such as Brushfield's spots (trisomy 21) and colobomas. Examine for the red reflex of the retina. Leukocoria can be caused by glaucoma (cloudy cornea), cataract, or tumor (retinoblastoma). Infants at risk for chorioretinitis (congenital viral infection) should undergo a formal retinal examination with pupils dilated prior to nursery discharge or as an outpatient.

Nose

Examine the nose for size and shape. In utero compression can cause deformities. Because babies under 1 month of age are obligate nose breathers, any nasal obstruction (eg, bilateral choanal atresia or stenosis) can cause respiratory distress. Unilateral choanal atresia can be diagnosed by occluding each naris. Purulent nasal discharge at birth suggests congenital syphilis.

Ears

Malformed or malpositioned (low-set or posteriorly rotated) ears are often associated with other congenital anomalies. The tympanic membranes should be visualized.

Mouth

Epithelial (Epstein's) pearls are retention cysts along the gum margins and at the junction of the hard and soft palates. Natal teeth may be present and sometimes need to be removed to avoid the risk of aspiration. Check the integrity and shape of the palate; rule out cleft lip and cleft palate. A small mandible and tongue with cleft soft palate is seen with Pierre-Robin syndrome and can result in respiratory difficulty as the tongue occludes the airway. A prominent tongue can be seen in trisomy 21 and Beckwith-Wiedemann syndrome. Excessive drooling suggests esophageal atresia.

Neck

Redundant skin or webbing is seen in Turner's syndrome. Sinus tracts may be seen as remnants of branchial clefts. Check for masses: midline (thyroid), anterior to the sternocleidomastoids (branchial cleft cysts), within the sternocleidomastoid (hematoma, torticollis), and posterior to the sternocleidomastoid (cystic hygroma).

Chest & Lungs

Check for fractured clavicles (crepitus, bruising, and tenderness). Increased anteroposterior diameter (barrel chest) can be seen with aspiration syndromes. Check air entry bilaterally. Diminished breath sounds with respiratory distress suggest pneumothorax or a space-occupying lesion (eg, diaphragmatic hernia). Check the position of the mediastinum and heart tones. A shift is seen with pneumothorax (tension) or with a space-occupying lesion. With pneumomediastinum, the heart sounds are muffled. Expiratory grunting and decreased air entry are seen with hyaline membrane disease. Rales are not of clinical significance at this age.

Heart

Examination of the heart is described in detail in Chapter 18. *Note:* Murmurs are commonly present in the first hours and are most often benign. Severe congenital heart disease in the newborn may be present with no murmur at all. The two most common presentations of heart disease in the newborn are cyanosis and congestive heart failure with abnormalities of pulses. In hypoplastic left heart and critical aortic stenosis, pulses are diminished at all sites. In aortic coarctation and interrupted aortic arch, pulses are diminished in the lower extremities.

Abdomen

Check for softness, distention, and bowel sounds. If polyhydramnios was present or excessive oral secretions are noted, pass a soft catheter into the stomach to rule out esophageal atresia. Palpate for kidneys—most abdominal masses in the newborn are associated with kidney disorders (multicystic or dysplastic, hydronephrosis, etc). When the abdomen is relaxed, normal-sized kidneys may be felt but are not prominent. A markedly scaphoid abdomen plus respiratory distress suggests diaphragmatic hernia. Absence of abdominal musculature (prune belly syndrome) may occur in association with renal abnormalities. Check the size of the liver and the spleen. These organs are superficial and discernible by light palpation in the newborn. The outline of a distended bladder may be seen and palpated above the pubic symphysis.

Genitalia & Anus

Male and female genitals show characteristics according to gestational age (Table 2–2). In the female during the first few days, a whitish vaginal discharge with or without blood is normal. Check the patency and location of the anus.

Skeleton

Check for obvious anomalies—eg, the absence of a bone, clubfoot, fusion or webbing of digits, and extra digits. Examine for hip dislocation by attempting to dislocate the femur posteriorly and then abducting the legs to relocate the femur. Examine for extremity fractures and for palsies (especially brachial plexus injuries). Rule out myelomeningoceles and other spinal deformities (eg, scoliosis). Arthrogryposis (multiple joint contractures) is seen with chronic limitation of movement in utero because of lack of amniotic fluid or from a congenital neuromuscular disease.

Neurologic Examination

Observe resting tone (normal term newborns should exhibit flexion of the upper and lower extremities) and spontaneous movements. Look for symmetry of movements. Extension of extremities should result in spontaneous recoil to the flexed position. Assess the character of the cry; a high-pitched cry may be indicative of disease of the central nervous system (eg, hemorrhage). Hypotonia and a weak cry are indicative of systemic disease or a congenital neuromuscular disorder. Check for newborn reflexes:

(1) Rooting reflex: Head turns to the side of a facial stimulus.

(2) Sucking reflex in response to a nipple or the examiner's finger in the mouth.

(3) Traction response: The infant is pulled by the arms to a sitting position. Initially, the head lags, then with active flexion comes to the midline briefly before falling forward.

(4) Palmar grasp with placement of the examiner's finger in the palm.

(5) Deep tendon reflexes: Several beats of ankle clonus and an upgoing Babinski reflex may be normal.

(6) Placing: Rub the dorsum of one foot on the underside of a surface. The infant will flex the knee and bring the foot up.

(7) Moro (startle) reflex: Hold the infant and support the head. Allow the head to drop 1–2 cm suddenly. The arms will abduct at the shoulder and extend at the elbow. Adduction will follow. The hands show a prominent spreading or extension of the fingers.

Hegyi T et al: Blood pressure ranges in premature infants: I. The first hours of life. J Pediatr 1994;124:627.

Hegyi T et al: Blood pressure ranges in premature infants: II. The first weeks of life. Pediatrics 1996;97:336.

John RH, Schachner LA: Neonatal dermatologic challenges. Pediatr Rev 1997;18:86.

CARE OF THE NORMAL NEWBORN

The primary responsibility of the level 1 nursery is care of the well infant. This includes promoting mother–infant bonding, establishing feeding, and teaching the techniques of newborn care. Surveillance of the infant is a key function of the staff; they must be alert for the signs and symptoms of illness, including temperature instability, change in activity, refusal to feed, pallor, cyanosis, early or excessive jaundice, tachypnea and respiratory distress, delayed (beyond 24 hours) passage of first stool or voiding of urine, and bilious vomiting.

Several preventive measures are undertaken routinely in the normal newborn nursery.

Eye prophylaxis to prevent gonococcal ophthalmia is routinely administered within 1 hour after birth with either erythromycin ointment or silver nitrate 1% drops. Because of the severe chemical conjunctivitis caused by silver nitrate, erythromycin is preferred.

Vitamin K, 1 mg, is given intramuscularly or subcutaneously within 4 hours after birth to prevent hemorrhagic disease of the newborn. The area to be injected must be thoroughly cleansed before injection to prevent infection.

Hepatitis B vaccine is recommended for all infants with birth weights over 2000 g, and hepatitis B immune globulin (HBIG) is also administered if the mother is known to be surface antigen-positive. Follow-up injections of hepatitis B vaccine will be needed at 1–2 months and 6 months of age.

Cord blood is collected on all infants at birth and used for blood typing and Coombs' testing if the mother is type O or Rh-negative. Cord blood is useful also for other tests, such as toxicology screens. Blood from a doubly clamped cord can be used to check pH, base deficit, and lactate concentrations for up to 1 hour after delivery.

Rapid glucose testing should be performed in infants at risk for hypoglycemia (SGA, preterm, LGA, infant of a diabetic mother [IDM], stressed infant). Values less than 40 mg/dL should be confirmed by laboratory blood glucose testing.

Hematocrit should be measured at age 3–6 hours in infants at risk for or those who have symptoms of polycythemia or anemia.

The state-sponsored newborn genetic screen (for

inborn errors of metabolism such as phenylketonuria, galactosemia, sickle cell disease, hypothyroidism, and cystic fibrosis) is performed just prior to discharge, after 24–48 hours in hospital if possible. In many states, a repeat test is required at 8–14 days of age because the PKU test is often falsely negative when obtained at under 24 hours of age. In infants with prolonged hospital stays, the test should be performed by 1 week of age.

Infants should be positioned supine or lying on the right side with the dependent arm forward to minimize the risk of sudden infant death syndrome (SIDS).

FEEDING THE WELL NEWBORN INFANT

Indications that the baby is ready for feeding include (1) alertness and vigor, (2) absence of abdominal distention, (3) good bowel sounds, and (4) normal hunger cry. All of these usually occur within 6 hours after birth, but fetal distress or traumatic delivery may prolong this period.

The healthy term infant should be allowed to feed every 2–5 hours on demand. The first feeding usually occurs by 3 hours of life, often as early as in the delivery room. Breast milk or formula (20 kcal/oz) can be given. For formula-fed babies, the volume generally increases from 0.5–1 oz per feeding initially to 1.5–2 oz per feeding on day 3. By day 3, the average term newborn takes in about 100 mL/kg/d of milk.

Although a wide range of infant formulas can satisfy the nutritional needs of most neonates, breast milk is the standard on which formulas are based (see also Chapter 10). The distribution of calories in human milk is 55% fat, 38% carbohydrate, and 7% protein, with a whey to casein ratio of 60:40, allowing easy protein digestion. Despite the low concentrations of several vitamins and minerals, their bioavailability is high. All of the necessary nutrients, vitamins, minerals, and water are provided by human milk for the first 6 months of life except vitamin K (thus, 1 mg intramuscularly is administered at birth), vitamin D (200–300 IU/d if minimal sunlight exposure), fluoride (0.25 mg/d after 6 months if water supply not fluoridated), and vitamin B_{12} (0.3–0.5 mg/d if the mother is a strict vegetarian). Other advantages of breast milk include (1) the presence of immunologic, antimicrobial, and anti-inflammatory factors, including IgA, cellular, and protein or enzymatic components that decrease the incidence of upper respiratory and gastrointestinal infections in infancy; (2) the possibility that breast feeding may decrease the frequency and severity of childhood eczema and asthma; (3) promotion of mother-infant bonding; and (4) recent evidence that breast milk as a nutritional source improves neurodevelopmental outcomes.

Although approximately 55% of mothers in the United States initiate breast feeding, only 20% continue to breastfeed at 6 months. Hospital practices that facilitate the successful initiation of breast feeding include rooming-in, nursing on demand, and avoiding the use of pacifiers and supplemental formula (unless medically indicated). The nursery staff must be cognizant of problems associated with breast feeding and be able to provide help and support for mothers in the hospital. It is essential that an experienced professional observe and assist with at least one feeding to document good latch-on, important in preventing the common breast feeding problems of sore nipples, unsatisfied babies, engorgement, poor milk supply, and excessive hyperbilirubinemia ("lack-of-breast-milk jaundice"). Recommendations the nursing mother and health care provider can use to achieve successful breast feeding are presented in Table 2–6.

Neifert MR: The optimization of breast-feeding in the perinatal period. Clinics in Perinatol 1998;25:303.

Powers NG, Naylor AG, Wester RA: Hospital policies: Crucial to breastfeeding success. Semin Perinatol 1994;18:517.

Powers NG, Slusser W: Breastfeeding update 2: Clinical lactation management. Pediatr Rev 1997;18:147.

Slusser W, Powers NG: Breastfeeding update 1: Immunology, nutrition, and advocacy. Pediatr Rev 1997;18:111

EARLY NEWBORN DISCHARGE

The trend for several years has been toward shorter hospital stays for well mothers and infants, with typical stays in 1997 of 24 hours following a normal vaginal delivery and 48–72 hours following a cesarean section. Although there has been a growing consumer backlash against early discharge, culminating in the passage of the Newborns' and Mothers' Health Protection Act (effective January 1, 1998), it is unlikely that the typical length of stay for the normal newborn will increase substantially. Discharge at 24–36 hours of age appears safe and appropriate for most infants if there are no contraindications (Table 2–7) and a follow-up visit, either in the home with a visiting nurse or in the office, at 48–72 hours after discharge is ensured. Most infants with severe cardiorespiratory disorders and infections are identified in the first 6 hours of life. The exception would be the infant treated with intrapartum antibiotic prophylaxis for maternal group B streptococcal colonization or infection. The CDC and AAP have recommended that these infants be observed in hospital for 48 hours because of the possibility of "partial treatment" with delayed onset of symptoms of infection. Other problems such as jaundice and difficulties in breast feeding typically occur after 48 hours and can usually be dealt with on an outpatient basis provided good follow-up has been arranged.

The AAP recommends a follow-up visit within

Table 2–6. Guidelines for successful breast feeding.*

	First 8 Hours	8–24 Hours	Day 2	Day 3	Day 4	Day 5	Day 6 Onward
Milk supply		You may be able to express a few drops of milk.	Milk should come in between the second and fourth days.			Milk should be in. Breasts may be firm or leak milk.	Breasts should feel softer after feedings.
Baby's activity	Baby is usually wide-awake in the first hour of life. Put baby to breast within 30 minutes after birth.	Wake up your baby. Babies may not wake up on their own to feed.	Baby should be more cooperative and less sleepy.	Look for early feeding cues such as rooting, lip smacking, and hands to face.			Baby should appear satisfied after feedings.
Feeding routine	Baby may go into a deep sleep 2–4 hours after birth.	Feed your baby every 1½–3 hours or as often as wanted—at least 8–10 times a day.	Use chart to write down time of each feeding.			May go one longer interval (up to 5 hours between feeds) in a 24-hour period.	
Breast feeding	Baby will wake up and be alert and responsive for several more hours after initial deep sleep.	As long as Mom is comfortable, nurse at both breasts as long as baby is actively sucking.	Try to nurse both sides each feeding, aiming at 10 minutes per side. Expect some nipple tenderness.	Consider hand expressing or pumping a few drops of milk to soften the nipple if the breast is too firm for the baby to latch on.	Nurse a minimum of 10–15 minutes per side every 2–3 hours for the first few months of life.		Mom's nipple tenderness is improving or is gone.
Baby's urine output		Baby must have a minimum of one wet diaper in first 24 hours.	Baby must have at least one wet diaper every 8–11 hours.	You should see an increase in wet diapers (up to four to six) in 24 hours.	Baby's urine should be light yellow.	Baby should have six to eight wet diapers per day of colorless or light yellow urine.	
Baby's stool		Baby should have a black-green (meconium) stool.	Baby may have a second very dark (meconium) stool.	Baby's stools should be in transition from black-green to yellow.		Baby should have three or four yellow, seedy stools a day.	The number of stools may decrease gradually after 4–6 weeks of life.

*Modified, with permission, from Gabrielski L: Lactation support services. The Children's Hospital, Denver, 1994.

Table 2–7. Criteria for early newborn discharge.

Contraindications to early newborn discharge
1. Jaundice at ≤ 24 hours
2. Mother treated with antibiotics in labor for GBS prophylaxis
3. Known or suspected narcotic addiction or withdrawal
4. Physical defects requiring evaluation
5. Oral defects (clefts, micrognathia)

Relative contraindications to early newborn discharge (infants at high risk for feeding failure, excessive jaundice)
1. Prematurity or borderline prematurity (< 38 weeks' gestation)
2. Birth weight < 2700 g (6 lb)
3. Baby difficult to arouse for feeding; not demanding regularly in nursery
4. Medical or neurologic problems (Down's syndrome, hypotonia, cardiac problems)
5. Twins or higher multiples
6. ABO incompatibility or severe jaundice in previous child
7. Mother whose previous breast-fed infant gained weight poorly
8. Mother with breast surgery involving periareolar areas (if attempting to nurse)

Table 2–8. Guiidelines for early outpatient follow-up evaluation.

History
Rhythmic sucking and audible swallowing for at least 10 minutes total per feeding?
Baby wakes and demands to feed every 2–3 hours (at least eight to ten feedings per 24 hours)?
Do breasts feel full before feedings, and softer after?
Are there at least six noticeably wet diapers per 24 hours?
Are there yellow bowel movements (no longer meconium)—at least four per 24 hours?
Is baby still acting hungry after nursing (frequently sucks hands, rooting)?

Physical assessment
Weight, unclothed: should not be more than 8–10% below birth weight
Extent and severity of jaundice
Assessment of hydration, alertness, general well-being
Cardiovascular examination: murmurs, brachial and femoral pulses, respirations

48–72 hours for any newborn discharged before 48 hours of age. Infants who are small or slightly premature—especially if breast feeding—are at particular risk for inadequate intake. Suggested guidelines for the follow-up interview and physical examination are presented in Table 2–8. The optimal timing of discharge must be determined in each case based on medical, social, and financial factors.

CIRCUMCISION

Circumcision is an elective procedure to be performed only in healthy, stable infants. The procedure probably has medical benefits, including prevention of phimosis, paraphimosis, and balanoposthitis as well as a decreased incidence of cancer of the penis, cervical cancer (in partners of circumcised men), sexually transmitted diseases (including HIV), and urinary tract infection in male infants. Most parents, however, make the decision regarding circumcision for nonmedical reasons. The risks of the procedure include local infection, bleeding, removal of too much skin, and urethral injury. The incidence of these complications is less than 1%. Local anesthesia (dorsal penile nerve block with 1% lidocaine without epinephrine) or topical application of an anesthetic cream (eg, lidocaine-prilocaine cream) are safe and effective and should always be used. Techniques that allow visualization of the glans throughout the procedure (Plastibell and Gomco clamp) are preferred to a "blind" technique (eg, Mogen clamp) because of occasional amputation of the glans with the latter. Circumcision is contraindicated in infants with genital abnormalities (eg, hypospadias). Appropriate laboratory evaluation should be performed prior to the procedure in infants with a family history of bleeding disorders.

HEARING SCREENING

Normal hearing is critical to normal language development. All infants should be screened for risk of hearing loss by history (family history of congenital hearing loss or the possibility of congenital infection such as cytomegalovirus) and physical examination (abnormalities of external ear, preauricular pits or tags) and referred for testing if positive. Infants who have been significantly ill or who have received any potentially ototoxic drugs for more than 72 hours should be referred for screening. Universal screening by auditory brainstem evoked responses (ABRs) or evoked otoacoustic emissions (EOAE) as early as possible is endorsed by the AAP. Primary care providers and parents need to be alert to the possibility of hearing loss and offered ready referral in suspect cases.

American Academy of Pediatrics Committee on Fetus and Newborn: Hospital stay for healthy term newborns. Pediatrics 1995;96:788.
American Academy of Pediatrics Committee on Genetics: Newborn screening fact sheets. Pediatrics 1996;98:473.
American Academy of Pediatrics Joint Committee on Infant Hearing: Joint Committee on Infant Hearing position statement. Pediatrics 1995;95:152.
American Academy of Pediatrics Task Force on Infant Po-

sitioning and SIDS: Positioning and sudden infant death syndrome (SIDS): Update. Pediatrics 1996;98:1216.

American Academy of Pediatrics Vitamin K Ad Hoc Task Force: Controversies concerning vitamin K and the newborn. Pediatrics 1993;91:1001.

Braveman P et al: Early discharge of newborns and mothers: A critical review of the literature. Pediatrics 1995;96:716.

Britton JR et al: Early discharge of the term newborn: A continued dilemma. Pediatrics 1994;94:291.

Craig JC et al: Effect of circumcision on incidence of urinary tract infection in preschool boys. J Pediatr 1996;128:23.

Niku SD, Stock JA, Kaplan GW: Neonatal circumcision. Urol Clin North Am 1995;22:57.

Thilo EH, Townsend SF: Early newborn discharge: Have we gone too far? Contemp Pediatr 1996;13:29.

Thilo EH, Townsend SF, Merenstein GB: The history of policy and practice related to the perinatal stay. Clin Perinatol 1998;25:257.

Wiswell TE: Circumcision circumspection. N Engl J Med 1997;336:1244.

COMMON PROBLEMS IN TERM NEWBORNS

NEONATAL JAUNDICE

Jaundice is a common neonatal problem. Sixty-five percent of newborns develop clinical jaundice with a bilirubin level above 5 mg/dL during the first week of life. From an evolutionary standpoint, hyperbilirubinemia ought to confer some biologic advantage if it occurs so often. Bilirubin is a potent antioxidant and peroxyl scavenger that may help the newborn, who is deficient in most antioxidant substances such as vitamin E, catalase, and superoxide dismutase, to avoid oxygen toxicity in the days after birth. Hyperbilirubinemia can also be toxic, with high levels resulting in an encephalopathy known as kernicterus.

Metabolism of Bilirubin

Heme (iron protoporphyrin) is broken down by heme oxygenase to iron, which is conserved; carbon monoxide, which is exhaled; and biliverdin, which is then further metabolized to bilirubin by the enzyme bilirubin reductase. Each 1 g of hemoglobin breakdown results in the production of 34 mg of bilirubin (1 mg/dL = 17.2 μmol/L of bilirubin). Bilirubin is carried bound to albumin to the liver, where, in the presence of the enzyme uridyldiphosphoglucuronyl transferase (UDPGT; glucuronyl transferase), it is taken up by the hepatocyte and conjugated with two glucuronide molecules. The conjugated bilirubin is then excreted through the bile to the intestine. In the presence of normal gut flora, the conjugated bilirubin

is further metabolized to stercobilins and excreted in the stool. In the absence of gut flora—and with slow intestinal motility, as in the first few days of life—the conjugated bilirubin remains in the intestinal lumen, where a mucosal enzyme (β-glucuronidase) can cleave off the glucuronide molecules, leaving unconjugated bilirubin to be reabsorbed (the enterohepatic circulation of bilirubin).

Bilirubin Toxicity

The exact mechanism by which bilirubin is toxic to cells is not known. It is assumed that if the amount of lipid-soluble unconjugated bilirubin exceeds the available binding sites on albumin, there will then be "free" bilirubin that can enter neurons and damage them. The blood-brain barrier probably plays an important role in protecting an individual from brain damage, but its integrity is impossible to measure clinically. It is not known whether there is a level of bilirubin above which brain damage would always occur even in a healthy individual.

The syndrome of bilirubin encephalopathy was well described in the era before exchange transfusion as treatment for Rh isoimmunization (see below). The pathologic correlate is known as kernicterus, named for the yellow staining of the subthalamic nuclei ("kerns") seen at autopsy. The early symptoms of bilirubin encephalopathy consist of lethargy, hypotonia, and poor sucking, progressing to hypertonia, opisthotonos, and a high-pitched cry. Long-term sequelae include athetoid cerebral palsy, sensorineural deafness, limitation of upward gaze, and dental dysplasia. Whether or not bilirubin causes more subtle neurologic abnormalities remains debatable.

Bilirubin encephalopathy is very rare with current neonatal management. The only infant in which a specific bilirubin level (20 mg/dL [344 μmol/L] and above) has been associated with an increased risk of kernicterus is the Rh-isoimmunized infant. This observation—and the management strategy of keeping bilirubin under 20 mg/dL with exchange transfusion if needed—has been extended to other neonates with hemolytic disease despite an absence of data on the risk. The risk of bilirubin encephalopathy is probably very small for term infants without hemolysis even at bilirubin levels of 25 mg/dL (430 μmol/L) and above. Premature infants are probably at some increased risk because of associated illnesses that may affect the integrity of the blood-brain barrier and reduced albumin levels. For this reason, a lower level of bilirubin is generally assumed to represent the "exchange level" in these infants and is usually determined arbitrarily based on the infant's birth weight and gestational age. One common approach is to use 1% of the birth weight in grams as the "exchange level" in mg/dL (eg, 12 mg/dL for a 1200-g infant)—down to a low of 10 mg/dL. Many other approaches exist as well.

Causes of Unconjugated Hyperbilirubinemia

The causes of unconjugated hyperbilirubinemia can be grouped into two main categories: overproduction of bilirubin and decreased conjugation of bilirubin (Table 2–9).

A. Increased Bilirubin Production: Increased production of bilirubin results from an increased rate of red blood cell destruction (hemolysis) due to the presence of maternal antibodies against fetal cells (Coombs' test-positive), abnormal red cell membrane shape (ie, spherocytosis), or abnormal red cell enzymes (ie, glucose-6-phosphate dehydrogenase [G6PD] deficiency). The antibodies can be directed against the major blood group antigens (the type A or type B infant of a type O mother) or the minor antigens (the Rh system: D, E, C, d, e, c, Kell, Duffy, etc).

1. Antibody-mediated hemolysis (Coombs' test-positive)–ABO incompatibility is common,

Table 2–9. Etiology of jaundice secondary to unconjugated hyperbilirubemia.

Overproduction of bilirubin
1. Increased rate of hemolysis (reticulocyte count elevated)
   a. Patients with a positive Coombs' test
      Rh incompatibility
      ABO incompatibility
      Other blood group sensitizations
   b. Patients with a negative Coombs' test
      Abnormal red cell shapes
         Spherocytosis
         Elliptocytosis
         Pyknocytosis
         Stomatocytosis
      Red cell enzyme abnormalities
         Glucose-6-phosphate dehydrogenase deficiency
         Pyruvate kinase deficiency
         Hexokinase deficiency
         Other metabolic defects
   c. Patients with bacterial or viral sepsis
2. Nonhemolytic causes of increased bilirubin load:
   (Unconjugated bilirubin elevated, reticulocyte count normal.)
   a. Extravascular hemorrhage
      Cephalohematoma
      Extensive bruising
      Central nervous system hemorrhage
   b. Polycythemia
   c. Exaggerated enterohepatic circulation of bilirubin
      Gastrointestinal tract obstruction
      Functional ileus

Decreased rate of conjugation
   (Unconjugated bilirubin elevated, reticulocyte count normal)
   "Physiologic" jaundice
   Crigler-Najjar syndrome
      Type I glucuronyl transferase deficiency, autosomal recessive
      Type II glucuronyl transferase deficiency, autosomal dominant
   Gilbert's syndrome
   ?Galactosemia
   ?Hypothyroidism

usually not severe, and can accompany any pregnancy in a type O mother. The severity is not predictable because of variability in the amount of naturally occurring anti-A or anti-B IgG antibodies in the mother. Although 20% of pregnancies are the appropriate "set-ups" for ABO incompatibility (mother O, baby A or B), only about 33% of such infants are Coombs' test-positive and only about 20% of these develop jaundice. In addition to hyperbilirubinemia in the first days of life, these infants may develop a significant anemia over the first several weeks and on occasion may need to be transfused at a few weeks of age.

Rh isoimmunization is much less common and increases in severity with each immunized pregnancy because of an increased maternal IgG antibody production each time. Most Rh disease can be prevented by administering high-titer $Rh_o(D)$ immune globulin to an Rh-negative woman after any invasive procedure during pregnancy as well as after any miscarriage, abortion, or delivery of an Rh-positive infant. In severe cases, erythroblastosis fetalis (hydrops or generalized edema with heart failure related to severe anemia in the fetus) occurs, often resulting in fetal or neonatal death without appropriate antenatal intervention. In less severe cases, hemolysis is the main problem, with resultant hyperbilirubinemia and anemia. The cornerstone of antenatal management once isoimmunization has been diagnosed is transfusion of the fetus with Rh-negative cells, either directly into the umbilical vein via percutaneous cordocentesis or into the fetal abdominal cavity. Following delivery, phototherapy is usually started immediately, with exchange transfusion (see below) as needed. A 500 mg/kg dose of intravenous immunoglobulin (IVIG) given to the infant as soon after delivery as the diagnosis is made has recently been shown to decrease the need for exchange transfusion. Ongoing hemolysis will still occur until all maternal antibody is gone; therefore, these infants need to be followed carefully over the first 2 months for development of anemia severe enough to require transfusion. The role of erythropoietin therapy in treating late anemia is under investigation.

2. Nonimmune hemolysis (Coombs' test-negative)–Hereditary spherocytosis is the most common red cell membrane defect, resulting in hemolysis because of decreased red cell deformability. These infants may have hyperbilirubinemia severe enough to require exchange transfusion. Mild to moderate splenomegaly may be present. Diagnosis is suspected by peripheral blood smear and confirmed by red cell osmotic fragility study. A family history of anemia, jaundice, and gallstones may be elicited.

G6PD deficiency is the most common red cell enzyme defect resulting in hemolysis and should be suspected in a male (it is X-linked) of African, Mediterranean, or Asian descent, particularly when the onset of jaundice is later than usual.

3. Nonhemolytic increased bilirubin production–Enclosed hemorrhage, such as cephalohematoma, intracranial hemorrhage, or extensive bruising in the skin, can lead to jaundice as the red blood cells are broken down and removed. Polycythemia leads to jaundice by increased red cell mass, with increased numbers of cells reaching senescence daily. Ileus, either paralytic or mechanical, related to a bowel obstruction, leads to hyperbilirubinemia secondary to increased enterohepatic circulation.

B. Decreased Rate of Conjugation:

1. UDPGT deficiency–Crigler-Najjar syndrome type I (complete deficiency, autosomal recessive) and type II (partial deficiency, autosomal dominant) present as excessive and prolonged neonatal jaundice, but both forms are very rare.

Gilbert's syndrome is a mild autosomal dominant disorder affecting 3–6% of the population and characterized by decreased hepatic UDPGT levels. Mild unconjugated hyperbilirubinemia without other liver function abnormalities occurs after puberty. The possible relationship of this disorder to neonatal jaundice is under investigation.

C. Hyperbilirubinemia Caused by Unknown or Multiple Factors:

1. Physiologic jaundice–The contributing factors to physiologic jaundice include UDPGT inactivity at birth, a relatively high red cell mass even in the nonpolycythemic neonate, and an absence of intestinal flora, with initially slow intestinal motility leading to an active enterohepatic circulation of bilirubin. For jaundice to be "physiologic" rather than pathologic, the following criteria should be satisfied: (1) clinical jaundice appears after 24 hours of age; (2) total bilirubin rises by less than 5 mg/dL (86 μmol/L) per day; (3) peak bilirubin occurs at 3–5 days of age, with a total bilirubin of no more than 15 mg/dL (258 μmol/L); and (4) clinical jaundice is resolved by 1 week in the term infant and by 2 weeks in the preterm infant. Hyperbilirubinemia outside of these parameters—or jaundice that requires treatment—is not physiologic and must be further evaluated (see below).

2. High altitude–Infants at 3100 m (10,000 ft) have twice the incidence of bilirubin over 12 mg/dL (206 μmol/L) as infants at 1600 m (5200 ft) and four times that of infants at sea level: 39% versus 16% versus 8%, respectively. Possible mechanisms include increased bilirubin production secondary to increased hematocrit and decreased clearance caused by hypoxemia.

3. Racial differences–Asians are more likely than whites or blacks to have a bilirubin greater than 12 mg/dL (206 μmol/L): 23% versus 10–13% versus 4%, respectively.

4. Prematurity–Premature infants frequently have poor enteral intake, delayed stooling, and increased enterohepatic circulation. Even at 37 weeks' gestation, they are four times more likely than at 40 weeks to have a bilirubin greater than 13 mg/dL (224 μmol/L).

5. Breast feeding and jaundice–There are two syndromes of jaundice associated with breast feeding: breast milk jaundice and breast feeding–associated jaundice ("lack-of-breast-milk jaundice").

Breast milk jaundice is an uncommon syndrome of prolonged unconjugated hyperbilirubinemia believed to be caused by an inhibitor of conjugation present in the breast milk of some mothers. Suggested substances have included pregnanediol, free fatty acids, steroids, and β-glucuronidase. The hyperbilirubinemia peaks at 10–15 days of age, with a maximal level of 10–30 mg/dL (172–516 μmol/L), and declines slowly by 3–12 weeks of age. If nursing is interrupted for 24–48 hours, the bilirubin level falls precipitously and will not rebound to the same level when nursing is resumed.

Breast feeding–associated jaundice, also known as "lack-of-breast-milk jaundice," is a common entity. Breast-fed infants have a higher incidence (9%) of bilirubin over 13 mg/dL (224 μmol/L) than formula-fed infants (2%) and are more likely to have bilirubin over 15 mg/dL (258 μmol/L) than formula-fed infants: 2% versus 0.3%. The pathogenesis appears to be decreased enteral intake and increased enterohepatic circulation. No increase in bilirubin production is seen, as measured by carbon monoxide exhalation. Although rarely associated with bilirubin encephalopathy, this type of jaundice should be considered a sign of failure to establish an adequate milk supply and should prompt specific inquiries into this possibility (Table 2–10). If inadequate intake is present, the infant should receive supplementation with formula if needed, and the mother should be instructed to nurse more frequently and to pump her breasts with an electric breast pump every 2 hours to enhance milk production. A consultation with a certified lactation specialist should be considered, since many physicians feel inadequately prepared to handle these situations. Since hospital discharge of normal newborns occurs before the milk supply is established, a follow-up visit 2–3 days after discharge is of obvious importance.

These two entities may sometimes overlap in the same infant, since prolonged jaundice is common in breast-fed infants (20–30%), and many of those infants with high bilirubins in the first days also persist longest.

Table 2–10. Signs of inadequate breast milk intake.

Weight loss of > 8–10% from birth
Fewer than six noticeably wet diapers per day
Fewer than four stools per day
Nursing fewer than eight times per 24 hours for at least 10
  minutes each feed

D. Prolonged Hyperbilirubinemia: Causes of prolonged hyperbilirubinemia include hemolytic disease, breast milk jaundice, Crigler-Najjar syndrome, bowel obstruction, congenital hypothyroidism, and galactosemia. Galactosemia generally presents with hepatomegaly in an ill-appearing, often septic infant, and the hyperbilirubinemia is usually mixed.

Evaluation of Hyperbilirubinemia

Clinical jaundice appears at a bilirubin level of 5 mg/dL (86 μmol/L) and appears first on the head, progressing down the chest and abdomen as the level increases. By the time jaundice is noted on the distal extremities, the level is likely to be at least 15 mg/dL (258 μmol/L). Infants who develop clinical jaundice on the first day of life—or who develop excessive jaundice—require evaluation. The minimal evaluation consists of a feeding and elimination history, weight (and comparison with birth weight), examination for any source of excessive heme breakdown, and laboratory evaluation for blood type, Coombs' testing, CBC with smear, and total bilirubin level. A G6PD test should be considered if the infant is a male of African, Asian, or Mediterranean racial background, particularly if the jaundice presents later than usual. A fractionated bilirubin level should be obtained if the infant appears acutely ill, if jaundice is prolonged, or if there is dark urine with light stools.

Because of large interlaboratory variability, serial bilirubin levels should be obtained from a single laboratory whenever possible to make interpretation more accurate.

Treatment of Hyperbilirubinemia

A. Protoporphyrins: Tin and zinc protoporphyrin or mesoporphyrin (Sn-PP, Zn-PP; Sn-MP, Zn-MP) are inhibitors of heme oxygenase, the enzyme that begins the catabolism of heme (iron protoporphyrin). Studies are under way involving a single injection of these substances shortly after birth to prevent the formation of bilirubin. Although early results are promising, these drugs are still experimental.

B. Phototherapy: Phototherapy is used most commonly, since it is relatively noninvasive and safe. Light at a wavelength absorbed by bilirubin (blue or white spectrum) is used. The unconjugated bilirubin in the skin is converted by such light to a stereoisomer compound that is water-soluble and able to be excreted in the bile without conjugation. A minimum of 10–12 μW/cm^2 irradiance is required, and efficacy is dose-dependent. The dose can be raised by increasing the body surface area exposed to the light and by moving the lights closer to the baby. Fiberoptic blankets are effective. The infant's eyes should be shielded from the light to prevent damage to retinal cells. A frequent side effect of phototherapy is diar-

rhea, which is managed by feeding a non-lactose-containing formula for the duration of the treatment.

Phototherapy is started when the bilirubin level is approximately 5 mg/dL (86 μmol/L) lower than the "exchange level" for that infant (eg, at levels of 15–18 mg/dL [258–310 μmol/L] for a term infant), depending also on the age of the infant. Guidelines for the use of phototherapy in the term infant with and without ABO incompatibility are shown in Tables 2–11 and 2–12. Although phototherapy has been shown to decrease the likelihood of exchange transfusion, the long-term benefits of its use in infants with less severe jaundice are unknown.

C. Exchange Transfusion: Double-volume exchange transfusion (approximately 160–200 mL/kg body weight) remains necessary in the rare case of hemolysis resulting from Rh isoimmunization, ABO incompatibility, or hereditary spherocytosis. In addition to decreasing the bilirubin level by approximately 50% acutely, the exchange also serves to remove nearly 80% of the sensitized or abnormal red blood cells and offending antibody so that ongoing hemolysis will be decreased. The procedure is invasive and not without risk. The risk of mortality is greatest in the smallest, most immature, and otherwise unstable infants, but sudden death during the procedure can occur in any infant. Because of the rarity of the procedure and its inherent risk, it should be performed very cautiously, preferably at a referral center.

For the typical exchange transfusion, the umbilical vein is catheterized, and reconstituted whole blood with a hematocrit of approximately 50% is used in aliquots of 8–10 mL per pass. Hypocalcemia occurs during the procedure because of binding to the citrate-phosphate-dextrose anticoagulant and needs to be corrected periodically. Hypoglycemia is common following the procedure and requires close monitoring. Thrombocytopenia occurs because of the removal of platelets. The entire procedure should take 1–2 hours and should be performed using aseptic technique.

American Academy of Pediatrics Provisional Committee for Quality Improvement and Subcommittee on Hyperbilirubinemia: Practice parameter: Management of hyperbilirubinemia in the healthy term newborn. Pediatrics 1994;94:558.
Kappas A et al: Direct comparison of Sn-mesoporphyrin, an inhibitor of bilirubin production, and phototherapy

Table 2–11. Guidelines for treatment of the term infant with ABO incompatibility.

Phototherapy if–
Bilirubin ≥ 10 mg/dL at < 12 hours
Bilirubin ≥ 12–14 mg/dL at < 18 hours
Bilirubin ≥ 15 mg/dL at > 24 hours

Table 2–12. Guidelines for use of phototherapy in the term infant without hemolysis.

Bilirubin ≥ 15 mg/dL, age < 2 days: Evaluation, phototherapy
Bilirubin ≥ 18 mg/dL, age > 2–3 days: Evaluation, phototherapy
Bilirubin ≥ 20–22 mg/dL, age > 3–4 days: Evaluation, phototherapy; consider interruption of nursing and formula supplementation; have mother use electric breast pump during interruption of breast feeding
Bilirubin ≥ 25 mg/dL: As above, plus consider exchange transfusion

controlling hyperbilirubinemia in term and near-term newborns. Pediatrics 1995;95:468.

Martinez JC et al: Hyperbilirubinemia in the breast-fed newborn: A controlled trial of four interventions. Pediatrics 1993;91:470.

Newman TB, Maisels MJ: Evaluation and treatment of jaundice in the term newborn: A kinder, gentler approach. Pediatrics 1992;89:809.

Peterec SM: Management of neonatal Rh disease. Clin Perinatol 1995;22:561.

Rubo J et al: High-dose intravenous immune globulin therapy for hyperbilirubinemia caused by Rh hemolytic disease. J Pediatr 1992;121:93.

Watchko JF, Oski FA: Bilirubin 20 mg/dL = vigintiphobia. Pediatrics 1983;71:660.

HYPOGLYCEMIA

Blood glucose concentration in the fetus is approximately 15 mg/dL less than the maternal glucose concentration. Glucose concentration normally decreases in the immediate postnatal period, with concentrations below 35–40 mg/dL being considered indicative of hypoglycemia. By 3 hours, the glucose concentration in normal term babies stabilizes between 50 and 80 mg/dL. After the first few hours of life, concentrations below 40 mg/dL should be considered abnormal.

The two most commonly encountered groups of term newborn infants at high risk for neonatal hypoglycemia are IDMs and infants with IUGRs.

Infant of a Diabetic Mother (IDM)

The IDM baby has abundant glucose stores in the form of glycogen and fat but develops hypoglycemia because of hyperinsulinemia induced by maternal and fetal hyperglycemia. Other tissues also grow abnormally in utero, probably as a consequence of increased flow of nutrients from the maternal circulation. The result is a macrosomic infant who is at increased risk for trauma during delivery. Other problems related to the in utero metabolic environment include a cardiomyopathy (asymmetric septal hypertrophy), which can present as a murmur with or

without cardiac failure and respiratory distress, and, more rarely, microcolon, which presents as low intestinal obstruction. IDMs whose mothers have diabetes at conception are also at increased risk for congenital anomalies probably related to first-trimester glucose control. Other neonatal problems include a hypercoagulable state and polycythemia, a combination that predisposes the infant to large venous thromboses (eg, renal vein thrombosis). Finally, these infants are somewhat immature for their gestational age and are at increased risk for hyaline membrane disease, hypocalcemia, and hyperbilirubinemia.

Intrauterine Growth Restriction

The infant with IUGR has reduced glucose stores in the form of glycogen and body fat and therefore is prone to hypoglycemia despite relatively appropriate endocrine adjustments at birth. In addition to hypoglycemia, marked hyperglycemia and a transient diabetes mellitus–like syndrome may occasionally develop, particularly in the very preterm SGA infant. These problems can usually be handled by adjusting glucose intake, though insulin is sometimes needed transiently.

Other Causes of Hypoglycemia

Hypoglycemia occurs with disorders associated with islet cell hyperplasia (Beckwith–Wiedemann syndrome [macroglossia, omphalocele, macrosomia], erythroblastosis fetalis, nesidioblastosis), inborn errors of metabolism (glycogen storage disease, galactosemia), and endocrine disorders (panhypopituitarism, other deficiencies of counterregulatory hormones). It may also occur as a complication of birth asphyxia, hypoxia, or other stresses, including bacterial and viral sepsis. Prematures are also at risk for hypoglycemia because of decreased glycogen stores.

Clinical Findings

The signs of hypoglycemia in the newborn are relatively nonspecific and may be subtle: lethargy, poor feeding, irritability, tremulousness, jitteriness, apnea, and seizures. The disorder is most severe and resistant to treatment if due to hyperinsulinemia. Cardiac failure may occur in severe cases, particularly in IDM babies with cardiomyopathy. Infants with hyperinsulinemic states can experience the onset of hypoglycemia very early (within the first 30–60 minutes of life).

Blood glucose can be measured by heel stick using a bedside glucometer. All infants at risk should be screened, including IDMs, IUGRs, premature infants, and any infant with symptoms that could be due to hypoglycemia. All low or borderline values should be confirmed by direct measurement of blood glucose concentration determined in the laboratory. It is important to continue surveillance of glucose concentration until the baby has been on full enteral feedings without intravenous supplementation for a 24-hour period. Relapse of hypoglycemia thereafter is unlikely.

Infants with hypoglycemia requiring intravenous glucose infusions for more than 5 days should be evaluated for the less common causes of hypoglycemia. This workup should include evaluation for inborn errors of metabolism, hyperinsulinemic states, and deficiencies of counterregulatory hormones.

Treatment

Therapy is based on provision of glucose either enterally or intravenously. Suggested guidelines for treatment are presented in Table 2–13. In hyperinsulinemic states, boluses of glucose should be avoided and a higher glucose infusion rate used. After initial correction with a bolus of $D_{10}W$, 2 mL/kg, glucose infusion should be gradually increased as needed from a starting rate of 6 mg/kg/min. Finally, in both IDM and IUGR babies, those with high hematocrits and hypoglycemia are most likely to show clinical signs of hypoglycemia. In such infants, both the hypoglycemia and the polycythemia should be treated—with intravenous glucose infusion and partial exchange transfusion, respectively.

Prognosis

The prognosis of hypoglycemia is good if therapy

is prompt. Central nervous system sequelae are seen in infants with neonatal seizures resulting from hypoglycemia.

Hawdon JM et al: Prevention and management of neonatal hypoglycemia. Arch Dis Child Fetal Neonatal Ed 1994;70:F60.
Reece EA, Homko CJ: Infant of the diabetic mother. Semin Perinatol 1994;18:459.

RESPIRATORY DISTRESS IN THE TERM NEWBORN

Essentials of Diagnosis & Typical Features

- Tachypnea, respiratory rate > 60 breaths/min.
- Retractions (intercostal, sternal).
- Expiratory grunting.
- Cyanosis on room air.

General Considerations

Respiratory distress is among the most common symptom complexes seen in the newborn. It may result from both noncardiopulmonary and cardiopulmonary causes (Table 2–14). Chest radiography, arterial blood gases, and pulse oximetry are useful in assessing both the cause and the severity of the problem. It is important to consider the noncardiopulmonary causes listed in Table 2–14 because the natural tendency is to focus on the heart and lungs. Most of the noncardiopulmonary causes can be ruled out by the history, physical examination, and a few simple laboratory tests. The evaluation of cardiovascular disorders is discussed in a subsequent section.

The most common pulmonary causes of respiratory distress in the term infant are transient tachypnea, aspiration syndromes, air leaks, and congenital pneumonia.

A. Transient Tachypnea (Retained Fetal Lung Fluid): Respiratory distress is typically present from birth, usually associated with a mild to moderate oxygen requirement (25–50% O_2). The infant may be term or near-term, nonasphyxiated, following a short labor or cesarean section without labor. Chest x-ray shows perihilar streaking and fluid in interlobar fissures. Resolution usually occurs within 12–24 hours.

B. Aspiration Syndromes: The infant is typically term or near-term, frequently with some fetal distress prior to delivery or depression at delivery. Blood or meconium is usually present in the amniotic fluid, but occasionally the fluid is clear. Respiratory distress is present from birth, in many cases manifested by a barrel chest appearance and coarse breath sounds. An increasing O_2 need from pneumonitis may require intubation and ventilation. Chest x-ray shows coarse irregular infiltrates, hyperexpansion, and, in the worst cases, lobar consolidation.

When the amniotic fluid contains meconium or

Table 2–13. Hypoglycemia: Suggested therapeutic regimens.

Screening Test[1]	Presence of Symptoms	Action
20–40 mg/dL	No symptoms	Draw blood glucose;[2] if the infant is alert and vigorous, feed; follow with frequent glucose monitoring. If the baby continues to have blood glucose < 40 mg/dL, provide IV glucose at 6 mg/kg/min ($D_{10}W$ at 3.6 mL/kg/h).
< 40 mg/dL	Symptoms present	Draw blood glucose;[2] provide bolus of $D_{10}W$ (2 mL/kg) followed by an infusion of 6 mg/kg/min (3.6 mL/kg/h).
< 20 mg/dL	With or without symptoms	Draw blood glucose;[2] provide bolus of $D_{10}W$ followed by an infusion of 6 mg/kg/min. If IV access cannot be obtained immediately, an umbilical vein line should be utilized.

[1]Rapid bedside determination.
[2]Laboratory confirmation.

Table 2–14. Causes of respiratory distress in the newborn.[1]

Noncardiopulmonary
  Hypothermia or hyperthermia
  Hypoglycemia
  Polycythemia
  Metabolic acidosis
  Drug intoxications or withdrawal
  Insult to the central nervous system
    Asphyxia
    Hemorrhage
  Neuromuscular disease
  Phrenic nerve injury
  Asphyxiating thoracic dystrophy
Cardiovascular
  Left-sided outflow tract obstruction
    Hypoplastic left heart
    Aortic stenosis
    Coarctation of the aorta
  Cyanotic lesions
    Transposition of the great vessels
    Total anomalous pulmonary venous return
    Tricuspid atresia
    Right-sided outflow obstruction
Pulmonary
  Upper airway obstruction
    Choanal atresia
    Vocal cord paralysis
    Lingual thyroid
  Meconium aspiration
  Clear fluid aspiration
  Transient tachypnea
  Pneumonia
  Pulmonary hypoplasia
  Hyaline membrane disease
  Pneumothorax
  Pleural effusions
  Mass lesions
    Lobar emphysema
    Cystic adenomatoid malformation

[1]Reproduced, with permission, from Rosenberg AA: Neonatal adaptation. In: *Obstetrics: Normal and Problem Pregnancies.* Gabbe SG, Niebyl JR, Simpson JL (editors). Churchill Livingstone, 1996.

blood, suctioning of the infant's mouth and nose as the head is delivered and before delivery of the chest is recommended to prevent aspiration of these secretions with the onset of breathing. If the infant is depressed or shows signs of respiratory distress at birth, suctioning of the trachea under direct vision is recommended, especially prior to commencing resuscitation with positive-pressure ventilation. Although these procedures are recommended, they will not prevent all cases of meconium or blood aspiration. Aspiration often occurs in utero as the "stressed" infant gasps. Babies with aspirations are at risk of air leak (pneumothorax) because of uneven aeration with segmental overdistention and are at risk for persistent pulmonary hypertension (see Cardiac Problems, below). Standard treatment includes ventilatory support, antibiotics, and pressor support of systemic blood pressure.

C. Congenital Pneumonia: Infants may be of any gestational age, with or without a maternal history of rupture of the membranes > 12 hours or chorioamnionitis or maternal antibiotic administration. Onset of respiratory distress may be at birth or may be delayed for several hours. Chest x-ray may resemble that of retained lung fluid or hyaline membrane disease; rarely, there may be a lobar infiltrate

The lungs are the most common site of infection in the neonate. Most commonly, infections ascend from the genital tract before or during labor, with the vaginal or rectal flora the most likely infectious agents (group B streptococci, *E coli, Klebsiella*). Shock, poor perfusion, and absolute neutropenia (< 2000/μL) provide corroborating evidence for pneumonia. Gram's stain of tracheal aspirate may be helpful. Because no signs or laboratory findings can confirm the presence or absence of pneumonia with certainty, all infants with respiratory distress should receive a blood culture and broad-spectrum antibiotic therapy until the diagnosis of a bacterial infection can be ruled out.

D. Spontaneous Pneumothorax: Respiratory distress (primarily tachypnea) is present from birth, typically not severe, and requires mild to moderate supplemental O_2. Breath sounds may be decreased on the affected side; heart tones may be shifted toward the opposite side and may be distant. Chest x-ray will show pneumothorax or pneumomediastinum.

This entity occurs in 1% of all deliveries. The risk is increased by manipulations such as positive-pressure ventilation in the delivery room. Treatment usually consists of supplemental O_2 and watchful waiting. Breathing 100% O_2 for a few hours may accelerate reabsorption of the extrapulmonary gas by creating a diffusion gradient for nitrogen across the surface of the lung ("nitrogen washout" technique). This is effective only if the infant was breathing room air or O_2 at low concentration at the time of the pneumothorax. Drainage by needle thoracentesis or tube thoracostomy is occasionally required. There is a small increased risk of renal abnormalities associated with spontaneous pneumothorax. Therefore, a careful physical examination of the kidneys and observation of urine output are indicated. If pulmonary hypoplasia with pneumothorax is suspected, renal ultrasound would also be indicated.

E. Other Pulmonary Causes: The other pulmonary causes of respiratory distress are fairly rare. Bilateral choanal atresia should be suspected if there is no air movement when the infant breathes through the nose. These infants present in the delivery room with good color and heart rate while crying but become cyanotic and bradycardiac when they quiet down and resume normal breathing. Other causes of upper airway obstruction are usually characterized by some degree of stridor or poor air movement despite good respiratory effort. Pleural effusions can be suspected in hydropic infants (eg, those with erythroblastosis fetalis). Space-occupying lesions cause a shift of the mediastinum and asymmetric breath sounds and would be apparent on chest x-ray.

Treatment

Whatever the cause, the cornerstone of treatment of neonatal respiratory distress is provision of adequate supplemental oxygen to maintain a PaO_2 of 60–70 mm Hg and a saturation by pulse oximetry (SpO_2) of 92–96%. PaO_2 levels less than 50 mm Hg are associated with pulmonary vasoconstriction, which can exacerbate hypoxemia, while those greater than 100 mm Hg may increase the risk of oxygen toxicity without additional benefit. Oxygen should be warmed, humidified, and delivered through an air blender. Concentration should be measured with a calibrated oxygen analyzer. An umbilical or peripheral arterial line should be placed in any infant requiring more than 45% FIO_2 by 4–6 hours of life to allow frequent blood gas determinations. Noninvasive monitoring with a pulse oximeter should be used.

Other supportive treatment includes intravenous provision of glucose and water. Unless infection can be unequivocally ruled out, blood cultures should be obtained and broad-spectrum antibiotics started. Colloid solutions (eg, 5% albumin) can be given in infusions of 10 mL/kg over 30 minutes for low blood pressure, poor perfusion, and metabolic acidosis. Sodium bicarbonate (1–2 mEq/kg) is indicated for treatment of documented metabolic acidosis that has not responded to oxygen, ventilation, and volume. Specific workup should be pursued as indicated by the history and physical findings. In most cases, a chest x-ray study, blood gas measurements, complete blood count, and blood glucose allow a diagnosis.

Intubation and ventilation should be undertaken for signs of respiratory failure ($PaO_2 < 60$ mm Hg in 70–80% FIO_2 or $PaCO_2 > 60$ mm Hg). Peak pressures should be adequate to produce chest wall expansion and audible breath sounds (usually 18–24 cm H_2O). Positive end-expiratory pressure (4–6 cm H_2O) should also be used. Ventilation rates of 20–50 breaths per minute are usually required. The goal is to maintain a PaO_2 of 60–70 mm Hg and a $PaCO_2$ of 40–50 mm Hg.

Prognosis

Most of the respiratory conditions affecting the term infant are acute and resolve in the first several days. Meconium aspiration syndrome and congenital pneumonia are associated with significant long-term pulmonary morbidity (chronic lung disease) and mortality (approximately 10–20%). Mortality rates in these disorders have been reduced by use of high-frequency ventilation, inhaled nitric oxide (NO) to treat pulmonary hypertension, and extracorporeal membrane oxygenation (ECMO).

Brodsky L: Congenital stridor. Pediatr Rev 1996;17:408.

Greenough A: Meconium aspiration syndrome: Prevention and treatment. Early Hum Dev 1995;41:183.

Katz VL, Bowes WA: Meconium aspiration syndrome: Reflections on a murky subject. Am J Obstet Gynecol 1992;166:171.

Wiswell TE, Brent RC: Meconium staining and the meconium aspiration syndrome: Unresolved issues. Pediatr Clin North Am 1993;40:955.

HEART MURMURS
(See also section on Cardiac Problems.)

Heart murmurs are common in the first days of life and do not usually signify structural heart problems. If a murmur is present at birth, however, it should be considered a valvular problem until proved otherwise since the common benign transitional murmurs (eg, patent ductus arteriosus) are not audible until minutes to hours after birth.

If an infant is pink, well-perfused, and in no respiratory distress and has palpable and symmetric pulses (right brachial pulse no stronger than the femoral pulse), the murmur is most likely transitional. Transitional murmurs are soft (grade 1–3/6), heard at the left upper to midsternal border, and generally loudest during the first 24 hours. If the murmur persists beyond 24 hours, blood pressure in the right arm and a leg should be determined. If there is a difference of more than 15 mm Hg (arm > leg), cardiology consultation should be arranged to evaluate for coarctation of the aorta. If there is no difference, the infant can be discharged home with follow-up in 2–3 days for auscultation and evaluation for signs of congestive failure. If signs of failure or cyanosis are present, the infant should be referred for evaluation without delay. If the murmur persists without these signs, the infant can be referred for elective evaluation at 2–4 weeks of age.

Burton DA, Cabalka AK: Cardiac evaluation of infants: The first year of life. Pediatr Clin North Am 1994;41:991.

Sapin SO: Recognizing normal heart murmurs: A logic-based mnemonic. Pediatrics 1997;99:616.

BIRTH TRAUMA

Most birth trauma is associated with difficult delivery, particularly with a large infant, abnormal position, or fetal distress requiring rapid extraction. The most common injuries are soft tissue bruising, fractures (clavicle, humerus, or femur), and cervical plexus palsies, though skull fractures, intracranial hemorrhage (primarily subdural and subarachnoid), and cervical spinal cord injuries can also occur.

Fractures are often diagnosed by the obstetrician, who may feel and hear a snap during delivery. Clavicular fractures may cause decreased spontaneous movement of the arm, with tenderness and crepitus over the area. Humeral or femoral fractures may cause tenderness and swelling over the shaft with a diaphyseal fracture, with limited spontaneous extremity motion in all cases. Epiphyseal fractures are harder to diagnose radiographically owing to the cartilaginous nature of the epiphysis. After 8–10 days, callus appears and is visible on radiographs. Treatment in all cases is gentle handling, with immobilization for 8–10 days: the humerus against the chest with elbow flexed; the femur with a posterior splint from below the knee to the buttock.

Brachial plexus injuries may result from traction as the head is pulled away from the shoulder during delivery. Injury to the C5–C6 roots is most common and results in Erb-Duchenne palsy. The arm is limp, adducted and internally rotated, extended and pronated at the elbow, and flexed at the wrist ("waiter's tip posture"). Grasp is present. If the lower nerve roots (C8–T1) are involved, the hand is flaccid (Klumpke's palsy). Isolated involvement of these roots is rare. If the entire plexus is injured, the arm and hand are flaccid, with an associated sensory deficit.

Early treatment for brachial plexus injury is conservative, since function usually returns over several weeks. Referral should be made to a physical therapist so the parents can be instructed on range of motion exercises and splinting and for further evaluation if needed. Return of function begins in the deltoid and biceps, with recovery by 3 months in most cases.

Spinal cord injury can occur at birth, especially in difficult breech extractions with hyperextension of the neck, or in midforceps rotations where the body fails to turn with the head. Infants are flaccid, quadriplegic, and without respiratory efforts at birth, though facial movements are preserved. The long-term outlook for such infants is grim.

Facial nerve palsy is sometimes associated with forceps use but more often results from chronic in utero pressure of the baby's head against the mother's sacrum. The infant has asymmetric mouth movements and eye closure with poor movement on the affected side. Most cases resolve spontaneously within a few days to 3 weeks.

Eng GD: Neuromuscular disease. In: *Neonatology: Pathophysiology and Management of the Newborn.* Avery GB, Fletcher MA, MacDonald MG (editors). Lippincott, 1994.

Griffin PP: Orthopedics. In: *Neonatology: Pathophysiology and Management of the Newborn.* Avery GB, Fletcher MA, MacDonald MG (editors). Lippincott, 1994.

Ouzounian JG, Korst LM, Phelan JP: Permanent Erb palsy: A traction-related injury? Obstet Gynecol 1997;89:130.

INFANTS OF MOTHERS WHO ABUSE DRUGS

The problem of newborn infants born to mothers abusing drugs is increasing in all communities. The most common drugs are tobacco, alcohol, marijuana, and cocaine. Because these mothers may abuse many drugs and give an unreliable history of drug usage, it may be difficult to pinpoint which drug is causing the morbidity seen in a newborn infant. Early hospital discharge makes discovery of these infants based on physical findings and abnormal behavior much more difficult.

1. COCAINE

Cocaine is currently the most commonly abused illicit drug, identified in up to 20–40% of gravidas on urban delivery services; moreover, cocaine is often used in association with other drugs. The obstetric effects include maternal hypertension, decreased uterine blood flow, fetal hypoxemia, and uterine contractions. The rates of stillbirth, abruptio placentae, and preterm labor are increased two- to fourfold over nonusers, as is the rate of IUGR also. Other effects in the fetus include microcephaly, cerebral infarctions, and congenital malformations caused by vascular infarcts such as intestinal atresia. In high-risk populations (no prenatal care, placental abruptions, and preterm labor), urine toxicology screens should be performed in mothers and infants. Analysis of meconium enhances diagnosis by indicating cumulative drug use prior to delivery.

As with other illegal drugs, cocaine seems to have long-term neurobehavioral effects, but multiple drug use and environmental factors preclude assigning specific effects to cocaine with certainty. The risk of SIDS is increased three to seven times over the risk in nonusers (0.5–1% of exposed infants).

2. OPIOIDS

Essentials of Diagnosis & Typical Features

- Irritability, hyperactivity, incessant hunger and salivation.
- Vomiting, diarrhea, excessive weight loss.
- Tremors, seizures.
- Nasal stuffiness, sneezing.
- Often IUGR.

Clinical Findings

The withdrawal signs in infants born to mothers who are addicted to heroin or who have been in maintenance methadone programs are similar. The clinical findings in infants born to methadone-maintained mothers may actually be more severe and prolonged than those seen with heroin. Clinical manifestations begin usually within 1–2 days. The clinical picture is typical enough to suggest a diagnosis even if a maternal history of drug abuse has not been obtained, though onset may not occur prior to discharge at 24 hours. Confirmation should be attempted with urine toxicology, but results will be negative unless the last drug dose was within a few days before delivery. Meconium can also be tested for illicit drugs and is more likely to be positive since the substances accumulate throughout pregnancy.

Treatment

Careful observation of the infant is a requirement. If opioid abuse or withdrawal is suspected, the baby is not a candidate for early discharge. Supportive treatment includes swaddling the infant and providing a quiet, dimly lighted environment. In general, specific treatment should be avoided unless the infant has severe symptoms or excessive weight loss. There is no single drug that has been uniformly effective, and the first choice varies among nurseries. The drugs that have been used include phenobarbital at an initial loading dose of 15–20 mg/kg intramuscularly, followed by a maintenance dose of 5 mg/kg/d in two divided doses, usually given orally. Opioids, diazepam, and clonidine have also been used, though the present authors prefer phenobarbital because of its safety and predictability. Treatment can be tapered over several days to a week. Both handling and procedures in the nursery should be kept to a minimum.

Prognosis

These infants demonstrate long-term neurobehavioral handicaps. However, it is difficult to distinguish the effects of in utero drug exposure from those of environmental influences during upbringing. Infants of opioid abusers have a four- to fivefold increased risk of SIDS.

3. ALCOHOL

The effects of alcohol on the fetus and the newborn are roughly proportionate to the degree of ethanol abuse. Fetal growth and development are adversely affected, and infants can suffer withdrawal similar to that associated with maternal opioid abuse. Features observed are listed in Table 2–15.

Children with full-blown fetal alcohol syndrome demonstrate postnatal growth deficiency and mild to moderate mental retardation. Those with lesser effects are at increased risk for attention deficit disorder and subtle developmental delays.

4. TOBACCO SMOKING

Smoking has been shown to have a negative impact on the growth rate of the fetus. The more the mother smokes, the greater the degree of intrauterine growth restriction. More recently, smoking during pregnancy has been associated with mild neurodevel-

Table 2–15. Features observed in fetal alcohol syndrome and fetal alcohol effects.[1,2]

Common Features[3]	Associated Features
Growth	**Craniofacial**
Prenatal and postnatal growth deficiency	Ptosis
Decreased adipose tissue	**Skeletal**
Performance	Joint alterations, including camptodactyly, flexion contractures at elbows, congenital hip dislocations
Mental retardation	
Developmental delay	
Fine motor dysfunction	
Infant irritability, child hyperactivity, and poor attention span	Radioulnar synostosis
	Tapering terminal phalanges, hypoplastic fingernails and toenails
Speech problems	Cervical spine abnormalities
Poor coordination, hypotonia	Altered palm crease patterns
Craniofacial	Pectus excavatum
Microcephaly	**Cardiac**
Short palpebral fissures	Ventricular septal defect
Retrognathia in infancy	Atrial septal defect
Maxillary hypoplasia	Tetralogy of Fallot, great vessel anomalies
Hypoplastic long or smooth philtrum	**Other**
Thin vermilion of upper lip	Cleft lip, cleft palate
	Myopia, strabismus
Short, upturned nose	Epicanthal folds
Micrognathia in adolescence	Dental malocclusion
	Hearing loss, protuberant ears
	Abnormal thoracic cage
	Strawberry hemangiomas
	Hypoplastic labia majora
	Microphthalmia, blepharophimosis
	Small teeth with faulty enamel
	Hypospadias; small, rotated kidneys; hydronephrosis
	Hirsutism in infancy
	Hernias of diaphragm, umbilicus, or groin, diastasis recti

[1]Reproduced, with permission, from the American Academy of Pediatrics Committee on Substance Abuse: Fetal alcohol syndrome and fetal alcohol effects. Pediatrics 1993;91:1004.
[2]Principal and associated features observed in 245 affected individuals.
[3]Observed in over 50%.

opmental handicap. However, it is important to recognize that the possible effects of multiple drug abuse apply to this category as well, and the potential interaction of multiple factors on fetal growth and development must be considered.

5. TOLUENE EMBRYOPATHY

Solvent abuse (paint, lacquer, or glue sniffing) is relatively common. The active organic solvent in these agents is toluene. Features attributable to in utero toluene exposure include prematurity, intrauterine growth retardation, microcephaly, craniofacial abnormalities similar to those associated with in utero alcohol exposure (Table 2–15), nail hypoplasia, and renal anomalies. Long-term effects include postnatal growth deficiency and developmental delay.

6. OTHER DRUGS

There are two categories under which drugs and their effects on the newborn should be considered. In the first category are drugs to which the fetus is exposed because of its exposure to the mother. In many cases these are drugs prescribed for therapy of maternal conditions. The human placenta is relatively permeable, particularly to lipophilic solutes. Whenever possible, drug therapy of the mother should be postponed until after the first trimester. Drugs with potential fetal toxicity include antineoplastics, antithyroid agents, benzodiazepines, warfarin, lithium, ACE inhibitors (captopril, enalapril), and immunosuppressants.

In the second category are drugs the infant acquires from the mother during breast feeding. Most drugs taken by the mother at this time achieve some concentrations in breast milk, though they usually do not present a problem to the infant. If the drug is one that could have adverse effects on the baby, timing breast feeding to coincide with trough concentrations in the mother may be useful. The American Academy of Pediatrics (see first reference below) has recently reviewed drugs contraindicated in the breast-feeding mother.

American Academy of Pediatrics Committee on Drugs. Neonatal drug withdrawal. Pediatrics 1998;101:1079.
American Academy of Pediatrics Committee on Drugs: The transfer of drugs and other chemicals into human milk. Pediatrics 1994;93:137.
American Academy of Pediatrics Committee on Substance Abuse: Drug-exposed infants. Pediatrics 1995;96:364.
American Academy of Pediatrics Committee on Substance Abuse: Fetal alcohol syndrome and fetal alcohol effects. Pediatrics 1993;91:1004.
Pearson MA et al: Toluene embryopathy: Delineation of the phenotype and comparison with fetal alcohol syndrome. Pediatrics 1994;93:211.
Stromland K, Hellstrom A: Fetal alcohol syndrome: An ophthalmological and socioeducational prospective study. Pediatrics 1996;97:845.
Yaster M et al: The management of opioid and benzodiazepine dependence in infants, children, and adolescents. Pediatrics 1996;98:135.

MULTIPLE BIRTHS

Twinning has historically occurred as a demographic variation in one of 80 pregnancies (1.25%). The incidence of twinning in the United States in 1990, however, was 2.3% of pregnancies. A clear distinction should be made between dizygotic (fraternal) and monozygotic (identical) twins. Race, maternal parity, and maternal age affect the incidence only of dizygotic twinning. Drugs that induce ovulation, such as clomiphene citrate and gonadotropins, increase the incidence of dizygotic or polyzygotic twinning quite strikingly. Monozygotic twinning can be viewed as a birth defect; the incidence of malformations is also increased in identical twins and may affect only one of the twins. If a defect is found in one, the other should be examined carefully for lesser degrees of the same defect.

Examination of the placenta can help establish the type of twinning: Two amnionic membranes and two chorionic membranes are found in all cases of dizygotic twins and in one-third of monozygotic twins; a single chorionic membrane always indicates monozygotic twins.

Complications of Multiple Births

A. Intrauterine Growth Restriction: There is some degree of intrauterine growth restriction in most multiple pregnancies after 34 weeks. If prenatal care is good, however, the growth restriction is rarely significant. There are two exceptions: The first is the monochorial twin pregnancy in which there is an arteriovenous shunt from one twin's circulation to that of the other (twin–twin transfusion syndrome). The infant on the venous side becomes plethoric and considerably larger than the smaller anemic twin. Morbidity and mortality rates are considerable in twin–twin transfusion syndrome. Discordance in size—birth weights that are significantly different—can also occur when there are separate placentas. One placenta develops poorly, presumably because of a poor implantation site. In this instance, there is no fetal exchange of blood but there is a striking difference in the growth rates of the two infants.

B. Preterm Delivery: Gestation length tends to be inversely related to the number of fetuses. It is the prematurity that tends to increase the mortality or morbidity of twin pregnancies.

C. Obstetric Complications: Polyhydramnios, pregnancy-induced hypertension, premature rupture of membranes, abnormal fetal presentations, and prolapsed umbilical cord occur more frequently in women with multiple fetuses. In general, most of the complications can be avoided or minimized by good obstetric management. Multiple pregnancy should always be identified prenatally with ultrasound examinations; doing so allows the obstetrician and pediatrician or neonatologist to plan management jointly. The neonatal complications are usually related to prematurity. Prolongation of pregnancy, therefore, leads to a significant reduction in neonatal morbidity.

Follow-up studies of twin pregnancies have yielded conflicting results. In general, the studies do not suggest that twinning has a significant effect on later development, especially if prematurity is excluded as a separate risk factor.

D'Alton ME, Simpson LL: Syndromes in twins. Semin Perinatol 1995;19:375.

Houlihan C, Knuppel RA: Intrapartum management of multiple gestations. Clin Perinatol 1996;23:91.

Lopriore E et al: Twin-to-twin transfusion syndrome: New perspectives. J Pediatr 1995;127:675.

Powers WF, Kiely JL: The risks confronting twins: A national perspective. Am J Obstet Gynecol 1994;170:456.

NEONATAL INTENSIVE CARE

PERINATAL RESUSCITATION

Perinatal resuscitation consists of the steps taken by the obstetrician to support the infant during labor and delivery as well as the traditional resuscitative steps taken by the pediatrician after delivery. Intrapartum support includes maintaining maternal blood pressure with volume expanders if needed, maternal oxygen therapy, positioning the mother to improve placental perfusion, readjusting oxytocin infusions or administering a tocolytic if appropriate, minimizing trauma to the infant (particularly important in infants of very low birth weight), suctioning the nasopharynx upon delivery of the head if meconium is present in the amniotic fluid, obtaining all necessary cord blood samples, and completing an examination of the placenta.

Steps taken by the pediatrician or neonatologist focus on temperature support, initiation and maintenance of effective ventilation, maintenance of perfusion and hydration, and glucose regulation.

A number of conditions associated with pregnancy, labor, and delivery place the infant at risk for birth asphyxia: (1) maternal diseases such as diabetes, pregnancy-induced hypertension, heart and renal disease, and collagen-vascular disease; (2) fetal conditions such as prematurity, multiple births, growth retardation, and fetal anomalies; and (3) labor and delivery conditions, including fetal distress with or without meconium in the amniotic fluid and administration of anesthetics and opioid analgesics.

Physiology of Birth Asphyxia

Birth asphyxia can be the result of several mechanisms: (1) acute interruption of umbilical blood flow (eg, prolapsed cord with cord compression), (2) premature placental separation, (3) maternal hypotension or hypoxia, (4) chronic placental insufficiency, and (5) failure to execute newborn resuscitation properly.

The neonatal response to asphyxia follows a predictable pattern that has been demonstrated in a variety of species (Figure 2–2). The initial response to hypoxia is an increase in frequency of respiration and a rise in heart rate and blood pressure. Respirations then cease (primary apnea) as heart rate and blood pressure begin to fall. This initial period of apnea lasts 30–60 seconds. Gasping respirations (3–6/min) then begin, while heart rate and blood pressure gradually decline. Secondary or terminal apnea then ensues, with further decline in heart rate and blood pressure. The longer the duration of secondary apnea, the greater the risk for hypoxic organ injury. A cardinal feature of the defense against hypoxia is the underperfusion of certain tissue beds (eg, skin, muscle, kidneys, gastrointestinal tract), which allows the perfusion of core organs (ie, heart, brain, adrenals) to be maintained.

The response to resuscitation also follows a predictable pattern. During the period of primary apnea,

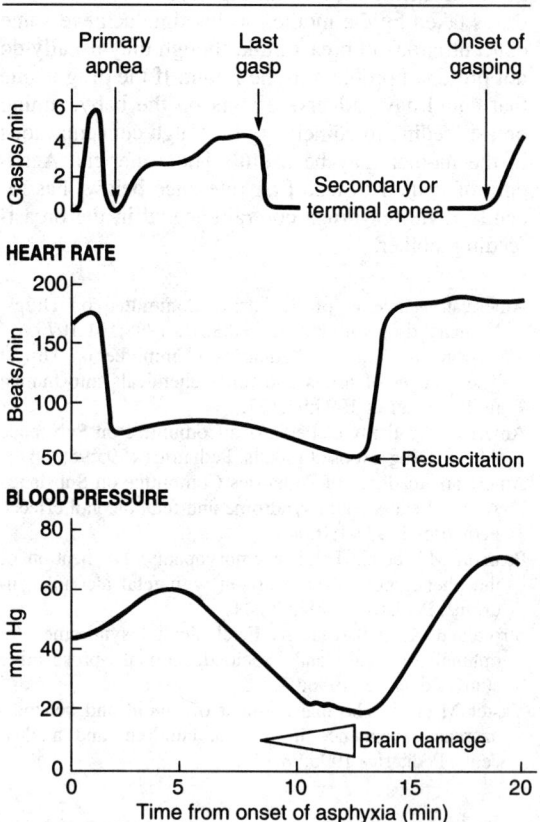

Figure 2–2. Schematic depiction of changes in rhesus monkeys during asphyxia and on resuscitation by positive-pressure ventilation. (Adapted and reproduced, with permission, from Dawes GS: *Fetal and Neonatal Physiology.* Year Book, 1968.)

almost any physical stimulus causes the baby to initiate respirations. Infants in secondary apnea require positive-pressure ventilation. The first sign of recovery is an increase in heart rate, followed by an increase in blood pressure with improved perfusion. The time required for rhythmic, spontaneous respirations to occur is related to the duration of the secondary apnea. As a rough rule, for each 1 minute past the last gasp, 2 minutes of positive-pressure breathing is required before gasping begins, and 4 minutes is required to reach rhythmic breathing. These times can vary depending on the degree and duration of intrauterine asphyxia. Not until some time later do spinal and corneal reflexes return. Muscle tone gradually improves over the course of several hours.

Delivery Room Management

When asphyxia is anticipated, a resuscitation team of two persons should be present—one to manage the airway and one to monitor the heartbeat and provide assistance. The necessary equipment and drugs are listed in Table 2–16.

A. **Steps in the Resuscitation:** (See Figure 2–3.)

1. Dry the infant well and place it under the radiant heat source.

2. Gently suction the mouth, then the nose.

3. Quickly assess the infant's condition. The best criteria are the infant's respiratory effort (apneic, gasping, regular) and heart rate (> 100 or < 100 beats/min). A depressed heart rate—indicative of hypoxic myocardial depression—is the single most reliable indicator of the need for resuscitation.

4. Infants who are breathing and have heart rates over 100 beats/min usually require no further intervention. Infants with heart rates less than 100/min and apnea or irregular respiratory efforts should be vigorously stimulated. The baby's back should be rubbed with a towel while oxygen is provided near the baby's face.

5. If the baby fails to respond to tactile stimulation within a few seconds, begin bag and mask ventilation, using a soft mask that seals well around the mouth and nose. For the initial inflations, pressures of 30–40 cm H_2O may be necessary to overcome surface-active forces in the lungs. Adequacy of ventilation is assessed by observing expansion of the infant's chest accompanied by an improvement in heart rate, perfusion, and color. After the first few breaths, lower the peak pressure to 15–20 cm H_2O. The baby's chest movement should resemble that of an easy breath rather than a deep sigh. The rate of bagging should be 40–60 breaths per minute.

6. Most neonates can be effectively resuscitated with a bag and mask. If the infant does not respond to bag and mask ventilation, try to reposition the head (slight extension), reapply the mask to achieve a good seal, consider suctioning the mouth and the oropharynx, and try ventilating with the mouth open.

Table 2–16. Equipment for neonatal resuscitation.*

Clinical Needs	Equipment
Thermoregulation	Radiant heat source with platform, mattress covered with warm sterile blankets, servo-control heating, temperature probe
Airway management	**Suction:** Bulb suction, mechanical suction with sterile catheters (6F, 8F, 10F), meconuim aspirator **Ventilation:** Manual infant resuscitation bag connected to manometer or with a pressure-release valve capable of delivering 100% oxygen, appropriate masks for term and preterm infants, oral airways, stethoscope. **Intubation:** Neonatal laryngoscope with No. 0 and No. 1 blades; endotracheal tubes (2.5, 3.0, 3.5 mm OD with stylet): extra bulbs and batteries for laryngoscope; scissors, adhesive tape, gloves
Gastric decompression	Nasogastric tube: 8F with 20-mL syringe
Administration of drugs and volume replacement	Sterile umbilical catheterization tray, umbilical catheters (3.5F and 5F), volume expanders (Ringer's lactate, 5% albumin or normal saline), drug box[1] with appropriate neonatal vials and dilutions, sterile syringes, needles, and alcohol sponges
Transport	Warmed transport isolette with oxygen source

*Modified, with permission, from Rosenberg AA: Neonatal adaptation. In: *Obstetrics: Normal and Problem Pregnancies.* Gabbe SG, Niebyl JR, Simpson JL (editors). Churchill Livingston, 1996.
[1]Epinephrine 1:10,000; naloxone hydrochloride 1 mg/mL; sodium bicarbonate 4.2% (5 mEq/10 mL); 10% dextrose.

If the infant does not respond within 30 seconds, intubation is appropriate.

Failure to respond to intubation and ventilation can result from (1) mechanical difficulties (Table 2–17), (2) profound asphyxia with myocardial depression, and (3) inadequate circulating blood volume.

Quickly rule out the mechanical causes listed in Table 2–17. Check to be sure the endotracheal tube passes through the vocal cords. Occlusion of the tube should be suspected when there is resistance to bagging and no chest wall movement. Very few neonates (approximately 0.1%) require either cardiac massage or drugs during resuscitation. Almost all newborns respond to ventilation with 100% oxygen if done effectively.

7. If mechanical causes are ruled out and the heart rate remains below 80/min and is not increasing after intubation and positive-pressure ventilation for 30 seconds, cardiac compression should be initiated.

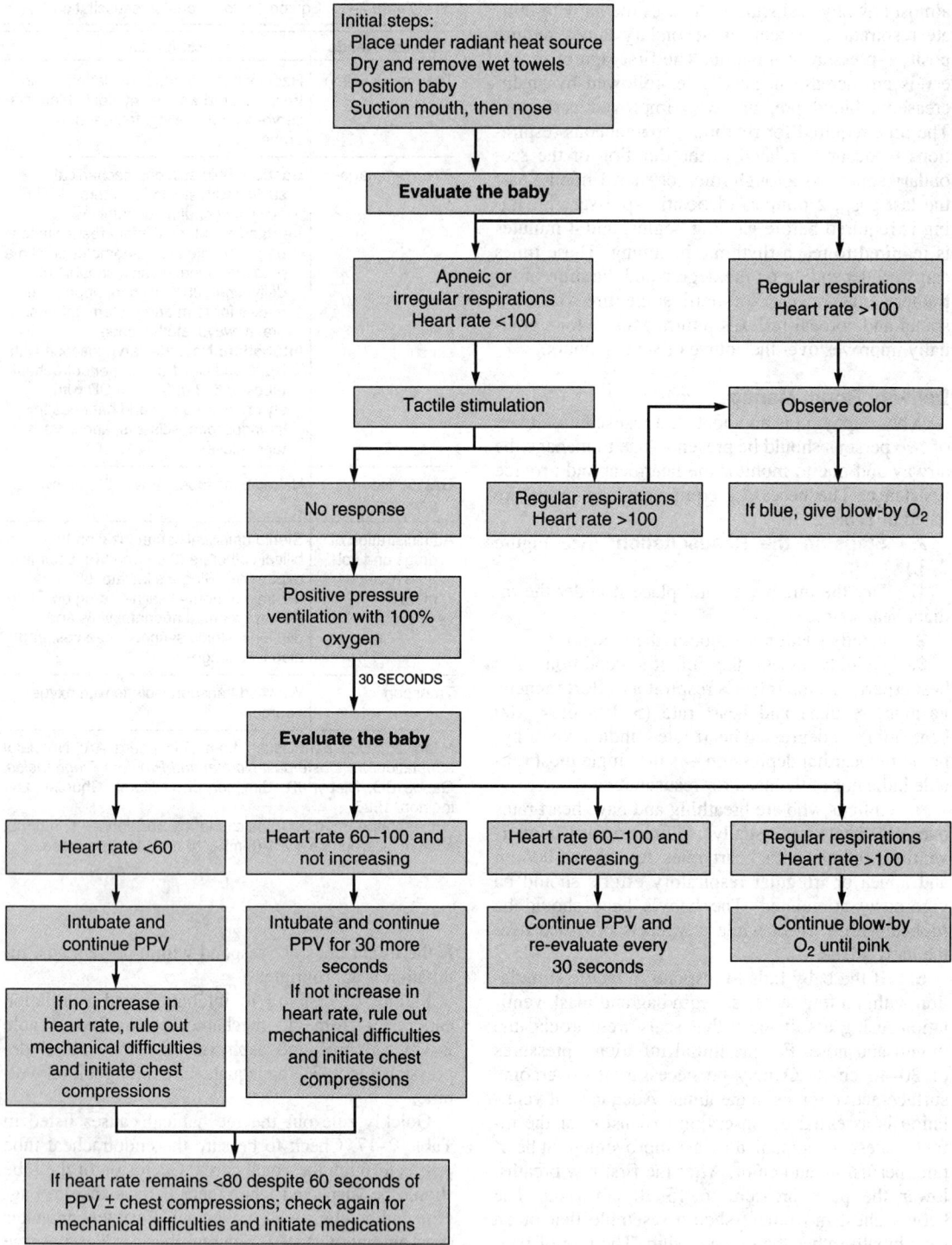

Figure 2–3. Delivery room management.

Table 2–17. Mechanical causes of failed resuscitation.[1]

Etiology	Examples
Equipment failure	Malfunctioning bag, oxygen not connected or running
Endotracheal tube malposition	Esophagus, right main stem bronchus
Occluded endotracheal tube	
Insufficient inflation pressure to expand lungs	
Space-occupying lesions in the thorax	Pneumothorax, pleural effusions, diaphragmatic hernia
Pulmonary hypoplasia	Extreme prematurity, oligohydramnios

[1]Reproduced, with permission, from Rosenberg AA: Neonatal adaptation. In: *Obstetrics: Normal and Problem Pregnancies*. Gabbe SG, Niebyl JR, Simpson JL (editors). Churchill Livingstone, 1996.

Simultaneous delivery of chest compressions and positive-pressure ventilation is likely to decrease the efficiency of ventilation. Therefore, chest compressions should be interspersed with ventilation at a 3:1 ratio (90 compressions and 30 breaths per minute).

8. If drugs are needed (rarely), the drug and dose of choice is epinephrine, 1:10,000 solution, 0.1–0.3 mL/kg given via the endotracheal tube or through an umbilical venous line. Some children and adults who do not respond to standard doses will respond to high-dose epinephrine (ten times the ineffective amount), but the safety and efficacy of such a dose have not been adequately evaluated in the newborn and it is thus not currently recommended. Sodium bicarbonate, 1–2 mEq/kg of the neonatal dilution (0.5 mEq/mL), can be used in prolonged resuscitation efforts in which the response to other measures is poor. If volume loss is suspected, 10 mL/kg of a volume expander (5% albumin, normal saline) should be administered through an umbilical vein line.

B. Continued Resuscitative Measures: The appropriateness of continued resuscitative efforts should be reevaluated in an infant who fails to respond to the above efforts. In current practice, resuscitative efforts are made even in "apparent stillbirths," ie, infants whose Apgar score at 1 minute is 0–1. Modern resuscitative techniques have led to an increasing survival rate for these infants, with 60% of survivors showing normal development. It is clear from a number of studies that initial resuscitation of these infants should proceed; however, subsequent continued support must depend on response to resuscitation. All studies emphasize that if the Apgar score is not improving markedly over the first 10–15 minutes of life, the mortality rate and the incidence of severe developmental handicaps among survivors are high.

C. Special Considerations:

1. Preterm infants–

a. Minimizing heat loss improves survival, so prewarmed towels should be available. The environmental temperature of the delivery suite should be raised to > 25 °C (especially for infants weighing < 1500 g).

b. In the extremely low birth weight infant (< 1000 g), proceed quickly to intubation.

c. Volume expanders and sodium bicarbonate (if needed) should be infused slowly to avoid rapid swings in blood pressure and serum osmolality.

2. Narcotic depression–In the case of opioid administration to the mother during labor, perform the resuscitation as described above. When the baby is stable with good heart rate, color, and perfusion but still has poor respiratory effort, a trial of naloxone (0.1 mg/kg intramuscularly, subcutaneously, intravenously, or intratracheally) is indicated. Naloxone should not be administered in place of positive-pressure ventilation. Naloxone should not be used in the infant of an opioid-addicted mother as it will precipitate withdrawal.

3. Meconium-stained amniotic fluid–

a. The obstetrician carefully suctions the oropharynx and the nasopharynx after delivery of the head with a suction apparatus attached to wall suction.

b. The delivery is then completed, and the baby is given to the resuscitation team.

c. If the baby is active and breathing, requiring no resuscitation, and if obstetric suctioning has been performed, the airway need not be inspected—only further suctioning of the mouth and nasopharynx is required.

d. The airway of any depressed infant requiring ventilation must be checked and cleared (by passage of a tube below the vocal cords) before positive-pressure ventilation is instituted. Special adapters are available for use with regulated wall suction to allow suction to be applied directly to the endotracheal tube.

4. Universal precautions should always be observed in the delivery room.

Management of the Asphyxiated Infant

Asphyxia is manifested by multiorgan dysfunction, seizures and hypoxic-ischemic encephalopathy, and metabolic acidemia. The infant who has suffered a significant episode of perinatal hypoxia and ischemia is at risk for dysfunction of multiple end organs (Table 2–18). The organ of greatest concern is the brain.

The clinical features of hypoxic-ischemic encephalopathy progress over time: birth to 12 hours, decreased level of consciousness, poor tone, decreased spontaneous movement, periodic breathing or apnea, and possible seizures; 12–24 hours, more

Table 2–18. Signs and symptoms caused by asphyxia.

Hypoxic-ischemic encephalopathy
Respiratory distress due to aspiration or secondary
  surfactant deficiency
Persistent pulmonary hypertension
Hypotension due to cardiac failure
Transient tricuspid valve insufficiency
Anuria or oliguria due to acute tubular necrosis
Feeding intolerance; necrotizing enterocolitis
Elevated aminotransferases due to liver injury
Disseminated intravascular coagulation
Hypocalcemia
Hypoglycemia

seizures, apneic spells, jitteriness, and weakness; after 24 hours, decreased level of consciousness, further respiratory abnormalities (progressive apnea), onset of brain stem signs (oculomotor and pupillary disturbances), poor feeding, and hypotonia.

The severity of clinical signs and the length of time the signs persist correlate with the severity of the insult. Other evaluations helpful in assessing severity in the term infant include EEG, CT scan, and evoked responses. As experience in the use of magnetic resonance imaging is gained, this technique may also prove useful. Markedly abnormal EEGs with voltage suppression and slowing evolving into a burst-suppression pattern are seen with severe clinical symptomatology. A CT scan early in the course may demonstrate diffuse hypodensity, whereas later scans may demonstrate brain atrophy and focal ischemic lesions. Visual and somatosensory evoked potentials provide information about function. In most instances, it is not necessary to use all of these tests, but some are obtained to confirm an ominous prognosis. Management is directed at supportive care and treatment of specific abnormalities. Fluids should be restricted initially to 60–80 mL/kg/d; oxygenation should be maintained (with mechanical ventilation if necessary); blood pressure should be supported with judicious volume expansion (if hypovolemic) and pressors; and glucose should be in the normal range of 40–100 mg/dL. Hypocalcemia, coagulation abnormalities, and metabolic acidemia should be corrected and seizures treated with intravenous phenobarbital (20 mg/kg as loading dose, with total initial 24-hour dosing up to 40 mg/kg). Other anticonvulsants should be reserved for refractory seizures.

Birth Asphyxia: Long-Term Outcome

Fetal heart rate tracings, cord pH, and 1-minute and 5-minute Apgar scores are imprecise predictors of long-term outcome. Apgar scores of 0–3 at 5 minutes in term infants result in an 8% risk of death in the first year of life and a 1% risk of cerebral palsy

among survivors. A 10-minute Apgar score of 0–3 predicts death in the first year in 18% of cases and cerebral palsy among survivors in 5%; at 15 minutes, 48% and 9%, respectively; and at 20 minutes, 59% and 57%, respectively. The single best predictor of outcome is the severity of clinical hypoxic-ischemic encephalopathy (severe symptomatology carries a 75% chance of death and a 100% rate of neurologic sequelae among survivors). The major sequela of hypoxic-ischemic encephalopathy is cerebral palsy with or without associated mental retardation and epilepsy. Other prognostic features include prolonged seizures refractory to therapy, markedly abnormal EEGs, and CT scans with evidence of major ischemic injury. Other clinical features required to support perinatal hypoxia as the cause of cerebral palsy include the presence of fetal distress prior to birth, a low cord pH of < 7.00, and evidence of other end organ dysfunction.

American Heart Association and American Academy of Pediatrics: *Textbook of Neonatal Resuscitation.* American Heart Association/American Academy of Pediatrics, 1994.

Carpenter TC, Stenmark KR: High-dose epinephrine is not superior to standard-dose epinephrine in pediatric in-hospital cardiopulmonary arrest. Pediatrics 1997;99:403.

Committee on Fetus and Newborn, American Academy of Pediatrics, and Committee on Obstetric Practice, American College of Obstetricians and Gynecologists: Use and abuse of the Apgar score. Pediatrics 1996;98:141.

Greenough A: Meconium aspiration syndrome: Prevention and treatment. Early Hum Dev 1995;41:183.

Nelson KB et al: Uncertain value of electronic fetal monitoring in predicting cerebral palsy. N Engl J Med 1996;334:613.

Perlman JM: Intrapartum hypoxic-ischemic cerebral injury and subsequent cerebral palsy: medicolegal issues. Pediatrics 1997;99:851.

Perlman JM, Risser R: Cardiopulmonary resuscitation in the delivery room: Associated clinical events. Arch Pediatr Adolesc Med 1995;149:20.

Robertson CMT, Finer NN: Long-term follow up of term neonates with perinatal asphyxia. Clin Perinatol 1993;20:483.

THE PRETERM INFANT

Premature infants account for the majority of high-risk newborns. The preterm infant faces a variety of physiologic handicaps:

(1) The ability to suck, swallow, and breathe in a coordinated fashion is not achieved until 34–36 weeks of gestation. Therefore, enteral feedings must be provided by gavage. Furthermore, preterm infants frequently have gastroesophageal reflux and an immature gag reflex, which increases the risk of aspiration of feedings.

(2) Decreased ability to maintain body temperature.

(3) Pulmonary immaturity–surfactant deficiency, often with structural immaturity in infants of less than 26 weeks' gestation. Their condition is complicated by the combination of noncompliant lungs and a compliant chest wall.

(4) Immature control of respiration, leading to apnea and bradycardia.

(5) Persistent patency of the ductus arteriosus, leading to further compromise of pulmonary gas exchange because of overperfusion of the lungs.

(6) Immature cerebral vasculature, predisposing the infant to subependymal or intraventricular hemorrhage and periventricular leukomalacia.

(7) Impaired substrate absorption by the gastrointestinal tract, compromising nutritional management.

(8) Immature renal function (including both filtration and tubular functions), complicating fluid and electrolyte management.

(9) Increased susceptibility to infection.

(10) Immaturity of metabolic processes, predisposing to hypoglycemia and hypocalcemia.

Delivery Room Care

See under Perinatal Resuscitation, above.

Care in the Nursery

A. Thermoregulation: Maintaining a stable body temperature is a function of heat production and conservation balanced against heat loss. Heat production in response to cold stress can occur through voluntary muscle activity, involuntary muscle activity (shivering), and thermogenesis not caused by shivering. Newborns produce heat mainly through the last of these three mechanisms. This metabolic heat production depends on the quantity of brown fat present, which is very limited in the preterm infant. Heat loss to the environment can occur through the following mechanisms: (1) radiation—transfer of heat from a warmer to a cooler object not in contact; (2) convection—transfer of heat to the surrounding gaseous environment, influenced by air movement and temperature; (3) conduction—transfer of heat to a cooler object in contact; and (4) evaporation—cooling secondary to water loss through the skin. Heat loss in the preterm newborn is accelerated because of a high ratio of surface area to body mass, reduced insulation of subcutaneous tissue, and water loss through the immature skin.

The thermal environment of the preterm neonate must be carefully regulated. The infant can be kept warm in an isolette, in which the air is heated and convective heat loss is minimized. Alternatively, the infant can be kept warm on an open bed with a radiant heat source. Although evaporative and convective heat losses are greater when the radiant warmer is used, this system allows easy access to a critically ill neonate. Ideally, the infant should be kept in a neutral thermal environment (Figure 2–4). The neutral thermal environment allows the infant to maintain a stable core body temperature with a minimum of metabolic heat production through oxygen consumption. The neutral thermal environment for a given infant depends on size, gestational age, and postnatal age. The neutral thermal environment (for either isolette or radiant warmer care) can be obtained by maintaining an abdominal skin temperature of 36.5 °C. Generally, when infants reach 1700–1800 g, they can maintain temperature while bundled in a bassinet.

B. Monitoring the High-Risk Infant: Care of the high-risk preterm infant requires sophisticated monitoring techniques. At a minimum, equipment to monitor heart rate, respirations, and blood pressure should be available. Oxygen saturation can be assessed continuously using pulse oximetry. This determination can be correlated with arterial oxygen tension (PaO_2) as needed. Transcutaneous PO_2 and PCO_2 can also be utilized to assess oxygenation and ventilation. Finally, arterial blood gases, electrolytes, glucose, calcium, bilirubin, and other chemistries must be measured on small volumes of blood. Early in the care of a sick preterm infant, the most efficient way to sample blood for tests as well as to provide fluids and monitor blood pressure is through an umbilical arterial line. Once the infant is stable and the need for frequent blood samples is reduced (usually 4–7 days), the umbilical line should be removed. All indwelling lines are associated with morbidity from thrombosis or embolism, infection, and bleeding.

C. Fluid and Electrolyte Therapy: Fluid requirements in preterm infants are a function of (1) insensible losses (skin and respiratory tract), (2) urine output, (3) stool output (< 5% of total), and (4) others, such as nasogastric losses. In most circumstances, the fluid requirement is determined largely by insensible losses plus urine losses. The major contribution to insensible water loss is evaporative skin loss. The rate of water loss is a function of gestational age (body weight), environment (losses are greater under a radiant warmer than in an isolette), and the use of phototherapy. Respiratory losses are minimal when infants are breathing humidified oxygen. The renal contribution to water requirement is influenced by the decreased ability of the preterm neonate to concentrate the urine and conserve water.

Electrolyte requirements are minimal for the first 24–48 hours until there is excretion in the urine. Basal requirements are as follows: sodium, 3 mEq/kg/d; potassium, 2 mEq/kg/d; chloride, 2–3 mEq/kg/d; and bicarbonate, 2–3 mEq/kg/d.

In the infant of gestational age less than 30 weeks, sodium and bicarbonate losses in the urine are frequently elevated, increasing the infant's requirement for these electrolytes.

Initial fluid management after birth is determined by the infant's size. Infants weighing more than 1500 g should start at 80–100 mL/kg/d of 10% dextrose in water ($D_{10}W$), whereas those weighing less should

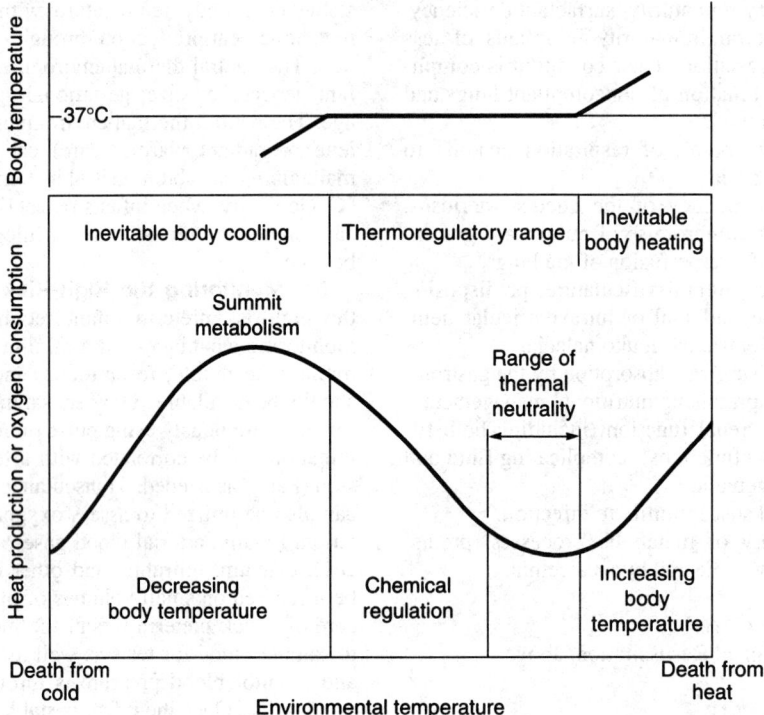

Figure 2–4. Effect of environmental temperature on oxygen consumption and body temperature. (Adapted and reproduced, with permission, from Klaus MH, Fanaroff AA, Martin RJ: The physical environment. In: *Care of the High-Risk Neonate,* 3rd ed. Klaus MH, Fanaroff AA [editors]. Saunders, 1986.)

start at 100–120 mL/kg/d of either $D_{10}W$ or 5% dextrose in water (D_5W) (infants < 800 g and < 26 weeks often become hyperglycemic on $D_{10}W$). The most critical issue in fluid management is monitoring. Measurements of body weight, urine output, fluid and electrolyte intake, serum and urine electrolytes, and glucose allow fairly precise determinations of the infant's water, glucose, and electrolyte needs. Parenteral nutrition should be started early and continued until an adequate enteral intake is achieved.

D. Nutritional Support: The average caloric requirement for the growing premature infant is 120 kcal/kg/d. Expected weight gain for the adequately nourished preterm infant is 10–30 g/d.

Infants initially require intravenous glucose infusions to maintain blood glucose concentration in the range of 60–100 mg/dL. Infusions of 5–7 mg/kg/min (approximately 80–100 mL/kg/d of a 10% dextrose solution) are usually needed. Nutritional support in the very low-birth-weight infant generally is started at 24–48 hours of age with parenteral alimentation solutions given either peripherally or centrally via an umbilical vein line or Silastic catheter (Table 2–19). Small-volume trophic feeds with breast milk or 20

kcal/oz premature formula should be started by gavage at 10–25% of the infant's nutritional needs as soon as possible and slowly advanced to full caloric needs over 3–7 days once the infant is stable. Intermittent bolus feedings are preferred because these appear to stimulate the release of gut-related hormones and may accelerate maturation of the gastrointestinal tract. The more rapid advancement schedule is used for infants weighing over 1500 g and the slowest schedule in the infant weighing less than 1000 g. *Note:* In the extremely low-birth-weight infant (< 1000 g) or the postsurgical neonate, continuous-drip feeds are sometimes better-tolerated.

In general, long-term nutritional support for infants of very low birth weight consists either of breast milk supplemented to increase protein, caloric density, and mineral content or of infant formulas modified for preterm infants. In all of these formulas, protein concentrations (approximately 2 g/dL) and caloric concentrations (approximately 24 kcal/oz) are relatively high. In addition, premature formulas contain some of the fat as medium-chain triglycerides—which do not require bile for emulsification—as an energy source. Increased amounts of calcium and phosphorus are provided to enhance bone mineraliza-

Table 2–19. Use of parenteral alimentation solutions.

	Volume (mL/kg/d)	Carbohydrate (g/dL)	Protein (g/kg)	Lipid (g/kg)	Calories (kcal/kg)
Peripheral: Short-term (7–10 days)					
Starting solution	100–150	$D_{10}W$	1	1	46–64
Target solution	150	$D_{12.5}W$	2.5	3	102
Central: Long-term (>10 days)					
Starting solution	100–150	$D_{10}W$	1	1	46–64
Target solution	130	$D_{20}W$	3–3.5	3	123

Notes:
1. Protein calories should be no more than 10% of total calories.
2. Advance dextrose in central hyperalimentation as tolerated by 2.5% per day as long as blood glucose remains normal.
3. Advance lipids by 0.5 g/kg/d as long as triglycerides are normal. Use 20% concentration.
4. Total water should be 100–150 mL/kg/d, depending on the child's fluid tolerance.

Monitoring:
1. Blood glucose two or three times a day when changing dextrose concentration, then daily.
2. Electrolytes daily, then twice a week when the child is receiving a stable solution.
3. Every other week blood urea nitrogen and serum creatinine; total protein and serum albumin; serum calcium, phosphate, magnesium, direct bilirubin, and CBC with platelet counts.

tion. The infant should be gradually advanced to feedings of higher caloric density after the full volume of either breast milk or formula (20 kcal/oz) is tolerated. Success of feedings is assessed by passage of feeds out of the stomach, abdominal examination free of distention, and normal stool pattern.

When the preterm infant approaches term, the nutritional source for the bottle-fed infant can be changed to a transitional formula (22 kcal/oz) until 6–9 months of age. Iron supplementation (2–4 mg/kg/d) is recommended for premature infants, beginning at about 2 months of life. This can be provided by iron-supplemented formulas. In some infants, iron supplementation may be indicated earlier. In particular, infants treated with erythropoietin (epoetin alfa) for prevention of anemia of prematurity require supplemental iron at a dosage of 4–8 mg/kg/d.

Als H et al: Individualized developmental care for the very low-birth-weight infant. JAMA 1994;272:853.
Bauer K et al: Body temperatures and oxygen consumption during skin-to-skin (kangaroo) care in stable preterm infants weighing less than 1500 grams. J Pediatr 1997;130:240.
Bell EF, Oh W: Fluid and electrolyte management. In: *Neonatology: Pathophysiology and Management of the Newborn.* Avery GB, Fletcher MA, MacDonald MG (editors). Lippincott, 1994.
Berseth CL: Minimal enteral feedings. Clin Perinatol 1995;22:195.
Gunn TR, Gluckman PD: Perinatal thermogenesis. Early Hum Dev 1995;42:169.
Kjartansson S et al: Water loss from the skin of term and preterm infants nursed under a radiant heater. Pediatr Res 1995;37:233.
LeBlanc MH: Thermoregulation: Incubators, radiant warmers, artificial skins, and body hoods. Clin Perinatol 1991;18:403.
Morley R, Lucas A: Nutrition and cognitive development. Brit Med Bull 1997;53:123.
Neu J (editor): Neonatal gastroenterology. Clin Perinatol 1996;23(2).
Pereira GR: Nutritional care of the extremely premature infant. Clin Perinatol 1995;22:61.
Schanler RJ: Suitability of human milk for the low-birth-weight infant. Clin Perinatol 1995;22:207.
Silvestre MAA et al: A prospective randomized trial comparing continuous versus intermittent feeding methods in very low birth weight neonates. J Pediatr 1996;128:748.
Troche B et al: Early minimal feedings promote growth in critically ill premature infants. Biol Neonate 1995;67:172.

1. APNEA IN THE PRETERM INFANT

Essentials of Diagnosis & Typical Features
- Respiratory pause of sufficient duration to result in cyanosis or bradycardia.
- Most common at under 34 weeks of gestation with onset at less than 2 weeks of age.
- Methylxanthines (eg, caffeine) provide effective treatment for apnea of prematurity.

General Considerations
In preterm infants, recurrent apneic episodes are a common problem. Apnea is defined as a respiratory pause lasting more than 20 seconds—or any pause accompanied by cyanosis and bradycardia. Shorter respiratory pauses associated with cyanosis or brady-

cardia also qualify as significant apnea but must be differentiated from periodic breathing, which is common in term as well as preterm infants. Periodic breathing is defined as regularly recurring ventilatory cycles interrupted by short pauses not associated with bradycardia or color change. Although apnea in premature infants is often not associated with a predisposing factor, there are a variety of processes that may precipitate apnea (Table 2–20). These processes should at least be considered before a diagnosis of apnea of prematurity can be established.

Apnea of prematurity is the most frequent cause of apnea. Most apnea of prematurity is mixed apnea characterized by a centrally (brain stem) mediated respiratory pause preceded or followed by airway obstruction. Less common is pure central or pure obstructive apnea. Apnea of prematurity is the result of immaturity of both the central respiratory regulatory centers and protective mechanisms that aid in maintaining airway patency.

Clinical Findings

Onset, typically during the first 2 weeks of life, is gradual, with the frequency of spells increasing over time. Pathologic apnea can be suspected in an infant with a sudden onset of frequent or very severe apneic spells. Apnea presenting from birth or on the first day of life is unusual but can occur in the preterm infant who does not require mechanical ventilation for respiratory distress syndrome. In the term or near-term infant, this presentation can suggest acute (asphyxia or birth trauma) or chronic (congenital hypotonia, structural central nervous system lesion, etc) neuromuscular abnormality.

The workup depends on the clinical presentation. All infants—regardless of the severity and frequency of apnea—require a minimum screening evaluation, including a general assessment of well-being (eg, tolerance of feedings, stable temperature, normal physi-

cal examination), a check of the association of spells with feeding, measurement of PaO_2 or SaO_2, blood glucose, hematocrit, and a review of the drug history. Infants with severe apnea of sudden onset may require a more extensive evaluation, including a workup for infection. Other specific tests are dictated by relevant signs, eg, evaluation for necrotizing enterocolitis in an infant with apnea and abdominal distention.

Treatment

The physician should first address any underlying cause. If the apnea is due simply to prematurity, treatment is dictated by the frequency and severity of apneic spells. Apneic spells frequent enough to interfere with other aspects of care (eg, feeding) or severe enough to necessitate bag and mask ventilation to relieve cyanosis and bradycardia require treatment. First-line therapy is with methylxanthines. Caffeine citrate (20 mg/kg as loading dose and then 5–10 mg/kg/d) is the drug of choice because of once-daily dosing and fewer side effects than theophylline (5 mg/kg load; 1–2 mg/kg every 6–12 hours). Side effects of methylxanthines include tachycardia, feeding intolerance, and (with overdosing) seizures. The dose used should be the smallest dose necessary to decrease the frequency of apnea and eliminate severe spells. Desired drug levels are usually in the range of 5–10 µg/mL for theophylline and 10–20 µg/mL for caffeine. Intravenous doxapram infused at a dose of 1 mg/kg/h for 48 hours is effective in some cases of methylxanthine-refractory apnea. Nasal CPAP (continuous positive airway pressure), by treating the obstructive component of apnea, can be effective treatment for some infants. Intubation and ventilation can eliminate apneic spells but carry risks of long-term endotracheal intubation.

Prognosis

In the majority of premature infants, apneic and bradycardiac spells cease by 34–36 weeks postconception. Occasionally the episodes last longer, and outpatient therapy with methylxanthines may be indicated. Whether to provide home monitoring for such infants is controversial. Apneic and bradycardiac episodes in the nursery are not predictors of later SIDS. However, home monitoring in infants still experiencing apnea and bradycardia at the time of hospital discharge may be indicated. The incidence of SIDS is slightly increased in preterm infants. Recent work in term infants has shown an increased incidence of SIDS in infants who sleep in the prone position. Whether or not this can be extrapolated to the preterm infant (in particular those with gastroesophageal reflux or persistent respiratory symptoms) is unclear. When possible, a sleeping position on the side (right side down) or, preferable, supine seems prudent unless contraindicated by reflux or respiratory symptoms.

Table 2–20. Causes of apnea in the preterm infant.

Temperature instability—both cold and heat stress
Response to passage of a feeding tube
Gastroesophageal reflux
Hypoxemia
   Pulmonary parenchymal disease
   Patent ductus arteriosus
   ?Anemia
Infection
   Sepsis (viral or bacterial)
   Necrotizing enterocolitis
Metabolic causes
   Hypoglycemia
   Hyponatremia
Intracranial hemorrhage
Posthemorrhagic hydrocephalus
Seizures
Drugs (eg, morphine)
Apnea of prematurity

2. HYALINE MEMBRANE DISEASE

Essentials of Diagnosis & Typical Features

- Tachypnea, cyanosis, and expiratory grunting.
- Poor air movement despite increased work of breathing.
- Chest x-ray showing atelectasis and air bronchograms.

General Considerations

The most common cause of respiratory distress in the preterm infant is hyaline membrane disease. The incidence increases from 5% at 35–36 weeks to more than 50% of infants of 26–28 weeks of gestation. This condition is caused by a deficiency of surfactant. Surfactant decreases surface tension in the alveolus during expiration, allowing the alveolus to remain partly expanded and in that way maintaining a functional residual capacity. The absence of surfactant results in poor lung compliance and atelectasis. The infant must expend a great deal of effort to expand the lungs with each breath, and respiratory failure ensues (Figure 2–5).

Clinical Findings

Infants with hyaline membrane disease demonstrate all the clinical signs of respiratory distress. On auscultation, air movement is diminished despite vigorous respiratory effort. Chest x-ray demonstrates diffuse bilateral atelectasis, causing a "ground-glass" appearance. Major airways are highlighted by the atelectatic air sacs, creating air bronchograms. In the

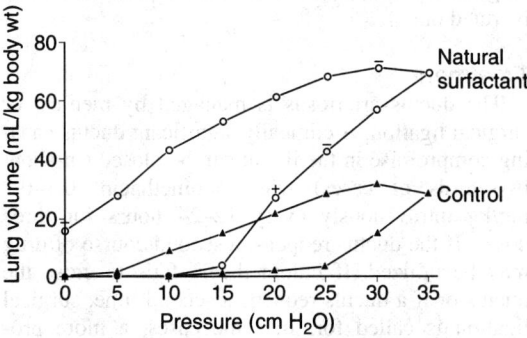

Figure 2–5. Pressure-volume relationships for the inflation and deflation of surfactant-deficient and surfactant-treated preterm rabbit lungs. (Reproduced, with permission, from Jobe AH: The developmental biology of the lung. In: *Neonatal-Perinatal Medicine: Diseases of the Fetus and Infant,* 5th ed. Fanaroff AA, Martin RJ [editors]. Mosby, 1992.)

unintubated child, there is doming of the diaphragms and underexpansion.

Treatment

Supplemental oxygen, early intubation and ventilation, and placement of umbilical artery and vein lines are the initial interventions required. A ventilator that can deliver breaths synchronized with the infant's respiratory efforts (synchronized intermittent mandatory ventilation; SIMV) should be utilized if available. High-frequency ventilators are also available for rescue of infants doing poorly on conventional ventilation with air leak problems.

Two exogenous surfactants (colfosceril palmitate [Exosurf Neonatal] and beractant [Survanta]) are approved in the United States by the Food and Drug Administration for use in infants with hyaline membrane disease. Surfactant replacement therapy, used both in the delivery room as prophylaxis and with established hyaline membrane disease as rescue, has been shown to decrease the mortality rate in preterm infants and to decrease air leak complications of the disease. Ventilator settings and oxygen requirements are significantly less in surfactant-treated infants than in controls during the acute course. The dose of the artificial surfactant Exosurf is 5 mL/kg intratracheally, while that of the bovine-derived Survanta is 4 mL/kg. The usual dosing schedule when the first dose is given in the delivery room to prevent hyaline membrane disease is a total of two or three doses given 8–12 hours apart as long as the infant remains ventilated on over 30–40% inspired oxygen concentration. Rescue surfactant is given as two to four doses 8–12 hours apart. The first dose is administered as soon as possible after birth, preferably before 2–4 hours of age. As the disease process evolves, proteins that inhibit surfactant function leak into the air spaces, making surfactant replacement less effective. The second dose should be administered to infants who continue to require ventilation and more than 30% inspired oxygen concentration. A prophylactic strategy may offer some advantage in those infants of 26 weeks' gestation or less. For infants over 26 weeks, early rescue therapy (as soon as a diagnosis of surfactant deficiency can be made) is the strategy of choice. The availability of surfactant replacement therapy has encouraged earlier intubation of infants with hyaline membrane disease. Surfactant replacement has also been used with some success in term infants with secondary surfactant deficiency resulting from pneumonia or meconium aspiration.

Antenatal administration of corticosteroids to the mother is an important strategy utilized by obstetricians to accelerate lung maturation. Infants whose mothers were given corticosteroids more than 24 hours prior to preterm birth have less respiratory distress syndrome and a lower mortality rate. Antenatal corticosteroids and exogenous surfactant administration after birth appear to have a synergistic effect on outcome.

3. CHRONIC LUNG DISEASE OF THE PREMATURE

Chronic lung disease of the premature, defined as respiratory symptoms, oxygen requirement, and chest x-ray abnormalities at 1 month of age, occurs in about 20% of infants ventilated for surfactant deficiency. The incidence is higher at lower gestational ages. The development of chronic lung disease is a function of lung immaturity at birth and exposure to high oxygen concentrations and ventilator barotrauma. The use of surfactant replacement therapy has, in general, diminished the severity of the chronic lung disease. The mortality rate from this complication is now very low, but significant morbidity still exists secondary to reactive airway symptoms, hospital readmissions during the first 2 years of life for intercurrent respiratory infection, and systemic hypertension. The management of infants who go on to develop chronic lung disease has been enhanced by the use of dexamethasone (0.5 mg/kg) to decrease lung inflammation. Dexamethasone is most effective when started in chronically ventilated infants at 10 days to 3 weeks of age. Dosing schedules used have varied from a 5-day course to intermittent 3- to 5-day bursts to an initial 3–5 days at full dose followed by a gradual wean in dosage over 4–6 weeks. Other treatments employed in the management of chronic lung disease include diuretics, inhaled β_2-adrenergic bronchodilators, and inhaled corticosteroids. After hospital discharge, some of these infants will continue to require oxygen at home. This can be monitored by pulse oximetry with a target SaO_2 of 94–96%.

American Academy of Pediatrics Task Force on Infant Positioning and SIDS: Positioning and sudden infant death syndrome (SIDS) update. Pediatrics 1996;98:1216.

Barrington KJ, Finer N, Li D: Predischarge respiratory recordings in very low-birth-weight newborn infants. J Pediatr 1996;129:934.

Brozanski BS et al: Effect of pulse dexamethasone therapy on the incidence of chronic lung disease in the very low-birth-weight infant. J Pediatr 1995;126:769.

Cleary JP et al: Improved oxygenation during synchronized intermittent mandatory ventilation in neonates with respiratory distress syndrome: A randomized crossover study. J Pediatr 1995;126:407.

Collaborative Dexamethasone Trial Group: Dexamethasone therapy in neonatal chronic lung disease: an international placebo-controlled trial. Pediatrics 1991;88:421.

Durand M et al: Effects of early dexamethasone therapy on pulmonary mechanics and chronic lung disease in very low-birth-weight infants: A randomized controlled trial. Pediatrics 1995;95:584.

Halliday HL: Overview of clinical trials comparing natural and synthetic surfactants. Biol Neonate 1995;67(Suppl 1):32.

Holtzman RB, Frank L (editors): Bronchopulmonary dysplasia. Clin Perinatol 1992;19:3.

Hunt CE: Prone sleeping in healthy infants and victims of sudden infant death syndrome. J Pediatr 1996;128:594.

Jobe AH: Pulmonary surfactant therapy. N Engl J Med 1993;328:861.

Larsen PB et al: Aminophylline versus caffeine citrate for apnea and bradycardia prophylaxis in premature neonates. Acta Paediatr 1995;84:360.

Miller MJ, Martin RJ: Apnea of prematurity. Clin Perinatol 1992;19:789.

National Institutes of Health Consensus Development Conference on Infantile Apnea and Home Monitoring. Pediatrics 1987;79:292.

Padbury JF, Ervin G, Polk DH: Extrapulmonary effects of antenatally administered steroids. J Pediatr 1996:128;167.

Wright L (editor): Effect of corticosteroids for fetal maturation on perinatal outcomes. Am J Obstet Gynecol 1995;173(Suppl):253.

4. PATENT DUCTUS ARTERIOSUS

Clinically significant patent ductus arteriosus usually presents on days 3–7 as the respiratory distress from hyaline membrane disease is improving. Presentation can be on day 1 or 2, especially in infants of less than 28 weeks' gestation and in those treated with surfactant replacement therapy. The signs include a hyperdynamic precordium, increased peripheral pulses, and a widened pulse pressure with or without a systolic heart murmur. Early presentations are not uncommonly manifested by systemic hypotension without a murmur or hyperdynamic circulation. These signs are often accompanied by an increase in respiratory support. The presence of significant patent ductus arteriosus can be confirmed by echocardiography. Before undertaking medical or surgical ligation, other structural heart disease must be ruled out.

Treatment

The ductus arteriosus is managed by medical or surgical ligation. A clinically significant ductus causing compromise in the infant can be closed (in about two-thirds of cases) with indomethacin, 0.1–0.2 mg/kg intravenously every 12–24 hours for three doses. If the ductus reopens, a second course of drug may be utilized. If indomethacin fails to close the ductus or if a ductus reopens a second time, surgical ligation is called for. In some cases, a more prolonged course of indomethacin is being utilized to prevent recurrences. In addition, in the extremely low-birth-weight infant (< 1000 g) who is at very high risk of developing a symptomatic ductus, a prophylactic strategy starting indomethacin on the first day of life can be used. The major side effect of indomethacin is transient oliguria, which can be managed by fluid restriction until urine output improves. Transient decreases in intestinal and cerebral blood flow caused by indomethacin can be ameliorated by giving the drug as a slow infusion over 1 hour. The drug should not be used if the infant is hyperkalemic, if the creatinine is greater than 2 mg/dL, or if the platelet count is less than 50,000/μL.

Causer RJ et al: Prophylactic indomethacin therapy in the first twenty-four hours of life for the prevention of patent ductus arteriosus in preterm infants treated prophylactically with surfactant in the delivery room. J Pediatr 1996;128:631.

Clyman RI: Recommendations for the postnatal use of indomethacin: An analysis of four separate treatment strategies. J Pediatr 1996;128:601.

Hammerman C et al: Continuous versus multiple rapid infusions of indomethacin: Effects on cerebral blood flow velocity. Pediatrics 1995;95:244.

5. NECROTIZING ENTEROCOLITIS

Essentials of Diagnosis & Typical Features

- Feeding intolerance with gastric aspirates or vomiting.
- Bloody stools.
- Abdominal distention and tenderness.
- Pneumatosis intestinalis on abdominal x-ray.

General Considerations

Necrotizing enterocolitis is the most common acquired gastrointestinal emergency in the newborn; it most often affects preterm infants, with an incidence of 10% in infants of birth weight less than 1500 g. In term infants, it is seen in association with polycythemia, congenital heart disease, and birth asphyxia. The pathogenesis of the disease is a multifactorial interaction between an immature gastrointestinal tract, mucosal injury, and potentially injurious factors in the lumen. Previous intestinal ischemia, bacterial or viral infection, and immunologic immaturity of the gut are felt to play a role in the genesis of the disorder. In up to 20% of affected infants, the only risk factor is prematurity.

Clinical Findings

The most common presenting sign is abdominal distention. Other signs include vomiting or increased gastric residuals, heme-positive stools, abdominal tenderness, temperature instability, increased apnea and bradycardia, decreased urine output, and poor perfusion. The complete blood count may show an increased white blood cell count with an increased band count or, as the disease progresses, absolute neutropenia. Thrombocytopenia is often seen along with stress-induced hyperglycemia and metabolic acidosis. Diagnosis is confirmed by the presence of pneumatosis intestinalis (air in the bowel wall) on x-ray. There is a spectrum of disease, and milder cases may exhibit only distention of bowel loops with bowel wall edema (thickened-appearing walls on x-ray).

Treatment

A. Medical Treatment: Necrotizing enterocolitis is managed by decompression of the gut by nasogastric tube, maintenance of oxygenation, mechanical ventilation if necessary, and intravenous fluids (colloid and normal saline) to replace third-space gastrointestinal losses. Enough fluid should be given to restore a good urine output. Other measures consist of broad-spectrum antibiotics (including anaerobic coverage), close monitoring of vital signs, physical examination, and laboratory studies (blood gases, white blood cell count, platelet count, and x-rays).

B. Surgical Treatment: Indications for surgery are evidence of perforation (free air present on a left lateral decubitus film), a fixed dilated loop of bowel on serial x-rays, abdominal wall cellulitis, or progressive deterioration despite maximal medical support. All of these signs are indicative of necrotic bowel. In the operating room, necrotic bowel is removed and ostomies are created. Reanastomosis is performed after the disease is resolved and the infant is bigger (usually > 2 kg).

Course & Prognosis

Infants managed either medically or surgically should not be refed until the disease is resolved (normal abdominal examination, resolution of pneumatosis on x-ray), usually in 10–14 days. Nutritional support during this time should be provided by total parenteral nutrition.

Death occurs in 10% of cases. Surgery is needed in less than 25% of cases. Long-term prognosis is determined by the amount of intestine lost. Infants with short bowel require long-term support with intravenous nutrition and therefore have very long hospitalizations. Even for those infants, however, the outcome is favorable because of improved parenteral nutrition formulations. Late strictures—about 3–6 weeks after initial diagnosis—occur in 8% of patients whether treated medically or surgically. Some of these strictures are severe enough to require operative management.

Kanto WP et al: Recognition and medical management of necrotizing enterocolitis. Clin Perinatol 1994;21:335.

MacKendrick W, Caplan M: Necrotizing enterocolitis: New thoughts about pathogenesis and potential treatments. Pediatr Clin North Am 1993;40:1047.

Major CA et al: Tocolysis with indomethacin increases the incidence of necrotizing enterocolitis in the low-birth-weight neonate. Am J Obstet Gynecol 1994;170:102.

Stoll BJ: Epidemiology of necrotizing enterocolitis. Clin Perinatol 1994;21:205.

6. ANEMIA OF THE PREMATURE

In the premature infant, the hemoglobin reaches its nadir at approximately 8–12 weeks and is 2–3 g/dL lower than that in the term infant. The lower nadir in the premature appears to be the result of a decreased erythropoietin response to the low red cell mass. Symptoms of anemia include poor feeding, lethargy, increased heart rate, poor weight gain, and perhaps apnea. The decision to transfuse is based on the presence of clinical symptoms. Transfusion is not indicated in an asymptomatic infant simply because of an arbitrary hematocrit number. Most infants become symptomatic if the hematocrit drops below 20%. With risks of transfusion, alternative therapies have been explored. Epoetin alfa, 150–250 units/kg subcutaneously three times per week, has been shown to increase hematocrit and reticulocyte count and to decrease the frequency and volume of transfused blood. This treatment should be reserved for the highest-risk infants (those less than 28–30 weeks' gestational age and below 1000–1200 g). For optimal effect, supplemental iron at a dosage of 4–8 mg/kg/d should be given. Treatment should start when infants are taking at least two-thirds of their nutrition enterally and should continue through 34–36 weeks postconception.

Doyle JJ: The role of erythropoietin in the anemia of prematurity. Semin Perinatol 1997;21:20.
Maier RF et al: The effect of epoetin beta (recombinant human erythropoietin) on the need for transfusion in very-low-birth-weight infants. N Engl J Med 1994; 330:1173.
Shannon K: Recombinant human erythropoietin in neonatal anemia. Clin Perinatol 1996;22:627.
Soubasi V et al: Follow-up of very low birth weight infants after erythropoietin treatment to prevent anemia of prematurity. J Pediatr 1995;127:291.

7. INTRAVENTRICULAR HEMORRHAGE

Essentials of Diagnosis & Typical Features

- Large bleeds are accompanied by hypotension, metabolic acidosis, and altered neurologic status. Smaller bleeds can be asymptomatic.
- Routine cranial ultrasound scanning is essential for diagnosis in infants less than 32 weeks of gestation.

General Considerations

Periventricular-intraventricular hemorrhage is seen almost exclusively in premature infants. The incidence is 20–30% in infants of less than 31 weeks' gestation and birth weight of less than 1500 g. The highest incidence is seen in babies of the lowest gestational age (< 26 weeks). Bleeding is most commonly seen in the subependymal germinal matrix (a region of undifferentiated cells). Bleeding can extend into the ventricular cavity. The proposed pathogenesis of bleeding is presented in Figure 2–6. The critical event is probably ischemia with reperfusion injury to the capillaries in the germinal matrix that occurs in the immediate perinatal period. The actual amount of bleeding is also influenced by a variety of factors that affect the pressure gradient across the injured capillary wall. This pathogenetic scheme applies also to intraparenchymal bleeding (venous infarction in a region rendered ischemic) and periventricular leukomalacia (ischemic white matter injury in a watershed region of arterial supply). Periventricular leukomalacia has a peak incidence in babies born between 28 and 32 weeks of gestation and appears to be associated with maternal chorioamnionitis.

Clinical Findings

Up to 50% of hemorrhages occur at less than 24 hours of age, and virtually all occur by the fourth day. The clinical syndrome ranges from rapid deterioration (coma, hypoventilation, decerebrate posturing, fixed pupils, bulging anterior fontanelle, hypotension, acidosis, acute drop in hematocrit) to a more gradual deterioration with more subtle neurologic changes to absence of any specific physiologic or neurologic signs.

The diagnosis can be confirmed by real-time ultrasound scan. This can be performed whenever bleeding is clinically suspected. If symptoms are absent, routine scanning should be done at 10–14 days in all infants of less than 30 weeks' gestation. Hemorrhages are graded as follows: grade I, germinal matrix hemorrhage only; grade II, intraventricular bleeding without ventricular enlargement; grade III, intraventricular bleeding with ventricular enlargement; and grade IV, any infant with intraparenchymal bleeding. The amount of bleeding is minor (grade I or II) in 75% of infants and major in the remainder.

Follow-up ultrasound examinations are based on the results of the initial scan. Infants with no bleeding or germinal matrix hemorrhage require only a single late scan at 4–6 weeks of age to look for periventricular leukomalacia. Any infant with blood in the ventricular system is at risk for posthemorrhagic ventriculomegaly. This is usually the result of impaired absorption of cerebrospinal fluid, but it can also occur secondary to obstructive phenomena. An initial follow-up scan should be done at 1–2 weeks after the initial scan. Infants with intraventricular bleeding and ventricular enlargement should be followed very 7–10 days until ventricular enlargement stabilizes or decreases. Infants without ventriculomegaly should have one additional scan at 4–6

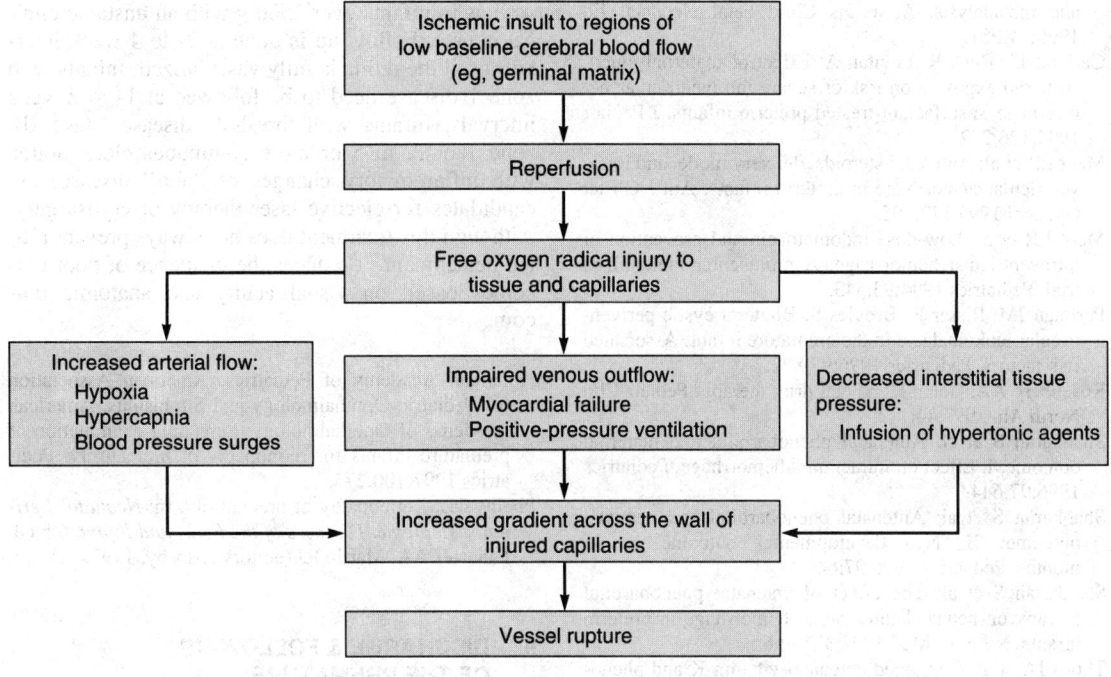

Figure 2–6. Pathogenesis of periventricular and intraventricular hemorrhage.

weeks. In addition, all infants born between 30 and 32 weeks of gestation should have at least a late scan (4–6 weeks) to look for ventriculomegaly, and periventricular leukomalacia.

Treatment

During acute hemorrhage, supportive treatment (including restoration of volume and hematocrit, oxygenation, and ventilation) should be provided to avoid further cerebral ischemia. Progressive posthemorrhagic hydrocephalus (if it develops) can sometimes be controlled by decreasing the production of cerebrospinal fluid (furosemide, 1 mg/kg/d, plus acetazolamide in increasing doses from 25–100 mg/kg/d) or by removal of cerebrospinal fluid (daily lumbar punctures). The process is usually self-limited and spontaneously resolves; placement of a ventriculoperitoneal shunt is usually not needed. Early treatment with medications or serial spinal taps does not appear to influence whether a shunt will ultimately be needed but may contribute to an improved long-term neurologic outcome.

Although the incidence and severity of intracranial bleeding have decreased in prematures, strategies to prevent this complication are still needed. Use of antenatal corticosteroids appears to be important in decreasing this complication, while phenobarbital may have a role in the mother who has not been "prepared" with steroids and is delivering at under 28 weeks of gestation. The route of delivery may also play a role, with babies delivered by cesarean section showing a decreased rate of intracranial bleeds, but this issue remains controversial. Postnatal strategies appear less promising, but early indomethacin may have some benefit.

Prognosis

There are no deaths as a result of grade I and grade II hemorrhages, whereas grade III and grade IV hemorrhages carry a mortality rate of 10–20%. Posthemorrhagic ventricular enlargement is rarely seen with grade I hemorrhages but is seen in 54–87% of grade II–IV hemorrhages. Very few of these infants will require a ventriculoperitoneal shunt. Long-term neurologic sequelae are seen no more frequently in infants with grade I and grade II hemorrhages than in preterm infants without bleeding. In infants with grade III and grade IV hemorrhages, severe sequelae occur in 20–25% of cases, mild sequelae in 35% of cases, and no sequelae in 40% of cases. The presence of severe periventricular leukomalacia, large parenchymal bleeds, and progressive ventriculomegaly greatly increases the risk of neurologic sequelae.

Batton DG et al: Current gestational age-related incidence of major intraventricular hemorrhage. J Pediatr 1994;125:623.

Fowlie PW: Prophylactic indomethacin: Systematic review

and metanalysis. Arch Dis Child Fetal Neonatal Ed 1996;74:F81.

Garland JS, Buck R, Levitan A: Effect of maternal glucocorticoid exposure on risk of severe intraventricular hemorrhage in surfactant-treated preterm infants. J Pediatr 1995;126:272.

Ment LR et al: Antenatal steroids, delivery mode, and intraventricular hemorrhage in preterm infants. Am J Obstet Gynecol 1995;172:795.

Ment LR et al: Low-dose indomethacin and prevention of intraventricular hemorrhage: A multicenter randomized trial. Pediatrics 1994;93:543.

Perlman JM, Risser R, Broyles S: Bilateral cystic periventricular leukomalacia in the premature infant: Associated risk factors. Pediatrics 1996;97:822.

Rosenberg AA, Galan HC: Fetal drug therapy. Pediatr Clin North Am 1997;44:113.

Shankaran S et al: Antenatal phenobarbital and maternal outcome: I. Effect on intracranial hemorrhage. Pediatrics 1996;97:644.

Shankaran S et al: Antenatal phenobarbital and neonatal outcome: II. Neurodevelopmental outcome at 36 months. Pediatrics 1996;97:649.

Shankaran S et al: The effect of antenatal phenobarbital therapy on neonatal intracranial hemorrhage in preterm infants. N Engl J Med 1997;337:466.

Thorp JA et al: Combined antenatal vitamin K and phenobarbital therapy for preventing intracranial hemorrhage in newborns less than 34 weeks gestation. Obstet Gynecol 1995;86:1.

Verma U et al: Obstetric antecedents of intraventricular hemorrhage and periventricular leukomalacia in the low-birth-weight neonate. Am J Obstet Gynecol 1997;176:275.

8. RETINOPATHY OF PREMATURITY

Retinopathy of prematurity occurs only in the incompletely vascularized retina of the premature. The incidence of any acute retinopathy in infants under 1250 g is 66%, whereas only 6% have retinopathy severe enough to warrant intervention. The incidence is highest in babies of the lowest gestational age. The condition appears to be triggered by an initial injury to the developing retinal vessels. Hypoxia, shock, asphyxia, vitamin E deficiency, and light exposure have been associated with this initial injury. After the initial injury, normal vessel development may follow, or abnormal vascularization may occur with ridge formation on the retina. The process can still regress at this point or may continue, with growth of fibrovascular tissue into the vitreous associated with inflammation, scarring, and retinal folds or detachment. The disease is graded by stages of abnormal vascular development and retinal detachment (I–V), by the zone of the eye involved (1–3, with zone 1 the posterior region around the macula), and by the amount of the retina involved in "clock hours."

Initial eye examination should be performed at 6 weeks of age in infants with a birth weight under 1500 g or with a gestational age under 28 weeks as well as in infants over 1500 g with an unstable clinical course. Follow-up is done at 2- to 4-week intervals until the retina is fully vascularized. Infants with zone 1 disease need to be followed at 1- to 2-week intervals. Infants with threshold disease (stage III, zone 1 or 2, in 5 or more continuous clock hours, with inflammatory changes of "plus" disease) are candidates for elective laser therapy or cryosurgery. Although this treatment does not always prevent retinal detachment, it reduces the incidence of poor outcomes based on visual acuity and anatomic outcomes.

American Academy of Pediatrics, American Association for Pediatric Ophthalmology and Strabismus, American Academy of Ophthalmology: Screening examination of premature infants for retinopathy of prematurity. Pediatrics 1997;100:273.

Phelps DL: Retinopathy of prematurity. In: Neonatal-Perinatal Medicine. Diseases of the Fetus and Infant, 6th ed. Fanaroff AA, Martin RJ (editors). Mosby, 1997.

9. DISCHARGE & FOLLOW-UP OF THE PREMATURE

Hospital Discharge

Medical criteria for discharge of the premature include the ability to maintain temperature in an open crib, nippling all feeds and gaining weight, and the absence of apneic and bradycardiac spells requiring intervention. Infants going home on supplemental oxygen should not desaturate too badly (< 80%) in room air or should demonstrate the ability to arouse in response to hypoxia. Factors such as support for the mother at home and the stability of the family situation play a role in the timing of discharge. Home nursing visits and early physician follow-up can be utilized to hasten discharge.

Follow-Up

With advances in obstetric and maternal care, survival for infants under 28 weeks' gestation or with birth weights as low as 1000 g is now better than 90%. Eighty percent or more survive at 26–27 weeks and birth weights of 800–1000 g. Survival at gestational age 25 weeks and birth weight 700–800 g is nearly 70%, with a considerable drop off below this level (Figure 2–7).

These high rates of survival do come with a price in terms of morbidity. Major neurologic sequelae, including cerebral palsy, cognitive delay, and hydrocephalus, is reported in 10–25% of survivors with birth weights under 1500 g. The rate of these sequelae tends to be higher in infants with lower birth weights. In addition to a higher incidence of severe neurologic sequelae, infants with birth weights under 1000 g have an increased rate of lesser disabilities, including learning and behavior problems. Risk fac-

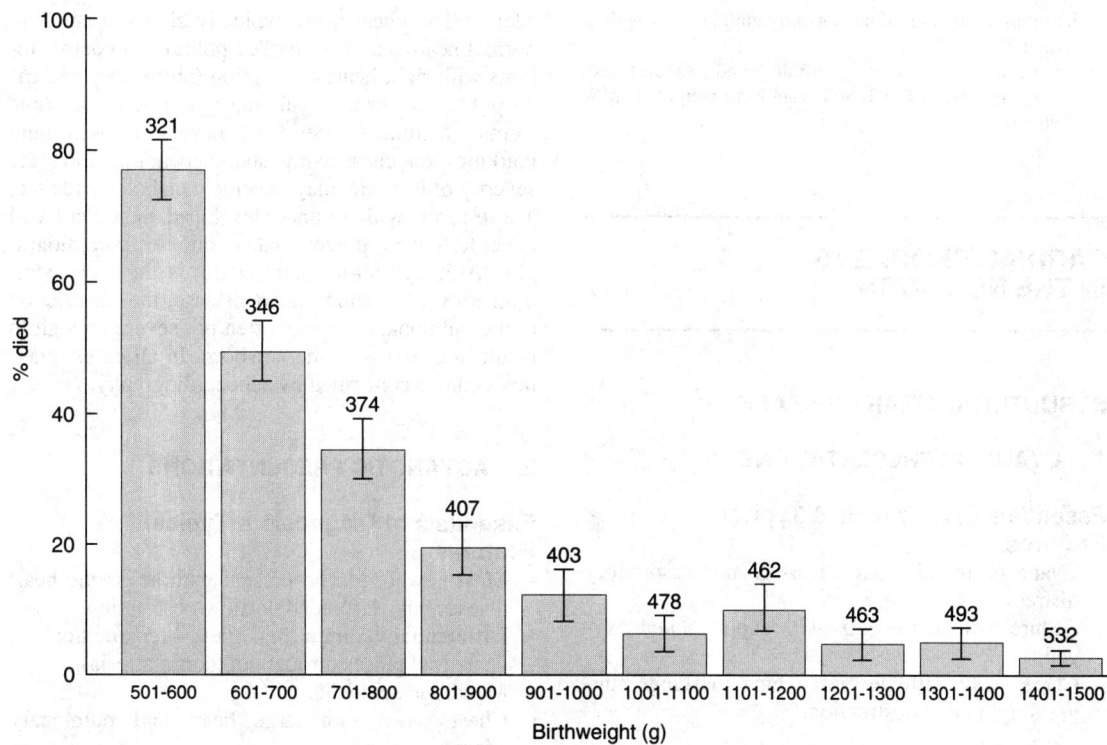

Figure 2–7. Mortality rates before discharge by 100-gram birth weight subgroups with 95% confidence intervals. (Reproduced, with permission, from Fanaroff AA et al: Very-low-birth-weight outcomes of the National Institute of Child Health and Human Development Neonatal Research Network, May 1991 through December 1992. Am J Obstet Gynecol 1995;173:1423.)

tors for neurologic sequelae include seizures, grade 3 or 4 intracranial hemorrhage, periventricular leukomalacia, severe intrauterine growth restriction, poor early head growth, need for mechanical ventilation, and low socioeconomic class. In addition, maternal fever and chorioamnionitis have been associated with an increased risk of cerebral palsy. Other morbidities in these infants include chronic lung disease and reactive airway disease, resulting in an increased risk from respiratory infections and hospital readmissions in the first 2 years, retinopathy of prematurity, hearing loss, and growth failure. All of these issues require close multidisciplinary outpatient follow-up.

Allen MC, Alexander GR: Using motor milestones as a multistep process to screen preterm infants for cerebral palsy. Develop Med Child Neurol 1997;39:12.

American Academy of Pediatrics Committee on Fetus and Newborn and American College of Obstetricians and Gynecologists Committee on Obstetric Practice: Perinatal care at the threshold of viability. Pediatrics 1995;96:974.

Fanaroff AA et al: Very-low-birth-weight outcomes of the National Institute of Child Health and Human Development Neonatal Research Network, May 1991 through December 1992. Am J Obstet Gynecol 1995;173:1423.

Giacoia GP et al: Follow-up of school-age children with bronchopulmonary dysplasia. J Pediatr 1997;130:400.

Hack M et al: School-age outcomes in children with birth weights under 750 grams. NEJM 1994;331:753.

Hack M et al: Very-low-birth-weight outcomes of the National Institute of Child Health and Human Development Neonatal Network, November 1989 to October 1990. Am J Obstet Gynecol 1995;172:457.

Hack M, Friedman H, Fanaroff AA: Outcomes of extremely low birth weight infants. Pediatrics 1996;98:931.

Hack M, Weissman B, Borawski-Clark E: Catch-up growth during childhood among very low-birth-weight children. Arch Pediatr Adolesc Med 1996;150:1122.

Halsey CL, Collin MF, Anderson CL: Extremely low-birth-weight children and their peers: A comparison of school-age outcomes. Arch Pediatr Adolesc Med 1996;150:790.

McCarton CM et al: Results at age 8 years of early intervention for low-birth-weight premature infants. JAMA 1997;277:126.

Morgan AM, Aldag JC: Early identification of cerebral palsy using a profile of abnormal motor patterns. Pediatrics 1996;98:692.

Strauss RS, Dietz WH: Effects of intrauterine growth retardation in premature infants on early childhood growth. J Pediatr 1997;130:95.

Tyson JE et al: Viability, morbidity and resource use among newborns of 501–800 gram birth weight. JAMA 1996;276:1645.

CARDIAC PROBLEMS IN THE NEWBORN

STRUCTURAL HEART DISEASE

1. CYANOTIC PRESENTATIONS

Essentials of Diagnosis & Typical Features

- Cyanosis, initially without associated respiratory distress.
- Failure to increase PaO_2 with supplemental oxygen.
- Chest x-ray with decreased lung markings suggests right heart obstruction.

General Consideration

The causes of cyanotic heart disease that present in the newborn period are transposition of the great vessels (TOGV), total anomalous pulmonary venous return (TAPVR), truncus arteriosus (some types), tricuspid atresia, and pulmonary atresia or critical pulmonary stenosis.

Clinical Findings

Infants with these disorders present with early cyanosis. The hallmark of many of these lesions is cyanosis in an infant without associated respiratory distress. In most, tachypnea does develop over time either because of increased pulmonary blood flow or secondary to metabolic acidemia from progressive hypoxemia. Diagnostic aids include comparing the blood gas or oxygen saturation in room air to that in 100% FIO_2. Failure of PaO_2 or SaO_2 to increase suggests cyanotic heart disease. Other useful aids are chest x-ray, electrocardiography, and echocardiography.

Transposition of the great vessels is the most common form of cyanotic heart disease presenting in the newborn period. Examination generally reveals a systolic murmur and single S_2. Chest x-ray shows a generous heart size and a narrow mediastinum with normal or increased lung markings. There is little change in PaO_2 or SaO_2 with supplemental oxygen. Total anomalous pulmonary venous return, in which venous return is obstructed, presents early with severe cyanosis and tachypnea because the pulmonary venous return is obstructed, resulting in pulmonary edema. The chest x-ray typically shows a small to normal heart size with marked pulmonary edema. Infants with right heart obstruction (pulmonary and tricuspid atresia, critical pulmonary stenosis, and some forms of truncus arteriosus) have decreased lung markings on chest x-ray and, depending upon the severity of hypoxia, may develop metabolic acidemia. Those forms with an underdeveloped right heart will have left-sided predominance on electrocardiography. Although tetralogy of Fallot is the most common form of cyanotic heart disease, the obstruction at the pulmonary valve is often not severe enough to result in cyanosis in the newborn. In all cases, diagnosis can be confirmed by echocardiography.

2. ACYANOTIC PRESENTATIONS

Essentials of Diagnosis & Typical Features

- Most newborns who present with acyanotic heart disease have left-sided outflow obstruction.
- Differentially diminished pulses (coarctation) or decreased pulses throughout (aortic atresia).
- Metabolic acidemia.
- Chest x-ray with large heart and pulmonary edema.

General Considerations

Newborn infants who present with serious acyanotic heart disease usually have congestive heart failure secondary to left-sided outflow tract obstruction. Infants with left-to-right shunt lesions (eg, ventricular septal defect) may have murmurs in the newborn period, but clinical symptoms do not occur until pulmonary vascular resistance drops enough to cause significant shunting and subsequent congestive heart failure (usually 3–4 weeks of age).

Clinical Findings

Infants with left-sided outflow obstruction generally do well the first day or so until the ductus arteriosus—the source of all or some of the systemic flow—narrows. Tachypnea, tachycardia, congestive heart failure, and metabolic acidosis develop. On examination, all of these infants have abnormalities of the pulses. In aortic atresia and stenosis, pulses are all diminished, whereas in coarctation syndromes, differential pulses (diminished or absent in the lower extremities) are evident. Chest x-ray films in these infants show a large heart and pulmonary edema. Diagnosis is confirmed with echocardiography.

Treatment

Early stabilization includes supportive therapy as needed (eg, intravenous glucose, oxygen, ventilation for respiratory failure, pressor support). Specific therapy includes infusions of prostaglandin E_1, 0.025–0.1 μg/kg/min, to maintain ductal patency. In some cyanotic lesions (eg, pulmonary atresia, tricuspid atresia, critical pulmonary stenosis) in which lung blood flow is ductus-dependent, this improves pulmonary blood flow and PaO_2 by allowing shunting through the ductus to the pulmonary artery. In left-sided outflow tract obstruction, systemic blood flow is ductus-dependent; prostaglandins improve systemic perfusion and resolve the acidosis. Further specific management—including palliative surgical and cardiac catheterization procedures—is discussed in Chapter 18.

PERSISTENT PULMONARY HYPERTENSION OF THE NEWBORN

Persistent pulmonary hypertension results when the normal decrease in pulmonary vascular resistance after birth does not occur. Most infants so affected are full-term or postterm, and many have experienced perinatal asphyxia. Other clinical associations include hypothermia, meconium aspiration syndrome, hyaline membrane disease, polycythemia, neonatal sepsis, chronic intrauterine hypoxia, and pulmonary hypoplasia.

There are three causes of persistent pulmonary hypertension: (1) acute vasoconstriction resulting from perinatal hypoxia, (2) prenatal increase in pulmonary vascular smooth muscle development, and (3) decreased cross-sectional area of the pulmonary vascular bed because of inadequate vessel number. In the first, an acute perinatal event leads to hypoxia and failure of the pulmonary vascular resistance to drop. In the second, abnormal muscularization of the pulmonary resistance vessels results in persistent hypertension after birth. The third category includes infants with pulmonary hypoplasia (eg, diaphragmatic hernia).

Clinical Findings

Clinically, the syndrome is characterized by onset on the first day of life, usually from birth. Respiratory distress is prominent, and PaO_2 is usually poorly responsive to high concentrations of inspired oxygen. Many of the infants have associated myocardial depression with resulting systemic hypotension. Echocardiography reveals right-to-left shunting at the level of the ductus arteriosus or foramen ovale (or both). Chest x-ray usually shows lung infiltrates related to associated pulmonary pathology (eg, meconium aspiration, hyaline membrane disease). If the majority of right-to-left shunt is at the ductal level, pre- and postductal differences in PaO_2 and SaO_2 will be seen.

Treatment

Therapy for persistent pulmonary hypertension involves supportive therapy for other postasphyxia problems (eg, anticonvulsants for seizures, careful fluid and electrolyte management for renal failure). Intravenous glucose should be provided to maintain normal blood sugar, and antibiotics should be administered for possible infection. Specific therapy is aimed both at increasing systemic arterial pressure and decreasing pulmonary arterial pressure to reverse the right-to-left shunting through fetal pathways. First-line therapy includes oxygen and ventilation (to reduce pulmonary vascular resistance) and colloid or crystalloid infusions (10 mL/kg, up to 30 mL/kg) to improve systemic pressure. Ideally, systolic pressure should be greater than 60 mm Hg. With compromised cardiac function, systemic pressors can be used as second-line therapy (eg, dopamine, 5–20 µg/kg/min; dobutamine, 5–20 µg/kg/min; or both). If oxygenation is still not adequate (PaO_2 < 55 mm Hg), a trial of alkalosis by hyperventilation is indicated. Many babies improve as the pH rises above 7.5–7.6. Since alkalosis seems to be helpful, any base deficit should be corrected with sodium bicarbonate to allow less vigorous hyperventilation. Recent studies using the inhaled gas nitric oxide (NO), which is identical or very similar to endogenous endothelium-derived relaxing factor, have shown it to be a very promising and specific pulmonary vasodilator. In addition, use of high-frequency oscillatory ventilation has proved effective in many of these infants, particularly those with severe associated lung disease.

Infants for whom conventional therapy is failing (poor oxygenation despite maximum support) may require ECMO. The infants are placed on bypass, with blood exiting the baby from the right atrium and returning to the aortic arch after passing through a membrane oxygenator. The lungs are essentially at rest during the procedure, and with resolution of the pulmonary hypertension the infants are weaned from ECMO back to conventional ventilator therapy. This therapy can save infants who might otherwise die but has major side effects that must be considered prior to its institution. Neurodevelopmental outcome among survivors of ECMO is similar to that of infants with persistent pulmonary hypertension managed without the procedure. Approximately 10–15% of survivors have significant neurologic sequelae, with cerebral palsy or cognitive delays. Other sequelae such as chronic lung disease, sensorineural hearing loss, and feeding problems have also been described in this population.

ARRHYTHMIAS

Irregularly irregular heart rates, commonly associated with premature atrial contractions and less commonly with premature ventricular contractions, are noted often in the first days of life of well newborns. These arrhythmias are benign and of no consequence. Clinically significant bradyarrhythmias are seen in association with congenital heart block. Heart block can be seen in an otherwise structurally normal heart (associated with maternal lupus) or with structural cardiac abnormalities. Treatment is with isoproterenol (starting dose: 0.1 µg/kg/min) to improve cardiac output or with temporary pacing. On electrocardiography, tachyarrhythmias can be either wide complex (eg, ventricular tachycardia) or narrow complex (eg, supraventricular tachycardia). Supraventricular tachycardia is the most common tachyarrhythmia in the neonate and may be a sign of structural heart disease, myocarditis, left atrial enlargement, and aberrant conduction pathways. Acute treatment is ice to the face and, if unsuccessful, adenosine given intravenously at a dose of 75–100 µg/kg. If there is no response, the dose can be increased up to 300 µg/kg. Long-term therapy is with digoxin or propranolol. Digoxin should not be used in cases with Wolff-Parkinson-White syndrome. Cardioversion is rarely needed for supraventricular tachycardia but is needed acutely for hemodynamically unstable ventricular tachycardia.

Bernbaum J et al: Survivors of extracorporeal membrane oxygenation at 1 year of age: The relationship of primary diagnosis with health and neurodevelopmental sequelae. Pediatrics 1995;96:907.

Gerstmann DR et al: The Provo multicenter early high-frequency oscillatory ventilator trial: Improved pulmonary and clinical outcome in respiratory distress syndrome. Pediatrics 1996;98:1044.

Glass P et al: Neurodevelopmental status at age five years of neonates treated with extracorporeal membrane oxygenation. J Pediatr 1995;127:447.

Kanto WP: A decade of experience with neonatal extracorporeal membrane oxygenation. J Pediatr 1994;124:335.

Kinsella JP, Abman SH: Recent developments in the pathophysiology and treatment of persistent pulmonary hypertension of the newborn. J Pediatr 1995;126:853.

Kinsella JP et al: Randomized, multicenter trial of inhaled nitric oxide and high frequency oscillatory ventilation in severe persistent pulmonary hypertension of the newborn. J Pediatr 1997;131:55.

Roberts JD et al: Inhaled nitric oxide and persistent pulmonary hypertension of the newborn. N Engl J Med 1997;336:605.

Rosenberg AA et al: Longitudinal follow-up of a cohort of newborn infants treated with inhaled nitric oxide for persistent pulmonary hypertension. J Pediatr 1997;131:70.

Rosenfeld LE: The diagnosis and management of cardiac arrhythmias in the neonatal period. Semin Perinatol 1993;17:135.

GASTROINTESTINAL & ABDOMINAL SURGICAL CONDITIONS IN THE NEWBORN (See also Chapter 19.)

ESOPHAGEAL ATRESIA & TRACHEOESOPHAGEAL FISTULA

Essentials of Diagnosis & Typical Features

- Polyhydramnios.
- Baby with excessive drooling and secretions, choking with attempted feeding.
- Unable to pass an orogastric tube to the stomach.

General Considerations

These associated conditions are characterized by a blind esophageal pouch and a fistulous connection between the proximal or distal esophagus (or both) and the airway. In 85% of affected infants, the fistula is between the distal esophagus and the airway. Polyhydramnios is common because of the high level of gastrointestinal obstruction.

Clinical Findings

Infants present in the first hours of life with copious secretions, choking, cyanosis, and respiratory distress. Diagnosis can be confirmed with chest x-ray after careful placement of a nasogastric tube to the point at which resistance is met. On chest x-ray, the tube will be seen in the blind pouch. If a tracheoesophageal fistula is present to the distal esophagus, gas will be present in the bowel. In cases of esophageal atresia without tracheoesophageal fistula, there is no gas in the bowel.

Treatment

The tube in the proximal pouch should be placed on continuous suction to drain secretions and prevent aspiration. The head of the bed should be elevated to prevent reflux of gastric contents through the distal fistula into the lungs. Intravenous glucose and fluids should be provided and oxygen administered as needed. Definitive treatment is by operation and depends on the distance between the segments of esophagus. If the distance is not too great, the fistula can be ligated and the ends of the esophagus anastomosed. In instances in which the ends of the esophagus cannot be brought together, the initial surgery entails fistula ligation and a gastrostomy for feeding. Echocardiography should be performed prior to surgery to rule out a right-sided aortic arch. In those cases, a left-sided thoracotomy would be preferred.

Prognosis

Prognosis is determined primarily by the presence or absence of associated anomalies. Vertebral, anal, cardiac, renal, and limb anomalies are also seen (VACTERL association). Evaluation for associated anomalies should be done early.

INTESTINAL OBSTRUCTION

A history of polyhydramnios is common and the fluid, if bile-stained, can easily be confused with thin meconium staining. The higher the obstruction in the intestine, the earlier the infant will present with vomiting and the less prominent the distention will be. The opposite is true for lower intestinal obstructions. Most obstructions are bowel atresias, believed to be caused by an ischemic event during development. Approximately 30% of cases of duodenal atresia are associated with Down's syndrome. Meconium ileus is a distal small bowel obstruction caused by the exceptionally viscous meconium produced by fetuses with cystic fibrosis. Hirschsprung's disease is due to a failure of neuronal migration to the myenteric plexus of the distal bowel so that the distal bowel lacks ganglion cells, causing a lack of peristalsis in that region with a functional obstruction.

Malrotation with midgut volvulus is a surgical emergency that presents in the first days to weeks as bilious vomiting without distention or tenderness. If malrotation is not treated promptly, torsion of the intestine around the superior mesenteric artery will lead to necrosis of the entire small bowel. For this reason, bilious vomiting in the neonate always demands immediate attention and evaluation.

Clinical Findings

Diagnosis of intestinal obstructions depends on plain abdominal radiographs with either upper GI series (high obstruction suspected) or contrast enema (lower obstruction apparent) to define the area of obstruction. Table 2–21 summarizes the findings expected.

All infants with meconium ileus are presumed to have cystic fibrosis. Infants with pancolonic Hirschsprung's disease, colon pseudo-obstruction syndrome, or colonic dysgenesis or atresia may also present with meconium impacted in the distal ileum. Definitive diagnosis of cystic fibrosis is by the sweat chloride test (Na^+ and Cl^- concentration > 60 mEq/L) or by genetic testing. Approximately 10–20% of infants with cystic fibrosis present with meconium ileus. Infants with cystic fibrosis and meconiumileus generally have a normal immunoreactive trypsinogen test because of the associated severe exocrine pancreatic insufficiency in utero.

Any in utero perforation results in meconium peritonitis with residual intra-abdominal calcifications. Many of these are completely healed at birth. If the infant has no signs of obstruction, no further immediate evaluation is needed. A sweat test to rule out cystic fibrosis should be done at a later date.

Low intestinal obstruction may present with delayed stooling (> 24 hours in term infants is abnormal) with mild distention. X-ray findings of gaseous distention should prompt contrast enema to diagnose (and treat) meconium plug syndrome. If no plug is

Table 2–21. Intestinal obstruction.

Site of Obstruction	Clinical Findings	Plain Radiographs	Contrast Study
Duodenal atresia	Down syndrome (30%); early vomiting, sometimes bilious	"Double bubble" (dilated stomach and proximal duodenum, no air distal)	Not needed
Malrotation and volvulus	Bilious vomiting with onset anytime in the first few weeks	Dilated stomach and proximal duodenum; paucity of air distally (may be normal gas pattern)	UGI shows displaced duodenojejunal junction with "corkscrew" deformity of twisted bowel
Jejunoileal atresia, meconium ileus	Bilious gastric contents > 25 mL at birth; progressive distention and bilious vomiting	Multiple dilated loops of bowel; intra-abdominal calcifications if in utero perforation occurred (meconium peritonitis)	Barium or osmotic contrast (eg, meglumine diatrizoate [Gastrografin]) enema shows microcolon; contrast refluxed into distal ileum may demonstrate and relieve meconium obstruction (successful in about 50%)
Meconium plug syndrome; Hirschsprung's disease	Distention, delayed stooling (>24 hours)	Diffuse bowel distention	Barium or osmotic contrast enema outlines and relieves plug; may show transition zone in Hirschsprung's disease; delayed emptying (> 24 hours) suggests Hirschsprung's disease

found, the diagnosis may be small left colon syndrome (seen in infants of diabetic mothers) or Hirschsprung's disease. Rectal biopsy will be required to make this diagnosis. Imperforate anus should be apparent on physical examination, though a rectovaginal fistula with a mildly abnormal-appearing anus can occasionally be confused with normal.

Treatment

Nasogastric suction to decompress the bowel, intravenous glucose, fluid and electrolyte replacement, and respiratory support as necessary should be instituted. Antibiotics are usually indicated. The definitive treatment for most of these conditions (with the exception of meconium plug syndrome, small left colon syndrome, and some cases of meconium ileus) is surgery.

Prognosis

Up to 10% of infants with meconium plug syndrome are subsequently found to have cystic fibrosis or Hirschsprung's disease. For this reason, some surgeons advocate performance of a sweat chloride test and rectal biopsy in all of these infants before discharge. The infant with meconium plug syndrome who is still symptomatic after contrast enema should have a rectal biopsy.

In cases of duodenal atresia associated with Down syndrome, the prognosis will depend on associated anomalies (eg, heart defects) and the severity of prestenotic duodenal dilation. Otherwise, these conditions usually carry an excellent prognosis after surgical repair.

ABDOMINAL WALL DEFECTS

1. OMPHALOCELE

Omphalocele is a membrane-covered herniation of abdominal contents into the base of the umbilical cord. There is a high incidence of associated anomalies (cardiac, gastrointestinal, chromosomal—eg, trisomy 13). The sac may contain liver and spleen as well as intestine.

Acute management of omphalocele involves covering the defect with a sterile dressing soaked with warm saline to prevent fluid loss, nasogastric decompression, intravenous fluids and glucose, and antibiotics. If the contents of the omphalocele will fit into the abdomen, a primary surgical closure is done. If not, a staged closure is performed, with gradual reduction of the omphalocele contents into the abdominal cavity and a secondary closure. Postoperatively, third-space fluid losses may be extensive; fluid and electrolyte therapy, therefore, must be carefully monitored.

2. GASTROSCHISIS

In gastroschisis, the intestine extrudes through an abdominal wall defect lateral to the umbilical cord. There is no membrane or sac and no liver or spleen outside the abdomen. Gastroschisis is associated with no anomalies except intestinal atresia. The herniation is thought to occur as a rupture through an ischemic portion of the abdominal wall.

Therapy is as described for omphalocele; however, primary closures can be successfully performed more frequently.

DIAPHRAGMATIC HERNIA

This congenital malformation consists of herniation of abdominal organs into the hemithorax (usually left) through a posterolateral defect in the diaphragm. It presents in the delivery room as severe respiratory distress in an infant with poor breath sounds and scaphoid abdomen. The rapidity and severity of presentation—as well as ultimate survival—are dependent on the degree of pulmonary hypoplasia, which is a result of compression by the intrathoracic abdominal contents in utero. Affected infants are prone to development of pneumothorax.

Treatment includes intubation and ventilation as well as decompression of the gastrointestinal tract with a nasogastric tube. An intravenous infusion of glucose and fluid should be started. Chest x-ray confirms the diagnosis. Surgery to reduce the abdominal contents from the thorax and to close the diaphragmatic defect is performed after the infant is stabilized. The postoperative course is often complicated by severe pulmonary hypertension, requiring therapy with high-frequency ventilation, inhaled NO, or ECMO. The mortality rate for this condition is 50%, with survival dependent on the degree of pulmonary hypoplasia.

GASTROINTESTINAL BLEEDING

Upper Gastrointestinal Bleeding

Upper gastrointestinal bleeding is not uncommon in the newborn nursery. Old blood (coffee-ground material) may be either swallowed maternal blood or infant blood from a bleeding gastric irritation such as gastritis or stress ulcer. Bright red blood from the stomach is most likely acute bleeding, again due to gastritis. Treatment generally consists of gastric lavage (a sample can be sent for Apt testing to determine if it is mother's or baby's blood) and antacid medication. If the volume of bleeding is large, intensive monitoring, fluid and blood replacement, and endoscopy are indicated (see Chapter 19).

Lower Gastrointestinal Bleeding

Rectal bleeding is less common than upper gastrointestinal bleeding in the newborn and may be seen with infections (eg, *Salmonella* acquired from the mother perinatally), milk intolerance (blood streaks with diarrhea), or, in stressed infants, necrotizing enterocolitis. An abdominal x-ray should be obtained to rule out pneumatosis intestinalis (air in the wall of the bowel) or other abnormalities in gas pattern (eg, obstruction). If the x-ray is negative and the examination is benign, a protein hydrolysate or "predigested" formula should be tried or the mother instructed to avoid all dairy products in her diet if nursing. If the amount of rectal bleeding is large or persistent, endoscopy will be needed.

GASTROESOPHAGEAL REFLUX

All people reflux occasionally, and physiologic regurgitant reflux is extremely common in infants. Reflux is pathologic and should be treated when it results in failure to thrive owing to excessive regurgitation, poor intake due to dysphagia and irritability, apnea or cyanotic episodes (acute life-threatening events), or chronic respiratory symptoms of wheezing and recurrent pneumonias.

Diagnosis is clinical, with confirmation by barium swallow or pH probe study.

Initial steps in treatment include prone positioning, with thickened feeds (rice cereal, 1 tbsp/oz of formula) for those with frequent regurgitation and poor weight gain. Gastric acid suppressants such as ranitidine (2 mg/kg twice a day) or cimetidine, along with a prokinetic agent such as cisapride (0.2 mg/kg three times daily), should also be used. Cisapride should be used with caution in premature infants, infants with existing heart disease, and ill infants on multiple drugs because of the risk of prolonged QT interval and other cardiac arrythmias. Since most infants improve by 12–15 months, surgery is reserved for the most severe cases, especially those with chronic neurologic or respiratory conditions that exacerbate reflux and those who have life-threatening events caused by reflux.

Adra AM et al: The fetus with gastroschisis: Impact of route of delivery and prenatal ultrasonography. Am J Obstet Gynecol 1996;174:540.

Bohn DJ et al: Postnatal management of congenital diaphragmatic hernia. Clin Perinatol 1996;23:843.

Cummings WA, Williams JL: Neonatal gastrointestinal imaging. Clin Perinatol 1996;23:387.

Kays DW: Surgical conditions of the neonatal intestinal tract. Clin Perinatol 1996;23:353.

Orenstein SR: Gastroesophageal reflux. Pediatr Rev 1992;13:174.

INFECTIONS OF THE NEWBORN

The fetus and the newborn infant are very susceptible to infections. There are three major routes of perinatal infection: (1) blood-borne transplacental infection of the fetus (eg, cytomegalovirus, rubella, syphilis); (2) ascending infection with disruption of the barrier provided by the amniotic membranes (eg, bacterial infections after 12–18 hours of ruptured membranes); and (3) infection upon passage through an infected birth canal or exposure to infected blood at delivery (eg, herpes simplex, hepatitis B, bacterial infections).

Susceptibility of the newborn to infection is related to immaturity of both the cellular and humoral immune systems at birth. This feature is particularly evident in the preterm neonate. Passive protection against some organisms is provided by transfer of IgG across the placenta during the third trimester of pregnancy. Preterm infants, especially those born at less than 30 weeks, do not have the benefit of the full amount of this passively acquired antibody.

BACTERIAL INFECTIONS

1. BACTERIAL SEPSIS

The incidence of early-onset (< 5 days) neonatal bacterial infection is 4–5 per 1000 live births. If there is rupture of the membranes more than 24 hours prior to delivery, the infection rate increases to 1 per 100 live births. If there is early rupture of membranes with chorioamnionitis, the infection rate increases further to 1 per 10 live births. Irrespective of membrane rupture, infection rates are five times higher in preterm than in term infants.

Early-onset bacterial infection presents most commonly on day 1 of life, with the majority of cases at less than 12 hours. Respiratory distress due to pneumonia is the most common presenting sign. Other features include unexplained low Apgar scores without fetal distress, poor perfusion, and hypotension. Late-onset bacterial infection (at more than 5 days of age) presents in a more subtle manner, with poor feeding, lethargy, hypotonia, temperature instability, altered perfusion, new or increased oxygen requirement, and apnea. Late-onset bacterial sepsis is more often associated with meningitis or other localized infections.

Low total white counts, absolute neutropenia (< 1000/μL), and elevated ratios of immature to mature neutrophils are suggestive of neonatal bacterial infection. Thrombocytopenia is also a common feature. Other laboratory signs are hypoglycemia or hyperglycemia with no change in glucose administration and unexplained metabolic acidosis. In early-onset bacterial infection, pneumonia is invariably present; chest x-ray films show infiltrates, but these infiltrates cannot be distinguished from those resulting from other causes of neonatal lung disease. Definitive diagnosis is made by positive cultures from blood, cerebrospinal fluid, etc.

Early-onset infection is most often caused by group B β-hemolytic streptococci (GBS) and gram-negative enteric pathogens (most commonly *Escherichia coli*). Another organism to consider is *Haemophilus influenzae.* Late-onset sepsis is caused by coagulase-negative staphylococci (most common in infants with indwelling central venous lines), *Staphylococcus aureus,* GBS, *Enterococcus, Pseudomonas,* and other gram-negative organisms.

Treatment

A high index of suspicion is important in the diagnosis and treatment of neonatal infection. Table 2–22 presents guidelines for the evaluation and management of term infants with risk factors or clinical signs of infection. Because the risk of infection is greater in the preterm infant and because respiratory disease is a common sign of infection, any preterm infant with respiratory disease requires blood cultures and broad-spectrum antibiotic therapy for 48–72 hours

Table 2–22. Guidelines for evaluation of neonatal bacterial infection in the term infant.

Risk Factor	Clinical Signs of Infection	Evaluation and Treatment
Delivery 12–18 hours after rupture of membranes	None	Observation
Delivery > 12–18 hours after rupture of membranes, chorioamnionitis	None	CBC, blood culture, broad-spectrum antibiotics for 48–72 hours[3]
Delivery > 12–18 hours after rupture of membranes, chorioamnionitis, maternal antibiotics[1]	None	CBC, blood culture, broad-spectrum antibiotics for 48–72 hours[3]
With or without risk factors	Present	CBC, blood and CSF cultures, perhaps urine culture (see below); broad-spectrum antibiotics[2]

[1]Early newborn discharge (< 48 hours) is contraindicated in these infants even if observation without treatment is elected.
[2]Irrespective of age at presentation, any infant who appears infected by clinical criteria should undergo cerebrospinal fluid examination. Urine culture is indicated in the evaluation of infants who were initially well but have developed symptoms after 2–3 days of age.
[3]If clinical signs are absent, close observation without treatment may be sufficient.

pending the results of cultures. An examination of cerebrospinal fluid should be performed when infection is highly suspected on a clinical basis (eg, associated hypotension, persistent metabolic acidosis, neutropenia). Antibiotic coverage should be directed initially toward suspected organisms. Early-onset sepsis is usually caused by GBS or gram-negative enteric organisms; broad-spectrum coverage, therefore, should include ampicillin plus an aminoglycoside or third-generation cephalosporin—eg, ampicillin, 100 mg/kg/d divided every 12 hours, and gentamicin, 2.5 mg/kg/dose every 12–24 hours (depending upon gestational age), or cefotaxime, 100 mg/kg/d divided every 12 hours. Late-onset infections can also be caused by the same organisms, but coverage may need to be expanded to include staphylococci. In particular, the preterm infant with an indwelling line is at risk for infection with coagulase-negative staphylococci, for which vancomycin is the drug of choice in a dosage of 10 mg/kg every 8–24 hours depending upon gestational and postnatal ages. Other supportive therapy includes the administration of intravenous immune globulin (500–750 mg/kg) to infants with known overwhelming infection. The duration of treatment for proved sepsis is 10–14 days of intravenous antibiotics. In addition, recombinant human granulocyte colony-stimulating factor (rhG-CSF) is under investigation for treatment of neutropenia in the septic infant. In sick infants, the essentials of good supportive therapy should be provided: intravenous glucose, colloid volume support, use of pressors as needed, and oxygen and ventilator support.

Prevention of neonatal GBS infection has been achieved with intrapartum administration of penicillin to selected maternal GBS carriers identified antepartum or intrapartum who have associated risk factors (preterm labor, premature rupture of the membranes before 37 weeks, rupture of the membranes beyond 18 hours at any gestational age, multiple births, maternal fever). If maternal GBS status is unknown, chemoprophylaxis may be indicated for one or more of the risk factors listed above (Figure 2–8). Figure 2–9 presents a suggested strategy for the infant born to a mother who received intrapartum prophylaxis.

2. MENINGITIS

Any newborn with bacterial sepsis is also at risk for meningitis. The incidence is low in infants with early-onset sepsis but much higher in infants with late-onset infection. The workup for any newborn with signs of infection should include a spinal tap. Diagnosis is suggested by a CSF protein greater than 150 mg/dL, glucose less than 30 mg/dL, more than 25 leukocytes/μL, and a positive Gram's stain. The diagnosis is confirmed by culture. The most common

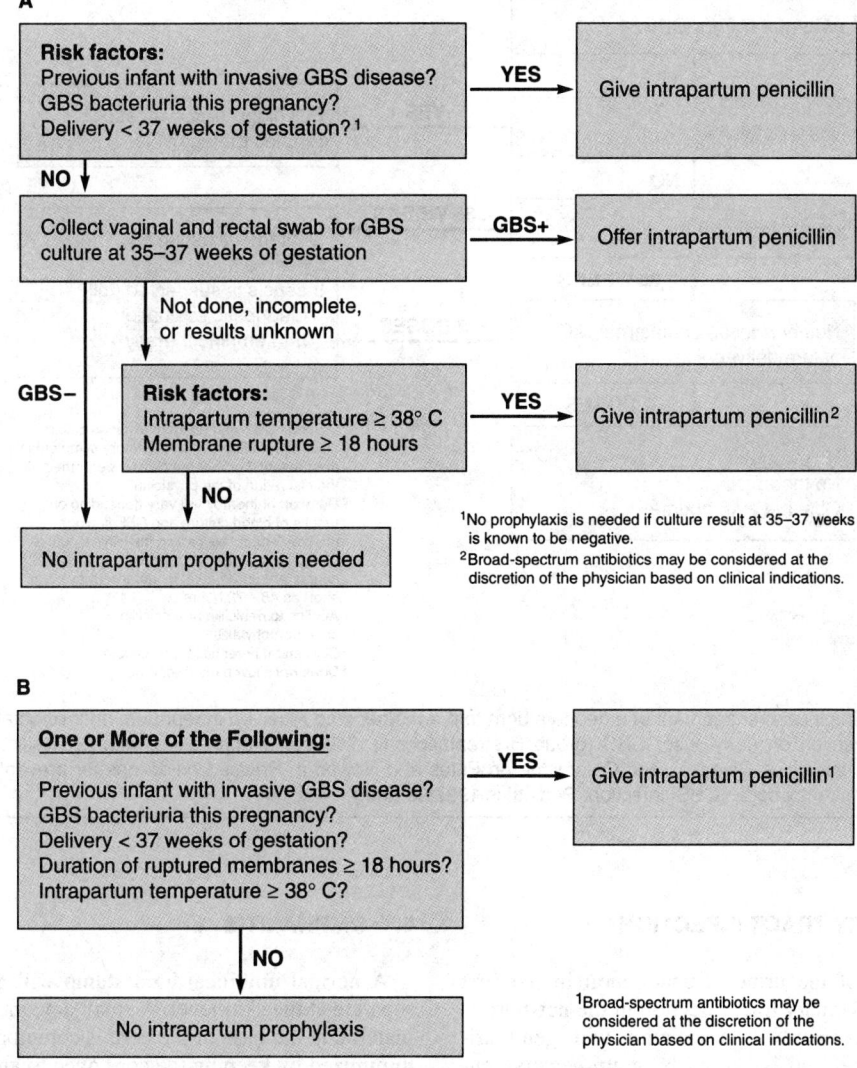

Figure 2–8. Algorithms for the intrapartum prevention of GBS (group B streptococcal) infection. **A:** Based on screening culture. **B:** Based on risk factor assessment. (Reproduced, with permission, from AAP Committee on Infectious Diseases and Committee on Fetus and Newborn: Revised guidelines for prevention of early-onset group B streptococcal [GBS] infection. Pediatrics 1997;99:489.)

organisms are GBS and gram-negative enteric bacteria. While sepsis can be treated with antibiotics for 10–14 days, meningitis should be treated for 21 days. The mortality rate of neonatal meningitis is approximately 25%, with significant neurologic morbidity present in one-third of the survivors. Use of dexamethasone has not been studied in neonates.

3. PNEUMONIA

The respiratory system can be infected in utero or upon passage through the birth canal. Early-onset neonatal infection is usually associated with pneumonia. Pneumonia should also be suspected in older neonates with a recent onset of tachypnea, retractions, and cyanosis. In infants already receiving respiratory support, an increase in the requirement for oxygen or ventilator support may indicate pneumonia. Not only common bacteria but also viruses (cytomegalovirus, respiratory syncytial virus, adenovirus, influenza, herpes simplex, parainfluenza) and *Chlamydia* can cause the disease. In infants with pre-existing respiratory disease, intercurrent pulmonary infections may contribute to the ultimate severity of chronic lung disease.

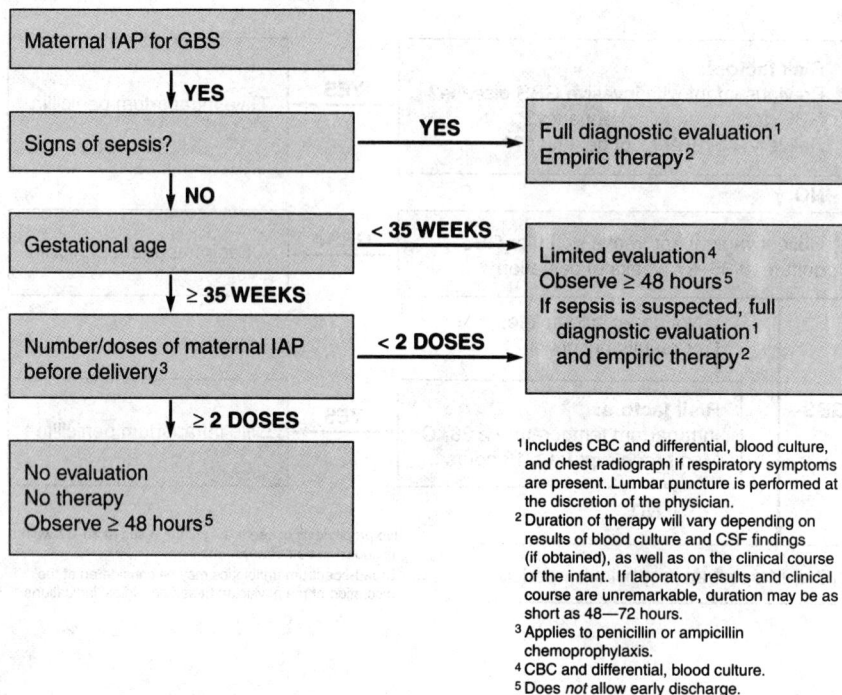

Figure 2–9. Empirical management of a neonate born to a a mother who received intrapartum antimicrobial prophylaxis (IAP) for prevention on early-onset GBS (group B streptococcal) disease. (Reproduced, with permission, from AAP Committee on Infectious Diseases and Committee on Fetus and Newborn. Revised guidelines for prevention of early-onset group B streptococcal [GBS] infection. Pediatrics 1997;99:489.)

4. URINARY TRACT INFECTION

Infection of the urine is uncommon in the first days of life. Urinary tract infection in the newborn is seen most commonly in association with genitourinary anomalies and is caused by gram-negative enteric pathogens. Urine should be evaluated as part of the workup for late-onset infection. Culture should be obtained either by suprapubic aspiration or bladder catheterization. Antibiotic therapy is continued intravenously for 10–14 days. Evaluation for genitourinary anomalies, starting with an ultrasound examination and a voiding cystourethrogram, should be done subsequently.

5. OTITIS MEDIA

Otitis media occurs in a significant number of long-term nursery occupants. It is particularly common in infants who have had prolonged endotracheal intubation or an indwelling nasogastric feeding tube. Evaluation for infection in such an infant is not complete without an ear examination. Gram-negative enteric pathogens are more commonly found infecting agents in nursery occupants than in outpatients.

6. OMPHALITIS

A normal umbilical cord stump will atrophy and separate at the skin level. A small amount of purulent material at the base of the cord is common but can be minimized by keeping the cord open to air and cleaning the base with alcohol several times a day. The cord can become colonized with streptococci, staphylococci, or gram-negative organisms that can cause local infection. Infections are more common in cords manipulated for venous or arterial lines. Omphalitis is diagnosed when redness and edema develop in the soft tissues around the stump. Local and systemic cultures should be obtained. Treatment is with broad-spectrum intravenous antibiotics. Complications are determined by the degree of infection of the cord vessels and include septic thrombophlebitis, hepatic abscess, necrotizing fasciitis, and portal vein thrombosis. Surgical consultation should be obtained because of the potential for necrotizing fasciitis.

American Academy of Pediatrics, Committee on Infectious Disease and Committee of Fetus and Newborn: Revised guidelines for prevention of early-onset group B streptococcal (GBS) infection. Pediatrics 1997;99:489.

Carr R, Modi N: Haemopoietic colony stimulating factors

for preterm neonates. Arch Dis Child Fetal Neonatal Ed 1997;76:F128.

Gotoff SP, Boyer KM: Prevention of early-onset neonatal group B streptococcal disease. Pediatrics 1997;99:866.

Stoll BJ et al: Early-onset sepsis on very low birth weight neonates: A report from the National Institute of Child Health and Human Development Neonatal Research Network. J Pediatr 1996;129:72.

Stoll BJ et al: Late-onset sepsis in very low birth weight neonates: A report from the National Institute of Child Health and Human Development Neonatal Research Network. J Pediatr 1996;129:63.

Wiswell TE et al: No lumbar puncture in the evaluation for early neonatal sepsis: Will meningitis be missed? Pediatrics 1995;95:803.

FUNGAL SEPSIS

With the survival of smaller, sicker infants, infection with *Candida* species has become more common. Infants of low birth weight with central lines who have had repeated exposures to broad-spectrum antibiotics are at highest risk. For infants of birth weight less than 1500 g, colonization rates of 27% have been demonstrated, with many of these infants developing cutaneous lesions. A much smaller percentage (2–5%) develop systemic disease.

Clinical features of fungal sepsis can be indistinguishable from those of late-onset bacterial sepsis but may be more subtle. Thrombocytopenia may be the earliest and only sign. Deep organ involvement (renal, eye, endocarditis) is commonly associated with systemic candidiasis. Treatment is with amphotericin B. In severe infections, flucytosine can be added for synergistic coverage. (See Chapter 37.)

Malassezia furfur is also seen in infants with central lines receiving intravenous fat emulsion. To eradicate this organism, as well as *Candida* species, it is necessary to remove the indwelling line.

Ng PC: Systemic fungal infections in neonates. Arch Dis Child Fetal Neonatal Ed 1994;71:F130.

CONGENITAL VIRAL & PARASITIC INFECTIONS
(See also Chapters 34 and 37.)

1. CYTOMEGALOVIRUS INFECTION

Cytomegalovirus (CMV) is the most common virus transmitted in utero. The incidence of congenital infection ranges from 0.2% to 2.2% of live births. Transmission of CMV can occur during either primary or reactivated infection in the mother. An important source of infection is children (especially those in a day care setting), who transmit the virus to parents and workers. The incidence of primary infection in pregnancy is 1–4%, with a 40% transplacental

transmission rate to the fetus. Of these infants, 85–90% are asymptomatic at birth, whereas 10–15% have clinically apparent disease—hepatosplenomegaly, petechiae, small size for gestational age, microcephaly, direct hyperbilirubinemia, thrombocytopenia, intracranial calcifications, and chorioretinitis. The risk of neonatal disease is higher when the mother acquires the infection in the first half of pregnancy. The incidence of reactivated infection in pregnancy is less than 1%, with an incidence of clinically apparent disease of 0–1%. Diagnosis in the neonate should be confirmed by culture of the virus from urine. Rapid diagnosis is possible with antigen detection techniques and identification of viral DNA by polymerase chain reaction (PCR) testing. Diagnosis can also be confirmed in utero from an amniocentesis specimen. Although experimental and not routinely recommended, ganciclovir therapy has been used in some severely ill neonates.

The mortality rate in patients with symptomatic congenital CMV may be as high as 20%. Sequelae such as hearing loss, mental retardation, delayed motor development, chorioretinitis and optic atrophy, seizures, language delays, and learning disability occur in 90% of symptomatic survivors. The incidence of complications is 5–15% in asymptomatic infants; the most frequent complication is hearing loss, which can be progressive.

Perinatal infection can also occur with acquisition of virus around the time of delivery. These infections are generally asymptomatic and without sequelae. Postnatal infection is usually asymptomatic but can cause hepatitis, pneumonitis, and neurologic illness in compromised seronegative prematures. The virus can be acquired postnatally through transfusions or ingestion of CMV-infected breast milk. Transfusion risk can be minimized by using frozen, washed red blood cells or CMV antibody-negative donors.

2. RUBELLA

Congenital rubella infection occurs as a result of rubella infection in the mother during pregnancy. The frequency of infection and damage in the fetus is as high as 80% in mothers infected during the first trimester. Fetal infection rates decline in the second trimester before increasing again in the third trimester. Fetal damage generally does not occur in infections acquired after 18 weeks of gestation. Clinical features of congenital rubella include adenopathy, bone radiolucencies, encephalitis, cardiac defects (pulmonary arterial hypoplasia and patent ductus arteriosus), cataracts, retinopathy, growth retardation, hepatosplenomegaly, thrombocytopenia, and purpura. Affected infants can be asymptomatic at birth but develop clinical sequelae during the first year of life. The diagnosis should be suspected in cases of a characteristic clinical illness in the mother (rash, adenopathy, arthritis) confirmed by serologic testing. Diagnosis can be confirmed by culture of pharyngeal secretions in the baby. Congenital rubella is now rare because prevention is possible with immunization.

3. VARICELLA

Congenital varicella is rare (< 5% after infection acquired during the first or second trimester) but may cause a constellation of findings including limb hypoplasia, cutaneous scars, microcephaly, cortical atrophy, chorioretinitis, and cataracts. Perinatal exposure (5 days before to 2 days after delivery) can cause severe to fatal disseminated varicella in the infant. If maternal varicella develops within this perinatal risk period, 1.25 mL of varicella immune globulin should be given to the newborn. If this has not been done, the illness can be treated with intravenous acyclovir (30 mg/kg/d divided every 8 hours).

Hospitalized premature infants of at least 28 weeks' gestation whose mothers have no history of chickenpox—and all infants of less than 28 weeks' gestational age—should receive varicella immune globulin following any postnatal exposure. Susceptible women of childbearing age should be immunized with varicella vaccine.

4. TOXOPLASMOSIS

Toxoplasmosis is caused by the protozoan *Toxoplasma gondii*. Maternal infection occurs in 0.1–0.5% of pregnancies and is usually asymptomatic. When primary infection occurs during pregnancy, up to 40% of the fetuses become infected, of whom 15% have severe damage. The sources of transmission include exposure to cat feces and ingestion of raw or undercooked meat. Although the risk of transmission increases to 90% near term, fetal damage is most likely to occur when maternal infection occurs in the second to sixth months of gestation.

Clinical findings include growth retardation, chorioretinitis, seizures, jaundice, hydrocephalus, microcephaly, cerebral calcifications, hepatosplenomegaly, adenopathy, cataracts, maculopapular rash, thrombocytopenia, and pneumonia. The majority of affected infants are asymptomatic at birth but show evidence of damage (chorioretinitis, blindness, low IQ, hearing loss) at a later time. Serologic tests, first for IgG and then for the specific IgM antibody, make the diagnosis. Infants with suspected infection should have an eye examination and CT scan. Organism isolation and PCR tests are also available for diagnosis in the neonate and from amniocentesis specimens.

Treatment of the acutely infected pregnant woman may prevent transmission to the fetus. Neonatal treatment using pyrimethamine and sulfadiazine with folinic acid can improve long-term outcome. (See Chapter 37.)

PERINATALLY ACQUIRED VIRAL INFECTIONS

1. HERPES SIMPLEX (See also Chapter 34.)

Herpes simplex virus (HSV) infection is most commonly acquired at the time of birth during transit through an infected birth canal. The mother may have either primary or reactivated secondary infection. Primary maternal infection, because of the high titer of organism and the absence of maternal antibodies, poses the greatest risk to the infant. The risk of neonatal infection with vaginal delivery in this setting is 33–50%. Seventy percent of mothers with primary herpes at the time of delivery are asymptomatic. The risk to an infant born to a mother with recurrent herpes simplex is much lower (< 3–5%). Time of presentation of localized (skin, eye, mouth) or disseminated disease (pneumonia, shock, hepatitis) in the infant is usually 5–14 days of age. Central nervous system disease usually presents at 14–28 days with lethargy and seizures. In about one-third of patients, localized skin, eye, and mouth disease is the first indication of infection. In another third, disseminated or central nervous system disease precedes skin, eye, and mouth findings, while the remaining third have disseminated or central nervous system disease in the absence of skin, eye, and mouth disease. Preliminary diagnosis can be made by scraping the base of a vesicle and finding multinucleated giant cells. Viral culture from vesicles, usually positive in 24–72 hours, makes the definitive diagnosis. In some cases, newer polymerase chain reaction DNA technology may assist in diagnosis.

Acyclovir (30–60 mg/kg/d given every 8 hours) is the drug of choice for neonatal herpes infection. Treatment improves survival of neonates with central nervous system and disseminated disease and prevents the spread of localized disease. Prevention is possible by not allowing delivery through an infected birth canal (eg, by cesarean section within 6 hours after rupture of the membranes). However, antepartum cervical cultures are poor predictors of the presence of virus at the time of delivery. Furthermore, given the low incidence of infection in the newborn in secondary maternal infection, cesarean section is not indicated for asymptomatic mothers with a history of herpes. In most settings, cesarean sections are still performed in mothers with active lesions (either primary or secondary) at the time of delivery. Infants born to mothers with a history of HSV infection but no active lesions can be observed closely after birth. Cultures should be obtained and acyclovir treatment initiated only for clinical signs consistent with herpesvirus infection. Infants born to mothers with active lesions—irrespective of the route of delivery—should be cultured (eye, oropharynx, umbilicus, rectum) 24 hours after delivery. If the infant is colonized (positive cultures) or if symptoms consistent with herpes infection develop, treatment with acyclovir should be started. In cases of maternal primary infection at the time of vaginal delivery, the infant should be cultured and started on acyclovir pending the results of cultures. The major problem facing perinatologists is the high percentage of asymptomatic primary maternal infection. In these cases, infection in the neonate is currently not preventable. Therefore, any infant who presents at the right age with symptoms consistent with neonatal herpes should be cultured and started on acyclovir pending the results of those cultures.

The prognosis is good for localized skin and mucosal disease that does not progress. The mortality rate for both disseminated and central nervous system herpes is high, with significant rates of morbidity among survivors despite treatment.

2. HEPATITIS B & C
(See also Chapter 20.)

Infants can be infected with hepatitis B at the time of birth. Clinical illness is rare in the neonatal period, but infants exposed in utero are at high risk of becoming chronic HBsAg carriers, developing chronic active hepatitis and, later, hepatocellular carcinoma. The presence of HBsAg should be determined in all pregnant women. If the result is positive, the infant should receive HBIG and hepatitis B vaccine as soon as possible after birth, followed by two subsequent vaccine doses at 1 and 6 months of age. If HBsAg has not been tested prior to birth in a mother at risk, the test should be run after delivery and hepatitis B vaccine given within 12 hours after birth. If the mother is subsequently found to be positive, HBIG should be given as soon as possible (preferably within 48 hours, but not later than 1 week after birth). Subsequent vaccine doses should be given at 1 and 6 months of age. The CDC and AAP recommend universal immunization of all newborns with hepatitis B vaccine at birth, at 1–2 months, and at 6–18 months. *Note:* In low-birth-weight infants, the initial vaccine should be given when the infant reaches a weight of 2000 g. In prematures born to HBsAg-positive mothers, vaccine and HBIG should be given at birth, but a three-vaccine hepatitis B series should be given after a weight of 2000 g is attained.

Hepatitis C perinatal transmissions occur in about 5% of infants born to mothers who carry the virus. At the present time, no prevention strategies exist.

3. ENTEROVIRAL INFECTION

Enteroviral infections occur with greatest frequency in the late summer and early fall. Infection is usually acquired in the perinatal period. There is often a history of maternal illness (fever, diarrhea, rash) in the week prior to delivery. The illness presents in the infant in the first 2 weeks of life. The illness is most commonly characterized by fevers, lethargy, irritability, diarrhea, and rash but is not severe. More severe forms occasionally occur, including meningoencephalitis and myocarditis, as well as a disseminated illness with hepatitis, pneumonia, shock, and disseminated intravascular coagulation. Diagnosis can be confirmed by culture (rectum, cerebrospinal fluid, blood) or by the more rapid PCR techniques.

There is no therapy of proved efficacy. The prognosis is good for all symptom complexes except severe disseminated disease, which carries a high mortality rate.

4. HIV INFECTION
(See also Chapter 35.)

Human immunodeficiency virus (HIV) can pass transplacentally, can be acquired at the time of delivery, or can be transmitted postpartum via breast milk. The prevalence of HIV infection among women of childbearing age in the United States is 1.5:1000. Transmission of virus occurs in about 30% of births. Administration of zidovudine during pregnancy, intrapartum, and for 6 weeks in the newborn period at a dosage of 2 mg/kg orally four times a day decreases vertical transmission to 8%. The risk of transmission is increased in mothers with advanced disease, low CD4 counts, and p24 antigenemia. Prematurity, vaginal delivery, ruptured membranes over 4 hours, and chorioamnionitis also increase the transmission rate. Diagnosis is based on clinical, immunologic, and serologic findings. Newborns with congenitally acquired HIV are often free of symptoms. Jaundice, neonatal giant cell hepatitis, and thrombocytopenia have been reported at birth. Failure to thrive, lymphadenopathy, hepatosplenomegaly, oral thrush, chronic diarrhea, bacterial infections with common organisms, and an increased incidence of upper and lower respiratory diseases, including lymphoid interstitial pneumonitis, may appear early in life or may be delayed for months to years.

The presence of maternal antibody acquired transplacentally confuses diagnosis in the neonate. The presence of anti-HIV antibody is not diagnostic of infection until after 18 months of age. An infant who is not infected should remain healthy, and the titer of antibody should decline during the first year of life. Diagnosis can be made in infants in the first few months of life by culture or detection of HIV

DNA sequences by polymerase chain reaction. These tests should be done at birth and repeated at 1–2 months and 4 months of age. An infant who is 4 months of age with no positive culture, PCR, or p24 antigen has a greater than 95% chance of not being infected. Follow-up should document antibody disappearance. An HIV-exposed infant is considered uninfected when there are no physical findings of HIV, immunologic tests are normal, virologic studies are negative, and two HIV antibody tests are negative.

Protection of health care workers is an important issue. Testing should be performed in all pregnant women. Because such testing will fail to identify some infected patients, however, universal precautions should be used. Gloves should be worn during all procedures involving blood and blood-contaminated fluids, intubation, and any invasive procedures using needles. When a splash exposure is possible (eg, in the delivery room), a mask and eye covers should be used.

OTHER INFECTIONS

1. CONGENITAL SYPHILIS

The infant is usually infected in utero by transplacental passage of *Treponema pallidum*. Active primary and secondary maternal syphilis leads to fetal infection in nearly 100%; latent disease, in 40%; and late disease, in 10%. Fetal infection is rare at under 18 weeks of gestation. Fetal infection can result in stillbirth or prematurity. Findings consistent with early congenital syphilis (presentation at under 2 years) include mucocutaneous lesions, lymphadenopathy, hepatosplenomegaly, bony changes, and hydrops. However, in the newborn period, infants are often asymptomatic, so that diagnosis is based on maternal and infant serologic testing and is only presumptive. Later manifestations (at over 2 years of age) include Hutchinson's teeth and mulberry molars, keratitis, chorioretinitis, glaucoma, hearing loss, saddle nose, saber shins, and mental retardation. An infant should be evaluated for congenital syphilis if it is born to a mother with positive nontreponemal tests confirmed by a positive treponemal test but without documented adequate treatment (parenteral penicillin G), including the expected fourfold decrease in nontreponemal antibody titer. Evaluation should include physical examination, a quantitative nontreponemal serologic test for syphilis, cerebrospinal fluid examination, long bone x-rays, and antitreponemal IgM. A definitive diagnosis can be made on rare occasions when the organism is identified by darkfield microscopy or pathologic examination of the placenta. Guidelines for therapy are presented in Table 2–23. Infants should be treated for congenital syphilis if they have proved or probable disease: (1) physical or x-ray evidence, (2) quantita-

Table 2–23. Recommended antimicrobial treatment of neonates (≤ 4 weeks of age) with proved or possible congenital syphilis.[1]

Clinical Status	Antimicrobial Therapy
I. Proved or highly probable disease	Aqueous crystalline penicillin G, for 10–14 d[2]
II. Asymptomatic, normal CSF and radiographic examination plus **maternal** history of the following:	
A. No therapy or inadequate penicillin treatment;[3] no documentation of therapy; failed therapy or reinfected	Aqueous crystalline penicillin G, IV, for 10–14 days,[3] or clinical and serologic follow-up, and benzathine penicillin G, 50,000 units/kg IM as single dose[4]
B. Adequate therapy but administered less than 1 month before delivery; response to therapy not demonstrated by a fourfold decrease in titer of a nontreponemal serologic test; erythromycin therapy	Clinical and serologic follow-up and benzathine penicillin G, 50,000 units/kg IM, as single dose[4]

[1]Modified, with permission, from Peter G, Hall CB, Orenstein WA (editors): *1997 Red Book: Report of the Committee on Infectious Diseases,* 24th ed. American Academy of Pediatrics, 1997.
[2]If more than 1 day of therapy is missed, the entire course should be restarted.
[3]See *Redbook* 1997 for definition (includes those in whom sequential serologic tests on the mother do not demonstrate a fourfold or greater decrease in nontreponemal antibody titer).
[4]Some experts recommend aqueous crystalline penicillin G as for proved or highly probable disease. Others would follow up the infant without giving antibiotic therapy if both clinical and serologic follow-up can be ensured.

tive nontreponemal antibody titers four times higher than the mother, (3) elevated cerebrospinal fluid protein or cell count or positive VDRL, or (4) a positive antitreponemal IgM test. Asymptomatic infants should be treated if the mother did not receive adequate treatment for syphilis.

2. TUBERCULOSIS
(See also Chapter 36.)

Congenital tuberculosis is rare but may occur in the infant of a mother with hematogenously spread tuberculosis or by aspiration of infected amniotic fluid in cases of tuberculous endometritis. Women with pulmonary tuberculosis are not likely to infect the fetus until after delivery. Postnatal acquisition is the most common mechanism of neonatal infection.

Management in these cases is based on the mother's evaluation.

(1) Mother with a positive skin test and negative chest x-ray, or mother with an abnormal chest x-ray but no evidence of acute disease: Investigate family contacts. Treat the mother with isoniazid (INH).

(2) Mother has an abnormal chest x-ray: Mother and infant should be separated until the mother is evaluated. If active tuberculosis is found, maintain separation until the mother is receiving antituberculosis therapy. Investigate family contacts.

(3) Mother with clinical or x-ray evidence of acute and possibly contagious tuberculosis: Evaluate the infant for congenital tuberculosis (skin test, chest x-ray, lumbar puncture, cultures) and HIV. Treat the mother and infant and separate them until the mother is felt to be noncontagious.

If congenital tuberculosis is suspected, multidrug therapy should be initiated.

3. CONJUNCTIVITIS

Neisseria gonorrhoeae may colonize an infant during passage through an infected birth canal. Gonococcal ophthalmitis presents at 3–7 days with purulent conjunctivitis. The diagnosis can be suspected when gram-negative intracellular diplococci are seen on a Gram-stained smear and confirmed by culture. Treatment is with intravenous or intramuscular ceftriaxone, 25–50 mg/kg (not to exceed 125 mg) given once. Prophylaxis at birth is with 1% silver nitrate or 0.5% erythromycin ointment. Infants born to mothers with known gonococcal disease should also receive a single dose of ceftriaxone.

Chlamydia trachomatis is another important cause of conjunctivitis, presenting at 5 days to several weeks of age with congestion, edema, and minimal discharge. The organism is acquired at birth after passage through an infected birth canal. Acquisition occurs in 50% of infants born to infected women, with a 25–50% risk of conjunctivitis. Prevalence in pregnancy is over 10% in some populations. Diagnosis is by isolation of the organism or by rapid antigen detection tests. Treatment is with oral erythromycin (30 mg/kg/d in divided doses every 8–12 hours) for 14 days. Topical treatment alone will not eradicate nasopharyngeal carriage, leaving the infant at risk for the development of pneumonitis. Infants born to mothers with untreated chlamydial infection should also be treated with oral erythromycin.

Aleixo LF, Goodenow MM, Sleasman JW: Zidovudine administered to women infected with human immunodeficiency virus type I and to their neonates reduces pediatric infection independent of an effect on levels of maternal virus. J Pediatr 1997;130:906.

American Academy of Pediatrics: Committee on Pediatric AIDS: Evolution and medical treatment of the HIV-exposed infant. Pediatrics 1997;99:909.

Annunziato PW, Gershon A: Herpes simplex infections. Pediatr Rev 1996;17:415.

Beeram MR et al: Lumbar puncture in the evaluation of possible asymptomatic congenital syphilis in neonates. J Pediatr 1996;128:125.

Blanche S et al: Relation of the course of HIV infection in children to the severity of the disease in their mothers at delivery. N Engl J Med 1994;330:308.

Boppana SB et al: Neuroradiographic findings in the newborn period and long term outcome in children with symptomatic congenital cytomegalovirus infection. Pediatrics 1997;99:409.

Connor EM et al: Reduction of maternal-infant transmission of human immunodeficiency virus type 1 with zidovudine treatment. N Engl J Med 1994;331:1173.

Enders G et al: Consequences of varicella and herpes zoster in pregnancy: Prospective study of 1739 cases. Lancet 1994;343:1548.

Evans HE (editor): Perinatal AIDS. Clin Perinatol 1994;21(1).

Fowler KB et al: Progressive and fluctuating hearing loss in children with asymptomatic congenital cytomegalovirus infection. J Pediatr 1997;130:624.

Gibbs RS, Amstey MS, Lezotte DC: Role of cesarean delivery in preventing neonatal herpes virus infection. JAMA 1993;270:94.

Glaser JH: Centers for Disease Control and Prevention guidelines for congenital syphilis. J Pediatr 1996;129:488.

Ivarsson SA, Lernmark B, Svanberg L: Ten-year clinical, developmental, and intellectual follow-up of children with congenital cytomegalovirus infection with neurologic symptoms at one year of age. Pediatrics 1997;99:800.

Landesman SH et al: Obstetrical factors and the transmission of human immunodeficiency virus type I from mother to child. N Engl J Med 1996;334:1617.

Lynfield R, Guerina NE: Toxoplasmosis. Pediatr Rev 1997;18:75.

McFarlin BL et al: Epidemic syphilis: Maternal factors associated with congenital infection. Am J Obstet Gynecol 1994;170:535.

Nigro G et al: Ganciclovir therapy for symptomatic congenital cytomegalovirus infection in infants: A two-regimen experience. J Pediatr 1994;124:318.

Pastuszak AL et al: Outcome after maternal varicella infection in the first 20 weeks of pregnancy. N Engl J Med 1994;330:901.

Peckham C, Gibb D: Mother-to-child transmission of the human immunodeficiency virus. N Engl J Med 1995;333:298.

Peter G, Hall CB, Orenstein WA (editors): *1997 Red Book: Report of the Committee on Infectious Diseases,* 24th ed. American Academy of Pediatrics, 1997.

Roizen N et al: Neurologic and developmental outcome in treated congenital toxoplasmosis. Pediatrics 1995;95:11.

Sperling RS et al: Maternal viral load, zidovudine treatment, and the risk of transmission of human immunodeficiency virus type I from mother to infant. N Engl J Med 1996;335:1621.

St. Louis ME et al: Risk for perinatal HIV-1 transmission according to maternal immunologic, virologic, and placental factors. JAMA 1993;269:2853.

Stamos JK, Rowley AH: Timely diagnosis of congenital infections. Pediatr Clin North Am 1994;41:1017.

Stoll BG, Weisman LE: Infections in perinatology. Clin Perinatol 1997;24(1).

HEMATOLOGIC DISORDERS IN THE NEWBORN

BLEEDING DISORDERS

Neonatal coagulation is discussed in Chapter 25. Bleeding in the newborn may result from inherited clotting deficiencies (eg, factor VIII deficiency) or acquired disorders—hemorrhagic disease of the newborn, disseminated intravascular coagulation (DIC), liver failure, and thrombocytopenia.

1. HEMORRHAGIC DISEASE OF THE NEWBORN

This disorder is caused by the deficiency of the vitamin K-dependent clotting factors (II, VII, IX, and X). Bleeding occurs in 0.25–1.7% of newborns who do not receive vitamin K prophylaxis after birth, generally in the first 5 days to 6 weeks in an otherwise well infant. Sites of ecchymoses and surface bleeding include the gastrointestinal tract, umbilical cord, circumcision site, and nose, though devastating intracranial hemorrhage can occur. Bleeding from vitamin K deficiency is more likely to occur in infants of mothers taking hydantoin anticonvulsants or warfarin—and in breast-fed infants because of very low amounts of vitamin K in breast milk, with slower and more restricted intestinal colonization. Differential diagnosis includes DIC and hepatic failure, both occurring in ill infants (Table 2–24).

Treatment consists of 1 mg of vitamin K subcutaneously or intravenously. Intramuscular injections should be avoided in infants who are bleeding.

2. THROMBOCYTOPENIA

Infants with thrombocytopenia have generalized petechiae (not just on the presenting part) and platelet counts under 150,000/μL (usually < 50,000/μL, may be < 10,000/μL).

Neonatal thrombocytopenia can be isolated or may occur in association with a deficiency of clotting factors. The differential diagnosis for thrombocytopenia with distinguishing clinical features is presented in Table 2–25. Treatment of neonatal thrombocytopenia is transfusion of platelets (10 mL/kg of platelets in-

Table 2–24. Features of infants bleeding from hemorrhagic disease of the newborn (HDN), disseminated intravascular coagulation (DIC), or liver failure.

	HDN	DIC	Liver Failure
Clinical	Well infant; no prophylactic vitamin K	Sick infant; hypoxia, sepsis, etc.	Sick infant; hepatitis, inborn errors of metabolism, shock liver
Bleeding	Gastrointestinal tract, umbilical cord, circumcision, nose	Generalized	Generalized
Onset	2–3 days	Any time	Any time
Platelet count	Normal	Decreased	Normal or decreased
Prothrombin time (PT)	Prolonged	Prolonged	Prolonged
Partial thromboplastin time (PTT)	Prolonged	Prolonged	Prolonged
Fibrinogen	Normal	Decreased	Decreased
Factor V	Normal	Decreased	Decreased

creases the platelet count by approximately 70,000/μL). Indications for transfusion in the term infant are clinical bleeding or a total platelet count less than 10,000–20,000/μL. In the preterm infant at risk for intraventricular hemorrhage, transfusion is indicated for counts less than 40,000–50,000/μL.

Isoimmune thrombocytopenia (analogous to Rh isoimmunization, with a PLA-1-negative mother and PLA-1-positive fetus) requires transfusion of maternal platelets, since 98% of the random population will also be PLA-1-positive. The mother would be the most readily available known PLA-1-negative donor. Treatment with steroids has been disappointing. Treatment with IVIG infusion, 1 g/d for 3 days or until the platelet count has doubled or is over 50,000/μL, is recommended. Antenatal therapy of the mother with IVIG with or without steroids is also beneficial, since 20–30% of infants with isoimmune thrombocytopenia will suffer from intracranial hemorrhage, half of them before birth.

Infants born to mothers with idiopathic thrombocytopenic purpura are at low risk for serious hemorrhage despite the thrombocytopenia, and treatment is usually unnecessary. If bleeding does occur, a 1- to 2-week course of prednisone, 2 mg/kg/d, is recommended. If severe hemorrhage is present, IVIG can also be used.

Table 2–25. Differential diagnosis of neonatal thrombocytopenia.

Disorder	Clinical Tips

Immune
  Passively acquired anti-
  body; idiopathic throm-
  bocytopenic purpura,
  systemic lupus erythe-
  matosus, drug-induced
	Proper history, maternal thrombocytopenia

Isoimmune sensitization to PLA-1 antigen	No rise in platelet count from random donor platelet transfusion. Positive antiplatelet antibodies in baby's serum, sustained rise in platelets by transfusion of mother's platelets

Infections
  Bacterial infections
  Congenital viral infections
	Sick infants with other signs consistent with infection

Syndromes
  Absent radii
  Fanconi's anemia
	Congenital anomalies, associated pancytopenia

Disseminated intravascular coagulation (DIC)	Sick infants, abnormalities of clotting factors
Giant hemangioma	
Thrombosis	Hyperviscous infants, vascular catheters
High-risk with respira- tory distress syndrome, pulmonary hypertension, etc	Isolated decrease in platelets is not uncommon in sick infants even in the absence of DIC (? localized trapping)

ANEMIA

The newborn infant with anemia from acute blood loss presents with signs of hypovolemia (tachycardia, poor perfusion, hypotension), with an initially normal hematocrit that falls after volume replacement. Anemia from chronic blood loss presents as pallor without signs of hypovolemia, with an initially low hematocrit and reticulocytosis.

Anemia can be caused by hemorrhage, hemolysis, or failure to produce red blood cells. Anemia presenting in the first 24–48 hours of life is the result of hemorrhage or hemolysis. Hemorrhage can occur in utero (fetoplacental, fetomaternal, or twin-to-twin), perinatally (cord rupture, placenta previa, incision through placenta at cesarean section), or internally (intracranial hemorrhage, cephalohematoma, ruptured liver or spleen). Hemolysis is caused by blood group incompatibilities, enzyme or membrane abnormalities, infection, and DIC, and is accompanied by significant hyperbilirubinemia.

Initial evaluation should include a review of the perinatal history, assessment of the infant's volume status, and a complete physical examination. A Klei-

haur-Betke test for fetal cells in the mother's circulation should be done. A complete blood count, blood smear, reticulocyte count, and direct and indirect Coombs' tests should be performed. This simple evaluation should suggest a diagnosis in most infants. It is important to remember that hemolysis related to blood group incompatibility will continue for weeks after birth. Serial hematocrits should be followed.

POLYCYTHEMIA

Polycythemia in the newborn is manifested by plethora, cyanosis, mild respiratory distress with tachypnea and oxygen need, hypoglycemia, poor feeding, emesis, and lethargy. The capillary hematocrit is > 68%, the venous hematocrit > 65%.

Elevated hematocrits occur in 2–5% of live births. Although 50% of polycythemic infants are AGA, the prevalence of polycythemia is greater in the SGA and LGA populations. Causes of increased hematocrit include (1) twin–twin transfusion, (2) maternal-fetal transfusion, (3) intrapartum transfusion from the placenta, and (4) chronic intrauterine hypoxia (SGA infants, LGA infants of diabetic mothers).

The consequence of polycythemia is hyperviscosity with decreased perfusion of the capillary beds. Clinical symptomatology can affect several organ systems (Table 2–26). Screening can be done by measuring a capillary (heel stick) hematocrit. If the value is greater than 68%, a peripheral venous hematocrit should be measured. Values greater than 65% should be considered consistent with hyperviscosity.

Treatment is recommended for symptomatic infants. Treatment for asymptomatic infants based strictly on hematocrit is controversial. Definitive treatment is accomplished by an isovolumic partial exchange transfusion with 5% albumin or normal saline, effectively decreasing the hematocrit. The

Table 2–26. Organ-related symptoms of hyperviscosity.

Central nervous system	Irritability, jitteriness, seizures, lethargy
Cardiopulmonary	Respiratory distress, secondary to congestive heart failure, or persistent pulmonary hypertension
Gastrointestinal	Vomiting, heme-positive stools, distention, necrotizing enterocolitis
Renal	Decreased urinary output, renal vein thrombosis
Metabolic	Hypoglycemia
Hematologic	Hyperbilirubinemia, thrombocytopenia

amount to exchange (in milliliters) is calculated using the following formula:

$$\frac{(PVH~[\%] - DH~[\%]) \times BV~(mL/kg) \times Wt~(kg)}{PVH~(\%)}$$

where PVH = peripheral venous hematocrit, DH = desired hematocrit, BV = blood volume, and Wt = weight.

Blood is withdrawn at a steady rate from an umbilical venous line while the replacement solution is infused at the same rate through a peripheral intravenous line over 15–30 minutes. The desired hematocrit value is 50–55%; the assumed blood volume is 80 mL/kg.

American Academy of Pediatrics Vitamin K Ad Hoc Task Force: Controversies concerning vitamin K and the newborn. Pediatrics 1993;91:1001.

Andrew M: The relevance of developmental hemostasis to hemorrhagic disorders of newborns. Semin Perinatol 1997;21:70.

Blanchette VS, Rand ML: Platelet disorders in newborn infants: Diagnosis and management. Semin Perinatol 1997;21:53.

Burrows RF, Kelton JG: Perinatal thrombocytopenia. Clin Perinatol 1995;22:779.

Bussel JB et al: Fetal alloimmune thrombocytopenia. N Engl J Med 1997;337:22.

Greer FR: Vitamin K deficiency and hemorrhage in infancy. Clin Perinatol 1995;22:759.

Johnson JM et al: Prenatal diagnosis and management of neonatal alloimmune thrombocytopenia. Semin Perinatol 1997;21:45.

Matsunaga AT, Lubin BH: Hemolytic anemia in the newborn. Clin Perinatol 1995;22:803.

Menell JS, Bussel JB: Antenatal management of the thrombocytopenias. Clin Perinatol 1994;21:591.

Werner EJ: Neonatal polycythemia and hyperviscosity. Clin Perinatol 1995;22:561.

RENAL DISORDERS IN THE NEWBORN

Renal function is dependent on postconceptional age. The glomerular filtration rate (GFR) is 20 mL/min/1.73 m^2 in term neonates and 10–13 mL/min/1.73 m^2 in infants 28–30 weeks of gestation. The velocity of maturation after birth is also dependent on postconceptional age. Creatinine can be used as a clinical marker of GFR. Values in the first month of life are shown in Table 2–27. Creatinine at birth reflects the maternal level and should decrease slowly over the first 3–4 weeks. An increasing serum creatinine is never normal. The ability to concentrate

Table 2–27. Normal values of serum creatinine (mg/dL).

Gestational Age at Birth (weeks)	Postnatal Age (days)	
	0–2	28
< 28	1.2	0.7
29–32	1.1	0.6
33–36	1.1	0.45
36–42	0.8	0.3

urine and retain sodium is also dependent on gestational age. Infants under 28–30 weeks of gestation are compromised in this respect and if not observed carefully can become dehydrated and hyponatremic. Preterm infants also have an increased bicarbonate excretion and a low tubular maximum for glucose (approximately 120 mg/dL).

RENAL FAILURE

Renal failure is most commonly seen in the setting of birth asphyxia, hypovolemia, or shock from any cause. The normal rate of urine flow is 1–3 mL/kg/h. After a hypoxic or ischemic insult, acute tubular necrosis may ensue. Typically, there are 2–3 days of anuria or oliguria associated with hematuria, proteinuria, and a rise in serum creatinine. The period of anuria or oliguria is followed by a period of polyuria and then gradual recovery. During the polyuric phase, excessive urine sodium and bicarbonate losses may be seen.

The initial step in management is restoration of the infant's volume status with colloid as needed. Thereafter, restriction of fluids to insensible water loss (40–60 mL/kg/d) without added electrolytes, plus milliliter-for-milliliter urine replacement, should be instituted. Serum and urine electrolytes and body weights should be followed frequently. These measures should be continued through the polyuric phase. After urine output has been reestablished, urine replacement should be decreased to between 0.5 and 0.75 mL for each milliliter of urine output to see if the infant has regained normal function. If that is the case, the infant can be returned to maintenance fluids.

Finally, many of these infants experience fluid overload and should be allowed to lose enough water through urination to return to birth weight. Hyperkalemia, which may become life-threatening, may occur in this situation despite the lack of added intravenous potassium. If the serum potassium reaches 7–7.5 mEq/L, therapy should be started with glucose and insulin infusion, giving 1 unit of insulin for every 3 g of glucose administered, plus binding resins. Calcium gluconate (100 mg/kg bolus) can also be helpful for arrhythmia resulting from hyper-kalemia.

Peritoneal dialysis is occasionally needed for the management of neonatal acute renal failure.

URINARY TRACT ANOMALIES

Abdominal masses in the newborn are most frequently caused by renal enlargement. Most common is a multicystic or dysplastic kidney; congenital hydronephrosis is second in frequency. Chromosomal abnormalities and syndromes with multiple anomalies frequently include renal abnormalities. An ultrasound examination is the first step in diagnosis. In pregnancies associated with oligohydramnios, renal agenesis or obstruction secondary to posterior urethral valves should be considered. Only bilateral disease or disease in a solitary kidney is associated with oligohydramnios, significant morbidity, and death. Such infants will generally also have pulmonary hypoplasia and die from pulmonary rather than renal insufficiency.

Prenatal ultrasonography identifies infants with renal anomalies (most often hydronephrosis) prior to birth. Postnatal evaluation of these infants should include renal ultrasound and a voiding cystourethrogram at about 1 week of age. Until genitourinary reflux is ruled out, these infants should receive antibiotic prophylaxis with low-dose penicillin or ampicillin.

RENAL VEIN THROMBOSIS

Renal vein thrombosis is seen most frequently in infants of diabetic mothers and in the context of dehydration and polycythemia. Of particular concern is the IDM infant who is also polycythemic. If fetal distress is superimposed on these problems, prompt reduction in blood viscosity is indicated. Thrombosis usually begins in intrarenal venules and can extend into larger veins. Clinically, there may be an enlarged kidney, with blood and protein in the urine. With bilateral renal vein thrombosis, anuria ensues. Diagnosis can be confirmed with an ultrasound examination that includes Doppler flow studies of the kidneys. Treatment involves correcting the predisposing condition and systemic heparinization for the thrombosis. Use of thrombolytics for this condition is controversial. Prognosis for a full recovery is uncertain. Some infants will go on to develop significant atrophy of the affected kidney and systemic hypertension.

Bueva A, Guignard J-P: Renal function in preterm neonates. Pediatr Res 1994;36:572.

Dudley JA et al: Clinical relevance and implications of an-tenatal hydronephrosis. Arch Dis Child Fetal Neonatal Ed 1997;76:F31.

Gloor JM: Management of prenatally detected fetal hydronephrosis. Mayo Clin Proc 1995;70:145.

Schmidt B: The etiology, diagnosis, and treatment of thrombotic disorders in newborn infants: A call for international and multi-institutional studies. Semin Perinatol 1997;21:86.

Sonntag J, Prankel B, Waltz S: Serum creatinine concentration, urinary creatinine excretion and creatinine clearance during the first 9 weeks in preterm infants with a birth weight below 1500 grams. Eur J Pediatr 1996;155:815.

NEUROLOGIC PROBLEMS IN THE NEWBORN

SEIZURES

Newborns rarely have well-organized tonic-clonic seizures because of their incomplete cortical organization and a preponderance of inhibitory synapses. The most common type of seizure is characterized by a constellation of findings, including horizontal deviation of the eyes with or without jerking; eyelid blinking or fluttering; sucking, smacking, drooling, and other oral-buccal movements; swimming, rowing, or paddling movements; and apneic spells. Strictly tonic or multifocal clonic episodes are also seen.

Clinical Findings

The differential diagnosis of neonatal seizures is presented in Table 2–28. Most neonatal seizures occur between 12 and 48 hours of age. Later-onset seizures suggest meningitis, benign familial seizures, or hypocalcemia. Information regarding antenatal drug use, the presence of birth asphyxia or trauma, and family history (regarding inherited disorders) should be obtained. Physical examination focuses on neurologic features, other signs of drug withdrawal, concurrent signs of infection, dysmorphic features, and intrauterine growth. Screening workup should include blood glucose, ionized calcium, and electrolytes in all cases. Further workup is dependent on diagnoses suggested by the history and physical examination. If there is any suspicion of infection, a spinal tap should be done. Hemorrhages and structural disease of the central nervous system can be addressed with real-time ultrasound and CT scan. Metabolic workup should be pursued when appropriate. EEG should be done; the presence of spike discharges must be noted and the background wave pattern evaluated. Not infrequently, correlation between EEG changes and clinical seizure activity is absent.

Table 2–28. Differential diagnosis of neonatal seizures.

Diagnosis	Comment
Hypoxic-ischemic encephalopathy	Most common cause (60%) onset in first 24 hours
Intracranial hemorrhage	Up to 15% of cases, periventric-ular-intraventricular hemorrhage, subdural or subarachnoid bleeding, stroke
Infection	12% of cases
Hypoglycemia	Small for gestational age, infant of a diabetic mother (IDM)
Hypocalcemia, hypomagnesemia	Infant of low birth weight, IDM
Hyponatremia	Rare, seen with syndrome of inappropriate secretion of antidiuretic hormone (SIADH)
Disorders of amino and organic acid metabolism, hyperammonemia	Associated acidosis, altered level of consciousness
Pyridoxine dependency	Seizures refractory to routine therapy; cessation of seizures after administration of pyridoxine
Developmental defects	Other anomalies, chromosomal syndromes
Drug withdrawal	
No cause found	10% of cases
Benign familial neonatal seizures	

Treatment

Adequate ventilation and perfusion should be ensured. Hypoglycemia should be treated immediately with a 2 mL/kg infusion of $D_{10}W$ followed by 6 mg/kg/min of $D_{10}W$ (100 mL/kg/d). Other treatments such as calcium or magnesium infusion and antibiotics are indicated to treat hypocalcemia, hypomagnesemia, and suspected infection. Electrolyte abnormalities should be corrected. Phenobarbital, 20 mg/kg intravenously, should be administered to stop seizures. Supplemental doses of 5 mg/kg can be used if seizures persist, up to a total of 40 mg/kg. In most cases, phenobarbital controls seizures. If seizures continue, therapy with phenytoin, sodium valproate, or lorazepam may be indicated. For refractory seizures, a trial of pyridoxine is indicated.

Prognosis

Outcome is related to the underlying cause of the seizure. The outcomes for hypoxic-ischemic encephalopathy and intracranial hemorrhage have been discussed. In these settings, seizures that are difficult to control carry a poor prognosis for normal development. Seizures resulting from hypoglycemia, infection of the central nervous system, some inborn errors of metabolism, and developmental defects also have a high rate of poor outcome. Seizures caused by hypocalcemia or isolated subarachnoid hemorrhage generally resolve without sequelae.

HYPOTONIA

One should be alert to the diagnosis of congenital hypotonia when a mother has polyhydramnios and a history of poor fetal movement. For a discussion of causes and evaluation, see Chapter 22.

INTRACRANIAL HEMORRHAGE*

1. SUBDURAL HEMORRHAGE

Subdural hemorrhage is related to birth trauma; the bleeding is caused by tears in the veins that bridge the subdural space. Prospective studies relating incidence to specific obstetric complications are not available.

The most common site of subdural bleeding is rupture of superficial cerebral veins with blood over the cerebral convexities. These hemorrhages can be asymptomatic or may cause seizures, with onset on days 2–3 of life, vomiting, irritability, and lethargy. Associated findings include retinal hemorrhages and a full fontanelle. The diagnosis is confirmed by CT scan.

Specific treatment entailing needle drainage of the subdural space is rarely necessary. Most infants survive, with 75% normal on follow-up.

2. PRIMARY SUBARACHNOID HEMORRHAGE

Primary subarachnoid hemorrhage is the most common type of neonatal intracranial hemorrhage. In the term infant, it can be related to trauma of delivery, whereas subarachnoid hemorrhage in the preterm infant is seen in association with germinal matrix hemorrhage. Clinically, these hemorrhages can be asymptomatic or can present with seizures and irritability on day 2 or, rarely, a massive hemorrhage with a rapid downhill course. The seizures associated with subarachnoid hemorrhage are very characteristic—usually brief, with a normal examination interictally. Diagnosis can be suspected on

---

*Intraventricular hemorrhage is discussed above in the section on care of the premature.

spinal tap and confirmed with CT scan. Long-term follow-up is uniformly good.

3. NEONATAL STROKE

Focal cerebral ischemic injury can be seen in the context of intraventricular hemorrhage in the premature and hypoxic ischemic encephalopathy. Neonatal stroke has also been described in the context of underlying disorders of thrombolysis and maternal drug use (cocaine). In some cases, the origin is unclear. The injury often occurs antenatally. The most common clinical presentation of an isolated cerebral infarct is with seizures, and diagnosis can be confirmed with CT scan. The most frequently described distribution is that of the middle cerebral artery.

Treatment is directed at controlling seizures. Long-term outcome is variable, ranging from normal to hemiplegias and cognitive deficits.

Bernes SM, Kaplan AM: Evolution of neonatal seizures. Pediatr Clin North Am 1994;41:1069.

Estan J, Hope P: Unilateral neonatal cerebral infarction in full term infants. Arch Dis Child Fetal Neonatal Ed 1997;76:F88.

Koelfen W, Freund M, Varnholt V: Neonatal stroke involving the middle cerebral artery in term infants: Clinical presentation, EEG and imaging studies, and outcome. Devel Med Child Neurol 1995;37:204.

Rennie JM: Neonatal seizures. Eur J Pediatr 1997;156:83.

METABOLIC DISORDERS IN THE NEWBORN*

HYPERGLYCEMIA

Hyperglycemia may develop in preterm infants, particularly those of very low birth weight who are also SGA. Glucose concentrations may exceed 200–250 mg/dL, particularly in the first few days of life. This transient diabetes-like syndrome usually lasts approximately 1–2 weeks.

Management may include simply reducing glucose intake while continuing to provide supplemental calories with intravenous amino acids and lipids, coupled with small milk feedings by gavage. Insulin infusions intravenously have also been used to permit a larger intravenous glucose intake without hyperglycemia. This is usually reserved for infants in whom it has not been possible to begin any gavage

---

*Hypoglycemia is discussed above in the section on common problems in the term newborn.

milk feedings and in whom caloric intake in the form of amino acids and lipids is small. However, this approach requires careful direct monitoring of blood glucose concentrations. Hyperglycemia can also be a problem in infants treated with dexamethasone for chronic lung disease.

HYPOCALCEMIA

Calcium concentration in the immediate newborn period decreases in all newborn infants. The concentration in fetal plasma is higher than that of the neonate or adult. Hypocalcemia is usually defined as a total serum concentration less than 7 mg/dL (equivalent to a calcium activity of 3.5 mEq/L), though the physiologically active fraction, ionized calcium, should be measured whenever possible. Ionized calcium is usually normal even when total calcium is as low as 6–7 mg/dL. An ionized calcium of greater than 0.9 mmol/L (1.8 mEq/L; 3.6 mg/dL) is not likely to be detrimental.

Clinical Findings

The clinical signs of hypocalcemia and hypocalcemic tetany include a high-pitched cry, jitteriness, tremulousness, and seizures.

Hypocalcemia tends to occur at two different times in the neonatal period. Early-onset hypocalcemia occurs in the first 2 days of life and has been associated with prematurity, maternal diabetes, asphyxia, and, rarely, maternal hypoparathyroidism. Late-onset hypocalcemia occurs at approximately 7–10 days of age and is seen in infants receiving modified cow's milk rather than infant formula (high phosphorus intake) or in infants with hypoparathyroidism or hypomagnesemia. Mothers in third-world countries often suffer from vitamin D deficiency, which can also contribute to late-onset hypocalcemia.

Treatment

A. Oral Calcium Therapy: The oral administration of calcium salts is a preferred method of treatment for chronic forms of hypocalcemia resulting from hypoparathyroidism but is rarely used in early-onset hypocalcemia. Calcium in the form of calcium gluconate can be given as a dilute solution or added to formula feedings several times a day. A dose of 0.5–1 g/kg/d provides approximately 45–90 mg of elemental calcium per kilogram per day. If a 10% solution of calcium gluconate is used, the dose is 5–10 mL/kg/d given in divided doses every 4 hours or every 6 hours.

B. Intravenous Calcium Therapy: Intravenous calcium therapy is usually needed for infants with symptomatic hypocalcemia or an ionized calcium less than 0.9 mmol/L. A number of precautions must be observed when calcium gluconate is given intravenously. The infusion must be given slowly so that there is no sudden increase in calcium concentration of blood entering the right atrium, which could cause severe bradycardia and even cardiac arrest. Furthermore, the infusion must be carefully observed, as an intravenous infiltrate containing calcium can cause full-thickness skin necrosis requiring grafting. For these reasons, intravenous calcium therapy should be given judiciously and through a central venous line if possible. Intravenous administration of 10% calcium gluconate is usually given as a bolus of 100–200 mg/kg over approximately 10–20 minutes, followed by a continuous infusion (0.5–1 g/kg/d) over 1–2 days. Ten percent calcium chloride (35–70 mg/kg per dose) may result in a larger increment in ionized calcium and greater improvement in mean arterial blood pressure in sick hypocalcemic infants and thus may have a role in the newborn. *Note:* Calcium salts cannot be added to intravenous solutions that contain sodium bicarbonate because they precipitate as calcium carbonate.

Prognosis

The prognosis is good for neonatal seizures entirely caused by hypocalcemia that is promptly treated.

INBORN ERRORS OF METABOLISM

The individual inborn errors of metabolism are rare, but collectively all such disorders create significant clinical problems. The diseases are considered in detail in Chapter 30, but the diagnoses should be entertained in infants who were initially well that present with sepsis-like syndromes, recurrent hypoglycemia, neurologic syndromes (seizures, altered levels of consciousness), and unexplained acidosis.

In the immediate neonatal period, urea cycle disorders commonly present as altered level of consciousness secondary to hyperammonemia. A clinical clue that supports this diagnosis is hyperventilation with primary respiratory alkalosis. The other major diagnostic category to consider consists of infants with severe acidemia secondary to organic acidemias.

Burton BK et al: Inborn errors of metabolism: The clinical diagnosis in early infancy. Pediatrics 1987;79:359.

Goodman ST, Greene CL: Inborn errors as causes of acute disease in infancy. Semin Perinatol 1991;15(Suppl 1):31.

Suleiman MY, Zaloga GP: How and when to manage ionized hypocalcemia in critically ill patients. J Crit Illness 1993;8:372.

REFERENCES

Briggs GG et al (editors): *Drugs in Pregnancy and Lactation,* 4th ed. Williams & Wilkins, 1994.

Fanaroff AA, Martin RJ (editors): *Neonatal-Perinatal Medicine. Diseases of the Fetus and Infant,* 6th ed. Mosby, 1997.

Gabbe SG, Niebyl JR, Simpson JL (editors): *Obstetrics: Normal and Problem Pregnancies,* 3rd ed. Churchill Livingstone, 1996.

Goldsmith JP, Karotkin EH (editors): *Assisted Ventilation of the Neonate,* 3rd ed. Saunders, 1996.

Jones KL (editor): *Smith's Recognizable Patterns of Human Malformation,* 5th ed. Saunders, 1997.

Jones MD Jr, Gleason CA, Lipstein SN (editors): *Hospital Care of the Recovering NICU Infant.* Williams & Wilkins, 1991.

Long WA (editor): *Fetal and Neonatal Cardiology.* Saunders, 1990.

Remington JS, Klein JO (editors): *Infectious Diseases of the Fetus and Newborn Infant,* 4th ed. Saunders, 1995.

Volpe JJ (editor): *Neurology of the Newborn,* 3rd ed. Saunders, 1995.

Young TE, Mangum OB (editors): *Neofax 97. A Manual of Drugs Used in Neonatal Care,* 10th ed. Ross Laboratories, 1997.

Developmental Disorders & Behavioral Problems

3

Edward Goldson, MD

Behavioral and developmental variations and disorders encompass a wide range of issues of importance to pediatricians. Most of the problems discussed in this chapter are familiar to the practitioner. However, with increasing knowledge of the neurologic and behavioral organization of children, newer concepts of these disorders are evolving and different approaches to their diagnosis and management are emerging.

Variations in children's behavior probably reflect a blend of intrinsic biologic characteristics and the environment with which the child interacts. This chapter will focus on two distinct areas. It will first address some of the more common complaints about behavior encountered by those who care for children. These behavioral "disorders" are by and large normal variations in behavior, a reflection of each child's individual biologic and temperament traits and the parents' responses. There are no "cures" for these behaviors, but management strategies are available that can enhance the parents' understanding of the child and its relationship to the environment and facilitate the parents' care of the growing infant and child.

The second part of this chapter discusses developmental delays involving cognitive and social competence—complex disorders with wide-ranging consequences for the child and its family. Management of these conditions requires a comprehensive and often multidisciplinary approach. The health care provider can play a major role in diagnosis, in coordinating the child's evaluation, in interpreting the results to the family, and in providing reassurance and support.

Capute AJ, Accardo PJ (editors). *Developmental Disabilities in Infancy and Childhood,* 2nd ed. Volume I: *Neurodevelopmental Diagnosis and Treatment.* Volume II: *The Spectrum of Developmental Disabilities.* Brookes, 1996.

Greydanus DE, Wolraich ML (editors): *Behavioral Pediatrics.* Springer, 1992.

Levine MD, Cary WB, Crocker AC (editors): Developmental-Behavioral Pediatrics, 2nd ed. Saunders, 1992.

Parker S, Zuckerman B (editors). *Behavioral and Developmental Pediatrics: A Handbook for Primary Care.* Little, Brown, 1995.

Wolraich ML (editor): *Disorders of Development and Learning: A Practical Guide to Assessment and Management,* 2nd ed. Mosby, 1996

Wolraich ML, Felice ME, Drotar D: *The Classification of Child and Adolescent Mental Diagnoses in Primary Care: Diagnostic and Statistical Manual for Primary Care (DSM-PC) Child and Adolescent Version.* American Academy of Pediatrics, 1996.

NORMALITY & TEMPERAMENT

The physician confronted by a disturbance in physiologic function is usually in little doubt about what is abnormal. Variations in temperament and behavior are not so straightforward. By labeling such variations as "disorders," we assume and imply that a disease entity exits. In this chapter the behaviors described are viewed as part of a continuum of responses by the child to a variety of internal and external experiences.

An associated phenomenon to be considered when confronting variations in temperament has been of interest to philosophers and writers since ancient times. The Greeks developed a concept of four temperament types: choleric, sanguine, melancholic, and phlegmatic. In more recent times, the accepted folk wisdom defined temperament as a genetically influenced behavioral disposition that is stable over time. Although there are a number of proposed models of temperament, the one usually used by pediatricians in clinical practice is that of Thomas and Chess.

Thomas & Chess Model

These authors describe temperament as being the "how" of behavior as distinguished from motivation (the "why") and ability (the "what"). Temperament is an independent psychologic attribute that is expressed as a response to an external stimulus. The influence of temperament is bidirectional—ie, the effect of a particular experience will be influenced by

The work of the previous authors, Drs Camp and Kozleski is very much appreciated.

Table 3–1. Theories of temperament.

Thomas and Chess	Temperament is an independent psychologic attribute, biologically determined, which is expressed as a response to an external stimulus. It is the child's behavioral style: an interactive model.
Rothbart	Temperament is a a function of biologically based individual differences in reactivity and self-regulation. It is subsumed under the concept of "personality" and goes beyond mere "behavioral style."
Buss and Plomin	Temperament is a set of genetically determined personality traits that appear early in life and are different from other inherited and acquired personality traits.
Goldsmith and Campos	Temperament is the individual's differences in the probability of experiencing emotions and arousal.

the child's temperament, and the child's temperament will influence the responses of those in the child's environment. Temperament is the style with which the child interacts with the environment. The perceptions and expectations of parents must always be taken into consideration when a child's behavior is evaluated. A child that one parent might describe as hyperactive would not be so characterized by another. This truism can be expanded to include all the dimensions of temperament. Thus, the concept of "goodness of fit" comes into play. For example, if the parents want and expect their child to be predictable but that is not in accord with the child's behavioral style, what emerges is a lack of "goodness of fit" and a potential source of tension. The parents may perceive the child as being "bad" or having a "behavioral disorder" rather than as having a developmental variation. An appreciation of this phenomenon is important because the physician may be able to enhance the parents' understanding of the child and influence their responses to the child's behavior. When there is "goodness of fit," there will be more harmony and a greater potential for healthy development not only of the child but also of the family. When "goodness of fit" is not present, tension and stress can result in parental anger, disappointment, frustration, and conflict with the child.

Other models of temperament include those of Rothbart, Buss and Plomin, and Goldsmith and Campos (Table 3–1). All models seek to identify intrinsic behavioral characteristics that lead the child to respond to the world in particular ways. One child may be highly emotional and another less so ("calmer") in response to a variety of experiences, stressful or pleasant. A child may be perceived as "hyperactive" by one parent but not by the other. One child may tolerate change easily, while another may have great difficulty in adapting to change. One child may toler-

ate discomfort more easily than another. One child may be sociable, another reclusive. The clinician must recognize that each child brings some intrinsic, biologically based traits to its environment and that such characteristics are neither good nor bad, right nor wrong, normal nor abnormal—they are simply part of the child. Thus, as one looks at variations in development, one should abandon the illness model and consider this construct as an aid to understanding the nature of the child's behavior and its influence on the parent–child relationship.

Barr RG: Normality: A clinically useless concept. The case of infant crying and colic. J Dev Behav Pediatr 1993;14:264.
Goldsmith HH et al: Roundtable: What is temperament? Four approaches. Child Dev 1987;58:505.
Prior M: Childhood temperament. J Child Psychol Psychiatry 1992;33:249.
Thomas A, Chess S: *Temperament and Development.* Brunner/Mazel, 1977.

COMMON DEVELOPMENTAL CONCERNS

COLIC

What is understood as colic consists of severe and paroxysmal crying that occurs mainly in the late afternoon. The infant's knees are drawn up, flatus is expelled, the facies is "pained," the fists are clenched, and there is minimal response to attempts at soothing. Studies in the United States have shown that among middle-class infants, crying takes up about 2 hours per day at 2 weeks of age, about 3 hours per day by 6 weeks, and gradually decreases to about 1 hour per day by 3 months. Crying can usually be modulated somewhat by a sensitive caretaker's intervention.

The word "colic" is derived from Greek *kolikos* ("pertaining to the colon"). While colic has traditionally been attributed to gastrointestinal disturbances, this has never been proved. Colic is a behavioral sign or symptom that begins in the first few weeks of life and usually peaks at 2 or 3 months. In about 30–40% of cases, colic continues into the fourth and fifth months.

The most common definition of colic is the one used by Wessel: "A colicky infant is one who is healthy and well fed but cries for more than 3 hours a day, for more than 3 days a week, and for more than 3 weeks"—commonly referred to as the "rule of threes." The important word in this definition is "healthy." The infant with colic has no definable physiologic disorder. Thus, before the diagnosis of colic can be made, the pediatrician must rule out diseases that might be causing the symptom. With the exception of the few infants who respond to elimination of cow's milk from its own or from the mother's diet, there has been little firm evidence of an association of colic with gastrointestinal disorders. There have been attempts to eliminate gas with simethicone and to slow gut motility with dicyclomine. Simethicone has not been shown to ameliorate colic. Dicyclomine has been associated with apnea in infants and is contraindicated.

This then leaves characteristics intrinsic to the child (ie, temperament) and parental caretaking patterns as contributing to colic. Behavioral states have three features: (1) they are self-organizing—ie, they are maintained until it is necessary to shift to another one; (2) they are stable over several minutes; and (3) the same stimulus elicits a state-specific response that is different from other states. There are (among others) a crying state, a quiet alert state, an active alert state, a transitional state, and a state of deep sleep. The states of importance with respect to colic are the crying state and the transitional state. During transition from one state to another, infant behavior may be more easily influenced. Once an infant is in a stable state (eg, crying), it becomes more difficult to bring about a change (eg, to soothe). How these transitions are accomplished is probably influenced by the infant's temperament as well as its neurologic maturity. Some infants move from one state to another easily and can be easily diverted; other infants sustain a particular state and are resistant to change.

The other component that needs to be considered with the colicky infant is the feeding and handling behavior of the caretaker. Colic is a behavioral phenomenon that involves interaction between the infant and the caretaker. Different caretakers perceive and respond to crying behavior differently. If the caretaker perceives the crying infant as being spoiled and demanding and is not sensitive to or knowledgeable about the infant's cues and rhythms—or is hurried and "rough" with the baby—the infant's ability to organize and soothe itself or respond to the caretaker's attempts at soothing may be compromised. Alternatively, if the temperament of an infant with colic is understood and the rhythms and cues deciphered, crying can be anticipated and the caretaker can intervene before the behavior becomes "organized" in the crying state and more difficult to extinguish.

Management

There are a number of approaches to the management of the infant with colic.

(1) Parents may need to be educated about the developmental characteristics of crying behavior and made aware that crying increases normally into the second month and abates by the third to fourth month.

(2) Parents may need reassurance, based on a complete history and physical examination, that the infant is not sick. Although these behaviors are stressful, they are a normal variant and usually self-limited. This discussion can be facilitated by having the parent keep a diary of crying and weight gain. If there is a diurnal pattern and adequate weight gain, an underlying disease process is less likely to be present. Parental anxiety must be relieved, as it may be a factor contributing to the problem.

(3) For the parents to be able to soothe and comfort the infant, they need to understand the baby's cues. The pediatrician can help by observing the infant's behavior and devising interventions aimed at calming both the infant and the parents. One can encourage a quiet environment without excessive handling. Rhythmic stimulation such as gentle swinging or rocking, soft music, drives in the car, or walks in the stroller may be helpful, especially if the parents are able to anticipate the onset of crying. Another approach is to change the feeding habits so that the infant is not rushed, has ample opportunity to burp, and, if necessary, to be fed more frequently so as to decrease gastric distention if that seems to be contributing to the problem.

(4) Medications such as phenobarbital elixir and dicyclomine have been found to be somewhat helpful, but their use is to be discouraged because of the risk of adverse reactions and overdosage.

(5) For colicky babies refractory to behavioral management, a trial of changing the feedings, eliminating cow's milk from the formula, or from the mother's diet if she is nursing, may be indicated.

Barr RG: Colic and gas. In: *Pediatric Gastrointestinal Disease: Pathophysiology, Diagnosis, and Management.* Walker WA et al (editors). BC Decker, 1991.

Barr RG, Geertsma MA: Colic: The pain perplex. In: *Pain in Infants, Children and Adolescents.* Schechter NL, Berde CB, Yaster M (editors). Williams & Wilkins, 1993.

Carey WB: "Colic": Primary excessive crying as an infant–environmental interaction. Pediatr Clin North Am 1984;31:993.

Miller AR, Barr RG: Infantile colic: Is it a gut issue? Pediatr Clin North Am 1991;38:1407.

FEEDING DISORDERS IN INFANTS & YOUNG CHILDREN

Children have feeding problems for various reasons. The common denominator, however, is usually food refusal. Infants and young children may refuse to eat because they find eating aversive (eg, it hurts or is frightening); they may have had unpleasant experiences (emotional or physiologic) associated with eating; they may be depressed; or they may be engaged in a developmental conflict with the caretaker that is being played out in the arena of feeding. The infant may refuse to eat if the rhythm of the feeding experience with the caretaker is not harmonious. The child who has had an esophageal atresia repair and has a stricture may find eating uncomfortable or even painful. The very young infant with severe oral candidiasis may refuse to eat because of pain. The child who has had a choking experience associated with feeding may be terrified to eat (oral motor dysfunction or aspiration). The child who is forced to eat by a maltreating parent or an overzealous caretaker may refuse feeds, as may the child who is physically threatened.

Depression in children may be expressed through food refusal. Food refusal may develop when the infant's cues around feeding are not correctly interpreted by the parent. The baby who needs to burp more frequently or who needs time between bites but instead is rushed will often passively refuse to eat. Some will be more active refusers, turn their heads away to avoid the feeder, spit out food, or push food away.

Chatoor and coworkers have adopted a developmental and interactive construct of the feeding experience. The stages through which the child normally progresses are establishment of homeostasis (0–2 months), attachment (2–6 months), and separation and individuation (6 months to 3 years). During the first stage, feeding can be most easily accomplished when the parent allows the infant to determine the timing, amount, pacing, and preference of food intake; during the attachment phase, allowing the infant to control the feeding permits the parent to engage the infant in a positive manner. This sets the table for the separation and individuation phase.

When there is a disturbance in the parent–child relationship at any of these developmental levels, difficulty in feeding may ensue, with both the parent and the child contributing to the dysfunctional interaction. One of the most striking manifestations of food refusal occurs during the stage of separation and individuation. Conflict may arise if the parent seeks to dominate the child by intrusive and controlling feeding behavior at the same time the child is striving to achieve autonomy. The scenario then observed is of the parent forcing food on the child while the child refuses to eat. This often leads to extreme parental frustration and anger, and the child may be inadequately nourished and developmentally and emotionally thwarted. When the pediatrician is attempting to sort out the factors contributing to a complaint of food refusal, it is essential first to obtain a complete history, including a social history. This should include information concerning the parents' perception of the child's behaviors and their expectations of the child.

Second, a complete physical examination should be performed, with emphasis on oral-motor behavior and other clues suggesting neurologic, anatomic, or physiologic abnormalities that could make feeding difficult. The child's emotional state and developmental level must be determined. This is particularly important if there is concern about depression or a history of developmental delays. If evidence of oral-motor difficulty is elicited, evaluation by an occupational therapist is warranted.

Third, the feeding interaction needs to be observed live, if possible.

Finally, the physician needs to help the parent understand that infants and children may have different styles of eating and different food preferences and may refuse foods they do not like. This is not necessarily abnormal but reflects temperamental differences and variations in the child's way of processing olfactory, gustatory, and tactile stimuli.

Management

The goal of intervention is to identify factors contributing to the disturbance and to work to overcome the difficulties. The parents may be taught to view the child's behavior differently and try not to impose their expectations and desires. Or the child's behavior may need to be modified so that the parent can provide adequate nurturing.

When the chief complaint is failure to gain weight or failure to thrive, a different approach is required. The differential diagnosis should include not only food refusal but also medical disorders and maltreatment. The most common reason for failure to gain weight is inadequate caloric intake. Excessive losses may be due to vomiting or diarrhea, to malabsorption, or to a combination of these factors. A complete history and physical examination must be performed, along with a comprehensive psychosocial and developmental history and observation of the feeding experience in the clinic or hospital or at home.

Laboratory studies include a complete blood count, erythrocyte sedimentation rate, urinalysis and urine culture, blood urea nitrogen, serum electrolytes and creatinine, and stool examination for ova and parasites and to look for evidence of malabsorption. Some practitioners also include liver and thyroid profiles.

Because of the complexity of the problem, a team approach to the diagnosis and treatment of failure to thrive may be most appropriate. The team should include a physician, nurse, social worker, and dietitian as well as occupational and physical therapists, developmentalists, and psychologists as required.

The goals of management of the child with poor weight gain are to establish a normal pattern of weight gain and to establish better family functioning. Guidelines to accomplishing these goals include the following:

(1) Establish a comprehensive diagnosis that considers all factors contributing to poor weight gain.

(2) Monitor the feeding interaction and ensure appropriate weight gain.

(3) Monitor the developmental progress of the child and the changes in the family dynamics that fa-

cilitate optimal weight gain and psychosocial development.

(4) Provide support to the family as they seek to help the child.

Chatoor I et al: Non-organic failure to thrive: A developmental perspective. Pediatr Ann 1984;13:829.

Frank D, Zeisel SH: Failure to thrive. Pediatr Clin North Am 1988;35:1187.

Macht J: *Poor Eaters.* Plenum, 1990.

Stevenson RD: Failure to thrive. In: *Behavioral Pediatrics.* Greydanus DE, Wolraich ML (editors). Springer, 1992.

SLEEP DISORDERS

Sleep is a complex physiologic process influenced by intrinsic biologic properties, individual temperamental characteristics, cultural norms and expectations, and environmental conditions. It is estimated that 20–30% of children experience sleep problems severe enough to cause concern. These problems usually fall into three groups: (1) nighttime attacks (parasomnias), (2) sleeplessness (insomnias or dyssomnias), and (3) excessive sleepiness during the day. Parasomnias and dyssomnias are discussed here.

Two sleep stages have been identified clinically and with the use of polysomnography (electroencephalography, electro-oculography, and electromyelography): rapid eye movement (REM) and nonrapid eye movement (NREM) sleep. In REM sleep, muscle tone is relaxed, the sleeper may twitch and grimace, and the eyes move erratically beneath closed lids. In adults, REM cycles occur during the night but are most frequent during the latter half of the night and last about 90 minutes.

NREM sleep is further divided into four stages. In the process of falling asleep, the individual enters stage 1, light sleep, characterized by reduced bodily movements, slow eye rolling, and sometimes opening and closing of the eyelids. Stage 2 sleep is characterized by slowing of eye movements, slowing of respirations and heart rate, and relaxation of the muscles but with repositioning of the body. Some dreaming may occur in this stage. Most mature individuals spend about half of their sleep time in this stage. Stages 3 and 4 (also called delta or slow wave sleep) are similar. These are the deepest NREM sleep stages, during which the body is relaxed, breathing is slow and shallow, and the heart rate is slow. Nighttime sleep consists of alternating episodes of NREM and REM sleep.

The onset of sleep occurs when the individual enters NREM stage 1 sleep. The individual then progresses to NREM stage 2 and on to NREM stages 3 and 4. The deepest NREM sleep occurs during the first 1–3 hours after going to sleep, with transitions to NREM stage 2 sleep and brief awakenings. REM and NREM stage 2 sleep cycles occur during the latter part of the night and are also interspersed with brief awakenings. Parasomnias occur during deep NREM sleep. Dreams and nightmares occur during REM sleep.

1. PARASOMNIAS

Parasomnias, consisting of arousal from deep NREM sleep are probably the most frightening for parents. They include night terrors (pavor nocturnus), sleepwalking (somnambulism), and nocturnal seizures.

Night Terrors

Night terrors commonly occur within 2 hours after falling asleep, during the deepest stage of NREM sleep, and are often associated with sleepwalking. They are reported in about 3% of children. During a night terror, the child may sit up in bed screaming and thrashing about, with rapid breathing, tachycardia, and sweating. The child often has a glazed look in its eyes, is essentially incoherent, and is unresponsive to comforting. The attack may last up to half an hour, after which the child goes back to sleep and has no memory of the event the next day. The parents must be reassured that the child is not in pain and that they should let the episode run its course.

Management of night terrors is by reassurance of the parents plus measures to avoid emotional and psychosocial stressors that might be contributing to the problem. Since sleepwalking can result in injury, the parents should determine if possible when the attacks usually occur and awaken the child to full arousal about 15 minutes before that time. After 4–5 minutes, the child is allowed to return to sleep. The waking is discontinued once the terrors stop, which is usually within a week.

In severe cases, pharmacologic interventions may be needed temporarily. Imipramine (25–50 mg at bedtime) may be useful. However, behavioral approaches to increase the total amount of sleep and to address the sources of anxiety and stress are of more long-term benefit.

Nightmares

Nightmares are frightening dreams during REM sleep, typically followed by awakening and occurring usually in the latter part of the night. The peak occurrence is in the age group from 3 to 5 years, with an incidence between 25% and 50%. A child who awakens during these episodes is usually alert. He or she can often describe the frightening images, recall the dream, and talk about it during the day. The child seeks and will respond positively to parental reassurance. The child will often have difficulty going back to sleep and will want to stay with the parents. By and large, nightmares are self-limited and need little treatment. However, if the child has recurrent nightmares, the pediatrician may have to make a more extensive investigation. Nightmares are often associated with stressful or frightening daytime events or anxieties that may include frightening television programs, traumatic life events, and chronic stresses in the family. In severe cases, a psychologist or psychiatrist may need to be consulted.

2. DYSSOMNIAS

The second group of disturbances consists of the dyssomnias, ie, problems of going to sleep and nighttime awakenings. While parasomnias are frightening to most parents, dyssomnias tend to be only annoying and frustrating. They can result in daytime fatigue of both the parents and the child, parental discord about management, and family disruption. A number of factors contribute to disturbances of sleep. The quantity and timing of feeds in the first years of life will influence nighttime awakening. Most infants beyond 6 months of age can go through the night without being fed. Thus, under normal circumstances, night waking for feeds is probably a learned behavior and is a function of the child's arousal and the parents' response to that arousal.

Co-sleeping can play a role in night waking. In many cultures, co-sleeping is accepted behavior. It is inappropriate behavior when it intrudes on the parents' rest and their sexual relationship.

Bedtime habits can influence settling in for the night as well as nighttime awakening. If the child learns that going to sleep is associated with pleasant parental behavior such as rocking, singing, reading, or nursing, going back to sleep after nighttime arousal may be difficult.

The child's temperament is another factor contributing to sleep. It has been reported that children with low sensory thresholds and less rhythmicity are more prone to night waking.

Children who have had perinatal difficulties, such as intracranial hemorrhage or hyaline membrane disease, have a greater incidence of night waking and difficulties returning to sleep.

Finally, psychosocial stressors can play a role in night waking.

Management

A complete medical and psychosocial history should be obtained and a physical examination performed. A detailed sleep history and diary should be maintained to which both parents contribute. Some clinicians use polysomnography to complete the evaluation. Problems often arise when parents try to put the child down before it is biologically ready. The child might then lie awake and cry.

In managing sleeping difficulties, the child's individual sleep behavior characteristics must be taken into account and parents' expectations and fears must be identified and addressed. Counseling is then provided on the following premises:

(1) Sleep is a highly active and organized process that matures during the first years of life. One-week-old infants sleep about 16 hours a day, 6 of those hours during the daylight hours. A 2-year-old sleeps a total of 13 hours a day, only 1 hour during the day.

(2) Individual circadian rhythms do not change immediately and require consistency and regularity over a period of time before change will occur.

(3) The duration of sleep for a given individual does not vary significantly from day to day, but there is a wide range of normal.

(4) The duration of nighttime sleep is inversely correlated with daytime sleep, and bedtimes and awakening times are positively correlated with each other.

(5) Night waking occurs in 40–60% of infants and young children. If the child does not cry or wake up the parents, such behavior should not be considered a sleep disturbance.

Parents need to set limits for the child while acknowledging the child's individual biologic rhythms. They should resist the child's attempts to put off bedtime or to engage them during nighttime awakenings. Putting a child to bed after prolonged rocking, feeding, or when the child has already fallen asleep frequently results in disturbances of settling down at night or going back to sleep after a nighttime awakening. The goal is to establish clear bedtime rituals, to put the child to bed while still awake, and to create a quiet, secure bedtime environment.

For the child who has a delayed sleep phase—difficulty in falling asleep and waking at desired times but no difficulty at a later hour—a regular schedule and consistent, nonstimulating bedtime rituals must be provided. Approaches used to alter the child's behavior include having the parents withdraw the attention elicited by the wakeful child and by positive reinforcement of the desired behavior. Another strategy to alter this sleep pattern is to gradually move the bedtime to an earlier hour and awaken the child earlier in the morning. However, there is nothing intrinsically normal or abnormal in the delayed sleep phase. It only becomes a problem when it differs from parental expectations.

Some children are afraid to go to sleep. The parent needs to help the child identify what is frightening about going to sleep and may need to stay near the child, reassuring him that he is safe and that Mommy and Daddy will not let anything happen to him. Over a period of time, the child can be reassured and the parent may not need to be so involved. This also applies to nighttime awakenings.

The key to management of children who have difficulty going to sleep or who awaken during the night and disturb others is to recognize that both the child and the parent play significant roles in initiating and sustaining what may be an undesirable behavior.

Thus, it becomes important for the physician and parents to understand normal sleep patterns, the parents' responses that inadvertently reinforce undesirable sleep behavior, and the child's individual temperament traits.

Adair RH, Bauchner H: Sleep problems in childhood. Curr Probl Pediatr 1993;23:147.

Dahl RE: The pharmacologic treatment of sleep disorders. Psychiatr Clin North Am 1992;15:161.

Ferber R: Sleeplessness, night awakening, and night crying in the infant and toddler. Pediatr Rev 1987;9:69.

Lozoff B, Zuckerman B: Sleep problems in children. Pediatr Rev 1988;10:17.

Mahowald MW, Rosen GM: Parasomnias in children. Pediatrician 1990;17:21.

Richman N: Recent progress in understanding and treatment of sleep disorders. Adv Dev Behav Pediatr 1986;7:45.

Sladkin K, Brown LW: Sleep disorders in children and adolescents. In: *Behavioral Pediatrics*. Greydanus DE, Wolraich ML (editors). Springer, 1992.

TEMPER TANTRUMS & BREATH-HOLDING SPELLS

1. TEMPER TANTRUMS

Temper tantrums are common between 12 months and 4 years of age, occurring about once a week in 50–80% of children in this age group. The child may throw himself down, kick and scream, strike out at people or objects in the room, and hold his breath. These behaviors may be considered normal as the young child seeks to achieve autonomy and mastery over the environment. They are often a reflection of immaturity as the child strives to accomplish age-appropriate developmental tasks and meets with difficulty because of inadequate motor and language skills, impulsiveness, or parental restrictions. In the home, these behaviors may be annoying. In public, they are embarrassing.

Some children tolerate frustration well, are able to persevere at tasks, and cope with difficulties easily; others have a much greater problem dealing with experiences above their developmental level. Tantrums can be minimized by understanding the child's temperament and what it is trying to communicate. There must also be a commitment to supporting the child's drive to master its feelings.

Management

Appropriate intervention can provide an opportunity for enhancing the child's growth. It should be remembered that the tantrum is a loss of control on the child's part and a blow to the self-image, which is frightening for the child. Therefore, the parent and the physician need to view these behaviors within the child's developmental context rather than from a negative, adversarial, angry viewpoint.

Several suggestions can be offered for parents and physicians in managing tantrums:

(1) Minimize the need to say "no" by "childproofing" the environment so that fewer restrictions need be enforced.

(2) Use distraction when frustration increases; direct the child to other, less frustrating activities; and reward the positive response.

(3) Present options within the child's capabilities so that it can achieve mastery and autonomy.

(4) Fight only those battles that need to be won and avoid those that arouse unnecessary conflict.

(5) Do not abandon the preschool child when a tantrum occurs. Stay nearby during the episode without intruding. A small child may need to be restrained. An older child can be asked to go to his or her room. Threats serve no purpose and should not be used.

(6) Do not use negative terms when the tantrum is occurring. Instead, point out that the child is out of control and give praise when it regains control.

(7) Never let a child hurt itself or others.

(8) Do not "hold a grudge" after the tantrum is over. However, the child's demands leading to the tantrum should not be granted.

(9) Seek to maintain an environment that provides positive reinforcement for desired behavior. Do not overreact to undesired behavior but set reasonable limits and provide responsible direction for the child.

(10) Approximately 5–20% of young children have severe temper tantrums which are frequent and disruptive. Such tantrums result from a disturbance in the parent–child interaction, poor parenting skills, lack of limit-setting, and permissiveness. They may be part of a larger behavioral or developmental disorder or may emerge under adverse socioeconomic conditions, in circumstances of maternal depression and family dysfunction, or when the child is in poor health. Referral to a psychologist or psychiatrist is appropriate while the pediatrician continues to support and work with the family.

2. BREATH-HOLDING SPELLS

While temper tantrums can be frustrating to parents, breath-holding spells can be terrifying. The name for this behavior may be a misnomer in that it connotes prolonged inspiration. In fact, it occurs during expiration and is reflexive—not volitional—in nature. It is a paroxysmal event occurring in 0.1–5% of healthy children aged 6 months to 6 years. The spells usually start during the first year of life, often in response to anger or a mild injury. The child is provoked, starts to cry—briefly or for a considerable time—and then falls silent. This is followed by a color change. Spells have been described as either pallid (acyanotic) or cyanotic, with the latter usually associated with anger and the former with an injury such as a fall. The spell may resolve spontaneously or the child may lose consciousness. In severe cases, the child may become limp and progress to opisthotonos, body jerks, and urinary incontinence. Only rarely does a spell proceed to asystole or a seizure.

For the child with frequent spells, underlying disorders such as seizures, orthostatic hypotension, obstructive sleep apnea, abnormalities of the central nervous system, tumors, familial dysautonomia, and Rett's syndrome need to be considered. There is an association between breath-holding spells, pica, and iron deficiency anemia. These conditions can be ruled out on the basis of the history, physical examination, and laboratory studies. Once it has been determined that the child is healthy, the focus of treatment is behavioral. Parents should be taught to handle the spells in a matter-of-fact manner and monitor the child for any untoward events. The reality is that parents cannot completely protect their child from upsetting and frustrating experiences and probably should not try to do so. Just as in temper tantrums, parents need to help the child control responses to frustration. They need to be careful not to be too permissive and submit to the child's every whim for fear the child might have a "spell." If a syncopal event should occur, the child should be placed in a lateral recumbent position to protect against head injury and avoid aspiration. Maintaining a patent oral airway is essential, but cardiopulmonary resuscitation should be avoided. There are no prophylactic medications. Atropine, 0.01 mg/kg given subcutaneously, has been used with some benefit in spells accompanied by bradycardia or asystole.

DiMario FJ Jr: Breath-holding spells in childhood. Am J Dis Child 1992;146:125.

Needlman R, Howard B, Zuckerman B: Temper tantrums: When to worry. Contemp Pediatr 1989;6:12.

Needlman R, Stevenson J, Zuckerman B: Psychosocial correlates of severe temper tantrums. J Dev Behav Pediatr 1991;12:77.

DEVELOPMENTAL DISORDERS

The developmental disorders include problems in the development of cognitive and social competence. Competence is defined by comparing performance levels of an individual child with norms accumulated from observation and testing of children of the same age. Other standards of competence compare the child's performance level with that of the adult norm or compare the child's present skills with skills needed to accomplish a given task or engage in a specific activity.

The measurement of developmental competence is patterned on concepts of measuring intelligence. Assessment of competence shows not only (1) that children are able to perform increasingly more complex and difficult tasks as they grow older but (2) that when groups of children of about the same age are tested, they are found to be at about the same developmental stage. Such assessments provide the basis for deriving an intelligence quotient and anticipating school performance and may also have implications for understanding social behavior.

Intelligence tests may be thought of as measures of general competence that attempt to determine what a child has learned from exposure to an environment. This assumes that informal opportunities for learning are similar within the culture. Anything that limits the breadth, depth, and variety of experiences or the ability of a child to profit from them may place limits on the learning a given child will achieve in a given period. Anything that increases systematic exposure or increases breadth, depth, and variety of exposure potentially enhances learning.

Many biologic and psychosocial factors influence a child's performance on developmental tests, and assessment of a child's general developmental or intellectual standing relative to other children sheds no light on the cause of the child's performance. Consequently, it is important to determine whether an intelligence test gives a representative estimate of the child's usual functioning and whether other information might explain low scores. Differences in experiential background may account for low scores of children from nondominant cultures given standard intelligence tests. Such explanations, however, do not necessarily alter the predictive value of scores from intelligence tests.

A variety of delays or deficiencies in the development of cognitive competence have also been identified and may be associated with deficiencies in general competence. The most significant of these are failure to acquire basic academic skills such as reading, writing, and arithmetic. Specific measures of competence are usually measures of achievement in areas where systematic instruction has been given (eg, music lessons, arithmetic lessons). Here again, both biologic and psychosocial factors (eg, "musical talent," "math aptitude") may facilitate or interfere with development of competence. Measures of relative standing in specific areas of achievement correlate well with measures of intelligence. This correlation provides the basis for determining a child's expected level of achievement, whereas the discrepancy between expected and actual levels of achievement is a key factor in defining developmental problems.

Traditionally, social and emotional aspects of development have not been conceptualized and tested as separate dimensions of competence. However, it is increasingly recognized that social competence is an important concept for assessing some aspects of social and emotional development. This is particularly true for aspects of behavior and social interaction such as empathy, distractibility, activity level, and aggression, which show strong, regular progression with age and which are associated with what has traditionally been termed cognitive development.

GENERAL PRINCIPLES IN EVALUATING COGNITIVE & SOCIAL COMPETENCE

Developmental evaluation should be based on (1) data defining a child's level of cognitive and social competence, (2) data that will assist in making an etiologic diagnosis, and (3) data relevant to planning management. These objectives are best achieved by a multidisciplinary team. In addition to the pediatrician, the team usually includes a psychologist, a social worker, an education specialist, and a speech and language specialist. Specialists in nursing, physical therapy, occupational therapy, ophthalmology, audiology, nutrition, and dentistry may also be required. Where a functioning team is not available, the primary care physician can achieve similar results by requesting consultations from various other professionals and obtaining information from school personnel and other community sources. The following discussion presents suggestions to assist the primary care physician in developing a database through use of questionnaires and screening tests when assistance from other professionals is limited or unavailable.

History

A. Medical History: The medical history should focus on aspects of pregnancy, labor, and delivery that might compromise the patient's central nervous system (eg, use of drugs or x-rays during pregnancy; neonatal infections, asphyxia, elevated bilirubin levels). Later evidence of central nervous system insults or injury, failure to thrive, chronic illnesses, hospitalizations, or abuse may also significantly influence the assessment of a child's performance at school age. Neonatal records are often an important source of information, since they may reveal information forgotten by or unknown to the parents.

B. Developmental History: The developmental history should include information about the age at which various milestones were achieved, especially those pertaining to speech and language. Inability to use meaningful words other than "dada," "mama," "bye-bye," and "hello" by 18 months and inability to speak in short sentences by 24 months are considered to reflect developmental delays. Development of motor skills is also important, particularly in

assessing mental retardation, but deviance or delay in motor development may also be present in conditions such as cerebral palsy and neuromuscular disorders not necessarily associated with mental retardation.

C. Family History: Information regarding central nervous system disorders, mental retardation, epilepsy, or evidence of school problems or specific learning disabilities in other family members should be included. Details of the mother's pregnancy history, including stillbirths, deaths, and other problems, may be helpful in defining physical causes of abnormal development.

D. Educational and Learning History: In preschool children, considerable information can be obtained from a description of what the child has learned in an informal setting. If the child has been placed in a formal preschool setting, information should be obtained regarding the type of preschool and the child's relationships with other children and especially with teachers, who can report on the child's performance and behavior in the classroom. Such assessments may be helpful in anticipating later problems.

After a child has reached school age, the educational history should include such details as grade placement, special education evaluation, and repetition of grades. Most school systems routinely test students at intervals using standardized tests. These tests, which are typically administered to whole classes in the spring of the academic year, measure academic progress in reading, math, science, and social studies. Student performance is then compared with a representative sample of peers across the country. Achievement scores are reported in terms of grade level attainment. For example, a 3.2 grade level means that a student is working in a particular curriculum area at the third grade, second month level. Achievement scores may also be reported as percentiles, where a student's performance is measured against a population of other students of the same age or grade level.

Although group-administered standardized tests measure student skills in academic areas, they are rarely of great value in identifying an individual student's specific areas of academic strength or weakness. When group-administered achievement scores differ by more than 1 year from a student's grade placement—or where achievement scores show a scatter of more than 1 year between scores—it may be advisable to consider further testing to better define the student's deficiencies.

Although a child's achievement scores can indicate that a school problem is occurring, that does not necessarily mean the child has a learning disability. Issues such as how instruction is being provided, whether the method is appropriate for the child's learning needs, and whether the content is concordant with the student's experience must be addressed in order to determine what action should be taken.

Information about the child's academic achievement should include learning patterns, ability to perform tasks, motivation to learn new material, interest areas, and preferences for learning activities. Furthermore, when test scores are available, it is critical to determine whether the test was group or individually administered. Information regarding the student's emotional reactions to school situations should focus on whether the behavior is appropriate to the social as well as academic contexts of school. In the absence of a psychologist or education specialist, direct contact with school personnel is imperative for the primary care physician.

E. Psychosocial History: Family problems and parental characteristics often interfere with development of cognitive and social competence and foster deviant behavior. Children of hostile, rejecting, authoritarian parents tend to be the most severely affected. Parents who provide little nurturance or sense of belonging, who are too lax or too harsh in punishment, or who fail to supervise their children tend to have children who show early evidence of aggressive behavior problems that persist into adolescence and adulthood. Children of nurturing parents who are firm and verbal in providing guidance and setting standards without being rigidly authoritarian show advanced competence that increases with age.

A good psychosocial history is an essential part of any developmental evaluation because childhood developmental problems are often provoked by problems within the family or a lack of family support for developing new skills. The history should include assessment of the family's ability to promote cognitive and social development, including information about the parents' language and cultural background, the quality of verbal interaction, disciplinary practices (use of positive reinforcement, reliance on physical punishment or limited use of reasoning), and the ability to set standards. The history should also include an evaluation for neglect, parenting practices that inhibit development, family instability, marital discord, a hostile attitude toward the child, limitations in cognitive and social competence, depression, signs of maladjustment (eg, alcoholism, chronic unemployment, criminal or psychiatric problems), and general stress in the parents and chaos in the family.

In examining only the child, it is often difficult to distinguish behavior disorders from developmental disorders. This difficulty has resulted in diagnosis by exclusion—psychosocial assessment is used to determine whether there are social or emotional factors that can account for the observed learning or behavior problems. This is a practical approach in middle-class families since it is often possible to ascertain that the family is reasonably stable and able to provide adequate support and stimulation to the child. Diagnosis of an organic disorder by exclusion of the possible psychosocial causes is an unsatisfactory approach for dealing with children from disadvantaged

families. The need for accurate assessment of these children is particularly acute, since they often have delays in both social and cognitive development and combinations of developmental delays and behavior problems. The importance of psychosocial issues cannot be overemphasized, since 90% of children who later show mental or emotional disorders are normal at birth and appear to be casualties of inadequate or pathologic environments.

At present, the most commonly used approach to family assessment is a social history. Some of this information is usually included in the history obtained by the primary care physician. However, if the child is undergoing a team evaluation, a social worker will provide the most thorough and complete analysis. In preschool children, it is often helpful to supplement the usual clinical social history with the HOME (Home Observation for Measurement of the Environment) interview assessment of Bradley and Caldwell. This is the most thoroughly studied instrument for the systematic evaluation of the growth-promoting aspects of the child's environment. This interview, which requires a home visit, is used to identify families unlikely to support development in their children. It may be performed by any trained person but is usually done by a social worker or nurse. A shorter questionnaire version of the HOME interview, the Home Screening Questionnaire (HSQ), provides most of the information obtained from the longer interview version and can be administered and scored by the pediatrician during a clinic or office visit. Neither scale is expected to be useful in evaluating children from middle or upper socioeconomic families.

Badger E, Burne D, Vietze P: Maternal risk factors as predictors of development outcome in early childhood. Infant Ment Health J 1981;2:33.

Bradley RH, Caldwell BM: Pediatric usefulness of home assessment. In: *Advances in Behavioral Pediatrics,* vol 2. Camp BW (editor). JAI Press, 1981.

Coons CE et al: *The Home Screening Questionnaire Reference Manual.* LADOCA, 1981.

Physical & Neurologic Examination

It is essential that a thorough physical and neurologic examination be performed. A number of children will demonstrate neurologic soft signs, such as clumsiness, right–left confusion, disordered temporal orientation, overflow phenomena, choreiform movements, and finger agnosia. Although soft signs are commonly associated with school learning and behavior problems, the significance of these signs is controversial because they are also found in children who have no other problems and because most appear to represent delay in maturation rather than dysfunction.

Recent studies linking minor physical anomalies with behavior disorders in childhood have prompted physicians to examine for the presence of dysmorphic features such as abnormal palmar creases, syndactyly, unruly hair, malformed ears, skin tags, and facial abnormalities. Although these features are commonly seen in children with mental retardation, the implications of their presence in nonretarded children are not fully understood.

Sensory Evaluation

All children in whom developmental delay or mental retardation is suspected should be examined for visual and auditory problems. In infants and young children, sensory deficits may be mistaken for retardation. Retarded children often have sensory deficits in addition to their retardation, and this increases the complexity of their problem. In most nonretarded school-age children, vision and hearing can be satisfactorily evaluated by the usual screening methods and referral made to a specialist for further evaluation of children with abnormal screening results.

A variety of vision problems have been proposed as causes of reading problems, most without substantial research support. Learning to read can be accomplished quite satisfactorily with limited visual acuity. Although it is important that visual defects be corrected to improve the child's overall functioning, it is generally agreed that learning problems are seldom linked to refractive errors. Difficulty with convergence at near point, however, may interfere significantly with the process of reading and should receive careful evaluation.

Hearing loss has a significant impact on language development and may be associated with severe learning and behavior problems. Deaf children are often mistakenly labeled retarded. Losses in the high-frequency range may be associated with problems in discriminating speech sounds necessary for school learning. Others may have problems differentiating speech sounds despite normal hearing.

Evaluation of Emotional & Social Behavior

Although some information can be obtained directly from the child through interviews, play, and projective testing, one must usually rely on interviews with parents and reports from school personnel to obtain a picture of the child's social competence. This information may also be obtained by social workers, psychologists, or psychiatrists.

A scale for recording teacher and parent ratings of general behavior is also useful for identifying children with deviant behavior other than distractibility and hyperactivity and for assessing the degree and amount of prosocial behavior. Several such scales are available for assessing children as young as 2 years of age. The most commonly used scale with both parent and teacher forms is the Child Behavior Checklist (Achenbach).

General adaptation and development of self-help are often included in developmental assessments of preschool children. Beginning around age 4 years (when abstract reasoning becomes the dominant factor in measures of cognitive development), it becomes increasingly important to include some assessment of general adaptation in the differential diagnosis of mental retardation. Children from minority cultures who perform poorly on IQ tests often appear less retarded when general adaptation is evaluated.

Rating scales of behavior, such as ACTeRS (ADD-H: Comprehensive Teachers Rating Scale) (Table 3–2) for identifying children with attention deficit disorder with or without hyperactivity, are important tools for assessing school behavior. ACTeRS has been designed to identify clusters of problems in the areas of attention, hyperactivity, social skills, and oppositional behavior. Norms to assess the degree of deviance are available. This scale is acceptable to teachers and can be used by primary care physicians to assess the need for and response to stimulant medication.

Evaluation of Family & Social Resources

The type, extent, and cost of educational and counseling services available to the child and family and the family's ability to carry through with treatment plans should be assessed early in the evaluation. These factors often limit or modify the treatment plan. Sixty percent of families with children evaluated for learning problems have clear-cut social and emotional problems. Much of this information will be derived from the psychosocial history. In addition, however, the primary care physician should become familiar with community resources for family assessment and counseling.

Evaluation of Intelligence

Intelligence tests usually present progressively more difficult questions testing general knowledge, reasoning, judgment, and analytic skills that are expected to develop through experiences encountered in the process of growing up. Where children have experiences grossly different from those in the standard population, their scores may be expected to vary. Originally, the IQ score obtained from such tests represented the percentage of expected growth a child had reached at a given age. This was derived by the following equation:

$$\frac{\textbf{Mental age determined by testing}}{\textbf{Chronologic age}} \times \textbf{100}$$

Scores on most modern tests can still be reported in terms of mental age ÷ chronologic age, but the most widely used tests yield IQ scores that represent a

Table 3–2.

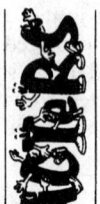

Rina K. Ullmann, M.Ed.
Esther K. Sleator, M.D.
Robert L. Sprague, Ph.D.

2nd Edition

Below are descriptions of behavior. Please read each item and compare the child's behavior with that of his or her classmates. Circle the number that most closely corresponds with your evaluation. Transfer the total raw score for each of the four sections to the profile sheet to determine normative percentile scores.

Child's Name: Elaine Sample
Rater: Mrs. Betsy J. Smith
ID #: 892772
Date: 11-15-93

ATTENTION

	Almost Never				Almost Always
1. Works well independently	(1)	2	3	4	5
2. Persists with task for reasonable amount of time	(1)	2	3	4	5
3. Completes assigned task satisfactorily with little additional assistance	(1)	2	3	4	5
4. Follows simple directions accurately	1	(2)	3	4	5
5. Follows a sequence of instructions	1	(2)	3	4	5
6. Functions well in the classroom	(1)	2	3	4	5

ADD ITEMS 1-6 AND PLACE TOTAL HERE __8__

HYPERACTIVITY

	Almost Never				Almost Always
7. Extremely overactive (out of seat, "on the go")	1	2	3	(4)	5
8. Overreacts	1	2	3	(4)	5
9. Fidgety (hands always busy)	1	2	3	(4)	5
10. Impulsive (acts or talks without thinking)	1	2	3	(4)	5
11. Restless (squirms in seat)	1	2	3	(4)	5

ADD ITEMS 7-11 AND PLACE TOTAL HERE __20__

SOCIAL SKILLS

	Almost Never				Almost Always
12. Behaves positively with peers/classmates	1	2	(3)	4	5
13. Verbal communication clear and "connected"	1	2	3	4	(5)
14. Nonverbal communication accurate	1	2	3	(4)	5
15. Follows group norms and social rules	1	2	(3)	4	5
16. Cites general rule when criticizing ("We aren't supposed to do that")	1	2	3	(4)	5
17. Skillful at making new friends	1	(2)	3	4	5
18. Approaches situations confidently	1	(2)	3	4	5

ADD ITEMS 12-18 AND PLACE TOTAL HERE __23__

OPPOSITIONAL

	Almost Never				Almost Always
19. Tries to get others into trouble	1	(2)	3	4	5
20. Starts fights over nothing	1	(2)	3	4	5
21. Makes malicious fun of people	1	(2)	3	4	5
22. Defies authority	1	(2)	3	4	5
23. Picks on others	1	(2)	3	4	5
24. Mean and cruel to other children	1	(2)	3	4	5

ADD ITEMS 19-24 AND PLACE TOTAL HERE __12__

MetriTech, Inc.

Copyright © 1986, 1988, 1991 by MetriTech, Inc.
111 North Market Street, Champaign, Illinois.

No portion of this form may be copied in any way without written permission.

(continued)

Table 3-2. (continued)

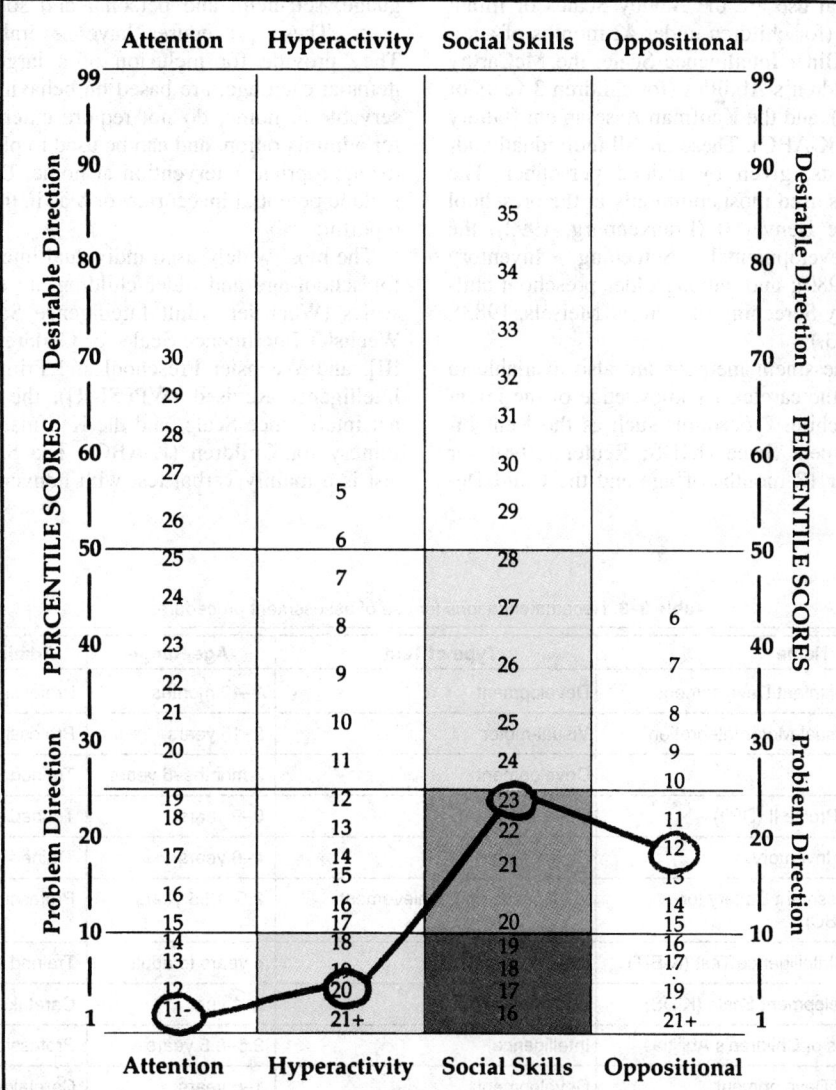

ACTeRS PROFILE—Girls' Form

Circle the raw scores in each of the four middle columns and determine percentile equivalents in the far left or right (boldface) columns. Note that some raw scores represent a range of percentiles (e.g., for Hyperactivity, the perfect score of 5 represents the range from the 56th percentile up).

Copyright © 1986, 1988, 1991 by MetriTech, Inc., Champaign, Illinois child's relative distance from the average child in standard score units.

In the preschool period, the principal diagnostic tests in general use are the Bayley Scales of Infant Development (for children under 42 months of age), the Stanford-Binet Intelligence Scale, the McCarthy Scales of Children's Abilities (for children 3 years of age and older), and the Kaufman Assessment Battery for Children (K-ABC). These are all individually administered tests, given by trained personnel. The screening tests used most commonly in the preschool period are the Denver II (Frankenburg, 1992); the Revised Developmental Screening Inventory (Knobloch, 1980); and, among older preschool children, the Early Screening Inventory (Meisels, 1983). (See Table 3–3.)

Several assessment methods are also available to capitalize on the caretaker's knowledge of the infant or preschool child. Procedures such as the Kent Infant Development Scale (KIDS; Reuter, 1990) for children under 12 months of age and the Child Development Inventory (Ireton, 1995) for children over 15 months of age use the caretaker's report to assess cognitive, gross motor, fine motor, expressive language, self-help, and personal and social development. These procedures have several advantages. They provide for inclusion of a large number of items at each age, are based on behavior readily observable at home, do not require extensive training for administration, and can be used to plan and monitor appropriate intervention at home. Disadvantages include potential inaccuracy or bias in the caretaker's reporting.

The most widely used individual intelligence tests for school-age and older children are the Wechsler scales (Wechsler Adult Intelligence Scale [WAIS], Wechsler Intelligence Scale for Children III [WISC-III], and Wechsler Preschool and Primary Scale of Intelligence–Revised [WPPSI-R]), the Stanford-Binet Intelligence Scale, and the Kaufman Assessment Battery for Children (K-ABC). The Stanford-Binet test is a mainly verbal test with nonverbal items in-

Table 3–3. Recommendations for use of assessment procedures.

Name	Type of Test	Age Range	Administered By
Bayley Scales of Infant Development	Development	1–42 months	Professional
Beery Test of Visual-Motor Integration	Visual-motor	2–15 years	Professional
Denver II	Development	3 months–6 years	Trained screener
Developmental Profile II (DPII)	Development	0–9 years	Trained screener
Early Screening Inventory	Development	4–6 years	Trained screener
Kaufmann Assessment Battery for Children (K-ABC)	Intelligence and achievement	2.5–12.5 years	Professional
Kaufmann Brief Intelligence Test (K-BIT)	Intelligence	4 years to adult	Trained screener
Kent Infant Development Scale (KIDS)	Development	0–1 year	Caretaker response
McCarthy Scales of Children's Abilities	Intelligence	2.5–8.5 years	Professional
Minnesota Child Development Inventory (MCDI)	Development	1–6 years	Caretaker response
Scales of Independent Behavior	Adaptive behavior	All ages	Professional
Slosson Intelligence Test	Intelligence	4.5 years to adult	Trained screener
Stanford-Binet Intelligence Scale	Intelligence	2 years to adult	Professional
Vineland Adaptive Behavior Scales	Adaptive behavior	All ages	Professional
Wechsler Preschool & Primary Scale of Intelligence–Revised (WPPSI-R)	Intelligence	3 years to 7 years, 3 months	Professional
Wechsler Intelligence Scale for Children–III (WISC-III)	Intelligence	6–16 years	Professional
Wide Range Achievement Test 3	Achievement: reading, spelling, math, visual-perceptual	5 years to adult	Trained screener
Woodcock-Johnson Psych-Educational Battery	Aptitude and achievement	3 years to adult	Professional

termingled. The Wechsler scales are subdivided into six verbal and six nonverbal tests so that a verbal IQ and performance IQ can be obtained as well as an IQ based on the full test (full-scale IQ). The Kaufman Battery is designed to assess differences in simultaneous and sequential processing of information as well as differences between aptitude and achievement. It is commonly thought that intelligence tests can reveal the potential for higher functioning, especially when scatter (the pattern of high and low scores) is examined. Both the K-ABC and the Wechsler scales are well-suited to this task.

The standardized, individually administered tests of intelligence discussed above are usually administered by psychologists. The Kaufman Brief Intelligence Test (K-BIT), the Slosson Intelligence Test, and the Peabody Picture Vocabulary Test are screening tests designed for use by nonspecialists, including office assistants and primary care physicians.

Evaluation of Achievement

Achievement usually refers to performance in school-related subject areas in which a child has received instruction. In the preschool period, achievement is seldom distinguished from general development. By the time the child enters kindergarten, a variety of procedures are available for assessing readiness. In a child with a mental age of 6 years, two of the best indicators of school readiness are the ability to engage in sustained task-oriented behavior and the knowledge of letter names and their sounds. A number of procedures are available to assess school readiness, and in recent years testing programs have been specifically designed for early identification of children with learning disabilities. Most of the early identification assessments are designed for use in schools or by psychologists. Several procedures are also available for use by primary care physicians in screening for school readiness at the time of well child visits in the age range from 4 to 5 years. These include the developmental screening tests described previously and the preschool portions of the Wide Range Achievement Test 3 (WRAT-3).

For school-age children, the scores of group-administered achievement tests done at school should be included in the education history. When low scores are obtained, individual testing should be performed before accepting the results as representative of the child's ability. Many school systems with special education services can administer individual tests of achievement and, with permission from the parents, give the test scores to the primary care physician. However, test scores alone do not constitute evidence of developmental disorders unless they have been interpreted carefully by an education specialist or school psychologist. Individually administered achievement tests such as the Woodcock-Johnson Psychoeducational Battery–Revised (Woodcock, 1990) are used to analyze a learner's performance.

The usefulness of complex tools such as the Woodcock-Johnson test and the validity of the results depend largely on the skills of the examiner in interpreting test performance and scores on as many as 27 subtests.

Three components of cognition appear to be particularly important for school learning and achievement: attention, memory, and the coordination of these processes. The ability to focus and sustain attention on events or tasks that are prescribed in school is a fundamental academic skill. Some children fail to sustain attention because of emotional factors. For others, failure to attend appears related to inability to determine what the task is and what procedures are required to complete it. In other words, they have difficulty in problem-solving. These children may have deficits in several areas critical to problem solving: (1) problem identification, (2) organization of strategies, (3) generalization from other similar situations, (4) attainment of logical solutions, and (5) critical analysis and evaluation. Inability to attend simultaneously to the task, to monitor one's performance, and to allot attention appropriately to various elements of the task is a source of difficulty for many of these learners.

Children may have trouble in cognitive development because of limited ability to store or retrieve information. Cognitive psychologists discuss this problem in terms of storage capacity, or how much information an individual can maintain in either short-term or long-term memory banks. Where capacity is not at issue, retrieval may pose a stumbling block. Children may lack a complex semantic retrieval system that would enable them to access stored information from multiple avenues. Teachers often say, "I know he knows it—he could do it all last week. But this week it's as if he never saw it before." Additional problems arise if attention, processing, and retrieval are not well coordinated. Patterns of performance on tests that assess these cognitive abilities may indicate that the child has a specific disability in one or more cognitive functions.

Individually administered achievement tests, in conjunction with measures of intelligence, are used to identify discrepancies between academic achievement and individual potential and to determine whether these discrepancies may be attributable to some form of learning disability.

Academic achievement is dependent also on environmental factors that are not necessarily measured by means of achievement tests. These factors include cultural background and experience, motivation to achieve, expectation of success, and instruction that accounts for these variables. A thorough diagnostic evaluation should address these concerns.

Evaluation of Adaptive Behavior

Assessment of adaptive behavior is seldom addressed directly in children unless a child is suspected of being mentally retarded. Because poor performance on a cognitive test may result from many factors, the accuracy of low scores must be confirmed by assessment of the functional level in everyday living. Instruments such as the Vineland Adaptive Behavior Scales and the Scales of Independent Behavior are questionnaires and structured interviews for assessing the child's developmental level in areas such as social interaction, communication, personal interactions, and community living skills.

Evaluation of Perceptual-Motor Function

Children with delays in copying and drawing skills also have problems in learning to read. These problems have been variously termed visual-perceptual and visual-motor problems, and their presence in children beyond 7–9 years of age may indicate central nervous system dysfunction, though this inference is controversial. Although there appears to be a relationship between visual-perceptual problems and reading problems in the early school years, as children get older reading achievement is found to be more related to intelligence even when the perceptual problems persist.

Because performance on tests of copying skills is highly correlated with intelligence, such tests are most useful when there is a discrepancy between the developmental level demonstrated on visual-perceptual tests and general intelligence. Methods for assessing the degree of this discrepancy are not as sophisticated as those for assessing the discrepancy between IQ and achievement. At a practical level, however, these problems may be severe enough to interfere with learning the skills of printing and cursive writing. Several visual-perceptual tests, such as the Beery Test of Visual-Motor Integration, are commonly used to examine copying skills per se.

Evaluation of Speech & Language

Speech and language delays are common in mentally retarded children but may also occur in children with average or above-average intelligence. Children who appear to have specific learning problems may on closer evaluation show evidence of delay in language development or an articulation problem. These problems can limit academic achievement in areas that depend on verbal skills (eg, reading). Speech and language delays in preschool children and methods for evaluating them are discussed in Chapter 1.

Evaluation of Motivation

Clinical assessment of motivation has received little attention despite mounting evidence that it is a key factor in determining how a child will use whatever time and help are available for learning new skills. Two main individual types can be identified: (1) those who are motivated to succeed as moderately difficult tasks and (2) those who are motivated mainly to avoid failure. The latter will attempt only very easy tasks, in which failure is unlikely, or very difficult ones, in which failure carries no stigma. One of the major shifts that occurs in the age range from 5 to 7 years is from motivational dependence on social and external rewards to internal motivation for mastery of skills. Some children do not make this shift and fail to learn in the usual academic climate, which emphasizes competition. Children who are motivated mainly to avoid failure need support from external sources (praise, concrete incentives) just for trying. Although motivational immaturity is seldom the principal problem, it is often a major determinant of how well a child will progress in school.

Achenbach TM: *The Child Behavior Checklist.* University of Vermont Press, 1991.

Beery KE: *Revised Administration, Scoring, and Teaching Manual for the Developmental Test of Visual-Motor Integration.* Modern Curriculum Press, 1982.

Bruininks RH et al: *Scales of Independent Behavior.* DLM Teaching Resources, 1984.

Frankenburg WK: The Denver II: A major revision and restandardization of the Denver Developmental Screening Test. Pediatrics 1992;89:91.

Ireton H: *Child Development Inventory.* Behavior Science Systems, 1995.

Knobloch H, Steven F, Malone AF: *Manual of Developmental Diagnosis.* Harper, 1980.

Meisels SJ, Wiske MS: *Early Screening Inventory.* Teachers College, 1983.

Reuter J, Bickett L: *The Kent Infant Development Scale.* Kent Developmental Metrics, 1990.

Sparrow SS et al: *Vineland Adaptive Behavior Scales: Interview Edition, Survey Form Manual.* American Guidance Service, 1984.

Wilkinson GS: *Wide Range Achievement Test 3.* Jastak, 1993.

Woodcock R: *Woodcock-Johnson Psychoeducational Battery–Revised.* Teaching Resources, 1990.

EVALUATING THE DISCREPANCY BETWEEN INTELLIGENCE & ACHIEVEMENT

The differential diagnosis of competence problems necessitates evaluation of the discrepancy between expected achievement based on measures of general competence (intelligence) and actual achievement in specific areas of academic performance.

The United States Office of Education defines the discrepancy between achievement and IQ as significant when achievement is less than 50% of expected grade level.

DISORDERS IN DEVELOPMENT OF COGNITIVE COMPETENCE (Table 3–4)

SPECIFIC LEARNING DISORDERS

Specific learning disorders may occur in any area of academic achievement, but the most common involve reading (dyslexia). Less common problems are arithmetic (dyscalculia) or writing (dysgraphia). Intelligence is usually average or above average. The key to diagnosis is a discrepancy between actual and expected achievement in an isolated area.

Descriptive Classification

A. Reading and Spelling Disorders (Developmental Dyslexia): Dyslexia is the most common specific learning disorder. It occurs more frequently in boys than in girls (3:1), and in 34% of cases there is a family history, especially among male relatives. Language problems and problems in sequencing are the most common causes of reading disorders. A variety of developmental problems such as clumsiness and incoordination, directional confusion, right-left confusion, disordered spatial orientation, and difficulties in naming colors and in recognizing the meaning of pictures have been reported in children with specific reading problems. A history of delays in speech and language development is present in at least one-third of cases.

Traditionally, the definition of specific reading disorder (dyslexia) included failure to learn to read despite adequate sensory apparatus, conventional instruction, average intelligence, and sociocultural opportunity. Such diagnosis by exclusion was an attempt to distinguish between "unexpected" reading failure and reading failure that could be explained by a more general or pervasive factor, such as mental subnormality, cultural or educational deprivation, sensory handicaps, or emotional disturbance. With this approach, most children with reading problems tend to be excluded from the diagnosis of specific reading disorder—ie, their reading problems are attributed to being slightly below average in intelligence, coming from economically disadvantaged homes, or having emotional and behavior problems. Yet many in this large group show reading achievement below expectancy for their mental age.

Current thinking endorses the concept that subtypes of reading disability should be described in terms of clear-cut characteristics irrespective of etiologic considerations. One approach attempts to distinguish among subtypes by analysis of reading and spelling errors. This has led to subtyping into two groups based on whether performance indicates heavier reliance on auditory-sequential-phonologic skills (auditory reader) or on visual-spatial-imagery (visual reader). A second approach uses associated disabilities in language, perceptual-motor skills, and memory to distinguish the following subtypes: (1) a language disorder group with defects in understanding and expression of oral language; (2) a dyscoordination group with defects in speech articulation, copying skills, and understanding of oral language; (3) a visual-spatial-perceptual disorder group with visual-constructive problems but intact oral language; and (4) a group with difficulty sequencing sounds (dysphonemic group).

B. Mathematics Disorders (Developmental Dyscalculia): Mathematics disorders have been studied primarily in relation to the Gerstmann syndrome (dyscalculia, right-left disorientation, and finger agnosia) and often have been considered to be part of a reading disorder. However, limited studies of school children who demonstrate a discrepancy between actual and expected achievement in arithmetic suggest that a specific syndrome of mathematical disability does exist and affects approximately 6% of the population. Developmental disorder is distinguished from acquired disorder by the absence of clearly defined brain damage and neurologic findings in the former.

Several types have been described and are characterized by difficulty in verbalizing, writing, reading, manipulating, or understanding mathematical operations. In individuals whose difficulties are confined to performance on numerical tests, signs of neurologic abnormalities tend to be few. In those who are unable to read or write numbers, the disorder may be associated with general disorders in reading and writing as well as mathematics, so that a learning disorder specific to mathematics may be difficult to demonstrate.

C. Writing Disorders (Developmental Dysgraphia): Children with reading problems often have illegible handwriting and spelling problems. In younger children, problems due to immature perceptual-motor development (eg, mirror writing, reversal of letters, and poor construction of letters) are common. Some children have problems confined to illegible handwriting, inaccurate copying, or inability to transmit sequences of verbal information onto paper. In some of these instances, illegibility is associated with deficits in fine motor coordination. Whether encountered alone or in combination with reading or math disability, specific training is often required to correct the penmanship problems.

A common syndrome seen in students during late elementary and junior high school involves not only elements of poor handwriting (slow, illegible, poor spatial organization) but also deficits in memory, expressive language, organization of ideas, and fluency. This has been termed "developmental output failure"; it is usually manifested by overall reduced pro-

Table 3–4. Differential diagnosis of learning problems.

Type of Learning Problem	Characteristics	Treatment Issues
Disorders with IQ-achievement discrepancy	Achievement is below IQ in an isolated area. The disorder is not caused by sensory impairment. Other areas are at level of expectancy.	Individualized instruction (often tutoring) in area of weakness should be provided. Normalized educational experiences in other areas are indicated.
Reading/spelling (dyslexia)	Achievement is below expectancy only in reading/spelling.	Specific instruction in reading/spelling/language arts is indicated. The child often exhibits generalized deficits in language processing. The child may have problems in math because of reading.
Arithmetic (dyscalculia)	Achievement is below expectancy only in arithmetic.	Specific instruction in math is indicated. Dsycalculia may be difficult to separate from a reading or writing disorder.
Writing (dysgraphia)	Achievement is below expectancy in written work.	Status of visual functioning must be clarified. Specific treatment for handwriting skills is indicated. Dysgraphia is often difficult to separate from dyslexia.
Hyperflexia	The child begins reading at a very early age (eg, 2 years). The child may appear autistic or show unusual discrepancies in abilities.	Comprehensive assessment and treatment in several areas of weakness is necessary. The prognosis for the autistic child is relatively good.
Nonspecific learning disorders: Underachievement	Achievement is below IQ in several areas. Underachievement may be caused by environmental, behavioral (eg, ADHD), motivational, or situational problems, or school absence.	The child often has emotional/behavior problems as well.
Generalized learning disability	Achievement is below IQ in several areas. The disability is not caused by sensory impairment. The disability is often accompanied by evidence of visual/perceptual/motor difficulties. Associated environmental, emotional/behavioral, or motivational problems are often present.	Unusual combinations of discrepant functioning may be a reflection of abnormal brain functioning.
Disorders without IQ-achievement discrepancy Slow learner	IQ and achievement are commensurate but at low-normal to below-normal levels.	Learning is slow but steady with appropriate programming.
Mental retardation	Both IQ and achievement are more than 2 SD below average.	
Educable	IQ is usually 50–70.	The child is capable of achieving rudiments of literacy.
Trainable	IQ is usually below 50.	The child is capable of acquiring preacademic and vocational skills.

ductivity, with refusals to complete work, failure to submit assignments, and "forgetting" to do homework.

Left-handed children deserve special attention because they have frequently had poor instruction. In most instances, their problems in penmanship will improve with appropriate instruction. Despite common belief to the contrary, there is little evidence associating left-handedness with any cognitive deficiency.

Etiologic Classification of Learning Disabilities

Both psychobiologic and sociopsychologic factors appear to play a major causative role in learning disabilities. Children who fail to learn despite conventional instruction, adequate familial-cultural opportunity, and adequate intelligence are thought to represent an idiopathic or genetic syndrome. This group is distinguished from children with emotional, educational, or cultural limitations or those with disorders secondary to sensory defects, brain damage, or mental retardation.

In the idiopathic group, the term "minimal brain dysfunction (MBD)" is often used when neurologic soft signs, poor motor coordination, and distractibility are present along with learning problems in children of average or above-average intelligence. Because research has failed to confirm neurologic dysfunction and because many of the characteristics taken singly are common in preschool children and tend to be present only in younger learning-disabled children, many commentators have abandoned the concept of minimal brain damage in favor of the view that the problem is one of immaturity.

Clinical Findings

A family history often turns up affected family members, especially among the males. With the exception of soft signs, the physical examination is usually normal. Behavior problems may be present. Intelligence test results often indicate average or above-average intelligence on nonverbal tests and may show some decrease in verbal IQ. In contrast, achievement in the affected area of learning is significantly below nonverbal intelligence and sometimes below verbal intelligence. Achievement in nonaffected areas tends to progress normally. Vision and hearing are usually normal, though deficits in processing auditory sequential information are often noted on extensive testing. Etiologic diagnosis is more difficult. The most important distinction is whether there is a strong family history, inadequate educational background, sociocultural disadvantage, or evidence of neurologic disease.

Treatment

Claims that instruction should be tailored to the subtype of reading disorder are not supported by research. There are basically three approaches to teaching children to read. First, many special educators use a bottom-up approach to developing reading skills—ie, children learn to identify letters, to match sounds and letters, to develop a basic sight word vocabulary, to apply sound and letter matches to novel words, and finally to read words in textual matter. This approach has been favored by special educators on the assumption that breaking down reading into simpler discrimination tasks that lend themselves to routinized drills will increase the learner's success rate.

A second approach assumes that learning to read is a language development task and therefore follows the same developmental sequence that occurs when young children learn to speak. Thus, reading is taught from a holistic perspective in which teachers help children make the connection between spoken words that describe the world around them to printed words and phrases. Children are exposed to repeated readings of simple books and encouraged to read along with the teacher. Comprehension rather than word recall is stressed. This approach also emphasizes the concurrent development of writing, since writing is the expressive aspect of reading. Rather than focusing on the mechanics of spelling, children are urged to write using invented spelling to understand the notion of written or printed words as visual referents to spoken words.

There is no statistical difference between the effectiveness of these two approaches. Thus, a careful assessment of individual needs should dictate the strategies used to help a child learn to read. A third approach, which combines emphasis on phonics with the semantic and experiential elements of comprehension, may be the most efficient means of teaching a child to read.

With the variety of approaches available, selection of the best approach for a particular child may require a series of learning trials. Most children will begin to demonstrate learning after four to six lessons. General principles for ensuring progress include introduction of phonics or word attack skills at some level of teaching, mastery of less difficult material before proceeding to more difficult material, and continuation of instruction over a long enough period for results to be long-lasting.

A minority of children fail to learn how to read despite individual instruction. For these children, a focus on goals that will ensure maximal independence as adults is vital even in the primary grades. Special education efficacy studies (eg, Kavale, 1982; Shepard, 1983) suggest that much of special education has inadequately addressed outcomes for the community (ie, employment and independent living), for individuals (ie, heightened self-esteem, community membership status), and for schools (ie, efficient delivery of services).

Prognosis

With or without individual instruction, only a minority of children remain nonreaders into adulthood. There are, however, many adolescents and adults who read poorly. The ultimate skill level usually depends on intelligence, the type and amount of individual instruction provided, the age at which remediation is started, motivation, and the child's general emotional state. In some adults, poor spelling may be the only stigma of a childhood reading problem, whereas other adults may continue to have problems in reading and general language skills as well. Even with individual instruction, progress is often slow—sometimes slower than progress being made by children described as slow learners. In children with specific learning disorders, however, progress in unaffected areas of achievement tends to proceed at a normal pace.

Kavale KA, Glass GV: The efficacy of special education interventions and practices: A compendium of meta-analysis findings. Focus Except Child 1982;15:1.

Kosc L: Developmental dyscalculia. J Learn Disab 1974;7:164.

Myklebust HR (editor): *Progress in Learning Disabilities,* vols 1–5. Grune & Stratton, 1983.

Rutter M (editor): *Developmental Neuropsychiatry.* Guilford, 1983.

Shepard LA, Smith LA, Vojir CP: Characteristics of pupils identified as learning disabled. J Spec Educ 1983;16:73.

Stahl S, Miller P: Whole language and language experience: Approaches for beginning reading: A quantitative research synthesis. Rev Educ Res 1989;59:87.

Pennington BF: Diagnosing Learning Disorders: A Neuropsychological Framework. Guilford Press, 1991.

THE SLOW LEARNER

The average IQ of children in this group tends to be in the 80s. Approximately 11% have neurologic dysfunction, 25% show questionable neurologic findings, and 60% have difficulty in copying geometric figures. Clumsiness, motor impersistence, and right-left confusion are twice as common in slow learners as in children with specific learning disorders. Forty percent have at least one sign of language delay (eg, first phrases after 24 months). The frequency of neurodevelopmental problems increases in children with lower IQs.

Clinical Findings

The most important characteristic of the slow learner is lack of a significant discrepancy between intelligence and achievement. These children are often low-average to borderline in intelligence, and achievement is slow but commensurate with mental age. The child is most often slow in all areas of achievement, but achievement in one area may be slower than in others. The lower the child's intelligence, the more one is likely to find evidence of neurodevelopmental problems and associated behavior problems. The history often reveals evidence of developmental delays, especially in the language area. A family history of school problems may be present. In the absence of a positive family history, problems during the pregnancy, advanced maternal age, or difficulties in the newborn period are often cited as possible causes of early brain damage that might explain the presence of such a child in a well-educated family.

Treatment

Educational programming that uses the community, school, and family for planning the curriculum often makes more sense for slow learners than the traditional academic curriculum. Families should be asked to participate in curriculum planning by identifying what they would like their child to be able to do in 3 years. By including the family in educational planning, recognition and acceptance of the child's capacities is made easier. Counseling or short-term psychotherapy can assist the family in dealing with feelings of denial or guilt. The school may have developed an appropriate educational plan for the child, and treatment needs to be directed toward helping the family accept the school's plan.

Prognosis

Given an opportunity to progress at their own rate, slow learners tend to make steady progress commensurate with their mental age. In many instances, long-term follow-up shows that these children make better progress in their areas of deficiency than do children with specific learning disorders.

NONSPECIFIC & EMOTIONALLY BASED LEARNING DISORDERS

Included in this group are the large numbers of children with learning disorders in association with psychiatric disorders, familial-cultural problems of motivation, and neurologic disorders such as epilepsy, structural brain abnormalities, and head injury. A significant discrepancy between intelligence and achievement may exist in one or more areas, or the child may be generally slow. Family problems are usually apparent, and children frequently come from culturally disadvantaged homes and large families. These children have many of the same educational needs as children with specific learning disorders, but they have been excluded from federally supported services for education of the learning disabled.

Differential Diagnosis

Differentiation from specific learning disabilities is made primarily on the basis of identifying motivational and emotional problems in the absence of specific learning problems in children with average or above-average intelligence. Slow learners or mentally retarded children with emotional problems may be indistinguishable. The most difficult differential diagnosis is between specific reading disabilities in an emotionally disturbed child and an emotionally based learning disability concentrated in the language area.

Children with head injury or brain damage may not present a diagnostic problem. Often, however, the pattern of performance on psychologic tests—particularly those that are sensitive to disturbances in cortical functioning—may be the only evidence pointing to brain dysfunction. Neurologic tests such as EEGs or CT scans are seldom of diagnostic usefulness.

Treatment

School systems in the United States are required by federal law to provide services to students who, through school-based diagnostic procedures, are labeled as emotionally disturbed. Services range from the development and implementation of behavior modification programs to full-day classes that serve students with these disorders. Curriculum components generally include manipulations of the instructional environment such as shortened or simplified academic task and cooperative learning groups. A second curriculum component focus is on the management of aggressive or out-of-control behaviors through cognitive behavior modification and behavior control training. In addition, a curriculum that addresses the development of social and affective skills should be a component of programming. A final ingredient in programs for students with emotional problems is counseling. The effectiveness of these programs is generally related to the skill of the multidisciplinary team assigned to the program. Services should reflect the needs of the student rather than a generic approach that treats all children with emotional disturbances in a similar fashion.

MENTAL RETARDATION

Mental retardation is defined as significantly subaverage intellectual functioning existing concurrently with deficits of adaptive behavior manifested in early life. Significantly subaverage intelligence is defined as 2 SD or more below average (IQ < 70 on the Wechsler scales or < 69 on the Stanford-Binet test) and affects approximately 2–3% of the general population. Another 6% are considered borderline in intelligence (IQ 70–79). Adaptive deficiency is less easily evaluated.

About 10% of the retarded population are identified during infancy and early childhood. Most fall in the moderate to profound retardation group (IQ below 50), and most have clear-cut evidence of brain damage, genetic disorder, or other pathologic conditions. Moderate to profound retardation is distributed equally among different socioeconomic groups but is more common in males than in females.

The remaining 90% of the retarded population tend to be mildly retarded (IQ 50–69), and most are not identified before entering school, partly because of insufficient efforts at earlier identification. The great majority of those with mild handicaps are diagnosed as cultural-familial retardates. They come from families characterized by low intelligence and low socioeconomic status. Many who are mildly handicapped and identified primarily during the school years eventually blend into society and become at least marginally adequate citizens.

Mildly retarded children (IQ 50–69) are considered educable and in many instances can function without major supportive services. Moderately retarded children (IQ 30–49) are considered trainable but require protective care (sheltered workshops, guardians, group homes). More recently, public schools in the United States have been required to provide services to members of this group. Severely to profoundly retarded children (IQ < 30) usually require continuous care. This group includes the most severely deformed, nonambulatory, and minimally communicative individuals. Educational programs at all levels of disability stress providing an appropriate education in the least restrictive environment possible.

Etiologic Considerations

A. Genetic:

1. Inborn errors of metabolism–Aminoacidopathies, cerebral lipidoses, mucopolysaccharidoses, disorders of carbohydrate metabolism.

2. Chromosome disorders–Autosomal disorders, sex chromosome disorders such as fragile X syndrome.

B. Intrauterine: Congenital infections, placental-fetal malfunction, complications of pregnancy (maternal malnutrition, preeclampsia-eclampsia, use of drugs or radiation, intrauterine growth retardation).

C. Perinatal: Prematurity, postmaturity, metabolic disorders (hypoglycemia, hyperbilirubinemia).

D. Postnatal: Endocrinopathies, metabolic disorders, trauma, infections, poisoning, maltreatment.

E. Cultural-Familial: Low family intelligence, environmental deprivation.

Clinical Findings

A. History: In infants and preschool children with developmental delays, there may be evidence of a genetic syndrome or factors in the prenatal or perinatal period that can account for delay. There may also be evidence of maternal deprivation or neglect, particularly among children who are only mildly or moderately delayed. The older the child at the time of diagnosis, the more likely it is that retardation will be explained by deficiencies in early experience or by familial-cultural factors. Even when there are other family members with similar problems, a genetic basis for the retardation often cannot be established. Mentally retarded children who are not diagnosed as such until after entering school often have a history of normal development in the first 2 years, and siblings may show a similar decline in relative competency as they grow older. Children who come from nondominant cultural backgrounds often show adequate functioning on measures of adaptation despite poor performance on standard intelligence tests.

If disruptive and antisocial behavior problems are absent, children who show relatively good adaptability tend to blend into society after leaving school despite subnormal intelligence.

B. Symptoms and Signs: In mental retardation, the developmental or intellectual performance is at least 2 SD below the mean, and there is evidence of limitation in adaptability. In preschool children, delay diagnosed on developmental screening tests may be the principal finding. Sensory defects are also common, as are speech and language problems, motor handicaps, neurodevelopmental delays, seizure disorders, and behavior problems. Signs of significant developmental delay, including deficiencies in adaptation, will often be evident by age 2 years.

Once the child reaches school age, general adaptation and achievement in all areas tend to be low but commensurate with mental age. Children with low IQs who are not retarded on measures of adaptation should not be diagnosed as mentally retarded. Occasionally, a mildly retarded or borderline child will show a significant discrepancy between actual and expected achievement in one academic area more than in others. This may technically represent a specific learning disability; however, if the child's overall intelligence is low enough (IQ < 70), special education will be indicated in any case. Maltreatment and other negative family experiences may result in bizarre behavior and emotional disturbance that are difficult to distinguish from autistic or psychotic behavior. Mentally retarded children often mirror disturbances going on within the family. The appearance of unusual behavior, sexual acting out, or bizarre activity in an otherwise stable retarded child is often an indication of a disturbance in the family.

C. Special Studies: General rules for ordering tests include laboratory testing for diagnosis of treatable conditions when an etiologic diagnosis is unknown (eg, amino acid or organic acid screen) and other tests such as electroencephalography, skull films, and chromosome studies if clinical findings suggest specific diseases or syndromes.

Differential Diagnosis

After a descriptive diagnosis is made of mental retardation, the database should provide enough information so that a decision can be made on how far to pursue an etiologic diagnosis. It is particularly important to distinguish the deaf, blind, and orthopedically handicapped from the mentally retarded. This is often difficult, since many retarded children also have sensory and orthopedic handicaps. It is also difficult to differentiate between autism and retardation in very young children since there can be overlap between the two.

Management

Mental retardation usually is diagnosed after a significant period of developmental delay has been ob-

served. The older the child at the time of diagnosis, the less the likelihood of reversing retardation even when a treatable cause is identified. Prevention is therefore the only significant approach to treatment. A screening program for early detection of inborn errors of metabolism and institution of treatment before significant damage to the nervous system can occur represents the model approach. This same model has been used in developing preventive programs for children at risk for familial-cultural retardation. Controlled studies of stimulation programs for infants in sociocultural groups with high rates of mental retardation have shown significant long-range results after termination of the program in the following circumstances: (1) when the parents have been involved in the program, (2) when the infant participated in the program frequently (once every 2 weeks or more), and (3) when the program continued for at least 2 years. The Head Start Program for preschool children has been shown to decrease the number of children in special education classes and to increase the number of children from high-risk populations who remain in school.

In most instances, management of the retarded child does not involve treatment of the retardation per se but must be directed toward assessing the impact on the family and on providing support and psychotherapy, protection for the child, education and rehabilitation to maximize the child's potential, and treatment of associated medical, emotional, and behavior problems.

A. Impact on the Family: The diagnosis of mental retardation is an event for which few families are prepared. Parents can often assess the mental age of their child within a few months but still refuse to accept the implications of this information. The tact and sensitivity with which the initial discussion of developmental delay is broached can determine how early appropriate treatment, education, and rehabilitation can be started. The primary care physician should be alert to parents' initial questions about developmental delays and pursue their initial concerns. A second opinion or repeated evaluation is almost mandatory when the impression of significant developmental delay arises unexpectedly from screening tests or school observations. After the diagnosis is confirmed, the family will need continued assistance and support in adjusting to the diagnosis and in making contact with community resources.

Retarded children and adults can usually remain within the family but may require help from family and community support services. These often include municipal social service agencies, infant education programs, occupational and physical therapy programs, and services for handicapped infants that can be started as early as the newborn period. In school-age children, most services are organized through public school systems, but the primary care physician may be called on to assist at times of crisis.

Once a severely handicapped child is "accepted" by the family, family resources may be totally consumed by the child's needs, often to the detriment of normal siblings. Professionals involved with these families should provide help in developing priorities and alleviating parental guilt at being unable to do everything everyone suggests for the child. Less severely handicapped children are often less apt to be accepted by the family, with resulting conflict and emotional disturbance as parents attempt to deny the evidence of retardation or seek more comfortable explanations for the child's delays. Parent support groups have been particularly helpful to families with retarded children.

B. Protection, Education, and Rehabilitation: The schools have responsibility for providing educational services to mentally retarded students ages 3–21 years in the least restrictive, most normalized environment in which the individual can reasonably be expected to receive educational benefit. Regardless of the extent of the disability, the judicial system has interpreted the provisions of the Individuals With Disabilities Act (IDEA), Part B of Public Law 101 to mean that all children—even those with the most profound mental retardation—must be served through the local public school system. Students with disabilities who are enrolled in private or parochial schools are also entitled to receive services through the local public school system. As a result, most metropolitan, suburban, and small school districts provide services for these students. Multidisciplinary teams trained to work with these individuals have responsibility for such health care procedures as catheterization, tube feeding, and so on. Motor and language therapists work in concert with special education teachers to provide programs that focus on increasing levels of personal care, daily living skills, social interaction, and communication. Many schools provide opportunities for interaction with nondisabled peers to increase the quality of life and natural supports for individuals with profound disabilities and to increase the capacity of children without disabilities to understand and appreciate the spectrum of human diversity. Where children with mental retardation have additional cognitive capacities, the opportunities for interaction with typical peers are increased. However, the curriculum continues to focus on developing functional independent living skills.

As children with mental retardation become adolescents, school personnel are required by law to plan for their transition from school to adult life. Multidisciplinary teams must identify specific goals that address support or independent work and residential needs into individualized educational plans. Adult human service agencies must be involved in these transition plans by the time the student reaches the age of 16 years. Passed in 1990, the Americans With Disabilities Act (ADA) ensures that employers must make accommodations for workers with disabilities, including individuals with mental retardation. Furthermore, ADA specifies that transportation systems and businesses that serve the public must provide access and services to individuals with all types of disabilities. Human services agencies funded to provide resources and services to adults with developmental disabilities, including mental retardation, continue to serve more and more profoundly disabled individuals in nonsheltered environments.

C. Treatment of Associated Medical, Emotional, and Behavior Problems: Sensory, motor, and orthopedic handicaps and other medical problems should be treated appropriately. The most controversial area of management concerns the use of psychotropic medication for treatment of emotional and behavior problems, especially in institutionalized retarded children. In the past phenothiazines have been the most commonly used medications. Currently, taking into consideration the misuse and overuse of such medications, this class of drugs is currently being avoided in favor of mood stabilizers, antidepressants, and selective serotonin reuptake inhibitors. To ensure the success of psychotropic medication in the mentally retarded—or any child considered for such treatment—an appropriate drug and dosage should selected on the basis of an accurate emotional or behavioral diagnosis, and the patient's response to the medication should be carefully monitored through direct observation.

MOTOR HANDICAPS

An estimated 6–7% of the population shows clumsiness, awkwardness, choreiform movements, or generally poor coordination but with no signs of systemic disease except for an increased incidence of other soft signs on neurologic examination. Many children in this group also show evidence of learning problems, and the motor problems have been cited as evidence of a neurologic basis for the learning problems. However, as with soft signs in general, this interpretation is controversial.

Clumsiness and awkwardness have also been reported in association with attention deficit disorder. In this instance, treatment with stimulant medications has frequently been accompanied by improvement in motor coordination. Occupational and physical therapy are often recommended for these children, though there are no adequately controlled studies to support the efficacy of these approaches for improving educational achievement. There is clear evidence that instruction in reading is better than perceptual-motor training in improving reading ability irrespective of the child's motor status. The area of mild motor disability has received so little formal scrutiny that much is yet to be learned about ways of identifying and ameliorating developmental impairments in motor skills.

Guralnick M: *The Effectiveness of Early Intervention.* Brooks, 1997.

Hagerman RJ: Medical follow-up and pharmacology. In: *Fragile X Syndrome: Diagnosis, Treatment and Research.* Hagerman RD, Cronister A (editors). Johns Hopkins University Press, 1996.

Rapin I: Autism. N Engl J Med 1997;337:97.

Schater FF, Stone RK (editors): *Practical Concerns About Siblings: Bridging the Research-Practice Gap.* Haworth Press, 1987.

Zigler E, Muenchow S: *Head Start: The Inside Story of America's Most Successful Educational Experiment.* Basic Books, 1992.

DEVELOPMENTAL & ADAPTATIONAL PROBLEMS

Developmental and adaptational problems are behavior problems that in normal children decline steadily with age. Manifestations include fears, distractibility, hyperactivity, destructiveness, lying, negativism, temper tantrums, enuresis, and thumb-sucking. Children with these manifestations rarely show maladjustment later in life. Absence of these manifestations, however, does not rule out later maladjustment. The gradual decline in these behavior problems is associated with maturation of cognitive competence, including not only intelligence but moral maturity and ego development as well. When deficiencies in social character and cognitive adaptability persist beyond the early school years, the prognosis for improvement is less favorable. The most common of these problems is attention deficit hyperactivity disorder.

ATTENTION DEFICIT HYPERACTIVITY DISORDER

Attention deficit hyperactivity disorder (ADHD) is characterized by distractibility, short attention span, and impulsiveness. The incidence is about 5%, and the disorder is more common in boys than in girls. Most of the children previously labeled hyperactive or said to have minimal brain dysfunction are children with ADHD. Attention span and ability to concentrate on cognitive tasks usually increase throughout childhood. The ability of preschool children to engage in sustained task-oriented behavior is one of the most reliable predictors of later school performance. Some evidence suggests that even in infants, attention span may be an early indication of later cognitive performance. In older children, attentiveness is one of the major characteristics of competent children with good peer relations.

The child who continues to have immature attentional behavior after age mates have matured is noticeably out of phase in cognitively and socially stressful situations, particularly at school. Such children may engage in aimless activity. Some display hyperactive behavior at home, on the playground, and in the physician's office as well as in the classroom. Some children with ADHD are described as hypoactive rather than hyperactive but are inattentive nevertheless.

The causes of attention deficit hyperactivity disorder are not well understood, though there is evidence of a genetic or constitutional basis for the problem in many children. The diagnosis is largely descriptive, but it implies that specific causes of distractibility and short attention span (eg, neurologic injury, emotional trauma, psychosis, depression) have been eliminated. Immaturity in development of the central nervous system is one of the most likely underlying causes of the problem. However, most children with ADHD have no neurologic abnormalities or abnormal findings on electroencephalography. The presence of neurodevelopmental signs has not been consistently related to treatment outcome.

Clinical Findings

A. History: The most important diagnostic information comes from a description of behavior in the classroom and teacher ratings on a scale such as ACTeRS (Table 3–2). Ratings on this scale that fall below the tenth percentile on attention, hyperactivity, or both, regardless of ratings on the other scales, are usually indicative of attention deficit hyperactivity disorder. If problems with attention or hyperactivity are not evident at school, it is very unlikely that the child has ADHD. Physicians worried about teacher bias in completing the rating should seek evaluations from several teachers. Teacher ratings are usually in agreement, whereas parental assessments often differ. It is useful to review information about oppositional behavior and social skills and obtain information about intelligence and academic performance, because many children with ADHD also show other behavior or learning problems. The most common behavior problem is aggressive or oppositional defiant disorder. The family history often reveals similar problems in other members, particularly males. Children with attention deficit disorder are frequently described as having been active, colicky infants, and parents typically report distractibility and hyperactivity in the preschool period. However, ADHD is usually first recognized as a problem after a child enters school. The diagnosis can sometimes be made with great confidence in preschool children, but the children's behaviors reflect a lack of adequate parental management or the presence of affective disturbances.

B. Symptoms and Signs: The neurologic examination may show signs of neurologic immaturity.

There are usually no sensory impairments, but a significant number of these children have learning problems that may be general or specific. ADHD occurs at all intellectual levels, but achievement is often adequate among children of average intelligence with behavior problems confined to ADHD despite teacher complaints that the child is "not learning." When a learning problem accompanies a behavior problem, the problems need to be addressed concurrently. Family problems may contribute to ADHD and increase the difficulty of treatment, especially in children who show aggressive behavior. ADHD is excluded when a diagnosis of childhood psychotic disorder has been made, but ADHD may occur in mentally retarded children.

C. Special Studies: Tests measuring continuous performance or vigilance have been widely used in research on children with ADHD. These tests usually require that the child look for occurrences of one specified design among many, either on a page or sequentially flashed on a screen. Two such vigilance tests (with norms) are commercially available for electronic administration. Nevertheless, the clinical application of these procedures is incompletely worked out. No other special tests aid in diagnosis. If there is a question of seizure disorder or clear evidence of neurologic disorder, investigation of these conditions is indicated.

Treatment

Treatment of ADHD may require both behavior modification and drugs. Stimulant drugs such as methylphenidate, dextroamphetamine, and pemoline are widely used. Tricyclic antidepressants, antianxiety drugs, and selective serotonergic reuptake inhibitors are also used. Drug treatment, if effective, tends to have more dramatic results than behavior modification. Drugs can be used effectively in combination.

Approximately 50–80% of children with ADHD respond to stimulant drug therapy. Dose-response studies on methylphenidate suggest that a dosage of 0.3 mg/kg/d produces optimal cognitive improvement (concentration) as well as significant improvement in social behavior. Greater improvement in social behavior can be achieved with higher doses, but this occurs at the expense of some loss in concentration and the increased risk of side effects such as anorexia and insomnia. Peak action usually occurs 2 hours after ingestion, and most effects have dissipated after 6 hours. The usual regimen is to start with an early morning dose, followed by a dose at noon if needed. Morning activities often require the most concentration, and the noon dose may be unnecessary. If problems at home are severe, a third dose may be given in the late afternoon. Dextroamphetamine and methylphenidate are similar in onset and duration of action, and most children who respond to one will respond to the other. Pemoline appears to have a later onset of action, and dosage often requires adjustment over a longer period of time.

The most common adverse reactions to stimulant drug therapy are decreased appetite, headache, stomachache, emotional lability, and insomnia. When these side effects appear early in the course of treatment, they are often transient or respond to dosage reduction. It is sometimes difficult to determine whether they are indeed medication-related; however, when in doubt, the best approach is to stop or change the medication. All of the stimulants have the potential for exacerbating motor and phonic tics and Tourette's syndrome but do not cause these disorders. Dextroamphetamine is contraindicated and methylphenidate is used cautiously in the presence of hypertension. Pemoline is contraindicated in patients with impaired hepatic function. Pemoline has also been linked to a hypersensitivity reaction that may result in jaundice and an elevation of liver enzymes. There had been concern that stimulant medications might lead to growth retardation, but this has not been confirmed. Nevertheless, linear growth and weight gain should be closely monitored.

Monitoring for side effects should be continuous. Weekly teacher reports (ACTeRS) during the first month are helpful for monitoring and evaluating treatment. The child should be reevaluated at 1 month to determine whether the response is sufficient to justify continuing with medication.

Prognosis

With or without treatment, the long-term outcome is better in the more intelligent children with stable families and uncomplicated ADHD. These children may only require short-term treatment (usually 2 years or less). In recent years, increasing emphasis has been placed on recognizing and treating adolescents and adults who continue to be symptomatic.

American Academy of Pediatrics Committee on Children With Disabilities and Committee on Drugs: Medication for child attentional disorders. Pediatrics 1996;98:301.

Baren M: ADHD: Do we finally have it right. Contemp Pediatr 1994(Nov);11:96.

Baren M: Managing ADHD. Contemp Pediatr 1994(Dec);11:29.

Ingersoll B: *Your Hyperactive Child: A Parent's Guide to Coping With Attention Deficit Disorders.* Doubleday, 1988.

Wender PH: *The Hyperactive Child, Adolescent, and Adult.* Oxford Univ Press, 1987.

4

Adolescence

David W. Kaplan, MD, MPH, & Kathleen A. Mammel, MD

Adolescence is a period of rapid physical, emotional, cognitive, and social growth and development. Generally, adolescence begins at age 11–12 years and ends between ages 18 and 21. Most teenagers complete puberty by 16–18 years; in Western society, however, for educational and cultural reasons, the adolescent period is prolonged to allow for further psychosocial development before the individual assumes adult responsibilities.

The developmental passage from childhood to adulthood encompasses the following steps: (1) completing puberty and somatic growth; (2) developing socially, emotionally, and cognitively—moving from concrete to abstract thinking; (3) establishing an independent identity and separating from the family; and (4) preparing for a career or vocation.

DEMOGRAPHY

In the United States in 1997, there were 19 million adolescents between the ages of 15 and 19 years and 17.3 million between 20 and 24 years of age. Adolescents and young adults (15–24 years of age) constitute 14% of the U.S. population.

MORTALITY DATA

There has been a remarkable decrease in the mortality rate among 15- to 24-year-olds during this century. Deaths resulting from infectious diseases such as tuberculosis, influenza, and pneumonia, which were common at the beginning of the century, are rare today. For the adolescent population, cultural and environmental rather than organic factors pose the greatest threats of early demise. The three leading causes of death in the adolescent population (ages 15–19 years) in 1995 were unintentional injury (42.7–78% of all unintentional injuries were caused by motor vehicle crashes), suicides (14.4%), and homicides (22.3%). These three causes of violent death accounted for 78%

of all adolescent deaths among 15- to 19-year-olds. Homicide is the leading cause of death for black adolescents aged 15–19 years, accounting for 49.2% of all deaths. Deaths resulting from homicide among black 15- to 19-year-olds increased 260% between 1983 and 1995. In 1995, 39.7% of all deaths among adolescent males aged 15–19 years were due to homicide and suicide. Although deaths from automobile crashes have decreased over the last few years, alcohol use remains the underlying cause of most teenage motor vehicle deaths. Almost two-thirds of motor vehicle deaths involving young drinking drivers occur on Friday, Saturday, or Sunday, and 70% occur between 8:00 PM and 4:00 AM.

MORBIDITY DATA

Demographic and economic changes in the American family since the mid 1970s have had a profound effect on children and adolescents. Between 1955 and 1990, the divorce rate rose from about 400,000 to nearly 1.2 million a year. Between 1960 and 1990, the number of children involved in divorce each year increased from 460,000 to 1.1 million. From 1990 to 1995, 20.8% of children and adolescents under the age of 18 years in the United States were living below the poverty level, compared with 12% in 1970. In 1995, 41.9% of black, 40% of Hispanic, and 16.2% of white children under 18 years of age lived in families with incomes below the poverty level.

The major causes of morbidity during adolescence are psychosocial: unintended pregnancy, sexually transmitted disease (STD), substance abuse, smoking, dropping out of school, depression, running away from home, physical violence, and juvenile delinquency. High-risk behavior in one area is often associated with problems in another (Figure 4–1). For example, teenagers who live in a dysfunctional family (eg, problems related to drinking or physical or sexual abuse) are much more likely than other teenagers to be depressed. A depressed teenager is at greater risk for

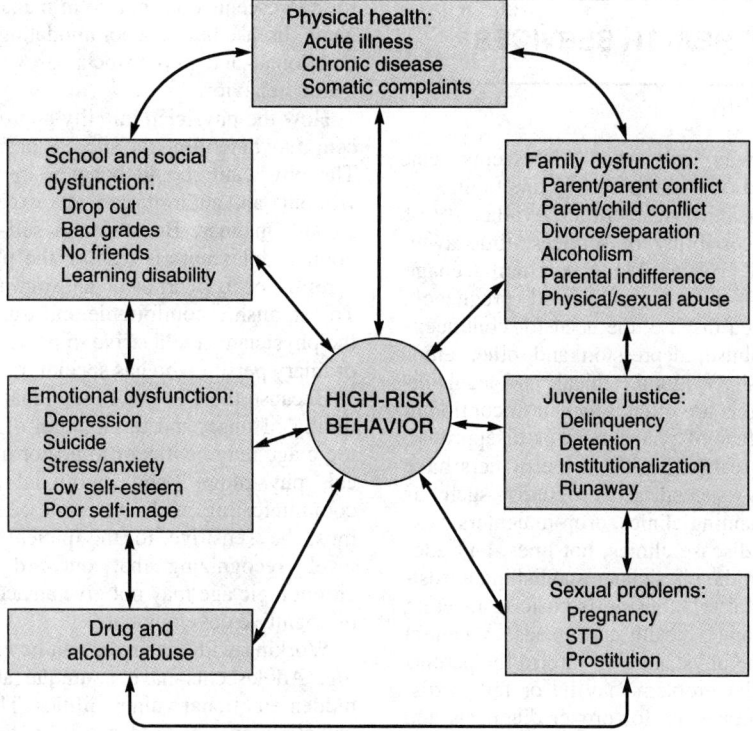

Figure 4–1. Interrelation of high-risk adolescent behavior.

drug and alcohol abuse, academic failure, inappropriate sexual activity, STDs, pregnancy, and suicide.

Early identification of the teenager at risk for these problems is important to prevent immediate complications and future associated problems. The early indicators of high risk for problems related to depression include the following:

(1) Decline in school performance.

(2) Excessive school absences or cutting class.

(3) Frequent or persistent psychosomatic complaints.

(4) Changes in sleeping or eating habits.

(5) Difficulty in concentrating or persistent boredom.

(6) Signs or symptoms of depression, extreme stress, or anxiety.

(7) Withdrawal from friends or family, or change to a new group of friends.

(8) Unusually severe violent or rebellious behavior, or radical personality change.

(9) Conflict with parents.

(10) Sexual acting-out.

(11) Conflicts with the law.

(12) Suicidal thoughts or preoccupation with themes of death.

(13) Drug and alcohol abuse.

(14) Running away from home.

American Academy of Pediatrics Committee on Adolescence: Firearms and adolescents. Pediatrics 1992;89: 784.

Hechinger FM: *Fateful Choices: Healthy Youth for the 21st Century.* Carnegie Corporation of New York, 1992.

Monthly Vital Statistics Report, Births and Deaths: United States, 1996. Centers for Disease Control and Prevention/National Center for Health Statistics, 1997;46 (Suppl 2):1.

Monthly Vital Statistics Report, Report of Final Mortality Statistics, 1995. Centers for Disease Control and Prevention/National Center for Health Statistics, 1997;45 (Suppl 2):11.

Ozer EM et al: *America's Adolescents: Are They Healthy?* San Francisco, California, University of California, San Francisco, National Adolescent Health Information Center, 1997.

Millstein SG, Petersen AC, Nightingale EO: *Promoting the Health of Adolescents: New Directions for the Twenty-First Century.* Oxford Univ Press, 1993.

Resnick MD et al: Protecting adolescents from harm: Findings from the national longitudinal study on adolescent health. JAMA 1997;

Stella CW, Blum R: Morbidity and mortality among US adolescents: An overview of data and trends. Am J Public Health 1996;86:513.

Wood DL et al: Access to medical care for children and adolescents in the United States. Pediatrics 1990;86:666.

DELIVERY OF HEALTH SERVICES

How, where, why, and when adolescents seek health care depend on a number of factors: ability to pay, distance to health care facilities, availability of transportation, accessibility of services, time away from school, and privacy. Many common teenage health problems—such as unintended pregnancy, sexually transmitted disease, the need for contraception, substance abuse, depression and other emotional problems—have moral, ethical, and legal implications. Teenagers are often reluctant to confide in their parents for fear of punishment or disapproval. Recognizing this reality, health care providers have established many specialized programs such as teenage family planning clinics, drop-in centers, sexually transmitted disease clinics, hot lines, and adolescent clinics. For the physician, establishing a trusting and confidential relationship is basic to meeting an adolescent patient's health care needs. A patient who senses that the physician will inform the parents about a confidential problem may lie or fail to disclose information essential for proper diagnosis and treatment.

GUIDELINES FOR ADOLESCENT PREVENTIVE SERVICES

The AMA guidelines for adolescent preventive services (GAPS) cover health screening and guidance, immunization, and health care delivery. The goals are (1) to deter adolescents from participating in behaviors that jeopardize health; (2) to detect physical, emotional, and behavioral problems early and intervene promptly; (3) to reinforce and encourage behaviors that promote healthful living; and (4) to provide immunization against infectious diseases. The guidelines recommend that adolescents between the ages of 11 and 21 have annual routine health visits. Health services should be developmentally appropriate and culturally sensitive, and confidentiality between patient and physician should be ensured. A complete schedule of the recommended guidelines is shown in Figure 4–2A.

RELATING TO THE ADOLESCENT PATIENT

Adolescence is one of the physically healthiest periods in an individual's life. The challenge of caring for adolescents does not lie in managing complex organic disease but in accommodating to the cognitive, emotional, and psychosocial growth that influences health behavior.

How the physician initially approaches the adolescent may determine the success or failure of the visit. The physician should behave simply and honestly, without an authoritarian or excessively "professional" manner. Because the self-esteem of many young adolescents is fragile, the physician must be careful not to overpower and intimidate the patient. To establish a comfortable and trusting relationship, the physician should strive to present the image of an ordinary person who has special training and skills.

Because there is great individual variability in the timing of onset and termination of puberty, chronologic age may be a poor indicator of expected physical, physiologic, and emotional development. In communicating with an adolescent, the physician must be sensitive to the patient's developmental level, recognizing that outward appearance and chronologic age may not give an accurate assessment of cognitive development.

Working with teenagers can be emotionally draining. Adolescents have a unique ability to identify hidden emotional vulnerabilities. The physician who has a personal need to control patients or foster dependency may be disappointed in caring for teenagers. Because teenagers are consumed with their own emotional needs, they rarely provide the physician with the ego rewards that younger or older patients do.

The physician should be sensitive to the issue of countertransference, the emotional reaction elicited in the physician by the adolescent. How the physician relates to the adolescent patient often depends on personal characteristics of the physician. This is especially true of physicians treating families with parent-adolescent conflicts. It is common for young physicians to overidentify with the teenage patient and for older physicians to see the conflict from the parents' perspective. Overidentification with the parents is readily sensed by the teenager, who is likely to view the physician as just another authority figure who cannot understand the problems of being a teenager. Assuming a parental-authoritarian role may jeopardize the establishment of a working relationship with the patient. In the case of the young physician, overidentification with the teenager may cause the parents to become defensive about their parenting role and discount the experience and ability of the physician.

THE SETTING

Adolescents respond positively to a setting and services that communicate a sensitivity to their age. A pediatrician's waiting room with toddlers' toys and

Preventive Health Services by Age and Procedure

Adolescents and young adults have a unique set of health care needs. The recommendations for Guidelines for Adolescent Services (GAPS) emphasize annual clinical preventive services visits that address both the developmental and psychosocial aspects of health, in addition to traditional biomedical conditions. These recommendations were developed by the American Medical Association with contributions from a Scientific Advisory Panel, comprised of national experts, as well as representatives of primary care medical organizations and the health insurance industry. The body of scientific evidence indicates that the periodicity and content of preventive services can be important in promoting the health and well-being of adolescents.

Procedure	Age of Adolescent										
	Early				Middle			Late			
	11	12	13	14	15	16	17	18	19	20	21
Health Guidance											
Parenting*		• (12–13)			• (15–16)						
Development	•	•	•	•	•	•	•	•	•	•	•
Diet and Physical Activity	•	•	•	•	•	•	•	•	•	•	•
Healthy Lifestyle**	•	•	•	•	•	•	•	•	•	•	•
Injury Prevention	•	•	•	•	•	•	•	•	•	•	•
Screening											
History											
Eating Disorders	•	•	•	•	•	•	•	•	•	•	•
Sexual Activity***	•	•	•	•	•	•	•	•	•	•	•
Alcohol and Other Drug Use	•	•	•	•	•	•	•	•	•	•	•
Tobacco Use	•	•	•	•	•	•	•	•	•	•	•
Abuse	•	•	•	•	•	•	•	•	•	•	•
School Performance	•	•	•	•	•	•	•	•	•	•	•
Depression	•	•	•	•	•	•	•	•	•	•	•
Risk for Suicide	•	•	•	•	•	•	•	•	•	•	•
Physical Assessment											
Blood Pressure	•	•	•	•	•	•	•	•	•	•	•
BMI	•	•	•	•	•	•	•	•	•	•	•
Comprehensive Exam		• (12–13)			• (15–16)				• (19–20)		
Tests											
Cholesterol	—— 1 ——				—— 1 ——			—— 1 ——			
TB	—— 2 ——				—— 2 ——			—— 2 ——			
GC, Chlamydia, Syphilis, & HPV	—— 3 ——				—— 3 ——			—— 3 ——			
HIV	—— 4 ——				—— 4 ——			—— 4 ——			
Pap Smear	—— 5 ——				—— 5 ——			—— 5 ——			
Immunizations											
MMR	— • —										
Td	— • —				—— O ——						
HepB	— • —				—— 6 ——			—— 6 ——			
Hep A	—— 7 ——				—— 7 ——			—— 7 ——			
Varicella	—— 8 ——				—— 8 ——			—— 8 ——			

1. Screening test performed once if family history is positive for early cardiovascular disease or hyperlipidemia.
2. Screen if positive for exposure to active TB or lives/works in high-risk situation, eg homeless shelter, jail, health care facility.
3. Screen at least annually if sexually active.
4. Screen if high risk for infection.
5. Screen annually if sexually active or if 18 years or older.
6. Vaccinate any adolescent not previously vaccinated.
7. Vaccinate if at risk for hepatitis A infection.
8. Offer vaccine if no reliable history of chickenpox or previous immunization.
* A parent health guidance visit is recommended during early and middle adolescence.
** Includes counseling regarding sexual behavior and avoidance of tobacco, alcohol, and other drug use.
*** Includes history of unintended pregnancy and STD.
O Do not give if administered in last five years.

A

Figure 4–2. A: Guidelines for preventive health services. (Reproduced, with permission, from AMA Guidelines for Adolescent Preventive Services: Recommendations and Rationale. American Medical Association, 1995.)

TEEN HEALTH HISTORY

This information is *strictly confidential.* Its purpose is to help your caregiver give you better care. We request that you fill out the form completely, but you may skip any question that you do not wish to answer.

NAME _____ DATE _____
       FIRST   MIDDLE INITIAL   LAST

BIRTHDATE _____ AGE _____ GRADE _____ Name that you like to be called _____

1. Why did you come to the clinic today? _____
_____
_____

STRICTLY CONFIDENTIAL

Medical History
2. Are you allergic to any medicines? . . . . YES NO
   Name of medicines _____
3. Are you taking any medicines now? . . . . YES NO
   Name of medicines _____
4. Do you have any long-term health conditions? . . . . YES NO
   Conditions _____
5. Date or age at your last tetanus (or dT) shot _____

School Information
6. What grade do you usually make in English? _____
   (Example: A, B, C, D, E, F)
7. What grade do you usually make in Math? _____
8. How many days were you absent from school last semester? _____
9. How many days were you absent last semester because of illness? _____
10. How do you get along at school? _____

| 1 | 2 | 3 | 4 | 5 | 6 | 7 |
| TERRIBLE | | | | | | GREAT |

11. Have you ever been suspended? . . . . YES NO
12. Have you ever dropped out of school? . . . . YES NO
13. Do you plan to graduate from high school? . . . . YES NO

Job/Career Information
14. Are you working? . . . . YES NO
   If YES, What is your job? _____
   How many hours do you work per week? _____
15. What are your future plans or career goals? _____

Family Information
16. Who do you live with? (Check all that apply.)
   _____ Both natural parents   _____ Stepmother   _____ Brother(s)-ages: _____
   _____ Mother   _____ Stepfather   _____ Sister(s)-ages: _____
   _____ Father   _____ Guardian   _____ Other:Explain _____
   _____ Adoptive parents   _____ Alone
17. Have there been any changes in your family? Check all that apply.
   _____ a. Marriage   _____ d. Serious illness   _____ g. Births
   _____ b. Separation   _____ e. Loss of job   _____ h. Deaths
   _____ c. Divorce   _____ f. Move to new home   _____ i. Other
18. Father's/stepfather's occupation or job: _____
   Mother's/stepmother's occupation or job: _____

B

Figure 4–2. B: Adolescent medical history questionnaire.

19. How do you get along at home?   **STRICTLY CONFIDENTIAL**

| 1 | 2 | 3 | 4 | 5 | 6 | 7 |
| TERRIBLE | | | | | | GREAT |

20. Have you ever run away from home?   . . . .   YES NO
21. Have you ever lived in foster care or an institution?   . . . .   YES NO

Self Information
22. On the whole, how do you like yourself?

| 1 | 2 | 3 | 4 | 5 | 6 | 7 |
| NOT VERY MUCH | | | | | | A LOT |

23. What do you do best?_____
24. If you could, what would you like to change about yourself? _____

_____

25. List any habits you would like to break. _____

_____

26. Do you feel people expect too much from you?   . . . .   YES NO
27. How do you get along with your friends/peers?

| 1 | 2 | 3 | 4 | 5 | 6 | 7 |
| TERRIBLE | | | | | | GREAT |

28. Do you feel you have friends you can count on?   . . . .   YES NO
29. Have you ever felt really sad or depressed for more than 3 days in a row? . .   YES NO
30. Have you ever thought of suicide as a solution to your problems? . . . .   YES NO
31. Have you gotten into any trouble because of your anger/temper? . . . .   YES NO

Health Concern
32. On a scale of 1–7, how would you rate your general health?

| 1 | 2 | 3 | 4 | 5 | 6 | 7 |
| TERRIBLE | | | | | | GREAT |

33. Do you have any questions or concerns about any of the following? (Check those that apply.)

____ Height/weight	____ Skin rash	____ Family violence/physical abuse
____ Blood pressure	____ Arms, legs/muscle or joint pain	____ Feeling down or depressed
____ Head/headaches		____ Dating
____ Dizziness/passing out	____ Frequent or painful urination	____ Sex
____ Eyes/vision		____ Worried about VD/STD
____ Ears/hearing/earaches	____ Wetting the bed	____ Masturbation
____ Nose/frequent colds	____ Sexual organs/genitals	____ Sexual abuse/rape
____ Mouth/teeth	____ Trouble sleeping	____ Having children/parenting/adoption
____ Neck/back	____ Tiredness	
____ Chest/breathing/coughing	____ Diet food/appetite	____ Cancer/or dying
____ Breasts	____ Eating disorder	____ Other (explain) _____
____ Heart	____ Smoking/drugs/alcohol	_____
____ Stomach/pain/vomiting	____ Future plans/jobs	
____ Diarrhea/constipation	____ Worried about parents	

Health Behavior Information
34. Have you lost or gained any weight in the last year? . . . .   YES NO
    Gained (   ) How much? _____
    Lost (   ) How much? _____
35. In the past year, have you tried to lose weight or control your weight by vomiting, taking diet pills or laxatives, or starving yourself? . . . .   YES NO
36. Do you ever drive after drinking or when high? . . . .   YES NO
37. Do you ever smoke cigarettes or use snuff or chewing tobacco? . . . .   YES NO
38. Do you ever smoke marijuana? . . . .   YES NO
39. Do you ever drink alcoholic beverages? . . . .   YES NO
40. Do you ever use street drugs (speed, cocaine, acid, crack, etc.)? . . . .   YES NO
41. Does anyone in your household smoke? . . . .   YES NO
42. Does anyone in your family have a problem with drugs or alcohol? . . . .   YES NO

Figure 4–2. B: (continued)

STRICTLY CONFIDENTIAL

43. Have you ever been in trouble with the police or the law? .... YES NO
44. Have you begun dating? .... YES NO
45. Do you currently have a boyfriend or girlfriend? .... YES NO
    If YES, how old is he/she? _____
46. Do you think you might be gay/lesbian/homosexual? .... YES NO
47. Have you ever had sex (sexual intercourse)? .... YES NO
48. Are you interested in receiving information on preventing pregnancy? ...... YES NO
49. If you have had sex, are you (or your partner) using any kind of birth control? YES NO
50. If you have had sex, have you ever been treated for gonorrhea or chlamydia
    or any other sexually transmitted disease? .... YES NO

For males only
51. Have you been taught how to use a condom correctly? .... YES NO
52. If you have had sex, do you use a condom every time or almost every time? YES NO
53. Have you ever fathered a child? .... YES NO

For females only   _____
54. How old were you when your periods began? .... _____
55. What date did your last period start? ....
56. Are your periods regular (once a month)?............................ YES NO
57. Do you have painful or excessively heavy periods? .... YES NO
58. Have you ever had a vaginal infection or been treated for a female disorder? YES NO
59. Do you think you might be pregnant? .... YES NO
60. Have you ever been pregnant? .... YES NO

Everyone
61. Do you have any other problems you would like to discuss with the caregiver? YES NO

Past Medical History
62. Were you born prematurely or did you have any serious problems as an infant? YES NO
63. Are you allergic to any medicines? .... YES NO
    If YES, what? _____

64. List any medications that you are taking and the problems for which the
    medication was given:

MEDICATION	REASON	HOW LONG
_____	_____	_____
_____	_____	_____
_____	_____	_____

65. Have you ever been hospitalized? .... YES NO
    If YES, describe your problem and your age at the time.

AGE	PROBLEM
_____	_____
_____	_____
_____	_____

66. Have you had any injuries? .... YES NO
    If YES, describe the injury and your age when it occurred.

AGE	KIND OF INJURY
_____	_____
_____	_____

67. Have you had any serious illnesses? .... YES NO
    If YES, state the kind of illness and your age when it started.

AGE	ILLNESS
_____	_____
_____	_____

Figure 4–2. B: (continued)

STRICTLY CONFIDENTIAL

Family History

Have any members of your family, alive or dead (parents, grandparents, uncles, aunts, brothers or sisters), had any of the following problems? If YES, please state the age of the person when the condition occurred and the person's relationship to you.

PROBLEM	YES	NO	DON'T KNOW	AGE	RELATIONSHIP
A. Seizure disorder Epilepsy					
B. Mental retardation Birth defects					
C. Migraine headaches					
D. High blood pressure High cholesterol					
E. Heart attack or stroke at less than age 60					
F. Lung disease Tuberculosis					
G. Liver or intestinal disease					
H. Kidney disease					
I. Allergies Asthma Eczema					
J. Arthritis					
K. Diabetes					
L. Endocrine problems Other glandular problems					
M. Obesity Eating disorder					
N. Cancer					
O. Blood disorders Sickle cell anemia					
P. Emotional problems Suicide					
Q. Alcoholism Drug problems					

Figure 4–2. B: (continued)

examination tables too short for a young adult make adolescent patients feel they have outgrown the practice. Similarly, a waiting room filled with geriatric or pregnant patients can make a teenager feel out of place.

It is not uncommon to see a teenage patient who has absolutely no interest in being there, especially when brought in for evaluation of drug and alcohol use, parent–child conflict, school failure, depression, or a suspected eating disorder. Even in cases of acute physical illness, the adolescent may feel anxiety about having a physical examination. If future visits are to be successful, the physician must spend time on the first visit to foster a sense of trust and an opportunity to feel comfortable.

CONFIDENTIALITY

It is helpful at the beginning of the visit to talk with the adolescent and the parents about what to expect. The physician should address the issue of confidentiality, telling the parents that two meetings—one with the teenager alone and one with only the parents—will take place. Adequate time must be spent with both the patient and the parents, or important information may be missed. At the beginning of the interview with the patient, it is useful to say, "I am likely to ask you some personal questions. This is not because I am trying to pry into your personal affairs but because these questions may be important to your health. I want to assure you that what we talk about is confidential, just between the two of us. If there is something I feel we should discuss with your parents, I will ask your permission first unless I feel it is life-threatening."

THE STRUCTURE OF THE VISIT

Caring for adolescents is a time-intensive process. In many adolescent practices, a 40–50% no-show rate is not unusual. Because of issues related to confidentiality, the chief complaint may conceal the patient's real concern. For example, a 15-year-old girl may walk in with a complaint of sore throat but actually be worried about being pregnant.

By the age of 11 or 12, patients should be seen alone. This gives them an opportunity to ask questions they may be embarrassed to ask in front of a parent. Because of the physical changes that take place in early puberty, some adolescents are too self-conscious to undress in front of a parent. If an adolescent comes in willingly, either for an acute illness or a routine physical examination, it may be helpful to meet with the adolescent and parent together to obtain the history. In the case of angry adolescents, brought in against their will, it is useful to meet with the parents and patient just long enough to have the parents describe the conflict and voice their concerns. This meeting should last no longer than 3–5 minutes, and the adolescent should then be seen alone. This approach conveys that the physician is primarily interested in the adolescent patient, yet gives the physician an opportunity to acknowledge the parents' concerns

The Interview

The first few minutes may dictate the success of the visit—whether or not a trusting relationship can be established. A few minutes just getting to know the patient is time well spent. For example, immediately asking, "Do you smoke marijuana?" when a teenager is brought in for suspected marijuana use confirms the adolescent's negative preconceptions about the physician and the purpose of the visit.

It is preferable to spend a few minutes asking non-threatening questions. "Tell me a little bit about yourself so I can get to know you." "What do you like to do most?" "Least?" "What are your friends like?" Neutral questions help defuse some of the patient's anger and anxiety. Toward the end of the interview, the physician can ask more directed questions about psychosocial concerns.

Medical history questionnaires for the patient and the parents are useful in collecting historical data (Figure 4–2B).

The history should include an assessment of progress with psychodevelopmental tasks and of behaviors potentially detrimental to health. The review of systems should include questions about the following:

(1) Nutrition: Number and balance of meals; calcium, iron, cholesterol intake.

(2) Sleep: Number of hours, problems with insomnia or frequent waking.

(3) Seat belt or helmet: Regularity of use.

(4) Self-care: Knowledge of testicular or breast self-examination, dental hygiene, and exercise.

(5) Family relationships: Parents, siblings, relatives.

(6) Peers: Best friend, involvement in group activities, gangs, boyfriends, girlfriends.

(7) School: Attendance, grades, activities.

(8) Educational and vocational interests: College, career, short-term and long-term vocational plans.

(9) Tobacco: Use of cigarettes, snuff, chewing tobacco.

(10) Substance abuse: Frequency, extent, and history of alcohol and drug use.

(11) Sexuality: Sexual activity, contraceptive use, pregnancies, history of sexually transmitted disease, number of sexual partners, risk for HIV infection.

(12) Emotional health: Signs of depression and excessive stress.

The physician's personal attention and interest is

likely to be a new experience for the teenager, who has probably received medical care only through a parent. The teenager should leave the visit with a sense of having a personal physician.

Physical Examination

During early adolescence, many teenagers may be shy and modest, especially with a physician of the opposite sex. The examiner should address this concern directly, because it can be allayed by acknowledging the uneasiness verbally and explaining the purpose of the examination—for example, "Many boys that I see who are your age are embarrassed to have their penis and testes (balls) examined. This is an important part of the examination for a couple of reasons. First, I want to make sure that there aren't any physical problems, and second, it helps me determine if your development is proceeding normally." This also introduces the subject of sexual development for discussion.

A pictorial chart of sexual development (Figures 4–3 and 4–4) is useful in showing the patient how development is proceeding and what changes to expect. The chart shows the relationship between height, breast development, menstruation, and pubic hair growth in the female and between height, penis and testes development, and pubic hair growth in the male. Many teenagers do not openly admit that they are interested in this subject, but they are usually attentive when it is raised. This discussion is particularly useful in counseling teenagers who lag behind their peers in physical development.

Because teenagers are sensitive about their changing bodies, it is useful to comment during the examination: "Your heart sounds fine. I feel a small lump under your right breast. This is very common during puberty in boys. It is called gynecomastia and should disappear in 6 months to a year. Don't worry, you are not turning into a girl."

If a teenage girl has not been sexually active and has no gynecologic complaints or abnormalities, a pelvic examination is usually not necessary until

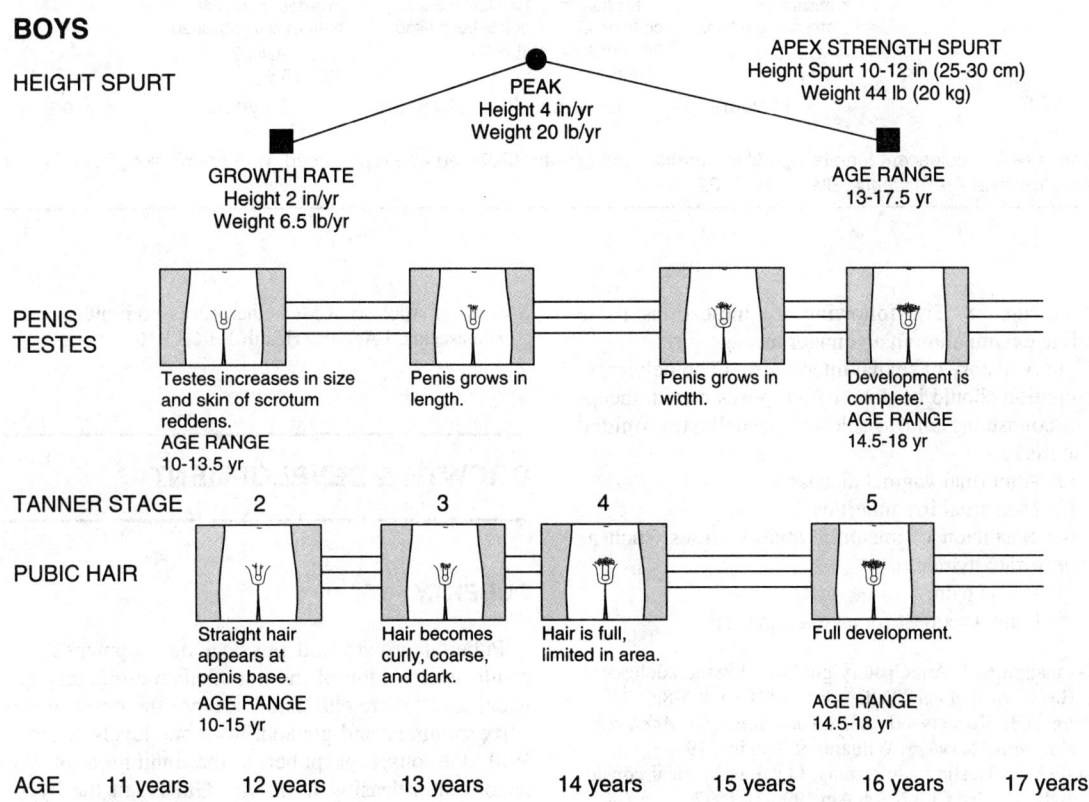

Figure 4–3. Adolescent male sexual maturation and growth. (Adapted and reproduced, with permission, from Tanner JM: *Growth at Adolescence.* Blackwell, 1962.)

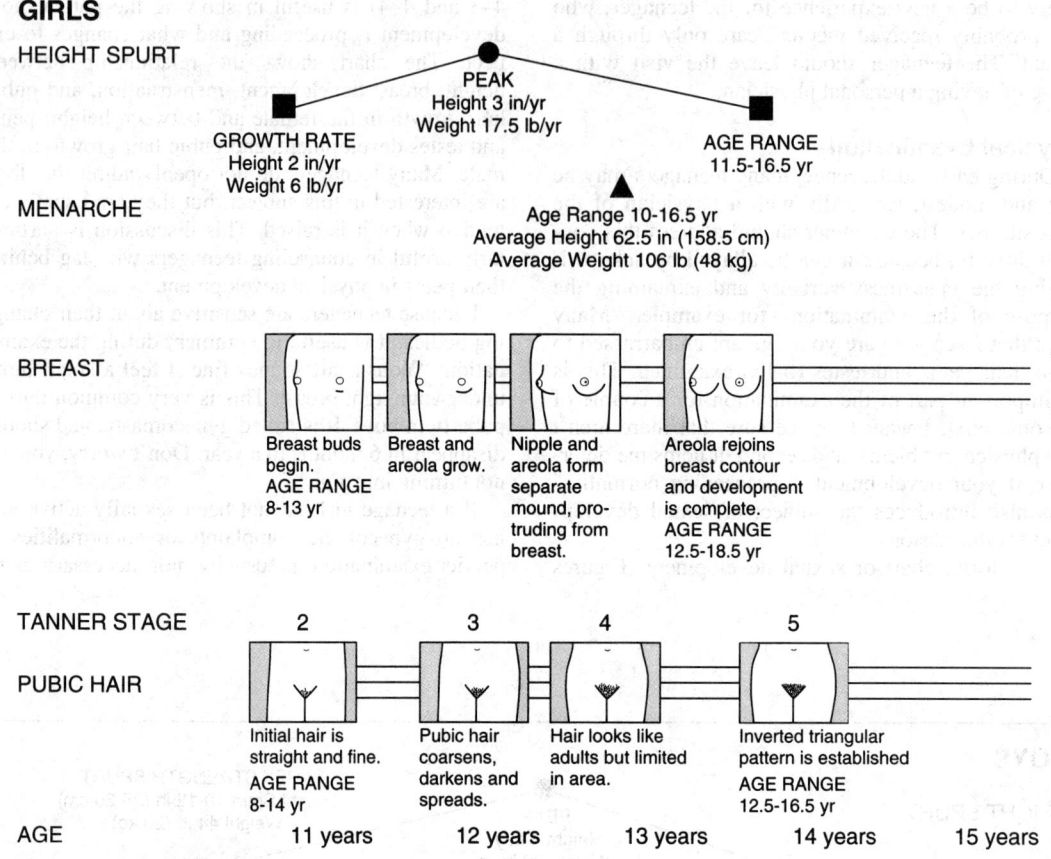

GIRLS

HEIGHT SPURT

PEAK
Height 3 in/yr
Weight 17.5 lb/yr

GROWTH RATE
Height 2 in/yr
Weight 6 lb/yr

AGE RANGE
11.5-16.5 yr

MENARCHE

Age Range 10-16.5 yr
Average Height 62.5 in (158.5 cm)
Average Weight 106 lb (48 kg)

BREAST

Breast buds
begin.
AGE RANGE
8-13 yr

Breast and
areola grow.

Nipple and
areola form
separate
mound, pro-
truding from
breast.

Areola rejoins
breast contour
and development
is complete.
AGE RANGE
12.5-18.5 yr

TANNER STAGE   2   3   4   5

PUBIC HAIR

Initial hair is
straight and fine.
AGE RANGE
8-14 yr

Pubic hair
coarsens,
darkens and
spreads.

Hair looks like
adults but limited
in area.

Inverted triangular
pattern is established
AGE RANGE
12.5-16.5 yr

AGE   11 years   12 years   13 years   14 years   15 years

Figure 4–4. Adolescent female sexual maturation and growth. (Adapted and reproduced, with permission, from Tanner JM: *Growth at Adolescence.* Blackwell, 1962.

about age 18. The following are indications for a pelvic examination in a younger teenage girl:

(1) A history of sexual intercourse. (The pelvic examination should be done for purposes of contraceptive counseling and to rule out sexually transmitted disease.)

(2) Abnormal vaginal discharge.

(3) Menstrual irregularities.

(4) Suspicion of anatomic abnormalities, such as imperforate hymen.

(5) Pelvic pain.

(6) Patient request for an examination.

Cavanaugh RM: Anticipatory guidance for the adolescent: Has it come of age? Pediatr Rev 1994;15:485-8.

Elster AB, Kuznets NJ: *AMA Guidelines for Adolescent Preventive Services.* Williams & Wilkins, 1994.

English A: Treating adolescents: Legal and ethical considerations. Med Clin North Am 1990;74:1097.

Green M (editor): *Bright Futures: Guidelines for Health Supervision of Infants, Children, and Adolescents.* National Center for Education in Maternal and Child Health, 1994.

Society for Adolescent Medicine: Access to health care for adolescents. J Adolesc Health 1991;13:162.

GROWTH & DEVELOPMENT

PUBERTY

Pubertal growth and physical development are a result of activation of the hypothalamic-pituitary-gonadal axis in late childhood. Before the onset of puberty, pituitary and gonadal hormone levels are low. With the onset of puberty, the inhibition of gonadotropin-releasing hormone (GnRH) in the hypothalamus is removed, allowing pulsatile production and release of the gonadotropins: luteinizing hormone (LH) and follicle-stimulating hormone (FSH). In early to mid adolescence, there is an increase in pulse frequency and amplitude of LH and FSH secretion, which stimulates the gonads to produce sex steroids (estrogen or testosterone). In the female, FSH stimulates ovarian maturation, granulosa cell function, and estradiol secretion. LH is important in ovulation and is involved also in corpus luteum formation and progesterone secretion. Initially, estradiol has an inhibitory effect on the release of LH and FSH. Eventually, estradiol becomes stimulatory, and the secretions of LH and FSH become cyclic. There is a progressive increase in estradiol, resulting in maturation of the female genital tract and breast development.

In the male, LH stimulates the interstitial cells of the testes, which produce testosterone. FSH stimulates the production of spermatocytes in the presence of testosterone. The testes also produce inhibin, a Sertoli cell protein that also inhibits the secretion of FSH. During puberty, circulating testosterone increases more than 20-fold. Levels of testosterone correlate with the physical stages of puberty and the degree of skeletal maturation.

PHYSICAL GROWTH

During adolescence, a teenager's weight almost doubles, and height increases by 15–20%. During puberty, major organs double in size with the exception of lymphoid tissue, which decreases in mass. Before puberty, there is little difference in muscular strength between boys and girls. The body's musculature increases both in size and strength during puberty, with maximal strength lagging behind the increase in size by many months. Boys attain greater strength and mass, and strength continues to increase into late puberty. Although motor coordination lags behind growth in stature and musculature, it continues to improve as strength increases.

The pubertal growth spurt begins nearly 2 years earlier in girls than in boys. Girls reach their peak height velocity (PHV) between 11½ and 12 years of age; boys, between 13½ and 14 years of age. Linear growth at peak velocity is 9.5 cm/y ± 1.5 cm for boys and 8.3 cm/y ± 1.2 cm for girls. Pubertal growth usually takes 2–4 years and continues longer in boys than in girls. By age 11 years in girls and age 12 in boys, 83–89% of ultimate height has been attained. An additional 18–23 cm in females and 25–30 cm in males will be achieved during further pubertal growth. Following menarche, growth is rarely more than 5–7.5 cm.

In boys, the quantity of body fat increases before onset of the height spurt. They then lose fat until the growth spurt has finished and gradually again increase in fat. Muscle mass doubles between ages 10 and 17 years. Girls, by contrast, gradually store fat from about age 6 and do not decrease the quantity of fat, though its location changes, with an increase of subcutaneous fat in the region of the pelvis, breasts, and upper back.

SEXUAL MATURATION

Tanner's scale of sexual maturation is useful clinically to categorize genital development. Tanner staging includes age ranges of normal development and specific descriptions for each stage of pubic hair growth, penis and testis development in boys, and breast maturation in girls. Figures 4–3 and 4–4 graphically represent this chronologic development with reference to each Tanner stage. Tanner stage I is prepuberty; stage V, adult maturity. In stage II there is sparse, fine, nonpigmented, downy pubic hair; in stage III, the hair becomes pigmented and curly and increases in amount; and in stage IV, the hair is adult in texture but limited in area. The appearance of pubic hair precedes that of axillary hair by more than 1 year. Male genital development begins with stage II, in which the testes become larger and the scrotal skin reddens and coarsens. In stage III, the penis lengthens; and in stage IV, the penis enlarges in overall size and the scrotal skin becomes pigmented.

Female breast development follows a predictable sequence. Small, raised breast buds appear in stage II. In stage III, there is general enlargement and elevation of breast and areolar tissue. The areola and papilla (nipple) form a separate mound from the breast in stage IV, and in stage V the areola assumes the same contour as the breast.

Great variability exists in the timing and onset of puberty and growth, and psychosocial development does not necessarily parallel physical changes. Because of this variability, chronologic age is a poor indication of physiologic and psychosocial development. Skeletal maturation correlates well with growth and pubertal development.

Teenagers have been entering puberty at increasingly earlier ages during the last century because of better nutrition and improved socioeconomic conditions. In the United States, the average age at menarche is 12¾ years. Among girls reaching menarche, the average weight is 48 kg, and the average height is 158.5 cm. However, menarche may be delayed until age 16 or may begin as early as age 10. Although the first measurable sign of puberty in girls is the beginning of the height spurt, the first conspicuous sign usually is development of breast buds between the ages of 8 and 11 years. Although breast development usually precedes the growth of pubic hair, in some girls the sequence may be reversed. A common concern for girls at this time is whether the breasts will be of the right size and shape, especially since it is not unusual for one breast to grow faster than the other. Among girls, the growth spurt starts at about age 9 years and reaches a peak at age 11½, usually at stage III–IV breast development and stage III pubic hair development. The spurt usually ends by age 14. Girls who mature early will reach their peak height velocity sooner and attain their final height earlier. Girls who mature late will attain a greater ultimate height because of the longer period of growth before the growth spurt. Final height is related to skeletal age at onset of puberty as well as genetic factors. The height spurt correlates more closely with breast developmental stages than with pubic hair stages.

The first sign of puberty in the male, usually between the ages of 10 and 12, is scrotal and testicular growth. Pubic hair usually appears early in puberty but may do so any time between ages 10 and 15 years. The penis begins to grow significantly a year or so after the onset of testicular and pubic hair development, usually between the ages of 10 and 13½. The first ejaculation usually occurs about 1 year after initiation of testicular growth, but its timing is highly variable. About 90% of boys have this experience between the ages of 11 and 15 years. Gynecomastia, a hard nodule under the nipple, occurs in a majority of boys, with a peak incidence between ages 14 and 15 years. Gynecomastia usually disappears within 6 months to 2 years. The height spurt begins at age 11 but increases rapidly between the ages of 12 and 13, with the PHV reached at age 13½ years. The period of pubertal development lasts much longer in boys and may not be completed until age 18 years. The height velocity is higher in males (8–11 cm/y) than females (6½–9½ cm/y). The development of axillary hair, deepening of the voice, and the development of chest hair in boys usually occurs in mid puberty, about 2 years after onset of growth of pubic hair. Facial and body hair begin to increase at ages 16–17 years.

Litt IF: Pubertal and psychosocial development: Implications for pediatricians. Pediatr Rev 1995;16:243.

Tanner JM, Davies PW: Clinical longitudinal standards for height and height velocity for North American children. J Pediatr 1985;107:317.

PSYCHOSOCIAL DEVELOPMENT

Adolescents are struggling to find out who they are, what they want to do in the future, and, in relation to that goal, what their personal strengths and weaknesses are. These questions arise primarily because teenagers are in the process of establishing their own identity. Adolescence is a period of progressive individuation and separation from the family. Because of the rapid physical, emotional, cognitive, and social growth occurring during adolescence, it is useful to divide the period into three sequential phases of development. Early adolescence occurs roughly between ages 10 and 13; middle adolescence, between ages 14 and 16; and late adolescence, at age 17 and later.

Early Adolescence

Early adolescence (ages 10–13) is characterized by rapid growth and development of secondary sex characteristics. Because of the rapid physical changes during this period, body image, self-concept, and self-esteem fluctuate dramatically. Concerns about how personal growth and development deviate from that of peers may be a great worry, especially short stature in boys and delayed breast development or delayed menarche in girls. Although there is a certain curiosity about sexuality, young adolescents tend to feel more comfortable with members of the same sex. Peer relationships become increasingly important. Young teenagers still think concretely and cannot easily conceptualize about the future. They may have vague and unrealistic professional goals, such as becoming a lead singer in a rock group or a movie star.

Middle Adolescence

During middle adolescence (14–16 years), as the rapid pubertal growth rate subsides, teenagers become more comfortable with their "new" bodies. Intense emotions and wide swings in mood are typical. Although some teenagers go through this experience relatively peacefully, others struggle desperately. Cognitively, teenagers move from concrete thinking to formal operations and develop the ability to think abstractly. With this new mental power comes a sense of omnipotence and a belief that the world can be changed by merely thinking about it. Sexually active teenagers may believe they do not need to worry about using contraception because they "can't get pregnant—it won't happen to me." Sixteen-year-old drivers believe they are the best drivers in the world and think the insurance industry is conspiring against them by charging such high rates for automobile insurance. With the onset of the ability to think abstractly, teenagers begin to see themselves as others see them and may become extremely self-centered. Because they are establishing their own identities, relationships with other people, including peers, are primarily narcissistic, and experimenting with different images is quite common. Peers determine the standards for identification, behavior, activities, and fashion and provide emotional support, intimacy, empathy, and the sharing of guilt and anxiety during the struggle for autonomy. The struggle for independence and autonomy is often a difficult and stressful period for both the teenager and the parents.

As sexuality increases in importance during this time, adolescents may begin dating and experimenting with sex. Relationships usually tend to be one-sided and narcissistic.

Late Adolescence

During late adolescence (age 17 years and older), the young person generally becomes less self-centered and begins caring more about others. Social relationships shift from the peer group to the individual. Dating becomes much more intimate. By age 18, nearly half of American girls and two thirds of boys have had sexual intercourse. The older adolescent becomes more independent from the family. The ability to think abstractly allows older adolescents to think more realistically in terms of future plans, actions, and careers. Older adolescents have rigid concepts of what is right or wrong. This is a period of idealism.

Homosexuality in Adolescence

Sexual orientation develops during early childhood. One's gender identity is established by age 2, and a sense of masculinity or femininity usually solidifies by age 5 or 6. Homosexual adults describe homosexual feelings during late childhood and early adolescence, years before engaging in overt homosexual acts.

Although only 5–10% of American young people acknowledge having had homosexual experiences and only 5% feel that they are or could be gay, homosexual experimentation is common, especially during early and middle adolescence. Experimentation may include mutual masturbation and fondling the genitals and does not by itself cause or lead to adult homosexuality. Theories about the etiology of homosexuality include genetic, hormonal, environmental, and psychologic models.

The development of homosexual identity in adolescence commonly progresses through two stages. The adolescent feels "different," develops a crush on a person of the same sex without clear self-awareness of a gay identity, and then goes through a "coming-out" phase in which the homosexual identity is defined for the individual and revealed to others. The coming-out phase may be a very difficult period for the young person and the family. The young adolescent is afraid of society's bias and seeks to reject homosexual feelings. This struggle with identity may include episodes of both homosexual and heterosexual promiscuity, sexually transmitted disease, depression, substance abuse, attempted suicide, school avoidance and failure, running away from home, and other crises.

In a clinical setting, the issue of homosexual identity most often surfaces as a result of a teenager being seen for a sexually transmitted disease, family conflict, school problem, attempted suicide, or substance abuse rather than as a result of a consultation about sexual orientation. Pediatricians should be aware of the psychosocial and medical implications of homosexual identity and be sensitive to the possibility of these problems in gay adolescents. Successful management depends on the physician's ability to gain the trust of the gay adolescent and on a knowledge of the wide range of medical and psychologic problems for which gay adolescents may be at risk. Pediatricians must be nonjudgmental in posing sexual questions if they are to be effective in encouraging the teenager to share concerns. Physicians who for religious or other personal reasons cannot be objective must refer the homosexual patient to another professional for treatment and counseling.

American Academy of Pediatrics Committee on Adolescence: Homosexuality and adolescence. Pediatrics 1993;92:631.

Ghai K, Rosenfeld RL: Disorders of pubertal development: Too early, too much, too late, or too little. Adolescent Medicine: State of the Art Reviews 1994;5:19.

Levine M et al (editors): *Developmental Behavioral Pediatrics,* 2nd ed. Saunders, 1992.

Milstein SG et al: Health-risk behaviors and health concerns among young adolescents. Pediatrics 1992;3:422.

Rowlett JD, Greydanus DE: Homosexuality in adolescence. Adolescent Medicine: State of the Art Reviews 1994;5:509.

Vaughan VC, Litt IF: *Child and Adolescent Development: Clinical Implications.* Saunders, 1990.

BEHAVIOR & PSYCHOLOGIC HEALTH

It is not unusual for adolescents to seek medical attention for seemingly minor complaints. During early adolescence, teenagers may worry about normal developmental changes such as gynecomastia. They may present with vague symptoms whereas the hidden agenda may be concerns about pregnancy or a sexually transmitted disease. Adolescents with emotional disorders often present with somatic symptoms—eg, abdominal pain, headaches, dizziness or syncope, fatigue, sleep problems, chest pain—that appear to have no biologic cause. The emotional basis of such complaints may be varied: somatoform disorder, depression, or stress and anxiety.

PSYCHOPHYSIOLOGIC SYMPTOMS & CONVERSION REACTIONS

The most common somatoform disorders during adolescence are conversion disorders or conversion reactions. (A conversion reaction is a psychophysiologic process in which unpleasant feelings, especially anxiety, depression, and guilt, are communicated through a physical symptom.) Psychophysiologic symptoms result when anxiety activates the autonomic nervous system, resulting in tachycardia, hyperventilation, and vasoconstriction. The emotional feeling may be threatening or unacceptable to the individual, who expresses it as a physical symptom rather than verbally. This process is unconscious, and the anxiety or unpleasant feeling is dissipated by the somatic symptom. The degree to which the conversion symptom lessens anxiety, depression, or the unpleasant feeling is referred to as "primary gain." Conversion symptoms not only diminish unpleasant feelings but also release the adolescent from conflict or an uncomfortable situation. This is referred to as "secondary gain." Secondary gain may intensify the symptoms, especially with increased attention from concerned parents and friends. Adolescents with conversion symptoms tend to have overprotective parents and become increasingly dependent on their parents as the symptom becomes the major focus concern in the family.

Clinical Findings

The symptom may appear at times of stress. Nervous, gastrointestinal, and cardiovascular symptoms are common: paresthesias, anesthesia, paralysis, dizziness, syncope, hyperventilation, abdominal pain, nausea and vomiting. Specific symptoms may reflect existing or previous illness (eg, pseudoseizures in adolescents with epilepsy) or modeling of a close relative's symptom (eg, chest pain in a boy whose grandfather died of a heart attack).

Conversion symptoms are more common in girls than boys. They occur in patients from all socioeconomic levels; however, the complexity of the symptom may vary with the sophistication and cognitive level of the patient.

Differential Diagnosis

The history and physical findings are usually inconsistent with anatomic and physiologic concepts. Conversion symptoms are exhibited most frequently at times of stress and in the presence of individuals meaningful to the patient. The patient often exhibits a characteristic personality pattern, including egocentricity, emotional lability, and dramatic and attention-seeking behaviors.

Conversion reactions must be differentiated from hypochondriasis, which is a preoccupation with developing or having a serious illness despite medical reassurance that there is no evidence of disease. Over time, the fear of one disease may give way to concern about another. In contrast to patients with conversion symptoms, who seem relieved if an organic cause is considered, patients with hypochondriasis become more anxious when such a cause is considered.

Malingering is uncommon during adolescence. The malingering patient consciously and intentionally produces false or exaggerated physical or psychologic symptoms. Such patients are motivated by external incentives such as avoiding work, evading criminal prosecution, obtaining drugs, or obtaining financial compensation. These patients may be hostile and aloof. Parents of patients with conversion disorders and malingering have a similar reaction to illness. They have an unconscious psychologic need to have sick children and reinforce their child's behavior.

Somatic delusions are physical symptoms, often bizarre, that accompany other signs of mental illness. Examples are visual or auditory hallucinations, delusions, incoherence or loosening of associations, rapid shifts of affect, and confusion.

Treatment

The physician must emphasize from the onset that both physical and emotional causes of the symptom need to be considered. The relationship between physical causes of emotional pain and emotional causes of physical pain should be described to the family, using examples such as stress causing an ulcer or making a severe headache worse. The patient should be encouraged to understand that the symptom may persist and that at least a short-term goal is to continue normal daily activities. Medication is rarely helpful. If the family will accept it, psychologic referral is often the best initial step toward psychotherapy. If the family resists psychiatric or psychologic referral, the pediatrician may need to begin to deal with some of the emotional factors responsible for the symptom while building rapport with the patient and family. Regular appointments should be scheduled. During the sessions, the teenager should be seen first and encouraged to talk about school, friends, the relationship with the parents, and the stresses of life. Discussion of the symptom itself should be minimized; however, the physician should be supportive and must never suggest that the pain is not real. As the parents gain further insight into the cause of the symptom, they will become less indulgent of the complaints, facilitating the resumption of normal activities. If management is successful, the adolescent will acquire increased coping skills and become more independent, with decreasing secondary gain.

If the symptom continues to interfere with daily activities and if the patient and parents feel that no progress is being made, psychologic referral is indicated. A psychotherapist experienced in treating adolescents with conversion reactions is in the best position to establish a strong therapeutic relationship with the patient and family. After referral is made, the pediatrician should continue to follow the patient to ensure compliance with psychotherapy.

American Psychiatric Association: *Diagnostic and Statistical Manual of Mental Disorders,* 4th ed. American Psychiatric Press, 1994.

Prazer G: Conversion reactions in adolescents. Pediatr Rev 1987;8:279.

DEPRESSION
(See also Chapter 6.)

Symptoms of clinical depression (lethargy, loss of interest, sleep disturbances, decreased energy, feelings of worthlessness, and difficulty concentrating) are common during adolescence. The intensity of feelings, often in response to seemingly trivial events such as a poor grade on an examination or not being invited to a party, makes it difficult to differentiate severe depression from normal sadness or dejection. In less severe depression, sadness or unhappiness associated with problems of everyday life is generally short-lived. The symptoms usually result in only minor impairment in school performance, social activities, and relationships with others. Symptoms respond to support and reassurance.

Clinical Findings

The presentation of serious depression in adolescence may be similar to that in adults, with vegetative signs such as depressed mood, crying spells or inability to cry, discouragement, irritability, a sense of emptiness and meaninglessness, negative expectations of oneself and the environment, low self-esteem, isolation, a feeling of helplessness, diminished interest or pleasure in activities, weight loss or weight gain, insomnia or hypersomnia, fatigue or loss of energy, feelings of worthlessness, and diminished ability to think or concentrate. However, it is not unusual for a serious depression to be masked because the teenager cannot tolerate the severe feelings of sadness. Such a teenager may present with recurrent or persistent psychosomatic complaints, such as abdominal pain, chest pain, headache, lethargy, weight loss, dizziness and syncope, or other nonspecific symptoms. Other behavioral manifestations of masked depression include truancy, running away from home, defiance of authorities, self-destructive behavior, vandalism, drug and alcohol abuse, sexual acting out, and delinquency.

Differential Diagnosis

A complete history and physical examination, including a careful review of the patient's past medical and psychosocial history, should be performed. The family history should be explored for psychiatric problems.

The teenager should be questioned about the symptoms of depression listed above, and specifically about suicidal ideation or preoccupation with thoughts of death. The history should include an assessment of school performance, looking for signs of academic deterioration, excessive absence or cutting class, changes in work or other outside activities, and changes in the family (eg, separation, divorce, serious illness, loss of employment by a parent, a recent move to a new school, increasing quarrels or fights with parents, the death of a close relative). The teenager may have withdrawn from friends or family or switched allegiance to a new group of friends. The physician should seek to develop a history of drug and alcohol abuse, conflicts with the police, sexual acting out, running away from home, unusually vio-

lent or rebellious behavior, or radical personality changes. Patients with vague somatic complaints or concerns about having a fatal illness may have an underlying affective disorder.

Adolescents presenting with symptoms of depression require a thorough medical evaluation to rule out any contributing or underlying medical illness. Among the medical conditions associated with affective disorders are eating disorders, organic disorders of the central nervous system (tumors, vascular lesions, closed head trauma, and subdural hematomas), metabolic and endocrinologic disorders (systemic lupus erythematosus, hypothyroidism, hyperthyroidism, Wilson's disease, hyperparathyroidism, Cushing's syndrome, Addison's disease, premenstrual syndrome), infections (infectious mononucleosis, syphilis), and mitral valve prolapse. Marijuana use, phencyclidine abuse, amphetamine withdrawal, and excessive caffeine intake can cause symptoms of depression. Common prescription and over-the-counter medications, including birth control pills, anticonvulsants, and beta-blockers, may cause depressive symptoms.

Some routine laboratory studies are indicated in the depressed patient to rule out organic disease: a complete blood count and sedimentation rate, urinalysis, serum electrolytes, blood urea nitrogen (BUN), serum calcium, thyroxine and thyroid-stimulating hormone, VDRL or rapid plasma reagin (RPR), and liver enzymes. Although metabolic markers such as abnormal secretion of cortisol, growth hormone, and thyrotropin-releasing hormone have been useful in confirming major depression in adults, these neurobiologic markers are less reliable in adolescents.

The risk of depression appears to be greatest in families with a history of early onset and chronic depression. Depression of early onset and bipolar illness are more likely to occur in families with a strong multigenerational history of depression. The lifetime risk of depressive illness in first-degree relatives of adult depressed patients has been estimated to be between 18% and 30%.

Treatment

The primary care physician may be able to counsel adolescents and parents if depression is mild or is the result of an acute personal loss or frustration and if the patient is not contemplating suicide or other life-threatening behaviors. If there is evidence of a long-standing depressive disorder, suicidal thoughts, or psychotic thinking—or if the physician does not feel competent or has no interest in counseling the patient—psychologic referral should be made.

Counseling involves establishing and maintaining a positive supportive relationship; following the patient at least weekly; remaining accessible to the patient at all times; encouraging the patient to express emotions openly, defining the problem and clarifying negative feelings, thoughts, and expectations; setting realistic goals; helping to negotiate interpersonal crises; teaching assertiveness and social skills; reassessing the depression as it is expressed; and staying alert to the possibility of suicide.

Patients with a clinical course consistent with bipolar disease or who have a significant depression that is unresponsive to supportive counseling should be referred to a psychiatrist for evaluation of antidepressant medication.

Brent DA: Depression and suicide in children and adolescents. Pediatr Rev 1993;14:380.

Hodgman CH, McAnarney ER: Adolescent depression and suicide: Rising problems. Hosp Pract (Off Ed) 1992;27;73.

Jensen PS, Ryan ND, Prien R: Psychopharmacology of child and adolescent major depression: Present status and future directions. J Child Adolesc Psychopharmacol 1992;2:31.

ADOLESCENT SUICIDE
(See also Chapter 6.)

In 1995, there were 4784 suicides among people 15–24 years of age: 1890 suicides among those 15–19 and 2894 among those 20–24. In the younger group, males had a rate 5.6 times higher than females, and white males had the highest rate, 18.4 per 100,000. The incidence of unsuccessful suicide attempts is three times higher in females than in males. The estimated ratio of attempted suicides to actual suicides is estimated to be 100:1–50:1. Firearms account for 67% of suicide deaths in both males and females.

With the normal mood swings of adolescence, short periods of depression are common, and a teenager may have thoughts of suicide. Normal mood swings during this period rarely interfere with sleeping, eating, or participating in normal activities. Acute depressive reactions (transient grief responses) to the loss of a family member or friend may result in depression lasting for weeks or even months. An adolescent who is unable to work through this grief can become increasingly depressed. A teenager who is unable to keep up with schoolwork, does not participate in normal social activities, withdraws socially, has sleep and appetite disturbances, and has feelings of hopelessness and helplessness should be considered to be at increased risk for suicide.

Another group of suicidal adolescents is composed of angry teenagers attempting to influence others by their actions. They may be only mildly depressed and may not have a long-standing wish to die. Teenagers in this group, usually females, may "attempt suicide" or make a "suicidal gesture" as a way of getting back at someone or gaining attention by frightening another person.

The last group at risk for suicide are adolescents with a serious psychiatric problem such as acute schizophrenia or a true psychotic depressive disorder.

Risk Assessment

The physician must determine the extent of the teenager's depression and assess the risk of inflicting self-harm. The evaluation should include interviews with both the teenager and the family. The history should include the medical, social, emotional, and academic background. (See Table 6–16: Clinical Interview to Assess Suicide Risk.) The physician should inquire about (1) common signs of depression; (2) recent events that could be the cause of an underlying depression; (3) evidence of long-standing problems in the home, at school, or with peers; (4) drug or substance use and abuse; (5) signs of psychotic thinking, such as delusions or hallucinations; and (6) evidence of masked depression, such as rebellious behavior, running away from home, reckless driving, or other acting-out behavior.

When seeing depressed patients, the physician should always inquire about thoughts of suicide: "Are things ever so bad that life doesn't seem worth living?" If the response is affirmative, a more specific question should be asked: "Have you thought of taking your life?" If the patient has thoughts of suicide, the immediacy of risk can be assessed by determining if there is a concrete, feasible plan. Although patients who are at greatest risk have a concrete plan that can be carried out in the near future—especially if they have rehearsed the plan—the physician should not dismiss the potential risk of suicide in the adolescent who does not describe a specific plan. The physician should pay attention to "gut feelings." There may be subtle nonverbal signs that the patient is at greater risk than may be apparent.

Treatment

The primary care physician is often in a unique position to identify an adolescent at risk for suicide, because many teenagers who attempt suicide seek medical attention in the weeks preceding the attempt. These visits are often for vague somatic complaints. If there is evidence of depression, the physician must assess the severity of the depression and suicidal risk. The pediatrician should always seek emergency psychologic consultation for any teenager who is severely depressed, psychotic, or acutely suicidal. It is the psychologist's or psychiatrist's responsibility to assess the seriousness of suicidal ideation and decide whether hospitalization or outpatient treatment is most appropriate. Adolescents with mild depression and at low risk for suicide should be followed closely, and the extent of the depression should be assessed on an ongoing basis. If at any point it appears that the patient is worsening or the teenager is not responding to supportive counseling, referral should be made.

American Academy of Pediatrics Committee on School Health: The potentially suicidal student in the school setting. Pediatrics 1990;86:481.

Blumenthal SJ: Youth suicide: The physician's role in suicide prevention. JAMA 1990;264:3194.

Crumley FE: Substance abuse and adolescent suicidal behavior. JAMA 1990;263:3051.

Kellerman AL et al: Suicide in the home in relation to gun ownership. N Engl J Med 1992;327:467.

Shaffer D et al: Preventing teenage suicide: A critical review. J Am Acad Child Adolesc Psychiatry 1988;27: 675.

SUBSTANCE ABUSE

Substance abuse is a complex problem for adolescents and the broader society. See Chapter 5 for an in-depth look at this issue.

EATING DISORDERS
(See also Chapter 6.)

The prevalence of anorexia nervosa among adolescents has steadily risen over the past 4 decades. At a rate of 0.48% for 15- to 19-year-olds, anorexia nervosa is now the third leading chronic condition of female adolescents after obesity and asthma. During the 1980s, 1–5% of adolescent girls met strict *DSM-III-R* criteria for bulimia nervosa. There are many more teens with disordered eating who do not meet full *DSM-IV* (Table 4–1) criteria for anorexia nervosa or bulimia nervosa—because weight is not a full 15% below expected weight, or because menses have ceased for less than 3 months, or because the subjects purge but do not binge—but who have no less emotional distress than those who meet the strict diagnostic criteria. The preponderance of eating disorders among higher socioeconomic groups is changing, and the disorders are now being found in all social classes. The causes remain unclear. Psychosocial and cultural factors include the current emphasis on thinness and the "superwoman" image. The genetic component and the neuroendocrine-hypothalamic role are being investigated.

A teenager with anorexia is unlikely to present to the physician of her own accord, because denial of illness a component of the syndrome. She may present because of fatigue, abdominal pain, nausea, fainting spells, hair loss, amenorrhea, or at the urgings of an astute school nurse or coach. Bulimics, however, may present on their own and may feel relieved to share their burden with someone.

Clinical Findings
A. Symptoms & Signs: The diagnosis of anorexia nervosa or bulimia nervosa is based largely on the history; specific diagnostic criteria are set forth in Table 4–1; however, the clinician is cautioned to have a low threshold of suspicion so that the opportunity for early intervention in subclinical cases will not be missed. The history needs to include the presenting symptoms; weight history, including desired weight; dietary intake, unusual eating behaviors, or avoided foods; history of any compensatory behaviors, such as vomiting, excessive exercise, or use of diet pills, diuretics, emetics, or laxatives; and menstrual history for irregular cycles, secondary amenorrhea, or delay in anticipated menarche. The social history may provide clues to a perfectionistic drive in anorexics, impulsiveness in bulimics (eg, substance abuse, sexual promiscuity), or family dysfunction. Review of systems should focus on symptoms of possible complications of the above behaviors and on symptoms of other diseases in the differential diagnosis. Use of the Eating Attitudes Test (EAT) and the Eating Disorder Inventory (EDI) may aid in diagnosis.

The physical examination is most often normal, but this does not rule out the diagnosis of an eating disorder. The anorexic may hide under layers of bulky clothing, but the loss of subcutaneous tissue becomes apparent when the patient disrobes. The anorexic's weight is the indicator of actual loss. Hypothermia, bradycardia, or hypotension may be evident when the anorexic's vital signs are assessed. Other findings in anorexia include dry skin, presence of fine, downy hair on the body or an increase in pigmentation of body hair, limpness and loss of sheen of the scalp hair, excoriation over the sacral spine from excessive sit-ups, prominent ribs, atrophied breasts, scaphoid abdomen, palpable hard stool in the rectal vault, cold extremities with acrocyanosis, squaring off of the convergence of the thighs, or edema of the extremities. Bulimics are usually of normal weight or within 4.5 kg (under or over) of normal. In patients

Table 4–1. Diagnostic criteria for eating disorders.[1]

Anorexia nervosa
  Weight loss or failure to gain weight during growth such that weight is 15% below norm for age and height
  Fear of weight gain or obesity despite being underweight
  Disturbed body image: feels all or part of body is fat even when severely underweight, or self-evaluation overly influenced by body image
  Interruption of menstrual cycles for at least 3 months

Bulimia nervosa
  Repeated binge eating (excessive number of calories in short period of time accompanied by the perception that one lacks control over eating)
  Recurrent compensatory behaviors to prevent weight gain (self-induced emesis; use of laxatives, diuretics, or emetics; excessive exercise, or severely restricted intake)
  Binge eating and compensatory behaviors both occurring at least twice a week for 3 months or more
  Self-evaluation overly influenced by body image
  Not occurring exclusively as part of anorexia nervosa

[1]Modified and reproduced from American Psychiatric Association: *Diagnostic and Statistical Manual of Mental Disorders,* 4th ed. APA Press, 1994.

with self-induced emesis, there may be loss of tooth enamel, particularly on the posterior aspect of the front teeth, or calluses on the dorsum of the fingers.

B. Laboratory Findings: The goal of laboratory tests is to exclude other diagnoses and assess the patient's status. Most laboratory studies do not change until late in the disease. It is useful to obtain a complete blood count to assess nutritional status, a sedimentation rate to help exclude inflammatory bowel disease or collagen-vascular disease, and electrolyte studies to detect the presence of hypochloremic alkalosis and hypokalemia due to vomiting or of metabolic acidosis due to laxative abuse. A urinalysis may show concentrated urine or, late in anorexia nervosa, loss of urine concentrating ability. Serum total protein and albumin are usually normal until late. Prealbumin, transferrin, or C3 complement levels can help assess the degree of malnutrition. Bone densitometry should be done at baseline for severely malnourished teens, especially those with a prolonged history or delayed growth. Serum calcium, phosphorus, and magnesium should be closely followed during refeeding, since these electrolytes may quickly become depleted, resulting in a medical emergency. Other laboratory studies, such as thyroid function tests, chest x-ray, electrocardiography, upper gastrointestinal series, or CT scan of the head need only be done as indicated by the presentation.

Differential Diagnosis

The causes of weight loss are legion. Causes such as cancer, collagen-vascular disease, diabetes mellitus, hyperthyroidism, malabsorptive syndromes, inflammatory bowel disease, or chronic renal, pulmonary, or cardiac disease warrant consideration in the suspected anorexic; however, in patients with these disorders there may be weight loss but no associated disturbance of body image or fear of obesity. Several psychiatric disturbances, including depression, may be associated with loss of appetite and weight loss. Some unusual central nervous system disorders may present like bulimia, but again there is no distorted body image or overconcern with body shape or weight.

Complications

Eating disorders can result in severe consequences to nearly every system of the body (Table 4–2). The most common complications, however, are fluid and electrolyte abnormalities and constipation. Recently, reduced bone mineral density and cortical atrophy of the brain have been appreciated as significant early consequences of anorexia nervosa in adolescents; long-term implications are still under investigation. Growth retardation can also occur. In addition, there may be long-term difficulties with eating and weight management.

Table 4–2. Complications of eating disorders.[1]

Cardiovascular	Hematologic
Bradycardia	Leukopenia
Postural hypotension	Anemia
Arrhythmia, sudden death	Thrombocytopenia
Congestive heart failure (during refeeding)	↓ESR
Pericardial effusion	Impaired cell-mediated immunity
Mitral valve prolapse	**Metabolic**
ECG abnormalities (prolonged QT, low voltage, T-wave abnormalities, conduction defects)	Dehydration
	Acidosis
	Hypokalemia
Endocrine	Hyponatremia
↓LH, FSH	Hypochloremia
↓T_3,↑rT_3; normal T_4, TSH	Hypochloremic alkalosis
Irregular menses	Hypocalcemia
Amenorrhea	Hypophosphatemia
Hypercortisolism	Hypomagnesemia
Growth retardation	Hypercarotenemia
Short stature	**Neurologic**
Delayed puberty	Cortical atrophy
Gastrointestinal	Peripheral neuropathy
Dental erosion	Seizures
Parotid swelling	Thermoregulatory abnormalities
Esophagitis, esophageal tears	↓REM and slow-wave sleep
Delayed gastric emptying	**Renal**
Gastric dilatation (rarely rupture)	Hematuria
Pancreatitis	Proteinuria
Constipation	↓Renal concentrating ability
Diarrhea (laxative abuse)	**Skeletal**
Superior mesenteric artery syndrome	Osteopenia
Hypercholesterolemia	Fractures
↑Liver function tests (fatty infiltration of the liver)	

[1]ESR = erythrocyte sedimentation rate; REM = rapid eye movement.

Treatment

First, the diagnosis must be discussed with the patient and her parents. The patient needs to know that the clinician understands what she is going through, aims to restore her to health, will not let her become fat, and will help her to regain control of her eating habits. The parents need to understand that eating disorders are symptoms of underlying conflicts, often a family problem, and that the family is important to the solution. They need to see that although the presenting symptoms are physical, eating disorders are psychiatric phenomena and require the intervention of mental health practitioners. With this age group, it is important to have a mental health practitioner who is skilled in family therapy and has experience with adolescents (see Chapter 6).

Restoration of the nutritional and physiologic state is an early goal of treatment because the patient may need to gain weight before she can deal effectively with her fear of obesity or other issues. A dietitian is helpful in establishing a refeeding program. The patient may be in no metabolic danger at the time of presentation, and provided the weight can be stabilized she may require not hospitalization but regular outpatient visits with medical and mental health professionals. An individualized contract can be drawn up and signed by the patient. This contract addresses such issues as long-term weight goals, rate of weight gain, amount of exercise, frequency of visits and of laboratory tests, minimal weight signaling the need for hospitalization, and consequences of failed weight goals. At each medical visit, the patient should be weighed in nothing but a gown after she voids. Body mass index (BMI) can be followed over time. The long-term goal is to achieve a weight at which menstruation can take place; in general, 90% of ideal body weight is required—but not alone sufficient—to restore menstruation. Vital signs and chest and abdominal examinations should also be conducted at each visit, and the height and the triceps skinfold should be monitored over time.

Most often, the patient can eat enough to replace nutrient deficits and to gain weight. High-calorie fluid supplements may be added to the diet if weekly weight goals are missed. It is best not to tell the patient that she must take in a certain number of calories, because she is already fixated on calories. Rather, plans can be developed with the assistance of the dietitian; the planned diets contain sufficient calories to gain 0.2–0.9 kg/wk (0.9–1.4 kg/wk for inpatients). In extremely malnourished and noncompliant hospitalized patients, nasogastric tube feedings or hyperalimentation may be necessary initially. With severe anorexics, one must watch for congestive heart failure caused by refeeding too rapidly. In addition, serum phosphate levels should be followed since there may be a shift from serum to cells during conversion to anabolic metabolism.

Drug therapy—including appetite stimulants or suppressants, antidepressants, anxiolytics, and anticonvulsants—has been investigated in a number of studies, but the results to date are equivocal. Antidepressants may be helpful in selected patients but need to be carefully monitored in cachectic patients. Selective serotonin reuptake inhibitors are often helpful in medically stable anorexics and have been shown to reduce the frequency of bingeing and purging—as well as obsessive thinking about food—in bulimics.

Hospitalization may become necessary for medical or psychiatric reasons (Table 4–3). Furthermore the patient may require hospitalization not because she is medically unstable or in emotional crisis but because she is out of control or making no progress as an outpatient and thus requires more intensive treatment.

Prognosis

Outcome is difficult to predict because there have been few long-term studies and there is little standardization of criteria and variables. It appears that 40–60% of significantly ill anorexics will make a

Table 4–3. Indications for hospitalization of an adolescent with an eating disorder.

Medical
  Weight < 75% of ideal body weight
  Severe metabolic disturbance
    Heart rate < 40 beats/min
    Temperature < 36 °C
    Systolic blood pressure < 70 mm Hg
    Serum K^+ < 2.5 mEq/L despite oral K^+ replacement
    Severe dehydration
  Cardiac arrhythmia
  Arrested growth and development
  Acute food refusal
  Severe binging and purging
  Failure to respond to outpatient treatment
Psychiatric
  Severe depression or risk of suicide
  Psychosis
  Family crisis
  Failure to comply with a therapeutic contract, or
    inadequate response to outpatient treatment

good physical and psychosocial recovery and that 75% will gain weight. The mortality rate ranges from nil to 19% and is at least 5% in those receiving therapy. The literature pertaining to bulimia is even more sparse, and the outcome appears less favorable. As few as 40–50% of treated bulimics are felt to be cured, and there is a greater likelihood of serious medical complications, death, and risk of suicide than for anorexics who do not manifest bulimic behavior. Recently, however, as the lay public has become more aware of the problem of eating disorders, the disease is being recognized earlier than before.

American Psychiatric Association: *Diagnostic and Statistical Manual of Mental Disorders,* 4th ed. American Psychiatric Press, 1994.

FBNC Study Group: Fluoxetine in the treatment of bulimia nervosa: A multicenter, placebo-controlled, double-blind trial. Arch Gen Psychiatry 1992;49:139.

Fisher M et al: Eating disorders in adolescents: A background paper. J Adolesc Health 1995;16:420.

Harper G: Eating disorders in adolescence. Pediatr Rev 1994;15:72.

Kaye WH: An open trial of fluoxetine in patients with anorexia nervosa. J Clin Psychiatry 1991;52:464.

Kreipe RE: Eating disorders among children and adolescents. Pediatr Rev 1995;16:370.

Kreipe RE et al: Eating disorders in adolescents: A position paper of the Society for Adolescent Medicine. J Adolesc Health 1995;16:476.

Romeo F: Adolescent boys and anorexia nervosa. Adolescence 1994;29:643.

Woodside DB: A review of anorexia nervosa and bulimia nervosa. Curr Probl Pediatr 1995;25:67.

EXOGENOUS OBESITY

Body weight is most commonly used to quantitate obesity; however, this disorder is a function of age, sex, height, frame, and Tanner stage. A body weight 20% above that appropriate for height is considered obesity. In adolescents, body weight alone tends to overestimate fatness. Underwater weights are the most accurate measure of lean body mass. Triceps skinfold thickness is the most practical way to measure obesity in teenagers. A triceps skinfold measurement of more than 1 SD above the mean (85th percentile) defines obesity, and one at the 95th percentile indicates superobesity. The BMI (weight [kg] divided by height squared [m^2]), used to assess obesity in adults, correlates less well with the percentage of body fat in children and adolescents (Figure 4–5)

Background

Obesity is the most common nutritional disorder of children in the United States, and the prevalence of obesity increases significantly between the elementary and high school years. If a child enters adolescence obese, the odds are 4:1 against later achievement of normal weight; but if a child leaves adolescence obese, the odds are 28:1 against later normal weight. The National Children and Youth Fitness Study, parts I and II, completed in 1987, demonstrated a decline in fitness of fifth through twelfth graders and first through fourth graders, respectively. Between 1973 and 1994, the weights of children and adolescents ages 5 to 24 years old increased by over 0.2 kg/yr. The prevalence of obesity, defined as greater than 85th percentile on the weight-for-height curve, in 1973 increased twofold by 1994. The reduction in fitness has paralleled a rise in hours of television watched by children. Factors known to increase the risk of a child's being obese include having obese parents and being an only child. The associated medical risks of obesity include hypertension, elevated triglyceride levels, cerebrovascular accidents, diabetes mellitus, gallbladder disease, slipped capital-femoral epiphyses, degenerative arthritis, and pregnancy complications. The psychosocial hazards of obesity tend to be the greatest consequence for adolescents, who may experience alienation, distorted peer relations, poor self-esteem, guilt, depression, or altered body image.

Diagnosis

A triceps skinfold measurement of more than 1 SD above the mean or weight 20% over ideal body weight indicates obesity. An adolescent with a BMI above the 85th percentile is considered to be at risk of overweight; weight above the 95th percentile is considered overweight. Patients can be identified as at risk for obesity based on current weight relative to height, growth and weight trend, and weight of family members. The history should include onset of obesity, eating and exercise habits, amount of time spent in sedentary activities such as watching television, previous successful and unsuccessful attempts at weight loss, and family history of obesity. In addition, one needs to assess a patient's readiness to lose weight—whether the patient is aware of or denies a weight problem; recognizes the relationship between food, activity, and weight; and recognizes that contributory factors can be controlled. When obesity is diagnosed, the following database can be collected: height; weight; BMI; blood pressure; triceps skinfold measurement; fat distribution; examination of the skin, thyroid, heart, and abdomen; hematocrit; and urinalysis. Endocrine causes, such as hypothyroidism or Cushing's disease, can generally be excluded on the basis of the history and physical examination. If an adolescent is healthy and has no delay of growth or sexual maturation, an underlying endocrinologic, neurologic, or genetic cause is unlikely.

Treatment

For poorly motivated patients, it is probably best—so as not to set the patient up for failure—to provide some basic information about weight control and make oneself available for future visits. For the more highly motivated patient, treatment should be appropriate to age and developmental level and should produce a significant reduction in body weight. The adolescent should be taught appropriate eating and exercise habits to maintain weight reduction yet meet nutritional needs for growth and development.

Anorexiant drugs, fasting, and bypass surgery have no role in the management of obese adolescents. An age-appropriate behavior modification program incorporating good dietary counseling and exercise is optimal (Table 4–4). Diet or exercise alone is not nearly as effective. Guidelines that group foods in categories according to their caloric density may be appreciated by adolescents who hate to count calories. Lifestyle activity recommendations, such as walking and taking the stairs, may be more effective in the long run than regimented exercise programs. Behavior modification components—such as recording one's eating and activity in a notebook, receiving systematic reinforcement for behavior changes, and restructuring how one sees oneself or plans for success—are especially helpful. Behavioral treatment involving parents has been shown to improve long-term maintenance of weight loss in children. Unfortunately, no program of weight reduction has been proved effective.

Bandini LG: Obesity in the adolescent. Adolescent Medicine: State of the Art Reviews 1992;3:459.

Dietz WH: Critical periods in childhood for the development of obesity. Am J Clin Nutr 1994;59:955.

Epstein LH et al: Ten-year follow-up of behavioral, family-based treatment for obese children. JAMA 1990;264:2519.

Freedman DS et al: Secular increases in relative weight and adiposity among children over two decades: The Bogalusa heart study. Pediatrics 1997;99:420.

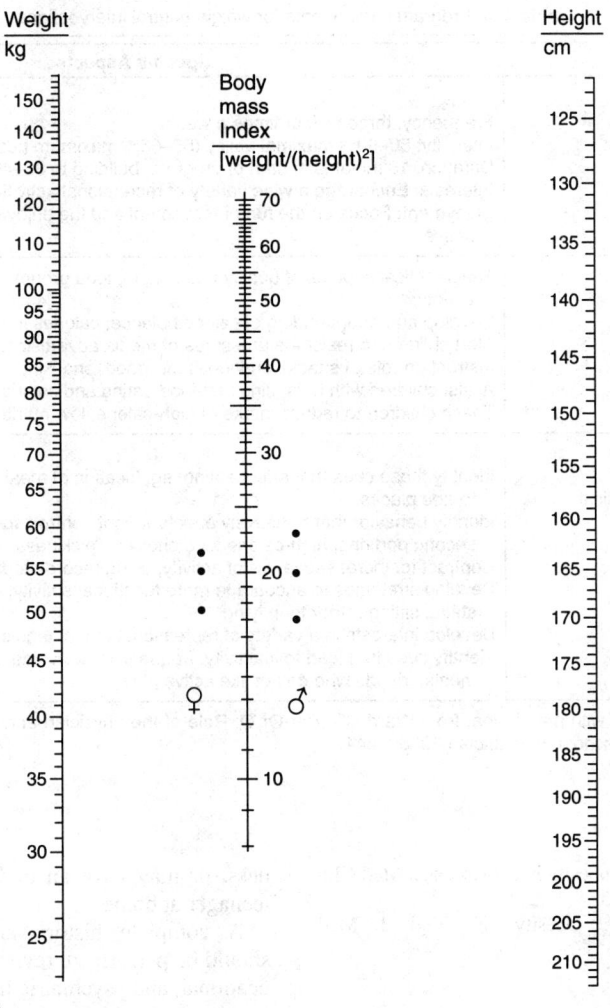

A

AGE	MALES							FEMALES						
(yr)	5th	10th	25th	50th	75th	90th	95th	5th	10th	25th	50th	75th	90th	95th
6	13.0	13.6	14.4	15.3	16.0	17.7	18.7	12.8	13.5	14.0	15.0	16.0	16.9	17.3
7	13.3	13.9	14.7	15.7	16.7	18.5	19.9	13.1	13.8	14.5	15.6	16.8	18.4	19.2
8	13.6	14.2	15.1	16.1	17.4	19.4	21.1	13.5	14.2	15.1	16.2	17.7	19.9	21.1
9	14.0	14.5	15.5	16.6	18.1	20.4	22.3	13.9	14.6	15.6	16.9	18.7	21.3	23.0
10	14.5	14.9	15.9	17.1	18.9	21.3	23.4	14.4	15.1	16.2	17.5	19.6	22.7	24.8
11	15.0	15.3	16.4	17.6	19.7	22.2	24.5	14.9	15.5	16.7	18.2	20.4	23.8	26.3
12	15.5	15.8	16.9	18.2	20.4	23.1	25.5	15.3	16.0	17.3	18.8	21.2	24.8	27.7
13	16.0	16.3	17.4	18.8	21.1	24.0	26.5	15.8	16.4	17.8	19.3	21.9	25.6	28.8
14	16.5	16.9	18.0	19.4	21.9	24.8	27.3	16.2	16.8	18.2	19.9	22.5	26.1	29.6
15	17.0	17.5	18.7	20.1	22.5	25.6	28.0	16.6	17.2	18.6	20.3	23.0	26.5	30.2
16	17.4	18.0	19.2	20.8	23.2	26.3	28.6	16.9	17.5	18.9	20.7	23.5	26.7	30.6
17	17.8	18.5	19.8	21.4	23.8	26.9	29.2	17.1	17.8	19.2	21.0	23.8	26.9	30.9
18-20	18.6	19.7	21.0	23.0	25.3	28.4	30.5	17.6	18.4	19.7	21.6	24.3	27.2	31.2
21-23	19.0	20.0	21.4	23.6	26.0	29.0	31.2	17.7	18.5	19.8	21.8	24.4	27.7	31.5

B

Figure 4–5. A: Nomogram for determining body mass index (BMI) from height and weight. A straight-edge connecting weight and height allows one to read BMI (weight in kg [height in m²]). The three dots on the left side of the BMI line represent 50th percentile values for females aged 20 years (top), 15 years (middle), and 10 years (bottom). The dots on the right side are for similar-aged males. **B:** Percentile values for BMI (kg/m²). (A and B reproduced, with permission, from Forbes GR: Nutrition and growth. In: *Textbook of Adolescent Medicine.* McAnarney ER et al [editors]. Saunders, 1992.)

Table 4–4. Program components for weight control interventions.

Component	Specific Aspects
Physical activity 1. Cardiovascular fitness 2. High-calorie equivalent	Frequency: three or four times a week. Intensity: 50–60% maximal ability (55–65% maximum heart rate). Duration: 15 minutes at start of program, building to 30–40 minutes. Interests: Encourage a wide variety of recreational activities. Enjoyment: Focus on the fun of movement and the enjoyment of being physically active.
Nutritional education	Teach critical aspects of quality nutrition, ie, food groups, serving requirements, and variety. Develop an understanding of caloric balance; calories in versus calories out. Alert children to resist the pressures of media advertising. Instruct on role of snacks and ideas for "good" snacking. Assist children with balancing fast-food eating and caloric intake. Teach children to reduce intake of high-calorie, low-nutrition foods.
Behavior modification 1. Change eating habits 2. Increase habitual physical activity	Identify those cues that affect eating, eg, location of meals, size of plates, food in easy-to-see places. Identify behavior that negatively affects weight control: speed of eating, chronic second portions, high-calorie food choices, "pickiness." Contract for increased levels of activity, using record cards or activity contracts. Develop strategies to encourage more functional activity, eg, walking to school, taking stairs, sitting rather than lying. Develop interests in a variety of recreational areas: tennis, dancing, skating. Identify cues that lead to inactivity: frequent TV watching, lying down after school or meals, friends who do not like active play.

[1]Modified and reproduced, with permission, from Ward DS, Bar-Or O: Role of the physician and physical education teacher in the treatment of obesity at school. Pediatrician 1986:13:44.

Rees JM: Management of obesity in adolescence. Med Clin North Am 1990;74:1275.

Rosenbaum MD et al: Obesity. N Engl J Med 1997;337:396.

SCHOOL AVOIDANCE

Any teenager who has missed more than 1 week of school for a physical illness or symptom—and whose clinical picture is inconsistent with a serious illness—should be suspected of harboring primary or secondary emotional factors that contribute to the absence. Investigation of absences may show a pattern, such as missing morning classes or missing the same days at the beginning or end of the week. Emotional factors for school absenteeism are usually attributed to physical symptoms in this age group.

School avoidance should be suspected in children who are consistently absent in spite of parents' and professionals' attempts to encourage school attendance. Adolescents with school avoidance problems often have a history of excessive absences or separation difficulties as a younger child. There may also be a record of recurrent somatic complaints. Parents of a school avoider often feel at a loss about how to compel their adolescent to attend school, may lack the sophistication to distinguish malingering from ill-

ness, or may have an underlying need to keep the teenager at home.

A complete history and physical examination should be performed, reviewing the past medical, educational, and psychiatric history. Signs of emotional problems should be explored. After obtaining permission from the patient and parents, the physician may find it helpful to speak directly with school officials and some key teachers. There may be problems with particular teachers or subjects or adverse environmental factors at the school (eg, school yard bullying, an intimidating instructor). Some students get so far behind academically that they see no way of catching up and feel overwhelmed. Separation anxiety, sometimes of long duration, may be manifested in subconscious worries that something may happen to the mother while the teenager is at school.

The school nurse may give useful information, including the number of visits to the nurse during the last school year. An important part of the history is how the parents respond to the absences and somatic complaints. There may be a subconscious attempt to keep the adolescent at home, which may be coupled with secondary gains (increased parental attention) for remaining at home.

Treatment

The importance of going back to school after a period of school avoidance in the next 2 or 3 days needs to be emphasized. The pediatrician should facilitate this process by offering to speak with school officials to excuse missed examinations, homework, and papers. The pediatrician should speak directly with teachers who are punitive. The objective is to make the transition back to school as easy as possible. The longer adolescents stay out of school, the more anxious they may become about returning and the more difficult the return becomes. If an illness or symptom becomes so severe that an adolescent cannot go to school, both the patient and the parents must be informed that a visit to a medical office is necessary. The physician focuses visits on the parents as much as on the adolescent to alleviate any parental guilt about sending the child to school. If the adolescent cannot stay in school, hospitalization should be recommended for an in-depth medical and psychiatric evaluation. Parents should be cautioned about the possibility of relapse after school holidays, summer vacation, or an acute illness.

Klerman LV: School absence: A health perspective. Pediatr Clin North Am 1988;35:1253.

SCHOOL FAILURE

When children graduate from grade school to middle school or junior high school, the amount and complexity of course work increase significantly. This occurs at about the same time as the rapid physical, social, and emotional changes of puberty. To perform well academically, young adolescents must have the necessary cognitive capacity, study habits, concentration, motivation, interest, and emotional focus. Academic failure presenting at adolescence has a broad differential: (1) limited intellectual abilities, (2) specific learning disabilities, (3) depression or emotional problems, (4) physical causes such as visual or hearing problems, (5) excessive school absenteeism secondary to chronic disease such as asthma or neurologic dysfunction, (6) lack of ability to concentrate, (7) attention deficit disorder, (8) lack of motivation, and (9) drug and alcohol problems. Each of these possible causes must be explored in depth (Table 4–5). Evaluation of this differential requires a careful history, physical examination, and appropriate laboratory tests as well as standardized educational and psychologic testing.

Treatment

Treatment depends on the cause. Management must be individualized to address specific needs, foster strengths, and implement a feasible program. For children with specific learning disabilities, an individual prescription for regular and special education courses, teachers, and extracurricular activities is important. Counseling helps these adolescents gain cop-

ing skills, raise self-esteem, and develop socialization skills. If there is a history of hyperactivity or attention deficit disorder along with poor ability to concentrate, a trial of stimulant medication (eg, methylphenidate, dextroamphetamine) may be useful. If the teenager appears to be depressed or if other serious emotional problems are uncovered, further psychologic evaluation should be recommended.

Goldman LS et al: Diagnosis and treatment of attention-deficit/hyperactivity disorder in children and adolescents. JAMA 1998;279:1100.
Kube DA, Shapiro BK: Persistent school dysfunction: Unrecognized comorbidity and suboptimal therapy. Clin Pediatr (Phila) 1996;45:571.
Shapiro BK, Gallico RP: Learning disabilities. Pediatr Clin North Am 1993;40:491.
Shaywitz BA, Fletcher JM, Shaywitz SE: Attention-deficit/hyperactivity disorder. Adv Pediatr 1997;44:331.
Shaywitz SE: Dyslexia. N Engl J Med 1998;338:307.

BREAST DISORDERS

The breast examination should become part of the routine physical examination in girls as soon as breast budding occurs. The preadolescent thus comes to accept breast examination as a routine part of health care, and the procedures serves as an opportunity to offer reassurance about any concerns she may have. The breast examination begins with inspection of the breasts for symmetry and Tanner stage. Asymmetric breast development is common and generally transient in adolescents. Unusual causes of breast asymmetry include unilateral breast hypoplasia, amastia, absence of the pectoralis major muscle, and unilateral virginal hypertrophy (massive enlargement of the breast during puberty).

Palpation of the breasts can be performed with the patient in the supine position and the patient's ipsilateral arm placed behind her head. The examiner palpates the breast tissue with the flat of the fingers in concentric circles from the sternum, clavicle, and axilla in to the areola. The areola should be gently compressed to check for discharge.

Instructions for breast self-examination and its purpose can be given to older adolescents during this portion of the physical examination, and the patient should be encouraged to begin monthly self-examination after each menstrual flow.

BREAST MASSES

Most breast masses in adolescents are benign (Table 4–6); however, approximately 150 cases of

Table 4–5. A classification of common developmental dysfunctions in adolescence.

Dysfunction	Subtypes	Frequent Manifestations[1]
1. Attention deficits	a. Primary b. Secondary (to anxiety or poor information processing) c. Situational (only evident in certain settings)	Weak attention to detail; distractibility; impulsivity, restlessness; task impersistence; performance inconsistency; organizational problems; reduced working capacity
2. Memory impairments	a. Generalized retrieval problems b. Modality-specific retrieval problems c. Attention-retention deficiencies	Deficient, undependable, or slow recall of data from long- or short-term memory Problems with revisualization or auditory, motor, or sequential recall Poor recall associated with superficial initial registration
3. Language disorders	a. Receptive b. Expressive	Poor verbal and reading comprehension; poor listening; trouble following directions and explanations Problems with word finding, sentence formulation Difficulty with written expression
4. Higher order cognitive disabilities	a. Inferential weakness b. Poor verbal reasoning c. Poor nonverbal reasoning d. Difficulty with abstraction, symbolization e. Weak generalization and rule application	Problems understanding and assimilating new concepts; tendency to think "concretely" delays in mathematics, reading comprehension, science, social studies
5. Fine motor incoordination	a. Eye:hand coordination problems b. Impaired propriokinesthetic feedback c. Dyspraxia d. Motor memory impairment	Slow, labored, sometimes illegible writing; awkward pencil grip; dyssynchrony between cognitive tempo and writing speed; output failure—reduced productivity
6. Organizational deficiencies	a. Temporal-sequential disorientation b. Material disarray c. Integrative dysfunction d. Resynthesis problems e. Attentional disorganization	Problems with time allocation, schedules, planning, arranging ideas in writing Tendency to lose, misplace, forget books, papers; trouble organizing notebook Varying inability to integrate data from multiple sources or sensory modalities Trouble extracting most salient details, retelling and adapting data to current demands Impulsivity, erratic tempo, poor self-monitoring, careless errors
7. Socialization disabilities	a. Wide range of subtypes, including conduct disorder, social impulsivity, impaired social cognition or feedback, egocentricity	Antisocial behaviors; delinquency; withdrawal; excessive dependency on peer support

Modified and reproduced, with permission, from Levine MD, Zallen BG: Learning disorders of adolescence. Pediatr Clin North Am 1984;31:2.
[1]Manifestations are likely to vary somewhat depending on compensatory strengths, quality of educational experience, and motivation.

Table 4–6. Breast masses in adolescent females.[1]

Most common	Rare
Benign fibroadenoma	Lymphangioma
Breast cyst	Hemangioma
Less common	Neurofibromatosis
Giant (juvenile) fibroadenoma	Dermatofibromatosis
Virginal (juvenile) hypertrophy	Papillomatosis
Breast abscess	Papilloma sarcoidosis
Lipoma	Nipple adenoma
Hematoma	Nipple keratoma
Malignant potential	Mammary duct estasia
Adenocarcinoma	Intraductal granuloma
Invasive ductal carcinoma	Galactocele
Intraductal papilloma	Metastatic disease
Cystosarcoma phyllodes	Other

[1]Reproduced, with permission, from Beach RK: Breast disorders. In: McAnarney ER et al: *Textbook of Adolescent Medicine.* Saunders, 1992.

adenocarcinoma of the breast are reported each year in the United States in women under 25 years of age. Fibroadenomas account for 90% of breast lumps in teenagers seen in referral clinics; the remainder are cysts. In general practice, cysts may account for as many as 60% of breast masses

Fibroadenoma

Fibroadenoma presents as a rubbery, well-demarcated, slowly growing, nontender mass that may occur in any quadrant but is most commonly found in the upper outer quadrant of the breast. Most are less than 5 cm in diameter. In 25% of cases, there are multiple or recurrent lesions. Quiescence can be expected after the teenage years.

Cysts

Breast cysts are generally tender and spongy, with exacerbation of symptoms premenstrually and abatement just after. Often they are multiple. Spontaneous regression occurs over two or three menstrual cycles in about 50% of cases.

It is reasonable to follow breast masses that are consistent with fibroadenoma or cyst in adolescents for two or three menstrual cycles. About 25% of fibroadenomas become smaller, and about 50% of cysts resolve. If there is no change in a presumed fibroadenoma after this time, ultrasound study will differentiate a solid tumor from a cyst. Patients with solid tumors over 2.5 cm in diameter should be referred for excisional biopsy. Those with tumors less than 2.5 cm in diameter may be followed every 3–6 months, since many will shrink or remain the same. Persistent cystic lesions may be drained by needle aspiration. Patients with suspicious lesions should be referred immediately to a breast surgeon (Table 4–7).

Fibrocystic Breasts

Fibrocystic breasts (or fibrocystic breast disease)

Table 4–7. Breast lesions.

Adenocarcinoma	Hard, nonmobile, well-circumscribed, painless mass; generally indolent clinical course; occurs also in males but less frequently.
Cystosarcoma phyllodes	Firm, rubbery mass that may suddenly enlarge; associated with skin necrosis; most often benign.
Giant juvenile fibroadenoma	Remarkable large fibroadenoma with overlying dilated superficial veins; accounts for 5–10% of fibroadenomas in adolescents; benign but requires excision to prevent breast atrophy and for cosmetic reasons.
Intraductal papilloma	A cylindric tumor arising from the ductal epithelium; often subareolar but may be in the periphery of the breast in adolescents, with associated nipple discharge. Most are benign but require excision for cytologic diagnosis.
Fat necrosis	Localized inflammatory process in one breast; follows trauma in about half of cases. Subsequent scarring may be confused with cancer.
Virginal or juvenile hypertrophy	Massive enlargement of both breasts or less often, one breast; attributed to end-organ hypersensitivity to normal hormonal levels just before or within a few years after menarche.
Miscellaneous	Fibroma, galactocele, hemangioma, intraductal granuloma, interstitial fibrosis, keratoma, lipoma, granular cell myoblastoma, papilloma, sclerosing adenosis.

is sometimes seen in older adolescents but is more common in women in the third and fourth decades. It is characterized by cyclic tenderness and nodularity bilaterally and is believed to be influenced by the estrogen-progesterone balance.

Reassuring the young woman about the benign nature of the process and emphasizing the importance of breast self-examination may be all that is needed. Oral contraceptives reduce the risk of fibrocystic breast disease and may be appropriate for the sexually active female with a personal history of breast cyst or family history of fibrocystic breasts. Studies have shown no association between methylxanthines and fibrocystic breasts; however, some women report reduced symptoms when they discontinue caffeine intake. The efficacy of vitamin E is unknown.

Breast Abscess

The female with a breast abscess usually complains of unilateral breast pain, and examination reveals overlying inflammatory changes. Often the examination is misleading in that the infection may extend much deeper than suspected. A palpable mass is found only late in the course. Although breast feeding is the most common cause of mastitis, trauma and eczema involving the areola are frequent factors in teenagers. *Staphylococcus aureus* is the most common cause, but other aerobic and anaerobic organisms have also been implicated.

Cyclic mastodynia, fibrocystic disease, or chest wall pain may also be causes of breast pain, but there should be no associated inflammatory signs.

Fluctuant abscesses should be surgically incised and drained. Oral antibiotics with appropriate coverage (dicloxacillin or a cephalosporin) should be given for 2–4 weeks. Ice packs for the first 24 hours and heat thereafter may relieve symptoms.

GALACTORRHEA

In teenagers, galactorrhea is most often benign; however, a careful history and workup are necessary. Prolactinomas are the most common pathologic cause of galactorrhea in adolescents of both sexes and generally present as failure of sexual maturation. Hypothyroidism is the second most common cause in the adolescent years but has been reported only in girls, usually prepubertally.

Galactorrhea may be present after spontaneous or induced abortions as well as postpartum. Numerous prescribed and illicit drugs are associated with galactorrhea (Table 4–8). In addition, stimulation of the intercostal nerves (following surgery or due to herpes zoster), stimulation of the nipples, endocrine disorders (hypothyroidism, pituitary prolactinoma), central nervous system disorders (hypothalamic injury), or significant emotional distress may produce galactorrhea.

Table 4–8. Drugs associated with breast symptoms (galactorrhea, gynecomastia, pain, mass).[1]

Street drugs (illicit or abused)
  Amphetamines
  Marijuana
  Mebrobamate
  Opioids
    Codeine
    Heroin
    Morphine
Hormones or related drugs
  Bromocriptine withdrawal
  Estrogens
  Human chorionic gonadotropin
  Methyltestosterone
  Oral contraceptives
  Tamoxifen
Cancer drugs
  Busulfan
  Vincristine
Prescription medications
  Amitriptyline
  Chlordiazepoxide
  Chlorpromazine
  Cimetidine
  Diazepam
  Digoxin
  Fluphenazine
  Haloperidol
  Imipramine
  Isoniazid
  Mesoridazine
  Methylodopa
  Perphenazine
  Phenothiazines
  Reserpine
  Spironolactone
  Thiethylperazine
  Thioxanthines
  Tricyclic antidepressants
  Trifluoperazine
  Trimeprazine

[1]Modified and reproduced, with permission, from Beach RK: Routine breast exams: A chance to reassure, guide, and protect. Contemp Pediatr 1987;4:70.

Clinical Findings

If there is no history of pregnancy or drug use, thyroid-stimulating hormone (TSH) and serum prolactin levels should be determined. An elevated TSH confirms the diagnosis of hypothyroidism. An elevated prolactin and normal TSH, often accompanied by amenorrhea, suggest a hypothalamic or pituitary tumor, and CT scan or MRI is indicated. When the prolactin level is normal, uncommon causes such as adrenal, renal, or ovarian tumors should be considered. The female with a negative workup and persistent galactorrhea may be followed with menstrual history and serum prolactin level every 6–12 months. In many cases, symptoms resolve spontaneously and no diagnosis is made. The female with an elevated serum prolactin concentration but negative prolactinoma workup may be treated with bromocriptine if her symptoms are bothersome or may be observed

with CT scan or MRI every 18 months for several years. Males with a negative workup and normal puberty need to be intensively followed. Males with elevated prolactin levels require a CT scan or MRI every 12–18 months even if the galactorrhea resolves, as there is a significant risk of harboring a pituitary adenoma.

Treatment

Treatment depends on the underlying cause. Prolactinomas may be surgically removed or suppressed with bromocriptine. Bromocriptine may also be beneficial to some amenorrheic females with normal serum prolactin levels.

GYNECOMASTIA

Gynecomastia is a common concern of male adolescents, most of whom (60–70%) develop transient subareolar breast tissue during Tanner stages II and III. Proposed causes include testosterone-estrogen imbalance, increased serum prolactin level, or abnormal serum protein binding levels.

Clinical Findings

In type I idiopathic gynecomastia, the adolescent presents with a unilateral (20% bilateral) tender, firm mass beneath the areola. More generalized breast enlargement is classified as type II. Pseudogynecomastia is the term for excessive fat tissue or prominent pectoralis muscles.

Differential Diagnosis

Gynecomastia may be drug-induced (see Table 4–9). Testicular, adrenal, or pituitary tumors, Klinefelter's syndrome, primary hypogonadism, thyroid or

Table 4–9. Drugs associated with gynecomastia

Antibiotics	**Drugs and substances of abuse**
Isoniazid	Alcohol
Ketoconazole	Amphetamines
Metronidazole	Marijuana
Anti-ulcer	Opiates
Cimetidine	**Hormones or related agents**
Omeprazole	Anabolic steroids
Ranitidine	Estrogens
Cardiovascular drugs	Chorionic gonadotropin
Captopril	**Psychoactive medications**
Digoxin	Tricyclic antidepressants, eg,
Enalapril	amitriptyline
Methyldopa	Antipsychotics, eg,
Reserpine	chlorpromazine, fluphena-
Verapamil	zine, haloperidol
Chemotherapeutic drugs	Anxiolytics, eg, chlordiaze-
Busulfan	poxide, diazepam
Vincristine	

hepatic dysfunction, or malnutrition may also be associated with gynecomastia (Table 4–10).

Treatment

If gynecomastia is idiopathic, reassurance about the common and benign nature of the process can be given. Resolution may take several months to 2 years. Medical reduction has been achieved with pharmacotherapeutic agents, such as dihydrotestosterone, danazol, clomiphene, and tamoxifen, but these agents should be reserved for patients in whom there is no decrease in breast size after 2 years. Surgery is reserved for those with significant psychologic trauma or severe breast enlargement.

Braunstein GD: Gynecomastia. N Engl J Med 1993;328:490.
Hindle WH, Pan EY: Breast disorders in female adolescents. AM:STARS 1994;5:123.
Neinstein LS: Review of breast masses in adolescents. Adolesc Pediatr Gynecol 1994;7:119.

GYNECOLOGIC DISORDERS IN ADOLESCENCE

PHYSIOLOGY OF MENSTRUATION

The menstrual cycle is divided into three consecutive phases: follicular (the first 14 days), ovulatory (midcycle), and luteal (days 16–28). During the follicular phase, pulsatile gonadotropin-releasing hormone (GnRH) stimulates anterior pituitary secretion of FSH and luteinizing hormone (LH). Under the influence of FSH and LH, a dominant follicle emerges by days 5–7 of the menstrual cycle, and the others become atretic. Rising estradiol levels cause proliferation of the endometrium. By the midfollicular

Table 4–10. Disorders associated with gynecomastia.

Klinefelter's syndrome
Traumatic paraplegia
Male pseudohermaphroditism
Testicular feminization syndrome
Reifenstein's syndrome
17-Ketosteroid reductase deficiency
Endocrine tumors (seminoma, Leydig cell tumor, teratoma, feminizing adrenal tumor, hepatoma, leukemia, hemophilia, bronchogenic carcinoma, leprosy, etc)
Hypothyroidism
Hyperthyroidism
Cirrhosis
Herpes zoster
Friedreich's ataxia

phase, FSH is beginning to decline secondary to estradiol-mediated negative feedback, while LH continues to rise as a result of estradiol-mediated positive feedback.

LH receptors on the follicle increase in number in the late follicular phase, increasing the estradiol secreted by the follicle. This amplifies endometrial proliferation. The rising LH initiates progesterone secretion and luteinization of the granulosa cells of the follicle. Progesterone in turn further stimulates LH and FSH. This leads to the LH surge, which causes the follicle to rupture and expel the oocyte.

During the luteal phase, the pulsatile release of GnRH occurs less frequently, and LH and FSH gradually decline. The corpus luteum secretes progesterone and 17-hydroxyprogesterone. The endometrium enters the secretory phase in response to rising levels of estrogen and progesterone, with maturation 8–9 days after ovulation. If there is no pregnancy or placental human chorionic gonadotropin (hCG), luteolysis begins; estrogen and progesterone levels decline; and the endometrial lining is shed as menstrual flow (Figure 4–6).

PELVIC EXAMINATION

A pelvic examination may be indicated to evaluate abdominal pain or menstrual disorders or to detect a suspected sexually transmitted disease in the adolescent. By 16–18 years of age, a routine pelvic examination should be performed to obtain the first Papanicolaou (Pap) smear and to evaluate reproductive anatomy. The adolescent may be apprehensive about the first examination. It should not be rushed, and an explanation of the procedure and its purpose should precede it. The patient can be encouraged to relax by slow, deep breathing and by relaxation of her lower abdominal and inner thigh muscles. A young adolescent may wish to have her mother present during the examination, but the history should be taken privately. A female chaperone should be present with male examiners.

The pelvic examination begins by placing the patient in the dorsal lithotomy position after equipment and supplies are ready (Table 4–11). The examiner inspects the external genitalia, noting the pubic hair maturity rating, the size of the clitoris (2–5 mm is normal), Skene's glands just inside the urethral meatus, and Bartholin's glands at 4 o'clock and 8 o'clock outside the hymenal ring. In cases of alleged sexual abuse or assault, the horizontal measurement of the relaxed prepubertal hymenal opening should be recorded and the presence of any lacerations, bruises, scarring, or synechiae about the hymen, vulva, or anus should be noted.

A vaginal speculum of the appropriate size is then inserted at a 45-degree twist and angled 45 degrees downward. (A medium Pedersen speculum is most

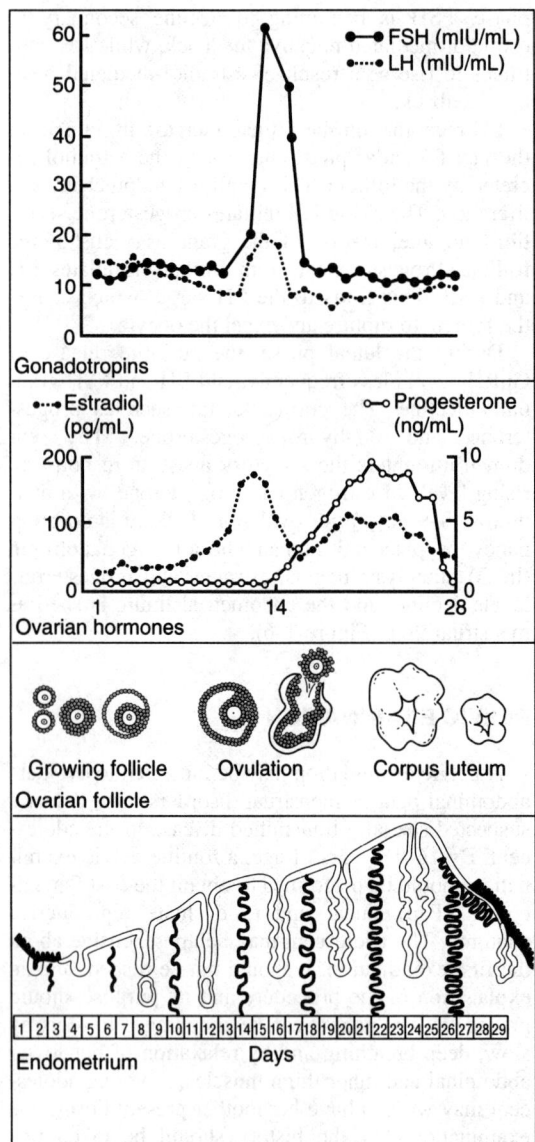

Figure 4–6. Physiology of the normal ovulatory menstrual cycle; gonadotropin secretion, ovarian hormone production, follicular maturation, and endometrial changes during one cycle. FSH = follicle-stimulating hormone, LH = luteinizing hormone. (Reproduced, with permission, from Emans SJH, Goldstein DP: *Pediatric & Adolescent Gynecology,* 3rd ed. Little, Brown, 1990.)

often used in sexually experienced patients; a narrow Huffman is used for virginal patients. A pediatric speculum may be necessary in examining children.) The vaginal walls are inspected for estrinization, inflammation, or lesions. The cervix should be dull pink. Cervical ectropion is commonly seen in adoles-

Table 4–11. Items for pelvic exam tray.

Medium and virginal speculums (warm)
Gloves
Applicator sticks, sterile
Sigmoidoscopy swabs to remove excess discharge
Cervical spatulas, cervical brushes
Microscope slides and cover slips (frosted and labeled)
Centrifuge tube or test tube (if swab is to be placed in drop of saline and slide prepared later)
NaCl dropper bottle
KOH dropper bottle
Slide container to send to lab
Gonorrhea culture plate (room temperature)
Chlamydia culture tube or antigen detection kit
Lubricant
Kleenex
Hemoccult cards
pH paper

cents; the columnar epithelium extends outside the cervical os onto the face of the cervix until later adolescence, when it recedes.

Specimens are obtained, including a wet preparation for leukocytes, trichomonads, and "clue cells"; potassium hydroxide preparation for yeast; cervical swab for gonorrhea culture; endocervical and cervical (transition zone from columnar to squamous epithelium) samples for Papanicolaou smear; and, last, a cervical swab for *Chlamydia* antigen detection testing. A cervical brush provides a higher yield of cells for the endocervical Papanicolaou slide. Papanicolaou smears should be interpreted by a cytopathologist at a laboratory employing the Bethesda system of classification.

The speculum is then removed, and bimanual examination is performed to assess uterine size and position, adnexal enlargement or tenderness, or cervical motion tenderness. Bimanual examination may reveal beading in the adnexa secondary to endometriosis.

MENSTRUAL DISORDERS

1. AMENORRHEA

Amenorrhea is the lack of onset of menses when normally anticipated. Primary amenorrhea is delay in menarche such that there are no menstrual periods or secondary sex characteristics by 14 years of age or no menses in the presence of secondary sex characteristics by 16 years of age. Constitutional delay is normal pubertal progression at a delayed onset or rate. Secondary amenorrhea is defined as the absence of menses for at least three cycles after regular cycles have been present. In some instances, evaluation should begin immediately, without waiting for the specified age or duration of lapsed periods, such as in patients with suspected pregnancy, short stature with the stigmas of Turner's syndrome, or an anatomic defect.

Evaluation for Primary Amenorrhea

Primary amenorrhea may be the result of anatomic abnormalities, chromosomal deviations, or physiologic delay (Table 4–12).

The history should include whether puberty has commenced, level of exercise, nutritional intake, presence of stressors, and the age at menarche for female relatives. A careful physical examination should be done, noting the percentage of ideal body weight for height and age, Tanner stage, vaginal patency, presence of the uterus (assessed through rectoabdominal examination or ultrasonography if pelvic examination is not appropriate), signs of virilization (acne, clitoromegaly of > 5 mm, hirsutism), or stigmas of Turner's syndrome (< 152 cm tall, shield-like chest, widely spaced nipples, increased carrying angle of the arms, webbed neck). The examiner keeps in mind that adrenal androgens are largely responsible for axillary and pubic hair and that estrogen is responsible for breast development; maturation of the external genitalia, vagina, and uterus; and menstruation. If pelvic examination reveals normal female external genitalia and pelvic organs, the physician may order a vaginal smear for estrogen influence or a challenge of medroxyprogesterone, 10 mg orally twice daily for 5 days (Figure 4–7). If the vaginal smear shows estrogen influence or if withdrawal bleeding occurs within 5–7 days after administration of medroxyprogesterone, normal anatomy and adequate estrogen effect are implied. Determination of serum LH level helps to rule out polycystic ovary syndrome; if this test is normal, reassurance may be given and the developmental process followed every few months. If estrogen is insufficient (atrophic vaginal smear or no withdrawal bleeding), serum gonadotropin levels (FSH and LH) should be determined. Low levels of gonadotropins indicate a more severe hypothalamic suppression, perhaps due to anorexia nervosa, chronic disease, or a central nervous system tumor. Involvement of a gynecologist and endocrinologist is helpful at this point. If gonadotropin levels are high, ovarian failure or gonadal dysgenesis is implied, and karyotype should clarify the cause. Absence of any sign of puberty by 14 years of age indicates inadequate estrogen, and the physician should check FSH, LH, and karyotype first before testing for estrogen effect.

If signs of virilization are present (Figure 4–8), determining levels of serum testosterone, free testosterone, and dehydroepiandrosterone sulfate (DHEAS) will help to distinguish polycystic ovaries from adrenal causes of virilization and amenorrhea. Although elevation of testosterone and DHEAS occurs in virilized patients with polycystic ovaries, it is not

Table 4–12. Causes of amenorrhea.

Hypothalamic pituitary axis
  Hypothalamic repression
    Emotional stress
    Depression
    Chronic disease
    Weight loss
    Obesity
    Severe dieting
    Strenuous athletics
    Drugs (post birth control pills, phenothiazines)
  CNS lesion
    Pituitary lesion: adenoma, prolactinoma
    Craniopharyngioma and other brainstem, parasellar tumors
    Head injury with hypothalamic contusion
    Infiltrative process (sarcoidosis)
    Vascular disease (hypothalamic vasculitis)
  Congenital conditions[1]
    Kallmann's syndrome
Ovaries
  Gonadal dysgenesis[1]
    Turner's syndrome (XO)
    Mosaic (XX/XO)
  Injury to ovary
    Autoimmune disease (may include thyroid, adrenal, islet cells)
    Infection (mumps, oophoritis)
    Toxins (alkylating chemotherapeutic agents)
    Irradiation
    Trauma, torsion (rare)
  Polycystic ovary syndrome (Stein-Leventhal) (virilization may be present)
  Ovarian failure
    Premature menopause (may result from causes of ovarian injury)
    Resistant ovary
    Variant of gonadal dysgenesis (mosaic)
Uterovaginal outflow tract
  Müllerian dysgenesis[1]
    Congenital deformity or absence of uterus, uterine tubes, or vagina
  Imperforate hymen, transverse vaginal septum, vaginal agenesis, agenesis of the cervix[1]
  Testicular feminization (absent uterus)[1]
  Uterine lining defect
    Asherman's syndrome (intrauterine synechiae postcurettage or endometritis)
    TB, brucellosis
Defect in hormone synthesis or action (virilization may be present)
  Adrenal hyperplasia[1]
  Cushing's disease
  Adrenal tumor
  Ovarian tumor (rare)
  Drugs (steroids, ACTH)

[1]Indicates condition that usually presents as primary amenorrhea.

as dramatic as with androgen-producing adrenal or ovarian tumors, adrenal hyperplasia, or Cushing's syndrome or disease. Endocrinologic consultation will assist in differentiating the latter causes. Polycystic ovaries is a spectrum of disorders not necessarily accompanied by classic symptoms of obesity, hirsutism, oligomenorrhea, and infertility. Although

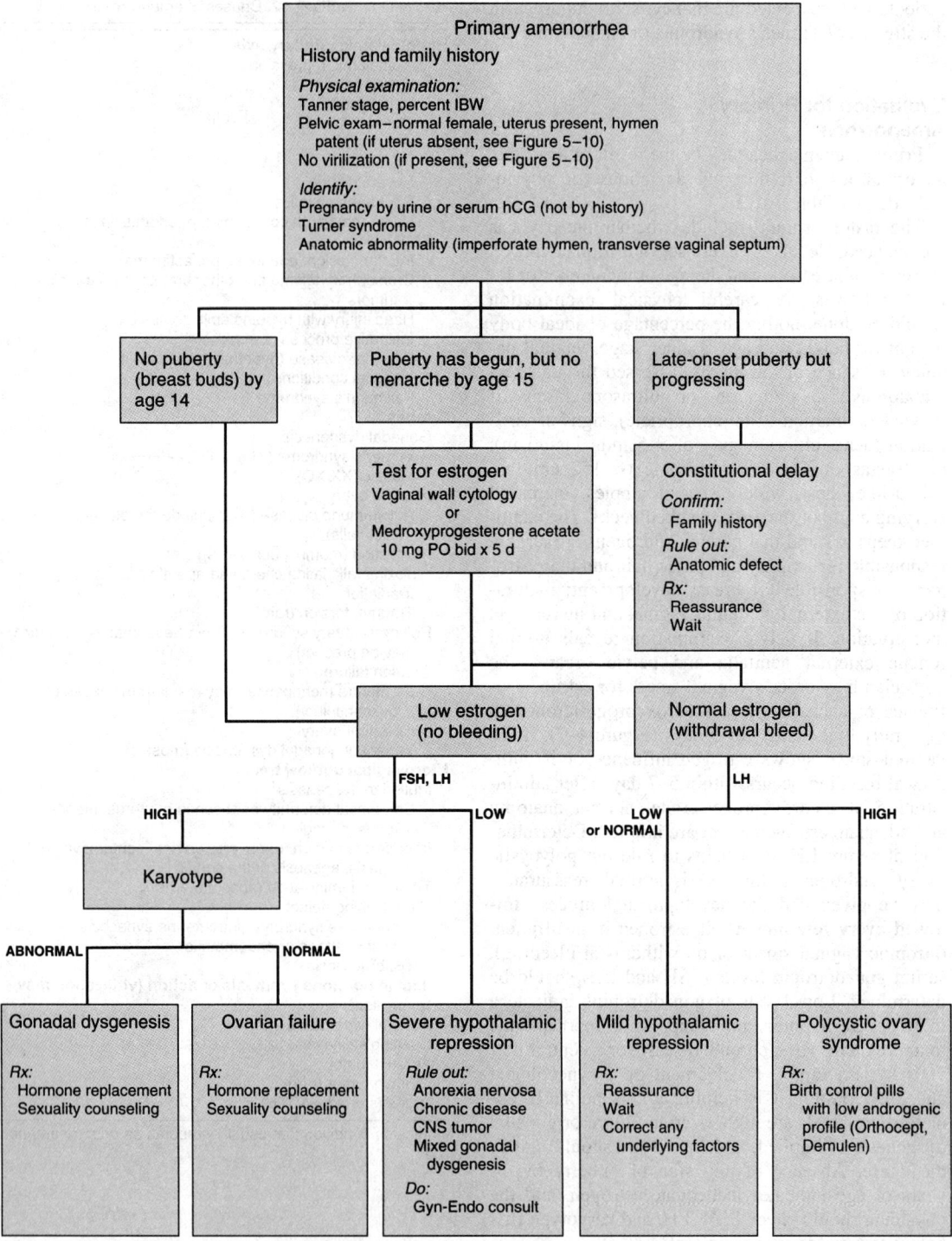

Figure 4–7. Evaluation of primary amenorrhea in a normal female. FSH = follicle-stimulating hormone, IBW = ideal body weight, LH = luteinizing hormone.

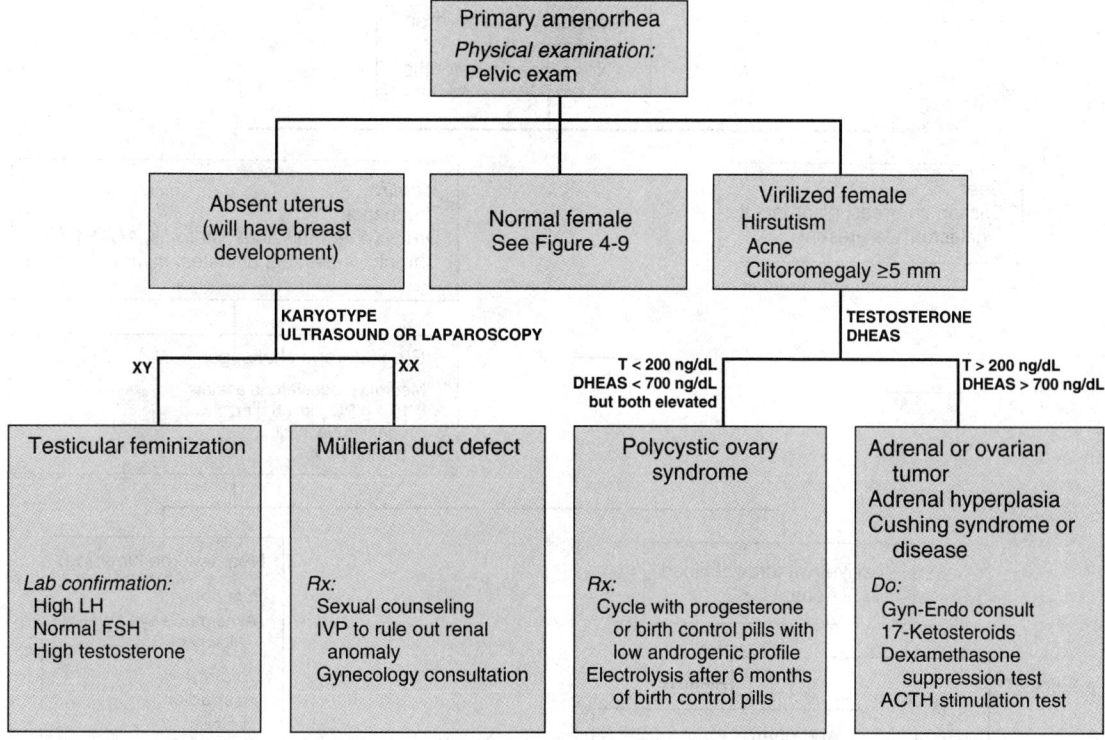

Figure 4–8. Evaluation of primary amenorrhea in a female without a uterus or with virilization.

a classic LH:FSH ratio of 3:1 is described in polycystic ovary syndrome, up to 40% of patients do not have elevated LH levels. Because of insufficient FSH, androstenedione cannot be converted to estradiol in the ovarian follicle, and anovulation and production of excess androgens result. If there is hirsutism and the ovaries are normal in size, these patients can be given progesterone, 10 mg daily, for the first 10 days of each month to allow withdrawal flow. Oral contraceptive pills containing a less androgenic progestin (Demulen, Orthocept) are an alternative treatment. Hirsute patients should have androgen levels determined (as above) and a lipid profile checked. Oral contraceptives may reduce hair diameter, but antiandrogens (spironolactone) are more effective. Weight loss in obese patients should suppress ovarian androgen production. Smoking cessation is indicated to avoid elevated androstenedione levels.

If physical examination reveals an absent uterus (Figure 4–8), karyotyping should be performed to differentiate testicular feminization from müllerian duct defect, because these two entities are managed differently.

Evaluation & Treatment of Secondary Amenorrhea

Secondary amenorrhea results when there is unopposed estrogen, maintaining the endometrium in the proliferative phase. The most common causes are pregnancy, stress, or polycystic ovary syndrome. The history should focus on issues of stress, chronic illness, drugs, weight change, strenuous exercise, sexual activity, and contraceptive use. A review of systems should include questions about headaches, visual changes, and galactorrhea. Physical examination should include ophthalmoscopic and visual field examination, palpation of the thyroid, determination of blood pressure and heart rate, compression of the areola to check for galactorrhea, and a search for signs of androgen excess (eg, hirsutism, clitoromegaly, severe acne, ovarian enlargement).

The first laboratory study obtained is a pregnancy test, even if the patient denies sexual activity. If there is no pregnancy, a progesterone challenge (medroxyprogesterone, 10 mg orally twice daily for 5 days) should be done to determine whether the patient has an estrogen-primed uterus that will respond with withdrawal bleeding 5–7 days later (Figure 4–9).

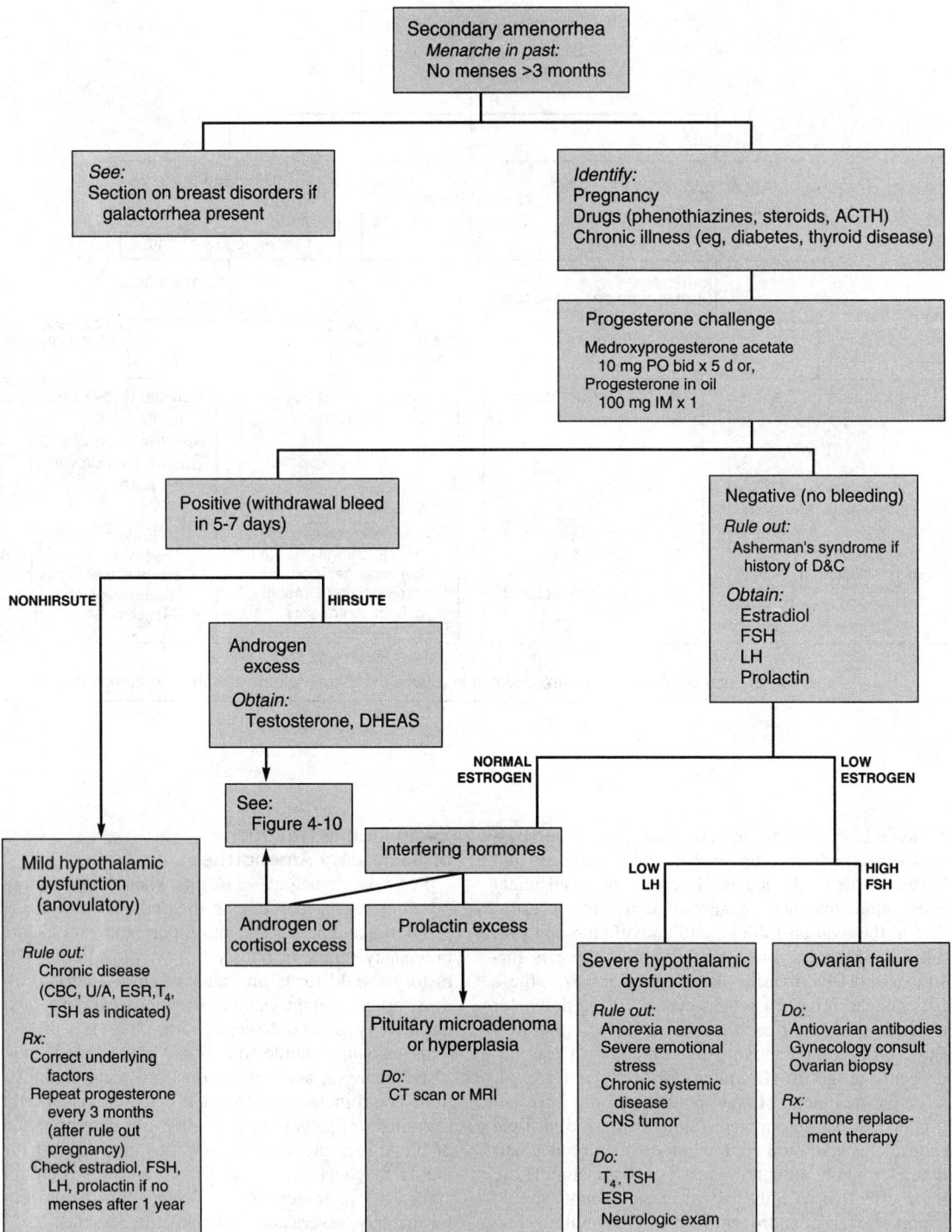

Figure 4–9. Evaluation of secondary amenorrhea. ACTH = adrenocorticotropic hormone, ESR = erythrocyte sedimentation rate, FSH = follicle-stimulating hormone, LH = luteinizing hormone, TSH = thyroid-stimulating hormone, U/A = urinalysis. (Modified from Mammel KA: Secondary amenorrhea. In: *Pediatric Decision Making,* 3rd ed. Berman S [editor]. Decker, 1995.)

Most patients who have withdrawal flow after progesterone have mild hypothalamic suppression due to weight change, athletics, stress, or illness; however, disorders such as polycystic ovary syndrome, adrenal disorders, ovarian tumors, thyroid disease, and diabetes mellitus should be excluded by history and physical examination and appropriate laboratory studies. (See the section on primary amenorrhea and Figure 4–9.)

If there is no withdrawal flow after the progesterone challenge (see Figure 4–9), serum levels of estradiol, FSH, LH, and prolactin should be checked. An elevated FSH level accompanied by a low estrogen level implies ovarian failure, in which case blood for antiovarian antibodies should be obtained and laparoscopy considered. If gonadotropin levels are low or normal and the estradiol level is low, hypothalamic amenorrhea is likely; however, one must consider the possibilities of a central nervous system tumor (prolactinoma), pituitary infarction from postpartum hemorrhage or sickle cell anemia, uterine synechiae, or chronic disease. Further evaluation may be necessary.

2. DYSMENORRHEA

Dysmenorrhea is the most common gynecologic complaint of adolescent girls, with an incidence of about 60%. Yet many teenage girls do not seek help from a physician, relying instead on female relatives, friends, and the media for advice. Therefore, the physician should ask about "menstrual cramps" when taking a review of systems.

Dysmenorrhea can be divided into primary and secondary dysmenorrhea on the basis of whether or not there is underlying pelvic disease.

Primary dysmenorrhea, in which no pelvic disease is detectable, can be further subdivided into primary spasmodic dysmenorrhea and psychogenic dysmenorrhea (Table 4–13). Primary spasmodic dysmenorrhea accounts for 80% of cases of adolescent dysmenorrhea and most often affects women under 25 years of age.

Pelvic examination is normal in females with primary spasmodic or psychogenic dysmenorrhea. The pelvic examination has diagnostic benefits and provides an opportunity to educate and reassure the patient about her normal reproductive function. However, if the patient has never been sexually active and the history is consistent with primary spasmodic dysmenorrhea, a trial of a prostaglandin inhibitor is justified. If the patient is sexually active or if there is no response to a prostaglandin inhibitor, pelvic examination is indicated.

Secondary dysmenorrhea is menstrual pain due to an underlying pelvic lesion (Table 4–13). Although uncommon in adolescents, when present it is most often due to infection or endometriosis. Endometriosis is not limited to adults, as once thought; in one study of adolescent females with chronic pelvic pain, more than 40% who had not received a definitive diagnosis by the third visit were found to have endometriosis.

The clinician evaluating a patient with secondary dysmenorrhea should take a sexual history and conduct a pelvic examination even if the patient is not sexually active. Culture for gonococci, a *Chlamydia* antigen detection test, a CBC and sedimentation rate, and a pregnancy test should be done. Gynecologic consultation is indicated to look for endometriosis or congenital problems by ultrasonography, hysteroscopy, or laparoscopy. Treatment depends on the cause (Table 4–13).

3. DYSFUNCTIONAL UTERINE BLEEDING

Dysfunctional uterine bleeding may consist of hypermenorrhea or polymenorrhea. It results when an endometrium that has proliferated under unopposed estrogen stimulation finally begins to slough, but incompletely, causing irregular, painless bleeding. The unopposed estrogen stimulation occurs during anovulatory cycles, common in younger adolescents who have not been menstruating for long but occurring also in older adolescents during times of stress or illness.

Clinical Findings

Typically, the adolescent has had several years of regular cycles and then begins to have menses every 2 weeks, or complains of bleeding for 2–3 weeks after 2–3 months of amenorrhea. A past history of painless, irregular periods at intervals of less than 3 weeks may also be elicited. Bleeding for more than 10 days should be considered abnormal. Dysfunctional uterine bleeding must be considered a diagnosis of exclusion (Table 4–14).

Management

A pregnancy test and pelvic examination with appropriate cultures should be performed in sexually active patients. A CBC, including a platelet count, should also be obtained. The history and physical findings may suggest the need for additional coagulation or hormonal studies. Coagulation studies should be done if the patient presents with severe bleeding or within 1 year after menarche. Management depends on the severity of the problem (Table 4–15). It is important to treat for a minimum of 3–4 months to progressively reduce the endometrium to baseline height.

4. MITTELSCHMERZ

Mittelschmerz is midcyle pain caused by irritation of the peritoneum due to spillage of fluid from the

Table 4–13. Dysmenorrhea in the adolescent.

Primary Dysmenorrhea—no pelvic pathology

	Etiology	Onset and Duration	Symptoms	Pelvic Exam	Treatment
Primary spasmodic	Excessive amount of prostaglandin F2α, which attaches to myometrium causing uterine contractions, hypoxia, and ischemia. Also, directly sensitizes pain receptors.	Begins with onset of flow or just prior and lasts 1–2 days. Does not start until 6–18 months after menarche, when cycles become ovulatory.	Lower abdominal cramps radiating to lower back and thighs. Associated nausea, vomiting diarrhea, and urinary frequency also due to excess prostaglandins.	Normal. May wait to examine if never sexually active and history is consistent with primary spasmodic dysmenorrhea.	Mild—heating pad, warm baths, nonprescription analgesics. Moderate—severe: prostaglandin inhibitors at onset of flow or pain. Oral contraceptives for sexually active patients.
Psychogenic	May have history of sexual abuse or may have difficulty adjusting to womanhood. May have secondary gain from school or work avoidance.	Starts at menarche. Pain begins with anticipation of menses and lasts throughout flow.	Abdominal cramps.	Normal.	Educate regarding normal menstrual function. Reassure that pain does not indicate pathology. Relaxation techniques and biofeedback. Counseling to understand underlying issues.

Secondary Dysmenorrhea—underlying pathology present. (Always perform pelvic exam if secondary dysmenorrhea suspected or patient is sexually active. Gonorrhea culture, test for *Chlamydia*, CBC, and ESR should be obtained.)

	Etiology	Onset and Duration	Symptoms	Pelvic Exam	Treatment
Infection	Most often due to a sexually transmitted disease such as chlamydia or gonorrhea.	Recent onset of pelvic cramps.	Pelvic cramps, excessive bleeding, intermenstrual spotting or vaginal discharge.	Mucopurulent or purulent discharge from cervical os, cervical friability, cervical motion tenderness, adnexal tenderness, positive culture for STD.	Appropriate antibiotics.
Endometriosis	Aberrant implants of endometrial tissue in pelvis or abdomen; may result from reflux.	Generally starts more than 2 years after menarche.	Pelvic pain, may occur intermenstrually.	Two thirds are tender on exam especially during late luteal phase.	Hormonal suppression by oral contraceptives or danazol. Surgery may be necessary for extensive disease.
Complication of pregnancy	Spontaneous abortion, ectopic pregnancy.	Acute onset.	Pelvic cramps associated with a delay in menses.	Positive hCG, enlarged uterus or adnexal mass.	Immediate gynecologic consult.
Congenital anomalies	Transverse vaginal septum, septate uterus, or cervical stenosis.	Onset at menarche.	Pelvic cramps.	Underlying congenital anomaly may be apparent. May require exam under anesthesia.	Gynecologic consult for ultrasound, hysteroscopy, or laparoscopy.
IUD	Increased uterine contractions, or increase risk for pelvic infection.	Onset after placement of IUD or acutely if due to infection.	Pelvic cramps, heavy menstrual bleeding, may have vaginal discharge.	Normal, or see infection earlier.	Prostaglandin inhibitors of mefenamic acid may be drug of choice because it also reduces flow. Appropriate antibiotics and consider removal of IUD if infection is present.
Pelvic adhesions	Previous abdominal surgery or pelvic inflammatory disease.	Delayed onset after surgery or PID.	Abdominal pain, may or may not be associated with menstrual cycles; possible alteration in bowel pattern.	Variable.	Surgery.

Table 4–14. Differential diagnosis of dysfunctional uterine bleeding in adolescents.[1]

Pelvic inflammatory disease or cervicitis
Complication of pregnancy: ectopic pregnancy, threatened abortion, incomplete abortion, missed abortion
Breakthrough bleeding on oral contraceptives
Blood dyscrasias: iron deficiency, thrombocytopenia, coagulaopathy, von Willebrand's disease, leukemia
Endocrine disorders: hypothyroidism, hyperthyroidism, diabetes mellitus, adrenal disease, hyperprolactinemia
Trauma
Foreign body
Uterine, vaginal, ovarian, abnormalities: carcinoma, fibroids, adenosis from DES, premature menopause

[1]Reproduced, with permission, from Merenstein GB, Kaplan DW, Rosenberg AA (editors): *Handbook of Pediatrics,* 17th ed. Appleton & Lange, 1994.

ruptured follicular cyst at the time of ovulation. The patient presents with a history of midcycle, unilateral dull or aching abdominal pain lasting a few minutes or as long as 8 hours. This pain rarely mimics the abdominal findings of acute appendicitis, torsion or rupture of an ovarian cyst, or ectopic pregnancy. The patient should be reassured and treated symptomatically. If the findings are severe enough to warrant consideration of the above diagnoses, laparoscopy may be done to rule them out.

5. PREMENSTRUAL SYNDROME

Premenstrual syndrome (PMS) refers to a cluster of physical and psychologic symptoms that are temporally related to the week preceding menstruation and are alleviated by the onset of menses. It should be distinguished from common premenstrual symp-

Table 4–15. Management of dysfunctional uterine bleeding.[1,2]

	Mild	Moderate	Severe
	Hct > 33% or Hb > 11 g/dL Shortened intervals or heavy flow	Hct 27–33% or Hb 9–11 g/dL Moderately heavy and prolonged cycles, or persistently short intervals	Hct < 27% or Hb < 9 g/dL (or dropping); orthostatic symptoms and signs Heavy vaginal bleeding
Acute treatment	Menstrual calendar Iron supplementation Nonsteroidal anti-inflammatory drug with menses may help reduce flow Consider oral contraceptive pills if patient is sexually active and desires contraception (standard once-daily dose)	Oral contraceptive pills (1/35) up to four pills per day and taper over 2–3 weeks; may need antiemetic. Bleeding should stop in a few days. Expect withdrawal flow a few days after last dose.	Fluids, blood transfusion as needed, admit to hospital **For hemostasis, consider:** conjugated estrogens (Premarin), 25 mg IV every 4–6 hours for 24 hours or until bleeding stops. Provide antiemetic medication. **Then:** oral contraceptive pills (1/35) cycle: 4 pills per day for 4 days 3 pills per day for 4 days 2 pills per day for 17 days withdrawal bleeding for 7 days[3]
Long-term management	Monitor menstrual calendar and hemoglobin Follow-up in 2 months	Cycle with either: (1) Medroxyprogesterone acetate, 10 mg orally twice a day for 10 days starting on day 14 of each cycle for 3–6 months, or– (2) Oral contraceptive pills (1/35)[4] for 3–6 months beginning the Sunday after withdrawal bleeding starts. Provide iron supplementation. Monitor hemoglobin Follow-up within 2–3 weeks and every 3 months	**Next:** Oral contraceptive pills (1/50)[5] cycle (using 28-day packs) for 3 months Begin the Sunday after withdrawal bleeding begins. Length of use dependent on resolution of anemia. Monitor hemoglobin Follow-up within 2–3 weeks and every 3 months

[1]Modified from Blythe M: Common menstrual problems. Part 3. Abnormal uterine bleeding. Adolescent Health Update 1992;4:1.
[2]Diagnosis: Prolonged (> 8 days) painless menses; heavy flow (> 6 tampons/pads per day); short cycles (< 21 days); no cause found.
[3]This schedule will use three 21-day packages.
[4]Triphasic oral contraceptive pills are acceptable.
[5]Use pill with 50 μg of ethinyl estradiol for first 3 months, then 30–35 μg monophasic or triphasic pill.

toms (fluid retention, breast tenderness), depression, idiopathic cyclic edema, premenstrual dysphoric disorder, fibromyalgia, chronic fatigue syndrome, and psychosomatic disorders. This may be difficult because of the diversity of symptoms ascribed to PMS and the variability from month to month in the same patient. Premenstrual symptoms most commonly cited include emotional lability, anxiety, poor concentration, impaired judgment, gastrointestinal symptoms, hot flushes, and hypoglycemic symptoms. Previously thought to be a disorder limited to adult women, recent studies indicate that adolescents also experience premenstrual symptoms. Although a number of causes have been proposed (progesterone deficiency, hyperprolactinemia, estrogen excess or imbalance of the estrogen:progesterone ratio, vitamin B_{12} deficiency, fluid retention, low levels of endorphins and prostaglandins, hypoglycemia, psychosomatic factors), none has been proved. There may be some hormonal role; women who have undergone hysterectomy but not oophorectomy may have cyclic symptoms resembling PMS, whereas postmenopausal women have no such symptoms. Several treatments have been advocated but without consistent benefits. Oral contraceptives or prostaglandin inhibitors may be beneficial for some women. Sertraline (50–100 mg) has been shown to be significantly better than placebo for treatment of premenstrual dysphoria.

6. OVARIAN CYSTS

Functional cysts account for 20–50% of ovarian tumors in adolescents and are a result of the normal physiologic process of ovulation. They may be asymptomatic or may cause menstrual irregularity, constipation, or urinary frequency. Functional cysts, unless large, rarely cause abdominal pain; however, torsion or hemorrhage of an ovarian cyst may present as an acute or subacute abdomen. **Follicular cysts** account for the majority of ovarian cysts. They are produced every cycle but occasionally are not resorbed. Follicular cysts are unilateral, usually not larger than 4 cm in diameter, and resolve spontaneously. If the patient is asymptomatic, she can be given oral contraceptives containing 50 mg of estrogen for suppression of ovulation and examined monthly. The patient should be referred to a gynecologist for laparoscopy if she is premenarcheal; if the cyst has a solid component or is larger than 5 cm by ultrasonography; if there are symptoms or signs suggestive of hemorrhage or torsion; or if the cyst fails to regress after two or three menstrual cycles. **Lutein cysts** occur less commonly and may be 5–10 cm in diameter. The patient may have associated amenorrhea or, as the cyst becomes atretic, heavy vaginal bleeding. The patient may be monitored on suppression with oral contraceptives for 3 months but should

have a laparoscopy if the cyst is larger than 5 cm or if there is pain or bleeding from the cyst.

7. ENDOMETRIOSIS

See Secondary Dysmenorrhea, above.

Braverman PK, Sondheimer SJ: Menstrual disorders. Pediatr Rev 1997;18:17.
Davis GD, Thillet E, Lindemann J: Clinical characteristics of adolescent endometriosis J Adolesc Health 1993;14:362.
Emans SJH: *Pediatric and Adolescent Gynecology*. Little, Brown, 1997.
Hillard PA: Abnormal uterine bleeding in adolescents. Contemp Pediatr 1995;12:79-90.
Murray S, London S: Management of ovarian cysts in neonates, children, and adolescents. Adolesc Pediatr Gynecol 1995;8:64.
National Cancer Institute Workshop: The 1988 Bethesda system for reporting cervical/vaginal cytological diagnoses. JAMA 1989;262:931.
Sanfilippo JS: Hyperandrogenemia: Clinical perspectives. AM:STARS 1994;5:143.
Yonkers KA et al: Symptomatic improvement of premenstrual dysphoric disorder with sertraline treatment. JAMA 1997;278:983

CONTRACEPTION

Fifty percent of teen pregnancies in the United States occur in the first 6 months after sexual activity begins. Unfortunately, sexually active adolescent females wait an average of 12 months after onset of sexual activity to seek contraceptive advice.

Abstinence & Decision Making

Many adolescents have given little thought to how they feel about their developing sexuality or how they will handle sexual situations. By talking with teenagers about sexual intercourse and its implications—and alternatives to intercourse—physicians can help them make informed decisions before they find themselves with unwanted pregnancy.

Teenagers need to be aware that 50% of all teenagers do not engage in sexual intercourse. If an adolescent chooses to remain abstinent, the clinician should reinforce that decision. It is also prudent to encourage adolescents to use contraception when they do engage in sexual intercourse.

Emergency Postcoital Contraception

A discussion of emergency postcoital contraception, which could potentially prevent 50–90% of unintended pregnancies and elective abortions, should be part of anticipatory guidance given to teenagers. The pregnancy rate after postcoital contraception is 1.8%, compared with 6.8% without such intervention. (See Table 4–16 for dosages.) Postcoital contraception must be started within 72 hours after unprotected intercourse, and it should be verified that other instances of unprotected intercourse beyond 72 hours have not occurred. It should not be used in patients with contraindications for routine use of oral contraceptives. An antiemetic may be given 30 minutes prior to the second dose if nausea results from the first dose, and a spare dose of antinausea pills may be provided to be used if vomiting occurs within 3 hours after a dose. A follow-up appointment should be scheduled in 2–3 weeks for pregnancy test, STD screening, and contraceptive counseling.

Condoms & Spermicides

The use of condoms has gained popularity—even among adolescents—as a result of the educational and marketing efforts driven by the AIDS epidemic. In 1988, 55% of sexually active 15- to 19-year-old males reported using a condom at first intercourse, and 57% at last intercourse—compared with about 20% of 17- to 19-year-old males in 1979. Regardless of whether another method is used, all sexually active adolescents should be counseled to use condoms. Condoms also offer protection against sexually transmitted diseases by preventing the transmission of gonococci, chlamydiae, spirochetes, hepatitis virion particles, and HIV. Spermicides containing nonoxynol-9 have virucidal and bactericidal effects. Aside from the diaphragm and cervical cap, barrier methods do not require a medical visit or prescription and are widely available (Table 4–16). The polyurethane vaginal pouch, or "female condom," is now available as well. Although it has pregnancy and sexually transmitted disease prevention properties similar to those of the male condom, its higher cost and greater difficulty of insertion make it unlikely to appeal to adolescents.

Table 4–16. Emergency postcoital contraception regimens.

Pill	Dosage[1,2]	Each Dose Achieves:
Levlen	Four tablets orally and repeat in 12 hours	Levonorgestrel 0.6 mg
Nordette	Four tablets orally and repeat in 12 hours	Levonorgestrel 0.6 mg
Lo-Ovral	Four tablets orally and repeat in 12 hours	Norgestrel 1.2 mg
Ovral[3]	Two tablets orally and repeat in 12 hours	Norgestrel 1.0 mg

[1]First dose must be given within 72 hours after unprotected intercourse.
[2]An antiemetic drug taken 30 minutes before the dose may help reduce nausea.
[3]Traditional method but may not be readily available.

Oral Contraceptives

Oral contraceptives have a three-pronged mechanism of action: (1) suppression of ovulation; (2) thickening of the cervical mucus, thereby making sperm penetration more difficult; and (3) atrophy of the endometrium, which diminishes the chance of implantation. The latter two actions are progestin effects.

A. Combination Oral Contraceptives: Combination oral contraceptives contain both estrogen and progestin. Ethinyl estradiol is the estrogen currently used in nearly all oral contraceptives in the United States. A number of progestins are used in oral contraceptives and differ in their estrogenic, antiestrogenic, and androgenic effects. Triphasic oral contraceptives were introduced in the United States in 1984. Their main advantage is a 35–39% lower progestin dose over the course of the month, resulting in fewer progestin-related metabolic effects such as those on lipids, blood pressure, and carbohydrate metabolism. Disadvantages include confusion due to the multiple pill colors and a breakthrough bleeding rate that is comparable to or somewhat greater than that of low-dose monophasic agents. As estrogen doses decreased in oral contraceptives, the androgenic side effects of progestins became more apparent, leading to the development of two progestins (desogestrel and norgestimate). These "new" progestins in combination with ethinyl estradiol are now available in the United States (after about 10 years of use in Europe). To date, clinical evaluations show virtually identical efficacy rates in pregnancy prevention, very similar metabolic and side effects, and the same noncontraceptive benefits as previous combination pills. A pill containing 30–35 μg of ethinyl estradiol with norgestimate, desogestrel, or ≤ 0.5 mg norethindrone is recommended for adolescents beginning oral contraceptives. These lower androgenic pills may especially benefit patients with polycystic ovary syndrome.

B. Minipill: Minipills contain progestins found in combination oral contraceptives—but in smaller doses—and no estrogen. Their chief use is in women who experience unacceptable estrogen-related side effects with combination oral contraceptives. Their lack of estrogen, however, is also responsible for the main side effect—less predictable menstrual patterns. For this reason, and because minipills are not as effective as combination oral contraceptives, they are a poor choice for adolescents. Their mechanism of action relies on the progestin-mediated actions, and ovulation is suppressed in only 15–40% of cycles.

C. Indications and Contraindications: Combined oral contraceptives may be the method of choice for sexually active adolescents, who frequently have unplanned intercourse; however, the patient must be able to comply with a daily dosing regimen. Most states allow oral contraceptives to be prescribed to minors confidentially. Ideally, it is best to wait until six to twelve regular menstrual cycles have occurred before beginning oral contraceptives; however, if the teenager is already sexually active, the medical and social risks of pregnancy probably outweigh the risks of oral contraceptives.

Oral contraceptives may also be used to treat dysmenorrhea (see above).

Contraindications to combined oral contraceptives can be categorized as absolute and relative (Table 4–17). When use of estrogenic agents is contraindicated, progestin-only pills and medroxyprogesterone are alternatives.

D. Beginning Birth Control Pills and Follow-Up: Before a patient begins taking oral contraceptives, a careful menstrual history, medical history, and family medical history should be taken. In addition, baseline weight and blood pressure should be established, breast and pelvic examination should be performed, and specimens for urinalysis, Papanicolaou smear, gonococcal culture, and chlamydial culture or antigen detection test should be obtained.

If there are no contraindications (see Table 4–17), the patient may begin her first pack of pills with her next menstrual period (either the first Sunday after flow begins or the first day of flow, depending on the brand). A triphasic or a low-dose combined oral contraceptive of low androgenic profile is used for those without contraindications to use of estrogen. With adolescents, it is wise to use 28-day packs rather than 21-day packs to reduce the chance of missing pills. The patient should be instructed on the use of her pills and on the possible risks and side effects and their warning signs. To ensure protection, she should use a back-up method, such as condoms and foam, for the first 2 weeks. In addition, the patient should be advised to use condoms at every intercourse to prevent sexually transmitted diseases. A follow-up visit in 1 month and then every 2–3 months for the first year may improve compliance, since teenagers often discontinue birth control pills because of nonmedical reasons or minor side effects. Teenagers may need reassurance about the safety of birth control pills and their added benefits (Table 4–18).

E. Management of Side Effects: A different type of combined oral contraceptive should be tried if a patient has a persistent minor side effect for more than the first 2–3 months. Adjustments should be made on the basis of hormonal effects desired (Table 4–19). Changes are most often made for persistent breakthrough bleeding not related to missed pills.

Injectable Hormonal Contraceptives

The depot form of medroxyprogesterone acetate (DMPA) is a long-acting injectable progestational contraceptive. It is given as a deep intramuscular injection of 150 mg into the gluteal or deltoid muscle every 12 weeks. The first injection should be given within the first 5 days of the menstrual cycle to ensure immediate contraceptive protection. DMPA works chiefly by blocking the LH surge, thereby suppressing ovulation, but it also thickens cervical mucus and alters the endometrium to inhibit blastocyst implantation. With a failure rate of less than 0.3%, minimal compliance issues, long-acting nature, reversibility, lack of interference with intercourse, and lack of estrogen-related side effects, it may be an attractive contraceptive for many adolescents, particularly for those who consider its 50% rate of amenorrhea at 1 year of use a desirable side effect or for

Table 4–17. Contraindications to combined birth control pills.

Absolute contraindications
  History of thrombophlebitis, thromboembolic disorder, cerebrovascular disease, ischemic heart disease
  Known or suspected carcinoma of the breast or estrogen-dependent neoplasia
  Known or suspected pregnancy
  History of benign or malignant liver tumor
  Undiagnosed abnormal vaginal bleeding
Strong relative contraindications
  Severe vascular or migraine headaches
  Hypertension
  Diabetes
  Active gallbladder disease
  Mononucleosis, acute phase
  Sickle cell disease or sickle C disease
  Upcoming major surgery
  Long-leg cast or major injury to lower leg
  Known impaired liver function at present time
  Completion of term pregnancy within past 10–14 days

Modified and reproduced, with permission, from Breedlove B, Judy B, Martin N (editors): *Contraceptive Technology 1988–1989*, 14th rev ed. Irvington Publishers, 1988.

Table 4–18. Noncontraceptive health benefits of oral contraceptive pills.

Protection against life-threatening conditions
Ovarian cancer
Endometrial cancer
Pelvic inflammatory disease
Ectopic pregnancy
Morbidity and mortality due to unintended pregnancies

Alleviate conditions affecting quality of life
Iron deficiency anemia
Benign breast disease
Dysmenorrhea
Irregular cycles
Functional ovarian cysts
Premenstrual syndrome

Mounting evidence
Improved bone density

Table 4–19. Pill side effects: hormone etiology.[1]

Estrogen Excess	Progestin Excess	Androgen Excess	Estrogen Deficiency	Progestin Deficiency
1. Nausea, dizziness	1. Increased appetite and weight gain (noncyclic)	1. Increased appetite and weight gain (noncyclic)	1. Irritability, nervousness	1. Late breakthrough bleeding and spotting
2. Edema and abdominal or leg pain with cyclic weight gain, bloating	2. Tiredness, fatigue, and weakness	2. Hirsutism	2. Hot flushes, vasomotor symptoms	2. Heavy menstrual flow and clots
3. Leukorrhea	3. Depression	3. Acne	3. Uterine prolapse, pelvic relaxation symptoms	3. Delayed onset of menses
4. Increased leiomyoma size	4. Decreased libido	4. Oily skin, rash	4. Early and midcycle spotting	4. Dysmenorrhea
5. Chloasma	5. Oily scalp, acne	5. Increased libido	5. Decreased amount of menstrual flow	5. Weight loss
6. Uterine cramps	6. Loss of hair	6. Cholestatic jaundice	6. No withdrawal bleeding	
7. Irritability, depression	7. Cholestatic jaundice	7. Pruritus	7. Decreased libido	
8. Increased fat deposition	8. Decreased length of menstrual flow		8. Diminished breast size	
9. Cervical extrophia	9. Hypertension?		9. Dry vaginal mucosa, atrophic vaginitis, and dyspareunia	
10. Poor contact lens fit	10. Headaches between pill packages		10. Headaches	
11. Telangiectasia	11. Candidal vaginitis/cervicitis		11. Depression	
12. Vascular-type headache	12. Increased breast size (alveolar tissue)			
13. Hypertension?	13. Breast tenderness			
14. Lactation suppression	14. Decreased carbohydrate tolerance			
15. Headaches while taking the Pill	15. Dilated leg veins			
16. Cystic breast changes	16. Pelvic congestion syndrome			
17. Breast tenderness				
18. Increased breast size (ductal and fatty tissue and fluid retention)				
19. Thrombophlebitis				
20. Cerebrovascular accidents				
21. Myocardial infarction				
22. Hepatic adenoma				
23. Cyclic weight gain				

[1]Adapted and reproduced, with permission, from: Dickey RP: Medical approaches to reproductive regulation: The pill. ACOG Semin Fam Plan 1974; Table II:21; Dickey RP: *Managing Contraceptive Pill Patients,* 4th ed. Creative Infomatics, 1984; and Hatcher RA et al: *Contraceptive Technology, 1986–1987,* 13th rev ed. Irvington, 1987.

whom estrogens are contraindicated. Patients should be warned about unpredictable menstrual patterns, the possibility of weight gain or mood changes, and the potential for decreased bone density, which remains under investigation. DMPA may reduce intravascular sickling and increase hemoglobin and red cell survival in patients with sickle cell disease. Moreover, DMPA may be the preferred method for patients with seizure disorders, since it has been found to reduce the number of seizures in some. Studies have shown no increased risk of liver cancer, breast cancer, or invasive squamous cell cervical cancer among users of DMPA, and the risk of endometrial and ovarian cancers is reduced.

The levonorgestrel-containing nonbiodegradable subdermal implant (Norplant System), which is inserted under the skin of the upper arm using a trocar, is highly effective for 5 years, with pregnancy rates ranging from 0.04 per 100 woman-years in the first year of use to 1.1 per 100 woman-years in the fifth year. It acts through ovulation inhibition and thickening of the cervical mucus. Menstrual irregularities (including prolonged bleeding, intermenstrual spotting, and amenorrhea) are the most common side effects, though headache, acne, weight gain or loss, and depression may occur as well. Its ease of use, lack of compliance issues, high efficacy, and long-term protection make the subdermal implant an ideal contraceptive for adolescents who can tolerate the menstrual irregularities.

Contraceptive Methods Not Usually Recommended for Teenagers

Adolescents should understand the menstrual cycle and be taught either that there is no "safe" period or that ovulation occurs 2 weeks before the next menstrual period and may be difficult to predict. Because teenagers frequently have irregular cycles and because sexual intercourse is often spontaneous and unplanned, the rhythm or calendar method is not effective for them. Adolescents also need to be taught that withdrawal is not a reliable method of contraception. Diaphragms and cervical caps require professional fitting and skill with insertion and are not popular among teenagers. Nulligravidity and behaviors that impose a risk of sexually transmitted disease are contraindications to the use of IUDs. Sterilization is rarely appropriate for adolescents.

American Academy of Pediatrics Committee on Adolescence: Contraception and adolescents. Pediatrics 1990;86:134.

American Academy of Pediatrics Committee on Adolescence: Condom availability for youth. Pediatrics 1995;95:281.

Beach RK: Contraception for adolescents: Part 1. Adolesc Health Update 1994;7(1):1.

Beach RK: Contraception for adolescents: Part 2. Adolesc Health Update 1995;7(2):1.

Cromer BA et al: A prospective study of adolescents who choose among levonorgestrel implant (Norplant), medroxyprogesterone acetate (Depo-Provera), or the combined oral contraceptive pills as contraception. Pediatrics 1994;94:687.

Derman SG, Peralta LM: Postcoital contraception: Present and future options. J Adolesc Health 1995;16:6.

Dickey RP: *Managing Contraceptive Pill Patients.* Creative Infomatics, 1997.

Earl DT, David DJ: Depo-Provera: An injectable contraceptive. Am Fam Physician 1994;49:891.

Hatcher RE et al: The pill: Combined oral contraceptives. In: *Contraceptive Technology,* 16th ed. Irvington, 1994.

Holder AR: Legal issues in adolescent sexual health. AM:STARS 1992;3:257.

Stevens-Simon C: Reproductive health care for your adolescent female patients. Contemp Pediatr 1997;35.

PREGNANCY

More than 1 million teenage girls become pregnant in the United States each year. The 1994 birth rate among teenagers 15–19 years of age was 5% lower than the recent high in 1991. Despite this recent decline, the 1994 rate was still higher than in any year during the period from 1974 to 1989. About 45% of 15- to 19-year-old females are sexually active, and more than one-third of these become pregnant within 2 years after onset of sexual activity. More than 80% of these pregnancies are unintended,

and about 68% of pregnancies in women under 20 years of age are out of wedlock.

Young maternal age and associated maternal risk factors have been linked to adverse neonatal outcome, including higher rates of low-birth-weight babies (< 2500 g) and neonatal mortality. The psychosocial consequences for the teenage mother and her infant are listed in Table 4–20. Teenagers who are pregnant require additional support from their caregivers, and clinics for young mothers may be the best providers.

Presentation

Adolescents may present with delayed or missed menses or may even request a pregnancy test, but often they present with an unrelated concern or have a hidden agenda. Because of the high level of denial, they may come in with complaints of abdominal

Table 4–20. Psychosocial consequences of pregnancy for the adolescent mother and her infant.

Mother	Infant
Increased morbidity related to pregnancy	**Greater health risks**
Greater risk of toxemia, anemia, prolonged labor, premature labor	Increased chance of low birth weight or prematurity
Increased chance of miscarriages, stillbirths	Increased risk of infant death
Increased change of maternal mortality	Increased risk of injury and hospitalization by age 5
Decreased educational attainment	**Decreased academic achievement**
Less likely to get high school diploma, go to college, or graduate	Lower cognitive scores
	Decreased development
Lower occupational attainment and prestige	Greater chance of being behind grade or needing remedial help
Less chance of stable employment (some resolution over time)	Lower chance of advanced academics
Lower job satisfaction	Lower academic aptitude as a teenager and perhaps a higher probability of dropping out of school
Lower income/wages	
Greater dependence on public assistance	
Less stable marital relationships	**Psychosocial consequences**
Higher rates of single parenthood	Greater risk of behavior problems
Earlier marriage (though less common than in the past)	Poverty
	Higher probability of living in a nonintact home while in high school
Accelerated pace of marriage, separation, divorce, and remarriage	Greater risk of adolescent pregnancy
Faster pace of subsequent childbearing	
High rate of repeat unintended pregnancy	
More births out of marriage	
Closer spacing of births	
Larger families	

pain, urinary frequency, dizziness, or other nonspecific symptoms and have no concern about pregnancy. A history of symptoms such as weight gain, engorged breasts, an unusually light or mistimed period, and urinary frequency can be sought, but the adolescent may not have noted these signs of pregnancy. Denial also contributes to the delay in seeking prenatal care. Only about one-third of adolescents receive prenatal care in the first trimester. Clinicians need to have a low threshold for suspicion of pregnancy. If there is any suspicion, a urine pregnancy test should be obtained.

Diagnosis

The history and physical examination may assist in making the diagnosis. Bluish coloring and softening of the cervix may be noted on speculum examination. The uterine fundus may be palpable on abdominal examination if sufficient time has elapsed. If uterine size on bimanual examination does not correspond to dates, one must consider ectopic pregnancy, incomplete or missed abortion, twin gestation, or inaccurate dates.

Enzyme-linked immunoassay test kits specific for the βhCG subunit and sensitive to less than 50 mIU/mL of hCG can be performed on urine (preferably the first morning voided specimen, because it is more concentrated) in less than 5 minutes and are accurate within 12 days after conception. Serum radioimmunoassay is also specific for the beta subunit, is accurate within 7 days after conception, and is helpful in ruling out ectopic pregnancy or threatened abortion.

The timing of pregnancy tests is important, since hCG levels rise initially after conception, peak at about 60–70 days, then drop to levels not detected by routine office slide tests after 16–20 weeks.

Special Issues in Management

When an adolescent presents for pregnancy testing, it is wise, before performing the test, to find out what she hopes the result will be and what she thinks she will do if the test is positive. If she wants to be pregnant and the test is negative, further counseling about the implications of teen pregnancy should be offered. For those who do not wish to be pregnant, this is a good time to begin contraception because teens who present for a pregnancy test that is negative have a high risk of pregnancy in the next 2 years.

If the adolescent is pregnant, the physician must discuss her support systems and her options with her (abortion, adoption, raising the baby). Many teenagers need help in telling and involving their parents. It is important to remain available for further assistance with decision making. If the patient knows what she wants to do, she should be referred to the appropriate resources. Since teenagers are often ambivalent about their plans and may have a high level of denial, it is prudent to follow up in 1 week to be

certain that a decision has been made and to help the patient obtain prenatal care if she has chosen to continue the pregnancy.

Maternal age alone is not responsible for low birth weight and poor fetal outcome; rather, low maternal prepregnancy weight, poor weight gain, delay in prenatal care, and low socioeconomic status also are contributing factors. The poor nutritional status of some teenagers and their erratic diets, smoking, drinking, or substance abuse, and high incidence of sexually transmitted diseases play a role. Teenagers are also at greater risk of eclampsia-preeclampsia, iron deficiency anemia, cephalopelvic disproportion, prolonged labor, premature labor, and maternal death. Early prenatal care and good nutrition can make a difference with a number of these problems.

Because of the high risk of a second unintended pregnancy within the next 2 years, postpartum contraceptive counseling and follow-up are imperative. Pregnancy prevention is the most cost-effective means of reducing the consequences of teenage pregnancy. Sexual decision making, contraceptive counseling, and close follow-up of sexually active adolescents of both sexes can make a difference. Adolescents who receive sexuality and contraceptive education are not more likely to have intercourse but are less likely to become pregnant than their counterparts who do not receive such instruction.

Ammerman S, Shafer MA, Snyder D: Ectopic pregnancy in adolescents: A clinical review for pediatricians. J Pediatr 1990;117:677.

Bluestein D, Starling ME: Helping pregnant teenagers. West J Med 1994;161:140.

Jaskiewicz JA, McAnarney ER: Pregnancy during adolescence. Pediatr Rev 1994;15:32.

Stevens-Simon C, Fullar SA, McAnarney ER: Teenage pregnancy: Caring for adolescent mothers with their infants in pediatric settings. Clin Pediatr 1989;28:282.

VULVOVAGINITIS

Vaginitis may be due to pathogens or to indigenous flora after a change in milieu of the vagina. Candidal vulvovaginitis and bacterial vaginosis (formerly called *Gardnerella, Haemophilus,* or nonspecific vaginitis) may occur in patients who are not sexually active. These are examples of indigenous flora that may cause infection. Bacterial vaginosis, however, is more prevalent in those who are sexually active. In sexually active patients, *Trichomonas* infection or cervicitis due to sexually transmitted pathogens must be considered (see Chapter 38). For this reason, sexually active patients or suspected victims of sexual abuse should have appropriate specimens taken to detect sexually transmitted disease even if yeast forms are present or bacterial vaginosis is identified.

1. PHYSIOLOGIC LEUKORRHEA

Leukorrhea is the normal vaginal discharge that begins around the time of menarche. The discharge is typically clear or whitish, and its consistency may vary according to cyclic hormonal influences. There should be no odor. Girls in early adolescence may have concerns about such a discharge and need reassurance that it is normal. This may be a good time to tell girls that there is no need for douching. If a vaginal wet preparation is examined, a few squamous epithelial cells may be revealed, but there should be fewer than five polymorphonuclear cells per high-power field.

2. CANDIDAL VULVOVAGINITIS

Candidal vulvovaginitis is caused by yeast. It typically occurs after a course of antibiotics, after which the normal perineal flora are altered and yeast is allowed to proliferate. Diabetics, patients with compromised immune systems, and those who are pregnant or receiving oral contraceptives are more prone to develop candidal infections.

Clinical Findings

The patient usually complains of vulvar pruritus or dyspareunia and a cheesy vaginal discharge, frequently beginning the week prior to menses. Examination of the vulva reveals an erythematous mucosa, sometimes with excoriation, and a thick, white, cheesy discharge. The discharge may be adherent to the walls of the vagina, which will also be inflamed if the infection is internal. Leukocytes may be seen on a wet preparation, and a potassium hydroxide preparation may reveal budding yeast or mycelia. The vaginal preparations are often not helpful, and the patient should be treated on the basis of the clinical examination. Vaginal culture for yeast is usually unnecessary.

Treatment

Butoconazole, clotrimazole, miconazole, terconazole, or tioconazole vaginal creams or suppositories designed for three or seven nightly doses are effective in most patients. Some patients require a longer course of treatment. Fluconazole (150 mg once orally) is also effective and may be beneficial on a monthly prophylactic basis for women with recurring infections. Patients with recurrent episodes should be given prophylactic treatment whenever they take antibiotics. It may be helpful to simultaneously treat the partners of sexually active patients with recurrent candidal infections.

3. BACTERIAL VAGINOSIS

Bacterial vaginosis may be caused by any of the indigenous vaginal flora, such as *Gardnerella, Bacteroides, Peptococcus,* or lactobacilli.

Clinical Findings

The patient generally complains of a malodorous mild discharge. On examination, a thin, homogeneous, grayish-white discharge is found adherent to the vaginal wall with diffuse vaginal erythema. A whiff test, in which a drop of potassium hydroxide is added to a smear of the discharge on a slide, results in the release of amines, causing a fishy odor. Wet preparation reveals an abundance of "clue cells" (vaginal epithelial cells stippled with adherent bacteria) and small pleomorphic rods.

Treatment

Treatment for bacterial vaginosis is with metronidazole (500 mg orally twice a day for 7 days) or clindamycin (300 mg orally twice a day for 7 days). Topical metronidazole or clindamycin may also be effective. Ampicillin (500 mg orally four times a day for 7 days) is the alternative for pregnant patients.

4. OTHER CAUSES OF VULVOVAGINITIS

Sexually Transmitted Diseases

Sexually transmitted diseases are an important cause of vaginal discharge in adolescents. (See Chapter 38.) One should obtain appropriate cultures whenever an adolescent complains of vaginal discharge even when the cervix appears normal.

Foreign Body Vaginitis

Foreign bodies—most commonly retained tampons—cause extremely malodorous vaginal discharges. Treatment consists of removal, for which ring forceps may be useful. Further treatment is generally not necessary.

Allergic or Contact Vaginitis

Bubble baths, feminine hygiene sprays, or vaginal contraceptive foams or suppositories may cause chemical irritation of the vaginal mucosa. Discontinuing use of the offending agent is indicated.

REFERENCES

Dryfoos JG: *Adolescents at Risk: Prevalence and Prevention.* Oxford University Press, 1990.

Emans SJH: *Pediatric and Adolescent Gynecology.* Little, Brown, 1997.

Friedman SB, Fisher M, Schonberg SK (editors): *Comprehensive Adolescent Health Care.* Quality Medical Publishing, 1992.

Greydanus DE: *Caring for Your Adolescent, Ages 12 to 21.* Bantam, 1991.

Guidelines for Adolescent Preventive Services: American Medical Association, 1992.

Hatcher RA et al: *Contraceptive Technology,* 16th ed. Irvington, 1994.

Hechinger FM: *Fateful Choices: Healthy Youth for the 21st Century.* Carnegie Corporation of New York, 1992.

Hofman A, Greydanus DE: *Adolescent Medicine,* 3rd ed. Appleton & Lange, 1997.

Holmes KK et al (editors): *Sexually Transmitted Diseases,* 2nd ed. McGraw-Hill, 1997.

McAnarney ER et al (editors): *Textbook of Adolescent Medicine.* Saunders, 1992.

Millstein SG, Petersen AC, Nightingale EO: *Promoting the Health of Adolescents: New Directions for the Twenty-First Century.* Oxford Univ Press, 1993.

Neinstein LS: *Adolescent Health Care: A Practical Guide,* 3rd ed. Williams & Wilkins, 1996.

5 Substance Abuse in Pediatrics

Catherine Stevens-Simon, MD

The use and abuse of mood-altering substances—alcohol, marijuana, opioids, cocaine, amphetamines, sedative-hypnotics, hallucinogens, inhalants, nicotine, and anabolic steroids—is a serious public health problem. The short- and long-term health, social, emotional, legal, and behavioral consequences of substance abuse are particularly damaging during childhood and adolescence. Not only does early substance use portend chronic, severe polysubstance abuse later in life, but substance use may also compromise physical, cognitive, and psychosocial aspects of adolescent development if this maladaptive behavior becomes the preferred response to environmental stressors.

Substance abuse tends to be a chronic, progressive disease. The first or **initiation stage**—from nonuser to user—is such a common feature of becoming an American adult that many authorities call it "normative" behavior. At this stage, substance use is typically limited to experimentation with tobacco or alcohol ("gateway" substances). During adolescence, young people are expected to establish an independent, autonomous identity by "trying out" a variety of behaviors within the safety of their family circles and peer groups. This process often involves experimentation with psychoactive substances, usually in culturally acceptable circumstances. Progression to the second or **continuation stage** of substance abuse is a nonnormative "risk" behavior with the potential to compromise adolescent development. The American Psychiatric Association criteria listed in Table 5–1 can be used to judge the severity of substance use that progresses beyond the experimentation stage to **substance abuse** or **substance dependency.** Maintenance and progression within a class of substances (eg, from beer to liquor) and progression across classes of substances (eg, from alcohol to marijuana) represent the third and fourth stages of substance abuse. Individuals at these stages are polysubstance abusers, and most manifest one or more of the symptoms of dependency listed in Table 5–1.

The transition from one stage to the next is typically a cyclic process of **regression, cessation,** and **relapse.** Common symptoms and physiologic effects of **intoxication** (which can occur at any stage) and **withdrawal** (a symptom of dependency) for the major classes of substances are presented in Tables 5–2 and 5–3.

Diagnostic and Statistical Manual of Mental Disorders, 4th ed. American Psychiatric Association, 1994.

Kandel D, Yamaguchi K: From beer to crack: Developmental patterns of drug involvement. Am J Pub Health 1993;83:851.

Schonberg SK: Substance use and abuse. In: *Textbook of Adolescent Medicine.* McAnarney ER et al (editors). Saunders, 1992.

US Department of Health and Human Services. Healthy People 2000: National Health Promotion and Disease Prevention Objectives. Government Printing Office, 1991; DHHS Publication No.(PHS) 91-50213.

SCOPE OF THE PROBLEM

The best source of information about the prevalence of substance abuse among American children and adolescents is the annual "Monitoring the Future" survey, which tracks health-related behaviors in a sample of 45,000 eighth, tenth, and twelfth graders in over 420 public and private schools across the United States. This study probably understates the magnitude of the problem of substance abuse because it excludes two of the most abuse-prone groups of young people—school dropouts and runaways. While the exclusion of these youngsters may only moderately minimize prevalence estimates for the entire population, errors in estimating drug use among subgroups with high rates of school dropout (eg, urban minority youths) are thought to be substantial.

Data from this survey and others show that alcohol is the most frequently abused substance in our society. Experimentation with alcohol typically begins in or before middle school, is more common among boys than girls, and is most common among whites, less common among Hispanics and Native Americans, and least common among blacks and Asians. Over 50% of children consume alcohol before high school, and over 90% do so before graduation. Over 25% of eighth graders and over 50% of high school

Table 5–1. Substance abuse and substance dependency.[1]

Diagnostic criteria for substance abuse
A. A maladaptive pattern of substance use leading to clinically significant impairment or distress, as manifested by one (or more) of the following occurring within a 12-month period:
  1. Recurrent substance use resulting in a failure to fulfill major role obligations at work, school, or home (eg, repeated absences or poor work performance related to substance use; substance-related absences, suspensions, or expulsions from school; neglect of children or household).
  2. Recurrent substance use in situations in which the substance use is physically hazardous (eg, driving an automobile or operating a machine when impaired by substance use).
  3. Recurrent substance-related legal problems (arrests for substance-related disorderly conduct).
  4. Continued substance use despite having persistent or recurrent social or interpersonal problems caused or exacerbated by the effects of the substance (eg, arguments with spouse about consequences of intoxication, physical fights).
B. Symptoms that have never met criteria for substance dependence for this class of substance.

Diagnostic criteria for substance dependency
A maladaptive pattern of substance use, leading to clinically significant impairment or distress, as manifested by three or more of the following, occurring at any time in the same 12-month period:
  1. Tolerance, as defined by either of the following:
    a. Need for markedly increased amounts of the substance to achieve intoxication or desired effect.
    b. Markedly diminished effect with continued use of the same amount of the substance.
  2. Withdrawal, as manifested by either of the following:
    a. The characteristic withdrawal syndrome for the substance (criteria A and B of the criteria for withdrawal from the specific substance).
    b. The same (or closely related) substance taken to relieve or avoid withdrawal symptoms.
  3. The substance often taken in larger amounts or over a longer period than was intended.
  4. A persistent desire or unsuccessful efforts to cut down or control substance use.
  5. A great deal of time spent in activities necessary to obtain the substance (eg, visiting multiple doctors, driving long distances), use the substance (chain-smoking), or recover from its effects.
  6. Important social, occupational, or recreational activities given up or reduced because of substance use.
  7. Continued substance use despite knowledge of having a persistent or recurrent physical or psychological problem that is likely to have been caused or exacerbated by the substance (eg, current cocaine use despite recognition of cocaine-induced depression, or continued drinking despite recognition that an ulcer was made worse by alcohol consumption).

[1]Reprinted, with permission, from the *Diagnostic and Statistical Manual of Mental Disorders*, 4th ed. Copyright 1994 American Psychiatric Association.

Table 5–2. Physiologic effects of commonly abused mood-altering substances.[1]

EYES/PUPILS	
Mydriasis	Amphetamines or other stimulants, cocaine, glutethimide, jimsonweed, LSD* Withdrawal from alcohol and opioids
Miosis	Alcohol, barbiturates, benzodiazepines, opioids, PCP*
Nystagmus	Alcohol, barbiturates, benzodiazepines, inhalants, PCP
Conjunctival injection	LSD, marijuana
Lacrimation	Inhalants, LSD. Withdrawal from opioids.
CARDIOVASCULAR	
Tachycardia	Amphetamines or other stimulants, cocaine, LSD, marijuana, PCP. Withdrawal from alcohol, barbiturates, benzodiazepines.
Hypertension	Amphetamines or other stimulants, cocaine, LSD, marijuana, PCP. Withdrawal from alcohol, barbiturates, benzodiazepines.
Hypotension	Barbiturates, opioids. Orthostatic: marijuana. Withdrawal from depressants.
Arrhythmia	Amphetamines or other stimulants, cocaine, inhalants, opioids, PCP
RESPIRATORY	
Depression	Opioids, depressants
Pulmonary edema	Opioids, stimulants
CORE BODY TEMPERATURE	
Elevated	Amphetamines or other stimulants, cocaine, PCP. Withdrawal from alcohol, barbiturates, benzodiazepines, opioids.
Decreased	Alcohol, barbiturates, benzodiazepines, opioids
PERIPHERAL NERVOUS SYSTEM RESPONSE	
Hyperreflexia	Amphetamines or other stimulants, cocaine, LSD, marijuana, methaqualone, PCP Withdrawal from alcohol, barbiturates, benzodiazepines
Hyporeflexia	Alcohol, barbiturates, benzodiazepines, inhalants, opioids
Tremor	Amphetamines or other stimulants, cocaine, LSD Withdrawal from alcohol, barbiturates, benzodiazepines, cocaine
Ataxia	Alcohol, amphetamines or other stimulants, barbiturates, benzodiazepines, inhalants, LSD, PCP
CENTRAL NERVOUS SYSTEM RESPONSE	
Hyperalertness	Amphetamines or other stimulants, cocaine
Sedation, somnolence	Alcohol, barbiturates, benzodiazepines, inhalants, marijuana, opioids
Seizures	Alcohol, amphetamines or other stimulants, cocaine, inhalants, methaqualone, opioids (particularly meperidine, propoxyphene) Withdrawal from alcohol, barbiturates, benzodiazepines
Hallucinations	Amphetamines or other stimulants, cocaine, inhalants, LSD, marijuana, PCP Withdrawal from alcohol, barbiturates, benzodiazepines
GASTROINTESTINAL	
Nausea, vomiting	Alcohol, amphetamines or other stimulants, cocaine, inhalants, LSD, opioids, peyote Withdrawal from alcohol, barbiturates, benzodiazepines, cocaine, opioids

[1]Adapted with permission from: Schwartz B, Alderman EM: Substance abuse. Pediatr Rev 1997;18:215. *LSD = lysergic acid diethylamide PCP = phencyclidine hydrochloride

Table 5–3. Effects of commonly abused mood-altering substances.

Substance	Pharmacology	Intoxication	Withdrawal	Chronic Use
Alcohol (ethanol)	Depressant; 10 g/drink Drink: 12 oz beer, 4 oz wine, 1½ oz liquor; one drink increases blood level by approximately 0.025 g/dL (varies by weight)	Legal: 0.05–0.1 g/dL (varies by state) Mild: < 0.1 g/dL; disinhibition, euphoria, mild sedation and impaired coordination Moderate: 0.1–0.2 g/dL; impaired mentation and judgment, slurred speech ataxia Severe: > 0.3 g/dL; confusion, stupor; > 0.4 g/dL; coma, depressed respiration	Mild: headache, tremors, nausea and vomiting ("hangover") Severe: fever, sweaty, seizure, agitation, hallucination, hypertension, tachycardia Delirium tremens (chronic use)	Hepatitis, cirrhosis, cardiac disease, Wernicke's encephalopathy, Korsakoff's syndrome
Marijuana (cannabis)	Delta-9-tetrahydrocannabinol (THC); 4–6% in marijuana; 20–30% in hashish	Low: euphoria, relaxation, impaired thinking High: mood changes, depersonalization, hallucinations Toxic: panic, delusions, paranoia, psychosis	Irritability, disturbed sleep, tremor, nystagmus, anorexia, diarrhea, vomiting	Cough, gynecomastia, low sperm count, infertility, amotivational syndrome, apathy
Cocaine	Stimulant; releases biogenic amines; concentration varies with preparation and route of administration	Hyperalert, increased energy, confident, insomnia, anxiety, paranoia, dilated pupils, tremors, seizures, hypertension, arrhythmia, tachycardia, fever, dry mouth Toxic: coma, psychosis, seizure, myocardial infarction, stroke, hyperthermia, rhabdomyolysis	Drug craving, depression, dysphoria, irritability, lethargy, tremors, nausea, hunger	Nasal septum ulceration, epistaxis, lung damage, intravenous drug use
Opioids (heroin, morphine, codeine, methadone, opium, fentanyl, meperidine, propoxyphene)	Depressant; binds central opioid receptor; variable concentrations with substance	Euphoria, sedation, impaired thinking, low blood pressure, pinpoint pupil, urinary retention Toxic: hypotension, arrhythmia, depressed respiration, stupor, coma, seizure, death	Only after > 3 weeks of regular use: drug craving, rhinorrhea, lacrimation, muscle aches, diarrhea, anxiety, tremors, hypertension, tachycardia.	IV drug use: cellulitis, endocarditis, embolisms, HIV
Amphetamines	Stimulant; sympathomimetic	Euphoria, hyperalert state, hyperactive, hypertension, arrhythmia, fever, flushing, dilated pupils, tremor, ataxia, dry mouth Toxic: coma, circulatory collapse, hypertensive crisis, cerebral hemorrhage	Lethargy, fatigue, depression, anxiety, nightmares, muscle cramps, abdominal pain, hunger	Paranoia, psychosis
Sedative-hypnotics (barbiturates, benzodiazepines, methaqualone)	Depressant	Sedation, lethargy, slurred speech, pinpoint pupils, hypotension, psychosis, seizures Toxic: stupor, coma, cardiac arrest, seizure, pulmonary edema, death	Only after weeks of use: agitation, delirium, psychosis, hallucinations, fever, flushing, hyper- or hypotension, death	Paranoia

(continued)

Table 5–3. Effects of commonly abused mood-altering substances. (continued)

Substance	Pharmacology	Intoxication	Withdrawal	Chronic Use
Hallucinogens (LSD, peyote, mescaline, mushrooms, nutmeg, jimsonweed)	Inhibition of serotonin release	Illusions, depersonalization, hallucination, anxiety, paranoia, ataxia, dilated pupils, hypertension, dry mouth Toxic: coma, terror, panic, "crazy feeling"	None	Flashbacks
Phenycyclidine	Dissociative anesthetic	Low dose (< 5 mg): illusions, hallucinations, ataxia, hypertension, flushing Moderate dose (5–10 mg): hyperthermia, salivation, myoclonus High dose: (> 10 mg): rigidity, seizure, arrhythmia, coma, death	None	Flashbacks
Inhalants (toluene, benzene, hydrocarbons and fluorocarbons)	Stimulation progressing to depression	Euphoria, giddiness, impaired judgment, ataxia, rhinorrhea, salivation, hallucination Toxic: respiratory depression, arrhythmia, coma, stupor, delirium, sudden death	None	Permanent damage to nerves, liver, heart, kidney, brain
Nicotine	Releases dopamine, 1 mg nicotine per cigarette	Relaxation, tachycardia, vertigo, anorexia	Drug craving, irritability, anxiety, hunger, impaired concentration	Permanent damage to lung, heart, cardiovascular system
Anabolic steroids[1]	Bind steroid receptor. Stacking: use many types simultaneously; pyramiding: increase dosage	Increased muscle bulk, strength, endurance, increased drive, hypogonadism, low sperm count, gynecomastia, decreased libido, virilization, irregular menses, hepatitis, early epiphysial closure, aggressiveness	Drug craving, dysphoria, irritability, depression	Tendon rupture, cardiomyopathy, atherosclerosis, peliosis hepatis (orally active C17 derivatives of testosterone are especially hepatotoxic)

[1]Despite conventional assumptions, scientific studies show that anabolic steroids do not improve aerobic athletic performance and improve strength only in athletes trained in weight lifting before they begin using steroids who continue to train and take a high-protein diet.

students seen in an average American pediatric practice have used alcohol within the last 30 days, and half have consumed five or more drinks on at least one occasion.

Use of tobacco, marijuana, and other mood-altering substances is less common (Table 5–4). Marijuana is the most commonly used illicit drug in the United States. In 1994, more that 65 million Americans (31% of the population) had tried marijuana at least once and almost 18 million (9%) had used marijuana within the past year. First experiences with marijuana and the substances listed in Table 5–4 typically occur during middle school and early high school. Initiation of substance abuse is rare after 20 years of age.

The level of substance abuse among American youth is high compared with use prior to 1965 and is among the highest in the Western industrialized world. The decline in the prevalence of illicit drug use that began in the early 1980s apparently reached its nadir in the early 1990s, and the use of all mood-altering substances has been increasing since 1993. The use of any illicit drug in the past year (annual use) by eighth graders almost doubled between 1991 and 1995 (from 11% to 21%). Similarly, the annual rate of substance use among high school seniors increased from 27% in 1991 to 39% in 1995—after a steady decline from a peak of 54% in 1979. Marijuana use has shown the most striking increase, with lifetime use increased from 6% to 16% among eighth graders and from 24% to 35% among twelfth graders between 1991 and 1995. The age at initiation of alco-

Table 5–4. Prevalence of pediatric substance use and abuse.[1]

Substance	Percent Users or Abusers by Grade Level		
	8th Graders	10th Graders	12th Graders
Alcohol			
Lifetime	54.5	70.5	80.7
Annual	45.3	63.5	73.7
30-day	24.6	38.8	51.3
Daily	0.7	1.7	3.5
Marijuana, hashish			
Lifetime	19.9	34.1	41.7
Annual	15.8	28.7	41.7
30-day	9.1	17.2	21.2
Daily	0.8	2.8	4.6
Cocaine			
Lifetime	4.2	5.0	6.0
Annual	2.6	3.5	4.0
30-day	1.2	1.7	1.8
Daily	0.1	0.1	0.2
Crack cocaine			
Lifetime	2.7	2.8	3.0
Annual	1.6	1.8	2.1
30-day	0.7	0.9	1.0
Daily	< 0.05	< 0.05	0.1
Heroin			
Lifetime	2.3	1.7	1.6
Annual	1.4	1.1	1.1
30-day	0.6	0.6	0.6
Daily	< .05	< .05	0.1
Stimulants			
Lifetime	13.1	17.4	15.3
Annual	8.7	11.9	9.3
30-day	4.2	5.3	4.0
Daily	0.2	0.2	0.3
Hallucinogens			
Lifetime	5.2	9.3	12.7
Annual	3.6	7.2	9.3
30-day	1.7	3.3	4.1
Daily	0.1	0.1	0.2
Inhalants			
Lifetime	21.6	19.0	17.4
Annual	12.8	9.6	8.0
30-day	6.1	3.5	3.2
Daily	0.2	0.1	0.1
Cigarettes (any use)			
Lifetime	46.4	57.6	64.2
30-day	19.1	27.9	33.5
Daily	9.3	16.3	21.6
> ½ pack per day	3.4	8.3	12.4
Steroids			
Lifetime	2.0	2.0	2.3
Annual	1.0	1.2	1.5
30-day	0.6	0.6	0.7
Daily	< 0.05	0.1	0.2

[1]Monitoring the Future Survey (1995).

hol and other substance abuse is dropping precipitously, and inhalant abuse is rapidly becoming a predominantly pediatric disease. These statistics are particularly worrisome because early-onset substance use is one of the best predictors of persistent abuse later in life.

Chen K, Kandel D: The natural history of drug use from adolescence to the mid-thirties in a general population sample. Am J Pub Health 1995;85:41.

Johnston LD, O'Malley APM, Bachman JG: National survey results on drug use from the Monitoring the Future Study, 1975–1995. (DHHS Publication No. NIH 94-0000).

Pierce JP, Gilpin E: How long will today's new adolescent smoker be addicted to cigarettes? Am J Pub Health 1996;86:253.

Swaim R et al: The effect of school dropout rates on estimates of adolescent substance use among three racial/ethnic groups. Am J Pub Health 1997;87:51.

MORBIDITY ASSOCIATED WITH SUBSTANCE ABUSE

Environmental substance exposure is a major cause of morbidity and mortality among American children. It is estimated that close to 10% of the total annual pediatric medical expenditure is attributable to the impact of parental smoking on medical conditions such as low birth weight, sudden infant death syndrome, bronchiolitis, asthma, otitis media, and fire-related injuries. Children who live in environments in which substance abuse is common are at increased risk for both accidental and nonaccidental trauma.

The leading causes of death among American teenagers are accidents, homicide, and suicide. Approximately half of all fatal motor vehicle accidents and of all homicides, as well as a substantial proportion of suicides, drowning, and fatal falls, are associated with the use of alcohol or other mood-altering substances. Because most preteens and teens are still socially immature and cognitively unsophisticated, they make errors in judgment even when cognition is only slightly impaired by drugs or alcohol. There is a correlation between substance use and both consensual and nonconsensual sexual activity, and most "date rapes" are associated with substance use by one or both individuals. Substance abuse at parties is associated with risk taking, delinquency, and violent confrontations. During intervals of depression and low self-esteem, substance abuse increases the risk of suicide and other self-destructive behavior.

Although few pediatric patients show manifestations of chronic substance abuse, the potential for serious, permanent physical harm should not be overlooked. Health care professionals are familiar with the risks associated with tobacco, alcohol, and cocaine but may not be aware that the active ingredient in marijuana (tetrahydrocannabinol; THC), can damage or destroy nerve cells in the hippocampus, changing the way information is processed and impairing functions crucial for learning and perhaps predisposing to an "amotivational syndrome." Daily use of one to three marijuana cigarettes produces as much lung damage as smoking a pack of cigarettes.

Aligne CA, Stoddard JJ: Tobacco and children: An economic evaluation of the medical effects of parental smoking. Arch Pediatr Adolesc Med 1997;151:648.

Committee on Sports Medicine and Fitness for the American Academy of Pediatrics: Adolescents and anabolic steroids: A subject review. Pediatrics 1997;99:904.

Dukarm CP et al: Illicit substance use, gender, and the risk of violent behavior among adolescents. Arch Pediatr Adolesc Med 1996;150:797.

Hansen WB, O'Malley PM: Drug use. In: *Handbook of Adolescent Health Risk Behavior.* DiClemente R, Hansen W, Ponton L (editors). Plenum, 1996.

Lieber C: Medical disorders of alcoholism. N Engl J Med 1995;333:1058.

Pope HG, Yurgelun-Todd D: The residual cognitive effects of heavy marijuana use in college students. JAMA 1996;275:521.

Windle M, Shope JT, Bukstein O: Alcohol use. In: *Handbook of Adolescent Health Risk Behavior.* DiClemente R, Hansen W, Ponton L (editors). Plenum, 1996.

RESPONSE TO THE PROBLEM

Federal and state legislatures and local governments have enacted measures prohibiting the use of psychoactive substances and ordinances intended to reduce the associated risks (eg, nighttime driving curfews). Large sums have been spent on school- and community-based prevention and treatment programs, but until recently little thought had been given to the role of primary pediatric health care providers. The American Academy of Pediatrics (AAP) has now recommended that all pediatric health care providers should (1) be alert for signs that predispose to progression from the initiation phase to the continuation phase of substance use, and (2) develop prevention plans for their nonusing patients and diagnosis and treatment plans for their substance-abusing patients.

Alderman E, Schonberg K, Cohen M: The pediatrician's role in the diagnosis and treatment of substance abuse. Pediatr Rev 1992;13:314.

Committee on Injury and Poison Prevention for The American Academy of Pediatrics: The teenage driver. Pediatrics 1996;98:987.

Committee on Substance Abuse for the American Academy of Pediatrics: Alcohol use and abuse: A pediatric concern. Pediatrics 1995;95:439.

DiFranza J, Savageau J, Aisquith B: Youth access to tobacco: The effects of age, gender, vending machine locks, and "It's the Law" programs. Am J Pub Health 1996;86:221.

Elster AB, Kuznets NJ (editors): *AMA Guidelines for Adolescent Preventive Services (GAPS).* Williams & Wilkins, 1994.

PREVENTING THE PROGRESSION FROM USE TO ABUSE

Most adolescents who use mood-altering substances do so only intermittently or experimentally. However, a substantial minority experience serious problems as a consequence of even limited use of drugs and alcohol. The challenge to the pediatric health care provider is to be alert to the warning signs, to identify patients early, and to intervene in an effective and timely fashion.

Male sex, young age at first use, and association with drug-using peers are the best predictors of ethanol and drug abuse. It is still unclear why only a minority of the young people who exhibit the high-risk characteristics listed in Table 5–5 go on to abuse substances. Substance abuse is a symptom of personal and social maladjustment as often as it is a cause. Since there is a direct relationship between the number of risk factors listed in Table 5–5 and the frequency of substance abuse, a combination of risk factors is the best indicator of risk. Even so, most teenagers who exhibit multiple risk characteristics never develop a substance abuse problem, presumably because the protective factors listed in Table 5–5 give them enough resiliency to deal with stress in more socially adaptive ways.

Being aware of the risk domains listed in Table 5–5 will help identify youngsters most apt to need counseling about substance abuse. Theories concerning the mechanisms responsible for the association between the risk factors listed in Table 5–5 and substance abuse are listed in Table 5–6. These theories provide a framework for understanding why individual patients may be at risk for progressing from occasional to established or compulsive substance abuse. Most of the theories emphasize social influences because during childhood and adolescence, associating with cigarette-smoking or substance-abusing peers is the most reliable predictor of both the onset and the progression of substance abuse. For example, most teenage smokers report smoking at home and cite smoking parents or relatives as excuses to continue smoking.

"Problem behavior theory" is one of the most frequently referenced concepts in the substance abuse literature. Its main argument is that socially disapproved behaviors tend to cluster and to resist intervention because they have both negative and positive consequences for the individual. "Expectancy theory," which takes up where problem behavior theory leaves off, proposes a potentially modifiable mechanism by which learning experiences influence substance abuse. Measuring alcohol- and drug-related expectancies has been found to provide a more accurate assessment of risk than any of the factors listed

Table 5–5. Factors that influence the progression from substance use to substance abuse.

Enabling Risk Factors	Potentially Protective Factors
SOCIETAL AND COMMUNITY	
Experimentation encouraged by media	Regular involvement in church activities
Illicit substances available	Support for norms and values of society
Extreme economic deprivation	Strict enforcement of laws prohibiting substance
Neighborhood disorganization, crowding	Use among minors and abuse among adults
Tolerance of licit and illicit substance use	Neighborhood resources, supportive adults
SCHOOL	
Lack of commitment to school or education	Strong commitment ot school or education
Truancy	Future oriented goals
Academic failure	Achievement-oriented
Early, persistent behavior problems	
FAMILY	
Models of substance abuse and other unconventional behavior	Models of convnetional behavior
Dysfunctional parenting styles; excessive authority or permissiveness	Attachment to parents
HIgh family conflict; low bonding	Cohesive family
	Nurturing parenting styles
PEERS	
Peer rejection in elementary grades	Popular with peers
Substance use prevalent among peers	Abstinent friends
Peer attitudes favorable to substance abuse and unconventional behavior	Peer attitudes favor conventional behavior
INDIVIDUAL	
Genetic predisposition	Positive self-concept, good self-esteem
Psychological diagnoses (attention deficit disorder; antisocial personality)	Intolerance of deviance
Depression and low self-esteem	Internally motivated, takes charge of problems
Alienation and rebelliousness	
Sexual or physical abuse	
Early onset of deviant behavior or delinquency	
Early onset of sexual behavior	
Aggressive	

in Table 5–5. Expectancies about the effects of substances are important determinants of social and psychologic reactions to them. Furthermore, expectancies are longitudinally related to different patterns of substance abuse. For example, within homogeneous groups of nondrinkers, low-risk drinkers, and high-risk drinkers, outcome expectancies differ significantly both at entry into college and 3 years later. Higher-risk drinkers expect more positive outcomes from drinking. Thus, data showing that close to 75% of eighth grade students believe that alcohol can contribute to desired changes in affect should be particularly worrisome to pediatric health care providers. Evidence that negative experiences with alcohol transform some high-risk freshmen drinkers into nondrinking seniors suggests that it may be possible to influence indulgence patterns by altering expectancies.

Early and effective intervention is critical if occasional use is to be stopped in its tracks. Without guidance, most youngsters do not draw sober conclusions from their negative experiences with drugs and alcohol. Despite serious accidents and socially unrewarding experiences, positive expectancies about the effects of alcohol tend to increase rather than decrease during the first 3 years of college.

Donaldson S, Graham J, Hansen W: Testing the generalizability of intervening mechanism theories: Understanding the effects of adolescent drug use prevention interventions. J Behav Med 1994;17:195.

Escobedo L, Reddy M, DuRant R: Relationship between cigarette smoking and health risk and problem behaviors among United States adolescents. Arch Pediatr Adolesc Med 1997;151:66.

Jessor R: Risk behavior in adolescence: A psychosocial framework for understanding and action. J Adolesc Health 1991;12:597.

Middleman AB et al: High-risk behaviors among high school students in Massachusetts who use anabolic steroids. Pediatrics 1995;96:268.

Miller NS, Fine J: Current epidemiology of comorbidity of psychiatric and addictive disorders. Psychiatr Clin North Am 1993;16:1.

Werner M, Walker L, Greene J: Relation of alcohol expectancies to changes in problem drinking among college students. Arch Pediatr Adolesc Med 1995;49:733.

Wolin SJ, Wolin S: The Resilient Self: How Survivors of Troubled Families Overcome Adversity. Villard Books, 1993.

PREVENTION OF SUBSTANCE ABUSE

The prevention of substance abuse and its sequelae has to be considered at both the population and the

Table 5–6. Theories accounting for the progression from substance use to substance abuse.[1]

Theory	Key Constructs and Assumptions	Major Protagonist
Problem Behavior	Socially problematic behaviors,[2] co-occur reflect a common underlying cause. The common antecedent is the result of the interaction among individual personality traits (eg, unconventionality), the perceived environment (eg, models of deviance), and a nondominant pattern of socialization (eg, low value on education).	Jessor R, Jessor R: Problem *Behavior and Psychosocial Development.* Academic Press, 1977.
Social Learning	Problem Behavior Theory plus a scheme to explain reinforcement of these behaviors. The risk of problem behavior increases when youngsters have the opportunity skillfully in unconventional settings and are rewarded for doing so.	Bandura A: *Social Learning Theory.* Prentice-Hall, 1977.
Reasoned Action	Behavior is determined by the interaction between perceived consequences attitudes toward those consequences. The risk of problem behavior increases when the perceived costs are low or the perceived benefits high.	Ajzen I, Fishbein M: *Understanding Attitudes and Predicting Behavior.* Prentice-Hall, 1980.
Health Belief	Health behaviors reflect assessments of perceived risk or harm, potential to avoid that harm through alternative behaviors, and ability to access requisite resources. The risk of unhealthy behavior increases when perceived health risk is low or the ability to avoid that risk is perceived to be low or unrelated to the behavior.	Becker MH: The health belief model and personal health behavior. Health Education Monograph 1974;2:324.
Social Control	Behavior is determined by the bonds an individual establishes with society. The risk of problem behavior increases when attachment to those who express conventional values is weak, commitment ot participation in conventional activities is low and little time is spent in these activities, and the central value system of society is not fully accepted.	Hirschi T: *Causes of Delinquency.* Univ California Press; 1969.
Peer Cluster	The socialization process that accompanies adolescent development results in the formation of peer clusters. Family sanctions, religious identifications, and school adjustment affect behavior indirectly through their effects on peer clusters.	Oetting ER, Beauvais F: Peer cluster theroy. J Counseling Psychology. 1987;34:205.
Expectancy	Problem Behavior and Reasoned Action Theory plus a mechanism by which lerning experiences exert an influence on future behavior. The risk of problem behavior increases when experiences reinforce preexisting positive expectancies.	Werner MJ: Relation of alcohol expectancies to change in problem drinking among college students. Arch Pediatr Adolesc Med 1995;149:733.
Self-medication	Individuals are predisposed to addiction when they suffer from painful affective states or psychiatric disorders; symptom relief perpetuates the use of specific substances.	Khantzian EJ: The self-medication hypothesis. Am J Psychiatry 1985;142:1259.

[1]Ordered by frequency of citation in the literature.
[2]A problem behavior is defined as any behavior compromising the accomplishment of normal developmental tasks of adolescence; most are hard to change because they also serve functions central to the psychosocial development of adolescents who lack conventional alternatives.

individual levels and at three stages: (1) primary—preventing the initiation phase of substance use; (2) secondary—preventing progression from the initiation to the continuation and maintenance phases; and (3) tertiary—preventing the morbid consequence of this progression.

Prevention at the Population Level

Prevention of substance abuse at the population level is a public health priority for the year 2000. The aim of these programs is to prevent substance abuse by changing the cultural attitudes and values that foster positive expectancies about substance use as a means of relieving stress and improving social skills. Programs designed to achieve this end typically focus on educating middle school and high school students about the adverse consequences of substance abuse and enabling them to resist peer pressures. The "Drug Awareness and Resistance Education" ("DARE") program is a familiar example of a primary prevention program.

Secondary programs target populations at increased risk for substance use. The aim is to prevent progression by individualized intervention to reduce the risk and enhance the protective factors listed in Table 5–5. This approach enables the provider to focus scarce resources on those who are most likely to benefit. Programs designed to prevent substance abuse among the children of alcoholic parents typify secondary prevention efforts.

Tertiary prevention programs target young people who have been identified as substance abusers. The aim is to prevent the morbid consequences of substance use. Identifying adolescents who misuse alcohol and drugs at parties and providing them with a safe ride home is one example. Since prevention efforts are more effective if they are targeted at reducing the risk of initiating substance use than at decreasing use, tertiary prevention is the least effective approach.

Pediatric health care providers who are asked to give advice about the selection of prevention programs should be aware that few such programs have been subjected to scientifically rigorous evaluation. Even so, there is broad consensus that interactive social skills training programs—designed to eliminate the psychologic factors and social influences that promote substance use—are more effective than noninteractive programs, which teach about the dangers associated with substance use; and resistance training programs, which teach youngsters to refuse explicit drug offers (ie, to "Just say no"). Indeed, during the last decade, when the latter approach was widely trumpeted, resistance training programs such as "DARE" were associated with a *decrease* in the proportion of middle and high school students who perceived illicit drug and alcohol use as dangerous and an increase in substance use. Since 1991, the percentage of high school seniors who think that regular marijuana use could harm them dropped from 79% to 61%, and annual marijuana use has risen from 24% to 35%. Even when knowledge- and resistance-based programs do increase student understanding of adverse consequences, there is no evidence of changed attitudes or abuse rates. Indeed, the reverse appears to be true.

The failure of resistance education programs has fostered interest in a potentially more useful type of program, exemplified by the "Adolescents Training and Learning to Avoid Steroids" (ATLAS) program. This program is designed to reduce prevalence estimates about the use of steroids by peers and to teach youngsters alternative dietary and exercise regimens. Pediatric health care providers should promote developmentally appropriate prevention programs like this one that address the social and psychologic problems predisposing youngsters to substance abuse.

Programs of the ATLAS model have been shown to be effective in randomized controlled trials. Parents and others should understand that most adolescents who abuse alcohol and drugs do not do so just for the "high." Rather, these behaviors are often purposeful, developmentally appropriate coping strategies. To the extent that these behaviors meet young peoples' developmental needs, they are not apt to be abandoned unless equally attractive alternatives are available. For example, even though many teenagers cite stress and anxiety as reasons for smoking, teen-oriented smoking cessation programs rarely address the young smoker's need for alternative coping strategies by offering stress management training. Similarly, for the average youngster growing up in an impoverished urban environment, the real costs of substance abuse may be too low and the rewards too high to be influenced by talk and "knowledge" alone. Since it is unreasonable to expect a talk-based intervention to change attitudes and behaviors in a direction that is opposite to the rest of the world, the efficacy of even the most promising prevention models and interventions is apt to decay over time unless talk is accompanied by changes in the social environment that provide substance-abusing children and adolescents with alternative ways to meet their developmental needs.

Botvin GJ et al: Long-term follow-up results of a randomized drug abuse prevention trial in a white middle-class population. JAMA 1995;273:1106.

Bruvold WH: A meta-analysis of adolescent smoking prevention programs. Am J Pub Health 1993;83:872.

Ennett S et al: How effective is drug abuse resistance education? A meta-analysis of project dare outcome evaluations. Am J Pub Health 1994;84:1394.

Goldberg L et al: Effects of a multidimensional anabolic steroid prevention intervention. JAMA 1996;276:1555.

Diagnosis & Prevention at the Individual Level

Since pediatric health care providers typically have the advantage of long-standing relationships with children and their families, they are in an ideal position to help families identify and address conditions that may predispose children to substance abuse. Screening and intervention should be started early in childhood, when family standards and values are being assimilated and at a time when the child's behavioral repertoire is still malleable.

A general psychosocial assessment is the best way to screen for substance abuse. Interviewing and counseling techniques and methods for taking a psychosocial history are discussed in Chapter 4. If reliable information is to be obtained, an atmosphere of trust and confidentiality must be established and maintained. By gradually shifting from a parent-based to a predominantly patient-based style of care before the struggle over autonomy begins, the pediatric health care provider can help parents perceive the change in orientation of health maintenance visits as a positive, growth-promoting step rather than as a challenge to their authority.

The universal screening approach outlined in the AMA guidelines for adolescent preventive services (GAPS) is critical given the high incidence of substance abuse and the subtlety of its early signs and symptoms. Few children and adolescents will have been abusing substances long enough to have developed overt signs and symptoms. Clues to possible substance abuse may include truancy, failing grades, problems with interpersonal relationships, delinquency, depressive affect, chronic fatigue, recurrent abdominal pains, chest pains or palpitations, headache, chronic cough, persistent nasal discharge, and recurrent complaints of sore throat. To avoid missing the early stages of substance abuse, clinicians treating pediatric patients must maintain a high index of suspicion and include substance abuse in the differential diagnosis of all behavioral, family, psychosocial, and medical problems they treat.

Fuller P, Cavanaugh R: Basic assessment and screening for substance abuse in the pediatrician's office. Pediatr Clin North Am 1995;42:295.
Werner M, Adger JH: Early identification, screening, and brief intervention for adolescent alcohol use. Arch Pediatr Adolesc Med 1995;149:1241.

Diagnostic Interview

When the psychosocial history suggests the possibility of substance use, the primary tasks of the diagnostic interview are the same as the evaluation of other medical problems (see Table 5–7).

First, specific information about the extent of the problem must be gathered. Eliciting multiple choice answers is a useful technique. For example,

Q: "Has anything really good ever happened to you when you are high?"
A: Halting or evasive reply.

versus–

Q: "Some of my patients like to get high because they feel good; others find it helps them relax and be

sociable with friends; and some find it helps them forget their problems. Are any of these things true for you?"
A: "Well, yes, I do feel . . . "

Second, the provider needs to determine why the patient has progressed from the initiation to the continuation or maintenance phase of substance abuse. The cause may be different at different periods of development. While peer group characteristics are one of the best predictors of substance use among early and middle adolescents, this is not so among older adolescents and young adults.

Brief questionnaires can be used if time does not allow more detailed investigation. Two instruments that have been rigorously evaluated in primary care settings are the CAGE questionnaire and the Perceived Benefits of Drinking Scale. CAGE is a mnemonic (acronym) derived from the first four questions listed in Table 5–8. Although a positive response to CAGE questions is not diagnostic of substance abuse, a score of 2 or more is highly suggestive. The Perceived Benefits of Drinking Scale consists of the next five statements listed in Table 5–8. Patients who endorse more than three statements deserve further evaluation. Since CAGE is more predictive of substance use problems among males and the Perceived Benefits of Drinking Scale is more predictive among females, many clinicians combine the two scales. Adding an additional ques-

Table 5–7. Diagnostic interview for substance abuse.

I. **Define the extent of the problem by determining:**
  Age at onset of substance use
  Which substances are being used
  Circumstances of use
    Where?
    When?
    With whom?
  To what extent substances are being used
    How frequently?
    How much (quantity)?
    With what associated symptoms (eg, tolerance, withdrawal)?
  With what result?
    What does the patient gain from becoming high?
    Does the patient get into risky situations while high?
    Does the patient engage in behaviors which are later regretted while high?
II. **Define the cause of the problem by developing a differential diagnosis**

Table 5–8. Substance abuse screening questionnaires.

Cage Questionnaire[1]

CUT DOWN: Have you ever felt you ought to cut down on your drinking (drug use)?
ANNOYED: Have people annoyed you by criticizing your drinking (drug use)?
GUILTY: Have you ever felt bad about your drinking (drug use)?
EYE OPENER: Have you ever had a drink (used drugs) to steady your nerves in the morning?

(Score 1 point for each positive answer; refer if total points ≥ 2)

[1]Ewing JE: Detecting alcoholism: The CAGE questionnaire. JAMA 1984;252:1905.

Perceived Benefits Scales[2]

1. Drinking (drug use) helps me forget my problems.
2. Drinking (drug use) helps me be friendly.
3. Drinking (drug use) helps me feel good about myself.
4. Drinking (drug use) helps me relax.
5. Drinking (drug use) helps me be friends with others who drink (use drugs).

(Score 1 point for each positive answer; refer if total points ≥ 3)

[2]Petchers MK, Singer MI: Perceived-Benefit-of-Drinking Scale. J Pediatr 1987;110:977.

tion about use of tobacco and a question about his or her best friend's use of mood-altering substances further enhances the diagnostic accuracy of these screening tools.

Although constructed as screening tools for alcohol abuse, the questions in Table 5–8 can be adapted to elicit similar information about use of other mood-altering substances and their use by close contacts (eg, parents and older siblings). Finally, clinicians may find it helpful to use these questionnaires to stimulate discussion of the patient's self-perception of his or her substance use. For example, if an adolescent admits to a previous attempt to cut down on drinking, this provides an opportunity to inquire about events that may have occasioned the attempt.

Additional screening instruments include the following: (1) The Personal Experience Inventory is a comprehensive, standardized 260-item self-report measure of chemical involvement and the psychosocial aspect of substance use. (2) The Personal Experience Screening Questionnaire is a quick, 38-item screen that evaluates the severity of the problem and associated psychosocial risks. (3) The Adolescent Diagnostic Interview is a structured interview based on the American Psychiatric Association's diagnostic criteria for substance abuse. (See Table 5–1.) Although these instruments may be too time-consuming for routine office use, they may prove helpful in the evaluation of patients who pose diagnostic or therapeutic dilemmas.

Armentano ME: Assessment, diagnosis, and treatment of the dually diagnosed adolescent. Pediatr Clin North Am 1995;42:479.
Kaminer Y: *Adolescent Substance Abuse: A Comprehensive Guide to Theory and Practice.* Plenum, 1994.

Pharmacologic Screening

The use of urine and blood testing in the detection of substance abuse is controversial. The consensus is that pharmacologic screening should be reserved for situations where behavioral dysfunction is of sufficient concern to outweigh the practical and ethical drawbacks of testing. The AAP recommends voluntary or even involuntary screening under certain circumstances (eg, an inexplicably obtunded patient in the emergency department) but discourages routine screening for the following reasons: (1) Voluntary screening programs are rarely truly voluntary owing to the negative consequences for those who decline to participate (eg, members of an athletic team who refuse testing); (2) infrequent users or individuals who have not used substances recently may be missed; and (3) confronting substance-abusing individuals with objective evidence of their use has little or no impact on their behavior. Finally, the AAP reminds providers that their role is counseling and treatment, not law enforcement, so that drug testing should not be done for the purpose of detecting illegal use. If testing is to be performed, the provider should discuss the plan for screening with the patient, explain the reasons for it, and obtain informed consent. The AAP does not consider parental permission sufficient justification for involuntary screening of mentally competent minors.

Beyond the ethical concerns associated with laboratory screens for substance abuse are the practical concerns. If testing is to be performed, it is imperative that it be done accurately and that the limitations of testing be clearly understood by all parties. Tests range from simple, inexpensive, chromatographic spot tests, which are convenient because they can be performed in the office, to sophisticated methods such as gas chromatography and mass spectrometry, which require specialized laboratory equipment and are usually reserved for forensic investigations. Most commercial medical laboratories use the enzyme multiplication immunoassay technique (EMIT), in which a sample of the fluid to be tested is added to a test reagent consisting of a known quantity of the radiolabeled index drug (ie, the drug being tested for). If the index drug is also present in the patient's urine or serum, it competes with the radiolabeled drug for binding sites on the test kit antibody. The unbound or excess drug can then be quantified with a spectrophotometer. Most of the commonly abused mood-altering substances (with the exception of solvents and inhalants) can be detected by this method.

Caution is necessary in interpreting results because false positives may be obtained as a result of antibody cross-reactions with the licit medications and substances listed in Table 5–9 or from passive exposure to illicit substances. The most common cause of false-negative tests is infrequent use. Table 5–10 shows that the duration of detectability in the urine after last use varies by class of substance and duration of use, ranging from a few hours for alcohol

Table 5–9. Causes of false-positive drug screens.

Opioids
  Poppy seeds
  Dextromethorphan
  Chlorpromazine
  Diphenoxylate
Amphetamines
  Ephedrine
  Phenylephrine
  Pseudophedrine
  N-Acetylprocainamide
  Chloroquine
  Procainamide
Phencyclidine
  Dextromethorphan
  Diphenhydramine
  Chlorpromazine
  Doxylamine
  Thioridazine

Table 5–10. Duration of urine positivity for selected drugs.[1]

Drug Class	Detection Time
Amphetamines	< 48 hours
Barbiturates	Short-acting: 1 day Long-acting: 2–3 weeks
Benzodiazepines	Single dose: 3 days Habitual user: 4–6 weeks
Cocaine metabolites	Acute use: 2–4 days Habitual user: 2 weeks
Ethanol	2–14 hours
Methadone	Up to 3 days
Opioids	Up to 2 days
Propoxyphene	6–48 hours
Cannabinoids	Moderate use: 5 days Habitual use: 10–20 days
Methaqualone	2 weeks
Phencyclidine	Acute use: 1 week Habitual use: 3 weeks
Anabolic steroids	Days to weeks

[1]Woolf A, Shannon M: Clinical toxicology for the pediatrician. Pediatr Clin North Am 1995;42:317.

to several weeks for chronic, daily marijuana use. False-negative results can also be obtained if the patient intentionally alters or adulterates the specimen, either by drinking a large volume of fluids or adding a substance such as bleach, vinegar, or golden seal powder to the specimen. (Teenagers should be advised that despite street lore, *ingesting* these compounds is an ineffective and potentially dangerous way to "clean up" their urine.) Close observation during collection and pretesting the temperature, specific gravity, and pH of urine samples may circumvent such deception.

Woolf A, Shannon M. Clinical toxicology for the pediatrician. Pediatr Clin North Am 1995;42:317.
Committee on Substance Abuse for the American Academy of Pediatrics: Testing for drugs of abuse in children and adolescents. Pediatrics 1996;98:305.

Beyond Primary Prevention

While primary prevention is preferable, children and adolescents are often brought to the office or emergency department intoxicated, experiencing an adverse drug reaction ("bad trip"), or requiring treatment for injuries sustained while intoxicated. It then becomes necessary to intervene at the secondary or tertiary level. Individuals experiencing acute effects, overdoses, and withdrawal exhibit the constellations of symptoms summarized in Tables 5–2 and 5–3.

(See also Chapter 11.) These acute situations serve as an opportunity to document substance abuse at a time when youngsters and their families may be acutely aware of the need for change and thus more receptive to help.

Ludwig S, Selbst SM, Lavelle J: Adolescent emergency conditions. In: *Textbook of Adolescent Medicine.* McAnarney ER et al (editors). Saunders, 1992.

OFFICE-BASED TREATMENT & REFERRAL

The AMA and the AAP recommend that all children and adolescents receive counseling about the dangers of substance use and abuse from their primary health care providers. By offering confidential health care services and routinely counseling about the risks associated with drug abuse, pediatricians can help most of their patients avoid the consequences of experimentation with mood-altering substances. However, more is required for youngsters in disadvantaged environments where substance abuse may be regarded as acceptable recreational behavior. Because substance use is often deeply embedded in the fabric of these young peoples' lives, most have little interest in prevention or treatment. Counseling strategies appropriate for patients who wish to change their behavior may be ineffective for a patient who does not consider use of mood-altering substances to be a problem. It may therefore be preferable to begin discussions about treatment by helping youngsters consider alternative ways of meeting the needs that substance use is currently meeting. The clinician may in this way help the patient devise alternatives that are more attractive than substance use. Realistically, few substance-abusing teenagers will choose to quit because of a single conversation with even a highly respected health care provider. The message is most effective when offered repeatedly from a variety of sources—family, peers, guidance counselors, and teachers.

Since an assessment of the patient's readiness to change is the critical first step in office-based, clinicians should consider the construct presented in Table 5–11. In theory, individuals pass through this series of stages in the course of changing problem behaviors. Thus, to be maximally effective, providers should tailor their counseling messages to the patient's stage of readiness to change.

Once it has been established that a patient is prepared to act on information about treatment, the next step is to select the program that best fits individual needs. Most drug treatment programs fail to individualize the approach to address vulnerabilities predisposing the patient to substance abuse. When programs are individualized, even brief (5- to 10-minute) counseling sessions will promote reductions in cigarette smoking and drinking. This strategy

Table 5–11. Stages of change and intervention tasks.

Patient Stage	Motivation Tasks
Precontemplation	Create doubt, increase the patient's awareness of risks and problems with current patterns of substance use
Contemplation	Help weigh the relative risks and benefits of changing substance use, evoke reasons to change and risks of not changing, strengthen the patient's self-efficacy for changing current use
Determination	Help patient determine the best course of action to change substance use from among available alternatives
Action	Help patient establish a clear plan of action toward changing substance use
Maintenance	Help the patient identify and use strategies to prevent relapse
Relapse	Help the patient renew the process of change starting at contemplation

[1]Reprinted from Werner MJ: Principles of brief intervention for adolescent alcohol, tobacco, and other drug use. Pediatr Clin North Am 1995;42:295. With permission of the publisher.

appears to be most effective when the health care provider's message is part of an office-wide program so that the entire staff reinforces the cessation message with every patient. Specific steps to help youngsters quit smoking are discussed in the next section and summarized in Table 5–12. These same strategies and principles can be applied to the treatment of drug and alcohol problems.

Intervention to Promote Smoking Cessation

Although more than half of adolescents who smoke regularly say they want to quit and have tried to quit, only a minority report that they have been advised or helped to do so by a health care provider. This is because for want of training the practitioner may feel unprepared to treat the problem. Lack of training fosters the misconception that smoking cessation interventions are time-consuming, nonreimbursable, and impractical in a busy office. In reality, studies conducted by the National Cancer Institute indicate that health care providers can help their patients stop smoking with short office interventions. Some of the most effective smoking cessation interventions are self-help programs consisting of a series of short (typically under 5 minutes) interventions by the pediatrician reinforced by the entire office staff using the simple protocol outlined in Table 5–12.

The first step is motivational. One should begin by providing patients with a list of reasons for quitting (see Table 5–13) or suggesting that they call 1-800-4CANCER to obtain the National Cancer Institute

Table 5–12. How to help your patients stop smoking.

Ask about smoking at every opportunity.
1. Do you smoke? How old were you when you started?
2. How much?
3. How soon after waking do you have your first cigarette?
4. Do you have friends who smoke? family members? relatives? role models?
5. Are you interested in stopping smoking?
6. Have you ever tried to stop before? If so, what happened?

Advise all smokers to stop.
1. State your advice clearly, for example: "As your physician, I must advise you to stop smoking now."
2. Personalize the message to quit. Refer to the patient's clinical condition, smoking history, family history, personal interests, or social roles (see Table 5–13).

Assist the patient in stopping.
1. Set a quit date. Help the patient pick a date within the next 4 weeks, acknowledging that no time is ideal.
2. Provide self-help materials. The smoking cessation coordinator or support staff member can review the materials with the patient.
3. Discuss the importance of a smoke-free environment.
4. Rehearse through role-playing how to respond to social situations where others are smoking.
5. Elicit support of parents and relatives; encourage them to stop smoking with their teen.
6. Encourage participation in activities that are incompatible with smoking.
7. Consider prescribing replacement therapy (patch or gum) for highly addicted patients (those who smoke a pack or more daily or who smoke their first cigarette within 30 minutes after waking).
8. Consider signing a stop-smoking contract with the patient.
9. If the patient is not willing to quit now, provide motivating literature and flag the chart and so remember to ask again at the next visit.

Arrange follow-up visits.
1. Set a follow-up visit within 1–2 weeks after the quit date.
2. Have a member of the office staff call or write the patient within 7 days after the initial visit, reinforcing the decision to stop and reminding the patient of the quit date.
3. At the first follow-up visit, ask about the patient's smoking status to provide support and help prevent relapse.
4. Set a second follow-up visit in 1 month.
5. Remind the teen that relapse is common—indeed the norm. When it happens, discuss the circumstances and encourage the patient to think of alternative responses and to try again.

[1]Adapted from Glynn T, Manley M: *How to Help Your Patients Stop Smoking: A National Cancer Institute Manual for Physicians.* National Institutes of Health, 1989.

"Quit for Good" or "Why Do You Smoke?" pamphlets and materials.

However, motivation alone is not enough. Learning to use coping skills to prevent relapse and avoiding discouragement at the time of relapse are the keys to success. Smoking cessation is a process that takes place over time. Relapse must be regarded as a normal part of quitting rather than evidence of per-

Table 5–13. Good reasons to stop smoking.[1]

For all teens
  Bad breath
  Stained teeth
  Cost
  Lack of independence—controlled by cigarettes
  Sore throats
  Ulcers
  Frequent respiratory infections; miss time at school and
    work
  Cough
  Impaired sports performance due to compromised respira-
    tory function and dyspnea
  Improved ability to play sports
  Feel better
  Live longer
  Easier to stop now than when older
For pregnant teens
  Increased rate of spontaneous abortion and fetal death
  Increased risk of low birth weight
For teen parents
  Increased coughing and respiratory infections among
    children of smokers
  Poor role model for child

[1]Adapted from Glynn T, Manley M: *How to Help Your Patients Stop Smoking: A National Cancer Institute Manual for
Physicians.* National Institutes of Health, 1989.

Table 5–14. Factors to consider prior to referral.

Duration and frequency of substance use
The type of substances being used
Presence of other psychologic disorders
  Attention deficit disorder
  Depression
  Antisocial personality
Presence of other social morbidities
  School failure
  Delinquency
  Homelessness
  Ongoing or past physical or sexual abuse

sonal failure or a reason to avoid further attempts. Patients can benefit from relapses if they are helped to identify the circumstances that led to the relapse and to devise strategies to avoid them or respond to them in a different manner. Since nicotine is a physically and psychologically addictive substance, replacement therapy may relieve withdrawal symptoms. There are two types of nicotine replacement systems available by prescription: nicotine polacrilex gum and transdermal nicotine patches. Nicotine replacement therapy increases smoking cessation rates and provides relief from withdrawal symptoms. Providers who do not wish to prescribe and monitor these pharmacologic therapies should limit their involvement with smoking patients to those who do not exhibit signs of nicotine dependency (eg, patients who smoke less than a pack of cigarettes a day or do not feel the need to smoke their first cigarette within 30 minutes after awakening). Most recently, a sustained-release form of the antidepressant bupropion has been shown in randomized trials to help smokers quit.

Referral

There is no consensus about which substance-abusing patients can be adequately treated in the office, which require referral, and which require hospitalization. Factors to be considered are summarized in Table 5–14. When doubt exists about the seriousness of the problem or the advisability of office management, consultation with a specialist should be sought.

Although most primary pediatric providers will not assume responsibility for the treatment of substance-abusing youngsters, clinicians can be instrumental in motivating their patients to seek treatment and in guiding them to appropriate treatment resources. Substance-abusing teenagers must be treated in teen-oriented treatment facilities. Despite the similarities between adult and adolescent substance abuse, adult programs are usually developmentally inappropriate and ineffective for adolescents. As discussed in Chapter 4, many adolescents are concrete thinkers. Their inability to reason deductively, especially about emotionally charged issues, makes it difficult for them to understand the abstract concepts (such as "denial") that are an integral component of most adult-oriented programs. This invariably frustrates counselors who misinterpret lack of comprehension as resistance to therapy and concrete responses as evidence of deceit.

Treatment programs range from low-intensity, outpatient, school-based student assistance programs that rely heavily on peers and nonprofessionals to residential, hospital-based programs staffed by psychiatrists and other professionals. Outpatient counseling programs are most appropriate for motivated patients who do not have significant mental health or behavioral problems and are not at risk for withdrawal. Some investigators have raised the concern that in pediatric settings, low-problem users may actually experience a strengthening of the drug subculture by associating with high-problem users in group therapy. More intensive day treatment programs are available for those who require a structured environment. Inpatient treatment should be considered for patients who need medical care and detoxification in addition to counseling, education, and family therapy. Finally, special "dual diagnosis" facilities are available to treat substance-abusing patients who also have other psychologic conditions. Mood and conduct disorders are common among substance-abusing children and adolescents; depression, attention deficit disorder, and antisocial personality are especially so. These patients are difficult to diagnose and treat because it is often unclear whether their symptoms are a consequence of substance use or a symptom of a comorbid psychologic disorder. Recognition of such disorders is critical because these patients must be treated in programs that include psychiatric expertise.

Approaches to the treatment of substance-abusing children and adolescents are typically modeled after adult treatment programs. Most notable are the "twelve-step programs" modeled after Alcoholics Anonymous. These programs are attractive because they demand total abstinence and acknowledge that substance abuse is a chronic disease requiring a lifelong commitment to abstinence and long-term support from family, peers, and community. Although treatment is usually effective, relapse is common. Since efficacy research has lagged behind practice and implementation (especially among low-intensity programs), there is little empirical evidence upon which to base recommendations for one program or another. Various forms of treatment appear to have the potential to be effective. Thus, in practice, referral recommendations should be based on the significance of the problem for the individual and the availability of affordable programs in the community.

Fleming M et al: Brief physician advice for problem alcohol drinkers. JAMA 1997;277:1039.

Henningfield J: Nicotine medications for smoking cessation. N Engl J Med 1995;333:1196.

Hurt RD et al: A comparison of sustained-release bupropion and placebo for smoking cessation. N Engl J Med 1997;337:1195.

Wall M et al: Pediatric office-based smoking intervention: Impact on maternal smoking and relapse. Pediatrics 1995;96:622.

Psychosocial Aspects of Pediatrics & Child & Adolescent Psychiatric Disorders

6

Donald W. Bechtold, MD, & R. Barkley Clark, MD

FAMILY LIFE

FAMILY FUNCTIONS

The structure of families has changed in recent years with the increase in the number of single-parent homes, reconstituted families, alternative lifestyles such as gay and lesbian parents, and the decline in the number of extended families living together. Despite these changes, the nuclear family continues to play a vital role in meeting the needs of society and of individual family members. The family serves the following functions: (1) rearing offspring to become autonomous adults and eventually competent parents and (2) meeting the needs of family members for nurturing, protection, feedback, recognition (mirroring), promoting adaptive behaviors, and emotional closeness and support. Evidence suggests that the lifestyle preferences of the parent figures are less important to healthy development than is the parents' ability of to serve parental functions consistently.

THE PARENTAL UNIT

The cornerstone of family functioning is the parental unit, which must serve as the source of leadership and authority. The parental unit must satisfy the emotional and physical needs of other, more dependent family members while at the same time defining the norms of behavior that will lead to independent adaptive functioning in the future. In short, the ways in which the parental unit exercises its leadership roles determine in large part the health or sickness of the family and its individual members.

Parenthood is emotionally and physically draining, and parents must have their own source of support to function as providers and setters of limits for the family. In the case of a two-parent unit, the partners provide the necessary emotional support, respite, and adult companionship for each other. The "women's movement" has helped men expand their parental roles and personal identities to include more nurturing activities. Because single parents often have no in-house source of adult support, the child is at risk of becoming a pseudoadult companion, thus completing the parental unit.

The lack of a solid partnership can be an important factor in virtually any child-centered problem. To function successfully as a parental unit, the couple must find the marriage mutually satisfying through mutual nurturing and affirmation, trust and respect, conflict recognition and resolution, and intimacy and sexual satisfaction.

When the parental unit is weakened by dissatisfaction or by persistent conflict, children are at risk of becoming the focus of parental attention and concern, thus displacing the conflict within the marriage unit onto the child. Concern about the child distracts the parents from their own marital problems, and the child ends up functioning as a buffer between the combatants, Questions designed to screen the quality of the marital and parental relationship are outlined in the section on screening for psychosocial problems and disorders.

Barker P: Healthy families and their development. In: *Basic Family Therapy.* Oxford Univ Press, 1992.

Martin A: *The Lesbian and Gay Parents' Handbook.* HarperCollins, 1993.

Miller DA: *Coping When a Parent Is Gay.* Rosen Publishing Group, 1993.

ISSUES IN PARENTHOOD

In rearing children, parents undertake a potentially rewarding but often tiring and frustrating task. Physical and emotional exhaustion as well as unfulfilled expectations about having children can be avoided or mitigated if both partners share the parenting responsibilities. Primary caregivers are also partly replenished emotionally by the child's positive responses and by memories of their own positive experiences as children. Children who are developmentally disabled or temperamentally difficult may be less responsive and rewarding. A mild consequence may be a state of tension in the family. In extreme forms child abuse and neglect may result.

Parents naturally want their children to be healthy, competent, and happy. Some parents have unrealistic fantasies about the children that may reflect their own unmet needs. Children with illnesses, disabilities, or temperamental difficulties call for modified expectations so the parents can meet the special needs implied.

Each new phase of child development presents unique challenges. The infancy years are a time of irregular sleep–wake cycles and a need for almost constant care and attendance. During the toddler years, the child's strivings for autonomy and independence must be endured without anger and without letting the child become the family tyrant. In the later preschool years, parents are faced with competitive challenges, requiring a balanced respect for the child's wishes to be "big" while still setting limits that maintain boundaries between the private lives of the parents (eg, the parents' bedroom) and children.

During the elementary school years, parents must let their children experience the challenges that await them outside the home. Parental support of skill development must be balanced with realistic definitions of success. Persistent separation anxiety on the part of parents and unrealistic standards of performance can contribute to a child's anxiety during school years.

The early adolescent has unpredictable changes of mood, intense attachment to peers, and a self-centered point of view, all of which deprive parents of the positive feedback they once enjoyed. Not since infancy and the toddler years have parents received so little gratitude for their efforts. Like parents of toddlers, the parents of young adolescents need to support autonomy while preventing tyranny and disaster.

The sexual interests of the middle adolescent can elicit parental reactions related to the parents' own concerns about sexuality, ranging from pride to fear to envy to sexual stimulation.

Finally, as the late adolescent prepares to leave home, parents face the sense of loss and grief associated with the emancipation of offspring going out into the world.

PSYCHOSOCIAL ASSESSMENT OF CHILDREN & FAMILIES

Five to 15 percent of children in the United States have psychiatric disorders, and nearly 50% of pediatric office visits are related to psychosocial or developmental problems. These statistics underscore the importance of psychosocial problems in children and their families.

SCREENING FOR PSYCHOSOCIAL PROBLEMS & PSYCHIATRIC DISORDERS WITHIN THE CONTEXT OF HEALTH MAINTENANCE VISITS

The most efficient indicator in screening for psychosocial problems is the history provided by caregivers. Psychosocial information can be obtained from three sources: checklists, general questioning, and direct questioning.

The 35-item pediatric symptom checklist (Table 6–1) screens children 6–12 years of age for psychosocial dysfunction. The checklist is to be completed in the waiting room by a parent or other caregiver. Each item is rated by the parents as "often present" (2 points), "sometimes present" (1 point), or "never present" (0 points). The information can be used in two ways: first, as a psychosocial review of symptoms and point of departure for the discussion of problems that "often" or "sometimes" occur; and second, as a general screening device, with a total score of 28 or higher indicating a need for in-depth psychosocial evaluation of the child.

Five questions forming the mnemonic "PSYCH" can be addressed to parents as a means of uncovering areas of concern. The questions can be slightly rephrased and then directed to children as well.

(1) Parent–child interaction: How are things going with you and your child?

(2) School: How are things going in school? (Academically and behaviorally.)

(3) Youth: How are things going with peer relationships?

(4) Casa: How are things going at home? (Including siblings, the marriage, and parents as individuals.)

(5) Happiness: How would you describe your child's mood? (Comfortable and happy versus tense and unhappy.)

Directed questions regarding age-appropriate behavior norms can then be reviewed. Concerns about infant attachment, "the terrible twos," childhood fears, school problems, and adolescent behavioral problems can in this way be brought into the open for further discussion.

ASSESSMENT OF PSYCHOSOCIAL SIGNS & SYMPTOMS

When an emotional or behavioral sign or symptom is present, a thorough psychosocial evaluation is indicated. Data must be collected from caregivers, the

Table 6–1. Pediatric symptom checklist.[1]

	Never	Sometimes	Often
1. Complains of aches or pains			
2. Spends more time alone			
3. Tires easily, little energy			
4. Fidgets, is unable to sit still			
5. Has trouble with a teacher			
6. Is less interested in school			
7. Acts as if driven by a motor			
8. Daydreams too much			
9. Is distracted easily			
10. Is afraid of new situations			
11. Feels sad, unhappy			
12. Is irritable, angry			
13. Feels hopeless			
14. Has trouble concentrating			
15. Has less interest in friends			
16. Fights with other children			
17. Is absent from school			
18. Experiences a drop in school grades			
19. Is down on himself or herself			
20. Visits doctor, with doctor finding nothing wrong			
21. Has trouble with sleeping			
22. Worries a lot			
23. Wants to be with you more than before			
24. Feels he or she is bad			
25. Takes unnecessary risks			
26. Gets hurt frequently			
27. Seems to be having less fun			
28. Acts younger than children the same age			
29. Does not listen to rules			
30. Does not show feelings			
31. Does not understand other people's feelings			
32. Teases others			
33. Blames others for his or her troubles			
34. Takes things that belong to others			

[1]Parents are asked to indicate which category—Never, Sometimes, or Often—best fits their child, with 0, 1, or 2 points assigned to each answer, respectively. For interpretation of scores, see text. Modified and reproduced, with permission, from Murphy JM, Jellinek M: Screening for psychosocial dysfunction in economically disadvantaged and minority children: Further validation of the pediatric symptom checklist. Am J Orthopsychiatry 1988;58:450. Copyright © 1988 by the American Orthopsychiatric Association.

child, and sometimes school personnel and others acquainted with the child's functioning. At least 30 minutes should be scheduled to cover the items listed in Table 6–2.

It is useful to see both parents and the patient first together, then the parents alone, and then the child alone. This sequence enables the physician to observe interactions among family members and gives the parents and the child an opportunity to talk confidentially about their concerns. Parents and children often feel shame and guilt about some personal inadequacy they perceive to be causing the problem. The physician can ease that burden and facilitate the assessment by acknowledging that the family is trying to cope and that the ultimate task of assessment is to seek solutions and not to assign blame. An attitude of nonjudgmental inquiry can be struck in supportive statements such as, "Let's see if we can figure out what might be happening here."

History of the Presenting Problem

First, obtain a detailed description of the problem. When did it start? Were there unusual stresses at that time? How is the child's life and the family's functioning affected? What does the child say about the problem? What attempts have been made to alleviate the problem? Do the parties have any opinions about the cause of the problem? Questions to screen for other psychosocial problems, listed in Table 6–2, can be asked when additional information is sought.

Interviewing the Preschool Child

Preschool children should be interviewed with the parents. As the parents discuss their concerns, the physician can look for the following behaviors:

(1) Does the child use the parent as a source of security and support?

(2) Does the 2- to 5-year-old warm up to the strange environment and begin to explore the

---

Table 6–2. Screening for psychosocial problems.

Developmental history
1. Review the landmarks of psychosocial development
2. Summarize the child's temperamental traits
3. Review stressful life events and the child's reactions to them
   a. Separations
   b. Losses
   c. Marital conflict
   d. Illnesses, injuries, and hospitalizations
4. Obtain details of past mental health problems and their treatment

Family history
1. Marital history
   a. Overall satisfaction with the marriage
   b. Conflicts or disagreements within the relationship
   c. Quantity and quality of time together away from children
   d. Whether the child comes between or is a source of conflict between the parents
   e. Marital history prior to having children
2. Parenting history
   a. Feelings about parenthood
   b. Whether parents feel united in dealing with the child
   c. "Division of labor" in parenting
   d. Parental energy or stress level
   e. Sleeping arrangements
   f. Privacy
   g. Attitudes about discipline
   h. Interference with discipline from outside the family (eg, ex-spouses, grandparents)
3. Stresses on the family
   a. Problems with employment
   b. Financial problems
   c. Changes of residence
   d. Illness, injuries, and deaths
4. Family history of mental health problems
   a. Depression? Who?
   b. Suicide attempts? Who?
   c. Psychiatric hospitalizations? Who?
   d. "Nervous breakdowns"? Who?
   e. Substance abuse or problems? Who?
   f. Nervousness or anxiety? Who?

Observation of parents
1. Do they agree on the existence of the problem or concern?
2. Are they uncooperative or antagonistic about the evaluation?
3. Does the parent appear depressed or overwhelmed?
4. Can the parents present a coherent picture of the problem and their family life?
5. Do the parents accept some responsibility for the child's problems, or do they blame forces outside the family and beyond their control?
6. Do they appear burdened with guilt about the child's problem?

Observation of the child
1. Does the child acknowledge the existence of a problem or concern?
2. Does the child want help?
3. Is the child uncooperative or antagonistic about the assessment?
4. What is the child's predominant mood or attitude?
5. What does the child wish could be different (eg, "three wishes")?
6. Does the child display unusual behavior (activity level, mannerisms, fearfulness)?
7. What is the child's apparent cognitive level?

Observation of parent–child interaction
1. Do the parents show concern about the child's feelings?
2. Does the child control or disrupt the joint interview?
3. Does the child respond to parental limits and control?
4. Do the parents inappropriately answer questions addressed to the child?
5. Is there obvious tension between family members?

Data from other sources
1. Waiting room observations by office staff
2. School (teacher, nurse, social worker, counselor)
3. Department of social services

room and even interact with the physician from a distance?

(3) How does the child relate to toys that are offered?

(4) What is the child's activity level?

(5) Does the child display unusual mannerisms (eg, intense clinging, stereotypical motor behaviors)?

(6) Does the child disrupt or attempt to control the interview?

(7) Does the parent attempt to place appropriate limits on behavior? How does the child respond?

It is helpful to have toy human figures available that the child can use to portray emotional states and interpersonal interactions. After hearing the history from the parents and after observing the child, the physician may question the 3- to 5-year-old about toy figures who appear to be feeling sad, worried, angry, or bossy. Children aged 3–5 are frequently able to confirm important interpersonal relationships and attitudes in such symbolic play activities.

Interviewing the School-Age Child

Most school-age children have mastered separation anxiety sufficiently to tolerate at least a brief interview with the physician. In addition, they may have important information to share about their own worries.

The child should be told beforehand by the parents or physician (or both) that the doctor will want to talk to the child about his or her feelings. School-age children understand and even appreciate parental concern about unhappiness, worries, and difficulty in getting along with people.

At the outset, it is useful to confirm that the purpose of the interview is to explore the child's own opinions about certain issues raised by the parents. Rapport can be enhanced by asking if the child has ever talked with anyone else about how he or she feels. If the answer is affirmative, the child may explain more about what he or she liked or did not like about that discussion. If the child has never before talked about personal feelings with a professional, the physician can acknowledge that it is often not easy to talk with "a stranger" about some kinds of problems.

The physician should then ascertain whether the child agrees that a problem exists (eg, unhappiness, worry, "not getting along"). If that is so, the physician should ask what the child can say about the magnitude of the problem, how it affects the child and the family, and what seems to be the cause.

Asking directly about how mom and dad get along can yield information about parental conflicts. A kinetic family drawing—"Draw your family and have everyone doing and saying something"—can provide clues to how the child fits into the family and how members of the family interact. Questions about school can yield information about life outside the home and with peers. Questions about worries, unhappy feelings, and what makes the child angry can access clues to the child's emotional life. Asking a child to make "three wishes" can uncover important concerns that may not have been apparent from the history: "Let's pretend you could have anything or change anything. What would you wish for and why?"

At the end of the child interview, it is important to share or reiterate the salient points derived from the interview and to state that the next step is to talk with the parents about ways to make things better for the child. At that time, it is good to discuss any concerns or misgivings the child might have about sharing information with parents so that the child's right to privacy is not arbitrarily violated. Most children want to make things better and thus will allow the physician to share appropriate concerns with the parents.

Interviewing the Adolescent

Because the developmental task of adolescence is to fashion an identity separate from that of the parents, the physician must show respect for the patient's point of view. That process begins with the patient participating in the format for the evaluation—meeting first alone with the physician, together with the parents, or after the physician has talked further with the parents. The parents need to be told why this is necessary, and the patient is then informed of the parents' expressed concern and the physician's wish to help the family determine whether a problem does in fact exist.

The issue of confidentiality must be approached forthrightly at the first interview. A good policy is to say, "What we talk about today is between you and me unless we decide someone should know or unless it appears to me that you might be in a potentially dangerous situation."

The interview might then start with a restatement of the parents' concern. The patient is then encouraged to describe the situation in his or her own words. The physician should then ask questions about:

(1) Predominant mood state.

(2) Nature of relationships with family members.

(3) Level of satisfaction with school and peer relationships.

(4) Plans for the future.

(5) Drug and alcohol use.

(6) Sexual activity.

(7) Worries or concerns.

(8) Biggest "stumbling block" in the adolescent's life.

(9) What the adolescent would like to be different.

In terminating the interview, the physician should review the salient points and discuss a plan either for further investigation or for ways of dealing with the problem.

Murphy JM et al: Screening for psychosocial dysfunction in pediatric practice. Clin Pediatr 1992;31:660.

Prugh DG: *The Psychosocial Aspects of Pediatrics.* Lea & Febiger, 1983.

DIAGNOSTIC FORMULATION & INTERPRETATION OF FINDINGS

Diagnosis starts with a description of the presenting problem, which is then scrutinized in the context of the child's age, developmental needs and tasks, temperament, the stresses and strains on the child and the family, and the functioning of the family system. The physician then develops an etiologic hypothesis by consideration of the following perspectives:

(1) The behavior falls within the range of normal given the child's developmental level.

(2) The behavior is a temperamental variation.

(3) The behavior is the result of nervous system dysfunction.

(4) The behavior is a normal reaction to stressful circumstances (eg, medical illness, change in family structure, loss of a loved one).

(5) The problem is primarily a reflection of family dysfunction (eg, the child is the "symptom bearer," or "scapegoat," or the "identified patient" for the family).

(6) The problem is a manifestation of a psychiatric disorder.

(7) Some combination of the above.

It can be seen that the physician's first task is to decide whether a "problem" exists. For example, how hyperactive must a 5-year-old be before he is too hyperactive? Functional impairment may be the single best marker of the difference between symptomatology and normal variation. When a child's function in such major domains of life as learning, peer relationships, family relationships, authority relationships, and recreation are impaired—or when there is a substantial deviation from the trajectory of normal developmental tasks—a differential diagnosis should be sought based upon the symptom profile. The physician's interpretation is then presented to the family. The interpretive process includes the following components: (1) an explanation of how the presenting problem or symptom is a reflection of a suspected cause; (2) a suggested plan of intervention based upon the presumed cause; and (3) a discussion of any further evaluation necessary to establish or refine a diagnosis.

A joint plan—physician, parents, and child—is then negotiated to address the child's special and developmental needs in light of the family structure and stresses. If a plan cannot be developed with reasonable effort, the question of referral to a mental health practitioner should be raised.

DEVELOPMENTAL DISTURBANCES & CONCERNS

Developmental disturbances are variations in normal child development that cause distress or concern. Parents frequently contact their physicians with questions about the "terrible twos," childhood fears and anxieties, and adolescent rebellion. The health care provider is faced with making the correct diagnosis, educating the parents about normal developmental variations, and then (when needed) developing strategies to help the parents facilitate normal parent–child interaction.

THE PUSHY PRESCHOOLER

The push for independence and autonomy that begins in the second year of life can pose problems for parents who are insecure in the parental role. Preschool children typically want to have their way even when it poses a danger or breaches generational boundaries. Children may try to decide when and what the family eats, what time is bedtime, and who sleeps in which bed—all as part of their rudimentary push to become independent.

The parents' task is to respect the child's wish for self-determination while setting limits and providing guidance so that the child does not become tyrannical or out of control. Parents who are having difficulty placing limits on behavior will come in with one of the following types of complaints:

(1) "Discipline won't work with this child."

(2) "I can't get her to do what I ask without getting mad."

(3) "He says, 'I don't have to do it if I don't want to.'"

(4) "She won't sleep in her own bed."

(5) "Other children his age don't like him. He always wants his way."

(6) "Is this child hyperactive?"

Parents who have difficulty saying "no" may just be emotionally drained or may believe that "confrontation" must be avoided. In the former case, parental depression or emotional exhaustion from working and single parenthood is common. In the latter case, the parent typically overidentifies with the frustrated child's distress and is then reminded of painful conflicts or unhappiness in his or her own life. Keeping the child "happy" (ie, avoiding conflict) keeps the parent from feeling distressed and unhappy.

In planning interventions, the physician must educate the parents about the sometimes pushy nature of children who are "flexing their muscles." With that explanation comes the need for external limits, because a child's judgment and self-control are as yet underdeveloped. Parents need to know that a child's disappointment and frustration with limits do not mean poor parenting or an unhappy child.

Parents who are emotionally depleted or depressed need to be cared for themselves, either through rest, emotional support, and assistance with parenting or through professional care for their depression.

In the case of a parent who avoids conflict, the physician should suggest addressing one or two discipline problems. For example, if toys are not picked up after a reminder, they are put away out of the child's reach for some announced period of time. Likewise, if a meal is not eaten within a reasonable and specified time limit, the food is taken away and snacks are withheld until the next meal. As the parent begins to feel more comfortably in control, the child's behavior typically becomes less oppositional; at this point, the parent should use positive reinforcement, such as, "I like the way you picked up your toys—let's read a story together."

Lieberman AF: The challenges of being (and raising) a toddler. In: *The Emotional Life of the Toddler.* Free Press, 1993.

CHILDHOOD FEARS & ANXIETIES

Childhood is a time of both excitement and worry—the latter manifested by fears and anxieties. In a study of nearly 500 randomly selected families, mothers reported that about 43% of their children had displayed at least seven fears or worries between 6 and 12 years of age. The vast majority of childhood fears are not associated with psychologic disorders; in fact, the fearful stimuli tend to evolve and change with age in a developmental sequence (see Table 6–3) and, overall, tend to decrease in frequency with age.

Although the manifestations of many developmental anxieties, such as separation distress and fear of the dark may wax and wane over months or years, most specific childhood fears are transient (days to weeks in duration) and not associated with substantial interference with daily life. In most cases, all that is needed is to reassure the parents about the developmental nature of fears; the parents, in turn, can then reassure their children that they will be fine even though they feel frightened at times. Fears become a source of greater concern to health care providers when they appear outside the normal developmental sequence of fears; when they are persistent; when they cause severe distress; or when they interfere with adaptive functioning, such as poor attendance at school or avoidance of peer relationships.

Table 6–3. Sequence of developmental anxieties.

Age at First Appearance	Source of Anxieties
Early infancy	Sudden loud noises, unpredictable stimuli, loss of postural support, heights
1 year	Stranger, unfamiliar situations and objects. Beginning of separation distress.
2–6 years	Animals, darkness, imaginary creatures (ghosts and monsters)
School age	Bodily injury, physical danger. Fear of loss of loved one.
Teens and adulthood	Fear of failure (eg, test anxiety), concerns about social acceptance, loss of a loved one, physical danger, natural disasters

Approximately 2–3% of children have fears troublesome enough to require specific mental health interventions such as referral to a child and adolescent psychiatrist.

Fraiberg SH: *The Magic Years: Understanding and Handling the Problems of Early Childhood.* Scribner, 1959.
Spence SH, McCathie H: The stability of fears in children: A two-year prospective study: A research note. J Child Psychol Psychiatry 1993;34:579.

ADOLESCENT REBELLION & TURMOIL

General theoretic impressions and sampling bias at one time tended to exaggerate the turmoil of normal adolescence. A longitudinal study of normal suburban middle-class boys through their high school years identified only 21% as experiencing tumultuous unrest. On closer examination, this segment was distinguished from the remainder of the sample by lower socioeconomic status, more overt marital conflicts in the family, and a higher than normal incidence of mental illness in the family. Overall, approximately 20% of normal adolescents have a stormy course; another 20% progress continuously and smoothly through adolescence; and the remainder show normal overall adjustment but have transient difficulties during times of stress.

When behavioral deviance or a clearly psychopathologic disorder is identified in adolescence, those problems tend not to remit with time. Continuity does, therefore, seem to exist between adolescent and adult psychopathology for many conditions.

PSYCHIATRIC DISORDERS

Psychiatric disturbances are classified on the basis of descriptive and phenomenologic data rather than presumed or hypothesized etiologic mechanisms. (See reference below.)

A psychiatric disorder is defined as a characteristic cluster of signs and symptoms (eg, emotions, behaviors, psychologic states) that are associated with subjective distress or maladaptive behavior. This definition presumes, therefore, that the individual's symptoms are of such intensity, persistence, and duration that the ability to adapt to life's challenges is compromised.

Psychiatric disorders have their origins in neurobiologic, psychologic (life experience), or environmental sources. The neurobiology of childhood disorders is today one of the most active areas of investigation in child and adolescent psychiatry. While much remains to be clarified, data from genetic studies point to heritable transmission of attention deficit hyperactivity disorder, schizophrenia, mood and anxiety disorders, pervasive developmental disorders, learning disorders, and tic disorders, among others. About 10% of children and adolescents are personally affected by psychiatric disorders and will benefit from psychiatric treatment

American Psychiatric Association: *Diagnostic and Statistical Manual of Mental Disorders,* 4th ed. American Psychiatric Press, 1994.

DISTURBANCES IN PARENT–INFANT INTERACTION

Primary Caregiver Dysfunction

Primary caregiver dysfunction can be defined as a failure to provide parenting functions (usually, but not necessarily, by the mother) because of parental vulnerability or disability. Although these parents have no single psychiatric diagnosis (and may not be formally diagnosable at all), they can manifest anxiety, distress, exhaustion, anger, or indifference in relation to the demands of child care. Caregiver dysfunction can result in a number of symptoms in the child, usually within the first 6 months of life (Table 6–4).

These individuals frequently have difficult psychosocial histories, find themselves currently without emotional or physical support, and have unmet personal needs (see Table 6–5). Characteristics of the child may also contribute to the parent's failure to "tune in and turn on" to the child's needs. Risk factors include prematurity, perinatal complications,

Table 6–4. Signs and symptoms suggesting primary caregiver dysfunction.

Failure to thrive
Feeding problems
Delays in development
Signs of abuse
Frequent physician visits, especially for nonspecific concerns
Excessive parental worry about illness in the child
Inadequate physical care
Child perceived as "difficult to deal with"
Sleep problems

birth defects, multiple births, and a difficult temperament. These characteristics frequently define the child as different, defective, or disappointing in the parent's eyes.

Clinical Findings

The diagnosis of caregiver dysfunction is made by interviewing the parents and observing the interaction between parent and child. The child should be evaluated for organic disorders that could explain the presenting symptoms.

A history directed toward identification of specific parental risk factors should be obtained directly from the parent (Table 6–5), with emphasis on feelings of stress or of being overwhelmed by the needs of the child or the demands of daily life. Attention should be paid to the parent's description of the child and to parental symptoms of anxiety or depression manifested by tension, irritability, fatigability, tearfulness, sleep disturbance, and a wish to avoid or withdraw from daily activities.

In observing the parent–child interaction, the physician should look for reciprocity, mutual enthusiasm, and enjoyment in the relationship, as opposed

Table 6–5. Parental risk factors contributing to primary caregiver dysfunction.

History of inadequate relations with own mother
Isolation from an adult support system (eg, single parent)
Psychiatric disorders (particularly acute or chronic depression)
Chronic psychosocial or cognitive dysfunctions (eg, unstable relationships, school problems, legal problems, employment problems)
Unresolved grief over past losses
Marital discord
Poverty or financial problems
Personal or family illnesses
Unwanted or difficult pregnancy
Current life stresses (eg, loss of a relationship, recent illness, job loss)

to pathologic signs of tension, irritability, or apathy on either side of the relationship.

Differential Diagnosis

Physical disorders that may explain the presenting symptoms must be ruled out, but it should also be noted that caregiver dysfunction and organic disease not infrequently coexist.

Complications

Parental dysfunction can result in disorders of attachment, nonorganic failure to thrive, child abuse, later behavioral problems in the child, and another generation of children who may themselves display caregiver dysfunction as parents.

Treatment

Treatment is focused primarily on supporting and educating the parents. The physician should empathize, explaining that being a parent is difficult and tiring work and that it requires health, energy, and emotional support. The task is to help the parent feel well physically and emotionally and then to facilitate the development of appropriate child care skills. Any underlying medical or psychiatric disorder of the parent should be treated, and a social support system should be found through friends and family. Parenting skills are taught and positively reinforced over time.

Prognosis

The prognosis depends greatly on the ability of the parent to view professional support and education as helpful rather than critical or indifferent.

Lieberman AF, Zeanah CH: Disorders of attachment in infancy. Child Adolesc Psychiatr Clin North Am 1995;4:571.

Zeanah CH, Boris NW, Larrieu JA: Infant development and developmental risk: A review of the past 10 years. J Am Acad Child Adolesc Psychiatry 1997;36:165.

PERVASIVE DEVELOPMENTAL DISORDERS & SCHIZOPHRENIA

Pervasive developmental disorders and childhood schizophrenia are most likely distinct groups of early-onset, severe neuropsychiatric disorders that were once referred to as childhood psychoses. The pervasive disorders (including autism) are now distinguished from childhood schizophrenia on the basis of clinical differences and family histories. The term "pervasive developmental disorder" denotes a group of disorders with the common findings of impairment of socialization skills and characteristic behavioral abnormalities. Speech and language deficits are common as well.

1. AUTISTIC DISORDER

Essentials of Diagnosis & Typical Features

- Severe deficits in social responsiveness and interpersonal relationships.
- Abnormal speech and language development.
- Behavioral peculiarities such as ritualized, repetitive, or stereotyped behaviors; rigidity; and poverty of age-typical interests and activities.
- Onset in infancy or early childhood (before age 3).

General Considerations

Autism is uncommon, with an incidence of approximately 4:10,000 school-age children. More boys than girls are affected (3–4:1).

Although the cause of autism is not known, central nervous system dysfunction is suggested by its higher incidence in populations affected by perinatal disorders: rubella, phenylketonuria, tuberous sclerosis, infantile spasms, encephalitis, and fragile X syndrome. Studies of twins reveal over 90% concordance for autism in monozygotic twins compared with 24% in dizygotic twins. No consistent psychopathologic pattern has been reported in the parents of autistic children, though 25% of families with an autistic child have other family members with language-related disorders.

Clinical Findings

Severe deficits in reciprocal social interaction—eg, delayed or absent social smile, failure to anticipate interaction with caregivers, and a lack of attention to a primary caregiver's face—are often evident even in the first year of life. In toddlers, findings include deficiencies in imitative play and a relative lack of interest in interactions with others. Language development is often quite delayed. In fact, children are often first referred for audiologic evaluation because of failure to respond to voices. When speech does begin to develop, it may be echolalic or nonsensical.

Autistic children often display peculiar interests, bizarre responses to sensory stimuli; repetitive, stereotypical motor behaviors (eg, twirling, hand flapping); odd posturing; self-injurious behavior; abnormal patterns of eating and sleeping; and unpredictable mood changes. Thematic "pretend" play is often impaired. An intense preoccupation with an age-unusual interest (such as power poles) may replace the usual broad range of interests of the child's age-mates. About 70% of autistic children have IQs under 70.

Differential Diagnosis

Although most autistic children function at the mentally retarded level, the vast majority of mentally retarded children do not show the essential characteristics of autism. A hearing or visual impairment must be ruled out with appropriate screening. Children with developmental speech and language disorders typically show better interpersonal interactions than autistic children. Evaluation should include investigations for metabolic disorders and fragile X syndrome.

Complications

Approximately 25% of autistic individuals eventually develop a seizure disorder. Some autistic adolescents who have higher cognitive skills become depressed as they become partially aware of their deficits.

Treatment

Behaviorally oriented special education classes or day treatment programs are vital in helping the autistic child acquire more appropriate social, linguistic, self-care, and cognitive skills.

Pharmacotherapy is aimed at reduction of specific target symptoms. Antipsychotic medications (eg, haloperidol, 0.5–4 mg/d) may modify a variety of disruptive symptoms, including hyperactivity, aggressiveness, and negativism, making the child more accessible to education. Fenfluramine may help the subset of autistic children with low serotonin. Other psychostimulants may benefit concurrent ADHD symptoms but can sometimes make the symptoms of autism more severe. Antidepressants (especially the SSRIs) may benefit both mood symptoms and symptoms of excessive rigidity or obsessive behavior. Mood stabilizers may ameliorate irritability, lability, or episodic dyscontrol. Naltrexone may help control self-injurious behavior or stereotypies.

Parents and families need strong support as well as education in coping with the disorder.

Prognosis

Autism is a lifelong disorder with a poor prognosis. Approximately one-sixth of autistic children become gainfully employed as adults, and another one-sixth are able to function in sheltered workshops and halfway houses. The remainder need ongoing supervision and support, often in a milieu-based therapeutic environment. The best prognosis is in children who have normal intelligence and have developed symbolic language skills by age 5 years.

Klin A, Volkmar FR: Autism and the pervasive developmental disorders. Child Adolesc Psychiatr Clin North Am 1995;4:617.

Mauk JE: Autism and pervasive developmental disorders. Pediatr Clin North Am 1993;40:567.

2. NONAUTISTIC PERVASIVE DEVELOPMENTAL DISORDERS

Essentials of Diagnosis & Typical Features

- Substantial social impairment, either primary or representing a loss of previously acquired social skills.
- Abnormalities in speech and language development or behavior similar to what is seen in autistic disorder.
- Onset by early childhood (may be as late as age 9 in childhood disintegrative disorder).

General Considerations

Children with nonautistic pervasive developmental disorders display a wide range of deficits in social, language, and behavioral skills that are similar to those in children with autism. Nonetheless, these children deviate from the diagnostic criteria for autistic disorder by failing to meet all the necessary diagnostic criteria, failing to fulfill severity threshold (ie, milder functional impairment), manifestation of atypical symptomatology (eg, the characteristic "hand-wringing" or gender distribution in Rett's disorder), or by later age at onset. In the past, many of these children would have been classified in the group manifesting "atypical development." Children with nonautistic pervasive developmental disorders probably outnumber autistic children by as much as 2–3:1.

Clinical Findings

These autistic-like children include those with Asperger's disorder, childhood disintegrative disorder, Rett's disorder, and pervasive developmental disorder not otherwise specified (PDD NOS) (see Table 6–6).

Differential Diagnosis

Specific developmental speech and language disorders should be distinguished. Hearing impairment should be ruled out with appropriate screening.

Treatment

The backbone of treatment for Asperger's disorder and PDD NOS is an adaptive behavioral approach aimed at inculcating and reinforcing more appropriate social and language skills and behaviors. Rett's disorder and childhood disintegrative disorder have much worse prognoses and call for multidisciplinary, often milieu-based interventions (as for autistic disorder). In all cases, family education and support are important.

Some children may benefit from treatment for depression as they become aware of their deficits. Psychoactive medications may be helpful for specific target symptoms as described for autistic disorder, above.

Table 6–6. Characteristics of nonautistic pervasive developmental disorders.

Disorder	Age at Onset	Clinical Features
Asperger's syndrome	Early childhood	"Odd" individuals (probably more common in males) with normal intelligence, motor clumsiness, eccentric interests, and a limited ability to appreciate social nuances
Childhood disintegrative disorder	3–4 years	Profound deterioration to severe autism
Rett's syndrome	5 months	Females with reduced head circumference and loss of social relatedness who develop stereotyped hand movements and have impaired language and mental functioning
Pervasive developmental disorder	Preschool years	Two to three times more common than autism, with similar but less severe symptoms

Prognosis

These are lifelong diagnoses. The prognosis is variable depending on the severity of social and language deficits.

Klin A, Volkmar FR: Autism and the pervasive developmental disorders. Child Adolesc Psychiatr Clin North Am 1995;4:617.

Towbin KE: PDD, NOS: A review and guidelines for clinical care. Child Adolesc Psychiatr Clin North Am 1994;3:149.

Wing L: Asperger's syndrome: A clinical account. Psychol Med 1981;11:115.

3. CHILDHOOD SCHIZOPHRENIA

Essentials of Diagnosis & Typical Features

- Rambling or illogical speech patterns.
- Bizarre thought content.
- Hallucinations, delusions, or both.

General Considerations

Childhood schizophrenia is probably the more severe form of the spectrum of schizophrenic disorders. It affects only one or two children in every 10,000 of the population under 15 years of age, and boys outnumber girls by approximately 2:1. Childhood schizophrenia appears to be genetically related to the adult type of schizophrenia.

Clinical Findings

Affected children display many of the symptoms of adult schizophrenia. Hallucinations or delusions, bizarre and morbid thought content, and rambling and illogical speech are typical. These children tend to withdraw into an internal world of fantasy and may then equate fantasy with external reality. They generally have difficulty with school work and with peer relationships. The vast majority of childhood schizophrenics have had nonspecific psychiatric symptoms or symptoms of delayed development for months or years prior to the onset of their overtly psychotic symptoms.

Differential Diagnosis

Psychotic symptoms in children under 8 years of age must be differentiated from manifestations of normal vivid fantasy life. Rambling speech and bizarre thought content are distinguishing features, as well as learning disabilities. In psychotic adolescents, mania is differentiated by high levels of energy, excitement, and irritability. Any youngster presenting with new psychotic symptoms requires a medical evaluation that includes physical and neurologic examinations (including MRI and EEG), drug screen, and metabolic screen for endocrinopathies, Wilson's disease, and delirium.

Treatment

The treatment of childhood schizophrenia focuses on four main areas: (1) ameliorating active psychotic symptoms, (2) inculcating social and cognitive skills, (3) reducing the risk of relapse of psychotic symptoms, and (4) providing support and education to parents and family members. Antipsychotic medications and a supportive, reality-oriented focus in relationships can help in a lessening of hallucinations, delusions, and frightening thoughts and reverse the tendency toward social withdrawal. Teaching life skills is probably best accomplished in a special education program or a day treatment setting. Support for the family emphasizes the importance of clear, focused communication and an emotionally calm climate in preventing recurrences of overtly psychotic symptoms.

Prognosis

Childhood schizophrenia is a chronic disorder with exacerbations and remissions of psychotic symptoms. It is generally believed that earlier onset (prior to age 13 years) and poor premorbid functioning (oddness or eccentricity) presage a poorer out-come.

Caplan R: Childhood schizophrenia: Assessment and treatment. Child Adolesc Psychiatr Clin North Am 1994;3:15.

Fish B et al: Infants at risk for schizophrenia: Sequelae of a genetic neurointegrative defect. Arch Gen Psychiatry 1992;49:221.

Volkmar, FR: Childhood and adolescent psychosis: A review of the past 10 years. J Am Acad Child Adolesc Psychiatry 1996;35:843.

Werry JS, McClellan JM: Predicting outcome in child and adolescent (early onset) schizophrenia and bipolar disorder. J Am Acad Child Adolesc Psychiatry 1992;31:147.

MOOD DISORDERS

1. DEPRESSION IN CHILDREN & ADOLESCENTS

Essentials of Diagnosis & Typical Features

- Dysphoric mood or depressed appearance, persisting for days to months at a time.
- Characteristic "neurovegetative" signs and symptoms (Table 6–7).

General Considerations

The term "depression" can denote an emotional state, a symptom, or a clinical syndrome. All three are now well-recognized entities in children and adolescents. The incidence of depression in children increases with age, from 1–3% before puberty to 3–6% of adolescents. The incidence of depression in chil-dren is higher when other family members have been affected by depressive disorders. The sex incidence is equal.

Clinical Findings

Clinical depression can be defined as a persistent state of unhappiness or misery that interferes with pleasure or productivity. The signs and symptoms of depression are surprisingly constant from early child-hood to adolescence and adulthood (Table 6–7). The dysphoria of depression in children and adolescents is as likely to be an irritable mood state as it is to be a down mood.

Typically, a child or adolescent with depression begins to look unhappy and may make comments such as, "I have no friends . . . Life is boring . . . There is nothing I can do to make things better . . . I wish I were dead." There is usually a change in be-havior patterns that includes social isolation, deterio-ration in schoolwork, loss of interest in usual activi-ties, and flashes of anger and irritability. Sleep and appetite patterns frequently change, and the child may complain of tiredness and nonspecific pain such as headaches or stomachaches.

Differential Diagnosis

Clinical depression can be identified by asking about the symptoms. Children are often more accu-rate than their caregivers in assessing their own mood state. When symptoms are numerous, persis-tent (2 weeks or more), and severe, a diagnosis of major depressive disorder is appropriate. When symptoms are fewer and of lesser severity but have persisted for months or years, a diagnosis of dys-thymic disorder is justified. Milder symptoms of short duration in response to some stressful life event warrant a diagnosis of adjustment disorder with de-pressed mood.

Children with attention deficit disorders, conduct disorders, and developmental disabilities can become quite "demoralized" or "reactively depressed" by their chronic difficulties in life. There are also sub-stantial rates of comorbidity of depression with atten-tion deficit hyperactivity disorder, conduct disorder, anxiety disorders, eating disorders, and substance abuse disorders. Medically ill patients also have an increased incidence of depression. Every child and adolescent with a depressed mood state should be asked about child physical and sexual abuse. De-pressed adolescents should be screened for hypothy-roidism and substance abuse.

Complications

Because the emotional pain associated with severe depression can be intensely distressing, suicide may be considered. In addition, adolescents have a propensity to avoid the pain of depression through substance abuse or excitement-seeking behaviors (eg,

Table 6–7. Clinical manifestations of depression in children and adolescents.

Depressive Symptom	Clinical Manifestations
Dysphoric mood	Tearfulness; sad, downturned expres-sion; unhappiness; slumped posture; quick temper; irritability; anger
Anhedonia	Loss of interest and enthusiasm in play, socializing, school, and usual ac-tivities; boredom; loss of pleasure
Fatigability	Lethargy and tiredness; no play after school
Morbid ideation	Self-deprecating thoughts, state-ments; thoughts of disaster, abandon-ment, death, suicide, or hopeless-ness
Somatic symptoms	Changes in sleep or appetite pat-terns; difficulty in concentrating; bod-ily complaints, particularly headache and stomachache

"partying," negativism and defiance, reckless behavior).

Treatment

Treatment consists of ameliorating the symptoms and helping the caregivers to respond more effectively to the patient's emotional needs. Efforts are made to resolve conflicts between family members and to increase the opportunity for enjoyable time spent together. Attitudes, expectations, and disciplinary methods are evaluated. The child is encouraged to become involved in activities and to pursue opportunities for maximizing skills and talents. Individual psychotherapy aimed at identifying pervasively negative thoughts and correcting negativistic cognitive distortions can increase the patient's awareness of care and concern on the part of adults. It also helps the young person to identify, label, and verbalize feelings and misperceptions.

When the symptoms of depression are severe and persistent and causing functional impairment, antidepressant medications can help, especially when there is a family history of depressive disorder responding to these agents. Controlled studies have generally not shown tricyclic antidepressants to be superior to placebo in children and adolescents with major depression. One recent study has demonstrated the superiority of fluoxetine to placebo in this population.

Prognosis

Depression in children and adolescents is a chronic condition that requires monitoring over time. Approximately one-third of preadolescents with major depression manifest bipolar disorder at 2-year follow-up.

Ambrosini PJ et al: Antidepressant treatments in children and adolescents: Affective disorders. J Am Acad Child Adolesc Psychiatry 1993;32:1.

Biederman J et al: Psychiatric comorbidity among referred juveniles with major depression: Fact or artifact? J Am Acad Child Adolesc Psychiatry 1995;34:579.

Birmaher B et al: Childhood and adolescent depression: A review of the past 10 years. Part I. J Am Acad Child Adolesc Psychiatry 1996;35:1427.

Birmaher B et al: Childhood and adolescent depression: A review of the past 10 years. Part II. J Am Acad Child Adolesc Psychiatry 1996;35:1575.

Emslie G, Rush AJ, Weinberg AW: A double-blind, randomized placebo-controlled trial of fluoxetine in depressed children and adolescents. Arch Gen Psychiatry [In press, 1998.]

Geller B et al: Rate and predictors of prepubertal bipolarity during follow-up of 6 to 12 year old depressed children. J Am Acad Child Adolesc Psychiatry 1994;33:461.

Kovacs M et al: Childhood onset dysthymic disorder: Clinical features and prospective naturalistic outcome. Arch Gen Psychiatry 1994;51:365.

McCauley E et al: Depression in young people: Initial presentation and clinical course. J Am Acad Child Adolesc Psychiatry 1993;32:714.

McCracken JT: The epidemiology of child and adolescent mood disorders. Psychiatr Clin North Am 1992;1:53.

Mood disorders in children and adolescence. The Harvard Mental Health Lett 1993;10(4 and 5).

Rao U et al: Unipolar depression in adolescents: Clinical outcome in adulthood. J Am Acad Child Adolesc Psychiatry 1995;34:566.

2. BIPOLAR DISORDER

Essentials of Diagnosis & Typical Features

- Periods of abnormally and persistently elevated, expansive, or irritable mood and heightened levels of energy and activity.
- Not caused by prescribed or illicit drugs.
- Associated symptoms: grandiosity, diminished need for sleep, pressured speech, racing thoughts, impaired judgment.

General Considerations

Bipolar disorder (previously referred to as manic-depressive disorder) is an episodic mood disorder manifested by alternating periods of manic—or hypomanic, as in bipolar II disorder—and depressive episodes or, less commonly, manic episodes alone. Children and adolescents often present with a variable course of mood instability combined with problems with conduct and impulse control. At least 20% of bipolar adults experience onset of symptoms before age 20. Onset of bipolar disorder before puberty is thought to be infrequent, while the lifetime prevalence of bipolar disorder in mid to late adolescence appears to approach 1%.

Clinical Findings

In about 70% of patients, the first symptoms are primarily those of depression; in the remainder, manic, hypomanic, or mixed states dominate the presentation. Manic patients present a variable pattern of elevated, expansive, or irritable mood along with more rapid speech, higher energy levels, some difficulty in sustaining concentration, and a decreased need for sleep. Patients often do not acknowledge any problem with their mood or behavior. The clinical picture can be quite dramatic, with florid psychotic symptoms of delusions and hallucinations (a full-blown manic psychosis), more subtle changes and lability in mood or behavior (cyclothymia), or milder symptoms of psychomotor activation (hypomania).

Differential Diagnosis

Diagnostic considerations include an acute organic process, particularly substance abuse disorder. Individuals with manic psychosis may resemble those with schizophrenia, but in bipolar disorder the thought disorder should clear with resolution of the mood symptoms, which should also be prominent. Hyperthyroidism should be ruled out. In prepubescent children, mania may be difficult to differentiate from ADHD and other disruptive behavior disorders. Intense and prolonged rages or dysphoria and some periodicity of symptom activity suggest bipolar disorder. Table 6–8 further defines points of differentiation between bipolar disorder, ADHD, and conduct disorder.

Complications

The poor judgment associated with manic episodes predisposes to dangerous, impulsive, and sometimes criminal activity. Affective disorders are associated with a 30-fold greater incidence of successful suicide. Substance abuse may be a further complication, often representing an attempt at self-medication for the mood problem.

Treatment & Prognosis

Most patients with bipolar disorder respond to pharmacotherapy with lithium, carbamazepine, or valproate—either alone or, in severe cases, in combination); supportive psychotherapy; and education about the recurrent nature of the illness.

Fristad MA et al: Bipolar disorder in children and adolescents. Child Adolesc Psychiatr Clin North Am 1992;1:13.
Kafantaris V: Treatment of bipolar disorder in children and adolescence. J Am Acad Child Adolesc Psychiatry 1995;34:732.
Kovacs M, Pollock M: Bipolar disorder and comorbid conduct disorder in childhood and adolescence. J Am Child Adolesc Psychiatry 1995;34:715.
Lewinsohn PM et al: Bipolar disorder in a community sample of older adolescents: Prevalence, phenomenology, comorbidity, and course. J Am Acad Child Adolesc Psychiatry 1995;34:454.
Wozniak J et al: Mania-like symptoms suggestive of childhood onset bipolar disorder in clinically referred children. J Am Acad Child Adolesc Psychiatry 1995;34:867.

CONDUCT DISORDERS

Essentials of Diagnosis & Typical Features

A persistent pattern of behavior that includes the following:

- Defiance of authority.
- Violating the rights of others or of society's norms.
- Aggressive behavior toward persons, animals, or property.

General Considerations

Disorders of conduct affect approximately 9% of males and 2% of females under the age of 18 years. This is a very heterogeneous population, and there is overlap with ADHD, learning and other neuropsychi-

Table 6–8. Differentiating behavior disorders.

	ADHD[1]	Conduct Disorder	Bipolar Disorder
School problems	Yes	Yes	Yes
Behavior problems	Yes	Yes	Yes
Defiant attitude	Occasional	Constant	Episodic
Motor restlessness	Constant	May be present	May wax and wane
Impulsivity	Constant	May be present	May wax and wane
Distractibility	Constant	May be present	May wax and wane
Anger expression	Short-lived (minutes)	Plans revenge	Intense rages (minutes to hours)
Thought content	May be immature	Blames others	Morbid or grandiose ideas
Sleep disturbance	May be present	No	May wax and wane
Self-deprecation	Briefly, with criticism	No	Prolonged, with or without suicidal ideation
Obsessed with ideas	No	No	Yes
Hallucinations	No	No	Diagnostic, if present
Family history	May be a history of school problems	May be a history of antisocial behavior	May be a history of mood disorders

[1]ADHD = attention deficit hyperactivity disorder.

atric disorders, mood disorders, and family dysfunction. Many of these individuals have "difficult temperaments" and come from broken homes where domestic violence, child abuse, drug abuse, shifting parental figures, and poverty are environmental risk factors. Harsh parental discipline with physical punishment appears to lead to more aggressive behavior in children and adolescents. While social learning partly explains this correlation, the genetic heritability of aggressive conduct and antisocial behaviors is currently under investigation.

Clinical Findings

The typical child with conduct disorder is a boy with tempestuous social and academic difficulties. Defiance of authority, fighting, tantrums, running away, school failure, and destruction of property are common symptoms. With increasing age, fire setting and theft may occur, followed in adolescence by truancy, vandalism, and substance abuse. Sexual promiscuity, sexual perpetration, and other frankly criminal behaviors may develop. Hyperactive, aggressive, and uncooperative behavior patterns in the preschool and early school years tend to predict conduct disorder in adolescence with a high degree of accuracy, especially when attention deficit hyperactivity disorder goes untreated. A history of reactive attachment disorder is an additional childhood risk factor. The risk for conduct disorder increases with inconsistent and severe parental disciplinary techniques, parental alcoholism, and parental antisocial behavior.

Differential Diagnosis

Young people with conduct disorders—especially those with more violent histories—have an increased incidence of neurologic signs and symptoms, psychomotor seizures, psychotic symptoms, mood disorders, ADHD, and learning disabilities. Efforts should be made to identify these associated disorders (Table 6–8) since they may suggest specific therapeutic interventions. Conduct disorder is best conceptualized as a final common pathway emerging from a variety of underlying neuropsychiatric conditions.

Treatment

Treatment is difficult and often not very effective. Efforts should be made to stabilize the environment and improve functioning within the home, particularly as it relates to disciplinary techniques. Any associated neurologic, psychiatric, or educational disorders should be treated specifically. In severe cases, residential treatment may be needed—often through the juvenile justice system.

Prognosis

The prognosis is generally poor, especially for children who present with onset before age 10 years; those who display a diversity of antisocial behaviors

across multiple settings; and those who are raised in an environment characterized by parental antisocial behavior, alcoholism, and conflict. Nearly half of such children become antisocial as adults. Antisocial behavior in childhood tends to predict a diagnosable psychiatric disorder in adulthood.

Kazdin AE: *Conduct Disorders in Childhood and Adolescence,* 2nd ed. Sage, 1995.

Weiss B et al: Some consequences of early harsh discipline: Child aggression and a maladaptive social information processing style. Child Dev 1992;63:1321.

ANXIETY DISORDERS

1. ANXIETY-BASED SCHOOL REFUSAL (SCHOOL AVOIDANCE)

Essentials of Diagnosis & Typical Features

- A persistent pattern of school avoidance related to symptoms of anxiety.
- Somatic symptoms on school mornings, with symptoms resolving if the child is allowed to remain at home.
- No organic medical disorder that accounts for the symptoms.
- High levels of parental anxiety are commonly observed.

General Considerations

Anxiety-based school refusal is a persistent behavioral symptom rather than a diagnostic entity. It refers to a pattern of school nonattendance resulting from anxiety, which may be related to a dread of leaving home (separation anxiety), a fear of some aspect of school ("true" school phobia), or a fear of feeling exposed or embarrassed at school (social phobia). In all cases, a realistic cause of the fear (eg, an intimidating teacher or a playground bully) should be ruled out. In most cases, anxiety-based school refusal is the prototype of developmentally inappropriate separation anxiety. The sex incidence is about equal, and there appear to be peaks of incidence at ages 6 and 7 years, again at 10–11 years, and in early adolescence.

Clinical Findings

In the preadolescent years, school refusal often begins after some precipitating stress in the family. The child's anxiety is then manifested either as somatic symptoms or in displacement of anxiety onto some aspect of the school environment. The somatic manifestations of anxiety include dizziness, nausea, and stomach distress. Characteristically, the symptoms become more severe as the time to leave for school approaches and then remit if the child is allowed to remain at home for the day. In older children, the onset is more insidious and often associated with social withdrawal and depression. There is an increased incidence of anxiety and mood disorders in these families.

Differential Diagnosis

The differential diagnosis of school nonattendance is set forth in Table 6–9. Medical disorders that may be causing the somatic symptoms must be ruled out. Children with learning disorders may wish to stay home to avoid the sense of failure they experience at school. Otherwise normal children may also have transient episodes of wanting to stay at home while they struggle with some internal conflict. The onset of school avoidance in mid or late adolescence may herald the onset of schizophrenia or other psychotic disorder. Finally, malingerers or truants are to be differentiated on the basis of their chronic noncompliance with adult authority and their preference for being with peers rather than at home.

Complications

The longer a child remains out of school, the more difficult it is to return and the more strained the relationship between child and parent becomes. Many parents of nonattending children feel tyrannized by their defiant, clinging child. Children often feel accused of "making up" their symptoms, leading to further antagonism between the child, parents, and medical caregivers.

Treatment

The goal of treatment is to help the child confront anxiety and overcome it by returning to school. This requires a strong alliance between the parents and the health care provider. The parent must understand that no underlying medical disorder exists; that the child's symptoms are a manifestation of anxiety; and that the basic problem is anxiety that must be faced to be overcome. Parents must be reminded that being good parents in this case means helping a child to face a distressing experience. Children must be reassured that their symptoms are caused by "worry" and that they will be overcome upon return to school.

A plan for returning the child to school is then developed with parents and school personnel. Firm "insistence" upon full compliance with this plan is essential. The child is brought to school by someone not likely to "give in"—eg, the father or an older sibling. If symptoms develop at school, the child should be checked by the school nurse and then returned to class after a brief rest. The parents must be reassured that school staff will handle the situation at school and that school personnel can reach the primary health care provider if any questions arise.

In cases in which the parents are unable to enter into that kind of treatment contract, in-depth mental health assistance must be provided. For children with very severe symptoms of separation or panic anxiety or major depression, tricyclic antidepressants, SSRIs, or a brief course of a high-potency benzodiazepine (eg, clonazepam) may be an important adjunct to the behavioral treatment.

Prognosis

Although the vast majority of preadolescent children can be returned to school, long-term outcomes are not uniformly favorable. A history of school refusal is more frequent in adults with "neuroticism," panic anxiety, and agoraphobia than in the general population.

Bell-Dolan D, Brazeal T: Separation anxiety disorder, overanxious disorder, and school refusal. Child Adolesc Psychiatr Clin North Am 1993;2:563.

Berg I: Absence from school and mental health. Br J Psychiatry 1992;161:154.

Kutcher S et al: Pharmacotherapy: Approaches and applications. In: *Anxiety Disorders in Children and Adolescents.* March JS (editor). Guilford, 1995.

Table 6–9. Differential diagnosis of school nonattendance.[1]

I. **Emotional or anxiety-based refusal[2]**
  A. Separation anxiety disorder (50–80% of anxious refusers)
  B. Generalization anxiety disorder
  C. Mood/depressive disorder (with or without combined anxiety)
  D. Social phobia
  E. Specific phobia
  F. Panic disorder
  G. Psychosis ("voices" say not to attend)
II. **Truancy[3] behavior disorders**
  A. Oppositional defiant disorder, conduct disorder
  B. Substance abuse disorders
III. **"Realistic" school refusal**
  A. Learning disability, unaddressed or undetected
  B. Marauding students (including gangs)
  C. Psychologically abusive teacher
  D. Family-sanctioned nonattendance
    1. For companionship
    2. For child care
    3. To care for the parent (role-reversal)
    4. To supplement family income
  E. Socioculturally sanctioned nonattendance (school is not valued)
  F. Homosexual attraction, gender concerns
IV. **Undiagnosed medical condition (including pregnancy)**

[1]Medically unexplained absence of more than 2 weeks.
[2]Subjectively distressed child who generally stays at home.
[3]Nonsubjectively distressed and not at home.

2. THE OVERLY ANXIOUS CHILD

Transient developmental fears are common in early childhood. Therefore, the person evaluating the

Table 6–10. Signs and symptoms of anxiety in children.

Direct manifestations of anxiety
  Psychologic manifestations:
    Fears and worries
    Uneasiness and apprehension
    Frightening themes in play and fantasy
  Psychomotor manifestations:
    Motoric restlessness and hyperactivity
    Sleep disturbances
    Decreased concentration
  Psychophysiologic manifestations:
    Autonomic hyperarousal
    Dizziness and lightheadedness
    Palpitations
    Shortness of breath
    Flushing, sweating, dry mouth
    Nausea and vomiting
    Panic
    Headaches and stomachaches
Indirect manifestations of anxiety
  Increased dependence on home and parents
  Avoidance of anxiety-producing stimuli
  Decreased school performance
  Increased self-doubt and irritability
  Ritualistic behaviors (eg, washing, counting)

Table 6–11. Anxiety disorders in children and adolescents.

Disorder	Major Clinical Manifestations
Separation anxiety disorder	Developmentally inappropriate wish to maintain proximity with caretakers; morbid worry of threats to family integrity or integrity of self upon separation; intense homesickness
Generalized anxiety disorder	Intense, disproportionate or irrational worry, often about future events
Social phobia	Painful shyness or self-consciousness; fear of humiliation with public scrutiny
Specific phobia	Avoidance of specific feared stimuli
Panic disorder	Unprovoked, intense fear with sympathetic hyperarousal, and often palpitations or hyper-ventilation
Posttraumatic stress disorder	Fear of a recurrence of an intense, anxiety-provoking traumatic experience, causing sympathetic hyperarousal, avoidance or reminders, and the reexperiencing of aspects of the traumatic event

clinical significance of anxiety symptoms in children must consider the age of the child, the developmental fears that can normally be expected at that age, the form of the symptoms and their duration, and the degree to which the symptoms disrupt the child's life.

Anxiety can be manifested either directly or indirectly as shown in Table 6–10. The characteristics of anxiety in childhood are listed in Table 6–11. Community-based studies of school-age children and adolescents suggest that nearly 10% of children have some type of anxiety disorder. The differential diagnosis of symptoms of anxiety is presented in Table 6–12.

The child's family and school environment should be evaluated for marital discord, family violence, harsh or inappropriate disciplinary methods, and emotional overstimulation. The child's experience of anxiety and its relationship to life events are explored, and the child is taught specific cognitive and behavioral techniques needed to confront the anxiety. Finally, when severe separation or panic anxiety appears to play a prominent role or when the child has persistent obsessive-compulsive disorder, psychopharmacologic agents may be helpful. Selective serotonin reuptake inhibitors may be helpful across a broad spectrum of anxiety symptoms. The long-term prognosis for these disorders is largely unknown; however, there appears to be continuity between high levels of childhood anxiety and anxiety disorders in adulthood.

Bernstein GA, Borchardt CM, Perwien AR: Anxiety disorders in children and adolescents: A review of the past 10

Table 6–12. Differential diagnosis of symptoms of anxiety.

I. **Normal developmental anxiety**
   A. Stranger anxiety (5 months to 2½ years, with a peak at 6–12 months)
   B. Separation anxiety (7 months to 4 years, with a peak at 18–36 months)
   C. The child is fearful or even phobic of the dark and monsters (3–6 years)
II. **"Appropriate" anxiety**
   A. Anticipating a painful or frightening experience
   B. Avoidance of a reminder of a painful or frightening experience
   C. Child abuse
III. **Anxiety disorder (see Table 6–11), with or without other comorbid psychiatric disorders**
IV. **Substance abuse**
V. **Medications and recreational drugs**
   A. Caffeinism (including colas and chocolate)
   B. Sympathomimetic agents
   C. Idiosyncratic drug reactions
VI. **Hypermetabolic or hyperarousal states**
   A. Hyperthyroidism
   B. Pheochromocytoma
   C. Anemia
   D. Hypoglycemia
   E. Hypoxemia
VII. **Cardiac abnormality**
   A. Dysrhythmia
   B. High-output state
   C. Mitral valve prolapse

years. J Am Acad Child Adolesc Psychiatry 1996;35:1110.

Birmaher B et al: Fluoxetine for childhood anxiety disorders. J Am Acad Child Adolesc Psychiatry 1994;33:993.

March JS (editor): *Anxiety Disorders in Children and Adolescents.* Guilford, 1995.

March JS, Leonard HL: Obsessive-compulsive disorder in children and adolescents: A review of the past 10 years. J Am Acad Child Adolesc Psychiatry 1996; 34:1265.

Popper CW: Psychopharmacologic treatment of anxiety disorders in adolescents and children. J Clin Psychiatry 1993;54(Suppl):52.

3. POSTTRAUMATIC STRESS DISORDER

Essentials of Diagnosis & Typical Features

- Signs and symptoms of autonomic hyperarousal.
- Avoidant behaviors and numbing of responsiveness.
- Flashbacks to a traumatic event, or other symptoms of "recurrence."
- All of the above following the experience of traumatic events such as natural disasters, unexpected personal tragedies, and ongoing interpersonal violence.

General Considerations

Long-overdue attention is now being paid to the horrific effects of family and community violence on the psychologic development of children and adolescents. About 40% of urban adolescents report having experienced or witnessed frightening violent events. As many as 25% of young people exposed to violence develop symptoms of posttraumatic stress.

Clinical Findings

Children who have been psychologically traumatized show persistent evidence of fear and anxiety and are hypervigilant to the possibility of repetition. They regress developmentally and experience fears of strangers, of the dark, and of being alone, and avoid reminders of the traumatic event.

Children also frequently reexperience elements of the events in dreams and flashbacks. In their symbolic play, one can often notice a monotonous repetition of some aspect of the traumatic event.

Treatment

The cornerstone of treatment for posttraumatic stress disorder is education of the child and family regarding the nature of posttraumatic stress disorder so that the child's emotional reactions and regressive behavior are not mistakenly viewed as "crazy" or "manipulative." Support, reassurance, repeated explanations, and understanding are needed. Specific fears will wane with time, and behavioral desensitization may help. A supportive relationship with a caregiving adult is essential. For children with more severe symptoms, a variety of psychoactive medications, including mood stabilizers, clonidine, propranolol, and antidepressants (singly or in combination), can be helpful.

Prognosis

Children who have experienced psychic trauma often harbor emotional scars. At 4- to 5-year follow-up investigations, many children continue to have vivid and frightening memories and dreams and a pessimistic view of the future. Evidence is growing to support a connection between victimization in childhood and unstable personality and mood disorders in later life.

Amaya-Jackson L, March JS: Posttraumatic stress disorder. In: *Anxiety Disorders in Children and Adolescents.* March JS (editor). Guilford, 1995.

Pynoos RS: Traumatic stress and developmental psychopathology in children and adolescents. Rev Psychiatry 1993;12:205.

Singer MI et al: Adolescents' exposure to violence and associated symptoms of psychological trauma. JAMA 1995;273:477.

Terr LC: Childhood trauma: An outline and review. Am J Psychiatry 1991;148:10.

SOMATOFORM DISORDERS

Essentials of Diagnosis & Typical Features

- A symptom suggesting physical dysfunction.
- No physical disorder accounting for the symptom.
- Symptoms causing distress, dysfunction, or both.
- Symptoms not voluntarily created or maintained, as in malingering.

Clinical Findings

Somatoform disorders suggest the presence of physical illness or disability for which no organic cause can be ascertained, though neither the patient nor the caregiver is consciously fabricating the symptoms. The category includes conversion disorder, hypochondriasis, somatization disorder, somatoform pain disorder, and body dysmorphic disorder (see Table 6–13).

Conversion symptoms most frequently occur in school-age children and adolescents. The exact incidence is unclear, but in pediatric practice they are probably more often seen as transient symptoms rather than as chronic disorders requiring help from mental health practitioners. A conversion symptom is thought to be an expression of underlying psychologic conflict. The specific symptom may be "symbolically determined" by the underlying conflict. Furthermore, the symptom may "resolve" the dilemma created by the underlying wish or fear (eg, a "paralyzed" child need not fear expressing his underlying rage or aggressive retaliatory impulses). Al-

Table 6–13. Somatoform disorders in children and adolescents.

Disorder	Major Clinical Manifestations
Conversion disorder	Symptom onset follows psychologically stressful event; symptoms express unconscious feelings and result in secondary gain
Hypochondriasis	Preoccupation with worry that physical symptoms manifest unrecognized and threatening condition; medical assurance does not provide relief from worry
Somatization disorder	Long standing preoccupation with multiple somatic symptoms
Somatoform pain disorder	Preoccupation with pain that results in distress or impairment beyond what would be expected from physical findings
Body dysmorphic disorder	Preoccupation with an imagined defect in personal appearance

though children can present with a variety of symptoms, many presentations initially suggest a disorder of neurologic or sensory origin. Children with conversion disorder may be surprisingly unconcerned about the substantial "disability" deriving from their symptoms. Symptoms include unusual sensory phenomena, paralysis, and movement or seizure-like disorders.

In the classic case of conversion disorder, the child's symptom complex and examination are not consistent with the clinical manifestations of any organic disease process. In addition, the symptoms frequently begin as an intercurrent illness within the context of a family experiencing stress, such as serious illness, a death, or family discord. On closer examination, the child's symptoms are often found to resemble symptoms present in other family members. Children with conversion symptoms often have some secondary gain associated with their symptoms.

A number of reports have pointed to the increased association of conversion symptoms with sexual overstimulation or sexual abuse. Health care providers should always keep that possibility in mind.

Differential Diagnosis

It is sometimes not possible to be sure that the symptoms are not due to disease. Follow-up observation is required to see whether further symptoms evolve.

Somatic symptoms can be prominent in children with anxiety and depressive disorders (Table 6–13). The child's mood state and associated symptoms of avoidance are helpful in determining whether such disorders are present. Occasionally, psychotic children present with somatic preoccupations and even somatic delusions.

Treatment & Prognosis

In most cases, conversion symptoms resolve quickly when the child and family are reassured that the symptom is a way of reacting to stress. The child is encouraged to continue with normal daily activities, knowing that the symptom will abate when the stress is resolved.

If the symptom does not resolve with reassurance, further investigation by a mental health professional is indicated. When the more chronic somatoform disorders evolve in children and adolescents, treatment with psychopharmacologic agents may be helpful.

Hollander E: Pharmacologic treatment of obsessive-compulsive spectrum disorders. Psychiatr Times 1993;10:36.

Nemzer ED: Somatoform disorders. In: *Child and Adolescent Psychiatry: A Comprehensive Textbook.* Lewis M (editor). Williams & Wilkins, 1991.

ADJUSTMENT DISORDERS

The most frequent and most disturbing stresses for children and adolescents are marital discord or dissolution, family illness, the loss of a loved one, or a change of residence.

When faced with stress, children can manifest many different symptoms, including changes in mood, changes in behavior, anxiety symptoms, and physical complaints. Key findings include the following: (1) the precipitating event or circumstance is identifiable; (2) the symptoms have appeared within 3 months after the occurrence of the stressful event; (3) although the child experiences distress or some functional impairment, the reaction is not severe or disabling; and (4) the reaction does not persist more than 6 months after the stressor has terminated. The range of symptoms of patients with adjustment disorders are listed in Table 6–14.

Differential Diagnosis

When symptoms are a reaction to an identifiable stressor but are severe, persistent, or disabling, de-

Table 6–14. Signs and symptoms of adjustment reactions.

Irritable, angry mood
Anxious, worried mood
Unhappy, depressed mood
Angry resistance to authority
Fatigue
Aches and pains
Decreased school performance
Social withdrawal
Any combination of the above

pressive disorder, anxiety disorder, and conduct disorders must be considered.

Treatment

The mainstay of treatment is the doctor's assurance that the emotional or behavioral change is a predictable consequence of the stressful event. This validates the child's reaction and encourages the child to talk about the stressful occurrence and its aftermath. Parents are asked to understand the child's reaction and encourage appropriate verbal expression of feelings, while also defining boundaries for behavior that prevent the child from feeling out of control.

Prognosis

The duration of symptoms in adjustment reactions depends on the severity of the stress, the child's personal sensitivity to stress and vulnerability to anxiety, depression, and other psychiatric disorders, and the available support system.

Tomb DA: Adjustment disorder. In: *Child and Adolescent Psychiatry: A Comprehensive Textbook.* Lewis M (editor). Williams & Wilkins, 1991.

ELIMINATION DISORDERS

1. ENURESIS

Essentials of Diagnosis & Typical Features

- Urinary incontinence in a child 5 years of age (or developmental equivalent) or older.
- No medication or general medical condition causing the urinary incontinence.

General Considerations

Enuresis is the passage of urine into bedclothes or undergarments, whether involuntary or intentional. At least 90% of enuretic children have primary nocturnal enuresis—ie, they wet only at night during sleep and have never had a sustained period of dryness. Diurnal enuresis (daytime wetting) is much less common, as is secondary enuresis, which develops after a child has had a sustained period of bladder control. The latter two varieties are much more frequently associated with emotional stress, anxiety, and psychiatric disorders. Primary nocturnal enuresis is most often a parasomnia, a deep-sleep (stage III or stage 4) event. Etiologically, it is generally viewed as a developmental disorder or maturational lag that children will outgrow. Only infrequently is it associated with a serious psychopathologic disorder.

Clinical Findings

Primary nocturnal enuresis is common (Table 6–15). The incidence is three times higher in boys than in girls. Most children with enuresis become

Table 6–15. Incidence of enuresis in children.

Age (years)	Primary Nocturnal Enuresis (%)	Occasional Daytime Enuresis (%)
5	15	8
7–8	7	—
10	3–5	—
12	2–3	1
14	1	—

continent by adolescence or earlier. The family history in such cases frequently reveals other members—especially fathers—who have had prolonged nighttime bed-wetting problems.

Although the cause of primary nocturnal enuresis is not established, it appears to be related to maturational delay of sleep and arousal mechanisms or to delay in development of increased bladder capacity.

Daytime wetting most often occurs in timid and shy children or in children with attention deficit disorder. It occurs with about equal frequency in boys and girls, and 60–80% of daytime wetters also wet at night.

Secondary enuresis typically follows a stressful event, such as the birth of a sibling, a loss, or discord within the family. The symptom can be seen as the result of regression in response to stress or as a more symbolic expression of the child's feelings.

Differential Diagnosis

The differential diagnosis includes urinary tract infections, neurologic diseases, seizure disorders, diabetes mellitus, and structural abnormalities of the urinary tract. Urinalysis and urine culture and observing the child's urinary stream can rule out the majority of organic causes of enuresis. Daytime wetting can occur in children with "difficult" temperaments or overt depression.

Complications

The most common complication of enuresis is low self-esteem in response to criticism from caregivers.

Treatment

Treatment should emphasize that the symptom is a developmental lag and will be outgrown even without treatment. If the child chooses to pursue treatment in any case, a program of bladder exercises can be prescribed: holding urine as long as possible during the day and then starting and stopping the stream at the toilet bowl. The child is instructed also to practice getting up from bed and going to the bathroom at bedtime before sleep. The child lies down, counts to 50, gets up, goes to the bathroom, and tries to urinate, and repeats this procedure 10–20 times each night. These procedures are helpful in perhaps 30–40% of children with nighttime wetting. For the remainder, an alerting buzzer that sounds early in the bed-wetting process is helpful for about 70% of children. The child is instructed to get up and go to the bathroom and finish emptying the bladder if the alarm goes off.

For others, a trial of imipramine is worthwhile at dosages of 25–50 mg at bedtime for children under 12 years of age and 50–75 mg for older children. Because many patients relapse once the drug is stopped, its primary use is for camp or overnight visits. Desmopressin acetate, 20–40 μg intranasally at bedtime, can result in complete remission of nocturnal enuresis in 50% of children as long as they continue the treatment.

Mental health treatment is more often needed for children with daytime wetting or secondary enuresis. The focus is on the verbal expression of feelings that may be associated with perpetuation of the symptom.

Howe AC, Walker CE: Behavioral management of toilet training, enuresis, and encopresis. Pediatr Clin North Am 1992;39:413.

Reiner WG: Enuresis in child psychiatric practice. Child Adolesc Psychiatr Clin North Am 1995;4:453.

2. ENCOPRESIS

Essentials of Diagnosis & Typical Features

- Fecal incontinence in a child 4 years of age (or developmental equivalent) or older.
- Not due to medication or medical disorder.

General Considerations

Functional encopresis is defined as the repeated passage of feces in inappropriate places in a child of at least the developmental equivalent of 4 years of age. It may be either involuntary or intentional, though most often it is involuntary. It affects approximately 1–1.5% of school-age children—boys four times as commonly as girls. Functional fecal incontinence is rare in adolescence.

Clinical Findings

Functional encopresis can be divided into four types: retentive, continuous, discontinuous, and "toilet phobia."

In **retentive encopresis**—also called psychogenic megacolon—the child withholds bowel movements, leading to the development of constipation, fecal impaction, and the seepage of soft or liquid feces around the margins of the impaction into the underclothing. Marked constipation and painful defecation often contribute to a vicious circle of withholding → larger impaction → further seepage. These children

often have a history of crossing their legs to resist the urge to defecate and of infrequent bowel movements large enough to stop up the toilet, and they are found on examination to have large fecal masses in their rectal vaults. Most of these children are distressed by the soiling that occurs.

Children with **continuous encopresis** have never gained primary control of bowel function. The bowel movement is usually randomly deposited in underclothing without regard to social norms. Typically, the family structure does not encourage organization and skill training, and for that reason the child has never had adequate bowel training. These children and their parents are more apt to be socially or intellectually disadvantaged.

Children with **discontinuous encopresis** have a history of normal bowel control for an extended period. Loss of control often occurs in response to a stressful event, such as the birth of a sibling, a separation, family illness, or marital disharmony. These children then begin to put feces in "irritating places" as an expression of anger or of a wish to be perceived as younger. They typically display relative indifference to the symptom.

In the infrequent case of **"toilet phobia,"** a young child views the toilet as a frightening structure to be avoided. These children may view the bowel movement as an extension of themselves, which is then swept away in a frightening manner. They may think that they, too, may be swept away "down the toilet."

Differential Diagnosis

Differential diagnosis includes the medical causes of constipation and retentive encopresis. Hirschsprung's disease can be ruled out with reasonable certainty by the history of passing large-caliber bowel movements in the past and by the presence of palpable stool in the rectal vault. Neurologic disorders, hypothyroidism, hypercalcemia, and diseases of smooth muscle must be considered as well. The child should be examined for anal fissures, which tend to encourage the withholding of bowel movement.

In addition, fecal soiling can be a presenting symptom in childhood depression and is sometimes a concomitant finding in children with attention deficit hyperactivity disorder. When fecal smearing is present, an underlying psychotic disorder should be considered.

Treatment

Identifying the type of encopresis is important in treatment planning. Another important variable is the child's own concern about the symptom. Children who display denial or indifference are much harder to treat. Children with coexisting depression or ADHD need to be treated for those conditions before focusing treatment on soiling.

With the most common type of encopresis—the retentive type—efforts are made to soften stool so that constipation and painful defecation do not perpetuate the behavior. These children are then taught to adopt a regular schedule of postprandial sessions on the toilet. A system of positive reinforcement can be added in which the child is rewarded for each day with no soiled underclothes. The responsibility for rinsing soiled clothing and depositing it in the appropriate receptacle rests with the child. In the case of continuous fecal soiling, the family is taught to train the child. For toilet phobia, a progressive series of rewarded desensitization steps is necessary. Children with discontinuous soiling that persists over a number of weeks often need psychotherapy to help them recognize and express their anger and wish to be dependent verbally rather than through fecal soiling.

Prognosis

While the ultimate prognosis is excellent, parental distress and parent–child conflict may be great prior to the cessation of symptoms. The natural history of soiling is that it resolves by adolescence in all but the most severely disturbed teenagers.

Howe AC, Walker CE: Behavioral management of toilet training, enuresis, and encopresis. Pediatr Clin North Am 1992;39:413.

Mikkelson EJ: Modern approaches to enuresis and encopresis. In: *Child and Adolescent Psychiatry: A Comprehensive Textbook.* Lewis M (editor). Williams & Wilkins, 1991.

SUICIDE IN CHILDREN & ADOLESCENTS

Suicide has become the third leading cause of death among United States inhabitants 15–24 years of age. The suicide rate among adolescents 15–19 years of age quadrupled—from approximately 2.7 to 11.3 per 100,000—over the last 40 years. For children 14 years of age and younger, the rate of completed suicide is low but increased by 120%—from 0.8 to 1.7 per 100,000—from 1980 to 1992.

Adolescent girls make three to four times as many suicide attempts as boys of the same age, but the number of completed suicides is three to four times greater in boys. Firearms are the most commonly used method in successful suicides, accounting for 40–60% of cases; hanging, carbon monoxide poisoning, and drug overdoses each account for approximately 10–15%. Each year, approximately 25% of high school students seriously consider suicide; 15% make a plan; 8% make some type of attempt; and 2% come to medical attention because of a suicide attempt.

Suicide is associated with psychopathologic disorder and should not be viewed as a philosophic choice about life or death or as a predictable response to overwhelming stress. Most commonly it is an angry, impulsive, and retaliatory act of aggression in an individual with a long history of behavior disorder and academic difficulties. Other suicide victims are high achievers who are temperamentally anxious and "high-strung" and who commit suicide impulsively after a failure or rejection, either real or only perceived. Mood disorders (in both sexes, but especially in females), substance abuse disorders (especially in males), and conduct disorders are commonly diagnosed at psychologic autopsy in adolescent suicide victims. Some adolescent suicides reflect an underlying psychotic disorder, with the young person usually committing suicide in response to an auditory hallucinatory command to do so.

The vast majority of young people who commit suicide give some clue to their distress or their tentative plans to commit suicide. Most show signs of dysphoric mood (anger, irritability, anxiety, or depression). Over 60% make comments such as "I wish I were dead" or "I just can't deal with this any longer" within the 24 hours prior to death. In one study, nearly 70% of subjects experienced a crisis event such as a loss (eg, rejection by girlfriend), a failure, or an arrest prior to completed suicide.

Assessment of Suicide Risk

Assessment of suicide risk calls for a high index of suspicion and a direct interview with the patient and significant others such as family members, peers, and teachers. A format for the interview is provided in Table 6–16.

The highest risk of suicide is among older white adolescent boys who express an intention to die, especially when away from other family members. High-risk factors include previous suicide attempts, a suicide note, a viable plan for suicide with the availability of lethal means, close personal exposure to suicide, conduct disorder, and substance abuse. Similar clues are signs and symptoms of major depression or dysthymia, a family history of suicide, a recent death in the family, and a view of death as a relief from the pain in their lives. Persons who have little or no family support, are facing a crisis in their lives at work or school, or refuse to agree not to commit suicide are also at high risk.

Principles of Intervention

Any suicide attempt must be considered a serious matter. The patient should not be left alone, and one should show understanding of the young person's pain and convey a desire to help. The physician should meet with the patient and the family, both alone and together, and listen carefully to their problems and perceptions. It should be made clear that

Table 6–16. Clinical interview to assess suicide risk.

1. An observation or change has been noted.
2. How have you been feeling (inside, emotionally)?
3. Have you had periods of feeling down or discouraged?
   a. How often?
   b. How long?
   c. How severe?
4. Do they interfere with your life?
   a. Daily activities?
   b. School or work?
   c. Sleep or appetite? Both?
   d. Family life?
5. Do you have feelings of–
   a. Self-criticism or worthlessness?
   b. Helplessness?
   c. Hopelessness?
   d. Wanting to give up?
6. Are the feelings ever so strong that life does not seem worth living? Have you had thoughts of suicide?
   a. Are you having thoughts of suicide now?
   b. How persistent are they?
   c. How much effort does it take to resist?
   d. Can you tolerate the pain you are feeling?
7. Have you made any plans to carry out suicide?
   a. What are the plans?
   b. Have you taken any tentative action (eg, obtaining a gun or rope, stockpiling pills)?
   c. As you have thought about suicide, how have you viewed the idea of death?
8. What deters you from trying suicide?
9. If the suicidal feelings are subsiding, could you resist the feelings if they returned?
10. Is there someone you can turn to for help at those times? Who?
11. Has the idea of suicide come up in the past?
    a. How often?
    b. When and under what circumstances?
    c. What has happened at those times?
12. Can you tolerate the pain that you are feeling right now?

with the assistance of mental health professionals, solutions can be found.

These patients should be hospitalized if there appears to be a high potential for suicide, if they are severely depressed or intoxicated, if the family does not appear appropriately concerned, or if there are practical limitations on providing supervision and support or to the ability to ensure safety.

Any decision to send the patient home without hospitalization should be made only after consultation with a mental health expert. The decision should rest on a perceived lessening of the risk of suicide and assurance of the family's ability to provide 24-hour supervision. The patient's home must be "sterilized" of guns, pills, knives, and razor blades, and the patient should be restricted from driving for at least the first 24 hours. The focus is on providing support and easing the emotional strain. Phone contact must be available, and the family must be committed to a plan for mental health treatment.

Finally, the physician should be aware of his or her own emotional reactions to dealing with potentially suicidal adolescents and their families. Because the assessment takes considerable time and energy, the physician should be on guard against becoming tired, irritable, or angry. The parents should not be blamed. The physician need not be afraid of precipitating suicide by direct and frank discussions of suicidal risk.

Gould MS et al: Psychosocial risk factors of child and adolescent completed suicide. Am J Psychiatry 1996;53:1155.

Hendin H: Psychodynamics of suicide, with particular reference to the young. Am J Psychiatry 1991;148:1150.

Rotheram MJ: Evaluation of imminent danger for suicide among youth. Am J Orthopsychiatry 1987;57:102.

Shaffer D et al: Psychiatric diagnosis in child and adolescent suicide. Arch Gen Psychiatry 1996;53:3398.

Suicide among children, adolescents, and young adults: United States, 1980–1992. (Editorial.) JAMA 1995;274:451.

THE CHRONICALLY ILL CHILD

Reactions to Chronic Illness or Disability

Five to 10 percent of individuals experience a prolonged period of illness or disability during childhood, and the psychosocial effects for the child and the family are often profound. Although the specific impact of illness on children and their families depends on the characteristics of the illness, the age of the child, and premorbid functioning, it can be expected that both the child and the parents will go through predictable stages toward eventual acceptance of the disease state. Shock and disbelief at the time of diagnosis give way in time to anger and to mourning the loss of the normal, healthy child. It may take months for a family to accept the disease, to cope with the stresses, and to resume normal life to the extent possible. These stages resemble those that follow the loss of a loved one. If anxiety and guilt remain prominent within the family, a pattern of overprotection can evolve. Likewise, when the illness is not accepted as a reality to be dealt with, a pattern of denial may become prominent. The clinical manifestations of these patterns of behavior are set forth in Table 6–17.

Assistance From Health Care Providers

A. Educate the Patient and Family: Children and their families should be given information about the illness, including its course and treatment, at frequent intervals. Factual, open discussions minimize

Table 6–17. Patterns of coping with chronic illness.

Overprotection
  Persistent anxiety or guilt
  Few friends and peer activities
  Poor school attendance
  Overconcern with somatic symptoms
  Secondary gain from the illness
Effective coping
  Realistic acceptance of limits imposed by illness
  Normalization of daily activities with peers, play, and school
Denial
  Lack of acceptance of the illness
  Poor medical compliance
  Risk-taking behaviors
  Lack of parental follow-through with medical instructions
  General pattern of acting-out behavior

anxieties. The explanation should be comprehensible to all, and time should be set aside for questions and answers. The setting can be created with the invitation, "Let's take some time together to review the situation again."

B. Prepare the Child for Changes and Procedures: The physician should explain what can be expected with a new turn in the illness or with upcoming medical procedures. This explanation enables the child to anticipate and in turn to master the new development and promotes trust between the patient and the health care providers.

C. Encourage Normal Activities: The child should attend school and play with peers as much as the illness allows. At the same time, parents should be encouraged to apply the same rules of discipline and behavior to the ill child as are applied to well siblings.

D. Encourage Compensatory Activities, Interests, and Skill Development: For example, a child whose athletic development has been interrupted by the disability might pursue the acquisition of computer skills.

E. Promote Self-Reliance: The health care provider should guide and encourage parents in helping ill children assume responsibility for some aspects of their medical care.

F. Periodically Review Family Coping: From time to time, the physician should ask, "How is everyone doing with this?" The feelings of the patient, the parents, and other children in the family are explored, as well as concerns about finances and the status of the marriage. Feelings of fear, guilt, anger, and grief should be watched for and accepted as normal reactions to difficult circumstances.

G. Recommend Support Groups: Lay support groups for the patient and family should be used to the fullest extent.

Long-Term Coping

The process of coping with a chronic illness is an ongoing one. Each change in the course of the illness and each new developmental stage for the child presents new challenges. With each step comes the need for new and painful acceptance of the disease and its limitations.

Lavigne JV, Faier-Routman J: Psychological adjustment to pediatric physical disorders: A meta-analytic review. J Pediatr Psychol 1992;17:133.
McGrath PJ, McAlpine L: Psychological perspectives on pediatric pain. J Pediatr 1993;122(Suppl):2.

THE TERMINALLY ILL CHILD

The diagnosis of fatal illness in a child is a severe blow even to families who have reason to suspect that outcome. Most parents accept the news of a fatal illness as the worst experience of their lives, and although parents want and need to know the truth, they are best told in piecemeal fashion beginning with temporizing phrases such as, "The news is not good—it's a life-threatening illness." The parents' reactions and questions can then be scrutinized for clues to how much they want to be told at any one time. Parents' reactions then proceed in a grief sequence including initial shock and disbelief lasting days to weeks, followed by anger, despair, and guilt over weeks to months, and ending in acceptance of the loss.

Although children probably do not fully understand the permanency of death until about 8 years of age, most ill children experience a sense of danger and doom that is associated with death before that age. Even so, the question of whether to tell a child about the fatal nature of a disease should in most cases be answered in the affirmative unless the parents object. Refusal of the adults to tell the child—especially when the adults themselves are very sad—leads to a "conspiracy of silence" that increases fear of the unknown in the child and leads to feelings of loneliness and isolation at the time of greatest need. In fact, children who are able to discuss their illness with family members are less depressed, have fewer behavior problems, have higher self-esteem, feel closer to their families, and adapt better to the rigors of their disease and its treatment.

Children are very observant and intuitive when it comes to understanding their illness and its general prognosis. At the same time, their primary concerns are the effects of the illness on everyday life, feeling sick, and limitations on normal activities. Children are also keenly aware of the family's reactions and are reluctant to bring up issues they know are upsetting to their parents. Whenever possible, parents should be encouraged to discuss the child's illness and to answer questions openly and honestly, including exploration of the child's fears and fantasies. Such interactions promote closeness and relieve the child's sense of isolation. Even with these active attempts to promote effective sharing between the child and the family, ill children frequently experience fear, anxiety, irritability, and anger over their illness and guilt over causing family distress. Sleep disturbances, tears, and clinging, dependent behavior are not infrequent or abnormal.

The siblings of dying children are also affected by the stress imposed on the family. They feel neglected and deprived because of the time their parents must spend with the sick child. Anger and jealousy then give rise to feelings of guilt over having such "bad" feelings about their sick sibling.

After the child dies, the period of bereavement may last up to 3 years. Family members may need outside help in dealing with their grief through supportive counseling services.

Grollman EA: *Talking About Death: A Dialogue Between Parent and Child.* Beacon, 1990.
Leach P: Will I die? Parenting 1993 (April):105.

EFFECTS OF MARITAL DISSOLUTION

Currently, about 40% of marriages will end in dissolution. Seventy-five percent of divorced parents remarry, and another 50% divorce a second time. Approximately 90% of single parents are mothers, and in about half of such cases the children have little or no contact with the father.

Clinical Effects of Marital Dissolution

The adverse emotional effects of divorce are far-reaching for both adults and children. Many women who have been through a divorce report that it takes 3 years for a sense of order and stability to return.

Effects on the parent–child relationship include a decrease in parenting capacity manifested by irregularity of schedules, flares of temper, lessening of emotional sensitivity and support of the child, inconsistent discipline, and decreased pleasure in the parent-child relationship. A tendency exists for the divorced parent to look to the child as a source of emotional support or even as a "surrogate spouse." Younger children become inappropriately close to their parents by acting as "little helpers" and parental advisors. Adolescents, on the other hand, may rebel in order to distance themselves from the emotional needs of their distressed parents.

The effects of divorce on children are seen most dramatically in the 2 years following dissolution of the marriage. Few children experience the dissolution of even turbulent marriages as a relief, because the breakup of the nuclear family is perceived as a loss of the structure that provides for their safety and support. Children would rarely choose divorce as a solution for their parents' problems.

The effects of divorce on children vary with the child's age and developmental level. Most preschoolers display symptoms of behavioral regression, expressing fears of separation at night and when they are with babysitters, sleep disturbances, and irritability. Children aged 5–8 express their grief with sadness and weeping. These children are heartbroken and wish for reconciliation of the parents. Approximately 50% experience a decrease in school performance. Children aged 9–12 respond with anger and blame and are at greatest risk of becoming a surrogate companion. In adolescence, anger is accompanied by depression. Teenagers become pessimistic about their own future involvement in intimate relationships.

Outcome

The most favorable outcome is for the parents to put aside old conflicts and resume caregiving relationships with their children in a collaborative manner. Children cannot develop in a setting of unremitting marital strife. Younger children actually fare best, particularly when they have a support network (eg, siblings, grandparents) while the parents are preoccupied with their own problems.

At 5-year follow-up, nearly 33% of children of divorced parents are moderately depressed. At 10-year follow-up, 40% of such children report worry, underachievement, self-deprecation, and lingering anger. Upon reaching adulthood, most survivors of divorce fear repeating their parents' unhappy marriages. In short, the impact of divorce upon children may be far-reaching in scope and long-term in duration.

Wallerstein JS: The long-term effects of divorce on children: A review. J Am Acad Child Adolesc Psychiatry 1991;30:349.

OVERVIEW OF PEDIATRIC PSYCHOPHARMACOLOGY

As with any medication, the risks as well as the benefits of administering psychoactive medications must be discussed with the child's guardian. Drug therapy is warranted only if the disorder is interfering with psychosocial development, interpersonal relationships, daily functioning, or the patient's sense of personal well-being. Informed consent should be given by the guardian and noted in the record. Psychopharmacologic agents are seldom the only treatment for a psychiatric disorder—most often they are best used adjunctively along with other therapeutic interventions.

A good rule when considering the use of psychoactive medications in children and adolescents is first to identify target symptoms that can be followed to evaluate the efficacy of treatment. When initiating treatment, start with low doses and increase slowly in divided doses, monitoring for side effects along with therapeutic effects. When drugs are discontinued, dosages should be tapered over 2–4 weeks in order to minimize withdrawal effects. When multiple choices of drug exist, one should select the medication with the fewest and least ominous risks and side effects. Polypharmacy should be avoided by choosing one drug that might ameliorate most or all of the target symptoms before considering the simultaneous administration of two or more agents.

Table 6–18 presents an overview of the clinical conditions for which psychopharmacologic agents might be considered. In the column of "probable" indications are listed agents whose efficacy has been established in controlled drug trials or after substantial clinical experience. The column of "possible" indications lists agents for which uncontrolled preliminary clinical investigations have suggested some therapeutic efficacy.

In the text that follows, the major classes of psychopharmacologic agents with probable clinical indications in child and adolescent psychiatry are represented. The more commonly prescribed drugs from each class are reviewed with reference to indications, relative contraindications, initial medical screening procedures (in addition to a general pediatric examination), dosage, adverse effects, drug interactions, and medical follow-up recommendations.

PSYCHOSTIMULANTS

Psychostimulants are the drugs of first choice for treating ADHD in children and adolescents. Approximately 75% of ADHD children exhibit improved attention span, decreased hyperactivity, and decreased impulsivity when given stimulant medications. Up to 75% of children with ADHD who do not respond favorably to one stimulant will respond to another. ADHD children and adolescents without prominent

Table 6–18. Indications for psychopharmacologic interventions in children and adolescents.

Condition	Probable	Possible
Attention deficit hyperactivity disorder	Psychostimulants, tricyclics, clonidine, bupropion	Neuroleptics, guanfacine, venlafaxine
Anorexia nervosa		SSRIs
Autistic disorder	Haloperidol, clomipramine, clonidine	Other neuroleptics, naltrexone
Bipolar disorder	Lithium, neuroleptics	Carbamazepine, valproate
Bulimia nervosa	SSRI's tricyclics	
Major depressive disorder		SSRIs, tricyclics, buproprion, lithium, venlafaxine
Nonspecific sedation	Diphenhydramine	
Panic disorder	SSRIs, tricyclics	High-potency benzodiazepines
Posttraumatic stress disorder		SSRIs, beta blockers, clonidine, lithium, carbamazepine, high-potency benzodiazepines, tricyclics
Obsessive-compulsive disorder	Clomipramine, SSRIs	
Schizophrenia	Neuroleptics	Atypical neuroleptics
Self-injurious behavior	Naltrexone	Neuroleptics, SSRIs
Separation anxiety disorder	Tricyclics	High-potency benzodiazepines, SSRIs
Severely aggressive behavior	Neuroleptics, lithium, carbamazepine	Beta blockers, clonidine
Tourette's disorder	Haloperidol, risperidone	Clonidine, tricyclics, clomipramine, SSRIs, guanfacine

hyperactivity (ADHD, predominantly inattentive type) are also likely to be responsive to stimulant medications.

Methylphenidate

A. Indications: See above.

B. Relative Contraindications: Use cautiously in individuals with a personal or family history of motor tics or Tourette's syndrome or if there is a personal or family history of substance abuse or addictive disorders.

C. Initial Medical Screening: One should search for a personal or family history of motor tics or Tourette's syndrome. The child should be observed for involuntary movements. Height, weight, pulse, and blood pressure should be recorded.

D. Dosage: Give initially 0.2–0.5 mg/kg per dose (usually 5–20 mg) before school and at noon, with or without another dose at 4 PM. The dose is then titrated upward weekly, checking for clinical effects. Administration on weekends and during vacations is determined by the need at those times. The duration of action is approximately 3–4 hours. The sustained-release preparation is not as effective in some children, and the duration of action may not be as long as the equivalent of 10 mg of methylphenidate in the morning and at noon.

E. Adverse Effects: Often dose-related and time-limited.

1. Common adverse effects–Anorexia, weight loss, abdominal distress, headache, insomnia, dysphoria and tearfulness, irritability, lethargy or "zombie-like" appearance, mild tachycardia, mild elevation in blood pressure.

2. Less common effects–Interdose rebound of ADHD symptoms, emergence of motor tics or Tourette's syndrome, behavioral stereotypy, seizures, tachycardia or hypertension, depression, mania, psychotic symptoms. Reduced growth velocity is seen only during active administration. Growth rebound occurs during periods of discontinuation. There is usually no noticeable compromise of ultimate height. Psychostimulants do not appear to predispose to future substance abuse.

F. Drug Interactions: Additive stimulant effects are seen with sympathomimetic amines (ephedrine, pseudoephedrine).

G. Medical Follow-Up: Pulse, blood pressure, height, and weight should be recorded every 3–4 months and at times of dosage increases. Assess for abnormal movements at each visit.

Dextroamphetamine Sulfate

The dosage is 2.5–10 mg twice daily before school and at noon, with or without another dose at 4 PM. A sustained-release preparation may have clinical effects for up to 8 hours. Other remarks are as for methylphenidate.

Pemoline

A. Indications: As above.

B. Relative Contraindications: As for methylphenidate, plus history of hepatic dysfunction or disease.

C. Initial Medical Screening: As for methylphenidate, plus liver function tests.

D. Dosage: The longer half-life of pemoline allows for the administration of a single dose each morning. The usual starting dose of 37.5 mg is increased weekly by 18.75 mg to the desired clinical effect or to a maximum daily dose of 112.5 mg. The onset of clinical effect may be delayed for 3–4 weeks.

E. Adverse Effects: Generally as for methylphenidate, but with fewer cardiovascular effects and less interdose rebound. Elevated liver enzymes occur in 1–3% of children receiving pemoline; hepatotoxic effects appear generally to be reversible with drug discontinuation; however, rare cases of liver failure have been reported. Consequently, pemoline is no longer recommended as first-line treatment for ADHD.

F. Drug Interactions: As for methylphenidate.

G. Medical Follow-Up: As for methylphenidate, plus liver function tests prior to initiation and every 3 months thereafter.

TRICYCLIC ANTIDEPRESSANTS

Imipramine

A. Indications: Imipramine is the most frequently prescribed antidepressant in children and adolescents. It has clinical efficacy in the treatment of ADHD, panic disorder, anxiety-based school refusal, separation anxiety disorder, bulimia, primary nocturnal enuresis, night terrors, and sleepwalking. It may be helpful in major depression in children and adolescents.

B. Relative Contraindications: Known cardiac disease or arrhythmia, undiagnosed syncope, known seizure disorder, family history of sudden cardiac death or cardiomyopathy, known electrolyte abnormality (with bingeing and purging).

C. Initial Medical Screening: The family history should be searched for sudden cardiac death and the patient's history for cardiac disease, arrhythmias, syncope, seizure disorder, or congenital hearing loss (associated with prolonged QT interval). Other screening procedures include serum electrolytes and BUN (with patients who have eating disorders), cardiac examination, and a baseline ECG.

D. Dosage: Daily dosage requirements vary considerably with different clinical disorders. Enuresis and sleep disorders can generally be treated with 25–75 mg of imipramine at bedtime depending on the size of the child. Treatment for ADHD often requires 1–3 mg/kg/d in two divided doses. Major depressive disorder and the anxiety disorders in children and adolescents frequently require 3–5 mg/kg/d in two divided doses. The onset of clinical effect may take 4–6 weeks to occur.

The starting dose is 1 mg/kg/d. Dosage increases of 25% are made every 4 or 5 days as tolerated to 3 mg/kg/d. Regular cardiovascular and electrocardiographic monitoring is required with each dosage increase above 3 mg/kg/d. Antidepressant effect is maximal with steady state plasma levels of imipramine plus desipramine (see below) ranging between 150 and 300 ng/mL.

E. Adverse Effects:

1. Cardiotoxic effects–The cardiotoxic effects of tricyclic antidepressants appear to be more frequent in children and adolescents than in adults. In addition to anticholinergic effects, tricyclic antidepressants have quinidine-like effects that result in slowing of cardiac conduction. Increased plasma levels appear to be weakly associated with an increased risk of cardiac conduction abnormalities. Steady state plasma levels of desipramine or of desipramine plus imipramine should therefore not exceed 300 ng/mL. In addition, each dosage increase above 3 mg/kg/d must be carefully monitored with pulse, blood pressure, and repeat ECGs. Upper limits for cardiovascular parameters when administering tricyclic antidepressants to children and adolescents are listed in Table 6–19.

2. Anticholinergic effects–Tachycardia, dry mouth, stuffy nose, blurred vision, constipation, sweating, vasomotor instability, withdrawal syndrome (gastrointestinal distress and psychomotor activation).

3. Other effects–Orthostatic hypotension, lowered seizure threshold, increased appetite and weight gain, sedation, irritability and psychomotor agitation, rash (often associated with yellow dye No. 5), headache, abdominal complaints, sleep disturbance and nightmares, mania.

F. Drug Interactions: Tricyclic antidepressants may potentiate the effects of central nervous system depressants and stimulants; barbiturates and

cigarette smoking may decrease plasma levels; phenothiazines, methylphenidate, and oral contraceptives may increase plasma levels; tachycardia may be more pronounced with marijuana.

G. Medical Follow-Up: Pulse and blood pressure with each dosage increase up to 3 mg/kg/d; pulse, blood pressure, and ECG with each dosage increase above 3 mg/kg/d; height, weight, pulse, blood pressure, and ECG every 3–4 months at steady state.

Desipramine

Other remarks as for imipramine.

A. Indications: As for imipramine, but often preferred over that drug because of fewer anticholinergic side effects. Suppression of tics in Tourette's syndrome has recently been reported.

B. Dosage: As for imipramine. Steady state plasma levels of desipramine should be between 150 and 300 ng/mL. Plasma levels above 300 ng/mL or total doses greater than 5 mg/kg/d should be avoided. Attention must be paid to pulse, blood pressure, and ECG with dosage increases above 3 mg/kg/d.

C. Adverse Effects: As for imipramine, except less prominent anticholinergic effects. There has also been concern about five unexplained instances of sudden cardiac death in children taking desipramine. The evidence to date does not support a causal link.

Nortriptyline

Other remarks as for imipramine.

A. Dosage: For major depressive disorder, 0.5–2 mg/kg/d in two divided doses. Therapeutic antidepressant effects appear to be associated with plasma levels between 60 and 100 ng/mL in children.

B. Adverse Effects: Fewer anticholinergic effects than imipramine. Daily doses should not exceed 2 mg/kg/d, and plasma levels should not exceed 150 ng/mL.

C. Medical Follow-Up: Careful cardiac monitoring with dosage increases.

Clomipramine

Other remarks as for imipramine.

A. Indications: Obsessive-compulsive disorder in children and adolescents, resulting in moderate to marked symptomatic improvement in 75% of individuals by week 5 of treatment. These effects appear to be independent of the drug's antidepressant effect. Clomipramine appears to be helpful also in reducing the ritualized repetitive behaviors of some autistic children.

B. Initial Medical Screening: As for imipramine, plus liver function tests.

C. Dosage: The initial daily dose of 1 mg/kg/d is advanced gradually to a target dose of approximately 3 mg/kg/d (with a maximum daily dose of 200 mg/d). Prepubertal children should receive the drug in two divided doses. Therapeutic blood levels are not yet established.

Table 6–19. Upper limits of cardiovascular parameters with tricyclic antidepressants.

Heart rate	130/min
Systolic blood pressure	130 mm Hg
Diastolic blood pressure	85 mm Hg
PR interval	0.2 s
QRS interval	0.12 s, or no more than 30% over baseline
QT corrected	0.45 s

E. Adverse Effects: As for imipramine. Some hepatotoxicity has been noted. Clomipramine appears to be as well tolerated as desipramine or imipramine.

SELECTIVE SEROTONIN REUPTAKE INHIBITORS (SSRIs)

Fluoxetine

A. Indications: Major depressive disorder in adolescents, particularly when there may be a high risk of drug overdose. Appears to be helpful also in child and adolescent anxiety disorders (especially obsessive-compulsive disorder) and eating disorders.

B. Relative Contraindications: Known liver disease or bipolar disorder.

C. Initial Medical Screening: General medical examination only.

D. Dosage: The major metabolites of fluoxetine have half-lives of approximately 1 week. This allows for once-daily or even alternate-day dosing. The initial daily dose of 5–10 mg is increased by 5–10 mg every 1–2 weeks as tolerated to a maximum dose of 40 mg/d. Antidepressant response is generally achieved by the sixth week in adolescents receiving daily doses of 20–40 mg. Fluoxetine is usually administered as a single morning dose but may be divided into morning and noon doses if side effects are a concern

E. Adverse Effects: Often dose-related and time-limited: gastrointestinal distress, nausea, headache, tremulousness, anorexia and weight loss, insomnia. Irritability, social disinhibition, restlessness, and emotional excitability can occur in approximately 20% of children taking SSRIs.

F. Drug Interactions: All SSRIs inhibit the efficiency of the hepatic P450 microsomal enzyme system. This can lead to higher than expected blood levels of other drugs, including antidepressants, antiarrhythmics, antipsychotics, beta blockers, opioids, and the antihistamine astemizole. Tryptophan may result in a serotonergic syndrome of psychomotor agitation and gastrointestinal distress.

G. Medical Follow-Up: General medical examination with weight and blood pressure.

Sertraline, Paroxetine, & Fluvoxamine

Other remarks as for fluoxetine.

A. Indications: Sertraline and paroxetine—as for fluoxetine; fluvoxamine—for obsessive-compulsive disorder.

B. Relative Contraindications: As for fluoxetine.

C. Initial Medical Screening: General medical examination.

D. Dosage: All three drugs have shorter half-lives than fluoxetine, whose half-life is approxi-

mately 1 week; the half-lives of sertraline and paroxetine are approximately 1–2 days, and that of fluvoxamine is approximately 16 hours. Sertraline and paroxetine are generally given once daily, usually in the morning. Fluvoxamine is generally given in divided doses, with the largest dose given at bedtime. Therapeutic doses of sertraline range from 50 to 150 mg/d and of paroxetine from 10 to 40 mg/d; the therapeutic dose range of fluvoxamine has not been established for children and adolescents; however, it should be less than the generally stated adult dosage range of 100–300 mg/d.

E. Drug Interactions: As for fluoxetine, but sertraline may inhibit cytochrome P450 hepatic enzymes less than fluoxetine or paroxetine.

OTHER ANTIDEPRESSANTS

Bupropion

A. Indications: Bupropion is a nontricyclic antidepressant that is receiving favorable attention for its therapeutic effects with major depressive disorder in adolescents and with ADHD in children and adolescents. Like the SSRIs, bupropion has very few anticholinergic or cardiotoxic effects.

B. Relative Contraindications: History of seizure disorder or eating disorder.

C. Initial Medical Screening: General medical examination if there is a history of seizures.

D. Dosage: The dosage is not established, but the range is thought to be from 150 to 450 mg/d in two or three divided doses. The maximum daily dosage in adolescents should be less than 450 mg. Because of the seizure potential, no dose should exceed 150 mg, and doses should be no closer together than 4 hours, preferably with at least 6 hours between doses.

E. Adverse Effects: Psychomotor activation (agitation or restlessness), headache, gastrointestinal distress, nausea, anorexia with weight loss, insomnia, tremulousness, precipitation of mania, and induction of seizures with doses above 450 mg/d. Teratogenic effects are uncertain.

F. Drug Interactions: Uncertain.

G. Medical Follow-Up: General medical examination.

Venlafaxine

A. Indications: Venlafaxine is a nontricyclic, non-SSRI antidepressant that inhibits reuptake of serotonin and norepinephrine. It appears to be a useful antidepressant in children and adolescents and perhaps also in ADHD.

B. Relative Contraindications: None known.

C. Initial Medical Screening: No specific issues.

D. Dosage: Not well established for children;

50–200 mg/d in two divided doses is probably appropriate.

E. Adverse Effects: Fewer anticholinergic, antihistaminic, and antiadrenergic side effects than the tricyclic antidepressants. The most common adverse effects are nausea, nervousness, and sweating. Like other antidepressants, venlafaxine can induce a manic switch in depressed bipolar patients.

F. Drug Interactions: Weak inhibitor of hepatic cytochrome P450 enzymes

G. Medical Follow-Up: General medical examination.

NEUROLEPTICS

The neuroleptics—also known as antipsychotics—are most clearly indicated for psychotic symptoms in patients with schizophrenia. They are also used for acute mania and as adjuncts to antidepressants in the treatment of psychotic depression (with delusions or hallucinations). They may be used very cautiously in refractory ADHD, in refractory obsessive-compulsive disorder, and in individuals with markedly aggressive behavioral problems unresponsive to other interventions.

Haloperidol

A. Indications: Haloperidol can also suppress tics in Tourette's syndrome and specific target symptoms in autistic disorder.

B. Relative Contraindications: Haloperidol is contraindicated in patients with a history of poorly controlled seizures, cardiac arrhythmias, agranulocytosis, previous neuroleptic malignant syndrome, or tardive dyskinesia.

C. Initial Medical Screening: One should observe and examine for abnormal movements and establish baseline CBC and liver function tests. An ECG should be taken if there is a history of cardiac disease or arrhythmia.

D. Dosage: Conservative treatment starts with 0.5–1 mg/d in two divided doses, increasing by 0.5 mg every 3–5 days to clinical effect, side effects, or a maximum daily dose of 4 mg. Daily doses above 4 mg should be reserved for the most disturbed and refractory patients. Antipsychotic effects may take 2–3 weeks to become fully apparent.

E. Adverse Effects: The two most troublesome adverse effects are cognitive slowing resulting from sedation and extrapyramidal syndromes. The high-potency neuroleptics (eg, haloperidol) cause less sedation but a greater frequency of extrapyramidal effects. The low-potency neuroleptics (eg, thioridazine) can cause greater sedation but fewer extrapyramidal effects. In any case, sedation, cognitive slowing, and extrapyramidal effects all tend to be dose-related. Because of the risk of tardive dyskinesia, neuroleptic medications should be reserved for

children and adolescents for whom less potentially harmful treatments are not available.

1. Extrapyramidal syndromes–Acute dystonic reactions are tonic muscle spasms, often of the tongue, jaw, or neck, which may result in such dramatically distressing symptoms as oculogyric crisis, torticollis, and even opisthotonos. The onset usually occurs within days after a dosage change and may occur in up to 25% of children treated with neuroleptics. Thioridazine is much less frequently associated with dystonic reactions. Acute neuroleptic-induced dystonias are quickly relieved by anticholinergics such as diphenhydramine.

2. Pseudoparkinsonism–Pseudoparkinsonism is usually manifested 1–4 weeks after the start of treatment. It presents as muscle stiffness, cogwheel rigidity, masked facies, bradykinesia, drooling, and occasionally pill-rolling tremor. Anticholinergic medications or dosage reductions are helpful.

3. Akathisia–Akathisia is usually manifested after 1–6 weeks of treatment. It presents as a very unpleasant feeling of driven motor restlessness that ranges from vague muscular discomfort to a markedly dysphoric agitation with frantic pacing. Anticholinergic agents or beta blockers are sometimes helpful.

4. Neuroleptic malignant syndrome–This is a medical emergency manifested by severe muscular rigidity, altered sensorium, hyperpyrexia, autonomic lability, and myoglobinemia. Mortality rates as high as 30% have been reported.

5. "Rabbit syndrome–This is a rare parkinsonism-like tremor of the mouth that develops late, presenting as rapid chewing-like movements similar to what is observed in rabbits.

6. Withdrawal symptoms–Dyskinesias are reversible movement disorders that appear following withdrawal of neuroleptic drugs. They occur in up to 25% of children exposed to neuroleptics for 1 year and in approximately 50% of those exposed for $2\frac{1}{2}$ years. Dyskinetic movements develop within 1–4 weeks after withdrawal of the drug and may persist for months.

7. Tardive dyskinesias–Tardive dyskinesias are irreversible movement disorders that appear after long-term use of neuroleptic medications. Choreoathetoid movements of the tongue and mouth are most common, but the extremities and trunk may also be involved. The risk of tardive dyskinesia is thought to be small in patients exposed to neuroleptics for less than 6 months. There is no effective treatment.

8. Other adverse effects of neuroleptics–Orthostatic hypotension, cardiac arrhythmias, anticholinergic effects, weight gain, irregular menses, gynecomastia (even galactorrhea), sexual dysfunction, photosensitivity, rashes, lowered seizure threshold, hepatic dysfunction, blood dyscrasias.

F. Drug Interactions: Potentiation of central nervous system depressant effects or the anticholinergic effects of other drugs may occur as well as increased plasma levels of antidepressants.

G. Medical Follow-Up: One should examine the patient at least every 3 months for signs of tardive dyskinesia.

Thioridazine

Thioridazine is effective in the treatment of psychotic disorders and severely aggressive disorders. It is not helpful for Tourette's syndrome.

The dose ranges from 20 to 200 mg/d in two divided doses. The adverse effects resemble those listed above for haloperidol, though thioridazine is considered less likely to cause acute dystonic reactions and pseudoparkinsonism. In doses above 800 mg/d, thioridazine is associated with retinitis pigmentosa.

Other comments as for haloperidol.

ATYPICAL NEUROLEPTICS

Risperidone

Risperidone blocks type 2 serotonin in addition to type 2 dopamine receptors. Adult schizophrenics given 2–8 mg/d of risperidone had better symptom relief and fewer side effects than those treated with conventional neuroleptics. Anecdotal reports suggest that similar results may be obtained in adolescents with schizophrenia. Risperidone has also demonstrated good clinical efficacy in the treatment of Tourette's syndrome. The initial dose is 1–6 mg/d in two divided doses.

Other comments as for haloperidol.

Clozapine

Clozapine blocks type 2 dopamine receptors weakly and is virtually free of extrapyramidal side effects, apparently including tardive dyskinesia. It was very effective in about 40% of chronic adult schizophrenics who did not respond to conventional neuroleptics. Non-dose-related agranulocytosis occurs in 0.5–2% of subjects. Of 200 subjects who developed agranulocytosis, seven died. There are case reports of benefit from clozapine in child and adolescent schizophrenics resistant to other treatment.

Relative contraindications are concurrent treatment with carbamazepine and any history of leukopenia. Initial medical screening is with CBC and liver function tests. The daily dose is 200–600 mg in two divided doses. Because of the risk of neutropenia, patients taking clozapine must be registered with the Clozapine Registry and a white blood cell count must be obtained weekly before a 1-week supply of the drug is dispensed. If the white count falls below 3000/μL, clozapine is usually discontinued. Other side effects include sedation, weight gain, and increased salivation. The incidence of seizures increases with doses above 600 mg/d.

MOOD STABILIZERS

Lithium Carbonate

A. Indications: Lithium remains a front-line drug in the treatment of bipolar mood disorder. It may be helpful also in the treatment of patients with severe aggressive symptoms, emotionally unstable behavior disorders, and behaviorally disturbed children whose parents are known lithium responders. Lithium has sometimes been shown to have an augmenting effect when combined with SSRIs in individuals with treatment-resistant depression and obsessive-compulsive disorder.

B. Relative Contraindications: Lithium is contraindicated in patients with known renal, thyroid, or cardiac disease; those at high risk for dehydration and electrolyte imbalance (eg, vomiting and purging); and those at risk of pregnancy (teratogenic effects).

C. Initial Medical Screening: General medical screening with pulse, blood pressure, height, and weight; CBC; serum electrolytes, BUN, and creatinine; and thyroid function tests with TSH.

D. Dosage: Oral doses of lithium up to 1800 mg/d are frequently necessary to maintain therapeutic blood levels of 1–1.5 mEq/L. The drug is generally given in three divided doses—or two doses with sustained-release lithium preparations. Blood samples should be drawn 12 hours after the last dose.

E. Adverse Effects:

1. Lithium toxicity–Lithium has a low therapeutic index—ie, blood levels required for therapeutic effect are close to associated with toxic symptoms. Mild toxicity—increased tremor, gastrointestinal distress, neuromuscular irritability, and altered consciousness—can be seen with blood levels above 1.5 mEq/L. Moderate to severe symptoms of lithium toxicity are associated with blood levels above 2 mEq/L.

2. Common lithium side effects–Intention tremor, gastrointestinal distress (including nausea and vomiting and sometimes diarrhea), polyuria and polydipsia, drowsiness, malaise, weight gain, acne, granulocytosis.

3. Uncommon lithium side effects–Hypothyroidism, chronic renal disease; unknown effects on developing bone.

F. Drug Interactions: Excessive salt intake and salt restriction should be avoided. Thiazide diuretics and nonsteroidal anti-inflammatory agents (except aspirin and acetaminophen) lead to increased lithium levels. Precautions against dehydration are required in hot weather and with vigorous exercise.

G. Medical Follow-Up: Serum lithium levels should be measured 5–7 days following a change in dosage and then monthly at steady state; serum creatinine and TSH concentrations should be determined every 3–4 months.

Valproate

A. Indications: Valproate is a front-line medication for bipolar disorder in adults. Its efficacy in acute mania equals that of lithium, but it is generally better tolerated. Valproate is more effective than lithium in patients with rapid bipolar cycling (more than four cycles per year) and in patients with mixed states (coexisting symptoms of depression and mania). Valproate may be more effective than lithium in adolescents with bipolar disorder because they often have rapid cycling and mixed states.

B. Relative Contraindications: Liver dysfunction.

C. Initial Medical Screening: CBC and liver function tests.

D. Dosage: Usually starts at 15 mg/kg/d and is increased in increments of 5–10 mg/kg/d every 1–2 weeks to a range of 500–1500 mg/d in two or three divided doses. Trough levels in the range of 80–120 μg/mL are thought to be therapeutic.

E. Adverse Effects: Ten to 20 percent of patients experience sedation or anorexia, especially early in treatment or if the dose is increased too rapidly. Gastrointestinal upset occurs in 25% of patients and, when severe, can usually be treated with cimetidine. Increased appetite and weight gain can be troublesome for adolescents. Blurred vision, headache, hair loss, and tremor occur occasionally. Slight elevations in aminotransferases are frequent. Severe idiosyncratic hepatitis, pancreatitis, and agranulocytosis occur only rarely.

F. Medical Follow-Up: Serum alanine aminotransferase should be checked every 3–4 weeks for 3–4 months. Subsequently, alanine aminotransferase, CBC, and trough valproate levels should be obtained every 3–4 months.

Carbamazepine

A. Indications: Similar to lithium and valproate, Carbamazepine may be effective for bipolar disorder or for the target symptoms of mood instability, irritability, or behavioral dyscontrol. Some data suggest that it is more effective than valproate for the depressive phases of a bipolar disorder. This may relate to its similarities with the tricyclic antidepressants.

B. Relative Contraindications: History of previous bone marrow depression or history of adverse hematologic reaction to another drug; history of sensitivity to a tricyclic antidepressant.

C. Initial Medical Screening: CBC with platelets, reticulocytes, serum iron, and BUN; liver function tests; urinalysis.

D. Dosage: Usually starts at 10–20 mg/kg/d in two divided doses in children younger than 6 years; 100 mg twice daily in children 6–12 years; and 200 mg twice daily in children over 12 years. Doses may be increased weekly to effective symptom control. Total daily doses should not exceed 35 mg/kg/d in children younger than 6 years; 1000 mg/d in children 6–15 years; and 1200 mg/d in adolescents older than 15 years. Plasma levels in the range of 4–12 μg/mL are thought to be therapeutic.

E. Adverse Effects: Aplastic anemia and agranulocytosis are rare. Leukopenia and thrombocytopenia are more common, and if present should be monitored closely for evidence of bone marrow depression. These effects usually occur early and transiently and then spontaneously revert toward normal. Hepatic damage, renal impairment, and ocular changes may also be seen. Nausea, dizziness, sedation, headache, dry mouth, diplopia, and constipation reflect the drug's mild anticholinergic properties.

F. Medical Follow-Up: Conservative management suggests that hematologic, hepatic, and renal parameters should be followed at least every 3 months for the first year. White counts below 3000/μL or absolute neutrophil counts below 1000/μL call for discontinuation and referral for hematology consultation.

ALPHA-ADRENERGIC AGONISTS

Clonidine

A. Indications: Clonidine is a nonselective alpha-adrenergic agonist that has been found to be clinically useful in decreasing states of hyperarousal. It seems to be particularly helpful as an adjunct to methylphenidate in children with ADHD when the history is of very early onset of marked hyperactivity, aggression, and oppositional behavior. Bedtime doses of clonidine can be helpful with the delayed onset of sleep that can be seen with ADHD or stimulant medication effects. It is also frequently effective in the treatment of ADHD and tics in Tourette's syndrome and in states of hyperarousal associated with posttraumatic stress disorder. Clonidine also appears helpful with ADHD-like symptoms in some autistic children.

B. Relative Contraindications: Clonidine is contraindicated in patients with known renal or cardiovascular disease and those with a family or personal history of depression.

C. Initial Medical Screening: The pulse and blood pressure should be recorded and a baseline ECG taken.

D. Dosage: Initial dosage of clonidine is 0.05 mg at bedtime; that dose is increased after 3–5 days by giving 0.05 mg also in the morning; and further dosage increases are made by adding 0.05 mg first in the morning, then at noon, and then in the evening every 3–5 days to a maximum total daily dose of 0.3 mg (3–5 μg/kg/d) in three or four divided doses per day. The half-life of clonidine is in the range of 3–4 hours. Although a clinical response generally becomes apparent by about 4 weeks, treatment effects may increase over 2–3 months. Therapeutic doses of methylphenidate can frequently be decreased by 30–50% when used in conjunction with clonidine.

Transdermal administration of clonidine using a skin patch can be quite effective but may result in skin irritation in 40% of cases. Patches are generally changed every 5 days.

E. Adverse Effects: Sedation can be prominent. Other side effects include fatigability, mild hypotension, increased appetite and weight gain, headache, sleep disturbance, gastrointestinal distress, skin irritation with transdermal administration, and rebound hypertension with abrupt withdrawal. Bradycardia can occasionally be marked.

F. Drug Interactions: Increased sedation with central nervous system depressants; possible cardiotoxicity with cocaine; increased anticholinergic toxicity.

G. Medical Follow-Up: Pulse and blood pressure should be recorded every 2 weeks for 2 months and then every 3 months. The discontinuation of clonidine should occur gradually—at a rate of 0.05 mg every 3 days—to avoid rebound hypertension. Blood pressure should be monitored during withdrawal.

Guanfacine

Guanfacine is a selective agonist for α_2-adrenergic receptors with advantages over the nonselective agonist clonidine. Guanfacine is less sedating and less hypotensive and has a longer half-life, allowing for twice-daily dosing. Case reports find guanfacine effective in ADHD and Tourette's syndrome with comorbid ADHD.

Relative contraindications are as for clonidine. Initial medical screening should record pulse and blood pressure. The dosage is 2–4 mg/d in two or three divided doses. Adverse effects include transient headaches and stomachaches in 25% of patients. Sedation and hypertension are mild. For medical follow-up, pulse and blood pressure should be checked every 1–2 weeks for 2 months and then at 3-month intervals.

BETA-ADRENERGIC BLOCKERS

Propranolol

A. Indications: Propranolol is a nonselective beta-adrenoceptor blocking agent that reduces peripheral autonomic tone and in that way ameliorates the somatic symptoms of anxiety, including palpitations, tremulousness, sweating, and blushing. Propranolol appears to have clinical efficacy in the treatment of performance anxiety (stage fright), post-traumatic stress disorder, episodic outbursts of rage, lithium-induced tremor, and neuroleptic-induced akathisia.

B. Relative Contraindications: Propranolol should not be given to patients with a history of dia-

betes, cardiovascular disease, reactive airway disease, or depression.

C. Initial Medical Screening: Pulse and blood pressure should be recorded, as well as fasting blood sugar in patients with a family history of diabetes.

D. Dosage: Daily doses range from 10 to 120 mg/d for prepubertal children and from 20 to 300 mg/d for adolescents. Blood pressure should be kept above 90/60 mm Hg in adolescents, and the pulse should be kept above 60/min. The drug is usually given in three divided doses.

E. Adverse Effects: Sedation, fatigue, bradycardia, hypotension, bronchospasm, depression, sleep disturbance, hypoglycemia in diabetics, sexual dysfunction.

F. Drug Interactions: Propranolol may inhibit the action of sympathomimetics and xanthines.

G. Medical Follow-Up: Pulse and blood pressure must be closely monitored.

OPIOID ANTAGONIST

Naltrexone

Naltrexone is helpful in some cases of autistic disorder and in the management of self-injurious behavior in autistic and mentally retarded individuals. A single daily dose of 0.5–1.5 mg/kg has been found to decrease self-injurious behavior, social withdrawal, hyperactivity, and stereotypy. The only adverse effect is sedation.

Alvir J et al: Clozapine induced agranulocytosis. N Engl J Med 1993;329:162.

Barrickman LL et al: Bupropion vs. methylphenidate in the treatment of ADHD. J Am Acad Child Adolesc Psychiatry 1995;34:649.

Biederman J et al: Estimation of the association between desipramine and the risk for sudden death in 5–14 yr old children. J Clin Psychiatry 1995;56:87.

Birmaher B et al: Fluoxetine for childhood anxiety disorders. J Am Acad Child Adolesc Psychiatry 1994;33:993.

Campbell M et al: Lithium in hospitalized aggressive children with conduct disorder: A double blind and placebo-controlled study. J Am Acad Child Adolesc Psychiatry 1995;34:445.

Chappel PB et al: Guanfacine treatment of comorbid ADHD and Tourette's syndrome: Preliminary clinical experience. J Am Acad Child Adolesc Psychiatry 1995;34:140.

Crewe HK et al: The effects of SSRI's on cytochrome P4502D6 (CYP2D6) activity in human liver microenzymes. Br J Clin Pharmacol 1992;34:262.

Frankhauser MP et al: A double-blind, placebo controlled study of the efficacy of transdermal clonidine in autism. J Clin Psychiatry 1992;53:77.

Gordon CT et al: A double-blind comparison of clomipramine, desipramine, and placebo in the treatment of autistic disorder. Arch Gen Psychiatry 1993;50:441.

Green WH: *Child and Adolescent Psychopharmacology.* Williams & Wilkins, 1995.

Hunt RD et al: An open trial of guanfacine in the treatment

of ADHD. J Am Acad Child Adolesc Psychiatry 1995;34:50.

Leonard HL et al: Pharmacology of the selective serotonin reuptake inhibitors in children and adolescents. J Am Acad Child Adolesc Psychiatry 1997;36:725.

Morton WA et al: Venlafaxine: A structurally unique and novel antidepressant. Ann Pharmacother 1995;29:387.

The P450 family. Biol Ther Psychiatry Newsl 1995;18:29.

Pickar D, Hsiao JK: Clozapine treatment of schizophrenia. JAMA 1995;274:981.

Quintana H, Keshavan M: Case study: Risperidone in children and adolescents with schizophrenia. J Am Acad Child Adolesc Psychiatry 1995;34:1292.

Remschmidt H et al: An open trial of clozapine in 36 adolescents with schizophrenia. J Child Adolesc Psychopharmacol 1994;4:31.

Riddle MA (editor): Pediatric psychopharmacology I. Child Adolesc Psychiatr Clin North Am 1995;4(1).

Riddle MA (editor): Pediatric psychopharmacology II. Child Adolesc Psychiatr Clin North Am 1995;4(2).

Risperidone. Biol Ther Psychiatry Newsl 1993;16:45.

Settle EC: Bupropion: Update 1993. Int Drug Ther Newsl 1993;28:29.

Tierney E et al: Sertraline for major depression in children and adolescents: Preliminary clinical experience. J Child Adolesc Psychopharmacol 1995;5:13.

Venlafaxine offers an alternative to stimulants. Clin Psychiatry News 1995 (July):5.

West SA et al: An open trial of valproate in the treatment of adolescent mania. J Child Adolesc Psychopharmacol 1994;4:263.

Wilens T et al: Clonidine for sleep disturbances associated with ADHD. J Am Acad Child Adolesc Psychiatry 1994;33:424.

Wilens T et al: Nortriptyline in the treatment of ADHD: A chart review of 58 cases. J Am Acad Child Adolesc Psychiatry 1993;32:343.

Child Abuse & Neglect

7

Richard D. Krugman, MD, & Andrew P. Sirotnak, MD

The problem of child abuse and neglect, barely recognized as a significant problem in the early editions of this textbook, has grown to a problem of such serious proportions that in 1990 the United States Advisory Board on Child Abuse and Neglect called the present state of the nation's ability to protect children a "national emergency". Seven years later, the emergency is still with us. What Dr Henry Kempe and his colleagues first called "battered child syndrome" was thought to affect 749 children in the United States in 1960. The best data now available suggest that 1–1.5% of American children are abused or neglected annually. In 1995 there were an estimated 3 million reports of abuse and neglect, which translates to an approximate national maltreatment rate of 25 victims per 1000 children. One million of these cases were substantiated by child protective service agencies. At least 1000 children are victims of fatal child abuse each year. This dramatic increase in cases has resulted from increased recognition of the problem by professionals, partly in response to statutory reporting mandates; a broadening of the definitions of abuse and neglect from the original "battered child" concept; and changes in the demography and social structure of families and neighborhoods over the past several decades.

Abuse and neglect of children is best considered in an ecologic perspective which recognizes the individual, family, social, and psychologic influences that come together to contribute to the problem. For most pediatric health care professionals, however, their involvement will be limited to individual cases. This chapter focuses on the knowledge necessary for the recognition, intervention, and follow-up of the more common forms of child maltreatment and to highlight the role of pediatric professionals in prevention.

FORMS OF CHILD MALTREATMENT

Child maltreatment may occur either within or outside the family. The proportion of intrafamilial to extrafamilial cases varies with the type of abuse as well as the gender and age of child. Each of the following conditions may exist as separate or concurrent diagnoses.

Physical Abuse

Physical abuse of children is most often inflicted by a caretaker or family member but occasionally by a stranger. The most common manifestations include bruises, burns, fractures, head trauma, and abdominal injuries. A small but significant number of unexpected pediatric deaths, particularly in infants and very young children (eg, SIDS), are related to physical abuse.

Sexual Abuse

Sexual abuse is defined as the engaging of dependent, developmentally immature children in sexual activities that they do not fully comprehend and to which they cannot give consent or activities which violate the laws and taboos of a society. It includes all forms of incest, sexual assault or rape, and pedophilia. This includes fondling, oral-genital contact, all forms of intercourse or penetration, exhibitionism, voyeurism, exploitation or prostitution, and the involvement of children in the production of pornography.

Emotional Abuse

Emotional or psychologic abuse has been defined as the rejection, ignoring, criticizing, isolation, or terrorizing of children, all of which have the effect of eroding their self-esteem. The most common form is verbal abuse or denigration. Children who witness domestic violence should be considered emotionally abused.

Physical Neglect

Physical neglect is the failure to provide the necessary food, clothing, shelter, and a safe environment in which children can grow and develop. Although often associated with poverty or ignorance, physical neglect involves a more serious problem than just lack of resources. There is often a component of emotional neglect and either a failure or an inability,

195

intentionally or otherwise, to recognize and respond to the needs of the child.

Emotional Neglect

The most common feature of emotional neglect is the absence of normal parent–child attachment and a subsequent inability to recognize and respond to an infant's or child's needs. A common manifestation of emotional neglect in infancy is nutritional (nonorganic) failure to thrive.

Medical Care Neglect

Medical care neglect is failure to provide the needed treatment to infants or children with life-threatening illness or other serious or chronic medical conditions.

Munchausen Syndrome by Proxy

This is a relatively unusual disorder in which a caretaker, usually the mother, either simulates or creates the symptoms or signs of illness in a child. The child can present with a long list of medical problems or often bizarre recurrent complaints. Fatal cases have been reported.

RECOGNITION OF ABUSE & NEGLECT

The most common features suggesting a diagnosis of child abuse are summarized in Tables 7–1 and 7–2. There may be obvious signs of injury, sexual abuse, or neglect. Classic radiographic and laboratory findings are discussed below. Psychosocial factors may indicate risk for or confirm child maltreatment.

Recognition of any form of abuse and neglect of children can only occur if the possibility is entertained in the differential diagnosis of the child's presenting medical condition. The approach to the family should be supportive, nonaccusatory, and empathetic. The individual who brings the child in for care may not have any involvement in the abuse. Approximately one-third of child abuse incidents occur in extrafamilial settings. Nevertheless, the assumption that the caretaker is "nice," combined with failure to consider the possibility of abuse, can be costly and even fatal. Raising the possibility that a child has been abused is not the same as accusing the caretaker of being the abuser. The health professional who is examining the child can explain to the family that there are several possibilities which might explain the injuries or abuse-related symptoms with which the child has presented. If the family or presenting caretaker is not involved in the child's maltreatment, they will welcome the necessary report and investigation.

History

The medical diagnosis of **physical abuse** is based

Table 7–1. Common historical features in child abuse cases.

Discrepant history
Delay in seeking care
Event or behavior by child that triggers a loss of control of caretaker
History of abuse in the caretaker's childhood
Inappropriate affect of the caretaker
Pattern of increasing severity if no intervention
Social or physical isolation of the child or caretaker
Stress or crisis in the family or the caretaker
Unrealistic expectations of caretaker for the child

on the presence of a "discrepant history." The history offered by the caretaker is not consistent with the clinical findings. The "discrepancy" may exist because the history is absent, partial, changing over time, or simply illogical or improbable. The presence of a discrepant history should prompt a request for consultation with a multidisciplinary child protection team or a report to the child protective services agency. This agency is mandated by state law to investigate reports of suspected child abuse and neglect. Investigation by social services and possibly law enforcement officers, as well as a home visit, may be required to sort out the circumstances of the child's injuries. Other common historical features in child abuse cases are listed in Table 7–1.

Sexual abuse may present to the clinician in different ways: (1) The child may be brought in for routine care or for an acute problem, and sexual abuse

Table 7–2. Presentations of sexual abuse.

General or direct statements about sexual abuse
Sexualized play or behavior in developmentally immature children
Sexual abuse of other children by the victim
Behavioral changes
  Sleep disturbances (eg, nightmares and night terrors)
  Appetite disturbances (eg, anorexia, bulimia)
  Depression, social withdrawal, anxiety
  Aggression, temper tantrums, impulsiveness
  Neurotic or conduct disorders, phobias or avoidant behaviors
  Guilt, low self-esteem, mistrust, feelings of helplessness
  Hysterical or conversion reactions
  Suicidal, runaway threats or behavior
  Excessive masturbation
Medical conditions
  Recurrent abdominal pain or frequent somatic complaints
  Genital, anal, or urethral trauma
  Recurrent complaints of genital or anal pain, discharge, bleeding
  Enuresis or encopresis
  Sexually transmitted diseases
  Pregnancy
Promiscuity or prostitution, sexual dysfunction, fear of intimacy
School problems or truancy
Substance abuse

may be suspected by the medical professional as a result of the history or the physical examination. (2) The parent or caretaker, suspecting that the child may have been sexually abused, may bring the child to the health care provider and request an examination to "rule in or rule out" abuse. (3) The child may be referred by child protective services or the police for an evidentiary examination following either disclosure of sexual abuse by the child or an allegation of abuse by a parent or third party. Table 7–2 lists the presentations of child sexual abuse. It should be emphasized that with the exception of acute trauma, certain sexually transmitted diseases, or forensic laboratory evidence, none of these presentations are specific. The presentations listed should arouse suspicion of the possibility of sexual abuse and lead the practitioner to ask the appropriate questions—again, in a compassionate and nonaccusatory manner. The American Academy of Pediatrics has published guidelines for the evaluation of child sexual abuse as well as other guidelines relating to child maltreatment.

Emotional abuse may cause nonspecific symptoms in children. Loss of self-esteem or self-confidence, sleep disturbances, somatic symptoms (eg, headaches, stomachaches), hypervigilance, or avoidant or phobic behaviors (eg, school refusal, running away) may be presenting complaints. These complaints may also be seen in children who experience domestic violence. Emotional abuse can occur in the home or day care, school, sports team, or other settings.

Even though in 1995 there were twice as many reports of neglect of children than of physical abuse, it is not easily documented on history. **Physical neglect**—which must be differentiated from the deprivations of poverty—will be present even after adequate social services to families in need have been provided. **Emotionally neglectful parents** appear to have an inability to recognize the physical or emotional states of their children. For example, an emotionally neglectful parent may ignore the cry of an infant that may be incorrectly perceived as an expression of anger. This misinterpretation leads to inadequate nutrition and failure to thrive. The clinician must evaluate the psychosocial history and family dynamics when neglect is a consideration, and a careful social services investigation may be required.

The history offered in cases of **failure to thrive** is often discrepant with the physical findings. Infants who have experienced a significant deceleration in growth are probably not receiving adequate amounts or appropriate types of food despite the dietary history provided. Medical conditions causing poor growth in infancy and early childhood can be ruled out with a detailed history and minimal laboratory tests. A psychosocial history may reveal maternal depression, family chaos or dysfunction, or other previously unknown social risk factors (eg, substance abuse, violence, poverty, psychiatric illness). Placement of the child with another caregiver or hospitalization of the severely malnourished patient is usually followed by a dramatic weight gain.

Physical Findings

The findings upon examination of physically abused children may include abrasions, alopecia, bites, bruises, burns, dental trauma, fractures, lacerations, ligature marks, or scars. Injuries may be in multiple stages of healing. Bruises in physically abused children are sometimes patterned (eg, belt marks, looped cord marks, grab or pinch marks) and are typically found over the soft tissue areas of the body. Toddlers or older children typically sustain accidental bruises over bony prominences such as shins and elbows. Any bruise in an infant not developmentally mobile should be viewed with concern. (Other child abuse emergencies are listed in Table 7–3). Lacerations of the frenulum or tongue and bruising of the lips may be associated with force feeding. Pathognomonic burn patterns include stocking or glove distribution; immersion burns of the buttocks, sometimes with a "doughnut hole" area of sparing; and branding burns such as with cigarettes or hot objects (eg, grill, curling iron, or lighter). The absence of splash marks or a pattern consistent with spillage may be helpful in differentiating accidental from nonaccidental scald burns.

Head and abdominal trauma may present with signs and symptoms consistent with those injuries. Inflicted head trauma ("shaken baby syndrome") and abdominal injuries may be associated with no visible findings on examination. The finding of retinal hemorrhages in an infant without an appropriate medical condition (eg, leukemia, congenital infection, clotting disorder) should arouse concern about possible inflicted head trauma. Retinal hemorrhages are not commonly seen after CPR in either infants or children.

The genital and anal findings of **sexually abused** children, as well as the normal developmental

Table 7–3. Potential child abuse medical emergencies.

Any infant with bruises (especially head, facial, or abdominal), burns, or fractures

Any infant or child under 2 years of age with a history of suspected "shaken baby" head trauma or other inflicted head injury

Any child who has sustained suspicious or known inflicted abdominal trauma

Any child with burns in stocking or glove distribution or in other unusual patterns, burns to the genitalia, and any unexplained burn injury

Any child with disclosure or sign of sexual assault within 48–72 hours after alleged event if the possibility of acute injury is present or if forensic evidence exists changes and variations in prepubertal female hymens, have been described in recent atlases. The majority of victims of sexual abuse have no physical findings. The reasons for this include delay in disclosure by the child, abuse that may cause no physical trauma (eg, fondling, oral-genital contact, exploitation by pornographic photography), or rapid healing of minor injuries such as labial, hymenal, or anal abrasions, contusions, or lacerations. Nonspecific abnormalities of the genital and rectal regions such as erythema, rashes, and irritation) may not suggest sexual abuse in the absence of a corroborating history, disclosure, or behavioral changes. Finally, some medical conditions may be misdiagnosed as sexual abuse (eg, lichen sclerosus, dermatitis, labial adhesions, congenital urethral or vulvar disorders, Crohn's disease, and accidental straddle injuries to the labia) and can be ruled out by careful history and examination.

Certain sexually transmitted diseases (STDs) should strongly suggest sexual abuse. *Neisseria gonorrhoeae* or the stigmas of syphilis beyond the perinatal period are diagnostic of sexual abuse. *Chlamydia trachomatis,* herpes simplex virus type 2, trichomoniasis, and human papillomavirus (HPV) are all sexually transmitted, though the course of these perinatally acquired infections may be protracted. In the case of HPV, an initial appearance venereal warts beyond the toddler age should raise concerns about sexual abuse. Finally, sexual abuse must be considered with the diagnosis of HIV infection when other modes of transmission (eg, transfusion, perinatal acquisition) have been ruled out. The CDC and sexual abuse atlases both list guidelines for the screening of STDs in sexually abused children and adolescents.

Infants and children with nonorganic **failure to thrive** have a relative absence of subcutaneous fat in the cheeks, buttocks, and extremities. Other conditions associated with poor nutrient and vitamin intake may be present. If the condition has persisted for some time, they may also appear and act depressed. Older children who have been emotionally neglected on a chronic basic may also have short stature ("deprivation dwarfism"). The head circumference is usually normal in nonorganic failure to thrive. Microcephaly may signify a prenatal condition, congenital disease, or chronic nutritional deprivation and increases the likelihood of more serious and possibly permanent developmental delay.

Children with **Munchausen syndrome by proxy** may present with the signs and symptoms of whatever illness is factitiously produced or simulated. They may be actually ill or reported to be ill and have a normal clinical appearance. Among the most common reported presentations are recurrent apnea, dehydration from induced vomiting or diarrhea, sepsis when contaminants are injected into a child, change in mental status, fever, gastrointestinal bleeding, and seizures.

Radiologic & Laboratory Findings

Certain radiologic findings are strong indicators of physical abuse: Examples are metaphysial "corner" or "bucket handle" fractures of the long bones in infants, spiral fracture of the extremities in nonambulatory infants, rib fractures, spinous process fractures, and fractures in multiple stages of healing. Skeletal surveys in children 3 years of age or younger should be performed when a suspicious fracture is diagnosed. CT or MRI findings of subdural hemorrhage in infants are highly correlated with abusive head trauma, especially after the advent of infant seat restraint laws that have reduced the incidence of head trauma in infants. Abdominal CT is the preferred test in suspected abdominal trauma. Any infant or very young child with suspected abuse-related head or abdominal trauma should be evaluated immediately by an emergency physician or trauma surgeon.

Coagulation studies and CBC with platelets are useful in children who present with multiple or severe bruising in different ages of healing. Coagulopathy conditions may confuse the diagnostic picture but can be excluded with a careful history, examination, laboratory screens, and hematologic consultation if necessary

The differential diagnosis of other forms of physical abuse can be considered in the context of a detailed trauma history, family medical history, radiographic findings, and laboratory testing. The diagnosis of osteogenesis imperfecta or other collagen-vascular disorders, for example, may be considered in the child with skin and joint findings or multiple fractures with or without the classic radiographic presentation and is best made in consultation with a geneticist, an orthopedic surgeon, and a radiologist. Trauma—accidental or inflicted—leads the differential diagnosis list for subdural hematomas. Coagulopathy, disorders of copper metabolism, amino acid or organic acid metabolism (eg, Menkes' syndrome, glutaric acidemia type 1, methylmalonic acidemia), chronic or previous central nervous system infection, birth trauma, or congenital central nervous system malformation (eg, arteriovenous malformations, cerebrospinal fluid collections) may need to be ruled out in some cases. It should be recognized, however, that children with these rare disorders can also be abuse victims.

The **forensic evaluation** of sexually abused children should be performed in a setting that prevents further emotional distress. If from the history there is a possibility that the child may have had contact with the ejaculate of a perpetrator within 72 hours, an examination looking for semen or its markers (eg, acid phosphatase) should be performed according to established protocols. More importantly, if there is a history of possible sexual abuse within the past 48–72 hours and the child reports a physical complaint or a sign is observed (eg, genital or anal bleeding or discharge), the child should be examined for signs of trauma. The laboratory and serologic evaluation of sexually transmitted diseases should be guided by the type of contact reported and the epidemiology of these infections in the community.

Children with failure to thrive or malnutrition should not have an extensive workup. Complete blood count, urinalysis, electrolyte panel, and liver function tests are sufficient screening. Newborn screening should be documented as normal. Other tests should be guided by any clinical history that points to a previously undiagnosed condition (eg, thyroid, metabolic studies). A skeletal survey may be helpful in the case where concurrent physical abuse is suspected. The best "test," however, is placement in a setting in which the child can be fed and monitored. Hospital or foster care placement may be required. Weight gain may not occur for several days to a week in severe cases.

Any child with recurrent polymicrobial sepsis (especially in children with indwelling catheters), recurrent apnea, chronic dehydration of unknown cause, or other highly unusual, unexplained laboratory findings should raise the suspicion of Munchausen syndrome by proxy.

MANAGEMENT & REPORTING OF CHILD ABUSE & NEGLECT

Physical abuse injuries, sexually transmitted diseases, and medical sequelae of neglect should of course be treated immediately. Children with failure to thrive related to emotional and physical neglect need to be placed in a setting where they can be fed and cared for. Likewise, the child in danger of recurrent abuse needs to placed in a safe environment.

In every state, clinicians and many other professionals who come in contact with children are "mandated reporters." If abuse or neglect is suspected, a report must be made to the local or state agency designated to investigate such matters. In most cases, this will be the child protective services agency. Law enforcement agencies may also receive such reports. The purpose of the report is to permit professionals to gather the information needed to determine whether the child's environment (eg, home, school, day care setting, foster home) is safe. Many hospitals and communities make child protection teams or consultants available when there are questions about the diagnosis and management in a child abuse case.

A listing of pediatric consultants in child abuse is available form the American Academy of Pediatrics.

Except in extreme cases, the reporting of emotional abuse is not likely to generate a response from child protection agencies. Practitioners can encourage parents to get involved with parent effectiveness training programs (eg, Parents as First Teachers, or Parents Anonymous) or seek mental health consultation. Support for the child may also include mental health counseling or age-appropriate peer activities either in school or the community.

PREVENTION OF CHILD ABUSE & NEGLECT

Physical abuse is preventable in many cases. Extensive experience and evaluation of high-risk families has shown that the provision of "home visitor" services to families at risk can prevent physical abuse of children. These services can be provided by public health nurses or trained paraprofessionals, though there are more data available describing public health nurse intervention. This makes it as easy for the family to pick up the telephone and ask for help before they abuse a child as it is for a neighbor or physician to report an episode of abuse after it has occurred. Parent education and anticipatory guidance may also be helpful, particularly with respect to handling situations that stress parents (eg, colic, crying, toilet training), age-appropriate discipline, and general developmental issues. Prevention of abusive injuries perpetrated by nonparent caretakers (eg, babysitters, nannies, unrelated adults in the home) may be addressed by education and counseling of mothers about safe child care arrangements.

The prevention of sexual abuse is more difficult. Most efforts in this area involve teaching children to protect themselves and their "private parts" from harm or interference. These programs are useful but are in general not as efficacious as they are necessary. The age of toilet training is a good anticipatory guidance time to encourage parents to consider this discussion. The most rational approach is to place the burden of responsibility of prevention on the adults that supervise the child rather than on the children themselves.

Efforts to prevent emotional abuse of children have been undertaken through extensive media campaigns. No data are available to assess the effectiveness of this approach.

REFERENCES

American Academy of Pediatrics: Adolescent assault victim needs: A review of issues and a model protocol. Pediatrics 1996;98:991.

American Academy of Pediatrics: Distinguishing sudden infant death syndrome from child abuse fatalities. Pediatrics 1994;94:124.

American Academy of Pediatrics: Guidelines for the evaluation of sexual abuse of children. Pediatrics 1991;87:254-260.

American Academy of Pediatrics: Investigation and review of unexpected infant and child deaths. Pediatrics 1993;92:734.

American Academy of Pediatrics: Shaken baby syndrome: Inflicted cerebral trauma. Pediatrics 1993;92:872.

American Medical Association: *Diagnostic and Treatment Guidelines on Domestic Violence.* American Medical Association, 1992.

American Medical Association: *Diagnostic and Treatment Guidelines on Child Sexual Abuse.* American Medical Association, 1992.

Briere J et al: *The APSAC Handbook on Child Maltreatment.* Sage, 1996.

Giardino AP, Christian CW, Giardino ER (editors): *A Practical Guide to the Evaluation of Child Abuse and Neglect.* Sage, 1997.

Heger A, Emans SJ (editors): *Evaluation of the Sexually Abused Child: A Medical Textbook and Photographic Atlas.* Oxford Univ Press, 1992.

Helfer ME, Kempe RS, Krugman RD (editors): *The Battered Child,* 5th ed. Univ Chicago Press, 1997.

Kleinman PK (editor): *Diagnostic Imaging of Child Abuse,* 2nd ed. Williams & Wilkins, 1998.

Olds D et al: Long-term effects of home visitation on maternal life course and child abuse and neglect. JAMA 1997;278:637.

Reece RM (editor): *Child Abuse: Medical Diagnosis and Management.* Lea & Febiger, 1994.

Rosenberg DA: Web of deceit: A literature review of Munchausen syndrome by proxy. Child Abuse Negl 1987;11:547.

Ambulatory Pediatrics

8

Robert M. Brayden, MD & Roxann M. Headley, MD

Pediatric outpatient services provide a child or adolescent with comprehensive longitudinal care and emphasize preventive health care. This chapter discusses common elements of ambulatory visits and offers guidance in the conduct of the health supervision visit, chronic disease follow-up, and consultations. Special attention is paid to the problems of telephone triage, fever, and growth deficiency.

PEDIATRIC HISTORY

The pediatric history is unique in that children do not usually provide their own history. Instead, the parent describes the child's complaints and behavior to the physician, who then interprets what the parent says. The sometimes vague exposition of complaints offered by parents can leave unclear the nature of the symptoms and the sequence in which they appeared. Vague complaints may be statements of the parent's own concerns about the child's progress. Instead of reporting that a child has had a "warm, red, tender, swollen knee for 2 days," the parent may say that the child has "not played well for about a week" or that he "no longer wants to play on the soccer team." Many visits are occasioned by problems at school, such as low grades or troublesome peer relationships. To distinguish organic illness from emotional or behavioral conditions and to intervene appropriately without subjecting the child to unnecessary testing, the physician must understand the family and its hopes for and concerns about the child. It is often necessary to ask specifically what problems the parent wishes to address in order to determine what really prompted the office visit.

It is essential also to obtain as much of the history as possible directly from the patient. Direct histories not only provide firsthand information but also give the child a degree of control over a potentially threatening situation and may reveal important information about the family.

Obtaining a comprehensive pediatric history is time-consuming. Many offices provide questionnaires for parents to complete before the clinician sees the child. Data from questionnaires should make an outpatient visit more productive, allowing the physician to address problems in detail while reviewing and dismissing areas that are not of concern. According to some recent studies, questionnaires may be more productive than face-to-face interviews in revealing sensitive parts of the history. However, failure to study and assimilate this information prior to the interview may cause the distraught parent to feel that the time and effort have been wasted.

Those elements of the history that will be of interest over time must be readily accessible in the medical record. In some practices, such information is accumulated on a summary sheet, as illustrated in Figure 8–1, which may contain demographic data, a problem list, information about chronic medications, allergies, and previous hospitalizations, and the names of other physicians providing care for the patient. It is usually not feasible to maintain immunization data on the front sheet because of the documentation requirements of the National Childhood Vaccine Injury Act. A second page for immunization data is preferable.

The components of a comprehensive pediatric history are listed in Table 8–1. Ideally, these components should be obtained at the first office visit. The first seven items are included on the summary pages. Items 8 and 9 are dealt with during each episodic care visit. The entire list should be reviewed and augmented with relevant updates at each health supervision visit.

PEDIATRIC PHYSICAL EXAMINATION

In approaching the child, time must be taken to allow the patient to become familiar with the examiner. Interactions and instructions help the child under-

Name _____ Nickname _____ D.O.B. _____
Mother _____ Father _____ Sibs _____
S.S. # _____ Insurance _____

Chronic Problems			Chronic Medications		
Date of onset	Description	Date resolved	Start date		Stop date
			Allergies:		
Date	Hospitalizations/Injuries/Procedures		Date	Consultants	

Figure 8–1. Use of a summary sheet such as this at the front of the record facilitates reorienting the caregiver and his or her partners to the patient. Some practices keep track of health supervision visits on this sheet to tell the physician whether the child is likely to have received the appropriate preventive services. Previously, many practices recorded the administration of immunizations on this sheet. However, a second page that lists data required by the National Childhood Vaccine Injury Act may be more useful. When an allergy with potential for anaphylaxis is identified, the patient should wear a medical alert bracelet and obtain an epinephrine kit, if appropriate.

stand what is occurring and what is expected. A gentle, friendly manner and a quiet voice help establish a setting that yields a nonthreatening physical examination. The order in which the child's organ systems are examined should take into consideration the need for a quiet child, the extent of trust established, and the imminence of pain or emotional response. Painful or unpleasant procedures should be deferred until the

end of the examination. Whether or not the physician can establish rapport with the child, the process should proceed efficiently, quickly, and systematically.

Because young children may perceive the examination as fearsome and become fussy, simple inspection is very important. The examiner should make observations throughout the visit, paying special at-

Table 8–1. Components of the pediatric historical database.[1]

1. Demographic data	Patient's name and nickname, date of birth, social security number, sex, race, parents' names (first and last), siblings' name, and payor mechanism
2. Problem list	Major or significant problems, including dates of onset and resolution
3. Allergies	Offending agent, nature of the reaction, treatment needed, and date allergy diagnosed
4. Chronic medications	Name, concentration, dose, and frequency of chronically used medications
5. Birth history	Maternal health during pregnancy, medications, street drugs used, complications of pregnancy; duration and ease of labor; form of delivery; analgesics and anesthetics used; need for monitoring; and labor complications. Infant's birth weight, gestational age, Apgar scores, and problems in the neonatal period
6. Screening procedures	Results of all screening procedures and actions taken should be maintained as a distinct part of the medical record, including newborn screening, vision and hearing screening, any health screen, or screening laboratory tests. (Developmental screening results are maintained in the development section; see 14, below.)
7. Immunizations	Date of each immunization administered, vaccine manufacturer and lot number, and name of the person administering the vaccine; previous reaction and contraindication to immunization (eg, immunodeficiency or an evolving neurologic problem)
8. Reasons for visit	The patient's or parents' concerns, stated in their own words, serve as the focus for the visit
9. Present illness	A concise chronologic summary of the problems necessitating a visit, including the duration, progression, exacerbating factors, ameliorating interventions, and associations
10. Past history state of health	A statement regarding the child's functionality and general well-being, including a summary record of past significant illnesses, injuries, hospitalizations, and procedures
11. Diet	Eating patterns, likes and dislikes, use of vitamins, and relative amounts of carbohydrates, fat, and protein in the diet
12. Family history	Information about the illnesses of relatives, preferably in the form of a family tree
13. Social history	Family constellation, relationships, parents' educational background, religious preference, and the role of the child in the family; socioeconomic profile of the family to identify resources available to the child, access to services that may be needed, and anticipated stressors
14. Development	(1) Attainment of developmental milestones (including developmental testing results); (2) social habits and milestones (toilet habits, play, major activities, sleep patterns, discipline, peer relationships); (3) school progress and documentation of specific achievements and grades
15. Sexual history	Family's sexual attitudes, sex education, sexual development, sexual activity, sexually transmitted diseases, and birth control measures
16. Review of systems (ROS)	This area tends to be overlooked because of the work required to obtain a complete ROS and integrate data into the patient's problems list and care plan. A focused ROS is essential if any problem is to be addressed adequately.

[1]The components of this table should be included in a child's medical record and structured to allow easy review and modification.

tention to how the child interacts with the environment. Observation also affords the examiner a chance to assess parent–child interactions.

Clothing should be removed slowly and gently to avoid chilling or threatening the child. A parent or the child itself is usually the best person to do this. Modesty should always be respected, and drapes should be provided. Examinations of adolescents should be chaperoned whenever a stressful or painful procedure must be performed.

Examination tables are convenient, but a parent's lap is a safe haven for a young child. For most pur-

poses, an adequate examination can be conducted on a "table" formed by the parent's and examiner's legs as they sit facing each other.

The nature of the physical examination changes as the child develops. Table 8–2 sets forth the differences in examination of a 2-month-old child compared with a 14-year-old.

Bates B et al: *A Guide to Physical Diagnosis,* 6th ed. Lippincott, 1995.

Zitelli BJ, David HW (editors): *Atlas of Pediatric Physical Diagnosis,* 2nd ed. Mosby, 1992.

Table 8–2. The focused physical examination, comparing the emphasis for examinations of a 2-month-old and a 14-year-old.

	2-Month-Old	14-Year-Old
Growth	Length, weight, head circumference	Height, weight
Head, eye, ear, nose, & throat	Fontanelles, sutures, intact palate, red reflex, tear ducts, ear pits/deformities	Fundi, dentition
Skin	Birthmarks	Acne, distribution of hair, sequelae of sun exposure
Neck	Sinus tract, residua of torticollis	Thyroid
Chest		Breast development[1]
Cardiovascular	Murmurs, pulses	Blood pressure
Extremities	Physical deformities, proportion	Muscular development
Genitalia	Normal anatomy, descent of testes	Tanner staging[1]
Neurologic	Body position, tone, reflexes	Coordination, abstract reasoning

[1]Some physicians teach breast and testicular self-examination during the physical examination.

PREVENTIVE HEALTH CARE SERVICES

One of several timetables for preventive care services (from the Committee on Practice and Ambulatory Medicine, American Academy of Pediatrics) is illustrated in Figure 8–2. In areas where efficacy data are lacking, expert opinion has been used as the basis for these plans. For example, whereas immunizations are universally understood to be effective and necessary, there is disagreement about whether universal screening for certain metabolic diseases is warranted. The guidelines are no more than that—the practitioner should individualize decisions about services according to the child's needs.

The preventive services visit should be structured to review acute and chronic problems, conduct a complete physical examination, order appropriate screening tests, and anticipate future developments. New historical information should be elicited through an interval history. Development should be subjectively assessed at each visit. Developmental surveillance is further facilitated through the systematic use of a variety of parent questionnaires or screening tests. Vision and hearing should be assessed at each visit, with objective assessments at intervals. Hematocrit, blood lead level, urinalysis, and metabolic screening may also be part of the visit. The examination in the first year of life focuses on possible congenital anomalies. After the first year, the examination focuses on physical development, the progress of any existing disease, and alterations in growth. At each visit, growth is carefully docu-

mented and the growth chart is brought up to date (see Chapter 1).

A major portion of the health maintenance visit is anticipatory guidance. This portion of the visit enables the health care provider to address behavioral, developmental, safety, and nutritional issues that will arise before the next well child care visit.

American Academy of Pediatrics, Committee on Psychosocial Aspects of Child and Family Health: *Guidelines for Health Supervision III,* 3rd ed. American Academy of Pediatrics, 1996.

Green M: *Bright Futures: Guidelines for Health Supervision of Infants, Children, and Adolescents.* National Center for Education in Maternal and Child Health, 1994.

Report of the US Preventive Services Task Force: *Guide to Clinical Preventive Services,* 2nd ed. International Medical Publishing, 1996.

Schmitt BD, Brayden RM, Kempe A: Parent handouts: Cornerstone of a health education program. Contemp Pediatr 1997;14:120.

HEALTH SUPERVISION VISITS

GROWTH PARAMETERS

Height, weight, and head circumference are carefully measured and plotted at each visit during the first 3 years. (Growth charts are presented in Chapter 1.) To ensure accurate weight measurements for longitudinal comparisons, infants should be undressed

Committee on Practice and Ambulatory Medicine

Each child and family is unique; therefore, these **Recommendations for Preventive Pediatric Health Care** are designed for the care of children who are receiving competent parenting, have no manifestations of any important health problems, and are growing and developing in satisfactory fashion. **Additional visits may become necessary** if circumstances suggest variations from normal.

These guidlines represent a consensus by the Committee on Practice and Ambulatory Medicine in consultation with national committees and sections of the American Academy of Pediatrics. The Committee emphasizes the great importance of **continuity of care** in comprehensive health supervision and the need to avoid **fragmentation of care.**

A **prenatal visit** is recommended for parents who are at high risk, for first-time parents, and for those who request a conference. The prenatal visit should include anticipatory guidance and pertinent medical history. Every infant should have a newborn evaluation after birth.

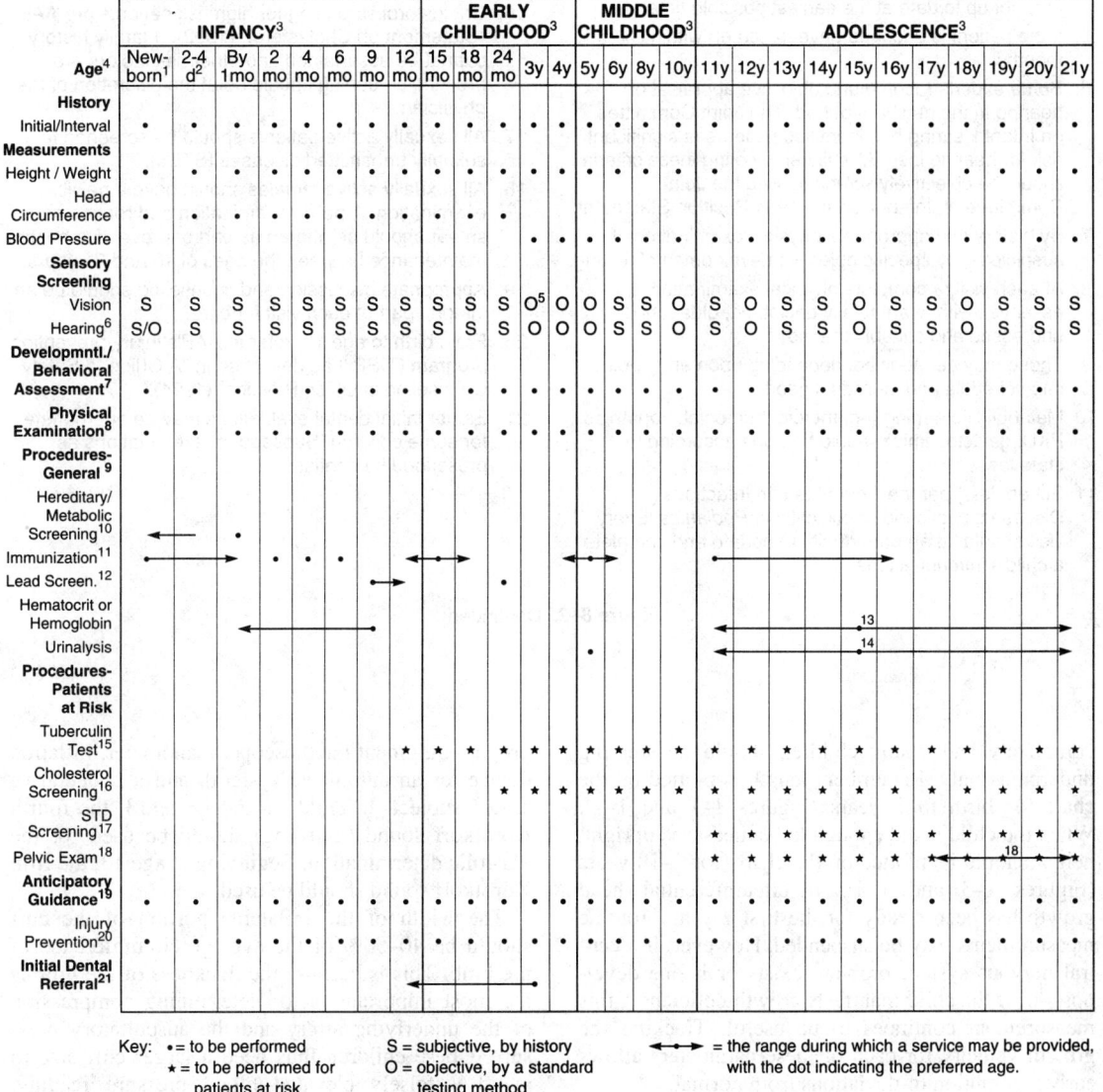

Key: • = to be performed
      ★ = to be performed for patients at risk

S = subjective, by history
O = objective, by a standard testing method

◄—•—► = the range during which a service may be provided, with the dot indicating the preferred age.

NB: Special chemical, immunologic, and endocrine testing is usually carried out upon specific indications. Testing other than newborn (eg. inborn errors of metabolism, sickle disease, etc.) is discretionary with the physician.

The recommendations in this publication do not indicate an exclusive course of treatment or serve as a standard of medical care. Variations, taking into account individual circumstances, may be appropriate.

Figure 8–2. Recommendations for preventive health care.

1. Breastfeeding encouraged and instruction and support offered.
2. For newborns discharged in less than 48 hours after delivery.
3. Developmental, psychosocial, and chronic disease issues for children and adolescents may require frequent counseling and treatment visits separate from preventive care visits.
4. If a child comes under care for the first time at any point on the schedule, or if any items are not accomplished at the suggested age, the schedule should be brought up to date at the earliest possible time.
5. If the patient is uncooperative, rescreen within six months.
6. Some experts recommend objective appraisal of hearing in the newborn period. The Joint Committee on Infant Hearing has identified patients at significant risk for hearing loss. All children meeting these criteria should be objectively screened. See the Joint Committee on Infant Hearing 1994 Position Statement.
7. By history and appropriate physical examination: if suspicious, by specific objective developmental testing.
8. At each visit, a complete physical examination is essential, with infant totally unclothed, older child undressed and suitably draped.
9. These may be modified, depending upon entry point into schedule and individual need.
10. Metabolic screening (eg. thyroid, hemoglobinopathies, PKU, galactosemia) should be done according to state law.
11. Schedule(s) per the Committee on Infectious Diseases, published periodically in *Pediatrics*. Every visit should be an opportunity to update and complete a child's immunizations.
12. Blood lead screen per AAP statement "Lead Poisoning: From Screening to Primary Prevention" (1993).
13. All menstruating adolescents should be screened.
14. Conduct dipstick urinalysis for leukocytes for male and female adolescents.
15. TB testing per AAP statement "Screening for Tuberculosis in Infants and Children" (1994). Testing should be done upon recognition of high risk factors. If results are negative but high risk situation continues, testing should be repeated on an annual basis.
16. Cholesterol screening for high risk patients per AAP "Statement on Cholesterol" (1992). If family history cannot be ascertained and other risk factors are present, screening should be at the discretion of the physician.
17. All sexually active patients should be screened for sexually transmitted diseases (STDs).
18. All sexually active females should have a pelvic examination. A pelvic examination and routine pap smear should be offered as part of preventive health maintenance between the ages of 18 and 21 years.
19. Appropriate discussion and counseling should be an integral part of each visit for care.
20. From birth to age 12, refer to AAP's injury prevention program (TIPP[3]) as described in "A Guide to Safety Counseling in Office Practice" (1994).
21. Earlier initial dental evaluations may be appropriate for some children. Subsequent examinations as prescribed by dentist.

Figure 8–2. Continued

completely and young children should be wearing underpants only. Recumbent length is plotted on the chart for birth to 3 years (Figures 1–1 and 1–2). When the child is old enough to be measured upright, height should be plotted on the charts for 2–18 years (Figures 1–3 and 1–4). If circumferential head growth has been steady for the first 2 years, routine measurements may be suspended. However, if a central nervous system problem exists or if one develops—or if the child manifests growth deficiency, this measurement continues to be useful. Tracking the growth velocity for each of these parameters allows early recognition of deviations from normal.

BLOOD PRESSURE

Blood pressure screening at well child visits should be started at 3 years of age. If the child has a renal or cardiac abnormality, a blood pressure reading should be obtained at each visit regardless of age. Accurate determination of blood pressure requires proper equipment (stethoscope, manometer, inflation device, or an automated system), and a cooperative seated subject. In children under age 13, the fourth Korotkoff sound (muffling) should be used for the diastolic determination. Beginning at age 13, the fifth Korotkoff sound should be used.

The width of the inflatable portion of the cuff should be 40–50% of the average circumference of the limb. This is because the thickness of the limb is the most important factor determining compression of the underlying artery and the auscultatory pressure. Obese children thus need a larger cuff size to avoid a falsely elevated blood pressure reading. Cuffs that are too narrow will overestimate and those that are too wide will underestimate the true blood pressure.

Blood pressure norms are given in Table 18–5.

Park MK: Physical examination. In: *Pediatric Cardiology for Practitioners*, 3rd ed. Mosby Year Book, 1996.
Perloff D et al: Human blood pressure determination by sphygmomanometry. Circulation 1993;88:2460.

VISION & HEARING

The neonate's eyes should be equal in size. The anterior chamber should be inspected for evidence of bleeding that may have been the result of birth trauma. The presence of bilateral red reflexes on ophthalmoscopic examination rules out opacification from congenital cataracts or retinoblastoma. Photophobia, excessive tearing, or clouding of the cornea may be signs of glaucoma. By 1 month of age, infants should focus on a face. From infancy until age 3 years, the parents should be queried for evidence that the child has satisfactory vision. Beginning at 3 years of age, office screening of vision using Allen cards or the Snellen tumbling E chart should be attempted. Each eye is tested separately. Credit is given for any line on which the child gets more than 50% correct. A child who is unable to follow the instructions should be tested again in 6 months. Because visual acuity improves with age, results of the test are interpreted using the cutoff values in Table 8–3; however, a two-line discrepancy between the two eyes should prompt evaluation of visual acuity by an ophthalmologist or optometrist. Throughout the preschool years, the clinician should screen for undetected strabismus (ocular misalignment) and amblyopia (loss of vision from disuse). The corneal light reflex test, the cover test, and visual acuity testing are described further in Chapter 14.

Audiometric screening for all newborns using evoked otoacoustic emissions is a subject of controversy. All neonates at high risk for hearing loss, however, should be tested (see Chapter 16). During infancy and toddlerhood, hearing can be assessed by asking the parent and by using simple office tools such as shaking rattles or snapping the fingers. Pure tone audiometry in the office is feasible beginning at 3 years of age. The clinician should become familiar with the numerous risk factors associated with hearing loss and screen individuals with these conditions as appropriate. (See Chapter 16 for further details.)

US Public Health Service: Vision screening in children. Am Fam Physician 1994;50:587.

Table 8–3. Age-appropriate visual acuity.[1]

Age (years)	Minimal Acceptable Acuity
3	20/40
4	20/30
5	20/20

[1]Refer to an ophthalmologist if minimal acuity is not met at a given age or if there is a difference in scores of two or more lines between the eyes.

DEVELOPMENTAL & BEHAVIORAL ASSESSMENT

At each visit, the parent should be interviewed about all aspects of the child's development. Questionnaires or formal screening tests such as the Denver II may help to objectively document development. Other helpful tests are the Denver Articulation Screening Examination, the Early Language Milestone Scale, and the Parents' Evaluations of Developmental Status (PEDS). The school-age child's cognitive function is assessed indirectly through academic achievement, and his or her emotional well-being is screened by interview and observation. Behaviors appropriate for age are reviewed at each visit. These behaviors include feeding, sleep, elimination, self-stimulating behaviors (thumbsucking, rocking, head-banging, masturbation), and recurrent pain syndromes (headache, chest pain, abdominal pain, limb pain). Observation of parent–child interactions (eg, feeding, compliance tasks) may provide the clinician with important information to help shape behavioral counsel. The child's temperament and the family's disciplinary techniques are important considerations before providing advice.

LABORATORY SCREENING

Newborn Screening

Use of screening tests for relatively common or early-onset and severe inborn errors of metabolism is commonly called "newborn screening." Blood is collected from the newborn infant before hospital discharge, and the results are usually available within a week. In some states, newborn screens are repeated at outpatient visits within the first 2 weeks of life.

All 50 states in the USA mandate newborn screening for phenylketonuria and congenital hypothyroidism. Without diagnosis, both diseases result in severe mental retardation, but early treatment maintains cognitive function in the normal range. Other diseases for which screening is required by law vary from state to state, but the lists may include galactosemia, homocystinuria, biotinidase deficiency, adrenal hyperplasia, cystic fibrosis, hemoglobinopathies, maple syrup urine disease, tyrosinemia, and toxoplasmosis. Although some of the diseases are rare, the burden of suffering they cause is heavy, and the effectiveness of early intervention is, for the most part, quite good. Screening tests are usually accurate but false negatives and false positives do occur. If symptoms of a disease are present despite a negative screening test, the infant should be tested further. Because cutoff levels for normal values of the test are established to reduce false negatives and because of administrative or laboratory errors, false positives are often more common than true positives. If the screening test is reported as positive, a confirmatory test must be sent and parental anxiety addressed.

Lead Toxicity

The developing infant and child are at special risk for lead exposure. Blood lead levels over 55 µg/dL can produce multiorgan system effects such as colic, nausea, nephritis, muscle aches, encephalopathy, seizures, headache, and anemia. Children with low levels (10–25 µg/dL) may have more behavior problems, more learning disabilities, and lower IQs than cohorts with levels below 10 µg/dL—and these effects persist into later life. The primary source of lead exposure in this country remains lead-based paint, even though most of its uses have been banned since 1977. Probably because of environmental controls such as the elimination of leaded gasolines and paints as well as public service educational efforts, lead levels have declined nationally from a mean of 16 µg/dL in 1976 to about 5 µg/dL today. However, considerable variation exists in different parts of the United States.

Caregivers of children between the ages of 6 months and 6 years may be screened by questionnaire for possible environmental risk factors for lead exposure (Table 8–4). If risks factors are present, a blood lead level should be obtained. In some states and communities, routine screening of blood lead levels should be performed at 9–12 months and at 2 years of age regardless of the presence of risk factors. In other locations, blood lead screening is recommended only for targeted groups of children. Targeted screening is recommended in communities where less than 12% of children have blood lead levels above 10 µg/dL or where <27% of the houses were built before 1950. In all states, public health authorities are responsible for setting policy on lead screening.

A venous sample is preferred over a capillary specimen. Blood lead levels below 10 µg/dL are acceptable. The cognitive development of children with confirmed blood levels over 14 µg/dL should be

Table 8–4. Lead exposure screening questionnaire.[1]

Does your child—
1. Live in or regularly visit a house with peeling or chipping paint built before 1960? This could include a day care center, preschool, the home of a babysitter or relative, etc.
2. Live in or regularly visit a house built before 1960 with recent, ongoing, or planned renovation or remodeling?
3. Have a brother or sister, housemate, or playmate being followed up or treated for lead poisoning (ie, blood level ≥ 15 µg/dL)?
4. Live with an adult whose job or hobby involves exposure to lead?
5. Live near an active lead smelter, battery recycling plant, or other industry likely to release lead?

[1]From the Centers for Disease Control and Prevention.

evaluated and attempts made to identify the environmental source. Iron deficiency should be treated if present. Chelation of lead should be considered for levels above 25 µg/dL and is urgently required for levels of 70 µg/dL or more. As more data are collected, low-risk communities may be identified where routine blood lead screening is unnecessary.

Anemia

Iron deficiency is the most common cause of anemia in young children, though the incidence has declined in recent years due, in large part, to the use of iron-fortified formulas in the first year. Risk factors for iron deficiency include prematurity, small for gestational age (SGA) status, multiple pregnancy, iron deficiency in the mother, use of nonfortified formula or cow's milk before 12 months, chronic illness, restricted diet, and extensive blood loss. Asymptomatic iron deficiency anemia in the young child has been associated with behavioral and developmental problems, and deficits persist into school age despite correction of the anemia.

Primary prevention of iron deficiency should be achieved through dietary means including feeding infants iron-containing cereals by six months of age, the avoidance of low-iron milks during infancy, and the limiting of cow's milk to 24 ounces per day in children aged 1–5 years. Recommendations for screening for iron deficiency vary with the presence of the above risk factors. A screening hemoglobin or hematocrit for high-risk children between the ages of 6 and 12 months is recommended and should be considered annually through age 5 years. Therefore, screening of infants at 9 months of age seems reasonable. A screening hematocrit is recommended for pregnant teenagers.

Hypercholesterolemia & Hyperlipidemia

The benefits and risks of screening for hypercholesterolemia and hyperlipidemia in children are at present undecided. If either parent has a cholesterol level above 240 mg/dL, it may be prudent to screen children older than age 2 years. If there is a history of cardiovascular disease before age 55 in a parent or grandparent, a complete lipoprotein analysis (fasting cholesterol, high-density lipoproteins, low-density lipoproteins, triglycerides) is recommended. For all children, a prudent diet is advised (see below).

Bacteriuria

There is controversy also about screening asymptomatic children for bacteriuria. For infant males, the prevalence of asymptomatic bacteriuria is 2–4%, and for girls in the early grade school years it is 5–6%. It is assumed (though not proved) that detection and treatment of asymptomatic bacteriuria may prevent pyelonephritis and the possible subsequent development of renal scarring. The dipstick urinalysis, including a nitrite test for bacteriuria and a leukocyte esterase test for pyuria, is an inexpensive screening test, but the 20% false-positive rate indicates that children must be rescreened or the urine must be cultured, thus increasing the cost substantially. The United States Preventive Services Task Force recommends not screening for asymptomatic bacteriuria in children.

Tuberculosis

In 1996 in the USA, 1372 new cases of tuberculosis were reported in children under 15 years of age. Well child care should include assessment of risk for exposure to tuberculosis, and tuberculosis screening should be based on high-risk status. High-risk infants, children, and adolescents include those with infectious or high-risk contacts; those who are immunosuppressed, including HIV–positive persons; those who have resided in or traveled to areas of high prevalence (Asia, Pacific Islands, Middle East, Africa, Latin America); those with a chest radiograph suggesting disease; and those with clinical symptoms. The Mantoux test is the recommended screening test beginning as early as 3 months of age and repeated annually if the risk persists. The tine test should not be used.

Screening of Adolescent Patients

Screening adolescents for blood cholesterol, tuberculosis, and HIV should be offered based on high-risk criteria outlined in this chapter and in Chapter 35. During routine visits, adolescents should be sensitively questioned about sexually transmitted disease risk factors (eg, multiple partners; early onset of sexual activity, including child sexual abuse), and STD symptoms (eg, genital discharge, infectious lesions, pelvic pain). Teenage girls who are sexually active and all girls regardless of sexual experience aged 18 years and over should have a Papanicolaou smear. This test should be performed at least every 3 years thereafter and more frequently in patients with STD risk factors. Because females with STDs are often not symptomatic, gonococcal and chlamydial cultures and screening tests for syphilis, human papillomavirus infection, and trichomoniasis are appropriate at the time of each Papanicolaou smear.

American Academy of Pediatrics, Committee on Environmental Health: Screening for elevated blood lead levels. Pediatrics 1998;101:1072.

American Academy of Pediatrics, Committee on Genetics: Issues in newborn screening. Pediatrics 1992;89:345.

American Academy of Pediatrics, Committee on Infectious Diseases: Update on tuberculosis skin testing in children. Pediatrics 1996;97:282.

American Medical Association, Department of Adolescent Health: *Guidelines for Adolescent Preventive Services Recommendations Monograph,* 2nd ed. American Medical Association, 1995.

Centers for Disease Control and Prevention. Recommendations to Prevent and Control Iron Deficiency in the United States. MMWR 1998;47(RR-3):1–29.

Table 8–5. Preventive handouts for health supervision visits.[1]

Age	Suggested Topics
2 weeks	Sleep problems: Prevention
2 months	Passive smoking
4 months	Weaning problems: Prevention
6 months	Teething
12 months	Temper tantrums
18 months	Toilet training basics
2 years	Time-out technique
3 years	Spoiled children: Prevention
4 years	Sex education for preschoolers
5 years	Television: Reducing the negative impact
6 years	School work: Preventing problems
8 years	Siblings' arguments and quarrels
10 years	R-rated movies
12 years	Adolescents: Dealing with normal rebellion

[1]Adapted and reproduced, with permission, from *Contemporary Pediatrics*. The guides listed here are available on request as a set containing a single photocopy of each guide, which you may duplicate for distribution to families in your practice without permission. Please request by letter to Parent Guides, Contemporary Pediatrics, 5 Paragon Drive, Montvale, NJ 07645, enclosing five dollars to defray the cost of postage and handling. Allow several weeks for delivery.

Peter G, Hall CB, Orenstein WA (editors): *1997 Red Book: Report of the Committee on Infectious Diseases,* 24th ed. American Academy of Pediatrics, 1997.

Report of the US Preventive Services Task Force: Guide to Clinical Preventive Services, 2nd ed. International Medical Publishing, 1996.

ANTICIPATORY GUIDANCE

A major portion of the health supervision visit is anticipatory guidance. This feature of the visit enables the clinician to direct the parent's or the older child's attention to issues that may arise in future. Guidance must be appropriate to age and should focus on—but not be limited to—any concerns expressed by the parent or patient. Anticipatory guidance should focus in depth on issues most relevant to that child rather than run through a number of issues superficially. A combination of oral and printed presentations may be used. Handouts are an important supplement to anticipatory guidance. A routine schedule for preventive handouts is shown on Table 8–5. Areas of concern include diet, injury prevention, developmental and behavioral issues, and health promotion. Injury prevention is discussed below; other topics are found in other sections of this book.

Injury Prevention

Injuries are the leading cause of death in children and adolescents after the first year of life (Figure 8–3). For young people aged 15–24 years, injuries are responsible for more than 75% of deaths. Each year, 16 million visits to emergency departments are occasioned by injuries to children and adolescents, and more than 500,000 of these patients are hospitalized.

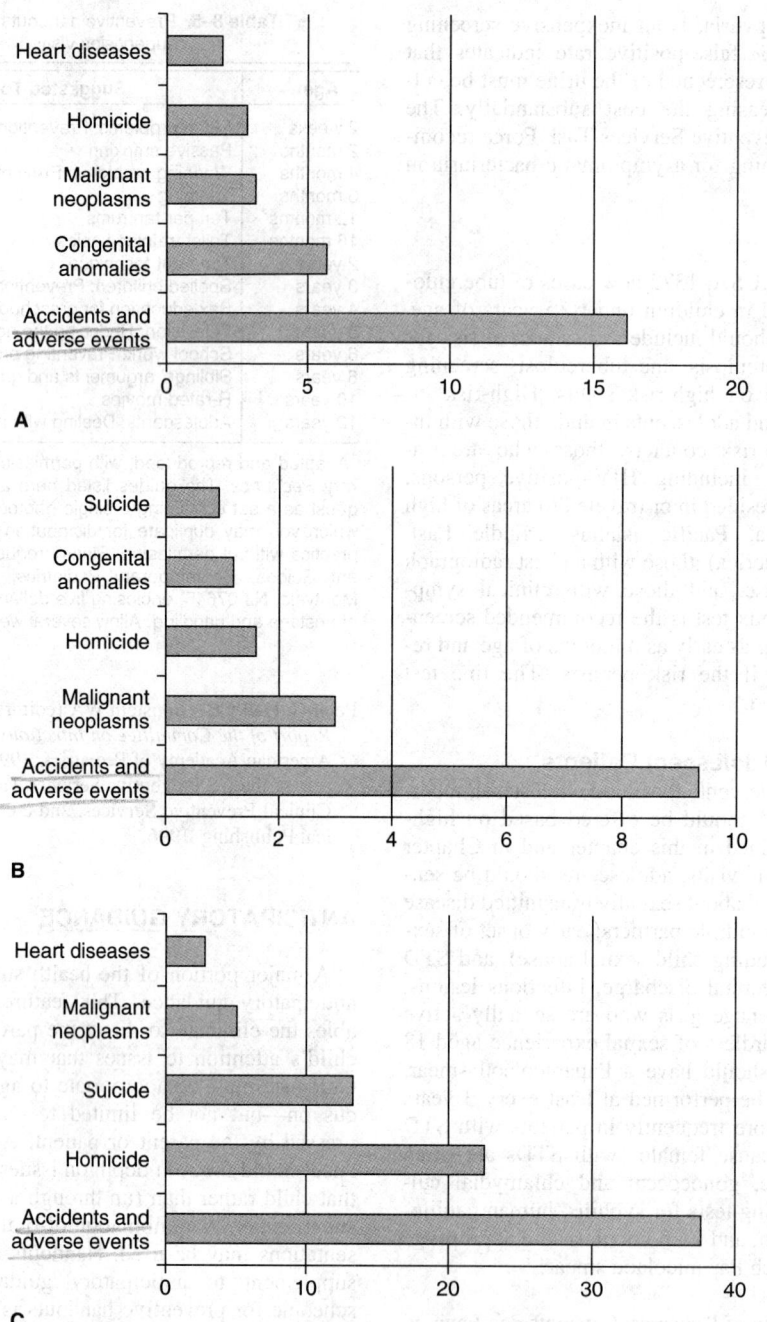

Figure 8–3. Leading causes of death in children **(A)** at 1–4 years, **(B)** at 5–14 years, and **(C)** at 15–24 years of age (the 1992 rate per 100,000 population). (From the National Center for Health Statistics.)

In the case of physical injury to a young child, the physician must recognize that some injuries may be intentional or the result of parental neglect.

Injury prevention counseling should be part of each health supervision visit and can be reinforced at episodic visits. Counseling should focus on problems that are frequent and age-appropriate. Passive strategies of prevention should be emphasized, as these are more effective than active strategies; for example, encouraging the use of childproof cupboard latches to prevent poisoning will be more effective than instructing parents to watch their children closely.

A questionnaire to assess the safety of the home, such as The Injury Prevention Program (TIPP),* can be completed in the waiting room. Advice can then be tailored to the specific needs of each family, with reinforcement from age-specific TIPP handouts.

Advocacy on behalf of children and adolescents for safety legislation and community safety programs should involve the entire community. A community program in Seattle to promote the use of bicycle helmets has resulted in an increase in helmet use from 2% to nearly 40%. The primary care provider is in an ideal position to identify high-risk situations and intervene before injury occurs. For example, if a teenager has emotional problems (eg, depression) and history of driving violations, the clinician should consider interventions that could prevent a motor vehicle accident.

A. Motor Vehicle Injuries: The foremost killer and crippler of children in the United States is the motor vehicle. Car safety seats for children are required in this country, and their use could reduce vehicle-associated fatalities and hospitalizations by at least 50%. The type of safety seat to be used depends on the child's weight: less than 20 lb, rear-facing infant seat, avoiding seats with airbags; 20–40 lb, forward-facing toddler seat; 40–60 lb, shield booster seat with lap belt. For children over 60 lb, a regular lap belt should be used. When children are over 4 feet, a shoulder strap with lap belt should be used.

When a child is a passenger in a car crash, the case fatality rate is 1%; for children hit by cars, the risk of fatality increases threefold.

Using a cellular telephone while driving is associated with a fourfold increase in motor vehicle accidents. Parents and others should be advised of this risk.

B. Bicycle Injuries: Head trauma accounts for three-fourths of all bicycle-related fatalities. More than 85% of brain injuries can be prevented through the use of bicycle helmets.

C. Firearm Injuries: In the United States, an average of 14 children and adolescents are killed every day by firearms. Injuries from firearms are more frequent for young people aged 15–24 years than for any other age group, and black males are especially vulnerable. Some gun deaths may be accidental, but most are the result of homicide or suicide. A gun in the home doubles the likelihood of a lethal suicide attempt. Although handguns are often kept in homes for protection, a gun is more likely to kill a family member or a friend than an intruder. The most effective way to prevent firearm injuries is to remove guns from the home. However, if families keep firearms at home, they should be advised to store them in a locked cabinet or drawer and to store ammunition separately.

*Available from the American Pediatric Association, Publications Department, 141 Northwest Point Blvd, PO Box 927, Elk Grove Village, IL 60007; phone 1-800-433-9016).

D. Drowning and Near Drowning: Children between the ages of 1 and 3 years have the highest rate of drowning. In some warm weather states (especially Arizona, California, and Florida), drowning deaths exceed the number of deaths caused by motor vehicle or pedestrian accidents. For every death by drowning, six children are hospitalized for near drowning, and up to 10% of survivors suffer severe brain damage. Children under 1 year of age are most likely to drown in the bathtub; for children 1–4 years of age, drowning or near drowning occurs most often in home swimming pools; and for school-age children and teens, drowning occurs most often in bodies of water. Home pools must be securely fenced, and parents should know how to perform cardiopulmonary resuscitation. School-age children should be taught to swim, but recreational swimming should always be supervised.

E. Burn Injuries: Burns are the leading cause of injury-related deaths in the home. Categories of burn injury include smoke inhalation, flame contact, scalding, and electrical, chemical, and ultraviolet burns, with scalding being the most common type in children. Most scalds involve foods and beverages, but nearly one-fourth of scalds are with tap water, and for that reason it is recommended that hot water heaters be set to less than 54 °C (130° F). The greatest number of fire-related deaths result from smoke inhalation. Smoke detectors can prevent 85% of the injuries and deaths caused by fires in the home. Families should practice emergency evacuation from the home.

Committee on Injury and Poison Prevention: Office-based counseling for injury prevention. Pediatrics 1994; 94:566.

Hazinski MF et al: Pediatric injury prevention. Ann Emerg Med 1993;22:456.

Monthly Vital Statistics Report: National Center for Health Statistics, Centers for Disease Control and Prevention, 1997, page 39. (www.cdc.gov/nchswww/fastats/volodex1.htm)

PRUDENT DIET

Iron-fortified formula or breast milk should be used for the first year of life, after which whole cow's milk can be given. Because of continued rapid growth and high energy needs, children should continue to drink whole milk until 2 years of age. Baby foods are generally introduced around 6 months of age.

By 2 years of age, a prudent diet consists of diverse food sources, encourages high-fiber foods (eg, fruits, vegetables, and grain products), and limits sodium and fat intake. Specific nutrient guidelines include the following:

Carbohydrates: about 55% of total calories
Protein: about 15–20% of total calories
Total fat: < 30% of total calories

Saturated fat: < 10% of total calories
Cholesterol: < 300 mg/d

IMMUNIZATIONS

A child's immunization status can easily be monitored in the medical record database. Parents also should keep an immunization record book. Immunization schedules and other details are presented in Chapter 9.

To improve immunization rates, clinicians should screen records and administer required immunizations at every type of visit, including acute care visits for minor illnesses. Clinicians should administer all needed vaccinations simultaneously and should develop recall and reminder systems to prompt vaccination visits. Flexible appointment scheduling, nurse administration protocols, short waiting times, and repeated emphasis on the importance and timing of immunizations can remove some of the barriers to early and complete vaccination.

OTHER TYPES OF OFFICE VISITS

ACUTE CARE VISITS

The acute care visit must be an efficient, structured routine. Office personnel should determine the reason for the visit, obtain a brief synopsis of the child's symptoms, and list known drug allergies. The physician should document the events related to the presenting problem together with a physical examination. The record should include a diagnosis and supporting laboratory data. Treatments and follow-up instructions must be recorded, including when to return to the office if the problem is not ameliorated. Immunization status should be screened and appropriate vaccinations given.

PRENATAL VISITS

Ideally, a couple's first trip to a physician's office should take place before the birth of the baby. A prenatal visit goes a long way toward establishing trust and enables the physician to learn about a family's expectations, concerns, and fears regarding the anticipated birth of a child. If the infant develops a problem during the newborn period, the physician who has not already met the family may have difficulty establishing rapport. Prenatal visits should be conducted in a relaxed atmosphere, with both parents present if possible.

A prenatal visit provides an easy way to acquaint parents with how the practice is conducted, its hours of operation, after-hours coverage, appointment scheduling, and billing. Parents want to know whom they will speak to when they call the office, when they may bring in children for acute care visits, and how their concerns will be dealt with.

PRESCHOOL VISITS

Development, elimination patterns, social behavior, and diet should be assessed at preschool visits between 3 and 5 years of age. Development and social behavior will affect the child's adjustment to school. Control of bladder and bowel functions is important to successful school entry, and vision and hearing should be screened at this time. Families should be advised of the goals of a "preschool" visit and should be encouraged to come in prior to having their child "out of the home" whether the reason be the start of kindergarten or day care.

SPORTS PHYSICALS

The purpose of the preparticipation health evaluation is to determine whether a child can safely participate in organized sports activity. Attention should be directed toward those parts of the body that are most vulnerable to the stresses of sports. The history and physical examination should focus on the following systems: cardiovascular (stenotic lesions, hypertension, surgery), respiratory (asthma), vision, genitourinary (absence or loss of function of one organ), gastrointestinal (hepatosplenomegaly, hernia), skin (infection), musculoskeletal (inflammation, dysfunction), and neurologic (concussions, uncontrolled seizures). The sports physical should include counseling about medication usage (eg, diuretic, steroid, and beta-blocker abuse, changes in insulin requirements), protective equipment, proper supervision and instruction, injury management, and the emotional aspects of competition and teamwork. The physician may wish to suggest sports that will be compatible with the child's size, strength, endurance, and agility. The potential for mild menstrual irregularities should be explained to the adolescent female athlete. The athlete with moderate to severe menstrual irregularities should be referred for endocrinologic evaluation. Anticipatory guidance should address nutritional needs to maintain growth, cessation of activity when pain occurs, and fluid and electrolyte availability to avoid dehydration.

CHRONIC DISEASE FOLLOW-UP

A chronic illness is defined as one that has been present for more than 3 months. When both the history from the parent and the physical examination are used to find cases of chronic disease, rates are 25% for children and 35% for adolescents. Only about 10% of children with chronic conditions will have a functional impairment.

The family's emotional responses to the child with chronic illness should be addressed, and referrals to counselors should be offered if needed. Specialty referrals need to be monitored and results recorded in the chart in an organized manner. Chronic problems often mean chronic medications and the need to monitor their use. Notes should be made in the chart whenever a prescription is refilled. A medication summary page in the chart allows easy access to the drug history and is a convenient place to make notes such as when the anticonvulsant level was last checked and what it was at that time (Figure 8–4). Children with medical appliances such as gastrostomy tubes and indwelling intravenous and bladder catheters need advice on their management. Nutritional intake is often complicated and must be closely and carefully monitored.

Ludder-Jackson P, Vessey JA: *Primary Care of the Child with a Chronic Condition,* 2nd ed. Mosby Year Book, 1990.

COUNSELING

Topics amenable to office counseling include family upheavals such as separation, divorce, or remarriage; behavioral issues such as negativism and noncompliance, temper tantrums, oppositional behavior, biting, attention deficit disorder, childhood fears, and feeding disorders; school problems; deaths of family members or close friends; and parenting. Forty-five minutes is usually enough time for the therapeutic process to evolve, and this time should be protected from interruption. The young child is usually interviewed with the parent; school-age children and adolescents benefit from time alone with the physician. After assessing the situation in one or two sessions, the primary care physician must decide whether the

Medication: _____

Date	Tablet Size or Liquid Concentration	Sig.	Disp.	Number of Refills	Approved by	Called by	Pharmacy and Phone No.

Figure 8–4. Medication summary sheet.

child's and family's needs are within his or her area of expertise or whether referral to another professional such as a psychologist or a education specialist would be appropriate.

CONSULTATIONS*

Referring Source

Children may be referred to a general pediatrician for consultation by a parent who desires a second opinion regarding a specific problem; by another physician, such as a subspecialist or family physician; by other professionals, such as school officials, nurses, psychologists, or social workers; or by an insurance company wanting a second opinion. Consultations usually require one or two 45- to 60-minute appointments. When the patient is referred to a pediatric consultant, the number of visits and the extent of service should be specified. A screening questionnaire, completed in advance by a parent, should delineate the patient's physical, intellectual, and emotional problems and serve as an initial database.

A. Evaluation Only: The consultant can conduct a diagnostic evaluation and tell the parents only that the findings will be conveyed to the primary care physician. Parents generally do not like this approach. They are paying for the consultation, and they want to hear something from the expert.

B. Evaluation and Interpretation: After the evaluation is completed, the consultant may discuss the diagnosis and the causes of the problems with the family. Recommendations for therapy can be reviewed in general terms and with the clear understanding that the referring physician will be coordinating the therapy. A specific return appointment date with the referring physician should be scheduled. The consultant may be called on periodically to reassess the response to therapy and to offer revised recommendations.

C. Evaluation and Treatment of an Isolated Problem: The referring physician usually wants the consultant to assume responsibility for management of the problem that is the subject of the referral. In most cases, treatable problems such as recurrent headaches, encopresis, and growth deficiency will require only two to four visits. The consultant should clearly reinforce the referring physician's role as the continuing provider of health supervision and acute illness care during this interval. When the problem is resolved, the patient should be returned to the referring physician for resumption of all health care.

Communication With the Referring Source

Communication is the key to a satisfactory referral process. The pediatric consultant may send the referral source a brief note acknowledging the referral and requesting additional information. The final consultation report should be sent promptly, with content appropriate for the referring source. School officials usually want to know only whether the patient is physically healthy or, if not, what their responsibility is. A referring physician expects a full report. Recommendations should be specific (drugs, dosages, other forms of therapy, duration of therapy, specific laboratory tests, etc). A copy of or reference to a recent review article on the subject will also be appreciated.

A medical evaluation should contain a factual summary of the history, physical examination, laboratory, and radiologic findings. Families are grateful if a copy is sent to them for their information and records. Some cases require a brief telephone interaction in addition to the written report. Examples would be situations in which the patient needs to return to the referring physician before a consultation report can be sent, the patient needs to be referred to another specialist or needs laboratory or imaging studies, or a question exists about proper disposition.

At the end of the consultation, the parents should be told when the patient should see the primary physician—usually in 1–2 weeks. Positive comments about the referring physician's competence and judgment serve to support the primary physician-patient relationship. The parents must feel confident that the primary physician can provide the necessary followup care. If the referring physician had tentatively made the correct diagnosis prior to referral, the consultant's corroboration should be made clear to the parents and included in the consultation report.

Bailie MD et al: Making consultation and referrals count. Contemp Pediatr 1988;5:96.

TELEPHONE TRIAGING & ADVICE*

The physician is the person best qualified to give medical advice, both in the office and over the phone. However, most questions require only routine answers and can be handled by a trained office nurse. Office policies about medical advice over the phone should be standardized. Routine instructions for handling minor infections, minor injuries, reactions to immunizations, infant feeding problems, newborn care, and prescription refills are easy to communicate to parents if they are written in an office protocol book. The protocol book should also specify the point at which each problem requires an office visit. This decision depends on (1) the type and duration of the symptom, (2) the age of the patient, (3) whether or not the patient acts "very sick," (4) an assessment of the calling caregiver's anxiety, and (5) the presence of any underlying chronic disease. (For example, most patients under 1 year of age with diarrhea

---

*Contributed by Barton D. Schmitt, MD.

*Contributed by Barton D. Schmitt, MD.

and vomiting need to be seen.) After telephone base-line data are gathered, the nurse must be able to decide whether the child needs to be seen immediately, should be seen later by appointment, or can be safely cared for at home. In doubtful cases, the nurse should err on the side of seeing the patient. For all calls, pertinent telephone data should be recorded and saved. In most cases, it does not need to be entered into the patient's chart.

Parents should understand that during office hours nurses will manage all calls except emergency calls and that weekend, evening, and nighttime calls should be restricted to emergencies or urgent problems that cannot wait until the next office day. Many calls are from anxious, inexperienced parents who need reassurance and acceptance, not criticism. Their interaction with the nurse should help to build confidence. Parents can be asked what they had considered doing, and that plan of action should be endorsed if possible. As parents become more confident and independent, unnecessary calls and visits will be less frequent. However, the nurse should convey the impression that telephone calls are indeed important and that the parent should not hesitate to call whenever he or she is concerned.

The physician accepts some calls: (1) true emergencies, (2) calls from physicians and other professionals, (3) calls regarding hospitalized patients, (4) calls from a parent who demands to talk to the physician, and (5) calls about problems the nurse is uncertain how to manage. Telephone calls that come after the office is closed may be handled in the same way. A nurse—either one from the practice or one under contract with a commercial telephone service—can take the call initially. A physician must be available as backup to the nurse.

There are four other methods of dealing with telephone calls, none of which serves as an acceptable alternative to having an office nurse screen calls and give telephone advice: (1) The physician can accept calls at any time throughout the day. These interruptions are unacceptable to most physicians and to most families who are in the office at the time. (2) The physician can have a "telephone hour" at the beginning, middle, and end of the day and accept only emergency calls at other times. The disadvantages of this approach are that some parents must then wait for answers to urgent questions, and the physician lengthens his or her day with many routine calls. (3) The physician may charge for telephone advice. This decreases the number of calls but may discourage important calls and thus inhibit preventive pediatrics. (4) The physician can permit nonmedical office personnel to accept telephone calls. This approach would result in inconsistent medical advice and could be dangerous. The physician is of course legally liable for any harm to a patient caused by improper advice given over the phone by employees.

Another option is recorded telephone advice. Commercial services are available that allow the caller to choose from a list of hundreds of recorded health topics. A dedicated phone line or menu allows the caller to access the messages. These technologies can be used to inform families about infectious illnesses present in the community, their home management, and symptoms that should cause the parent to seek medical care for the child.

Schmitt BD: *Pediatric Telephone Protocols,* 4th ed. Decision Press, 1997.

FEVER*

Pediatricians are called on daily to evaluate children with fever, defined as a rectal temperature over 38 °C, an oral temperature over 37.5 °C, or an axillary temperature over 37.2 °C.

Body temperature normally fluctuates during the day and may be 0.5 °C below normal in the morning, progressing to 0.5 °C above normal in the evening. Mild elevations of 1–1.5 °C can be caused by exercise, excessive clothing, a hot bath, or hot weather. Warm food or drink can elevate an oral temperature; therefore, if one of these causes is suspected, the temperature should be taken again in 30 minutes.

Fever occurs when there is a rise in the hypothalamic set-point (caused by infection, malignancy, collagen-vascular disease, some drugs, etc), when the body's heat production or environmental heat exceeds heat loss mechanisms (as in malignant hyperthermia, excessive environmental heat), or when heat loss mechanisms are defective (as in ectodermal dysplasia). The vast majority of fevers are caused by viral infections and last no longer than 3 days. There is little relationship between fever magnitude and serious bacterial infection until the temperature exceeds 40.6 °C. Teething does not cause fever over 38.4 °C.

Fever causes no harm, such as brain damage, when it is less than 41.7 °C. Fortunately, the brain's thermostat keeps untreated fevers resulting from infection below 41.1 °C. While all children have fever on occasion, only 4% develop a febrile convulsion. The febrile seizure itself is generally harmless, but it does indicate the need to rule out a serious condition, especially meningitis.

Guidelines for Evaluating Children With Fever

A. **See Immediately If:**
(1) The child is less than 3 months old.
(2) The fever is over 40.6 °C.
(3) The child is crying inconsolably or whimpering.
(4) The child cries when moved or even touched.
(5) The child is difficult to awaken.

---

*Contributed by Barton D. Schmitt, MD.

(6) The neck is stiff.

(7) Purple spots or dots are present on the skin.

(8) Breathing is difficult, and no better after the nasal passages are cleared.

(9) The child is drooling saliva and is unable to swallow anything.

(10) A convulsion has occurred.

(11) The child acts or looks "very sick."

B. See Within 24 Hours If:

(1) The child is 3–6 months old (unless fever occurs within 48 hours after a DTP vaccination and the infant has no other serious symptoms).

(2) The fever exceeds 40 °C (especially if the child is under 3 years old).

(3) Burning or pain occurs with urination.

(4) The fever has been present for more than 24 hours without an obvious cause or identified site of infection.

(5) The fever subsided for more than 24 hours and then returned.

(6) The fever has been present for more than 72 hours.

Types of Thermometers

Glass (with mercury) thermometers are inexpensive, but they record the temperature slowly, are often hard to read, and must be disinfected after each use. Oral temperatures are accurate provided no hot or cold drinks or foods have been consumed in the preceding 20 minutes. Axillary temperatures are the least accurate but better than no measurement. Rectal temperatures are uncomfortable and embarrassing for children and are now rarely taken. The thermometer must be left in place for 2 minutes for rectal, 3 minutes for oral, and 5–6 minutes for axillary temperatures.

Digital thermometers measure quickly and, in some studies, have been more accurate than glass thermometers. Tympanic thermometers read the temperature of the eardrum and are probably as accurate as the rectal temperature if used properly. Temperatures are measured in less than 2 seconds without discomfort, and the cooperation of the child is not essential.

Liquid crystal strips applied to the forehead are inaccurate and miss fevers in many children. Touching the forehead also tends to miss mild fevers.

Treatment of Fever

A. "Fever Phobia" and the Overtreatment of Fever: "Fever phobia" is a term that describes the parents' anxious response to the fevers that all children experience. Schmitt's study (1980) found that 80% of parents thought fevers between 40 and 41.1 °C cause brain damage. About 20% of parents thought that if they did not treat the fever, it would keep going higher. Neither of these beliefs is warranted by the facts. Because of these misconceptions, many parents treat low-grade fevers unnecessarily.

Teaching parents about fever can reduce the number of telephone calls and visits to the doctor.

B. Acetaminophen: Acetaminophen is indicated for children older than 2 months of age if the fever is over 39 °C or the child is uncomfortable. It can be given every 4–6 hours and will reduce the fever by 1–2 °C within 2 hours. Antipyretics do not bring the temperature down to normal unless the fever was low-grade to begin with.

C. Liquid Ibuprofen: Ibuprofen and acetaminophen are similar in safety and in their ability to reduce fever. Ibuprofen lasts 6–8 hours, compared with 4–6 hours for acetaminophen. Parents should be cautioned that the milligram-per-kilogram dosing and the concentration of these drugs are different.

D. Cautions About Aspirin: Aspirin should not be used for fever because several studies have linked its use during viral illnesses (especially chickenpox and influenza) to Reye's syndrome.

E. Sponging for Fever: Indications for immediate sponging with lukewarm water (never alcohol) are febrile delirium, a febrile seizure, or any fever over 41.1 °C. For other children, sponging is rarely necessary. Acetaminophen should always be given 30 minutes prior to sponging. Until acetaminophen has taken effect, sponging will only cause shivering, which may ultimately raise the temperature. Heat stroke requires immediate cold water sponging (antipyretics are not beneficial).

F. Other Measures: Extra fluids should be encouraged. Body fluids are lost during fever because of sweating, and the increased respiratory rate associated with fever means increased insensible losses through respiratory vapors.

Beach P, McCormick D: Fever and tympanic thermometry. Clin Pediatr 1991;30(Suppl):1.

Schmitt BD: Fever phobia: Misconceptions of parents about fever. Am J Dis Child 1980;134:176.

EVALUATION OF THE FEBRILE INFANT & TODDLER

Every day, febrile children are evaluated by clinicians. Those at increased risk for serious bacterial illness must be identified and treated appropriately. Children under the age of 3 years who present with fever but no obvious source of infection present a challenge to physicians. Both minor illnesses and serious bacterial infections—sepsis, meningitis, urinary tract infections, pneumonia, septic arthritis or osteomyelitis, enteritis—are common at this age.

Bacterial pathogens most commonly seen in the infant under 2 months of age are group B streptococci and *Escherichia coli*. *Streptococcus pneumo-*

niae is more commonly encountered in older children. The incidence of *Haemophilus influenzae* type b infection has declined dramatically since the availability of Hib vaccination for infants. Other pathogens responsible for invasive disease include *Staphylococcus aureus, Salmonella* species, and other gram-negative organisms.

In general, as the height of the fever increases, the risk of serious bacterial infection increases. In infants younger than 30 days, the rate was found to be 4.4% for temperatures of 38.1–39 °C, 7.6% for 39.1–39.9 °C, and 18% for temperatures of 40 °C or more. Various studies report the risk of occult bacteremia in children 3–36 months of age with fever without source to be from 3–11%.

Management

The management of infants and toddlers with fever without a recognized source is controversial. Useful guidelines can be offered as follows:

(1) Hospitalize any child who appears toxic.

(2) Newborns under 4 weeks of age should be hospitalized and receive a sepsis workup even though the risk of serious bacterial infection—if they meet the low-risk criteria set forth in Table 8–6—is quite small. Hospitalized infants are usually given parenteral antibiotics pending culture results; however, they could also be observed in the hospital without antibiotics.

(3) Identify the "low-risk" febrile infant (1–3 months of age). (See Table 8–6.) Because the probability of serious bacterial infection is 0.2%, these infants can be managed on an outpatient basis with one of two options: (1) Culture urine and reevaluate in 24 hours; or (2) culture blood, urine, and cerebrospinal fluid, administer ceftriaxone (50 mg/kg), and reevaluate in 24 hours. Parenteral antibiotics are more effective than oral antibiotics.

(4) Hospitalize the toxic febrile infant.

(5) Determine the temperature of the previously healthy child 3 months to 3 years of age. If the fever is below 39 °C, use antipyretics and follow up. If the temperature is 39 °C or above, obtain a white blood cell count. If the count is at least 15,000/μL, obtain a blood culture and treat with ceftriaxone, 50 mg/kg. Males under 6 months of age and females under 2 years of age should also have a urine specimen, collected either by catheterization or suprapubic tap, sent for culture. Chest x-rays and cerebrospinal fluid and stool cultures are useful only if indicated by the history or examination.

Follow-Up

Infants and children with positive blood or cerebrospinal fluid cultures should be admitted to a hospital and given parenteral antibiotics. If the blood culture grows nonresistant *S pneumoniae* and the child is afebrile at the follow-up visit, outpatient therapy with oral amoxicillin or penicillin is adequate. Urinary tract infections may also be treated on an outpatient basis with oral antibiotics (based on sensitivity studies) if the child is afebrile.

Baraff LJ et al: Practice guidelines for the management of infants and children 0 to 36 months of age with fever without source. Pediatrics 1993;92:1.

Bonadio WA, Romine K, Gyuro J: Relationship of fever magnitude to rate of serious bacterial infections in neonates. J Pediatr 1990;116:733.

Kramer MS, Shapiro ED: Management of the young febrile child: A commentary on recent practice guidelines. Pediatrics 1997;100:128.

GROWTH DEFICIENCY (Failure to Thrive)

Growth deficiency—formerly termed failure to thrive—is deceleration of growth velocity resulting in crossing two major percentile lines on the growth chart. The diagnosis is warranted also if a child under 6 months of age has not grown for 2 consecutive months or if a child over 6 months of age has not grown for 3 consecutive months. Growth deficiency is present in about 8% of the pediatric population.

In cases historically termed *nonorganic* failure to thrive, undernutrition is a result of environmental factors and aberrant caregiver–child interaction. For cases previously termed *organic* failure to thrive, undernutrition occurs as a result of major organ system disease (eg, renal failure, congenital heart disease, hypothyroidism).

Specific patterns of growth deficiency suggest different causes. In type I growth deficiency, the head circumference is preserved while the weight is depressed more than the height. This most common type results from inadequate caloric intake, excessive loss of calories, excessive utilization of calories, or

Table 8–6. Identification of the febrile infant 1–3 months of age at low risk for serious bacterial infection.

Nontoxic
Previously healthy
No bacterial focus on examination (except otitis media)
Good social situation
White blood cell count 5000–15,000/μL and fewer than 1500 band forms/μL[1]
Urinalysis with fewer than five white blood cells per high-power field
If diarrhea is present, fewer than five white blood cells per high-power field in stool

[1]In general, the higher the white count or the absolute neutrophil count, the greater the likelihood of bacteremia. When the white count exceeds 15,000/μL, the probability of bacteremia increases fivefold.

inability to use calories peripherally. Most such cases result from inadequate delivery of calories. This may be the result of poverty, lack of caregiver understanding, poor caregiver-child interaction, abnormal feeding patterns, or a combination of factors. Type II growth deficiency, which is associated with genetically determined short stature, endocrinopathies, constitutional growth delay, or various forms of skeletal dysplasias, is characterized by normal head circumference and proportionate diminution of height and weight. In type III growth deficiency, all three parameters of growth—head circumference, weight, and height—are lower than normal. This pattern is associated with central nervous system abnormalities, chromosomal defects, and in utero or perinatal insults.

Clinical Findings

A. Initial Evaluation: The history and physical examination will identify the cause of growth reduction in the vast majority of cases. The history includes the following:

(1) Birth history: Newborn screening result. Rule out intrauterine growth retardation, anoxia, congenital infections.

(2) Feeding and nutrition: Difficulty sucking, chewing, swallowing. Feeding patterns. Intake of formula, milk, juice, solids.

(3) Stooling and voiding of urine: Diarrhea, constipation, vomiting, poor urine stream.

(4) Growth pattern: Several points on the growth chart are crucial.

(5) Recurrent infections.

(6) Hospitalizations.

(7) HIV risk factors.

(8) Developmental history.

(9) Social and family factors: Family composition, financial status, supports, stresses. Heritable diseases, heights and weights of relatives.

(11) Review of systems.

The physical examination should focus on signs of organic disease or evidence of abuse or neglect: dysmorphic features, skin lesions, neck masses, adventitial breath sounds, heart murmurs, abdominal masses, and neuromuscular tone and strength. Throughout the evaluation, one should observe the caregiver-child interaction and the level of family functioning. Developmental screening and laboratory screening tests (complete blood count, BUN, creatinine, electrolytes, urinalysis, and urine culture) complete the initial office evaluation.

B. Further Evaluation: A prospective 3-day diet record should be a standard part of the evaluation. This has utility in assessing undernutrition even when organic disease is present. The diet history is evaluated by a pediatric dietitian for calories, protein, and micronutrients as well as for the pattern of eating. Additional laboratory tests should be ordered based on the history and physical examination. For

Table 8–7. Acceptable weight gain by age.

Age (months)	Weight Gain (g/d)
Birth to 3	20–30
3–6	15–20
6–9	10–15
9–12	6–11
12–18	5–8
18–24	3–7

example, stool collection for fat determination is indicated if a history of diarrhea suggests malabsorption. Moderate or high amounts of proteinuria should prompt workup for nephrotic syndrome. Vomiting should suggest a gastrointestinal, metabolic, neurologic, infectious, or renal cause. The tempo of evaluation should be based on the severity of symptoms and the magnitude of growth failure.

Treatment

A successful treatment plan addresses the child's diet and eating patterns, the child's development, family or caregiver strengths and weaknesses, and any organic disease. High-calorie diets and frequent monitoring (every 1 or 2 weeks initially) are essential. Acceptable weight gain varies by age (Table 8–7).

The child with growth deficiency may also be developmentally delayed because of living in an environment that fails to promote development or from the effect on the brain of nutrient deprivation. Restoring nutrition does not fully reverse the deficit but does reduce the long-term consequences.

Education in nutrition and child development as well as psychosocial support of the primary caregiver are essential. If family dysfunction is mild, behavior modification and counseling will be useful. Day care may benefit the child by providing a structured environment for all activities, including eating. If family dysfunction is severe, the local department of social services can help provide structure and assistance to the family. Rarely, the child may need to be temporarily or permanently removed from the home.

Previously, the child with growth deficiency was separated from the mother, hospitalized, and then returned home without modifying the environment. Hospitalization today is reserved for management of dehydration, for cases in which home therapy has failed to result in expected growth, for children who show evidence of abuse or willful neglect, for management of an illness that compromises a child's ability to eat, or for care pending foster home placement.

Maggioni A, Lifshitz F: Nutritional management of failure to thrive. Pediatr Clin North Am 1995;42:791.

Weston JA: Growth deficiency. In: *Pediatric Decision Making,* 3rd ed. Berman S (editor). Mosby Year Book, 1996.

Immunization

9

Eric A.F. Simoes, MD, DCH

Immunization is used either to prevent primary infection or to prevent the secondary consequences of an infection. Any assessment of the benefits of a proposed immunization program must take into account the likelihood of occurrence of infection in a defined population or specific individual and the likelihood that the vaccination will prevent that infection. The anticipated benefit of immunization must be weighed against the risk to the individual of adverse consequences. The physician must present this information to the parents so they can give informed consent to immunization.The immunization recommendations outlined in this chapter are current but will change as technology evolves and our understanding of the epidemiology of vaccine-preventable diseases changes. The most useful sources for current information about immunization are listed below:

(1) Morbidity and Mortality Weekly Report. Published weekly by the Centers for Disease Control and Prevention (CDC), Atlanta, GA 30333. MMWR contains recommendations of the United States Public Health Service Advisory Committee on Immunization Practices (ACIP).

(2) *The Red Book: Report of The Committee on Infectious Diseases.* Published at 2- to 3-year intervals by The American Academy of Pediatrics. The *1997 Red Book* is available from The American Academy of Pediatrics (AAP). Updates are published in the journal *Pediatrics*.

STANDARDS FOR PEDIATRIC IMMUNIZATION PRACTICES

Although 97–98% of children in the United States are vaccinated by or shortly after school entry, between 37% and 56% of the more than 8 million 2-year-olds in this country are not fully immunized. Low immunization coverage has been attributed to difficulties in reaching the urban poor and racial and ethnic mi-

norities. However, the health care delivery system also contributes to low immunization coverage. Parents seeking immunization for their children face significant barriers; not all providers take advantage of opportunities to administer vaccines, and inadequate or absent third-party payment for immunizations further reduces coverage. The contraindications and precautions relating to immunization presented in Table 9–1 reflect the current recommendations of the Advisory Committee on Immunization Practices and the Committee of Infectious Diseases of the American Academy of Pediatrics.

1997 Red Book: Report of the Committee on Infectious Diseases, 24th ed. American Academy of Pediatrics, 1997.
Status Report on the Childhood Immunization Initiative: National, state, and urban area vaccination coverage levels among children aged 19–35 months—United States, 1996. MMWR Morb Mortal Wkly Rep 1997;46(29): 658.

SAFETY OF IMMUNIZATION

VACCINE FACTORS

The safety standards for all vaccines licensed for use in the United States are established by the Food and Drug Administration (FDA) and involve regular examination of manufacturing techniques as well as production lots of vaccine. There have been no incidents of bacterial or viral contamination of vaccines at the factory level in the United States for decades.

FACTORS RELATED TO VACCINE ADMINISTRATION

The use of disposable syringes and needles or some other form of single-dose delivery of vaccine is

Table 9–1. Guide to contraindications and precautions to vaccinations (January, 1997).[1]

GENERAL FOR ALL VACCINES (DTP or DTaP, OPV, IPV, MMR, Hib, HBV, Var)

Contraindications	Not contraindications
Anaphylactic reaction to a vaccine contraindicates further doses of that vaccine	Mild to moderate local reaction (soreness, redness, swelling) following a dose of an injectable antigen
Anaphylactic reaction to a vaccine constituent contra-indicates the use of vaccines containing that substance	Low-grade or moderate fever following a prior vaccine dose
Moderate or severe illnesses with or without a fever	Mild acute illness with or without low-grade fever
	Current antimicrobial therapy
	Convalescent phase of illnesses
	Prematurity (same dosage and indications as for normal, full-term infants)
	Recent exposure to an infectious disease
	History of penicillin or other nonspecific allergies or family history of such allergies
	Pregnancy of mother or household contact
	Unvaccinated household contact

DTP or DTaP[2]

Contraindication	Not contraindications
Encephalopathy within 7 days of administration of previous dose of DTP or DTaP	Family history of convulsions[3]
Precautions[2]	Family history of sudden infant death syndrome
Fever of ≥ 40.5 °C (105 °F) within 48 hours after vaccination with a prior dose of DTP or DTaP	Family history of an adverse event following DTP or DTaP administration
Collapse or shocklike state (hypotonic-hyporesponsive episode) within 48 hours after receiving a prior dose of DTP or DTaP	
Seizures within 3 days of receiving a prior dose of DTP or DTaP (see footnote 3 regarding management of children with a personal history of seizures at any time)	
Persistent, inconsolable crying lasting ≥ 3 hours within 48 hours of receiving a prior dose of DTP or DTaP	
Guillain-Barré syndrome (GBS) within 6 weeks after a dose[4]	

OPV[5]

Contraindications	Not contraindications
Infection with HIV or a household contact with HIV	Breast feeding
Known immunodeficiency (hematologic and solid tumors; congenital immunodeficiency, and long-term immunosuppressive therapy)	Current antimicrobial therapy
Immunodeficient household contact	Mild diarrhea
Precaution[2]	
Pregnancy	

IPV[2]

Contraindication
Anaphylactic reaction to neomycin or streptomycin
Precaution[2]
Pregnancy

MMR[2]

Contraindications	Not contraindications
Anaphylactic reactions to neomycin	Tuberculosis or positive PPD
Pregnancy	Simultaneous TB skin testing[7]
Known immunodeficiency (hematologic and solid tumors; congenital immunodeficiency; severe HIV infection, and long-term immunosuppressive therapy)	Breast feeding
Anaphylactic reaction to gelatin	Pregnancy of mother or recipient
Precautions[1,6]	
Recent (within 3–11 months depending upon product and dose) immune globulin administration	Immunodeficient family member or household contact
Thrombocytopenia or history of thrombocytopenic purpura	Infection with HIV
	Nonanaphylactic reactions to eggs or neomycin

Hib

Contraindications
None identified

Hepatitis B

Contraindications	Not contraindication
Anaphylactic reaction to baker's yeast	Pregnancy

(continued)

Table 9–1. (continued)

Varicella

Contraindications	**Not contraindications**
Anaphylactic reaction to neomycin and to gelatin	Immunodeficiency in a household contact
Infection with HIV	Household contact with HIV
Known altered immunodeficiency (hematologic and solid tumors; congenital immunodeficiency; and long-term immunosuppressive therapy)	
Precautions[2]	
Recent (within 5 months)	
IG administration[9]	
Family history of immunodeficiency[10]	

[1]From Peter G, Hall CB, Orenstein WA (editors): *1997 Red Book: Report of the Committee on Infectious Diseases*, 24th ed. American Academy of Pediatrics, 1997.

[2]The events or conditions listed as precautions, although not contraindications, should be carefully reviewed. The benefits and risks of administering a specific vaccine to an individual under the circumstances should be considered. If the risks are believed to outweigh the benefits, the immunization should be withheld; if the benefits are believed to outweigh the risks (eg, during an outbreak or foreign travel), the immunization should be given. Whether and when to administer DTaP or DTP to children with proved or suspected underlying neurologic disorders should be decided on an individual basis. On theoretical grounds it is prudent to avoid vaccinating pregnant women. However, if immediate protection against poliomyelitis is needed, OPV, not IPV, is recommended.

[3]Acetaminophen given prior to administering DTaP or DTP and thereafter every 4 hours for 24 hours should be considered for children with a personal or family history of convulsions in siblings or parents.

[4]The decision to give additional doses of DTaP or DTP should be based on consideration of the benefit of further vaccination versus the risk of recurrence of GBS. For example, completion of the primary series in children is justified.

[5]A theoretical risk is that the administration of multiple live virus vaccines (eg, OPV and MMR) within 30 days of one another if not given on the same day will result in a suboptimal immune response. No data to substantiate this, however.

[6]Measles vaccination may temporarily suppress tuberculin reactivity. MMR vaccine may be given after or on the same day as TB testing. If MMR has been given recently, postpone the TB test until 4–6 weeks after administration of MMR. If giving MMR simultaneously with tuberculin skin test, use the Mantoux test and not multiple puncture test, because the latter requires confirmation if positive, which would have to be postponed 4–6 weeks.

[7]An anaphylactic reaction to egg ingestion formerly was considered a contraindication unless skin testing and, if indicated, desensitization had been performed: However, skin testing is no longer recommended. For further information, see recommendations of AAP in the 1997 *Red Book* and of ACIP.

[8]The decision to vaccinate should be based on consideration of the benefits of immunity to measles, mumps, and rubella versus the risk of recurrence or exacerbation of thrombocytopenia following vaccination, or from natural infections of measles or rubella. In most instances, the benefits of vaccination will be much greater than the potential risks and justify giving MMR, particularly in view of the even greater risk of thrombocytopenia following measles or rubella disease. However, if a prior episode of thrombocytopenia occurred in close temporal proximity to vaccination, not giving a subsequent dose may be prudent.

[9]Varicella vaccine should not be given for at least 5 months after administration of blood (except washed red blood cells), or plasma transfusions, immune globulin, or VZIG. Immune globulin or VZIG should not be given for 3 weeks following vaccination unless the benefits exceed those of the vaccination. In such cases, the vaccinee should either be revaccinated 5 months later or tested for immunity 6 months later and revaccinated if seronegative.

[10]Varicella vaccine should not be given to a member of a household with a family history of immunodeficiency until the immune status of the recipient and other children in the family is documented.

preferred to minimize the opportunity for contamination. If reusable glass syringes are used, they must be thoroughly cleaned and autoclaved after each use. If autoclaving is not possible, either dry heat at 170 °C for 2 hours or boiling for 30 minutes is an acceptable alternative. A 70% solution of alcohol is appropriate for disinfection of the stopper of the vaccine container and of the skin at the injection site.

The manufacturer's recommendations for route and site of administration of injectable vaccines are critical for safety and efficacy. All vaccines containing an adjuvant must be administered intramuscularly to avoid granuloma formation or necrosis. Such injections should be given into the anterolateral thigh (not intragluteally) in infants (< 18 months of age) and may be given in the deltoid or triceps in older children. A 22-gauge needle 1–1¼ inches long is rec-

ommended for children, but a 25-gauge ⅝-inch needle may be sufficient for young infants. Aqueous vaccines may be administered intramuscularly, subcutaneously, or intradermally. For subcutaneous or intradermal injections, a 25-gauge ¾- to ⅝-inch needle is recommended. Good injection technique, including aspiration prior to injection, must always be practiced. A separate syringe and needle should be used for each vaccine.

It is safe to administer many combinations of vaccines simultaneously without increasing the risk of adverse effects. (See individual preparations below for further discussion.) Inactivated vaccines (with the exception of cholera and yellow fever) can be given simultaneously or at any time after a different vaccine. Whenever possible, live-virus vaccines, if not administered on the same day, should be given at least 30 days apart. Lapses in the immunization schedule do not call for reinstitution of the series. If an immunoglobulin has been administered, live-virus vaccination should be delayed 6–10 months to avoid interference with the immune response.

HOST FACTORS

Healthy Children

Minor acute illnesses, with or without low-grade fever, are not contraindications to vaccination, since there is no evidence that vaccination under these conditions increases the rate of adverse effects or decreases efficacy. A moderate to severe febrile illness may be a reason to postpone vaccination. Routine physical examination and taking temperatures are not necessary before vaccinating apparently healthy infants and children.

Children With Chronic Illnesses

Most chronic diseases are not contraindications to vaccination; in fact, children with chronic diseases may be at greater risk of complications from vaccine-preventable diseases, such as influenza and pneumococcal infections. Premature infants are a good example. They should be immunized according to their chronologic, not gestational, age. Vaccine doses should not be reduced for preterm or low-birth-weight infants. The one exception to this rule may be children with progressive central nervous system disorders. Vaccination may be deferred or avoided entirely for such children, whereas children with static central nervous system diseases are candidates for vaccination.

Immunodeficient Children

Congenitally immunodeficient children should not be immunized with live-virus or live-bacteria vaccines. Depending on the nature of the immunodeficiency, other vaccines are safe. However, these may fail to evoke an immune response. Children with cancer and children being treated with corticosteroids or other immunosuppressive agents should not be vaccinated with live-virus or live-bacteria vaccines. This contraindication does not apply if the malignancy is in remission and chemotherapy has not been administered for at least 90 days. Live virus vaccines may also be administered to previously healthy children being treated with low to moderate doses of corticosteroids for less than 14 days; children receiving low to moderate doses of alternate-day corticosteroids; children being maintained on physiologic corticosteroid therapy without other immunodeficiency; and children using only topical, inhaled, or intra-articular corticosteroids. These guidelines apply also to children with documented HIV infection, with the proviso that live measles, mumps, and rubella vaccinations are recommended whereas oral poliovirus and varicella vaccinations are not. (Severely immunocompromised children

with HIV infection should not receive the measles vaccine.) Siblings and household contacts of a child who is immunodeficient should not receive oral poliovirus vaccine unless the immunodeficient child has been successfully immunized against poliomyelitis. If that is not the case, the siblings should receive inactivated poliovirus vaccine (IPV). Measles, mumps, and rubella (MMR) vaccines are not contraindicated under these circumstances.

Allergic or Hypersensitive Children

Hypersensitivity reactions are rare following vaccination. They are generally attributable to a trace component of the vaccine rather than to the antigen itself. MMR, IPV, and varicella-zoster vaccine (VZV) contain microgram quantities of neomycin, and IPV also contains trace amounts of streptomycin and polymyxin B. Children with known anaphylactic responses to these antibiotics should not be given these vaccines. Trace quantities of egg antigens may be present in influenza and yellow fever vaccines. Children who have had anaphylactic reactions to eggs should not be given these vaccines. Children with less serious reactions to eggs may generally be safely immunized with these products as well as with MMR. If doubt exists about the nature of a child's egg sensitivity, a skin testing procedure is outlined in the *Red Book.* Some vaccines (MMR, varicella, and yellow fever) contain gelatin, a substance to which persons with known food allergy may develop an anaphylactic reaction. Skin testing before vaccination may be an option in such cases.

Recommendations of the Advisory Committee on Immunization Practices (ACIP). MMWR Morb Mortal Wkly Rep 1994;43:RR-1.
American Academy of Pediatrics, Committee on Pediatric AIDS: Evaluation and medical treatment of the HIV-exposed infant. Pediatrics 1997;99:909.
1997 Red Book: Report of the Committee on Infectious Diseases, 24th ed. American Academy of Pediatrics, 1997.

THE COMPOSITION OF IMMUNIZING AGENTS

ACTIVE IMMUNIZATION

The immune response to immunization is variable, and a small proportion of children receiving certain antigens simply do not mount a response that is capable of conferring protection. For this reason, every vaccine has a definable failure rate.

The immunogen is suspended or dissolved in sterile

water or saline, or in more complex media such as tissue culture medium, which may contain constituents from the biologic system used to produce the immunogen. Most vaccines contain preservatives such as mercurials, and trace amounts of antibiotics such as neomycin may be incorporated to prevent bacterial overgrowth. Some vaccines contain adjuvants such as aluminum hydroxide and aluminum phosphate that also help to retain the immunogen in a "depot site" for a prolonged time, thus increasing the antigenic stimulation.

Finally, despite rigorous testing and high standards of mechanical and biologic purity and stability, vaccines may contain unwanted and undetectable antigens and other materials. Although the prospect is unlikely, vaccine administration could have unforeseen adverse consequences. Thus, vaccines should be administered where there is ready access to emergency resuscitative equipment and drugs (epinephrine, antihistamines).

PASSIVE IMMUNIZATION

Immune globulin (IG) is derived from pooled donations of large numbers of individuals (more than 1000 per lot). IG is prepared by alcohol fractionation, is sterile, and will not transmit any infectious agents (including hepatitis B and C viruses and HIV). IG is a 16.5% solution consisting primarily of immunoglobulin G with very small amounts of immunoglobulins A and M.

ROUTINE CHILDHOOD & ADOLESCENT IMMUNIZATIONS

Table 9–2 sets forth a schedule of routine immunizations for normal infants and children. Even if the interval elapsed between doses in a series of immunizations is longer than recommended, that series can be resumed as if no interruption had taken place—it is not necessary to begin the series again. Children whose vaccination status is unknown should be considered unprotected. Table 9–3 presents recommended schedules for children who did not start vaccination at the recommended time during the first year of life. Variations from these schedules may be necessitated by epidemiologic or individual clinical circumstances. Recently, in order to reduce vaccine-preventable diseases in adolescents, the AAP, AFP, and AMA have recommended routine considerations of adolescent vaccinations. Their recommendations are presented in Table 9–4.

Safe Handling of Vaccines

The numerous vaccines and other immunologic substances, such as antibody preparations and immunoglobulins for routine use by the practitioner, vary in correct storage temperatures. Vaccines that require routine freezing are varicella and oral polio-vaccine. Yellow fever vaccine may also be stored frozen. Product package inserts should be consulted for detailed information on vaccine storage conditions and shelf life.

American Academy of Pediatrics, Committee on Infectious Diseases: Recommended childhood immunization schedule—United States, January–December 1997. Pediatrics 1997;99:136.
American Academy of Pediatrics, Committee on Infectious Diseases: Immunization of adolescents: Recommendations of the Advisory Committee on Immunization Practices, the American Academy of Pediatrics, the American Academy of Family Physicians, and the American Medical Association. Pediatrics 1997;99:479.

DIPHTHERIA

Diphtheria toxoid is prepared by the formaldehyde inactivation of diphtheria toxin. The toxoid content of the several available preparations varies and is measured in limit of flocculation (Lf) units. The protective efficacy of diphtheria toxoid has never been measured on a mass scale but is estimated to be greater than 85%.

Preparations Available

(1) Diphtheria toxoid is used only when tetanus toxoid and pertussis vaccine are both contraindicated. It contains 10–12 Lf units per immunizing dose.

(2) Diphtheria-tetanus (DT) (pediatric) is used when pertussis vaccine is contraindicated. DT contains 6.7–12.5 Lf units of diphtheria toxoid per dose. Pediatric DT should not be used in adults because of potentially severe adverse reactions.

(3) Tetanus-diphtheria (Td) (adult) is for use in persons 7 years of age or older and contains 2 Lf units or less of diphtheria toxoid. It is less likely to produce local reactions while still eliciting a good immunogenic response in this population.

(4) Diphtheria-tetanus-pertussis (DTP) was the standard immunizing agent for healthy children and contains 6.7–12.5 Lf units of diphtheria toxoid per dose. Diphtheria-tetanus-acellular pertussis (DTaP) contains 6.7–12.5 Lf units of diphtheria toxins per dose and is recommended for diphtheria immunization.

Diphtheria-tetanus-pertussis and *Haemophilus* D conjugate vaccine (DTP-Hib) contains 6.7–12.5 Lf units of diphtheria toxin and may be used in place of DTP and Hib vaccine.

Dosage & Schedule of Administration

The above preparations are administered intramuscularly in a dose of 0.5 mL. Administration of these adsorbed preparations by jet injection may be associated with more local reactions. See Table 9–3 for the routine schedule and Table 9–4 for immunization of

Table 9–2. Recommended childhood vaccinations—United States, January–December 1998.[1,2]
Vaccines[2] are listed under the routinely recommended ages. Heavy borders indicate ranges of acceptable ages for immunization. Catch-up immunizations should be given during any visit when feasible. Shaded boxes indicate vaccines to be assessed and given if necessary during the early adolescent period.

Vaccine	Birth	1 mo	2 mos	4 mos	6 mos	12 mos	15 mos	18 mos	4–6 yrs	11–12 yrs	14–16 yrs
Hepatitis B[3]	Hep B-1										
			Hep B-2			Hep B-3				Hep B[4]	
Diphtheria and tetanus toxoids and pertussis vaccine[5]			DTP	DTP	DTP		DTaP or DTP[5]		DTP or DTaP	Td	
Haemophilus influenzae type b[6]			Hib	Hib	Hib	Hib					
Poliovirus[7]			Polio	Polio		Polio[7]			Polio		
Measles-mumps-rubella[8]						MMR			MMR	MMR[8]	
Varicella-zoster virus[9]						Var				Var[9]	

[1]Approved by the Advisory Committee on Immunization Practices (ACIP), the American Academy of Pediatrics (AAP), and the American Academy of Family Physicians (AAFP).

[2]This schedule sets forth the recommended ages for routine administration of currently licensed vaccines for childhood immunizations. Some combination vaccines are available and may be used whenever administration of all components of the vaccine is indicated. Providers should consult the manufacturers' package inserts for detailed recommendations.

[3]*Infants born to HBsAg-negative mothers* should receive 2.5 μg of Merck vaccine (Recombivax HB) or 10 μg of SmithKline Beecham (SB) vaccine (Engerix-B). The second dose should be administered ≥ 1 month after the first dose. The third dose should be given at least 2 months after the second but not before 6 months of age.

Infants born to HBsAg-positive mothers should receive 0.5 mL of hepatitis B immune globulin (HBIG) within 12 hours after birth and either 5 μg of Merck vaccine (Recombivax HB) or 10 μg of SB vaccine (Engerix-B) at a separate site. The second dose is recommended at age 1–2 months and the third dose at age 6 months.

Infants born to mothers whose HBsAg status in unknown should receive either 5 μg of Merck vaccine (Recombivax HB) or 10 μg of SB vaccine (Engerix-B) within 12 hours after birth. The second dose of vaccine is recommended at age 1 month and the third dose at age 6 months. Blood should be drawn at the time of delivery to determine the mother's HBsAg status; if it is positive, the infant should receive HBIG as soon as possible (no later than 1 week of age). The dosage and timing of subsequent vaccine doses should be based on the mother's HBsAg status.

[4]Children and adolescents who have not been vaccinated against hepatitis B in infancy may begin the series during any visit. Those who have not previously received three doses of hepatitis B vaccine should initiate or complete the series at age 11–12 years, and unvaccinated older adolescents should be vaccinated whenever possible. The second dose should be administered at least 1 month after the first dose, and the third dose should be administered at least 4 months after the first dose and at least 2 months after the second dose.

[5]DTaP (diphtheria and tetanus toxoids and acellular pertussis vaccine) is the preferred vaccine for all doses in the vaccination series, including completion of the series in children who have received one or more doses of whole cell DTP vaccine. Whole cell DTP is an acceptable alternative to DTaP. The fourth dose (DTP or DTaP) may be administered as early as 12 months of age provided 6 months have elapsed since the third dose and if the child is unlikely to return at age 15–18 months. Td (tetanus and diphtheria toxoids) is recommended at 11–12 years of age if at least 5 years have elapsed since the last dose of DTP, DTaP, or DT. Subsequent routine Td boosters are recommended every 10 years.

[6]Three *H influenzae* type b (Hib) conjugate vaccines are licensed for infant use. If PrP-OMP (PedvaxHIBG [Merck]) is administered at 2 and 4 months of age, a dose at 6 months is not required.

[7]Two poliovirus vaccines are currently licensed in the United States: inactivated poliovirus vaccine (IPV) and oral poliovirus vaccine (OPV). The following schedules are all acceptable to the ACIP, AAP, and AAFP. Parents and providers may choose among these options.
 (1) Two doses of IPV followed by two doses of OPV.
 (2) Four doses of IPV.
 (3) Four doses of OPV.
The ACIP recommends two doses of IPV at 2 and 4 months of age followed by two doses of OPV at 12–18 months and 4–6 years of age. IPV is the only poliovirus vaccine recommended for immunocompromised persons and their household contacts.

[8]The second dose of MMR is recommended routinely at 4–6 years of age but may be administered during any visit provided at least 1 month has elapsed since receipt of the first dose and that both doses are administered beginning at or after 12 months of age. Those who have not previously received the second dose should complete the schedule no later than at the 11- to 12-year-old visit.

[9]Susceptible children may receive varicella vaccine (Var) at any visit after the first birthday, and those who lack a reliable history of chickenpox should be immunized during the 11- to 12-year-old visit. Susceptibles 13 years of age or older should receive two doses at least 1 month apart.

Table 9–3. Recommended immunization schedules for children not immunized in the first year of life.[1,2]

Recommended Time or Age	Immunizations[3,4,5]	Comments
YOUNGER THAN 7 YEARS		
First visit	DTaP (or DTP), Hib,[6] HBV, MMR, OPV[7]	If indicated, tuberculin testing may be done at same visit. If child is 5 years of age or older, Hib is not indicated in most circumstances.
Interval after first visit 1 month (4 weeks)	DTaP (or DTP), HBV, Var[8]	The second dose of OPV may be given if accelerated poliomyelitis vaccination is necessary, such as for travelers to areas where polio is endemic.
2 months	DTaP (or DTP), Hib,[6] OPV[7]	Second dose of Hib is indicated only if the first dose was received when younger than 15 months.
≥ 8 months	DTaP (or DTP), HBV, OPV[7]	OPV and HBV are not given if the third doses were given earlier.
Age 4–6 (at or before school entry)	DTaP (or DTP), OPV,[7] MMR[9]	DTaP (or DTP) is not necessary if the fourth dose was given after the fourth birthday; OPV is not necessary if the third dose was given after the fourth birthday.
Age 11–12 years	See Table 9–4.	
7–12 YEARS		
First visit	HBV, MMR, Td, OPV[7]	
Interval after first visit 2 months (8 weeks)	HBV, MMR,[9] Var,[8] Td, OPV[7]	OPV also may be given 1 month after the first visit if accelerated poliomyelitis vaccination is necessary.
8–14 months	HBV,[10] Td, OPV[7]	OPV is not given if the third dose was given earlier.
Age 11–12 years	See Table 9–4.	

[1]Peter G, Hall CB, Orenstein WA (editors): *1997 Red Book: Report of the Committee on Infectious Diseases, 24th ed.* American Academy of Pediatrics, 1997.

[2]The table is not consistent with all package inserts. For products used, also consult manufacturer's package insert for instructions on storage, handling, dosage, and administration. Biologicals prepared for different manufacturers may vary, and package inserts of the same manufacturer may change from time to time. Therefore, the physician should be aware of the contents of the current package insert.

[3]If all needed vaccines cannot be administered simultaneously, priority should be given to protecting the child against those diseases that pose the greatest immediate risk. In the United States, these diseases for children younger than 2 years usually are measles and *Haemophilus influenzae* type b infection; for children older than 7 years, they are measles, mumps, and rubella. Before 13 years of age, immunity against hepatitis B and varicella should be ensured.

[4]DTaP, HBV, Hib, MMR, and Var can be given simultaneously at separate sites if failure of the patient to return for future immunizations is a concern.

[5]For further information on pertussis and poliomyelitis immunization, see text.

[6]See text.

[7]IPV is also acceptable. However, for infants and children starting vaccination late (ie, after 6 months of age), OPV is preferred in order to complete an accelerated schedule with a minimum number of injections (see text).

[8]Varicella vaccine can be administered to susceptible children any time after 12 months of age. Unvaccinated children who lack a reliable history of chickenpox should be vaccinated before their 13th birthday.

[9]Minimal interval between doses of MMR is 1 month (4 weeks).

[10]HBV may be given earlier in a 0-, 2-, and 4-month schedule.

Vaccine abbreviations: HBV, hepatitis B virus vaccine; Var, varicella vaccine; DTP, diphtheria and tetanus toxoids and pertussis vaccine; DTaP, diphtheria and tetanus toxoids and acellular pertussis vaccine; Hib, *Haemophilus influenzae* type b conjugate vaccine; OPV, oral poliovirus vaccine; IPV, inactivated poliovirus vaccine; MMR, live measles-mumps-rubella vaccine; Td, adult tetanus toxoid (full dose) and diphtheria toxoid (reduced dose), for children ≥ 7 years and adults.

children not appropriately immunized during the first year of life.

Adverse Effects

No significant adverse reactions have been associated with diphtheria toxoid alone.

Antibody Preparations

Equine diphtheria antitoxin is available for the treatment of diphtheria. Dosage depends on the size and location of the diphtheritic membrane and an estimate of the patient's level of intoxication. Before using this preparation, the presence or absence of

Table 9–4. Recommended schedule of vaccinations for adolescents ages 11–12 years.[1]

Immunobiologic	Indications	Name	Dose	Frequency	Route
Hepatitis A vaccine	Adolescents who are at increased risk of hepatitis A infection or its complications	HAVRIX[2]	720 EL.U.[3]/0.5 mL[4]	A total of two doses at 0,[5] 6–12 months	IM
		VAQTA[2]	25 units/0.5 mL	A total of two doses at 0, 6–12 months	IM
Hepatitis B vaccine	Adolescents not vaccinated previously for hepatitis B	Recombivax HB[2]	5 μg/0.5 mL	A total of three doses at 0, 1–2, 4–6 months	IM
		Engerix-B[2]	10 μg/0.5 mL	A total of three doses at 0, 1–2, 4–6 months	IM
Influenza vaccine	Adolescents who are at increased risk for complications caused by influenza or who have contact with persons at increased risk for these complications	Influenza virus vaccine[6]	0.5 mL	Annually (September to December)	IM
Measles, mumps, and rubella vaccine (MMR)	Adolescents not vaccinated previously with two doses of measles vaccine at ≥ 12 months of age	MMR[2,6]	0.5 mL	One dose	SC
Pneumococcal polysaccharide vaccine	Adolescents who are at increased risk for pneumococcal disease or its complications	Pneumococcal vaccine polyvalant[6]	0.5 mL	One dose	IM or SC
Tetanus and diphtheria toxoids (Td)	Adolescents not vaccinated within the previous 5 years	Tetanus and diphtheria toxoids, absorbed (for adult use)[6]	0.5 mL	Every 10 years	IM
Varicella virus vaccine	Adolescents not vaccinated and who have no reliable history of chickenpox	VARIVAX[2]	0.5 mL	One dose[7]	SC

[1]Peter G, Hall CB, Orenstein WA (editors): *1997 Red Book: Report of the Committee on Infectious Diseases*, 24th ed. American Academy of Pediatrics, 1997.
[2]Manufacturer's product name.
[3]Enzyme-linked immunosorbent assay (ELISA) unit.
[4]Alternative dosage and schedule of 360 EL.U./0.5 mL and a total of three doses administered at 0, 1, and 6–12 months.
[5]0 months represents timing of the initial dose, and subsequent numbers represent months after the initial dose.
[6]Generic name.
[7]Adolescents ≥ 13 years of age should be administered a total of two doses (0.5 mL/dose) subcutaneously at 0 and 4–8 weeks.

equine serum sensitivity must be determined using 0.02 mL of intradermal (1:1000 dilution) tests. If the test is positive, desensitization must be undertaken. If negative, the following doses are suggested:

Site	Duration of Lesion	Toxic?	Dose (units)
Pharyngeal or laryngeal	≤ 48 hours	—	20,000–40,000
Nasopharyngeal	—	—	40,000–60,000
Extensive or brawny swelling of the neck	≥ 72 hours	Yes	80,000–100,000
Cutaneous	—	—	20,000–40,000

As of January 1997, diphtheria antitoxin is no longer commercially available in the USA but may be obtained from the CDC.

Toxigenic *Corynebacterium diphtheriae*—Northern Plains Indian Community, August–October 1996. MMWR Morb Mortal Wkly Rep 1997;46(22):507.

TETANUS

Tetanus toxoid is prepared by inactivating the toxin with formaldehyde. Its activity is measured in Lf units and the dosage is generally 4–10 Lf units per immunizing dose for adsorbed products and 4–5 Lf units per dose for the fluid product. The protective efficacy of tetanus toxoid has never been measured in any large study, but it is believed to be high.

Preparations Available

(1) Tetanus toxoid (fluid) is used rarely—only when rapid immunization is desirable.

(2) Tetanus toxoid adsorbed on aluminum phosphate is the standard single-antigen "booster" toxoid.

(3) Tetanus-diphtheria (pediatric DT and adult Td) is discussed above.

(4) Diphtheria-tetanus-pertussis (DTP).

(5) Diphtheria-tetanus-acellular pertussis (DTaP).

(6) Diphtheria-tetanus-pertussis-*Haemophilus influenzae* b (DTP-Hib) is discussed later in the section on Hib.

Dosage & Schedule
of Administration

The above preparations are administered intramuscularly in a dose of 0.5 mL. See Table 9–2 for the routine schedule and Table 9–3 for vaccination of children not appropriately immunized during the first year of life. A booster dose of tetanus-diphtheria (Td) should be scheduled at 11–12 years of age or at 14–16 years of age and every 10 years thereafter to protect against tetanus and diphtheria.

Adverse Effects

Significant reactions to tetanus toxoid, historically an extremely safe preparation, are very unusual. Anaphylaxis, Guillain-Barré syndrome, and brachial neuritis related to tetanus toxoid are extremely rare.

Antibody Preparations

Tetanus immune globulin (TIG) (human) is indicated in the management of tetanus-prone wounds in individuals who have had an uncertain number or fewer than three tetanus immunizations. Persons immunized within 10 years need not receive TIG regardless of the nature of their wound. The dose is 300–600 units (one or two vials) intramuscularly. Part of the dose may be infiltrated locally.

Tetanus Surveillance—United States, 1991–1994. MMWR Morb Mortal Wkly Rep 1997;46(SS-2):15.

PERTUSSIS

Pertussis vaccines currently used in the United States for initial immunization are killed whole-cell preparations and three FDA-licensed acellular formulations of DTP (DTaP). The DTP preparations have a protective efficacy of about 70–90% after three doses depending on the source. Further epidemiologic evidence of the efficacy of pertussis vaccine is provided by the observation of a large increase in reported pertussis cases in Great Britain and Japan after those two countries reduced or abandoned use of the vaccine.

Preparations Available

(1) Pertussis vaccine (adsorbed) is manufactured by the Division of Biologic Products, Michigan Department of Public Health, for use within that state. It may be obtained for other use by consultation with the department.

(2) Diphtheria-tetanus-pertussis (DTP).

(3) Diphtheria-tetanus-acellular pertussis (DTaP)

(4) Diphtheria-tetanus-pertussis-*Haemophilus influenzae* b (DTP-Hib).

Dosage & Schedule
of Administration

Each of the available preparations is administered in a dose of 0.5 mL intramuscularly. See Table 9–2 for the routine schedule and Table 9–3 for vaccination of those children not appropriately immunized during the first year of life.

Adverse Effects

A large number of adverse reactions have been attributed to pertussis vaccine. These can be divided into three categories: local reactions, mild to moderate systemic reactions (that occur in up to half of children), and severe systemic reactions. The estimated rates of these reactions within the first 48 hours after vaccination are shown below. The only absolute contraindications to the further use of pertussis vaccine are an anaphylactic reaction to the vaccine or a severe acute neurologic illness within 7 days after vaccination (see Table 9–2). Precaution is urged for the following associations: a convulsion within 3 days (1:1750); persistent, severe, inconsolable screaming or crying for over 3 hours (1:100); a hypotonic-hyporesponsive episode within 48 hours (1:1750); and an unexplained temperature rise to 40.5 °C within 48 hours (1:330).

Controversy continues regarding the causation of serious neurologic illness by pertussis vaccine. A reassessment of the only large-scale case-control study with enough statistical power to examine this issue—the British National Childhood Encephalopathy Study (NCES)—has led to a reappraisal of the relationship.

It was calculated that while the attributable risk for serious acute neurologic injury ranges from less than 1 per million to 1:140,000, the risk for permanent brain damage is even lower if indeed there is any risk at all. This reassessment, along with new studies, has led the American Academy of Pediatrics, the Canadian National Advisory Committee, and the British Pediatric Association to conclude that pertussis vaccine has not been proved to be the cause of brain damage and to reaffirm the safety and effectiveness of routine whole-cell pertussis vaccine in immunization programs for infants and children.

On July 3, 1991, the National Academy of Sciences Institute of Medicine released a report entitled *Adverse Effects of Pertussis and Rubella Vaccines.* The committee concluded that the vaccine was causally related to only four adverse effects: acute encephalopathy, the range of excess risk being nil to 10.5 per million immunizations; shock (and an unusual shocklike state), 3.5–291 cases per 100,000 immunizations; anaphylaxis, 2 cases per 100,000 injections of DTP; and protracted, inconsolable crying, 0.1–6% of recipients. Thus, although epidemiologic evidence may be consistent with a causal relationship, there is no plausible clinical evidence for a role of pertussis toxin in severe DTP reactions.

DIPHTHERIA-TETANUS-PERTUSSIS

Diphtheria and tetanus toxoids and pertussis vaccine (DTP) has been used for the vaccination of healthy infants against the three diseases for more than 40 years. It has the combined clinical efficacy of the three single-dose preparations, and the efficacy of pertussis vaccine may even be enhanced by the adjuvant effect of the diphtheria and tetanus toxoids. It can be safely and effectively administered simultaneously with OPV or IPV, MMR, HBV, and the *Haemophilus influenzae* type b vaccines.

Preparations Available

Each dose of combined diphtheria and tetanus toxoids and whole-cell pertussis vaccine contains 6.7–12.5 Lf units of diphtheria toxoid, 5 Lf units of tetanus toxoid, and not more than 16 opacity units of pertussis vaccine adsorbed with one of several adjuvants (alum, aluminum phosphate, or aluminum hydroxide, depending on the manufacturer).

Dosage & Schedule of Administration

DTP is administered in a dose of 0.5 mL intramuscularly. See Table 9–2 for the routine schedule and Table 9–3 for children not appropriately immunized during the first year of life.

Adverse Effects; Antibody Preparations

See above with the individual component vaccines.

American Academy of Pediatrics, Committee on Infectious Diseases: The relationship between pertussis vaccine and central nervous system sequelae: Continuing assessment. Pediatrics 1996;97:279.

Blumberg DA et al: Severe reactions associated with diphtheria-tetanus-pertussis vaccine: Detailed study of children with seizures, hypotonic-hyporesponsive episodes, high fevers, and persistent crying. Pediatrics 1993;91:1158.

Institute of Medicine: DPT vaccine and chronic nervous system dysfunction, a new analysis. National Academy Press, 1997.

Onorato IM et al: Efficacy of whole-cell pertussis vaccine in preschool children in the United States. JAMA 1992;267:2745.

Pertussis vaccination: Use of acellular pertussis vaccines among infants and young children: Recommendations of the Advisory Committee on Immunization Practices (ACIP). MMWR Morb Mortal Wkly Rep 1997;46(RR-7):1.

DIPHTHERIA-TETANUS & ACELLULAR PERTUSSIS VACCINE

Two basic types of acellular (DTaP) vaccines have been studied. The T-type vaccines are produced by extraction and purification of B pertussis cultures. In contrast, the B-type vaccines contain combinations of pertussis toxin (PT), filamentous hemagglutinin (FHA), pertactin (Prn), and fimbriae (Fim). It has been hypothesized that immunity against PT alone may be sufficient to protect against pertussis, but this view has been challenged, and it has been claimed that FHA, Prn, and Fim antibodies may be required for optimal protection.

Efficacy trials of various acellular pertussis vaccines in Sweden, Germany, Italy, and Senegal have established a two- to tenfold lesser frequency of "minor" adverse events and reduced rates of more serious events (hypotonic-hyporesponsive episodes, persistent crying, temperatures higher than 40 °C, and seizures) compared with the whole-cell vaccine, good immunogenicity, and a protective efficacy ranging from 59% to 89%. On the basis of those trials and smaller ones in the United States, the FDA has licensed use of three DTaP vaccines for use in the routine immunization schedule for infants at 2, 4, and 6 months. DTaP is preferred over DTP for all doses. During the transition period, DTP is an acceptable alternative to any of the five doses. DTP-Hib is also an acceptable alternative. For children with adverse reactions in the "precaution" category to DTP, DTaP may be substituted. In those with a true contraindication, DTP/DTaP should not be used.

Preparations Available

(1) Diphtheria-tetanus-acellular pertussis (Wyeth/Lederle) contains 9 Lf units of diphtheria toxoid, 5 Lf units of tetanus toxoid, and 300 hemagglutinating units of Takeda acellular pertussis component (34.3 μg of FHA, 3.2 μg of inactivated PT, 1.6 μg of Pn, and 0.8 μg of Fim type 2), adsorbed to aluminum hydroxide and aluminum phosphate.

Diphtheria-tetanus-acellular pertussis (Pasteur-Mérieux-Connaught) contains 6.7 Lf units of diphtheria toxoid, 5 Lf units of tetanus toxoid, 23.4 μg of inactivated PT, and 23.4 μg of FHA, absorbed to aluminum potassium sulfate.

Diphtheria-tetanus-acellular pertussis (SmithKline Beecham) contains 25 Lf of diphtheria toxoid, 10 Lf of tetanus toxoid, 25 μg of PT, 25 μg FHA, 8 μg Pn absorbed to aluminum hydroxide.

Diphtheria-tetanus-acellular pertussis-Hib (Pasteur-Mèrieux-Connaught) has been licensed for use as the fourth dose (booster) in the DPT immunization series.

Dosage & Schedule of Administration

DTaP is administered in a dose of 0.5 mL intramuscularly. See Table 9–2 for the routine schedule and Table 9–3 for the procedure in children not immunized during the first year.

Whenever feasible, the same brand of DTaP should be used for all doses.

Adverse Effects

Local reactions, fever, and other mild systemic effects occur with one-fourth to two-thirds the frequency noted following whole-cell DTP vaccination. Moderate to severe systemic effects, including fever of 40.5 °C, persistent inconsolable crying lasting 3 hours or more, and hypotonic-hyporesponsive episodes, are less frequent than with whole-cell DTP. These are without sequelae. Severe neurologic effects have not been temporally associated with DTaP vaccinations in limited use in the United States.

American Academy of Pediatrics, Committee on Infectious Diseases: Acellular pertussis vaccine: Recommendations for use as the initial series in infants and children. Pediatrics 1997;99:282.

Decker MD et al: Comparison of 13 acellular pertussis vaccines: Adverse reactions. Pediatrics 1995;96(Suppl): S557.

Greco D et al: A controlled trial of two acellular vaccines and one whole cell vaccine against pertussis. N Engl J Med 1996;334:341.

Gustafsson L et al: A controlled trial of a two-component acellular, a five-component acellular, and a whole cell pertussis vaccine. N Engl J Med 1996;334:349.

Pertussis vaccination: Use of acellular pertussis vaccines among infants and young children. MMWR Morb Mortal Wkly Rep 1997;46(RR-7):1.

Zepp F et al: Evidence for induction of polysaccharide specific B-cell-memory in the 1st year of life: Plain *Haemophilus influenzae* type b-PRP (Hib) boosters children primed with a tetanus-conjugate Hib-DTaP-HBV combined vaccine. Eur J Pediatr 1997;156:18.

POLIOMYELITIS

Vaccines directed against poliovirus infections have largely eliminated the naturally occurring disease in developed countries. In the United States, the number of reported cases of paralytic poliomyelitis has fallen from more than 18,000 in 1954 to 0–10 per year currently. Live attenuated oral poliovirus vaccine (OPV) and injectable poliovirus vaccine of enhanced potency (IPV-E), which has a higher content of antigens than the old IPV, are the only vaccines against poliomyelitis available in the United States.

IPV is incapable of causing poliomyelitis by virtue of being inactivated, whereas OPV can do so rarely. The rate of this in the United States is one case of paralytic disease per 760,000 first doses of OPV distributed. Ninety-three percent of recipient cases and 76% of all vaccine-associated paralytic poliomyelitis (VAPP) occur after administration of the first or second dose of OPV. The risk of paralysis in the immunodeficient recipient may be as much as 6800 times that in normals. IPV cannot multiply in the gut as OPV does—in theory, not protecting against intestinal infection with wild virus, as OPV does—and thus cannot produce "secondary vaccination" of close contacts of vaccinees. IPV, however, produces a much higher serologic response than OPV, a higher booster response at lower prevaccination levels, and an equivalent mucosal response. IPV has the practical advantage of not requiring freezing for storage, as OPV does. However, the mass administration of OPV requires no needles and syringes. The ACIP recommends a sequential dose of IPV for the first two doses followed by two doses of OPV. The virtues of this schedule are (1) the reduced rate of VAPP (two doses of IPV should protect recipients and allow immunodeficiencies to become manifest before the first OPV dose at 12–18 months); (2) the fact that OPV would provide mucosal immunity and community protection; and (3) the argument that the two doses of OPV would reduce the need for two more injections. The AAP, however, recognizes the logistic difficulties in giving two more injections and the fact that combination vaccines will soon be available and recommends that sequential IPV-OPV, IPV alone, or OPV alone are all acceptable. Exceptions include immunodeficient recipients (including HIV-positive persons), recipients who have immunodeficient persons or unimmunized adults in their households, and unvaccinated adults, all of whom should receive IPV. In addition, anyone who is informed of the risks and benefits of OPV should be permitted to elect to receive IPV if prepared to commit to a full schedule of vaccination with that preparation. Immunization with OPV alone is recommended when parents or providers prefer not to give additional injections (if IPV is used) and for children starting a vaccination schedule after 6 months of age (when compliance will be better with OPV).

Preparations Available

(1) Inactivated injectable poliovirus vaccine of enhanced potency (IPV-E) contains 40, 8, and 32 D-antigen units, respectively, of types 1, 2, and 3 poliovirus.

(2) Trivalent live attenuated oral poliovirus vaccine (OPV) contains at least 105.4, 104.5, and 105.2

TCID50 of attenuated Sabin strains of poliovirus types 1, 2, and 3, respectively.

Dosage & Schedule of Administration

A. IPV-E: This is the only vaccine preparation available and is administered in a dose of 0.5 mL subcutaneously. Combination DPT–IPV-E vaccines are not yet licensed in the United States.

B. OPV: A single thawed ampule is given orally for each dose. See Table 9–2 for the routine schedule and Table 9–3 for the procedure in children not appropriately immunized during the first year.

Adverse Effects

IPV has essentially no adverse effects associated with it other than possible rare hypersensitivity reactions to trace quantities of antibiotics. OPV carries a risk of vaccine-associated paralytic disease for immunodeficient recipients, immunodeficient contacts of recipients, and unvaccinated healthy adult contacts of recipients.

American Academy of Pediatrics, Committee on Infectious Diseases: Poliomyelitis prevention: Recommendations for use of inactivated poliovirus vaccine and live oral poliovirus vaccine. Pediatrics 1997;99:300.

Faden H et al: Long-term immunity to poliovirus in children immunized with live attenuated and enhanced-potency inactivated trivalent poliovirus vaccines. J Infect Dis 1993;168:453.

Poliomyelitis prevention in the United States: Introduction of a sequential vaccination schedule of inactivated poliovirus vaccine followed by oral poliovirus vaccine: Recommendations of the Advisory Committee on Immunization Practices (ACIP). MMWR Morb Mortal Wkly Rep 1997;46(RR-3):1.

Simoes EA, Abzug MJ: Enteroviruses: Issues in poliomyelitis immunization and perinatal enterovirus infections. Curr Opin Infect Dis 1993;6:547.

MEASLES

Routine measles vaccination was introduced in the United States in 1963. Since 1976, the Moraten strain vaccine has been used. In 1979, an improved stabilizer was added that made the vaccine more heat-stable.

After the introduction of measles vaccine, the annual number of reported cases in the United States decreased from about 500,000 in 1963 to 1497 in 1983. Between 1989 and 1991, there was a resurgence of measles, with 55,622 cases reported. The major reasons for the increase in cases and the resulting deaths are failure to provide vaccine to preschool children 15 months of age or older, the presence in the community of susceptible children under 15 months of age, and the accumulation of appropriately vaccinated but nonimmune individuals (primary vac-

cine failures: 2–10%) in schools and colleges. These reasons have led to recommendations for the routine revaccination of all children.

Given the efficacy rate of the current vaccine (> 95%), the elimination of indigenous measles from the United States is an attainable public health goal. Since 1991, measles coverage has increased to over 90% for the first dose and as much as 65% of school-age children who received a second dose, resulting in a sustained decline in measles cases with interruption of measles transmission.

Preparations Available

The Moraten strain is derived from the Edmonston B strain after multiple passages in chick embryo tissue culture and contains 1000–5000 TCID50 of the United States Reference Measles Virus. The Moraten strain is equally effective in combination—with mumps vaccine (MM), with rubella vaccine (MR), and with mumps and rubella vaccines (MMR).

Dosage & Schedule of Administration

A. Routine Vaccination: The first dose of measles vaccine should ordinarily be given as MMR to 12-month-old or 15-month-old children. A dose of 0.5 mL, whether alone or in combination, should be given subcutaneously. The recommended age for the second vaccination with MMR varies: 4–6 years (ACIP) or 11–12 years (AAP). The advantages of the former recommendation are that implementation is easy, there is no extra cost for physician visits, and elementary schools have an extensive tracking system to ensure compliance. The advantage of the later age of vaccination is that it has a rapid impact, since it is closer to the age when outbreaks occur. The individual practitioner can adopt either recommendation but may be preempted in this decision by laws mandating revaccination at school entry. Timing of MMR when immune globulin has been administered depends on the child's age as well as the type and route of administration. Consult the AAP *Red Book* for specific recommendations. The interval ranges between 3 and 11 months.

B. Vaccination in High-Risk Geographic Areas: A high-risk area has been defined by the ACIP as (1) a county with over five cases among preschool children during each of the last 5 years; (2) a county with a recent outbreak among preschool children; or (3) a city with a large unvaccinated population. In high-risk areas, age at primary vaccination may be lowered to 12 months, and the second dose should be administered at 4–6 or 11–12 years of age.

C. Revaccination Under Other Circumstances: Persons entering colleges and other institutions for education beyond high school, medical personnel beginning employment, and persons traveling abroad should have documentation of immunity to measles, defined as receipt of two doses of measles vaccine after their first birthday, birth before 1957, or a documented measles history or immunity. Children traveling to endemic areas should be immunized as if they were in an outbreak area (see next section).

D. Outbreak Control: An outbreak is defined in a community whenever a single case of measles is documented. Control depends on immediate protection of all susceptible persons (defined as persons who have no documented immunity to measles). In the case of unvaccinated individuals, the following recommendations hold: (1) 6–11 months of age, monovalent measles vaccine (or MMR) if cases are occurring in children less than 1 year old, followed by MMR at 15 months and again at 4–6 or 11–12 years; and (2) 12 months of age or older, MMR followed by revaccination at the recommended times.

A child with an unclear or unknown vaccination history should be reimmunized with MMR. Anyone with a known exposure who is not certain of receiving two doses of MMR should receive an additional dose. Measles vaccination is contraindicated in pregnant women, women intending to become pregnant within the next 90 days, immunocompromised persons (except those with HIV infection), and persons with anaphylactic egg or neomycin allergy. Children with minor acute illnesses (including febrile illnesses), nonanaphylactic egg allergy, or a history of tuberculosis should be immunized. Monovalent measles or MMR may be safely administered simultaneously with DTP and OPV.

Adverse Effects

Between 5% and 15% of vaccinees become febrile to 39.5 °C or higher about 1 week after vaccination, and 5% may develop a transient morbilliform rash. Encephalitis and other central nervous system conditions are reported to occur at a frequency of one case per 3 million doses in the United States. This rate is lower than the rate of these conditions in the general unvaccinated population, implying that the relationship between them and measles vaccination may not be causal. Recent reports have suggested that there may be a slightly increased risk for febrile convulsions in children with a family or personal history of seizures. A case of fatal measles vaccine strain pneumonia has been reported in an HIV-infected man who received MMR.

Antibody Preparations

If a child is seen within 72 hours after exposure, vaccination is the preferred method of protection. IG, given at a dose of 0.25 mL/kg (0.5 mL/kg in the immunocompromised) intramuscularly, is effective in preventing or modifying measles if it is given within 6 days after exposure.

American Academy of Pediatrics, Committee on Infectious Diseases: Recommended timing of routine measles immunization for children who have recently received immune globulin preparations. Pediatrics 1994;95:682.

Edmonson MB et al: Measles vaccination during the respiratory virus season and risk of vaccine failure. Pediatrics 1996;98:905.

Halsey NA: Increased mortality after high titer measles vaccines: Too much of a good thing. Pediatr Infect Dis J 1993;12:462.

James JM et al: Safe administration of the measles vaccine to children allergic to eggs. N Engl J Med 1995;332:1262.

Measles—United States, 1996, and the interruption of indigenous transmission. MMWR Morb Mortal Wkly Rep 1997;46(11):242.

Measles eradication: Recommendations from a meeting cosponsored by the World Health Organization, the Pan American Health Organization, and CDC. MMWR Morb Mortal Wkly Rep 1997;46(RR-11):1.

Measles pneumonitis following measles-mumps-rubella vaccination of a patient with HIV infection, 1993. MMWR Morb Mortal Wkly Rep 1996;45:603.

MUMPS

Mumps vaccine has dramatically reduced the incidence of this infection and its complications in the United States, from 152,000 cases in 1968 to a low of 2982 cases in 1985. The incidence has remained at about 1500 cases a year after a minor resurgence in 1986–1987.

Preparations Available

The Jeryl Lynn Strain is the only preparation available as monovalent vaccine. It is prepared from virus isolated from a child and passaged in embryonated eggs and in chick embryo tissue culture. It contains the equivalent of over 20,000 TCID50 of the United States Reference Mumps Virus. The Jeryl Lynn vaccine is also available in combination with measles vaccine (MM), with rubella vaccine, and with measles and rubella vaccines (MMR).

Dosage & Schedule of Administration

Mumps vaccine is given to children in the combination vaccine MMR at the age of 15 months and again at 4–6 or 11–12 years of age. Despite the over 95% efficacy of the mumps vaccine, outbreaks have been reported in highly vaccinated populations. Most cases were attributed to primary vaccine failure. It is hoped that the two-dose schedule will prevent these outbreaks. As monovalent vaccine, it is safe and effective if given after the first birthday. The dose of either monovalent or MMR vaccines is 0.5 mL subcutaneously. Use of the monovalent vaccine is limited to susceptibles with proved immunity to the other constituents of MMR. Revaccination with mumps vaccine or any of the vaccines in MMR is not harmful. Anyone with an unclear vaccination history should therefore be immunized. The same recommendations and contraindications apply to mumps vaccine as to measles vaccine (see above).

Adverse Effects

Reactions after mumps vaccination are rare and include parotitis, low-grade fever, and orchitis. In 1989, a nationwide surveillance of neurologic complications after mumps vaccine was conducted in Japan. There were at least 311 cases of mild aseptic meningitis (96 had vaccine-type mumps virus in the cerebrospinal fluid) among 630,157 recipients. There were no sequelae. Aseptic meningitis may be more common than was previously suspected (1–4 cases per 10,000 vaccinations).

Fujinaga T et al: A prefecture-wide survey of mumps meningitis associated with measles, mumps and rubella vaccine. Pediatr Infect Dis J 1991;10:204.

King JC et al: Measles, mumps and rubella antibodies in vaccinated Baltimore children. Am J Dis Child 1993;147:558.

Mumps prevention. Recommendations of the Immunization Practices Advisory Committee (ACIP). MMWR Morb Mortal Wkly Rep 1989;38:388, 397.

RUBELLA

The use of rubella vaccine represents an important deviation from the public health philosophy underlying the other vaccines discussed in this chapter. It is not intended to protect individuals from the consequences of rubella infection but rather to prevent congenital rubella syndrome. In the United States, the approach has been to vaccinate young children. The intent is to reduce transmission to susceptible women of childbearing age via a herd immunity effect. Immunity lasts for at least 15 years. Other countries, notably the United Kingdom, vaccinate pubertal girls (aged 11–14). The relative efficacy of these two strategies in the prevention of congenital rubella syndrome is not clear.

With the use of rubella vaccines since 1970, rubella incidence rates have declined more than 95%. However, approximately 10% of young adults are now susceptible to rubella. Outbreaks have occurred in settings where adult susceptibles congregated (eg, prisons, colleges). In most cases, failure to vaccinate susceptible persons, not vaccine failure, was implicated.

Preparations Available

The RA 27/3 strain is the only vaccine available in the United States. It is grown in human diploid cells. Each dose contains more than 1000 TCID50 of the United States Reference Rubella Virus. The RA 27/3 strain is available in combined preparations with measles vaccine (MR), mumps vaccine, and measles and mumps vaccines (MMR).

Dosage & Schedule of Administration

Either the monovalent or combined forms should be administered subcutaneously in a dose of 0.5 mL. Current practice is to use MMR vaccine at 15 months of age and at 4–6 or 11–12 years of age. A person can be considered immune only with documentation of either serologic immunity to rubella or vaccination with at least one dose of rubella vaccine after 1 year of age. A clinical diagnosis of rubella is unacceptable. Susceptible pubertal girls and postpubertal women identified by premarital or prenatal screening should also be immunized. All susceptible adults in institutional settings (including colleges), day care center personnel, military personnel, and hospital and health care personnel should be immunized. Whenever rubella vaccination is offered to a woman of childbearing age, pregnancy should be ruled out and the woman advised to prevent conception during the 90 days following vaccination.

It has been estimated that the risk of serious malformations attributable to giving the RA 27/3 vaccine to pregnant women is from nil to 1.6%. This is much less than the over 20% risk of congenital rubella syndrome after maternal infection in the first trimester of pregnancy.

Adverse Effects

In children, adverse effects from rubella vaccination are very unusual. Five to 15 percent of children develop rash, fever, or lymphadenopathy 5–12 days after vaccination. Rash also occurs alone or as a mild rubella illness in 2–4% of adults. Arthralgia and arthritis occur in 10–25% of adult vaccinees. Chronic arthritis may be causally related to RA 27/3 vaccinations. Rare complications include peripheral neuritis and neuropathy, transverse myelitis, and diffuse myelitis.

Herrmann KL: Rubella in the United States: Toward a strategy for disease control and elimination. Epidemiol Infect 1991;107:55.

Howson CP, Fineberg HV: Adverse events following pertussis and rubella vaccines. JAMA 1992;267:392.

HAEMOPHILUS INFLUENZAE TYPE b INFECTION

The first vaccine licensed against *Haemophilus influenzae* type b in the United States was composed of the capsular polysaccharide of *H influenzae* type b polyribosylribitol phosphate (PRP). This vaccine, which became available in 1985 for children between 2 and 5 years of age, was moderately effective in preventing *H influenzae* type b disease. Conjugation of the PRP with protein carriers confers T cell-dependent characteristics on the vaccine and enhances the immunologic response to PRP in infancy. Since

1994, four conjugate vaccines and a combination vaccine (DTP-Hib, Tetramune) have been licensed for children (Table 9–5).

Studies in infants aged 2–6 months demonstrated the immunogenicity of each of these vaccines except PRP-D, which is recommended for children over 12 months of age. A geometric mean titer (GMT) of 1 μg/mL of antipolysaccharide antibody 3 weeks postvaccination has correlated with long-term protection from invasive disease. After three doses at ages 2, 4, and 6 months, each of the three vaccines—HbOC, PRP-OMP, and PRP-T—produces protective levels of antibody. Regardless of the vaccine used in the primary series, booster vaccination of children over age 12 months with any licensed vaccine elicits an adequate response. Furthermore, each vaccine is immunogenic as a single dose given after 15 months of age. Limited information on interchangeability of different Hib vaccines suggests that any combination of the three doses of Hib conjugate vaccines will provide adequate protection.

Clinical trials for all three conjugate vaccines among infants 2–6 months of age have been published. These studies form the basis for the FDA approval of vaccine use and recommendations by the American Academy of Pediatrics and the Immunization Practices Advisory Committee on the use of *Haemophilus* type b conjugate vaccines. Because of the differences in the immunogenic response and the different regimens used in these trials, the recommendations for use of HbOC, PRP-T, and PRP-OMP differ and are summarized in Table 9–6.

The FDA has licensed HbOC-DTP (Tetramune) and recently PRP-OMP-hepatitis B (Comvax) for use in infants as young as 2 months of age. Antibody responses are comparable to HbOC and DTP or PRP-OMP and hepatitis B administered separately. If the exact conjugate vaccine previously administered is unknown, it is recommended that at least three doses of conjugate vaccine be administered to children between 2 and 6 months of age. Unvaccinated or partially vaccinated children younger than 24 months of age who experience invasive *H influenzae* type b disease should receive a complete series of vaccinations. Children over the age of 24 months mount an adequate immune response to invasive *H influenzae* type b disease and do not require further vaccinations. Unimmunized children 5 years of age or older with a chronic illness known to be associated with invasive *H influenzae* type b disease, such as sickle cell anemia and asplenia, should be given a single dose of any of the licensed conjugate vaccines. Regardless of the regimen implemented, it is crucial to complete the series, since cases of invasive *H influenzae* type b disease have been described in partially vaccinated children.

Preparations Available
See Table 9–6.

Dosage & Schedule of Administration
Regardless of which preparation is used, the dose is 0.5 mL intramuscularly.

Adverse Effects
These are the first vaccines for which the FDA requires active surveillance for adverse reactions after licensure. Fewer than 5% of those immunized develop systemic reactions (including fever) to the vaccine. About 25% of recipients develop local reactions. Adverse effects following the second dose of PRP-OMP are more frequent than following the first dose and more frequent following the third dose of

Table 9–5. *Haemophilus influenzae* type b conjugate vaccines for children.

Vaccine	Trade Name and Manufacturer	Polysaccharide	Linkage	Protein Carrier
PRP-D[1]	ProHIBIT (Connaught/Pasteur Mérieux)	Medium	Six-carbon	Diphtheria toxoid
HbOC	HibTITER (Wyeth-Lederle-Praxis)	Small	None	CRM[197] mutant *Corynebacterium diphtheriae* toxin protein
PRP-OMP	PedvaxHIB (Merck & Co.)	Medium	Thioether	*Neisseria meningitidis* outer membrane protein complex
PRP-T	ACTHIB OmniHIB (Connaught/ Pasteur Mérieux)	Large	Six-carbon	Tetanus toxoid
HbOC-DTP	Tetramune (Wyeth-Lederle-Praxis)	Small	None	See above for HbOC
PRP-OMP- Hepatitis B	Comvax (Merck & Co.)	Medium	Thioether	See above for PRP-OMP

[1]Limited to children over 12 months of age.

Table 9–6. Schedule for Hib conjugate vaccine administration.

Vaccine	Age at First Vaccination	Primary Series (Same Vaccine if Possible)	Booster (Any Conjugate Vaccine)
HbOC or PRP-T[1]	2–6 months	Three doses 2 months apart	12–15 months
	7–11 months	Two doses 2 months apart	12–19 months
	12–14 months	One dose	2 months later
	15–59 months	One dose	. . .
PRP-OMP[2]	2–6 months	Two doses 2 months apart	12–15 months
	7–11 months	Two doses 2 months apart	12–18 months
	12–14 months	One dose	2 months later
	15–59 months	One dose	. . .

[1]Tetramune may be administered by the same schedule for primary immunization as HbOC or PRP-T (when the series begins at 2–6 months of age). A booster dose of DTP or DTaP should be administered at 4–6 years of age, before kindergarten or elementary school. This booster is not necessary if the fourth vaccinating dose was administered after the fourth birthday.

[2]Comvax may be administered by the same schedule for primary immunization as PRP-OMP. It should only be used in infants of hepatitis B-negative mothers. If the series is started late, three doses should be given if started in infants (≤ 10 months), two doses if started at 11–14 months, and one dose if started at age 15–71 months. However, three doses of hepatitis B vaccine are required regardless of age of starting immunization.

HbOC than following the first two doses. There have been no reports of more severe reactions.

American Academy of Pediatrics, Committee on Infectious Diseases: *Haemophilus influenzae* type b conjugate vaccines: Recommendations for immunization with recently and previously licensed vaccines. Pediatrics 1993;92: 480.

Bewley KM et al: Interchangeability of *Haemophilus influenzae* type b vaccines in the primary series: Evaluation of a two-dose mixed regimen. Pediatrics 1996;98:898.

FDA approval for infants of a *Haemophilus influenzae* type b conjugate and hepatitis B (recombinant) combined vaccine. MMWR Morb Mortal Wkly Rep 1997; 46(5):107.

Greenberg DP et al: Enhanced antibody responses in infants given different sequences of heterogeneous *Haemophilus influenzae* type b conjugate vaccines. J Pediatr 1995;126:206.

Recommendations for use of *Haemophilus* b conjugate vaccines and a combined diphtheria, tetanus, pertussis, and *Haemophilus* b vaccine: Recommendations of the Advisory Committee on Immunization Practices (ACIP). MMWR Morb Mortal Wkly Rep 1993;42:1.

HEPATITIS A

In children, the hepatitis A virus (HAV) is transmitted primarily by the fecal-oral and rarely by other routes, such as sexual contact and blood-borne transmission during viremia. The major source of pediatric transmission is close personal contact with a person infected with HAV. The second most important cause is transmission in day care centers, where the index case is usually an adult such as a child care provider or a parent. International travelers acquire HAV, but the risk of transmission is less than in day care centers. Epidemiologically, high-risk populations for transmission of HAV are Native Americans, Alaskan Natives, Hispanics, and Hasidic Jews. In children, HAV causes anicteric hepatitis in about 90% of cases and is symptomatic in the remainder.

Preparations Available

HAV vaccines are prepared from supernatants of infected cell cultures by formalin inactivation and absorption to aluminum hydroxide.

Dosage & Route of Administration

Havrix (SmithKline Beecham) is available in two formulations: 360 EL.U. (ELISA units) administered in three doses of 0.5 mL separated by 1 and 6–12 months. A higher-dose preparation (720 EL.U.) can be given as two doses separated by 6–12 months.

Vaqta (Merck & Co.) contains 25 units (equivalent to 25 nanograms of virus protein) given as two 0.5 mL doses separated by 6–18 months.

Both vaccines should be stored and shipped at 2–8 °C and should not be frozen. They are licensed for use in children over 2 years of age.

Adverse Effects

Adverse reactions are mild and consist of pain at the injection site, headache, and fever. The vaccine should not be administered to children with hypersensitivity to alum or phenoxyethanol.

Antibody Preparations

Immune globulin (IG) for intramuscular injection can be used for preexposure prophylaxis for children under 2 years of age. The recommended dosages are 0.02 mL/kg in a single dose if the duration of exposure is likely to be less than 3 months, or 0.06 mL/kg if exposure is likely to be more than 3 months. For long-term prophylaxis, booster doses can be repeated every 5 months. For children older than 2 years, the HAV vaccine is preferred. IG may be used for postexposure prophylaxis usually within 14 days after exposure since the incubation period with HAV is 25–30 days. HAV vaccines can also be used within the 14 days of exposure, but extra doses will be needed.

American Academy of Pediatrics, Committee on Infectious Diseases: Prevention of hepatitis A infections: Guidelines for use of hepatitis A vaccine and immune globulin. Pediatrics 1996;96:1207.
Balcarek KB et al: Safety and immunogenicity of an inactivated hepatitis A vaccine in preschool children. J Infect Dis 1995;171(Suppl 1):S70.
McMahon BJ et al: Immunogenicity of an inactivated hepatitis A vaccine in Alaska native children and native and non-native adults. J Infect Dis 1995;171:676.
Prevention of hepatitis A through active or passive immunization: Recommendations of the Advisory Committee on Immunization Practices (ACIP). MMWR Morb Mortal Wkly Rep 1996;45(RR-15):1.

HEPATITIS B

Hepatitis B vaccine is 85% effective in preventing perinatally acquired infection and 80–95% effective in preventing most postnatally acquired infections.

In 1988, the American College of Obstetrics and Gynecology recommended that all pregnant women be routinely screened for hepatitis B surface antigen (HBsAg). Women with positive reactions are highly likely to transmit the infection to their offspring. The use of hepatitis B vaccine with hepatitis B immune globulin (HBIG) as postexposure prophylaxis is established as an effective means of interrupting mother-to-infant transmission—except for the 2–3% of infants who acquire hepatitis B in utero.

Several risk categories have been identified as target populations for preexposure vaccination. Those that are relevant to physicians caring for children include clients and staff in institutions for the developmentally delayed, clients and staff of hemodialysis units, recipients of clotting factor concentrates, homosexually active males, users of illicit injectable drugs, household contacts of chronic hepatitis B carriers, and all health care personnel. With the exception of high-risk neonates, all persons identified as being at high risk should be screened for markers of past infection and immunized if proved susceptible. Since vaccines consist of a purified inactive subunit of the virus and are not infectious, they are not contraindicated in immunosuppressed individuals or in pregnant women.

Each year about 300,000 persons in the United States are infected with hepatitis B virus; 50% of these develop clinical hepatitis, 10,000 are hospitalized, and an estimated 20,000–30,000 become chronic carriers. The risk of carriage varies inversely with age; thus, although only 1–3% of the infections occur in children under 5 years of age, they account for 20–30% of new carriers each year. Chronic carriers are at 12–300 times greater risk than noncarriers of developing primary liver cancer, and 25% develop chronic active hepatitis that progresses to cirrhosis over 5–20 years.

Hepatitis B vaccine is highly immunogenic in children and young adults, and higher antibody titers are obtained when vaccination is begun later in infancy or childhood and with longer intervals between the second and third doses. The protective efficacy of hepatitis B vaccine correlates well with antibody levels, and virtually all persons with 10 mIU/mL or more are protected in clinical trials.

Universal childhood vaccination with hepatitis B vaccine has recently been recommended both by the ACIP and the AAP. When resources are limited, the AAP recommends giving the highest priority to immunization of high-risk infants and children, followed by all infants, adolescents in high-risk areas, and, finally, all adolescents. The AAP has also published recommendations for the prevention of hepatitis B infections in school settings.

Optimally, three intramuscular doses of hepatitis B vaccine are needed. Increasing the interval between the first and second doses has little effect on immunogenicity, but longer intervals between the last two doses (4–12 months) result in higher titers of anti-HBs. Thus, adequate responses and seroconversion rates are achieved with doses administered at birth, 1 month, and 6 months; or birth, 2 months, and 6 months; or 2 months, 4 months, and 6 months. Simultaneous administration with other vaccines at different sites is safe and efficacious.

Preparations Available

Recombinant vaccine, licensed in 1986, is the only vaccine type available. It is immunologically indistinguishable from the HBsAg found in chronic carriers. Three vaccines, adsorbed with aluminum hydroxide and thimerosal, are licensed: Recombivax HB and Comvax (Merck & Co.), containing 10 µg/mL; and Engerix-B (SmithKline Beecham), containing 20 µg/mL.

Dosage & Schedule of Administration

Note: Hepatitis B vaccine should be given only in the deltoid muscle for adolescents and children and in the anterolateral thigh muscle for infants and neonates. Administration intradermally or in the buttocks has resulted in poor immune responses in some individuals, and these sites are not recommended.

A. Neonatal: Infants of HBsAg-positive mothers should be cleansed of blood in the delivery room. Both hepatitis B vaccine (see Table 9–7) and hepatitis B immune globulin (HBIG, 0.5 mL intramuscularly) should be administered simultaneously at different sites as soon as the baby is stable, preferably in the delivery room and within 12 hours after birth. The vaccine should be repeated at 1 month and 6 months. At 12–15 months of age, immunized infants should be tested for antibody to HBsAg (anti-HBs). If the anti-HBs is positive, vaccination has been effective. If negative, HBsAg should be tested for; if the result is positive, immunization has failed and the infant is a chronic carrier. If both HBsAg and anti-HBs are negative, the series should be repeated at 0, 1, and 6 months followed by repeat anti-HBs testing 1 month after the third dose.

For infants born to mothers of unknown HBsAg status, the same schedule should be followed except that HBIG be withheld until the HBsAg status is known. If she is HBsAg-positive, HBIG should be initiated as soon as possible but within 7 days after birth.

For infants born to HBsAg-negative mothers, the first dose should be administered in the newborn period—or, if this is not possible, at least before 2 months of age. The doses and the schedule for routine vaccination of these infants are set forth in Table 9–7. For preterm infants born to HBsAg-negative mothers with birth weights of less than 2000 g, initiation of hepatitis B vaccination should be delayed until the infant weighs 2000 g or more.

If maternal screening is not possible, the infant should receive the first dose within 12 hours after birth, the second at 1–2 months of age, and the third at 6 months.

B. Older Children and Adolescents: All children should receive hepatitis B vaccine as part of the routine schedule. Both the AAP and ACIP recommend vaccination of adolescents. Resources permitting, the universal immunization of all adolescents is recommended. (See Table 9–7 for dosages and schedules.)

C. Immunosuppressed Persons and Dialysis Patients: Hemodialysis patients and other immunocompromised persons should be vaccinated with larger doses or increased numbers of doses (or both) (see Table 9–7).

D. Lapsed Hepatitis B Immunization: The three-dose series can be completed regardless of the interval from the last vaccine dose. There is no need to start the series over or to test routinely for anti-HBs unless the child's mother is HBsAg-positive.

Vaccination in the perinatal period could prevent 22,000 cases of acute HBV infection and a maximum of 6000 chronic HBV infections annually. However, it is estimated that 300,000 persons become infected with HBV and 20,000–30,000 become chronic carriers annually. The dose of vaccine in children is half that of adolescents. Compliance with vaccination is better in infancy than in adolescence.

E. Postexposure Prophylaxis: Postexposure prophylaxis is indicated in individuals with inadvertent percutaneous or permucosal exposure to HBsAg-positive blood, sexual exposure to an HBsAg-positive individual, or household exposure of an

Table 9–7. Hepatitis B vaccine schedule and dosage.

	Vaccine Dose		
	Recombivax HB	Engerix-B	Schedule: Doses at Ages
Infants of HBsAg-negative mothers[1]	0.5 mL[2]	0.5 mL	0–2 days, 1–2 months, and 6–18 months
Older children < 11 years (not vaccinated at birth)	0.5 mL[2]	0.5 mL	1–2, 4, and 6–18 months[4]
Infants of HBsAg-positive mothers (HBIG 0.5 mL should also be given)	1.0 mL[2]	0.5 mL	Day 0, 1 month, and 6 months
Children and adolescents aged 11–19 years	0.5 mL[3]	1.0 mL	Day 0, 1 month, and 6 months; or day 0, 2 months, and 4 months
Immunosuppressed persons and dialysis patients	1.0 mL[5]	2.0 mL[6]	

[1]Infants of mothers with unknown HBsAg status should be tested at delivery. The infant should receive hepatitis B vaccine within 12 hours after birth in a dose appropriate for infants born to HBsAg-positive mothers. Preterm infants should receive vaccine at a weight of 2000 g or more.
[2]Pediatric formulation.
[3]Adult formulation.
[4]May be given along with routine vaccinations.
[5]Special formulation containing 40 mg/mL at day 0, 1 month, and 6 months.
[6]Two doses of 1 mL at one site in a four-dose schedule at day 0 and at 1, 2, and 6 months.

infant under 12 months of age to a caregiver with acute hepatitis B. Unvaccinated individuals should receive HBIG (0.06 mL/kg—maximum 5 mL—within 24 hours [its value after 7 days is unknown]) and the first dose of hepatitis B vaccine at a separate site or within 7 days after exposure. Previously vaccinated persons should be retested for anti-HBs. If levels are adequate (≥ 10 mIU/mL), no treatment is necessary. If levels are inadequate, a booster dose is required. In individuals who cannot be tested, a dose of HBIG should be given. A known nonresponder should receive either two doses of HBIG (1 month apart) or one dose of HBIG and one of vaccine. If the patient becomes a chronic carrier, all household contacts should also receive vaccination.

Adverse Effects

The overall rate of adverse effects is low and minor, and effects include fever (1–6%) and pain at the injection site (3–29%). Despite vaccination of approximately 2.5 million persons with recombinant vaccine, no excess risk of Guillain-Barré syndrome has been observed.

Antibody Preparations

HBIG is prepared from HIV-negative donors with high titers of HBs antibody and has an anti-HBs titer of greater than 1:100,000 by radioimmunoassay. The Cohn fractionation process used to prepare this product inactivates HIV, and there is no evidence for HIV transmission by HBIG. The use of HBIG is described above.

American Academy of Pediatrics, Committee on Infectious Diseases: Prevention of hepatitis B virus infection in school setting. Pediatrics 1993;91:848.
American Academy of Pediatrics, Committee on Infectious Diseases: Update on timing of hepatitis B vaccination for premature infants and for children with lapsed immunization. Pediatrics 1994;94:403.
FDA approval for infants of a *Haemophilus influenzae* type B conjugate and hepatitis B (recombinant) combined vaccine. MMWR Morb Mortal Wkly Rep 1997;46:107.
Greenberg DP et al: Pediatric experience with recombinant hepatitis B vaccines and relevant safety and immunogenicity studies. Pediatr Infect Dis J 1993;12:438.
Halsey NA et al: Discussion of Immunization Practices Advisory Committee/American Academy of Pediatrics recommendations for universal infant hepatitis B vaccination. Pediatr Infect Dis J 1993;12:446.
Woodruff BA et al: Progress toward integrating hepatitis B vaccine into routine infant immunization schedules in the United States, 1991 through 1994. Pediatrics 1995;97:798.

VARICELLA

About 4 million cases of varicella occur annually in the United States, mostly in children under 10 years of age. A live attenuated varicella-zoster vaccine (VZV) was developed in Japan in the 1970s and licensed in the United States by the FDA in 1995 for children over 12 months of age.

Preparations Available

A cell-free preparation of OKA strain VZV is produced and marketed in the United States (Merck & Co.). Each dose of VZV contains not less than 1350 plaque-forming units of VZV and trace amounts of neomycin in a lyophilized form. Storage in a freezer at a temperature of –15 °C or colder provides a shelf life of 15 months. VZV must be administered within 30 minutes after thawing and reconstitution.

Dosage & Schedule of Administration

In healthy children, a single dose of VZV results in a seroconversion rate of more than 95%. These antibodies persist for up to 20 years following immunization. One dose (0.5 mL) of VZV is recommended for immunization for all healthy children 12 months to 13 years of age who lack a history of varicella. Children over 13 years require two doses of VZV 1 month apart. VZV may be given simultaneously with MMR at separate sites. If not given simultaneously, the interval between administration of VZV and MMR must be greater than 1 month. Simultaneous VZV administration probably does not affect the immune response to other childhood vaccines, though further immunogenicity studies are needed.

Adverse Events

About 5% of children and 10% of adults develop a mild VZV-related maculopapular or varicelliform rash. Local reactions occur in 25% of patients and consist of transient pain, tenderness, or redness. Herpes zoster occurs no more frequently in patients who receive VZV than in those who had natural varicella. Spread of VZV strain virus to nonimmune contacts is uncommon, but spread has recently been documented from an immunized child to its pregnant mother. VZV should not be administered within at least 5 months after injection of immune globulin or other blood products.

Contraindications

Table 9–2 lists contraindications to VZV immunization, such as hypersensitivity or allergy to any VZV component, including neomycin. VZV is also contraindicated in children with cancers involving the bone marrow or in children with primary immunodeficiencies or those receiving immunosuppressive therapy. It is recommended that VZV be avoided during pregnancy and by individuals with active untreated tuberculosis. Because VZV is attenuated and produces mild disease, it has been suggested that VZV might actually be preferable in some immunocompromised groups.

Antibody Preparations

Varicella-zoster immune globulin (VZIG) is prepared from plasma harvested from persons known to have high titers of antivaricella antibody. It is indicated for high-risk susceptible persons who are exposed to varicella, eg, immunocompromised individuals without a history of chickenpox, susceptible pregnant women, newborns whose mothers develop varicella 5 days prior to delivery and within 48 hours after delivery, hospitalized premature infants of less than 28 weeks' gestational age, and hospitalized premature infants of less than 28 weeks' gestation whose mother had no history of chickenpox or seronegativity. Exposure is defined as a household contact or playmate contact (over 1 h/d), hospital contact (in the same or contiguous room or ward), intimate contact with a person with zoster deemed contagious, or a newborn contact. Susceptibility is defined as the absence of anti-VZV antibody by a sensitive test. VZIG must be administered within 96 hours after exposure. Newborns should be given one vial (125 units) intramuscularly. The dose for all others is 125 units/10 kg body weight intramuscularly (maximum dose, 625 units). VZIG should be readministered following reexposure of susceptible persons if more than 2 weeks has elapsed since a prior dose of VZIG.

American Academy of Pediatrics Committee on Infectious Diseases: Recommendations for the use of live attenuated varicella vaccine. Pediatrics 1995;95:79.
Gershon A: Varicella-zoster virus: Prospects for control. Adv Pediatr Infect Dis 1995;10:93.
Krause PR, Kleinman DM: Efficacy, immunogenicity, safety and use of live attenuated chickenpox vaccine. J Pediatr 1995;127:518.
Prevention of varicella: Recommendations of the Advisory Committee on Immunization Practice (ACIP). MMWR Morb Mortal Wkly Rep 1996;45(RR-11):1.

VACCINATIONS FOR SPECIAL SITUATIONS

INFLUENZA

Influenza occurs each winter and early spring, often associated with significant morbidity and mortality rates in certain high-risk persons. In pediatric practice, these include children with hemoglobinopathies and with chronic cardiac, pulmonary (including asthma), metabolic, renal, and immunosuppressive diseases. Children and teenagers receiving long-term aspirin therapy should also receive the vaccine, as well as household members (including children) of persons in high-risk groups. The vaccine may be administered to children over 6 months of age. Physicians should identify high-risk children in their practices and encourage parents to seek influenza vaccination for them each fall. In pandemic years, it may be important to advocate vaccination in all children regardless of their usual state of health. Influenza vaccination has a 65–80% efficacy in protecting against disease.

Each year, recommendations are formulated in the spring and summer regarding the constituents of influenza vaccine for the coming season. These recommendations are based on the results of surveillance in Asia and the southern hemisphere during the spring and summer. The vaccine each year is a trivalent inactivated vaccine containing antigens from two strains of influenza A and one strain of influenza B. Influenza vaccine virus is grown in eggs and formalin-inactivated. These whole-virus preparations may be further treated with detergents to produce split (subvirion) or purified surface antigen vaccines.

Influenza causes serious illness in very young children, especially because of the ear and sinopulmonary bacterial superinfections that often follow. Unfortunately, the trivalent inactivated vaccine may have limited efficacy in this age group. Protection is short-lived and often incomplete. Live attenuated influenza A and B vaccines are being produced by genetic reassortment. A live cold-adapted type A vaccine administered intranasally has been shown to be safe and immunogenic in children as young as 6 months of age. Studies are under way to determine whether combinations of live and inactivated vaccines are immunogenic in young children. A new nasal cold-adapted vaccine (Aviron), proved 93% effective in preventing influenza, awaits FDA approval. Influenza vaccine has been shown in some but not all studies to increase HIV-1 replication transiently. Nevertheless, the CDC currently recommends influenza vaccination for all HIV-infected persons.

Preparations Available

Several manufacturers produce similar vaccines each year. Whole virus vaccines produce unacceptably high rates of adverse reactions in children and are therefore contraindicated. Only split-virus (subvirion) or purified surface antigen preparations should be used. These are also effective in adults and adolescents.

Dosage & Schedule of Administration

Children under 6 months of age should not be routinely immunized. Two doses are recommended for children under 9 years of age who are receiving influenza vaccine for the first time. The dose for children 6–35 months of age is two doses of 0.25 mL intramuscularly given 4–6 weeks apart; for older children, 0.5 mL once intramuscularly. Split virus vaccine should be used for children under 12 years of age, and either split or whole virus vaccine after 12 years. The recommended site of vaccination is the anterolateral aspect of the thigh for younger children and the deltoid for older children. Since this vaccine is inactivated, pregnancy is not an absolute contraindication to its use.

The 1997–1998 vaccine will use the antigen equivalent strains: A/Johannesburg/82/96 (H1N1), A/Nanchang/933/95 (H3N2), and B/Harbin/07/94.

Adverse Effects

A small proportion of children will experience some systemic toxicity, consisting of fever, malaise, and myalgias. These symptoms generally begin 6–12 hours after vaccination and may last 24–48 hours. Cases of Guillain-Barré syndrome followed the swine influenza vaccination program in 1976–1977, but careful study showed no association with that vaccine in children and young adults—nor in any age with subsequent vaccines. In patients with anaphylactic egg allergies in whom influenza vaccination is indicated, a protocol for influenza vaccination has been referenced below.

Glesby MJ et al: The effect of influenza vaccination on human immunodeficiency virus type 1 load: A randomized, double-blinded, placebo-controlled study. J Infect Dis 1996;174:1332.

Gruber WC et al: Comparison of monovalent and trivalent live attenuated influenza vaccines in young children. J Infect Dis 1993;168:53.

Murphy KR, Strunk RC: Safe administration of influenza vaccine in asthmatic children sensitive to egg proteins. J Pediatr 1985;106:9313.

Prevention and control of influenza: Recommendations of the Advisory Committee on Immunization Practices (ACIP). MMWR Morb Mortal Wkly Rep 1997;46(RR-9):1.

Stuprans SL et al: Activation of virus replication after vaccination of HIV-1-infected individuals. J Exper Med 1995;182:1727.

PNEUMOCOCCAL INFECTIONS

Infections with *Streptococcus pneumoniae* cause significant morbidity and mortality in certain high-risk groups, including children with chronic cardiovascular, pulmonary, or liver diseases, anatomic and functional asplenia (and sickle cell disease), nephrotic syndrome, chronic renal failure, diabetes mellitus, cerebrospinal fluid leaks, and immunosuppression (including those with HIV infection complement deficiencies and organ transplants). Recent outbreaks of pneumococcal disease in Alaskan natives and certain Native American populations have led the ACIP to recommend routine pneumococcal vaccination for these groups. The vaccine is of limited efficacy in children under 2 years of age. It is not in-

dicated for children attending day care facilities or for those having only recurrent upper respiratory tract infections such as otitis media or sinusitis. The protective efficacy of the vaccine in high-risk children has not been well studied but is presumed to be about 60%, based on extrapolation from investigations in adults. In persons over 5 years of age, the overall efficacy has been estimated to be 57% (95% CI = 45–66%). The currently used 23-valent vaccine was licensed in 1983. Conjugate pneumococcal vaccines that may work in young children are undergoing clinical trials.

Preparations Available

The standard dose of currently available vaccines contains 25 μg each of the purified capsular polysaccharide antigen of 23 serotypes of *S pneumoniae*. These 23 types cause 88% of the bacteremic and meningitic pneumococcal disease in adults and nearly 100% of those in children in the United States—and nearly 85% of acute pneumococcal otitis media in children. Cross-reactive antibody responses may protect against an additional 8% of bacteremic serotypes in adults.

Dosage & Schedule of Administration

The dose is 0.5 mL, given intramuscularly or subcutaneously. If splenectomy or immunosuppression can be anticipated, the vaccine should be given at least 2 weeks previously. Routine revaccination is not indicated because of an increased risk of adverse reactions. Children who received their initial vaccination during chemotherapy for Hodgkin's disease should be revaccinated 3–4 months after cessation of chemotherapy. Revaccination may be considered after 3–5 years in children at high risk of fatal pneumococcal infection such as those with sickle cell anemia, nephrotic syndrome, renal failure, organ transplants, or asplenia. Pregnant women should generally not be vaccinated. Vaccination is not a substitute for antibiotic prophylaxis in certain high-risk children.

Adverse Effects

Fifty percent of all vaccine recipients develop pain and redness at the injection site. Fewer than 1% develop systemic side effects such as fever and myalgia. Anaphylaxis is rare.

Antibody Preparations

Most authorities recommend the routine use of IGIV in agammaglobulinemic patients and in some patients with HIV infection, in part to prevent pneumococcal disease.

Davidson M et al: The epidemiology of invasive pneumococcal disease in Alaska, 1986–1990: Ethnic differences and opportunities for prevention. J Infect Dis 1994;170:368.

Gessner BD et al: Risk factors for invasive disease caused by *Streptococcus pneumoniae* among Alaska native children younger than two years of age. Pediatr Infect Dis J 1995;14:123.

Keller DW et al: Preventing bacterial respiratory tract infections among persons infected with human immunodeficiency virus. Clin Infect Dis 1995;21(Suppl 1):S77.

Prevention of pneumococcal disease: Recommendations of the Advisory Committee on Immunization Practices (ACIP). MMWR Morb Mortal Wkly Rep 1997;46(RR-8):1.

RABIES

Human rabies has been rare in the United States over the last several decades, but animal rabies persists in many feral animal species throughout the country, and domestic animals may be secondarily infected. Travelers to developing countries, where dogs are a major vector, account for about 70% of cases of human rabies in the United States. The risk of rabies transmission is highly dependent on the nature of the animal-to-human contact (the risk of rabies after a bite from a rabid animal is 50 times the risk after a scratch), the species of animal involved (in the United States, 3–20% of bats and 12–70% of raccoons, skunks, or foxes are positive for rabies, but only 0.01% of rodents are positive), and the locale of the incident. Local public health officials are well versed in the epidemiology of animal rabies in their jurisdictions and should be consulted before postexposure rabies prophylaxis is undertaken. First, they can avert unnecessary vaccination. Second, they can assist in the proper handling of the animal if confinement or testing is appropriate. Third, they can supply needed biologicals that may not be routinely stocked in hospitals, offices, or pharmacies. In some jurisdictions, these biologicals are supplied at no expense to the recipient if the use is authorized by the appropriate public health official. In order to facilitate consultation, the physician should have the following information at hand: the species of animal, whether it is available for testing or confinement, the nature of the attack (provoked or unprovoked), and the nature of the exposure (bite, scratch, lick, aerosol of saliva, etc). Confinement and observation of the biting animal are appropriate only when that animal is either a dog or a cat and appears well.

Preexposure prophylaxis is indicated for veterinarians, animal handlers, and any persons, including children, whose work or home environment potentially places them in close contact with animal species in which rabies is endemic—bats, skunks, raccoons, and foxes. Travelers visiting foreign areas of enzootic rabies for over 30 days should also receive a primary course of vaccination. A recent study in Vietnam (where rabies is endemic) demonstrated

that DPT-IPV and rabies vaccine could be safely administered in a routine vaccination schedule.

Preparations Available

(1) Human diploid cell rabies vaccine (HDCV) is prepared from the Pitman-Moore strain of rabies virus grown in human diploid cell culture, concentrated by ultracentrifugation and inactivated with β-propiolactone. It is manufactured by Pasteur-Mérieux-Connaught and supplied in two forms: a single-dose vial of 1 mL, when reconstituted for intramuscular use; and a single-dose vial of 0.1 mL for intradermal use.

(2) Rabies vaccine, adsorbed (RVA), was licensed in March 1988 and is distributed by the Biologics Products Program, Michigan Department of Public Health. Available from SmithKline Beecham, it is produced from the Kissling strain of rabies virus, grown on fetal rhesus lung diploid cell culture, inactivated with β-propiolactone, and adsorbed to aluminum phosphate.

Dosage & Schedule of Administration

Both types are equally safe and efficacious for both preexposure and postexposure prophylaxis when given intramuscularly. Only the HDCV has been evaluated for the intradermal route.

A. Primary Preexposure Vaccination:

1. Intramuscular route–Three intramuscular injections in the deltoid area of 1 mL of HDCV or RVA on days 0, 7, and 21 or 28. The intragluteal route of administration is not recommended because of a poor immunologic response.

2. Intradermal route–An alternative mode of vaccination consisting of three intradermal doses of 0.1 mL of HDCV (RVA cannot be used) in the area over the deltoid on days 0, 7, and 21 or 28. *Note:* Concomitant chloroquine phosphate use (for malaria chemoprophylaxis) interferes with the antibody response to intradermal vaccination with HDCV but not with the intramuscular mode of vaccination. Thus, when simultaneous rabies and malaria prophylaxis is indicated, the intramuscular mode of vaccination is preferred.

B. Postexposure Prophylaxis:

1. In unvaccinated individuals–The wound should be immediately and thoroughly cleansed with soap and water. As soon as possible after exposure (and up to 7 days after the first dose of vaccine), administer 20 IU/kg of rabies immune globulin (RIG) intramuscularly. (If possible, half the dose should be infiltrated around the wound and the other half given intramuscularly in the gluteal area.) At a different site—also as soon as possible after exposure—administer the first dose of HDCV. Four subsequent doses of HDCV should be given on days 3, 7, 14, and 28. The World Health Organization (WHO) recommends an additional dose on day 90, but the ACIP does not concur.

2. In previously vaccinated individuals–The wound should be cleaned with soap and water. RIG is not necessary, and only two doses of HDCV or RVA, 1 mL intramuscularly on days 0 and 3, are needed.

C. Booster Vaccination:

1. Preexposure booster doses of vaccine–Travelers living or visiting (for more than 30 days) in areas where rabies is enzootic in dogs should have a serum sample tested for rabies antibody every 2 years. If the titer is less than 1:5 for complete neutralization by the rapid fluorescent focus inhibition test, a booster dose should be administered.

Adverse Effects

HDCV is relatively free of side effects. Approximately 30–74% of adults experience pain, swelling, or erythema at the injection site, 7% have headache, 5% have nausea, and 4% have fever. Children complain of side effects less frequently. Allergic reactions occur chiefly after booster doses. The rate of anaphylaxis is estimated to be 1:10,000 doses. An immune complex-like reaction occurs in about 6% of persons 2–21 days after receiving booster doses of HDCV.

Travelers to countries where rabies is enzootic in dogs may need rabies vaccine immediately and may have to use locally available vaccines and antisera. In many developing countries, the only vaccines readily available may be nerve tissue vaccines (NTV) derived from the brains of adult animals or suckling mice, and the antirabies sera may be of equine origin. While the antisera have complication rates of only 1–6%, the NTV may induce neuroparalytic reactions in 1:2000 to 1:200 vaccinees; this is a significant risk and may justify preexposure vaccination with HDCV prior to travel.

Antibody Preparations

Rabies immune globulin (RIG) is prepared from the plasma of human volunteers hyperimmunized with rabies vaccine. The rabies-neutralizing antibody content is 150 IU/mL, supplied in 2 mL or 10 mL vials. It is very safe. Usage is described above.

Dreesen DW et al: A global review of rabies vaccines for human use. Vaccine 1997;15(Suppl):S2.

Fishbein DB et al: Rabies. N Engl J Med 1992;329:1632.

Lang J et al: Randomised feasibility trial of pre-exposure rabies vaccination with DTP-IPV in infants. Lancet 1997;349:1663.

Rabies prevention: United States, 1991. MMWR Morb Mortal Wkly Rep 1990;40(RR-3):1.

Reid-Sanden FL et al: Administration of rabies vaccine in the gluteal area: A continuing problem. Arch Intern Med 1991;151:821.

World Health Organization Expert Committee on Rabies: Rabies vaccination. WHO Tech Rep Ser 1992;824:1.

TYPHOID FEVER

Typhoid vaccines have shown variable efficacy in field trials. Protection is inversely related to inoculum size in laboratory-based volunteer studies, which may be why some field trials have been disappointing. Three vaccines are available in the United States: a heat- and phenol-inactivated whole bacterial vaccine for parenteral use; a parental capsular polysaccharide vaccine purified Vi (virulence) antigen (Vi CPS); and a live attenuated vaccine for oral use (Ty21a). The vaccines have been in use for many years, and their protective efficacy ranges from 51–76% (heat- and phenol-inactivated) to 17–66% (Vi CPS and Ty21A) and the reaction rates have been low. Moderate protection against invasive *Salmonella typhi* has been demonstrated for 2–5 years following vaccination.

Routine typhoid vaccination is not recommended in the United States. It is indicated for use in children who reside in households with a proved typhoid carrier or in children who are going to reside in an endemic area. The oral vaccine is most commonly used. However, noncompliance with dosing instructions occurs frequently, and correct usage should be stressed or the Vi CPS vaccine used. Although the vaccine is not approved for use in children under 6 years of age, a liquid formulation was found to be safe and immunogenic (70% seroconversion) in children aged 2–6 years. Travelers should be advised, however, that since none of the vaccines offer total protection, careful selection of food and drink is imperative.

Preparations Available

Parenteral killed vaccine is a saline suspension of heat- and phenol-inactivated *S typhi* organisms at a concentration of not less than 10^9 bacteria per milliliter. It is supplied in multidose vials of 5, 10, or 20 mL.

Parenteral Vi CPS is a capsular polysaccharide vaccine containing purified Vi (virulence) antigen for intramuscular use.

(3) Oral live attenuated vaccine is supplied as enteric-coated capsules and contains the attenuated strain *S typhi* Ty21a.

Dosage & Schedule of Administration

The killed whole cell vaccine is given subcutaneously in a series of two injections of 0.5 mL each (for children ≥ 10 years of age) or 0.25 mL (children <10 years of age), 4 weeks or more apart, with booster doses every 3 years if residence in an endemic area continues. The booster dose is 0.5 mL (age > 10 years) or 0.25 mL (age < 10 years) subcutaneously or 0.1 mL intradermally.

The dose of Vi CPS is a single intramuscular dose with boosters needed every 2 years. The minimum age is 2 years.

The dose of the oral preparation is one capsule a day on alternate days to a total of four capsules, taken before meals. The capsules should be kept refrigerated. A full course of four capsules is recommended every 2–5 years if exposure continues. This vaccine is not approved for children under 6 years of age, and capsules should not be dispensed from a package that has been opened beforehand. A recent study has demonstrated that administration of proguanil inhibits the immune response to Ty21a This vaccine should not be administered when proguanil is being used.

Adverse Reactions

The parenteral vaccine produces 1–2 days of severe discomfort at the injection site in 6–40% of vaccinees, causing missed school or work in 13–24% of vaccinated individuals. Fever and other systemic reactions occur in 15–30% of vaccinees. The only contraindication is a previous severe reaction to parenteral typhoid vaccination. The vaccine can be used in immunocompromised individuals.

The Vi CPS and oral preparation rarely produce side effects (< 7%); the most common ones are abdominal discomfort, nausea, and vomiting. The Ty21a vaccine should not be used in immunocompromised individuals.

Cryz SJ et al: Safety and immunogenicity of *Salmonella typhi* Ty21a vaccine in young Thai children. Infect Immun 1993;61:1149.

Kollaritsch H et al: Safety and immunogenicity of live oral cholera and typhoid vaccines administered alone or in combination with antimalarial drugs, oral polio vaccine, or yellow fever vaccine. J Infect Dis 1997;174:871.

Rahman S et al: Use of oral typhoid vaccine strain Ty21a in a New York state travel immunization facility. Am J Trop Med Hyg 1993;48:823.

Typhoid immunization: Recommendations of the Immunization Practices Advisory Committee (ACIP). MMWR Morb Mortal Wkly Rep 1990;39(RR-10):1.

MENINGOCOCCAL DISEASE

A quadrivalent vaccine containing 50 µg each of purified bacterial polysaccharide antigen from capsular groups A, C, Y, and W135 is available in the United States. Since meningococcal infection is not endemic in the United States, routine use of this vaccine is unnecessary. However, functionally or anatomically asplenic children should be vaccinated, and vaccination should be considered also for complement-deficient children. Meningococcal vaccine will protect travelers to countries with hyperepidemic or endemic disease. The group A component is immunogenic in children over 3 months of age and the group C component in those over 24 months of age. The dose is 0.5 mL given once subcutaneously. In epidemic situations, children as young as 3 months of age have been vaccinated with two doses 3 months apart. In general, the vaccine should not be administered to such children before their second birthday. Adverse reactions are unusual, consisting of local pain and erythema at the injection site. The antibody levels decline after 5 years and are unaffected by booster doses. Sustained protection may require the development of vaccines that induce T cell memory.

Ceesay SJ et al: Decline in meningococcal antibody levels in African children 5 years after vaccination and the lack of an effect of booster immunization. J Infect Dis 1993;167:1212.

Control and prevention of meningococcal disease and control and prevention of serogroup C meningococcal disease: Evaluation and management of suspected outbreaks. Recommendations of the Advisory Committee of Immunization Practices (ACIP). MMWR Morb Mortal Wkly Rep 1997;46(RR-5):1..

Jackson LA et al: Serogroup C meningococcal outbreaks in the United States: An emerging threat. JAMA 1995;273:383.

Twumasi PA et al: A trial of a group A plus group C meningococcal polysaccharide-protein conjugate vaccine in African infants. J Infect Dis 1995;171:632.

CHOLERA

The currently available cholera vaccine is a phenol-killed whole bacterial cell preparation. Its use is limited because it has a maximum protective efficacy of only 50% with a duration of protection of only 3–6 months. Furthermore, it confers no protection against serotype O139, the currently circulating strain of *Vibrio cholerae*. It is no longer required by any country. Vaccination frequently results in redness and pain at the injection site, and fever, malaise, and myalgia occur approximately 1% of the time. The vaccine may be administered subcutaneously or intramuscularly. A primary series consists of two doses at least 1 week apart. Boosters may need to be given as frequently as every 6 months. For the quantity to be administered, see below. Vaccine should not be given to children under 6 months of age.

	Age at Immunization		
	6 months to 4 years	5–10 years	> 10 years
Dose	0.2 mL	0.3 mL	0.5 mL

Since *V cholerae* is not invasive and secretory IgA (sIgA) is crucial, the newer vaccines are administered orally. Two oral nonliving vaccines (one consisting solely of killed whole vibrios and the other in combination with the B subunit of cholera toxin) are safe and immunogenic. In field trials in Bangladesh, the protective efficacy was only 55–60% over 2 years of follow-up. Additional live oral vaccines are being developed against cholera (CVD 111, an El Tor *Vibrio cholerae* O1 vaccine strain, Peru 15, or subunit vaccines). These approaches show promise, and an improved oral vaccine may be available in the next few years.

Bergquist C, et al: Intranasal vaccination of humans with recombinant cholera toxin B subunit induces systemic and local antibody responses in the upper respiratory tract and the vagina. Infect Immun 1997;65:2676.

Imported cholera associated with a newly described toxigenic *Vibrio cholerae* 0139 strain—California, 1993. MMWR Morb Mortal Wkly Rep 1993;42:501.

Sack DA et al: Evaluation of Peru-15, a new live oral vaccine for cholera, in volunteers. J Infect Dis 1997;176:201.

Tacket CO et al: Volunteer studies investigating the safety and efficacy of live oral El Tor *Vibrio cholerae* 01 vaccine strain CVD 111. Am J Trop Med Hyg 1997;56:533.

PLAGUE

Plague vaccine is composed of inactivated whole bacteria (*Yersinia pestis*). It should be used in children who reside in or are traveling to endemic areas. It should be administered intramuscularly according to the following dosage schedule:

	Age (years)			
	< 1	1–4	5–10	> 10
Day 0	0.1 mL	0.2 mL	0.3 mL	0.5 mL
Day 30	0.1 mL	0.2 mL	0.3 mL	0.5 mL
Days 60–120	0.04 mL	0.08 mL	0.12 mL	0.2 mL

Booster doses in the amount of the last dose listed above should be given at 6-month intervals until five doses have been given, and boosters should then be given at intervals of 1–2 years as long as the child resides in the endemic area.

Plague vaccine. Recommendations of the Immunization Practices Advisory Committee (ACIP). MMWR Morb Mortal Wkly Rep 1997;46(RR-14):1.

TUBERCULOSIS

BCG vaccine consists of live attenuated *Mycobacterium bovis*. BCG is not currently indicated for mass use in the United States, chiefly because of doubts about its efficacy. BCG is useful only in tuberculin-negative infants or older children residing in house-holds where untreated or poorly treated individuals with active infection with isoniazid- and rifampin-resistant *M tuberculosis* also reside. BCG may be indicated in infants or children living under constant exposure without access to removal from continuous exposure, prophylaxis, and treatment. BCG reduces the risk of tuberculous meningitis and disseminated tuberculosis in pediatric populations. It is given intradermally in a dose of 0.05 mL for newborns and 0.1 mL for all other children. Mantoux testing is advised 2–3 months later, and revaccination is advised if the Mantoux test is negative. Adverse effects occur in 1–10% of healthy individuals and include local ulceration, regional lymph node enlargement, and lupus vulgaris. The vaccine is contraindicated in immunocompromised individuals, including those with HIV infection, because they can have disseminated or fatal infection. To ensure that those infected with tuberculosis are evaluated, a 5 mm or greater cutoff for a positive Mantoux test is taken. In immune-competent persons, the cutoff is 10 mm or above. BCG almost invariably causes its recipients to be tuberculin-positive. However, in a child with a history of BCG vaccination who is being investigated for tuberculosis as a case contact, a positive Mantoux test should be interpreted as indicating infection with *M tuberculosis,* essentially ignoring the history of BCG vaccination.

BCG is the most widely used vaccine in the world and has been administered to over 2.5 billion people with a low incidence of serious complications. It is cheap, can be given any time after birth, sensitizes the vaccinated individual for 5–50 years, and stimulates both B cell and T cell immune responses.

Cohn DL. Use of the bacille Calmette-Guérin vaccination for the prevention of tuberculosis: Renewed interest in an old vaccine. Am J Med Sci 1997;313:372.

Essential components of a tuberculosis prevention and control program. MMWR Morb Mortal Wkly Rep 1995:44(RR-11):1.

Guidelines for prevention of nosocomial pneumonia. MMWR Morb Mortal Wkly Rep 1997;46(RR-1):1.

Marsh BJ et al: The risks and benefits of childhood bacille Calmette-Guérin immunization among adults with AIDS. International MAC study groups. AIDS 1997;11:669.

Use of BCG vaccines in the control of tuberculosis: A joint statement by the ACIP and the Advisory Committee for Elimination of Tuberculosis (ACET). MMWR Morb Mortal Wkly Rep 1996;45(RR-4):1.

YELLOW FEVER

Immunization against yellow fever is indicated for children as young as 6 months of age traveling to endemic areas or to countries that require it for entry, but otherwise immunization should be delayed until age 9 months or older. Public health authorities maintain updated information on these requirements and must be consulted. Yellow fever vaccine is a live vaccine made from the 17D yellow fever attenuated virus strain grown in chick embryos. It is contraindicated in infants less than 4 months of age, in pregnant women, in persons with anaphylactic egg allergy, and in immunocompromised individuals. It can only be administered at licensed yellow fever vaccination locations (usually public health departments). The dose is standardized to 1000 mouse LD50 units by the WHO. The package insert must therefore be consulted to determine the appropriate volume to be administered (generally 0.5 mL). The vaccine is injected subcutaneously. The International Health Regulations require revaccination at 10-year intervals, but immunity may last 30–35 years and is probably lifelong. Adverse reactions are generally mild—consisting of fever, headache, and myalgia 5–10 days after vaccination—and are uncommon, occurring in 2–5% of vaccinees. Rarely, encephalitis occurs within 30 days following vaccination (two cases have been reported after more than 24 million doses given in the United States). This is more likely to occur in infants less than 6 months of age. Yellow fever and cholera vaccines, when given simultaneously or less than 3 weeks apart, each interfere with the immune response of the other. These two vaccines should therefore be administered at least 3 weeks apart. There is no contraindication to giving other live-virus vaccines simultaneously with yellow fever vaccine.

Robertson SE et al: Yellow fever: A decade of reemergence. JAMA 1996;276:1157.

Yellow fever vaccine: Recommendations of the Immunization Practices Advisory Committee (ACIP). MMWR Morb Mortal Wkly Rep 1990;39(RR-6):1.

PASSIVE IMMUNIZATION

Immune Globulin Intramuscular (IGIM)

Immune globulin is indicated as replacement therapy in antibody deficiency disorders at a dose of 0.6 mL/kg per month intramuscularly. It may prevent or modify infection with hepatitis A virus if administered in a dose of 0.02 mL/kg within 14 days after exposure. Measles infection may be prevented or modified in a susceptible person if IG is given in a dose of 0.25 mL/kg within 6 days after exposure. Special forms of include tetanus immune globulin (TIG), hepatitis B immune globulin (HBIG), rabies immune globulin (RIG), and varicella-zoster immune globulin (VZIG). These are obtained from donors known to have high titers of antibody against the organism in question. Their use has been described above.

IGIM must only be given intramuscularly. The dose varies depending on the clinical indication. Adverse reactions include pain at the injection site, headache, chills, dyspnea, nausea, and anaphylaxis, although all but the first are rare.

Immune Globulin Intravenous (IGIV)

The primary indications for IGIV are for replacement therapy in antibody-deficient individuals, for the treatment of Kawasaki disease, and for the treatment of some patients with idiopathic thrombocytopenic purpura and other autoimmune diseases. IGIV may be beneficial in some children with HIV infection. Specific antibody-enriched IGIV preparations have also been developed for the prevention and treatment of virus infections: cytomegalovirus immune globulin (CMVIG) for prevention and treatment of CMV disease and respiratory syncytial virus immune globulin (RSVIG) for prevention of RSV illness in high-risk children.

IGIV must only be given intravenously. Adverse reactions include headache, flushing, diaphoresis, hypotension, fever, nausea, vomiting, and anaphylaxis.

Antitoxins & Antivenins

Immune globulins of animal origin are available for use in certain specific situations. These include botulinum antitoxin, diphtheria antitoxin, and snake and spider antivenins. A variety of adverse reactions, including acute febrile responses, anaphylaxis, and serum sickness, may develop after use of these products. A schedule for hypersensitivity testing and desensitization for antisera of equine origin can be found in the *Red Book.*

LEGAL ISSUES IN IMMUNIZATION

The National Childhood Vaccine Injury Act of 1986 established two programs: the National Vaccine Program (NVP) and the National Vaccine Injury Compensation Program (NVICP). The purpose was to provide "no-fault" compensation for persons found to have been injured by certain vaccines. Under the terms of the Act, liability claims against those who administer or manufacture vaccines must go before a federal compensation board before a civil suit may be filed. Compensation may be sought for certain events following certain immunizations within specified time intervals. Legal representatives (parents, guardians) must reject the judgment rendered by this compensation board before a civil suit may be filed in either state or federal court. The compensation system is now funded by a continuing surcharge levied against the manufacturers for each dose sold of the specified vaccines.

To receive compensation for injury from vaccines, the injured person or his or her representative must (1) go through the NVICP; (2) present evidence of death or residual effects lasting longer than 6 months and expenses greater than $1000; (3) file a claim within 3 years after onset of the first symptoms or within 2 years after death; and (4) supply medical records or sworn affidavits in support of the claim.

Following a claim, the defendant—the Secretary of the Department of Health and Human Services—evaluates the petition. Compensation is recommended if there is no alternative cause and the injury is a listed reportable event (see revised Vaccine Injury Table effective March 10, 1995)—or, if the injury was not a reportable event, a vaccine was the proximate cause. Once a decision is made, the petitioner can accept or reject it within 90 days. If petitioner accepts the decision, no claim can thereafter be filed against the manufacturer or the vaccine provider. If the claim is not accepted, civil relief is available through the tort system, but the manufacturer cannot be sued for failure to warn the vaccinee of the risks associated with the product.

The Act imposes specific record-keeping and adverse reaction reporting duties on physicians who ad-minister vaccines. For each dose administered, the medical record of the vaccinee or some other permanent record maintained in the administrator's office must set forth (1) the date of administration; (2) the name of the manufacturer and lot number of the vaccine; and (3) the name, work address, and title of the person administering the vaccine. Physicians administering the specified vaccines are also obliged by the Act to report any of the specified reactions to the Vaccine Adverse Events Reporting System (VAERS)—call 1-800-822-7967 for forms. Compensation forms from the NVICP may be obtained by calling 1-800-338-2382. The Act provides no penalty for failure to report.

Vaccine information materials are available from the CDC to meet the requirements of the Act. There are separate short (1500- to 2000-word) forms for DTP, MMR, and poliovirus vaccines. Patients or parents are legally required to sign these forms if the vaccine is purchased on a federal contract. Informed consent is also needed for physicians who wish to be fully covered by the vaccine compensation program.

Evans G: National Childhood Vaccine Injury Act: Revision of the vaccine injury table. Pediatrics 1996;98:1179.

National Childhood Vaccine Injury Act: Requirements for permanent vaccination records and for reporting of selected events after vaccination. MMWR Morb Mortal Wkly Rep 1996;37:197.

10 Normal Childhood Nutrition & Its Disorders

Nancy F. Krebs, MD, MS, & K. Michael Hambidge, MB, BChir, ScD

NUTRITIONAL REQUIREMENTS

NUTRITION & GROWTH

The nutrient requirements of the child are influenced substantially by the rate of growth, body composition, and the composition of new growth. These factors vary with the age of the subject and are especially important during early postnatal life. Growth rates are higher in early infancy than at any other stage of the life cycle, including the peak of the adolescent growth spurt (Table 10–1). These rates decline rapidly starting in the second month of postnatal life (proportionately later in the premature infant). Because of a more rapid rate of growth in early infancy, nutrient requirements for males are slightly higher than those for females.

Nutrient requirements also depend on body composition. In the adult, the brain, which accounts for only 2% of body weight, contributes 19% to the total basal energy expenditure. In contrast, in a term neonate, the brain accounts for 10% of body weight and for 44% of total energy needs under basal conditions. Thus, in the young infant, total basal energy expenditure and the energy requirement of the brain are relatively high.

Composition of new weight gain is a third factor that influences nutrient requirements and changes the nutrient requirements with age. For example, fat accounts for about 40% of weight gain between birth and 4 months but for only 3% between 24 and 36 months. The corresponding figures for protein are 11% and 21%; for water, 45% and 68%. The high physiologic rate of fat deposition in early infancy has implications not only for energy requirements but also for the optimal composition of infant feeds.

Because of the high nutrient requirements for growth and the body composition, the young infant is especially vulnerable to undernutrition. Slowed physical growth rate is an early and prominent sign of undernutrition in the young infant. The limited fat stores of the very young infant mean that energy reserves are unusually restricted. The relatively large size and continued growth of the brain render the central nervous system especially vulnerable to the effects of malnutrition in early postnatal life.

Dewey KG et al: Growth of breast-fed infants deviates from current reference data: A pooled analysis of US, Canadian, and European datasets. Pediatrics 1995;96: 495.

ENERGY

The major determinants of energy expenditure are basal metabolism, metabolic response to food, physical activity, and growth. In addition, the efficiency of energy utilization may be a significant factor, and thermoregulation may contribute in extremes of ambient temperature if the body is inadequately clothed. Because adequate data on requirements for physical activity in infants and children are not available and because individual growth requirements are variable, recommendations have been based on calculations of actual intakes by healthy subjects. The distinct recent trend toward lower figures for infants reflects a move away from hypercaloric and possibly inappropriate feeding practices that were in vogue between 1930 and 1970, when the growth data giving rise to the National Center for Health Statistics (NCHS) standards were collected. Suggested guidelines for energy intake of infants and young children are given in Table 10–2. Also included in this table are carefully calculated energy intakes of fully breast-fed infants, which have been verified recently in a number of centers. Growth velocity of breast-fed infants during the first 3 months typically equals or exceeds the 50th percentile for the NCHS grids. The recommended energy intakes of the Food and Nutrition Board, National Academy of Sciences, National Research Council (10th edition), are not synonymous with requirements. Moreover, the RDAs do not take into account the rapid changes in requirements that occur over the course of infancy, especially in the first 6 months. For these reasons, this

Table 10–1. Changes in growth rate, energy required for growth, and body composition in infants and young child.

Age (months)	Growth Rate (g/d) Male	Growth Rate (g/d) Both	Growth Rate (g/d) Female	Energy Requirements for Growth (kcal/kg/d)	Body Composition[1] Water	Body Composition[1] Protein	Body Composition[1] Fat
0–0.25		0 (See note 2.)			75	11.5	11
0.25–1	40		35	50			
1–2	35		30	25			
2–3	28		25	16			
3–6		20		10	60	11.5	26
6–9		15					
9–12		12					
12–18		8					
18–36		6		2	61	16	21

[1]Data from Fomon SJ (editor): *Infant Nutrition,* 2nd ed. Saunders, 1974.
[2]Birth weight is regained by 10 d. Weight loss of more than 10% of birth weight indicates dehydration or malnutrition; this applies to both formula-fed and breast-fed infants.

source should be used cautiously for calculating energy requirements of infants.

After the first 4 years, energy requirements expressed on a body weight basis fall progressively to 40 kcal/kg/d by the end of adolescence. Approximate daily energy requirements can be calculated by adding 100 kcal/y to a base of 1000 kcal at 1 year of age. Appetite and growth are reliable indices of caloric needs of most healthy children, but intake also depends, to some extent, on the energy density of the formula. Individual energy requirements of normal infants and children vary considerably, and malnutrition and disease add enormously to this vari-

ation. Basal energy requirements for the premature infant are approximately 120 kcal/kg/d.

One method of calculating requirements for malnourished patients is to base these on the ideal body weight (IBW; ie, 50th percentile weight for patients length/height–age or 50th percentile weight-for-height) rather than actual weight. Alternatively, the extra requirement kcal/d for "catch-up" growth can be calculated as:

$$\frac{5 \times \text{Weight (g) deficit below IBW}}{\text{Interval (days) for correction of deficit}}$$

Table 10–2. Recommendations for energy and protein intake.[1]

	Energy (kcal/kg/d) Based on Measurements of Energy Expenditure	Energy (kcal/kg/d) Intake From Human Milk	Energy (kcal/kg/d) Guidelines for Average Replacement	Protein (g/kg/d) Intake From Human Milk	Protein (g/kg/d) Guidelines for Average Requirements
10 days to 1 month	—	105	120	2.05	2.5
1–2 months	110	110	115	1.75	2.25
2–3 months	95	105	105	1.36	2.25
3–4 months	95	75–85	95	1.20	2.0
4–6 months	95	75–85	95	1.05	1.7
6–12 months	85	70	90	—	1.5
1–2 years	85	—	90	—	1.2
2–3 years	85	—	90	—	1.1
3–5 years	—	—	90	—	1.1

[1]Compiled from Krebs NF et al: Growth and intakes of energy and zinc in infants fed human milk. J Pediatr 1994;124:32–9; Garza C, Butte NF: Energy intakes of human milk-fed infants during the first year. J Pediatr 1990;117:(S)124.

where 5 kcal is the energy cost of each gram of new tissue deposited.

These calculations should be adjusted on an ongoing basis according to the growth response.

Heining MJ et al: Energy and protein intakes of breast-fed and formula-fed infants during the first year of life and their association with growth velocity: The Darling Study. Am J Clin Nutr 1993;58:152.

World Health Organization: Report of a Joint FAO/WHO/UNO Expert Consultation: Energy and Protein Requirements. WHO Tech Rep Ser No. 724, 1985;724.

PROTEIN

Only amino acids and ammonium compounds are usable as sources of nitrogen in human nutrition. Amino acids are provided by dietary protein. Dietary protein is hydrolyzed by pepsin in the stomach and by pancreatic trypsin digestion in the lumen of the small intestine. This is followed by peptidase digestion by pancreatic and intestinal peptidases. Nitrogen is absorbed from the gut lumen as amino acids and via short-peptide carrier systems. Absorption of nitrogen is more efficient from synthetic diets that contain peptides in addition to amino acids. Some intact proteins can be absorbed in early postnatal life and may result in allergies to these proteins.

The liver plays a central role in amino acid metabolism, including regulation of the absorbed amino acids. Excess amino acids, including essential amino acids, are degraded in the liver—except for the branched-chain amino acids, which pass into the systemic circulation and are taken up primarily by muscle. Insulin stimulates this uptake and suppresses muscle protein catabolism. Protein turnover rates far exceed intake, indicating a marked reutilization of amino acids. However, some of these amino acids released from protein turnover are degraded. After removal of the amino group, the keto acids are either utilized directly for energy or converted to carbohydrate and fat. Nitrogen is excreted primarily via the kidney as urea.

All the body's protein plays a role in body structure or function. Because there are no true stores of body protein, a regular dietary supply is necessary, and any loss of protein decreases functional capacity. In infants and children, optimal growth depends on an adequate dietary protein supply. Relatively subtle effects of protein deficiency are now recognized—especially those affecting tissues with rapid protein turnover rates, such as the immune system and the gastrointestinal mucosa.

In relation to body weight, protein synthesis rates, protein turnover rates, and increments in body protein are exceptionally high in the infant, especially the premature infant. Eighty percent of the dietary protein requirement of the premature infant is uti-

lized for growth, compared with only 20% in the 1-year-old child. Protein requirements expressed on a body weight basis decline rapidly across infancy as growth velocity decreases. The figures given in Table 10–2, which are derived chiefly from the report of the Joint FAO/WHO/UNO Expert Committee and are similar to those published in *Recommended Dietary Allowances* (10th edition), deliver a comfortable margin above the quantity provided in breast milk. The recommendations for premature infants weighing less than 1500 g is 3 g/kg/d or more.

Protein requirements increase in the presence of unusual cutaneous or enteral losses, burns, trauma, and severe sepsis. Requirements also increase during times of catch-up growth accompanying recovery from malnutrition (approximately 0.2 g of protein per gram of new tissue deposited). In a young infant during rapid recovery, this could amount to as much as 1–2 g/kg/d of extra requirement. By 1 year of age, this is unlikely to be more than 0.5 g of protein/kg/d. Circumstances in which the intake of protein may be deficient include low-protein supplements (eg, fruit juices) in the breast-fed infant, protein malabsorption (cystic fibrosis), or the use of a low-protein weaning food (eg, cassava) as the dietary staple.

The quality of protein depends on its amino acid composition. Infants require 43% of protein as essential amino acids, and children require 36%. Eight essential amino acids cannot be synthesized by adults: isoleucine, leucine, lysine, methionine, phenylalanine, threonine, tryptophan, and valine. Histidine may be added to this list. Cysteine and tyrosine are considered partially essential because their rates of synthesis are limited and may be inadequate in certain circumstances. During early development, rates of synthesis of cysteine, tyrosine, and perhaps taurine do not provide sufficient amounts of these substances. Taurine is a substrate in the conjugation of bile acids, and taurine supplements have been reported to improve fat absorption in preterm infants and in infants with cystic fibrosis. Taurine supplements have been reported to improve auditory brain stem–evoked potentials in preterm infants. Lack of an essential amino acid leads to weight loss within 1–2 weeks. Wheat and rice are deficient in lysine, and legumes are deficient in methionine. Appropriate mixtures of vegetable protein are therefore necessary to achieve high protein quality.

Glutamine is another important example of a nonessential amino acid whose synthesis is inadequate under certain abnormal circumstances. The integrity of the enterocyte, for example, may be dependent on addition of glutamine to parenteral nutrition in infants who cannot tolerate any enteral intake.

Because the mechanisms for removal of excess nitrogen are efficient, moderate excesses of protein are not harmful and may help to ensure an adequate supply of certain micronutrients. Adverse effects of excessive protein intakes may include increased calcium losses in urine and, over a life span, increased loss of renal mass. A gross excess of protein may cause elevated blood urea nitrogen, acidosis, hyperammonemia, and, in the premature infant, failure to thrive, lethargy, and fever.

Souba WW: Intestinal glutamine metabolism and nutrition. J Nutr Biochem 1993;4:2.

LIPIDS

Fats are the main dietary energy source for infants and account for up to 50% of energy in human milk. Over 98% of these fats are in the form of triglycerides, which have an energy density of 9 calories per gram. Fats can be efficiently stored in adipose tissue with a minimal energy cost of storage. This is especially important in the young infant. Fats are required for the absorption of fat-soluble vitamins and for myelination of the central nervous system. Fat also provides essential fatty acids (EFAs) necessary for brain development, for phospholipids in cell membranes, and for the synthesis of prostaglandins and leukotrienes. The EFAs are polyunsaturated fatty acids derived from linoleic acid (18:2ω6, ie, 18 carbons and two double bonds with the first located six carbons from the methyl [omega] end) and linolenic acid (18:3ω3) by elongation and further desaturation. Among these are arachidonic acid (20:4ω6), which can be obtained from dietary linoleic acid and is present primarily in membrane phospholipids. Oxygenation of arachidonic acid through the lipoxygenase pathway yields leukotrienes, and oxygenation through the cyclooxygenase pathway yields prostaglandins. Important derivatives of linolenic acid are eicosapentaenoic acid (20:6ω3) and docosahexaenoic acid (22:6ω3), which is found in human milk and brain lipids. Visual acuity of formula-fed premature infants is improved with the addition of 20:6ω3, which is not derived readily from 18:3ω3.

Clinical features of EFA ω6 deficiency include growth failure, abnormal scaliness, erythematous skin lesions, decreased capillary resistance, increased fragility of erythrocytes, thrombocytopenia, poor wound healing, and increased susceptibility to infection. The clinical features of deficiency of ω3 fatty acids are less well defined, but dermatitis and neurologic abnormalities—including blurred vision, peripheral neuropathy, and weakness—have been reported. Marine oil–supplemented formula improves visual acuity of preterm infants through 4 months of age by improving docosahexaenoic acid status. Fatty fish are the best dietary source of ω3 fatty acids. A high intake of fatty fish is associated with a decrease in platelet adhesiveness and decreased inflammatory response.

Up to 5–10% of fatty acids in human milk are polyunsaturated. Most of these are ω6 series, but long-chain ω3 fatty acids are also present. Breast milk also contains about 40% of fatty acids as monounsaturates, primarily oleic acid (18:1) and up to 10% of total fatty acids as medium-chain triglycerides (MCT). In general, the percentage of calories derived from fat is a little lower in infant formulas than in human milk. Typically, these formulas contain a relatively high percentage of linoleic acid but very little long-chain ω3. The American Academy of Pediatrics recommends that infants receive a minimum of 30% of calories from fat, including a minimum of 1.7% of total calories from ω6 fatty acids and 0.5% of calories from ω3. Providing up to 40–50% of energy requirements as fats is desirable at this age. In contrast, children older than 2 years should be switched gradually to a diet containing approximately 30% of total calories from fat, with no more than 10% of calories either from saturated fats or polyunsaturated fats.

Triglycerides are hydrolyzed to monoglycerides, free fatty acids, and glycerol in the lumen of the gut. Substantial hydrolysis of triglycerides in milk formulas occurs in the stomach by the action of lingual and gastric lipases. Pancreatic lipases and bile salt levels are relatively low in early postnatal life, but breast milk contains a bile salt–stimulated lipase that is effective in the lumen of the duodenum. Bile salts promote the formation of the colipase-lipase complex, which adheres to the triglycerides prior to hydrolysis. Bile salts also have a major role in the emulsification of fatty acids, allowing their passage through the unstirred water layer to the surface of the mucosal cell. After passage into the enterocyte, long-chain ($\geq C_{12}$) fatty acids and monoglycerides are reesterified to triglycerides and are packaged with phospholipids, cholesterol, and protein into chylomicrons, which are transported in the lymphatics to the systemic circulation. At the capillary endothelial surfaces in adipose and muscle tissue, lipoprotein lipase (LPL) hydrolyzes triglycerides from chylomicrons, releasing free fatty acids and glycerol, which are taken up by the adjacent cells. LPL also hydrolyzes triglycerides synthesized in the liver and transported to peripheral tissues as very low density lipoproteins.

β-Oxidation of fatty acids takes place in the mitochondria of muscle and liver. Carnitine is necessary for oxidation of the fatty acids, which must cross the mitochondrial membranes as acylcarnitine. Carnitine is synthesized in the human liver and kidney from lysine and methionine. Carnitine needs of infants are met by breast milk or formulas, and carnitine has recently been added to soy-based formulas but is not present in intravenous infusates. In the liver, substantial quantities of fatty acids are converted to ketone bodies, which are then released into the circulation and provide an important source of fuel for the brain in the young infant.

Medium-chain triglycerides (MCTs C_8 and C_{10}, ie, energy density 7.6 kcal/g) are sufficiently soluble that micelle formation is not required for them to diffuse through the unstirred water layer. They are much more readily absorbed than long-chain triglycerides and are then transported directly to the liver via the portal circulation. MCTs are rapidly metabolized in the liver, undergoing β-oxidation or ketogenesis. They do not require carnitine to enter the mitochondria. Ketones are formed from MCT even when provided orally. MCTs are useful for patients with luminal phase defects (eg, cirrhosis), absorptive defects (eg, short bowel syndrome), and chronic inflammatory bowel disease. The potential side effects of MCT administration include diarrhea when they are given in large quantities, high octanoic acid levels in patients with cirrhosis, and, if they are the only source of lipids, deficiency of EFA.

Nettleton JA: Are n-3 fatty acids essential nutrients for fetal and infant development? J Am Diet Assoc 1993;93:58.

CARBOHYDRATES

The energy density of carbohydrate is 4 kcal/g. Approximately 40% of caloric intake in human milk is in the form of lactose, or "milk sugar." The percentage of energy from lactose in cow's milk is only 20%, but infant formulas generally provide a somewhat higher percentage of energy from carbohydrates than does human milk.

After the first 2 years of life, 60% or more of energy requirements should be derived from carbohydrates, including no more than 10% from simple sugars. These dietary guidelines are, unfortunately, not reflected in the diets of North American children, who typically derive 25% of energy from sucrose and less than 20% from complex carbohydrates. Diets high in complex carbohydrates are, however, typical for most of the world's population of children.

The rate at which lactase hydrolyzes lactose to glucose and galactose in the brush border determines how quickly milk carbohydrates are absorbed. Lactase levels are highest in young infants, declining by more than 50% later in the first year. Lactase levels decline further with age, especially in children who are not of northern European descent. Many black and Hispanic children cannot consume large amounts of dairy products without some evidence of lactose intolerance, such as flatulence and loose stools. Lactase is located predominantly at the tip of the intestinal villi, where it is especially vulnerable to the effects of gastroenteritis or malnutrition. Thus, it may be helpful to avoid giving lactose-containing foods to children recovering from gastroenteritis or malnutrition, though this is not universally necessary. Galactose is preferentially converted to glycogen in the liver prior to conversion to glucose for subsequent oxidation. Infants with galactosemia, an inborn metabolic disease caused by deficient galactose-1-phosphate uridyltransferase, require a lactose-free diet starting in the neonatal period.

Starch is broken down in the lumen of the gut into disaccharides and oligosaccharides, which are hydrolyzed into glucose by maltase, isomaltase, and glucoamylase in the brush border. Glucoamylase, which hydrolyzes oligosaccharides of 4–9 glucose units, is located predominantly at the base of the villi, where it may be protected from partial villus atrophy. Glucose polymers of this length are used extensively in special infant formulas and for caloric supplementation. Advantages include a relatively low osmolar effect in the lumen of the intestine as well as relatively easy hydrolysis by the compromised mucosa. Glucose and galactose are absorbed actively with sodium. This provides the theoretic basis for the composition of oral rehydration solutions in the management of diarrhea. The glucose enhances the absorption of sodium (and thus of water) and also supplies some energy.

During and immediately following a meal, plasma glucose levels are maintained by glucose absorption. If less than 10% of dietary energy is provided by carbohydrate, ketosis results. Within 2–4 hours after a meal, maintenance of plasma glucose depends increasingly on utilization of hepatic glycogen stores. These provide only 100–150 g glucose in the adult and only 6 g in the neonate. Subsequently, until the next meal, there is progressive dependence on gluconeogenesis. Glucose is the principal fuel for the brain and is a necessary energy source for certain other tissues, including red and white blood cells.

Children and adolescents in North America consume large quantities of sucrose (table sugar) in such items as soft drinks, candy, syrups, and sweetened breakfast cereals. A high intake of sucrose may predispose to obesity and is a major risk factor for dental caries. Sucrase hydrolyzes sucrose to glucose and fructose in the brush border of the small intestine. Fructose is absorbed more slowly than and independently of glucose by a facilitated diffusion process. This characteristic provides a distinct advantage. Neither fructose nor galactose stimulates insulin secretion. Fructose, however, is easily converted to hepatic triglycerides, which may be especially undesirable in malnourished subjects.

Dietary fiber can be classified into two major types: nondigested carbohydrate (β1–4 linkages) and noncarbohydrate (lignin). Insoluble fibers (cellulose, hemicellulose, and lignin) increase stool bulk and water content and decrease gut transit time. They may impair mineral absorption. Soluble fibers (pectins, mucilages, oat bran) bind bile acids and reduce lipid and cholesterol absorption. Pectins also slow gastric emptying and the rate of nutrient absorption. Fiber intakes are quite low in North America. Few data regarding the fiber needs of children are available.

Nicklas TA et al: Dietary fiber intake of children and young adults: the Bogalusa Heart Study. J Am Diet Assoc 1995;95:209.

MAJOR MINERALS

(See Table 10–3 for recommended intakes.)

Calcium

The major dietary sources of calcium are milk and other dairy products. Although some calcium is available from other sources, including legumes, broccoli, some green leafy vegetables, and fortified cereals, it is difficult to achieve an adequate intake of calcium if dairy products are excluded from the diet. In such cases, a calcium supplement may be desirable. Average calcium absorption, which depends on calcium status and intake, is 20–30%, but calcium absorption from human milk is 60%. Absorption is enhanced by lactose, glucose, and protein and is impaired by phytate, fiber, oxalate, and unabsorbed fat. Control of calcium absorption is exerted primarily by changes in levels of 1,25-dihydroxycholecalciferol, which are increased in response to an increase in circulating parathyroid hormone (PTH). PTH, which is secreted in response to a fall in plasma ionized calcium, also increases the release of calcium from bone. Calcium is excreted primarily via the kidney. It is the most abundant mineral in the body, and more than 99% is in the skeleton. Many vital cellular processes depend on calcium, especially changes in cytosolic free calcium levels. Changes in these levels also occur in various pathologic states and can grossly disturb intracellular metabolism. A deficiency in dietary calcium can occur in premature infants and lactating adolescents as a result of a restricted milk intake and also in patients with steatorrhea. The effect is a decrease in bone density, possibly progressing to rickets. Bone density increases with increasing calcium intake up to daily intakes of more than 1000 mg in adolescents. Maximizing bone density at this stage of the life cycle has important implications for achieving peak bone density and minimizing postmenopausal osteoporosis.

Kreipe RE: Bone mineral density in adolescents. Pediatr Ann 1995;24:308.
Rubin K et al: Predictors of axial and peripheral bone mineral density in healthy children and adolescents, with special attention to the role of puberty. J Pediatr 1993;123:863.

Phosphorus

Phosphorus is abundant in meats, eggs, dairy products, grains, legumes, and nuts. Phosphorus levels are high in processed foods and very high in colas and other soft drinks. Approximately 80% of dietary phosphorus is absorbed; the kidney is responsible for homeostatic control. PTH decreases tubular reabsorption of phosphorus. More than 85% of body phosphorus is in bone. Phosphorus is also a component of many organic compounds that have a vital

Table 10–3. Suggested dietary intakes of mineral and trace elements.

Nutrient	Premature Infant	Term Infant	Children > 1 Year
Sodium		50 mg/kg/d (2 mmol/kg/d)	250–500 mg/d (10–20 mmol/d)
Potassium		80 mg/kg/d (2 mmol/kg/d)	800 mg/d (20 mmol/d)
Chloride		70 mg/kg/d (2 mmol/kg/d)	700 mg/d (20 mmol/d)
Calcium	180 mg/kg/d	400 (200) mg/d[1]	800 mg/d
Phosphorus	150 mg/kg/d	300 (100) mg/d[1]	600 mg/d
Magnesium	15 mg/kg/d	40 mg/d	100 mg/d
Iron	2 mg/kg/d (after first 1 or 2 months)	1 mg/kg/d (≤ 0.1)[1]	10 mg/d (18 mg/d in adolescence)
Zinc	1.5 mg/kg/d	$4 \rightarrow 2$ ($2 \rightarrow 0.75$) mg/d[1]	2–10 mg/d
Copper	0.12 mg/kg/d	0.2–0.4 mg/d	0.5–2 mg/d
Selenium	0.003 mg/kg/d	0.01–0.03 mg/d	0.03–0.1 mg/d
Iodine	0.001 mg/kg/d	0.05 mg/d	0.07–0.15 mg/d

[1]Amounts in parentheses are for the fully breast-fed infant aged < 4–6 months.

role in metabolism, including ATP and 2,3-diphosphoglycerate. Many of the clinical effects of phosphorus depletion are attributable to cellular energy depletion from lack of ATP or to cellular anoxia secondary to impaired release of oxygen from hemoglobin. Other key compounds containing phosphorus include cell membrane phospholipids and nucleotides.

Nutritional phosphorus deficiency is rare but has been documented in very premature infants fed human milk—in whom it can cause osteoporosis and rickets—and in patients with severe protein-energy malnutrition. Nonnutritional causes of phosphorus depletion include diarrhea, Fanconi's tubulopathy, and the ingestion of phosphorus-binding antacids. Severe hypophosphatemia results from a deficiency together with an acute extracellular to intracellular shift in phosphorus. This shift can be triggered by a glucose load, by insulin, or during nutritional rehabilitation of the malnourished patient. Phosphorus deficiency affects most organ systems, including muscle (weakness progressing to rhabdomyolysis), cellular components of blood (both physiologic and functional changes), the gastrointestinal system, the central nervous system, and bone (bone pain, osteomalacia). Respiratory insufficiency may result from weakness of the diaphragm. Phosphate depletion in the premature infant can cause hypercalcemia. Phosphorus depletion can be treated with phosphorus salts or skim milk. Phosphorus excess may cause neonatal tetany due to decreased serum calcium. Phosphorus retention in chronic renal disease leads to metabolic bone disease.

Fouser L: Disorders of calcium, phosphorus and magnesium. Pediatr Ann 1995;24:38.

Magnesium

Two-thirds of dietary magnesium is derived from vegetables, cereals, and nuts. The kidney exerts very effective control of magnesium homeostasis. When intake is low, excretion is minimal, and intracellular levels are maintained very effectively. Magnesium is the second most abundant intracellular cation; 50% is in bone. Levels in the cell cytosol are 10 times those of the extracellular fluids and are especially high in mitochondria. Magnesium activates many enzymes, especially phosphorus-hydrolyzing and transferring enzymes involved in energy metabolism. Magnesium also plays major roles in nucleic acid metabolism.

Dietary magnesium deficiency is not recognized except as a component of protein-energy malnutrition, but magnesium depletion may occur secondary to renal disease or intestinal malabsorption. Clinical effects include increased neuromuscular excitability, muscle fasciculation and tremors, personality changes, neurologic abnormalities, and electrocardiographic changes (depression of ST segment and T waves). Disturbances of PTH metabolism can cause secondary hypocalcemia. Acute states of magnesium depletion can be treated with a 50% solution of $MgSO_4$ providing 0.3–0.5 mEq of magnesium per kilogram (3–6 mEq maximum) given intravenously over 3 hours and repeated over the remainder of a 24-hour period. Magnesium excess can cause respiratory depression, lethargy, and coma.

Sodium

In the United States and western Europe, only 10% of sodium intake is derived directly from food. Fifteen percent is derived from cooking and 75% from processed foods. The 10% derived from unprocessed foods is more than adequate to meet the normal requirement. Current dietary recommendations include a reduction from the typical intakes of North Americans, in which the ratio of sodium to potassium is 2:1; this ratio is 0.25:1 in other societies and in other mammalian species. High sodium:potassium ratios have been implicated in the pathogenesis of hypertension, especially if the intake of dietary calcium is low. Fifteen percent of the population may be susceptible to adverse effects from high sodium:potassium ratios.

Excessive sweating or cystic fibrosis may increase sodium requirements. Sodium deficiency, which occurs most commonly as a result of diarrhea and vomiting, causes dehydration. Anorexia, vomiting, and mental apathy may result from chronic depletion of sodium chloride. Hyponatremic and hypernatremic dehydration are discussed in Chapter 39.

Severe malnutrition and severe stress or hypermetabolism can disturb the ionic gradient across cell membranes and lead to an excess in intracellular sodium, which can adversely affect cellular metabolism. Sodium should be administered only with great caution in these circumstances.

Avner ED: Clinical disorders of water metabolism: Hyponatremia and hypernatremia. Pediatr Ann 1995;24:23.

Chloride

The intake and homeostasis of dietary chloride are closely linked with those of sodium. However, chloride is itself important in the physiologic mechanisms of the kidney and of the gut. Active chloride transport in the ascending loop of Henle is necessary for the passive reabsorption of sodium. Thus, a deficiency of chloride leads to a decrease in the absorption of sodium in the ascending loop of Henle and an increase in the amount of sodium presented to the lumen of the distal tube. This sodium is exchanged for H^+ and K^+, which can result in hypokalemic alkalosis.

Infants fed formulas low in chloride have experienced a nutritional deficiency of chloride. Other causes of chloride deficiency include cystic fibrosis, pyloric stenosis and other causes of vomiting, familial chloride diarrhea, chronic diuretic (furosemide) therapy, and Bartter's syndrome. Chloride deficiency has been associated with failure to thrive and may especially affect head growth. Other clinical features may include anorexia, lethargy, muscle weakness, vomiting, dehydration, and hypovolemia. Laboratory features include hypochloremia, hypokalemia, metabolic alkalosis, and hyperreninemia. Urine chloride levels depend on the cause of the depletion.

Potassium

Potassium is readily available in unprocessed foods, including nuts, whole grains, meats and fish, beans, bananas, and orange juice. Relatively high potassium intakes are encouraged except in the presence of renal failure. The kidneys control potassium homeostasis via the aldosterone-renin-angiotensin endocrine system. Potassium is the principal intracellular cation. The amount of total body potassium, therefore, depends on lean body mass. Potassium deficiency occurs in protein-energy malnutrition and, if not aggressively treated during the acute management stage, can be a cause of sudden death from cardiac failure. Because of loss of lean body mass, excessive potassium is excreted in the urine in any catabolic state. Again, this requires aggressive replenishment during recovery. In acidosis, intracellular potassium is exchanged for H^+. Potassium, thus shifted into the extracellular fluid, is subsequently lost in the urine, and total body potassium is depleted (eg, in diabetic ketoacidosis) despite normal or elevated levels of plasma potassium. Other prominent causes of potassium deficiency include diarrhea and the use of diuretics. The effects of potassium deficiency are muscle weakness, mental confusion, and sudden death from arrhythmias. Electrocardiographic findings include depression of the ST segment and low T waves. Hyperkalemia may result from renal insufficiency.

TRACE ELEMENTS

Trace elements that have a recognized role in human nutrition are iron, iodine, zinc, copper, selenium, manganese, molybdenum, chromium, cobalt (as a component of vitamin B_{12}), and fluoride. Dietary requirements of trace elements are summarized in Table 10–3. Iron deficiency is discussed in Chapter 20. In general, good dietary sources of trace elements include human milk, meats, shellfish, legumes, nuts, and whole-grain cereals. Fish are a good source of selenium. Absorption of iron, zinc, copper, and probably other trace elements from human milk is especially favorable; the breast-fed infant does not normally require other sources of trace elements, including iron, for the first 4–6 months. Factors affecting the absorption of trace elements include the quantity of that trace element in the diet; dietary factors that form insoluble complexes (phytate, fiber, phosphate, oxalate); factors affecting oxidation state (ascorbic acid increases iron absorption and decreases copper absorption); chemical form (heme versus nonheme iron); competitive inhibition at mucosal cell (interactions of iron, zinc, and copper); and host factors (including nutritional status, diarrhea, impaired mucosal function). The gastrointestinal tract is the major site of homeostatic control for iron and zinc, the liver for copper, the intestinal tract and liver for manganese, and the kidneys for selenium, chromium, and iodine.

Deficiencies of iron, zinc, and possibly copper occur in the free-living population; in certain geochemical areas, the same is true of iodine and selenium. Infants fed cow's milk are at risk for deficiencies in iron and copper. Excessive losses, factors impairing absorption, or iatrogenic factors can cause deficiencies of iron, zinc, or copper. Deficiencies in these elements, as well as selenium, chromium, manganese, and molybdenum, have been associated with the use of synthetic diets, especially intravenous feeding. Protein-energy malnutrition may be complicated by deficiencies in iron, zinc, copper, selenium, or chromium. Finally, deficiencies in zinc, copper, iron, and molybdenum occur as a result of specific inborn metabolic diseases affecting the metabolism of these elements.

Krebs NF, Hambidge KM: Trace elements in human nutrition. In: *Nutrition in Pediatrics,* 2nd ed. Walker WA, Watkins JB (editors). BC Decker, 1997.

Zinc

Zinc is a component of many enzymes, plays multiple roles in nucleic acid metabolism and protein synthesis, and is important for membrane structure and function. Causes of zinc deficiency include diets low in available zinc during periods of rapid growth in infancy and childhood, synthetic oral or intravenous diets lacking adequate zinc supplements, diseases associated with impaired absorption (eg, regional enteritis) or excessive losses (eg, chronic diarrhea) of zinc, and one or more inborn diseases of zinc metabolism. Zinc deficiency may be a factor of secondary importance in some cases of anorexia nervosa. Several recent large zinc supplementation trials have demonstrated significant reductions in the incidence of acute and persistent diarrhea in infants and young children. Improved zinc status in these populations has also been associated with improved immunocompetence and increased activity levels. Clinical effects of a mild deficiency include impaired growth and poor appetite. More severe cases are characterized by changes in mood, irritability, and lethargy. Impairment of the immune system, especially T cell function, has been linked to increased susceptibility to infection. The most severe cases are characterized by an acro-orificial skin rash, usually accompanied by diarrhea and alopecia. These features occur in patients with acrodermatitis enteropathica, an inborn error of zinc metabolism; in those undergoing intravenous feeding without adequate zinc supplements; and in some breast-fed infants whose mothers have a defect in the secretion of zinc by the mammary gland. Plasma zinc collected before breakfast is below 6 μmol/L (40 μg/dL) in cases of severe zinc deficiency and 6–9 μmol/L (40–60 μg/dL) in cases of moderate zinc deficiency. In cases of mild zinc deficiency, plasma zinc concentrations may be within the normal range (9–15 μmol/L). Moderate hypozincemia occurs in response to release of interleukin-1 and in pregnancy even when zinc intake is adequate.

Suspected dietary zinc deficiency can be treated with 1 mg/kg/d of zinc for 3 months (eg, 4.5 mg of $ZnSO_4 \cdot 7H_2O$ per kilogram per day), preferably administered separately from meals and from iron supplements. Sustained clinical remissions in acrodermatitis enteropathica are usually achieved with 30–50 mg Zn^{2+} per day, but larger quantities may be required.

Bentley ME et al: Zinc supplementation affects the activity patterns of rural Guatemalan infants. J Nutr 1997;127: 1333.

Goldenberg RL et al: Zinc supplementation in pregnancy increases birthweight and head circumference in infants. JAMA 1995;274:463.

Ruel MT et al: Impact of zinc supplementation on morbidity from diarrhea and respiratory infections among rural Guatemalan children. Pediatrics 1997;99:808.

Sazawal S et al: Effect of zinc supplementation on cell-mediated immunity and lymphocyte subsets in preschool children. Indian Pediatr 1997;34:589.

Copper

Copper is a vital component of several oxidative enzymes, including cytochrome c oxidase, the terminal oxidase in the electron transport chain; cytosolic and mitochondrial superoxide dismutases, which have key roles in the body defense against free radicals; lysyl oxidase, which is necessary for the cross-linking of elastin and collagen; and ferroxidases (including ceruloplasmin) necessary for the oxidation of ferrous storage iron to ferric iron prior to attachment to transferrin for transport to the red cell precursors in the bone marrow. Cu^{2+} is highly reactive and must be transported in the circulation tightly bound to ceruloplasmin so that its oxidative potential (when it is free or loosely bound) can be contained.

Copper deficiency may occur in the following circumstances: in premature infants fed milk preparations low in copper; in association with prolonged feeding with unmodified cow's milk; in association with more generalized malnutritional states; in patients maintained on prolonged total parenteral nutrition without copper supplementation; and secondary to intestinal malabsorption states or prolonged diarrhea.

Osteoporosis is an early finding. Later skeletal changes include enlargement of costochondral carti-

lages, cupping and flaring of long-bone metaphyses, and spontaneous fractures of the ribs. The radiologic findings must be distinguished from battering (not symmetric), rickets, and scurvy. Neutropenia and hypochromic anemia are other early manifestations. The anemia is unresponsive to iron therapy. Very severe central nervous system disease is present in Menkes' steely (kinky) hair syndrome, in which a profound copper deficiency state results from a specific X-linked inherited defect in cellular metabolism of copper.

A low plasma copper or ceruloplasmin level helps confirm the diagnosis of copper deficiency. However, these levels are normally very low in the young infant, especially the premature infant, and are higher than adult values in later infancy and early childhood. Hence, carefully age-matched normal data are necessary for comparison. Interleukin-1 grossly elevates ceruloplasmin and copper levels; these levels are also very high in pregnancy.

Copper deficiency can be treated with a 1% solution of copper sulfate (2 mg of the salt or 500 μg of elemental copper per day for infants).

Harris ED: Menkes' disease: Perspective and update in a fatal copper disorder. Nutr Rev 1993;51:235.

Selenium

Selenium is an essential component of glutathione peroxidase, which catalyzes the reduction of hydrogen peroxide to water in the cell cytosol by the addition of reducing equivalents derived from glutathione. Hence, selenium plays an important role in the body's defenses against free radicals.

Selenium deficiency is now recognized as the major etiologic factor in Keshan disease, an often fatal cardiomyopathy affecting primarily infants, children, and young women in a large area of China where there is a severe geochemical deficiency of selenium. Similar cases have been identified in the United States in patients maintained on long-term total parenteral nutrition without adequate selenium supplements. Other patients receiving parenteral nutritional support have manifested selenium deficiency with incapacitating skeletal muscle pain and tenderness. Macrocytosis and loss of hair pigment occur in milder states of selenium deficiency. Blood levels are especially low in premature infants with bronchopulmonary dysplasia. It appears that the selenium intake of infants, especially premature infants, is suboptimal and is likely to be increased in the near future.

A plasma selenium level less than 0.5 μmol/L (< 40 μg/L) is compatible with mild selenium deficiency; a level less than 0.12 μmol/L (< 10 μg/L) indicates a possible severe selenium deficiency.

Iodine

Endemic goiter resulting from iodine deficiency has been eradicated in North America by effective prophylactic measures but continues to be a major health problem in many developing countries. Goiter occurs when iodine intake or excretion in urine is less than 20 μg/d. Most goitrous persons are clinically euthyroid. Maternal iodine deficiency causes endemic cretinism in about 5–15% of neonates who develop endemic goiters.

"Neurologic" endemic cretinism, seen clinically in most regions, is characterized by severe mental retardation, deaf-mutism, spastic diplegia, and strabismus. Clinical evidence of hypothyroidism is usually absent, and it is thought that the neurologic damage may be due to a direct effect of fetal iodine deficiency or to an imbalance between T_4 (low) and T_3 (normal or elevated). "Myxedematous" endemic cretinism predominates in some central African countries. Signs of congenital hypothyroidism are seen in this type. Milder neurologic damage occurs in many other cases of endemic neonatal goiter.

In North American countries, the use of iodized salt has been highly effective in preventing goiter. In areas where endemic goiter occurs, intramuscular depot injections of iodized oil have also been used extensively for prevention.

Fluoride Supplementation

When fluoride is incorporated into the hydroxyapatite matrix of dentin, it affords an inexpensive and effective means of helping to prevent dental caries. Fluoride is most effectively administered in the drinking water, but in infancy and childhood, fluoride in vitamin preparations or tablets serves the same purpose. Ready-made formulas provide less than 0.3 ppm. The well-recognized benefits of topical fluoride supplementation must be viewed in light of an increasing incidence of fluorosis in US children. Fluorosis is characterized by an increased porosity (undermineralization) of the enamel and is evident clinically as discoloration of the teeth. Recommendations for fluoride supplementation in infants have recently been revised (Table 10–4). The American Academy of Pediatrics Committee on Nutrition favors supplementation initiated shortly after birth in breast-fed infants (0.25

Table 10–4. Supplemental fluoride recommendations (mg/d).[1]

Age	Concentration of Fluoride in Drinking Water		
	< 0.3 ppm	0.3–0.6 ppm	> 0.6 ppm
6 months to 3 years	0.25	0	0
3–6 years	0.5	0.25	0
6–16 years	1	0.5	0

[1]From Council on Dental Therapeutics, 1994.

mg/d), but recognizes the view that initiation of supplements at 6 months may provide adequate protection.

American Academy of Pediatrics Committee on Nutrition: *Pediatric Nutrition Handbook,* 3rd ed. American Academy of Pediatrics, 1993.
Fomon SJ: Fluoride. In: *Nutrition of Normal Infants.* Mosby, 1993.

VITAMINS

1. FAT-SOLUBLE VITAMINS

Because they are insoluble in water, the fat-soluble vitamins require digestion and absorption of dietary fat and a carrier system for transport in the blood. Deficiencies in these vitamins develop more slowly than deficiencies in water-soluble vitamins because the body accumulates stores of fat-soluble vitamins. Excessive intakes carry a considerable potential for toxicity (Table 10–5).

Udall JN, Greene HL: Vitamin update. Pediatr Rev 1992;13:185.

Vitamin A

Dietary sources of vitamin A include dairy products, fortified margarine, eggs, liver, meats, fish oils, and corn. The vitamin A precursor β-carotene occurs in abundance in yellow and green vegetables. Dietary retinyl palmitate requires hydrolysis by pancreatic and intestinal hydrolases. β-Carotene is cleaved in the intestinal mucosal cells by dioxygenase to yield two molecules of retinal (retinaldehyde), which is then reduced to retinol (vitamin A alcohol). Carotene appears to have an important physiologic role in its own right as a powerful antioxidant.

Retinol is reesterified in the mucosal cells and transported in chylomicrons to the liver, where it is stored. From the liver, vitamin A is transported to the rest of the body attached to retinol-binding protein complexed to prealbumin. Retinol-binding protein may be decreased in liver disease or in protein-energy malnutrition. Circulating retinol-binding protein may be increased in chronic renal failure.

Vitamin A has a critical role in the photochemical basis of vision. The photosensitive pigment rhodopsin is formed from retinal and a protein called opsin. Vitamin A also modifies differentiation and proliferation of epithelial cells, especially in the respiratory tract. Vitamin A is necessary for glycoprotein synthesis and for the integrity of the immune system and may affect gene expression. Retinol can be irreversibly oxidized to retinoic acid, which is effective in glycoprotein synthesis but is ineffective for vision.

Vitamin A deficiency occurs in premature infants, in association with intravenous nutrition with inade-

Table 10–5. Effects of vitamin toxicity.

Thiamin
(Very rare.) Anaphylaxis; respiratory depression
Riboflavin
None
Pyridoxine
Sensory neuropathy at doses > 500 mg/d
Niacin
Histamine release → cutaneous vasodilation; cardiac arrhythmias; cholestatic jaundice; gastrointestinal disturbance; hyperuricemia; glucose intolerance
Pantothenic acid
Diarrhea
Biotin
None
Folate
May mask B_{12} deficiency, hypersensitivity
Cobalamin
None
Vitamin C
Interference with copper absorption; decreased tolerance to hypoxia, increased oxalic acid excretion
Carnitine
None recognized
Vitamin A
(> 20,000 IU/d): Vomiting, increased intracranial pressure (pseudotumor cerebri); irritability; headaches; insomnia; emotional lability; dry, desquamating skin; myalgia and arthralgia; abdominal pain; hepatosplenomegaly; cortical thickening of bones of hands and feet
Vitamin D
(> 40,000 IU/d): Hypercalcemia; vomiting; constipation; nephrocalcinosis
Vitamin E
(? 25–100 mg/kg/d IV): Necrotizing enterocolitis and liver toxicity (but probably due to polysorbate 80 used as a solubilizer)
Vitamin K
Lipid-soluble vitamin K: Very low order of toxicity. *Water-soluble, synthetic vitamin K:* Vomiting, porphyrinuria; albuminuria; hemolytic anemia; hemoglobinuria; hyperbilirubinemia (do not give to neonates)

quate vitamin A supplements, and in association with protein-energy malnutrition, when the manifestations are frequently made more severe by measles. Other causes of vitamin A deficiency are cultural factors (failure to grow vegetables even when practical, eg, in Central America and the Philippines), fat malabsorption syndromes (including biliary atresia), giardiasis, and cystic fibrosis.

The classic features of vitamin A deficiency are primarily related to the eye and vision. Night blindness progresses to xerosis (dryness of cornea and conjunctiva), xerophthalmia (extreme dryness of the conjunctiva), Bitot's spots, keratomalacia (clouding and softening of the cornea), ulceration and perforation of the cornea, prolapse of the lens and iris, and eventually blindness. Vitamin A deficiency is the leading cause of irreversible blindness in children worldwide. Other features of vitamin A deficiency can include follicular hyperkeratosis (dry, thickened, rough skin), pruritus, growth retardation, increased

susceptibility to infection, anemia, and hepatosplenomegaly. Vitamin A treatment of children with measles in developing countries has been associated with reductions in morbidity and mortality.

Serum levels of retinol below 20 μg/dL are considered low; a level below 10 μg/dL indicates deficiency. A ratio of retinol:retinol-binding protein below 0.7 is also indicative of vitamin A deficiency.

Suggested intakes of vitamin A are summarized in Table 10–6. Therapy of xerophthalmia requires 50,000–100,000 IU orally or intramuscularly. The standard maintenance dose in fat malabsorption syndromes is 2500–5000 IU (800–1600 μg). Doses as high as 25,000–50,000 IU/d may be needed, but monitoring to avoid toxicity is essential. Vitamin A

Table 10–6. Suggested intakes of vitamins.

	Premature Infants[1] (per kg/d)	Term Infants[1] (per day)	Adults[2] (per day)
Thiamin (mg)	0.35	12	1.5
Riboflavin (mg)	0.2	0.5	1.7
Pyridoxine (mg)	0.2	0.6	2.0
Niacin (mg NE)[3]	7	17 (NE)	19 (NE)
Pantothenic acid (mg)	2	5	4–7
Biotin (μg)	6	20	30–100
Folic acid (μg)	50	140	400
Cobalamin (μg)	0.3	1	2.0
Vitamin A (μg RE)[4]	500	700	1000
Vitamin C (mg)	25	80	60
Vitamin D (μg) (cholecalciferol)	4 (160 IU)	10 (400 IU)	5
Vitamin E (mg) (α-tocopherol)	3 (See note 5.)	7	10
Vitamin K (μg)	80	20	80

[1]Based on recent recommendations for intravenous vitamins. (Green HL Hambige KM, Schanler R, Tsang RC: Guidelines for the use of vitamins, trace elements, calcium, magnesium, and phosphorus in infants and children receiving total parenteral nutrition: Report of the Subcommittee on Pediatric Parenteral Nutrient Requirements from the Committee on Clinical Practice Issues of The American Society for Clinical Nutrition. Am J Clin Nutr 1988;48:1324 © AM J Clin Nutr. American Society for Clinical Nutrition.)
[2]Based on *Recommended Dietary Allowances,* 10th ed. National Research Council, National Academy Press, 1989, (except for folate).
[3]NE = Niacin equivalents.
[4]RE = Retinol equivalents (1 μg of retinol or 6 mg of β-carotene = 1 RE; 1 IU = 0.3 μg of retinol).
[5]Oral doses up to 25 mg/d are now frequently used with the expectation that this may help to combat oxidant stress.

can be provided in these circumstances as a water-soluble preparation, Aquasol A (1 mL = 50,000 IU). The effects of vitamin A toxicity are summarized in Table 10–5.

American Academy of Pediatrics Committee on Infectious Diseases: Vitamin A treatment of measles. Pediatrics 1993;91:1014.

Fawzi WW et al: Vitamin A supplementation and child mortality: A meta-analysis. JAMA 1993;269:898.

Vitamin D

Vitamin D requirements are normally met primarily from ultraviolet radiation of dehydrocholesterol in the skin with the formation of cholecalciferol (vitamin D_3). Similarly, vitamin D_2, or ergocalciferol, is derived from radiation of ergosterol. Vitamin D is transported from the skin to the liver attached to a specific carrier protein. The primary dietary source is vitamin D–fortified milk and formulas. Egg yolk and fatty fish contain some vitamin D. Vitamin D absorption depends on normal fat absorption. Absorbed vitamin D is transported to the liver in chylomicrons. Vitamins D_2 and D_3 undergo 25-hydroxylation in the liver and then 1α-hydroxylation in kidney proximal tubules to yield 25-hydroxycholecalciferol and 1,25-dihydroxycholecalciferol, respectively. Parathyroid hormone activates the 1α-hydroxylase enzyme in the kidney. Calcifediol (25-hydroxycholecalciferol) is the major circulating form of vitamin D. Calcitriol (1,25-dihydroxycholecalciferol) is the biologically active form of vitamin D. Calcitriol stimulates the intestinal absorption of calcium and phosphate, the renal reabsorption of filtered calcium, and the mobilization of calcium and phosphorus from bone.

Vitamin D deficiency results from lack of adequate sunlight coupled with a low dietary intake. An infant requires only 30 minutes per week of total body sun exposure or 2 hours per week of head exposure to maintain adequate vitamin D status. The breast-fed infant can acquire sufficient vitamin D from human milk if the mother's vitamin D status is optimal. Otherwise, a vitamin D supplement is required to avoid risk of rickets. In the United States, cow's milk and infant formulas are routinely supplemented with vitamin D. Nutritional rickets may occur in older infants and children who are not exposed to the sun or whose skin is deeply pigmented and who do not drink vitamin D–fortified milk.

Vitamin D deficiency also occurs in fat malabsorption syndromes, including small intestinal disease, cholestasis, and lymphatic obstruction. Use of P450–stimulating drugs may decrease hydroxylated vitamin D, which can also be decreased by hepatic and renal disease and by inborn errors of metabolism. End-organ unresponsiveness to calcitriol may also occur.

The clinical effects of vitamin D deficiency are osteomalacia (adults) or rickets (children), in which there is an accumulation in bone of osteoid (matrix) with reduced calcification. Cartilage fails to mature and calcify. The effects include craniotabes, rachitic rosary, pigeon breast, bowed legs, delayed eruption of teeth and enamel defects, Harrison's groove, scoliosis, kyphosis, dwarfism, painful bones, fractures, anorexia, and weakness. X-ray findings include cupping, fraying, and flaring of metaphyses; the loss of sharp definition of bone trabeculae accounts for the general decrease in skeletal radiodensity. The diagnosis is supported by characteristic radiologic abnormalities of the skeleton, low serum phosphorus levels, high serum alkaline phosphatase levels, and high parathyroid hormone levels. The diagnosis can be confirmed by a low level of serum 25-hydroxycholecalciferol.

Rickets is treated with 1600–5000 IU/d of vitamin D_3 (1 IU = 0.25 µg). If this is poorly absorbed, 25-hydroxycholecalciferol, 2 µg/kg/d, or 1,25-dihydroxycholecalciferol, 0.05–0.2 µg/kg/d, is given. Renal osteodystrophy is treated with 1,25-dihydroxycholecalciferol (calcitriol).

Suggested dietary intakes for vitamin D are summarized in Table 10–6 and toxic effects in Table 10–5.

Fraser DR: Vitamin D. Lancet 1995;345:104.

Vitamin E

Vegetable oils provide the main dietary source of vitamin E. Coconut and olive oils, however, are low in vitamin E. Some vitamin E is present in cereals, dairy products, and eggs. Activity may decrease with processing, storage, or heating. Vitamin E is a family of compounds, the tocopherols. There are four major forms: alpha, gamma, beta, and delta; α-tocopherol has the highest biologic activity. Vitamin E can donate an electron to a free radical molecule to stop oxidant reactions. Oxidized vitamin E is then reduced by ascorbic acid or glutathione. The reduced tocopherol is able to "scavenge" another free radical. The nutrients that participate in antioxidant defenses include β-carotene, vitamin C, selenium, copper, manganese, and zinc. Vitamin E is located at specific sites in the cell to protect polyunsaturated fatty acids in the membrane lipids from lipid peroxidation and to protect thiol groups and nucleic acids. Vitamin E also functions as a cell membrane stabilizer, may function in the electron transport chain, and may modulate chromosomal expression.

Vitamin E deficiency may occur in the following circumstances: in the premature infant; in cholestatic liver disease, pancreatic insufficiency (including cystic fibrosis), abetalipoproteinemia, and short bowel syndrome; as an isolated inborn error of vitamin E metabolism; and perhaps as a result of increased utilization due to oxidant stress.

Vitamin E deficiency shortens red cell half-life and may cause hemolytic anemia. Chronic vitamin E deficiency secondary to malabsorption results in a progressive neurologic disorder with loss of deep tendon reflexes, loss of coordination, loss of perception of vibration and position sensation, abnormalities in eye movements, weakness, scoliosis, and degeneration of the retina. In premature infants, vitamin E deficiency may contribute to oxidant injury of the lung, retina, and brain (brain hemorrhage). These putative adverse effects in the premature infant require confirmation.

Vitamin E nutritional status can be partially assessed with serum vitamin E (normal range for children is 3–15 mg/mL). The ratio of serum vitamin E to total serum lipid is normally more than 0.8 mg/g. Hydrogen peroxide–induced hemolysis is also used as a test of vitamin E status.

Suggested intakes are summarized in Table 10–6. Requirements increase if dietary polyunsaturated fatty acids (PUFA) increase (there is a need for 0.4–0.5 mg of vitamin E per gram of PUFA in the diet). One international unit = 1 mg of dl-α-tocopheryl acetate.

Large oral doses (up to 100 IU/kg/d) of vitamin E correct the deficiency resulting from most malabsorption syndromes. Intramuscular injections (5–7 mg/kg/wk) may be necessary in some cases of cholestatic liver disease. For abetalipoproteinemia, 100–200 IU/kg/d of vitamin E are needed. Vitamin E therapy in ischemia-reperfusion injury and in the prevention of intracranial hemorrhage in the preterm infant remains experimental. Toxic effects of vitamin E are summarized in Table 10–5.

Meydani M: Vitamin E. Lancet 1995;345:170.

Vitamin K

Vitamin K_1 (phylloquinone) is obtained from leafy vegetables, soybean oil, fruits, seeds, and cow's milk. Vitamin K_2 (menaquinone), which has 60% of the activity of K_1, is synthesized by intestinal bacteria. K_2 may be a major source of vitamin K in infants and young children, but less is produced in the intestine of the breast-fed infant.

Vitamin K is necessary for the post-translational carboxylation of glutamic acid residues of the vitamin K–dependent coagulation proteins. Carboxylation allows these proteins to bind calcium, leading to activation of the clotting factors. Thus, vitamin K is necessary for the maintenance of normal plasma levels of coagulation factors II (prothrombin), VII, IX, and X and is also necessary for maintenance of normal levels of the anticoagulation protein C. Vitamin K deficiency occurs in newborns, especially those who are breast fed and who do not receive vitamin K prophylaxis at delivery. This deficiency results in hemorrhagic disease of the newborn. Later, vitamin K deficiency may result from fat malabsorption syndromes and the use of nonabsorbed antibiotics and anticoagulant drugs (eg, warfarin). Clinical features

are hemorrhage into the skin (purpura), gastrointestinal tract, genital urinary tract, gingiva, lungs, joints, and central nervous system, which may be fatal. Vitamin K status can be assessed with plasma levels of protein-induced vitamin K absence or by prothrombin time.

Vitamin K requirements are summarized in Table 10–6. Newborns require prophylactic intramuscular vitamin K (0.5–1 mg). For older children with acute bleeding, 3–10 mg of vitamin K is given intramuscularly or intravenously. For chronic malabsorption syndromes, 2.5 mg twice weekly to 5 mg/d is given orally. To reverse warfarin effect, 50–100 mg of intravenous vitamin K is given. Toxic effects are summarized in Table 10–5.

Shearer MJ: Vitamin K. Lancet 1995;345:229.

2. WATER-SOLUBLE VITAMINS

Deficiencies of water-soluble vitamins are much less common in the United States because infant formulas and many foods are fortified, particularly with B vitamins. Most bread and wheat products are now routinely fortified with B vitamins. There is now conclusive evidence that folic acid supplements (400 μg/d) during the periconceptional period provide a strong protective effect for neural tube defects. A good dietary intake of folate, which is likely to result from conformity with current dietary guidelines, also results in significant protection. A good dietary intake of folate as well as a multivitamin supplement in the periconceptional period may also afford protection against neuroectodermal brain tumors in young children.

The danger of toxicity from water-soluble vitamins is not as great because excesses can be excreted in the urine. However, deficiencies in these vitamins can also develop more quickly than deficiencies in fat-soluble vitamins because of the limited stores.

Additional salient details are summarized in Tables 10–6 to 10–11. Although dietary intake of the water-soluble vitamins on a daily basis is not necessary, these vitamins, with the exception of vitamin B_{12}, are not stored in the body.

Carnitine is synthesized in the liver and kidneys from lysine and methionine. In certain circumstances (Table 10–10), however, synthesis is inadequate, and carnitine can then be considered a vitamin. A dietary supply of other organic compounds, such as inositol, may also be required in certain circumstances.

Recommendations for use of folic acid to reduce number of spina bifida cases and other neural tube defects. MMWR Morb Mortal Wkly Rep 1992;41:1.

Table 10–7. Summary of biologic roles of water-soluble vitamins.

B vitamins involved in production of energy of metabolism

Thiamin (B_1)
  Thiamin pyrophosphate is coenzyme in oxidative decarboxylation (pyruvate dehydrogenase, α-ketoglutarate dehydrogenase, and transketolase)
Riboflavin (B_2)
  Coenzyme of several flavoproteins (eg, flavin mononucleotide [FMN] and flavin adenine dinucleotide [FAD]) involved in oxidative/electron transfer enzyme systems
Niacin
  Hydrogen-carrying coenzymes: nicotinamide-adenine dinucleotide (NAD), nicotinamide-adenine dinucleotide phosphate (NADP); decisive role in intermediary metabolism
Pantothenic acid
  Major component of coenzyme A
Biotin
  Component of several carboxylase enzymes involved in fat and carbohydrate metabolism

Hematopoietic B vitamins

Folic acid
  Tetrahydrofolate has essential role in one-carbon transfers. Essential role in purine and pyramidine synthesis; deficiency → arrest of cell division (especially bone marrow and intestine)
Cobalamin (B_{12})
  Methyl cobalamin (cytoplasm): synthesis of methionine with simultaneous synthesis of tetrahydrofolate (reason for megaloblastic anemia in B_{12} deficiency). Adenosyl cobalamin (mitochondria) is coenzyme for mutases and dehydratases.

Other B vitamins

Pyridoxine (B_6)
  Prosthetic group of transaminases, etc, involved in amino acid interconversions; prostaglandin and heme synthesis; central nervous system function; carbohydrate metabolism; immune development

Other water-soluble vitamins

L-Ascorbic acid (C)
  Strong reducing agent—probably involved in all hydroxylations. Roles include collagen synthesis; phenylalanine → tyrosine; tryptophan → 5-hydroxytryptophan; dopamine → norepinephrine; Fe^{3+}; folic acid → folinic acid; cholesterol → bile acids; leukocyte function; interferon production; carnitine synthesis. Copper metabolism; reduces oxidized vitamin E.
Carnitine
  Transfer of long-chain fatty acids from cytosol to mitochondria (necessary for β-oxidation)

Table 10–8. Major dietary sources of water-soluble vitamins.

Thiamin
  Whole grains, cereals (including fortification), lean pork, legumes
Riboflavin
  Dairy products, meat, poultry, wheat germ, leafy vegetables
Pyridoxine
  All foods
Niacin
  Meats, poultry, fish, legumes, wheat, all foods except fats, synthesized in body from tryptophan
Pantothenic acid
  Ubiquitous
Biotin
  Yeast, liver, kidneys, legumes, nuts, egg yolks (synthesized by intestinal bacteria)
Folic Acid
  Leafy vegetables (lost in cooking), fruits, whole grains, wheat germ, orange juice, beans, nuts
Cobalamin
  Eggs, dairy products, liver, meats; none in plants
Vitamin C
  Fresh fruits and vegetables
Carnitine
  Meats, dairy products, none in plants

logic factors in breast milk (including secretory IgA, lysozyme, lactoferrin, bifidus factor, and macrophages) help to provide protection against gastrointestinal and upper respiratory infections. In developing countries, lack of refrigeration and contaminated water supplies frequently make formula feeding especially hazardous. Allergic diseases are less common among infants who have been breast fed. Although formulas have improved progressively and are made to resemble breast milk as closely as possible, it is impossible to mimic the nutritional or immune composition of human milk. Additional differ-

Table 10–9. Circumstances in which the possibility of vitamin deficiencies merit particular consideration.

Circumstance	Possible Deficiency
Prematurity	All vitamins
Protein-energy malnutrition	B_1, B_2, folate, A
Synthetic diets (including total parenteral nutrition	All vitamins
Inherited disorders	Folate, B_{12} D, carnitine
Vitamin-drug interactions	B_6, biotin, folate, B_{12}, carnitine, fat-soluble vitamins
Fat malabsorbtion syndrome	Fat-soluble vitamins
Breast feeding	B_1,[1] folate,[2] B_{12},[3] D,[4] K[5]
Periconceptional	Folate

[1]Alcoholic or malnourished mother.
[2]Folate-deficient mother.
[3]Vegan mother.
[4]Infant not exposed to sunlight and mother's vitamin D status suboptimal.
[5]Maternal status poor; neonatal prophylaxis omitted.

INFANT FEEDING

BREAST FEEDING

Breast feeding, one of the most important influences on children's health worldwide, provides optimal nutrition for the normal infant during the early months of life. Numerous immunoactive immuno-

Table 10–10. Causes of deficiencies
in water-soluble vitamins.

Thiamin
Infantile beriberi; seen in infants breast fed by mothers with history of alcoholism or poor diet; has been described as complication of total parenteral nutrition (TPN); protein-energy malnutrition; prematurity
Riboflavin
General undernutrition; prematurity; inactivation in TPN solutions exposed to light
Pyridoxine
Prematurity (these infants may not convert pyridoxine → pyridoxal-5-P); B_6 dependency syndromes; drugs (isoniazid); heat-treated formulas (historical)
Niacin
Maize or millet diets (high leucine and low tryptophan intakes); prematurity
Pantothenic acid
None
Biotin
Suppressed intestinal flora and impaired intestinal absorption
Folic acid
Prematurity; seen in term breast-fed infants whose mothers are folate-deficient and in term infants fed unsupplemented processed cow's milk or goat's milk; kwashiorkor; chronic overcooking; malabsorption of folate because of a congenital defect; sprue; celiac disease; drugs (phenytoin)
Increased requirements: chronic hemolytic anemias, diarrhea, malignancies, hypermetabolic states, infections, extensive skin disease, cirrhosis, pregnancy
Cobalamin
Rare; seen in breast-fed infants of mothers with latent pernicious anemia or who are on an unsupplemented strict vegetarian diet; absence of luminal proteases; congenital malabsorption of B_{12}
Vitamin C
Prematurity; maternal megadoses during pregnancy → deficiency in infants; lack of fresh fruits or vegetables; seen in infants fed formula and pasteurized cow's milk (historical)
Carnitine
Seen in premature infants fed unsupplemented soy formula or fed intravenously; dialysis; inherited deficits in carnitine synthesis; organic acidemias; valproic acid

Table 10–11. Clinical features of deficiencies
in water-soluble vitamins.

Thiamin
Infantile beriberi (cardiac; aphonic; pseudomeningitic)
Riboflavin
Cheilosis; angular stomatitis; glossitis; soreness and burning of lips and mouth; dermatitis of nasolabial fold and genitals; ± ocular signs (photophobia → indistinct vision)
Pyridoxine
Listlessness; irritability; seizures; gastrointestinal disturbance; anemia; cheilosis; glossitis
Niacin
Pellagra (weakness; lassitude; dermatitis of exposed areas; diarrhea; dementia)
Pantothenic acid
Weakness; gastrointestinal disturbance; burning feet.
Biotin
Scaly dermatitis; alopecia; irritability; lethargy
Folate
Megaloblastic anemia; neutropenia; thrombocytopenia; growth retardation; delayed maturation of central nervous system in infants; diarrhea (mucosal ulcerations); glossitis; jaundice; mild splenomegaly; neural tube defects
Cobalamin
Megaloblastic anemia; neurologic degeneration
Vitamin C
Anorexia, irritability, apathy, pallor; fever; tachycardia; diarrhea; failure to thrive; increased susceptibility to infections; hemorrhages under skin, mucous membranes, into joints and under periosteum; long-bone tenderness; costochondral beading
Carnitine
Increased serum triglycerides and free fatty acids; decreasd ketones; fatty liver; hypoglycemia; genetic: progressive muscle weakness or cardiomyopathy or hypoglycemia

ences of physiologic importance continue to be identified. Furthermore, the relationship developed through breast feeding can be an important part of early maternal interactions with the infant and provides a source of security and comfort to the infant.

In the last decade, breast feeding has been reestablished as the predominant mode of feeding the young infant in the United States. Unfortunately, breast feeding rates remain low among several subpopulations of women, including low-income, minority, and young mothers; many mothers face obstacles in maintaining lactation once they return to work. Skilled use of a breast pump, particularly an electric one, may help to maintain lactation in these circumstances.

Absolute contraindications to breast feeding are rare. They include tuberculosis (in the mother) and

galactosemia (in the infant). Although breast milk may serve as a vehicle for transmission of HIV, preliminary evidence suggests this is not a major route of transmission. Current recommendations are that HIV-infected mothers in developed countries refrain from breast feeding because of the widely available, safe alternatives. In developing countries, the risk of HIV infection via breast milk is generally considered less than the known benefits of breast feeding, particularly when alternative feeding methods may be hazardous.

The premature infant under 1500 g may benefit from the addition of a milk fortifier, particularly to increase the density of protein, energy, calcium, and phosphorus. Breast-fed infants with cystic fibrosis may need an energy and protein supplement unless exogenous pancreatic enzymes are provided.

Management of Breast Feeding

Because most of today's grandmothers bottle-fed their children, the "art" of breast feeding is no longer automatically passed from mother to daughter. Hence, the role of the health professional in supporting and promoting breast feeding is of greater importance. Organizations such as the La Leche League have been effective in promoting breast feeding as well as in providing education and support for mothers and health professionals alike.

Perinatal hospital routines and follow-up pediatric care have a great impact on the successful initiation of breast feeding. Breast feeding is promoted by prenatal and postpartum education, frequent mother-baby contact after delivery, one-on-one advice about breast feeding technique, demand feeding, rooming-in, avoidance of bottle supplements, early follow-up after delivery, maternal confidence, family support, adequate maternity leave, and good advice about common problems such as sore nipples. Breast feeding is undermined by mother and baby separations, feeding babies in the nursery at night, routinely offering supplemental bottles, conflicting advice from staff, incorrect infant positioning and latch-on, scheduled feedings, lack of maternal confidence or support, delayed follow-up, early return to employment, and inaccurate advice for common breast feeding difficulties.

It is important for the mother to know that very few women are unable to nurse their babies. The newborn is generally fed ad libitum every 2–3 hours, with longer intervals (4–5 hours) at night. Thus, a newborn infant nurses at least eight to ten times a day, so that a generous milk supply is stimulated. This frequency is not an indication of inadequate lactation. Mothers also frequently need to be reassured about stooling pattern. In early stages, a loose stool is often passed with each feeding; later (at 3–4 months of age), there may be an interval of several days between stools. Failure to pass several stools a day in the early weeks of breast feeding suggests inadequate milk intake and supply.

Expressing milk may be indicated if the mother returns to her job or if the infant is premature, cannot suck adequately, or is hospitalized. Modern electric breast pumps are very effective and can be borrowed or rented.

Technique of Breast Feeding

Breast feeding can be started after delivery as soon as both mother and baby are stable. Correct positioning and breast feeding technique are necessary to ensure effective nipple stimulation and optimal breast emptying with minimal nipple discomfort.

If the mother wishes to nurse while sitting, the infant should be elevated to the height of the breast and turned completely to face the mother, so that their abdomens touch. The mother's arms supporting the infant should be held tightly at her side, bringing the baby's head in line with her breast. The breast should be supported by the lower fingers of her free hand, with the nipple compressed between the thumb and index fingers to make it more protractile. The infant's initial licking and mouthing of the nipple helps make it more erect. When the infant opens its mouth,

the mother should rapidly insert as much nipple and areola as possible.

Some breast-fed infants fail to thrive. The most common cause of early failure to thrive is poorly managed mammary engorgement, which rapidly decreases milk supply. Unrelieved engorgement can result from inappropriately long intervals between feeding, improper infant suckling, a nondemanding infant, sore nipples, maternal or infant illness, nursing from only one breast, and latching difficulties. The mother's ignorance of technique, inappropriate feeding routines, and inadequate amounts of fluid and rest for the mother all can be factors. Some infants are too sleepy to do well on an ad libitum regimen and, in particular, may need waking to feed at night. Primary lactation failure is rare but does occur. Some decline in weight-for-age percentiles after 3 months should not necessarily be interpreted as an indication of inadequate nutrition, because the commonly used percentile charts have been constructed primarily from data on infants who have been formula-fed.

Rigid time restrictions should not be imposed. Sensible guidelines are 5 minutes per breast at each feeding the first day, 10 minutes on each side at each feeding the second day, and approximately 15 minutes per side thereafter. A vigorous infant can obtain most of the available milk in 5–7 minutes, but additional sucking time ensures breast emptying and ongoing milk production and satisfies the infant's sucking urge. The side on which feeding is commenced should be alternated. The mother may break suction gently after nursing by inserting her finger between the baby's gums.

Follow-Up

Individualized assessment before discharge should identify the mothers and infants needing additional support. All cases require early follow-up after discharge. The onset of copious milk secretion between the second and fourth postpartum day is a critical time in the establishment of lactation. Failure to empty the breasts during this time can cause engorgement secondary to unrelieved pressure in the mammary gland, which quickly leads to diminished milk production.

Common Problems

Mild nipple tenderness requires attention to proper positioning of the infant and correct latch-on. Ancillary measures include nursing for shorter periods, beginning feedings on the less sore side, air drying the nipples well after nursing, and the application of lanolin cream. Severe nipple pain and cracking usually indicate improper infant attachment. Temporary pumping, which is well tolerated, may be needed.

Breast feeding jaundice is exaggerated physiologic jaundice associated with inadequate intake of breast milk, infrequent stooling, and unsatisfactory weight gain. If possible, the jaundice should be managed by increasing the frequency of nursing and, if necessary, augmenting the infant's sucking with regular breast pumping. Supplemental feedings may be necessary, but care should be taken not to decrease breast milk production further.

In a small percentage of breast-fed infants, breast milk jaundice is caused by an unidentified property of the milk that inhibits conjugation of bilirubin. In severe cases, interruption of breast feeding for 24–36 hours may be necessary. The mother's breast should be emptied with an electric breast pump during this period.

Maternal mastitis should be suspected when a nursing mother complains of a flu-like illness with local breast tenderness. Antibiotic therapy providing coverage against β-lactamase–producing organisms should be given for 10 days. Analgesics may be necessary, but breast feeding should be continued. Breast pumping may be a helpful adjunctive therapy.

Maternal Drug Use

Many factors play a role in determining the effects of maternal drug therapy on the nursing infant, including the route of administration, dosage, molecular weight, pH, and protein binding. In general, any drug prescribed therapeutically to newborns can be consumed via breast milk without ill effect. Very few therapeutic drugs are absolutely contraindicated; these include radioactive compounds, antimetabolites, lithium, diazepam, chloramphenicol, antithyroid drugs, and tetracycline. For up-to-date information, a regional drug center should be consulted.

Maternal use of illicit or recreational drugs is a contraindication to breast feeding. If a woman is unable to discontinue drug use, she should not breast-feed. Expression of milk for a feeding or two after use of a drug is not an acceptable compromise. The breast-fed infants of mothers taking methadone (but no alcohol or other drugs) as part of a treatment program have generally not experienced ill effects when the daily maternal methadone dose is under 40 mg.

Nutrient Composition

The nutrient composition of human milk is summarized and compared with that of cow's milk and formulas in Table 10–12. Outstanding characteristics include (1) the relatively low protein content, which is, however, quite adequate for the normal infant; (2) a generous but not excessive quantity of essential fatty acids; (3) the presence of long-chain unsaturated fatty acids of the ω3 series, of which docosahexaenoic acid is thought to be especially important; (4) a relatively low sodium and solute load; and (5) the lower concentration of calcium, iron, and zinc, which with the very favorable absorption provides adequate quantities of these nutrients to the normal breast-fed infant for 4–6 months despite the relatively low intakes. A source of iron, either from iron-fortified cereal, meat, or a supplement, should be introduced by age 6 months.

Weaning

Weaning can take place according to the needs and desires of both infant and mother. Gradual weaning, starting typically after 4–6 months, is preferred. Bottle feedings (or cup feedings) are increased progressively over a period of several weeks as breast feedings are omitted.

American Academy of Pediatrics Committee on Drugs: Transfer of drugs and other chemicals to human milk. Pediatrics 1994;93:137.

Beaudry M et al: Relation between infant feeding and infection during first six months of life. J Pediatr 1995;126:191.

Krebs NF et al: Growth and intakes of energy and zinc in infants fed human milk. J Pediatr 1994;124:32.

Lawrence RA: *Breastfeeding. A Guide for the Medical Profession.* Mosby-Year Book, 1994.

Losch M et al: Impact of attitudes on maternal decisions regarding infant feeding. J Pediatr 1995;126:507.

Neifert MA: Early assessment of the breastfeeding infant. Contemp Pediatr 1996:13:142.

Ryan AS: The resurgence of breastfeeding in the United States. Pediatrics 1997;99. (Electronic version): e12.http://www.pediatrics.org/ogi/content/full/99/4/e12. April 1997.

SPECIAL DIETARY PRODUCTS FOR INFANTS

Feeding During the Second 6 Months

The standard (iron-fortified) infant formulas are suitable for use in the second 6 months. These formulas are preferred to unmodified cow's milk, which may be introduced cautiously after 9 months of age.

Soy Protein Formulas

The major indication for the use of soy protein formulas is lactose intolerance. For example, it is reasonable to recommend a soy protein formula during recovery from acute gastroenteritis for a period of 2–4 weeks. A lactose-free cow's milk–based formula is also available (Lactofree, Mead Johnson). Soy protein formulas are also used frequently in cases of suspected intolerance to cow's milk protein. However, infants who have true cow's milk protein intolerance may also be intolerant of soy protein. Many infants in the United States are currently fed soy protein formulas without good reason.

Semielemental Formulas

These formulas include Pregestimil (Mead Johnson), Nutramigen (Mead Johnson), and Alimentum (Ross). The major nitrogen source of each of these products is casein hydrolysate, supplemented with

Table 10–12. The composition of milk (per 100 kcal).

Nutrient (unit)	Minimal Level Recommended[1]	Mature Human Milk	Typical Commercial Formula	Cow's Milk (mean)
Protein (g)	1.8 (See note 2.)	1.3–1.6	2.3	5.1
Fat (g)	3.3 (See note 3.)	5	5.3	5.7
Carbohydrate (g)	—	10.3	10.8	7.3
Linoleic acid (mg)	300	560	2300	125
Vitamin A (IU)	250	250	300	216
Vitamin D (IU)	40	3	63	3
Vitamin E (IU)	0.3 FT 0.7 LBW 1 g of linoleic	0.3	2	0.1
Vitamin K (μg)	4	2	9	5
Vitamin C (mg)	8	7.8	8.1	2.3
Thiamine (μg)	40	25	80	59
Riboflavin (μg)	60	60	100	252
Niacin (μg)	250	250	1200	131
Vitamin B_6 (μg)	15 μg of protein	15	63	66
Folic acid (μg)	4	4	10	8
Pantothenic acid (μg)	300	300	450	489
Vitamin B_{12} (μg)	0.15	0.15	0.25	0.56
Biotin (μg)	1.5	1	2.5	3.1
Inositol (mg)	4	20	5.5	20
Choline (mg)	7	13	10	23
Calcium (mg)	5	50	75	186
Phosphorus (mg)	25	25	65	145
Magnesium (mg)	6	6	8	20
Iron (mg)	1	0.1	1.5 in fortified	0.08
Iodine (μg)	5	4–9	10	7
Copper (μg)	60	25–60	80	20
Zinc (mg)	0.5	0.1–0.5	0.65	0.6
Manganese (μg)	5	1.5	5–160	3
Sodium (mEq)	0.9	1	1.7	3.3
Potassium (mEq)	2.1	2.1	2.7	6
Chloride (mEq)	1.6	1.6	2.3	4.6
Osmolarity (mOsm)	—	11.3	16–18.4	40

[1]Committee on Nutrition, American Academy of Pediatrics.
[2]Protein of nutritional quality equal to casein.
[3]Includes 300 mg of essential fatty acids.

selected amino acids. Each contains an abundance of EFA from vegetable oil; Pregestimil and Alimentum also provide substantial amounts of MCTs. Pregestimil contains corn syrup solids; Nutramigen contains sucrose, which also provides part of the carbohydrate content in Alimentum.

These formulas are invaluable in a wide variety of malabsorption syndromes, including short bowel syndromes and some cases of chronic diarrhea and cystic fibrosis. They are also effective in feeding infants who cannot tolerate cow's milk and soy protein.

Formula Supplements

The most useful formula supplements are MCT oil and Polycose (Ross), both of which may be used to increase the energy density of a formula. Often it is more appropriate, however, to increase the concentration of the formula and thus increase the density of all nutrients.

Special Formulas

Special formulas include those in which one component, often an amino acid, is reduced in concentration or removed for the dietary management of specific inborn metabolic diseases. Also included under this heading is Amin-Aid (American McGaw).

Complete information regarding the composition of these special formulas, the standard infant formulas, and special formulas for premature infants can be found in standard reference texts and in the manufacturer's literature.

PRUDENT DIET

A prudent diet should be encouraged for all children 2 years of age and older since children with high cholesterol levels tend to become adults with high cholesterol levels and are likely, therefore, to have an increased risk of coronary heart disease. Nutritional habits are formed early in life; dietary intervention may, therefore, be exceptionally effective when started in early childhood.

Salient features of a prudent diet include the following:

(1) Total fat should constitute less than 30% of caloric intake, with saturated fats and polyunsaturated fats providing less than 10% each. Thus, monounsaturated fats should provide 10% or more of caloric intake from fat.

(2) Cholesterol intake should be less than 100 mg/1000 kcal/d, to a maximum of 300 mg/d.

(3) Carbohydrates should provide 60% or more of daily caloric intake, with 50% or more in the form of complex carbohydrates (ie, no more than 10% in the form of simple sugars). A high-fiber diet is also recommended.

(4) The diet should be nutritionally complete, include a variety of foods, and be adequate for optimal growth and activity.

(5) A low salt intake is advised.

The consumption of lean cuts of meats and poultry should be encouraged. Fish should be broiled or baked. Skim milk, soft margarine, and vegetable oils (especially olive oil) should be used. Consumption of egg yolks should be limited to two or three occasions per week. Whole-grain bread and cereals and plentiful amounts of fruits and vegetables are recommended. The consumption of processed foods, soft drinks, desserts, and candy should be limited.

A prudent diet should be only one component of counseling on lifestyles for children. Other aspects are the maintenance of ideal body weight, a regular exercise program, avoidance of smoking, and screening for hypertension. Universal screening for total cholesterol is controversial. Current recommendations are to routinely screen those children who have a positive family history of premature cardiovascular disease, although this approach will identify only about 50% of those with significantly elevated cholesterol levels. If the result is high (≥200 mg/dL), a lipoprotein analysis should be obtained.

American Academy of Pediatrics Committee on Nutrition: Statement on cholesterol. Pediatrics 1992;90:469.

Kleinman RE et al: Dietary guidelines for children: U.S. Recommendations. J Nutr 1996;126:1028S.

Munoz KA et al: Food intakes of U.S. children and adolescents compared with recommendations. Pediatrics 1997;100:323.

Niinikoski H et al: Growth until 3 years of age in a prospective, randomized trial of a diet with reduced saturated fat and cholesterol. Pediatrics 1997;99:687.

Obarzanek E et al: Safety of a fat-reduced diet: The Dietary Intervention Study in Children (DISC). Pediatrics 1997;100:51.

INTRAVENOUS NUTRITION

INDICATIONS

Supplemental Peripheral Nutrition

Supplemental peripheral nutrition is indicated when complete enteral feeding is not possible or desirable (eg, in the premature infant of very low birth weight during the first few days of postnatal life or in the malnourished surgical patient during the early postoperative period). Short-term partial intravenous feeding via a peripheral vein is a preferred alternative to dextrose and electrolyte solutions alone. Because of the osmolality of the solutions required, it is usually impossible to achieve total parenteral nutrition via a peripheral vein.

Total Parenteral Nutrition

Total parenteral nutrition (TPN) should be provided only when clearly indicated. Apart from the expense, numerous risks are associated with this method of feeding (see below). In addition, the powerful homeostatic control mechanisms provided by the intestine and the liver are bypassed. Even when TPN is indicated, every effort should be made to provide at least a minimum of nutrients enterally to help preserve the integrity of the gastrointestinal mucosa and of gastrointestinal function.

The primary indication for TPN is the loss of function of the gastrointestinal tract that prohibits the provision of more than a small proportion of required nutrients by the enteral route. Important examples include short bowel syndrome, some congenital defects of the gastrointestinal tract, and prematurity.

CATHETER SELECTION & POSITION

The Broviac is the catheter of choice for long-term intravenous nutrition. For periods of up to 3–4 weeks, a percutaneous central venous catheter threaded into the superior vena cava from a peripheral vein can be used. For the infusion of dextrose concentrations higher than 12.5%, the tip of the catheter should be located in the superior vena cava or right atrium. After placement, a chest x-ray must be obtained to check this position. If the catheter is to be used for nutrition and medications, a double-line catheter should be inserted.

COMPLICATIONS

Mechanical Complications

A. Related to Catheter Insertion or to Erosion of Catheter Through a Major Blood Vessel:

There is an extensive list of complications involving trauma to adjacent tissues and organs, including damage to the brachial plexus, hydrothorax, pneumothorax, hemothorax, and cerebrospinal fluid penetration. The catheter may slip, especially if care is not taken at the time of dressing or tubing change. The patient may manipulate the line.

B. Clotting of the Catheter: Addition of heparin (1 unit/mL) to the solution is an effective means of preventing this complication. If a catheter does become occluded urokinase can be administered for clot lysis.

C. Related to Composition of Infusate: Calcium phosphate precipitation is a major problem if excess amounts of calcium or phosphorus are administered. The quantities of calcium and phosphate that can be added to the infusate vary widely, depending on the particular commercial amino acid source. Factors that increase the risk of calcium phosphate precipitation include increasing pH and decreasing concentrations of amino acids. Precipitation of medications incompatible with TPN or lipids can also cause clotting.

Septic Complications

Septic complications are the most common cause of nonelective catheter removal, but strict use of aseptic technique and once-daily entry into the catheter at tubing change can result in greatly reduced rates of line sepsis. For this reason, strict adherence to the standardized nursing protocol (for nurses and physicians) is mandatory.

Fever over 38–38.5 °C in a patient with a central catheter should be considered a line infection until proved otherwise. Cultures should be obtained and intravenous antibiotics empirically initiated.

Metabolic Complications

A wide variety of metabolic complications associated with TPN has been documented. Many of these have been related to deficiencies or excesses of specific nutrients. The incidence of these complications has decreased as a result of improvements in amino acid solutions and lipid emulsions and a better understanding of how to achieve appropriate intakes of most nutrients. However, specific deficiencies still occur, especially in the premature infant. Avoidance of deficiencies and excesses and of metabolic disorders requires careful attention to the nutrient balance, electrolyte composition, and delivery rate of the infusate and careful monitoring, especially when the composition or delivery rate is changed.

Currently, the most challenging metabolic complication is cholestasis, particularly common in premature infants of very low birth weight. The cause of TPN-associated cholestasis is not presently known. Patient and medical risk factors include prematurity, sepsis, hypoxia, major surgery (especially gastrointestinal surgery), absence of enteral feeds with associated atrophy of the intestinal mucosa and lack of biliary stimulation, and bacterial overgrowth in the small bowel. TPN-related risk factors include amino acid excess or imbalance, prolonged duration of TPN, and excessive feeding. Amino acid solutions with added cysteine decrease cholestasis. Practices that may minimize cholestasis include initiating enteral feedings (even trophic) as soon as feasible, avoiding sepsis by meticulous line care, avoiding overfeeding, using cysteine- and taurine-containing amino acid formulations designed for infants (eg, Trophamine), preventing or treating small bowel bacterial overgrowth, protecting TPN solutions from light, and avoiding hepatotoxic medications.

NUTRIENT REQUIREMENTS & DELIVERY

Energy

When patients are fed intravenously, no fat and carbohydrate intakes are unabsorbed, and no energy is used in nutrient absorption. These factors account for at least 7% of energy in the diet of the enterally fed subject. The intravenously fed patient also expends less energy in physical activity because of the impediment to mobility. Average energy requirements are therefore at least 7% lower in children fed intravenously, and the decrease in activity probably increases this figure to a total reduction of 10–15%. Caloric guidelines for the intravenous feeding of infants and young children are as follows:

Age (months)	Requirements (kcal/kg/d)
0–1	100–110
2–4	90–100
5–60	70–90
> 5 years	1500

These guidelines are averages; individuals vary considerably. A multitude of factors can significantly increase the energy requirement, including exposure to a cold environment, fever, sepsis, burns, trauma, cardiac or pulmonary disease, and "catch-up" growth after malnutrition.

With few exceptions, such as some cases of respiratory insufficiency, at least 60% of energy requirements is provided as glucose. Up to 40% of calories may be provided by intravenous fat emulsions.

Dextrose

The energy density of intravenous dextrose (monohydrate) is 3.4 kcal/g. Thus, a 10% solution of dextrose in water ($D_{10}W$) provides 0.34 kcal/mL. Dextrose is the main exogenous energy source provided by total intravenous feeding. Intravenous dextrose suppresses gluconeogenesis and provides a substrate that can be oxidized directly, especially by the brain, red and white blood cells, and wounds. Because of the high osmolality of dextrose solutions ($D_{10}W$ yields 505 mOsm/kg H_2O), concentrations greater than 10–12.5% cannot be delivered via a peripheral vein or improperly positioned central line.

The amount of glucose supplied is determined by the rate of administration as well as the dextrose concentration. Consequently, it is important to calculate the desired glucose load in planning dextrose infusions.

The standard initial quantity of dextrose administered is 10 g/kg/d, which provides 34 kcal/kg/d. This is typically provided as 100 mL/kg/d of $D_{10}W$. Tolerance to intravenous dextrose normally increases rapidly, primarily because hepatic production of endogenous glucose is suppressed. Dextrose can be increased by 2.5 g/kg/d. Standard final infusates for infants usually contain $D_{20}W$, but if necessary (especially at low flow rates), concentrations up to $D_{30}W$ or greater may be used. Such high concentrations should be delivered only into the superior vena cava or right atrium. Tolerance to intravenous dextrose loads is markedly diminished in the premature neonate and in patients in hypermetabolic states.

Problems associated with intravenous dextrose administration include hyperglycemia, hyperosmolality, and glucosuria (with osmotic diuresis and dehydration). Possible causes of unexpected hyperglycemia include the following: (1) inadvertent infusion of higher glucose concentrations than ordered; (2) uneven flow rate; (3) sepsis; (4) a stress situation; and (5) pancreatitis. Intravenous insulin reduces hyperglycemia but does not increase glucose oxidation rates; it may also decrease the oxidation of fatty acids, resulting in less energy for metabolism. Hence, insulin should be used very cautiously. A standard intravenous dose is 1 unit/4 g of carbohydrate, but much smaller quantities may be adequate.

Hypoglycemia may occur after an abrupt decrease in or cessation of intravenous glucose. When cyclic intravenous nutrition is provided, the intravenous glucose load should be decreased steadily for 1–2 hours prior to discontinuing the infusate. If the central line must be removed, the intravenous dextrose should be gradually tapered over several hours.

The maximum oxidation rate of infused dextrose in infants is 18 g/kg/d (less if given with ≥3 g of lipid/kg/d). The corresponding rates at 6 years, at 10 years, and in adult life are 13, 8, and 4.3 g/kg/d, respectively. The very low birth weight neonate seldom tolerates more than 8–12 g/kg/d. Quantities of exogenous dextrose in excess of maximal glucose oxidation rates are used initially to replace depleted glycogen stores; hepatic lipogenesis occurs thereafter. Excess hepatic lipogenesis may lead to a fatty liver. Lipogenesis results in release of carbon dioxide, which when added to the amount of carbon dioxide produced by glucose oxidation (which is 40% greater than that produced by lipid oxidation) may elevate the $PaCO_2$ and aggravate respiratory insufficiency or impede weaning from a respirator.

Lipids

The energy density of lipid emulsions (20%) is 10 kcal/g lipid or 2 kcal/mL infusate. The lipids are derived from either soybean or safflower oil. All consist of more than 50% linoleic acid and 4–9% linolenic acid. It is recognized that this high level of linoleic is NOT ideal except when small quantities of lipid are being given to prevent a deficiency in EFA. Ultimately, improved emulsions are anticipated. Because 10% and 20% lipid emulsions contain the same concentrations of phospholipids, a 10% solution delivers more phospholipid per gram of lipid than a 20% solution. Twenty percent lipid emulsions are preferred.

The level of LPL activity is the rate-limiting factor in the metabolism and clearance of fat emulsions from the circulation. LPL activity is inhibited or decreased by malnutrition, leukotrienes, immaturity, growth hormone, hypercholesterolemia, hyperphospholipidemia, and theophylline. LPL activity is enhanced by glucose, insulin, lipid, catecholamines, and exercise. Heparin releases LPL from the endothelium into the circulation and enhances the rate of hydrolysis and clearance of triglycerides. In small premature infants, low-dose heparin infusions may increase tolerance to intravenous lipid emulsion.

The advantages of using fat emulsions to provide up to 40% of caloric intake include the following:

(1) The high energy density allows more energy to be provided when fluid volume is restricted.

(2) The low osmolality (280 mosm/kg H_2O) is of special value when using a peripheral line.

(3) Deficiencies in EFA can be prevented.

(4) The production of CO_2 is 40% lower per unit of energy, an important consideration in cases of pulmonary insufficiency.

(5) The energy cost of fat storage is negligible.

(6) The risk of fatty liver is decreased because of decreased hepatic lipogenesis from dextrose.

Potential disadvantages of fat emulsions include the following:

(1) Impairment of function of lymphocytes, neutrophils, macrophages, and the reticuloendothelial system.

(2) Coagulation defects, including thrombocytopenia, elevated prothrombin time (PT), and partial thromboplastin time (PTT).

(3) Decrease in pulmonary oxygen diffusion.

(4) Competition by free fatty acids with bilirubin and drugs for albumin-binding sites.

(5) Increase in LDL cholesterol.

In general, these adverse effects can be avoided by starting with modest quantities and advancing cautiously in light of results of triglyceride monitoring and clinical circumstances. In cases of severe sepsis, special caution is required to ensure that the lipid is effectively metabolized. Monitoring with long-term use is also essential.

Start with 1 g/kg/d. Advance every 1–2 days by 0.5–1 g/kg/d up to 2.5 g/kg/d in an infant and 3.5 g/kg/d in a child. Check serum triglycerides before starting and before and after increasing dose. Request results the same day. As a general rule, do not increase the dose if the serum triglyceride is greater than 250 mg/dL during infusion (150 mg/dL in neonates) or if the trough level is greater than 150 mg/dL.

Note: Linoleic acid must constitute 2–3% of caloric intake (300 mg linoleic acid per 100 kcal) to avoid deficiency in EFA. Linolenic acid (1%) is also needed and is adequately supplied when linoleic acid needs are met. Administration of 2 g/kg of lipid three times per week will prevent EFA deficiency.

Nitrogen

One gram of nitrogen is yielded by 6.25 g of protein (1 g of protein contains 16% nitrogen). Caloric density of protein is equal to 4 kcal/g.

A. Protein Requirements: Protein requirements for intravenous feeding are the same as those for normal oral feeding (see Table 10–2).

B. Protein-Energy Interactions: There are important interactions between protein and energy requirements. A positive nitrogen balance cannot be achieved on a hypocaloric diet, because protein will be catabolized for energy. When energy intakes are low, the administration of some amino acid does, however, improve the severity of the negative nitrogen balance. Conversely, when nitrogen intake is low, the provision of calories improves nitrogen balance to some extent. In infants, the energy necessary to minimize nitrogen loss associated with an amino acid–free diet is approximately 70 kcal/kg/d. At this level of energy intake, positive nitrogen balance is dependent on the level of nitrogen intake and is independent of further increase in energy intake.

In infants receiving about 50 kcal/kg/d, increasing protein intake up to 3 g/kg/d improves the nitrogen balance. In these circumstances, therefore, a ratio of grams of nitrogen per kilocalorie as low as 1:100 can be advantageous. However, at higher levels of energy intake, ratios of 1:250 to 1:150 or more are optimal. Although these ratios provide a useful crude check, they are not usually the best means of determining protein requirements.

C. Intravenous Amino Acid Solutions: Nitrogen requirements can be met by one of the commercially available amino acid solutions. There is no clear advantage for any of the standard preparations over the others as sources of amino acids for older children and adults, but accumulating evidence suggests that the use of Trophamine (Kendall-McGaw) in infants, including premature infants, is associated

with a normal plasma amino acid profile, superior nitrogen retention, and a lower incidence of cholestasis. Trophamine contains 60% essential amino acids, is relatively high in branched-chain amino acids, contains taurine, and is compatible with the addition of cysteine within 24–48 hours after administration. The dose of added cysteine is 40 mg per gram of Trophamine. The relatively low pH of Trophamine is also advantageous for solubility of calcium and phosphorus.

Normally, the final infusate contains 2–3% amino acids, depending on the rate of infusion. In the severely malnourished infant, the initial amount should be 1 g/kg/d.

Because of the high osmolality of amino acid solutions, the concentration should not be advanced beyond 2% in peripheral vein infusates.

D. Monitoring: Monitoring for tolerance of the intravenous amino acid solutions should include routine blood urea nitrogen. Serum alkaline phosphatase, γ-glutamyltransferase, and bilirubin should be monitored to detect the onset of cholestatic liver disease.

E. Special Amino Acid Preparations: Some solutions are designed to provide high concentrations of branched-chain amino acids. These solutions are expensive and should not be ordered without a specific reason, which does not include their routine use in liver disease. They may be indicated in hepatic failure, especially in the presence of encephalopathy, and are also undergoing experimental use in multisystem organ failure. In this circumstance, the branched-chain amino acids are given as a source of metabolizable energy, providing up to 25% of energy intake. Solutions containing only essential amino acids have some application in the management of patients with renal failure.

F. Albumin: Albumin (0.5–1 g/kg per dose) can be added to the infusate when clinically indicated to restore blood volume or oncotic pressure. If the origin of hypoalbuminemia is considered to be primarily nutritional, however, the hypoalbuminemia should be managed by careful nutritional rehabilitation rather than by intravenous administration of albumin. Albumin is deficient in isoleucine and tryptophan and has too long a half-life (15–20 days) to be considered a useful nutritional source of amino acids.

Minerals & Electrolytes

A. Calcium, Phosphorus, and Magnesium: The intravenously fed premature and term infant should be given relatively high amounts of calcium and phosphorus. Current recommendations are as follows: calcium, 500–600 mg/L; phosphorus, 400–450 mg/L; and magnesium, 50–70 mg/L. After the age of 1 year, the recommendations are as follows: calcium, 200–400 mg/L; phosphorus, 150–300 mg/L; and magnesium, 20–40 mg/L. The calcium:phosphorus ratio should be 1.3:1 by weight or 1:1 by molar ratio.

These recommendations are deliberately presented on a per liter infusate basis to avoid inadvertent administration of concentrations of calcium and phosphorus that are high enough to precipitate in the tubing. During periods of fluid restriction, care must be taken not to inadvertently increase the concentration of calcium and phosphorus in the infusate. These recommendations assume an average fluid intake of 120–150 mL/kg/d and an infusate of 25 g of amino acid per liter. With lower amino acid concentrations, the concentrations of calcium and phosphorus should be decreased.

B. Electrolytes: Standard recommendations are given in Figure 10–1. After chloride requirements are met, the remainder of the anion required to balance the cation should be given as acetate to avoid the possibility of acidosis resulting from excessive chloride. The required concentrations of electrolytes depend to some extent on the flow rate of the infusate and must be modified if flow rates are unusually low or high and if there are specific indications in individual patients. Intravenous sodium should be administered very sparingly in the severely malnourished patient because of impaired membrane function and high intracellular sodium levels. Conversely, generous quantities of potassium are indicated. Replacement electrolytes and fluids should be delivered via a separate infusate.

C. Trace Elements: Recommended intravenous intakes of trace elements are given in Figure 10–1.

When intravenous nutrition is supplemental or limited to less than 2 weeks, only zinc need routinely be added.

Intravenous copper requirements are relatively low in the young infant because of the presence of hepatic copper stores. These are significant even in the 28-week fetus. Circulating levels of copper and manganese should be monitored in the presence of cholestatic liver disease. If monitoring is not feasible, temporary withdrawal of added copper and manganese is advisable. Copper and manganese are excreted primarily in the bile, but selenium, chromium, and molybdenum are excreted primarily in the urine. These trace elements, therefore, should be administered with caution in the presence of renal failure.

For patients being maintained on long-term parenteral nutrition, a dose of 1 µg/kg/d of iodine avoids any risk of iodine deficiency and does not increase the risk of toxicity from accidental absorption of topical iodine-containing preparations.

Although low doses of iron are routinely added in some centers to the intravenous infusate for infants and children, no official recommendation has been made because of the lack of adequate published data regarding compatibility. Iron added to the infusate should be in a diluted form of iron dextran in a concentration of 1 mg/L. After 2 months of age, maintenance intravenous iron requirements for the term infant are approximately 100 µg/kg/d intravenously. After the first month, the premature infant requires up to 200 µg/kg/d intravenously. Although overload is unlikely to occur during short-term parenteral nutrition, a surreptitious accumulation of extra iron could occur if parenteral nutrition is prolonged. This risk is enhanced if the patient has received blood transfusions. A second concern is that the potential for free iron is increased in malnourished infants with low transferrin levels. Excess iron is thought to enhance the risk of gram-negative septicemia. Iron has powerful oxidant properties and can enhance the demand for antioxidants, especially vitamin E. None of these concerns appear to preclude the routine use of iron supplements during intravenous nutrition, but they do emphasize the need for a conservative attitude in determining dosage schedules.

Vitamins

Recommendations for intravenous vitamin intakes are given in Table 10–6. MVI Pediatric (Armour) meets the guidelines for term infants. The recommended dose of MVI Pediatric for premature infants is 2 mL (40%) of a single-dose vial per kilogram per day. This formulation is not optimal (too little vitamin A, excessive amounts of water-soluble vitamins), but it is currently the best available.

Intravenous lipid preparations contain enough tocopherol to affect total blood tocopherol levels. The majority of tocopherol in soybean oil emulsion is γ-tocopherol, which has substantially less biologic activity than α-tocopherol, which is present in safflower oil emulsions.

A dose of 40 IU/kg/d of vitamin D (maximum 400 IU/d) is adequate for both term and preterm infants.

Fluid Requirements

The initial fluid volume and subsequent increments in flow rate are determined by basic fluid requirements, the clinical status of the patient, and the extent to which additional fluid administration can be tolerated and may be required to achieve adequate nutrient intake. Calculation of initial fluid volumes to be administered should be based on standard pediatric practice. Tolerance of higher flow rates must be determined on an individual basis. If replacement fluids are required for ongoing abnormal losses, these should be administered via a separate line.

Ordering

An example of a parenteral nutrition order form for pediatrics is given in Figure 10–1. Orders should be reviewed daily when changes are made and when the patient is acutely ill.

Monitoring

Vital signs should be checked on each shift.

With central catheter in situ and fever more than 38 °C, peripheral and central line blood cultures,

	Standard Order	Modifications To Standard Order	*Adjustments for Neonates and Premature Infants (Circle these when required and cross out corresponding items* under "standard order")

PEDIATRIC PARENTERAL NUTRITION (PN) ORDER FORM   Imprint Patient Plate

Weight of patient _____kg   Central line_____   Peripheral line _____   _____

Rate _____

Protein (as amino acid)* _____   g%   *Use trophamine and cysteine for patients in level II and III nurseries who have a central line or are on a day 6 of peripheral therapy.

Dextrose _____   g%

Na _____ 30 meq/L

K _____ 25 meq/L

Cl _____ 20 meq/L

Acetate _____ 45 meq/L

Ca (as gluconate) (10 mM Ca/L) _____ 20 meq/L

Mg (as sulfate) _____ 3 meq/L

P_____ 10 meq/L

MVI Pediatric _____ *5.0 mL/d   *2 mL/kg/d for patients < 2.5 kg

Zinc _____ *1.0 mg/L   *Zn: 400 µg/kg/d < 2 kg body weight 250 µg/kg/d others < 3 mo old

Copper _____ 200 µg /L

Manganese _____ 5.0 µg/L

Chromium _____ 2.0 µg/L

Selenium _____ 20.0 µg/L

Iodide _____ 10 µg /L

Heparin _____ 1000 Units/L

Cysteine (40 mg/g trophamine)* _____ mg/L   *Use only with trophamine

Pharmacy will automatically account for electrolytes provided in amino acid preparation.

Changes in Na or K to be made as: Cl only___, or Acetate only___, Cl: Acetate 1:1__, or other

Cl: Acetate ratio (specify_____).

Date:_____ Signature:_____M.D.

Figure 10–1. Example of pediatric parenteral nutrition order. Standard recommendations for minerals and trace elements are indicated.

urine cultures, complete physical examination, and examination of intravenous entry point are required. Instability of vital signs, elevated white blood cell count with left shift, and glycosuria suggest sepsis. Removal of the central venous catheter should be considered if patient is toxic or unresponsive to antibiotics (the patient must be weaned of high-dose dextrose prior to removal of the catheter).

A. Physical Examination: Monitor especially for hepatomegaly (differential diagnoses include fluid overload, congestive heart failure, steatosis, and hepatitis) and edema (differential diagnoses: fluid overload, congestive heart failure, hypoalbuminemia, thrombosis of superior vena cava).

B. Intake and Output Record: Calories and volume delivered should be calculated from previous day's intake and output sheets (that which was delivered rather than that which was ordered). The following should be recorded on flow sheets: intravenous, enteral, and total fluid (mL/kg/d); dextrose (g/kg/d); protein (g/kg/d); lipids (g/kg/d); energy (kcal/kg/d).

C. Growth, Urine, and Blood: Routine monitoring guidelines given in Table 10–13 are only a guide. These are minimum requirements, except in the very long-term stable patients. Individual variables should be monitored more frequently as indicated, as should additional variables or clinical indications. For example, a blood ammonia should be ordered in an infant with lethargy, pallor, poor growth, acidosis, azotemia, and elevated liver enzymes.

Beath SV et al: Parenteral nutrition-related cholestasis in postsurgical neonates: Multivariate analysis of risk factors. J Pediatr Surg 1996;31:604.

Greene HL et al: Guidelines for the use of vitamins, trace elements, calcium, magnesium, and phosphorus in infants and children receiving total parenteral nutrition: Report of the Subcommittee on Pediatric Parenteral Nutrient Requirements from the Committee on Clinical Practice Issues of the American Society for Clinical Nutrition. Am J Clin Nutr 1988;48:1324.

Heird WC: Amino acid and energy needs of pediatric patients receiving parenteral nutrition. Pediatr Clin North Am 1995;42:765.

INTENSIVE CARE NUTRITION

Severe stress of any kind (eg, large surface area and deep burns, major trauma, major surgery, sepsis) results in common metabolic changes that require special understanding and nutritional management. First, several hormones are increased, including thyroid hormone, catecholamines, cortisol, and glucagon. These hormones, acting directly on peripheral tissues or indirectly through an increase in peripheral insulin resistance (as a result, insulin concentration may actually increase), produce hypermetabolism, increased protein catabolism, and hyperglycemia. These effects develop rapidly, from seconds for the catecholamines, to minutes for insulin and glucagon, to hours for thyroid and cortisol. Rapid measurements of these hormones and their metabolic effects are not available for routine clinical management, so the clinician must know that their concentration changes and metabolic effects are going to be present, highly variable, and significant, requiring special management early in the course of stressful events to counter their adverse effects on fuel metabolism. Early and aggressive intravenous and enteral nutrition are essential, with an emphasis on providing an increased supply of amino acids, particularly the branched-chain amino acids. Trials of insulin infusion, including coinfusion of growth hormone and insulinlike growth factor–I, are under way. The goal of such aggressive, early treatment is to provide an excess of nonprotein calories (favoring lipids over glucose) and amino acids to preserve essential protein structures.

Table 10–13. Routine TPN monitoring summary.

Variables	Acute Stage	Long-Term

Growth
  Weight
  Length
  Head circumference
	
	Daily
	Weekly
	Weekly
		
		Weekly

Urine
  Glucose (dipstick)
  Specific gravity
  Volume
	
	With each void
	Void
	Daily
		
		With changes in intake or status

Blood
  Glucose
  Na⁺, K⁺, Cl⁻, CO₂, BUN
 	
  Ca²⁺, Mg²⁺, P
  Total protein, albumin, bilirubin, AST, and alkaline phosphatase
  Zinc and copper
  Triglycerides
  CBC
	
	4 hours after changes,[1] then daily × 2
	Daily for 2 days after changes,[1] then twice weekly
	Initially, then twice weekly
	Initially , then weekly
	
	Initially
	Initially, 1 day after changes,[1] then weekly
	Initially, then twice weekly; according to clinical indications (see text)
		
		Weekly
		Weekly
		
		Weekly
		Every other week
		
		Monthly
		Weekly
		Twice weekly

[1]Changes include alterations in concentration or flow rate.

Allison SP: Overview: Substrate and acute catabolism. In: *Organ Metabolism and Nutrition.* Kinney JM, Tucker HN (editors). Raven, 1994.

Provision of Nutrients in Hypermetabolic States

The most important principle is to continue enteral feeding whenever possible, so that the integrity of the enterocytes can be maintained. The increase in energy requirements varies according to the severity of hypermetabolism and its cause. Requirements are highest in burn patients, but major trauma and severe sepsis increase energy expenditure by 20–50%.

The uncontrolled muscle proteolysis and negative nitrogen balance that are characteristic of the hypermetabolic state cannot be counteracted totally by aggressive nutrition support, but the adverse effects can be attenuated. Negative nitrogen balance can be improved by providing 1½ to two times the basal protein requirement for that age. Larger quantities are unlikely to improve nitrogen balance, and they require substantial energy expenditure for oxidation and will increase CO_2 production. Additional amounts (up to 25% of caloric needs) of branched-chain amino acids (enteral or parenteral) are currently being used as an energy source for skeletal muscle.

Another major metabolic aberration in stress-induced, hypermetabolic states is persistent, uncontrolled hepatic gluconeogenesis, often producing markedly elevated blood glucose concentrations. Gluconeogenesis is not switched off—as would normally be expected—by the administration of intravenous dextrose; in fact, dextrose administration tends to aggravate hyperglycemia and increase hepatic lipogenesis. In some patients (especially those who develop multisystem organ failure), only very modest quantities (< 45% of energy requirements) will be tolerated. If severe hyperglycemia and glycosuria occur, temporary insulin therapy is necessary. However, the putative effects of insulin in hypermetabolic states are complex and not well clarified. Hypermetabolism is characterized by insulin resistance. Furthermore, insulin requires the simultaneous administration of greater-than-normal amounts (up to 25% of energy needs) of amino acids to limit or partially reverse the uncontrolled muscle catabolism and gluconeogenesis. Theoretically, insulin administration could decrease lipolysis and thus deprive the hypermetabolic patient of some of the major sources of utilizable endogenous fuel.

Although lipolysis is increased in hypermetabolic states, β-oxidation of fatty acids also is increased, at least initially. Intravenous lipids usually can be metabolized well in early stages, and up to 50% of energy may be provided as lipid. Metabolically, lipid is the preferred fuel in patients with severe sepsis. Lipid tolerance deteriorates in advanced multisystem organ failure.

The metabolic and nutritional advantages of lipid as a fuel must be balanced against potential adverse effects in the septic child. (See Intravenous Lipids, above.) It is important not to administer fat emulsion in excess of quantities that can be cleared effectively from the circulation.

Much interest recently has focused on the potential benefits of glutamine during acute stress. Glutamine is a nonessential amino acid which is an important source of nitrogen for nucleic acid synthesis. It becomes conditionally essential and serves as a preferred energy source for certain tissues, including enterocytes. Supplementation with glutamine, orally or parenterally, has been associated with lessened bacterial translocation from the gut, improved nitrogen balance, and improved tolerance to enteral feeds in critically ill patients. Although most studies have been undertaken in adults, trials in pediatric bone marrow transplant patients and in children with short bowel syndrome are under way.

McClave SA, Snider HL: Understanding the metabolic response to critical illness: Factors that cause patients to deviate from the expected pattern of hypermetabolism. New Horizons 1994;2:139.

Tremel H et al: Glutamine dipeptideósupplemented parenteral nutrition maintains intestinal function in the critically ill. Gastroenterology 1994;107:1595.

REFERENCES

Walker WA, Watkins JB (editors): *Nutrition in Pediatrics: Basic Science and Clinical Applications,* 2nd ed. BC Dekker, 1996.

11 Emergencies, Injuries, & Poisoning

F. Keith Battan, MD, Richard C. Dart, MD, PhD, & Barry H. Rumack, MD

I. EMERGENCIES & INJURIES

F. Keith Battan, MD

Pediatric emergency medicine is a subspecialty with fellowship training and board certification that has developed to provide resuscitation and urgent care of infants, children, and adolescents. The body of research literature in this field is substantial and growing rapidly. The EMS-C (Emergency Medical Services for Children) movement exists to enhance the spectrum of care of the severely ill or injured child: community injury prevention, prehospital care by emergency medical technicians and paramedics, emergency department-based stabilization and critical care, and rehabilitation. Specialists in pediatric emergency medicine are intimately involved in the care of injured patients, since trauma is the leading cause of death among children over 1 year of age.

Isaacman DJ, Davis HW: Pediatric emergency medicine: State of the art. Pediatrics 1993;91:587.
Lohr KN, Durch JS (editors): *Emergency Medical Services for Children, Report to the Nation from the Institute of Medicine, Committee on Pediatric Emergency Medical Services.* National Academy Press, 1993.

ADVANCED LIFE SUPPORT FOR INFANTS & CHILDREN

Children may present in cardiopulmonary failure from a wide variety of causes, mainly respiratory disorders. Regardless of the primary origin, a systematic approach allows rapid determination of the patient's physiologic status with concurrent initiation of resuscitative measures. The goal of rapid assessment and intervention is not necessarily to make a specific etiologic diagnosis but to determine the degree of physiologic derangement—Is there respiratory failure? Is there shock?—and then to intervene promptly to ensure adequate oxygenation, ventilation, and circulation. Once initial resuscitative measures are begun, consideration of the etiology of the arrest begins.

Children who become apneic, pulseless, and asystolic virtually never survive without neurologic devastation. When progressive deterioration leads to bradycardia and ultimately to asystole, sufficient hypoxic and ischemic insult to the brain and other vital organs has occurred to make neurologic recovery extremely unlikely, even if the child survives the arrest, which occurs in less than 1% of arrests. Children who respond to ventilation and oxygenation alone or to less than 5 minutes of advanced life support are much more likely to survive neurologically intact. Therefore, it is essential to recognize the child who is at risk for progressing to cardiopulmonary arrest and to provide aggressive intervention before progression to asystole occurs.

Note: Universal precautions must be maintained during resuscitation efforts.

THE ABCs OF RESUSCITATION

Severely ill children should be rapidly evaluated in a deliberate sequence of *a*irway patency, *b*reathing adequacy, and *c*irculation integrity. Derangement in each must be corrected before proceeding to the next function. Thus, if a child's airway is obstructed, one must open the airway (eg, by head positioning and the chin lift maneuver) before assessing breathing and then circulation.

Airway

Look, listen, and feel for airway patency: (1) *Look* for signs of obstruction such as inspiratory work or suprasternal retractions. A patient with significant airway obstruction will have an altered level of consciousness, such as agitation or unresponsiveness. (2) *Listen* for adventitious breath sounds such as stridor, snoring, or gurgling. (3) *Feel* for air movement with your face near the child's mouth and nose.

The airway is managed initially by noninvasive means such as oxygen administration, chin lift, suctioning, or bag-valve-mask ventilation, then by invasive maneuvers such as endotracheal intubation or cricothyroidotomy. If neck injury is suspected, the cervical spine must be immobilized. (See Approach to the Pediatric Trauma Patient, below.) The following discussion assumes that basic life support skills have been mastered.

Knowledge of pediatric anatomic differences will help assess and manage the airway. Infants are obligate nasal breathers; therefore, secretions or blood can cause significant distress. Children's tongues are large relative to their oral cavities, and the larynx is high and anteriorly located. In unconscious children,

prolapse of the tongue into the posterior pharynx is the most common cause of airway obstruction.

A. Place the head in the "sniffing position" (Figure 11–1). The neck should be slightly flexed and the head gently extended so as to bring the face forward. This position aligns the oral, pharyngeal, and tracheal planes (Figure 11–2). The head should be repositioned if airway obstruction persists after head tilt and jaw thrust. In an infant, the relatively large occiput puts the head in a sniffing position when supine; in an older child, more head extension is necessary. Avoid hyperextension of the neck, especially in infants.

B. Perform the chin lift or jaw thrust maneuver (Figure 11–3). Lift the chin upward while avoiding pressure on the submental triangle, or lift the jaw by traction upward on the angle of the jaw. Jaw thrust without head tilt should be done if cervical spine injury is possible.

C. Suction the mouth of secretions, blood, and foreign material.

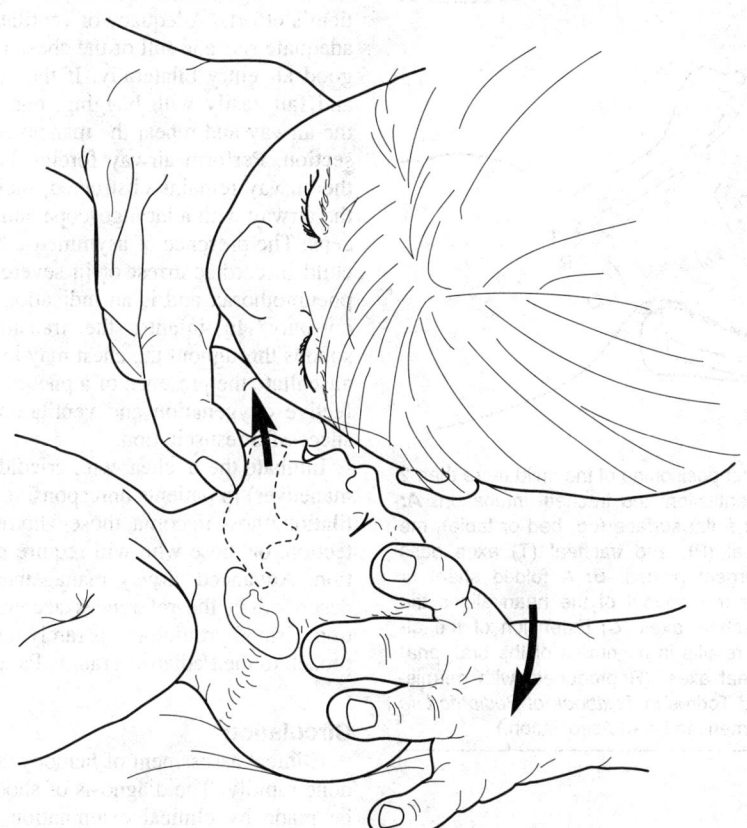

Figure 11–1. Opening the airway with the head tilt–chin lift maneuver. One hand is used to tilt the head, extending the neck. The index finger of the rescuer's other hand lifts the mandible outward by lifting on the chin. Head tilt should not be performed if cervical spine injury is suspected. (Reproduced, with permission, from *Textbook of Pediatric Life Support.* © 1997, American Heart Association.)

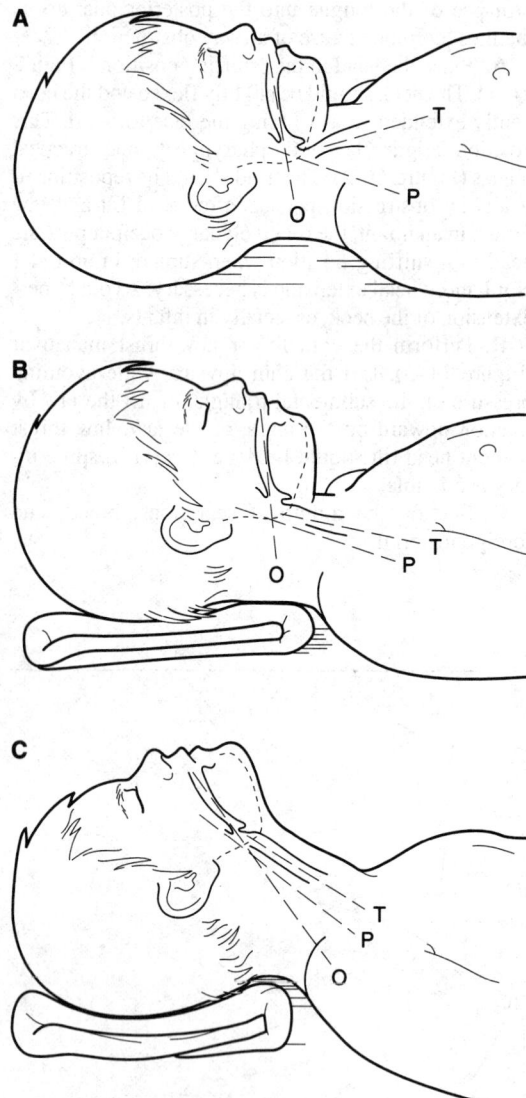

Figure 11–2. Correct positioning of the child more than 2 years of age for ventilation and tracheal intubation. **A:** With the patient on a flat surface (eg, bed or table), the oral (O), pharyngeal (P), and tracheal (T) axes pass through three divergent planes. **B:** A folded sheet or towel placed under the occiput of the head aligns the pharyngeal and tracheal axes. **C:** Extension of the atlanto-occipital joint results in alignment of the oral, pharyngeal, and tracheal axes. (Reproduced, with permission, from Cote and Todres in *Textbook of Pediatric Life Support.* © 1997, American Heart Association.)

D. Remove visible foreign bodies, using the fingers or a Magill forceps–visualizing by means of a laryngoscope if necessary. Blind finger sweeps should not be done.

E. Insert an oropharyngeal or, in the conscious patient, a nasopharyngeal airway to relieve upper airway obstruction due to prolapse of the tongue and mandibular block of tissue into the posterior pharynx (Figures 11–4 and 11–5). The correct size for an oropharyngeal airway is obtained by measuring from the upper central gumline to the angle of the jaw. Nasopharyngeal airways should fit snugly but not tightly within the nares and should be equal in length to the distance from the nares to the tragus.

Breathing

Assessment of respiratory status is largely accomplished by inspection. (1) *Look* for adequate and symmetric chest rise and fall, respiratory rate, increased work of breathing including retractions, flaring, and grunting, skin color, and tracheal deviation. Again note mental status. (2) *Listen* for adventitious breath sounds such as wheezing. Auscultate for air entry, symmetry of breath sounds, and rales. (3) *Feel* for subcutaneous crepitus.

If there is inadequate spontaneous breathing, or apnea, initiate positive-pressure ventilation with bag-mask ventilation and 100% oxygen. If some respiratory effort is present, coordinate bagging with the patient's efforts. Adequacy of ventilation is reflected in adequate rise and fall of the chest and auscultation of good air entry bilaterally. If the chest does not rise and fall easily with bagging, one should reposition the airway and repeat the maneuvers in the "airway" section. Perform airway foreign body maneuvers if the airway remains obstructed, including visualizing the airway with a laryngoscope and using Magill forceps. The presence of asymmetric breath sounds in a child in cardiac arrest or in severe distress suggests pneumothorax and is an indication for needle thoracostomy. In infants, the transmission of breath sounds throughout the chest may impair the ability to auscultate the presence of a pneumothorax. *Note:* Effective oxygenation and ventilation are the keys to successful resuscitation.

Intubate the trachea, with cricoid pressure (Sellick maneuver) in patients unresponsive to bag-mask ventilation, those in coma, those who require airway protection, or those who will require prolonged ventilation. Advanced airway management techniques are described in the references accompanying this section. Cricothyroidotomy is rarely necessary. (See Approach to the Pediatric Trauma Patient.)

Circulation

Clinical assessment of hemodynamic status can be done rapidly. The diagnosis of shock can and should be made by clinical examination before the blood pressure is measured.

A. Pulses: Check heart rate and adequacy of peripheral pulses. Pulses can be bounding in the early phases of septic shock, or weak and thready with severe hypovolemia. Tachycardia is a nonspecific sign

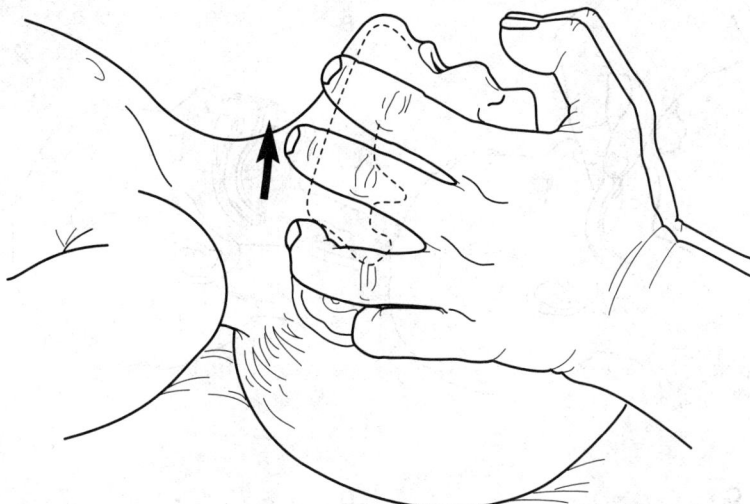

Figure 11–3. Opening the airway with the jaw-thrust maneuver. The airway is opened by lifting the angle of the mandible. The rescuer uses two or three fingers of each hand to lift the jaw while the remaining fingers guide the jaw upward and outward. (Reproduced, with permission, from *Textbook of Pediatric Life Support.* © 1994, American Heart Association.)

of distress, whereas bradycardia for age is a prearrest sign and necessitates aggressive resuscitation.

B. Extremities: If distal extremities are cool, locate the proximal point at which they become warm to assess the severity of shock. For example, a child whose extremities are cool distal to the elbows and knees is severely hypoperfused.

C. Capillary Refill Time: This is an important indicator of perfusion. A refill time longer than 2.0 seconds is abnormal unless the child is cold.

D. Mental Status: Hypoxia, hypercapnia, or ischemia will result in altered mentation.

E. Skin Color: Cyanosis is a late finding in children owing to their relative anemia. Compromised cardiopulmonary status can be reflected in pallor or in gray, mottled, or ashen skin colors.

F. Blood Pressure: Determination of blood pressure is not necessary to make the diagnosis of shock. It is important to remember that shock or inadequate perfusion of vital organs may be present before the blood pressure falls below the normal limits for age. As intravascular volume falls, peripheral vascular resistance increases so that blood pressure is maintained until there is 25–30% depletion of blood volume, followed by a precipitous and often irreversible deterioration into shock (Figure 11–6). Shock that occurs with signs of decreased perfusion (eg, tachycardia and delayed capillary refill time) but normal blood pressure is compensated shock. When blood pressure also falls, decompensated shock is present. The appropriate-sized cuff must be used to obtain an accurate blood pressure.

MANAGEMENT OF SHOCK

Intravenous access is essential but can be difficult to establish in the volume-contracted patient. First attempts should be for peripheral access, especially the antecubital veins, with attempts limited to 90 seconds. Central cannulation—depending on individual preference and expertise—follows quickly. Alternatives are percutaneous cannulation of femoral, subclavian, or internal or external jugular veins; cutdown at antecubital, femoral, or saphenous sites; or intraosseous lines (Figure 11–7). Consider intraosseous needle placement in any severely ill child when venous access cannot be rapidly established. Use short, wide-bore catheters to allow maximal flow rates. Children in shock and other severely ill children should have two intravenous sites started. In newborns, the umbilical veins may be cannulated.

Consider arterial access if beat-to-beat monitoring or frequent laboratory tests will be needed.

Differentiation of Shock States & Initial Therapy

Therapy for inadequate circulation is based on the cause of circulatory failure.

A. Hypovolemic Shock: The most common type of shock in the pediatric population is hypovolemic. Common causes include dehydration from vomiting and diarrhea, diabetes, or heat illness; hemorrhage; and loss of plasma from burns or trauma. Initial therapy is with isotonic crystalloid solution, that is, lactated Ringer's solution or normal saline so-

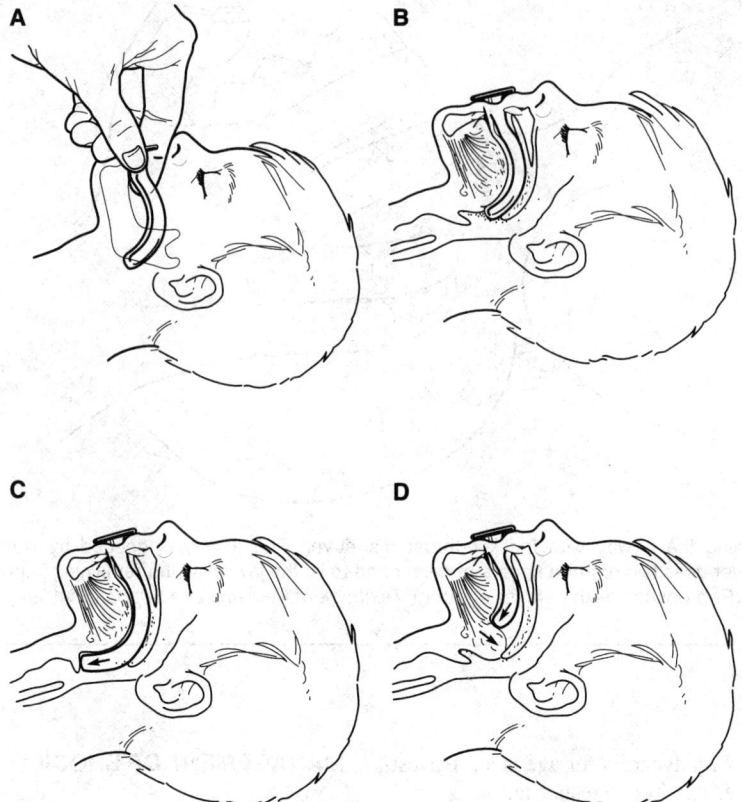

Figure 11–4. *A–D:* Proper airway selection. An airway of the proper size should relieve obstruction caused by the tongue without damaging laryngeal structures. The appropriate size can be estimated by holding the airway next to the child's face *(A).* The tip of the airway should end just cephalad to the angle of the mandible *(broken line),* resulting in proper alignment with the glottic opening *(B).* If the oral airway inserted is too large, the tip will align posterior to the angle of the mandible *(C)* and obstruct the glottic opening by pushing the epiglottis down *(arrow).* If the oral airway inserted is too small, the tip will align well above the angle of the mandible *(D)* and exacerbate airway obstruction by pushing the tongue into the oropharynx *(D, arrows).* (Adapted, with permission, from Cote and Todres in *Textbook of Pediatric Life Support.* © 1997, American Heart Association.)

lution. Give 20 mL/kg body weight, repeated as necessary, with frequent reassessments, until perfusion normalizes. Children tolerate large volumes of fluid replacement–up to and over the full circulating blood volume of 80 mL/kg can be given safely with appropriate monitoring. Blood product replacement may be necessary in trauma patients not responding to two boluses of crystalloid solution. Pressors are not required in simple hypovolemic states.

B. Distributive Shock: Distributive shock represents relative hypovolemia from increased vascular capacitance of circulating volume. Examples are sepsis, anaphylaxis, and spinal cord injury. Initial therapy is again by isotonic volume replacement, but pressors may be necessary if perfusion does not normalize after delivery of two 20 mL/kg boluses of fluid.

Children in distributive shock must be admitted to a pediatric intensive care unit.

C. Cardiogenic Shock: Cardiogenic shock can occur as a complication of congenital heart disease, myocarditis, arrhythmias, ingestions (eg, clonidine, tricyclic antidepressants), or as a sequela of prolonged shock due to any cause. The diagnosis is suggested by any of the following signs: abnormal cardiac rhythm, distended neck veins, rales, abnormal heart sounds such as an S_3 or S_4, friction rub, narrow pulse pressure, or hepatomegaly. Chest radiographs will show cardiomegaly and pulmonary edema—not seen in shock due to other causes. An initial bolus of crystalloid may be given, but dopamine or other pressors, and possibly agents to reduce afterload, are necessary to improve perfusion. Invasive cardiopulmonary monitoring is essential.

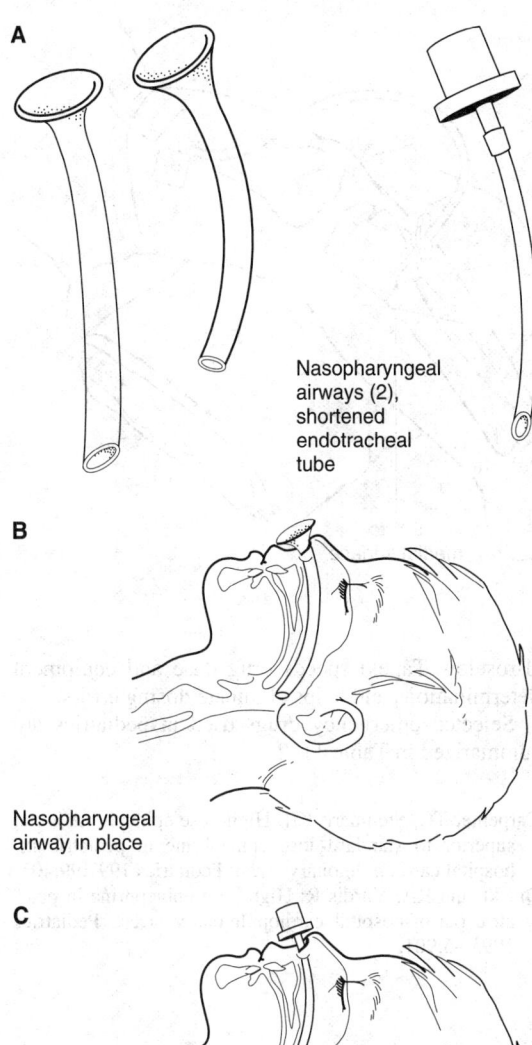

Figure 11–5. **A:** Nasopharyngeaal airway. A shortened endotracheal tube may be substituted (to reduce resistance). **B:** Placement of a nasopharyngeal airway. Note that the standard 15-mm adapter must be firmly reinserted into the endotracheal tube. **C:** Cut-off endotracheal tube used as a nasopharyngeal airway. (Reproduced, with permission, from *Textbook of Pediatric Life Support.* © 1997, American Heart Association.)

Children in cardiogenic shock must be admitted to a pediatric intensive care unit.

Observation & Further Management

Reassess perfusion immediately after each bolus of fluid to determine additional fluid needs. Serial central venous pressure determinations or a chest radiograph may aid clinical assessments to help determine volume status. Place a Foley catheter to monitor urine output.

Caution must be exercised with volume replacement if intracranial pressure is potentially elevated, such as in severe head injury, diabetic ketoacidosis, or meningitis. Even in such situations, however, intravascular volume must be restored, as reflected by adequate peripheral perfusion and mean arterial pressure, to achieve adequate cerebral perfusion pressure.

Summary of Cardiopulmonary Resuscitation

Assess the ABCs in sequential fashion, and begin interventions as soon as a derangement is detected—before assessing the next system. After each intervention, it is essential that each system be reassessed to ensure improvement and to avoid failing to recognize clinical deterioration.

Bell LM: Shock. In: *Textbook of Pediatric Emergency Medicine.* Fleisher GR, Ludwig S (editors). Williams & Wilkins, 1993.

Chameides L, Hazinski MF (editors): *Textbook of Pediatric*

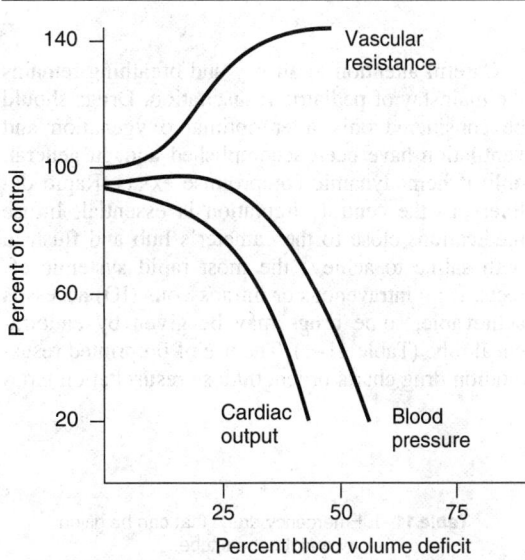

Figure 11–6. Model for cardiovascular response to hypovolemia from hemorrhage (based on normative data). (Reproduced, with permission, from *Textbook of Pediatric Life Support.* © 1997, American Heart Association.)

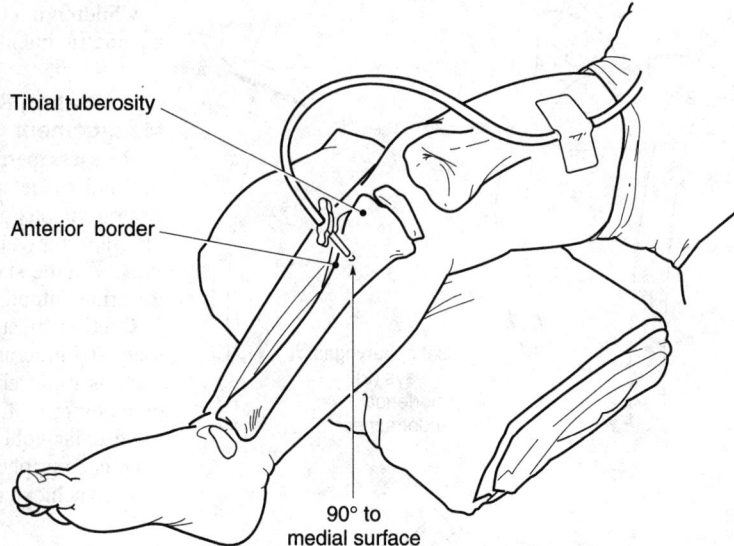

Figure 11–7. Intraosseous cannulation technique. (Reproduced, with permission, from *Textbook of Pediatric Life Support.* © 1997, American Heart Association.)

Labels in figure: Tibial tuberosity; Anterior border; 90° to medial surface

Advanced Life Support. American Heart Association/ American Academy of Pediatrics, 1997.

Silverman BK (editor): *Textbook of Advanced Pediatric Life Support.* APLS Joint Task Force: American College of Emergency Physicians/American Academy of Pediatrics, 1993.

EMERGENCY PEDIATRIC DRUGS

Careful attention to airway and breathing remains the mainstay of pediatric resuscitation. Drugs should be considered only after optimal oxygenation and ventilation have been accomplished and, in general, only if hemodynamic compromise exists. Rapid delivery to the central circulation is essential. Infuse medications close to the catheter's hub and flush in with saline to achieve the most rapid systemic effects. If no intravenous or intraosseous (IO) access is achievable, some drugs may be given by endotracheal tube (Table 11–1). The use of preprinted resuscitation drug charts or length/dose resuscitation tapes (Broselow Tapes) speeds drug dose and equipment determinations and helps eliminate dosing errors.

Selected emergency drugs used in pediatrics are summarized in Table 11–2.

Carpenter TC, Stenmark KR: High-dose epinephrine is not superior to standard-dose epinephrine in pediatric in-hospital cardiopulmonary arrest: Pediatrics 1997;99:403.

Dieckmann RA, Vardis R: High-dose epinephrine in pediatric out-of-hospital cardiopulmonary arrest. Pediatrics 1995;95:901.

APPROACH TO THE SERIOUSLY ILL CHILD

Often a child presents in cardiorespiratory failure of unknown cause. Occasionally, an unstable patient presents with a known diagnosis, such as a child known to have asthma in status asthmaticus and respiratory failure, or a child with known congenital heart disease. The initial approach is identical, however, and designed to rapidly identify and reverse life-threatening conditions.

Preparation for Emergency Management

Resuscitation of a severely ill child requires action simultaneously at two levels: rapid cardiopulmonary assessment, with indicated stabilizing measures, while venous access ("lifelines") is gained and moni-

Table 11–1. Emergency drugs that can be given by endotracheal tube.

Lidocaine
Epinephrine
Atropine
Naloxone

Table 11–2. Emergency pediatric drugs.

Drug	Indications	Dosage and Route[1]	Comment
Atropine	1. Bradycardia, especially cardiac in origin 2. Vagally mediated brady-cardia, eg, during laryn-goscopy and intubation 3. Anticholinesterase poisoning	0.01–0.02 mg/kg (minimum, 0.1 mg; maximum, 1–2 mg) IV, IO, ET. May repeat every 5 minutes.	Atropine may be useful in hemodynami-cally significant primary cardiac-based bradycardias. Because of paradoxic bradycardia sometimes seen in infants, a minimum dose of 0.1 mg is recom-mended by the American Heart Associ-ation. Epinephrine is the first-line drug in pediatrics for bradycardia caused by hypoxia or ischemia.
Bicarbonate	1. Documented metabolic acidosis 2. Hyperkalemia	1 meq/kg IV or IO; by arterial blood gas: 0.3 × kg × base deficit. May repeat every 5 minutes.	Infuse slowly. Sodium bicarbonate will be effective only if the patient is ade-quately oxygenated, ventilated, and per-fused. Some adverse side effects.
Calcium chloride 10%	1. Documented hypocalcemia 2. Calcium channel blocker overdose 3. Hyperkalemia, hypermagnesemia	10–30 mg/kg slowly IV, preferably centrally, or IO with caution.	Calcium is no longer indicated for asys-tole. Potent tissue necrosis results if in-filtration occurs. Use with caution.
Epinephrine	1. Bradycardia, especially hypoxic-ischemic 2. Hypotension (by infusion) 3. Asystole 4. Fine ventricular fibrillation refractory to initial defibrilla-tion 5. Pulseless electrical activity 6. Anaphylaxis	Bradycardia and first dose in arrests: 0.01 mg/kg of 1:10,000 solution IV or IO. Second and subsequent doses in arrests: 0.1–0.2 mg/kg of 1:1000 solution IV or IO. Repeat every 3 minutes. ET: 0.1 mg/kg of 1:1000 solution. SC: 0.01 mg/kg of 1:1000 solution (= 0.01 mL/kg) (anaphylactic shock). Max-imum dose: 0.3–0.5 mL. Constant infusion by IV drip: 0.1–1 µg/kg	Epinephrine is the single most impor-tant drug in pediatric resuscitation. Evi-dence from animal studies and small series of human subjects indicates that the present recommended dose may be insufficient and that doses of 0.1–0.3 mg/kg may be optimal. A random-ized controlled trial has not been done.
Glucose	1. Hypoglycemia 2. Altered mental status (em-pirical) 3. With insulin, for hyperkale-mia	0.5–1 g/kg IV or, IO. May repeat as necessary.	Neonates: 1 mL/kg $D_{10}W$. Older children: 2–4 mL/kg $D_{25}W$, 6–10 mL/kg $D_{10}W$.
Naloxone	1. Opioid overdose 2. Altered mental status (em-pirical)	0.1 mg/kg IV, IO, or ET; maximum dose, 1 mg. May repeat as necessary.	Side effects are few. A dose of 2 mg may be given in young children, Repeat as necessary, or give as constant infusion in opioid overdoses.

[1]ET = endotracheally, IO = intraosseously, IV = intravenously, SC = subcutaneously.

tored. The technique of accomplishing these concur-rent goals is outlined below.

A. If advance notice of the patient's arrival has been received from prehospital providers or via tele-phone, prepare a resuscitation room and summon ap-propriate personnel as needed, such as a neurosur-geon for an unresponsive child after severe head injury or a radiology technician for assessment of line and tube placement.

B. Assign team responsibilities, including a team leader plus others designated to manage the airway, perform chest compressions, achieve access, draw blood for laboratory studies, place monitors, gather additional historical data, and provide family sup-port.

C. Age-appropriate equipment should be made ready, including a cardiorespiratory monitor, pulse oximeter, and appropriate blood pressure cuff. Age- and weight-appropriate laryngoscope blades, endo-tracheal tubes, nasogastric tubes, and indwelling uri-nary catheter should be assembled for rapid access. See Table 11–3 for sizes.

Reception & Assessment

When the patient arrives, the team leader begins a rapid assessment as team members perform their preas-

Table 11–3. Equipment sizes and estimated weight by age.

Age (years)	Weight (kg)	Endotracheal Tube Size (mm)[1]	Laryngoscope Blade (Size)	Chest Tube (Fr)	Foley (Fr)
Premature	1–2.5	2.5 uncuffed	0	8	5
Term newborn	3	3.0	0–1	10	8
1	10	3.5–4.0	1	18	8
2	12	4.5	1	18	10
3	14	4.5	1	20	10
4	16	5.0	2	22	10
5	18	5.0–5.5	2	24	10
6	20	5.5	2	26	12
7	22	5.5–6.0	2	26	12
8	24	6.0 cuffed	2	28	14
10	32	6.0–6.5 cuffed	2–3	30	14
Adolescent	50	7.0 cuffed	3	36	14
Adult	70	8.0 cuffed	3	40	14

[1]Internal diameter.

signed tasks. If the patient is received from prehospital care providers, careful attention must be paid to their report, since they have information that they alone have observed. Interventions and medications should be ordered only by the team leader to avoid confusion, and the leader should refrain from personally performing distracting procedures. A complete record (with times) should be kept of events, including medications, interventions, and response to intervention.

A. All Cases: In addition to cardiac compressions and ventilation, ensure that the following are instituted.

(1) 100% high-flow oxygen.
(2) Cardiorespiratory monitoring.
(3) Pulse oximetry and end-tidal CO_2 monitor, if available.
(4) Intravenous (peripheral, intraosseous, or central) access within 90 seconds. Two lines preferred.
(5) Blood drawn and sent.
(6) Full vital signs obtained.
(7) Clothes removed.
(8) Foley catheter and nasogastric tube inserted.
(9) Complete history.
(10) Notify needed consultants.
(11) Family support.

B. As Appropriate:
(1) Immobilize neck.
(2) Have chest x-ray taken for line and tube placement.
(3) Insert CVP and arterial line.

APPROACH TO THE PEDIATRIC TRAUMA PATIENT

Injuries, including motor vehicle crashes, falls, burns, and immersions, account for the greatest number of deaths among children over 1 year of age. Pediatricians must be cognizant of this sobering statistic, become involved, and work with injury prevention specialists, prehospital providers, and emergency, critical care, and rehabilitation physicians and nurses to reduce this terrible loss.

A team approach to the severely injured child, using preassigned roles as above, will optimize outcomes. Accurate, timed records are invaluable. A calm atmosphere in the receiving unit will contribute to thoughtful care. Compiling a problem list helps determine priorities in timing of definitive care. Assignment of a pediatric trauma score assists in triage decisions and prognosis. Conscious children are terribly frightened by serious injury; constant reassurance can help alleviate anxiety. Analgesia and sedation can and should be given to appropriately stable patients. Parents often feel angry and guilty and require ongoing support from the services of social workers or Child Life workers (therapists knowledgeable about child development) whenever possible.

The past decade has seen the emergence of designated pediatric trauma centers, where dedicated teams of pediatric specialists in trauma surgery, orthopedics, neurosurgery, critical care, and emergency pediatrics combine to provide optimal multidisciplinary care. Because most children with severe injuries are not seen in these centers, however, pediatricians and others must be able to provide initial assessment and stabilization of the child with life-threatening injuries before transport to a verified pediatric trauma center.

Mechanism of Injury

The mechanism of injury dictates the evaluation. One should document the time of occurrence, the type of energy transfer to the child (eg, hit by a car, rapid deceleration), secondary injury at impact if the child was thrown by the initial impact, appearance of the child at the scene according to bystanders, interventions performed, and clinical condition during transport. The report of emergency service personnel is invaluable. All information of this type must be forwarded with the patient to the referral facility.

Trauma in children is predominantly blunt, though penetrating trauma does occur. Head and abdominal injuries are particularly important in the pediatric age group.

Initial Assessment & Management

Children die from injuries during three distinct time periods: at the scene, usually from irreparable central nervous system injury, disruption of major vessels, or airway compromise; within minutes to hours after the injury, usually from intracranial hemorrhage, hemopneumothorax, liver or spleen injury, or bleeding from multiple sites; and much later, usually in intensive care units, from multiorgan failure. It is this middle group that can benefit most from expeditious management—hence the term "golden hour" of trauma. Most (98%) children who reach a hospital survive until discharge, and most deaths from trauma in children are due to head injuries. Therefore, cerebral resuscitation must be the foremost consideration when treating seriously injured children. The ultimate measure of outcome is the child's eventual level of functioning.

There is a method for evaluating injured patients in a systematic way that provides a rapid assessment and stabilization phase, followed by a head-to-toe examination and definitive care phase. These are called the primary and secondary surveys, respectively.

PRIMARY SURVEY

The primary survey is designed to identify rapidly and treat immediately all physiologic derangements resulting from trauma. It is the resuscitation phase. Priorities are still airway, breathing, and circulation, but with important further considerations in the trauma setting:

Airway, with cervical spine control
Breathing
Circulation, with hemorrhage control
Disability (neurologic deficit)
Exposure (undress the patient completely and examine)

Evaluation and treatment of the ABCs are as discussed previously. Modifications in the trauma setting will be added here.

Airway

Failure to manage the airway appropriately is the most common cause of preventable death. Administer 100% high-flow oxygen to all patients. During assessment and management of the airway, one should provide cervical spine protection, initially by manual in-line immobilization (not traction). A hard cervical spine collar is then applied, and the head is taped to a backboard, surrounded by some means of cushioning (eg, rolled blankets) to further immobilize the head and allow log-rolling of the child in case of vomiting. The body must also be secured to the backboard.

Assess the airway for patency as before. Head positioning must avoid flexion or extension of the neck—eg, use jaw thrust rather than chin lift. Suction the mouth and pharynx free of blood, foreign material, or secretions, and remove loose teeth. Insert a nasopharyngeal or oropharyngeal airway if upper airway noises are heard or obstruction from posterior prolapse of the tongue occurs. A child with a depressed level of consciousness or a need for prolonged ventilation, hyperventilation, or operative intervention requires endotracheal intubation after bag-mask preoxygenation. Orotracheal intubation is the route of choice and is possible without cervical spine manipulation. Nasotracheal intubation may be possible in the children 12 years or older with spontaneous respirations—if not contraindicated by midfacial injury with the possibility of cribriform plate disruption. Rarely, if tracheal intubation cannot be accomplished—particularly in the setting of massive midfacial trauma—cricothyroidotomy may be necessary. Needle cricothyroidotomy using a large-bore catheter through the cricothyroid membrane is the procedure of choice in the younger patient (less than 12 years). Operative revision will be needed for formal controlled tracheostomy.

Breathing

Most ventilatory problems are adequately resolved by the airway maneuvers previously described and by positive-pressure ventilation. Breathing assessment is as described previously: One should assess for an adequate rate and for symmetric chest rise, increased work of breathing, color, tracheal deviation, crepitus, flail segments, deformity, or penetrating wounds. Sources of traumatic pulmonary compromise include pneumothorax, hemothorax, pulmonary contusion, flail chest, and central nervous system depression. Asymmetric breath sounds, particularly if tracheal deviation, cyanosis, or bradycardia is present, suggests pneumothorax, probably under tension. To evacuate the pneumothorax, insert a large-bore catheter-over-needle attached to a syringe over the fourth rib in the anterior axillary line into the pleural cavity and withdraw air. If a pneumothorax or hemothorax was present, place a chest tube to water seal. Insertion should be over the rib to avoid the neurovascular bundle. Open pneumothoraces can be treated temporarily by taping petrolatum-impregnated gauze on three sides over the wound, creating a flap valve. After airway and breathing have been stabilized, hemodynamic status may be addressed.

Circulation

Ongoing hemorrhage, external or internal, gives pediatric trauma some of its unique anxiety-provoking character. During the assessment of circulation, intravenous access should be achieved, preferably at two sites. If peripheral access is not readily available, a central line, cutdown, or intraosseous line should be established. A cardiorespiratory monitor should be applied early in the resuscitation. Peripheral perfusion and blood pressure should be should be recorded at frequent intervals. Determine hematocrit, blood type and cross-match, liver function tests, and serum amylase.

External hemorrhage can be controlled by direct pressure. To avoid damage to adjoining nerves and vessels, avoid placing hemostats on vessels, except in the scalp.

Determination of the site of internal hemorrhage can be challenging. Sites include the chest, abdomen, retroperitoneum, pelvis, and thighs. Bleeding into the intracranial vault rarely causes shock in children except in infants. The aid of an experienced pediatric trauma surgeon and radiologic studies—principally double-contrast computed tomography (CT) and ultrasound—help to locate the site of internal bleeding.

Suspect cardiac tamponade after penetrating or blunt injury to the chest if shock, narrowed pulse pressure, distended neck veins, hepatomegaly, or muffled heart sounds are present. Treat with rapid volume infusion and pericardiocentesis.

Treat signs of poor perfusion vigorously: A tachycardic child with a capillary refill time of 3 seconds is in shock and sustaining vital organ insults. Remember that hypotension is a late finding. Volume replacement is initially accomplished by rapid infusion of isotonic crystalloid at 20 mL/kg of body weight, followed by 10 mL/kg of packed red blood cells if perfusion does not normalize after two crystalloid bolus infusions.

Reassessment should be done rapidly following each bolus. If clinical signs of perfusion have not normalized, repeat the bolus. Lack of response or later signs of hypovolemia suggest the need for blood transfusion and possible surgical exploration. Blood loss at the scene and ongoing losses should be replaced on a 3:1 basis with crystalloid solution.

A common problem is the brain-injured child who is at risk for cerebral edema and intracranial hypertension and who is also hypovolemic. In such cases, circulating volume must be restored to ensure adequate cerebral perfusion; therefore, fluid replacement is required until perfusion normalizes and fluid restriction may be instituted thereafter.

Disability

A brief neurologic examination is performed to assess pupillary size and reaction to light and the level of consciousness. The level of consciousness can be reproducibly characterized by the AVPU system (Table 11–4). Pediatric Glasgow Coma Scale assessments should be done as part of the secondary survey (Table 11–5; see below). Changes in intracranial pressure or cerebral perfusion are eventually reflected in changes in these scales.

Exposure

Significant injuries can be missed unless the child is completely undressed and examined fully, front and back. Movement can be minimized by cutting away clothing as necessary. Because of their high ratio of surface area to body mass, infants and children cool rapidly. Because hypothermia compromises outcome except with isolated head injuries, it is necessary to continuously monitor the body temperature and use warming techniques as necessary.

Monitoring

Cardiopulmonary monitors with pulse oximetry and end-tidal CO_2 monitors should be put in place immediately. At the completion of the primary phase, additional "tubes" should be placed.

A. Nasogastric or Orogastric Tube: Children's stomachs should be assumed to be full at all times, and gastric distention from positive-pressure ventilation increases the chance of vomiting and aspiration.

B. Urinary Catheter: An indwelling urinary bladder catheter should be placed to monitor urine output. Contraindications are based on the risk of urethral transection; signs include blood at the mea-

Table 11–4. AVPU system for evaluation of level of consciousness.

A	Alert
V	Responsive to *Voice*
P	Responsive to *Pain*
U	*Un*responsive

Table 11–5. Glasgow Coma Scale.[1]

Eye opening response	
Spontaneous	4
To speech	3
To pain	2
None	1
Verbal response	
Oriented	5
Confused conversation	4
Inappropriate words	3
Incomprehensible sounds	2
None	1
Best upper limb motor response	
Obeys	6
Localizes	5
Withdraws	4
Flexion in response to pain	3
Extension in response to pain	2
None	1

[1]The appropriate number from each section is added to total between 3 and 15. A score <8 usually indicates CNS depression requiring positive pressure ventilation.

tus or in the scrotum or a displaced prostate detected on rectal examination. Urine should be tested for blood. Urine output should exceed 1 mL/kg/h.

SECONDARY SURVEY

After the resuscitation phase, a head-to-toe examination should be performed to reveal all injuries and determine priorities for definitive care.

Skin

Search for lacerations, hematomas, swelling, and abrasions. Remove foreign material, and cleanse as necessary. Cutaneous signs may indicate underlying pathology (eg, a flank hematoma overlying a renal contusion), though surface signs may be absent with significant internal injury. Skin changes may evolve. Make certain that the tetanus immunization status is current.

Head

Check for hemotympanum and for clear or bloody cerebrospinal fluid leak from the nares. Battle's sign and raccoon eyes are late signs of basilar skull fracture. Explore wounds, excluding foreign bodies and defects in galea or skull. Closed head injury is most commonly encountered. CT scan of the head is an integral part of evaluation for altered level of consciousness, seizure after trauma, or focal neurologic findings (see below).

Spine

Cervical spine injury must be ruled out in all children. The only exceptions to this rule are children with normal neurologic examinations who are able to deny neck pain or tenderness on palpation of the neck and who have no other painful injuries that might obscure the pain of a cervical spine injury.

Voluntary movement of the extremities must be observed. A cross-table neck radiograph is obtained initially, followed by anteroposterior and odontoid views. "Normal" studies do not exclude significant injury, which can be bony or ligamentous, or of the spinal cord itself. Therefore, an obtunded child should be maintained in cervical spine immobilization until the child has awakened and an appropriate neurologic examination can be performed. The entire thoracolumbar spine must be palpated and areas of pain or tenderness examined by radiography.

Chest

Pneumothoraces are detected and decompressed during the primary survey. Hemothoraces can occur with rib fractures and intercostal vessel injury, large pulmonary vessel injury, or pulmonary laceration. Tracheobronchial disruption is suggested by large continued air leak despite chest tube decompression. With large energy transfer, pulmonary contusion can occur, requiring ventilatory support. Myocardial contusions are unusual in children.

Abdomen

Blunt abdominal injury is very common in multisystem injuries. Significant injury can exist without cutaneous signs or instability of vital signs. Tenderness, guarding, distention, lack of bowel sounds, or hemodynamic instability mandates immediate evaluation by a pediatric trauma surgeon. Injury to solid viscera frequently can be managed nonoperatively in hemodynamically stable patients; however, in the absence of intestinal perforation or hypotension, operative treatment is indicated. Serial examinations, ultrasound, and CT scan—or, in unstable patients, diagnostic peritoneal lavage—provide diagnostic help. Elevated liver function tests have good specificity but only fair sensitivity for hepatic injury. Serum amylase will progressively rise with pancreatic injury, which may not be easily visualized by initial CT.

Pelvis

Pelvic fractures are classically manifested by pain, crepitus, and abnormal motion. Pelvic fracture is a relative contraindication to urethral catheter insertion. Perform a rectal examination, noting prostate position in boys, tone, and tenderness. Stool should be tested for blood. Orthopedic consultation is indicated if pelvic fracture is suspected.

Genitourinary System

If urethral transection is suspected (see above), perform a urethrogram before catheter placement. Diagnostic imaging of the child with hematuria is evolving, with CT scan becoming the modality of choice. Intravenous urograms are performed at some centers. Management of kidney injury is largely nonoperative except for renal pedicle injuries.

Extremities

Long bone fractures are common but rarely life-threatening. Test for pulses, perfusion, and sensation. Neurovascular compromise requires immediate orthopedic consultation. Careful palpation and serial examination will reveal orthopedic injuries requiring diagnostic imaging and treatment. Delayed diagnosis of fracture is not uncommon when children are comatose; reexamination is necessary to avoid missing previously missed fractures.

Central Nervous System

Because most deaths in children with multisystem trauma are from head injuries, neurointensive care is of primary importance in continued trauma management. Significant injuries include diffuse axonal injury, cerebral edema, subdural and epidural hematomas, parenchymal hemorrhages, and spinal cord injury. A full sensorimotor examination should be performed, noting pupillary size and extraocular movements. Deficits require immediate neurosurgical consultation. Extensor or flexor posturing represents intracranial hypertension (not seizure activity) until proved otherwise and should be treated with mild hyperventilation ($PaCO_2$ 35–38 mm Hg) adequate but not excessive volume resuscitation, and consideration of diuretics, usually mannitol. Normal peripheral perfusion must be assured before fluid restriction is started to optimize cerebral perfusion. Level of consciousness by the AVPU system or Glasgow Coma Scale (see Tables 11–4 and 11–5) should be serially assessed. Seizure activity warrants exclusion of significant intracranial injury. Acute spinal cord injury may benefit from high-dose methylprednisolone therapy. Corticosteroids are not indicated for head trauma.

American College of Surgeons, Committee on Trauma: *Textbook of Advanced Trauma Life Support.* American College of Surgeons, 1993.

Givens TG et al: Pediatric cervical spine injury: A three-year experience. J Trauma 1996;41:310.

HEAD INJURY

Closed head injuries range in severity from minor asymptomatic trauma without sequelae to intracranial hemorrhage leading to death. Head injury, including the shaken-baby syndrome, is common in cases of child abuse. Most deaths following multiple trauma are from head injury. Even following minor closed head injury, there can be neurologic sequelae, including subtle neuropsychiatric effects. Children may be classified clinically at the time of initial evaluation as

Table 11–6. Clinical classification of head-injured patients.[1]

Mild	No loss of consciousness or amnesia; alert and oriented. Asymptomatic or with only slight headache and dizziness.
Moderate	Possible findings: history of loss of consciousness, amnesia; posttraumatic seizures, vomiting, more than slight headache, listlessness, lethargy.
Severe	Possible findings: disoriented, unable to follow commands, decreasing level of consciousness, focal neurologic signs, penetrating skull injury or depressed skull fracture.

[1]Reproduced, with permission, from Rosenthal BW, Bergman I: Intracranial injury after moderate head trauma in children. J Pediatr 1989;115:346.

having mild, moderate, or severe head injury (Table 11–6).

Assessment

The considerations discussed above in the section on approach to the pediatric trauma patient apply here as well. The history should include the time and mechanism of injury. How far did the child fall and onto what surface? Was there loss of consciousness? Does the child remember events preceding, during, and following the injury? What have been the levels of consciousness and activity since the injury? Has there been vomiting, headache, ataxia, or visual disturbance?

The physical examination should be complete, including the spine, keeping in mind the mechanism of injury, and should include a detailed neurologic examination. Look for associated injuries such as mandibular fracture, scalp or skull injury, or cervical spine injury. Cerebrospinal fluid leak from the ears or nose, or the two later-appearing signs of periorbital hematomas (raccoon eyes) and Battle's sign, imply basilar skull fracture. In children over 3 years of age, obtain vital signs and assess the level of consciousness by the AVPU system (Table 11–4) or Glasgow Coma Scale (Table 11–5), noting irritability or lethargy; pupillary equality, size, and reaction to light; funduscopic examination; reflexes; body posture; and rectal tone. Always consider child abuse—the injuries observed should be consistent with the history.

Radiographic studies may be indicated. Plain films are useful only in cases of penetrating head trauma or for assessing depressed skull fractures and ruling out foreign bodies. Major morbidity does not follow from skull fracture per se but rather from the associated intracranial injury. The presence of a skull fracture on plain films increases the likelihood of finding a serious intracranial injury demonstrated by CT scanning. CT scan should be performed in the child with a history of significant impact, with persistent vomiting, or with an abnormal or lateralizing neurologic examination, including an abnormal mental status that does not quickly return to normal.

CONCUSSION

A concussion injury is defined as a brief loss or alteration of consciousness followed by a return to normal. Brain tissue is not damaged, and there are no focal findings on detailed neurologic examination. There may be pallor, amnesia, or several episodes of vomiting. Disposition is based on the clinical course and suitability of follow-up. The patient may be discharged when neurologically normal after a period of observation. Parents should assess the child at home every 3–4 hours for the first 24–36 hours and return if the child exhibits altered level of consciousness, persistent vomiting, gait disturbances, unequal pupils, seizures, or increasing headache, or if the parents have any concerns.

CONTUSION

A bruise of the brain matter is a contusion. There is a decrease in level of consciousness, and focal findings are present that correspond to the area of the brain that is injured. These patients require CT scan, a period of observation, and consideration of neurosurgical consultation.

ACUTE INTRACRANIAL HYPERTENSION

Close observation will detect early signs and symptoms of intracranial pressure elevation. Early recognition is essential to avoid disastrous outcomes. Serious intracranial pathology after closed head injury includes subdural or epidural hematomas, parenchymal hemorrhage, diffuse axonal injury, and cerebral edema. In addition to traumatic causes, intracranial pressure elevation with or without herniation syndromes may be seen in spontaneous intracranial hemorrhage, central nervous system infection, hydrocephalus, ruptured arteriovenous malformation, metabolic derangement (eg, diabetic ketoacidosis), or tumor. Symptoms include headache, diplopia, vomiting, agitation, gait difficulties, and a progressively decreasing level of consciousness. Other signs may include stiff neck, cranial nerve palsies, and progressive hemiparesis. Cushing's triad (bradycardia, hypertension, and irregular respirations) is a late and prearrest finding. Papilledema is also a late finding. Lumbar puncture should not be performed before CT scan if there is concern about intracranial pressure elevation because of the risk of precipitating herniation.

Therapy for intracranial pressure elevation must be swift and aggressive. Strict attention to the ABCs is paramount. Controlled rapid-sequence intubation with appropriate sedation, muscle relaxation, and agents to reduce the intracranial pressure elevation that accompanies intubation is followed by mild hyperventilation ($Paco_2$ lowered to 35–38 mm Hg) and avoidance of hypoperfusion and hypoxemia. Mannitol (0.5 g/kg intravenously), an osmotic diuretic, will reduce brain water, as will furosemide (0.1–0.2 mg/kg intravenously). These measures effectively reduce cerebral blood flow and acutely lower intracranial pressure. Normal arterial blood pressure and peripheral perfusion should be maintained by fluid infusion and pressors, if necessary. Adjunctive measures include elevating the head of the bed 30 degrees, treating hyperpyrexia and pain, and maintaining the head in a midline position. Obtain immediate neurosurgical evaluation. Further details about management of intracranial hypertension (cerebral edema) are presented in Chapter 12.

DISPOSITION FOR CHILDREN WITH CLOSED HEAD INJURY

Patients with mild head injury as defined in Table 11–6 may be discharged with detailed written instructions—after a period of brief observation—if the examination remains normal and parental supervision and follow-up are appropriate. Some children with moderate head injury will require admission or prolonged observation. If the patient responds to voice commands and mental status is gradually improving over a period of several hours, in-hospital observation may be done without further radiographic studies. If the mental status deteriorates, however, CT scan and neurosurgical consultation are indicated. If the CT scan is normal and if the physical findings normalize, these children may also be discharged after a period of observation.

Patients with severe head injury require cerebral resuscitation, evaluation by a neurosurgeon, and admission to hospital.

Bracken MB et al: A randomized, controlled trial of methylprednisolone or naloxone in the treatment of acute spinal cord injury. N Engl J Med 1990;322:1405.

Gnauck K et al: Emergency intubation of the pediatric medical patient: Use of anesthetic agents in the emergency department. Ann Emerg Med 1994;23:1242.

Kharasch SJ et al: The routine use of radiography and arterial blood gases in the evaluation of blunt trauma in children. Ann Emerg Med 1994;23:212.

Marion DW, Bouma GJ: The use of stable xenon-enhanced computed tomographic studies of cerebral blood flow to defines changes in cerebral carbon dioxide vasoresponsivity caused by a severe head injury. Neurosurgery 1991;29:869.

McGrory BJ et al: Acute fractures and dislocations of the

cervical spine in children and adolescents. J Bone Joint Surg 1993;75[Am]:988.

Orenstein JB et al: Delayed diagnosis of pediatric cervical spine injury. Pediatrics 1992;89:1185.

Pigula FA et al: The effect of hypotension and hypoxia on children with severe head injuries. J Pediatr Surg 1993;28:310.

Pons P: Head trauma. In: Rosen P et al (editors). Emergency Medicine: Concepts and Clinical Practice, 3rd ed. CV Mosby, 1996.

Rosenthal BW, Bergman I: Intracranial injury after moderate head trauma in children. J Pediatr 1989;115:346.

BURNS

Thermal injury is a major cause of accidental death and disfigurement in children. Pain, morbidity, the association with child abuse, and the preventable nature of burns constitute an area of major concern in pediatrics. Common causes include hot water or food, appliances, flames, grills, vehicle-related burns, and curling irons. Burns occur commonly in toddlers—in boys more frequently than in girls.

Electrical Burns

Even brief contact with a high-voltage source will result in a contact burn. If an arc is created with passage of current through the body, the pattern of the thermal injury will depend on the path of the current; therefore, a thorough search should be made for an exit wound and internal injuries. Extensive damage to deep tissues may occur. Current traversing the heart may cause nonperfusing arrhythmias. Neurologic effects of electrical burns can be immediate (eg, confusion, disorientation, peripheral nerve injury), delayed (eg, nerve damage in the thrombosed limb after compartment syndrome), or late (eg, impaired concentration or memory).

Electric cords are a common source of these injuries. Typically, an infant or toddler bites an electric cord, sustaining burns to the commissure of the lips that appear gray and necrotic, with surrounding erythema. Delayed coagulation around the mouth may occur, and as the burn heals, sloughing of eschar may lead to brisk bleeding.

EVALUATION OF THE BURNED PATIENT

Classification

Burns are classified clinically according to the nature of the burn and the extent and thickness; associated injuries are ascertained in the initial evaluation.

Superficial burns are easily recognized and treated. They are painful, dry, red, and hypersensitive. Sunburn is a common example. Healing occurs with minimal damage to epidermis. At the other end of the spectrum are **full-thickness** burns affecting all epidermal and dermal elements, leaving avascular

skin. The wound is dry, depressed, leathery in appearance, and without sensation. Unless skin grafting is provided, the scar will be hard, uneven, and fibrotic. **Partial-thickness** burns are further classified as superficial or deep, depending on appearance and healing time, with each subgroup treated differently. Superficial partial-thickness burns are red and may blister. Deep partial-thickness burns are white and dry, blanch with pressure, and have decreased sensitivity to pain.

Management

Burn management depends on the depth and extent of thermal injury. Burn extent can be classified as major or minor. Minor burns are less than 10% of the body surface area for superficial and partial-thickness burns, or less than 2% for full-thickness burns. Burns of the hands, feet, face, eyes, ears, and perineum are considered major.

A. Superficial and Partial-Thickness Burns: These injuries can generally be treated in the outpatient setting. Superficial burns are treated with cool compresses and analgesia. Treatment of partial-thickness burns with blisters consists of aseptic debridement, antiseptic cleansing, and topical antimicrobial coverage. Blisters appear early in deeper partial-thickness burns and if open should be debrided. After debridement, the wound should be cleansed with dilute (1–5%) povidone-iodine solution, thoroughly washed with normal saline, and covered with topical antibiotic, commonly silver sulfadiazine. The wound should be protected with a bulky dressing and reexamined within 24 hours and serially thereafter, depending on the course. Wounds with a potential for causing loss of function or scarring—especially wounds of the hand or digits—should be promptly referred to a burn surgeon.

B. Full-Thickness and Deep or Extensive Partial-Thickness Burns: Major burns place particular importance on the ABCs of trauma management. Early establishment of an artificial airway is critical with oral or nasal burns because of their association with inhalation injuries and critical airway narrowing.

Burn Resuscitation Protocol	
• Secure the airway	• Establish IV access
• Administer 100% oxygen	• Restore intravascular
• Assist ventilation if necessary	volume
• Remove all clothing	• Perform complete
• Stop the burning process	examination
• Irrigate chemical burns	

The trauma resuscitation protocol outlined previously in Primary Survey should be followed. There may be inhalation injury from carbon monoxide, cyanide, or other toxic products if flames were present. A nasogastric tube and bladder catheter should be placed. The secondary survey should ascertain whether any other injuries are present, including those suggestive of abuse.

Fluid administration is based on several principles. Capillary permeability is markedly increased. Fluid needs are based on percentage of body surface area burned, depth, and age. Maintaining normal intravascular pressure and replacing fluid losses are essential. Figure 11–8 shows percentages of body surface area by body part in infants and children. The Parkland

Infant Less Than One Year of Age

Name_____ Age_____ Ward_____

1st-degree erythema not to be included.

2nd-degree   3rd-degree

Variations From Adults Distribution in Infants and Children (in Percent).

	New-born	1 Year	5 Years	10 Years
Head	19	17	13	11
Both thighs	11	13	16	17
Both lower legs	10	10	11	12
Neck	2			
Anterior trunk	13			
Posterior trunk	13			
Both upper arms	8			
Both lower arms	6	These percentages		
Both hands	5	remain constant at		
Both buttocks	6	all ages		
Both feet	7			
Genitalia	1			
	100			

Figure 11–8. Lund and Browder modification of Berkow's scale for estimating extent of burns. (The table under the illustration is after Berkow.)

formula for fluid therapy is 4 mL/kg per percent of body surface area burned for the first 24 hours, with half in the first 8 hours, in addition to maintenance rates. Acutely, however, fluid resuscitation should be based on clinical assessment of volume depletion as described above.

Indications for admission include major burns as defined above; uncertainty of follow-up; suspicion of abuse; presence of upper airway injury; explosion, inhalation, electrical, or chemical burns; burns associated with fractures; or the need for parenteral pain control. Children with chronic metabolic or connective tissue diseases and infants deserve hospitalization.

Deitch EA: The management of burns. N Engl J Med 1990;323:1249.
Joffe MD: Burns. In: Textbook of Pediatric Emergency Medicine, 3rd ed. Fleisher G, Ludwig S (editors). Williams & Wilkins, 1993.
Powell EC, Tanz RR: Comparison of childhood burns associated with use of microwave ovens and conventional stoves. Pediatrics 1993;91:344.

DISORDERS DUE TO HIGH ENVIRONMENTAL TEMPERATURE

Disorders due to heat range from mild cramps to life-threatening heat stroke. Heat cramps are characterized by brief, severe cramping (not rigidity) of skeletal or abdominal muscles following exertion. Core temperature is normal or only slightly elevated. Heat cramps may be associated with a relative sodium deficiency. Mild cases can be treated with oral salt-containing solutions; more severe cases require intravenous infusion of normal saline solution. Heat exhaustion is manifested by constitutional symptoms after exposure to heat and humidity. Patients continue to sweat, and core temperature is again normal or only slightly increased. Patients with heat exhaustion have varying proportions of salt and water depletion. Presenting symptoms and signs include weakness, fatigue, headache, disorientation, pallor, thirst, nausea and vomiting, and occasionally muscle cramps. Shock may be present. There should be no major central nervous system dysfunction. Treat with intravenous fluids, modified by measured electrolyte levels. Both heat cramps and heat exhaustion can be avoided with acclimatization and liberal water and salt intake during exercise.

Heat stroke represents failure of thermoregulation and is life-threatening. The diagnosis is based on a rectal temperature of over 40 °C with associated neurologic signs in a patient with an exposure history.

Lack of sweating is not a necessary criterion. Symptoms are similar to those of heat exhaustion, but central nervous system dysfunction is more prominent. Patients with heat stroke are often incoherent and combative. In more severe cases, vomiting, shivering, coma, seizures, nuchal rigidity, and posturing may be present. Patients can have high, low, or normal cardiac output. Cellular hypoxia, enzyme denaturation and inactivation, and disrupted cell membranes lead to global end-organ derangements: rhabdomyolysis, myocardial necrosis, electrolyte abnormalities, acute tubular necrosis and renal failure, hepatic degeneration, adult respiratory distress syndrome, and disseminated intravascular coagulation. Consider sepsis, malignant hyperthermia, and neuroleptic malignant syndrome in the differential diagnosis.

Heat Stroke Management

A. Immediately cool body with cool water mist, ice, fans, or other cooling device.

B. If comatose, protect the airway, giving 100% oxygen.

C. Administer intravenous fluids: Isotonic crystalloid for hypotension, 5% dextrose/50% normal saline for maintenance. Consider central venous pressure determination.

D. Cardiac monitor, continuous rectal temperatures, Foley catheter, nasogastric tube.

E. Obtain laboratory tests: Complete blood count, electrolytes, glucose, creatinine, prothrombin time and partial thromboplastin time, creatine kinase, liver function tests, arterial blood gases, urinalysis, and serum calcium, magnesium, and phosphate.

F. Admit to pediatric intensive care unit.

Thompson AE: Environmental emergencies. In: *Textbook of Pediatric Emergency Medicine,* 3rd ed. Fleisher GR, Ludwig S (editors). Williams & Wilkins, 1993.
Yarbrough B: Heat illness. In: *Emergency Medicine: Concepts and Clinical Practice,* 3rd ed. Rosen P et al (editors). Mosby, 1996.

HYPOTHERMIA

Hypothermia in children, defined as core temperature less than 35 °C, is frequently associated with cold water submersion accidents. Many other disorders cause incidental hypothermia, including sepsis, metabolic derangements, ingestions, central nervous system disorders, and endocrinopathies. Neonates, trauma victims, intoxicated patients, and the chronically disabled are particularly at risk. Diagnosis requires maintaining a high index of suspicion, particularly in temperate climates. Mortality rates are high and are related to the underlying disorder.

As core temperature falls, a variety of mechanisms begin to conserve and produce heat. Peripheral vasoconstriction allows optimal maintenance of core temperature. Heat production can be increased by a hypothalamic-mediated increase in muscle tone and metabolism. When shivering begins, heat production increases to two to four times basal levels.

Clinical Findings

Clinical manifestations of hypothermia depend on the severity of body temperature depression. Severe cases (< 28 °C) mimic death: Patients are pale or cyanotic, pupils may be fixed and dilated, muscles are rigid, and there may be no palpable pulses. Heart rates as low as 4–6/min may provide adequate perfusion, however, because of the lowered metabolic needs in severe hypothermia. If these findings are primarily a result of hypothermia and not postmortem changes, the fact of death cannot be ascertained until the patient has been rewarmed and remains unresponsive to resuscitative efforts. Children with a core temperature as low as 19 °C have survived neurologically intact.

Treatment

A. General Supportive Measures: Management of patients with hypothermia is complex but largely supportive. Core body temperature must be documented by continuously monitoring with a low-reading indwelling rectal thermometer. Patients must be handled gently, since the hypothermic myocardium is exquisitely sensitive and prone to arrhythmias. Ventricular fibrillation may occur spontaneously or as a result of minor handling or invasive procedures. If asystole or ventricular fibrillation is present on the cardiac monitor, perform chest compressions and use standard pediatric advanced life support techniques and medications. Spontaneous reversion to sinus rhythm at 28–30 °C may occur as rewarming proceeds.

B. Rewarming:

1. Passive rewarming, such as covering with blankets, is appropriate only for mild cases (> 33 °C).

2. Active rewarming is achieved by external or core rewarming techniques. External rewarming methods include warming lights, thermal mattresses or electric warming blankets, immersion in warm baths, and hot water bottles or warmed bags of intravenous solutions. One must be aware of the potential for core temperature "afterdrop" as warmed peripheral acidemic blood is distributed to the core circulation. Core rewarming techniques are optimal and include the delivery of warmed, humidified oxygen and the use of warmed (to 40 °C) fluids for intravenous replacement, peritoneal dialysis, bladder irrigation, and mediastinal lavage. Hemodialysis and ex-

Table 11–7. Management of hypothermia.

General measures
Administer warmed and humidified 100% oxygen.
Monitor core temperature, heart and respiratory rates, and blood pressure continuously.
Consider central venous pressure determination.

Laboratory studies
Complete blood count and platelets
Serum electrolytes, glucose, creatinine, amylase
Prothrombin time, partial thromboplastin time
Arterial blood gases
Consider toxicology screen

Treatment
Correct hypoxemia, hypercapnia, pH < 7.2, clotting abnormalities, and glucose and electrolyte disturbances.
Start rewarming techniques: passive, active (core and external), depending on degree of hypothermia.
Replace intravascular volume with warmed intravenous normal saline or lactated Ringer's injection at 42 °C.
Treat asystole and ventricular fibrillation per PALS protocols. Cardiac massage should be continued at least until core temperature reaches 30 °C, when defibrillation is more likely to be effective.

tracorporeal blood rewarming achieve controlled core rewarming, can stabilize volume and electrolyte disturbances, and are maximally effective (Table 11–7).

Gentilello LM et al: Continuous arteriovenous rewarming: Rapid reversal of hypothermia in critically ill patients. J Trauma 1992;32:316.

Thompson AE: Environmental emergencies. In: *Textbook of Pediatric Emergency Medicine,* 3rd ed. Fleisher GR, Ludwig S (editors). Williams & Wilkins,1993.

Weinberg AD: Hypothermia. Ann Emerg Med 1993;22:370.

SUBMERSION INJURIES

Drowning is the second most common cause of death by unintentional injury among children. Water hazards are ubiquitous and include lakes and streams, swimming pools, bathtubs, and even toilets, buckets, and washing machines. Risk factors include epilepsy, alcohol, intentional trauma, and *lack of supervision.* Males predominate in submersion deaths, as in most other accidental deaths. All pediatric care providers must make efforts to prevent these needless tragedies.

Submersion incidents are classified according to outcome: drownings are those with death occurring within 24 hours; survival for over 24 hours constitutes near-drowning. Major morbidity stems from central nervous system and pulmonary insult. Fresh water aspiration results in pulmonary surfactant disruption and membrane leak, with subsequent pulmonary edema. Salt-water aspiration creates an osmotic gradient for the influx of water into the lungs. However, the type of water aspirated ultimately has little clinical significance. Laryngospasm or breath-holding may lead to loss of consciousness and cardiovascular collapse before aspiration can occur ("dry drowning").

Anoxia from laryngospasm or aspiration leads to irreversible central nervous system damage after only 4–6 minutes. A child must fall through ice or directly into icy water to allow cerebral metabolism to be sufficiently slowed by hypothermia to provide some protection from anoxic damage.

Cardiovascular changes include myocardial depression and arrhythmias. Electrolyte alterations are generally slight. Unless hemolysis occurs, hemoglobin concentrations also change only slightly.

Assessment & Management

Depending on the duration of submersion and any protective hypothermia effects, children may appear clinically dead or completely normal. Observation over time assists with prognosis. The child who has been rewarmed to at least 33 °C and is still apneic and pulseless in the emergency department will probably not survive to discharge or will be left with severe neurologic deficits. Until a determination of brain death can be made, however, aggressive resuscitation should be continued.

One should keep in mind possible associated injuries, such as neck injury from diving into shallow water. Core temperature should be monitored continuously with a low-reading rectal thermometer.

For children who appear well initially, observation for 12–24 hours will detect late decompensation in gas exchange. An abnormal chest radiograph, abnormal arterial blood gases, or hypoxemia by pulse oximetry indicates the need for treatment with supplemental oxygen, cardiopulmonary monitoring, and frequent reassessment. Serially assess the degree of respiratory distress and mental status. Signs of pulmonary infection may appear many hours after the submersion event.

Patients who are in coma and who require mechanical ventilation have a high risk of anoxic encephalopathy. The value of therapy with hyperventilation, corticosteroids, intentional hypothermia, and barbiturates remains unproved.

Bratton SL et al: Serial neurologic examinations after near drowning and outcome. Arch Pediatr Adolesc Med 1994;148:167.

Quan L: Drowning issues in resuscitation. Ann Emerg Med 1993;22(Part 2):366.

Spack L et al: Failure of aggressive therapy to alter outcome in pediatric near-drowning. Pediatr Emerg Care 1997;13:98.

BITES: ANIMAL & HUMAN

Bites account for a large number of visits to the emergency department. Most fatalities are due to dog bites. However, the majority of infected bite wounds are from human and cat bites.

DOG BITES

Boys are bitten more frequently than girls, and the dog is known by the victim in most cases. Younger children have a higher incidence of head and neck wounds, whereas school-age children are bitten most often on the upper extremities.

Dog bites are treated in somewhat the same way as other wounds: high-pressure, high-volume irrigation with normal saline, scrubbing, debridement of any devitalized tissue and removal of foreign matter, and tetanus prophylaxis. The risk of rabies is low in developed countries, but rabies prophylaxis should be considered when appropriate. Wounds should be sutured only if necessary for cosmetic reasons. Prophylactic antibiotics have not been shown to decrease rates of infection in low-risk dog bite wounds not involving the hands or feet. If a bite involves a joint, periosteum, or neurovascular bundle, prompt orthopedic surgery consultation should be obtained.

Pathogens that infect dog bites include *Pasteurella multocida,* streptococci, staphylococci, and anaerobes. Infected dog bites can be treated with penicillin for *P multocida,* and broad-spectrum coverage can be provided by amoxicillin and clavulanic acid. Complications of dog bites include scarring, central nervous system infections, septic arthritis, osteomyelitis, endocarditis, and sepsis.

CAT BITES

Cat-inflicted wounds occur more frequently in girls, and their principal complication is infection. Wound management is similar to that for dog bites. Cat wounds should not be sutured except when absolutely necessary for cosmetic reasons. Cat bites create a puncture-wound inoculum, and prophylactic antibiotics (penicillin plus cephalexin, or amoxicillin and clavulanic acid) are recommended. *P multocida* is the most common pathogen.

HUMAN BITES

Most human bites occur during fights. *P multocida* is not a known pathogen in human bites—cultures most commonly grow streptococci, anaerobes, staphylococci, and *Eikenella corrodens.* Hand wounds and deep wounds should be treated with coverage against *E corrodens* and gram-positive pathogens by a penicillinase-resistant penicillin. Wound management is the same as for dog bites. Only severe lacerations involving the face should be sutured. Other wounds can be managed by delayed primary closure or healing by second intention.

A major complication of human bite wounds is infection of the metacarpophalangeal joints. Clenched-fist injuries from human bites should be evaluated by a hand surgeon. Operative debridement is followed in many cases by intravenous antibiotics.

Hodge D, Tecklenburg FW: Bites and Stings. In: *Textbook of Pediatric Emergency Medicine.* Fleisher GR, Ludwig S (editors). Williams & Wilkins, 1993.

Leung AKC et al: Human bites in children. Pediatr Emerg Care 1992;8:255.

II. POISONING

Richard C. Dart, MD, PhD,
& Barry H. Rumack, MD

Poisonings result from the complex interaction of the agent, the child, and the family environment. The peak incidence is at age 2 years. Most ingestions occur in children under 5 years of age as a result of insecure storage of drugs, household chemicals, etc. Twenty-five percent of children will have a second episode of ingestion within 1 year following the first one. Repeated poisonings may require intervention on the child's behalf. Accidental poisonings are unusual after age 5 years. "Poisonings" in older children and adolescents usually represent manipulative behavior, chemical or drug abuse, or genuine suicide attempts.

Litovitz TL et al: 1995 annual report of the American Association of Poison Control Centers' Toxic Exposure Surveillance System. Am J Emerg Med 1996;14:487.

PREVENTING CHILDHOOD POISONINGS

Each year, children are accidentally poisoned by medicines, polishes, insecticides, drain cleaners, bleaches, household chemicals, and garage products. It is the responsibility of adults to make sure that children are not exposed to potentially toxic substances.

Here are some suggestions for parents:

(1) Insist on packages with safety closures and learn how to use them properly.

(2) Keep household cleaning supplies, medicines, garage products, and insecticides out of the reach and sight of your child. Lock them up whenever possible.

(3) Never store food and cleaning products together. Store medicine and chemicals in original containers and never in food or beverage containers.

(4) Avoid taking medicine in your child's presence. Children love to imitate. Always call medicine by its proper name. Never suggest that medicine is "candy"—especially aspirin and children's vitamins.

(5) Read the label on all products and heed warnings and cautions. Never use medicine from an unlabeled or unreadable container. Never pour medicine in a darkened area where the label cannot be clearly seen.

(6) If you are interrupted while using a product, take it with you—it takes only a few seconds for your child to get into it.

(7) Know what your child can do physically. For example, if you have a crawling infant, keep household products stored above floor level, not beneath the kitchen sink.

(8) Keep the phone number of your doctor, poison center, hospital, police department, and emergency medical system (EMS) near the phone.

PHARMACOLOGIC PRINCIPLES OF TOXICOLOGY

In the evaluation of the poisoned patient, it is important to compare the anticipated pharmacologic or toxic effects with the clinical presentation of the patient. If the history is that the patient ingested phenobarbital 30 minutes ago but the clinical examination reveals dilated pupils, tachycardia, dry mouth, absent bowel sounds, and active hallucinations—clearly anticholinergic toxicity—diagnosis and therapy should proceed accordingly. Knowledge of the pharmacoki-

netics of the toxic agent helps the physician to plan a rational approach to definitive care after necessary life-supporting measures have been instituted.

LD50

Estimates of the LD50 (the amount per kilogram of body weight of a drug required to kill 50% of a group of experimental animals) or MLD are of little clinical value in humans. It is usually impossible to determine with accuracy the amount swallowed or absorbed, the metabolic status of the patient, or in which patients the response to the agent will be atypical. Furthermore, these values are often not valid in humans even if the history is accurate.

Half-Life ($t_{1/2}$)

The $t_{1/2}$ of an agent must be interpreted carefully. Most published $t_{1/2}$ values are for therapeutic dosages. The $t_{1/2}$ may increase as the quantity of the ingested substance increases for many common intoxicants such as barbiturates, salicylates, and phenytoin. One cannot rely on the published $t_{1/2}$ for salicylate (2 hours) to assume rapid elimination of the drug. In an acute salicylate overdose (150 mg/kg), the apparent $t_{1/2}$ is prolonged to 24–30 hours.

Volume of Distribution (V_d)

The volume of distribution (V_d) of a drug is determined by dividing the amount of drug absorbed by the blood level. With theophylline, for example, this is 0.46 L/kg body weight, or 32 L in an adult. Ethchlorvynol, a lipophilic drug, on the other hand, distributes well beyond total body water. Because the calculation produces a volume above body weight (300 L in an adult, five times the body weight in children), this figure is frequently referred to as an apparent volume of distribution, a designation shared by many drugs (Table 11–8).

Table 11–8. Some examples of pK_a and V_d.[1]

Drug	pK_a	Diuresis	Dialysis	Apparent V_d
Amobarbital	7.9	No	No	200–300% body weight
Amphetamine	9.8	No	Yes	60% body weight
Aspirin	3.5	Alkaline	Yes	15–40% body weight
Chlorpromazine	9.3	No	No	40–50 L/kg (2800–3500% body weight)
Codeine	8.2	No	No	5–10 L/kg (350–700% body weight)
Desipramine	10.2	No	No	30–40 L/kg (2100–2800% body weight)
Ethchlorvynol	8.7	No	No	5–10 L/kg (350–700% body weight)
Glutethimide	4.5	No	No	10–20 L/kg (700–1400% body weight)
Isoniazid	3.5	Alkaline	Yes	61% body weight
Methadone	8.3	No	No	5–10 L/kg (350–700% body weight)
Methicillin	2.8	No	Yes	60% body weight
Phenobarbital	7.4	Alkaline	Yes	75% body weight
Phenytoin	8.3	No	No	60–80% body weight
Tetracycline	7.7	No	No	200–300% body weight

[1]See Table 40–2 for additional V_d values.

The V_d can be useful in predicting which drugs will be removed by dialysis or exchange transfusion. When a drug is differentially concentrated in body lipids or is heavily tissue- or protein-bound and has a high volume of distribution, only a small proportion of the drug will be in the free form and thus accessible to diuresis, dialysis, or exchange transfusion. On the other hand, a drug that is water-soluble and has a low volume of distribution may cross the dialysis membrane well and also respond to diuresis. In general, methods of extracorporeal elimination are not effective for toxic agents with a V_d greater than 1 L/kg.

Metabolism & Excretion

The route of excretion or detoxification is important for planning treatment. Methanol, for example, is metabolized to the toxic product, formic acid. This metabolic step may be blocked by ethanol. Secobarbital, a short-acting barbiturate, is poorly excreted in the urine and has a larger V_d, making forced diuresis ineffective.

Blood Levels

Care of the poisoned patient should never be guided solely by laboratory measurements. Treatment should be directed first by the clinical signs and symptoms, followed by more specific therapy based on laboratory determinations. Clinical information may speed the identification of a poison by the laboratory pathologist.

GENERAL TREATMENT OF POISONING

The telephone is often the first contact in pediatric poisoning. Proper telephone management can reduce morbidity and prevent unwarranted or excessive treatment. The decision to refer the patient is based on the identity and dose of the ingested agent, the age of the child, the time of day, the reliability of the parent, and whether child neglect or endangerment is suspected.

Initial Telephone Contact

Basic information that should be written down at the first telephone contact includes the patient's name, age, weight, address and telephone number, the agent and amount of agent ingested, the patient's present condition, and the time elapsed since ingestion or other exposure.

Use the history to evaluate the urgency of the situation and decide whether immediate emergency transportation to a health facility is indicated. If immediate danger does not exist, the physician should obtain more details about the suspected toxic agent. It may be difficult to obtain an accurate history. Obtain names of drugs or ingredients, manufacturers, prescription numbers, names and phone numbers of prescribing physician and pharmacy, and so on. Find out whether the substance was shared among several children, whether it had been recently purchased, who had last used it, how full it was, and how much was spilled. If one is unsure of the significance of an exposure, consultation with a certified Poison Control Center is recommended.

FIRST AID FOR POISONING (Advice for Parents)

Always keep syrup of ipecac in your home. Determine whether activated charcoal for home use is available in your area, and store it with the ipecac if obtainable. The ipecac is used to induce vomiting; the activated charcoal is used to bind poisons. Use them only as instructed by your Poison Control Center or doctor.

Inhaled Poisons

If smoke, gas, or fumes have been inhaled, immediately drag or carry the victim to fresh air. Then call the Poison Control Center or your doctor. Do not enter an area where there are poisonous fumes that have caused loss of consciousness. Too often the rescuer becomes a victim as well.

Poisons on the Skin

If the poison has been spilled on the skin or clothing, remove the clothing and flood the involved parts with water. Wash with soapy water and rinse thoroughly. Then call the Poison Control Center or your doctor.

Swallowed Poisons

If the substance swallowed is a medicine, give nothing. Milk or water should be immediately administered to any patient who has ingested a strongly acid or alkaline agent. Do not give more than 15 mL/kg (250 mL maximum in a child weighing 16 kg or more). Do not induce vomiting in patients who are comatose, convulsing, or who have lost the gag reflex. If emesis is induced on the way to the hospital, syrup of ipecac should be administered as described in the section below on prevention of absorption. (See page 294.) *Caution:* Antidote labels on products may be incorrect. Do not give salt, vinegar, or lemon juice. Call before doing anything else.

Poisons in the Eye

Rinse out the eye with plain water before the patient arrives at the emergency room. Use plain tap water—do not try to neutralize acids or alkalies. Pour water into the eye from a drinking glass or pitcher for 15–20 minutes. Then transport the patient to the hospital.

Bring the Poison to the Hospital

Everything in the vicinity of the patient that may be a cause of poisoning should be brought along.

OBTAINING INFORMATION ABOUT POISONS

Up-to-date data on ingredients of commercial products and medications can usually be obtained from a certified regional poison center and through the POISINDEX Information System. It is important to have the actual container at hand if the manufacturer is called. In some cases, the experience of the company physician may be of value in management. *Caution:* Antidote information on labels of commercial products or in the Physician's Desk Reference may be incorrect or inappropriate.

FOLLOW-UP

In over 95% of cases of ingestion of potentially toxic substances by children, a trip to the hospital is not required. In these cases, it is important to call the parent at 1 and 4 hours after an ingestion. If the child has actually ingested an additional unknown agent and develops symptoms, a change in management may be needed, including transportation to the hospital. An additional call should be made 24 hours after the ingestion to begin the process of poison prevention.

PREVENTION OF POISONING

A major goal of pediatricians is to reduce the number of accidental ingestions in the high-risk age group under 5 years of age. A systematic poison education effort should be part of the routine care of every patient. Parents of very young children should be encouraged to search the house and identify all hazardous substances that should be removed from the home or locked up. Pediatric or medical office staff can help families with poison prevention by telephone by asking a few simple questions about storage of hazardous substances in the home. The following is a partial list of potentially poisonous substances that must be stored safely if there are small children in the home: drain-cleaning crystals or liquid, dishwasher soap and cleaning supplies, paints and paint thinners, garden spray and other insecticide materials, automobile products (antifreeze, windshield wiper fluid, gasoline), and all medications.

If there are problems that may increase the risk of poisoning, the parents should be seen in person or a public health nurse sent to the home.

The section above entitled Preventing Childhood Poisonings may be copied from this book and given to parents along with a bottle of syrup of ipecac at the 6-month checkup. Reinforcement should occur at the 1-year checkup to make certain that adequate poison-proofing measures have been instituted and maintained.

INITIAL EMERGENCY DEPARTMENT CONTACT

Make Certain the Patient Is Breathing

As in all emergencies, the principles of treatment are attention to airway, breathing, and circulation. These are sometimes overlooked under the stressful conditions of a pediatric poisoning.

Treat Shock

Initial therapy of the hypotensive patient should consist of laying the patient flat and administering isotonic solutions by vein. Vasopressors should be reserved for poisoned patients in shock who do not respond to these standard measures.

Treat Burns

Burns may occur following exposure to strong acid or strong alkaline agents or petroleum distillates. Burned areas should be decontaminated by flooding with sterile saline solution or water. A burn unit should be consulted if more than minimal burn damage has been sustained. Skin decontamination should be performed in a patient with cutaneous exposure. Emergency department personnel in contact with a patient who has been contaminated (with an organophosphate insecticide, for example) should themselves be decontaminated if their skin or clothing becomes contaminated.

Take a Pertinent History

The history should be taken from the parents and all individuals present at the scene. It may be crucial to determine all of the kinds of poisons in the home. These may include drugs used by family members, chemicals associated with the hobbies or occupations of family members, or the purity of the water supply. Unusual dietary or medication habits or other clues to the possible cause of poisoning should also be investigated.

Assess Coma, Hyperactivity, & Withdrawal

It is useful to determine the level of coma, the degree of hyperactivity, or the severity of withdrawal symptoms as a means of assessing the efficacy of treatment.

A. Determine the Level of Coma: Coma is graded on a scale of 0–4:

0	Asleep but can be aroused and can answer questions
1	Withdraws from painful stimuli; reflexes intact
2	Does not withdraw from painful stimuli; most reflexes intact; no respiratory or circulatory depression
3	Most or all reflexes absent; no depression of respiration or circulation
4	Reflexes absent; respiratory depression with cyanosis, circulatory failure, or shock

B. Determine the Degree of Hyperactivity:

1+	Restlessness, irritability, insomnia, tremor, hyperreflexia, sweating, mydriasis, flushing
2+	Confusion, hyperactivity, hypertension, tachypnea, tachycardia, extrasystoles, sweating, mydriasis, flushing, mild hyperpyrexia
3+	Delirium, mania, self-injury, marked hypertension, tachycardia, cardiac arrhythmias, hyperpyrexia
4+	The above symptoms and signs plus convulsions, coma, and circulatory collapse

C. Determine the Severity of Narcotic Withdrawal Symptoms: Score the following findings on a scale of 0–2:

Diarrhea	Hyperactive bowel sounds
Insomnia	Restlessness
Dilated pupils	Tachycardia
Lacrimation	Hypertension
Gooseflesh	Yawning
Muscle cramps	

A score of 1–5 represents mild, 6–10 moderate, and 11–15 severe withdrawal symptoms.

Seizures, which are unusual in narcotic withdrawal, indicate severe withdrawal problems.

DEFINITIVE THERAPY OF POISONING

Prevention of Absorption

A. Emesis: Induced vomiting is *contraindicated* in patients who are comatose, convulsing, have lost the gag reflex, or have ingested strong acids, strong bases, some hydrocarbons, or sharp objects. In the case of hydrocarbons, vomiting should be induced if more than 1 mL/kg has been ingested or if the substance contains heavy metals.

1. Ipecac method–Adult dose, 30 mL; pediatric dose, 15 mL. Give orally and repeat once in 20 minutes if necessary. The procedure is as follows:

a. Give ipecac orally.

b. Follow with up to 6 oz of water or whatever fluid the child will drink.

c. Keep the patient ambulatory.

d. After 20 minutes, repeat the dose once if vomiting has not occurred.

2. Other emetics–The only approved oral emetic agent is syrup of ipecac. Use of sodium chloride may lead to lethal hypernatremia. Apomorphine should not be used because its depressant effect outlasts the duration of reversal by naloxone. Other emetic agents, such as mustard and soap, are not as effective as syrup of ipecac and should be avoided.

B. Lavage: If the patient is or is becoming unconscious, is convulsing, or has lost the gag reflex, gastric lavage following endotracheal or nasotracheal intubation should be performed rather than induction of vomiting. Lavage is less effective than emesis if a small (8–16F) tube is utilized but not if the recommended 28–36F Ewald tube is used. The tube should be inserted orally, and lavage should be with warm saline solution in a small child to avoid hyponatremia or hypothermia. Save the initial aspirate for laboratory determination and lavage until the returns have been clear for 1 liter. Monitor the amount of fluid given. The amount instilled should approximate the amount removed.

Emesis and lavage recover an average of about 30% of the stomach contents. Although these procedures may be helpful in reducing the amount of material available for absorption, approximately 70% of an ingested dose will remain. Additional measures such as charcoal and cathartics should be instituted to prevent further absorption.

C. Charcoal: Thirty grams of charcoal should be made into a slurry with a minimum of 240 mL of diluent. Give 1–2 g/kg (maximum, 100 g) per dose. The charcoal may be in an aqueous slurry or mixed with a saline cathartic or sorbitol.

Repeating the dose of activated charcoal may be useful for those agents that undergo enterohepatic circulation or those that slow passage through the gastrointestinal tract. When multiple doses of activated charcoal are given, repeated doses of sorbitol or saline cathartics must not be given. Repeated doses of cathartics may cause electrolyte imbalances and fluid loss. Charcoal dosing is repeated every 266 hours until charcoal is passed per rectum.

The patient may regurgitate some of the charcoal, but 70% is usually retained. Charcoal has been shown to reduce the half-life of an agent even when it is given after the intravenous administration of phenobarbital or theophylline.

D. Catharsis: *Caution:* Despite their widespread use, cathartics have not been shown to improve outcome. The use of cathartics should therefore be limited to patients in whom they can be safely used. In particular, do not give cathartics containing magnesium or phosphate to patients in renal failure. Pneumonitis may occur following aspiration of oil-based cathartics.

Acceptable cathartics include magnesium sulfate or sodium sulfate (250 mg/kg/dose orally [maximum, 30 g]); magnesium citrate (4 mL/kg/dose [maximum, 300 mL]); and sorbitol (1–1.5 g/kg/dose, of a 35% solution, for children over 1 year of age [maximum, 50 g/dose]). Sorbitol should be administered in a health care facility so that fluid and electrolyte status can be monitored, especially in children.

E. Whole Gut Lavage: Whole bowel lavage utilizes an orally administered, nonabsorbable hypertonic solution such as CoLyte or GoLYTELY. The use of this procedure in poisoned patients remains controversial. Preliminary recommendations for use of whole bowel irrigation include poisoning with sustained-release preparations, mechanical movement of items through the bowel (eg, cocaine packets, iron tablets), and poisoning with substances poorly absorbed by charcoal (lithium, iron). Underlying bowel pathology and intestinal obstruction are relative contraindications to its use.

Bond GR et al: Influence of time until emesis on the efficacy of decontamination using acetaminophen as a marker in a pediatric population. Ann Emerg Med 1993;22:1403.

Kulig K et al: Management of acutely poisoned patients without gastric emptying. Ann Emerg Med 1985;14:562.

Phillips S, Gomez H, Brent J: Pediatric gastrointestinal decontamination in acute toxin ingestion. J Clin Pharmacol 1993;33:497.

Enhancement of Urinary Excretion

Urinary excretion of certain substances can be hastened by urinary alkalinization or dialysis. In the past, forced diuresis or forced alkaline diuresis was used. While these have been abandoned because of their high complication rates, it is important to make certain that the patient is not volume-depleted. Volume-depleted patients should receive a normal saline bolus of 10–20 mL/kg, followed by sufficient intravenous fluid administration to maintain urine output at 2–3 mL/kg/h.

A. Urinary Alkalinization:

1. Alkaline diuresis–Urinary alkalinization should be chosen on the basis of the substance's pK_a, so that ionized drug will be trapped in the tubular lumen and not reabsorbed (see Table 11–8). Thus, if the pK_a is less than 7.5, urinary alkalinization is appropriate; if it is over 8.0, this technique is not usually beneficial. The pK_a is sometimes included along with general drug information. Urinary alkalinization can usually be achieved with sodium bicarbonate. It is well to observe for potassium depletion, caused by the shift of potassium intracellularly. Follow serum K^+ and observe for electrocardiographic (ECG) evidence of hypokalemia. If complications such as renal failure or pulmonary edema are present, hemodialysis or hemoperfusion may be required.

B. Dialysis: Hemodialysis (or peritoneal dialysis if hemodialysis is unavailable) is useful in the poisonings listed below. Dialysis should be considered part of supportive care if the patient satisfies any of the following criteria:

1. Clinical criteria–

a. Stage 3 or 4 coma or hyperactivity that is caused by a dialyzable drug and cannot be treated by conservative means.

b. Hypotension threatening renal or hepatic function that cannot be corrected by adjusting circulating volume.

c. Marked hyperosmolality or severe acid-base or electrolyte disturbances not responding to therapy.

d. Marked hypothermia or hyperthermia not responding to therapy.

2. Immediate dialysis–Immediate dialysis should be considered in ethylene glycol and methanol poisoning only if acidosis is refractory and blood levels of ethanol of 100 mg/dL are consistently maintained .

3. Dialysis indicated on basis of condition of patient–In general, dialyze if patient is in coma deeper than level 3. Peritoneal dialysis or exchange transfusion may be more useful than hemodialysis in small children—as much for ease of achieving fluid and electrolyte homeostasis as for poison removal. Other drugs not listed here may be dialyzable. Information should be verified prior to institution of dialysis.

Alcohols	Bromides	Paraldehyde
Amphetamines	Calcium	Potassium
Anilines	Chloral hydrate	Quinidine
Antibiotics	Fluorides	Quinine
Barbiturates (long-	Iodides	Salicylates
acting)	Isoniazid	Strychnine
Boric acid	Meprobamate	Thiocyanates

4. Dialysis not indicated except for support–

Antidepressants (tricyclics and MAO inhibitors)	Heroin and other opioids
	Methaqualone
Antihistamines	Methyprylon
Barbiturates (short-acting)	Oxazepam
Chlordiazepoxide	Phenothiazines
Diazepam	Synthetic anticholinergics
Digitalis and related drugs	and belladonna compounds
Diphenoxylate with atropine	

Hemoperfusion

Perfusion of blood through charcoal- or resin-filled devices has theoretical advantages for some poisons, but is often difficult to arrange on an emergent basis. Contact your nephrology service to determine availability and expertise in this modality.

MANAGEMENT OF SPECIFIC COMMON POISONINGS

ACETAMINOPHEN (Paracetamol)

Overdosage of acetaminophen can cause severe hepatotoxicity. The incidence of hepatotoxicity in adults and adolescents has been reported to be ten times higher than in children under 5 years of age. In the latter group, less than 0.1% develop hepatotoxicity after acetaminophen overdose.

Acetaminophen is normally metabolized in the liver. A small percentage of the drug goes through a pathway leading to a toxic metabolite. Normally, this nucleophilic reactant is removed harmlessly by conjugation with glutathione. In overdosage, the supply of glutathione becomes exhausted, and the metabolite may bind covalently to components of liver cells to produce necrosis.

Treatment

Treatment is to supply a surrogate glutathione by giving acetylcysteine. In the United States, it may only be given orally. Consultation on difficult cases may be obtained from the Rocky Mountain Poison Center (800-525-6115). Blood levels should be obtained as soon as possible after 4 hours and plotted on Figure 11–9. Acetylcysteine is administered to patients whose acetaminophen levels plot in the toxic range on the nomogram (see Figure 11–9). Acetylcysteine is effective even when given more than 24 hours after ingestion.

The dose of acetylcysteine is 140 mg/kg orally, diluted to a 5% solution in sweet fruit juice or carbonated soft drink. The primary problems associated with administration are nausea and vomiting. After this loading dose, 70 mg/kg should be administered orally every 4 hours for 72 hours. Aspartate aminotransferase (AST), alanine aminotransferase (ALT), serum bilirubin, and plasma prothrombin time should be followed daily. Significant abnormalities of liver function may not develop until up to 72 hours after ingestion. Repeated miscalculated overdoses given by parents to treat fever are the major source of toxicity in children under age 10 years, and parents are often unaware of the significance of symptoms of toxicity, thus delaying its prompt recognition and therapy.

Rivera-Penera T et al: Outcome of acetaminophen overdose in pediatric patients and factors contributing to hepatotoxicity. J Pediatr 1997;130:300.
Smilkstein M et al: Efficacy of oral *N*-acetylcysteine in the treatment of acetaminophen overdose. N Engl J Med 1988;319:1557.
Webster PA et al: Acetaminophen toxicity in children: Diagnostic confirmation using a specific antigenic biomarker. J Clin Pharmacol 1996;36:397.

ALCOHOL, ETHYL (Ethanol)

Alcoholic beverages, tinctures, cosmetics, and rubbing alcohol are common sources of poisoning in children. Concomitant exposure to other depressant drugs increases the seriousness of the intoxication. (Blood levels cited below are for adults; comparable figures for children are not available. In most states, alcohol levels of 50–80 mg/dL are considered compatible with impaired faculties, and levels of 80–150 mg/dL are considered evidence of intoxication.)

Blood Alcohol Level	Effects
50–150 mg/dL	Incoordination, slow reaction time, blurred vision.
150–300 mg/dL	Visual impairment, staggering, and slurred speech. Marked hypoglycemia may be present.
300–500 mg/dL	Marked incoordination, stupor, hypoglycemia, and convulsions.
> 500 mg/dL	Coma and death, except in individuals who have developed tolerance.

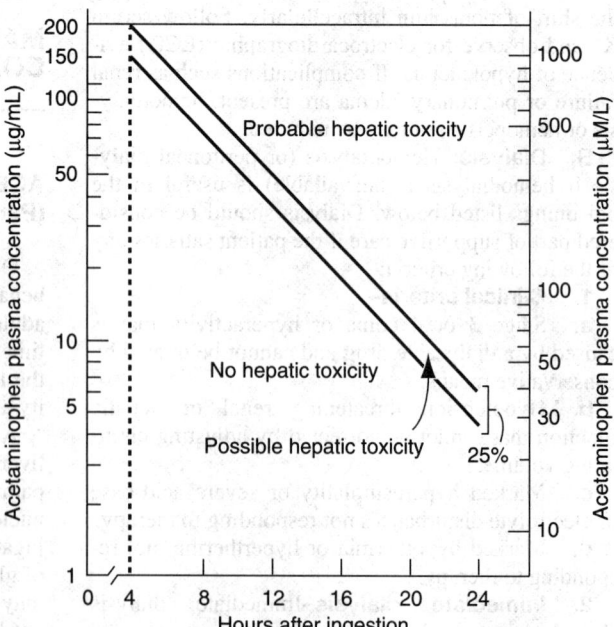

Figure 11–9. Semilogarithmic plot of plasma acetaminophen levels versus time. (Modified and reproduced, with permission, from Rumack BH, Matthew H: Acetaminophen poisoning and toxicity. Pediatrics 1975;55:871.)

Complete absorption of alcohol requires 30 minutes to 6 hours, depending upon the volume, the presence of food, the time spent in consuming the alcohol, etc. The rate of metabolic degradation is constant (about 20 mg/h in an adult). Less than 10% is excreted in the urine. Absolute ethanol, 1 mL/kg, results in a peak blood level of about 100 mg/dL in 1 hour after ingestion. Acute intoxication and chronic alcoholism increase the risk of subarachnoid hemorrhage.

Treatment

Management of hypoglycemia and acidosis is usually the only measure required. Start an intravenous drip of D_5W or $D_{10}W$ if blood glucose is under 60 mg/dL. Fructose has been suggested as an accelerator of metabolism, but it may cause vomiting, intensify lactic acidosis, and decrease blood volume via osmotic diuresis. Glucagon does not correct the hypoglycemia, because hepatic glycogen stores are reduced. Oxygen saturation should be measured and oxygen given in serious overdose because death is usually caused by respiratory failure. In severe cases, cerebral edema should be treated with dexamethasone, 0.1 mg/kg intravenously every 4–6 hours. Dialysis is indicated in life-threatening intoxication.

Leung AKC: Ethyl alcohol ingestions in children. Clin Pediatr (Phila) 1986;25:617.

Scherger DL et al: Ethyl alcohol (ethanol)-containing cologne, perfume, and aftershave ingestions in children. Am J Dis Child 1988;142:630.

AMPHETAMINES & RELATED DRUGS (Methamphetamine)

Clinical Presentation

A. Acute Poisoning: Amphetamine poisoning is common because of the widespread availability of "diet pills" and the use of "speed," "crank," "crystal," and "ice" by adolescents. (Care must be taken in the interpretation of slang terms because they have multiple meanings.) Symptoms include central nervous system stimulation, anxiety, hyperactivity, hyperpyrexia, hypertension, abdominal cramps, nausea and vomiting, and inability to void urine. Severe cases may include rhabdomyolysis. A toxic psychosis indistinguishable from paranoid schizophrenia may occur.

B. Chronic Poisoning: Chronic amphetamine users develop tolerance; more than 1500 mg of intravenous methamphetamine can be used daily. Hyperactivity, disorganization, and euphoria are followed by exhaustion, depression, and coma lasting 2–3 days. Heavy users, taking more than 100 mg/d, have restlessness, incoordination of thought, insomnia, nervousness, irritability, and visual hallucinations. Psychosis may be precipitated by the chronic administration of high doses. Depression, weakness, tremors, gastrointestinal complaints, and suicidal thoughts occur frequently.

Treatment

Standard decontamination procedures should be used: gastric emptying followed by charcoal in recent ingestions; activated charcoal alone if ingestion occurred hours earlier. The treatment of choice is diazepam. If this fails to reduce hyperactivity, chlorpromazine (0.5–1 mg/kg intravenously) may be given and repeated in 30 minutes. A maximum daily dose of 2.5–6 mg/kg may be used. Chlorpromazine may produce hypotension. In case of extreme agitation or hallucinations, droperidol (0.1 mg/kg/dose) or haloperidol (up to 0.1 mg/kg) parenterally has been used. When combinations of amphetamines and barbiturates (diet pills) are used, the action of the amphetamines begins first, followed by a depression caused by the barbiturates. In these cases, treatment with additional barbiturates is contraindicated because of the risk of respiratory failure.

Chronic users may be withdrawn rapidly from amphetamines. On the other hand, if amphetamine-barbiturate combination tablets have been used, the barbiturates must be withdrawn gradually to prevent withdrawal seizures. Psychiatric treatment should be provided.

Broscoe JG et al: Pemoline-induced choreoathetosis and rhabdomyolysis. Med Toxicol 1988;3:72.

Gary NE, Saidi P: Methamphetamine intoxication. Am J Med 1978;64:537.

Hong R, Matsuyama E, Nur K: Cardiomyopathy associated with the smoking of crystal methamphetamine. JAMA 1991;265:1152.

Jackson JG: The hazards of smokable methamphetamine. N Engl J Med 1989;321:907.

Stek AM et al: Maternal and fetal cardiovascular responses to methamphetamine in the pregnant sheep. Am J Obstet Gynecol 1993;169:888.

ANESTHETICS, LOCAL

Intoxication from local anesthetics may be associated with central nervous system stimulation, acidosis, delirium, ataxia, shock, convulsions, and death. Methemoglobinuria has been reported following local dental analgesia. The recommended dose for subcutaneous infiltration is 4.5 mg/kg. The temptation to exceed this dose in procedures lasting a long time is great and may result in inadvertent overdosage. Oral application of viscous lidocaine may produce toxicity. Hypercapnia may lower the seizure threshold to locally injected anesthetics.

Local anesthetics used in obstetrics cross the placental barrier and are not efficiently metabolized by the fetal liver. Mepivacaine, lidocaine, and bupivacaine can cause fetal bradycardia, neonatal depression, and death. Prilocaine causes methemoglobine-mia, which should be treated if levels in the blood exceed 40% or if the patient is symptomatic.

Accidental injection of mepivacaine into the head of the fetus during paracervical anesthesia has caused neonatal asphyxia, cyanosis, acidosis, bradycardia, convulsions, and death.

Treatment

If the anesthetic has been ingested, induced vomiting should be followed by activated charcoal. Mucous membranes should be carefully cleansed. Oxygen administration is indicated, with assisted ventilation if necessary. Methemoglobinemia is treated with methylene blue, 1%, 0.2 mL/kg (1–2 mg/kg/dose) intravenously over 5–10 minutes; this should promptly relieve the cyanosis. Acidosis may be treated with sodium bicarbonate, seizures with diazepam, bradycardia with atropine. Therapeutic levels of mepivacaine, lidocaine, and procaine are less than 5 μg/mL.

Amitai Y, Whitesell L, Lovejoy FH: Death following accidental lidocaine overdose in a child. N Engl J Med 1986;314:181.
Bozynski MEA, Rubarth LB, Patel JA: Lidocaine toxicity after maternal pudendal anesthesia in a term infant with fetal distress. Am J Perinatol 1987;4:164.

0.1–0.2 mg/kg intravenously, can be used to control seizures. Forced diuresis is not helpful. Exchange transfusion was reported to be effective in one case.

Cetaruk EW, Aaron CK: Hazards of nonprescription medications. Emerg Med Clin North Am 1994;12:483.
Rumack BH et al: Ornade and anticholinergic toxicity, hypertension, hallucinations and arrhythmia. Clin Toxicol 1974;7:573.
Tobin JR et al: Astemizole-induced cardiac conduction disturbances in a child. JAMA 1991;266:2737.

ARSENIC

Arsenic is commonly used in insecticides (fruit tree or tobacco sprays), rodenticides, weed killers, and wallpaper. It is well absorbed primarily through the gastrointestinal and respiratory tracts, but skin absorption may occur. Arsenic can be found in the urine, hair, and nails by laboratory testing.

Highly toxic soluble derivatives of this compound, such as sodium arsenite, are frequently found in liquid preparations and can cause death in as many as 65% of victims. The alkyl methanearsonates found in "persistent" or "preemergence"-type weed killers are relatively less soluble and less toxic. Poisonings with a liquid arsenical preparation that does not contain alkyl methanearsonate compounds should be consid-

nervous system depression, children often react paradoxically with excitement, hallucinations, delirium, ataxia, tremors, and convulsions followed by central nervous system depression, respiratory failure, or cardiovascular collapse. Anticholinergic effects such as dry mouth, fixed dilated pupils, flushed face, fever, and hallucinations may be prominent.

Antihistamines are widely available in allergy, sleep, cold, and antiemetic preparations, and many are supplied in sustained-release forms, which increases the likelihood of dangerous overdoses. They are absorbed rapidly and metabolized by the liver, lungs, and kidneys. A potentially toxic dose is 10–50 mg/kg of the most commonly used antihistamines, but toxic reactions have occurred at much lower doses.

Treatment

Activated charcoal should be used to reduce drug absorption. Emetics may be ineffective if the antihistamine is structurally related to phenothiazines. A cathartic is indicated for sustained-release preparations. Physostigmine, 0.5–2 mg slowly intravenously, dramatically reverses the central and peripheral anticholinergic effects of antihistamines, but it should be used only for diagnostic purposes. Diazepam,

Clinical Presentation

A. Acute Poisoning: Abdominal pain, vomiting, watery and bloody diarrhea, cardiovascular collapse, paresthesias, neck pain, and garlic odor on breath occur. Convulsions, coma, anuria, and exfoliative dermatitis are later signs. Inhalation may cause pulmonary edema. Death is the result of cardiovascular collapse.

B. Chronic Poisoning: Anorexia, generalized weakness, giddiness, colic, abdominal pain, polyneuritis, dermatitis, nail changes, alopecia, and anemia often develop.

Treatment

In acute poisoning, induce vomiting and administer activated charcoal. Then immediately give dimercaprol (BAL), 2.5 mg/kg intramuscularly, and follow with 2 mg/kg intramuscularly every 4 hours. The dimercaprol-arsenic complex is dialyzable. A second choice is succimer. The initial dose is 10 mg/kg every 8 hours for 5 days. A third choice is penicillamine, 100 mg/kg orally to a maximum of 1 g/d in four divided doses.

Chronic arsenic intoxication should be treated with succimer or penicillamine. Collect a 24-hour baseline urine specimen and then begin chelation. If the 24-hour urine arsenic level is greater than 50 mg, continue chelation for 5 days. After 10 days, repeat the 5-day cycle once or twice depending on how soon the urine arsenic level falls below 50 mg/24 h.

Cullen MN, Wolf LR, St Clair D: Pediatric arsenic ingestion. Am J Emerg Med 1995;13:432.

BARBITURATES

The toxic effects of barbiturates include confusion, poor coordination, coma, miotic or fixed dilated pupils, and respiratory depression. Respiratory acidosis is commonly associated with pulmonary atelectasis, and hypotension occurs frequently in severely poisoned patients. Ingestion of more than 6 mg/kg of long-acting or 3 mg/kg of short-acting barbiturates is usually toxic.

Treatment

If the patient is awake, vomiting should be induced and activated charcoal should be given. Careful, conservative management with emphasis on maintaining a clear airway, adequate ventilation, and control of hypotension is critical. Urinary alkalinization and the use of multiple-dose charcoal may decrease the elimination half-life of phenobarbital but have not been shown to alter the clinical course. Hemodialysis is not useful in the treatment of poisoning with short-acting barbiturates. Analeptics are contraindicated.

Amitai Y, Degani Y: Treatment of phenobarbital poisoning with multiple dose activated charcoal in an infant. J Emerg Med 1990;8:449.
Lindberg MC, Cunningham A, Lindberg NH: Acute phenobarbital intoxication. South Med J 1992;85:803.

BELLADONNA ALKALOIDS
(Atropine, Jimsonweed, Potato Leaves, Scopolamine, Stramonium)

The effects of anticholinergic compounds include dry mouth; thirst; decreased sweating with hot, dry, red skin; high fever; and tachycardia that may be preceded by bradycardia. The pupils are dilated, and vision is blurred. Speech and swallowing may be impaired. Hallucinations, delirium, and coma are common. Leukocytosis may occur, confusing the diagnosis.

Atropinism has been caused by normal doses of atropine or homatropine eye drops, especially in children with Down's syndrome. Many common plants and over-the-counter sleeping medications contain belladonna alkaloids.

Treatment

Emesis or lavage should be followed by activated charcoal and cathartics. Gastric emptying is slowed by anticholinergics, so that gastric decontamination may be useful even if delayed. Physostigmine, 0.5–2 mg slowly intravenously (can be repeated every 30 minutes as needed), dramatically reverses the central and peripheral signs of atropinism but should be used only as a diagnostic agent. Neostigmine is ineffective because it does not enter the central nervous system. High fever must be controlled. Catheterization may be needed if the patient cannot void.

Beech M, Hell C, Nightingale P: Central anticholinergic syndrome. Lancet 1987;1:1089.
Fitzgerald DA et al: Seizures associated with 1% cyclopentolate eyedrops. J Paediatr Child Health 1990;26:106.

CARBON MONOXIDE

The degree of toxicity correlates well with the carboxyhemoglobin level taken soon after acute exposure but not after oxygen has been given or when there has been some time since exposure. Onset of symptoms may be more rapid and more severe if the patient lives at a high altitude, has a high respiratory rate (ie, infants), is pregnant, or has myocardial insufficiency or lung disease. Normal blood may contain up to 5% carboxyhemoglobin.

The most prominent early symptom is headache. Proteinuria, glycosuria, elevated serum aminotransferase levels, or ECG changes may be present in the acute phase. Permanent cardiac, liver, renal, or central nervous system damage occasionally occurs. The outcome of severe poisoning may be complete recovery, vegetative state, or any degree of mental injury between these extremes. The primary mental deficits are neuropsychiatric.

Treatment

The biologic half-life of carbon monoxide on room air is approximately 200–300 minutes; on 100% oxygen, it is 60–90 minutes. Hyperbaric oxygen therapy at 2–2.5 atm of oxygen shortens the half-life to 30 minutes. After the level has been reduced to near zero, therapy is aimed at the nonspecific sequelae of anoxia. Dexamethasone, 0.1 mg/kg intravenously or intramuscularly every 4–6 hours, should be added if cerebral edema develops.

Thom SR et al: Delayed neuropsychologic sequelae after carbon monoxide poisoning: Prevention by treatment with hyperbaric oxygen. Ann Emerg Med 1995;25:474.
Roy B, Crawford R: Pitfalls in diagnosis and management of carbon monoxide poisoning. J Acad Emerg Med 1996;13:62.
Walker AR. Emergency department management of house fire burns and carbon monoxide poisoning in children. Curr Opin Pediatr 1996;8:239.

CAUSTICS

1. ACIDS
(Hydrochloric, Hydrofluoric, Nitric, & Sulfuric Acids; Sodium Bisulfate)

Strong acids are commonly found in metal and toilet bowl cleaners, batteries, and other products. Hydrofluoric acid is the most toxic and hydrochloric acid the least toxic of these household substances. However, even a few drops can be fatal if aspirated into the trachea.

Painful swallowing, mucous membrane burns, bloody emesis, abdominal pain, respiratory distress due to edema of the epiglottis, thirst, shock, and renal failure can occur. Coma and convulsions sometimes are seen terminally. Residual lesions include esophageal, gastric, and pyloric strictures as well as scars of the cornea, skin, and oropharynx.

Hydrofluoric acid is a particularly dangerous poison. Dermal exposure creates a penetrating burn that can progress for hours or days. Large dermal exposure or ingestion may produce life-threatening hypocalcemia as well as burn reactions.

Treatment

Emetics and lavage are contraindicated. Water or milk (< 15 mL/kg) are used to dilute the acid, because a heat-producing chemical reaction does not occur. Take care not to induce emesis by excessive fluid administration. Alkalies should not be used. Burned areas of the skin, mucous membranes, or eyes should be washed with copious amounts of warm water. Opioids for pain may be needed. An endotracheal tube may be required to alleviate laryngeal edema. Esophagoscopy should be performed if the patient has significant burns or difficulty in swallowing. Acids are likely to produce gastric burns or esophageal burns. Evidence is not conclusive, but corticosteroids have not proved to be of use.

Hydrofluoric acid burns on skin are treated with 10% calcium gluconate gel or calcium gluconate infusion. Severe exposure may require large doses of intravenous calcium. Therapy should be guided by calcium levels, the ECG, and clinical signs.

2. BASES
(Clinitest Tablets, Clorox, Drano, Liquid-Plumr, Purex, Sani-Clor)

Alkalies produce more severe injuries than acids. Some substances, such as Clinitest Tablets or Drano, are quite toxic, whereas the chlorinated bleaches (3–6% solutions of sodium hypochlorite) are usually not toxic. When sodium hypochlorite comes in contact with acid in the stomach, hypochlorous acid, which is very irritating to the mucous membranes and skin, is formed. Rapid inactivation of this substance prevents systemic toxicity. Chlorinated beaches, when mixed with a strong acid (toilet bowl cleaners) or ammonia, may produce irritating chlorine or chloramine gas.

Alkalies can burn the skin, mucous membranes, and eyes. Respiratory distress may be due to edema of the epiglottis, pulmonary edema resulting from inhalation of fumes, or pneumonia. Mediastinitis or other intercurrent infections or shock can occur. Perforation of the esophagus or stomach is rare.

Treatment

The skin and mucous membranes should be cleansed with copious amounts of water. A local anesthetic can be instilled in the eye if necessary to alleviate blepharospasm. The eye should be irrigated for at least 20–30 minutes. Ophthalmologic consultation should be obtained for all alkaline eye burns.

Ingestions should be treated with water as a diluent. Routine esophagoscopy is no longer indicated to rule out burns of the esophagus due to chlorinated bleaches unless an unusually large amount has been ingested or the patient is symptomatic. The absence of oral lesions does not rule out the possibility of laryngeal or esophageal burns following granular alkali ingestion. The use of corticosteroids is controversial but has not been shown to improve long-term outcome. Antibiotics may be needed if mediastinitis is likely, but they should not be used prophylactically. (See also Caustic Burns of the Esophagus in Chapter 19).

Gaudreault P et al: Predictability of esophageal injury from signs and symptoms: A study of caustic ingestion in 378 children. Pediatrics 1983;71:767.

Lovejoy FH Jr: Corrosive injury of the esophagus in children: Failure of corticosteroid treatment reemphasizes prevention. (Editorial.) N Engl J Med 1990;323:668.

Nuutinen M et al: Consequences of caustic ingestion in children. Acta Pediatr 1994;83:1200.

COCAINE

Most street cocaine is adulterated. Cocaine is absorbed intranasally or via inhalation or ingestion. Effects are noted almost immediately when the drug is taken intravenously or smoked. Peak effects are delayed for about an hour when the drug is taken orally or nasally. Cocaine prevents the reuptake of endogenous catecholamines, thereby causing an initial sympathetic discharge, followed by catechol depletion after chronic abuse.

Clinical Findings

A local anesthetic and vasoconstrictor, cocaine is also a potent stimulant to both the central nervous system and the cardiovascular system. The initial tachycardia, hyperpnea, hypertension, and stimulation of the central nervous system are often followed by coma, seizures, hypotension, and respiratory depression. In severe cases, various dysrhythmias may be seen, including sinus tachycardia, atrial arrhythmias, premature ventricular contractions, bigeminy, and ventricular fibrillation. If large doses are taken intravenously, cardiac failure, dysrhythmias, or hyperthermia may result in death.

Treatment

Testing for cocaine in blood or plasma is generally not clinically useful, but a qualitative analysis of the urine may aid in confirming the diagnosis. For severe cases, an ECG is indicated. When a teenager is suspected of being a "body packer," x-rays of the gastrointestinal tract are warranted. Cocaine is usually smoked or taken intranasally or intravenously; for this reason, decontamination is seldom possible. When cocaine is taken orally, lavage may be indicated, depending on the potential for seizures or loss of gag reflex. Activated charcoal may also be indicated. For body packers, whole bowel lavage may be useful in passing the packets quickly. Seizures may be treated with intravenous diazepam titrated to response or intravenous phenytoin (loading dose 10–15 mg/kg, maintenance 4–7 mg/kg/24 h). Hypotension may be treated with standard agents. However, because cocaine abuse may deplete norepinephrine, an indirect agent such as dopamine may be less effective than a direct agent such as norepinephrine. Agitation is best treated with diazepam.

Azuma SD, Chasnoff IJ: Outcome of children prenatally exposed to cocaine and other drugs: A path analysis of three-year data. Pediatr 1993;92:396.

Durand DJ, Espinoza AM, Nickerson BT: Association between prenatal cocaine exposure and sudden infant death syndrome. J Pediatr 1990;117:909.

Fitzmaurice LS et al: TAC use and absorption of cocaine in a pediatric emergency department. Ann Emerg Med 1990;19:515.

King TA et al: Neurologic manifestations of in utero cocaine exposure in near-term and term infants. Pediatrics 1995;96:259.

Mott SH, Packer RJ, Soldin SJ. Neurologic manifestations of cocaine exposure in childhood. Pediatr 1994;93:557.

CONTRACEPTIVE PILLS

The only known toxic effects following acute ingestion of oral contraceptive agents are nausea, vomiting, and vaginal bleeding in girls.

COSMETICS & RELATED PRODUCTS

The relative toxicities of commonly ingested products in this group are listed in Table 11–9.

Permanent wave neutralizers may contain bro-

Table 11–9. Relative toxicities of cosmetics and similar products.

High toxicity	Low toxicity
Permanent wave neutralizers	Perfume
	Hair removers
	Deodorants
Moderate toxicity	Bath salts
Fingernail polish	
Fingernail polish remover	**No toxicity**
Metallic hair dyes	Liquid makeup
Home permanent wave lotion	Vegetable hair dye
	Cleansing cream
Bath oil	Hair dressing
Shaving lotion	(nonalcoholic)
Hair tonic (alcoholic)	Hand lotion or cream
Cologne, toilet water	Lipstick

mates, peroxides, or perborates. Bromates have been removed from most products because they can cause nausea, vomiting, abdominal pain, shock, hemolysis, renal failure, and convulsions. Perborates can cause boric acid poisoning. Four grams of bromate salts is potentially lethal.

Poisoning is treated by induced emesis or gastric lavage with 1% sodium thiosulfate followed by demulcents to relieve gastric irritation. Sodium bicarbonate, 2%, in the lavage fluid may reduce hydrobromic acid formation. Sodium thiosulfate, 1%, 100–500 mL, can be given intravenously, but methylene blue should not be used to treat methemoglobinemia in this situation, because it increases the toxicity of bromates. Dialysis is indicated in renal failure but does not enhance excretion of bromate.

Fingernail polish removers used to contain toluene, but now usually have an acetone base, which does not require specific treatment other than monitoring central nervous system status.

Cobalt, copper, cadmium, iron, lead, nickel, silver, bismuth, and tin are sometimes found in metallic hair dyes. In large amounts, they can cause skin sensitization, urticaria, dermatitis, eye damage, vertigo, hypertension, asthma, methemoglobinemia, tremors, convulsions, and coma. Treatment for ingestions is to administer demulcents and, only with large amounts, the appropriate antidote for the heavy metal involved.

Home permanent wave lotions, hair straighteners, and hair removers usually contain thioglycolic acid salts, which cause alkaline irritation and perhaps central nervous system depression.

Shaving lotion, hair tonic, hair straighteners, cologne, and toilet water contain denatured alcohol, which can cause central nervous system depression and hypoglycemia.

Deodorants usually consist of an antibacterial agent in a cream base. Antiperspirants are aluminum salts, which frequently cause skin sensitization. Zirconium oxide can cause granulomas in the axilla with chronic use.

Fischer H, Caurdy-Bess L: Scalp burns from a permanent wave product. Clin Pediatr (Phila) 1990;29:53.

CYCLIC ANTIDEPRESSANTS

Cyclic antidepressants (eg, amitriptyline, imipramine) have a very low toxic:therapeutic ratio, and even a moderate overdose can have serious effects. Cyclic antidepressant overdosage causes dysrhythmias, coma, convulsions, hypertension (and, later, hypotension), and hallucinations. These may be life-threatening and require rapid intervention. One agent, amoxapine, differs in that it causes fewer cardiovascular complications, but it has a higher incidence of seizures.

Treatment

An ECG should be taken in all patients. If dysrhythmias are demonstrated, the patient should be admitted and monitored until free of irregularity for 24 hours. Another indication for monitoring is persistent tachycardia of more than 110 beats/min plus additional findings of anticholinergic toxicity. The onset of dysrhythmias is rare beyond 24 hours after ingestion.

Alkalinization with sodium bicarbonate, 0.5 meq/kg intravenously, or hyperventilation may dramatically reverse ventricular dysrhythmias and narrow the QRS interval. Phenytoin or lidocaine may be added for treatment of arrhythmias. Sodium bicarbonate should be administered to all patients with significant dysrhythmias to achieve a pH of 7.5–7.6. Forced diuresis is contraindicated. A QRS interval greater than 100 ms specifically identifies patients at risk to develop dysrhythmias. Diazepam should be given for convulsions.

Hypotension is a major problem. Cyclic antidepressants block the reuptake of catecholamines, thereby producing initial hypertension followed by hypotension. Treatment with physostigmine is not effective. Vasopressors are generally effective. Dopamine is the agent of choice because it is readily available. If dopamine is ineffective, norepinephrine (0.1–1 mg/kg/min, titrated to response) should be added. Diuresis and hemodialysis are not effective. Decontamination should include gastric lavage and administration of activated charcoal.

Ellison DW, Pentel PR: Clinical features and consequences of seizures due to cyclic antidepressant overdose. Am J Emerg Med 1989;7:5.

Lavoie RW, Gansert CG, Weiss RE: Value of initial ECG findings and plasma drug levels in cyclic antidepressant overdose. Ann Emerg Med 1990;19:696.

Liebelt EL, Francis PD, Woolf AD: ECG lead aVR versus QRS interval in predicting seizures and arrhythmias in acute tricyclic antidepressant toxicity. Ann Emerg Med 1995;26:195.

DIGITALIS & OTHER CARDIAC GLYCOSIDES

Clinical features include nausea, vomiting, diarrhea, headache, delirium, confusion, and, occasionally, coma. Cardiac irregularities such as atrial fibrillation, paroxysmal atrial tachycardia, and atrial flutter often occur. Death usually is the result of ventricular fibrillation. Transplacental intoxication by digitalis has been reported.

Treatment

If vomiting has not occurred, induce emesis or provide lavage followed by charcoal and cathartics. Potassium should not be given in acute overdosage unless there is laboratory evidence of hypokalemia. In acute overdosage, hyperkalemia is more common.

The patient must be monitored carefully for electrocardiographic changes. Every type of dysrhythmia has been reported in digitalis intoxication. The correction of acidosis better demonstrates the degree of potassium deficiency present. Bradycardias have been treated with atropine. Phenytoin, lidocaine, magnesium salts (not in renal failure), amiodarone, and bretylium have been used to correct arrhythmias.

Definitive treatment is with digoxin immune fab (ovine) (Digibind). Indications for its use include ventricular dysrhythmias and progressive bradydysrhythmia. Techniques of determining dosage are described in product literature.

Antman EM et al: Treatment of 150 cases of life-threatening digitalis intoxication with digoxin-specific Fab antibody fragments. Circulation 1990;81:1744.

Kaufman J et al: Use of digoxin Fab immune fragments in a seven-day-old infant. Pediatr Emerg Care 1990;6:118.

DIPHENOXYLATE WITH ATROPINE (Lomotil)

Lomotil contains diphenoxylate hydrochloride, a synthetic narcotic, and atropine sulfate. Small amounts are potentially lethal in children; it is contraindicated in children under age 2 years. Early signs of intoxication with this preparation are due to its anticholinergic effect and consist of fever, facial flushing, tachypnea, and lethargy. However, the miotic effect of the narcotic predominates. Later, hypothermia, increasing central nervous system depression, and loss of the facial flush occur. Seizures are probably secondary to hypoxia.

Treatment

Prolonged monitoring (24 hours) with pulse oximetry is sufficient in most cases. If respiratory depression occurs, an airway should be established with an endotracheal tube. Gastric lavage and administration of activated charcoal may be useful because of the prolonged delay in gastric emptying time.

Naloxone hydrochloride (0.4–2 mg intravenously in children and adults) should be given. A transient improvement in respiration may be followed by respiratory depression. Repeated doses may be required because the duration of action of diphenoxylate is considerably longer than that of naloxone. The anticholinergic effects do not usually require treatment.

McCarron MM, Challoner KR, Thompson GA: Diphenoxylate-atropine (Lomotil) overdose in children: An update. Pediatrics 1991;87:694.

DISINFECTANTS & DEODORIZERS

1. NAPHTHALENE

Naphthalene is commonly found in mothballs, disinfectants, and deodorizers. Naphthalene's toxicity is often not fully appreciated. It is absorbed not only when ingested but also through the skin and lungs. It is potentially hazardous to store baby clothes in naphthalene, because baby oil is an excellent solvent that may increase dermal absorption.

Metabolic products of naphthalene may cause severe hemolytic anemia, similar to that due to primaquine toxicity, 2–7 days after ingestion. Other physical findings include vomiting, diarrhea, jaundice, oliguria, anuria, coma, and convulsions. The urine may contain hemoglobin, protein, and casts.

Treatment

Induced vomiting should be followed by activated charcoal and a cathartic. Urinary alkalinization may prevent blocking of the renal tubules by acid hematin crystals. Anuria may persist for 1–2 weeks and still be completely reversible.

Ostlere L, Amos R, Wass JAH: Haemolytic anaemia associated with ingestion of naphthalene-containing anointing oil. Postgrad Med J 1988;64:444.
Picchioni AL: Mothball poisoning in children. Am J Hosp Pharm 1960;17:303.

2. p-DICHLOROBENZENE, PHENOLIC ACIDS, & OTHERS

Disinfectants and deodorizers containing p-dichlorobenzene or sodium sulfate are much less toxic than those containing naphthalene. Disinfectants containing phenolic acids are highly toxic, especially if they contain a borate ion. Phenol precipitates tissue proteins and causes respiratory alkalosis followed by metabolic acidosis. Some phenols cause methemoglobinemia.

Local gangrene occurs after prolonged contact with tissue. Phenol is readily absorbed from the gas-trointestinal tract, causing diffuse capillary damage and, in some cases, methemoglobinemia. Pentachlorophenol, which has been used in terminal rinsing of diapers, has caused infant fatalities.

The toxicity of alkalies, quaternary ammonium compounds, pine oil, and halogenated disinfectants varies with the concentration of active ingredients. Wick deodorizers are usually of moderate toxicity. Iodophor disinfectants are the safest. Spray deodorizers are not usually toxic, because a child is not likely to swallow a very large dose.

Manifestations of acute quaternary ammonium compound ingestion include diaphoresis, strong irritation, thirst, vomiting, diarrhea, cyanosis, hyperactivity, coma, convulsions, hypotension, abdominal pain, and pulmonary edema. Acute liver or renal failure may develop later.

Treatment

Activated charcoal may be used prior to gastric lavage. Castor oil dissolves phenol and may retard its absorption. This property of castor oil, however, has not been proved clinically. Mineral oil and alcohol are contraindicated because they increase the gastric absorption of phenol. A cathartic may be useful. The metabolic acidosis must be carefully managed. Anticonvulsants or measures to treat shock may be needed.

Because phenols are absorbed through the skin, exposed areas should be irrigated copiously with water. Undiluted polyethylene glycol may be a useful solvent as well.

Mucklow ES: Accidental feeding of dilute antiseptic solution (chlorhexidine 0.05% with cetrimide 1%) to five babies. Hum Toxicol 1988;7:567.
Pegg SP, Campbell DC: Children's burns due to cresol. Burns 1985;11:294.
Van Berkel M, de Wolff FA: Survival after acute benzalkonium chloride poisoning. Hum Toxicol 1988;7:191.

DISK BATTERY

Small, flat, smooth disk-shaped batteries measure between 10 and 25 mm in diameter. About 69% of them pass through the gastrointestinal tract in 48 hours and 85% in 72 hours. Some may become entrapped. These batteries contain caustic materials and heavy metals.

Batteries impacted in the esophagus may cause symptoms of refusal to take food, increased salivation, vomiting with or without blood, and pain or discomfort. Aspiration into the trachea may also occur. Fatalities have been reported in association with esophageal perforation.

When a history of disk battery ingestion is obtained, x-rays of the entire respiratory tract and gastrointestinal tract should be taken so that the battery can be located and the proper therapy determined.

Treatment

If the disk battery is located in the esophagus, it must be removed immediately. If the battery has been in the esophagus for more than 24 hours, the risk of caustic burn is greater.

Location of the disk battery below the esophagus has been associated with tissue damage, but the course has been benign in most cases. Perforated Meckel's diverticulum has been the major complication. It may take as long as 7 days for spontaneous passage to occur, and lack of movement in the gastrointestinal tract may not require removal in an asymptomatic patient. Some have suggested repeated x-rays and surgical intervention if passage of the battery pauses, but this approach may be excessive. Batteries that have opened in the gastrointestinal tract have been associated with some toxicity due to mercury, but the patients have recovered.

Emesis is ineffective in removal of the battery from the stomach. Asymptomatic patients may simply be observed and stools examined for passage of the battery. If the battery has not passed within 7 days or if the patient becomes symptomatic, x-rays should be repeated. If the battery has come apart or appears not to be moving, a purgative, enema, or nonabsorbable intestinal lavage solution should be administered. If these methods are not successful, surgical intervention may be required. Levels of heavy metals (mainly of mercury) should be measured in patients in whom the battery has opened or symptoms have developed.

Litovitz TL Schmitz BF: Ingestion of cylindrical and button batteries: an analysis of 2382 cases. Pediatrics 1992; 89:747.

HYDROCARBONS (Benzene, Charcoal Lighter Fluid, Gasoline, Kerosene, Petroleum Distillates, Turpentine)

Ingestion may cause irritation of mucous membranes, vomiting, blood-tinged diarrhea, respiratory distress, cyanosis, tachycardia, and fever. Although a small amount of certain hydrocarbons (10 mL) is potentially fatal, patients have survived ingestion of several ounces of other petroleum distillates. The more aromatic a hydrocarbon and the lower its viscosity rating, the more potentially toxic it is. Benzene, gasoline, kerosene, and red seal oil furniture polish are the most dangerous. A dose exceeding 1 mL/kg is likely to cause central nervous system depression. A history of coughing or choking, as well as vomiting, suggests aspiration with resulting hydrocarbon pneumonia. This is an acute hemorrhagic

necrotizing disease that usually develops within 24 hours of the ingestion and resolves without sequelae in 3–5 days. However, several weeks may be required for full resolution of a hydrocarbon pneumonia. Pneumonia may be caused by the aspiration of a few drops of petroleum distillate into the lung or by absorption from the circulatory system. Pulmonary edema and hemorrhage, cardiac dilatation and dysrhythmias, hepatosplenomegaly, proteinuria, and hematuria can occur following large overdoses. Hypoglycemia is occasionally present. A chest film may reveal pneumonia within hours after the ingestion. An abnormal urinalysis in a child with a previously normal urinary tract suggests a large overdose.

Treatment

Both emetics and lavage should be avoided when only a small amount has been ingested. It is impossible to do a "cautious gastric lavage" unless a cuffed endotracheal tube is inserted. Under these circumstances, gastric lavage may be done using saline. Following lavage, magnesium or sodium sulfate should be left in the stomach. (Mineral oil should not be given, because it is capable of causing a low-grade lipoid pneumonia.)

Emetics are probably preferable to gastric lavage if massive ingestion has occurred. Epinephrine should not be used with halogenated hydrocarbons because it may affect an already sensitized myocardium. Analeptic drugs are contraindicated. The usefulness of corticosteroids is debated, and antibiotics should be reserved for patients with infections. Oxygen and mist are helpful. Extracorporeal membrane oxygenation has been successful in at least two cases of failure with standard therapy.

Anas N, Namasonthi V, Ginsburg C: Criteria for hospitalizing children who have ingested products containing hydrocarbons. JAMA 1981;246:840.
Bysani GK, Rucoba RJ, Noah ZL: Treatment of hydrocarbon pneumonitis. High frequency jet ventilation as an alternative to extracorporeal membrane oxygenation. Chest 1994;106:300.
Weber TR et al: Prolonged extracorporeal support for non-neonatal respiratory failure. J Pediatr Surg 1992;27:1100.

IBUPROFEN

Most exposures in children do not produce symptoms. In one study, for example, children ingesting up to 2.4 g remained asymptomatic. When symptoms occur, the most common are abdominal pain, vomiting, drowsiness, and lethargy. In rare cases, apnea (especially in young children), seizures, metabolic acidosis, and central nervous system depression leading to coma have occurred.

Treatment

If a child has ingested less than 100 mg/kg, dilution with water or milk may be all that is necessary to minimize the gastrointestinal upset. In children, the volume of liquid used for dilution should be less than 4 oz. When the ingested amount is more than 400 mg/kg, there is a potential for seizures or central nervous system depression; therefore, gastric lavage may be preferred to emesis. If the ingested amount is between 100 and 400 mg/kg, emesis may be of equal value. Activated charcoal and a cathartic may also be of some value. There is no specific antidote. Neither alkalinization of the urine nor hemodialysis has been proved helpful.

Hall AH, Rumack BH: Treatment of patients with ibuprofen overdose. Ann Emerg Med 1988;17:185.
Hall AH et al: Ibuprofen overdose: A prospective study. West J Med 1988;148:653.
Lesko SM, Mitchell AA: An assessment of the safety of pediatric ibuprofen. A practitioner-based randomized clinical trial. JAMA 1995;273:929.

INSECT STINGS
(Bee, Wasp, & Hornet)

Insect stings are painful but not usually dangerous; however, death from anaphylaxis may occur. Bee venom, has hemolytic, neurotoxic, and histamine-like activities that can on rare occasions cause hemoglobinuria and severe anaphylactoid reactions.

Treatment

The physician should remove the stinger, taking care not to squeeze the attached venom sac. For allergic reactions, epinephrine 1:1000 solution, 0.01 mL/kg, should be administered intravenously or subcutaneously above the site of the sting. Three to four whiffs from an isoproterenol aerosol inhaler may be given at 3- to 4-minute intervals as needed. Corticosteroids (hydrocortisone), 100 mg intravenously, and diphenhydramine, 1.5 mg/kg intravenously, are useful ancillary drugs but have no immediate effect. Ephedrine or antihistamines may be used for 2 or 3 days to prevent recurrence of symptoms.

A patient who has had a potentially life-threatening insect sting should be desensitized against the Hymenoptera group, because the honey bee, wasp, hornet, and yellow jacket have common antigens in their venom.

For the more usual stings, cold compresses, aspirin, and diphenhydramine 1 mg/kg orally, are sufficient.

Barsky HE: Stinging insect allergy: Avoidance, identification, and treatment. Postgrad Med J 1987;82:157.
Reisman RE, Livingstone A: Late-onset allergic reactions, including serum sickness after insect stings. J Allergy Clin Immunol 1989;84:331.

INSECTICIDES

The petroleum distillates or other organic solvents used in these products are often as toxic as the pesticide. Unless otherwise indicated, induced vomiting or gastric lavage after insertion of an endotracheal tube is warranted.

DePalma AE, Kwalich DS, Zukerberg N: Pesticide poisoning in children. JAMA 1970;211:1979.
Rumack BH, Spoerke DG, Smolinske SC (editors): POISINDEX Information System. Micromedex, Inc, Denver, Colorado. [Published quarterly.]

1. CHLORINATED HYDROCARBONS (Aldrin, Carbinol, Chlordane, DDT, Dieldrin, Endrin, Heptachlor, Lindane, Toxaphene, etc)

Signs of intoxication include salivation, gastrointestinal irritability, abdominal pain, vomiting, diarrhea, central nervous system depression, and convulsions. Inhalation exposure causes irritation of the eyes, nose, and throat; blurred vision; cough; and pulmonary edema.

Chlorinated hydrocarbons are absorbed through the skin, respiratory tract, and gastrointestinal tract. Decontamination of skin with soap and evacuation of the stomach contents are critical. All contaminated clothing should be removed. Castor oil, milk, and other substances containing fats or oils should not be left in the stomach because they increase absorption of the chlorinated hydrocarbons. Convulsions should be treated with diazepam, 0.1–0.3 mg/kg intravenously. Epinephrine should not be used because it may cause cardiac arrhythmias.

2. ORGANOPHOSPHATE (CHOLINESTERASE-INHIBITING) INSECTICIDES (Chlorthion, Co-Ral, DFP, Diazinon, Malathion, Paraoxon, Parathion, Phosdrin, TEPP, Thio-TEPP, etc)

Dizziness, headache, blurred vision, miosis, tearing, salivation, nausea, vomiting, diarrhea, hyperglycemia, cyanosis, sense of constriction of the chest, dyspnea, sweating, weakness, muscular twitching, convulsions, loss of reflexes and sphincter control, and coma can occur.

The clinical findings are the result of cholinesterase inhibition, which causes an accumulation of acetylcholine. The onset of symptoms occurs within 12 hours of the exposure. Red cell cholinesterase levels should be measured as soon as possible. (Some normal individuals have a low serum cholinesterase level.) Normal values vary in different laboratories. In general, a decrease of red cell cholinesterase to below 25% of normal indicates significant exposure.

Repeated low-grade exposure may result in sudden, acute toxic reactions. This syndrome usually occurs after repeated household spraying rather than agricultural exposure.

Although all organophosphates act by inhibiting cholinesterase activity, they vary greatly in their toxicity. Parathion, for example, is 100 times more toxic than malathion. The toxicity is influenced by the specific compound, the type of formulation (liquid or solid), the vehicle, and the route of absorption (lungs, skin, or gastrointestinal tract).

Treatment

Atropine plus a cholinesterase reactivator, pralidoxime, is an antidote for organophosphate insecticide poisoning. After assessment and management of the ABCs, large doses of atropine should be given and repeated every few minutes until signs of atropinism are present. An appropriate starting dose of atropine is 2–4 mg intravenously in an adult and 0.05 mg/kg in a child. The patient should receive enough atropine to stop secretions (approximately 10 times the normal dose). Severe poisoning may require gram quantities of atropine per 24 hours.

Because atropine antagonizes the muscarinic parasympathetic effects of the organophosphates but does not affect the nicotinic receptor, it does not improve muscular weakness. Pralidoxime should also be given immediately in more severe cases and repeated every 6–12 hours as needed (25–50 mg/kg diluted to 5% and infused over 5–30 minutes at a rate of no more than 500 mg/min). Pralidoxime should be used in addition to—not in place of—atropine if red cell cholinesterase is less than 25% of normal. Pralidoxime is most useful within 48 hours after the exposure but has shown some effects 2–6 days later. Morphine, theophylline, aminophylline, succinylcholine, and tranquilizers of the reserpine and phenothiazine types are contraindicated. Hyperglycemia is common in severe poisonings.

Decontamination of skin, nails, hair, and clothing with soapy water is extremely important. Decontamination must be done carefully to avoid abrasions, which increase organophosphate absorption.

Bardin PG, Van Eeden SF: Organophosphate poisoning: Grading the severity and comparing treatment between atropine and glycopyrrolate. Crit Care Med 1990;8:956.

Borowitz SM: Prolonged organophosphate toxicity in a 26-month-old child. J Pediatr 1988;112:302.

Chaturvedi AK et al: Toxicological evaluation of a poisoning attributed to ingestion of malathion inspect spray and correlation with in vitro inhibition of cholinesterases. Hum Toxicol 1989;8:11.

3. CARBAMATES (Carbaryl, Sevin, Zectran, Etc)

Carbamate insecticides are reversible inhibitors of cholinesterase. The signs and symptoms of intoxication are similar to those associated with organophosphate poisoning but are generally less severe. Atropine titrated to effect is sufficient treatment. Pralidoxime should not be used with carbaryl poisoning but is of value with other carbamates. In combined exposures to organophosphates, give atropine but reserve pralidoxime for cases in which the red cell cholinesterase is depressed below 25% of normal or marked effects of nicotinic receptor stimulation are present.

Harris LW et al: The relationship between oxime induced reactivation of carbamylated acetylcholinesterase and antidotal efficacy against carbamate intoxication. Toxicol Appl Pharmacol 1989;98:128.

4. BOTANICAL INSECTICIDES (Black Flag Bug Killer, Black Leaf CPR Insect Killer, Flit Aerosol House & Garden Insect Killer, French's Flea Powder, Raid, etc)

Allergic reactions, asthma-like symptoms, coma, and convulsions have been seen. Pyrethrins, allethrin, ryania, and rotenone do not commonly cause signs of toxicity. Antihistamines, short-acting barbiturates, and atropine are helpful as symptomatic treatment.

IRON

Five stages of intoxication occur following iron intoxication: (1) Hemorrhagic gastroenteritis, which occurs 30–60 minutes after ingestion and may be associated with shock, acidosis, coagulation defects, and coma. This phase usually lasts 4–6 hours. (2) Phase of improvement, lasting 2–12 hours, during which patient looks better. (3) Delayed shock, which may occur 12–48 hours after ingestion and is usually associated with a serum iron level greater than 500 mg/dL. Metabolic acidosis, fever, leukocytosis, and coma may also be present. (4) Liver damage with hepatic failure. (5) Residual pyloric stenosis, which may develop about 4 weeks after the ingestion.

Once iron is absorbed from the gastrointestinal tract, it is not normally eliminated in feces but may be partially excreted in the urine, giving it a red color prior to chelation. A reddish discoloration of the urine suggests a serum iron level greater than 350 mg/dL.

Treatment

Gastrointestinal decontamination is based on clinical assessment. Syrup of ipecac may be administered at home, with appropriate follow-up, provided the history does not warrant an emergency department visit. The patient should be referred to a health care facility if symptomatic or if the history indicates toxic amounts. Gastric lavage and whole bowel irrigation should be considered in these patients.

Shock must be treated in the usual manner. Sodium bicarbonate or Fleet's Phospho-Soda left in the stomach to form the insoluble phosphate or carbonate have not shown clinical benefit and have caused lethal hypernatremia or hyperphosphatemia. Deferoxamine, a specific chelating agent for iron, is a useful adjunct in the treatment of severe iron poisoning. It forms a soluble complex that is excreted in the urine. It is contraindicated in patients with renal failure unless dialysis can be used. Institute intravenous deferoxamine chelation therapy if the patient is symptomatic and a serum iron determination cannot be readily obtained, or if the peak serum iron exceeds 400 μg/dL (62.6 μmol/L) at 4–5 hours after ingestion.

Deferoxamine should not be delayed until serum iron levels are available in serious cases of poisoning. Intravenous administration is indicated if the patient is in shock, in which case it should be given at a dosage of 15 mg/kg/h. Infusion rates up to 35 mg/kg/h have been used in life-threatening poisonings. Rapid intravenous administration can cause hypotension, facial flushing, urticaria, tachycardia, and shock. Deferoxamine, 90 mg/kg intramuscularly every 8 hours (maximum, 1 g), may be given if intravenous access cannot be established, but the procedure is painful. The drug should not be given orally. The indications for discontinuation of deferoxamine have not been clearly delineated. Generally, it can be stopped after 12–24 hours if the acidosis has resolved and the patient is improving.

Hemodialysis, peritoneal dialysis, or exchange transfusion can be used to increase the excretion of the dialyzable complex. Urine output should be monitored and urine sediment examined for evidence of renal tubular damage. Initial laboratory studies should include blood typing and cross-matching; total protein; serum iron, sodium, potassium, and chloride; P_{CO_2}; pH; and liver function tests. Serum iron levels fall rapidly even if deferoxamine is not given.

After the acute episode, liver function studies and an upper gastrointestinal series are indicated to rule out residual damage.

Chyka DA, Butler AY: Assessment of acute iron poisoning by laboratory and clinical observations. Am J Emerg Med 1993;11:99.

Mann KV et al: Management of acute iron overdose. Clin Pharm 1989;8:428.

LEAD

Lead poisoning causes vague symptoms, including weakness, irritability, weight loss, vomiting, personality changes, ataxia, constipation, headache, and colicky abdominal pain. Late manifestations consist of retarded development, convulsions, and coma associated with increased intracranial pressure. The latter is a medical emergency.

Plumbism usually occurs insidiously in children under 5 years of age. The most likely sources of lead include flaking leaded paint, artist's paints, fruit tree sprays, solder, brass alloys, home-glazed pottery, and fumes from burning batteries. Only paint containing less than 1% lead is safe for interior use (furniture, toys, etc). Repetitive ingestions of small amounts of lead are far more serious than a single massive exposure. Toxic effects are likely to occur if more than 0.5 mg of lead per day is absorbed.

Blood lead levels are used to assess the severity of exposure. A complete blood count and serum ferritin concentration should be obtained; iron deficiency increases absorption of lead. Glycosuria, proteinuria, hematuria, and aminoaciduria occur frequently. Blood lead levels usually exceed 80 μg/dL in symptomatic patients. Abnormal blood lead levels should be repeated in asymptomatic patients to rule out laboratory error. Specimens must be meticulously obtained in acid-washed containers. A normocytic, slightly hypochromic anemia with basophilic stippling of the red cells and reticulocytosis may be present in plumbism. Stippling of red blood cells is absent in cases involving only recent ingestion.

The cerebrospinal fluid protein is elevated, and the white cell count is usually less than 100 cells/μL. Cerebrospinal fluid pressure may be elevated in patients with encephalopathy; lumbar punctures must be performed cautiously to prevent herniation.

Treatment

Standard gastrointestinal decontamination is indicated if an acute ingestion has occurred or lead is noted on the abdominal x-ray. Succimer is an orally administered chelator approved for use in children and reported to be as efficacious as calcium edetate. Treatment for children with blood lead levels of 20–45 μg/dL has not been determined. Succimer should be initiated at blood lead levels over 45 μg/dL. The initial dose is 10 mg/kg (350 mg/m²) every 8 hours for 5 days. The same dose is then given every 12 hours for 14 days. At least 2 weeks should elapse between courses. Blood lead levels increase somewhat ("rebound") after discontinuation of therapy. Courses of dimercaprol (4 mg/kg/dose) and calcium edetate may still be used but are no longer the preferred method, except in cases of lead encephalopathy.

Anticonvulsants may be needed. Mannitol or corticosteroids and volume restriction are indicated in patients with encephalopathy. A high-calcium, high-phosphorus diet and large doses of vitamin D may remove lead from the blood by depositing it in the bones. A public health team should evaluate the source of the lead. Necessary corrections should be completed before the child is returned home.

American Academy of Pediatrics Committee on Drugs: Treatment guidelines for lead exposure in children. Pediatrics 1995;96:155.

Chisholm J et al: Recognition and management of children with increased lead absorption. Arch Dis Child 1979; 54:249.

Glotzer DE, Weitzman M: Commonly asked questions about childhood lead poisoning. Pediatr Ann 1995;24:630.

Graziano JG et al: Controlled study of *meso*-2,3-dimercaptosuccinic acid for the management of childhood lead intoxication. J Pediatr 1992;120:133.

Needleman HL et al: The long term effects of exposure to low doses of lead in childhood: An 11-year follow-up report. N Engl J Med 1990;322:83.

MUSHROOMS

Toxic mushrooms are often difficult to distinguish from edible varieties. Symptoms vary with the species ingested, time of year, stage of maturity, quantity eaten, method of preparation, and interval since ingestion. A mushroom that is toxic to one individual may not be toxic for another. Drinking alcohol and eating certain mushrooms may cause a reaction similar to that seen with disulfiram and alcohol. Cooking destroys some toxins but not the deadly one produced by *Amanita phalloides,* which is responsible for 90% of deaths due to mushroom poisoning. Mushrooms toxins are absorbed relatively slowly. Onset of symptoms within 2 hours of ingestion suggests muscarinic toxin, whereas a delay of symptoms for 6–48 hours after ingestion strongly suggests *Amanita* (amanitin) poisoning. Patients who have ingested *A phalloides* may relapse and die of hepatic or renal failure following initial improvement.

Mushroom poisoning may be manifested by muscarinic symptoms (salivation, vomiting, diarrhea, cramping abdominal pain, tenesmus, miosis, and dyspnea), coma, convulsions, hallucinations, hemolysis, and delayed hepatic and renal failure.

Treatment

Induce vomiting and follow with activated charcoal and a saline cathartic. If the patient has muscarinic signs, give atropine, 0.05 mg/kg intramuscularly (0.02 mg/kg in toddlers), and repeat as needed (usually every 30 minutes) to keep the patient atropinized. Atropine, however, is only used when there are cholinergic effects and not for all mushrooms. Hypoglycemia is most likely to occur in patients with delayed onset of symptoms. Try to identify the mushroom if the patient is symptomatic. Local botanical gardens, university departments of botany, and societies of mycologists may be able to help. Supportive care is usually all that is needed except in the case of *A phalloides,* where penicillin, silibinin, or hemodialysis may be indicated.

Lampe KF, McCann MA: Differential diagnosis of poisoning by North American mushrooms, with particular emphasis on *Amanita phalloides*-like intoxication. Ann Emerg Med 1987;16:956.

Spoerke DG, Rumack BH (editors): *Mushroom Poisoning, Diagnosis and Treatment,* 2nd ed. CRC Press, 1994.

NITRITES, NITRATES, ANILINE, PENTACHLOROPHENOL, & DINITROPHENOL

Nausea, vertigo, vomiting, cyanosis (methemoglobinemia), cramping abdominal pain, tachycardia, cardiovascular collapse, tachypnea, coma, shock, convulsions, and death are possible manifestations of nitrite or nitrate poisoning.

Nitrite and nitrate compounds found in the home include amyl nitrite, butyl nitrates, isobutyl nitrates, nitroglycerin, pentaerythritol tetranitrate, sodium nitrite, nitrobenzene, and phenazopyridine. Pentachlorophenol and dinitrophenol, which are found in wood preservatives, produce methemoglobinemia and high fever because of uncoupling of oxidative phosphorylation. Headache, dizziness, and bradycardia have been reported. High concentrations of nitrites in water or spinach have been the most common cause of nitrite-induced methemoglobinemia. Symptoms do not usually occur until 15–50% of the hemoglobin has been converted to methemoglobin. A rapid test is to compare a drop of normal blood with the patient's blood on a dry filter paper. Brown discoloration of the patient's blood indicates a methemoglobin level of more than 15%.

Treatment

Induce vomiting, administer activated charcoal, and follow with a cathartic. Decontaminate affected skin with soap and water. Oxygen and artificial respiration may be needed. If the blood methemoglobin level exceeds 30%, or if levels cannot be obtained and the patient is symptomatic, give a 1% solution of methylene blue, 0.2 mL/kg intravenously over 5–10 minutes. Avoid perivascular infiltration, because it causes necrosis of the skin and subcutaneous tissues. A dramatic change in the degree of cyanosis should occur. Transfusion is occasionally necessary. Epinephrine and other vasoconstrictors are contraindicated. If reflex bradycardia occurs, atropine should be used.

Bardoczky GI, Wathieu M, D'Hollander A: Prilocaine-induced methemoglobinemia evidenced by pulse oximetry. Acta Anaesthesiol Scand 1990;34:162.

Caudill L, Walbridge J, Kuhn G: Methemoglobinemia as a cause of coma. Ann Emerg Med 1990;19:677.

Kaplan A et al: Methaemoglobinaemia due to accidental

sodium nitrite poisoning: Report of 10 cases. S Afr Med J 1990;77:300.

OPIOIDS
(Codeine, Heroin, Methadone, Morphine, Propoxyphene)

Opioid-related medical problems may include drug addiction, withdrawal in a newborn infant, and accidental overdoses. Unlike other narcotics, methadone is readily absorbed from the gastrointestinal tract. Most opioids, including heroin, methadone, meperidine, morphine, and codeine, are excreted in the urine within 24 hours and can be readily detected.

Adolescent narcotic addicts often have other medical problems, including cellulitis, abscesses, thrombophlebitis, tetanus, infective endocarditis, HIV infection, tuberculosis, hepatitis, malaria, foreign body emboli, thrombosis of pulmonary arterioles, diabetes mellitus, obstetric complications, nephropathy, and peptic ulcer.

Treatment of Overdosage
Opioids can cause respiratory depression, stridor, coma, increased oropharyngeal secretions, sinus bradycardia, and urinary retention. Pulmonary edema rarely occurs in children; deaths usually result from aspiration of gastric contents, respiratory arrest, and cerebral edema, singly or in combination. Convulsions may occur with propoxyphene overdosage.

Although suggested doses for naloxone hydrochloride range from 0.01 to 0.1 mg/kg, it is generally unnecessary to calculate the dosage on this basis. This extremely safe antidote should be given in sufficient quantity to reverse opioid binding sites. For children under 1 year of age, 1 ampule (0.4 mg) should be given initially; if there is no response, give five more ampules (2 mg) rapidly. Older children should be given 0.4–0.8 mg, followed by 2–4 mg if there is no response. An improvement in respiratory status may be followed by respiratory depression, because the depressant action of narcotics may last 24–48 hours but the antagonist's duration of action is less than 1 hour. Neonates poisoned in utero may require 10–30 mg/kg to reverse the effect.

Withdrawal in the Addict
Diazepam, 10 mg every 6 hours orally, has been recommended for the treatment of mild narcotic withdrawal in ambulatory adolescents. Management of withdrawal in the confirmed addict may be accomplished with the administration of clonidine, by substitution with methadone, or with reintroduction of the original addicting agent, if available through a supervised drug withdrawal program. A tapered course over 3 weeks will accomplish this goal. Death rarely, if ever, occurs. The abrupt discontinuation of narcotics (cold turkey method) is not recommended and may cause severe physical withdrawal signs.

Withdrawal in the Newborn
A newborn infant in opioid withdrawal is usually small for gestational age and demonstrates yawning, sneezing, decreased Moro reflex, hunger but uncoordinated sucking action, jitteriness, tremor, constant movement, a shrill protracted cry, increased tendon reflexes, convulsions, vomiting, fever, watery diarrhea, cyanosis, dehydration, vasomotor instability, seizure, and collapse. The onset of symptoms commonly begins in the first 48 hours but may be delayed as long as 8 days depending upon the timing of the mother's last fix and her predelivery medication. The diagnosis can be easily confirmed by identifying the narcotic in the urine of the mother and baby.

Several methods of treatment have been suggested for narcotic withdrawal in the newborn. Phenobarbital, 8 mg/kg/d intramuscularly or orally in four doses for 4 days and then reduced by one third every 2 days as signs decrease, may be continued for as long as 3 weeks. Methadone may be necessary in those infants with congenital methadone addiction who are not controlled in their withdrawal by large doses of phenobarbital. Dosage should be 0.5 mg/kg/d in two divided doses but can be gradually increased as needed. Slow tapering off may be necessary over 4 weeks for methadone addiction.

It is not clear whether prophylactic treatment with these drugs decreases the complication rate. The mortality rate of untreated narcotic withdrawal in the newborn may be as high as 45%.

Bradberry JC, Raebel MA: Continuous infusion of naloxone in the treatment of narcotic overdose. Drug Intell Clin Pharm 1981;15:945.
American Academy of Pediatrics Committee on Drugs: Naloxone dosage and route of administration for infants and children: Addendum to emergency drug doses for infants and children. Pediatrics 1990;86:484.

PHENOTHIAZINES
(Chlorpromazine, Prochlorperazine, Trifluoperazine)

Clinical Presentations
A. Extrapyramidal Crisis: Episodes characterized by torticollis, stiffening of the body, spasticity, poor speech, catatonia, and inability to communicate although conscious are typical manifestations. These episodes usually last a few seconds to a few minutes but have rarely caused death. Extrapyramidal crises may represent idiosyncratic reactions and are aggravated by dehydration. The signs and symptoms occur most often in children who have received prochlorperazine. They are commonly mistaken for psychotic episodes.

B. Overdose: Lethargy and deep prolonged coma commonly occur. Promazine, chlorpromazine, and prochlorperazine are the drugs most likely to cause respiratory depression and precipitous drops in blood pressure. Occasionally, paradoxic hyperactivity and extrapyramidal signs as well as hyperglycemia and acetonemia are present. Seizures are uncommon.

Treatment

Extrapyramidal signs are alleviated within minutes by the slow intravenous administration of diphenhydramine, 1–2 mg/kg (maximum, 50 mg), or benztropine mesylate, 1–2 mg intravenously (1 mg/min). No other treatment is usually indicated.

Patients with overdoses should be treated conservatively. Vomiting should be induced with ipecac followed by administration of activated charcoal. Emetics are often unsuccessful because phenothiazines are potent antiemetics; gastric lavage may be the only practical way to remove gastric contents. Hypotension may be treated with standard agents, starting with isotonic saline administration. Agitation is best treated with diazepam. Neuroleptic malignant syndrome may be treated with dantrolene, 1 mg/kg (maximum, 50 mg) every 12 hours.

Baker PB et al: Hyperthermia, hypertension, hypertonia, and coma in massive thioridazine overdose. Am J Emerg Med 1988;6:346.

Sanders KM, Minnema AM, Murray GB: Low incidence of extrapyramidal symptoms in treatment of delirium with intravenous haloperidol and lorazepam in the intensive care unit. J Intens Care Med 1989;4:201.

PLANTS

Many common ornamental, garden, and wild plants are potentially toxic. Only in a few cases will small amounts of a plant cause severe illness or death. Table 11–10 lists the most toxic plants, symptoms and signs of poisoning, and treatment.

Table 11–10. Poisoning due to plants.[1]

	Symptoms and Signs	Treatment
Arum family: *Caladium, Dieffenbachia,* calla lily, dumbcane (oxalic acid)	Burning of mucous membranes and airway obstruction secondary to edema caused by calcium oxalate crystals.	Accessible areas should be thoroughly washed. Corticosteroids relieve airway obstruction. Apply cold packs to affected mucous membranes.
Castor bean plant (ricin—a toxalbumin) Jequinty bean (abrin—a toxalbumin)	Mucous membrane irritation, nausea, vomiting, bloody diarrhea, blurred vision, circulatory collapse, acute hemolytic anemia, convulsions, uremia.	Fluid and electrolyte monitoring. Saline cathartic. Forced alkaline diuresis will prevent complications due to hemagglutination and hemolysis.
Foxglove, lily of the valley, and oleander[2]	Nausea, diarrhea, visual disturbances, and cardiac irregularities (eg, heart block).	See treatment for digitalis drugs in text.
Jimsonweed: See Belladonna Alkaloids	Mydriasis, dry mouth, tachycardia, and hallucinations.	Activated charcoal
Larkspur (ajacine, *Delphinium,* delphinine)	Nausea and vomiting, irritability, muscular paralysis, and CNS depression.	Symptomatic. Atropine may be helpful.
Monkshood (aconite)	Numbness of mucous membranes, visual disturbances, tingling, dizziness, tinnitus, hypotension, bradycardia, and convulsions.	Activated charcoal, oxygen. Atropine is probably helpful.
Poison hemlock (coniine)	Mydriasis, trembling, dizziness, bradycardia. CNS depression, muscular paralysis, and convulsions. Death is due to respiratory paralysis.	Symptomatic. Oxygen and cardiac monitoring equipment are desirable. Assisted respiration is often necessary. Give anticonvulsants if needed.
Rhododendron (grayanotoxin)	Abdominal cramps, vomiting, severe diarrhea, muscular paralysis, CNS and circulatory depression. Hypertension with very large doses.	Atropine can prevent bradycardia. Epinephrine is contraindicated. Antihypertensives may be needed.
Yellow jessamine (active ingredient, geisemine, is related to strychnine)	Restlessness, convusions, muscular paralysis, and respiratory depression.	Symptomatic. Because of the relation to strychnine, activated charcoal and diazepam for seizures are worth trying.

[1]Many other plants cause minor irritation but are not likely to cause serious problems unless large amounts are ingested. See Lampe KF, McCann MA: *AMA Handbook of Poisonous and Injurious Plants.* American Medical Association, 1985. See also Rumack BH, Spoerke DG (editors): POISINDEX® information System. Micromedex, IAC, Denver, Colorado. [Published quarterly.]
[2]Done AK: Ornamental and deadly. Emerg Med (April) 1973;5:255.

Frohne D, Pfander HJ: *A Colour Atlas of Poisonous Plants.* Wolfe, 1984.

Lampe KF, McCann MA: *AMA Handbook of Poisonous and Injurious Plants.* American Medical Association, 1985.

PSYCHOTROPIC DRUGS

Psychotropic drugs consist of four general classes: stimulants (amphetamines, cocaine), depressants (eg, narcotics, barbiturates), antidepressants and tranquilizers, and hallucinogens (eg, LSD, PCP).

Clinical Presentations

The following clinical findings are commonly seen in patients abusing drugs. See also other entries discussed in alphabetic sequence in this chapter.

A. Stimulants: Agitation, euphoria, grandiose feelings, tachycardia, fever, abdominal cramps, visual and auditory hallucinations, mydriasis, coma, convulsions, and respiratory depression.

B. Depressants: Emotional lability, ataxia, diplopia, nystagmus, vertigo, poor accommodation, respiratory depression, coma, apnea, and convulsions. Dilatation of conjunctival blood vessels suggests marijuana ingestion. Narcotics cause miotic pupils and, occasionally, pulmonary edema.

C. Antidepressants and Tranquilizers: Hypotension, lethargy, respiratory depression, coma, and extrapyramidal reactions.

D. Hallucinogens and Psychoactive Drugs: Belladonna alkaloids cause mydriasis, dry mouth, nausea, vomiting, urinary retention, confusion, disorientation, paranoid delusions, hallucinations, fever, hypotension, aggressive behavior, convulsions, and coma. **Psychoactive drugs** such as LSD cause mydriasis, unexplained bizarre behavior, hallucinations, and generalized undifferentiated psychotic behavior.

Management of the Patient Who Abuses Drugs

Only a small percentage of the persons using drugs come to the attention of physicians; those who do are usually suffering from adverse reactions such as panic states, drug psychoses, homicidal or suicidal thoughts, or respiratory depression.

Even with cooperative patients, an accurate history is difficult to obtain. The user often does not really know what drug has been taken or how much. "Street drugs" are almost always adulterated with one or more other compounds. Multiple drugs are often taken together, making it impossible to clinically define the type of drug. Friends may be a useful source of information. A drug history is most easily obtained in a quiet spot by a gentle, nonthreatening, honest examiner.

The general appearance, skin, lymphatics, cardiorespiratory status, gastrointestinal tract, and central nervous system should be stressed during the physical examination, because they often provide clues suggesting drug abuse. A drug history should not be taken from an adolescent in the parents' presence.

Hallucinogens are not life-threatening unless the patient is frankly homicidal or suicidal. A specific diagnosis is usually not necessary for management; instead, the presenting signs and symptoms are treated. Does the patient appear intoxicated? In withdrawal? "Flashing back?" Is some illness or injury (eg, head trauma) being masked by a drug effect? (Remember that a known drug user may still have hallucinations from meningoencephalitis.)

The signs and symptoms in a given patient are a function of not only the drug and the dose but also the level of acquired tolerance, the "setting," the patient's physical condition and personality traits, the potentiating effects of other drugs, and many other factors.

A common drug problem is the "bad trip," which is usually a panic reaction. This is best managed by "talking the patient down" and minimizing auditory and visual stimuli. Sitting with a friend while the drug effect dissipates may be the best treatment that can be offered. This may take several hours. The physician's job is not to terminate the drug effect but to help the patient over the bad experience.

Drug therapy is often unnecessary and may complicate the clinical course of a patient with a panic reaction. Although phenothiazines have been commonly used to treat "bad trips," they should be avoided if the specific drug is not known, because they may enhance toxicity or produce unwanted side effects. Diazepam is the drug of choice if a sedative effect is required. Physical restraints are rarely indicated and usually increase the patient's panic reaction.

For treatment of life-threatening drug abuse, consult the section on the specific drug elsewhere in this chapter and the section on general management at the beginning of the chapter.

After the acute episode, the physician must decide whether psychiatric referral is indicated; in general, patients who have made suicidal gestures or attempts and adolescents who are not communicating with their families should be referred.

Dar KJ, McBrien ME: MDMA induced hyperthermia: Report of a fatality and review of current therapy. Intensive Care Med 1996;22:995.

SALICYLATES

The use of childproof containers and publicity regarding accidental poisoning have reduced the incidence of acute salicylate poisoning. Nevertheless, serious intoxication still occurs and must be regarded as an emergency.

Salicylates uncouple oxidative phosphorylation, leading to increased heat production, excessive sweating, and dehydration. They also interfere with glucose metabolism and may cause hypoglycemia or hyperglycemia. Respiratory center stimulation occurs early.

Patients usually have signs of hyperventilation, sweating, dehydration, and fever. Vomiting and diarrhea sometimes occur. In severe cases, disorientation, convulsions, and coma may develop.

The severity of acute intoxication can in some measure be judged by serum salicylate levels. High levels are always dangerous irrespective of clinical signs, and low levels may be misleading in chronic cases. Other laboratory values usually indicate metabolic acidosis despite hyperventilation; low serum K$^+$ values; and often abnormal serum glucose levels.

Salicylate poisoning is classified as mild when plasma pH is greater than 7.4 and urine pH is greater than 6.0; as moderate when plasma pH is greater than 7.4 and urine pH is less than 6.0; and as severe when plasma pH is less than 7.4 and urine pH is less than 6.0.

In mild and moderate poisoning, stimulation of the respiratory center produces respiratory alkalosis. In severe intoxication (seen in severe acute ingestion with high salicylate levels and in chronic toxicity with lower levels), respiratory response is unable to overcome the metabolic overdose.

Once the urine becomes acidic, progressively smaller amounts of salicylate are excreted. Until this process is reversed, the half-life will remain prolonged, because metabolism contributes little to the removal of salicylate.

Chronic severe poisoning may be seen as early as 3 days after a regimen of salicylate is begun. Findings usually include vomiting, diarrhea, and dehydration.

Treatment

Charcoal binds salicylates well and, after emesis or lavage, should be given for acute ingestions. Mild poisoning may require only the administration of oral fluids and confirmation that the salicylate level is falling. Moderate poisoning is reflected by moderate dehydration and depletion of potassium. Fluids must be administered to correct dehydration and produce urine with a pH of greater than 7.0 at a rate of 2–3 mL/kg/h. Initial intravenous solutions should be isotonic, with sodium bicarbonate constituting half the electrolyte content. Once the patient is rehydrated, the solution can contain more free water and approximately 40 meq of potassium per liter.

Severe ingestion is marked by major dehydration in cases of chronic poisoning. Symptoms may be confused with those of Reye's syndrome, encephalopathy, and metabolic acidosis. Salicylate levels may even be in the "therapeutic range." Major fluid correction of dehydration is required. Once this has been accomplished, hypokalemia must be corrected and sodium bicarbonate given. Usual requirements are sodium bicarbonate, 1–2 mEq/kg/h over the first 6–8 hours, and K$^+$, 20–40 mEq/L. A urine flow of 2–3 mL/kg/h should be established.

Vitamin K should be administered, although bleeding is rare except in severely poisoned patients. Renal failure or pulmonary edema is an indication for dialysis. Hemodialysis is most effective and peritoneal dialysis relatively ineffective. Acetazolamide should not be used.

Yip L, Dart RC, Gabow PA: Concepts and controversies in salicylate toxicity. Emerg Med Clin North Am 1994;12:351.

SCORPION STINGS

Scorpion stings are common in arid areas of the southwestern USA. Scorpion venom is more toxic than most snake venoms, but only minute amounts are injected. Although neurologic manifestations may last a week, most clinical signs subside within 24–48 hours.

The most common scorpions in the USA are members of the *Vejovis, Hadrurus, Androctonus,* and *Centruroides* species. Stings by the first three produce edema and pain. Stings by *Centruroides* cause tingling or burning paresthesias that begin at the site of the sting; other findings include hypersalivation, restlessness, muscular fasciculation, abdominal cramps, opisthotonos, convulsions, urinary incontinence, and respiratory failure.

Treatment

Sedation is the primary therapy. In severe cases, the airway may become compromised by secretions and weakness of respiratory muscles. Endotracheal intubation may be required. Patients may require treatment for seizures, hypertension, or tachycardia.

The prognosis is good as long as the airway is managed appropriately.

Bond GR. Antivenin administration for *Centruroides* scorpion sting: Risks and benefits. Ann Emerg Med 1992;21:788

Rachesky IJ et al: Treatments for *Centruroides exilicauda* envenomation. Am J Dis Child 1984;138:1136.

SNAKEBITE

Despite the lethal potential of venomous snakes, human morbidity and mortality rates are surprisingly low. The outcome depends on the size of the child, the site of the bite, the degree of envenomation, the type of snake, and the effectiveness of treatment.

Ninety-eight percent of poisonous snakebites in the USA are caused by pit vipers (rattlesnakes, water moccasins, and copperheads). A few are caused by elapids (coral snakes), and occasional bites occur from cobras and other nonindigenous exotic snakes kept as pets. Snake venom is a complex mixture of enzymes, peptides, and proteins that may have predominantly cytotoxic, neurotoxic, hemotoxic, or cardiotoxic effects but other effects as well. Up to 25% of bites by pit vipers do not result in venom injection.

Pit viper venom is predominantly caused by a severe local reaction with pain, discoloration, and edema, as well as hemorrhage.

Swelling and pain occur soon after rattlesnake bite and are a certain indication that envenomation has occurred. During the first few hours, swelling and ecchymosis extend proximally from the bite. The bite is often obvious as a double puncture mark surrounded by ecchymosis. Hematemesis, melena, hemoptysis, and other manifestations of coagulopathy develop in severe cases. Respiratory difficulty and shock are the ultimate causes of death. Even in fatal rattlesnake bite, there is usually a period of 6–8 hours between the bite and death; there is, therefore, usually enough time to start effective treatment.

Coral snake envenomation causes little local pain, swelling, or necrosis, and systemic reactions are often delayed. The signs of coral snake envenomation include bulbar paralysis, dysphagia, and dysphoria; these may appear in 5–10 hours and may be followed by total peripheral paralysis and death in 24 hours.

Treatment

Children in snake-infested areas should wear boots and long trousers, should not walk barefoot, and should be cautioned not to explore under ledges or in holes.

The treatment of snakebite envenomation is controversial, but the following approach seems most useful.

A. Emergency (First Aid) Treatment: The most important first aid measure is transportation to a medical facility. Splint the affected extremity and minimize the patient's motion. Tourniquets and ice packs are contraindicated. Incision and suction are not useful for either crotalid or elapid snake bite. High vacuum suction (Extractor) has been shown to remove venom in a rabbit model and is now commercially available.

B. Definitive Medical Management: Blood should be drawn for hematocrit, clotting time and platelet function, and serum electrolyte determinations. Establish two secure intravenous sites for the administration of antivenin and other medications.

Specific antivenin is indicated when signs of progressive envenomation are present. Polyvalent pit viper antivenin and eastern coral snake antivenin (Wyeth Laboratories) are available from hospital pharmacies. There is no antivenin for the western coral snake. If horse serum sensitivity tests are negative, antivenin should be given intravenously over 1 hour. For pit vipers, give 5–8 vials for minimal, 8–15 vials for moderate, and 15 or more vials for severe envenomation. Dilute each vial to 50–200 mL. (Antivenin should not be given intramuscularly or subcutaneously.) Epinephrine, 0.3 mL of 1:1000 solution, should be drawn up in a syringe before antivenin is administered. Hemorrhage, pain, and shock are rapidly diminished by adequate amounts of antivenin. For coral snakes, give three to five vials of antivenin in 250–500 mL of isotonic saline solution. An additional three to five vials may be required.

Codeine, 1–1.5 mg/kg per dose orally, or meperidine, 0.6–1.5 mg/kg per dose orally or intramuscularly, is necessary to control pain. Cryotherapy is contraindicated because it commonly causes additional tissue damage. Early physiotherapy minimizes contractures. In rare cases, fasciotomy to relieve pressure within muscular compartments is required. The evaluation of function as well as of pulses will better predict the need for fasciotomy. Corticosteroids (hydrocortisone, 1–2 g intravenously every 4–6 hours) are useful in the treatment of serum sickness or anaphylactic shock. Antibiotics are not needed unless clinical signs of infection occur. Tetanus status should be evaluated and treated, if needed.

Kitchens CS, Van Mierop LHS: Envenomation by the eastern coral snake *(Micrurus fulvius):* A study of 39 victims. JAMA 1987;258:1615.

Russell FE: *Snake Venom Poisoning.* Scholium International, 1983.

SOAPS & DETERGENTS

1. SOAPS

Soap is made from salts of fatty acids. Some toilet soap bars contain both soap and detergent. Ingestion of soap bars may cause vomiting and diarrhea, but they have a low toxicity. Induced emesis is unnecessary.

2. DETERGENTS

Detergents are nonsoap synthetic products used for cleaning purposes because of their surfactant properties. Commercial products include granules, powders, and liquids. Dishwasher detergents are very alkaline and can cause caustic burns. Low concentrations of bleaching and antibacterial agents as well as enzymes are found in many preparations. The pure compounds are moderately toxic, but the concentration used is too small to alter the product's toxicity significantly, although occasional primary or allergic irritative phenomena have been noted in housewives and in employees manufacturing these products.

Cationic Detergents (Ceepryn, Diaperene, Phemerol, Zephiran)

Cationic detergents in dilute solutions (0.5%) cause mucosal irritation, but higher concentrations (10–15%) may cause caustic burns to mucosa. Clinical effects include nausea, vomiting, collapse, coma, and convulsions. As little as 2.25 g of some cationic agents have caused death in an adult. In four cases, 100–400 mg/kg of benzalkonium chloride caused death. Cationic detergents are rapidly inactivated by tissues and ordinary soap.

Because of the caustic potential and rapid onset of seizures, emesis is not recommended. Activated charcoal and a cathartic should be administered. Anticonvulsants may be needed.

Anionic Detergents

Most common household detergents are anionic. Laundry compounds have water softener (sodium phosphate) added, which is a strong irritant and may reduce ionized calcium. Anionic detergents irritate the skin by removing natural oils. Although ingestion causes diarrhea, intestinal distention, and vomiting, no fatalities have been reported.

The only treatment usually required is to discontinue use if skin irritation occurs and replace fluids and electrolytes. Induced vomiting is not indicated following ingestion of electric dishwasher detergent, because of its alkalinity. Dilute with water or milk.

Nonionic Detergents (Brij Products; Tritons X-45, X-100, X-102, & X-144)

These compounds include lauryl, stearyl, and oleyl alcohols and octyl phenol. They have a minimal irritating effect on the skin and are almost nontoxic when swallowed.

Deichmann WB, Gerarde HW: Hazards of alkaline laundry detergents. JAMA 1972;220:1014.
Enzyme detergents. (Editorial.) Br Med J 1970;1:518.
Jeven JE: Severe dermatitis and "biological" detergents. Br Med J 1970;1:299.

SPIDER BITES

Most medically important bites in the USA are caused by the black widow spider (*Latrodectus mactans*) and the North American brown recluse (violin) spider (*Loxosceles reclusa*). It is helpful if positive identification of the spider can be made, since many spider bites may mimic those of the brown recluse spider.

Black Widow Spider

The black widow spider is endemic to nearly all areas of the United States. The initial bite causes sharp fleeting pain. Local and systemic muscular cramping, abdominal pain, nausea and vomiting, and shock can occur. Convulsions are more commonly seen in small children. Systemic signs of black widow spider bite may be confused with other causes of acute abdomen. Although paresthesias, nervousness, and transient muscle spasms may persist for weeks in survivors, recovery from the acute phase is generally complete within 3 days. In contrast to popular opinion, death is extremely rare.

Most authors recommend calcium gluconate as initial therapy (50 mg/kg intravenously per dose, up to 250 mg/kg/24 h), although it is often not effective and the effects are of short duration. Methocarbamol (15 mg/kg orally) or diazepam titrated to effect is useful. Morphine or barbiturates may occasionally be needed for control of pain or restlessness, but they increase the possibility of respiratory depression. Antivenin is available but should be reserved for severe cases in which the above therapies have failed. Local treatment of the bite is not helpful.

Brown Recluse Spider (Violin Spider)

The North American brown recluse spider is most commonly seen in the central and midwestern areas of the United States. Its bite characteristically produces a localized reaction with progressively severe pain within 24 hours. The initial bleb on an erythematous ischemic base is replaced by a black eschar within 1 week. This eschar separates in 2–5 weeks, leaving an ulcer that heals slowly. Systemic signs include cyanosis, morbilliform rash, fever, chills, malaise, weakness, nausea and vomiting, joint pains, hemolytic reactions with hemoglobinuria, jaundice, and delirium. Fatalities are rare. Fatal disseminated intravascular coagulation has been reported.

Although of unproved efficacy, the following therapies have been used: dexamethasone, 4 mg intravenously four times a day, during the acute phase; polymorphonuclear leukocyte inhibitors, such as dapsone or colchicine, and oxygen applied to the bite site; and total excision of the lesion to the fascial level.

Alario A et al: Cutaneous necrosis following a spider bite: A case report and review. Pediatrics 1987;79:618.
Clark RF et al: Clinical presentation and treatment of black widow spider envenomation: A review of 163 cases. Ann Emerg Med 1992;21:782.
Wasserman GS, Anderson PC: Loxoscelism and necrotic arachnidism. J Tox Clin Toxicol 1984;21:451.
Yarbrough BE: Current treatment of brown recluse spider bites. Curr Concepts Wound Care 1987;4:1.

THYROID PREPARATIONS
(Thyroid Desiccated,
Sodium Levothyroxine)

Ingestion of the equivalent of 50–150 g of desiccated thyroid can cause signs of hyperthyroidism, including irritability, mydriasis, hyperpyrexia, tachycardia, and diarrhea. Maximal clinical effect occurs about 9 days after ingestion—several days after the protein-bound iodine level has fallen dramatically.

Induce vomiting. If the patient develops clinical signs of toxicity, propranolol, 0.01–0.1 mg/kg (maximum, 1 mg), is useful because of its antiadrenergic activity.

Golightly LK et al: Clinical effects of accidental levothyroxine ingestion in children. Am J Dis Child 1987;141:1025.

Gorman RL et al: High anxiety—low toxicity: A massive T_4 ingestion. Pediatrics 1988;82:666.

VITAMINS

Accidental ingestion of excessive amounts of vitamins rarely causes significant problems. Occasional cases of hypervitaminosis A and D do occur, however, particularly in patients with poor hepatic or renal function. The fluoride contained in many multivitamin preparations is not a realistic hazard, because a 2- or 3-year-old child could eat 100 tablets, containing 1 mg of sodium fluoride per tablet, without producing serious symptoms. Iron poisoning has been reported with multiple vitamin tablets containing iron. Pyridoxine abuse has caused neuropathies; nicotinic acid, myopathy.

Dalton K, Dalton MJT: Characteristics of pyridoxine overdose neuropathy syndrome. Acta Neurol Scand 1987;76:8.

Dean BS, Krenzelok EP: Multiple vitamins and vitamins with iron: Accidental poisoning in children. Vet Hum Toxicol 1988;30:23.

DiPalma JR, Ritchie DM: Vitamin toxicity. Ann Rev Pharm Tox 1977;17:133.

Litin SC, Anderson CF: Nicotinic acid-associated myopathy: A report of three cases. Am J Med 1989;86:481.

WARFARIN

Warfarin is used as a rodenticide. It causes hypoprothrombinemia and capillary injury. It is readily absorbed from the gastrointestinal tract but is absorbed poorly through the skin. A dose of 0.5 mg/kg of warfarin may be toxic in a child. A prothrombin time is helpful in establishing the severity of the poisoning.

Treatment consists of induced vomiting followed by a saline cathartic. If bleeding occurs or the prothrombin time is prolonged, give 1–5 mg of vitamin K_1 (phytonadione) intramuscularly or subcutaneously. For large ingestions with established toxicity, 0.6 mg/kg may be given.

A new group of long-acting anticoagulant rodenticides (brodifacoum, difenacoum, bromadiolone, diphacinone, pinone, valone, and coumatetralyl) have been a more serious toxicologic problem than warfarin. They also cause hypoprothrombinemia and a bleeding diathesis that responds to phytonadione, though the anticoagulant activity may persist for periods ranging from 6 weeks to several months. Treatment with vitamin K_1 may be needed for weeks.

REFERENCES

Baselt RC, Cravey RH: *Disposition of Toxic Drugs and Chemicals in Man,* 3rd ed. Year Book, 1989.

Bresinsky A, Besl H: *A Colour Atlas of Poisonous Fungi: A Handbook for Pharmacists, Doctors, and Biologists.* Wolfe, 1990.

Clayton GD, Clayton FE: *Patty's Industrial Hygiene and Toxicology,* vol 2, 4th ed, Wiley-Interscience, 1993.

Finkel AJ (editor): *Hamilton & Hardy's Industrial Toxicology,* 4th ed. Publishing Sciences Group, 1983.

Goldfrank LR et al: *Goldfrank's Toxicologic Emergencies,* 5th ed. Appleton & Lange, 1998.

Haddad LM, Shanmnon MW, Winchester JF: *Clinical Management of Poisoning and Drug Overdose,* 3rd ed. Saunders, 1998.

Grant WM: *Toxicology of the Eye,* 3rd ed. Thomas, 1986.

Koren G: *Maternal-Fetal Toxicology: A Clinician's Guide,* 2nd ed. Dekker, 1994.

Lampe KF, McCann MA: *AMA Handbook of Poisonous and Injurious Plants.* American Medical Association, 1985.

Olson KR (editor): *Poisoning and Drug Overdose.* Appleton & Lange, 1990.

Rumack BH, Spoerke DG, Smolinske SC (editors): POISINDEX Information System. Micromedex, Inc, Denver, Colorado. [Published quarterly.]

12

Critical Care

Emily L. Dobyns, MD, Anthony G. Durmowicz, MD,
Desmond B. Henry, Jr., MD, Stanley L. Loftness, MD, & Kurt R. Stenmark, MD

Pediatric critical care is a subspecialty devoted to the understanding of the pathophysiology of life-threatening diseases and the development of technical facilities for monitoring and treating these patients. The patients often require the attention of multiple specialized services such as an emergency transport service, stabilization in the emergency department, operative treatment, and nutritional support. It is this high level of interdisciplinary collaboration and communication that has improved patient survival in the ICU.

Children are resilient and have tremendous recovery potential, in many cases recovering from injuries that adults would not survive. They may, however, be nonverbal, uncooperative, and unable to understand their illness or the hospital environment, and thus may require the services provided by social workers, psychiatrists, physical therapists, and speech therapists to help their families and themselves cope with their illness. The dynamic features of continuing growth and development must also be factored into patient and family needs.

The pediatric ICU provides the specialized environment, equipment, and specialists needed to evaluate, diagnose, and treat critically ill patients on a 24-hour basis. This unit permits close observation by experienced team members, thereby permitting rapid responses to changes in the patients' acuity. In many cases, these changes can be anticipated and management plans altered accordingly.

American Academy of Pediatrics, Committee on Hospital Care: Guidelines and levels of care for pediatric intensive care units. Crit Care Med 1993;21:1077.
Hazinski MF: Physician-nurse interaction in the paediatric intensive care unit. In: *Textbook of Pediatric Critical Care.* Holbrook PR (editor). Saunders, 1993.
Pollack MM: Outcome analysis. In: *Textbook of Pediatric Critical Care.* Holbrook PR (editor). Saunders, 1993.

ACUTE RESPIRATORY FAILURE

Respiratory failure is defined as inability of the respiratory system to deliver adequate oxygen or to remove CO_2 from the circulation, leading to arterial hypoxia, hypercapnia, or both. It accounts for approximately 50% of deaths of children under 1 year of age. Infants are at higher risk for respiratory failure because their thoracic cage is soft and provides an unstable base for the ribs. Intercostal muscles are poorly developed, so children cannot achieve the "bucket handle" motion that characterizes adult breathing. Furthermore, the diaphragm is less effective in infants because it is relatively flat and short and has fewer type I muscle fibers. During rapid eye movement (REM) sleep, the ventilatory movements of the rib cage become uncoordinated and out of phase with those of the diaphragm. The infant's trachea is only one-third the diameter of the adult trachea, so a 1-mm thickening of the respiratory mucosa causes a 75% reduction in cross-sectional area in the infant airway, compared to only a 20% reduction in the adult airway. Finally, children's alveoli are smaller and have a greater tendency to collapse and cause atelectasis.

Respiratory failure can be classified into two types, which usually coexist in variable proportion. The Pa_{O_2} is low in both, while the Pa_{CO_2} is high only in type II patients (Table 12–1). Type I is the failure of the lung to oxygenate the blood and occurs in three situations: (1) The most common is a **ventilation/perfusion defect** ($\dot{V}/\dot{Q}$ mismatch), which occurs when blood flows to parts of the lung that are poorly ventilated or underventilated. (2) **Diffusion defects** are caused by thickened alveolar membrane or a buildup of interstitial fluid at the alveolar-capillary junction. (3) **Intrapulmonary shunt** occurs when blood flows through areas of the lung that are never ventilated.

Type II respiratory failure generally results from alveolar hypoventilation and is usually secondary (Table 12–1). Hypoxemia is not always related to respiratory failure. Right-to-left cardiac shunts, high altitude with its low ambient oxygen concentration, and the production of methemoglobin all may produce severe hypoxemia with normal respiratory function.

Clinical Findings

A. Symptoms and Signs: The clinical find-

Table 12–1. Types of respiratory failure.

Findings	Causes	Examples
Type I Hypoxia Decreased PaO_2 Normal $PaCO_2$	Ventilation/perfusion defect	Positional (supine in bed), adult respiratory distress syndrome (ARDS), atelectasis, pneumonia, pulmonary embolus, bronchopulmonary dysplasia
	Diffusion impairment	Pulmonary edema, ARDS, interstitial pneumonia
	Shunt	Pulmonary arteriovenous malformation, congenital adenomatoid malformation
Type II Hypoxia Hypercapnia Decreased PaO_2 Increased $PaCO_2$	Hypoventilation	Neuromuscular disease (polio, Guillain-Barré syndrome), head trauma, sedation, chest wall dysfunction (burns), kyphosis, severe reactive airways

ings in respiratory failure are caused by the low PaO_2, high $PaCO_2$, and pH changes affecting the lungs, heart, kidneys, and brain. Clinical features of progressive respiratory failure are summarized in Table 12–2. Hypercapnia depresses the central nervous system, and the resulting acidemia depresses myocardial function. Patients in respiratory failure can exhibit significant changes in central nervous system and cardiac function (Table 12–2). Features

Table 12–2. Clinical criteria for respiratory failure.

Respiratory
  Wheezing
  Expiratory grunting
  Decreased or absent breath sounds
  Flaring of alae nasi
  Retractions of chest wall
  Tachypnea, bradypnea, or apnea
  Cyanosis
Cerebral
  Restlessness
  Irritability
  Headache
  Confusion
  Convulsions
  Coma
Cardiac
  Bradycardia or excessive tachycardia
  Hypotension or hypertension
General
  Fatigue
  Sweating

of respiratory failure are not always clinically evident, and some signs or symptoms may have nonrespiratory causes. Furthermore, a strictly clinical assessment of arterial hypoxemia or hypercapnia is not reliable. Thus, precise assessment of oxygenation and ventilatory adequacy must be based on both clinical and laboratory data.

B. Laboratory Findings: Laboratory findings are often helpful in gauging the severity and acuity of respiratory failure. Arterial oxygen saturation can be measured continuously and noninvasively by pulse oximetry. Readings may be affected by poor perfusion, hyperbilirubinemia, severe anemia, methemoglobinemia, and hypercapnia. Nevertheless, oximetry should be used in the assessment and management of all patients with suspected respiratory failure. Capnography provides a continuous noninvasive measure of $PaCO_2$. End-tidal CO_2 ($ETCO_2$) approximates alveolar CO_2. $ETCO_2$ may be falsely lowered in severe respiratory disease as a result of increased dead space. Despite this limitation, $ETCO_2$ provides a trend for assessing the disease process over time. Because of this discrepancy and the ongoing need to assess the acid-base status of the patient, **arterial blood gas measurement** remains the best means for assessment of acute respiratory failure. Arterial blood gases give information on the acid-base status (with a measured pH and calculated bicarbonate level) as well as the PaO_2 and $PaCO_2$) in the patient. The $PaCO_2$ is a sensitive measure of ventilation and is inversely related to the minute ventilation (Figure 12–1). Knowing the arterial blood gas values and the

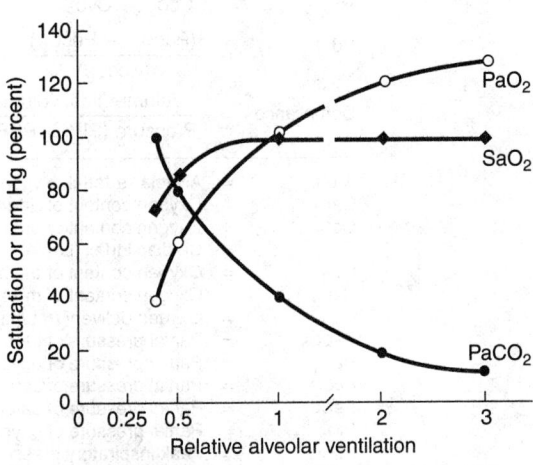

Figure 12–1. Relationship between alveolar ventilation, arterial oxygen saturation (SaO_2), and partial pressures of oxygen and CO_2 in the arterial blood (PaO_2 and $PaCO_2$, respectively). (Reproduced, with permission, from Pagtakhan RD, Chernicic V: Respiratory failure in the pediatric patient. Pediatr Rev 1982;3:244.)

inspired oxygen concentration enables one to calculate several parameters that may be helpful in determining the efficiency of gas exchange. The difference between alveolar oxygen concentration and the arterial oxygen value is the **alveolar-arterial oxygen difference** ($AaDO_2$). The $AaDO_2$ is less than 15 mm Hg under normal conditions, and it increases with increasing inspired oxygen concentrations to about 100 mm Hg in normal patients breathing 100% oxygen. Diffusion impairment, shunts, and $\dot{V}/Q$ mismatches all cause increased $AaDO_2$ (Table 12–3).

In addition to the calculation of the $AaDO_2$, assessment of the intrapulmonary shunting (that percentage of pulmonary blood flow which passes through nonventilated areas of the lung) may be helpful. Normal individuals have less than a 5% physiologic shunt from bronchial, thebesian, and coronary circulations. Shunt fractions greater than 15% usually indicate the need for aggressive respiratory support. When intrapulmonary shunt reaches 50% of pulmonary blood flow, PaO_2 does not increase regardless of the amount of supplemental oxygen used.

Dead space ventilation is that part of the breath in the conducting air passages plus the alveolar volume which is ventilated but not perfused by the pulmonary circulation. Dead space ventilation is increased in bronchopulmonary dysplasia, $\dot{V}/Q$ mismatches, pulmonary interstitial emphysema, pulmonary embolism, and many other entities. Decreasing dead space ventilation depends on its cause, but such methods as tracheostomy in patients with chronic respiratory failure or streptokinase therapy in persons with pulmonary emboli are examples.

Treatment

A. Oxygen Supplementation: Patients with hypoxemia induced by respiratory failure may respond to supplemental oxygen administration alone (Table 12–4). Those with hypoventilation and diffusion defects respond better than patients with shunts or $\dot{V}/Q$ mismatches. Severe $\dot{V}/Q$ mismatches often do not respond to anything but aggressive airway management and mechanical ventilation. Patients with a decreased functional residual capacity (FRC)—the amount of air left in the lungs at the end of passive expiration—often respond to the delivery of continuous positive airway pressure (CPAP), 5–10 cm H_2O by either mask or endotracheal tube. This improves oxygenation by increasing FRC to above closing capacity (closing capacity is the combination of the ex-

Table 12–3. Pulmonary status equations.

PiO_2 = (barometric pressure – 47) × % inspired oxygen concentration
$AaDO_2$ = PiO_2 – ($PaCO_2$/R) – PaO_2 (normal = 5–15 mm Hg)
CO_2 = (1.34 × hemoglobin × SaO_2) + (0.003 × PaO_2)
DO_2 = CaO_2 × CI × 10 (normal 620 ± 50 mL/min/m^2)
Oxygen consumption ($\dot{V}O_2$) = (CaO_2 – CvO_2) × CI × 10 (normal 120–200 mL/min/m^2)

$$\frac{Qs}{Qt} = \frac{CcO_2 - CaO_2}{CcO_2 - CvO_2} \qquad \text{(normal < 5\%)}$$

$$Vd = \frac{(PaCO_2 - PeCO_2)}{(PcCO_2)} \qquad \text{(normal approximately 2 mL/kg)}$$

$$\text{Compliance} = \frac{\text{Volume (tidal volume)}}{\text{Pressure (PIP – PEEP)}} \qquad \text{(normals vary with age)}$$

$AaDO_2$	=	Alveolar-arterial oxygen difference (mm Hg)
CaO_2	=	Oxygen content of arterial blood (mL/dL)
CcO_2	=	Oxygen content of pulmonary capillary blood (mL/dL)
CI	=	Cardiac index (L/min)
CO_2	=	Oxygen content of the blood (mL/dL)
CvO_2	=	Oxygen content of mixed venous blood (mL/dL)
DO_2	=	Oxygen delivery (mL/min)
$PaCO_2$	=	Partial pressure of carbon dioxide in arterial blood (mm Hg)
PaO_2	=	Partial pressure of oxygen in arterial blood (mm Hg)
$PcCO_2$	=	Partial pressure of carbon dioxide in capillary blood (mm Hg)
$PeCO_2$	=	Partial pressure of carbon dioxide in expired air (mm Hg)
PiO_2	=	Partial pressure of oxygen in inspired air (mm Hg)
PIP	=	Peak inspiratory pressure
Qs/Qt	=	Intrapulmonary shunt (in patients without cardiac shunt) (%)
R	=	Respiratory quotient (usually 0.8)
SaO_2	=	Arterial oxygen saturation (fractional)
Vd	=	Physiologic dead space (anatomic dead space + alveolar dead space) (mL)
Ve	=	Expiratory minute volume (L/min)
VO_2	=	Oxygen consumption per minute

Table 12–4. Supplemental oxygen therapy.

Source	Maximum % O_2	Range of Flow Rates	Advantages	Disadvantages
Nasal cannula	35–40%	0.125–4 L/min	Easily applied, relatively comfortable	Uncomfortable at higher flow rates, requires open nasal airways, easily dislodged, lower % O_2, nosebleeds
Simple mask	50–60%	5–10 L/min	Higher % O_2, good for mouth breathers	Uncomfortable, dangerous for patients with poor airway control and at risk for emesis, hard to give airway care, unsure of % O_2
Face tent	40–60%	8–10 L/min	Higher % O_2, good for mouth breathers, less restrictive	Uncomfortable, dangerous for patients with poor airway control and at risk for emesis, hard to give airway care, unsure of % O_2
Rebreathing mask	80–90%	5–10 L/min	Higher % O_2, good for mouth breathers, highest O_2 concentration	Uncomfortable, dangerous for patients with poor airway control and at risk for emesis, hard to give airway care, unsure of % O_2
Oxyhood	90–100%	5–10 L/min (mixed at wall)	Stable and accurate O_2 concentration	Temperature regulation, hard to give airway care

piratory reserve volume and closing volume and represents the volume that the FRC must exceed during tidal breathing to prevent closure of airways). Patients with severe hypoxemia, hypoventilation, or apnea require assistance with bag and mask ventilation until the airway is intubated. Ventilation may be maintained for some time with a mask of the proper size, but gastric distention, emesis, and inadequate tidal volumes are possible complications. An artificial airway may be lifesaving for patients who fail to respond to simple oxygen supplements.

B. Intubation: Intubation of the trachea in infants and children requires experienced personnel and the right equipment. A patient in respiratory failure whose airway must be stabilized should first be properly positioned to facilitate air exchange while supplemental oxygen is given. The sniffing position is used in infants. Head extension with jaw thrust is used in older children without neck injuries. If obstructed by secretions or vomitus, the airway must be cleared by suction. When not obstructed by a foreign body or epiglottitis, airways should open easily with proper positioning and placement of an oral or nasopharyngeal airway of the correct size. Conscious patients tolerate nasal airways better than oral airways. As each step is taken, it is imperative to monitor changes in chest movement, airway and breath sounds, skin color, and mental status. Patients with a normal airway may be intubated under intravenous anesthesia by experienced physicians (Table 12–5). Patients with obstructed upper airways (eg, patients with croup, epiglottitis, foreign bodies, or subglottic stenosis) should be awake when intubated unless trained airway specialists decide otherwise.

The size of the endotracheal tube is of critical importance in pediatrics (see Table 11–3 for sizes). Too large a tube can cause pressure necrosis of the tissues in the subglottic region. (This is the narrowest portion of the upper airway in children—in contrast to the glottis in adults.) The scarring that follows necrosis can cause permanent stenosis of the subglottic region, requiring tracheostomy or cricoid split for repair. Too small an endotracheal tube can result in inadequate pulmonary toilet and excessive air leak around the endotracheal tube, making optimal ventilation and oxygenation difficult. Two useful methods to calculate the size of the endotracheal tube that is appropriate for a child are (1) measuring the height with a Broselow tape and then reading the endotracheal tube size off the tape or (2) in children over 2 years of age, tube size = $(16 + \text{age in years}) \div 4$. Patients under 8 years of age should have uncuffed endotracheal tubes.

After placement of the endotracheal tube, breath sounds should be evaluated for bilateral equality. One should then check for a leak between the endotracheal tube and the larynx. To do this, connect a pressure-monitored anesthesia bag to the circuit and allow it to inflate, creating positive pressure. Check for the leak by auscultating over the throat, noting the pressure at which air escapes around the endotracheal tube. Leaks of 15–20 cm H_2O are acceptable. Larger leaks (> 20 cm H_2O) are acceptable only in patients having severe lung disease and poor compliance and requiring high pressures to achieve ventilation. In this situation, one must be aware of the possible postextubation complications of subglottic stenosis in the patient. A chest x-ray is necessary for final assessment of endotracheal tube placement.

Table 12–5. Drugs commonly used for controlled intubation.

Drug	Dose (mg/kg)	Advantages	Disadvantages
Atropine	0.02; minimum of 0.1	Blocks bradycardia, dries secretions	Tachycardia, fever, histamine release, seizures, coma
Thiopental	3–5	Fast onset, short duration of action	Vascular irritant, negative inotropic, no analgesic properties, histamine release (avoid in asthma), rarely induces porphyria
Ketamine	1–2 IV 4–8 IM	Fast onset, positive inotropic	Increased bronchorrhea, increased pulmonary and systemic vascular resistance, increased intracranial pressure, emergence problems
Succinylcholine (depolarizing muscle relaxant)	1–2	Fast onset, short duration of action	Bradycardia (premedicate with atropine); fasciculations; contraindicated in burns, hyperkalemia, massive trauma, and various neurologic disorders
Pancuronium (nondepolarizing muscle relaxant)	0.1	Lasts 40–60 min, can be given by continuous infusion, reversible	Slow onset (2–3 minutes), tachycardia
Vecuronium (nondepolarizing muscle relaxant)	0.1	Lasts 20–30 min, can be given by continuous infusion, reversible	Slow onset (2–3 minutes)

Artigas A, Bernara GR, Carlet J, et al: The American–European Consensus Conference on ARDs, Part 2. Am J Respir Crit Care Med 1998;157:1332.

Demling RH, Knox JB: Basic concepts of lung function and dysfunction: Oxygenation, ventilation, and mechanics. New Horizons 1993;1:362.

Durmowicz AG, Stenmark KR: Acute respiratory failure. In: *Kendig's Disorders of the Respiratory Tract in Children,* 6th ed. Chernick V and Boat TF (editors). Saunders, 1998.

Prevoznik SJ: Intubation of the trachea. In: *Introduction to Anesthesia,* 7th ed. Dripps RD, Eckenhoff JE, Vandam LD (editors). Saunders, 1988.

Ring JC, Stidham GL: Novel therapies for acute respiratory failure. Pediatr Clin North Am 1994;41:1325.6.

Sachdeva RC, Guntupalli KK: Acute respiratory distress syndrome. Crit Care Clin 1997;13:503.

MECHANICAL VENTILATION

The increased compliance of an infant's chest wall, the increasing number of alveoli until approximately the age of 8, the small size of the airways, and the lack of collateral ventilation make pediatric ventilation challenging. Mechanical ventilators are designed to facilitate movement of air into and out of the lungs and to deliver oxygen. They use either positive pressure to "pump" the lungs full of gas or negative pressure to "suck" air into the lungs, much like the diaphragm does. This section deals with the more commonly used positive-pressure mechanical ventilators that are most appropriate for acute situations.

Pressure Ventilators

Pressure-limited, time-cycled ventilation is increasingly used to ventilate older children and adults to minimize barotrauma. In pressure-limited ventilators, air flow is generated at the start of the inspiratory cycle and continues until a preset pressure is reached. Pressure is maintained until, at the end of the inspiratory time, the exhalation valve opens. Pressure ventilators provide intermittent mandatory ventilation (IMV) so that, when set to 15 breaths per minute, the machine delivers a breath every 4 seconds. Newer ventilators can provide synchronized pressure-limited ventilation. The advantages of pressure-limited ventilators lie in their ability to support spontaneous respirations with continuous gas flow, their avoidance of barotrauma by limiting the pressure of breaths, and their relatively simple operation. The main disadvantages are the possibility of inadequate tidal volumes, especially during periods of rapidly changing lung compliance.

Volume Ventilators

Reduced working volumes and low-compliance ventilator tubing now allow volume ventilators to be used in patients of any age. With these ventilators, a standard tidal volume is set (10–15 mL/kg), and the inspiratory time is set either to an absolute value (0.3–1.5 seconds) or to a percentage of the respiratory cycle. In contrast to pressure-limited ventilators, volume-limited ventilators deliver a preset tidal volume. The pressure generated in response to a preset tidal volume will therefore change as lung compliance changes. There is usually a pressure limit dial where a preset pressure can be set above which the ventilator breath will be halted. This is a safety mechanism to avoid dangerously high lung inflation pressures. These ventilators may function in either an intermittent (IMV) or synchronized (SIMV) fashion. SIMV allows a window of time during which a patient's inspiratory effort will initiate the delivery of a tidal volume and is often helpful in patients breathing spontaneously. Volume ventilators are volume-limited and either volume-cycled or time-cycled. They may provide either continuous flow through the system, allowing uninterrupted access of fresh gas to the patient (which decreases the work of breathing, especially in young infants) or flow that is held in check until an inspiratory effort opens a demand valve.

Volume ventilators may have as added variables an inspiratory hold, volume support, or pressure support. The advantages of volume ventilators include ensured delivery of a preset volume, compliance measurements, and availability of SIMV. Disadvantages of some volume ventilators include possible increased barotrauma from excessive delivery pressure and lack of a continuous flow system.

Positive End-Expiratory Pressure

All mechanical ventilators open their expiratory limbs at the end of inspiration until a preset pressure is achieved; this is the positive end-expiratory pressure (PEEP) value. During ventilation of normal lungs, "physiologic" PEEP is felt to be 2–4 cm H_2O pressure. In disease states, a higher PEEP may increase the FRC, open previously collapsed alveoli, increase mean airway pressure (MAP), and improve oxygenation. A higher PEEP, though often valuable, may cause CO_2 retention, barotrauma with extrapleural air leaks, decreased central venous return, decreased cardiac output, and increased intracranial pressure. Continuous positive airway pressure (CPAP) is the lowest expiratory pressure a spontaneously breathing patient achieves and for practical purposes is synonymous with PEEP. PEEP and CPAP have an optimal setting for each individual patient, maximally improving FRC and $\dot{V}/Q$ mismatches while not causing the problems associated with excessive intrathoracic pressure (see earlier). Multiple parameters have been proposed with varying success to define optimal PEEP. Variables that should be considered in determining appropriate PEEP include PaO_2, central venous pressure, and cardiac output. PEEP should be decreased for pulmonary leak and cerebral edema and may need to be increased for pneumonia, pulmonary edema, and adult respiratory distress syndrome.

Ventilator Management

Mechanical ventilators affect both ventilation and oxygenation. Ventilation is related to alveolar minute volume. On a pressure ventilator, the minute volume is directly related to rate and peak inspiratory pressure; on a volume ventilator, it is related to rate and tidal volume. Thus, increased rate, tidal volume, or peak inspiratory pressure will increase ventilation and should decrease the $PaCO_2$. Changes in oxygenation other than those resulting from the concentration of delivered oxygen depend in part on the variables that determine MAP or the average of all the pressures experienced by the lung in one respiratory cycle. These include PEEP, inspiratory time, and the peak inspiratory pressure delivered. By increasing any of these settings, one achieves an elevation in MAP and, up to a point, an increase in oxygenation. One must remember that increasing these settings can worsen $\dot{V}/Q$ mismatches, decrease cardiac output, and decrease oxygen delivery to the tissue. Therefore, the changes resulting in elevated MAP do not always improve arterial oxygenation or oxygen delivery.

The intubated patient deserves attention directed toward improving comfort and decreasing anxiety. Chloral hydrate, benzodiazepines, and narcotics have been used. Continuous infusions of the short-acting benzodiazepines and opioids create a steady state of sedation. Occasionally, patients are so agitated that ventilation and oxygenation suffer. In these cases, muscle paralysis may facilitate oxygenation and ventilation. The nondepolarizing neuromuscular blocking agents pancuronium bromide and vecuronium bromide are most commonly used for this purpose. They may be given as necessary or as continuous infusions. When giving muscle relaxants, one must be prepared to provide, by mechanical means, ventilation and oxygenation to the patient who previously breathed spontaneously; in most cases, ventilatory support must be increased.

Monitoring the Ventilated Patient

Ventilated patients must be monitored for respiratory rate and activity, chest wall movement, and quality of breath sounds. Oxygenation should be measured either by arterial blood gases or by transmission oximetry with lightweight digital or earlobe probes. O_2 (PtO_2) or CO_2 ($PtCO_2$) can be measured transcutaneously with sufficient accuracy in younger patients with good skin perfusion. $PaCO_2$ may also be assessed by monitoring end-tidal CO_2 ($PetCO_2$). This is done by placing a gas-sampling port on the endotracheal tube and analyzing expired gas for $PetCO_2$. This technique appears to be more valuable in patients with large tidal volumes, and its accuracy improves with more proximal sampling, ie, closer to the airways. $PetCO_2$ values may differ from measured $PaCO_2$ and are most useful for following relative fluctuations in $PaCO_2$.

The ventilator itself has many variables. The most common are tidal volume, minute ventilation, peak inspiratory pressure, and inspiratory and expiratory time. MAP should be monitored in mechanically ventilated patients and maintained as low as possible to achieve adequate oxygenation and ventilation. Work of breathing and oxygen consumption may also be measured; these measurements may be helpful in making ventilator changes in chronically ventilated patients. While technologic advances in monitoring provide more data, they do not substitute for the physical examination and good clinical judgment.

Alternative Methods of Ventilation

High-frequency jet ventilation with passive expiration (300–3000/min) and high-frequency oscillation with active expiration (300–1800/min) have been used to manage select groups of neonates and older pediatric patients, including those suffering from major pulmonary barotrauma (air leaks, pulmonary interstitial emphysema), respiratory distress syndrome, and congenital diaphragmatic hernia. These techniques have also been used to manage patients who have undergone operative procedures on airway structures, so that MAP can be maintained with lower peak inspiratory pressure, thus helping prevent postoperative air leaks at the surgical site.

Pressure-controlled inverse ratio ventilation and permissive hypercapnia have also been used successfully to manage severe respiratory failure such as that seen in adult respiratory distress syndrome. These techniques allow maintenance of high MAP while reducing peak inspiratory pressure and the incidence of barotrauma to as low a level as possible.

Fluorocarbon-based liquids instilled into the lung to fill the FRC have been used to improve oxygenation and lung compliance in children with severe respiratory failure on ECMO. This treatment has been associated with the occurrence of pneumothorax. More extensive evaluation of liquid ventilation is presently under way.

Betit P, Thompson JE, Benjamin PK: Mechanical ventilation. In: *Neonatal and Pediatric Respiratory Care,* 2nd ed. Koff PB, Eitzman D, Neu J (editors). Mosby–Year Book, 1993.

Gowski DT, Miro AM: New ventilatory strategies in acute respiratory failure. Crit Care Nurs Q 1996;19:1.

Martin LD: New approaches to ventilation in infants and children. Curr Opin Pediatr 1995;7:250.3.

ADULT RESPIRATORY DISTRESS SYNDROME (ARDS)

ARDS is a syndrome of acute respiratory failure characterized by increased pulmonary capillary permeability and pulmonary edema that results in refractory hypoxemia, decreased lung compliance, and bilateral diffuse alveolar infiltrates on chest radiography. ARDS accounts for approximately 1% of PICU admissions.

ARDS may be precipitated by a variety of insults (Table 12–6), of which infection is the most common. Despite the diversity of causes, the clinical presentation is remarkably similar in most cases.

Table 12–6. Adult respiratory distress syndrome risk factors.

Direct Lung Injury	Indirect Lung Injury
Aspiration of gastric contents	Sepsis syndrome
Inhalation of toxic fumes	Multiple trauma
Near-drowning	Multiple transfusions
Oxygen toxicity	Fat embolism
Pulmonary contusion	Shock
Pneumonia: bacterial, viral, other	Pancreatitis
	Drug overdoses (especially aspirin, opioids, tricyclic antidepressants, barbiturates)
	Burns

An expanded definition of ARDS or acute lung injury has been developed to define the clinical features better. First, the severity of acute lung injury is scored through assessments of arterial oxygenation (PaO_2/FIO_2), chest radiographs, static lung compliance, and the level of PEEP required. Second, because the clinical disorder or disorders that led to the development of acute lung injury clearly influence the patient's prognosis for recovery, precise definition of the underlying problem becomes important. For instance, although the average mortality rate in this population is 45–60%, the rate is quite variable and dependent on the associated clinical disorder, with mortality rates of 90% in ARDS associated with sepsis and only 10% in ARDS associated with fat embolism. The third part of the definition specifies the failure of organs other than the lung. Nonpulmonary organ failure is of major importance in the outcome of the ARDS patient. For instance, concomitant hepatic failure and ARDS are associated with an almost 100% mortality rate. In fact, any combination of three organs that have failed for more than 7 days carries a 98% mortality rate.

Thus, a more quantitative definition of pulmonary and nonpulmonary organ failure, including the associated clinical disorders, is critical for establishing the actual incidence of ARDS and for determining the prognosis for recovery.

Clinical Presentation & Pathophysiology

ARDS can be roughly divided into four clinical phases (Table 12–7). In the earliest phase, the patient may exhibit dyspnea and tachypnea with a relatively normal PO_2 and a hyperventilation-induced respiratory alkalosis. No significant abnormalities are noted on physical or radiologic examination of the chest. Experimental studies suggest that neutrophils accumulate in the lungs at this stage and that their products damage lung endothelium. Over the next few hours, hypoxemia increases and respiratory distress becomes clinically apparent, with cyanosis, tachycardia, irritability, and dyspnea. Radiographic evidence of early parenchymal change is noted by "fluffy" alveolar in-

Table 12–7. Pathophysiologic changes of modern adult respiratory distress syndrome (low-pressure pulmonary edema).[1]

Radiographic Change	Clinical Findings	Physiologic Change	Pathologic Change
Phase 1 (early changes)			
Normal radiograph	Dyspnea, tachypnea, normal chest examination	Mild pulmonary hypertension, normoxemic or mild hypoxemia, hypercapnia	Neutrophil sequestration, no clear tissue damage
Phase 2 (onset of parenchymal changes)[2]			
Patchy alveolar infiltrates beginning in dependent lung No perivascular cuffs (unless a component of high-pressure edema is present) Normal heart size	Dyspnea, tachypnea, cyanosis, tachycardia, course rales	Pulmonary hypertension, normal wedge pressure, increased lung permeability, increased lung water, increasing shunt, progressive decrease in compliance, moderate to severe hypoxemia	Neutrophil infiltration, vascular congestion, fibrin strands, platelet clumps, alveolar septal edema, intra-alveolar protein, white cells, type I epithelial damage
Phase 3 (acute respiratory failure with progression, 2–10 days)			
Diffuse alveolar infiltrates Air bronchograms Decreased lung volume No bronchovascular cuffs Normal heart	Tachypnea, tachycardia, hyperdynamic state, sepsis syndrome, signs of consolidation, diffuse rhonchi	Phase 2 changes persist. Progression of symptoms, increasing shunt fraction, further decrease in compliance, increased minute ventilation, impaired oxygen extraction of hemoglobin.	Increased interstitial and alveolar inflammatory exudate with neutrophil and mononuclear cells, type II cell proliferation, beginning fibroblast proliferation, thromboembolic occlusion
Phase 4 (pulmonary fibrosis, pneumonia with progression, > 10 days)[3]			
Persistent diffuse infiltrates Superimposed new pneumonic infiltrates Recurrent pneumothorax Normal heart size Enlargement with pulmonale	Symptoms as above, recurrent sepsis, evidence of multiple organ system failure	Phase 3 changes persist. Recurrent pneumonia, progressive lung restriction, impaired tissue oxygenation, impaired oxygen extraction. Multiple organ system failure.	Type II cell hyperplasia, interstitial thickening; infiltration of lymphocytes, macrophages, fibroblasts; loculated pneumonia or interstitial fibrosis; medial thickening and remodeling of arterioles

[1]Modified slightly and reproduced, with permission, from Demling RH: Adult respiratory distress syndrome: Current concepts. New Horizons 1993;1:388.
[2]The process is readily reversible at this stage if the initiating factor is controlled.
[3]Multiple organ system failure is common. The mortality rate is greater than 80% at this stage, since resolution is more difficult.

filtrates initially appearing in dependent lung fields, indicative of pulmonary edema. The edema fluid typically has a high concentration of protein (75–95% of plasma protein concentration) which is characteristic of an increased-permeability edema and differentiates it from cardiogenic or hydrostatic pulmonary edema. Epithelial injury in ARDS lowers the threshold for alveolar edema and impairs gas exchange. If patients can reabsorb the alveolar edema within 12 hours of formation, alveolar epithelial function remains reasonably intact and there is an excellent chance for recovery. In contrast, patients who have no change in edema fluid content or protein concentration in the first 12 hours after onset of mechanical ventilation have a much higher mortality rate. Pulmonary hypertension, decreases in lung compliance, and increases in airway resistance are also noted. Clinical studies suggest that airway resistance may be increased in 50% of patients with ARDS.

Type II cell and fibroblast proliferation occur in the interstitium of the lung during the subacute phase of ARDS (5–10 days after lung injury). Decreased lung volumes and signs of consolidation are noted clinically and radiographically. Worsening of the hypoxemia with an increasing shunt fraction as well as a further decrease in lung compliance are noted. Some patients develop an accelerated fibrosing alveolitis in which there is a marked increase in fibroblasts and collagen formation in the interstitium. The mechanisms responsible for these changes are not clear. Current investigation centers on the role of growth and differentiation factors such as transforming growth factor b and platelet-derived growth factor released by resident and nonresident lung cells such as alveolar macrophages, mast cells, neutrophils, alveolar type II cells, and fibroblasts.

During the chronic phase of ARDS (10–14 days after lung injury), there is fibrosis, emphysema, and pulmonary vascular obliteration. Patients usually do not have as severe an oxygenation defect as they did in the acute phase, and the requirements for PEEP may decline. Patients have large amounts of dead space and may require a high minute ventilation. Their compliance remains low, perhaps because of pulmonary fibrosis and insufficient surface-active material.

Secondary infections are common in the subacute and chronic phases of ARDS and significantly influence the outcome. The mechanisms responsible for increased host susceptibility to infection during this phase are not well understood.

The mortality rates in the late phase of ARDS exceed 80%. Death is usually caused by multiple organ failure and systemic hemodynamic instability rather than by hypoxia.

Treatment

A. Ventilatory Support: An FIO_2 greater than 50% over 24 hours can cause lung injury to ARDS patients, so positive-pressure ventilation and PEEP are used to improve oxygenation. Ventilation is best on a volume ventilator because of rapidly changing compliance of the lungs. Poor compliance may result in high peak inspiratory pressure. PEEP is used to open collapsed alveoli, reduce shunting, and increase FRC above the closing volume. All these measures decrease dead space ventilation and may improve oxygenation. The PEEP that provides the best combination of oxygenation, lung compliance, cardiac output, and lowered intrapulmonary shunt is found by increasing the PEEP by increments (2–3 cm H_2O every 30 minutes) until pulmonary and hemodynamic measurements fit the patient's requirements. PEEPs of 15–25 cm H_2O have been used successfully in some patients. Before increasing PEEP, one should optimize conditions by making sure that the intravascular volume is appropriate, the endotracheal tube does not leak, and the patient is well sedated or paralyzed. A Qs/Qt of less than 15%, oxygen saturations greater than 90% while being ventilated with an FIO_2 of less than 60%, and a good cardiac output may signal the end point of PEEP adjustments.

Blood gases (PaO_2 and $PaCO_2$) should not be normalized at the cost of injuring the lung with high pressures and high concentrations of oxygen. Permissive hypercapnia in the face of normal blood pH is acceptable. Newer ventilator strategies (discussed above in the section on Alternative Methods of Ventilation) are also being tried in an attempt to decrease lung injury. These include primarily a switch from volume-controlled to pressure-controlled ventilation, or high-frequency oscillatory ventilation (HFOV).

B. Hemodynamic Support: Hemodynamic support is directed toward increasing perfusion and oxygen delivery. Volume expansion is achieved by giving packed red blood cells to maintain the hematocrit between 40% and 50% and by giving colloid or crystalloid solutions to nonanemic volume-depleted patients. There is no one recommendation on the type of fluid to give the nonanemic patient. Certainly, colloids should be used in patients with low intravascular oncotic pressures as estimated by reduced total protein or albumin concentrations. In all other ARDS patients, however, the optimal fluid resuscitation has not been well established. Use of inotropic drugs is often necessary. The most effective inotropic dosages should be determined by monitoring blood pressure, urinary output, cardiac output, pulmonary and systemic vascular resistances, and the patient's gas exchange.

C. Control of Infection: Prevention or early treatment of infection is an extremely important aspect of the management of ARDS.

D. Pharmacotherapy: Drug therapies have not proved particularly successful. Clinical studies have not shown that steroids, ibuprofen, or indomethacin benefit ARDS patients. Vasodilators such as nitroglycerin, sodium nitroprusside, prostaglandin E_1 and I_2, and calcium channel blockers have all been used to combat pulmonary vasoconstriction, but their use is frequently limited by the development of systemic hypotension. As yet, there is no clear evidence suggesting that these drugs have beneficial effects. Some enthusiasm exists for the treatment of patients with antibodies specific to circulating mediators of sepsis and lung injury. In a number of carefully controlled clinical trials of anticytokine agents, it has not been possible to demonstrate any significant difference in outcomes. A recent trial of adults with ARDS treated with liposomal prostaglandin E_1 demonstrated an improvement in oxygenation, lung compliance, and decrease in number of days on mechanical ventilation. Further evaluation is needed.

E. Monitoring: Multiorgan system monitoring is needed in patients with ARDS. Ventilation can be assessed by monitoring arterial blood gases, oxygen saturation, and end-tidal CO_2. Lung compliance should be known as increases in PEEP or tidal volume are made. Obtaining chest films daily is important for patients receiving vigorous support because severe ARDS is associated with a 40–60% incidence of air leaks. Hemodynamic monitoring should include, at a minimum, central venous monitoring to determine volume status; if PEEPs greater than 12 cm H_2O are used, a pulmonary artery catheter is recommended. Surveillance for infection or sepsis—by monitoring with cultures (blood, urine, tracheal aspirate, cerebrospinal fluid) and following the temperature curve and white blood cell count—is important because secondary infections are common and increase the mortality rate strikingly. Renal, liver, and gastrointestinal function need close attention because of the great likelihood of multiple organ dysfunction.

F. Alternative Management: New techniques have evolved in the respiratory treatment of ARDS. High-frequency ventilation has proved helpful only in patients with large air leaks, although more and better trials evaluating the efficacy of high-frequency oscillatory or jet ventilation are needed. Surfactant replacement therapy has been tried with some success in patients with ARDS. Surfactant replacement, in some instances, improves lung compliance and allows patients' lungs to be ventilated at a smaller FIO_2, with weaning from mechanical ventilation earlier than in nontreated patients. In randomized trials of surfactant, there were no differences in outcome (death, length of ventilation or hospitalization), but there was some evidence of decreased inflammation. Pediatric patients with severe ARDS who received extracorporeal membrane oxygenation (ECMO) have better survival rates than historical controls. Other less invasive methods such as HFOV or inhaled nitric oxide are being used earlier and more frequently than in the past with some anecdotal success. This has made further prospective randomized studies of ECMO difficult to complete. ECMO remains a rescue therapy for patients with severe ARDS unresponsive to other modalities. Criteria for selecting which patients should receive these new therapies have not been established. Very recent reports have demonstrated that inhaled nitric oxide may be beneficial in ARDS. This effect is based on the ability of NO to reduce pulmonary artery pressure and to improve the matching of ventilation with perfusion without producing systemic vasodilation. Patient selection and efficacy of these new therapies have yet to be established, but many of them are being documented in prospective randomized clinical trials.

G. Follow-Up: The follow-up of pediatric ARDS patients is limited. One report of 10 children followed 1–4 years after severe ARDS showed 3 still symptomatic and 7 with hypoxemia at rest. Until further information is available, all patients with a history of ARDS need close follow-up of pulmonary function.

Abraham E et al: Liposomal prostaglandin E$_1$ in acute respiratory distress syndrome: A placebo-controlled, randomized, double-blind, multicenter clinical trial. Crit Care Med 1996;24:10.

Chollet-Martin S et al: Alveolar neutrophil functions and cytokine levels in patients with the adult respiratory distress syndrome during nitric oxide inhalation. Am J Respir Crit Care Med 1996;153:985.

Demling RH: Adult respiratory distress syndrome: Current concepts. New Horizons 1993;1:388.

Gattinoni L et al: Effects of positive end-expiratory pressure on regional distribution of tidal volume and recruitment in adult respiratory distress syndrome. Am J Respir Crit Care Med 1995;151:1807.

MacNaughton PD, Evans TW: Management of adult respiratory distress syndrome. Lancet 1992;339:469.

Walmrath D et al: Direct comparison of inhaled nitric oxide and aerosolized prostacyclin in acute respiratory distress syndrome. Am J Respir Crit Care Med 1996;153:991.

Weiner-Kronish JP, Gropper MA, Matthay MA: The adult respiratory distress syndrome: Definition and prognosis, pathogenesis and treatment. Br J Anaesth 1990;65:107.

ASTHMA (LIFE-THREATENING)

Status asthmaticus may be defined as reversible small airway obstruction that is refractory to sympathomimetic and anti-inflammatory agents and which may progress to respiratory failure without prompt and aggressive intervention. Life-threatening asthma is caused by severe bronchospasm, excessive mucous secretion, inflammation, and edema of the airways (Chapter 17). Reversal of these mechanisms is the key to successful treatment. Status asthmaticus remains a common diagnosis among children admitted to the ICU, and asthma continues to be associated with a surprisingly high mortality rate.

The physical examination helps determine the severity of illness. Accessory muscle (sternocleidomastoid) use correlates well with an FEV$_1$ and peak expiratory flow rates (PEFRs) less than 50% of normal predicted values. A paradoxic pulse of over 22 mm Hg has been correlated with elevated PaCO$_2$ levels. The absence of wheezing may be misleading because, in order to produce a wheezing sound, the patient must take in a certain amount of air. The arterial blood gas remains the single most important laboratory determination in the evaluation of a child in severe status asthmaticus. Patients with severe respiratory distress, signs of exhaustion, alterations in consciousness, elevated PaCO$_2$, or acidosis should be admitted to the PICU.

Treatment

Because of inadequate minute ventilation and $\dot{V}/\dot{Q}$ mismatching, severe asthmatics are almost always hypoxemic and should receive supplemental humidified oxygen immediately.

A. Pharmacotherapy:

1. Nebulized β$_2$-agonist therapy such as with albuterol or terbutaline remains first-line therapy to reverse acute bronchoconstriction. If the patient is in severe distress and has poor inspiratory flow rates, thus preventing adequate delivery of nebulized medication, subcutaneous injection of epinephrine or terbutaline may be required. The frequency of β$_2$-agonist administration varies according to the severity of the patient's symptoms and the occurrence of adverse side effects. Albuterol may be given continuously by nebulization, usually without serious side effects. However, the heart rate and blood pressure of these patients should be closely monitored, as excessive tachycardia and ventricular ectopy may occur.

2. Theophylline confers additional benefit when given with steroids and β$_2$ agonists. Besides bronchodilation, it decreases mucociliary inflammatory mediators and reduces microvascular permeability. When the decision to add theophylline to high-dose β$_2$-agonist therapy for severe status asthmaticus is being weighed, the increased risk of serious side effects such as tachycardia and cardiac arrhythmias must be considered.

3. **Systemic corticosteroids,** by decreasing inflammation, stabilizing mast cells, and increase β$_2$-agonist receptors, speed the resolution of severe asthma exacerbations refractory to bronchodilator therapy and should be given to all patients admitted to the hospital with severe asthma. The optimal dose is not known, although a frequently used dosage is 1 mg/kg of intravenous methylprednisolone every 6 hours. The acute complications of corticosteroid usage include gastrointestinal bleeding and perforations.

4. Nebulized **anticholinergic agents** are also recommended, at least as a trial, in severe asthmatics. In some patients, cholinergic-related bronchoconstriction is more marked than in others, so not all patients respond. Nebulized ipratropium bromide is the drug of choice. Atropine has more potential side effects than ipratropium bromide, for example, tachycardia, urinary retention, and pupillary dilation, but can be given up to every 6 hours.

5. **Terbutaline,** a relatively specific β_2 agonist, is used intravenously in children with severe airway obstruction and impending respiratory failure. Owing to its relative specificity for β_2 receptors, terbutaline has fewer cardiac side effects than previously available intravenous beta agonists. Patients receiving intravenous beta-agonist therapy should have indwelling arterial lines for continuous pressure and blood gas monitoring and have cardiac enzymes monitored for signs of myocardial damage.

B. Specific Drugs and Dosages:

1. Give humidified oxygen Try to keep O_2 saturations at 90% or higher.

2. Beta-sympathomimetic therapy Albuterol or terbutaline by nebulization (albuterol, 0.1 mg/kg per nebulization, up to 2.5 mg; or terbutaline, 0.1–0.2 mg/kg per nebulization, up to 4 mg). Albuterol may be given continuously at a dose of 0.5 mg/kg/h to a maximum of 15 mg/h.

3. Corticosteroids–Methylprednisolone, 2 mg/kg intravenously as a loading dose, then 1 mg/kg intravenously every 6 hours.

4. Intravenous aminophylline–Each 1 mg/kg of aminophylline given as a loading dose will increase the level by approximately 2 mg/dL. In a patient who has not previously received aminophylline or oral theophylline preparations, load with 7–8 mg/kg of aminophylline in an attempt to achieve a level of 15 mg/dL; then start a continuous infusion of aminophylline at a dosage of 0.8–1 mg/kg/h. Watch closely for toxicity (gastric upset, tachycardia, seizures) and follow levels closely, trying to maintain steady-state levels of 12–16 mg/dL.

5. Anticholinergic therapy–Atropine, 0.025–0.05 mg/kg per dose up to 2 mg every 6–8 hours by nebulization, or ipratropine bromide, 60–80 mg by metered-dose inhaler or 250 mg by nebulization every 6 hours, is useful in some patients.

6. Intravenous beta-sympathomimetic therapy–This should be used only in patients who have not responded to the preceding steps and have worsening respiratory failure. Give **terbutaline,** 10 mg/kg over 10 minutes as a loading dose, and then start an infusion at 0.1 mg/kg/min, increasing by increments of 0.1 mg/kg/min every 30 minutes until a response

is achieved or side effects (tachycardia, tremor, nausea) become apparent.

7. Intravenous administration of magnesium sulfate–This has been reported as an effective bronchodilator in adults with severe status asthmaticus. Its smooth muscle relaxation properties are probably caused by interference with calcium flux in the bronchial smooth muscle cell.

C. Mechanical Ventilation: If the above aggressive management fails to result in significant improvement, mechanical ventilation may be necessary. In general, if there is steady deterioration (increased acidosis, rising $PaCO_2$), despite intensive therapy for asthma, the patient should be intubated and mechanically ventilated. Mechanical ventilation in asthmatics is difficult and by no means simplifies treatment. The goal of mechanical ventilation in an intubated asthmatic is to maintain adequate oxygenation and ventilation with the least amount of barotrauma until other therapies become effective. Airway obstruction from persistent bronchoconstriction remains a major problem because the constricted bronchus is lined with smooth muscle, and paralyzing drugs affect only skeletal muscle. The patient, once intubated, should remain paralyzed and sedated. A volume ventilator is necessary to deliver a reasonable tidal volume in patients with poor lung compliance. Expiratory time should be prolonged to avoid air trapping. The IMV rate may need to be lowered to allow sufficient expiration time. PEEP should be kept low. There are isolated reports of patients who require greater PEEP, but these are the exception. Aerosolized beta agonists may be given through the ventilator circuit and should be administered as close to the endotracheal tube as possible.

Weaning the very ill asthmatic from ICU therapy should begin with ventilatory support followed by the aggressive drug therapy. Changes should be made slowly, because patients can rebound and worsen quickly.

D. Metabolic Changes in the Severe Asthmatic: Metabolic disorders may occur in the severe asthmatic. Hypercapnia, hypoxia, and a poor perfusion may lead to acidosis. Slow intravenous sodium bicarbonate therapy (1 mEq/kg for pH < 7.20) in the ventilated patient is a reasonable treatment of metabolic acidosis, although it may raise the $PaCO_2$. Hypokalemia is also a complication of beta-agonist therapy, and serum potassium needs to be monitored, especially in patients receiving nebulized beta-agonist drugs continuously.

E. Monitoring: Severe asthmatics should be monitored for heart rate, blood pressure, O_2 saturation, and arterial pH and $PaCO_2$. Ventilator monitoring must be meticulous, because increases in peak inspiratory pressure or decreases in pulmonary compliance may signal worsening bronchoconstriction or an extrapleural air leak. In addition, if the patient is mechanically ventilated and paralyzed, the degree of nerve block should be monitored using an electrical stimulator, as nondepolarizing agents given with corticosteroids can cause prolonged paralysis and muscle weakness. Chest films of ventilated asthmatics should be obtained daily.

Brugman SM, Larsen GL: Asthma in infants and small children. Clin Chest Med 1995;16:637.

DeNicola LK et al: Treatment of critical status asthmaticus in children. Pediatr Clin North Am 1994;41:1293.

Dhand R, Tobin MJ: Inhaled bronchodilator therapy in mechanically ventilated patients. Am J Respir Crit Care Med 1997;156:3.

Koff PB, Durmowicz AG: Pharmacology. In: *Neonatal and Pediatric Respiratory Care,* 2nd ed. Koff PB, Eitzman D, Neu J (editors). Mosby Year Book, 1993.

Manthous CA: Management of severe exacerbations of asthma. Am J Med 1995;99:298.

National Asthma Education Program, Expert Panel Report: *Guidelines for the Diagnosis and Management of Asthma 1991.* National Heart, Lung, and Blood Institute, 1991.

POSTOPERATIVE CARDIAC MANAGEMENT

The outcome for pediatric patients undergoing cardiac surgery has been improved by advances in surgical technique, myocardial preservation, and postoperative care. A clear understanding of the preoperative anatomy and dysfunction (eg, the existence of pulmonary hypertension in lesions associated with high pulmonary blood flow), the operative repair, the intraoperative events, and the postoperative hemodynamic and metabolic conditions is necessary for postoperative care.

Cardiopulmonary bypass and deep hypothermic arrest affect the function of multiple organs. Some of the effects most pertinent to postoperative care include increased total body water, transient myocardial dysfunction, gas exchange abnormalities, coagulation abnormalities, and hormonal and stress responses. In addition, general anesthesia is associated with atelectasis and decreased functional reserve capacity. Postoperative management seeks to minimize these adverse effects. Close monitoring of the patient allows early recognition and response to changing hemodynamic, respiratory, and metabolic status. Physical assessment of heart and breath sounds is helpful in detecting cardiac tamponade, pneumothorax, and signs of congestive heart failure.

Ventricular function is determined by measuring systemic arterial pressure and waveform, heart rate, skin color, extremity perfusion, peripheral pulses, urinary output, core temperature, and acid-base status. In some cases, cardiac output is measured by thermodilution with a pulmonary artery catheter. The factors that influence cardiac output (preload or end-diastolic volume, afterload or systolic wall tension, contractility,

heart rate, rhythm) are assessed and manipulated as needed. If cardiac output is inadequate, the first approach should be to increase the blood volume so as to increase cardiac filling. A second approach is to reduce the cardiac afterload with a vasodilator such as nitroprusside. Inotropic agents (dopamine, dobutamine) are added if these initial adjustments fail.

Conduction abnormalities are common in the postoperative period. They can be related to electrolyte abnormalities, rewarming following hypothermia, or injury to the conduction pathways. Since heart rate and rhythm can affect cardiac output, cardiac rhythm is continuously monitored by electrocardiography to detect arrhythmias rapidly. Tachycardia can be particularly detrimental, because it shortens diastolic filling (decreasing preload and reducing coronary artery perfusion) and increases myocardial oxygen demand. Treatment is directed first to the cause (eg, normalizing temperature and electrolytes, pain control) and may require specific antiarrhythmics or pacing.

Following surgery, the right ventricle can be small and stiff. Its function can be improved by reducing pulmonary vascular resistance (PVR). Pulmonary vascular tone can be reduced by giving oxygen or inhaled nitric oxide and by manipulating gas exchange, pH, and lung volumes with mechanical ventilation. PVR can also be lowered by inducing a respiratory alkalosis by alterations in both ventilatory rate and volume. Maintaining appropriate lung volumes, especially FRC, is critical to reducing PVR. Compression of the pulmonary microvasculature by atelectasis and compression of the capillaries in the alveolar septum by hyperinflation are both associated with elevation of the PVR. Both of these extremes should be avoided by appropriate manipulation of tidal volume, PEEP, and inspiratory pressure. Postoperative pain management is easier in patients whose ventilation is mechanically maintained. This is needed to reduce stress and labile hemodynamic responses to pain. The patient's primary lesion and postoperative complications dictate how aggressively the patient can be weaned from the ventilator. Extubation is considered when the patient is hemodynamically stable, arrhythmias are controlled, reoperation is not planned, and the patient can maintain an airway with satisfactory gas exchange.

Castaneda AR, Mayer JE, Jonas RA: The neonate with critical congenital heart disease. Repair: A surgical challenge. J Thorac Cardiovasc Surg 1989;98:869.

Wieman DS et al: Perioperative respiratory management in cardiac surgery. Clin Chest Med 1993;14:283.

Zaloga GP et al: Pharmacologic cardiovascular support. Crit Care Clin 1993;9:335.

SHOCK

Shock may be defined as failure of the cardiovascular system to deliver critical substrates and to remove toxic metabolites. This failure leads to anaerobic metabolism in cells and ultimately to irreversible cellular damage. Shock has been categorized into a series of recognizable stages: compensated, uncompensated, and irreversible. Patients in compensated shock have relatively normal cardiac output and normal blood pressures, but they have alterations in the microcirculation that increase flow to some organs and reduce flow to others. In infants, compensatory increases in cardiac output are achieved primarily by tachycardia rather than by increases in stroke volume. Heart rates of 190–210/min are common in infants with compensated shock, but heart rates over 220/min raise the possibility of supraventricular tachycardia. In older patients, cardiac contractility (stroke volume) and heart rate increase to improve cardiac output. Blood pressure remains normal initially because of peripheral vasoconstriction and increased systemic vascular resistance. Thus, hypotension occurs late and is more characteristic of the uncompensated stage of shock. In the uncompensated stage, there is further deterioration of the oxygen and nutrient supply to the cells with subsequent cellular breakdown and release of toxic substances, causing further redistribution of flow. At this point, the patient is hypotensive, with poor cardiac output. Irreversible shock involving organ damage of the brain and heart is terminal.

The causes of shock are hypovolemic, cardiogenic, and distributive. Often, two or three of these occur together. **Hypovolemic shock** is caused by decreased circulating blood volume. This may result from loss of whole blood or plasma or from fluid loss from the kidney or gut. These patients usually have intact compensatory mechanisms which maintain normal blood pressure by increasing cardiac output and shunting blood away from certain organs. All these responses serve to protect blood flow to the heart and brain. Untreated, hypovolemic shock can progress to an irreversible stage.

Cardiogenic shock is an ominous state of decreased substrate delivery secondary to "pump failure." The causes include congenital heart disease, cardiac surgery (following cardioplegia and ventriculotomy), cardiomyopathy secondary to infection or toxins, and ischemic-reperfusion injuries. The patient's compensatory efforts (eg, release of catecholamines with increases in blood pressure, heart rate, and systemic vascular resistance) often have deleterious effects on an already stressed and injured myocardium.

"Distributive shock" is a catchall phrase for those cases that involve arterial and capillary shunting past tissue beds with an increase in venous capacitance. Examples include anaphylaxis and septic shock. Gram-negative septic shock appears to be mediated by endotoxins (lipopolysaccharides) and subsequent formation of cytokines (tumor necrosis factor, interleukin-1 [IL-1], IL-10), eicosanoid products, brady-

kinin, and endorphins. These agents can directly mediate many of the manifestations of septic shock, and they also amplify the injury by attracting granulocytes and macrophages—cells that cause further epithelial injury, activate additional cells, and release mediators. Vasodilators (prostaglandin I_2, endorphins) predominate early, causing a drop in systemic vascular resistance. Cardiac output generally is increased to compensate for the decreased systemic vascular resistance. This phase has been described as "warm shock," since the skin remains well perfused and warm. As septic shock progresses, the heart is no longer able to maintain such a high output, and vasoconstrictors (thromboxane, leukotrienes, endothelin) predominate, with resultant decreased peripheral perfusion. Extremities become cool, urine output decreases, and oxygen delivery falls. The speed with which distributive shock progresses varies according to the cause; it can be quite fast in anaphylaxis and insidious in cases associated with gram-positive cocci.

Other Organ Involvement

Organ dysfunction during and after an episode of shock is common. Systems most often affected include the kidney, the blood coagulation system, the lungs, the central nervous system, the liver, and the gastrointestinal tract. The kidney responds to hypotension by increasing plasma renin and angiotensin concentrations, causing a decrease in glomerular filtration rate and urine output. This can progress to damage of the energy-consuming renal parenchyma, causing acute tubular necrosis. Coagulopathies may exist in any type of shock but are especially common in septic shock. They result from the release of mediators that activate the clotting cascade, leading ultimately to a consumptive coagulopathy. The central nervous system dysfunction is related to decreased cerebral perfusion pressure and thus to decreased substrate delivery to the brain. Liver dysfunction commonly occurs after shock and may be manifested by increases in liver enzymes or a bleeding diathesis. Gastrointestinal problems include ileus, bleeding (eg, gastritis, ulcers), and necrosis with sloughing of intestinal mucosa. These organ system complications should be aggressively searched for after an episode of shock. Multiple organ system failure secondary to shock greatly increases the mortality rates.

Monitoring

Both noninvasive and invasive monitoring of the patient in shock provides information on the severity, progression, and response to treatment. Extremely valuable information can be derived from examination of the cardiovascular, central nervous, renal, musculoskeletal, and mucocutaneous systems.

A. Clinical Findings:

1. Cardiovascular system—Tachycardia is not always present even in profound hypotension. Hypotension occurs late in pediatric shock (mean systolic blood pressure for a child over 2 years of age can be estimated by adding 90 mm Hg to twice the age in years). An important part of the cardiovascular examination is simultaneous palpation of distal and proximal pulses. An increase in the amplitude difference of pulses between proximal arteries (carotid, brachial, femoral) and distal arteries (radial, posterior tibial, dorsalis pedis) can be palpated in early shock and reflects increased systemic vascular resistance. Distal pulses may be thready or absent even in the presence of normal blood pressure because of poor stroke volume compensated by tachycardia and increased systemic vascular resistance. In uncompensated shock, hypotension is present and proximal pulses are also diminished. Early shock causes peripheral cutaneous vasoconstriction, which preserves flow to vital organs.

2. Skin–Because of peripheral vasoconstriction, the skin is gray or ashen in newborns and pale and cold in older patients. Capillary refilling after blanching is slow (> 3 seconds). Mottling of the skin may also be observed.

3. Musculoskeletal system–Decreased oxygen delivery to the musculoskeletal system produces hypotonia. Decreased spontaneous motor activity, flaccidity, and prostration are observed.

4. Urinary output–Urine output is directly proportionate to renal blood flow and the glomerular filtration rate. Catheterization of the bladder is necessary to give accurate and continuous information. (Normal urine output is ≥ 1 mL/kg/h; outputs < 0.5 mL/kg/h are considered significantly decreased.)

5. Central nervous system–The patient's level of consciousness reflects the adequacy of cortical perfusion. When this is severely impaired, the infant or child fails to respond first to verbal stimuli, then to light touch, and finally to pain. Lack of motor response and failure to cry in response to venipuncture or lumbar puncture should alert the clinician to the severity of the situation. In uncompensated shock in the presence of hypotension, brain stem perfusion may be decreased. Poor thalamic perfusion can result in loss of sympathetic tone. Finally, poor medullary flow produces irregular respirations followed by gasping, apnea, and respiratory arrest.

B. Invasive Monitoring: Patients with poor cardiac output who are hypovolemic often need invasive monitoring for diagnostic and therapeutic reasons. Arterial catheters give constant blood pressure readings, and, to an experienced interpreter, the shape of the waveform is helpful in evaluating cardiac output. Central venous pressure monitoring gives useful information about relative changes in volume status as therapy is given. Central venous pressure monitoring does not provide information about absolute volume status because intravascular volume, which is considered preload, is most accurately inferred from left ventricular end-diastolic pressures. Therefore, intravascular volume is more accurately assessed by monitoring pulmonary capillary wedge pressure or left atrial pressure. Measurements of pulmonary capillary wedge pressure can be obtained with a pulmonary artery catheter. The pulmonary artery catheter provides additional valuable information on volume and cardiac status (Table 12–8) but is associated with a higher complication rate than central venous pressure lines. Measurements of arterial and mixed venous oxygen saturations, along with cardiac output data, are useful in calculating oxygen delivery, consumption, and extraction. Oxygen consumption is frequently reduced long before hypotension is present. With the use of a pulmonary artery catheter, the effects of manipulating hemoglobin, oxygen saturation, and cardiac output (the determinants of oxygen consumption and delivery) can be followed in attempts to achieve independence of oxygen delivery and consumption. Patients receiving significant inotropic or ventilatory support may also benefit from the placement of a pulmonary artery catheter.

Table 12–8. Hemodynamic parameters.[1]

Parameter	Formula[2]	Normal Values	Units
Cardiac output	$CO = HR \times SV$	Wide age-dependent range	L/min
Cardiac index	$CI = CO/BSA$	3.5–5.5	$L/min/m^2$
Stroke index	$SI = SV/BSA$	30–60	mL/m^2
Systemic vascular resistance	$SVR = 79.9 \dfrac{(MAP - CVP)}{CI}$	800–1600	dyne s/cm^{-5}/m^2
Pulmonary vascular resistance	$PVR = 79.9 \dfrac{(MPAP - PCWP)}{CI}$	80–240	dyne s/cm^{-5}/m^2

[1]Formulas and normals from Katz RW, Pollack M, Weibley R: Pulmonary artery catheterization in pediatric intensive care. Adv Pediatr 1984;30:169.
[2]HR = heart rate, SV = stroke volume, BSA = body surface area, MAP = mean arterial pressure, CVP = central venous pressure, MPAP = mean pulmonary artery pressure, PCWP = pulmonary capillary wedge pressure.

Treatment

A. Fluid Resuscitation: A timely infusion of fluids may reverse the shock in patients with hypovolemic and distributive shock. Patients with cardiogenic shock, however, may worsen when given intravenous fluids unnecessarily because of the diminished ability of the left ventricle to handle volume.

Initially, most patients tolerate crystalloid (salt solution), which is readily available and inexpensive. However, 4 hours after a crystalloid infusion, only 20% of the solution remains in the intravascular space. Patients with serious capillary leaks and ongoing plasma losses (eg, burn cases) should initially receive crystalloid, because in these cases colloid (protein and salt solution) leaks into the interstitium. The protein draws intravascular fluid into the interstitium, thus increasing ongoing losses. Patients with hypoalbuminemia or those with intact capillaries who need to retain volume in the intravascular space (eg, patients at risk for cerebral edema) probably benefit from colloid infusions. Experience with dextran (a starch compound dissolved in salt solution) is limited. The amount of fluids given should be governed by physical examination, cardiovascular status, and laboratory results. Patients with normal heart function tolerate increased volume better than those with poor function.

B. Pharmacotherapy: Inotropic support may be needed in patients unable to meet the increased demand for cardiac output. Dopamine can increase renal, coronary, and cerebral blood flow by its action on beta receptors and dopaminergic receptors. At higher doses (15 mg/kg/min), alpha-vasoconstrictor actions predominate. Dobutamine is often added to dopamine. Indeed, dobutamine may be the drug of choice in low cardiac output states because—unlike dopamine—it increases stroke volume and therefore cardiac output while decreasing left ventricular wall tension and myocardial oxygen consumption. Norepinephrine can be used to increase peripheral vasoconstriction, especially in septic shock. Epinephrine should be used with caution because it increases heart rate and afterload, neither of which may be well tolerated in the failing heart. Patients with increased systemic vascular resistance receiving cardiotonic drugs may benefit from a direct vasodilator to reduce the systemic vascular resistance or afterload and increase cardiac contractility (Table 12–9).

The role of inflammation in the pathogenesis of shock continues to be defined. Infusion of endotoxin and other mediators into animals or humans has reproduced many of the pathophysiologic features of sepsis. Drugs that block these mediators appear to be beneficial when given early to animals. Human studies of these same blockers have failed to demonstrate a clear benefit. The discrepancies may result from the low-affinity binding and insufficient neutralizing of lipopolysaccharide by these antibodies. The molecular mechanisms by which lipopolysaccharide activates cells are becoming better understood, which may assist in the development of effective therapies. The roles of inflammatory mediators and how they interact to injure or benefit the host are understood less well. Ibuprofen, with its ability to block cyclooxygenase (cyclo-oxygenase metabolites are known inflammatory mediators), has shown a trend toward stabilizing patients with septic shock, and clinical trials are planned. Recently, excess production of NO has been demonstrated to contribute to the hypotension and poor perfusion seen in shock. Analogs of L-arginine (L-NMA) have been used to block the production of NO in animal models of septic shock with some improvement in survival. Anecdotal use in adults with severe septic shock has demonstrated some success.

Corticosteroids, by virtue of their action on many mediators, are thought to play a role in shock and—based on positive results in animal models of septic shock—have been advocated for treatment of shock. Clinical trials of steroids in sepsis showed no difference in mortality rates between steroid-treated and placebo-treated groups. Two exceptions appear to be children with meningococcal meningitis and AIDS patients with Pneumocystis pneumonia. Both groups have shown improvement in oxygenation and a trend toward improved survival when treated with corticosteroids.

ECMO has been considered in the treatment of shock in patients with recoverable cardiac and pulmonary function who require both pulmonary and cardiac support. Eight of ten neonates with fulminant septic shock not responsive to conventional treatment survived after treatment. Further data are needed to determine the role of this modality in the treatment of shock.

Bernard GR: Sepsis trials. Am J Respir Crit Care 1995; 152:4.

Bone RC, Balk RA, Cerra FB, and the ACCP/SCCM Consensus Conference Committee: Definitions for sepsis and organ failure and guidelines for the use of innovative therapies in sepsis. Chest 1992;101:1644.

Groenveld ABJ, Kolkman JJ: Splanchnic tonometry: A review of physiology, methodology, and clinical applications. J Crit Care 1994;9:198.

Herbert PC et al for the Canadian Critical Care Trial Group: Transfusion requirement in critical care: A pilot study. JAMA 1995;273:1439.

Marsh CB, Wewers MD: The pathogenesis of sepsis: Factors that modulate the response to gram-negative bacterial infection. Clin Chest Med 1996;17:183.

Shoemaker WC: Oxygen transport and oxygen metabolism in shock and critical illness: Invasive and non-invasive monitoring of circulatory dysfunction and shock. Crit Care Clin 1996;12:939.

Warren HS: Strategies for the treatment of sepsis. N Engl J Med 1997;336:952.

Weikert LE, Bernard GR: Pharmacotherapy of sepsis. Clin Chest Med 1996;17:289.

Table 12–9. Pharmacologic support of the shock patient.

Drug	Dose	Alpha-Adrenergic Effect[1]	Beta-Adrenergic Effect[1]	Vasodilator Effect	Actions and Advantages	Disadvantages
Dopamine	1–20 µg/kg/min	+ to +++ (dose-related)	+ to +++ (dose-related)	At low doses, renal vasodilation occurs (dopaminergic receptors)	Moderate inotrope, wide and safe dosage range, short half-life	May cause worsening of pulmonary vasoconstriction
Dobutamine	1–10 µg/kg/min	0	+++		Moderate inotrope, less chronotropic, fewer dysrhythmias than with isoproterenol or epinephrine	Marked variation among patients
Epinephrine	0.05–1 µg/kg/min	++ to +++ (dose-related)	+++		Significant increases in inotropy, chronotropy, and systemic vascular resistance	Tachycardia, dysrhythmias, renal ischemia, systemic and pulmonary vascular resistance
Isoproterenol	0.05–1 µg/kg/min	0	+++	Peripheral vasodilation	Significant increase in inotropy and chronotropy. Systemic vascular resistance can drop, and pulmonary vascular resistance should not increase and may decrease.	Significant myocardial oxygen consumption increases, tachycardia, dysrhythmia
Norepinephrine	0.05–1 µg/kg/min	+++	+++		Powerful vasoconstrictor (systemic and pulmonary); rarely used except possibly in patients with very low systemic vascular resistance or in conjunction with vasodilator	Reduced cardiac output if afterload is too high, renal ischemia
Nitroprusside	0.05–8 µg/kg/min	0	0	Arterial and venous dilation (smooth muscle relaxation)	Decreases systemic and pulmonary vascular resistance, very short-acting. Blood pressure returns to previous levels within 1–10 minutes after infusion is stopped.	Toxicities (thiocyanates and cyanide), increased intracranial pressure and ventilation/perfusion mismatch, methemoglobinemia, increased intracranial pressure

[1]0 = no effect, + = small effect, ++ = moderate effect, +++ = potent effect.

INDICATIONS FOR CENTRAL VENOUS & ARTERIAL CANNULATION

Placement of catheters into the central venous or arterial circulation may be justified for continuous assessment of intravascular volume, cardiac function, blood drawing for lab work or administration of volume, drugs, or hyperalimentation.

General Rules for Equipment Selection & Technique

(1) Vascular access equipment should be selected based on evaluation of the following: material; tendency to burr, buckle, or crimp; patient comfort; thrombogenicity; resistance to bacterial colonization; and price.

(2) Greater consistency and success can be achieved by restricting the variety, number of kits, and equipment.

(3) Open the kit and examine all components. This includes feeding the wire through the needle and filling all lines with normal saline to prevent air from entering the circulation.

(4) In the awake or sedated patient, greater success can be achieved if two people perform the procedure (in addition to those occupied with restraining or positioning the patient).

(5) Apply EMLA cream (eutectic mixture of lidocaine 2.5% and prilocaine 2.5%) to the area of punc-

ture (45 minutes before the procedure) or infiltrate with an appropriate local anesthetic before prepping and draping the skin.

(6) Sterilize and drape the area around the point of entry.

(7) When searching for the vessel, make straight passes while maintaining slight negative pressure. Advance and withdraw the needle at the same speed. Frequently, the blood return will occur during withdrawal.

(8) Once there is free flow of venous blood into the syringe, remove the syringe without moving the needle and, if using the Seldinger technique, pass the J wire through the needle. When appropriate, watch the ECG for arrhythmias, since they are frequently seen when the J wire touches the right side of the heart.

(9) Withdraw the needle over the J wire and clean the wire of blood.

(10) Make a nick with a No. 11 blade at the point where the J wire enters the skin. Pass the introducer or the intravascular catheter (or both) over the J wire.

(11) With the catheters in place, remove the wire along with the introducer.

(12) Check to make sure that blood can be drawn easily through the new line.

(13) Verify the position of the line on x-ray.

Points of Entry for Venous Line Placement

(1) External jugular vein: Place a soft cloth roll beneath the patient's shoulder and turn the head to the contralateral side (Figure 12–2). Valsalva's maneuver, Trendelenburg position, or occlusion of the vessel at the clavicular level are ways of temporarily increasing jugular distention and visibility. To overcome the problems of this vessel's mobility and thick wall, apply cephalic retraction of the skin over the vessel superior to the point of needle entry. Maintain gentle negative pressure in the syringe attached to the needle as it is advanced toward the vessel. Needle entry into the vessel lumen is usually signaled by a change in resistance followed by appearance of venous blood in the hub of the needle. Lay the needle along the side of the vessel and advance it a few more millimeters to ensure that the bevel of the needle is completely in the vessel lumen. Remove the syringe without moving the needle and pass a soft J wire into the vessel lumen. With manipulation, the J wire should pass into the central circulation. Remove the needle and pass the central line over the J wire.

(2) Internal jugular vein: Once the patient has been prepped, draped, and positioned as shown in Figure 12–3, feel for the trachea halfway between the angle of the jaw and the suprasternal notch and then feel lateral to the trachea for the carotid pulse. Just lateral to the carotid pulse, at a 30-degree angle from horizontal, insert a finder needle (25-gauge), aiming

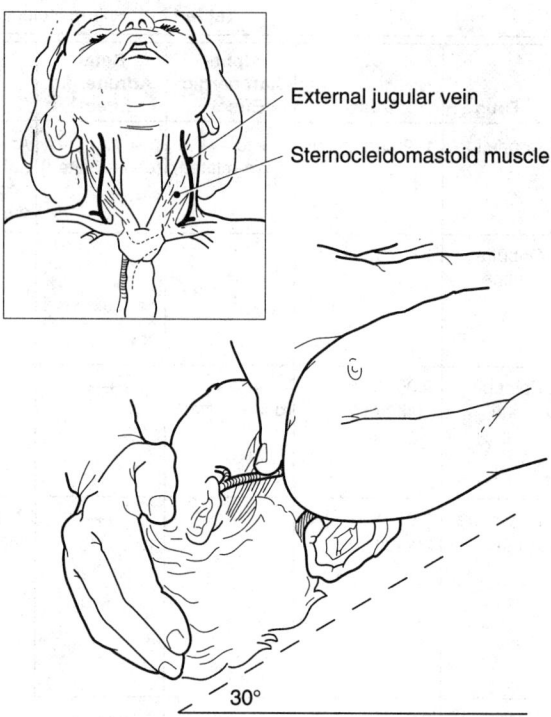

External jugular vein

Sternocleidomastoid muscle

30°

Figure 12–2. External jugular vein technique. (Reproduced, with permission, from Chameides L: *Textbook of Pediatric Advanced Life Support.* American Heart Association, 1988.)

between the ipsilateral nipple and shoulder. Once venous return is established, remove the finder needle and repeat the procedure with the appropriate-size larger needle.

(3) Subclavian vein: After the patient has been prepped, draped, and positioned (Figure 12–4), move the needle flat along the chest, entering along the inferior edge of the clavicle just lateral to the midclavicular line and aiming for the suprasternal notch. Once venous return is established, use the Seldinger technique.

(4) Femoral vein: With the patient's leg slightly abducted (Figure 12–5), find the femoral artery 3–4 cm below the inguinal ligament. The femoral vein is just medial and parallel to the femoral artery. Insert the needle at a 30- to 45-degree angle. Once venous return is established, use the Seldinger technique.

(5) Antecubital vein: "PIC" (peripherally inserted catheter) lines (2.8F–4F) are long, soft Silastic styleted catheters most commonly threaded from an antecubital vessel to the right atrium. These lines are not difficult to insert and are easy to dress and keep clean. They are suited for long-term use because they are less thrombogenic, tolerable for the patient, and good for infusion of hyperalimentation and drugs. In

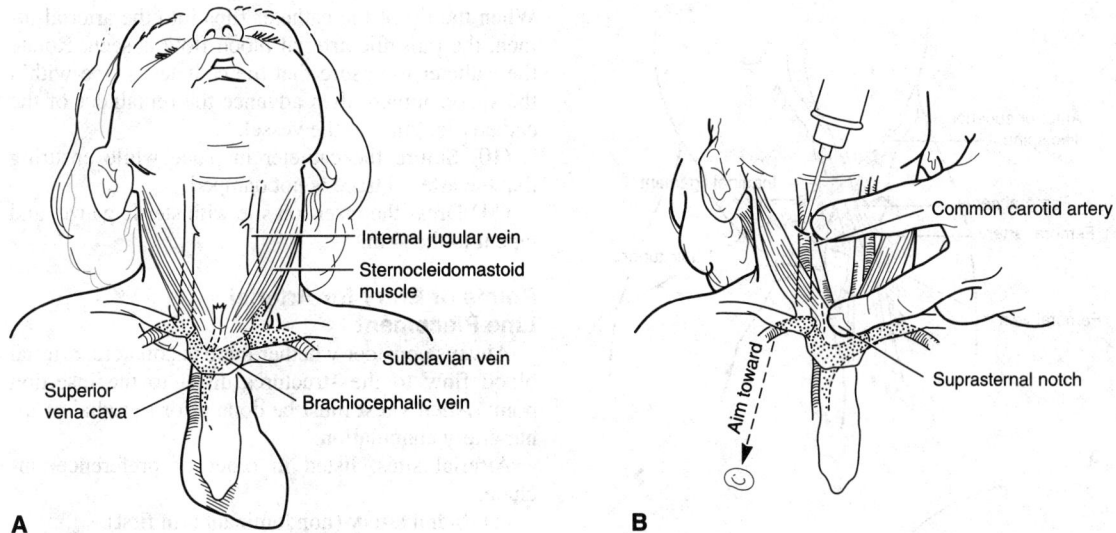

Figure 12–3. A: The internal jugular vein and its relationship to the surrounding anatomy. **B:** Technique of anterior internal jugular cannulation. (Reproduced, with permission, from Chameides L: *Textbook of Pediatric Advanced Life Support.* American Heart Association, 1988.)

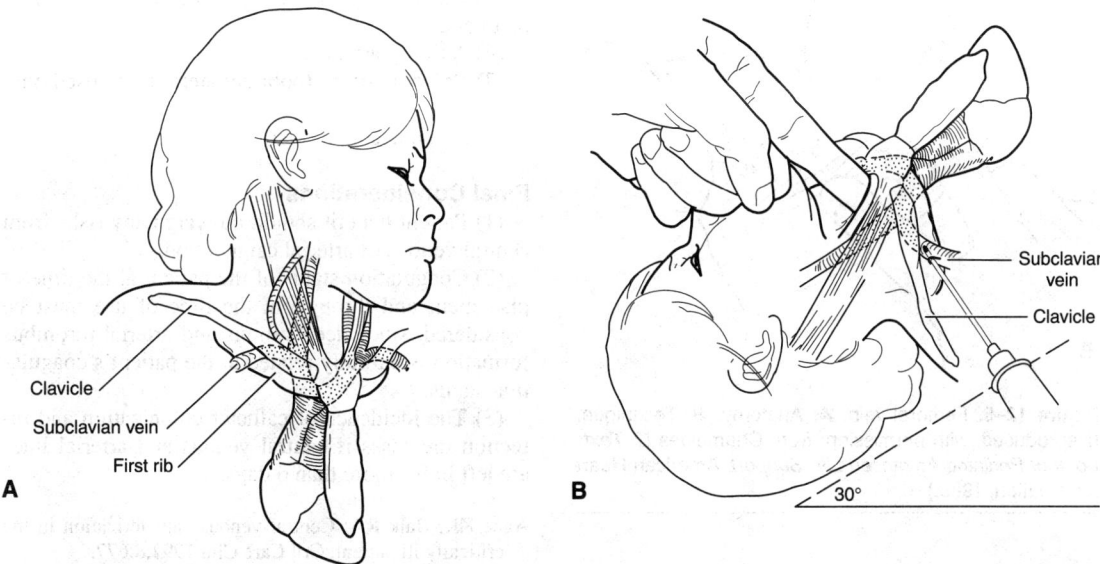

Figure 12–4. Subclavian artery. **A:** Anatomy. **B:** Technique. (Reproduced, with permission, from Chameides L: *Textbook of Pediatric Advanced Life Support.* American Heart Association, 1988.)

general, they are not suitable for obtaining blood for laboratory analysis.

General Rules for Cannulation of the Arterial System

(1) Rules 1–6 for the central venous system apply for the arterial system as well.

(2) The Seldinger technique can be applied for arterial tree cannulation.

(3) Most arteries can be cannulated percutaneously.

(4) Puncture the skin at the insertion site to eliminate any drag or resistance on the catheter advancement.

(5) Insert the cannula at a 30-degree angle to the skin surface, advancing at a slow rate toward the arterial pulse. Watch the hub of the cannula for a flash of arterial blood.

(6) When arterial flash is seen, lower the catheter to a 10-degree angle with the surface of the skin and advance the catheter into the lumen of the artery. If successful, pulsatile arterial flow will continue into

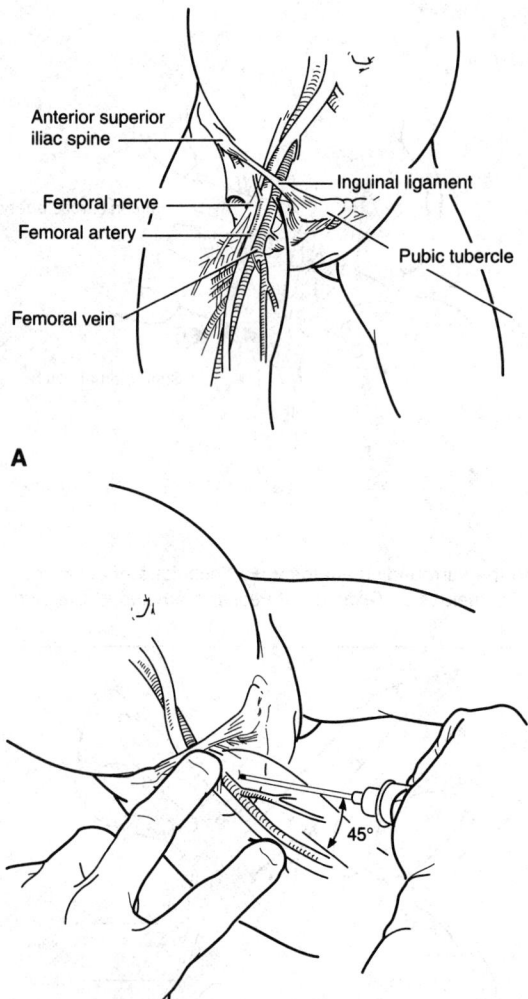

A

B

Figure 12–5. Femoral vein. **A:** Anatomy. **B:** Technique. (Reproduced, with permission, from Chameides L: *Textbook of Pediatric Advanced Life Support.* American Heart Association, 1988.)

the catheter. Advance an additional centimeter to make certain that the catheter is in the arterial lumen.

(7) Hold the catheter while removing the needle stylet. Arterial blood will pulse out of the catheter if the tip is in the arterial lumen.

(8) Advance the catheter into the lumen; attach a syringe containing normal saline with 1 unit/mL of heparin; aspirate to make certain that there are no bubbles; and then gently flush the catheter.

(9) If arterial flow into the needle stylet stops during catheter advancement, advance this unit an additional centimeter. Remove the needle stylet and place it on a sterile surface. Pull the catheter out slowly.

When the tip of the catheter flips into the arterial lumen, the pulsatile arterial blood flow is seen. Rotate the catheter to ensure that the catheter is free within the vessel lumen, then advance the remainder of the catheter length into the vessel.

(10) Suture the catheter in place while ensuring that the arterial trace is not damped.

(11) Dress the insertion site with sterile gauze, and tape it to the skin.

Points of Entry for Arterial Line Placement

Always consider whether there is collateral arterial blood flow to the structures distal to the insertion point. Allen's test must be done prior to radial or ulnar artery cannulation.

Arterial sites, listed in order of preference, include:

(1) Radial artery (nondominant arm first).

(2) Femoral artery (morbidity is the same as for the radial artery beyond the newborn period).

(3) Posterior tibial artery.

(4) Dorsalis pedis artery.

(5) Ulnar artery (if distal radial filling is present in that hand).

(6) Axillary artery.

(7) Brachial artery (poor collateral flow, used only during cardiac surgery in newborn-sized patients with arterial access limitations).

Final Considerations

(1) Patient benefit should outweigh any risks from central venous or arterial cannulation.

(2) Coagulation status of the patient at the time of placement and throughout the time of use must be considered, since deep venous and arterial thrombus formation is partially related to the patient's coagulation status.

(3) The incidence of catheter colonization and infection increases if central venous and arterial lines are left in for more than 6 days.

Agee KR, Balk RA: Central venous catheterization in the critically ill patient. Crit Care Clin 1992;8:677.

Allen EV: Thromboangiitis obliterans: Methods of diagnosis of chronic occlusive arterial lesions distal to the wrist with illustrative cases. Am J Med Sci 1929;178:237.

Clark VL, Kruse JA: Arterial catheterization. Crit Care Clin 1992;8:687.

Seldinger SI: Catheter placement of needle in percutaneous arteriography; a new technique. Acta Radiol 1953;39:368.

CEREBRAL EDEMA

Cerebral edema is a major cause of morbidity and mortality in the PICU. Cerebral edema is generally broken down into three types. **Cytotoxic edema** is caused by direct cellular injury, usually as a consequence of hypoxia or anoxia. Cellular energy stores are depleted, and ionic pumps of the cell cease activity, causing fluid to accumulate in the cell. **Vasogenic edema** is the result of direct injury to the blood–brain barrier. When the tight junctions of the endothelium are injured, water and protein can extravasate into the interstitium of the brain. In traumatic head injury, this may be a major cause of edema. **Interstitial edema** is caused by an imbalance of cerebrospinal fluid production and reabsorption and is treatable with ventricular shunting.

Much of the damage to the brain from traumatic head injury is a result of direct damage to neurons and therefore is not influenced by intensive therapy. The goal of ICU management is to decrease secondary injury to the brain resulting from hypoxia, hypoperfusion, and acidosis. The role of hypoxia and ischemia in causing damage is related to metabolic breakdown caused both by intracellular hypoxia and the cascade of events that follow cell reperfusion. Reperfusion injury in the ischemic region is believed to be related to free radical interaction with lipid membranes, DNA, and intracellular calcium, resulting in cellular damage.

Clinical Findings

A. Symptoms and Signs: Patients with elevations in intracranial pressure (ICP) may develop headaches, vomiting, diplopia, seizures, or a decrease in Glasgow Coma Score. Physical findings include alterations in mental status, alterations in muscle tone and deep tendon reflexes, bradycardia, hypertension, and a bulging fontanelle or increase in head circumference (< 12 months of age). Papilledema may take 8–12 hours to develop. The young patient may not demonstrate the Cushing reflex of hypertension, bradycardia, and decreased respirations.

B. ICP Monitoring: (Table 12–10.) The benefit of ICP monitoring is dependent on the cause of cerebral edema. ICP monitoring has shown potential benefit in acute head trauma and Reye's syndrome. Its

use in cerebral hemorrhage, meningitis, and encephalitis is more controversial. No benefit has been shown in hypoxic-ischemic injuries, such as near-drowning or sudden infant death syndrome (SIDS).

Treatment

Treatment for ICP should be started when clinical evidence of its presence exists. Therapies can be broken down into basic and advanced therapies.

A. Basic Therapies: These therapies do not require the presence of an ICP monitor.

1. Elevation of the head of the bed to 30 degrees, with the head maintained in the midline.

2. Ventilation of the patient to maintain a P_{O_2} greater than 80 mm Hg and a P_{CO_2} of 25–30 mm Hg.

3. Maintenance of the blood pressure in the normal range for age.

4. Avoidance of hyperthermia, which increases cerebral metabolic rate.

5. Avoidance of seizures, which increase cerebral oxygen consumption. Prophylactic anticonvulsants may be indicated, especially in head trauma.

6. Paralysis and sedation should be used only if necessary to control ventilation and patient movement.

7. Hypovolemia should be treated aggressively to maintain blood pressure. Raising the osmolality of the blood to between 300 and 310 mOsm/kg will help slow the formation of edema and reduce the ICP. This can be accomplished through the use of mannitol, furosemide, and/or moderate fluid restriction.

8. Lidocaine (1 mg/kg IV) given 1 minute before endotracheal tube suctioning blunts the ICP response to stimulation.

B. Advanced Therapies: These therapies are more controversial and require the continuous monitoring of ICP.

1. Maintenance of the cerebral perfusion pressure (CPP = MAP – ICP) at 60 mm Hg or higher. The optimal pressure has not been established. Positive inotropic agents may be required to maintain the pressure.

Table 12–10. Comparison of intracranial pressure monitoring techniques.

Type of Monitor	Placement	Advantages	Disadvantages
External (pressure-sensitive)	Over the skin of open anterior fontanelle	Noninvasive. Useful as trending device.	Very indirect measurement. Useful in limited age group.
Epidural (fiberoptic, hydraulic, and pneumatic)	Between skull and dura	Easy placement. Low risk of infection. Difficult to occlude.	Unable to draw off CSF. May create epidural bleeding.
Subarachnoid (hydraulic or fiberoptic)	Between dura and brain substance	Easy placement. Low risk of infection.	May be occluded by debris. Unable to draw off CSF. May give falsely low readings.
Intraventricular (hydraulic, fiberoptic)	Inside the lateral ventricle	Most direct measurement. Therapeutic if able to draw off CSF.	Requires adequately sized lateral ventricles. Increased risk of bleeding and infection.

2. Barbiturate coma has been shown to be effective in controlling ICP, but not necessarily in improving outcome. The barbiturates are all negative inotropes and vasodilators and may decrease CPP.

3. Moderate hypothermia and decompressive craniotomy have been shown to lower ICP, but not to improve outcome.

C. Experimental Therapies: Free radical scavengers and calcium channel blockers have been used to improve outcome following head trauma in animals. Specific amino acid excitatory neurotransmitters have been identified and implicated in neurologic injury and seizures. Specific antagonists are being investigated and may prove to be effective treatment. Human trials based on these experimental findings are being proposed.

Outcome

Pupillary response is an important prognostic indicator, with a mortality rate of 50% associated with an absent unilateral response and 90% with an absent response bilaterally.

Bullock R, Chesnut RM, Clifton G: Guidelines for the management of severe head injury. J Neurotrauma 1996;13:639.

Chesnut RM: Secondary brain insults after head injury: Clinical perspectives. New Horizons 1995;3:366.

Lang EW, Chesnut RM: Intracranial pressure and cerebral perfusion pressure in severe head injury. New Horizons 1995;3:400.

Marion DW et al: Treatment of traumatic brain injury with moderate hypothermia. N Engl J Med 1997;336:540.

Marshall LF, Marshall SB: Pharmacologic therapy: Promising clinical investigations. New Horizons 1995;3:573.

Robertson CS, Cormio M: Cerebral metabolic management. New Horizons 1995;3:410.

ETHICAL CONSIDERATIONS IN INTENSIVE CARE

Patient Autonomy

Although the pediatric patient is generally a minor, respect for the patient's rights and wishes should still play a part in the decision-making process. Whenever appropriate, the child should be included in discussions concerning the clinical problem and its management.

Organ Donation

Organ transplants are no longer experimental. The demand for organs has increased while organ procurement has remained unchanged.

The prospect of organ or tissue donation should be considered in all patients dying in the ICU. To be an organ donor, the patient must be brain-dead and have no exclusions for transplant. (Contact the Organ Procurement Organization in the area for exclusions.) Tissue (heart valves, corneas, skin, bone) can be obtained even if the patient does not meet brain death criteria. The Required Request Law mandates that health care professionals approach all donor-eligible families to inquire about organ procurement. The decision to donate must be made free of coercion, with informed consent, and without financial incentive.

Brain Death (See Chapter 22)

The limited pool of organ donation candidates and the increasing number of potential recipients has made the diagnosis of death prior to the cessation of physiologic function an imperative professional obligation. Currently, the diagnosis of brain death is fairly straightforward and accepted in all jurisdictions. It requires the following conditions:

(1) The absence of a primary remediable condition that might mimic brain death (eg, acute subdural hemorrhage). This generally requires a clear history or a CT scan.

(2) The absence of hypotension with consequent cerebral hypoperfusion that would alter cerebral activity.

(3) The absence of hypothermia, which would alter cerebral activity. Generally, this requires a temperature of greater than 35 °C.

(4) The absence of exposure to drugs or toxins that would mimic brain death. This generally requires a toxicology screen. Therapeutic levels of anticonvulsants and sedatives will not mimic brain death.

Once these conditions have been met, the brain death examination can be performed. This examination is designed to guarantee the absence of any cortical or brain stem activity. The following procedures must be performed:

(1) Assessment of cranial nerve function.

(2) Assessment of pain response.

(3) Assessment of respiratory drive. A 3-minute apnea test should be performed starting with a PCO_2 of 55 mm Hg, and with the patient on 100% oxygen during the test.

Discontinuance of Life Support

In spite of advances in medicine, ICU patients are frequently at the limits of the physician's ability to sustain life. In the interests of the quality of life for the patient and the family, it is often necessary to consider the limitation or discontinuance of life-sustaining treatments. Certain principles underlie the majority of such decisions:

(1) The patient should be considered terminal. Generally, this implies that continuation of life in the best of possible circumstances will be less than 1 year. In addition, some patients with no ability to meaningfully interact with their environment may also be considered.

(2) There must be single organ system failure that is not amenable to transplant (eg, the cerebral cortex) or multiple organ system failure.

(3) There must be a medical consensus among involved health care personnel as to these diagnoses. This requires the concurrence of at least two physicians as well as of nursing and social services personnel.

(4) The burden of continued existence—pain and suffering—should outweigh any potential gain of continued therapy.

(5) The patient, if appropriate and capable, and the patient's parents and guardians must be fully informed and in agreement with the course of action.

Hospital ethics committees may be of assistance in situations in which there is disagreement among health care providers.

Once the decision to limit or discontinue medical therapy has been agreed on, a course of action that is both humane and in compliance with good medical practice must be determined. All medical therapy may be considered to be extraordinary in certain circumstances.

These decisions cannot be considered irrevocable. If at any time the family or health care providers wish to reconsider the decision, full medical therapy should be reinstituted until the situation is clarified.

Arnold RM, Skiminoff LA, Frader JE: Ethical issues in organ procurement: A review for intensivists. Crit Care Clin 1996;12:29.

Brody H et al: Withdrawing intensive life-sustaining treatment: Recommendations for compassionate clinical management. N Engl J Med 1997;336:652.

Mejia RE, Pollack MM: Variability in brain death determination practices in children. JAMA 1995;274:550.

Nelson LJ, Nelson RM: Ethics and the provision of futile, harmful, or burdensome treatment to children. Crit Care Med 1992;20:427.

NUTRITIONAL SUPPORT AFTER INJURY

Trauma, sepsis, and significant injury are associated with a variety of profound metabolic and physiologic responses. Nutritional status has an impact on in-hospital morbidity rates and mortality outcomes. Inadequate nutrition can impair wound healing and immune function and prevent early weaning from mechanical ventilation. Stress in critically ill children induces more than simple starvation. The hypermetabolic response seen during severe stress results in increased energy usage and endogenous nutrient requirement, especially protein. The metabolic needs of critically ill children are largely managed by intravenous hyperalimentation, tailored to meet stress and hypercatabolic states (qv).

Manning EMC, Shenkin A: Nutritional assessment in the critically ill. Crit Care Clin 1995;11:603.

Soeters PB, Olde Damink SWM: Nutritional considerations in the critically ill. Curr Opin Crit Care 1996;2:153.

PAIN & ANXIETY CONTROL
(Table 12–11)

Anxiety control and pain relief are two of the most important responsibilities of the critical care physician. Earlier perceptions that children do not require pain relief have drastically changed in response to documented proof of improved outcomes in children receiving appropriate pain relief. The anxiety of children in the ICU is well known. These responses may interact to heighten fear and the perception of pain and may reach levels sufficient to cause deterioration in the patient's clinical condition. It is important to distinguish between anxiety and pain, since pharmacologic therapy may be directed at either one or both of these symptoms.

Sedation

Sedative (anxiolytic) drugs are used to induce calmness without producing sleep—although at high doses all anxiolytics will cause drowsiness and sleep. The five indications for the use of sedative drugs are (1) to allay fear and anxiety; (2) to manage acute confusional states; (3) to facilitate treatment or diagnostic procedures; (4) to facilitate mechanical ventilation; and (5) to obtund physiologic responses to stress, that is, reduce tachycardia, hypertension, or increases in intracranial pressure. In the ICU setting, a parenteral (intravenous bolus or infusion) preparation is essential to allow titration of clinical effects in the face of possible impaired organ dysfunction (cardiac, respiratory, hepatic, renal, etc). Sedatives fall into several classes, with the opioid and benzodiazepine classes serving as the mainstay of anxiety treatment in the ICU.

A. Benzodiazepines: Benzodiazepines possess anxiolytic, hypnotic, anticonvulsant, and skeletal muscle relaxant properties. Although their exact mode of action is not known, it appears to be located within the limbic system of the central nervous system and to involve the neuroinhibitory transmitter γ-aminobutyric acid. Most benzodiazepines are metabolized in the liver, with their metabolites subsequently excreted in the urine; thus, patients in liver failure are likely to have long elimination times.

Benzodiazepine overdosage can cause respiratory depression if given rapidly in high doses, and they potentiate the analgesic and respiratory depressive effects of opioids and barbiturates.

Three benzodiazepines with differing half-lives are presently used in the ICU setting.

1. Midazolam–Midazolam has the shortest half-life (1½–3½ hours) of the benzodiazepines and is the only benzodiazepine that should be administered as a continuous intravenous infusion. It produces excellent retrograde amnesia lasting for 20–40 minutes after a single intravenous dose. Therefore, it can be used either for short-term sedation or for "awake" procedures such as endoscopy or as a continuous in-

Table 12–11. Pain and anxiety control.

Drug	Dose and Method of Administration[1]	Advantages	Disadvantages	Usual Duration of Effect
Morphine	IV, 0.1 mg/kg; continuous infusion; 0.01–0.05 mg/kg/h	Excellent pain relief, reversible	Respiratory depression, hypotension, nausea, suppression of intestinal motility, histamine release	2–4 hours
Meperidine	IV, 1 mg/kg	Good pain relief, reversible	Respiratory depression, histamine release, nausea, suppression of intestinal motility	2–4 hours
Fentanyl	IV, 1–2 μg/kg; continuous infusion; 0.5–2 μg/kg/h	Excellent pain relief, reversible, short half-life	Respiratory depression, chest wall rigidity, severe nausea and vomiting	30 minutes
Diazepam	IV, 0.1 mg/kg	Sedation and seizure control	Respiratory depression, jaundice, phlebitis	1–3 hours
Lorazepam	IV, 0.1 mg/kg	Longer half-life, sedation and seizure control	Nausea and vomiting, respiratory depression, phlebitis	2–4 hours
Midazolam	IV, 0.1 mg/kg	Short half-life, only benzodiazepine given as continuous infusion	Respiratory depression	30–60 minutes

[1]IV administration is most common in the ICU. The effects of morphine, meperidine, and fentanyl are reversible by administration of naloxone (opioid antagonist).

fusion in the anxious, restless patient. The single intravenous dose is 0.1 mg/kg, while a continuous infusion should be started at a rate of 0.1 mg/kg/h after an initial loading dose of 0.1 mg/kg. The midazolam infusion dosage must be titrated upward to achieve the desired effect. Midazolam is not an analgesic, and if very high doses are being used without the proper effect and it is felt that analgesia is also needed, the dose of midazolam can usually be lowered by the concurrent use of small doses of an appropriate analgesic such as morphine or fentanyl. When administering midazolam or any other benzodiazepine, it is important to monitor cardiorespiratory status and have resuscitation facilities available.

2. Diazepam–Diazepam has a longer half-life than midazolam and can be given orally as well as by the intravenous route. Its disadvantage in the ICU is its intermediary metabolite, nordiazepam, which has a very long elimination half-life and may accumulate, causing prolonged sedation. It produces excellent anxiolysis and amnesia. Additionally, it is used to treat acute status epilepticus. The intravenous dose is 0.1 mg/kg and can be repeated every 15 minutes to achieve the desired effect or until undesirable side effects such as somnolence and respiratory depression occur.

3. Lorazepam–Lorazepam possesses the longest half-life of the three benzodiazepines discussed here and can be used to achieve sedation for as long as 6–8 hours. It has less effect on the cardiovascular and respiratory systems than other benzodiazepines

and can be given orally, intravenously, or intramuscularly, with the intravenous route the most effective in the ICU setting. The intravenous dosage is 0.1 mg/kg. Lorazepam can also be used to treat acute status epilepticus.

B. Other Drugs:

1. Chloral hydrate–Chloral hydrate is an enteral sedative and hypnotic agent frequently used in children. After either oral or rectal administration, it is rapidly metabolized by the liver to its active form trichloroethanol, which has an 8-hour half-life. A sedative dose is 6–20 mg/kg per dose, usually given every 6–8 hours, while the hypnotic dose is up to 50 mg/kg with a maximum dose of 1 g. The hypnotic dose is frequently used to sedate young children for outpatient radiologic procedures such as CT scanning and MRI. There is little effect on respiration or blood pressure with therapeutic doses of chloral hydrate. The drug is irritating to mucus membranes, however, and may cause gastric upset if administered on an empty stomach.

2. Ketamine–Ketamine is a phencyclidine derivative that produces a trance-like state of immobility and amnesia known as "dissociative anesthesia." After intramuscular or intravenous administration, it causes central sympathetic nervous system stimulation with resultant increases in heart rate, blood pressure, and cardiac output. Respiration is not depressed at therapeutic doses. However, salivary and tracheobronchial mucous gland secretions are increased, so atropine should be administered 20 minutes prior to the ketamine. A distinct disadvantage of its use is the occurrence of unpleasant dreams or hallucinations, although the incidence is decreased in children compared to adults and can be reduced even further by the concurrent administration of a benzodiazepine. Because of its inotropic properties, it is useful for the sedation of certain critically ill patients whose condition is unstable. It is given as an intravenous injection of 1–2 mg/kg over 60 seconds, with supplementary doses of 0.5 mg/kg being required every 10–30 minutes to maintain an adequate level of anesthesia. Alternatively, it can be administered as an intramuscular injection of 5–10 mg/kg, which usually produces the desired level of anesthesia within 3–4 minutes. If prolonged anesthesia is required, ketamine can be administered by intravenous infusion at doses of 3–20 mg/kg/h.

3. Antihistamines–The antihistamines **diphenhydramine** and **hydroxyzine** can be used as sedatives but are not as effective as the benzodiazepines. Diphenhydramine produces sedation in only 50% of those treated. It can be given intravenously, intramuscularly, or orally at a dose of 1 mg/kg. Hydroxyzine can be given either intramuscularly or orally. It is frequently used concurrently with morphine or meperidine, adding anxiolysis and potentiating the effects of the opioid. The sedative effects of both drugs can last from 4 to 6 hours following a single dose.

4. Propofol–Propofol is an anesthetic induction agent whose main advantage is a rapid recovery time and no cumulative effects resulting from its rapid hepatic metabolism. It has no analgesic properties, frequently causes pain on injection, and causes a dose-related fall in blood pressure because of decreases in systemic vascular resistance. It is available as a 1% concentration in 20% intravenous fat emulsion and thus should be included in considerations about nutritional replacement. Triglyceride levels should be followed. Propofol may be associated with microbial contamination and sepsis if sterile techniques for preparation and infusion are not strictly followed. Propofol as a continuous infusion for sedation in pediatrics is being compared with sedation with benzodiazepines in a randomized multicenter study. The drug is very expensive. The sedative dose is 1 mg/kg as an intravenous bolus followed by an infusion of 1 mg/kg/h.

5. Barbiturates–Barbiturates (phenobarbital, thiopental) can cause direct myocardial and respiratory depression and are, in general, poor choices for sedation of seriously ill patients. Phenobarbital has a very long half-life (up to 4 days), and recovery from thiopental, though it is a "short-acting" barbiturate, can be prolonged because remobilization of tissue stores occurs.

Analgesia

A. Opioid Analgesics: Opioid analgesics (morphine, fentanyl, codeine, meperidine) are the mainstays of therapy for most forms of acute severe pain as well as chronic cancer pain management. They possess both analgesic and dose-related sedative effects, although there is a range of plasma concentrations that produce analgesia without clouding of the sensorium. In addition, opioids can cause respiratory depression, nausea, pruritus, slowed intestinal motility, miosis, urinary retention, cough suppression, biliary spasm, and vasodilation. There is great individual variation in the dose of opioid required to produce adequate analgesia. Therefore, in the intensive care setting, a continuous infusion of morphine or fentanyl allows dosages to be easily titrated to achieve the desired effect.

In general, infants under 3 months of age are more susceptible to the respiratory depressant effects of opioids, and starting dosages for these patients should be about one-third to one-half the usual pediatric dose. Most opioids (except meperidine) have minimal cardiac depressive effects, and critically ill patients generally tolerate them well. Fentanyl does not cause the histamine release that morphine does and thus produces less vasodilation and drop in systemic blood pressure. Opioids are metabolized in the liver, with metabolites excreted in the urine. Thus, patients with hepatic or renal impairment may have a prolonged response to their administration. Patients who receive regular doses of opioids for 2 weeks or more frequently develop a physiologic dependence with the development of withdrawal symptoms (agitation, tachypnea, tachycardia, sweating, diarrhea) upon acute termination of the drug. In these patients, gradual tapering of the opioid dosage over a 5- to 10-day period will prevent withdrawal symptoms. As with any potent sedative or analgesic used in the ICU setting, appropriate patient monitoring (pulse oximetry, cardiorespiratory monitoring, blood pressure monitoring) should be used during the period of opioid administration, and equipment should be available to support prompt intervention if undesired side effects occur.

The ICU regimen for sedation and analgesia must be carefully modified when the patient is transferred to the ward or a lower vigilance area. Patients with baseline respiratory, hepatic, or renal insufficiencies are most predisposed to respiratory insufficiency from sedatives or opioid analgesics.

Patient-controlled analgesia (PCA) is a computer-controlled infusion pump for constant infusion or patient-controlled bolus infusion of opioid analgesics. The basal infusion mode is intended to provide a constant serum level of analgesic. The bolus mode allows the patient to self-administer, by pushing a button, additional doses for breakthrough pain. The patient is usually permitted six boluses an hour, with 10-minute blockouts. If the patient is using allotted hourly boluses, this usually means that the basal infusion rate is too low.

The patient must understand the concept of PCA in order to be a candidate for its use. There are circumstances in pediatrics in which it is appropriate for the nurse or parent to administer the bolus dose.

Naloxone reverses the analgesia, sedative, and respiratory depressive effects of opioid agonists. Its administration should again be titrated to achieve the desired effect (eg, reversal of respiratory depression, since full reversal using 0.01–0.02 mL/kg may cause acute anxiety, dysphoria, nausea, and vomiting). Furthermore, since the duration of effect of naloxone is shorter (30 minutes) than that of most opioids, the patient must be carefully observed for reappearance of the undesired effect.

B. Nonopioid Analgesics: Nonopioid analgesics used in the treatment of mild to moderate pain include acetaminophen, aspirin, and other nonsteroidal anti-inflammatory drugs (NSAIDs), such as ibuprofen and naproxen.

1. Acetaminophen–Acetaminophen is the most commonly used analgesic in pediatrics in the United States and is the drug of choice for mild to moderate pain because of its low toxicity and lack of effect on bleeding time. It is metabolized by the liver. Suggested doses are 10–15 mg/kg orally to approximately 10–20 mg/kg rectally every 4 hours.

2. Aspirin–Aspirin is also an effective analgesic for mild to moderate pain at doses of 10–15 mg/kg orally every 4 hours. However, its prolongation of bleeding time, association with Reye's syndrome, and propensity to cause gastric irritation limit its usefulness in pediatric practice. Aspirin and other NSAIDs are still useful, especially for pain of inflammatory origin, bone pain, and pain associated with rheumatic conditions.

3. Other NSAIDs–Ibuprofen and naproxen are both NSAIDs whose use has been limited in pediatrics to date. **Naproxen** is FDA-approved for children 2–12 years of age (5–7 mg/kg orally every 8–12 hours), while **ibuprofen** requires more frequent dosing intervals (4–10 mg/kg orally every 6–8 hours).

All of the NSAIDs have a therapeutic "ceiling"—ie, unlike opioids, which have a dose-related increase in potency, there is no increase in analgesic potency above the recommended dose. They all can cause gastritis and should be given with antacids or with meals. In addition, the analgesic effects of acetaminophen, aspirin, and other NSAIDs are additive to those of opioids. Thus, if additional analgesia is required, their use should be continued and an appropriate oral opioid (codeine, morphine) or parenteral opioid (morphine, fentanyl) begun.

American Academy of Pediatrics Committee on Drugs: Guidelines for monitoring and management of pediatric patients during and after sedation for diagnostic and therapeutic procedures. Pediatrics 1992;89:1110.

Barr J, Donner A: Optimal intravenous dosing strategies for sedatives and analgesics in the intensive care unit. Crit Care Clin 1995;11:827.

Mazzeo AJ: Sedation for the mechanically ventilated patient. Crit Care Clin 1995;11:937.

Tung A, Rosenthal M: Patients requiring sedation. Crit Care Clinic 1995;11:791.

Skin

13

Joseph G. Morelli, MD, & William L. Weston, MD

GENERAL PRINCIPLES OF DIAGNOSIS OF SKIN DISORDERS

Examination of the Skin

Examination of the skin requires that the entire surface of the body be palpated and inspected in good light. The onset and duration of each symptom should be recorded, together with a description of the primary lesion and any secondary changes, using the terminology set forth in Table 13–1).

GENERAL PRINCIPLES OF TREATMENT OF SKIN DISORDERS

TOPICAL THERAPY

Treatment should be simple and aimed at preserving normal skin physiology, keeping in mind that one is treating the child and not the anxious parent or grandparent. Topical therapy is often preferred because medication can be delivered in optimal concentrations to the desired site.

Water is an important therapeutic agent, and optimally hydrated skin is soft and smooth. This occurs at approximately 60% environmental humidity. Because water evaporates readily from the cutaneous surface, skin hydration (stratum corneum of the epidermis) is dependent on the water concentration in the air, and sweating contributes little. However, if sweat is prevented from evaporating (eg, in the axilla, groin), local humidity and hydration of the skin are increased. As humidity falls below 15–20%, the stratum corneum shrinks and cracks; the epidermal barrier is lost and allows irritants to enter the skin and induce an inflammatory response. Replacement of water will correct this condition if evaporation is prevented. Therefore, dry and scaly skin is treated by soaking the skin in water for 5 minutes and then adding a barrier to evaporation (Table 13–2). Oils and ointments prevent evaporation for 8–12 hours, so they must be applied once or twice a day. In areas already occluded (axilla, diaper area), ointments or oils will merely increase retention of water and should not be used.

Overhydration (maceration) can also occur. As environmental humidity increases to 90–100%, the number of water molecules absorbed by the stratum corneum increases and the tight lipid junctions between the cells of the stratum corneum are gradually replaced by weak hydrogen bonds; the cells eventually become widely separated, and the epidermal barrier falls apart. This occurs in immersion foot, diaper areas, axillae, etc. It is desirable to enhance evaporation of water in these areas by air drying.

WET DRESSINGS

By placing the skin in an environment where the humidity is 100% and allowing the moisture to evaporate to 60%, pruritus is relieved. Evaporation of water stimulates cold-dependent nerve fibers in the skin and this may prevent the transmission of the itching sensation via pain fibers to the central nervous system. It also is vasoconstrictive, thereby helping to reduce the erythema and also decreasing the inflammatory cellular response.

The simplest form of wet dressing consists of one set of wet underwear (eg, long johns) worn under a dry pair. The underwear should be soaked in warm (not hot) water and wrung out until no more drops come out. When covered by the dry layer, the wet dressings need to be changed only every 4–6 hours.

TOPICAL GLUCOCORTICOIDS

Twice-daily application of topical steroids is the mainstay of treatment for all forms of dermatitis

Table 13–1. Examination of the skin.

Clinical Appearance	Description and Examples[1]
Primary lesions (first to appear)	
Macule	Any circumscribed color change in the skin that is flat. *Examples:* White (vitiligo), brown (café au lait spot), purple (petechia).
Papule	A solid, elevated area less than 1 cm in diameter whose top may be pointed, rounded, or flat. *Examples:* Acne, warts, small lesions of psoriasis.
Plaque	A solid, circumscribed area more than 1 cm in diameter, usually flat-topped. *Example:* Psoriasis.
Vesicle	A circumscribed, elevated lesion less than 1 cm in diameter and containing clear serous fluid. *Example:* Blisters of herpes simplex.
Bulla	A circumscribed, elevated lesion more than 1 cm in diameter and containing clear serous fluid. *Example:* Bullous erythema multiforme.
Pustule	A vesicle containing a purulent exudate. *Examples:* Acne, folliculitis.
Nodule	A deep-seated mass with indistinct borders that elevates the overlying epidermis. *Examples:* Tumors, granuloma annulare. If it moves with the skin on palpation, it is intradermal; if the skin moves over the nodule, it is subcutaneous.
Wheal	A circumscribed, flat-topped, firm elevation of skin resulting from tense edema of the papillary dermis. *Example:* Urticaria.
Secondary changes	
Scales	Dry, thin plates of keratinized epidermal cells (stratum corneum). *Examples:* Psoriasis, ichthyosis.
Lichenification	Induration of skin with exaggerated skin lines and a shiny surface resulting from chronic rubbing of the skin. *Example:* Atopic dermatitis.
Erosion and oozing	A moist, circumscribed, slightly depressed area representing a blister base with the roof of the blister removed. *Examples:* Burns, bullous erythema multiforme. Most oral blisters present as erosions.
Crusts	Dried exudate of plasma on the surface of the skin following acute dermatitis. *Examples:* Impetigo, contact dermatitis.
Fissures	A linear split in the skin extending through the epidermis into the dermis. *Example:* Angular cheilitis.
Scars	A flat, raised, or depressed area of fibrotic replacement of dermis or subcutaneous tissue. *Examples:* Acne scar, burn scar.
Atrophy	Depression of the skin surface caused by thinning of one or more layers of skin. *Example:* Lichen sclerosis et atrophicus.
Color	The lesion should be described as red, yellow, brown, tan, or blue. Particular attention should be given to the blanching of red or lesions. Failure to blanch suggests bleeding into the dermis (petechiae).
Configuration of lesions	
Annular (circular)	Annular nodules represent granuloma annulare; annular papules are more apt to be caused by dermatophyte infections.
Linear (straight lines)	Linear papules represent lichen striatus; linear vesicles, incontinentia pigmenti; linear papules with burrows, scabies.
Grouped	Grouped vesicles occur in herpes simplex or zoster.
Discrete	Discrete lesions are independent of each other.
Distribution	Note whether the eruption is generalized, acral (hands, feet, buttocks, face), or localized to a specific skin region.

[1]Skin lesions are described in reverse order from the presentation here. Begin with distribution, then configuration, color, secondary changes, and primary changes. For example, guttate psoriasis could be described as generalized discrete, red, scaly papules.

Table 13–2. Bases used for topical preparations.

Base	Combined With	Uses
Liquids		Wet dressings: relieve pruritus, vasoconstrict
	Powder	Shake lotions, drying pastes: relieve pruritus, vasoconstrict
	Grease and emulsifier; oil in water	Cream: penetrates quickly (10–15 min) and thus allows evaporation
	Excess grease and emulsifier; water in oil	Emollient cream: penetrates more slowly and thus retains moisture on skin
Grease		Ointments: occlusive (hold material on skin for prolonged time) and prevent evaporation of water
Gel		Transparent, colorless, semisolid emulsion: nongreasy, more drying and irritating than cream
Powder		Enhances evaporation

Characteristics of bases for topical preparations:
1. Most greases are triglycerides (eg, Aquaphor, petrolatum, Eucerin).
2. Oils are fluid fats (eg, Alpha Keri, olive oil, mineral oil).
3. True fats (eg, lard, animal fats) contain free fatty acids that cause irritation.
4. Ointments (eg, Aquaphor, petrolatum) should not be used in intertriginous areas such as the axillae, between the toes, and in the perineum, because they increase maceration. Lotions or creams are preferred in these areas.
5. Oils and ointments hold medication on the skin for long periods and are therefore ideal for barriers or prophylaxis and for dried areas of skin. Medication gets into the skin more slowly from ointments.
6. Creams carry medication into skin and are preferable for intertriginous dermatitis.
7. Solutions, gels, or lotions should be used for scalp treatments.

(Table 13–3). Topical steroids can also be used under wet dressings. Wet dressings are removed every 4–6 hours, and a topical steroid is applied; the skin is then covered again with wet dressings. If treatment is applied throughout the 24-hour period, maximum benefit is obtained after 72 hours; if treatment is applied only at night, maximum benefit is obtained after 7 days. When the condition has improved, the wet dressings are discontinued and a steroid ointment is applied twice daily. Daily application of steroids is not to be continued for more than 1 month. Only low-potency steroids (Table 13–3) are applied to the face or intertriginous areas.

Table 13–3. Topical glucocorticoids.

	Concentrations
Low potency[1] = 1–9 Hydrocortisone	0.5% and 1%
Desonide	0.05%
Moderate potency = 10–99 Mometasone furoate	0.1%
Hydrocortisone valerate	0.2%
Fluocinolone acetonide	0.025%
Triamcinolone acetonide	0.01%
Amcinonide	0.1%
High potency = 100–499 Desoximetasone	0.25%
Fluocinonide	0.05%
Halcinonide	0.1%
Super potency = 500–7500 Betamethasone dipropionate	0.05%
Clobetasol propionate	0.05%

[1]1% hydrocortisone is defined as having a potency of 1.

Hepburn D, Yohn JJ, Weston WL: Topical glucocorticoid treatment in infants, children, and adolescents. Adv Dermatol 1994;9:225.

DISORDERS OF THE SKIN IN NEWBORNS

TRANSIENT DISEASES IN THE NEWBORN

Milia
Multiple white papules 1 mm in diameter scattered over the forehead, nose, and cheeks are present in up to 40% of newborn infants. Histologically, they represent superficial epidermal cysts filled with keratinous material associated with the developing pilosebaceous follicle. Their intraoral counterparts are called Epstein's pearls and are even more common than facial milia. All of these cystic structures spontaneously rupture and exfoliate their contents.

Sebaceous Gland Hyperplasia
Prominent yellow macules at the opening of each pilosebaceous follicle, predominantly over the nose, represent overgrowth of sebaceous glands in re-

sponse to the same androgenic stimulation that occurs in adolescence.

Acne Neonatorum

Open and closed comedones, erythematous papules, and pustules identical in appearance to adolescent acne may occur in infants over the forehead, cheeks, and chin. The lesions may be present at birth but usually do not appear until 4–6 weeks of age. Spontaneous resolution occurs over a period of 6 months to 1 year. Rarely, neonatal acne may be a manifestation of a virilizing syndrome.

Harlequin Color Change

A cutaneous vascular phenomenon unique to neonates in the first week of life occurs when the infant (particularly one of low birth weight) is placed on one side. The dependent half develops an erythematous flush with a sharp demarcation at the midline, and the upper half of the body becomes pale. The color changes usually subside within a few seconds after the infant is placed supine but may persist for as long as 20 minutes.

Mottling

A lace-like pattern of dilated cutaneous vessels appears over the extremities and often the trunk of neonates exposed to lowered room temperature. This feature is transient and usually disappears completely upon rewarming.

Erythema Toxicum

Up to 50% of term infants develop erythema toxicum. Usually at 24–48 hours of age, blotchy erythematous macules 2–3 cm in diameter appear, most prominently on the chest but also on the back, face, and extremities. These are occasionally present at birth. Onset after 4–5 days of life is rare. The lesions vary in number from two or three up to as many as 100. Incidence is much higher in term infants than in premature ones. The macular erythema may fade within 24–48 hours or may progress to formation of urticarial wheals in the center of the macules or, in 10% of cases, pustules. Examination of a Wright-stained smear of the lesion will reveal numerous eosinophils. This may be accompanied by peripheral blood eosinophilia of up to 20%. All of the lesions fade and disappear by 5–7 days. A similar eruption in black newborns, benign pustular melanosis, shows mostly neutrophils and leaves hyperpigmentation.

Sucking Blisters

Bullae, either intact or as an erosion with a blister base without inflammatory borders, may occur over the forearms, wrists, thumbs, or upper lip. These presumably result from vigorous sucking in utero. They resolve without complications.

Miliaria

Obstruction of the eccrine sweat ducts occurs often in neonates and produces one of two clinical pictures. Obstruction in the stratum corneum causes **miliaria crystallina,** characterized by tiny (1- to 2-mm), superficial grouped vesicles without erythema over intertriginous areas and adjacent skin (eg, neck, upper chest). More commonly, obstruction of the eccrine duct deeper in the epidermis results in erythematous grouped papules in the same areas and is called miliaria rubra. Rarely, these may progress to pustules. Heat and high humidity predispose the patient to eccrine duct pore closure. Removal to a cooler environment is the treatment of choice.

Subcutaneous Fat Necrosis

Reddish or purple, sharply circumscribed, firm nodules occurring over the cheeks, buttocks, arms, and thighs and occurring between day 1 and day 7 in infants represent subcutaneous fat necrosis. Cold injury is thought to play an important role. These lesions resolve spontaneously over a period of weeks, although—as in all instances of fat necrosis—they may calcify.

Weston WL, Lane AT, Morelli JG: *Color Textbook of Pediatric Dermatology,* 2nd ed. Mosby-Year Book, 1996.

PIGMENT CELL BIRTHMARKS, NEVI, & MELANOMA

Birthmarks may involve an overgrowth of one or more of any of the normal components of skin: pigment cells, blood vessels, lymph vessels, etc. A nevus is a hamartoma of highly differentiated cells that retain their normal function.

Mongolian Spot

A blue-black macule found over the lumbosacral area in 90% of Native American, black, and Asian infants is called a mongolian spot. These spots are occasionally noted over the shoulders and back and may extend over the buttocks. Histologically, they consist of spindle-shaped pigment cells located deep in the dermis. The lesions fade somewhat with time as a result of darkening of the overlying skin, but some traces may persist into adult life.

Café au Lait Macule

A café au lait macule is a light brown, oval macule (dark brown on black skin) that may be found anywhere on the body. Ten percent of white and 22% of black children have café au lait spots over 1.5 cm in greatest diameter. These lesions persist throughout life and may increase in number with age. The presence of six or more such lesions over 1.5 cm in greatest diameter may be a clue to neurofibromatosis 1 (NF-1). Patients with Albright's syndrome (Chapter

28) also have increased numbers of café au lait macules. Most newborns with NF-1 will acquire the macules later.

Spindle & Epithelioid Cell Nevus

A reddish-brown solitary nodule appearing on the face or upper arm of a child represents a spindle and epithelioid cell nevus. Histologically, it consists of pigment-producing cells of bizarre shape with numerous mitoses.

Junctional Nevus
& Compound Nevus

Dark brown or black macules, usually few in number at birth but becoming more numerous with age, represent junctional nevi. Histologically, these lesions are large clones of melanocytes at the junction of the epidermis and dermis. With aging, they may become raised (papules) and contain intradermal melanocytes, creating a compound nevus. Often the surface becomes irregular and roughened.

Brown to blue solitary papules with smooth surfaces represent intradermal nevi. When pigmentation is present deeper in the dermis, the lesions appear blue or blue-black and are called blue nevi.

Melanoma

Pigmented lesions with variegated colors (red, white, blue), notched borders, and nonuniform, irregular surfaces should arouse a suspicion of melanoma. Ulceration and bleeding are advanced signs of melanoma. If melanoma is suspected, excisional biopsy for pathologic examination should be done as the treatment of choice.

Giant Pigmented Nevus
(Bathing Trunk Nevus)

An irregular dark brown to black plaque over at least 5% of the body surface represents a giant pigmented nevus. Often the lesions are of such size as to cover the entire trunk (bathing trunk nevi). Histologically, they are compound nevi. Transformation to malignant melanoma has been reported in as many as 10% of cases in some series, though the true incidence is probably much lower. Malignant change may occur in the neonatal period or at any time thereafter.

Tissue expanders may be useful in excision of large lesions. The risk of melanoma and the potential for cosmetic improvement should be carefully evaluated for each patient.

Angelucci D et al: Rapid perinatal growth mimicking malignant transformation in a giant congenital melanocytic nevus. Hum Pathol 1991;22:297.

From L: Congenital nevi: Let's be practical. Pediatr Dermatol 1992;9:345.

Mackie RM: Nevi as risk factors for melanoma. Pediatr Dermatol 1992;9:340.

Swerdlow AJ, English JS, Qiao Z: The risk of melanoma in

patients with congenital nevi: A cohort study. J Am Acad Dermatol 1995;32:595.

Nassan A, al-Nafussi A, Quaba A: Cutaneous malignant melanoma in children and adolescents in Scotland, 1979–1991. Plast Reconstr Surg 1996;98:442.

VASCULAR BIRTHMARKS

Capillary Malformations

Flat vascular birthmarks can be divided into two types: those that are orange or light red (salmon patch) and those that are dark red or bluish-red (port wine stain).

The salmon patch is a light red macule found over the nape of the neck, upper eyelids, and glabella. Fifty percent of infants have such lesions over their necks. Eyelid lesions fade completely within 3–6 months; those on the neck fade somewhat but usually persist into adult life.

Port wine stains are dark red or purple macules appearing anywhere on the body. A bilateral port wine stain or one covering the entire half of the face may be a clue to Sturge-Weber syndrome, which is characterized by seizures, mental retardation, glaucoma, and hemiplegia (Chapter 22). Most infants with smaller, unilateral port wine stains do not have Sturge-Weber syndrome. Similarly, a port wine stain over an extremity may be associated with hypertrophy of the soft tissue and bone of that extremity (Klippel-Trenaunay syndrome). The pulsed dye laser is the treatment of choice for infants and children with port wine stains.

Morelli JG et al: Initial lesion size is a critical factor in determining the response of port wine stains in children treated with the pulsed (450 microsecond) dye (585 nanometer) laser. Arch Pediatr Adolesc Med 1995;149:1142.

Talman B et al: Portwine stains and the likelihood of ophthalmologic or CNS complications. Pediatrics 1991;87:323.

Hemangioma

A red, rubbery nodule with a roughened surface is a hemangioma. The lesion is often not present at birth but is represented by a permanent blanched area on the skin that is supplanted at 2–4 weeks of age by red nodules. Histologically, these are benign tumors of capillary endothelial cells. Hemangiomas may be superficial, deep, or mixed. The terms strawberry and cavernous are misleading and should not be used. The biologic behavior of a hemangioma is the same despite its location. Fifty percent resolve spontaneously by age 5, 70% by age 7, 90% by age 9, and the rest by adolescence, leaving redundant skin, hypopigmentation, and telangiectasia. Local complications include superficial ulceration and secondary pyoderma.

Complications that require immediate treatment are (1) thrombocytopenia resulting from platelet trapping within the lesion (Kasabach-Merritt syndrome); (2) airway obstruction (hemangiomas of the head and neck are often associated with subglottic hemangiomas); (3) visual obstruction (with resulting amblyopia); and (4) cardiac decompensation (high-output failure). In these instances, the treatment of choice is with prednisone, 1–2 mg/kg orally daily or every other day for 4–6 weeks. Interferon alfa-2a has been used to treat serious hemangiomas unresponsive to prednisone. If the lesion is ulcerated or bleeding, pulsed dye laser treatment may be helpful.

Eskowitz RAB, Mulliken JB, Folkman J: Interferon alfa-2a therapy for life-threatening hemangiomas of infancy. N Engl J Med 1992;326:1456.
Esterly NB: Hemangiomas in infants and children: Clinical observation. Pediatr Dermatol 1992;9:353.
Garden JM, Bakus AD, Paller AS: Treatment of cutaneous hemangiomas by the flashlamp-pumped pulsed dye laser: Prospective analysis. J Pediatr 1992;120:555.
Morelli JG et al: Management of ulcerated hemangiomas in infancy. Arch Pediatr Adolesc Med 1994;148:1104.

Lymphangioma

Lymphangiomas are rubbery, skin-colored nodules occurring in the parotid area (cystic hygromas) or on the tongue. They often result in grotesque enlargement of soft tissues. Surgical excision is the only treatment, though the results are not satisfactory.

EPIDERMAL BIRTHMARKS

Epidermal Nevus

Linear or groups of linear, warty, papular, unilateral lesions represent overgrowth of epidermis since birth. These areas may range from dirty yellow to brown or may be darkly pigmented. The histologic features of the lesions include thickening of the epidermis and elongation of the rete ridges and hyperkeratosis. Clinically, widespread lesions may be associated with focal motor seizures, mental subnormality, and skeletal anomalies.

Treatment once or twice daily with topical calcipotriene may improve the lesions.

Rogers M: Epidermal nevi and the epidermal nevus syndrome: A review of 233 cases. Pediatr Dermatol 1992;9:342.
Micali G, Nasca MR, Musumeci MI: Effect of topical calcipotriol on inflammatory linear verrucous epidermal nevus. (Letter.) Pediatr Dermatol 1995;12:386.

Nevus Comedonicus

The lesion known as nevus comedonicus consists of linear groups of widely dilated follicular openings plugged with keratin, giving the appearance of localized noninflammatory acne. The treatment of choice is surgical removal. If this is not feasible, topical retinoic acid is helpful.

Nevus Sebaceus

The nevus sebaceus of Jadassohn is a hamartoma of sebaceous glands and underlying apocrine glands that is diagnosed by the appearance at birth of a yellowish, hairless, smooth plaque in the scalp or on the face. The lesion may be contiguous with an epidermal nevus on the face and constitute part of the linear epidermal nevus syndrome.

Histologically, nevus sebaceus represents an overabundance of sebaceous glands without hair follicles. At puberty, with androgenic stimulation, the sebaceous cells in the nevus divide, expand their cellular volume, and synthesize sebum, resulting in a warty mass. Because 15% of these lesions become basal cell carcinomas after puberty, excision is recommended before puberty.

CONNECTIVE TISSUE BIRTHMARKS (Juvenile Elastoma, Collagenoma)

Connective tissue nevi are smooth, skin-colored papules 1–10 mm in diameter that are grouped on the trunk. A solitary, larger (5–10 cm) nodule is called a **shagreen patch** and is histologically indistinguishable from other connective tissue nevi that show thickened, abundant collagen bundles with or without associated increases of elastic tissue. Although the shagreen patch is a cutaneous clue to tuberous sclerosis (Chapter 22), the other connective tissue nevi occur as isolated events. These nevi remain throughout life and need no treatment.

HEREDITARY SKIN DISORDERS

The Ichthyoses

Ichthyosis is a term applied to several heritable diseases characterized by the presence of excessive scales on the skin. Major categories are listed in Table 13–4. Treatment consists of controlling scaling with Lac-Hydrin 12% applied once daily. Restoring water to the skin is also very helpful.

Paller AS: Laboratory tests for ichthyosis. Dermatol Clin 1994;12:99.

Epidermolysis Bullosa

The diagnostic feature of this group of diseases is the formation of blisters in response to slight trauma. They can be divided into scarring and nonscarring types (Table 13–5).

Treatment usually consists of systemic antibiotics for infection, protection of the skin with petrolatum, zinc oxide, or synthetic dressings and cooling the skin. If hands and feet are involved, reducing skin friction with 5% glutaraldehyde every 3 days is helpful.

Paller AS: The genetic basis of hereditary blistering disorders. Curr Opin Pediatr 1996;8:367.

Table 13–4. Four major types of ichthyosis.

Name	Age at Onset	Clinical Features	Genetic Defect	Inheritance
Ichthyosis with normal epidermal turnover				
Ichthyosis vulgaris	Childhood	Fine scales, deep palmar and plantar markings	Filaggrin/profilaggrin	Autosomal dominant
X-linked ichthyosis	Birth	Palms and soles spared; thick scales that darken with age; corneal opacities in patients and carrier mothers	Cholesterol sulfatase	X-linked
Ichthyosis with increased epidermal turnover				
Epidermolytic hyper-keratosis	Birth	Verrucous, yellow scales in flexural areas and palms and soles	Keratins 1 and 10	Autosomal dominant
Lamellar ichthyosis	Birth; collodion baby	Erythroderma, ectropion, large coarse scales; thickened palms and soles	Transglutaminase 1	Autosomal recessive

COMMON SKIN DISEASES IN INFANTS, CHILDREN, & ADOLESCENTS

ACNE

The common forms of acne in pediatric patients occur at two ages: in the newborn period and in adolescence. Neonatal acne is a response to maternal androgen, first appearing at 4–6 weeks of age and lasting until 4–6 months of age. The lesions are primarily on the face, upper chest, and back, in a distribution similar to that seen in adolescent acne. It has been hypothesized, but not proved, that infants who have severe neonatal acne will develop severe adolescent acne.

The onset of adolescent acne is between ages 8 and 10 in 40% of children. The early lesions are usually limited to the face and are primarily closed comedones (whiteheads; see below). Eventually, 85% of adolescents develop some form of acne.

Table 13–5. Types of epidermolysis bullosa.

Name	Age at Onset	Clinical Features	Genetic Defect	Inheritance
Nonscarring types				
Epidermolysis bullosa simplex	Birth	Hemorrhagic blisters over the lower legs; cooling prevents blisters	Keratins 5 and 14	Autosomal dominant
Recurrent bullous eruption of the hands and feet (Weber-Cockayne syndrome)	First few years of life	Blisters brought out by walking	Keratins 5 and 14	Autosomal dominant
Junctional bullous dermolysis (Herlitz's disease)	Birth	Erosions on legs, oral mucosa; severe perioral involvement	Laminin V	Autosomal recessive
Scarring types				
Epidermolysis bullosa dystrophica, dominant	Infancy	Numerous blisters on hands and feet; milia formation	Type VII collagen	Autosomal dominant
Epidermolysis bullosa dystrophica, recessive	Birth	Repeated episodes of blistering, secondary infection and scarring—"mitten hands and feet"	Type VII collagen	Autosomal recessive

Clinical Findings

Acne occurs in sebaceous follicles, which, unlike hair follicles, have large, abundant sebaceous glands and usually lack hair. They are located primarily on the face, upper chest, back, and penis. Obstruction of the sebaceous follicle opening produces the clinical lesion of acne. If the obstruction occurs at the follicular mouth, the clinical lesion is characterized by a wide, patulous opening filled with a plug of stratum corneum cells. This is the open comedo, or blackhead. Open comedones are the predominant clinical lesion in early adolescent acne. The black color is caused not by dirt but by oxidized melanin within the stratum corneum cellular plug. Open comedones do not often progress to inflammatory lesions. Closed comedones, or whiteheads, are caused by obstruction just beneath the follicular opening in the neck of the sebaceous follicle, which produces a cystic swelling of the follicular duct directly beneath the epidermis. The stratum corneum produced accumulates continuously within the cystic cavity. The resultant lesion is an enlarging sphere just beneath the skin surface. Most authorities believe that closed comedones are precursors of inflammatory acne. If open or closed comedones are the predominant lesions on the skin in adolescent acne, the condition is called comedonal acne.

In typical adolescent acne, several different types of lesions are present simultaneously, eg, open and closed comedones and inflammatory lesions such as papules, pustules, and cysts. Inflammatory lesions may also rarely occur as interconnecting, draining sinus tracts. Adolescents with cystic acne require prompt medical attention, since ruptured cysts and sinus tracts result in severe scar formation. New acne scars are highly vascular and have a reddish or purplish hue. Such scars return to normal skin color after several years. Acne scars may be depressed beneath the skin level, raised, or flat to the skin. In adolescents with a tendency toward keloid formation, keloidal scars can occur following acne lesions, particularly over the sternal area.

Differential Diagnosis

Consider rosacea, nevus comedonicus, flat warts, the angiofibromas of tuberous sclerosis, miliaria, and molluscum contagiosum.

Pathogenesis

The primary event in acne formation is obstruction of the sebaceous follicle. Ordinarily, the lining of such follicles contains one or two layers of stratum corneum cells, but in acne the stratum corneum is overproduced. This phenomenon is androgen-dependent in adolescent acne. The sebaceous follicles contain an enzyme, testosterone 5α-reductase, which converts plasma testosterone to dihydrotestosterone. This androgen is a potent stimulus for nuclear division of the follicular germinative cells and subsequently of excessive cell production. Thus, obstruction requires the presence of both circulating androgens and the converting enzyme. After the production or administration of androgens, there is a delay until cellular proliferation occurs and follicular obstruction subsequently appears.

The pathogenesis of inflammatory acne is not well understood. Undoubtedly, physical manipulation of a closed comedo could lead to rupture of the cavity contents into the dermis with a subsequent inflammatory response. Spontaneous inflammation also occurs in obstructed follicles, but the reason for this is unclear. An attractive hypothesis is that overgrowth of gram-positive bacteria in the obstructed follicle (either *Propionibacterium acnes* or *Staphylococcus epidermidis*) might stimulate factors that initiate inflammation. Overproduction of sebum and free fatty acid formation seem unlikely as causes of inflammation in acne as presently understood.

Adolescent acne may result from several external causes. Frictional acne caused by headbands, football helmets, or tight-fitting brassieres or other garments occurs predominantly underneath the area where the garment is worn. Oil-based cosmetics may be responsible for predominantly comedonal acne, and hair sprays may produce acne along the hair margin.

Drug-induced acne should be suspected in teenagers if all lesions are in the same stage at the same time and if involvement extends to the lower abdomen, lower back, arms, and legs. Drugs responsible for acne include corticotropin (ACTH), glucocorticoids, androgens, hydantoins, and isoniazid, each of which increases plasma testosterone.

Treatment

A. Topical Keratolytic Agents: The mainstay of acne therapy is the use of potent topical keratolytic agents applied to the skin to relieve follicular obstruction. The four most effective keratolytic agents are tretinoin (retinoic acid), benzoyl peroxide gel, azelaic acid, and adapalene. The agents may be used once daily, or the combination of retinoic acid cream, azelaic acid, and adapalene applied to acne-bearing areas of the skin once daily in the evening and a benzoyl peroxide gel applied once daily in the morning may be used. This regimen will control 80–85% of cases of adolescent acne.

B. Topical Antibiotics: Topical antibiotics are used to avoid the side effects caused by systemic antibiotics. Topical antibiotics are less effective than systemic antibiotics and at best are equivalent in potency to 250 mg of tetracycline orally once a day. One percent clindamycin phosphate solution is the most efficacious topical antibiotic. Some percutaneous absorption may occur rarely with this drug, resulting in diarrhea and colitis; 1.5% and 2% topical erythromycin solutions are effective; 1% topical tetracycline solution is minimally effective.

C. Systemic Antibiotics: Antibiotics that are

concentrated in sebum, such as tetracycline, minocycline, and erythromycin, are very effective in inflammatory acne. The usual dose of tetracycline or erythromycin is 0.5–1 g; of minocycline, 50–100 mg taken once or twice daily on an empty stomach (nothing to eat 1 hour before or after the medication). Treatment should be continued for 2–3 months until the acne lesions are suppressed.

D. Oral Retinoids: An oral retinoid, 13-*cis*-retinoic acid (isotretinoin; Accutane), is the most effective treatment for severe cystic acne. The precise mechanism of its action is unknown, but decreased sebum production, decreased follicular obstruction, decreased skin bacteria, and general anti-inflammatory activities have been described. The initial dosage is 40 mg once or twice daily. This drug is not effective in comedonal acne or other mild forms of acne. Side effects include dryness and scaliness of the skin, dry lips, and, occasionally, dry eyes and dry nose. Up to 10% of patients experience mild, reversible hair loss. Elevated liver enzymes and blood lipids have rarely been described. Isotretinoin is teratogenic—use in young women of childbearing age is not recommended unless strict adherence to the manufacturer's guidelines is ensured.

E. Other Acne Treatments: There is no convincing evidence that dietary management, mild drying agents, abrasive scrubs, oral vitamin A, ultraviolet light, cryotherapy, or incision and drainage have any beneficial effects in the management of acne.

F. Avoidance of Cosmetics and Hair Spray: Acne can be aggravated by a variety of external factors that result in further obstruction of partially occluded sebaceous follicles. Discontinuing the use of oil-based cosmetics, face creams, and hair sprays may alleviate the comedonal component of acne within 4–6 weeks.

Patient Education & Follow-Up Visits

The mechanism of acne formation and the treatment plan must be explained to adolescent patients. Time should be set aside at the first visit to answer questions. Explain that there will not be much improvement for 4–8 weeks. Establish guidelines for ideal control, and explain that the best result the patient can expect is the appearance of only one or two new pimples a month. No drug is available that will prevent an adolescent from ever having another acne lesion. A written education sheet is useful.

Follow-up visits should be made every 6–8 weeks. The criterion for ideal control is a few lesions every 4 weeks. Explain again what medications are being used and what the treatment is intended to achieve, and question the patient to determine whether the medications are being used properly.

Dahl MV (editor): *Perspectives: Current concepts in Acne and Rosacea.* A symposium at the American Academy of Dermatology, Orlando, Florida, July, 1996.

BACTERIAL INFECTIONS OF THE SKIN

Impetigo

Erosions covered by honey-colored crusts are diagnostic of impetigo. Staphylococci and group A streptococci are important pathogens in this disease, which histologically consists of superficial invasion of bacteria into the upper epidermis, forming a subcorneal pustule.

Patients should be treated with an antimicrobial agent effective against *Staphylococcus aureus* (β-lactamase–resistant penicillins or cephalosporins, clindamycin, amoxicillin-clavulanate) for 7–10 days. Topical mupirocin (three times daily) is also effective.

Shriner DL, Schwartz RA, Janninger CK: Impetigo. Cutis 1995;56:30.

Bullous Impetigo

All impetigo is bullous, with the blister forming just beneath the stratum corneum, but in "bullous impetigo" there is, in addition to the usual erosion covered by a honey-colored crust, a border filled with clear fluid. Staphylococci may be isolated from these lesions, and systemic signs of circulating exfoliatin are absent. "Bullous varicella" is a disorder that represents bullous impetigo as a superinfection in varicella lesions. Treatment with oral antistaphylococcal drugs for 7–10 days is effective. Application of cool compresses to debride crusts is a helpful symptomatic measure.

Ecthyma

Ecthyma is a firm, dry crust, surrounded by erythema, that exudes purulent material. It represents deep invasion by group A β-hemolytic streptococci through the epidermis to the superficial dermis. Treatment is with systemic penicillin.

Cellulitis

Cellulitis is characterized by erythematous, hot, tender, ill-defined, edematous plaques accompanied by regional lymphadenopathy. Histologically, this disorder represents invasion of microorganisms into the lower dermis and sometimes beyond, with obstruction of local lymphatics. Group A β-hemolytic streptococci and coagulase-positive staphylococci are the most common causes; pneumococci and *Haemophilus influenzae* are rare causes. Staphylococcal infections are usually more localized and more likely to have a purulent center; streptococcal infections spread more rapidly, but these characteristics cannot be used to specify the infecting agent. An entry site of prior trauma or infection (eg, varicella) is often present. Septicemia is common, and treatment is with an appropriate systemic antibiotic.

Sachs MK: Cutaneous cellulitis. Arch Dermatol 1991; 127:493.

Folliculitis

A pustule at a follicular opening represents folliculitis. If the pustule occurs at eccrine sweat orifices, it is correctly called poritis. Staphylococci and streptococci are the most frequent pathogens. Treatment consists of measures to remove follicular obstruction—either cool, wet compresses for 24 hours or keratolytics such as those used for acne.

Abscess

An abscess occurs deep in the skin, at the bottom of a follicle or an apocrine gland, and is diagnosed as an erythematous, firm, acutely tender nodule with ill-defined borders. Staphylococci are the most common organisms. Treatment consists of incision and drainage and systemic antibiotics.

Scalded Skin Syndrome

This entity consists of the sudden onset of bright red, acutely painful skin, most obvious perorally, periorbitally, and in the flexural areas of the neck, the axillae, the popliteal and antecubital areas, and the groin. The slightest pressure on the skin results in severe pain and separation of the epidermis, leaving a glistening layer (the stratum granulosum of the epidermis) beneath. The disease is caused by a circulating toxin (exfoliatin) elaborated by phage group II staphylococci. The site of action of the exfoliatin is the intracellular area of the granular layer, resulting in a separation of cells.

Scalded skin syndrome includes Ritter's disease of the newborn, toxic shock syndrome, and the mildest form, staphylococcal scarlet fever. (See also Bullous Impetigo, above.) In all of the forms of this entity, the causative staphylococci may be isolated not from the skin but rather from the nasopharynx, an abscess, sinus blood culture, etc. Treatment is with systemic antistaphylococcal drugs.

Gemmell CG: Staphylococcal scalded skin syndrome. J Med Microbiol 1995;43:318.

FUNGAL INFECTIONS OF THE SKIN

1. DERMATOPHYTE INFECTIONS

Dermatophytes become attached to the superficial layer of the epidermis, nails, and hair, where they proliferate. They grow mainly within the stratum corneum and do not invade the lower epidermis or dermis. Release of toxins from dermatophytes, especially those whose natural host is animals or soil—eg, *Microsporum canis* and *Trichophyton verrucosum*—results in dermatitis. Fungal infection should be suspected with any red and scaly lesion.

Classification & Diagnosis

A. Tinea Capitis: Thickened, broken-off hairs with erythema and scaling of underlying scalp are the distinguishing features (Table 13–6). In epidemic ringworm, hairs are broken off at the surface of the scalp, leaving a "black dot" appearance. Pustule formation and a boggy, fluctuant mass on the scalp occur in *M canis* and *Trichophyton tonsurans* infections. This mass, called a kerion, represents an exaggerated host response to the organism. Fungal culture should be performed in all cases of suspected tinea capitis.

B. Tinea Corporis: Tinea corporis presents either as annular marginated papules with a thin scale and clear center or as an annular confluent dermatitis. The most common organisms are *Trichophyton mentagrophytes* and *M canis*. The diagnosis is made by scraping thin scales from the border of the lesion, dissolving them in 20% KOH, and examining for hyphae.

C. Tinea Cruris: Symmetric, sharply marginated lesions in inguinal areas are seen with tinea cruris. The most common organisms are *Trichophyton rubrum*, *T mentagrophytes*, and *Epidermophyton floccosum*.

D. Tinea Pedis: The diagnosis of tinea pedis in a prepubertal child must always be regarded with skepticism; atopic feet or contact dermatitis is a more likely diagnosis in this age group. Tinea pedis is seen most commonly in postpubertal males with blisters on the instep of the foot. Fissuring between the toes is occasionally seen.

E. Tinea Unguium (Onychomycosis): Loosening of the nail plate from the nail bed (onycholysis), giving a yellow discoloration, is the first sign of fungal invasion of the nails. Thickening of the distal nail plate then occurs, followed by scaling and a crumbly appearance of the entire nail plate surface. *T rubrum* and *T mentagrophytes* are the most common causes. The diagnosis is confirmed by KOH examination and fungal culture. Usually only one or two nails are involved. If every nail is involved, psoriasis or lichen planus is a more likely diagnosis than fungal infection.

Table 13–6. Clinical features of tinea capitis.

Most Common Organisms	Clinical Appearance	Microscopic Appearance in KOH
Trichophyton tonsurans (90%)	Hairs broken off 2–3 mm from follicle; "black dot"; no fluorescence	Hyphae and spores within hair
Microsporum canis (10%)	Thickened broken-off hairs that fluoresce yellow-green with Wood's lamp[1]	Small spores outside of hair; hyphae within hair

[1]Select fluorescent hairs for examination in KOH and culture.

Treatment

The treatment of dermatophytosis is quite simple: If hair or nails are involved, griseofulvin is the treatment of choice. Topical antifungal agents do not enter hair or nails in sufficient concentration to clear the infection. The absorption of griseofulvin from the gastrointestinal tract is enhanced by a fatty meal; thus, whole milk or ice cream taken with the medication increases absorption. The dosage of griseofulvin is 20 mg/kg/d. With hair infections, cultures should be done every 4 weeks and treatment should be continued for 6–8 weeks following a negative culture. In nail infections, treat for a minimum of 3 months. The side effects are few, and the drug has been used successfully in the newborn period.

Tinea corporis, tinea pedis, and tinea cruris can be treated effectively with topical medication after careful inspection to make certain that the hair and nails are not involved. Treatment with clotrimazole (Lotrimin), miconazole (Micatin), econazole (Spectazole), or haloprogin (Halotex) applied twice daily for 3–4 weeks is recommended.

Goldgeier MH: Fungal infections of the skin, hair and nails. Pediatr Ann 1993;22:253.

Elewski BE, Hay RJ: International summit on cutaneous antifungal therapy. Pediatr Dermatol 1996;13:69

Lesher JL Jr: Recent developments in antifungal therapy. Dermatol Clin 1996;14:23.

2. TINEA VERSICOLOR

Tinea versicolor is a superficial infection caused by *Pityrosporum orbiculare* (also called *Malassezia furfur*), a yeast-like fungus. It characteristically causes polycyclic connected hypopigmented macules and very fine scales in areas of sun-induced pigmentation. In winter, the polycyclic macules appear reddish-brown.

Treatment consists of application of selenium sulfide (Selsun), 2.5% suspension, or topical antifungals. Selenium sulfide should be applied to the whole body and left on overnight. Treatment can be repeated again in 1 week and then monthly thereafter. It tends to be somewhat irritating, and the patient should be warned about this difficulty.

Savin R: Diagnosis and treatment of tinea versicolor. J Fam Pract 1996;43:127.

3. *CANDIDA ALBICANS* INFECTIONS (See Chapter 37.)

In addition to being a frequent invader in diaper dermatitis, *Candida albicans* also infects the oral mucosa, where it appears as thick white patches with an erythematous base (thrush); the angles of the mouth, where it causes fissures and white exudate (perlèche); and the cuticular region of the fingers, where thickening of the cuticle, dull red erythema, and distortion of growth of the nail plate suggest the diagnosis of candidal paronychia. *Candida* dermatitis is characterized by sharply defined erythematous patches, sometimes with eroded areas. Pustules, vesicles, or papules may be present as satellite lesions. Similar infections may be found in other moist areas, such as the axillae and neck folds. This infection is more common in children who have recently received antibiotics.

A topical imidazole cream is the drug of first choice for *C albicans* infections. In diaper dermatitis, the cream form can be applied every 3–4 hours. In oral thrush, nystatin suspension should be applied directly to the mucosa with the parent's finger or a cotton-tipped applicator, since it is not absorbed and acts topically. In candidal paronychia, the antifungal agent is applied over the area, covered with occlusive plastic wrapping, and left on overnight after the application is made airtight. Refractory candidiasis will respond to a brief course of oral fluconazole.

Thomas I: Superficial and deep candidiasis. Int J Dermatol 1993;32:778.

VIRAL INFECTIONS OF THE SKIN

Herpes Simplex

Grouped vesicles or grouped erosions suggest herpes simplex. The microscopic finding of epidermal giant cells after scraping the vesicle base with a No. 15 blade, smearing on a slide, and staining with Wright's stain (Tzanck smear) suggests herpes simplex or varicella-zoster. A rapid immunofluorescent test for HSV is available. In infants, lesions resulting from herpes simplex type 1 are seen on the gingiva and lips, periorbitally, or on the thumb in thumb suckers. Recurrent erosions in the mouth are usually aphthous stomatitis in children rather than recurrent herpes simplex. Herpes simplex type 2 is seen on the genitalia and in the mouth in adolescents. Cutaneous dissemination of herpes simplex occurs in patients with atopic dermatitis (**eczema herpeticum, Kaposi's varicelliform eruption**). The treatment of this and other herpesvirus infections is discussed in Chapter 34. In severe disseminated infection, oral acyclovir may be helpful.

Spruance SL: The natural history of recurrent oral-facial herpes simplex virus infection. Semin Dermatol 1992;11:200.

Varicella-Zoster

Grouped vesicles in a dermatome on the trunk or face suggest herpes zoster. Zoster in children may not be painful and usually has a mild course. In patients with compromised host resistance, the appearance of an erythematous border around the vesicles is a good prognostic sign. Conversely, large bullae without a tendency to crusting imply a poor host response to the virus. Varicella-zoster and herpes simplex lesions undergo the same series of changes: papule, vesicle, pustule, crust, slightly depressed scar. Varicella appears in crops, and many different stages of lesions are present at the same time.

Itching is usually the only symptom, and cool baths as frequently as necessary or drying lotions such as calamine lotion are sufficient to relieve symptoms. In immunosuppressed children, intravenous or oral acyclovir should be used.

Wharton M: The epidemiology of varicella-zoster virus infections. Infect Dis Clin North Am 1996;10:571.
Balfour HH Jr: Clinical aspects of chickenpox and herpes zoster. J Int Med Res 1994;22(Suppl)1:3A.

HIV Infection

The average time of onset of skin lesions after perinatally acquired HIV infection is 4 months; after transfusion-acquired infection, it is 11 months. Persistent oral candidiasis and recalcitrant candidal diaper rash are the most frequent cutaneous manifestations of infantile HIV infection. Severe or recurrent herpetic gingivostomatitis, herpes zoster, and molluscum contagiosum are seen. Recurrent staphylococcal pyodermas, tinea of the face, and onychomycosis are also observed. A generalized dermatitis with features of seborrhea is extremely common. In general, persistent, recurrent, or extensive skin infections should make one suspicious of HIV infection.

Prose NS: Cutaneous manifestations of pediatric HIV infections. Pediatr Dermatol 1992;9:326.
Smith KJ et al: Cutaneous findings in HIV-1 positive patients: A 42 month prospective study. J Am Acad Dermatol 1994;31:746.

Virus-Induced Tumors

A. Molluscum Contagiosum: Molluscum contagiosum consists of umbilicated, white or whitish-yellow papules in groups on the genitalia or trunk. They are common in sexually active adolescents as well as in infants and preschool children. Crushing a lesion between glass slides followed by microscopic examination after staining with Wright's stain will demonstrate epidermal cells with inclusions. Molluscum contagiosum is a poxvirus that induces the epidermis to proliferate, forming a pale papule.

Removal of the lesion with a sharp curette or knife is curative. This therapy may leave a small scar, and one must weigh the advantage of removal of lesions that will disappear in 2–3 years.

B. Warts: Warts are skin-colored papules with irregular (verrucous) surfaces. They are intraepidermal tumors caused by infection with human papillomavirus. This DNA virus induces the epidermal cells to proliferate, thus resulting in the warty growth.

No therapy for warts is ideal, and some types of therapy should be avoided because the recurrence rate of warts is high. Flat warts generally require no treatment. They may be considered a mild wart virus infection, and since they usually disappear within 6–9 months they are best left alone. This holds true especially for all flat warts on the face. A good response to 0.05% tretinoin (Retin-A) cream, applied once daily for 3–4 weeks, has been reported.

The best treatment for the solitary common ("vulgaris") wart is to freeze it with liquid nitrogen. The liquid nitrogen should be allowed to drip from the cotton-tipped applicator onto the wart without pressure. Pressure exaggerates cold injury by causing vasoconstriction and may produce a deep ulcer and scar. Liquid nitrogen is applied by drip until the wart turns completely white and stays white for 20–25 seconds. Large and painful plantar warts are treated most effectively by applying 40% salicylic acid plaster cut with a scissors to fit the lesion. The sticky brown side of the plaster is placed against the lesion, taped on securely with adhesive tape, and left on for 5 days. The plaster is then removed, and the white necrotic warty tissue can be gently rubbed off with the finger and a new salicylic acid plaster applied. This procedure is repeated every 5 days, and the patient is seen every 4 weeks. Most plantar warts resolve in 6–8 weeks when treated in this way.

Sharp scalpel excision, electrosurgery, and laser surgery should be avoided, since the resulting scar often becomes a more difficult problem than the wart itself and there may be recurrence of the wart in the area of the scar.

Venereal warts (condylomata acuminata) are best treated with 25% podophyllum resin (podophyllin) in alcohol or Podofilox, a lower concentration of purified podophyllin. These should be painted on the lesions and then washed off after 4 hours. Retreatment in 7–10 days may be necessary. A wart not on the vulvar mucous membrane but on the adjacent skin should be treated as a common wart and frozen.

For isolated warts and periungual warts, cantharidin (Cantharone, Verr-Canth) is effective and painless in children. It causes a blister and sometimes is difficult to control. An undesirable complication is the appearance of warts along the margins of the cantharidin blister. Cantharidin is applied to the skin, allowed to dry, and covered with occlusive tape such as Blenderm for 24 hours.

No wart therapy is immediately and definitively successful, and recurrences are reported in more than 30% of cases even with the best care.

Armstrong DK, Handley JM: Anogenital warts in prepubertal children: Pathogenesis, HPV typing and management. Int J STD AIDS 1997;8:78
Ordoukhanian E, Lane AT: Warts and molluscum contagio-

sum: Beware of treatments worse than the disease. Postgrad Med 1997:101:223

Siegfried EC: Warts on children: An approach to therapy. Pediatr Ann 1996;25:79.

INSECT INFESTATIONS

Scabies

Scabies is suggested by linear burrows about the wrists, ankles, finger webs, areolas, anterior axillary folds, genitalia, or face (in infants). Often there are excoriations, honey-colored crusts, and pustules from secondary infection. Identification of the female mite or her eggs and feces is necessary to confirm the diagnosis. Scrape an unscratched papule or burrow with a No. 15 blade and examine microscopically in immersion oil to confirm the diagnosis. In a child who is often scratching, scrape under the fingernails. Examine the parents for unscratched burrows.

Lindane (gamma benzene hexachloride; Kwell) and permethrin are excellent scabicides. However, since lindane is concentrated in the central nervous system, where toxicity from systemic absorption in infants has been reported, the following restricted use of this agent is recommended: (1) For adults and older children, one treatment of lindane lotion or cream applied to the entire body and left on for 4 hours, followed by showering, is sufficient. (2) Infants tend to have more organisms and many more lesions and may have to be retreated in 7–10 days. All family members should be treated simultaneously. Permethrin 5% cream (Elimite) may be substituted for lindane in infants.

Peterson CM, Eichenfield LF: Scabies. Pediatr Ann 1996;25:97.

Pediculoses
(Louse Infestations)

Excoriated papules and pustules with a history of severe itching at night suggest infestation with the human body louse. This louse may be discovered in the seams of underwear but not on the body. In the scalp hair, the gelatinous nits of the head louse adhere tightly to the hair shaft. The pubic louse may be found crawling among pubic hairs, or blue-black macules may be found dispersed through the pubic region (maculae ceruleae). The pubic louse is often seen on the eyelashes of newborns.

Lindane (gamma benzene hexachloride; Kwell) is recommended: For head lice, a shampoo preparation is left on the scalp for 5 minutes and rinsed out thoroughly. The hair is then combed with a fine-tooth comb to remove nits. This may be repeated in 7 days. Lindane cream or lotion applied to the body for 4 hours may be necessary for body lice, but boiling the clothing for 10 minutes followed by ironing the seams with a hot iron usually eliminates them. Per-

methrin 1% creme rinse also eliminates lice. Lindane cream or lotion applied to the pubic area for 24 hours is sufficient to treat pediculosis pubis. It may be repeated in 4–5 days.

Ibarr J, Hall DM: Head lice in school children. Arch Dis Child 1996;36:471.

Burgess IF: Human lice and their management. Adv Parasitol 1995;36:271.

Papular Urticaria

Papular urticaria is characterized by grouped erythematous papules surrounded by an urticarial flare and distributed over the shoulders, upper arms, and buttocks in infants. These lesions represent delayed hypersensitivity reactions to stinging or biting insects and can be reproduced by patch testing with the offending insect. Fleas from dogs and cats are the usual offenders. Less commonly, mosquitoes, lice, scabies, and bird and grass mites are involved. The sensitivity is transient, lasting 4–6 months. The logical therapy is to remove the offending insect. Topical corticosteroids and oral antihistamines will control symptoms.

Howard R, Frieden IJ: Papular urticaria in children. Pediatr Dermatol 1996;35:1.

DERMATITIS
(Eczema)

The terms "dermatitis" and "eczema" are currently used interchangeably in dermatology, though the etymologic implication of eczema is "a boiling over" and the term originally denoted an acute weeping dermatosis. All forms of dermatitis, regardless of cause, may present with acute edema, erythema, and oozing with crusting, mild erythema alone, or lichenification. Lichenification is diagnosed by thickening of the skin with a shiny surface and exaggerated, deepened skin markings. It is the response of the skin to chronic rubbing or scratching.

Although the lesions of the various dermatoses are histologically indistinguishable, clinicians have nonetheless divided the disease group called dermatitis into several categories based on known causes in some cases and differing natural histories in others.

1. ATOPIC DERMATITIS

Atopic dermatitis is not a clearly defined clinical entity but a general term for chronic superficial inflammation of the skin that can be applied to a heterogeneous group of patients. Many (not all) patients go through three clinical phases. In the first, infantile eczema, the dermatitis begins on the cheeks and scalp and frequently expresses itself as oval patches on the trunk, later involving the extensor surfaces of the extremities. The usual age at onset is 2–3 months, and this phase ends at age 18 months to 2 years. Only one-third of all infants with atopic eczema progress to phase 2—childhood or flexural eczema—in which the predominant involvement is in the antecubital and popliteal fossae, the neck, the wrists, and sometimes the hands or feet. This phase lasts from age 2 years to adolescence. Some children will have involvement only of the soles of the feet, with cracking, redness, and pain—so-called **atopic feet.** Only one-third of children with typical flexural eczema will progress to adolescent eczema, which is usually manifested by hand dermatitis only. Atopic dermatitis is quite unusual after age 30.

Atopic dermatitis has no known cause, and despite the high incidence of asthma and hay fever in these patients (30%) and their families (70%), evidence for allergy beyond this hereditary association is limited to testimonials. The case for food and inhalant allergens as specific causes of atopic dermatitis is not strong.

A few patients with atopic dermatitis have immunodeficiency with recurrent pyodermas, unusual susceptibility to herpes simplex and vaccinia virus, hyperimmunoglobulinemia E, defective neutrophil and monocyte chemotaxis, and impaired T lymphocyte function (see Chapter 27).

A faulty epidermal barrier may predispose the patient with atopic dermatitis to itchy skin. Inability to hold water within the stratum corneum results in rapid evaporation of water, shrinking of the stratum corneum, and "cracks" in the epidermal barrier. Such skin forms an ineffective barrier to the entry of various irritants—and, indeed, it may be clinically useful to regard atopic dermatitis as a primary irritant contact dermatitis and simply tell the patient, "You have sensitive skin." Chronic atopic dermatitis is frequently secondarily infected with *Staphylococcus aureus* or *Streptococcus pyogenes.*

Treatment

A. Acute Stages: Application of wet dressings and topical corticosteroids is the treatment of choice for acute, weeping atopic eczema. A topical steroid preparation is applied two times daily and covered with wet dressings as outlined at the beginning of this chapter. Systemic antibiotics chosen on the basis of appropriate skin cultures may be necessary, since lesions in the acute stages are often secondarily infected.

B. Chronic Stages: Treatment is aimed at avoiding irritants and restoring water to the skin. No soaps or harsh shampoos should be used, and the patient should avoid woolen or any rough clothing. Restoring water to the skin is accomplished by two baths daily, less than 5 minutes each, after which lubricating oils or ointments are applied. Moisturel is a useful lubricant. Plain petrolatum and lards are often

too greasy and may cause considerable sweat retention. Liberal use of Cetaphil lotion as a soap substitute four or five times a day is also satisfactory as a means of lubrication. A bedroom humidifier is often helpful. Topical corticosteroids should be limited to the less potent ones (see Table 13–3). Hydrocortisone ointment, 1% twice daily, is often sufficient. There is never any reason to use super- or high-potency corticosteroids in atopic dermatitis. In superinfected atopic dermatitis, systemic antibiotics for 10–14 days are necessary.

Treatment failures in chronic atopic dermatitis are most often the result of patient noncompliance. This is a frustrating disease for parent and child.

Kay J et al: The prevalence of childhood atopic dermatitis in a general population. J Am Acad Dermatol 1994;30:35.

Rothe MJ, Grant-Kels JM: Atopic dermatitis: An update. J Am Acad Dermatol 1996;35:1.

Williams HC et al: The UK Working Party's diagnostic criteria for atopic dermatitis. I. Derivation of a minimum set of discriminators for atopic dermatitis. Br J Dermatol 1994;131:383.

2. NUMMULAR ECZEMA

Nummular eczema is characterized by numerous symmetrically distributed coin-shaped patches of dermatitis, principally on the extremities. These may be acute, oozing, and crusted or dry and scaling. The disease lasts 9 months to 2 years. The differential diagnosis should include tinea corporis and atopic dermatitis.

The same topical measures should be used as for atopic dermatitis, though treatment is often more difficult.

3. PRIMARY IRRITANT CONTACT DERMATITIS (Diaper Dermatitis)

Contact dermatitis is of two types: primary irritant and allergic eczematous. Primary irritant dermatitis develops within a few hours, reaches peak severity at 24 hours, and then disappears. Allergic eczematous contact dermatitis (see below) has a delayed onset of 18 hours, peaks at 48–72 hours, and often lasts as long as 2–3 weeks even if exposure to the offending antigen is discontinued.

Diaper dermatitis, the most common form of primary irritant contact dermatitis seen in pediatric practice, is caused by prolonged contact of the skin with urine and feces, which contain irritating chemicals such as urea and intestinal enzymes. The diagnosis of diaper dermatitis is based on the picture of erythema and thickening of the skin in the perineal area and the history of skin contact with urine or feces. In 80% of cases of diaper dermatitis lasting more than 3 days, the affected area is colonized with *Candida albicans* even before appearance of the classic signs of a beefy red, sharply marginated dermatitis with satellite lesions.

Treatment consists of changing diapers frequently. Because rubber or plastic pants prevent evaporation of the contactant and enhance its penetration into the skin, they should be avoided as much as possible. Air drying is useful. Streptococcal perianal cellulitis should be included in the differential diagnosis. Treatment of long-standing diaper dermatitis should include application of nystatin or an imidazole cream with each diaper change.

4. ALLERGIC ECZEMATOUS CONTACT DERMATITIS (Poison Ivy Dermatitis)

Children often present with acute dermatitis with blister formation, oozing, and crusting. Blisters are often linear and of acute onset. Plants such as poison ivy, poison sumac, and poison oak cause most cases of allergic contact dermatitis in children.

Allergic contact dermatitis has all the features of delayed-type (T lymphocyte-mediated) hypersensitivity. Although many substances may cause such a reaction, nickel sulfate, potassium dichromate, and neomycin are the most common causes. The true incidence of allergic contact dermatitis in children is not known.

Treatment of contact dermatitis in localized areas is with topical corticosteroids. In severe generalized involvement, prednisone, 1–2 mg/kg/d orally for 10–14 days, can be used.

Marks JG Jr et al: Prevention of poison ivy and poison oak allergic contact dermatitis by quaternium-18 bentonite. J Am Acad Dermatol 1995;33:212.

McAlvany JP, Sheretz EF: Contact dermatitis in children and adolescents. Adv Dermatol 1994;9:205.

5. SEBORRHEIC DERMATITIS

Seborrheic dermatitis consists of an erythematous scaly dermatitis accompanied by overproduction of sebum occurring in areas rich in sebaceous glands, ie, the face, scalp, and perineum. This common condition occurs predominantly in the newborn and at puberty, the ages at which hormonal stimulation of sebum production is maximal. Although it is tempting to speculate that overproduction of sebum causes the dermatitis, the exact relationship is unclear.

Seborrheic dermatitis on the scalp in infancy is clinically similar to atopic dermatitis, and the distinction may become clear only after other areas are in-

volved. Psoriasis also occurs in seborrheic areas in older children and should be considered in the differential diagnosis.

Seborrheic dermatitis responds well to topical corticosteroids; 1% hydrocortisone cream three times daily is often sufficient.

6. DANDRUFF

Physiologic scaling or mild seborrhea, in the form of greasy scalp scales, may be treated by medicated dandruff shampoos.

7. DRY SKIN DERMATITIS (Asteatotic Eczema, Xerosis)

Newborns and older children who live in arid climates are susceptible to dry skin, characterized by large cracked scales with erythematous borders. The stratum corneum is dependent on environmental humidity for its water, and below 30% environmental humidity the stratum corneum loses water, shrinks, and cracks. These cracks in the epidermal barrier allow irritating substances to enter the skin, predisposing the patient to dermatitis.

Treatment consists of increasing the water content of the skin's immediate external environment. House humidifiers are very useful. Two 5-minute baths a day with immediate application of oils or ointments (petrolatum) after the bath will allow the skin to retain water. Frequent soaping of the skin impairs its water-holding capacity and serves as an irritating alkali, and all soaps should therefore be avoided. Frequent use of emollients (eg, Cetaphil, Eucerin, Lubriderm, Moisturel) should be a major part of therapy.

8. KERATOSIS PILARIS

Follicular papules containing a white inspissated scale characterize keratosis pilaris. Individual lesions are discrete and may be red. They are prominent on the extensor surfaces of the upper arms and thighs and on the buttocks and cheeks. In severe cases, the lesions may be generalized. Such lesions are seen frequently in children with dry skin and have also been associated with atopic dermatitis and ichthyosis vulgaris.

Treatment is with keratolytics such as topical retinoic acid, lactic acid, or urea creams followed by skin hydration.

9. PITYRIASIS ALBA

White, scaly macular areas with indistinct borders are seen over extensor surfaces of extremities and on the cheeks in children. Suntanning exaggerates these lesions. Histologic examination reveals a mild dermatitis. These lesions may be confused with tinea versicolor. There is no satisfactory treatment.

COMMON SKIN TUMORS

If the skin moves with the nodule on lateral palpation, the tumor is located within the dermis; if the skin moves over the nodule, it is subcutaneous. Table 13–7 lists the tumors according to these categories.

Epidermal Inclusion Cysts

Epidermal inclusion cysts are smooth, dome-shaped nodules in the skin that may grow to 2 cm in diameter. In infants, they may be found about the eyes and in older children and adolescents on the chest, back, or scalp. They are the most common superficial lumps in children. Treatment, if desired, is surgical excision.

Granuloma Annulare

Circles or semicircles of nontender intradermal nodules found over the lower legs and ankles, the dorsum of the hands and wrists, and the trunk, in that order, suggest granuloma annulare. Histologically, the disease appears as a central area of tissue death (necrobiosis) surrounded by macrophages and lymphocytes. No treatment is necessary. Lesions resolve spontaneously within 1–2 years in most children.

Pyogenic Granuloma

Rapid growth of a dark red papule with an ulcerated and crusted surface over 1–2 weeks following skin trauma suggests pyogenic granuloma. Histologically, this represents excessive new vessel formation with or without inflammation (granulation tissue). It is neither pyogenic nor granulomatous but should be regarded as an abnormal healing response. Pulsed dye laser and excision are the treatments of choice.

Keloids

Keloids are scars raised above the skin surface with many radial projections of scar tissue. They continue to enlarge over several years. They are often found on the face, earlobes, neck, chest, and back. Keloids show no racial predilection. Treatment includes intralesional injection with triamcinolone acetonide, 20 mg/mL, or excision and injection with corticosteroids.

PAPULOSQUAMOUS ERUPTIONS
(See Table 13–8.)

Papulosquamous eruptions comprise papules or plaques with varying degrees of scale.

1. PITYRIASIS ROSEA

Erythematous papules that coalesce to form oval plaques preceded by a large oval plaque with central clearing and a scaly border (the herald patch) establish the diagnosis of pityriasis rosea. The herald patch has the appearance of ringworm and is often treated as such. It appears 1–30 days before the onset of the generalized papular eruption. The oval plaques are parallel in their long axis and follow Langer's lines of skin cleavage. In whites, the lesions are primarily on the trunk, accentuated in the axillary and inguinal areas. In blacks, lesions are primarily on the extremities. This disease is common in school-age children and adolescents and is presumed to be viral in origin. Recently, HHV-7 has been demonstrated in the skin, plasma, and monocytes of pityriasis rosea patients. It lasts 6 weeks and may be pruritic the first 7–10 days. The major differential diagnosis is secondary syphilis, and a VDRL test should be done if syphilis is suspected. A chronic variant of this disease may last 2–3 years and is called **chronic parapsoriasis** or **pityriasis lichenoides chronicus.**

Exposing the skin to sunlight until a mild sunburn occurs (slight redness) will hasten the disappearance of lesions. Ordinarily, no treatment is necessary.

Table 13–7. Common skin tumors.

Intradermal
  Epidermal inclusion cyst
  Pilomatricoma
  Dermatofibroma
  Melanocytic nevus
  Pyogenic granuloma
  Neurofibroma
  Granuloma annulare
Subcutaneous
  Lipoma
  Rheumatoid nodule

Table 13–8. Papulosquamous eruptions in children.

Psoriasis
Pityriasis rosea
Secondary syphilis
Lichen planus
Chronic parapsoriasis
Pityriasis rubra pilaris
Tinea corporis
Dermatomyositis
Lupus erythematosus

Drago F et al: Human herpes virus 7 in pityriasis rosea. Lancet 1997;243:1367.

2. PSORIASIS

Psoriasis is characterized by erythematous papules covered by thick white scales. Guttate ("drop-like") psoriasis is a common form in children that often follows an episode of streptococcal pharyngitis by 2–3 weeks. The sudden onset of small papules (3–8 mm), seen predominantly over the trunk and quickly covered with thick white scales, is characteristic of guttate psoriasis. Chronic psoriasis is marked by thick, large scaly plaques (5–10 cm) over the elbows, knees, scalp, and other sites of trauma. Pinpoint pits in the nail plate are seen, as well as yellow discoloration of the nail plate resulting from onycholysis. Thickening of all 20 nails is an uncommon feature. The sacral and seborrheic areas are commonly involved.

Psoriasis has no known cause and demonstrates active proliferation of epidermal cells, with a turnover time of 3–4 days versus 28 days for normal skin. These rapidly proliferating epidermal cells are producing excessive stratum corneum, giving rise to thick, opaque scales. Papulosquamous eruptions that present problems of differential diagnosis are listed in Table 13–8.

Treatment

All therapy is aimed at diminishing epidermal turnover time. Sunlight or artificial ultraviolet light (UVL) alone will produce some improvement. Coal tar enhances the effect of UVL and hastens the disappearance of psoriatic lesions. Bathing with a bath product containing tar (eg, Balnetar) at night, followed by UVL the next day, may be sufficient in mild cases. In more severe psoriasis, 10% liquor carbonis detergens in petrolatum should be applied after the bath. The newer tar gels (Estar, PsoriGel) cause less staining and are most efficacious. They are applied twice daily for 6–8 weeks.

Crude coal tar therapy is messy and stains bedclothes, and patients may prefer to use topical corticosteroids. Penetration of topical corticosteroids through the enlarged epidermal barrier in psoriasis requires that more potent preparations be used, eg, fluocinonide 0.05% (Lidex) or fluocinolone acetonide 0.025% (Synalar) two or three times daily.

Anthralin therapy is also useful. Anthralin is applied to the skin for a short contact time (eg, 20 minutes once daily) and then washed off with a neutral soap (eg, Dove). A 6-week course of treatment is recommended. Topical calcipotriene (Dovonex) applied twice daily for 8 weeks is also an effective treatment.

Scalp care using a tar shampoo requires leaving the shampoo on for 5 minutes, washing it off, and then shampooing with commercial shampoo to remove scales. It may be necessary to shampoo daily until scaling is reduced.

More severe cases of psoriasis are best treated by a dermatologist.

Krueger GG, Duvic M: Epidemiology of psoriasis: Clinical issues. J Invest Dermatol 1994;102:145.
Ortonne JP: Aetiology and pathogenesis of psoriasis. Br J Dermatol 1996;135(Suppl):1.

HAIR LOSS (Alopecia)

Hair loss in children (Table 13–9) imposes great emotional stress on the patient and the parent. A 60% hair loss in a single area is necessary before hair loss can be detected clinically. Examination should begin with the scalp to determine whether there are color or infiltrative changes. Hairs should be examined microscopically for breaking and structural defects and to see whether growing or resting hairs are being shed. Placing removed hairs in mounting fluid (Permount) on a glass microscope slide makes them easy to examine. Three diseases account for most cases of hair loss in children: alopecia areata, tinea capitis, and trichotillomania.

Alopecia Areata

Loss of every hair in a localized area is called alopecia areata. This is the most common cause of hair loss in children. An immunologic pathogenic mechanism is suspected because dense infiltration of lymphocytes precedes hair loss. Ninety-five percent of children with alopecia areata completely regrow their hair within 12 months, although as many as 40% may have a relapse in 5–6 years. A rare and unusual form of alopecia areata begins at the occiput and proceeds along the hair margins to the frontal

Table 13–9. Other causes of hair loss in children.

Hair loss with scalp changes
  Nodules and tumors:
    Nevus sebaceus
    Epidermal nevus
  Thickening:
    Burn
  Atrophy:
    Lupus erythematosus
    Lichen planus
Hair loss with hair shaft defects (hair fails to grow out enough to require haircuts)
  Monilethrix—alternating bands of thin and thick areas
  Trichorrhexis nodosa—nodules with fragmented hair
  Trichorrhexis invaginata (bamboo hair)—intussusception of one hair into another
  Pili torti—hair twisted 180 degrees, brittle
  Pili annulati—alternating bands of light and dark pigmentation

scalp. This variety, called **ophiasis,** often results in total scalp hair loss (**alopecia totalis**). The prognosis for regrowth in ophiasis is poor.

No treatment is indicated for alopecia areata. Systemic corticosteroids given to suppress the inflammatory response will result in hair growth, but the hair will fall out again when the drug is discontinued. In children with alopecia totalis, a wig is most helpful.

Tobin DJ et al: Antibodies to hair follicles in alopecia areata. J Invest Dermatol 1994;102:721.
Sahn EE: Alopecia areata in childhood. Semin Dermatol 1995;14:9.

Trichotillomania

Traumatic hair pulling causes the hair shafts to be broken off at different lengths, an ill-defined area of hair loss, petechiae around follicular openings, and a wrinkled hair shaft on microscopic examination. This may be merely habit or the result of severe anxiety in the child. Eyelashes and eyebrows rather than scalp hair may be pulled out. If the behavior has a long history, psychiatric evaluation may be helpful. Oiling the hair to make it slippery is an aid to behavior modification.

Jaspers JP: The diagnosis and psychopharmacological treatment of trichotillomania: A review. Pharmacopsychiatry 1996;29:115.
Christiansen GA, Crow SJ: The characterization and treatment of trichotillomania. J Clin Psychiatry 1995;57(Suppl):42.

REACTIVE ERYTHEMAS

Erythema Multiforme

Erythema multiforme begins with papules that later develop a dark center and then evolve into lesions with central blisters and the characteristic target lesions (iris lesions) with three concentric circles of color change. Primary injury is to endothelial cells, with later destruction of epidermal basal cells and blister formation. Erythema multiforme has sometimes been diagnosed in patients with severe mucous membrane involvement, but **Stevens-Johnson syndrome** is the usual term when severe involvement of conjunctiva, oral cavity, and genital mucosa also occur.

Many causes are suspected, particularly herpes simplex virus, sulfonamide drugs, and *Mycoplasma* infections. Recurrent erythema multiforme is usually associated with reactivation of herpes simplex virus. In the mild form, spontaneous healing occurs in 10–14 days, but Stevens-Johnson syndrome may last 6–8 weeks.

Treatment is symptomatic in uncomplicated erythema multiforme. Removal of offending drugs is an obvious measure. Oral antihistamines such as hydroxyzine, 2 mg/kg/d orally, are useful. Cool compresses and wet dressings will relieve pruritus. Steroids have not been demonstrated to be effective.

Weston WL: What is erythema multiforme? Pediatr Ann 1996;25:106.
Weston JA, Weston WL: The overdiagnosis of erythema multiforme. Pediatrics 1992;89:802.
Weston WL et al: Herpes simplex virus in childhood erythema multiforme. Pediatrics 1992;89:32.

Drug Eruptions

Drugs may produce urticarial, morbilliform, scarlatiniform, or bullous skin eruptions. Urticaria may appear within minutes after drug administration, but most reactions begin 7–14 days after the drug is first administered. These eruptions may occur in patients who have received these drugs for long periods, and eruptions continue for days after the drug has been discontinued. Drugs commonly implicated in skin reactions are listed in Table 13–10.

Breathnach SM, Hintner H: *Adverse Reactions in the Skin.* Blackwell, 1992.
Breathnach SM: Management of drug eruption. (Two parts.) Australian Journal of Dermatology 1995;36:121, 187.

MISCELLANEOUS SKIN DISORDERS ENCOUNTERED IN PEDIATRIC PRACTICE

Aphthous Stomatitis

Recurrent erosions on the gums, lips, tongue, palate, and buccal mucosa are often confused with herpes simplex. A smear of the base of such a lesion stained with Wright's stain will aid in ruling out herpes simplex by the absence of epithelial multinucleate giant cells. A culture for herpes simplex is also

Table 13–10. Common drug reactions.

Erythema multiforme/toxic epidermal necrolysis
  Sulfonamides
  Nonsteroidal anti-inflammatory drugs
  Anticonvulsants
Urticaria
  Penicillins
  Sulfonamides
  Barbiturates
  Opioids
Morbilliform eruption
  Penicillins
  Cephalosporins
  Sulfonamides
  Anticonvulsants
Photodermatitis
  Psoralens
  Tetracyclines
  Thiazides
  Sulfonamides

useful in this difficult differential diagnostic problem. It has been shown that recurrence of aphthous stomatitis correlates positively with lymphocyte-mediated cytotoxicity.

There is no specific therapy for this condition. Rinsing the mouth with liquid antacids will provide relief in most patients. Topical corticosteroids in a gel base (eg, fluocinonide gel) may provide some relief. In severe cases that interfere with eating, prednisone, 1 mg/kg/d orally for 3–5 days, will suffice to abort an episode. Colchicine, 0.2–0.5 mg/d, sometimes reduces the frequency of attacks.

Jasmin JR et al: Local treatment of minor aphthous ulceration in children. Am J Dis Child 1993;60:26.

Rees TD, Binnie WH: Recurrent aphthous stomatitis. Dermatol Clin 1996;14:243.

Vitiligo

Vitiligo is characterized clinically by the development of areas of depigmentation. These are often symmetric and occur mainly on extensor surfaces. The depigmentation results from a destruction of melanocytes. The basis for this destruction is unknown, but immunologically mediated damage is likely and vitiligo sometimes occurs in individuals with selective IgA deficiency, graft-versus-host disease, or autoimmune endocrinopathies. Treatment is not very effective. Topical psoralens with UV irradiation are reserved for children over 12 years of age.

Jaisankar TJ, Baruah MC, Gorg BR: Vitiligo in children. Int J Dermatol 1992;31:621.

REFERENCES

Schachner L, Hansen R: *Pediatric Dermatology,* 2nd ed. Churchill Livingstone, 1996.

Weston WL, Lane AT, Morelli JG: *Color Textbook of Pediatric Dermatology,* 2nd ed. Mosby-Year Book, 1996.

Eye

Allan M. Eisenbaum, MD

The subspecialties within the general field of ophthalmology are oriented by structure, such as the retina, or disease, such as glaucoma. Pediatric ophthalmology is unique in that it encompasses the entire panoply of ophthalmic disease in the pediatric age group. As such, this branch of ophthalmology includes not only disease processes affecting the eye and its adnexa but also those that reflect systemic pathologic processes. In this chapter, the most important and most common pediatric ophthalmologic problems are presented with emphasis on diagnosis and treatment, organizing the topics both anatomically and by disease category.

COMMON NONSPECIFIC SIGNS & SYMPTOMS

Nonspecific signs and symptoms commonly occur as the chief complaint or as an element of the history of a child with eye disease. Five of these findings are presented below along with a sixth—leukocoria—which often has serious implications.

Redness

Redness (injection) of the bulbar conjunctiva or deeper vessels is a common presenting complaint. Causes include superficial or penetrating foreign bodies, infection, allergy, and conjunctivitis associated with systemic entities such as Stevens-Johnson syndrome or Kawasaki disease. Irritating noxious agents also result in injection. Subconjunctival hemorrhage may be traumatic or may be associated with hematopoietic disease, vascular anomalies, or inflammatory processes (Table 14–1).

Tearing

In infants, tearing is usually due to nasolacrimal obstruction, but tearing may also be associated with glaucoma, in which case photophobia and blepharospasm may also be present. Inflammation, allergic and viral diseases, and corneal irritation can also cause tearing.

Discharge

Purulent discharge is usually associated with bacterial conjunctivitis. Watery discharge occurs with viral infection, iritis, superficial foreign bodies, and nasolacrimal obstruction. Mucoid discharge may be a sign of allergic conjunctivitis or nasolacrimal obstruction. Histologically, a mucoid discharge due to allergy will probably show eosinophils; a purulent bacterial discharge will show polymorphonuclear leukocytes.

Pain

Pain in or around the eye may be due to foreign bodies, corneal abrasions, lacerations, acute infections of the globe or ocular adnexa, iritis, and glaucoma. Large refractive errors, poor accommodative ability, and sinus disease may manifest as headaches.

Photophobia

Acute aversion to light may occur with corneal abrasions, foreign bodies, and iritis. Photophobia is present in infants with glaucoma, albinism, and aniridia. Fair-skinned individuals may be light-sensitive. Photophobia is common after ocular surgery and after dilation of the pupil with mydriatic and cycloplegic agents.

Leukocoria

Although not a common sign or complaint, leukocoria (a white pupil) is associated with serious diseases and requires prompt ophthalmologic consultation. Causes of leukocoria include retinoblastoma, retinopathy of prematurity, pupillary membrane, cataract, vitreous opacities, retinal detachment, and retinal dysplasia (Figure 14–1).

REFRACTIVE ERRORS

Refractive error refers to the optical state of the eye. It is a physical characteristic such as height or weight and can be quantitated. Not all refractive errors require correction. There are three types: myopia, hyperopia, and astigmatism. Inequality of the refractive state between the two eyes (anisometropia) can cause ambly-

Table 14–1. Differential diagnosis of redness of the eye in pediatric patients.

	Acute Conjunctivitis	Acute Iritis	Acute Glaucoma[1]	Corneal Abrasion
Incidence	Very common	Uncommon	Rare	Fairly common
Etiology	Usually bacterial; may be viral, fungal, or allergic	Varied, trauma; may be associated with juvenile rheumatoid arthritis	Developmental defects or obstruction of aqueous drainage channels	Foreign body; abrasion
Redness	Diffuse injection of conjunctiva; greater toward fornices	Purple-red; circum-corneal injection	Often diffuse injection of bulbar conjunctiva	Diffuse injection of conjunctiva
Discharge	Moderate to heavy; mucoid or mucopurulent	None	None; tearing	Watery
Visual acuity	Normal	Decreased	Decreased	Decreased
Corneal transparency	Clear	Clear or some haze	Hazy; cornea enlarged in congenital form	Variable haze; positive fluorescein stain
Anterior chamber depth	Normal	Normal; cloudy	Shallow; deep in congenital form	Normal
Pupil size	Normal	Constricted	Dilated	Normal
Intraocular pressure	Normal	Usually normal; may be low or elevated	Elevated	Normal
Conjunctival smear results	Pathogens identified; numerous polymorphonuclear neutrophils in bacterial infection, mononuclear cells in viral infection	Normal	Normal	Normal

[1]Primary narrow-angle glaucoma is very rare in children. Congenital glaucoma may not produce redness of the eye.

opia (reduced vision with or without an organic lesion; see Amblyopia & Strabismus, below).

Myopia
(Nearsightedness)

For the individual with myopia, objects nearby are in focus; those at a distance are blurred. The onset is typically at about 8 years of age. A myopic person may squint to produce a pinhole effect, which improves distance vision. Headaches are common. Divergent lenses provide clear distance vision.

Hyperopia
(Farsightedness)

Saying that the hyperopic child is sighted for far (not near) is somewhat misleading, since the child can focus on near objects if the hyperopia is not excessive. Large amounts of uncorrected hyperopia can cause esotropia and amblyopia (see Amblyopia & Strabismus, below). Most children have a hyperopic refraction that begins to diminish at about 8 years of age and does not require correction.

Astigmatism

When either the cornea or the crystalline lens is not perfectly spherical, an image will not be sharply focused in one plane. Schematically, there will be two planes of focus either of which can be in front of or behind the retina. This refractive state is described as astigmatism. Large amounts of astigmatism not corrected at an early age can cause decreased vision

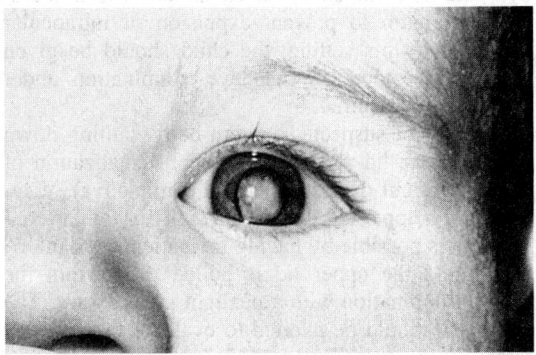

Figure 14–1. Leukocoria of left eye with mild microphthalmia caused by retrolental membrane (persistent hyperplastic primary vitreous).

from amblyopia, but proper refractive correction can prevent this.

EXAMINATION

Ophthalmic examination of the pediatric patient begins with a calm demeanor and reassuring voice. Having a parent present is invaluable. The examination includes a history, assessment of visual acuity, external examination, observation of ocular alignment and motility, and ophthalmoscopic examination. Intraocular pressure is less frequently measured. Testing of binocular status and near point is desirable.

Circumstances will dictate the use of ancillary procedures such as instilling fluorescein dye and radiologic tests (MRI and CT). Electroretinography and electro-oculography test retinal function. Visual evoked response testing assesses the function of the visual pathways. Visual field testing demonstrates the presence or absence of scotomas and visual field defects.

History

Evaluation begins by ascertaining the chief complaint and taking a history of the present illness. The past ocular history is obtained, as well as the perinatal and developmental history and any history of allergy. The family history should be explored for ocular disorders that may be familial or inherited.

Visual Acuity

Visual acuity testing is the single most important test of visual function and should be part of every general physical examination. The visual acuity should be tested and recorded after ocular trauma and before and after any ophthalmologic treatment. Acuity should be tested in each eye individually. If latent nystagmus is present, vision should be tested simultaneously in both eyes as well as in each eye individually (see below). Vision is recorded both without spectacles (uncorrected vision) and with spectacles in place (corrected vision). In older children who can cooperate, use of a pinhole will improve vision in children not wearing the appropriate spectacle prescription.

The type of test used to determine visual acuity is dictated by the age of the child. In the sleeping newborn, the presence of a blepharospastic response to bright light is an adequate response. At 6 weeks of age, eye-to-eye contact with slow following movements can be detected. By 3 months, the infant should demonstrate fixing and following ocular movements for objects at a distance of 2–3 feet. At 6 months of age, interest in movement across the room is the norm. Vision can be recorded for the presence or absence of fixing and following behavior and for whether vision is steady (unsteady when nystagmus

is present) and maintained. Vision should be tested and recorded for each eye. Visual acuity can be quantified in infants using other techniques such as the preferential looking technique or the pattern visual evoked response.

In the verbal child, the use of familiar icons will allow for a quantitative test. Allen cards with familiar pictures can be used to test children aged 2½–3 years. Four-year-olds are often ready to play the tumbling E game or HOTV letters. Literate children are tested with letters. Typical acuity levels in developmentally appropriate children are approximately 20/60 in 2½-year-olds, 20/40–20/30 in 3-year-olds, 20/30–20/25 in 4-year-olds, and 20/20 in literate 5-year-olds. Perhaps more important than the absolute visual acuity is the presence of a difference of acuity between the two eyes, which might be a sign of amblyopia, uncorrected refractive error, or disease.

The practitioner should be aware of two situations complicated by nystagmus. Children who require a face turn or torticollis to quiet the nystagmus will have poor visual acuity results when tested in the absence of the compensatory head posture.

When latent nystagmus is present, acuity testing is particularly challenging (see Nystagmus, below). Nystagmus appears or worsens when an eye is occluded, degrading central vision. To minimize the nystagmus, the occluder should be held about 12 inches in front of the eye not being tested. Testing both eyes simultaneously without occlusion often gives a better visual acuity measurement than when either eye is tested individually.

External Examination

Inspection of the anterior segment of the globe and its adnexa requires adequate illumination and often magnification. Immobilization of the child may be necessary. A drop of topical anesthetic may facilitate the examination. Assessment of the entire anterior segment except the trabecular meshwork is possible. In cases of suspected perforation of the globe, it may be best to keep the child at rest, patch and shield the eye, and hold the extent of examination to a necessary minimum to prevent expulsion of intraocular contents. In this setting, the child should be given nothing by mouth in case eye examination under anesthesia is required.

In cases of suspected foreign body, pulling down on the lower lid provides excellent visualization of the inferior cul-de-sac (palpebral conjunctiva). Visualizing the upper cul-de-sac and superior bulbar conjunctiva is possible by having the patient look inferiorly while the upper lid is pulled away from the globe. Illumination with a penlight is necessary. The upper lid should be everted to evaluate the superior tarsal conjunctiva (Figure 14–2).

When indicated for further evaluation of the cornea, a small amount of fluorescein solution should be instilled into the lower cul-de-sac. Blue light will

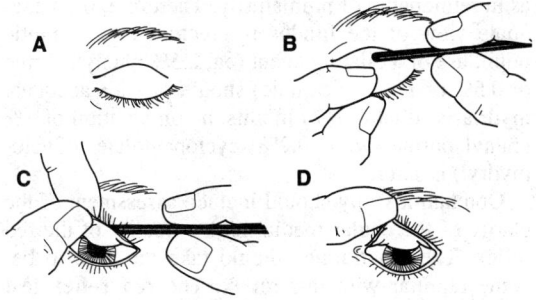

Figure 14–2. Eversion of the upper lid. ***A:*** The patient looks downward. ***B:*** The fingers pull the lid down, and a rod is placed on the upper tarsal border. ***C:*** The lid is pulled up over the rod. ***D:*** The lid is everted. (Redrawn and reproduced, with permission, from Liebman SD, Gellis SS [editors]: *The Pediatrician's Ophthalmology.* Mosby, 1966.)

Table 14–2. Function and innervation of each of the extraocular muscles.

Muscle	Function	Innervation
Medial rectus	Adductor	Oculomotor (third)
Lateral rectus	Abductor	Abducens (sixth)
Inferior rectus	Depressor Adductor Extorter	Oculomotor
Superior rectus	Elevator Adductor Intorter	Oculomotor
Inferior oblique	Elevator Abductor Extorter	Oculomotor
Superior oblique	Depressor Abductor Intorter	Trochlear (fourth)

stain defects yellow. Disease-specific staining patterns may be observed. For example, herpes simplex lesions of the corneal epithelium produce a dendrite. A foreign body lodged beneath the upper lid shows one or more vertical lines of stain on the cornea. Contact lens overwear produces a central staining pattern. A fine, scattered punctate pattern may be a sign of viral keratitis or medication toxicity. Punctate erosions of the inferior third of the cornea can be seen with staphylococcal blepharitis or exposure keratitis secondary to incomplete lid closure.

Alignment & Motility Evaluation

Alignment and motility should be tested, since amblyopia is associated with strabismus. Besides alignment, ocular rotations should be evaluated in the six cardinal positions of gaze (Table 14–2; Figure 14–3). A small toy is an interesting target for testing ocular rotations in infants; a penlight works well in older children.

Alignment can be assessed in several ways. In order of increasing accuracy, these methods are observation, the corneal light reflex test, and cover testing. Observation includes an educated guess about whether the eyes are properly aligned. Corneal light reflex evaluation (Hirschberg's test) is performed by shining a beam of a light at the patient's eyes, observing the reflections off each cornea, and estimating whether these "reflexes" appear to be properly positioned. If the reflection of light is noted temporally on the cornea, esotropia is suspected (Figure 14–4). Nasal reflection of the light suggests exotropia. Accuracy of these tests increases with increasing angles of misalignment.

Another way of evaluating alignment is with the cover test, in which the patient fixes on a target while

one eye is covered. If the uncovered eye is deviated inward (esotropia) or outward (exotropia), a corrective movement is made by the uncovered eye to refixate the target. The other eye is similarly tested. When the occluder is removed from the eye just uncovered, a refixation movement of that eye indicates a phoria, or latent deviation if alignment is reestablished. If the uncovered eyes picks up fixation and strabismus is still present, then that eye can be presumed to be dominant and the nonpreferred eye possibly amblyopic. If the eye remains deviated after the occluder is removed, a tropia is noted to be present (Figure 14–5).

Ophthalmoscopic Examination

A hand-held direct ophthalmoscope allows visualization of the ocular fundus. As the patient's pupil becomes more constricted, viewing the fundus be-

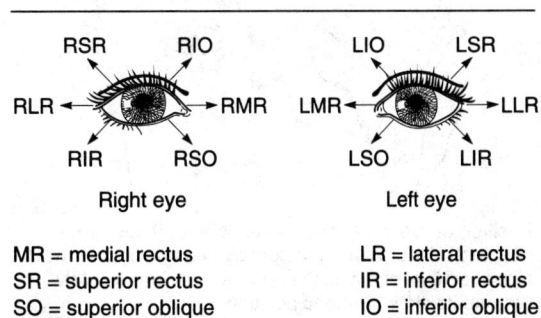

MR = medial rectus
SR = superior rectus
SO = superior oblique

LR = lateral rectus
IR = inferior rectus
IO = inferior oblique

Figure 14–3. Cardinal positions of gaze and muscles primarily tested in those fields of gaze. Arrow indicates position in which each muscle is tested.

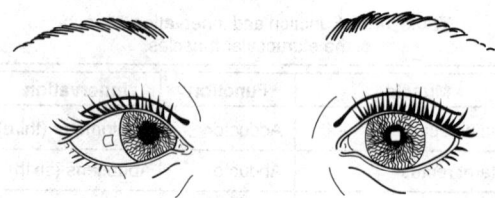

Figure 14–4. Temporal displacement of light reflection showing esotropia (internal deviation) of the right eye. Nasal displacement of the reflection would show exotropia (outward deviation).

comes more difficult. Although it is taught that pupillary dilation can precipitate an attack of angle-closure glaucoma in the predisposed adult, children are not predisposed to angle closure. Exceptions include those with a dislocated lens or an eye previously compromised by a retrolental membrane, such

as in retinopathy of prematurity. Therefore, if an adequate view of the fundus is precluded by a miotic pupil, use of a dilating agent (eg, 2.5% phenylephrine or 0.5% or 1% tropicamide) should provide adequate mydriasis (dilation). In infants, a combination of 1% phenylephrine with 0.2% cyclopentolate (Cyclomydryl) is safer.

Ophthalmoscopy should include assessment of the clarity of the ocular media, ie, the quality of the red reflex. The practitioner should take the time to become familiar with this reflex. The **red reflex test** (Brückner's test) is useful for identifying disorders such as media opacities, large refractive errors, and strabismus. A difference in quality of the red reflexes between the two eyes constitutes a positive Brückner test and requires referral to an ophthalmologist. A red reflex chart is available through the American Academy of Pediatrics. Structures to be observed include the optic disk, blood vessels, the macular reflex, and retinal changes as well as the clarity of the vitreous media. By increasing the amount of plus lens dialed into the instrument, the point of focus moves anteri-

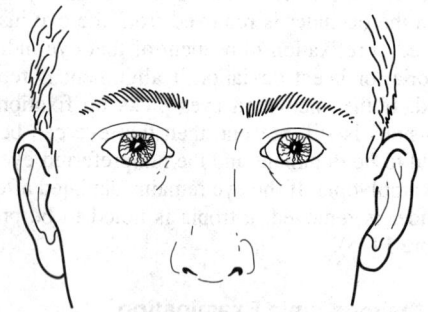

Eyes straight (maintained in position by fusion).

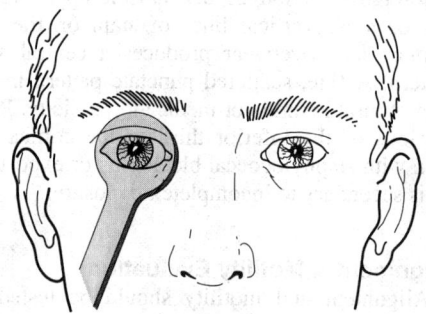

Position of eye under cover in orthophoria (fusion-free position). The right eye under cover has not moved.

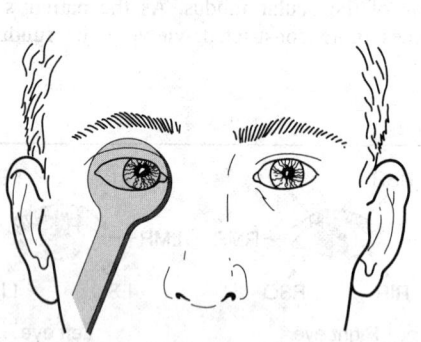

Position of eye under cover in esophoria (fusion-free position). Under cover, the right eye has deviated inward. Upon removal of cover, the right eye will immediately resume its straight-ahead position.

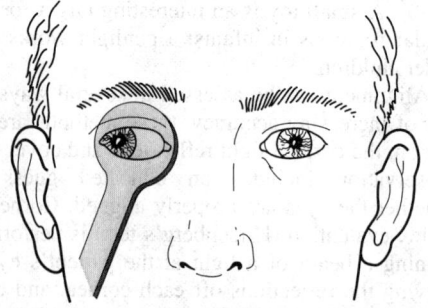

Position of eye under cover in exophoria (fusion-free position). Under cover, the right eye has deviated outward. Upon removal of the cover, the right eye will immediately resume its straight-ahead position.

Figure 14–5. Cover testing. The patient is instructed to look at a target at eye level 20 feet away. Note that in the presence of strabismus, the deviation will remain when the cover is removed. (From Vaughan DG, Asbury T, Riordan-Eva P [editors]: *General Ophthalmology,* 14th ed. Appleton & Lange, 1995.)

orly from the vitreous to the lens and finally to the cornea.

OCULAR TRAUMA

Foreign Bodies & Abrasions

Foreign bodies on the globe and palpebral conjunctiva usually cause discomfort and red eye. Magnification may be needed for inspection. Foreign bodies that lodge on the upper palpebral conjunctiva are best viewed by everting the lid on itself and removing with a cotton applicator. The lower lid presents no problem with visualization. After removal of a foreign body, no other treatment is needed if there is no corneal abrasion.

When foreign bodies are noted on the bulbar conjunctiva or cornea (Figure 14–6), removal is facilitated by using a topical anesthetic. If the foreign body is not too adherent, it can be dislodged with a stream of irrigating solution (Dacriose or saline) or with a cotton applicator after instillation of a topical anesthetic. Otherwise, a foreign body spud or needle is used to undermine the foreign body. This must be done with adequate magnification and illumination. An antibiotic ointment is then instilled. For corneal involvement, a gentle pressure patch is applied. Ferrous corneal bodies often have an associated rust ring, which is removed under slitlamp visualization.

Corneal abrasions are evaluated with fluorescein dye and treated with a topical antibiotic and a pressure patch. A drop of topical cycloplegic agent such as 5% homatropine or 0.25% scopolamine is useful to relieve the discomfort of ciliary spasm and iritis. Daily follow-up is required until healing is complete.

Suspected intraocular foreign bodies and corneal and scleral lacerations require emergency referral to an ophthalmologist. The diagnosis may be difficult if the signs of obvious corneal perforation—shallow anterior chamber with hyphema and irregular pupil—are not present (Figure 14–7). Furthermore, nonradiopaque materials such as glass will not be seen on x-ray.

INJURIES TO THE EYELIDS

Ecchymosis

Orbital and soft tissue trauma may produce "black eye," or ecchymosis (blue or purplish hemorrhagic areas) of the eyelids. The extent of the injury to the eye and orbit may not correlate fully with its appearance. Blowout fracture, which occurs from blunt trauma fracturing the walls of the orbit, must be suspected. Ocular motility must be assessed and the globe examined for injury and for increased intraocular pressure. Cold compresses are used in the first 24 hours after injury to reduce hemorrhage and swelling. Nonaccidental trauma needs to be considered when orbital injury is poorly explained.

Lacerations

The lids and lacrimal apparatus are susceptible to laceration. Except for superficial lacerations away from the globe, repair is best performed in the operating room under general anesthesia. Special consideration must be given to lacerations involving the lid margin, to through-and-through lacerations, and to lacerations that may involve the levator muscle in the upper lid or canaliculi.

Burns

Eyelid burns can occur in toddlers from contact with a lighted cigarette. The cornea is often involved

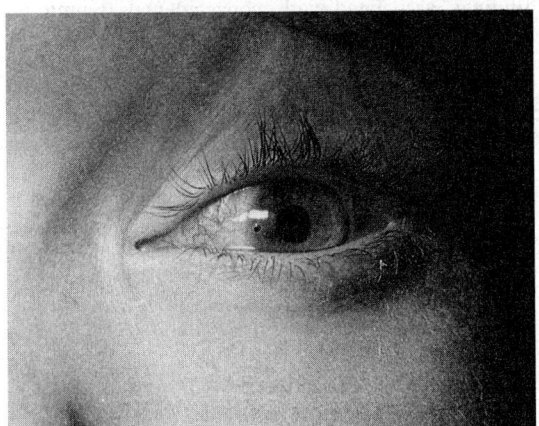

Figure 14–6. Corneal foreign body at the nasal edge of the cornea.

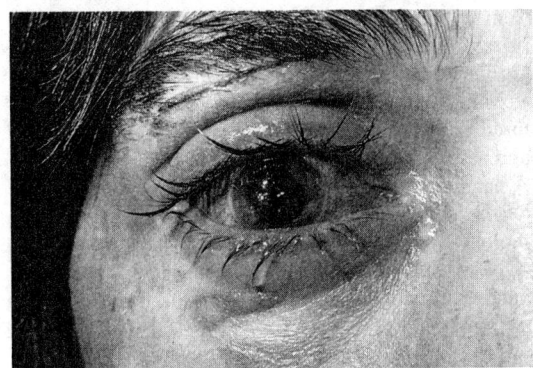

Figure 14–7. Corneal laceration with irregular pupil and vitreous loss.

as well. These burns usually heal following application of antibiotic ointment. Severe thermal or chemical burns can cause scars resulting in ectropion or entropion of the lid and scarring of the conjunctiva and cul-de-sac.

Burns of the conjunctiva and cornea may be thermal, radiant, or chemical. Superficial thermal burns cause pain, tearing, and injection. Management is with topical antibiotics and patching. Add a cycloplegic agent if corneal involvement is present, since ciliary spasm and iritis may accompany the injury.

Radiant energy causes ultraviolet keratitis. Typical examples are welder's burn or burns associated with skiing without goggles in bright sunlight. The fluorescein dye pattern will show a uniformly stippled appearance of the corneal epithelium. Antibiotic ointment, pressure patches, and a cycloplegic agent such as 5% homatropine are usually followed by recovery within 24 hours.

Chemical burns with strong acid and alkaline agents can be blinding. Examples are exploding batteries, spilled drain cleaner, and bleach. Alkali burns may not cause significant injection since the conjunctival vessels become damaged. Alkalis tend to penetrate deeper into ocular tissue than acids. Immediate treatment consists of copious irrigation as soon as possible after the injury. The patient should be referred to an ophthalmologist.

Cullom RD Jr, Chang B (editors): *The Wills Eye Manual Office and Emergency Room Diagnosis and Treatment of Eye Disease,* 2nd ed. Lippincott, 1994.

Hyphema

Blunt trauma to the globe may cause bleeding within the anterior chamber from a ruptured vessel located near the root of the iris or in the anterior chamber angle. Bleeding may be microscopic or may fill the entire anterior chamber (Figure 14–8). Blunt trauma severe enough to cause hyphema may be associated with other ocular injury, including iritis, retinal edema or detachment, and glaucoma. In patients with sickle cell anemia, even moderate elevations of intraocular pressure may quickly lead to optic atrophy. Therefore, these patients require extra vigilance in diagnosing and treating hyphema.

Management of hyphema in an otherwise uninjured patient should include testing of visual acuity and assessment of the integrity of the globe and orbit. A patch and shield should be placed over the eye, the head elevated, and arrangements made for ophthalmologic referral.

Nontraumatic causes of hyphema include juvenile xanthogranuloma, retinoblastoma, and blood dyscrasias.

Fong LP: Secondary hemorrhage in traumatic hyphema: Predictive factors for selective prophylaxis. Ophthalmology 1994;101:1583.

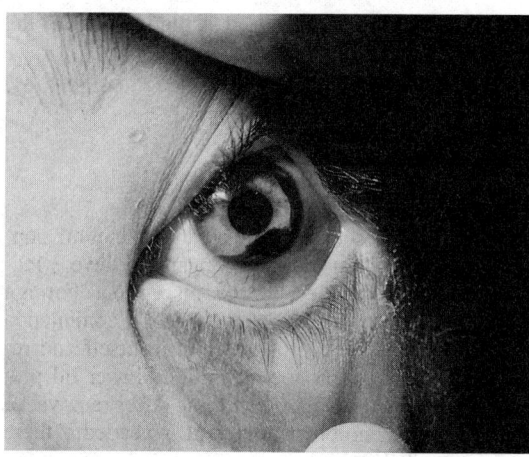

Figure 14–8. Hyphema filling approximately 20% of the anterior chamber.

Teboul BK et al: Clinical evaluation of aminocaproic acid for managing traumatic hyphema in children. Ophthalmology 1995;102:1646.

Nonaccidental Trauma & Shaken Baby Syndrome

From an ocular standpoint, in both nonaccidental trauma and shaken baby syndrome, the hallmark of diagnosis is retinal hemorrhage. Hemorrhages may be unilateral or bilateral and may be located in the posterior pole or periphery. Whereas retinal hemorrhages tend to resolve fairly quickly, those in the vitreous do not. If a blood clot lies over the macula, deprivation amblyopia may occur. Retinal and vitreous hemorrhages associated with intracranial hemorrhage from skull injury are known as Terson's syndrome. Retinal hemorrhages are rarely associated with cardiopulmonary resuscitation or seizures. Other ocular findings associated with nonaccidental trauma include lid ecchymosis, subconjunctival hemorrhage, and hyphema.

Koser M, DeRespinis PA: The association of vision threatening ocular injury with infant walker use. Arch Pediatr Adolesc Med 1995;149:1275.

Odom A, Christ E: Prevalence of retinal hemorrhages in pediatric patients after in-hospital cardiopulmonary resuscitation: A prospective study. Pediatrics 1997;99(6). URL: http://www.pediatrics.org/cgi/content/full.99/6/e3 (Pediatrics electronic pages.)

Sandramouli S: Retinal hemorrhages and convulsions. Arch Dis Child 1997;76:449.

Prevention of Ocular Injuries

Fireworks and air rifles should be avoided. Safety goggles should be used in laboratories and industrial arts classes and when operating snow blowers, power lawn mowers, and power tools and when using hammers and nails. Sports-related eye injuries can be prevented with protective eyewear. Sports goggles and visors of polycarbonate or CR-39 plastic will prevent injuries in games using fast projectiles or where opponents may swing elbows or poke at the eye.

The one-eyed individual should be specifically advised about eye protection and counseled to avoid high-risk activities such as the martial arts.

American Academy of Pediatrics Committee on Sports Medicine and Fitness and American Academy of Ophthalmology Committee on Eye Safety and Sports Ophthalmology: Protective eyewear for young athletes. Pediatrics 1996;98:311.

Committee on Injury and Poison Prevention, American Academy of Pediatrics: Firearm injuries affecting the pediatric population (RE9234). Pediatrics 1992;89:788.

Napier SM et al: Eye injuries in athletics and recreation. Surv Ophthalmol 1996;41:229.

Olson LM et al: Pediatrician's experience with and attitudes toward firearms: Results of a national survey. Arch Pediatr Adolesc Med 1997:151.

DISORDERS OF THE OCULAR STRUCTURES

Diseases of the Eyelids

Blepharitis is inflammation of the lid margin characterized by crusty debris at the base of the lashes, varying degrees of erythema at the lid margins, and, in severe cases, secondary corneal changes such as punctate erosions, vascularization, and ulcers. When conjunctival injection accompanies blepharitis, the condition is known as blepharoconjunctivitis. *Staphylococcus* is the most common bacterial cause. Treatment includes lid scrubs with a nonburning baby shampoo several times a week and application of a topical antibiotic ointment such as erythromycin or bacitracin at bedtime.

Pediculosis of the lids (phthiriasis palpebrarum) is caused by *Phthirus pubis*. Nits and adult lice can be seen on the eyelashes when viewed with a magnifying glass. Mechanical removal and application to the lid margins of phospholine iodide or 1% mercuric oxide ointment can be effective. Other bodily areas of involvement must also be treated if involved. Family members and contacts may also be infected.

Papillomavirus may infect the lid and conjunctiva. Warts may be recurrent, multiple, and difficult to treat. Treatment modalities include cryotherapy, cautery, and use of the carbon dioxide laser.

Localized staphylococcal infections of the glands of Zeis within the lid cause a sty (hordeolum). When the infection coalesces and points internally or externally, it may discharge itself or require incision. The lesion is tender and red. Warm compresses help to hasten the acute process. Some practitioners prescribe a topical antibiotic. Any coexisting blepharitis should be cleared up.

Chalazion is inflammation of the meibomian glands, which may produce a tender nodule over the tarsus of the upper or lower lid. In addition to localized erythema of the corresponding palpebral conjunctiva, there may be a yellow lipogranuloma (Figure 14–9). Treatment includes warm compresses for 5–10 minutes at a time four times a day for up to 6 weeks. If incision and curettage is needed, the child will require a general anesthetic.

Turow VD: Phthiriasis palpebrarum: An unusual course of blepharitis. Arch Pediatr Adolesc Med 1995;149:704.

Viral Lid Disease

Herpes simplex virus may involve the lids at the time of primary herpes simplex infection. Vesicular lesions with an erythematous base are seen. Treatment is with topical 1% trifluridine or 3% vidarabine. Herpes zoster causes vesicular disease in association

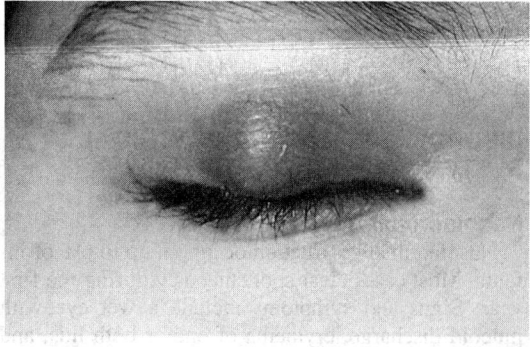

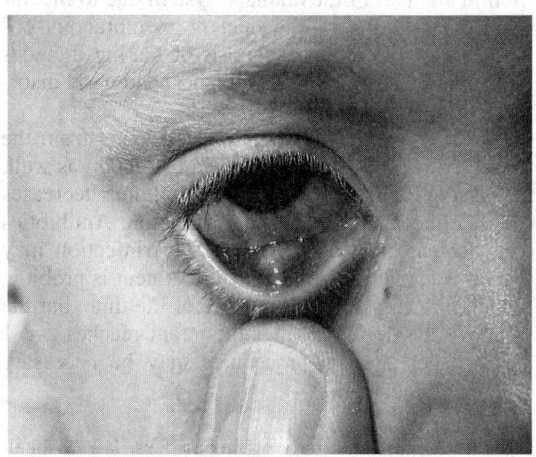

Figure 14–9. Chalazion. *A:* Right upper lid, external view. *B:* Right lower lid.

with a skin eruption in the dermatome of the ophthalmic branch of the trigeminal nerve. In older children, treatment of ophthalmic herpes zoster with oral acyclovir or valacyclovir within 5 days after onset may reduce the morbidity. When vesicles are present on the tip of the nose with herpes zoster (Hutchinson's sign), ocular involvement, including iritis, may develop. Herpes simplex or herpes zoster can be diagnosed by rapid viral culture (24–48 hours). Impetigo is in the differential diagnosis of vesicular lid disease.

Molluscum contagiosum lesions are typically umbilicated papules. If near the lid margin, the lesions may shed and cause conjunctivitis. Cautery or excision of lesions at the lid margin is useful.

Baum J: Infections of the eye. Clin Infect Dis 1995;21:479.

Lid Ptosis

Ptosis (droopy upper lid) may be congenital or acquired but is usually congenital in children owing to a defective levator muscle. Other causes of ptosis are Horner's syndrome, myasthenia gravis, lid injuries, and third nerve palsy. Surgical correction is indicated for moderate to severe ptosis. Mild cases less often require operative management. Ptosis may be associated with astigmatism and amblyopia.

DISORDERS OF THE NASOLACRIMAL SYSTEM

Nasolacrimal Duct Obstruction

Nasolacrimal obstruction occurs in up to 6% of infants. Most cases clear spontaneously during the first year. Signs and symptoms include a wet eye with mucoid discharge, erythema of one or both lids, and conjunctivitis (Figure 14–10). There may be obstruction in any part of the drainage system due to incomplete canalization of the duct or membranous obstructions. Differential diagnosis of tearing includes congenital glaucoma, foreign bodies, and nasal disorders.

Massage over the duct may clear debris from the nasolacrimal sac and perhaps the obstruction as well. Cleansing the lids and medial canthal area decreases the likelihood of infection and irritation. Antibiotics can decrease the discharge, but superinfection may occur. The mainstay of surgical treatment is probing, which is successful 80% or more of the time, but the success rate decreases after the infant reaches age 1 year. Other surgical procedures may be necessary when probings fail.

Kassoff J, Meyer D: Early office-based vs. late hospital-based nasolacrimal duct probing: A clinical decision analysis. Arch Ophthalmol 1995;113:1168.

Paul TD, Shepherd R: Congenital nasolacrimal duct obstruction: Natural history and the timing of optional intervention. J Pediatr Ophthalmol Strabismus 1994;31:362.

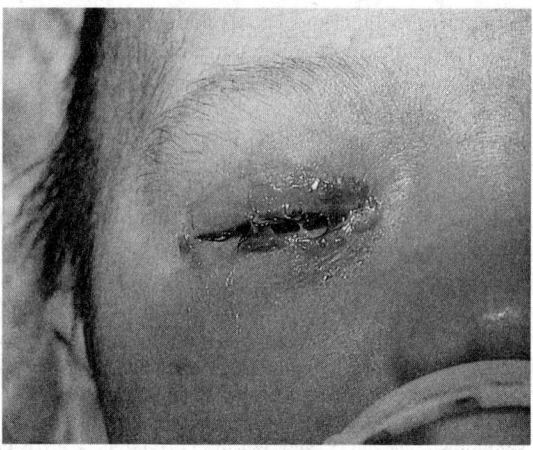

Figure 14–10. Nasolacrimal obstruction, right eye. Mattering on upper and lower lids.

Congenital Dacryocystocele

Congenital dacryocystocele is thought to be due to obstructions proximal and distal to the nasolacrimal sac. At birth, the nasolacrimal sac is distended and has a bluish hue that often leads to an erroneous diagnosis of hemangioma. The tense and swollen sac displaces the medial canthus superiorly. Massage and warm compresses are sometimes effective, but probing of the nasolacrimal system often is necessary. Repeated probings may be required.

Dacryocystitis

Acute and chronic dacryocystitis are typically bacterial and due to organisms such as *Staphylococcus aureus, Streptococcus pneumoniae, Streptococcus pyogenes,* viridans streptococci, *Moraxella catarrhalis,* and *Haemophilus* species. Attempts at identifying the offending organism by culture and staining should be made when possible. Acute dacryocystitis presents with inflammation, swelling, tenderness, and pain over the lacrimal sac (located inferior to the medial canthal tendon). There may also be fever. When the infection is organized, it may point externally (Figure 14–11). A purulent discharge and tearing can be expected, since the cause of infection is almost always nasolacrimal obstruction.

Signs of chronic dacryocystitis are mucopurulent debris on the lids and lashes, tearing, injection of the palpebral conjunctiva, and reflux of pus at the puncta when pressure is applied over the sac. Chronic dacryocystitis and recurrent episodes of low-grade dacryocystitis are due to nasolacrimal obstruction.

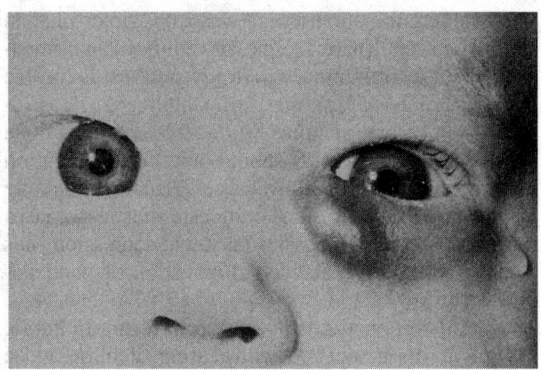

Figure 14–11. Acute dacryocystitis in an 11-week-old infant.

Treatment of severe acute dacryocystitis is with systemic antibiotics. Oral antibiotics can be tried in milder cases. Topical antibiotic administration is adjunctive and is also used with recurrent chronic infections. Warm compresses are beneficial. If a pointing lesion is present, it can be incised and drained, though a fistula can result. After the acute episode subsides—and in chronic cases—the nasolacrimal obstruction must be relieved surgically.

DISEASES OF THE CONJUNCTIVA

Conjunctivitis may be infectious, allergic, or associated with systemic disease (Table 14–3).

Ophthalmia Neonatorum

Ophthalmia neonatorum (conjunctivitis in the newborn) occurs during the first month of life. It is characterized by redness and swelling of the lids and conjunctiva and by discharge (Figure 14–12). Ophthalmia neonatorum may be due to inflammation resulting from silver nitrate prophylaxis, bacterial infection (gonococcal, staphylococcal, pneumococcal, chlamydial), or viral infection. In developed countries, chlamydia is the most common cause. Neonatal conjunctivitis is visually threatening if due to *Neisseria gonorrhoeae*. Herpes simplex is a rare but serious cause of neonatal conjunctivitis. Gram staining, Giemsa staining for elementary bodies, enzyme immunoassay for chlamydiae, and cultures aid in making an etiologic diagnosis.

While no single prophylactic medication can eliminate all cases of neonatal conjunctivitis, povidone-iodine may provide broader coverage against the organisms causing this disease than silver nitrate or erythromycin ointment. Silver nitrate is not effective against chlamydiae. The choice of prophylactic agent is often dictated by local epidemiology and cost considerations.

Treatment of these infections requires specific systemic antibiotics since they can cause serious infections in other organs. Parents should be examined and treated when a sexually associated pathogen is present.

Isenberg SJ, Apt L, Wood M: A controlled trial of povidone-iodine as prophylaxis against ophthalmia neonatorum. N Engl J Med 1995;332:562.
Isenberg SJ et al: Povidone-iodine for ophthalmia neonatorum prophylaxis. Am J Ophthalmol 1994;118:701.

Table 14–3. Clinical and laboratory features of conjunctivitis.[1]

	Viral	Bacterial	Chlamydial	Allergic
Itching	Minimal	Minimal	Minimal	Severe
Hyperemia	Generalized	Generalized	Generalized	Generalized
Tearing	Profuse	Moderate	Moderate	Moderate
Exudation	Minimal, mucoid	Profuse, purulent	Profuse; mucoid or mucopurulent	Minimal, slight mucus
Preauricular adenopathy	Common	Uncommon	Common only in inclusion conjunctivitis	None
Stained conjunctival smears and scrapings	Lymphocytes, plasma cells, multinucleated giant cells, eosinophilic intranuclear inclusions	Neutrophils, bacteria	Neutrophils, plasma cells, basophilic intracytoplasmic inclusions	Eosinophils
Associated sore throat and fever	Occasionally	Occasionally	Never	Never

[1]Modified from Vaughan D, Asbury T, Riordan-Eva P (editors): *General Ophthalmology,* 15th ed. Appleton & Lange, 1998.

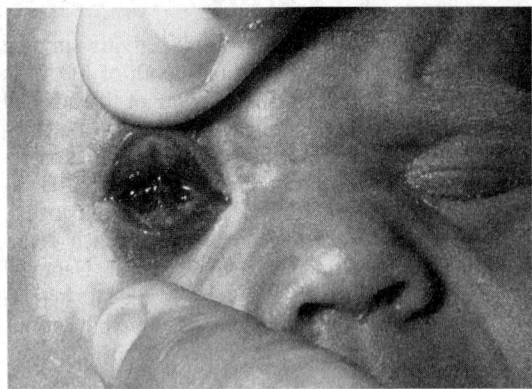

Figure 14–12. Ophthalmia neonatorum due to *Chlamydia trachomatis* infection in a 2-week-old infant. Note marked lid and conjunctival inflammation.

Bacterial Conjunctivitis

In general, bacterial conjunctivitis is accompanied by a purulent discharge and viral infection by a watery discharge. One or both eyes may be involved. Regional lymphadenopathy is not a common finding in bacterial conjunctivitis except in cases of oculoglandular syndrome due to *S aureus,* group A beta-hemolytic streptococci, *Mycobacterium tuberculosis* or atypical mycobacteria, *Francisella tularensis* (the agent of tularemia), and *Bartonella henselae* (the agent of cat-scratch fever).

Common bacterial causes of conjunctivitis in older children include nontypable *Haemophilus* species, *S pneumoniae, M catarrhalis,* and *S aureus.* If conjunctivitis is not associated with systemic illness, topical antibiotics such as erythromycin, polymyxin-bacitracin, sulfacetamide, tobramycin, and fluoroquinolones are usually adequate. Systemic therapy is recommended for conjunctivitis associated with *Chlamydia trachomatis, N gonorrhoeae,* and *N meningitidis.*

Baum J: Infections of the eye. Clin Infect Dis 1995;21:479.

Viral Conjunctivitis

Adenovirus infection is often associated with pharyngitis, a follicular reaction of the palpebral conjunctiva, and preauricular adenopathy (pharyngoconjunctival fever). Epidemic keratoconjunctivitis is also a frequent presentation. Treatment is supportive.

Herpes simplex virus may cause conjunctivitis or blepharoconjunctivitis. Treatment is with topical triflutidine 1%.

Allergic Conjunctivitis

In hay fever conjunctivitis, the eyes are red and itchy, with mucoid discharge. Symptomatic treatment is with a combination topical vasoconstrictor plus an antihistamine (naphazoline-antazoline); a nonsteroidal anti-inflammatory drug such as ketorolac tromethamine 0.5%; a mast cell stabilizer such as lodoxamide tromethamine 0.1%; or prednisolone 0.125%. Corticosteroids should be used with caution because their extended use causes glaucoma in some patients. Prolonged use of corticosteroids also causes cataracts. Central nervous system depression has been reported with accidental ingestion of naphazoline.

Vernal conjunctivitis is a seasonal form of allergic conjunctivitis associated with tearing, itching, and a stringy discharge. It is more common in males. In the palpebral form, dramatic changes of the superior palpebral conjunctiva occur, with cobblestone papillae (Figure 14–13). Corneal ulcers can occur. Topical treatments include a mast cell stabilizer such as 4% cromolyn sodium or 0.1% lodoxamide tromethamine and limited use of a topical corticosteroid. One form of vernal conjunctivitis presents with nodules at the limbus. Contact lens wear may induce a conjunctivitis that appears similar to the palpebral form of vernal conjunctivitis.

Tobias JD: Central nervous system depression following accidental ingestion of Visine Eye Drops. Clin Pediatr (Phila) 1996;35:539.

Mucocutaneous Diseases

Conjunctivitis and conjunctival changes are seen in a number of systemic syndromes. Examples are erythema multiforme-Stevens-Johnson syndrome (see Chapter 13), Reiter's syndrome (Chapter 38), and Kawasaki disease (Chapter 18), which is associated also with iritis. With Stevens-Johnson syn-

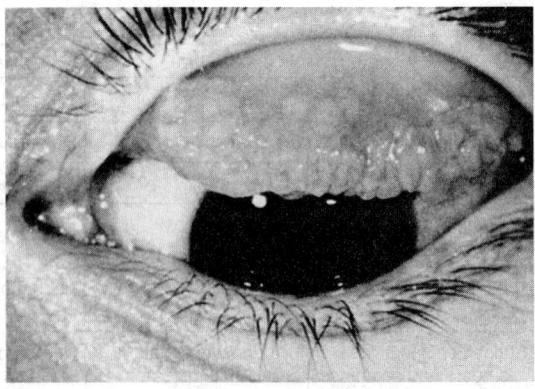

Figure 14–13. Vernal conjunctivitis. "Cobblestone" papillae in superior tarsal conjunctiva. (Reproduced, with permission, from Vaughan D, Asbury T, Riordan-Eva P [editors]: *General Ophthalmology,* 14th ed. Appleton & Lange, 1995.)

drome, conjunctival changes include erythema, vesicular lesions that frequently rupture, and symblepharon (adhesions) between the raw edges of the bulbar and palpebral conjunctiva. Management may include lubricants to provide comfort and a topical corticosteroid to prevent adhesions and dry eye in severe cases of erythema multiforme. Cycloplegic agents and topical corticosteroids are prescribed for iritis in Kawasaki disease.

Power WJ et al: Analysis of the acute ophthalmic manifestations of the erythema multiforme/Stevens-Johnson syndrome/toxic epidermal necrolysis disease spectrum. Ophthalmology 1995;102:1669.

DISORDERS OF THE IRIS

Iris Coloboma

Iris coloboma is a developmental defect due to incomplete closure of the anterior embryonal fissure. The pupil will have an elongated shape reminiscent of a keyhole or cat's eye (Figure 14–14). The affected area is located inferonasally but may extend posteriorly, involving the retina and choroid. The effect on visual acuity is variable. Iris coloboma may be an isolated defect or may be associated with a number of chromosomal abnormalities and syndromes.

Aniridia

Aniridia is a bilateral disorder that includes macular hypoplasia and absence of almost all of the iris (Figure 14–15). Cataract, corneal changes, and glaucoma are often seen. Photophobia and nystagmus occur.

Aniridia may occur as an autosomal dominant inheritance pattern or in a sporadic form that is associated with Wilms' tumor. Repeated examination and abdominal ultrasonography are thus indicated. The

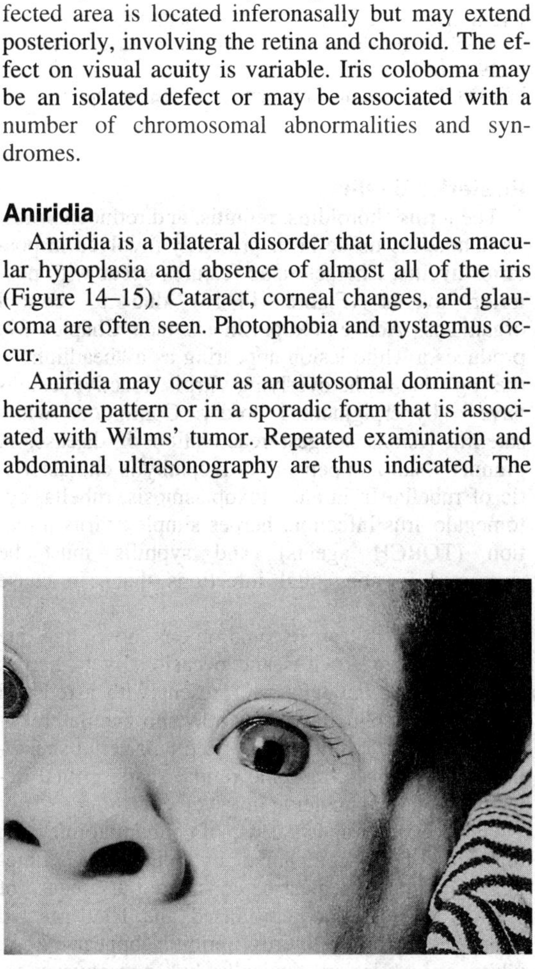

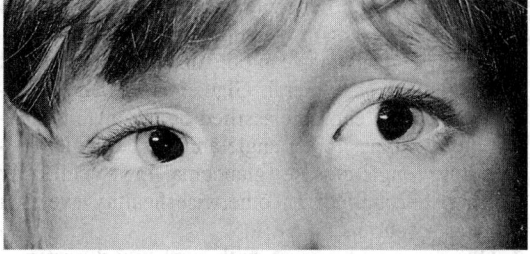

Figure 14–15. Bilateral aniridia. Iris remnants present temporally in each eye.

aniridia gene has been isolated to the 11p13 chromosome region. Aniridia, genitourinary abnormalities, and mental retardation have been linked to an 11p deletion.

Albinism

Albinism can have a profound effect on vision requiring low-vision aids. It may be ocular or oculocutaneous and is inherited by different modes depending on the type. Bleeding problems occur in individuals with Hermansky-Pudlak syndrome, in which oculocutaneous albinism is associated with a platelet abnormality.

Iris color in albinism varies according to type and severity of albinism as well as the individual's race. Iris transillumination may be obvious or may require slitlamp examination to detect focal areas of transillumination.

Other iris conditions include heterochromia of the irides, which can be seen in congenital Horner's syndrome, after iritis, or with tumors and nevi of the iris. Acquired iris nodules, known as Lisch nodules, are seen in type I neurofibromatosis. When seen on slitlamp examination, they are 1–2 mm in diameter and often beige in color, though their appearance can be variable. Iris xanthogranuloma occurring with juvenile xanthogranuloma can cause hyphema and glaucoma. Patients with juvenile xanthogranuloma should be evaluated by an ophthalmologist for ocular involvement.

Summers CG, King RA: Ophthalmic features of minimal pigment oculocutaneous albinism. Ophthalmology 1994;101:906.

GLAUCOMA

Glaucoma is increased intraocular pressure, which causes damage to ocular structures and loss of vision. Signs of glaucoma presenting within the first year of life include buphthalmos (enlargement of the globe) as well as tearing, photophobia, corneal enlargement

Figure 14–14. Iris coloboma located inferiorly.

and clouding due to edema, and optic nerve cupping. After age 2–3 years, only optic nerve changes occur.

Pediatric glaucomas can be congenital or acquired and unilateral or bilateral. Glaucoma may be inherited. Glaucoma can be classified on an anatomic basis into two types: open-angle and closed-angle. Precipitating angle-closure glaucoma in a child by dilating the pupil of an otherwise healthy eye is a very rare occurrence.

Glaucoma also occurs with ocular and systemic syndromes. Aniridia and anterior segment dysgenesis are examples. Systemic syndromes associated with glaucoma include Sturge-Weber syndrome, the oculocerebrorenal syndrome of Lowe, and the Pierre-Robin sequence. Glaucoma can also occur with hyphema, iritis, lens dislocation, intraocular tumor, and retinopathy of prematurity.

Treatment depends on the cause, but surgery is often the choice.

Ritch R, Shields MB, Krupin T (editors): *The Glaucomas,* 2nd ed. 3 vols. Mosby, 1996.

UVEITIS

Inflammation of the uveal tract can be subdivided according to the uveal tissue primarily involved (iris, choroid, retina) or by location, ie, anterior, intermediate, or posterior uveitis. Perhaps the most commonly diagnosed form of uveitis in childhood is traumatic iridocyclitis (iritis).

Anterior Uveitis

Iritis (anterior uveitis, iridocyclitis) is usually accompanied by injection, photophobia, pain, and blurred vision. An exception to this is iritis associated with juvenile rheumatoid arthritis (Chapter 24). The eye is quiet and asymptomatic, but slitlamp examination will reveal iritis.

Although iridocyclitis associated with juvenile rheumatoid arthritis occurs most often in girls with pauciarticular arthritis and a positive antinuclear antibody, all children with juvenile rheumatoid arthritis need to be screened. Treatment with a topical corticosteroid and a cycloplegic agent is aimed at quieting the inflammation and preventing or delaying the onset of cataract and glaucoma. Methotrexate is used in refractory cases.

Inflammatory bowel disease is also associated with iritis—perhaps more commonly with Crohn's disease than with ulcerative colitis. Other ocular findings of the anterior segment that can be associated with inflammatory bowel disease include conjunctivitis, episcleritis, and sterile corneal infiltrates. Posterior segment findings may include central serous retinochoroidopathy, panuveitis (inflammation of all uveal tissue), choroiditis, ischemic optic neuropathy, retinal vasculitis, neuroretinitis, and intermediate uveitis (see below).

Posterior subcapsular cataracts are seen in patients with or without ocular inflammation. Most if not all of these patients have been taking corticosteroids as part of the long-term treatment of inflammatory bowel disease. Children with Crohn's disease or ulcerative colitis should have routine periodic ophthalmologic examinations to rule out ocular inflammation, which may be asymptomatic, and cataracts associated with systemic corticosteroids.

Other causes of anterior uveitis in children include syphilis, tuberculosis, sarcoidosis, and Lyme disease, all but the latter also causing posterior uveitis. Juvenile spondyloarthropathies, including ankylosing spondylitis, Reiter's syndrome, and psoriatic arthritis, are also associated with anterior uveitis. A substantial percentage of cases are of unknown origin.

American Academy of Pediatrics Section on Rheumatology and Ophthalmology: Guidelines for ophthalmologic examinations in children with juvenile rheumatoid arthritis. Pediatrics 1993;92:295.

Rychwalski PJ, Cruz OA: Asymptomatic uveitis in young people with inflammatory bowel disease. JAAPOS 1997;1:111.

Winsett M: Inflammatory bowel disease in children and adolescents. Pediatr Ann 1997;26:227.

Posterior Uveitis

The terms choroiditis, retinitis, and retinochoroiditis denote the tissue layer primarily involved in posterior uveitis. Characteristic features occur with posterior uveitis (Figure 14–16) due to certain organisms. Active toxoplasmosis (see Chapter 37) produces a white lesion appearing as a "headlight in the fog" due to the overlying vitritis. Inactive lesions have a hyperpigmented border. Contiguous white satellite lesions suggest reactivation of disease. A granular "salt and pepper" retinopathy is characteristic of rubella. In infants, toxoplasmosis, rubella, cytomegalovirus infection, herpes simplex virus infection (TORCH agents), and syphilis must be suspected in congenital infections that can cause chorioretinitis.

Acute retinal necrosis syndrome is most often due to varicella-zoster virus and occasionally to herpes simplex virus. Patients may present with a red and painful eye. Ophthalmoscopy may show unilateral or bilateral patchy white areas of retina, arterial sheathing, vitreous haze, atrophic retinal scars, retinal detachment, and optic nerve involvement.

Cytomegalovirus is a cause of congenital infection that may be accompanied by retinitis. Cytomegalovirus infection must be considered as a cause of retinitis in immunocompromised and HIV-infected children. Cytomegalovirus retinitis appears as a white retinal lesion, typically but not always associated with hemorrhage, or as a granular, indolent-

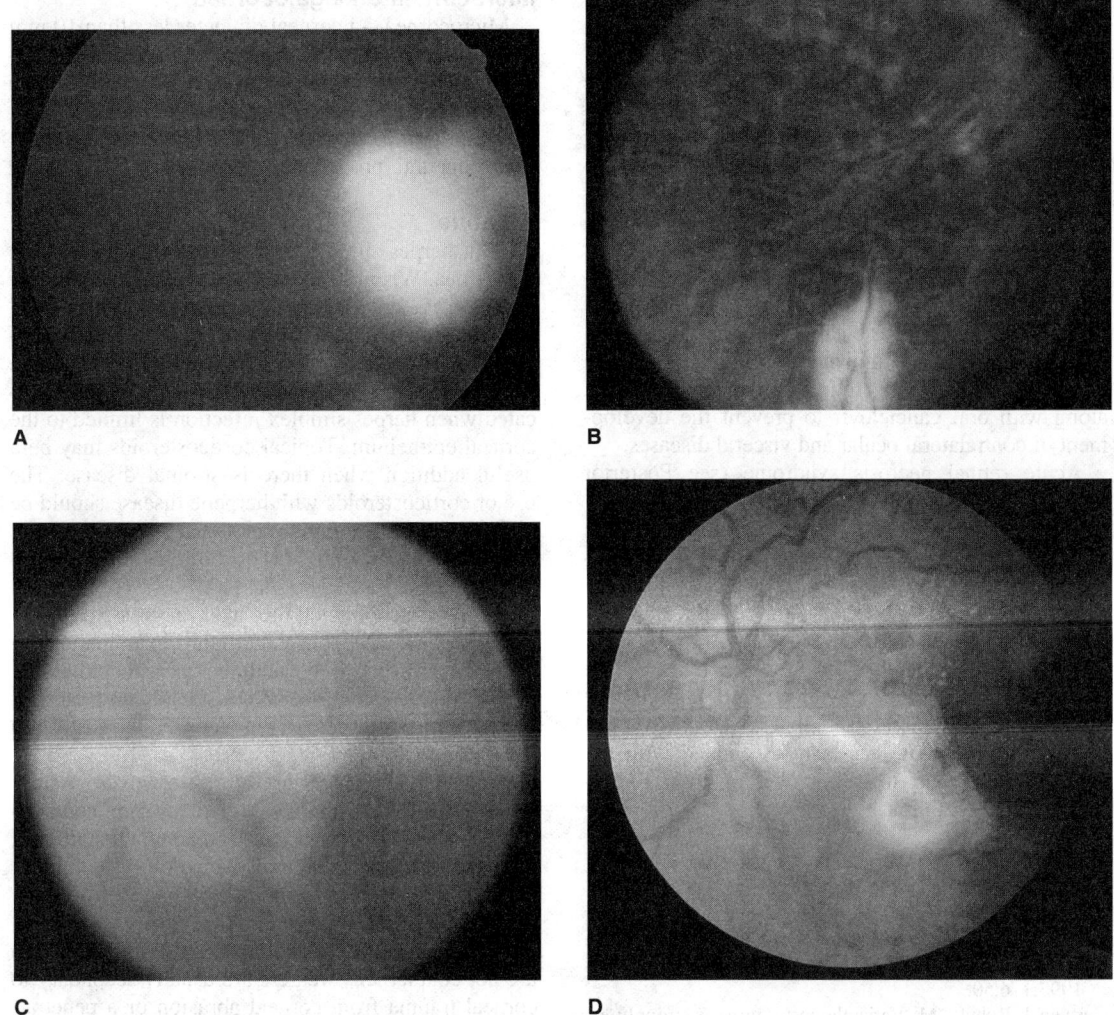

Figure 14–16. Posterior uveitis. **A:** Toxoplasmic retinochoroiditis. **B:** Cytomegalovirus retinitis. **C:** Acute retinal necrosis. **D:** *Toxocara* granuloma. (Courtesy of J Zilis.)

appearing lesion with hemorrhage and a white periphery. "Cotton wool spots" (nerve fiber layer infarcts) are also commonly seen in HIV-positive patients.

In toddlers and older youngsters, *Toxocara canis* or *Toxocara cati* infections ("ocular larva migrans"; see Chapter 37) occur from ingesting soil contaminated with parasite eggs. The disease is usually unilateral. Common presentations include a red injected eye, leukocoria, and decreased vision. Fundus examination may show endophthalmitis (vitreous abscess) or localized granuloma. Diagnosis is based on the appearance of the lesion and serologic testing utilizing the enzyme-linked immunosorbent assay

(ELISA) for *T canis* and *T cati*. Treatment options include periocular corticosteroid injections and vitrectomy.

Intermediate Uveitis

Pars planitis, often of uncertain cause, may present with vitreous floaters. Macular edema and decreased vision can result.

Toxocara infections with peripheral granuloma can be associated with intermediate uveitis, as can inflammatory bowel disease. Retinoblastoma and other neoplasms can imitate uveitis, causing a so-called "masquerade" syndrome.

AIDS & THE EYE

Ocular infections are important manifestations of AIDS (see Chapter 35). As CD4 T-lymphocyte counts fall below 200/μL, opportunistic infections increase in these patients. Important pathogens causing eye infection include *Toxoplasma gondii* and cytomegalovirus. Especially when CD4+ counts fall below 50/μL, the patient is at high risk for cytomegalovirus retinitis (see section on posterior uveitis) and blindness. Both foscarnet and ganciclovir are useful in treating cytomegalovirus infection, though recurrences occur with either drug. Ganciclovir intraocular implants also appear to be effective in controlling retinitis in the treated eye, along with oral ganciclovir to prevent the development of contralateral ocular and visceral diseases.

Acute retinal necrosis syndrome (see Posterior Uveitis) is a severe necrotizing retinitis in AIDS patients that often results in blindness. Most cases are thought to be due to herpes zoster. Other agents implicated are herpes simplex types 1 and 2 and occasionally cytomegalovirus. Therapy with antiviral agents is often ineffective.

Antiretroviral therapy with reverse transcriptase inhibitors (zidovudine, stavudine, and lamivudine) and protease inhibitors (saquinavir, ritonavir, indinavir, and nelfinavir) has been associated with the current leveling off in the number of cases of cytomegalovirus retinitis.

Cytomegalovirus (CMV) culture results, drug resistance, and clinical outcome in patients with AIDS and CMV retinitis treated with foscarnet or ganciclovir. Studies of ocular complications of AIDS (SOCA) in collaboration with AIDS Clinical Trial Group. J Infect Dis 1997;176:50.

Garweg J, Bohnke M: Varicella-zoster virus is strongly associated with atypical necrotizing herpetic retinopathies. Clin Infect Dis 1997;24:603..

Jabs DA, Bartlett JG: AIDS and ophthalmology: A period of transition. (Editorial.) Am J Ophthalmol 1997;124:227.

DISORDERS OF THE CORNEA

Corneal trauma is dealt with in the section on ocular trauma earlier in this chapter.

Conditions Causing Corneal Clouding

The differential diagnosis of corneal clouding in a newborn infant includes forceps trauma, congenital glaucoma, infection, congenital malformation, and tumor. In older children, corneal clouding may be seen with mucopolysaccharidoses, Wilson's disease, and cystinosis. Infiltrates occur with virus infections, staphylococcal lid disease, corneal dystrophies, and interstitial keratitis due to congenital syphilis.

Microcornea & Megalocornea

Microcornea—a corneal diameter less than 10 mm in a full-term infant or older child—may be associated with other anterior segment malformations or a microphthalmic globe. Megalocornea—diameter of 12.5 mm or greater—is regarded as due to congenital glaucoma until proved otherwise.

Keratitis

Both herpes simplex and herpes zoster can infect the cornea. When the epithelium breaks down, a dendritic or ameboid pattern can be seen with fluorescein staining. Corneal involvement with herpes simplex can be recurrent and lead to blindness. Topical antivirals such as trifluridine or vidarabine are indicated when herpes simplex infection is limited to the corneal epithelium. Topical corticosteroids may be a useful addition when there is stromal disease. The use of corticosteroids with herpetic disease should be undertaken by an ophthalmologist. Oral acyclovir started in the early phase (first 5 days) may be helpful in herpes zoster eye disease.

Adenovirus conjunctivitis may progress to keratitis 1–2 weeks after onset. Slitlamp examination reveals white infiltrates beneath the corneal epithelium. Vision may be decreased. In most cases no treatment is necessary since adenovirus keratitis is most often self-limiting.

Contact lens wearers are at risk of severe vision-threatening *Acanthamoeba* keratitis from contaminated contact lens solutions. Treatment is difficult and may require corneal transplantation.

Corneal Ulcers

Bacterial corneal ulcers in healthy children who are not contact lens wearers are usually secondary to corneal trauma from corneal abrasion or a penetrating foreign body. Decreased vision, pain, injection, a white corneal infiltrate (ulcer), and hypopyon (pus in the anterior chamber) may all be present. Prompt referral to an ophthalmologist is necessary for culture and antibiotic treatment.

DISORDERS OF THE LENS

Lens disorders involve abnormality of clarity or position. Lens opacification—cataract—can affect vision depending on its density, size, and position. Visual potential is also influenced by age at onset and the success of amblyopia treatment.

Cataracts

Cataracts in children may be unilateral or bilateral, may exist as isolated defects, or may be accompanied by other ocular disorders or systemic disease (Figure 14–17). Congenital and infantile cataracts may also be part of a chromosomal syndrome. Leukocoria, poor fixation, and strabismus or nystagmus (or both)

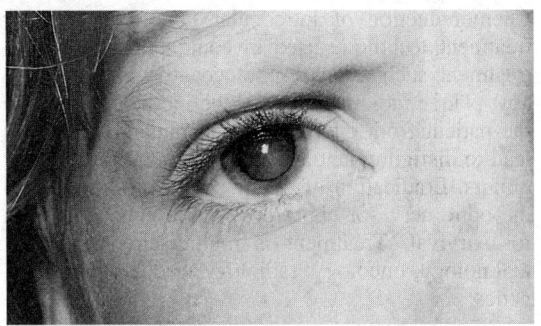

Figure 14–17. Cataract causing leukocoria.

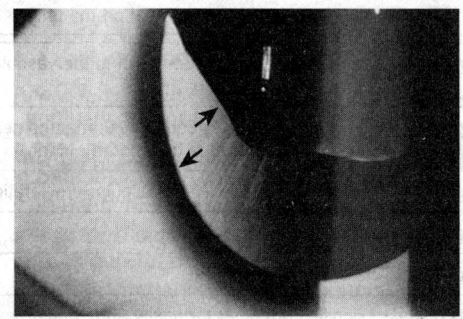

Figure 14–18. Subluxated lens. Lens dislocated superiorly. Arrows mark edge of lens and iris. (Reproduced, with permission, from *Pediatric Ophthalmology and Strabismus.* Section 6. Basic Clinical Science Course 1994. American Academy of Ophthalmology, 1995.)

may be the presenting complaints. In the newborn, absence of a red reflex should suggest the possibility of cataract, especially if examination is with a dilated pupil.

The appearance of the cataract may sometimes suggest its cause. Anterior capsular cataracts are developmental, not related to infection or metabolic problems. Laboratory investigation for infectious and metabolic causes is often indicated, eg, cultures or serologic tests for toxoplasmosis, rubella, cytomegalovirus infection, herpes simplex infection, and syphilis and evaluation for metabolic errors.

Early diagnosis and treatment are necessary to prevent deprivation amblyopia in children under 9 years of age, since they are visually immature. Cataracts that are visually significant require removal. Rehabilitation with an intraocular lens is becoming more commonplace, but contact lenses and spectacles still play a role, as does occlusion of the better-seeing eye to treat the amblyopia.

Dislocated Lenses

Lens dislocation is usually bilateral except when due to trauma. Subluxation causes refractive errors of large magnitude, difficult to correct. Other ophthalmologic concerns are pupillary block glaucoma and retinal detachment.

Dislocated lenses are associated with other ocular conditions and systemic syndromes, including Marfan's syndrome, homocystinuria, Weill-Marchesani syndrome, sulfite oxidase deficiency, hyperlysinemia, syphilis, and Ehlers-Danlos syndrome. Workup and treatment are multidisciplinary endeavors (Figure 14–18).

Ainsworth JR, Cohen S: Pediatric cataract management with variations in surgical technique and aphakic optical correction. Ophthalmology 1997;104:1096.

Wright KW (editor): Lens abnormalities. In: *Pediatric Ophthalmology and Strabismus.* Mosby Year Book, 1995.

DISORDERS OF THE RETINA

Retinopathy of Prematurity

The practitioner may encounter diseases of the retina in the newborn period or shortly after. Retinopathy of prematurity (ROP) continues to be a cause of blindness, especially for infants less than 28 weeks' gestation and weighing less than 1250 g. Premature infants with incomplete retinal vascularization are at risk for developing abnormal peripheral retinal vascularization, which may lead to retinal detachment in severe cases. However, most cases of ROP do not progress to retinal detachment and require no treatment.

The risk of developing visually threatening ROP is inversely proportionate to birth weight and gestational age. Infants less than 1500 g at birth may develop visually threatening ROP. The cause of this disorder—including the role of supplemental oxygen in the neonatal period—is still not fully understood. The duration of supplemental oxygen—but not the concentration of delivered oxygen—does correlate with the development of ROP. Other correlates are hyaline membrane disease, bronchopulmonary dysplasia, patent ductus arteriosus, apnea and bradycardia, intraventricular hemorrhage, and multiple births.

Screening guidelines and a uniform classification system have been adopted. The first retinal examination is recommended at 4–6 weeks of age (Table 14–4). Follow-up examinations depend on the findings and the risk of developing the disease. The treatment of stage III+ ROP (plus disease denotes arteriole tortuosity and venous dilation) with cryotherapy

Table 14–4. Stages of retinopathy of prematurity.

Stage I	Demarcation line or border dividing the vascular from the avascular retina
Stage II	Ridge. Line of stage I acquires volume and rises above the surface retina to become a ridge.
Stage III	Ridge with extraretinal fibrovascular proliferation
Stage IV	Subtotal retinal detachment
Stage V	Total retinal detachment

"Plus disease" signifies arteriolar tortuosity and venular dilation of posterior pole vessels.

or plus laser therapy has reduced the occurrence of visual loss by 50%. In spite of all treatment, there are still some cases that go on to develop blinding retinal detachment. Other findings associated with ROP include strabismus, amblyopia, myopia, and glaucoma.

American Academy of Pediatrics, the American Association for Pediatric Ophthalmology and Strabismus, and the American Academy of Ophthalmology. A joint statement. Screening examination of premature infants for retinopathy of prematurity. Pediatrics 1997;100:273.

Cryotherapy for Retinopathy of Prematurity Cooperative Group. The natural ocular outcome of premature birth and retinopathy: Status at 1 year. Arch Ophthalmol 1994;112:903.

Dobson V et al: Grating visual acuity in eyes with retinal residue of retinopathy of prematurity. Arch Ophthalmol 1995;113:1172.

Retinoblastoma

Retinoblastoma is the most common primary intraocular malignancy of childhood, with an incidence of up to 1:15,000 live births (see Chapter 26). Most patients present before 3 years of age, with bilateral cases presenting earlier than unilateral ones.

Both sporadic and inherited forms of retinoblastoma occur. Inheritance is autosomal dominant with high penetrance. The disease may present as a solitary mass or as multiple tumors in one or both eyes. Inherited cases and some unilateral cases are due to germinal mutation, whereas the unilateral cases with a solitary tumor are due to a somatic retinal mutation. In both cases, the mutation occurs in the region of the q14 band on chromosome 13. Individuals with a germinal mutation are at risk for the development of tumors other than retinoblastoma (pineal tumors, osteosarcoma, and other soft tissue sarcomas).

The most common presenting sign in a child with previously undiagnosed retinoblastoma is leukocoria (Figure 14–1). Others present with strabismus, red eye, glaucoma, or pseudohypopyon (appearance of pus in the anterior chamber).

Treatment of unilateral cases, especially of large tumors, usually has been enucleation, since at the time of presentation the eye is filled with tumor.

Chemoreduction of intraocular tumors is a newer treatment technique used in conjunction with local treatment such as laser photocoagulation, cryotherapy, plaque radiotherapy, and thermotherapy to spare the patient from enucleation and radiation that may lead to disfigurement and the induction of secondary tumors. Eradication of tumor before infiltration into the optic nerve or choroid carries a good prognosis for survival. Treatment is multidisciplinary—ophthalmology, oncology, radiology, pediatrics, and genetics.

Gallie BL et al: Chemotherapy with focal therapy can cure intraocular retinoblastoma without radiotherapy. Arch Ophthalmol 1997;114:1321.

Kingston JE et al: Results of combined chemotherapy and radiotherapy for advanced intraocular retinoblastoma. Arch Ophthalmol 1997;114:1339.

Murphree AL et al: Chemotherapy plus local treatment in the management of intraocular retinoblastoma. Arch Ophthalmol 1997;114:1348.

Shields CL et al: Chemoreduction in the initial management of intraocular retinoblastoma. Arch Ophthalmol 1997;114:1330.

Retinal Detachment

Retinal detachment occurs infrequently in children. Common causes are trauma and high myopia. Other causes in childhood are ROP, Marfan's syndrome, and Stickler's syndrome.

Symptoms of detachment are floaters, flashing lights, and loss of visual field. However, children often cannot appreciate or verbalize their symptoms. A detachment may not be discovered until the child is referred after failing a vision screening examination, strabismus supervenes, or leukocoria is noted.

Treatment of retinal detachment is surgical.

DISEASES OF THE OPTIC NERVE

Optic nerve function is evaluated by checking visual acuity, color vision, pupillary response, and visual fields. Poor optic nerve function results in decreased central or peripheral vision, strabismus, and nystagmus.

The "swinging flashlight test" is used to assess function of each optic nerve. It is performed by shining a light alternately in front of each pupil to check for an afferent pupillary defect. An abnormal response in the affected eye is pupillary dilation when the light is directed into that eye. This results from poorer conduction along the optic nerve of the affected eye, which in turn results in less pupillary constriction of both eyes than occurs when the light is shined into the noninvolved eye. Hippus—rhythmic dilating and constricting movements of the pupil—can be confused with an afferent pupillary defect, also known as a Marcus Gunn pupillary defect.

The optic nerve is evaluated as to size, shape,

color, and vascularity. Occasionally, myelinization past the entrance of the optic nerve head occurs. It appears white, with a feathered edge (Figure 14–19). Myelinization onto the retina can be associated with myopia and amblyopia. Anatomic defects of the optic nerve include colobomatous defects and pits.

Optic nerve hypoplasia may be associated with absence of the septum pellucidum and hypothalamic-pituitary dysfunction, which is known as septo-optic dysplasia, or de Morsier's syndrome. Children with septo-optic dysplasia and hypocortisolism are at risk for sudden death during febrile illness from thermoregulatory disturbance and dehydration from diabetes insipidus. Optic nerve hypoplasia may occur in infants of diabetic mothers and has also been associated with alcohol use or ingestion of quinine or phenytoin during pregnancy. Anatomically, the size of the involved optic nerve may range from absent (aplasia) to almost full size, with a segmental defect. However, the nerve often appears larger than it is because it is surrounded by a depigmented halo. Visual function with optic nerve hypoplasia ranges from mildly decreased to light perception only. If only one eye is involved, the child usually presents with strabismus. If both eyes are affected, nystagmus is usually the presenting sign.

Since the optic nerve is an outgrowth of the brain, changes in this structure often reflect central nervous system disease.

Papilledema

Papilledema is associated with increased intracra-nial pressure due to any cause, such as tumor or intracranial infection. This appears as an elevated disk with indistinct margins, increased vessel diameter, and increased capillarity, giving the disk a hyperemic appearance with surrounding hemorrhages (Figure 14–20). Observed changes may be subtle to striking. Nerve head changes are bilateral and generally symmetric. Papilledema (optic disk edema) occurs also with idiopathic intracranial hypertension—almost equally in boys and girls, and sometimes associated with obesity. Other associated causes are otitis media, viral infections, corticosteroid use and withdrawal, sinus infection, and trauma. Early in its course, the patient with papilledema may notice no change in vision, though there may be enlargement of the blind spot. Transient obscurations of vision (amaurosis fugax) may occur as the process becomes more long-standing. Further effects on vision will occur as the papilledema becomes chronic. Workup and treatment are directed toward finding the underlying systemic or central nervous system cause.

Papillitis

Papillitis, a form of optic neuritis seen on ophthalmoscopic examination as an inflamed optic nerve head, may have the same appearance as papilledema. However, papillitis may be unilateral, whereas papilledema is almost always bilateral. Papillitis can be differentiated from papilledema by an afferent pupillary defect (Marcus Gunn pupil); by its greater effect in decreasing visual acuity and color vision; and by

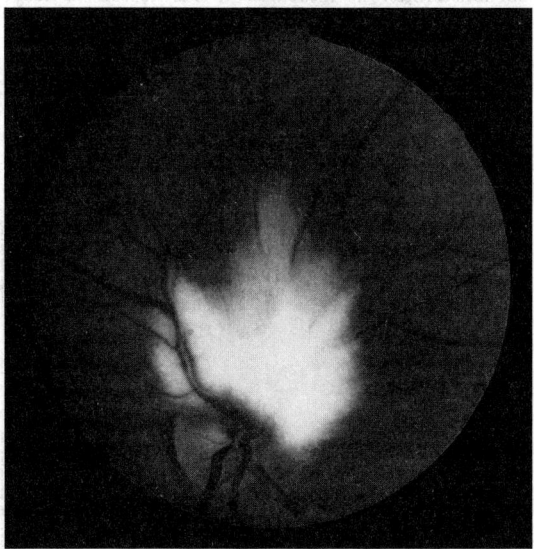

Figure 14–19. Myelinization extending from optic nerve superiorly onto the retina.

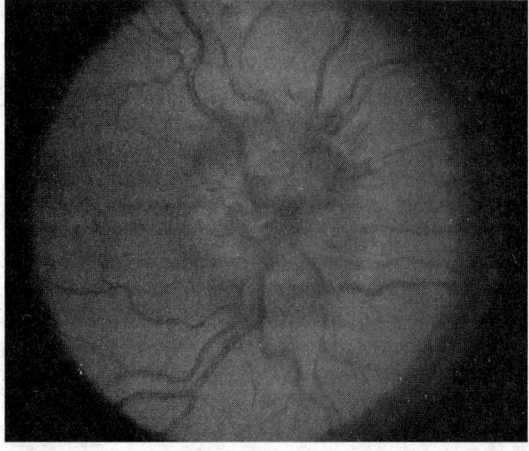

Figure 14–20. Florid papilledema. (Courtesy of J Zilis.)

the presence of a central scotoma. Papilledema that is not yet chronic will not have as dramatic an effect on vision. Since increased intracranial pressure can cause both papilledema and a sixth (abducens) nerve palsy, papilledema can be differentiated from papillitis if esotropia and loss of abduction are also present. In pseudopapilledema, a normal variant of the optic disk, the disk appears elevated, with indistinct margins and a normal vascular pattern. Not infrequently, pseudopapilledema is found in hyperopic individuals.

Optic Atrophy

Optic atrophy, noted as pallor of the nerve head with loss of capillarity, is most frequently seen in children after neurologic compromise during the perinatal period. An example would be a prematurely born infant who develops an intraventricular hemorrhage. Hydrocephalus, glioma of the optic nerve, craniostenosis, certain neurologic diseases, and toxins such as methyl alcohol can cause optic atrophy as well as certain inborn errors of metabolism.

Babikian P et al: Idiopathic intracranial hypertension in children: The Iowa experience. Child Neurol 1994;9:144.
Brodsky MC et al: Sudden death in septo-optic dysplasia. Arch Ophthalmol 1997;115:66.
Scott IU et al: Idiopathic intracranial hypertension in children and adolescents. Am J Ophthalmol 1997;124:253.

DISEASES OF THE ORBIT

Periorbital & Orbital Cellulitis

The fascia of the eyelids joins with the fibrous orbital septum to isolate the orbit from the lids. Infections arising external to the orbital septum are termed preseptal. Preseptal (periorbital) cellulitis, which indicates infection of the structures of the eyelid, is characterized by lid edema, swelling, pain, and mild fever. It usually arises from a local exogenous source such as an abrasion of the eyelid, from other infections (hordeolum, dacryocystitis, chalazion), or from infected varicella or insect bite lesions. *Staphylococcus aureus* and *Streptococcus pyogenes* are the most common pathogens from these sources. Preseptal infections in children under 3 years of age also occur from bacteremia, though this is much less common since *Haemophilus influenzae* immunization became available. *Streptococcus pneumoniae* is still an occasional cause of this infection. Children with periorbital cellulitis from presumed bacteremia must be examined for additional foci of infection.

Infection of the orbit almost always arises from contiguous sinus infection, since the walls of three sinuses make up portions of the orbital walls and infection can breach these walls or extend by way of bridging veins. The orbital contents can develop a phlegmon (orbital cellulitis), or frank pus can develop in the orbit (orbital abscess). When the orbit is infected, the signs of periorbital infection are joined by proptosis, restricted eye movement, and pain with eye movement. Fever is usually high and hectic. CT scanning or MRI is required to establish the extent of the infection within the orbit. Sinus imaging should be obtained at the same time. The etiologic agents are those of acute or chronic sinusitis—respiratory flora and anaerobes. *S aureus* is also frequently implicated.

Therapy of preseptal infection is with systemic antibiotics. Treatment of orbital infections often requires surgical drainage in conjunction with intravenous antibiotics. Drainage of infected sinuses is often part of the therapy.

Tole DM, Anderton LS, Hayward JM: Orbital cellulitis demands early recognition, urgent admission and aggressive management. J Accid Emerg Med 1995;12:151.

Craniofacial Anomalies

Craniofacial anomalies can affect the orbit and visual system. Examples of changes associated with craniofacial disease involving the orbits are proptosis, corneal exposure, hypertelorism, strabismus, amblyopia, and lid coloboma.

Orbital Tumors

Both benign and malignant orbital lesions occur in children. The most common tumor is capillary hemangioma (Figure 14–21). This type of tumor may be located superficially in the lid or deep in the orbit and can cause ptosis, refractive errors, and amblyopia. Deeper lesions may cause proptosis. Capillary hemangiomas in infants initially increase in size before involuting at about 5 years of age. Therapy with corticosteroids is indicated if the lesion is large enough to cause amblyopia.

Orbital dermoid cysts vary in size and are usually found temporally at the brow and orbital rim or superonasally. These lesions are firm, well-

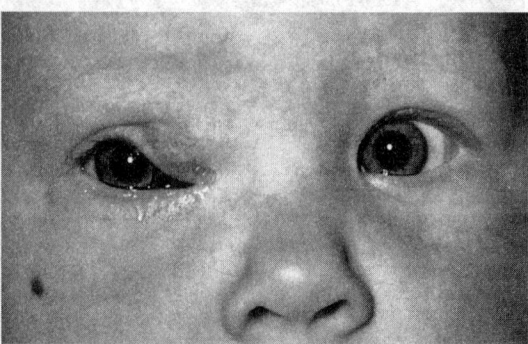

Figure 14–21. Right upper lid hemangioma causing ptosis.

encapsulated, and mobile. Rupture of the cyst causes a severe inflammatory reaction. Treatment is by excision. Lymphangioma occurring in the orbit is typically poorly encapsulated, increases in size with upper respiratory infection, and is susceptible to hemorrhage. Other benign tumors of the orbit are orbital pseudotumor, neurofibroma, teratoma, and tumors arising from bone, connective tissue, and neural tissue.

Of grave concern is orbital rhabdomyosarcoma, the most common primary orbital malignancy in childhood (see Chapter 26). This tumor grows rapidly and displaces the globe. The average age at onset is 7 years. The tumor is often initially mistaken for orbital swelling due to insignificant trauma. Radiation and chemotherapy are the mainstays of treatment after biopsy confirms the diagnosis. With expeditious diagnosis and proper treatment, the survival rate of patients with orbital rhabdomyosarcoma confined to the orbit approaches 90%.

Tumors metastatic to the orbit also occur, neuroblastoma being the most common. Presentation may be with proptosis, orbital ecchymosis ("raccoon eyes"), Horner's syndrome, or opsoclonus ("dancing eyes"). Ewing's sarcoma, leukemia, Burkitt's lymphoma, and the histiocytosis X group of diseases may involve the orbit.

Abramson DH, Notis CM: Visual acuity after radiation for orbital rhabdomyosarcoma. Am J Ophthalmol 1994;118:808.
Mannor GE et al: Multidisciplinary management of refractory orbital rhabdomyosarcoma. Ophthalmology 1997;104:1198.

NYSTAGMUS

Nystagmus is rhythmic oscillations of the eyes. It may be unilateral or bilateral, more pronounced in one eye, or gaze-dependent. Nystagmus may be associated with esotropia or may occur with ocular lesions that cause deprivation amblyopia (eg, media opacities) or conditions in which the visual pathways are hypoplastic. Both optic nerve hypoplasia and macular hypoplasia, which occurs with aniridia or ocular albinism, are associated with nystagmus. Nystagmus can also occur with normal ocular structures and seemingly normal central nervous system development. In the latter instance, the nystagmus may be blocked in certain positions of gaze, in which case a face turn or torticollis may develop. Latent nystagmus is seen when one eye is occluded. This type of nystagmus occurs in patients with congenital esotropia. There may also be an associated amblyopia.

Most nystagmus presenting in childhood is of ocular origin, but central nervous system disease and, less frequently, inner ear disease are other causes. A central nervous system cause is likely when the nystagmus is acquired. Fundus examination should seek optic nerve abnormalities and the presence of a macular reflex, since optic nerve hypoplasia and macular hypoplasia both can cause nystagmus.

Evaluation of nystagmus begins with the pediatric ophthalmologist, since associated ocular pathology is common. Some types of nystagmus can be treated, usually with surgery; less frequently, prisms are useful. Spasmus nutans, in which there is a rapid, shimmering disconjugate nystagmus with head bobbing and torticollis, is said to improve with time. Glioma of the hypothalamus can mimic spasmus nutans.

Arnoldi KA, Tychen L: Prevalence of intracranial lesions in children initially diagnosed with disconjugate nystagmus (spasmus nutans). J Pediatr Ophthalmol Strabismus 1995;32:296.

AMBLYOPIA & STRABISMUS

For visual development to proceed normally, a child must experience a normal visual environment with well-aligned eyes that are free of visually threatening disease and significant refractive errors. The consequences of not meeting these requirements during the sensitive period of visual development in the first decade of life are strabismus and decreased vision, or amblyopia.

Amblyopia

Amblyopia is a unilateral or bilateral reduction in central visual acuity due to the sensory deprivation of a well-formed retinal image that occurs with or without a visible organic lesion commensurate with the degree of visual loss. Amblyopia can occur only during the critical period of visual development in the first decade of life when the visual nervous system is plastic.

There are three types. **Strabismic amblyopia** may occur in the nondominant eye of a strabismic patient. **Refractive amblyopia** can occur in both eyes if significant refractive errors are untreated (ametropic or refractive amblyopia). Another type of refractive amblyopia may occur in the eye with the worse refractive error when there is imbalance between the eyes (anisometropic amblyopia). **Deprivation amblyopia** occurs when dense cataracts or complete ptosis prevents formation of a formed retinal image. Of the three types of amblyopia, this form of amblyopia results in the worst vision.

The earlier treatment is begun, the better the chance of improving visual acuity. Treatment is usually discontinued after age 9 years. Amblyogenic factors such as refractive errors are addressed. Because of the extreme sensitivity of the visual nervous system in infants, congenital cataracts and media opacities must be diagnosed and treated within the first few weeks of life. Visual rehabilitation and amblyopia treatment must then be started in order to foster visual development.

After eradicating amblyogenic factors, the mainstay of treatment is patching the sound eye, which causes the visual nervous system to process input from the amblyopic eye and in that way permits the development of useful vision. Other treatment modalities include "fogging" the sound eye with cycloplegic drops, lenses, and filters.

Keech RV, Kutschke PJ: Upper age limit for the development of amblyopia. J Pediatr Ophthalmol Strabismus 1995;32:89.

Strabismus

Strabismus is misalignment of the visual axes of the two eyes. Its prevalence in childhood is about 2–3%. Strabismus is categorized by the direction of the deviation and its frequency. Early diagnosis of strabismus and amblyopia provides the best chance of reaching full visual potential. Strabismus may cause or be due to amblyopia.

Misdiagnosis of strabismus—pseudostrabismus—can occur when relying on the corneal light reflex test. If the child has prominent epicanthal folds, pseudoesotropia may be erroneously diagnosed.

An infant destined to be well-aligned may appear intermittently esotropic, but this should occur less frequently over the first few months of life. By 5 or 6 months, the baby should be constantly well aligned. Children do not outgrow strabismus if it is truly present.

Beside its effect on visual development, strabismus may be a marker of other ocular or systemic disease. Twenty percent of patients with retinoblastoma present with strabismus. Patients with central nervous system disorders such as hydrocephalus, space-occupying lesions, and an amaurotic (blind) eye can also present with strabismus. In children under 3 or 4 years of age, blind eyes tend to assume a position of esodeviation, but after about age 4 an amaurotic eye tends to show an exotropic shift.

A. Esotropia: In esotropia, the visual axes of the eyes are excessively convergent. In terms of cause and treatment, esotropia can be categorized as to age at onset. Congenital esotropia (infantile esotropia) has its onset in the first year of life in healthy infants. The deviation is large. Surgery is the mainstay of treatment. To foster the development of binocular vision, good alignment should be achieved by age 2 years.

Esotropia beginning in the first year is also seen in infants born prematurely or in the child with a complicated perinatal history associated with central nervous system problems such as intracranial hemorrhage and periventricular leukomalacia. There are also syndromes with which esotropia is associated. In Möbius' syndrome (congenital facial diplegia), a sixth nerve palsy causing esotropia is associated with palsies of the seventh and twelfth cranial nerves and limb deformities. Duane's syndrome, which can affect both horizontal muscles, may be an isolated defect or may be associated with a multitude of systemic defects (eg, Goldenhar's syndrome). Children with unilateral paretic or restrictive causes of esotropia may develop face turns toward the affected eye.

The most frequent type of acquired esotropia is the accommodative type (Figure 14–22). Onset is usually between 2 and 5 years of age. The deviation is vari-

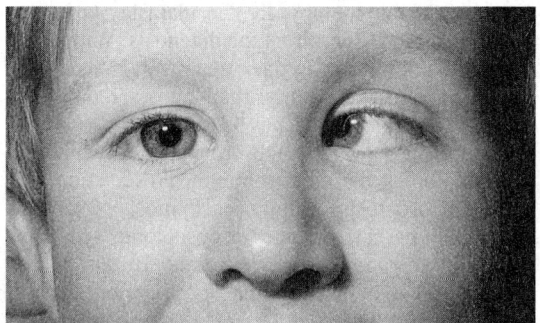

A

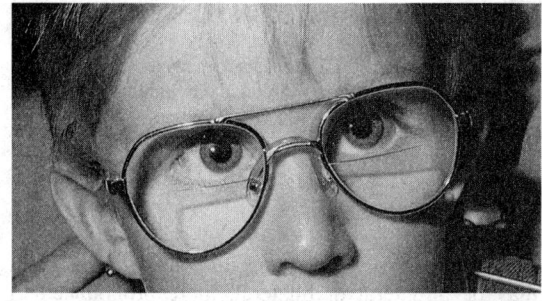

B

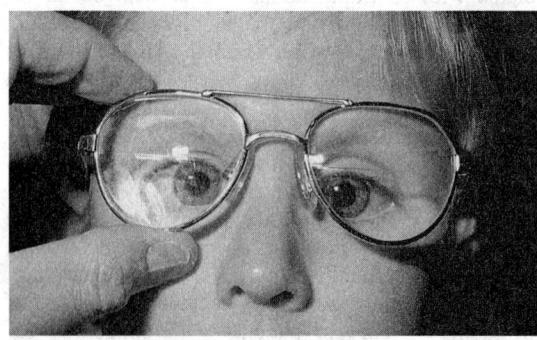

C

Figure 14–22. Accommodative esotropia. Without spectacles, esotropic (**A**). With spectacles, well-aligned at distance (**B**) and at near with bifocal correction (**C**).

able in magnitude and constancy and often accompanied by amblyopia. One type of accommodative esotropia is associated with a high hyperopic refraction. In another type, the deviation is worse with near than with distant vision. This type of esodeviation is independent of the refractive error. Management includes glasses, amblyopia treatment, and in some cases surgery. After age 5 years, any esotropia of recent onset should arouse suspicion of central nervous system disease. Infratentorial masses, hydrocephalus, and demyelinating diseases are causes of abducens palsy, which presents as an esotropia, lateral rectus paralysis or paresis, and face turn. The face turn is an attempt to maintain binocularity away from the field of action of the paretic muscle. Papilledema is present with increased intracranial pressure. Besides the vulnerability of the abducens nerve to increased intracranial pressure, it is susceptible to infection and inflammation. Otitis media and Gradenigo's syndrome (inflammatory disease of the petrous bone) can cause sixth nerve palsy. Less commonly, migraine and diabetes mellitus are considerations in children with sixth nerve palsy. Workup includes imaging studies and neurologic examination.

B. Exotropia: Exotropia does not usually offer as many diagnostic pitfalls as esotropia. The visual axes of the two eyes are deviated in a divergent position (Figure 14–23). The deviation most often begins intermittently and is seen after age 2 years. Congenital (infantile) exotropia is extremely rare in an otherwise healthy infant. Early-onset exotropia may be seen in infants and children with severe neurologic problems. Treatment is with surgery, patching, and occasionally glasses.

Pickering JD et al: Alignment success following medial rectus recessions in normal and delayed children. J Pediatr Ophthalmol Strabismus 1995;32:225.

Shauly Y, Prager TC, Mazow ML: Clinical characteristics and long term results in infantile esotropia. Am J Ophthalmol 1994;117:183.

UNEXPLAINED DECREASED VISION IN INFANTS & CHILDREN

Some infants with delayed visual development during the first few months of life who are otherwise normal neurologically will reach an appropriate level of visual maturation.

Occult causes of poor vision and blindness in children include Leber's congenital amaurosis, a childhood form of retinitis pigmentosa; achromatopsia, the absence of cones in the retina; and optic nerve abnormalities, including optic nerve hypoplasia and atrophy as well as night blindness.

Cerebral visual impairment, also known as cortical blindness, is manifested as decreased visual attentiveness of varying degree. Cerebral visual impair-

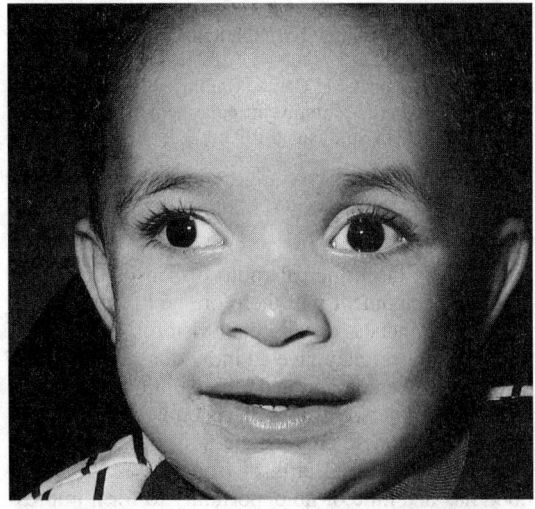

A

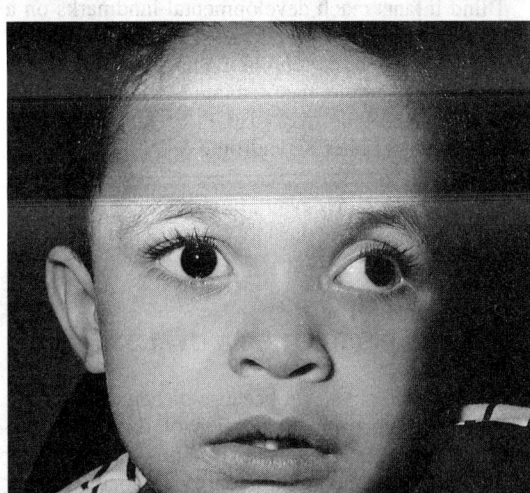

B

Figure 14–23. Exotropia. Fixation with left (*A*) and right eye (*B*).

ment can be congenital or acquired. Insults to the optic pathways and higher cortical visual centers are responsible. Asphyxia, trauma, and intracranial hemorrhage are some of the causes of cortical visual impairment.

Besides an ophthalmologic workup, electroretinography and visual evoked response testing may be required. Imaging studies of the brain and a pediatric neurologic evaluation may be useful. A low-vision assessment may be indicated. Low-vision aids enhance remaining vision. Devices used include magnifiers for both distance and near, closed-circuit television, and large-print reading materials.

Colenbrander A, Fletcher DC (guest editors): Low vision and vision rehabilitation. Ophthalmol Clin North Am 1994;27:27.

King KM, Cronin CM: Ocular findings in premature infants with grade IV intraventricular hemorrhage. J Pediatr Ophthalmol Strabismus 1993;30:84.

THE BLIND CHILD

Vision is the principal route of sensory input. A child's development will therefore be profoundly affected by blindness or very poor vision. Although acquired blindness may give an individual time to grow as a sighted person and make preparations for life as a nonsighted person if loss of vision is slow and predicted, psychologic consequences must be addressed. The child blind from birth or from very early childhood has had little or no opportunity to form impressions of the physical world with the benefit of sight.

Blind infants reach developmental landmarks on a different schedule from that of sighted children. In addition, some blind children are multiply handicapped. For example, the prematurely born child who is blind from ROP may also have cerebral palsy. Children with Usher's syndrome are both deaf and blind.

Blind children and their families should receive the benefit of knowledgeable therapists and support groups.

LEARNING DISABILITIES & DYSLEXIA

Visits to the physician because of educational difficulties are common. Evaluation of the child with learning disabilities and dyslexia should include ophthalmologic examination to identify any ocular disorders that could cause or contribute to poor school performance. Most children with learning difficulties have no demonstrable problems on ophthalmic examination.

A multidisciplinary approach as suggested by the American Academy of Pediatrics, the American Association for Pediatric Ophthalmology and Strabismus, and the American Academy of Ophthalmology is recommended in evaluating children with learning disabilities. Although many therapies directed at "training the eyes" exist, scientific support for such approaches is weak.

Menacker SJ et al: Do tinted lenses improve the reading performance of dyslexic children? A cohort study. Arch Ophthalmol 1993;111:213.

VISION SCREENING

Vision screening in the pediatric age group is a challenge, especially in younger and developmentally delayed children. Nevertheless, vision screening is consistent with the recommendations of the American Academy of Pediatrics. Early diagnosis of risk factors that should be screened for because they interfere with normal visual development and are amblyogenic include media opacities, strabismus, and both high and unequal (anisometropic) refractive errors.

The practitioner should have an understanding of the limitations of the screening test being administered. When possible, visual acuity of each eye and alignment of the two eyes should be assessed. (Acceptable acuities for different ages are set forth in the section on visual acuity.) A caveat to observe when testing monocular visual acuity is that because of the "crowding phenomenon," an amblyopic eye may score better when presented with single, isolated targets than when multiple targets on a line are presented. Preschool and young school-age children often test better when looking at a visual acuity chart at a 10-foot distance than at one placed at 20 feet or when looking into the type of machine typically used at a motor vehicles department.

When it is not possible to measure visual acuity or assess alignment in the preschool age group, random dot stereopsis testing is effective in screening for manifest strabismus and amblyopia, but this test may miss some cases of anisometropic (unequal refractive error) amblyopia and small-angle strabismus. This test is not necessarily designed to detect refractive errors.

An innovative technique that may prove useful for developmentally delayed children and perhaps infants is photoscreening or photorefraction, which evaluates the Brückner and corneal reflexes (see sections above on Alignment and Motility and on Ophthalmoscopy).

Birch E, Williams C: Random dot stereoacuity of preschool children. J Pediatr Ophthalmol Strabismus 1997;34:217.

Committee on Practice and Ambulatory Medicine and Section of Ophthalmology. Eye examination and vision screening in infants and young adults. Pediatrics 1996;98:153.

Simons K: Preschool vision screening: Rationale, methodology and outcome. Surv Ophthalmol 1996;41:3.

REFERENCES

American Academy of Ophthalmology: *Pediatric Ophthalmology and Strabismus. Basic and Clinical Science Course.* Section 6, 1996–1997.

Brodsky MC, Baker RS, Hamed LM: *Pediatric Neuro-Ophthalmology.* Springer, 1996.

Cullom RD Jr, Chang B (editors): *The Wills Eye Manual Office and Emergency Room Diagnosis and Treatment of Eye Disease,* 2nd ed. Lippincott, 1994.

Fraunfelder FT, Roy FH (editors): *Current Ocular Therapy 4.* Saunders, 1995.

Isenberg SJ (editor): *The Eye in Infancy,* 2nd ed. Mosby, 1994.

Nussenblatt RB, Whitcup SM, Palestine AG (editors): *Uveitis Fundamentals and Clinical Practice,* 2nd ed. Mosby, 1996.

Ritch R, Shields MB, Krupin T (editors): *The Glaucomas,* 2nd ed. 3 vols. Mosby, 1996.

Stewart WM (editor): *Surgery of the Eyelid, Orbit and Lacrimal System.* 3 vols. American Academy of Ophthalmology, 1993, 1994, 1995.

Tasman W, Jaeger EA (editors): *Duane's Clinical Ophthalmology.* 6 vols. Lippincott, 1994. (1995 edition on CD-ROM.)

Vaughan DG, Asbury T, Riordan-Eva P (editors): *General Ophthalmology,* 14th ed. Appleton & Lange, 1995.

Wright KW (editor): *Pediatric Ophthalmology and Strabismus.* Mosby Year Book, 1995.

15   Oral Medicine & Dentistry

William A. Mueller, DMD, & R.B. Abrams, DDS

In 1986, the American Academy of Pediatric Dentistry recommended that a child's first oral examination should be performed no later than 12 months of age. This position has remained consistent since that time. Recently, the AAPD has suggested that the infant oral health care visit should be the foundation for a lifetime of preventive education and dental care. The goal is to ensure optimal oral health through childhood and adolescence. Most oral disease in children is preventable. Oral examination, anticipatory guidance, and therapeutic intervention for the infant are essential for preventing oral disease in children.

Because of their knowledge of nursing caries and other types of caries and their familiarity with the effectiveness of sealants, fluorides, and cariology, pediatric dentists are the parents' best resource for help in rearing caries-free children, and they should be consulted before the onset of disease. Ideally, infant oral health should begin with prenatal oral health counseling. A postnatal oral evaluation should be scheduled within the first year, optimally within 6 months after eruption of the first tooth. This contact should consist of infant risk assessment and anticipatory guidance. This approach advances dental care past tooth monitoring to health promotion. In essence, the first infant oral health visit is a well child visit.

Infant risk assessment determines the danger for each child of developing oral disease. Specific examples are the child whose nursing habits increase susceptibility to nursing caries or the child in a nonfluoridated area who is at greater risk for caries. Anticipatory guidance is directed toward individualized cost-effective use of dental services. Based on the infant risk assessment, an individualized program can be fashioned for each baby.

The primary goals for an infant oral health program are as follows:

To establish with parents the goals of oral health
To inform parents of their role in reaching these goals
To motivate parents to learn and practice good preventive dental care

To initiate a long-term dental care relationship with parents

Current research is changing the traditional view of dental caries as the manifestation of caries activity (eg, "holes in the teeth"). Practitioners are now pursuing the more practical objective of diagnosing and treating the caries process itself. Viewing caries as cavitated teeth precludes this possibility. The traditional "cavity" is irreversible and requires surgical correction. "Filling cavities" does nothing to address the underlying pathologic process that caused them. Prevention, early diagnosis, and prompt intervention offer greater efficiency and better health outcomes with lower costs.

"Cariology" is the most current buzzword in pediatric dentistry. The basic tenets of this concept can be summarized as follows:

(1) Caries is the most common chronic disease of childhood.

(2) Caries is an infectious disease. It is transmissible and caused by colonization of *Streptococcus mutans.*

(3) Caries "competency" is established before age 3.

(4) Caries is a process present in all individuals. The expression of cavities is dependent upon its level of activity and the individual's resistance

(5) After establishment of *S mutans* in the oral cavity, caries is a dietary disease.

(6) Control of caries before age 3 is aimed at limiting the establishment of *S mutans* by reducing the number of episodes of direct transmission from highly infected mothers; reducing dietary support for *S mutans* (refined carbohydrate); and ensuring proper levels of fluoride exposure topically and systemically.

(7) Control of caries after age 3 is aimed at limiting the acidogenesis of oral flora by reducing the frequency of carbohydrate ingestion and maintaining a high frequency of fluoride exposures.

(8) There is a threshold of caries activity below which clinical disease does not develop.

ORAL EXAMINATION
OF THE NEWBORN & INFANT

The mouth of the normal newborn is lined with an intact, smooth, moist, and shiny mucosa. The alveolar ridges (Figure 15–1) are continuous and relatively smooth. Within the alveolar bone are numerous tooth buds which at birth are mostly primary teeth with a few permanent teeth just starting to calcify.

Teeth

The primary teeth begin to form at approximately 6 weeks of gestation, and their calcification starts in the second trimester. The permanent teeth are just beginning to develop at birth. There is enough development of permanent teeth to permit their damage by perinatal or antenatal insults such as anoxia, severe jaundice, or infection.

The primary teeth usually begin to erupt at approximately 6–7 months of age. However, on rare occasions (1:2000), teeth are present at birth (natal teeth) or erupt within the first month (neonatal teeth). These are most common in the anterior mandible and can be "real" primary teeth or supernumerary teeth. These can be differentiated radiographically. On occasion, these teeth must be removed to facilitate nursing, heal persistent ulceration of the tongue, or eliminate the risk of aspiration. Consultation with a pediatric dentist is advisable.

Frena

There should be noticeable but small maxillary and mandibular labial frena (Figure 15–2). There may also be several small accessory frena farther posteriorly. The extreme is multiple thick tightly bound frena, as in oral-facial-digital syndrome. Decisions about if and when a labial frenum should be surgically reduced are best left until adolescence. Many thick frena need not be corrected.

The tongue is connected to the floor of the mouth by the lingual frenum (Figures 15–1 and 15–3). This connection should not impede the free movement of the tongue. If the attachment is tight and high up on the alveolar ridge (Figure 15–4), it may restrict movement and cause periodontal damage. This condition is called ankyloglossia (tongue-tie). If it needs to be surgically corrected, earlier (3–4 years) is better than later, but there is usually no urgency for surgery in the neonatal period.

The Palate

The palate of the newborn should be intact and continuous from the alveolar ridge anteriorly to the uvula (Figure 15–1). Cleft lip and palate are common defects (1:700 live births). The cleft of the palate can be unilateral or bilateral (Figure 15–5). The cleft can involve just the alveolar ridge, as in Figure 15–5, or the ridge and entire palate. Clefts can also be isolated soft palate defects. This is common in the Pierre

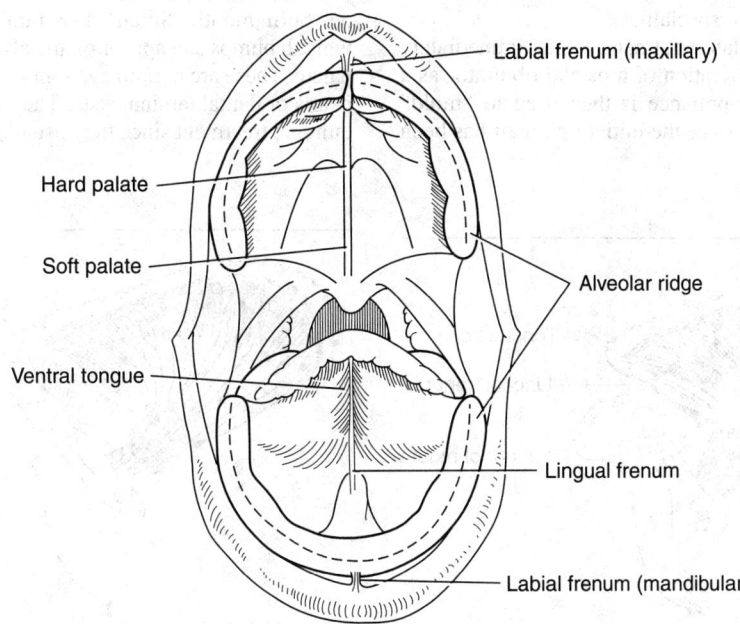

Figure 15–1. Normal anatomy of the newborn mouth.

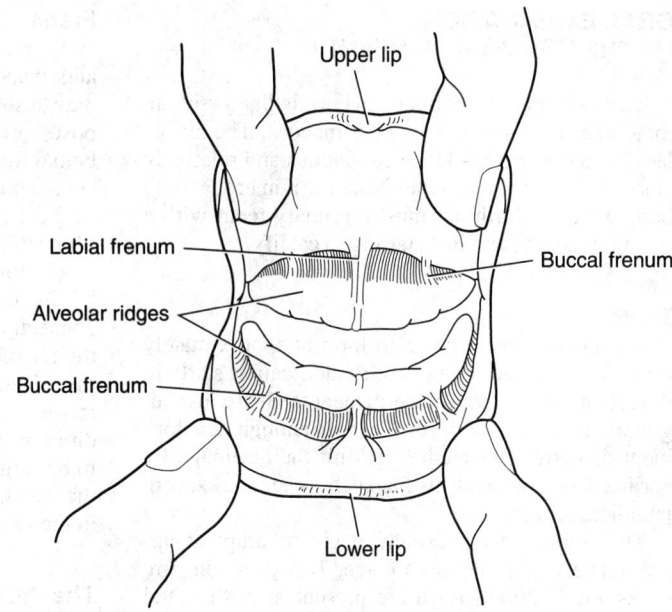

Figure 15–2. The frena.

Robin syndrome. A final classification of cleft palate is submucous cleft, which is harder to detect. This is a muscular problem in the soft palate with a notch in the bony component. Affected children sometimes have a bifid uvula.

Cleft lip and palate rehabilitation requires an extensive program involving many specialties and can be a lifelong endeavor. Owing to the complexity of the problem, children with cleft palate are best managed by a cleft palate team with coordinated care from all the relevant specialties.

Cleft lip and palate treatment begins immediately after birth with fabrication of a palatal obturator as a feeding aid. This appliance is then used to "mold" the alveolus closed once the initial lip repair has been accomplished. In the case of bilateral cleft lip and palate, the dentist will often apply extraoral orthopedic traction to guide the protruding premaxilla back into the oral cavity to facilitate surgical lip closure. Dental involvement in children with cleft palate is extensive and is coordinated by the cleft palate team.

Other Soft Tissue Variations

Other minor soft tissue variations can exist in the newborn mouth. Small (1–2 mm), round, smooth, whitish bumps can appear on the alveolar ridges or the palate. These are keratin cysts and are called Epstein's pearls or dental lamina cysts. They are benign and require no treatment since they usually disappear.

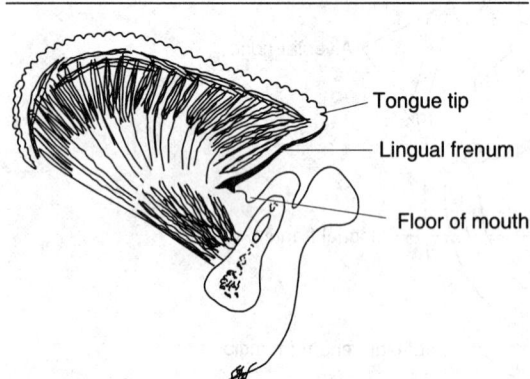

Figure 15–3. Normal position of lingual frenum.

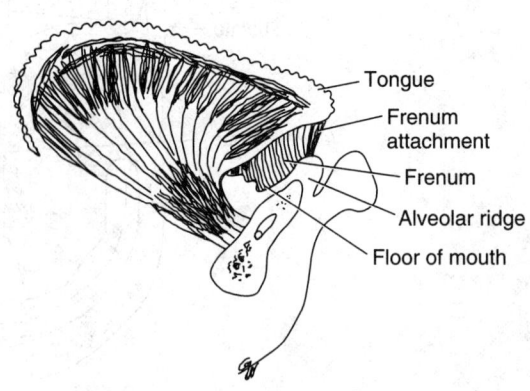

Figure 15–4. Ankyloglossia (tongue-tie).

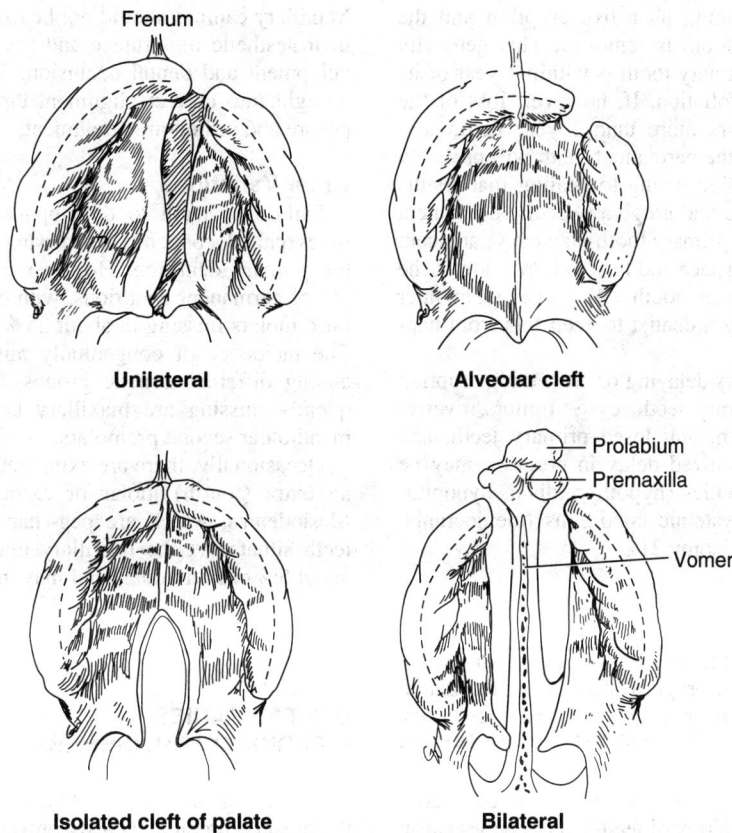

Figure 15–5. Types of clefts.

Some newborns may have small intraoral lymphangiomas on the alveolar ridge or the floor of the mouth. These and any other soft tissue variations that are more noticeable or larger than those just described should be evaluated by a dentist familiar with management of neonates.

ERUPTION OF THE TEETH

Normal Eruption

As the child grows and begins to develop teeth, problems of teething may occur. Primary teeth generally begin to erupt at about 6 months of age. They are usually mandibular incisors but can be maxillary first and appear as early as 3–4 months or as late as 12–16 months. Concerns about sequence or timing of eruption should be discussed with a dentist familiar with young children. There are many reported side effects from teething—diarrhea, drooling, fever, rash, and so on—but any real correlation is doubtful.

Common treatment for teething pain has been application of a topical anesthetic or "teething gel."

Most of these agents contain benzocaine or, less commonly, lidocaine. They can cause numbness of the entire oral cavity and pharynx, and suppression of the gag reflex can be a serious sequela. Systemic analgesia (acetaminophen or ibuprofen) is safer and more effective. Solid rubber or chilled fluid-filled teething toys are beneficial, if only for distraction purposes. Massaging the gums can be very soothing.

Occasionally, swelling of the gingiva is seen during teething. This condition can present as red to purple, round, raised, smooth lesions that may be symptomatic but usually are not. They can appear in the anterior or posterior alveolar ridge and are always on the crest. These "eruption cysts" or "eruption hematomas" are fluid-filled areas immediately overlying an erupting tooth and generally disappear spontaneously. Any decision about operative management is best left to a dental specialist.

Delayed Eruption

Premature loss of a primary tooth can cause either accelerated or delayed eruption of the underlying secondary tooth. Early eruption occurs if the permanent tooth is beginning its active eruption and the overlying primary tooth is removed. This generally occurs when the primary tooth is within 1 year of its normal time of exfoliation. If, however, loss of the primary tooth occurs more than 1 year before expected exfoliation, the permanent tooth will probably be delayed in eruption owing to healing that results in filling in of bone and gingiva over the permanent tooth. The loss of a primary tooth may cause adjacent teeth to tip into the space and lead to impaction of the underlying permanent tooth. A space maintainer should be placed by a dentist to keep this from happening.

Other local factors delaying or preventing eruption include supernumerary teeth, cysts, tumors, overretained primary teeth, ankylosed primary teeth, and impaction. A generalized delay in eruption may be due to endocrinopathies (hypothyroidism, hypopituitarism) or other systemic conditions (cleidocranial dysplasia, rickets, trisomy 21).

Ectopic Eruption

Ectopic eruption occurs when the position of an erupting tooth is abnormal. In severe instances, the order in which teeth erupt is affected. If the dental arch provides insufficient room, permanent teeth may erupt abnormally. In the mandible, lower incisors may be lingually placed to such an extent that the primary incisors do not exfoliate. The parents' concern about a "double row of teeth" may be the reason for the child's first dental visit. If the primary teeth are not loose, they may be removed by the dentist; if they are loose, they are generally allowed to exfoliate naturally. In the maxilla, inadequate room for eruption of the permanent first molar may cause abnormal resorption of the distal root structures of the second primary molar. If the problem is severe, the permanent molar may even become caught under the unresorbed enamel crown of the deciduous molar and thus require extraction of the primary tooth and orthodontic repositioning of the permanent first molar after it has erupted. If the first molar is not repositioned, the second premolar is likely to become impacted. If problems are detected early, the dentist may be able to redirect the permanent molar's eruption pathway so that it erupts correctly and the second primary molar is not lost.

Impaction

Impaction occurs when a tooth is prevented from erupting for any reason. The teeth most often affected are the third molars ("wisdom teeth") and the maxillary canines. Because patients with impacted third molars are at risk for developing ameloblastomas or dentigerous cysts, if these teeth are not surgically removed, the impacted third molar (along with its opposing third molar) should be removed after it has been determined that eruption cannot occur. This decision may not be possible until the late teens.

Maxillary canines should not be extracted because of their aesthetic importance and key role in facial development and dental occlusion. They can often be brought into correct alignment through surgical exposure and orthodontic treatment.

Other Variations

Failure of teeth to develop—a condition sometimes called congenitally missing teeth—is rare in the primary dentition. However, it occurs in about 5% of permanent dentitions, with one or more of the third molars missing in about 25% of all individuals. The incidence of congenitally missing teeth varies among different genetic groups, but the most frequently missing are maxillary lateral incisors and mandibular second premolars.

Occasionally, there are extra teeth—most typically an extra (fourth) molar or extra (third) bicuspid. Mesiodentes, which are peg-shaped supernumerary teeth situated at the maxillary midline, are seen in about 5% of individuals and may interfere with eruption of permanent incisors. Mesiodentes should be considered for removal even if they do not erupt.

DENTAL CARIES & PERIODONTAL DISEASE

Dental caries and periodontal disease are among the most common and easily preventable of all infectious diseases. Oral hygiene for the infant should start at birth. The gums can be gently cleaned with a moist soft cloth. Once the teeth begin to erupt, oral hygiene must be practiced in earnest. Again, a soft moist cloth can be used after feeding to gently rub the teeth. A very small, very soft toothbrush can be used as well. Toothpaste at the start is not necessary.

Figure 15–6 demonstrates the conditions that must be met for onset of dental caries. Once teeth are present, they can be attacked by acidogenic bacteria, especially *S mutans*. Dental plaque accumulates on the surface of the teeth as an adherent film. As plaque grows, bacteria accumulate within it in close proximity to the tooth. The third necessary ingredient is a substrate for the bacteria. In the case of dental caries, carbohydrate—especially refined carbohydrates such as sucrose—is the most active in that the bacteria metabolize sucrose and produce acid as a by-product. The acidic environment causes the enamel of the teeth to dissolve, which is the beginning of caries. After the decay process has penetrated the enamel, there is very little to keep it from affecting the vital tissues (nerve) of the tooth. The tooth subsequently becomes necrotic, and an abscess occurs (Figure 15–7). This process is not always symptomatic, but it can lead to severe pain, fever, and swelling.

In the early stages of decay, the tooth may be sensitive to temperature changes or especially sweets. At this point, the tooth can be repaired by removing the

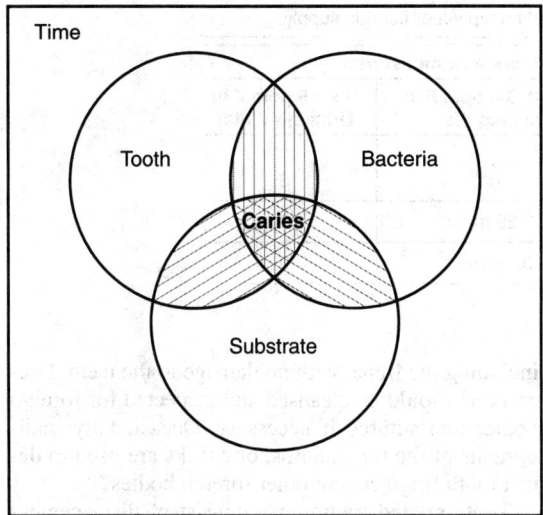

Figure 15–6. Conditions necessary for caries.

caries and "filling" the defect. As the decay progresses, more pain may be involved, and root canal therapy is usually necessary. Once an abscess has formed, with or without swelling, a choice must be made between root canal therapy and removal of the tooth. In the presence of cellulitis or facial space abscess, extraction is usually the treatment of choice.

Many people question the importance of the primary dentition. Baby teeth allow the child to eat properly, speak properly, have a good self-image, and preserve the space for the permanent dentition. Premature loss of primary teeth can cause major orthodontic and dental growth and development problems.

Preventing Dental Caries

To prevent dental caries, it is necessary to remove the bacteria on a regular basis. Brushing with a fluoride-containing toothpaste and flossing the teeth regularly (at least twice daily) will minimize the oral flora. A second step is to decrease the amount of substrate available to the bacteria. Limiting or eliminating refined carbohydrate is very effective (low-sugar diets), as is limiting exposures to refined carbohydrates, since each exposure produces an acidic environment for up to 30 minutes. The form of the substrate is important also. Caramels, licorice, raisins, gummy bears, and so on are concentrated sugar and because of their sticky texture will remain on the teeth much longer than the same sugar in liquid form. The primary care physician can play an invaluable role in disseminating this information and reinforcing these ideas.

Fluoride

Systemic fluoride, whether from water fluoridation or dietary supplementation, is incorporated into the crystalline structure of the enamel and creates a stronger, more acid-resistant covering. Topically applied fluoride is important in interfering with the metabolism of the oral flora and especially in remineralizing early carious lesions. Table 15–1 sets forth the current systemic fluoride dose recommended by the American Academy of Pediatrics and the American Academy of Pediatric Dentistry. It is important not to exceed these recommendations since doing so may lead to fluorosis, which is unsightly staining of the permanent teeth.

Daily topical fluoride therapy is used in addition to all other oral hygiene measures in certain high-risk children. Children allowed to take their bottle to bed and those who nurse at will and fall asleep nursing are at risk for nursing caries. This particular type of decay involves mostly the maxillary incisors. When a child is lying in bed sucking on a bottle, the contents of the bottle are "trapped" between the backs of the front teeth and the tongue. This allows for more concentrated damage to the teeth as the acid produced by bacteria fails to dissipate. In addition, as the child

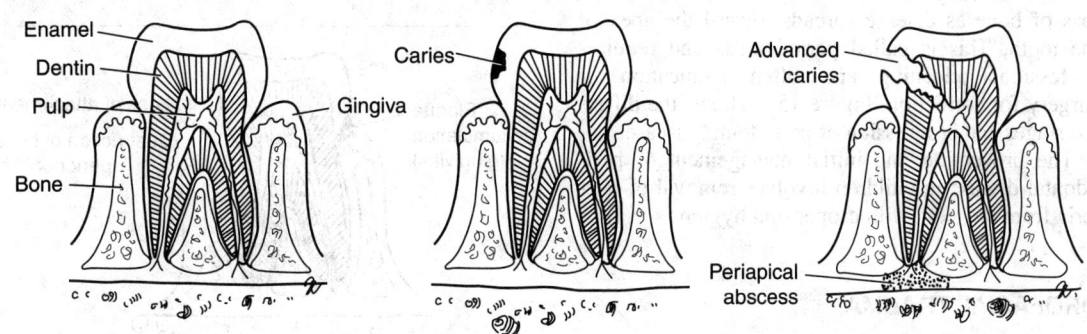

Figure 15–7. Tooth anatomy and progression of caries.

Table 15–1. Fluoride dosages based on tap water fluoride supply.

Age (years)	Dose of Fluoride Administered		
	If < 0.3 ppm F in Drinking Water	If 0.3–0.6 ppm F in Drinking Water	If > 0.6 ppm F in Drinking Water
6 months to 3 years	0.25 mg/d	0	0
3–6 years	0.5 mg/d	0.25 mg/d	0
6–16 years	1 mg/d	0.5 mg/d	0

falls asleep, salivary function decreases dramatically. This further endangers the teeth by eliminating the buffering capacity of saliva and its remineralizing potential. Topical fluoride may slow the decay process. In combination with eliminating high-risk nursing practices and instituting good oral hygiene, these infants may avoid serious dental problems.

Patients with chronically low oral pH may benefit from daily topical fluoride. This patient group includes those with gastroesophageal reflux, bulimia, or salivary dysfunction from radiation, graft-versus-host disease, or autoimmune disease. Saliva is the most effective oral cavity buffer there is. It also helps remineralize minor enamel dissolution. Xerostomia can lead to rampant caries. These children must have dental care more frequently than healthy children. Multiply handicapped children who cannot maintain proper oral hygiene can also benefit from additional topical fluoride. Any child with a serious medical problem or disability should be referred to a pediatric dentist as early as possible.

Periodontal Disease

Periodontal disease is a problem with the supporting structures: bone, gums, and ligaments. It begins as inflammation of the gum tissue adjacent to the tooth. Bacterial accumulation in the space between the tooth and gum (gingival sulcus) causes irritation that leads to inflamed tissue. This beginning phase is called gingivitis. As the inflammation spreads through the sulcus, there is more soft tissue involvement. Eventually, there is soft tissue destruction and loss of bone as disease spreads toward the apex of the tooth. This is called periodontitis and requires professional cleaning and often medication or surgery for correction. Figure 15–8 shows the different stages and progression of periodontal disease.

The prevention and initial management of periodontal disease in children involves removal of bacteria from the teeth with proper oral hygiene.

OROFACIAL TRAUMA

Orofacial trauma often consists only of abrasions or lacerations of the lips, gingiva, tongue, or mucosa, including the frena, with no damage to the teeth. Lacerations should be cleansed and inspected for foreign bodies and sutured if necessary. Occasionally, radiographs of the tongue, lips, or cheeks are used to detect tooth fragments or other foreign bodies.

Tooth-related trauma can consist of displacement (luxation), fracture, or loss of teeth (avulsion). Figure 15–9 demonstrates the different luxation injuries, and Figure 15–10 shows the different degrees of tooth fracture.

The most innocent luxation injury is mobility without displacement (subluxation). Unless mobility is extensive, this condition can be followed without active intervention. An intrusive luxation in the primary dentition is usually observed for a period of time to discern whether the tooth or teeth will reerupt (Figure 15–9). If this has not occurred after several months or if the area becomes infected, the teeth are usually removed. There is a chance of damage to permanent teeth with any intrusive injury of primary teeth. Permanent teeth intrusions are corrected with surgical or orthodontic repositioning of teeth and placement of a splint for 10–14 days. Root canal treatment may be necessary later. Lateral and extrusive luxations of permanent teeth are generally repositioned and splinted. Severe luxations in any direction in primary teeth are treated with extraction.

Avulsed primary dentition is not replanted. The area is investigated for fractured roots or foreign

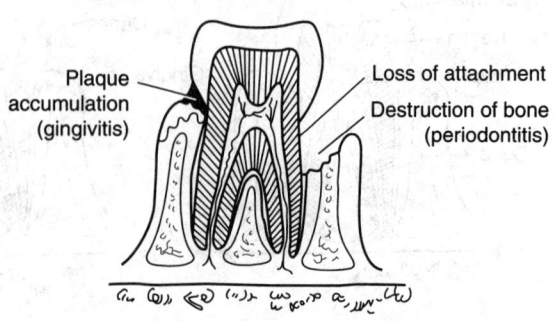

Figure 15–8. Periodontal disease.

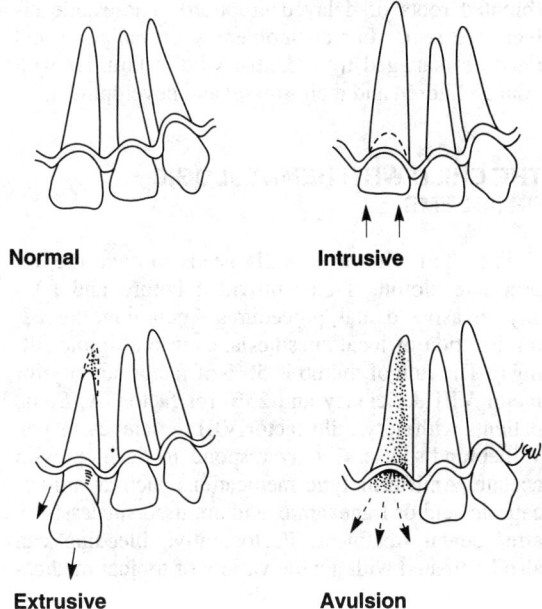

Figure 15–9. Patterns of luxation injuries.

bodies. Avulsed permanent teeth are gently cleansed and replanted with splinting. If replaced into the alveolar bone within 1 hour, these teeth have a good prognosis. The prognosis worsens rapidly with increased time outside of the mouth. Hank's solution is the best storage and transport medium for avulsed teeth that will be replanted. Milk, water, saline, or saliva can be used if Hank's solution is not accessible.

All luxated and replanted teeth need to be followed carefully and regularly by a dentist. These teeth can become abscessed or fused to the bone (ankylosed) at any time during the healing process.

A patient with fractured teeth should be seen promptly by a dentist. Fractured teeth often need to be protected quickly to avoid sensitivity, pain, or in-

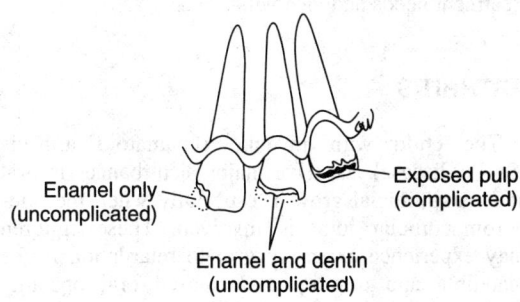

Figure 15–10. Patterns of crown fractures.

fection of exposed pulp. If the fracture is severe enough, it may require immediate root canal surgery.

All facial trauma needs to be evaluated for jaw fracture. Blows to the chin are among the most common childhood orofacial traumas. They are also a leading cause of condylar fracture in the pediatric population. One should be suspicious of pain or deviation when the jaw is opened.

DENTAL EMERGENCIES

Dental emergencies other than trauma usually present as pain or swelling due to advanced caries. Odontogenic pain usually responds to acetaminophen, ibuprofen, codeine, or, in severe cases, hydrocodone. As with teething, topical application of medicaments is of limited value.

Swelling confined to the gum tissue above or below the tooth is usually not an urgent situation. This "gumboil" or parulis represents infection that has spread outward from the root of the tooth through the bone and periosteum into the gum. Usually it will begin to drain and leave a fistulous tract. If the infection invades the facial spaces, cellulitis can occur. Swelling of the mid face—especially the bridge of the nose and the lower eyelid—is an urgent situation. All facial swelling needs to be evaluated by a dentist. Extraction of teeth or root canal therapy combined with antibiotics is the usual treatment. With extensive facial cellulitis, many young children require hospitalization and intravenous antibiotics.

ANTIBIOTICS IN PEDIATRIC DENTISTRY

The antibiotics of choice for odontogenic infection are amoxicillin and clindamycin.

Several patient groups require prophylactic antibiotic coverage prior to any invasive dental manipulation, including tooth cleaning. Cardiovascular patients at risk for subacute infective endocarditis are at the top of this list. The American Heart Association has made specific recommendations for premedication of cardiac patients. Immunosuppressed patients (oncology, HIV, posttransplant) also require coverage, as do children with indwelling central venous catheters. Patients with Broviac, Quinton, Hickman, etc, lines are routinely medicated prior to invasive dental treatment even though there are no reported dental-related catheter infections.

Children with a ventriculoperitoneal shunt should not receive prophylaxis because there is no circulatory connection to such a shunt and therefore no danger from bacteremia.

All of these children needing prophylaxis are premedicated using current American Heart Association guidelines.

THE PEDIATRIC ONCOLOGY PATIENT

The child with cancer should be evaluated by a dentist knowledgeable about pediatric oncology as soon after diagnosis as possible. The aim of the consultation is to eliminate all existing and potential sources of infection before the child receives chemotherapy and must undergo periods of significant neutropenia. Once chemotherapy begins, there is a brief interval before "counts" reach their nadir (7–10 days). Areas of concern to the dentist include abscessed teeth, teeth with extensive caries, teeth that will soon exfoliate, ragged or broken teeth or fillings, and orthodontic appliances. Once the child becomes neutropenic, abscessed, infected, or severely carious teeth can no longer be considered innocent even if asymptomatic. A loose tooth that will soon exfoliate can become a nidus for infection as well as a cause of bleeding if the patient becomes profoundly thrombocytopenic. Sharp, ragged teeth can be a source of irritation that can lead to infection. Chemotherapeutic drugs are cytotoxic to the oral mucosa. The oral mucosa becomes atrophic and ulcerates with ease (mucositis). This is painful and often leads to inadequate oral intake and nutrition. Once the mucosal barrier is breached by ulceration, the patient can become septic, especially with alpha-hemolytic streptococci and other mouth flora. Friction and damage to mucosa is the main concern with braces. Therefore, all orthodontic hardware is removed prior to chemotherapy.

The pediatric oncology patient should be monitored throughout cancer therapy to screen for infection, manage oral bleeding, and control oral pain. These children can experience spontaneous oral hemorrhaging, especially when platelet counts are below 20,000/μL. Poor oral hygiene or areas of irritation can increase the chances of bleeding.

Children receiving radiation therapy to the head and neck are prone to develop extensive salivary dysfunction (xerostomia) when salivary tissue is in the path of the primary beam of radiation. This should be managed aggressively to avoid rapid extensive destruction of dentition. Customized fluoride applicators are used in this situation combined with close follow-up.

Children undergoing bone marrow transplantation must be similarly screened. They may develop oral morbidity from an acute graft-versus-host reaction while they are in isolation before their marrow has become reconstituted. Long-term follow-up includes monitoring of growth, managing salivary dysfunction from total body radiation, and treatment of oral graft-versus-host disease.

The pediatric oncology patient also needs to be followed carefully after completion of therapy to manage oral and maxillofacial growth disturbances. Late effects of therapy include morphologic changes in tooth development (microdontia or extensive hypocalcification) and disturbances in eruption (blunted roots or delayed eruption). These side effects are seen after chemotherapy or radiation and must be managed by a dentist who is familiar with young children and their growth and development.

THE CHILD WITH HEMATOLOGIC PROBLEMS

The child with hemophilia needs to have the appropriate clotting factor provided before and after any invasive dental procedures (including the administration of local anesthesia, even for simple fillings). The rule of thumb is 50% of factor activity for factor VIII deficiency and 25% for factor IX. Some patients with very mild factor VIII deficiency or von Willebrand's disease may respond to desmopressin acetate. Antifibrinolytic medications such as aminocaproic acid or tranexamic acid are used successfully after dental treatment. Postoperative bleeding can also be treated with a wide variety of topical medications such as Gelfoam and thrombin.

The pediatric patient receiving anticoagulant therapy must undergo dosage adjustment before invasive dental treatment. This is a relatively simple matter when dealing with heparin, with its short half-life of 4–6 hours. It is a much more difficult problem with warfarin, which has a half-life of 40–70 hours.

DIABETIC PATIENTS

Children who are insulin-dependent are prone to dental problems. The diabetic child has an impaired capacity to heal, a higher incidence of periodontal disease, and a higher caries rate. These children need to be followed carefully on a routine basis. Care must be taken not to disturb the regular cycle of eating and insulin dosage. Anxiety associated with dental appointments can cause a major upset in the diabetic child's routine. Postoperative pain or pain from dental abscess can cause patients not to eat. Warnings about eating until the numbness wears off or until the filling gets hard can also create imbalances in the patient's normal schedule of food intake and insulin dosage. Insulin levels must be adjusted to conform to treatment needs and vice versa.

ARTHRITIS

The child with juvenile rheumatoid arthritis (Still's disease) can have major disturbances in oral and maxillofacial growth, especially when the temporomandibular joint is involved. These children may experience extensive growth retardation in the mandible and develop a decreased oral opening. Dental care can be very difficult to deliver. The arthritic child's medication regimen must also be considered prior to invasive dental treatment. Methotrexate (because of immune suppression) and aspirin and nonsteroidal anti-inflammatory agents (because of their antiplatelet effects) are of concern to the dental practitioner.

RENAL DISEASE

The pediatric patient with chronic renal disease usually has a greatly decreased incidence of dental caries. This is presumably due to increased salivary urea concentration. There is, however, an increased incidence of enamel hypoplasia and xerostomia. Uremic stomatitis was once a common finding in renal disease, but no longer. Oral ecchymosis and petechiae are common. The renal transplant child must be managed in light of its immunosuppressed status and should be monitored for complications secondary to immunosuppression.

REACTIVE AIRWAY DISEASE

The child with severe reactive airway disease can be a management problem for the dental practitioner.

Managing behavior and medications are the two major concerns. The stress of an invasive dental procedure can trigger a reactive airway episode. The patient receiving multiple medications, including corticosteroids, must be carefully managed through the stressful experience.

DENTAL REFERRAL

Referral to a dentist is appropriate whenever there is a question about a child's oral and maxillofacial health and development. Most pediatric dentists will want to see a child for a first visit by 12 months of age. The average child should be seen every 6 months for dental follow-up. This recommendation changes for any child with additional risk factors as described in this chapter—they should be seen earlier and more frequently.

Close cooperation between physicians and dentists can lead to improved outcomes for both the well child and the medically compromised child. Early intervention in the dental disease process will result in reduced morbidity and healthier children.

REFERENCES

Caulfield P, Cutter G, Dasanayake A: Acquisition of mutans streptococci by infants; Evidence of a discrete window of infectivity. J Dent Res 1993;72:37.

Krasner K, Rankou H: New philosophy for the treatment of avulsed teeth. Oral Surg Med Pathol 1995;79:616.

Mueller W: When baby teeth decay. Contemp Pediatr 1993;10:75.

Nowak A: What pediatricians can do to promote oral health. Contemp Pediatr 1993;10:90.

Stephen Berman, MD, & Kenny Chan, MD

I. THE EAR

INFECTIONS OF THE EAR

Infections of the ear represent a spectrum of diseases involving the structures of the outer ear (otitis externa), middle ear (otitis media), mastoid (mastoiditis), and inner ear (labyrinthitis).

1. OTITIS EXTERNA

Otitis externa is inflammation of the skin lining the ear canal and surrounding soft tissue. The most common cause is loss of the protective function of cerumen, leading to maceration of the underlying skin. Other causes are trauma to the ear canal from using cotton-tipped applicators for cleaning or from poorly fitted ear plugs while swimming; contact dermatitis due to hair sprays, perfumes, or self-administered ear drops; and chronic drainage from a perforated tympanic membrane. Infections due to *Staphylococcus aureus* or *Pseudomonas aeruginosa* may also occur.

Symptoms include pain and itching in the ear, especially with chewing or pressure on the tragus. Movement of the pinna or tragus causes considerable pain. Drainage may be minimal. The ear canal may be grossly swollen, and the patient may resist any attempt to insert an ear speculum. Debris is noticeable in the canal. It is often impossible to visualize the tympanic membrane. Hearing is normal unless complete occlusion has occurred.

Treatment

Topical treatment usually suffices. The crucial initial step is removal of desquamated epithelium and moist cerumen. This debris can be irrigated out or suctioned out using warm Burow's solution (one packet of Domeboro Powder to 250 mL tap water) or

normal saline. Once the ear canal is open, instill antibiotic-corticosteroid ear drops three or four times daily. The corticosteroid is needed to reduce the inflammatory response. If the canal is too edematous to allow the ear drop to get in, an ear wick for the first few days may be helpful. Oral antibiotics are indicated if any signs of invasive infection are present, such as fever, cellulitis of the auricles, or tender postauricular lymph nodes. Prescribe an antistaphylococcal antibiotic while awaiting the results of culture of the ear canal discharge. Systemic antibiotics alone without topical treatment may not clear up otitis externa. Analgesics may be required temporarily.

During the acute phase, the patient should avoid swimming. A cotton ear plug is not helpful and may prolong the infection. Schedule a follow-up visit in 1 week to document an intact tympanic membrane. Children who have intact tympanic membranes and are predisposed to this problem should instill 2 or 3 drops of a 1:1 solution of white vinegar and 70% ethyl alcohol into the ears before and after swimming.

2. OTITIS MEDIA

Classification & Clinical Findings

Otitis media (inflammation of the middle ear) is an infection associated with middle ear effusion (a collection of fluid in the middle ear space) or otorrhea (a discharge from the ear through a perforation in the tympanic membrane or ventilating tube). Otitis media can be further classified by its associated clinical symptoms, otoscopic findings, duration, frequency, and complications into acute otitis media, otitis media with effusion (residual or persistent effusion), unresponsive acute otitis media, recurrent otitis media, otitis media with complications, and chronic suppurative otitis media.

A. Acute Otitis Media: Acute otitis media is commonly defined as inflammation of the middle ear presenting with rapid onset of symptoms such as otalgia, fever, irritability, anorexia, or vomiting. Otoscopic findings of middle ear inflammation include decreased tympanic membrane mobility, a bulging tympanic membrane with impaired visibility of the ossicular landmarks, a yellow or red color, exudate on the membrane, and bullae. In acute otitis media, symptoms are nonspecific and often result from an associated viral upper respiratory infection. Therefore, the case definition of acute otitis media may be based on otoscopic findings of inflammation regardless of other symptoms. Approximately one-third of patients with otoscopic signs of inflammation and decreased mobility do not present with fever, pain, or irritability.

B. Otitis Media With Effusion: Otitis media with effusion is defined as an asymptomatic middle ear effusion that may be associated with a "plugged ear" feeling. Findings that suggest otitis media with effusion include visualization of air-fluid levels, clear or amber middle ear fluid, and diminished membrane mobility when the membrane is translucent or transparent. The presence of an effusion is associated with either a mild or moderate conductive hearing impairment of 15 dB or higher. Otitis media with effusion can also be associated with negative middle ear pressure, which is suggested by prominence of the lateral process, shortening of the long arm of the malleus with a more horizontal orientation, and better mobility with negative compared with positive pressure.

Otitis media with residual effusion is characterized by the presence of an asymptomatic middle ear effusion without otoscopic signs of inflammation 3–16 weeks following the diagnosis of acute otitis. After 16 weeks, this condition can be considered **otitis media with persistent effusion.**

Both acute otitis media and otitis media with effusion can be associated with decreased tympanic membrane mobility, a flat type B tympanogram, and conductive hearing loss. The distinguishing characteristics from acute otitis media are the absence of symptoms and inflammation of the membrane.

C. Unresponsive Acute Otitis Media: This type is characterized by clinical signs and symptoms associated with otoscopic findings of inflammation that continue beyond 48 hours of therapy.

D. Recurrent Acute Otitis Media: Defined as three new acute otitis media episodes within 6 months or four episodes during 1 year.

E. Otitis Media With Complications: This type involves damage to the middle ear structures such as tympanosclerosis, retraction pockets, adhesions, ossicular erosion, cholesteatoma, and perforations as well as other intratemporal and intracranial complications. Tympanosclerosis is caused by chronic inflammation or trauma that produces granulation tissue and hyalinization. The appearance of a small defect in the posterosuperior area of the pars tensa or in the pars flaccida suggests a retraction pocket. Retraction pockets occur when chronic inflammation and negative pressure in the middle ear

space produce atrophy and atelectasis of the tympanic membrane.

Continued inflammation can cause adhesions between the retraction pocket and the ossicles. This condition, referred to as *adhesive otitis,* predisposes to formation of a cholesteatoma or fixation and erosion of the ossicles. Erosion of the ossicles results from osteitis and compromise of the blood supply. Ossicular discontinuity produces a hearing loss with a 25- to 50-dB threshold. A tympanogram with very high compliance indicates ossicular discontinuity. The presence of a greasy-looking mass or debris seen in a retraction pocket or perforation suggests cholesteatoma regardless of the presence of discharge. When a perforation is present, the condition is usually painless. If no infection is present, the middle ear cavity generally contains normal mucosa. If infection is superimposed, serous or purulent drainage will be seen, and the middle ear cavity may contain granulation tissue or even polyps. A conductive hearing loss is usually present depending on the size and location of the perforation. The site of perforation is important. Central perforations are usually relatively safe from cholesteatoma formation. Peripheral perforations, especially in the pars flaccida, impose a risk for development of cholesteatoma because the ear canal epithelium adjacent to the perforation may invade it.

F. Chronic Suppurative Otitis Media: This type is defined as persistent otorrhea present longer than 6 weeks. Most often it occurs in children with tympanostomy tubes or tympanic membrane perforations. Occasionally, it is an accompanying sign of cholesteatoma. Visualization of the tympanic membrane, meticulous culture of the drainage, and appropriate antimicrobial therapy are keys to management of cases not related to cholesteatoma.

Pathogenesis

The pathogenesis of otitis media can be viewed as a contest between the pathogen and the host, with many factors influencing the outcome. The pathogen's chances of winning are increased when the infecting inoculum in the middle ear space is larger and the strain of the organism has virulence factors that promote attachment to the respiratory epithelium. The chances of the host's winning are increased when immune defenses and nonimmune defenses are fully functional.

A. Colonization: The pathogen gains a major advantage when the nasopharynx becomes heavily colonized with "otitis pathogens," ie, *Streptococcus pneumoniae, Haemophilus influenzae,* or *Moraxella catarrhalis.* Colonization with these organisms increases the risk of otitis as well as recurrent episodes. Colonization with normal flora such as viridans streptococci may prevent otitis episodes by inhibiting the growth of *H influenzae* and *S pneumoniae.* In older children, xylitol chewing gum, which reduces growth of *S pneumoniae*, prevented acute otitis media. Viral upper respiratory infections increase the colonization of the nasopharynx with *H influenzae* and other otitis pathogens, perhaps because of increased adherence to mucosa. Therefore, factors that increase the frequency of viral respiratory infections, such as child care attendance, later birth order, and absence of breast feeding, promote colonization with otitis pathogens and predispose to otitis.

B. Aspiration Into the Middle Ear Space: Aspiration of nasopharyngeal secretions containing an otitis pathogen into the middle ear space is promoted by factors that increase the positive pressure in the nasopharyngeal space (eg, nasal obstruction) or negative pressure in the middle ear space (eg, auditory tube dysfunction). Concurrent viral respiratory infection or the irritation associated with passive smoking also promotes attachment of the pathogen to respiratory epithelium in the middle ear space.

C. Host Immune Defenses: The host's immune response is the most effective defense against otitis. However, this response is a double-edged sword that damages normal tissue in the process of eradicating the pathogen. Children who experience recurrent or persistent otitis may have selective impairments of immune defenses against specific otitis pathogens.

D. Breast Feeding and Exposure to Passive Smoking: Two environmental factors that influence otitis are breast feeding and exposure to passive smoke. Breast feeding reduces the incidence of acute respiratory infections, prevents colonization with otitis pathogens through selective IgA antibody, and decreases the amount of contaminated secretions aspirated into the middle ear space. Passive smoking increases the risk of persistent middle ear effusion by enhancing attachment of the pathogen, prolonging the inflammatory response, and impeding drainage through the auditory tube. For infants 12–18 months of age, each additional pack of cigarettes smoked at home is associated with an 11% increase in the duration of a middle ear effusion.

Microbiology

The relative importance of viral versus bacterial infections in otitis media is controversial. Since viruses have been isolated as the sole agent in only 6% of middle ear aspirates from patients with acute otitis media, it appears that viruses promote bacterial superinfection by impairing auditory tube function and favoring nasopharyngeal bacterial overgrowth as well as by impairing host immune and nonimmune defenses.

The most common bacterial pathogens in acute otitis media are *S pneumoniae* and nontypable *H influenzae*—the same organisms most frequently associated with sinusitis and pneumonia. Others include *M catarrhalis, S pyogenes, S aureus*, gram-negative enteric organisms, and anaerobic organisms. The microbiologic causes of acute otitis media in early infancy differ from those in later life. The risk of gram-negative enteric infection is especially high in infants under 6 weeks of age who are or have been hospitalized in a neonatal intensive care nursery. In normal infants seen during the first 3 months of life, acute otitis media is caused by *S aureus* and *Chlamydia trachomatis* as well as *S pneumoniae, H influenzae,* and *M catarrhalis.*

Aspirates of residual and persistent middle ear effusions often grow pathogenic organisms, most commonly *H influenzae, S pneumoniae, M catarrhalis,* and *S pyogenes*. Most strains of *H influenzae* and *M catarrhalis* are β-lactamase-positive. The roles of *S epidermidis* and diphtheroids are unclear.

Chronic suppurative otitis media is often caused by resistant organisms, especially *Pseudomonas, S aureus,* anaerobes, and gram-negative enteric organisms.

Resistant *S pneumoniae* is a common pathogen in acute and unresponsive otitis as well as in persistent effusions and chronic suppurative otitis, especially in patients with ventilating tubes. Children with resistant strains tend to be younger than 18 months of age and to have had more unresponsive infections. Prior antibiotic treatment appears to increase the risk of harboring resistant pathogens. Resistance develops through alteration in the structure of the penicillin-binding proteins. Strains with intermediate penicillin resistance have MICs of 0.1–1 µg/mL. Strains with MICs higher than 1 µg/mL have a high level of resistance. The prevalence of resistant strains varies considerably among geographic areas. Susceptibility patterns also vary with respect to trimethoprim-sulfamethoxazole, cephalosporins, and macrolides. Ninety to 100 percent of highly resistant strains are susceptible to clindamycin and rifampin.

Nasopharyngeal culture correctly identifies the pathogen causing acute otitis in only 30% of cases because multiple organisms are often isolated. However, the absence of a potential pathogen from a nasopharyngeal specimen rules out that organism.

Diagnosis

A. Pneumatic Otoscopy: Acute otitis media is over diagnosed. Errors in diagnosis stem from physician and parental bias in favor of treating a sick child with antibiotics, the temptation to accept the diagnosis without removing enough cerumen to adequately visualize the membrane, and the mistaken belief that a red membrane with normal mobility establishes the diagnosis. In fact, a red membrane can be caused by a viral upper respiratory infection, the child's crying, or efforts to remove cerumen. Assuming that the clinician is using a pneumatic otoscope head and has an adequate view of the membrane (Figure 16–1), the reasons why clinicians have difficulty in assessing

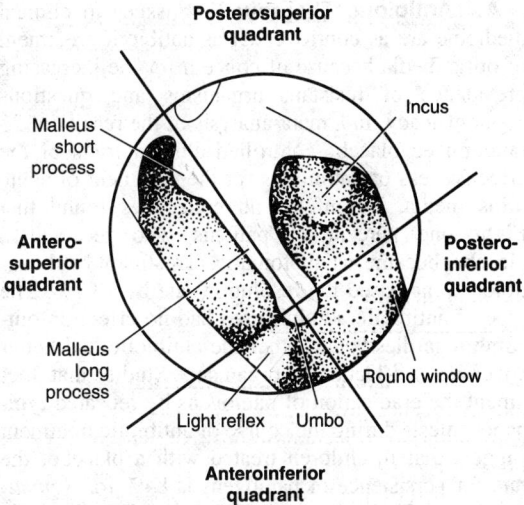

Figure 16–1. Schematic diagram of the left tympanic membrane. (Courtesy of the Department of Otolaryngology, University of Pittsburgh School of Medicine, and Eli Lilly and Co.)

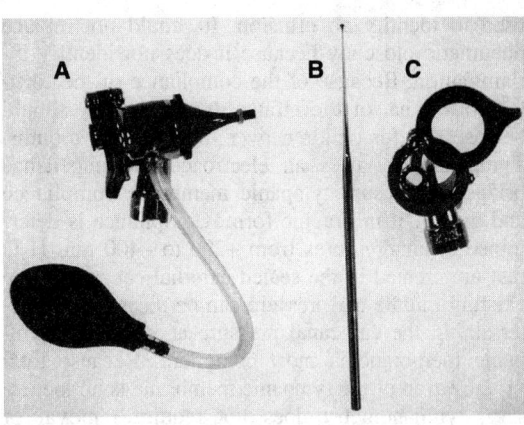

Figure 16–2. Equipment used to remove cerumen. **A:** Pneumatic otoscope with operating lens attached. **B:** Ear curette. **C:** Overlapping lateral (left) and overhead view of a pneumatic otoscope head with an additional operating lens attached.

membrane mobility include failure to achieve an adequate seal with the speculum, poor visualization due to low light intensity, and mistaking the ear canal wall for the membrane.

A pneumatic otoscope with a rubber suction bulb and tube is used to assess mobility of the tympanic membrane. The speculum inserted into the patient's ear canal must be large enough to provide an airtight seal. Placing a piece of rubber tubing 0.125–0.25 cm wide near the end of the ear speculum helps to create an adequate pneumatic seal. The tubing should be fit snugly on the speculum at a distance about 0.5 cm from its end (Figure 16–2). When the rubber bulb is squeezed, the tympanic membrane will move to and fro if no fluid is present (normal finding); if fluid is present in the middle ear space, the mobility of the tympanic membrane will be diminished. It is important to recognize that excessive pressures produced by the rubber bulb may cause mobility of an otherwise immobile tympanic membrane. The ability to assess mobility is compromised by low light intensity. Low light output is more likely due to weakness of the otoscope bulb than to battery failure.

B. Cerumen Removal: Cerumen removal is an essential skill for anyone who cares for children. Cerumen often prevents adequate visualization of the tympanic membrane. Impacted cerumen can also cause itching, pain, hearing loss, or otitis externa. Parents should be advised that earwax protects the ear (cerumen contains lysozymes and immunoglobulins that inhibit infection) and will come out by itself;

therefore, parents should never put anything into the ear canal to remove the ear wax.

Curetting of cerumen requires immobilization of the patient. The physician should remove cerumen under direct vision through the operating head of an otoscope. When an operating microscope is not available, an alternative method is to use a size 00 ear curette through a 3-mm speculum (for a 12-month-old) with a fiberoptic pneumatic otoscope head that has been modified with an additional attached operating lens as shown in Figure 16–2. Cerumen that obstructs the view of the tympanic membrane can often be pushed aside, the pneumatic seal reestablished, and mobility assessed without removing the speculum.

Irrigation can also be used to remove cerumen. Very hard cerumen may adhere to the wall of the ear canal and cause pain or bleeding if one attempts to remove it with a curette. This type of wax can be softened with Cerumenex or a few drops of detergent before irrigation is attempted. After 20 minutes, irrigation with a soft bulb syringe can be started with water warmed to 35–38 °C to prevent vertigo. A commercial jet tooth cleanser (eg, Water Pik) is also an excellent device for removing cerumen, but it is important to set it at low power (2 or less) to prevent damage to the intact tympanic membrane. A perforated tympanic membrane is a contraindication to any form of irrigation. In difficult cases, it may be necessary to use the expertise of an otolaryngologist.

C. Tympanometry: Tympanometry can be

used to identify an effusion. It should not replace pneumatic otoscopy because it does not identify inflammation. Because of the compliance of the cartilaginous canal of the infants, tympanometry should be reserved for children over the age of 6 months. Tympanometry uses an electroacoustic impedance bridge to measure tympanic membrane compliance and display it in graphic form. Compliance is determined at air pressures from +200 to –400 mm H_2O that are created in the sealed external ear canal. The existing middle ear pressure can be measured by determining the ear canal pressure at which the tympanic membrane is most compliant. Because total visualization of the tympanic membrane is not necessary, tympanometry does not require removal of cerumen unless the canal is completely blocked.

Tympanograms can be classified into three major patterns, as shown in Figure 16–3. The type A pattern, characterized by maximum compliance at normal atmospheric pressure, indicates a normal tympanic membrane, good auditory tube function, and absence of effusion. The type B pattern identifies a nonmobile tympanic membrane, which may be associated with middle ear effusion, perforation, patent ventilation tubes, or excessive and hard-packed cerumen. The type C pattern indicates an intact mobile tympanic membrane with poor auditory tube function and excessive negative pressure (> –150 mm H_2O air pressure) in the middle ear. Middle ear effusion is present in about 20% of patients with a type C pattern.

Treatment

An algorithm for the management of acute otitis media with effusion is presented in Figure 16–4. Drugs commonly used are listed in Table 16–1.

A. Antibiotic Therapy: Few issues in clinical medicine are as controversial as antibiotic treatment of otitis media because of concern for the increasing prevalence of resistant organisms and questions about efficacy. In a meta-analysis of the results of 33 randomized placebo-controlled clinical trials of the effectiveness of antibiotics for the treatment of acute otitis media, Rosenfeld and colleagues found that Eighty-one percent of patients who received a placebo became asymptomatic. Treatment with antibiotics increased the resolution rate by 13.7%. The type of antibiotic administered had no effect on outcome regardless of whether the antibiotic had better coverage of β-lactamase organisms. Studies that document the eradication of pathogens by repeated tympanocentesis during the course of antibiotic treatment suggest that in children treated with a placebo, the rate for persistence of pathogens is 84% for *S pneumoniae,* 64% for *M catarrhalis,* and 52% for nontypable *H influenzae.* While the clinical and bacteriologic success rates are significantly associated, the correlation is not good. For example, in cases where bacteriologic failure has been documented, 67% of the patients appeared to improve clinically. Conversely, in 32% of patients who did not appear to improve clinically, eradication of pathogens was demonstrated. The conclusion is that a child's clinical response may be influenced more by the course of the associated viral upper respiratory infection than by resolution of the acute otitis media. Persistence of symptoms without progression of otoscopic findings should not always indicate the need to switch antibiotics.

Although most clinicians routinely treat acute otitis with antibiotics, it is also reasonable to individualize this decision and involve the family in the

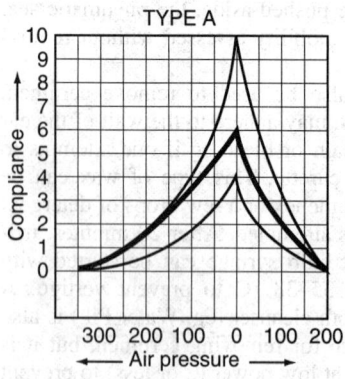 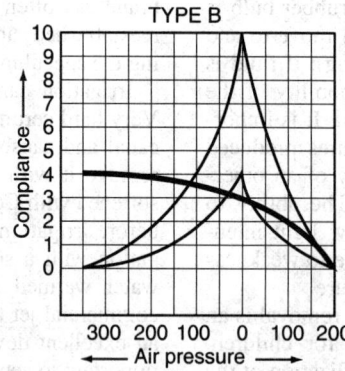 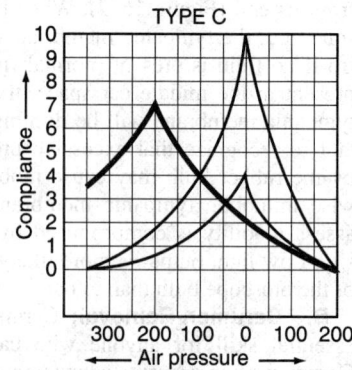

Figure 16–3. Type A tympanograms are characterized by maximum compliance at normal atmospheric pressure (0 mm H_2O air pressure). Type B tympanograms show little or no change in compliance of the tympanic membrane as air pressure in the external ear canal is varied. Type C tympanograms show near-normal compliance with significant negative middle ear pressures (typically more severe than –150 mm H_2O). (Reproduced, with permission, from Northern JL: Advanced techniques for measuring middle ear function. Pediatrics 1978;61:761.)

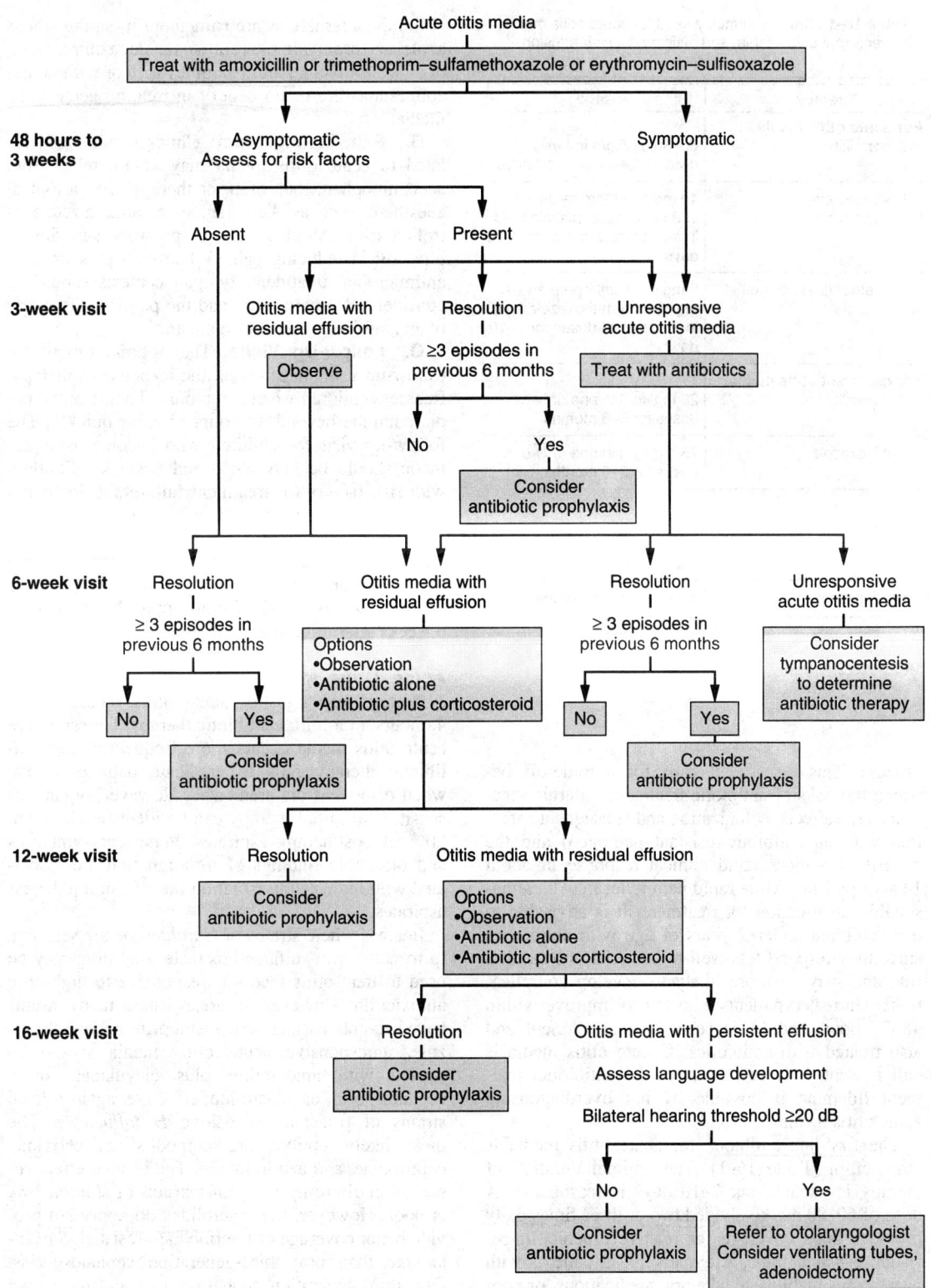

Figure 16–4. An algorithm for the management of otitis media. For prophylaxis in children with recurrent acute otitis media, see text. (From Berman S: Otitis media in children. N Engl J Med 1995;332:1561.)

Table 16–1. Drugs commonly used for acute otitis media, recurrent otitis media, and otitis media with effusion in children.[1]

Therapy	Dosage
For acute otitis media	
Amoxicillin	60–80 mg/kg/d in three divided doses for 7–10 days
Erythromycin-sulfisoxazole	40 mg of erythromycin and 150 mg of sulfisoxazole/kg/d in four divided doses for 7–10 days
Trimethoprim-sulfamethoxazole	8 mg of trimethoprim and 40 mg of sulfamethoxazole/kg/d in two divided doses for 7–10 days
For recurrent otitis media	
Amoxicillin	20 mg/kg/d in one or two doses for 3–6 months
Sulfisoxazole	75 mg/kg/d in one or two doses for 3–6 months
For otitis media with effusion	
Antibiotic agent	Give as for acute otitis media, but for 10–14 days
Prednisone or prednisolone	1 mg/kg/d in two divided doses for 7 days

[1]Adapted from Berman S: Otitis media in children. N Engl J Med 1995;332:1560.

process. This assessment calls for a trade-off between the risks of antibiotic treatment (allergic reactions, side effects, colonization and subsequent infection with an antibiotic-resistant pathogen) and the benefit of a more rapid clinical response in about 14% of patients. More rapid pain relief may be a reasonable justification for treatment. It is advisable to treat children under 2 years of age with antibiotics since they respond less well to bacterial polysaccharide and may be more likely to develop complications. Untreated patients who fail to improve within 48–72 hours should be seen for reassessment and also treated with antibiotics if acute otitis media is still present. It is best to avoid the antibiotic treatment dilemma if possible by not overdiagnosing acute otitis media.

The first-line antibiotic for acute otitis media is amoxicillin (Table 16–1). The optimal duration of therapy is unclear, but 7–10 days is reasonable. A dose of 60–80 mg/kg divided two or three times daily provides good coverage for relatively penicillin-resistant S pneumoniae. Alternatively, in patients with bacteremia, inability to take oral medications, or poor compliance, intramuscular ceftriaxone or procaine penicillin can be used. Procaine penicillin is similar to amoxicillin in its coverage of non-β-lactamase-producing H influenzae. In patients allergic to penicillin, the alternatives are trimethoprim-sulfamethoxazole, erythromycin plus sulfisoxazole, azithromycin, or clarithromycin. Antihistamines with or without decongestants are of no benefit in treating acute otitis media.

B. Pain Management: Children with pain related to acute otitis media may obtain relief from acetaminophen, ibuprofen, or therapy with a topical anesthetic such as Auralgan. In a randomized controlled trial, Auralgan ear drops were superior to olive oil in reducing pain. When pain persists after antimicrobial treatment, tympanocentesis should be considered for pain relief and the possible discovery of an antibiotic-resistant organism.

C. Follow-Up Visits: The optimal timing for follow-up visits depends on the response to therapy. Reassess children when symptoms of acute otitis media continue beyond 48 hours or recur quickly. The follow-up visit for children who become asymptomatic should be between 3 and 6 weeks. Children with risk factors for treatment failure should be examined 3 weeks after start of therapy. Risk factors include age under 15 months, a history of recurrent otitis media, or antibiotic-treated otitis media within the prior month. Follow-up visits for asymptomatic children without risk factors may be scheduled 6 weeks after initiating treatment.

D. Antibiotic Therapy for Unresponsive Acute Otitis Media: In about 10% of children, symptoms and signs of acute otitis media persist 48 hours after initial antibiotic therapy. Unresponsive acute otitis media occurs more frequently when antibiotic therapy fails to eradicate pathogens than when pathogens are eradicated. However, organisms sensitive to initial therapy can be identified in about 20% of posttherapy aspirates. Persistent symptoms and otoscopic findings of inflammation are associated with higher viral isolation rates from middle ear aspirates.

In areas where strains of H influenzae are sensitive to trimethoprim-sulfamethoxazole, that drug may be used to treat otitis media unresponsive to high-dose amoxicillin. However, in areas where many strains have become resistant to trimethoprim-sulfamethoxazole, unresponsive acute otitis media should be treated with amoxicillin plus clavulanate or a cephalosporin or macrolide effective against local strains of β-lactamase-positive H influenzae. The most likely options are cefpodoxime, cefixime, cefuroxime, and azithromycin. The in vivo effectiveness of clarithromycin against strains of H influenzae is poor. However, the macrolides do appear to provide better coverage of intermediate-resistant S pneumoniae than oral third-generation cephalosporins. Oral third-generation cephalosporins and the newer macrolides may provide improved coverage of S pneumoniae with intermediate resistance, but with the exception of ceftriaxone they offer minimal advantage in highly resistant strains. If unresponsive acute otitis media persists after a second course of antibiotics, consider ceftriaxone or myringotomy tympanocentesis, or both, in order to isolate the pathogen and drain the effusion.

E. Tympanocentesis or Myringotomy: Tympanocentesis is performed by placing a needle through the tympanic membrane and aspirating the middle ear fluid. Myringotomy involves making an incision in the drum with a myringotomy knife to drain the fluid. Indications for tympanocentesis or myringotomy are (1) acute otitis media in a hospitalized newborn, because the pathogens may be gramnegative; (2) acute otitis media in a patient with compromised host resistance, because the organism may be unusual; (3) painful bullae of the tympanic membrane; (4) a complete workup for presumed sepsis or meningitis; (5) unresponsive otitis media despite courses of two different antibiotics; and (6) acute mastoiditis.

The technique of tympanocentesis is as follows.

1. Premedication—In the conditions mentioned, the pain associated with tympanocentesis is only slightly greater than the pain that already exists from acute inflammation of the tympanic membrane. Therefore, no premedication is generally indicated. The patient who is extremely difficult to hold may be premedicated with meperidine, 1 mg/kg intramuscularly.

2. Restraint—The patient must be completely immobile while the incision is being made. A papoose board or a sheet can be used to immobilize the body. An extra attendant is required to hold the head steady.

3. Site selection—With an open-headed operating otoscope, the operator carefully selects a target. This is generally in the posteroinferior quadrant. This site prevents disruption of the ossicles during the procedure.

4. Aspiration—An 8.8 cm spinal needle (No. 18 or No. 20) with a short bevel is attached to a 1-mL syringe. The plunger is removed from the syringe, and a suction tube is placed over the syringe opening. The spinal needle is bent at a slight angle so that its end is out of the operator's line of vision. The operator moves the needle toward the posteroinferior quadrant, inserting it through the tympanic membrane, and aspirates the middle ear effusion into the syringe. Aspirate should be directly placed onto culture plates for maximum recovery.

F. Management of Recurrent Otitis: The decision to administer antibiotic prophylaxis to children who have experienced three documented episodes of acute otitis media in a 6-month period should be individualized and the risks and benefits reviewed with the parents. Antibiotic prophylaxis is as effective as ventilating tubes at preventing new otitis episodes. However, neither intervention appears to make a major clinical difference with respect to a placebo. Antibiotic prophylaxis is marginally effective in reducing the frequency of otitis episodes. A meta-analysis of nine randomized controlled trials with 958 subjects compared the difference in the rate of occurrence of acute otitis media per patient month while receiving antibiotic prophylaxis with that of placebo controls. Although antibiotic prophylaxis reduced the otitis rate by 44%, patients receiving antibiotics had only one fewer infection per year than the controls. These studies were carried out before the emergence of *S pneumoniae* resistant to penicillin and *H influenzae* resistant to trimethoprim-sulfamethoxazole. In areas with high prevalence of penicillin-resistant *S pneumoniae* and β-lactamase-positive *H influenzae,* amoxicillin prophylaxis does not appear to be effective. While the risk of acquiring resistant *S pneumoniae* while on prophylaxis appears to be increased, the sequelae of acquisition are not clear. Giving antibiotics at the onset of upper respiratory infection symptoms for 7–10 days rather than daily continuous therapy may be less likely to promote colonization with resistant *S pneumoniae* and may be as effective as continuous therapy.

Another approach to preventing recurrent otitis is active immunization. Clinical trials of the conjugate pneumococcal vaccine are under way. Consider immunizing children with recurrent otitis with influenza vaccine and in children older than 2 years with the 23-valent pneumococcal vaccine (Pneumovax).

Surgical options for the treatment of recurrent otitis media include tympanostomy with tube placement and adenoidectomy. One should consider referring children who have had five or more episodes of acute otitis media within 12 months for ventilating tubes. The decision to insert tubes should not be based solely on parental recall of the number of episodes. The benefit of ventilating tubes in preventing new infections is similar to that of antibiotic prophylaxis. However, the duration of each episode is markedly shortened. The benefit of adenoidectomy in preventing acute otitis has not been well documented, but there is evidence that some children with recurrent otitis have chronic adenoid infection.

G. Management of Otitis Media With Residual and Persistent Effusions: The main reason to treat otitis media with effusion is to avoid the adverse effect of prolonged conductive hearing impairment on language development and academic functioning. Although the available data document a causal relationship between severe congenital or acquired hearing loss (usually sensorineural) and language development, the data fail to establish a causal relationship between conductive hearing loss associated with otitis media and subsequent hearing-related developmental delays.

Residual middle ear effusions are part of the resolution continuum of acute otitis media, irrespective of antibiotic therapy. For example, about two-thirds of children with acute otitis media have a middle ear effusion or high negative middle ear pressure 1 month after diagnosis regardless of antibiotic ther-apy. The management options for otitis media with residual effusion for 6 weeks to 4 months include ob-servation, antibiotics alone, and combination antibi-otic and corticosteroid therapy. If combination ther-apy is selected, corticosteroid (prednisone) can be administered for 7 days combined with an antibiotic for 10–14 days. Unvaccinated children with no clear history of varicella who have been exposed in the preceding month should not receive prednisone be-cause of the potential risk of disseminated disease. Prednisone side effects are similar to those noted in treating asthmatic episodes with short corticosteroid courses: increased appetite, fluid retention, occa-sional vomiting, and, in rare cases, marked behav-ioral changes. If the patient clears the persistent mid-dle ear effusion unilaterally or bilaterally, follow the patient monthly and consider administering low-dose intermittent antibiotic prophylaxis with amoxicillin, 20 mg/kg/d, once or twice daily, or sulfisoxazole, 75 mg/kg/d, once or twice daily, for colds during the subsequent 3 months to prevent recurrence of otitis media.

The guideline recommendation developed by the Agency for Health Care Policy and Research for the management of otitis media with effusion is that ven-tilating tubes should be placed after the effusion has persisted for 4 months and is accompanied by a bilat-eral hearing impairment of 20 dB or greater. Earlier placement of ventilating tubes should depend on the child's developmental and behavioral status as well as on parental preference. The value of ventilating tubes for treating unilateral effusions in otherwise normal children is unclear.

In children who have otitis media with persistent effusion there is a higher than normal reported inci-dence of abnormalities such as cholesteatoma, adhe-sive otitis, retraction pockets, membrane atrophy, and persistent membrane perforation. However, the clini-cal usefulness of this association is limited, since there is no way to identify the small proportion of candidate children who will sustain damage to the middle ear and for whom insertion of ventilating tubes will prevent the damage.

H. Management of Otitis Media With Perfo-ration: Most perforations seen with acute otitis me-dia heal within 2 weeks. When perforations fail to heal after 3–6 months, surgical repair may be needed. Repair of the defect in the tympanic membrane is generally delayed until the child is older and auditory tube function has improved. Procedures include pa-per patch, fat myringoplasty, and tympanoplasty. Tympanoplasty is generally deferred until age 7–9 years. The perforated eardrum can be repaired earlier if the nonperforated drum remains free of infection and effusion for 1 year. Water activities should be limited to surface swimming, preferably with the use of an ear mold. Diving, jumping into the water, and underwater swimming should be interdicted.

I. Management of Chronic Suppurative Oti-tis Media: The successful treatment of chronic sup-purative otitis usually requires parenteral therapy with an antibiotic that covers *Pseudomonas* and anaerobes. The role of oral quinolone antibiotics ef-fective against *Pseudomonas* infection for outpatient management is unclear because of concern about possible side effects on growing cartilage in children.

When a cholesteatoma is associated with chronic suppurative otitis media, medical therapy is not ef-fective. If the discharge does not respond to 2 weeks of aggressive therapy, mastoiditis or cholesteatoma should be suspected. Serious central nervous system complications such as extradural abscess, subdural abscess, brain abscess, meningitis, labyrinthitis, or lateral sinus thrombophlebitis can occur with exten-sion of this process. Therefore, patients with facial palsy, vertigo, or other central nervous system signs should be immediately referred to an otolaryngolo-gist.

Berman S et al: Otitis media related antibiotic prescribing patterns, outcomes and expenditures in a pediatric Med-icaid population. Pediatrics 1997;100:585.

Berman S: Current concepts: Otitis media in children. N Engl J Med 1995;332:1560.

Brook I, Gober AE: Prophylaxis with amoxicillin or sul-fisoxazole for otitis media: Effect on the recovery of penicillin resistant bacteria from children. Clin Infect Dis 1996;22:143.

Byrns PJ et al: Utilization of services for otitis media by children enrolled in Medicaid. Arch Pediatr Adolesc Med 1997;151:407.

Craig WA, Andes D: Pharmacokinetics and pharmacody-namics of antibiotics in otitis media. Pediatr Infect Dis J 1996:15:255.

Dagan R et al: Antibiotic treatment in acute otitis media: In vivo demonstration of antibacterial activity. Clin Micro-biol Infect 1997;3(Suppl):S43.

Ey JL et al: Group Health Medical Associates: Passive smoke exposure and otitis media in the first year of life. Pediatrics 1995;95:670.

Gehanno P et al: Evaluation of nasopharyngeal cultures for bacteriologic assessment of acute otitis media in chil-dren. Pediatr Infect Dis J 1996:15:329.

Roark R, Berman S: Continuous twice daily or once daily amoxicillin prophylaxis compared with placebo for chil-dren with recurrent otitis media. Pediatr Infect Dis J 1997;16:376.

Rosenfeld RM et al: Clinical efficacy of antimicrobial drugs for acute otitis media: Metaanalysis of 5400 chil-dren from 33 randomized trials. J Pediatr 1994;124:355.

Rosenfeld RM: An evidence based approach to healing oti-tis media. Pediatr Clin North Am 1996;43:1165.

Uhare M et al: Xylitol chewing gum in the prevention of acute otitis media: A double blind randomized trial. Br Med J 1996;313:1180.

Williams RL et al: Use of antibiotics in preventing recur-rent acute otitis media and in treating otitis media with effusion. JAMA 1993;270:1344.

3. MASTOIDITIS

Infection of the mastoid antrum and air cells can be associated with an episode of acute otitis media. Mastoiditis is unusual before age 2 years, when air cells begin to develop. The most common etiologic agents are *S pyogenes, S pneumoniae,* and *S aureus. H influenzae* causes mastoiditis much less frequently than might be expected. Other agents that can cause this disease include *Pseudomonas, Mycobacterium,* enteropathic gram-negative rods, and *M catarrhalis.* Anaerobic organisms appear to play a role in chronic mastoiditis; however, no data are available on how frequently they cause acute mastoiditis.

Clinical Findings

The principal complaints of patients with mastoiditis are usually postauricular pain and fever. On examination, the mastoid area often appears swollen and reddened. In the late stage, it may be fluctuant. The earliest finding is severe tenderness upon mastoid percussion.

Acute otitis media is almost always present. Late findings are a pinna that is pushed forward by postauricular swelling and an ear canal that is narrowed in the posterosuperior wall because of pressure from the mastoid abscess. In infants under 1 year of age, the swelling occurs superior to the ear and pushes the pinna downward rather than outward. In the acute phase, there is diffuse inflammatory clouding of the mastoid cells as in every case of acute otitis media. Later, there is evidence of bony destruction and resorption of the mastoid air cells. The best way to determine the extent of disease is by CT scan.

Complications

Meningitis is a complication in up to 9% of cases of acute mastoiditis. This infection should be suspected when a child has high fever, stiff neck, severe headache, or other meningeal signs. Lumbar puncture should be performed for diagnosis. Brain abscess occurs in 2% of cases and may be associated with persistent headaches, recurring fever, or changes in sensorium.

Treatment

The patient with mastoiditis must be hospitalized because this disorder represents osteitis. Before therapy is initiated, tympanocentesis or myringotomy should be performed to obtain material for culture and to relieve the pressure in the middle ear-mastoid space.

The initial management of uncomplicated acute mastoiditis includes intravenous antibiotic therapy. Results of Gram-stained smears taken during tympanocentesis may help in the choice of antibiotics. Reasonable initial therapy is with ceftriaxone plus nafcillin or clindamycin. Indications for immediate surgery include clear evidence of a major complication such as meningitis, brain abscess, cavernous sinus thrombosis, acute suppurative labyrinthitis, or facial palsy. Some otolaryngologists consider the destruction of septation of the mastoid (coalescence) an indication for surgery as well. Duration of antibiotic therapy following mastoidectomy is dependent on the type of complication encountered. The prognosis is good if treatment is started early and continued until the process is inactive.

ACUTE TRAUMA TO THE MIDDLE EAR

Head injuries, a blow to the ear canal, sudden impact with water, blast injuries, or the insertion of pointed instruments into the ear canal can lead to perforation of the tympanic membrane or hematoma of the middle ear. One study reported that 50% of serious penetrating wounds of the tympanic membrane were due to parental use of a cotton-tipped swab.

Treatment of middle ear hematomas consists mainly of watchful waiting. Antibiotics are not necessary unless signs of superimposed infection appear. The prognosis for unimpaired hearing depends on whether or not the ossicles are dislocated or fractured in the process. The patient needs to be followed with audiometry until hearing has returned to normal.

Traumatic perforations of the tympanic membrane often do not heal spontaneously, in which case the patient should be referred to an otolaryngologist. Perforations caused by a foreign body must be attended to immediately, especially if accompanied by vertigo.

EAR CANAL FOREIGN BODY

Numerous objects can be inserted into the ear canal by a child. If the object is large, wedged into place, or difficult to remove with available instruments, the patient should be referred to an otolaryngologist early rather than risk traumatizing the ear canal and causing edema that will require removal under anesthesia.

HEMATOMA OF THE PINNA

Trauma to the earlobe can result in formation of a hematoma between the perichondrium and cartilage. The hematoma appears as a boggy purple swelling of the upper half of the earlobe. If this is not treated, it can cause pressure necrosis of the underlying cartilage and result in "cauliflower ear." To prevent this cosmetic deformity, physicians should refer patients to an otolaryngologist for aspiration and application of a carefully molded pressure dressing. Recurrent or persistent hematoma of the ear may require surgical drainage and insertion of a drain.

CONGENITAL EAR MALFORMATIONS

Agenesis of the external ear canal results in conductive hearing loss that requires evaluation in the first month of life by hearing specialists and an otolaryngologist.

"Lop ears" (Dumbo ears) lead to much teasing and ridicule. They can be surgically corrected at age 5 or 6 years—the ear is of approximately adult size by then, and there is little risk of affecting growth of the tissues.

An ear is low-set if the upper pole is below eye level. This condition is often associated with renal malformations (eg, Potter's syndrome), and renal ultrasound examination is helpful.

Preauricular tags, ectopic cartilage, fistulas, sinuses, and cysts require surgical correction, mainly for cosmetic reasons. Children with any of these findings should have their hearing tested. Most preauricular pits cause no symptoms. If one should become infected, the patient should receive antibiotic therapy and be referred to an otolaryngologist for eventual excision.

DETECTION & MANAGEMENT OF HEARING DEFICITS

Hearing deficits are classified as conductive, sensorineural, or mixed. **Conductive hearing loss** results from blockage of the transmission of sound waves from the external auditory canal to the inner ear and is characterized by normal bone conduction and reduced air conduction hearing. In children, conductive losses are most often caused by middle ear effusion. **Sensorineural hearing loss** occurs when the auditory nerve or cochlear hair cells are damaged. **Mixed hearing loss** is characterized by components of both conductive and sensorineural loss. The criteria for children are more stringent than for adults because normal hearing levels are lower in children than in adults, since children are in the process of learning language. In children, a hearing loss of 15–30 dB is considered mild, 31–50 dB moderate, 51–80 dB severe, and 81–100 dB profound.

Conductive Hearing Loss

By far the most important cause of conductive hearing loss during childhood is otitis media and its sequelae. Other causes include atresia, stenosis, or collapse of the ear canal; furuncle, cerumen, or foreign body in the ear; aural discharge; bony growths; otitis externa; perichondritis; and middle ear anomalies (eg, stapes fixation, ossicular malformation).

The average hearing loss due to middle ear effu-

sion (whether serous, purulent, or mucoid) is 27–31 dB, the equivalent of a mild hearing loss. This loss may be intermittent in nature and may occur in one or both ears.

The American Academy of Pediatrics recommends that hearing be assessed and language skills be monitored in children who have frequently recurring acute otitis media or middle ear effusion persisting longer than 3 months. The effects of hearing loss may be insidious and may not be discernible until the explosive phase of expressive language development occurs between 16 and 24 months of age; therefore, the optimal time for screening young children is between 18 and 24 months. An acceptable tool for language screening at this time is the Early Language Milestone (ELM) scale. Children 3, 4, and 5 years of age with recurring otitis media and effusion should also be screened for language delays.

To diminish the likelihood of communication disorder, the physician should inform the parents of a child with middle ear disease that the child's hearing may not be normal and should instruct the parents to (1) turn off sources of background noise (eg, televisions, radios, dishwashers) when speaking to the child; (2) focus on the child's face and gain his or her direct attention before speaking; (3) speak slightly louder than usual; and (4) have the teacher place the child in the front of the classroom.

Sensorineural Hearing Loss

Sensorineural hearing loss (SNHL) arises from a lesion in the cochlear structures of the inner ear or in the neural fibers of the auditory nerve (cranial nerve VIII). Most sensorineural losses in children are congenital, with an estimated incidence of 1:750–1000 live births. Causes can be classified as either congenital or postnatal and, within each classification, genetic or nongenetic. Common congenital genetic causes include inner ear dysplasias and sensorineural hearing loss with and without associated abnormalities (eg, Usher's syndrome). Postnatal onset of sensorineural hearing loss often occurs with associated genetic abnormalities (eg, Alport's syndrome and Klippel-Feil syndrome). Common congenital nongenetic causes are prenatal infections, teratogenic drugs, and perinatal injuries. Common postnatal nongenetic causes are infections, trauma, ototoxic drugs, metabolic disorders, neoplastic diseases, and autoimmune diseases. Prior to the introduction of Hib vaccine, meningitis was the most common cause of acquired hearing loss, with deafness occurring in about 10% of children with bacterial meningitis.

In the past, the effect of unilateral deafness on school performance was thought to be insignificant. Studies now show that more than one-third of affected children fail one or more grades in school. Therefore, merely recommending preferential classroom seating for these children is no longer sufficient; they should be referred for full evaluation of their hearing needs.

Acquisition of language skills is more severely affected by bilateral than by unilateral sensorineural hearing loss. The earlier the deafness occurs, the graver the consequences for language development; the earlier a sensorineural loss is detected and treated (by sound amplification and language habilitation), the better the chances of a good outcome.

Screening for Hearing Deficits

Screening procedures are established for early detection and diagnosis of hearing deficits. The need for identifying hearing impairment in infants was instituted in the 1970s with formation of the high-risk registry. The latest stage of evolution is the Joint Committee's 1994 Position Statement (see Screening of Newborns, below). It called for the use of auditory brain stem response screening, preferably before discharge from the hospital, for neonates identified as being at high risk. However, a Consensus Development Conference sponsored by the National Institutes of Health in 1993 recommended universal hearing screening of all neonates using evoked otoacoustic emission testing. The procedures listed in the following text are intended to serve as a guide, and confirmation of sensorineural hearing loss is dependent on audiologic testing.

A. Screening of Newborns: See Chapter 2.

B. Screening of Infants: The Joint Committee recommends hearing screening for infants (29 days to 2 years) if one of the following risk criteria is identified: (1) concerns regarding hearing, speech, language, or developmental delay; (2) bacterial meningitis; (3) neonatal risk factors (Chapter 2); (4) head trauma; (5) ototoxic drug use; (6) neurodegenerative disorders; and (7) childhood infectious diseases (eg, mumps, measles).

In the past, the parents' report of their infant's behavior was considered an adequate assessment of hearing. However, a deaf infant's behavior can appear normal and mislead the parents as well as the professional, especially if the infant has autosomal recessive deafness and is the firstborn child of carrier parents. The following office screening techniques should identify gross hearing losses but may or may not detect less severe losses due to otitis media.

1. Birth to 4 months–In response to a sudden loud sound (70 dB or more) produced by a horn, clacker, or special electronic device, the infant should show a startle reflex or blink the eyes.

2. Four months to 2 years–While the infant is distracted with a toy or bright object, a noisemaker is sounded softly outside the field of vision at the child's waist level. Normal responses are as follows: at 4 months, there is widening of the eyes, interruption of other activity, and perhaps a slight turning of the head in the direction of the sound; at 6 months, the head turns toward the sound; at 9 months or

older, the child is usually able to locate a sound originating from below as well as turn to the appropriate side; after 1 year, the child is able to locate sound whether it comes from below or above.

After responses to soft sounds are noted, a loud horn or clacker should be used to produce an eye blink or startle reflex. This last maneuver is necessary because deaf children are often visually alert and able to scan the environment so actively that their scanning can be mistaken for an appropriate response to the softer noise test. A deaf child will not blink in response to the loud sound. Consonant sounds such as "mama," "dada," "baba" should be present in speech by age 11 months. Children who fail to respond appropriately should be referred for audiologic assessment.

C. Screening of Older Children: When children reach 3 years of age, their hearing can be tested by earphones and pure tone audiometry. The test frequencies for screening are 1000 Hz, 2000 Hz, and 4000 Hz, with the same tone presented at each frequency. Normally, the screening level is 20 dB. If a soundproof room is not available, the screening may be done at 25 dB. If the child does not respond at any one of the test frequencies in either ear, the test should be repeated within 1 week. Failure on rescreening requires referral for audiologic evaluation.

High-risk categories in older children include osteogenesis imperfecta and syndromes associated with deafness, such as Waardenburg's syndrome, Hurler's syndrome, Alport's syndrome, Treacher Collins' syndrome, Klippel-Feil syndrome, and fetal alcohol syndrome. Children with these disorders should always receive audiologic evaluation. In addition, before any child is labeled as having mental retardation, autism, or severe behavior problems, the adequacy of hearing must be determined. If a developmental speech delay is diagnosed, hearing should be tested as the first step in evaluating the language problem.

Referral

In addition to the referrals for audiologic testing mentioned in the preceding text, a child with confirmed hearing loss should be referred to an otolaryngologist for evaluation and further management. Any child failing the language screen should be referred to a speech pathologist for language evaluation. Home language enrichment programs for children with mild language delays can be directed by the physician or by a speech pathologist. Programs for the deaf child vary from aural to total communication; the latter includes elements of aural programs plus signing. Each program should be thoroughly scrutinized for its relevance to the deaf child's age and hearing level.

Prevention

Appropriate care may treat or prevent conditions causing hearing deficits. Erythroblastosis fetalis can usually be prevented by the use of $Rh_o(D)$ immune globulin, and hyperbilirubinemia can be controlled by phototherapy and exchange transfusions. Congenital rubella infections can be prevented by the use of rubella vaccine, and immunizations for other childhood diseases (eg, mumps) effectively prevent hearing losses from those conditions. Aminoglycosides and diuretics, especially in combination, are potentially ototoxic and should be used judiciously and monitored carefully, especially in premature infants and in patients with renal insufficiency. Reduction of repeated exposure to loud noise in the child's environment—loud music, firecrackers, or shots from guns or cap pistols—will prevent high-frequency hearing losses.

Chan KH: Sensorineural hearing loss in children: Classification and evaluation. Otolaryngol Clin North Am 1994;27:473.

II. THE NOSE & PARANASAL SINUSES

ACUTE VIRAL RHINITIS (Common Cold)

The common cold is the most common pediatric infectious disease, and the incidence is higher in early childhood than in any other period of life. Children under age 5 have 6–12 colds per year. Upper respiratory infection may be caused by over 200 different viruses, including rhinovirus, coronavirus, adenovirus, influenza virus, parainfluenza virus, respiratory syncytial virus, and coxsackievirus.

Clinical Findings

The patient usually experiences a sudden onset of clear or mucoid rhinorrhea, nasal congestion, and fever. Mild sore throat and cough may also develop. Although the fever is usually low-grade in older children, in the first 5 or 6 years of life it can be as high as 40.6 °C without superinfection. The nose, throat, and tympanic membrane can appear red and inflamed.

Treatment

Treatment for the common cold is largely symptomatic. Acetaminophen or ibuprofen is helpful for fever, sore throat, or muscle aches. A stuffy, congested nose can be treated with normal saline nose drops (mix ½ tsp table salt with 6 oz of water), 3 drops in each nostril. After several minutes, a suction bulb can be used to remove the secretions of the infant unable to blow its nose. If this procedure fails af-

ter several attempts and the stuffy nose still interferes with feeding or sleep, consider long-acting xylometazoline or oxymetazoline 0.05% nose drops. Drops should be used only when the nose is congested and discontinued within 5 days to prevent rebound chemical rhinitis.

Antihistamines are not effective in relieving cold symptoms. In rhinoviral colds, increased levels of histamine are not observed. Antibiotics do not prevent superinfection and should not be used. Codeine and dextromethorphan should be discouraged because they do not alleviate the cough of the common cold. Parents should be instructed that fast breathing or difficult breathing with retraction is a sign of lower respiratory infection such as bronchiolitis or pneumonia.

The primary care physician can use the following guidelines when screening children with a cold for elective surgery. Surgery is usually postponed if fever or cough is present. Surgery can proceed if the child has only a runny nose, sore throat or ear infection. If anesthesia does not entail intubation, surgery may be permitted even when the child has a cough provided that chest radiograph is normal.

Taylor JA et al: Efficacy of cough suppressants in children. J Pediatr 1993;122:799.

SINUSITIS

1. ACUTE SINUSITIS

Acute bacterial infection of the paranasal sinuses is called sinusitis. The maxillary and ethmoidal sinuses are most commonly involved when mucociliary clearance and drainage are impaired by an upper respiratory infection or allergic rhinitis. The ethmoid sinus is the only one that is significantly developed at birth. The maxillary sinus is rudimentary at birth and visible on x-ray film by 6 months. The frontal sinus is not visible until the age 3–9 years. Clinical ethmoiditis does not usually occur until 6 months of age. About half of cases occur between 1 and 5 years of age, during which time the most common presenting sign is periorbital cellulitis. Maxillary sinusitis is seen clinically after 1 year of age. Frontal sinusitis is unusual before 10 years of age.

The pathogens that cause acute sinusitis are usually *S pneumoniae, H influenzae* (nontypable), *M catarrhalis,* and β-hemolytic streptococci. Rarely, anaerobic bacterial infections can cause fulminant frontal sinusitis. Viruses can be isolated in 10% of sinus aspirates, but their pathogenetic role is unclear.

Clinical Findings

The development of symptoms in acute sinusitis in children may be gradual or sudden. With gradual presentation, nasal discharge or postnasal drip and daytime cough persist longer than 10 days. In addition, a low-grade fever is often present in association with malodorous breath or intermittent, painless morning periorbital swelling. Older patients may complain of headache, a sense of facial fullness, or facial pain overlying the involved sinus. With the more sudden presentation, the patient presents with a high fever and more severe pain or periorbital inflammation. Ethmoiditis causes retro-orbital pain; maxillary sinusitis causes upper molar or zygomatic pain; and frontal sinusitis causes pain above the eyebrow.

Physical examination reveals inflamed nasal mucosa, usually associated with nasal or postnasal mucopurulent discharge. Occasionally, there is percussion tenderness overlying the sinusitis. In ethmoiditis, the tenderness is elicited by pressing medially on the inner canthus of the eye. Tenderness of the eyeball may be present also. Maxillary sinusitis is manifested by percussion tenderness on the maxillary bone, frontal sinusitis by tenderness in response to pressure upward on the floor of the supraorbital ridge. Periorbital swelling or mild discoloration may be present. The examination should identify exudative tonsillitis, a nasal foreign body, or dental caries and poor dental hygiene. Transillumination of the sinuses is difficult to perform and not very helpful unless it is grossly asymmetric.

Consider sinus aspiration for diagnostic purposes in patients with complications and in immunocompromised patients. Gram's stain or culture of nasal discharge does not correlate with cultures of sinus aspirates. If the patient is hospitalized because of complications, a blood culture should be obtained.

Imaging studies of the paranasal sinuses during acute illness are not indicated except for evaluation of complications. In the past, plain radiography was used to diagnose sinusitis when an air-fluid level or mucosal thickening greater than 4 mm was seen. CT should be ordered in children with complications or lack of resolution following adequate antibiotic therapy. Findings consistent with sinusitis may be found in asymptomatic patients with colds or nasal allergies. Because of sensitivity and specificity issues relating to plain radiography, CT scans are generally used in younger children and plain radiographs are reserved for older children and adolescents.

Complications

Complications are most apt to develop in the ethmoid sinus. Complications of ethmoiditis represent a continuum beginning with preseptal cellulitis, then postseptal cellulitis, subperiosteal abscess, orbital abscess, and cavernous sinus thrombosis. These complications are associated with decreased extraocular movement, proptosis, chemosis, and altered visual acuity. The most common complication of frontal sinusitis is osteitis of the frontal bone (Pott's puffy tumor). Intracranial extension leads to meningitis and to epidural, subdural, and brain abscesses. The most common max-illary complication is cellulitis of the cheek. Rarely, osteomyelitis of the maxilla can develop.

Treatment

Patients with evidence of invasive infection or any central nervous system complications should be hospitalized immediately. Intravenous therapy with nafcillin or clindamycin plus a third-generation cephalosporin such as cefotaxime should be initiated until culture results become available. Treat less severe cases of acute sinusitis with oral antibiotics for 10 days. Continue antibiotic treatment for another week if the patient has improved but is not totally asymptomatic. The usual antibiotic is amoxicillin, 60–80 mg/kg/d in three divided doses. In areas where β-lactamase-positive pathogens are common or when the patient is allergic to penicillin, use trimethoprim-sulfamethoxazole, a third-generation cephalosporin, a newer macrolide, or erythromycin plus sulfamethoxazole. Failure to improve after 48 hours suggests a resistant organism or potential complication. See the section on unresponsive acute otitis media for antibiotic recommendations, which are also appropriate for sinusitis.

Topical decongestants and oral combinations are frequently used in acute sinusitis to promote drainage. Their effectiveness has not been proved, and concern has been raised about potential adverse effects related to impaired ciliary function, decreased blood flow to the mucosa, and reduced diffusion of antibiotic into the sinuses. Patients with underlying allergic rhinitis may benefit from intranasal cromolyn or corticosteroid nasal spray. Vasoconstrictor nose drops and spray are associated with rebound edema if used for more than 5–7 days.

The patient may require acetaminophen, ibuprofen, or even codeine to permit sleep until drainage is achieved. The application of ice over the sinus may help to relieve pain.

2. RECURRENT OR CHRONIC SINUSITIS

Chronic or frequent episodes of sinusitis occur in very few patients. Recurrent and chronic sinusitis in infants and young children may be related to child care attendance. Important factors to consider include allergies, anatomy, and host immunity. Mucosal inflammation leading to obstruction is most commonly caused by allergic rhinitis and occasionally by nonallergic rhinitis. Rarely, chronic sinusitis is caused by anatomic variations such as septal deviation, polyp, or foreign body. In cases of chronic or recurrent pyogenic pansinusitis, poor host resistance (eg, an immune defect, Kartagener's syndrome, or cystic fibrosis)—though rare—must be ruled out by immunoglobulin studies, microscopic studies of respiratory cilia, and a sweat chloride test. Anaerobic and staphylococcal organisms are often responsible for chronic sinusitis. Evaluation by an allergist and an otolaryngologist may be useful in determining the underlying causes.

Surgical Treatment

A. Antral Lavage: Antral lavage, generally regarded as a diagnostic procedure, may have some therapeutic value. An aspirate or a sample irrigated from the maxillary sinus is retrieved either with a spinal needle or a curved-tip instrument under anesthesia. In the very young child, this may be the only procedure that can be performed.

B. Endoscopic Sinus Surgery: No data are available comparing the outcome of this procedure with traditional surgical drainage procedures. There are large variations in the reported uses of this procedure by otolaryngologists, especially in younger patients.

C. External Drainage: External ethmoidectomy and fronto-ethmoidectomy are used to manage complications arising from ethmoiditis and frontal sinusitis.

Dunham ME: New light on sinusitis. Contemp Pediatr 1994;11:102.

Gwaltney JM et al: Computed tomographic study of the common cold. N Engl J Med 1994;330:25.

Ueda D, Yoto Y: The ten day mark as a practical diagnostic approach for acute paranasal sinusitis in children. Pediatr Infect Dis J 1996;15:576.

CHOANAL ATRESIA

Choanal atresia occurs bilaterally in 25% of affected children and unilaterally in 75%. Bilateral cases cause severe respiratory distress at birth. Unilateral atresia generally presents with unilateral chronic nasal discharge and may be confused with sinusitis. An 8F soft rubber catheter should be passed through the nose and visualized in the oropharynx. If this procedure cannot be accomplished, a diagnosis of choanal atresia should be confirmed by radiographic study. The clinician should consider CHARGE syndrome association when choanal atresia is encountered. An oral airway should be used when a newborn has been diagnosed with bilateral choanal atresia. An otolaryngologist should be consulted for possible surgery to repair the atresia or bypass the upper airway obstruction. Unilateral atresia is generally not corrected until later in life.

Rothman G, Wood RA, Naclerio RM: Unilateral choanal atresia masquerading as chronic sinusitis. Pediatrics 1994;124:941.

RECURRENT RHINITIS

Recurrent rhinitis is frequently seen in the office practice of pediatrics. The child is brought in with the chief complaint that it "has one cold after another," has "constant colds," or "is always sick." Approximately two-thirds of these children have recurrent colds, and the remainder have either allergic rhinitis or recurrent sinusitis.

Allergic Rhinitis

The onset of "hay fever" is usually after a child is 2 years of age and has had adequate exposure to allergens. There is no fever or contagion among close contacts. The attacks include frequent sneezing, rubbing of the nose, and a profuse clear discharge. The nasal turbinates are swollen. The nasal smear demonstrates over 20% eosinophils. Nasal secretions should be collected only when the patient is symptomatic—between attacks or after treatment with antihistamines, the smear may be falsely negative. Use of vasoconstrictor nose drops beyond 5–7 days results in a rebound reaction and secondary nasal congestion (rhinitis medicamentosa). The offending nose drops should be discontinued. Concern has been raised about the effects of sedating antihistamines on school performance.

Cook PR, Nishioka GJ. Allergic rhinosinusitis in the pediatric population. Otolaryngol Clin North Am 1996; 29:39.

VASOMOTOR RHINITIS

Some children react to sudden changes in environmental temperature with prolonged congestion and rhinorrhea. Air pollution (especially tobacco smoke) may be a factor. Oral decongestants can be used to give symptomatic relief.

EPISTAXIS

The nose is an extremely vascular structure. In most cases, epistaxis (nosebleed) is due to mild trauma to the anterior portion of the nasal septum (Kiesselbach's area), usually due to vigorous nose rubbing, nose blowing, or nose picking. Less than 5% of children with recurrent epistaxis have a bleeding disorder. Examination of Kiesselbach's area usually reveals a red, raw surface with fresh clots or old crusts. Look for telangiectasia, hemangiomas, or varicosities.

Most patients do not need a hematologic workup, but bleeding tests are indicated if any of the following is present: a family history of a bleeding disorder, a past medical history of easy bleeding, spontaneous bleeding at other sites, bleeding that lasts for over 30 minutes or will not clot with direct pressure by the physician, onset before age 2 years, or a drop in hematocrit due to epistaxis. High blood pressure may also predispose to prolonged nosebleeds.

A nasopharyngeal angiofibroma may present as recurrent epistaxis. Adolescent boys are almost exclusively affected. CT scan of the nasal cavity and nasopharynx is diagnostic.

Treatment

The following approach can be carried out in the office or offered as phone advice: The patient should sit up and lean forward so as not to swallow the blood. The nasal cavity should be cleared of clots by blowing. The soft part of the nose is pinched firmly enough to elicit pain, with pressure over the bleeding site being maintained for 5 minutes by the clock. If bleeding continues, the bleeding site needs to be visualized. A small piece of gelatin sponge (Gelfoam) or collagen sponge (Surgicel) can be inserted over the bleeding site.

Friability of the nasal vessels can be decreased with daily application of either petroleum-based or water-based ointment by cotton-tipped applicator. The lubricant is applied daily until 5 days have passed without a nosebleed, then weekly for 1 month. Humidification of the patient's bedroom may be helpful. Aspirin should be avoided, as should vigorous blowing of the nose.

NASAL FURUNCLE

A nasal furuncle is an infection of a hair follicle in the anterior nares. Hair plucking or nose picking can provide a route of entry. The most common organism is *S aureus*. The diagnosis is made by finding an exquisitely tender, firm, red lump in the anterior naris. Treatment includes dicloxacillin or cephalexin orally for 5 days to prevent spread. The lesion should be gently incised and drained as soon as it points, usually with a needle. Topical bacitracin ointment may be of additional value. Since this lesion is in the drainage area of the cavernous sinus, the patient should be followed closely until healing is complete. Parents should be advised never to pick or squeeze a furuncle in this location—and neither should the physician. Associated cellulitis or spread requires hospitalization for administration of intravenous antibiotics.

NASAL SEPTUM SUBLUXATION

Newborn infants rarely have subluxation of the quadrangular cartilage of the septum. The top of the nose deviates to one side, and the inferior septal border deviates to the other. There is also leaning of the columella and instability of the nasal tip. This disorder must be distinguished from the more common transient flattening of the nose caused by the birth process. In the past, physicians were encouraged to reduce all subluxations in the nursery. Otolaryngolo-

gists are more likely to perform the reduction under anesthesia for more difficult cases.

NASAL FRACTURE

Most blows to the nose result in swallowing of blood and hematoma formation without fracture. A persistent nosebleed after trauma, crepitus or instability of the bones in the nasal bridge, and marked deviation of the nose to one side indicate fracture. However, septal injury can be ruled out only by careful intranasal examination. Patients with suspected nasal fractures should be referred to an otolaryngologist for definitive therapy. Resetting of the nasal fracture can be postponed up to 1 week without resulting in permanent deformity.

NASAL SEPTUM HEMATOMA

After nasal trauma, it is essential to examine the inside of the nose with a nasal speculum. Hematoma of the nasal septum imposes a considerable risk of pressure necrosis and resorption of the cartilage, leading to septal perforation or a saddle-back nose in adulthood. This diagnosis is confirmed by the abrupt onset of nasal obstruction following trauma and the presence of a boggy, widened nasal septum. The normal nasal septum is 2–4 mm thick.

Treatment consists of prompt referral to an otolaryngologist for evacuation of the hematoma and packing of the nose.

NASAL SEPTUM ABSCESS

A nasal septum abscess usually follows nasal trauma or a nasal furuncle. Examination reveals a fluctuant gray septal swelling, usually bilateral. The possible complications are the same as for nasal septum hematoma as well as spread of the infection to the central nervous system. Treatment consists of immediate hospitalization and incision and drainage by an otolaryngologist.

FOREIGN BODIES IN THE NOSE

There are many ways to remove nasal foreign bodies. The obvious first maneuver is vigorous nose blowing if the child is old enough. Nasal foreign body removal requires topical anesthesia, nasal decongestion, good lighting, correct instrumentation, and physical restraint. Topical tetracaine or lidocaine can be used in young children without aerodigestive tract compromise. Nasal decongestion can be achieved by topical pseudoephedrine or oxymetazoline. When the child is properly restrained, most nasal foreign bodies can be removed using a pair of alligator forceps through an operating head otoscope. If the object seems inaccessible, is wedged in, or is quite large, the patient should be referred to an otolaryngologist without worsening the situation through futile attempts at removal.

III. THE THROAT & ORAL CAVITY

ACUTE STOMATITIS

Recurrent Aphthous Stomatitis ("Canker Sore")

The main finding is one to three small ulcers (3–10 mm) on the insides of the lips or elsewhere in the mouth. There is usually no associated fever and no cervical adenopathy. The ulcers are very painful and last 1–2 weeks. They may recur numerous times throughout life. The cause is not known, though an allergic or autoimmune basis is suspected.

Treatment consists of coating the lesions with topical antacid or sucralfate four times daily. Topical corticosteroids, either in a dental paste such as triamcinolone acetonide 0.1% (Kenalog in Orabase) or in a mouthwash administered four times daily, also have efficacy. Pain can be reduced by a bland diet, avoiding salty or acid foods, switching from a bottle to a cup in infants, giving 2% viscous lidocaine prior to meals, and giving acetaminophen or even codeine at bedtime. If the child is not old enough to expectorate the lidocaine, it must not be used.

Herpes Simplex Gingivostomatitis

Approximately 1% of children who have their first encounter with the herpes simplex virus develop ten or more small ulcers (1–3 mm) of the buccal mucosa, anterior pillars, inner lips, tongue, and especially the gingiva. The lesions are often associated with fever, tender cervical nodes, and generalized inflammation of the mouth. Affected children are commonly under 3 years of age. Herpes simplex gingivostomatitis lasts 7–10 days. Severe dysphagia interferes with eating and drinking. Treatment is symptomatic, as described above for recurrent aphthous stomatitis, with the exception that corticosteroids are contraindicated because they may result in spread of the infection. Early in the course, consider prescribing oral acyclovir suspension (200 mg/5 mL), 10 mg/kg three times daily for 7 days. The patient must be followed closely. Dehydration occasionally ensues despite liberal offerings of cold fluids, in which case the patient must be hospitalized so that intravenous fluids can be administered. Herpetic laryngotracheitis is a rare complication.

Thrush

Oral candidiasis mainly affects infants and occasionally older children in a debilitated state. *Candida albicans* is a saprophyte that normally is not invasive unless the mouth is abraded. The use of broad-spectrum antibiotics and systemic or inhaled steroids may be contributing factors. The symptoms include soreness of the mouth and refusal of feedings. Lesions consist of white curd-like plaques predominantly on the buccal mucosa. These plaques cannot be washed away after a water feeding.

Specific treatment consists of nystatin oral suspension, 1 mL four times daily for 1 week, or miconazole gel. Treatment should be preceded by attempts to remove large plaques with a moistened cotton-tipped applicator or piece of gauze.

Hoppe JE and the Antifungal Study Group: Treatment of oropharyngeal candidiasis in immunocompetent infants: A randomized multicenter study of miconazole gel vs nystatin suspension. Pediatr Infect Dis J 1997;16:288.

Traumatic Oral Ulcers

Ulcers are a nonspecific response of the oral mucosa to trauma. Mechanical trauma most commonly occurs on the buccal mucosa secondary to accidentally biting with the molars. Thermal trauma, as from very hot foods, can also cause ulcerative lesions. Chemical ulcers can be produced by mucosal contact with aspirin, caustics, and the like. Oral ulcers can also occur with leukemia or on a recurrent basis with cyclic neutropenia. These lesions usually need no treatment. The pain subsides in 2 or 3 days.

ACUTE VIRAL PHARYNGITIS & TONSILLITIS

Over 90% of cases of sore throat and fever in children are due to viral infections. Most children develop associated rhinorrhea and mild cough. The findings seldom give any clue to the particular viral agent, but six types of viral pharyngitis are sufficiently distinctive to support an educated guess about the specific cause.

Clinical Findings

A. Infectious Mononucleosis: The findings are exudative tonsillitis, generalized cervical adenitis, and fever, usually in a teenage patient. A palpable spleen or axillary adenopathy adds weight to the diagnosis. The presence of more than 20% atypical lymphocytes on a peripheral blood smear or a positive mononucleosis spot test confirms the diagnosis, though the test is often falsely negative in children under 5 years old. This diagnosis is often not considered until a patient with a presumptive diagnosis of streptococcal pharyngitis has failed to respond to 48 hours of treatment with penicillin.

B. Herpangina: Herpangina ulcers, 2–3 mm in size, are found on the anterior pillars and sometimes on the soft palate and uvula. There are no ulcers in the anterior mouth, as there are in herpes simplex. Herpangina is caused by several members of the coxsackie A group of viruses, and a patient can have up to five bouts of herpangina in a lifetime.

C. Lymphonodular Pharyngitis: The classic finding is small, yellow-white nodules in the same distribution as the small ulcers in herpangina. In this condition, which is caused by coxsackievirus A10, the nodules do not ulcerate.

D. Hand, Foot, and Mouth Disease: This entity is caused by coxsackieviruses A5, A9, A10, and A16. Ulcers occur on the tongue and oral mucosa. Vesicles, which usually do not ulcerate, are found on the palms, soles, and interdigital areas.

E. Pharyngoconjunctival Fever: This disorder is caused by an adenovirus. Exudative tonsillitis, conjunctivitis, and fever are the main findings.

F. Rubeola: The prodrome of measles looks like any nonspecific viral respiratory infection until one closely examines the buccal mucosa and the inner aspects of the lower lip. Small white specks the size of salt granules on an erythematous base (Koplik's spots) found at these sites are pathognomonic of early measles.

Treatment

The treatment of acute viral pharyngitis is strictly symptomatic. Older children can gargle with warm saline solution or antacid solution. Younger children can suck on hard candy (especially butterscotch). Analgesics and antipyretics are sometimes helpful. Antibiotics are not helpful.

McMillan JA et al: Pharyngitis associated with herpes simplex virus in college students. Pediatr Infect Dis J 1993;12:280.

Nakayama M et al: Pharyngoconjunctival fever caused by adenovirus type 11. Pediatr Infect Dis J 1992;11:6.

ACUTE STREPTOCOCCAL PHARYNGITIS & TONSILLITIS

Approximately 10% of children with sore throat and fever have a streptococcal infection. Untreated streptococcal pharyngitis can result in acute rheumatic fever, glomerulonephritis, and suppurative complications (eg, cervical adenitis, peritonsillar abscess, otitis media, cellulitis, and septicemia). Vesicles and ulcers are suggestive of viral infection, whereas cervical adenitis, petechiae, a beefy-red uvula, and a tonsillar exudate suggest streptococcal infection; the only way to make a definitive diagnosis is by throat culture or rapid identification test. Rapid identification tests are very specific but lack sensitivity. Therefore, a positive test indicates *S pyo-*

genes infection, but a negative result requires confirmation with culture.

Treat cases of suspected or proved *S pyogenes* infection with a 10-day course of oral penicillin V potassium or a cephalosporin such as cephalexin, or with an intramuscular injection of penicillin G benzathine. Use erythromycin for patients with penicillin allergy. The treatment failure rate after 10 days of penicillin V administered three times daily varies from 6% to 23%. The small difference between the cure rates of penicillin and cephalosporins reported in the literature may represent eradication of the carrier state rather than treatment failure. Causes of treatment failure include unrecognized carriers, poor compliance, reacquisition of a different strain, inactivation of penicillin by β-lactamase, or the development of tolerance by *S pyogenes*. Approximately 5% of *S pyogenes* are resistant to erythromycin. Remember that trimethoprim-sulfamethoxazole is not an effective antibiotic for *S pyogenes*. Children should receive 24 hours of therapy before returning to school.

If the child has a history of recurrent streptococcal infection, one must document the presence of *S pyogenes* in an asymptomatic patient following a course of therapy. If compliance or the adequacy of antibiotic dosage was questionable, treat with intramuscular penicillin; otherwise, treat with an antibiotic effective against β-lactamase-producing organisms (amoxicillin plus clavulanate, a cephalosporin, or a macrolide). If this therapy fails to eradicate the organism, consider a course of clindamycin for 10 days.

In general, the carrier state is harmless, not contagious, and self-limited (2–6 months). An attempt to eradicate the carrier state is warranted only if the patient or another family member has frequent streptococcal infections or when a family member or patient has a history of rheumatic fever or glomerulonephritis.

Consider treatment also for carriers who live in closed or semiclosed community settings. If the patient has had three or more documented infections within 6 months, consider daily penicillin prophylaxis during the winter season. Refer patients for tonsillectomy only when they continue to have frequent episodes or when persistently enlarged tonsils cause chronic upper airway obstruction.

Other rare causes of acute nonviral pharyngitis are *Corynebacterium diphtheriae, Neisseria gonorrhoeae,* group C streptococci, meningococci, *Chlamydia, Francisella tularensis,* and *Mycoplasma pneumoniae.*

Denny FW: Tonsillopharyngitis 1994. Pediatr Rev 1994; 15:185.

Deutsch ES, Isaacson GC: Tonsils and adenoids: An update. Pediatr Rev 1995;16:17.

Tanz RR et al: Clindamycin treatment of chronic pharyngeal carriage of group A streptococci. J Pediatr 1991; 119:123.

Tarlow M: Macrolides in the management of streptococcal pharyngitis/tonsillitis. Pediatr Infect Dis J 1997;16:444.

RECURRENT PHARYNGITIS

School-age children are occasionally brought to a physician with a complaint of recurrent or persistent sore throat. Fever and other systemic manifestations are usually absent. There are three common causes of this problem: mouth breathing, postnasal drip, and school phobia.

Mouth breathing leads to dryness and irritation of the throat, especially in areas of low humidity. Occasionally, children complain even upon awakening that their lips are stuck to their teeth. The causes of mouth breathing should be investigated. Symptomatic treatment consists of good hydration and environmental humidification.

Postnasal drip due to chronic sinusitis can lead to constant irritation of the throat. Examination reveals mucopurulent secretions descending from the nasopharynx after the patient sniffs. The irritation is largely due to repeated clearing of the throat.

Children with **school attendance problems** are brought in repeatedly with complaints of sore throat, but physical examination reveals a normal oropharynx and tonsillar area. The diagnosis is made by asking the parent if the problem has been interfering with the child's school attendance. The answer will be affirmative and completely out of keeping with the symptoms.

PERITONSILLAR CELLULITIS OR ABSCESS
(Quinsy)

Tonsillar infection occasionally penetrates the tonsillar capsule, spreads to the surrounding tissues, and causes peritonsillar cellulitis. If untreated, necrosis occurs and a tonsillar abscess forms. This can occur at any age. The most common cause is β-hemolytic streptococcal infection. Other pathogens are group D streptococci, α-hemolytic streptococci, *S pneumoniae,* and anaerobes.

The patient complains of a severe sore throat even before the physical findings become marked. A high fever is usually present. The process is almost always unilateral. The tonsil bulges medially, and the anterior pillar is prominent. The soft palate and uvula on the involved side are edematous and displaced toward the uninvolved side. In severe cases, trismus, dysphagia, and, finally, drooling occur. The most serious complication of inadequately treated peritonsillar abscess is a lateral pharyngeal abscess. This causes fullness and tenderness of the lateral neck as well as torticollis. Without intervention, the lateral pharyngeal abscess threatens life by airway obstruction or carotid artery erosion.

It is often difficult to differentiate peritonsillar cellulitis from abscess. In adolescents, it is possible to aspirate the peritonsillar space to arrive at the diagnosis. However, it is reasonable to admit a child for 12–24 hours of intravenous antimicrobial therapy, since aggressive treatment in early cases of peritonsillar cellulitis usually prevents suppuration. Therapy with penicillin and clindamycin is appropriate. Failure to respond to therapy during the first 12–24 hours indicates a high probability of abscess formation. An otolaryngologist should be consulted for incision and drainage under general anesthesia.

Recurrent peritonsillar abscesses are so uncommon (7%) that routine tonsillectomy for a single bout is not indicated. Hospitalized patients can be discharged on oral antibiotics when fever has resolved for 24 hours and dysphagia has improved.

RETROPHARYNGEAL ABSCESS

Retropharyngeal nodes drain the adenoids, nasopharynx, and paranasal sinuses and can become infected. The most common causes are β-hemolytic streptococci and *S aureus*. If this pyogenic adenitis goes untreated, a retropharyngeal abscess forms. The process occurs most commonly during the first 2 years of life. Beyond this age, retropharyngeal abscess usually results from superinfection of a penetrating injury of the posterior wall of the oropharynx.

The diagnosis of retropharyngeal abscess should be strongly suspected in an infant with fever, respiratory symptoms, and neck hyperextension. Dysphagia, drooling, dyspnea, and gurgling respirations are also found and are due to impingement by the abscess. Prominent swelling on one side of the posterior pharyngeal wall confirms the diagnosis. Swelling usually stops at the midline because a medial raphe divides the prevertebral space. Lateral neck soft tissue films show the retropharyngeal space to be wider than the C4 vertebral body.

Although retropharyngeal abscess is a surgical emergency, frequently it cannot be distinguished from retropharyngeal adenitis. Immediate hospitalization and intravenous antimicrobial therapy with a semisynthetic penicillin or clindamycin is the first step for most cases. Immediate surgical drainage is required when a definite abscess is seen radiographically or when the airway is markedly compromised. In most instances, a period of 12–24 hours of antimicrobial therapy will help to differentiate the two entities. In the child with adenitis, fever will decrease and oral intake will increase. A child with retropharyngeal abscess will continue to deteriorate. A surgeon should incise and drain the abscess under general anesthesia to prevent its extension. The head should be kept down during incision to prevent aspiration of purulent material.

LUDWIG'S ANGINA

Ludwig's angina is a rapidly progressive cellulitis of the submandibular space. The submandibular space extends from the mucous membrane of the tongue to the muscular and fascial attachments of the hyoid bone. It is infrequently encountered in infants and children. The initiating factor in over 50% of cases is dental disease, including abscesses and extraction. Some patients have a history of lacerations and injuries to the floor of the mouth. Group A streptococci are the most common organisms identified, but other pathogens have been recovered.

The presenting symptoms are fever and tender swelling of the floor of the mouth. The tongue can become enlarged as well as tender and erythematous. Upward displacement of the tongue may cause dysphagia and drooling. Laboratory evaluation includes blood cultures and hypopharyngeal aspiration to attempt to identify the specific pathogen.

Treatment consists of giving high doses of intravenous clindamycin or ampicillin plus nafcillin until the results of cultures and sensitivity tests are available. Because the most common cause of death in Ludwig's angina is sudden airway obstruction, the patient must be monitored closely in the intensive care unit and intubation provided for progressive respiratory distress. Consult an otolaryngologist to identify and perform a drainage procedure.

ACUTE CERVICAL ADENITIS

Local infections of the ear, nose, and throat can spread to a regional node and cause a secondary inflammation there. The most commonly involved node is the jugulodigastric node, which drains the tonsillar area. The problem is most prevalent among preschool children.

The typical case involves a large, unilateral, solitary, tender node. About 70% of these cases are due to β-hemolytic streptococcal infection, 20% are due to staphylococci, and the remainder may be due to viruses. H influenzae type B or anaerobes have rarely been reported as a cause. Surgeons report a higher incidence of staphylococcal infection except in newborns, but they see a greater proportion of atypical cases that have failed to respond to penicillin therapy and thus require incision and drainage. The most common antecedent infection is pharyngitis or tonsillitis. Other entry sites for pyogenic adenitis include periapical dental abscess (usually producing a submandibular adenitis), facial impetigo (infected cuts or bug bites), infected acne, and otitis externa (usually producing a preauricular adenitis).

Early treatment with antibiotics prevents many cases of pyogenic adenitis from progressing to suppuration. However, once fluctuation occurs, antibiotic therapy alone is not sufficient. When fluctuation or pointing is present and the purified protein derivative (PPD) skin test is negative, needle aspiration may promote resolution and surgery may not be needed. If needle aspiration is not effective, the surgeon should incise and drain the abscess. Hospitalization is required only if the patient is toxic, dehydrated, dysphagic, dyspneic, or younger than 6 months of age.

Cat-scratch fever is frequently implicated in cases of chronic cervical adenopathy. The diagnosis is aided by the finding of a primary papule in approximately 61% of cases. In over 90% of cases, cat scratches are present or there is a history of contact with cats. The node is usually mildly tender. The cat-scratch skin test is helpful and relatively safe. Cat-scratch disease, caused by a pleomorphic gram-negative bacillus called *Bartonella henselae,* can be treated orally with rifampin (87% efficacy), ciprofloxacin (84% efficacy), or trimethoprim-sulfamethoxazole (58% efficacy). Intramuscular gentamicin is an acceptable alternative, which is about 73% effective.

Cervical lymphadenitis can be caused by nontuberculous mycobacterial species or *Mycobacterium avium* complex. The adenitis is often unilateral and indolent, developing over a prolonged period of time without systemic signs or much local pain. Atypical mycobacterial infections are often associated with PPD skin reactions less then 10 mm. A positive PPD can cause confusion regarding the possibility of tuberculosis. Fluctuant cervical nodes should be aspirated for Gram's stain and culture. Although treatment usually involves surgical excision, therapy with clarithromycin or rifampin may be tried.

Biaxin

Differential Diagnosis

A. Malignancy and Cervical Nodes: Malignant tumors usually are not suspected until the adenopathy persists despite treatment. Classically, the nodes are painless, nontender, and firm to hard in consistency. They may be fixed to underlying tissues. These nodes may occur as a single node, as unilateral multiple nodes in a chain, as bilateral cervical nodes, or as generalized adenopathy. Common malignancies that may present in the neck include Hodgkin's disease, non-Hodgkin's lymphoma, rhabdomyosarcoma, and thyroid carcinoma.

B. Imitators of Adenitis: Several structures in the neck can become infected and resemble a node. The first three masses are of congenital origin and are listed in order of frequency.

1. Thyroglossal duct cyst–When superinfected, this congenital malformation can become acutely swollen. Helpful findings are the fact that it is in the midline, located between the hyoid bone and suprasternal notch, and moves upward when the tongue is stuck out or during swallowing. Occasionally, the cyst develops a sinus tract and opening just lateral to the midline.

2. Branchial cleft cyst–When superinfected, this can become a tender mass 3–5 cm in diameter. Aids to diagnosis are the fact that the mass is located along the anterior border of the sternocleidomastoid muscle and is smooth and fluctuant, as a cyst should be. Occasionally, it is attached to the overlying skin by a small dimple or a draining sinus tract.

3. Cystic hygroma–Most of these lymphatic cysts are located in the posterior triangle just above the clavicle. The mass is soft and compressible and can be transilluminated. Over 60% of hygromas are noted at birth, and the remainder are usually seen by the time the child is 2 years of age. If cysts become large enough, they can compromise swallowing and breathing.

4. Parotitis–The most common pitfall in differential diagnosis of cervical adenopathy is mistaking parotitis for adenitis. However, a swollen parotid crosses the angle of the jaw, is associated with pre-auricular percussion tenderness, is bilateral in 70% of cases, and there is often a history of exposure to mumps and no mumps immunization. Submandibular parotitis can present a diagnostic dilemma.

5. Ranula–A ranula is a cyst in the floor of the mouth caused by obstruction of the ducts of the sublingual gland. A plunging ranula extends below the mylohyoid muscle and can present as a neck mass.

6. Sternocleidomastoid muscle hematoma–This cervical mass is noted at 2–4 weeks of age. On close examination, it is found to be part of the muscle body and not movable. An associated torticollis is usually confirmatory.

Bass JW, Vincent JM, Person DA: The expanding spectrum of *Bartonella* infections: II. Cat-scratch disease. Pediatr Infect Dis J 1997;16:163.

Chesney PJ: Cervical adenopathy. Pediatr Rev 1994; 15:276.

Gorenstein A, Somekh E: Suppurative cervical lymphadenitis: Treatment by needle aspirations. Pediatr Infect Dis J 1994;7:669.

SNORING, MOUTH BREATHING, & UPPER AIRWAY OBSTRUCTION

A child is sometimes brought in with complaints such as "he always breathes through his mouth," "he snores," or "he can't sleep at night." Large adenoids can be suspected in such cases if the typical "adenoid facies" is observed. The adenoids can be assessed by mirror examination, endoscopy, or radiographic studies. Severe cases of allergic rhinitis present like any other causes of nasal obstruction. History and physical examination will assist in the diagnosis. Nasal polyps appear as glistening, gray to pink, jelly-like masses that are prominent just inside the anterior nares and occur singly or in clusters. They occur in cystic fibrosis and severe allergic rhinitis. Do not mistake the turbinates for polyps. Persistent mouth breathing may be due to obstruction by nasopharyngeal tumor or by meningocele or encephalocele herniated into the nasal cavity. If unilateral nasal obstruction and epistaxis occur frequently, juvenile angiofibroma should be suspected.

Diagnosis

A lateral neck radiograph or fiberoptic nasopharyngoscopy will help assess the relative size of the adenoids. When episodes of hypopnea or obstructive apnea, poor weight gain, or clinical signs of cardiac disease are present, a chest radiograph and electrocardiogram should be obtained. Children with severe snoring may also develop obstructive sleep apnea or hypopnea, which can be identified by a sleep study polysomnogram. **Obstructive sleep apnea** is defined as periods when air flow stops for 6–10 seconds, associated with respiratory effort or bradycardia or with oxygen desaturation or termination with gasping and agitated arousal. **Hypopnea** is defined as loud snoring during sleep with periods of reduced airflow for 10 seconds or longer, associated with oxygen desaturation or arousal. (These are definitions for adults, since criteria for children are not established.) A sleep study polysomnogram measures heart rate, oxygen saturation, oronasal airflow, chest wall movement, and oronasal $PaCO_2$ along with electrocardiography and electroencephalography. The absence of oronasal airflow with the presence of chest wall movement, oxygen desaturation, and bradycardia is diagnostic of obstructive sleep apnea.

Demain JG, Goetz DW: Pediatric adenoidal hypertrophy and nasal airway obstruction. Otolaryngol Head Neck Surg 1991;105:427.

Everett AD, Koch WC, Saulsbury FT: Failure to thrive due to obstructive sleep apnea. Clin Pediatr 1987;26:90.

McBride JT: Snoring. Pediatr Rev 1993;14:445.

TONSILLECTOMY & ADENOIDECTOMY (T&A)

Tonsillectomy

The following conditions are indications for tonsillectomy with or without adenoidectomy: pulmonary conditions such as chronic hypoxia related to upper airway obstruction or hypopnea-obstructive sleep apnea, orofacial conditions such as mandibular growth abnormalities, dental malocclusion and swallowing disorders, speech abnormalities, and persistent or recurrent infections.

Chronic hypoxia related to upper airway obstruction can result in signs of right heart failure (cor pulmonale) or pulmonary hypertension. Obstructive sleep apnea presents with loud snoring during sleep with periods of respiratory pauses terminated with gasping and agitated arousal. In young children, sleep apnea should not be confused with restless sleep patterns, trained night feeders, and trained night crying. There is no consensus on the infectious criteria for tonsillectomy. Reasonable indications are four or more documented *S pyogenes* infections per year, a documented *S pyogenes* carrier state resistant to medical therapy, or six or more tonsillitis episodes per year or five or more per year for 2 years.

Adenoidectomy

The adenoids, composed of lymphoid tissue in the nasopharynx, are a component of Waldeyer's ring of lymphoid tissue with the palatine tonsils and lingual tonsils. Enlargement of the adenoids with or without infection can obstruct the upper airway, alter normal orofacial growth, and interfere with speech, swallowing, or auditory tube function. Most children with prolonged mouth breathing eventually develop dental malocclusion and what has been termed an adenoidal facies. The face is pinched and the maxilla narrowed because the molding pressures of the orbicularis oris and buccinator muscles are unopposed by the tongue. The role of hypertrophy and chronic infection in the pathogenesis of sinusitis is unclear.

Indications for adenoidectomy with or without tonsillectomy include pulmonary conditions such as chronic hypoxia related to upper airway obstruction, hypopnea, or obstructive sleep apnea; orofacial conditions such as mandibular growth abnormalities, dental malocclusion, and swallowing disorders; speech abnormalities; and persistent middle ear effusion. Children with suspected velopharyngeal insufficiency such as those with cleft palate should not have adenoidectomy except when there is a life-threatening obstruction.

Complications of T&A

The reported mortality rates associated with T&A vary from 4 to 6 per 100,000 procedures; the rate of hemorrhage has been reported to vary from 0.4 to 5 per hundred. Some children with previously normal speech develop hypernasal speech. The emotional hazards of hospitalization and surgery in a child under 5 years of age have been well documented.

Contraindications to T&A

A. Short Palate: Adenoids should not be removed in a child with a cleft palate or submucous cleft palate because of the risk of aggravating the velopharyngeal incompetence and causing hypernasal speech and nasal regurgitation. Occasionally, a "modified" adenoidectomy is performed in a child with marked obstructive sleep apnea who has a submucous cleft palate.

B. Bleeding Disorder: If a chronic bleeding disorder is present, it must be diagnosed and compensated for before T&A.

C. Acute Tonsillitis: An elective T&A should be postponed until acute tonsillitis is resolved. This guideline may prevent superinfection of the wound.

Deutsch ES, Isaacson GC: Tonsils and adenoids: An update. Pediatr Rev 1995;16:17.

Paradise JL et al: Efficacy of tonsillectomy for recurrent throat infection in severely affected children. N Engl J Med 1984;310:674.

DISORDERS OF THE LIPS

Labial Sucking Tubercle

A small baby may present with a small callus in the mid upper lip. It usually is asymptomatic and disappears after cup feeding is initiated.

Cheilitis

Dry, cracked, scaling lips are usually due to sun or wind exposure. Contact dermatitis from mouthpieces or various woodwind or brass instruments has also been reported. Licking the lips accentuates the process, and the patient should be warned of this. Liberal use of lip balms gives excellent results.

Inclusion Cyst

Inclusion (retention) cysts are due to the obstruction of mucous glands or other mucous membrane structures. In the newborn, they occur on the hard palate or gums and are called Epstein's pearls. These small cysts resolve spontaneously in 1–2 months. In older children, inclusion cysts usually occur on the palate, uvula, or tonsillar pillars. They appear as taut yellow sacs varying in size from 2 to 10 mm. Inclusion cysts that do not spontaneously resolve should undergo incision and drainage. Occasionally, a mucous cyst on the lower lip (mucocele) requires drainage for cosmetic reasons. Minor salivary glands are present at this site, and biting the lip may sever their ducts and initiate the problem.

DISORDERS OF THE TONGUE

Geographic Tongue (Benign Migratory Glossitis)

This condition of unknown cause is characterized by circular or elliptical smooth areas on the tongue devoid of papillae and surrounded by a narrow ring of hyperkeratosis. The pattern can change from day to day. The lesions are painless and may last months to years. This puzzling disorder is benign, uncommon after age 6, and requires no treatment.

Fissured Tongue (Scrotal Tongue)

This condition is marked by numerous irregular fissures on the dorsum of the tongue. It occurs in approximately 1% of the population and is usually a dominant trait. It is also frequently seen in children with trisomy 21 and other retarded patients who have the habit of chewing on a protruded tongue.

Coated Tongue (Furry Tongue)

The tongue normally becomes coated if mastication is impaired and the patient is taking a liquid or soft diet. Mouth breathing, fever, or dehydration can accentuate the process.

Macroglossia

Tongue hypertrophy and protrusion may be a clue to Beckwith-Wiedemann syndrome, glycogen storage disease, cretinism, Hurler's syndrome, lymphangioma, or hemangioma. Tongue reduction procedures should be considered in otherwise healthy subjects when macroglossia affects airway patency, eating, dental development, and normal mandibular growth. In trisomy 21, the normal-sized tongue protrudes because the oral cavity is small.

HALITOSIS

"Bad breath" is a puzzling and distressing complaint. In most cases, it is due to acute stomatitis, pharyngitis, or sinusitis. In children, there are two common causes of chronic halitosis: mouth breathing and thumb or blanket sucking. In older children and adolescents, halitosis can be one of the presenting symptoms of chronic sinusitis, gastric bezoar, bronchiectasis, and lung abscess. In older children, the presence of orthodontic devices or dentures can cause halitosis if good dental hygiene is not maintained. Halitosis can also be caused by decaying food particles embedded in cryptic tonsils. In adolescents, tobacco use is a common cause. Offensive skin odors (eg, dirty feet) of long duration can be absorbed and excreted through the lungs. Mouthwashes and chewable breath fresheners give limited improvement. The cause must be uncovered to help the patient with chronic halitosis.

SALIVARY GLAND DISORDERS

Suppurative Parotitis

Suppurative parotitis is an uncommon clinical disorder found chiefly in newborns and debilitated older patients. The parotid gland is swollen, tender, and often reddened. The diagnosis is made by expression of purulent material from Stensen's duct. The material should be smeared and cultured. Fever and leukocytosis may be present.

Treatment includes hospitalization and intravenous nafcillin because the most common causative organism is *S aureus*.

Recurrent Idiopathic Parotitis

Some children experience repeated episodes of parotid swelling that lasts 1–2 weeks and then resolves spontaneously. There is usually mild pain and often no fever. The process is most often unilateral, a fact that argues against an autoimmune process as the underlying cause and suggests instead some sort of obstructive process. Serum amylase is normal, which speaks against a diagnosis of viral parotitis, as can occur with mumps, parainfluenza infection, and other viral infections. As many as ten episodes may occur from age 2 years on. Antibiotic prophylaxis may reduce the number of episodes. The problem usually resolves spontaneously at puberty.

Treatment includes analgesics if pain is present. A 4-day course of corticosteroids can be recommended if it can be initiated early in an attack. A second attack of parotid swelling without fever should result in referral to an otolaryngologist for a sialogram to rule out calculus of Stensen's duct. The usual finding is sialectasia. The sialogram seems to improve as the recurrence rate diminishes.

Giglio MS, Landaeta M, Pinto ME: Microbiology of recurrent parotitis. Pediatr Infect Dis J 1997;16:386.

Tumors of the Parotid Gland

Mixed tumors, hemangiomas, and leukemia can present in the parotid gland as a hard or persistent mass. The patient should be referred to an oncologist and a surgeon.

Ranula

A ranula is a retention cyst of a sublingual salivary gland. It is found on the floor of the mouth to one side of the lingual frenulum. Ranula has been described as resembling a frog's belly because it is thin-walled and contains a clear bluish fluid. Referral to an otolaryngologist for excision of the cyst and associated sublingual gland is the treatment of choice.

CONGENITAL ORAL MALFORMATIONS

Tongue-Tie (Ankyloglossia)

The tightness of the lingual frenulum varies greatly among normal people. A short frenulum prevents both protrusion and elevation of the tongue. Puckering of the midline of the tongue occurring with tongue movement usually does not interfere with speech.

Treatment consists of reassurance. Although there is no evidence to support it, clipping of the frenulum is sometimes recommended if the tongue does not protrude beyond the teeth or gums. If this degree of tongue-tie is associated with impairment of rapid articulation, the patient should be referred to an otolaryngologist for correction. Casual frenulum clipping can result in significant bleeding.

Levy PA: Tongue tie: Management of a short sublingual frenulum. Pediatr Rev 1995;16:345.

Cleft Lip & Cleft Palate

Cleft lip, cleft palate, or both conditions are found in 1:800 live births. They are readily diagnosed in the newborn nursery. Treatment requires a multidisciplinary team approach—plastic surgeons, otolaryngologist, audiologists, speech therapists, orthodontists, and prosthodontists. Cleft lip repair is usually performed before 3 months of age. Cleft palate repair is usually performed at about 12 months of age and is essential to permit normal speech development, which should begin at this time. Approximately 90% of children with cleft palate have recurrent or persistent otitis media and must be carefully followed. Some otolaryngologists recommend prophylactic tympanoplasty tubes.

Bifid Uvula & Submucous Cleft Palate

A bifid uvula is present in 3% of healthy children. However, there is a close association (as high as 75%) between bifid uvula and submucous cleft palate. A submucous cleft can be diagnosed by noting a translucent zone in the middle of the soft palate. Palpation of the hard palate reveals absence of the posterior bony portion. Affected children have a 40% risk of developing persistent middle ear effusion. They are at risk also of incomplete closure of the palate, resulting in hypernasal speech. During feeding, some of these infants experience nasal regurgitation of food. Children with submucous cleft palate causing abnormal speech or nasal regurgitation of food need referral to a surgeon for repair.

High-Arched Palate

A high-arched palate is usually a genetic trait of no consequence. It is seen also in children who are chronic mouth breathers and in premature infants who undergo prolonged oral intubation. Some rare causes of high-arched palate are congenital disorders such as Marfan's syndrome, Treacher Collins' syndrome, and Ehlers-Danlos syndrome.

Robin (Pierre Robin) Sequence

This congenital malformation is characterized by the triad of micrognathia, cleft palate, and glossoptosis. Affected children present as emergencies in the newborn period because of infringement on the airway by the tongue. The main objective of treatment is to prevent asphyxia until the mandible becomes large enough to accommodate the tongue. In some cases, this objective can be achieved by leaving the child in a prone position while unattended. In severe cases, a tracheostomy is required. The child requires close observation and careful feeding until the problem is outgrown.

17 Respiratory Tract & Mediastinum

Gary L. Larsen, MD, Frank J. Accurso, MD, Robin R. Deterding, MD,
Ann C. Halbower, MD, & Carl W. White, MD

I. RESPIRATORY TRACT

Pediatric pulmonary diseases account for almost 50% of deaths in children under 1 year of age and about 20% of all hospitalizations of children under 15 years of age. Approximately 7% of children suffer some sort of chronic disorder of the lower respiratory system. Understanding the pathophysiology of many pediatric pulmonary diseases requires an appreciation of the normal growth and development of the lung. These matters are dealt with initially, followed by discussions of congenital and acquired diseases of the respiratory tract and mediastinum.

GROWTH & DEVELOPMENT

The lung derives from the foregut during the fourth week of gestation. Subsequent branching leads to development of the conducting airways (bronchial tree) by about 16 weeks. The terminal respiratory units—the gas-exchanging portion of the lung—develop from the latter third of gestation through the first few months after birth, when alveoli with adult morphology are formed. It is clear that alveoli increase in number throughout childhood, but the age at which this increase normally stops is controversial, with estimates ranging from 2 years to adolescence. Development of the pulmonary arterial system in general occurs with development of the airways, whereas capillary proliferation in the terminal respiratory units occurs with development of the alveoli.

At birth, the lung assumes the gas-exchanging function served by the placenta in utero, placing immediate stress on all components of the respiratory system. Abnormalities in the lung, respiratory mus-

cles, chest wall, airway, respiratory controller, or pulmonary circulation may therefore be present at birth. Survival after delivery depends, for example, on the development of the surfactant system to maintain airway stability and allow gas exchange. Immaturity of the surfactant system, often seen in infants of less than 35 weeks' gestational age, can result in severe respiratory morbidity in the immediate neonatal period as well as subsequent chronic lung disease. A lethal form of lung disease has recently been recognized in infants homozygous for abnormalities in the surfactant protein B gene. Persistent pulmonary hypertension of the newborn—failure of the normal transition to a low-resistance pulmonary circulation at birth—can complicate a number of neonatal respiratory diseases.

Several mechanical properties of the respiratory system in infants increase the risk of respiratory compromise. The upper airway in infants is smaller and less firm than the upper airway in adults; therefore, obstruction in response to infection, inflammation, or foreign body is more likely. The greater compliance of the infant's chest wall allows for collapse or labored breathing when respiration is obstructed. In addition, the infant has fewer fatigue-resistant diaphragmatic muscle fibers, so respiratory muscle fatigue may occur earlier in response to an increased load.

Infants' airways are now thought capable of responding to bronchoactive agents. The mechanisms responsible for this are not completely understood but probably include contractile elements in the airway that respond to neural stimuli. Recent studies also suggest that genetic and environmental factors play a role in the development of airway reactivity. Pulmonary defense mechanisms, including cough, mucociliary clearance, and local and circulating components of the immune system, are present at birth.

Merkus PJFM, ten Have-Opbroek AAW, Quanjer PH: Human lung growth: A review. Pediatr Pulmonol 1996; 21:383.

DIAGNOSTIC AIDS

PHYSICAL EXAMINATION OF THE RESPIRATORY TRACT

Assessing the rate, depth, ease, symmetry, and rhythm of respiration is critical to the detection of pulmonary disease. Attention should be paid to tracheal position and thoracic configuration. Auscultation should assess the quality of breath sounds and detect the presence of abnormal sounds such as fine or course crackles, wheezing, or rhonchi.

Extrapulmonary manifestations of pulmonary disease include growth failure, altered mental status (with hypoxemia or hypercapnia), cyanosis, clubbing, and osteoarthropathy. In a recent study of children with respiratory illnesses, abnormalities of attentiveness, consolability, respiratory effort, color, and movement had a good diagnostic accuracy in detecting hypoxemia. Evidence of cor pulmonale (loud pulmonic component of the second heart sound, hepatomegaly, elevated neck veins, and, rarely, peripheral edema) signifies advanced lung disease.

Respiratory disorders can be secondary to disease in other systems. It is therefore important to look for other conditions such as congenital heart disease (murmur, gallop), neuromuscular disease (muscle wasting, scoliosis), immunodeficiency (rash, diarrhea), and autoimmune disease or occult malignancy (arthritis, hepatosplenomegaly).

Accurso FJ, Eigen H, Loughlin GM: History and physical examination. In: *Respiratory Disease in Children: Diagnosis and Management.* Loughlin GM, Eigen H (editors). Williams & Wilkins, 1994.

Margolis PA et al: Accuracy of the clinical examination in detecting hypoxemia in infants with respiratory illness. J Pediatr 1994;124:552.

PULMONARY FUNCTION TESTS

Lung function tests can measure disease severity, define precipitants of symptoms, and evaluate therapy. They can help define the risks of anesthesia and surgery and assist in the planning of respiratory care in the postoperative period. However, the range of normal values for a test may be wide, and the predicted normal values change dramatically with growth. For this reason, serial determinations of lung function are often more informative than a single determination. Patient cooperation is essential for almost all physiologic assessments. Most children are not able to perform the necessary maneuvers before 5 years of age. Despite these problems, tests of lung function may still contribute to the care of children.

Spirometers are available on which forced vital capacity can be recorded either as a volume-time tracing (spirogram) or a flow-volume curve. The patient inhales maximally, holds the breath for a short period, and then exhales as fast as possible for at least 3 seconds. The tracing produced by the exhalation shows forced vital capacity (FVC), which is the total amount of air that is exhaled from maximum inspiration, and the forced expiratory volume (FEV) in the first second of the exhalation (FEV_1). The maximum midexpiratory flow rate (MMEF, or $FEF_{25-75\%}$), is the mean flow rate during the middle portion of the FVC maneuver. The FEV_1/FVC ratio is calculated from these absolute values; a ratio greater than 0.8 in children and young adults shows unlimited normal airflow.

These basic tests of lung function differentiate obstructive from restrictive processes. Examples of obstructive processes include asthma, chronic bronchitis, and cystic fibrosis; restrictive problems include chest wall deformities that limit lung expansion and interstitial processes due to collagen-vascular diseases, hypersensitivity pneumonitis, and interstitial fibrosis. Classically, diseases that obstruct airflow decrease the FEV_1 more than the FVC, so that the FEV_1/FVC ratio is low. In restrictive problems, however, the decreases in the FEV_1 and FVC are proportionate; thus, the ratio of FEV_1 to FVC is either normal or high. Clinical suspicion of a restrictive disease is usually an indication for referral to a specialist for evaluation.

The peak expiratory flow rate (PEFR), the maximal flow recorded during an FVC maneuver, can be assessed by hand-held devices and the results recorded. This practice may be helpful in following the course of various pulmonary disorders, especially those that are difficult to control and require multiple medications (eg, steroid-dependent asthma). These devices can also be used to give patients with poor perception of their disease an awareness of a decrease in lung function, thus facilitating earlier treatment.

Cross D, Nelson HS: The role of the peak flow meter in the diagnosis and management of asthma. J Allergy Clin Immunol 1991;87:120.

Wenzel SE, Larsen GL: Assessment of lung function: Pulmonary function tests. In: *Allergy, Asthma, and Immunology from Infancy to Childhood,* 3rd ed. Bierman CW et al (editors). Saunders, 1995.

ARTERIAL BLOOD GASES & NONINVASIVE ASSESSMENT OF OXYGEN TENSION & SATURATION

Arterial blood gas determination defines the balance between respiration at the tissue level and that in the lungs. Assessment of blood gases is essential in critically ill children and may be used also for determining the severity of lung involvement in chronic conditions. Blood gas measurements are affected by abnormalities of respiratory control, gas exchange, respiratory mechanics, and the circulation. In pediatrics, hypoxia (low PaO_2) most commonly results from mismatching of ventilation and perfusion. Hypercapnia (elevated $PaCO_2$) results from inadequate alveolar ventilation, ie, inability to clear the CO_2 produced. This is termed hypoventilation. Causes include decreased central respiratory drive, paralysis of respiratory muscles, or low tidal volume breathing as seen in restrictive lung diseases, severe scoliosis, or chest wall trauma. Table 17–1 gives normal values for arterial pH, PaO_2, and $PaCO_2$ at sea level and at 5000 feet.

Transcutaneous gas monitoring is a noninvasive assessment of PaO_2 and $PaCO_2$ using electrodes that measure gas tension at the skin surface. This allows continuous blood gas monitoring of patients prone to hypoventilation, eg, the critically ill or those with sleep apnea syndromes. However, transcutaneous monitoring can underestimate the $PaCO_2$ and overestimate the $PaCO_2$ unless skin perfusion is maximal. Thus, heating of the skin site is required and cardiac function should be stable. Low cardiac output, low blood pressure, or a hematocrit less than 30% reduces the reliability of this form of blood gas monitoring. The disadvantage of this system is the long calibration time, the lesser reliability in older children with thicker skin, and the need to move the electrode to avoid skin burns.

Pulse oximetry (measuring light absorption by transilluminating the skin) is the most reliable and easiest form of noninvasive monitoring of oxygenation. Oxygenated hemoglobin absorbs red light at certain wavelengths. Measurement during a systolic pulse allows estimation of arterial oxygen saturation as the machine corrects for the light absorbed at the tissue level between pulses. No heating of the skin is necessary. Values of oxygen saturation are reliable as low as 80%. The pulse oximeter has reduced reliability during conditions causing reduced arterial pulsation such as hypothermia, hypotension, or infusion of vasoconstrictor drugs. Carbon monoxide bound by hemoglobin results in higher than actual oxygen saturation readings.

Hay WW Jr, Thilo E, Curlander JB: Pulse oximetry in neonatal medicine. Clin Perinatol 1991;18:441.

Table 17–1. Normal arterial blood gas values on room air.

	pH	Pao₂ (mm Hg)	Paco₂ (mm Hg)
Sea level	7.38–7.42	85–95	36–42
5000 feet	7.36–7.40	65–75	35–40

Shapiro BA, Peruzzi WT: Transcutaneous gas monitoring In: *Clinical Application of Blood Gases,* 5th ed. Mosby, 1994.

CULTURE OF MATERIAL FROM THE RESPIRATORY TRACT

Expectorated sputum is rarely available from patients under 5–6 years of age. In older children, a Gram-stained smear of sputum showing significant numbers of organisms within neutrophils may identify a pathogen. Bacterial stains and cultures of nasopharyngeal secretions are frequently misleading.

Cultures from the lower respiratory tract can be obtained (1) by tracheal aspiration through an endotracheal tube or rigid or fiberoptic bronchoscope, (2) by transtracheal percutaneous aspiration, (3) by lung puncture, or (4) by the double-brush technique through a fiberoptic bronchoscope. The latter (preferred) technique can be used to obtain endobronchial secretions in older critically ill or debilitated children large enough to accommodate the large (4.9 mm) bronchoscope required.

Complications are most likely to occur with transtracheal percutaneous aspiration or lung puncture, and samples obtained by other means are more likely to be contaminated with oropharyngeal flora and may not be the best guide to therapy. Where thoracoscopic lung biopsy by a skilled operator is unavailable, lung puncture directed to an area of consolidation by CT scan or fluoroscopy may be the best approach for a child who deteriorates after initial antibiotic therapy or who is critically ill or immunocompromised. However, pneumothorax may complicate the picture. Open lung biopsy, though a major intervention, should be considered in the worsening or critically ill child when other approaches are unsuccessful. In skilled hands, thoracoscopic lung biopsy may obviate the open procedure and some of its potential complications. Thoracentesis should be performed when pleural fluid is present. Blood glucose and lactate dehydrogenase should be drawn simultaneously for comparison with pleural fluid levels. Blood cultures provide specific diagnoses and must be obtained in children with acute pneumonia.

Specimens obtained by invasive means should be studied for the following: (1) viruses, (2) *Mycoplasma pneumoniae*, (3) *Chlamydia*, (4) *Legionella pneumophila*, (5) *Bordetella pertussis*, (6) fungi (including *Pneumocystis carinii*), (7) acid-fast bacteria, and (8) anaerobes or other bacteria. These specimens should be studied for potential pathogens using rapid diagnostic techniques such as immunofluorescent antibody and enzyme-linked immunosorbent assay (ELISA). Counterimmunoelectrophoresis performed on pleural fluid, serum, or concentrated urine may help identify disease due to *Streptococcus pneumoniae* or *Haemophilus influenzae*. Because these tests can be performed quickly, they may obviate further, more invasive studies.

Alpert BE, O'Sullivan BP, Panitch HB: Nonbronchoscopic approach to bronchoalveolar lavage in children with artificial airways. Pediatr Pulmonol 1992;13:38.

Godfrey S et al: Yield from flexible bronchoscopy in children. Pediatr Pulmonol 1997;2:261.

Koumbourlis AC, Kurland G: Nonbronchoscopic bronchoalveolar lavage in mechanically ventilated infants: Technique, efficacy, and applications. Pediatr Pulmonol 1993;15:257.

IMAGING OF THE RESPIRATORY TRACT

The plain chest radiograph remains one of the most important techniques for investigating suspected lung disease. Both frontal and lateral views should be obtained. The radiograph is useful for evaluating air trapping caused by airway obstruction, volume loss caused by pneumonia, and interstitial problems such as pulmonary edema. Hyperaeration is best demonstrated in lateral views as flattening of the diaphragm. It is a common finding because young children commonly develop small airway obstruction and asthma. Parenchymal changes may cause increased interstitial markings, consolidation, air bronchograms, or loss of diaphragm or heart contours. When pleural fluid is suspected, lateral decubitus films may be helpful in determining the extent and mobility of the fluid. When a foreign body is suspected, forced expiratory films may demonstrate focal air trapping and shift of the mediastinum to the contralateral side. Lateral neck films can be useful in assessing the size of adenoids and tonsils and also in differentiating croup from epiglottitis, the latter being associated with the "thumbprint" sign.

Barium swallow is indicated for patients with suspected aspiration to detect swallowing dysfunction, tracheoesophageal fistula, gastroesophageal reflux, and achalasia. This technique is also important in detecting vascular rings and slings, because most of these abnormalities compress the esophagus. Airway fluoroscopy is another important tool for assessing both fixed airway obstruction (eg, tracheal stenosis) and dynamic airway obstruction (eg, tracheomalacia). Fluoroscopy or ultrasound of the diaphragm can detect paralysis by demonstrating paradoxic movement of the involved hemidiaphragm.

High-resolution computed tomography (CT scanning) is useful to evaluate diffuse infiltrative lung disease, metastatic disease, mediastinal masses, and chest wall disease. Characteristic patterns seen in interstitial lung disease (such as honeycombing in pulmonary fibrosis) or airway disease (such as bronchiectasis) are often missed on chest radiographs. MRI is useful for defining subtle or complex abnormalities and vascular rings. Ventilation/perfusion scans can provide information about regional ventilation and perfusion and can help detect vascular malformations and pulmonary emboli (rare in children). Pulmonary angiography is occasionally necessary to define the pulmonary vascular bed more precisely. Bronchography is rarely done in the United States but can be useful in the specific circumstance of contemplated lobectomy for suspected localized bronchiectasis.

Gibson AT et al: Imaging the neonatal chest. Clin Radiol 1997;52:172.

Kuhn JP: High resolution computed tomography of pediatric pulmonary disorders. Radiol Clin North Am 1993;31:453.

Newman B: The pediatric chest. Radiol Clin North Am 1993;31:453.

LARYNGOSCOPY & BRONCHOSCOPY

The indications for laryngoscopy include undiagnosed hoarseness, stridor, and symptoms of obstructive sleep apnea; indications for bronchoscopy include wheezing, suspected foreign body, pneumonia, atelectasis, chronic cough, hemoptysis, and placement of an endotracheal tube and assessment of patency. In general, the more specific the indication, the higher the diagnostic yield.

Pediatric bronchoscopy instruments are of either the flexible fiberoptic or rigid open tube type. The advantages of using a flexible bronchoscope include the following: (1) With sedation and topical anesthetics, the procedure can be done at the bedside; (2) evaluation of the upper airway can be done with little risk in patients who are awake; (3) the distal airways of intubated patients can be examined without removing the endotracheal tube; (4) the instrument can be used as an obturator to intubate a patient with a difficult upper airway; (5) endotracheal tube placement and patency can be checked; (6) assessment of airway dynamics is generally better; and (7) it is possible to examine more distal airways. The advantages of using a rigid instrument are (1) easier removal of foreign bodies (for this reason, rigid bronchoscopy remains the procedure of choice for suspected foreign body aspiration); (2) better airway control, which allows the patient to be ventilated through the bronchoscope; and (3) superior optics. The choice of procedures depends largely on the expertise available.

Bronchoalveolar lavage through a flexible bronchoscope is being used routinely in children to detect infection in both the immunocompetent and the immunocompromised host. Aspiration and hemorrhage are also suspected in the presence of lipid- and hemosiderin-laden macrophages, respectively. Transbronchial biopsy is being done often to look for infection and rejection in transplant patients and to diagnose other conditions such as sarcoidosis.

Green CG, Holinger LD, Gartlan MG: Technique. In: *Pediatric Laryngology and Bronchoesophagology.* Holinger LD, Lusk RP, Green CG (editors). Lippincott-Raven, 1997.

Schnellhase DE, Fan LL: Flexible endoscopy in the diagnosis and management of neonatal and pediatric airway and pulmonary disorders. Respir Care 1995;40:48.

GENERAL THERAPY OF PEDIATRIC LUNG DISEASES

OXYGEN THERAPY

Oxygen therapy in children with respiratory disease can reduce the work of breathing, resulting in fewer respiratory symptoms; relax the pulmonary vasculature, lessening the potential for pulmonary hypertension and congestive heart failure; and improve feeding. Patients breathing spontaneously can be treated by nasal cannula, head hood, or mask (including simple, rebreathing, nonrebreathing, or Venturi masks). The general goal of oxygen therapy is to achieve an arterial oxygen tension of 65–90 mm Hg or an oxygen saturation above 92%. The actual oxygen concentration achieved by nasal cannula or mask depends on the flow rate, the type of mask used, and the patient's age. Small changes in flow rate during oxygen administration by nasal cannula can lead to substantial changes in inspired oxygen concentration in young infants. The amount of oxygen required to correct hypoxemia may vary according to the child's activity. It is not unusual, for example, for an infant with chronic lung disease to require 0.75 L/min while awake but 1 L/min while asleep or feeding.

Although the head hood is an efficient device for delivery of oxygen in young infants, the nasal cannula is used more often because it allows the infant greater mobility. The cannula generally has nasal prongs that are inserted in the nares, but it can be modified by removing the prongs. This nasal catheter can then be taped under the nose or inserted in the nasopharynx. Flow through the nasal cannula should generally not exceed 3 L/min to avoid excessive drying of the mucosa. Even at high flow rates, oxygen by nasal cannula rarely delivers inspired oxygen concentrations greater than 40–45%. In contrast, partial rebreathing and non-rebreathing masks or head hoods achieve inspired oxygen concentrations as high as 90–100%.

Because the physical findings of hypoxemia are subtle, the adequacy of oxygenation should be measured as the arterial oxygen tension or by transcutaneous P_{O_2} monitoring. In addition, oxygen saturation can be determined by oximetry. The advantages of these latter noninvasive methods include the ability to obtain continuous measurements during various normal activities and to avoid artifacts caused by crying or breath holding during attempts at arterial puncture. For children with chronic cardiopulmonary disorders that may require supplemental oxygen therapy (eg, bronchopulmonary dysplasia or cystic fibrosis), frequent noninvasive assessments are essential to ensure the safety and adequacy of treatment.

Lester LA: Oxygen therapy. In: *Pediatric Respiratory Disease. Diagnosis and Treatment.* Hilman BC (editor). Saunders, 1993.

INHALATION OF BRONCHODILATORS

Airway obstruction that is at least partially reversed by a bronchodilator can be seen in cystic fibrosis, bronchiolitis, and bronchopulmonary dysplasia as well as in acute and chronic asthma.

The β-adrenergic agonists may be delivered by metered-dose inhaler (MDI), dry powder inhaler, or nebulizer. MDIs are convenient to use and are best combined with spacing devices for children who lack the ability to coordinate actuation of the MDI with inhalation. On the other hand, the nebulizer is a more effective method of delivering medication to infants and young children. Long-acting inhaled β_2-adrenergic agents relatively selective for the respiratory tract are now available (see Chapter 32). In the treatment of acute episodes of airway obstruction, the inhaled adrenergic agents have been shown to be as effective as the injectable agents. In addition, delivery of the drug by the aerosol route produces fewer side effects. These drugs can be safely administered at home as long as both the physician and the family realize that a poor response may signify the need for corticosteroids to help restore β-adrenergic responsiveness.

Anticholinergic agents may also acutely decrease airway obstruction. Furthermore, they may yield a longer duration of bronchodilation than do many adrenergic agents. Selected patients may benefit from receiving both β-adrenergic and anticholinergic agents. In general, this class of drugs is most effective in the treatment of chronic bronchitis.

Goren A et al: Assessment of the ability of young children to use a powder inhaler device (Turbuhaler). Pediatr Pulmonol 1994;18:77.

Nelson HS: Drug therapy: Beta-adrenergic bronchodilators. N Engl J Med 1995;333.

Shuh S et al: Efficacy of frequent nebulized ipratropium bromide added to frequent high-dose albuterol therapy in severe childhood asthma. J Pediatr 1995; 126:639.

PULMONARY PHYSIOTHERAPY

Chest physical therapy, with postural drainage, percussion, and forced expiratory maneuvers, has been widely used to improve the clearance of secretions even though there are few efficacy studies of the techniques used—chest physical therapy is not of proved efficacy in adults with uncomplicated pneumonias. Nevertheless, children with cystic fibrosis show less decline in pulmonary function if treated with traditional postural drainage and percussion than with directed coughing alone.

Postural drainage requires positioning of the patient to favor emptying each of the segmental bronchi. Percussion or vibration is used to loosen secretions and facilitate drainage. The positions and the technique of percussion should be carefully reviewed with the parents. In general, the patient spends 1–2 minutes in each of nine body positions (ie, 10–20 minutes for the duration of a treatment). Treatments may be given one to four times a day at home and sometimes more frequently in the hospital setting. Patients are encouraged to cough regularly during the procedure. Children who cannot be encouraged to cough may require pharyngeal suctioning by trained personnel.

"Blow bottles" that provide the patient feedback about respiratory efforts (incentive spirometry) may also encourage deep breathing. This technique is particularly useful in patients recovering from surgery.

Reisman JJ et al: Role of conventional physiotherapy in cystic fibrosis. J Pediatr 1988;113:632.

AVOIDANCE OF ENVIRONMENTAL HAZARDS

All parents or other caregivers should be counseled about environmental hazards to the lung. The list of potential hazards includes small objects that may be aspirated, allergens that can precipitate respiratory symptoms in atopic children, and cigarette smoke.

The harmful effects of smoking in the home deserve special emphasis. Children from families where the parents and others smoke have decreased lung growth as well as decreased pulmonary function in comparison with children raised in smoke-free homes. Exposure of children to tobacco smoke also leads to an increased frequency of lower respiratory tract infections and an increased incidence of respiratory symptoms, including recurrent wheezing. Health care providers must increase their efforts to educate patients and their families about the hazards of smoking.

Chilmonczyk BA et al: Association between exposure to environmental tobacco smoke and exacerbations of asthma in children. N Engl J Med 1993;328:1665.
Weitzman M et al: Maternal smoking and childhood asthma. Pediatrics 1990;85:505.

DISORDERS OF THE CONDUCTING AIRWAYS

The conducting airways (the nose, mouth, pharynx, larynx, trachea, bronchi, and bronchioles) direct inspired air to the gas exchange units of the lung; they do not participate in gas exchange themselves. Airflow obstruction in the conducting airways occurs by (1) external compression (eg, vascular ring, tumor), (2) abnormalities of the airway structure itself (eg, congenital defects, thickening of an airway wall due to inflammation), or (3) material in the airway lumen (eg, foreign body, mucus).

Airway obstruction can be fixed (airflow limited in both the inspiratory and the expiratory phases) or variable (airflow limited more in one phase of respiration than in the other). Variable obstruction is common in children because their airways are more compliant and susceptible to dynamic compression. With variable extrathoracic airway obstruction (eg, croup), airflow limitation is greater during inspiration, leading to inspiratory stridor. With variable intrathoracic obstruction (bronchomalacia), limitation is greater during expiration, producing expiratory wheezing. Thus, determining the phase of respiration in which obstruction is greatest may be helpful in localizing the site of obstruction.

EXTRATHORACIC AIRWAY OBSTRUCTION

Patients with abnormalities of the extrathoracic airway may present with snoring and other symptoms of obstructive apnea, hoarseness, brassy cough, or stridor. The course of the illness may be acute (eg, infectious croup), recurrent (eg, spasmodic croup), chronic (eg, subglottic stenosis), or progressive (eg, laryngeal papillomatosis). Significant risk factors are difficult delivery, ductal ligation, and intubation. Examination should determine if obstructive symptoms are present at rest or with agitation, if they are positional, or if they are related to sleep. The presence of agitation, air hunger, severe retractions, cyanosis, lethargy, or coma should alert the physician to a potentially life-threatening condition that may require immediate airway intervention. Helpful diagnostic studies in the evaluation of upper airway obstruction include chest and lateral neck films, airway fluoroscopy, and barium swallow. In patients who have symptoms of severe chronic obstruction, an ECG should be obtained to evaluate for right ventricular hypertrophy and pulmonary hypertension. Patients with obstructive sleep apnea should have polysomnography (measurements during sleep of the motion of the chest wall, airflow at the nose and mouth, heart rate, oxygen saturation, and selected electroencephalographic leads to stage sleep) to determine severity and to evaluate the need for tonsillectomy and adenoidectomy, oxygen, or continuous positive airway pressure (CPAP). In older children, pulmonary function tests can differentiate fixed from variable airflow obstruction and identify the site of variable obstruction. If noninvasive studies are unable to establish the cause, direct laryngoscopy and bronchoscopy remain the procedures of choice to establish the precise diagnosis. Treatment should be directed at relieving airway obstruction and correcting the underlying condition if possible.

Tan HKK, Holinger LD: How to evaluate and manage stridor in children. J Respir Dis 1994;15:245.

INTRATHORACIC AIRWAY OBSTRUCTION

Intrathoracic airway obstruction usually causes expiratory wheezing. The history should include the following: (1) age at onset; (2) precipitating factors (eg, exercise, upper respiratory illnesses, allergens, choking while eating); (3) course—acute (bronchiolitis, foreign body), chronic (tracheomalacia, vascular ring), recurrent (reactive airways disease), or progressive (cystic fibrosis, bronchiolitis obliterans); (4) presence and nature of cough; (5) production of sputum; (6) previous response to bronchodilators; (7) symptoms with positional changes (vascular rings); and (8) involvement of other organ systems (malabsorption in cystic fibrosis).

Physical examination should include growth measurements and vital signs. The examiner should look for cyanosis or pallor, barrel-shaped chest, retractions and use of accessory muscles, and clubbing. Auscultation should define the pattern and timing of respiration, detect the presence of crackles and wheezing, and determine whether findings are localized or generalized.

Routine tests include plain chest films, a sweat test, and pulmonary function tests in older children. Other diagnostic studies are dictated by the history and physical findings. Treatment should be directed toward the primary cause of the obstruction but generally includes a trial of bronchodilators.

CONGENITAL DISORDERS OF THE EXTRATHORACIC AIRWAY

LARYNGOMALACIA

Laryngomalacia is a benign congenital disorder in which the cartilaginous support for the supraglottic structures is underdeveloped. It is the most common cause of persistent stridor in infants and usually is seen in the first 6 weeks of life. Stridor has been reported to be worse in the supine position, with increased activity, with upper respiratory infections, and during feeding; however, the clinical presentation can be variable. Patients may have slight oxygen desaturation during sleep. Gastroesophageal reflux may also be associated with laryngomalacia requiring treatment. The condition usually improves with age and resolves by 2 years of age, but in some cases symptoms persist for years. The diagnosis is established by direct laryngoscopy, which shows inspiratory collapse of an "omega-shaped" epiglottis (with or without long, redundant arytenoids). In mildly affected patients with a typical presentation (those without stridor at rest or retractions), this procedure may not be necessary. No treatment is usually needed. However, in patients with severe symptoms of airway obstruction associated with feeding difficulties, failure to thrive, obstructive sleep apnea, or severe dyspnea, surgical epiglottoplasty may be necessary.

Mancuso RF: Stridor in neonates. Pediatr Clin North Am 1996;43:1339.
Roger G et al: Severe laryngomalacia: Surgical indications and results in 115 patients. Laryngoscope 1995;105:1111.

OTHER CONGENITAL PROBLEMS

Other rare congenital lesions of the larynx (laryngeal atresia, laryngeal web, laryngocele and cyst of the larynx, subglottic hemangioma, and laryngeal cleft) are best diagnosed by direct laryngoscopy. Laryngeal atresia obviously presents immediately after birth with severe respiratory distress and is usually fatal. Laryngeal web, representing fusion of the anterior portion of the true vocal cords, is associated with hoarseness, aphonia, and stridor. Surgical correction may be necessary depending on the degree of airway obstruction.

Congenital cysts and laryngoceles are believed to have similar origin. Cysts are more superficial, whereas laryngoceles communicate with the interior of the larynx. Cysts are generally fluid-filled, whereas laryngoceles may be air- or fluid-filled. Airway obstruction is usually prominent and requires surgery or laser therapy.

Subglottic hemangiomas are seen in infancy with signs of upper airway obstruction and are often associated with similar lesions of the skin. Although these lesions tend to regress spontaneously, airway obstruction may require laser surgical treatment or even tracheostomy.

Laryngeal cleft is a very rare condition resulting from failure of posterior cricoid fusion. Patients with this condition may have stridor but always aspirate severely, resulting in recurrent or chronic pneumonia and failure to thrive. Barium swallow is always positive for severe aspiration, but diagnosis can be very difficult even with direct laryngoscopy. Patients often require tracheostomy and gastrostomy, because surgical correction is not always successful.

Holinger LD: Congenital laryngeal abnormalities. In: *Pediatric Laryngology and Bronchoesophagology.* Holinger LD, Lusk RP, Green CG (editors). Lippincott-Raven, 1997.

Sie KCY, McGill T, Healy GB: Subglottic hemangioma; Ten years' experience with the carbon dioxide laser. Ann Otol Rhinol Laryngol 1994;103:167.

ACQUIRED DISORDERS OF THE EXTRATHORACIC AIRWAY

CROUP SYNDROME

Croup describes acute inflammatory diseases of the larynx including viral croup (laryngotracheobronchitis), epiglottitis (supraglottitis), and bacterial tracheitis. These are the main entities in the differential diagnosis for patients presenting with acute stridor, though spasmodic croup, angioneurotic edema, laryngeal or esophageal foreign body, and retropharyngeal abscess should be considered as well.

1. VIRAL CROUP

Viral croup generally affects younger children in the fall and early winter months and is most often caused by parainfluenza virus serotypes. Other organisms causing croup include respiratory syncytial virus, influenza virus, rubeola virus, adenovirus, and *Mycoplasma pneumoniae.* Although inflammation of the entire airway is usually present, edema formation in the subglottic space accounts for the predominant signs of upper airway obstruction.

Clinical Findings

A. Symptoms and Signs: There is usually a prodrome of upper respiratory tract symptoms followed by the development of a barking cough and stridor. Fever is usually absent or low-grade but may on occasion be as high as in patients with epiglottitis. Patients with mild disease may exhibit only stridor when agitated, but as obstruction worsens, symptoms may progress to stridor at rest, accompanied by retractions, air hunger, and cyanosis in severe cases. On examination, the presence of cough and the absence of drooling tend to favor the diagnosis of viral croup over epiglottitis.

B. Imaging: Lateral neck films can be diagnostically helpful by showing subglottic narrowing and a normal epiglottis. Although the matter is controversial, some authorities advocate direct inspection of the epiglottis when viral croup is suspected to reduce the possibility of missing a case of epiglottitis.

Treatment

Treatment of viral croup is based upon the symptoms. Mild croup, signified by a barking cough and no stridor at rest, requires supportive therapy with oral hydration and minimal handling. Mist therapy is used by some physicians, though clinical studies demonstrating its effectiveness are lacking. Conversely, patients with stridor at rest require active intervention. Oxygen should be administered to patients with oxygen desaturation. Nebulized racemic epinephrine (2.25% solution; 0.05 mL/kg to a maximum of 1.5 mL diluted in sterile saline) is commonly used because it has a rapid onset of action within 10–30 minutes. Both racemic epinephrine and epinephrine hydrochloride are effective in alleviating symptoms and decreasing the need for intubation. Once controversial, the efficacy of glucocorticoids in croup is now more firmly established. Dexamethasone, 0.6 mg/kg intramuscularly as one dose, has been shown to improve symptoms, reduce the duration of hospitalizations and intubations, and permit earlier discharge from the emergency room. Oral dexamethasone appears equally effective, and limited data suggest that lower doses of oral dexamethasone (0.15 mg/kg) may be as effective as the higher dose. Inhaled budesonide (2 mg) has been shown to improve symptoms and decrease hospital stay. Onset of action occurs within 2 hours, and this agent may be as effective as dexamethasone. If symptoms resolve after glucocorticoids and nebulized epinephrine, patients can safely be discharged to home after 3 hours of observation without fear of a sudden rebound in symptoms. If, however, recurrent nebulized epinephrine treatments are required or if respiratory distress persists, patients require hospitalization for close observation, supportive care, and nebulization treatments as needed. In patients with impending respiratory failure, an airway must be established (see below). Hospitalized patients with persistent symptoms over 3–4 days despite treatment should arouse suspicion of another cause of airway obstruction.

Patients with impending respiratory failure require an artificial airway. Intubation with an endotracheal tube of slightly smaller diameter than would ordinarily be used is reasonably safe. Extubation should be accomplished within 2–3 days to minimize the risk of laryngeal injury. If the patient fails extubation, tracheostomy may be required.

Prognosis

Most children with viral croup have an uneventful course and improve within a few days. There is evidence that patients with a history of croup may have airway hyperreactivity, but it has not been determined if this was present prior to the croup episode or if the croup episode itself altered airway function. Recurrence of croup occurs in some instances, implying airway hyperreactivity.

Boeck KD: Croup: A review. Eur J Pediatr 1995;154:432.

Godden CW et al: Double blind placebo controlled trial of nebulized budesonide for croup. Arch Dis Child 1997; 76:155.

Kairys SW, Olmstead EM, O'Connor GT: Steroid treatment of laryngotracheitis: A meta-analysis of the evidence from randomized trials. Pediatrics 1989;83:683.

Klassen TP, Rowe PC: Outpatient management of croup. Curr Opin Pediatr 1996;8:449.

Ledwith CA, Shea LM, Maureo RD: Safety and efficacy of nebulized racemic epinephrine in conjunction with oral dexamethasone and mist in the outpatient treatment of croup. Ann Emerg Med 1995;25:331.

McEniery J et al: Review of intubation in severe laryngotracheobronchitis. Pediatrics 1991;87:847.

2. EPIGLOTTITIS

Epiglottitis is a true medical emergency. In published case series, it is almost always caused by *Haemophilus influenzae* type B, though other organisms such as nontypeable *H influenzae*, *Streptococcus pneumoniae*, and groups A and C *Streptococcus pyogenes* have been implicated. Resulting inflammation and swelling of the supraglottic structures (epiglottis and arytenoids) can develop rapidly and lead to life-threatening upper airway obstruction. The incidence has decreased dramatically since *H influenzae* conjugate vaccine was introduced.

Clinical Findings

A. Symptoms and Signs: Typically, patients present with a sudden onset of fever, dysphagia, drooling, muffled voice, inspiratory retractions, cyanosis, and soft stridor. They often sit in a "sniffing dog" position, which gives them the best airway possible under the circumstances. Progression to total airway obstruction may occur and result in respiratory arrest. The definitive diagnosis is made by direct inspection of the epiglottis, a procedure that should be done by an experienced airway specialist under controlled conditions (usually the operating room). The typical findings are cherry-red and swollen epiglottis and arytenoids.

B. Imaging: Diagnostically, lateral neck films may be helpful in demonstrating a classic "thumbprint" sign. Obtaining films, however, may delay important airway intervention.

Treatment

Once the diagnosis of epiglottitis is made, endotracheal intubation should be performed immediately. Most anesthesiologists favor the use of general anesthesia (but not muscle relaxants) to facilitate intubation. After an airway is established, cultures of the blood and epiglottis should be obtained and the patient started on appropriate intravenous antibiotics to cover *H influenzae* (ceftriaxone sodium, 150 mg/kg/d in two divided doses, or equivalent cephalosporin).

Attention should be given to respiratory care of the intubated patient to prevent accidental extubation and tube obstruction. This includes adequate restraint, humidification, and frequent suctioning. Extubation can usually be accomplished in 24–48 hours, when direct inspection shows significant reduction in the size of the epiglottis. Some centers use resolution of fever as a criterion for extubation. Intravenous antibiotics should be continued for 2–3 days, followed by oral antibiotics to complete a 10-day course.

If a physician who has little experience in treating airway disorders and is located far from a pediatric care facility encounters a patient with epiglottitis, the following is recommended. Start the patient on oxygen and assemble all the airway equipment available. Manipulate the patient as little as possible, and allow the child to remain sitting up. Enlist the help of the most experienced airway person available, or call a transport team. Start an intravenous line and give antibiotics. If the patient obstructs completely and suffers a respiratory arrest, attempt to establish an airway by any means possible: bag and mask ventilation, intubation, transtracheal ventilation with a large-bore angiocatheter attached to a 3-mm endotracheal tube adapter and resuscitation bag, or tracheostomy.

Complications

Complications related to *H influenzae* infection in other sites include pneumonia, cervical adenitis, and septic arthritis. Meningitis is extremely rare.

Prognosis

Prompt recognition and appropriate treatment usually results in rapid resolution of swelling and inflammation. Recurrence is unusual.

Cressman WR, Myer CM: Diagnosis and management of croup and epiglottitis. Pediatr Clin North Am 1994; 41:265.

Valdepeña HG et al: Epiglottitis and *Haemophilus influenzae* immunization. The Pittsburgh experience—five-year review. Pediatrics 1995;96:424.

3. BACTERIAL TRACHEITIS

Bacterial tracheitis (pseudomembranous croup) is a severe form of laryngotracheobronchitis. The organism most often isolated is *Staphylococcus aureus,* but organisms such as *H influenzae,* group A *Streptococcus pyogenes, Neisseria* species, and others have been reported. The disease probably represents localized mucosal invasion of bacteria in patients with primary viral croup, resulting in inflammatory edema, purulent secretions, and pseudomembranes. Although cultures of the tracheal secretions are frequently positive, blood cultures are almost always negative.

Clinical Findings

A. Symptoms and Signs: The early clinical picture is similar to that of viral croup. However, instead of gradual improvement, patients develop high fever, toxicity, and progressive upper airway obstruction that is unresponsive to standard croup therapy. The incidence of sudden respiratory arrest or progressive respiratory failure is very high; in such instances, airway intervention is required.

B. Laboratory Findings: The white cell count is usually elevated, with left shift. Cultures of tracheal secretions usually demonstrate one of the causative organisms.

C. Diagnosis: Lateral neck films show a normal epiglottis but often severe subglottic and tracheal narrowing. Irregularity of the contour of the proximal tracheal mucosa can frequently be seen radiographically. Bronchoscopy showing a normal epiglottis, and the presence of copious purulent tracheal secretions confirms the diagnosis.

Treatment

Patients with suspected bacterial tracheitis should be managed in a fashion similar to management of epiglottitis. The incidence of respiratory arrest or progressive respiratory failure is high, so intubation is usually necessary. Because these patients often have thick, purulent tracheal secretions, humidification, frequent suctioning, and intensive care monitoring is required to prevent endotracheal tube obstruction. Intravenous antibiotics to cover *S aureus, H influenzae,* and the other organisms are indicated. Because thick secretions persist for several days, the required period of intubation is longer for bacterial tracheitis than for epiglottitis.

Despite the severity of this illness, the reported mortality rate is very low.

Britto J et al: Systemic complications associated with bacterial tracheitis. Arch Dis Child 1996;74:249.

Gallagher PG, Myer CM: An approach to the diagnosis and treatment of membranous laryngotracheobronchitis in infants and children. Pediatr Emerg Care 1991;7:337.

VOCAL CORD PARALYSIS

Unilateral or bilateral vocal cord paralysis may be congenital or, more commonly, may result from injury to the recurrent laryngeal nerves. Risk factors for acquired paralysis include difficult delivery (especially face presentation), neck and thoracic surgery (eg, ductal ligation, repair of tracheoesophageal fistula), trauma, mediastinal masses, pulmonary hypertension, and central nervous system disease (eg, Arnold-Chiari malformation). Patients usually present with varying degrees of hoarseness, aspiration, or high-pitched stridor. Unilateral cord paralysis is more likely to occur on the left because of the longer course of the left recurrent laryngeal nerve and its proximity to major thoracic structures. Patients with unilateral paralysis are usually hoarse but rarely have stridor. With bilateral cord paralysis, the closer to midline the cords are positioned, the greater the airway obstruction; the more lateral the cords are positioned, the greater the tendency to aspirate and experience hoarseness or aphonia. If partial function is preserved (paresis), the adductor muscles tend to operate better than the abductors, with a resultant high-pitched inspiratory stridor and normal voice. Airway intervention (intubation, tracheostomy) is rarely indicated in unilateral paralysis but is often necessary for bilateral paralysis. Recovery is related to the severity of nerve injury and the potential for healing.

Fan LL et al: Paralyzed left vocal cord associated with patent ductus arteriosus ligation. J Thorac Cardiovasc Surg 1989;98:611.

Zbar RI, Smith RJ: Vocal fold paralysis in infants twelve months of age and younger. Otolaryngol Head Neck Surg 1996;114:18.

SUBGLOTTIC STENOSIS

Subglottic stenosis may be congenital or, more commonly, may result from endotracheal intubation. Neonates and infants are particularly vulnerable to subglottic injury from intubation: The subglottis is the narrowest part of an infant's airway, and the cricoid cartilage, which supports the subglottis, is the only cartilage that completely encircles the airway. The clinical presentation may vary from totally asymptomatic to the typical picture of severe upper airway obstruction. Patients with signs of stridor who repeatedly fail extubation are likely to have subglottic stenosis. Subglottic stenosis should also be suspected in children with multiple, prolonged, or severe episodes of croup. As with other conditions, diagnosis is made by direct laryngoscopy and bronchoscopy. Tracheostomy is often required when airway compromise is severe. Although a number of surgical approaches to correct this problem have been tried, the failure rate is high. The most promising procedures are the "cricoid split," in which the cricoid cartilage is surgically opened (better for acquired than congenital lesions), and laryngotracheoplasty, in which a cartilage graft from another source (eg, rib) is used to expand the framework.

Couser RJ et al: Effectiveness of dexamethasone in preventing extubation failure in preterm infants at increased risk for airway edema. J Pediatr 1992;121:591.

Lesperance MM, Zalzal GH: Assessment and management of laryngotracheal stenosis. Pediatr Clin North Am 1996;43:1413.

LARYNGEAL TRAUMA

Injury to the larynx may result from external trauma, such as automobile accidents, snowmobile accidents (clothesline injury), and hanging; or internal trauma, such as noxious inhalation (burns and caustic substances) and intubation. External trauma can cause laryngeal fracture, which requires an emergency tracheostomy to prevent death. After appropriate airway intervention, attention should be directed to debridement and closure of lacerations. Reduction of laryngeal fractures should be performed as soon as the patient is stabilized.

Myers EN: Assessing and repairing laryngeal injuries. J Respir Dis 1982;3:43.

LARYNGEAL PAPILLOMATOSIS

Papillomas of the larynx are benign, warty growths that are difficult to treat and are the most common laryngeal neoplasm in children. Human papilloma viruses 6, 11, and 16 have been implicated as causative agents. A substantial percentage of mothers of patients with laryngeal papillomas have a history of genital condylomas at the time of delivery, so the virus may be acquired during passage through an infected birth canal.

The age at onset is usually 2–4 years, but the disease may present at any age. Patients usually develop hoarseness, croupy cough, or stridor that can lead to life-threatening airway obstruction. Diagnosis is by direct laryngoscopy.

Treatment is directed toward relieving airway obstruction, usually by surgical removal of the lesions. Tracheostomy is necessary when life-threatening obstruction or respiratory arrest occurs. Various surgical procedures (laser, cup forceps, cryosurgery) have been used to remove papillomas, but recurrences are the rule, and frequent reoperation may be needed. The lesions occasionally spread down the trachea and bronchi, making surgical removal more difficult. The use of interferon therapy remains controversial. Fortunately, spontaneous remissions do occur, usually by puberty, so that the goal of therapy is to maintain an adequate airway until remission occurs.

Bauman NM, Smith RJH: Recurrent respiratory papillomatosis. Pediatr Clin North Am 1996;43:1385.

Somers GR et al: Juvenile laryngeal papillomatosis in a pediatric population: A clinicopathologic study. Pediatr Pathol Lab Med 1997; 17:53.

CONGENITAL DISORDERS OF THE INTRATHORACIC AIRWAYS

TRACHEOMALACIA

Tracheomalacia exists when the cartilaginous framework of the trachea is inadequate to maintain airway patency. Because cartilage of the infant airway is normally "soft," all infants may have some degree of dynamic collapse of the trachea when pressure outside the trachea exceeds intraluminal pressure. In tracheomalacia, whether congenital or acquired, dynamic collapse leads to airway obstruction. The congenital variety may be isolated or associated with another developmental defect, such as tracheoesophageal fistula or vascular ring. It may be localized to part of the trachea or, more commonly, may involve the entire trachea as well as the remainder of the conducting airways. In severe cases, cartilage in the involved area may be missing or underdeveloped. The acquired variety has been associated with long-term ventilation of premature newborns that results in chronic tracheal injury.

Patients present with coarse wheezing, a prolonged expiratory phase, and a croupy cough, all of which increase with agitation and upper respiratory tract infections. Diagnosis can be made by cinefluoroscopy or bronchoscopy. Barium swallow may be indicated to rule out coexisting conditions. No treatment is usually indicated for the isolated condition, which generally improves over time. Coexisting lesions such as tracheoesophageal fistulas and vascular rings need primary repair. In severe cases of tracheomalacia, intubation or tracheostomy may be necessary, but this procedure alone is seldom satisfactory because airway collapse continues to exist below the tip of the artificial airway. Continuous positive airway pressure through an artificial airway can sometimes stabilize the collapsing airway.

Finder JD: Primary bronchomalacia in infants and children. J Pediatr 1997;130:59.

Paston F, Bye M: Tracheomalacia. Pediatr Rev 1996; 17:328.

VASCULAR RINGS & SLINGS

The commonest vascular anomalies to compress the trachea or esophagus are a double aortic arch, right aortic arch with left ligamentum arteriosum or patent ductus arteriosus, pulmonary sling, anomalous innominate or left carotid artery, and aberrant right subclavian artery. All but the latter are associated with tracheal compression and thus present in infancy with symptoms of chronic airway obstruction, including stridor, course wheezing, and croupy cough. Symptoms are often worse in the supine position. Respiratory compromise is most severe with double aortic arch and may lead to apnea, respiratory arrest, or even death. Esophageal compression, present in all but anomalous innominate or carotid artery, may result in feeding difficulties, including dysphagia and vomiting. Therefore, barium swallow demonstrating this esophageal compression is the mainstay of diagnosis. In the case of anomalous innominate or carotid artery, diagnosis is best established by cinefluoroscopy, MRI, or bronchoscopy.

Patients with significant symptoms require surgical correction, especially those with double aortic arch. Controversy exists about whether angiography is necessary to define the anatomy prior to surgery. Patients usually improve following correction but may have persistent but milder symptoms of airway obstruction due to associated tracheomalacia.

Edwards JE: Vascular rings and slings. In: *Fetal, Neonatal, and Infant Cardiac Disease.* Moller JH, Neal WA (editors). Appleton & Lange, 1990.

BRONCHOGENIC CYSTS

Bronchogenic cysts generally occur in the mid mediastinum (see Mediastinal Masses, below) near the carina and adjacent to the major bronchi but can be found elsewhere in the lung as well. Their sizes range from 2 to 10 cm. Cyst walls are thick and may contain pus, mucus, or blood. These develop from abnormal lung budding of the primitive foregut. They do not contain distal lung parenchyma and generally do not communicate with the airway.

Clinically, respiratory distress can appear acutely in early childhood or present as chronic wheezing, chronic cough, tachypnea, recurrent pneumonia, or stridor depending on the location and size of the cysts and the degree of airway compression. On physical examination, the trachea may deviate from the midline, and the percussion note over involved lobes may be hyperresonant. Breath sounds over such areas will also be decreased. Air trapping and hyperinflation of the affected lobes is found on chest x-ray film. Smaller lesions or those detected early may not be appreciated on chest x-rays or may appear spherical. Initial assessment of a suspected bronchogenic cyst usually includes barium swallow to demonstrate the presence of a mass. This study also helps determine whether the lesion communicates with the gastrointestinal tract. CT scans or ul-

trasonography can differentiate solid versus cystic mediastinal masses and define the cyst's relationship to the rest of the lung.

Treatment is by surgical resection. Postoperatively, vigorous pulmonary physiotherapy is required to prevent complications (atelectasis, infection of lung distal to the site of resection of the cyst).

Nuchtern JG, Harberg FJ: Congenital lung cysts. Semin Pediatr Surg 1994;3:233.

Ribet ME, Copin MC, Gosselin B: Bronchogenic cysts of the mediastinum. J Thorac Cardiovasc Surg 1995; 109:1003.

ACQUIRED DISORDERS OF THE INTRATHORACIC AIRWAYS

FOREIGN BODY ASPIRATION

Aspiration of a foreign body into the respiratory tract is a rarely observed event, so it is the abrupt onset of cough, choking, or wheezing—especially in children who have access to high-risk objects such as peanuts, hard candy, small toys—that suggests the diagnosis. Children between 6 months and 4 years of age are at particularly high risk, and many deaths are caused by respiratory obstruction each year

1. FOREIGN BODIES IN THE UPPER RESPIRATORY TRACT

The diagnosis is established by acute onset of cyanosis and choking along with inability to vocalize or cough (complete obstruction) or with drooling and stridor (partial obstruction).

Foreign bodies that lodge in the esophagus may compress the airway and cause respiratory distress. More typically, the foreign body lodges in the supraglottic airway, triggering protective reflexes that result in laryngospasm. Onset is generally abrupt, with a history of the child's running with food in its mouth or playing with seeds, small coins, toys, etc. Poor "child-proofing" in the home and cases in which an older sibling feeds age-inappropriate foods (eg, peanuts, hard candy, carrot slices) to the younger child are typical. If the obstruction is only partial, coughing, stridor, and the ability to vocalize may persist. If complete, an inability to cough or vocalize (aphonia) and cyanosis with marked distress are observed. Without treatment, progressive cyanosis, loss of consciousness, seizures, bradycardia, and cardiopulmonary arrest follow.

Treatment

The emergency treatment of upper airway obstruction due to foreign body aspiration is somewhat controversial. In general, it is recommended that if partial obstruction is present, children should be allowed to use their own cough reflex to extrude the foreign body. If after a brief observation period, the obstruction increases or the airway becomes completely obstructed, acute intervention is required. The AAP and AHA distinguish between children under or over 1 year of age. A choking infant under age 1 should be placed face-down over the rescuer's arm, with the head positioned below the trunk. Five measured back blows are delivered rapidly between the infant's scapulas with the heel of the rescuer's hand. If obstruction persists, the infant should be rolled over and five rapid chest compressions performed (similar to CPR). This sequence is repeated until the obstruction is relieved. In children over age 1 year, abdominal thrusts (Heimlich maneuver) may be performed, with special care in younger children because of concern about possible intra-abdominal organ injury.

In both groups, blind probing of the airway to dislodge a foreign body is discouraged because of the risk of impaction. The airway may be opened by jaw thrust, and if the foreign body can be directly visualized, careful removal with the fingers or instruments (Magill forceps) can be attempted. Patients with persistent apnea and inability to achieve adequate ventilation may require emergency intubation, tracheostomy, or needle cricothyrotomy—depending on the setting and the rescuer's skills.

Abman SH et al: Emergency treatment of foreign body obstruction of the upper airway in children. J Emerg Med 1984;2:7.

Chameides L, Hazinski MF (editors): *Textbook of Pediatric Advanced Life Support.* American Heart Association and American Academy of Pediatrics, 1990.

2. FOREIGN BODIES IN THE LOWER RESPIRATORY TRACT

Essentials of Diagnosis & Typical Features

- Sudden onset of coughing, wheezing, or respiratory distress.
- Asymmetric physical findings of decreased breath sounds or localized wheezing.
- Asymmetric radiographic findings, especially with forced expiratory view.

Clinical Findings

A. Symptoms and Signs: Respiratory symptoms and signs vary depending on the site of obstruction and the duration following the acute episode. For example, a large or central airway obstruction may cause marked distress. The acute cough or wheezing caused by a foreign body in the lower respiratory tract may diminish over time only to recur later and present as chronic cough or persistent wheezing. Thus, foreign body aspiration should be suspected in children with chronic cough, persistent wheezing, or recurrent pneumonia. Long-standing foreign bodies may lead to bronchiectasis or lung abscess. On physical examination, asymmetric breath sounds or localized wheezing also suggest the presence of a foreign body.

B. Imaging: Inspiratory and forced expiratory chest x-rays should be obtained if foreign body aspiration is suspected. The latter study can be obtained in young children by manually compressing the abdomen during expiration. The initial inspiratory view may show localized hyperinflation due to the ball-valve effect of the foreign body, causing distal air trapping. A positive forced expiratory study shows a mediastinal shift away from the affected side. If airway obstruction is complete, atelectasis and related volume loss will be the major radiologic findings. Chest fluoroscopy is an alternative approach for detecting air trapping and mediastinal shift.

Treatment

If the imaging is positive or if, despite negative imaging, clinical suspicion persists, further evaluation with bronchoscopy is indicated. Rigid bronchoscopy under general anesthesia is recommended. Flexible bronchoscopy may be helpful for follow-up evaluations (after the foreign object has been removed).

Children with suspected acute foreign body aspiration should be admitted to the hospital for evaluation and treatment. Chest postural drainage is no longer recommended because the foreign body may become dislodged and obstruct a major central airway. Bronchoscopy should not be delayed in children with respiratory distress but should be performed as soon as possible once the diagnosis is made—even in children with more chronic symptoms. Following the removal of the foreign body, β-adrenergic nebulization treatments followed by chest physiotherapy are recommended to help clear related mucus or bronchospasm. The relative dangers of missing a foreign body in the lower respiratory tract are much greater and include the development of bronchiectasis and lung abscess over time. This risk justifies an aggressive approach to suspected foreign bodies in undocumented but suspicious cases.

Martinot A et al: Indications for flexible versus rigid bronchoscopy in children with suspected foreign-body aspiration. Am J Respir Crit Care Med 1997;155:1676.

Wolach B et al: Aspirated foreign bodies in the respiratory tract of children: Eleven years experience with 127 patients. Int J Pediatr Otorhinolaryngol 1994;30:1.

BRONCHITIS

Essentials of Diagnosis & Typical Features

- Cough that usually progresses from dry to productive.
- Rhonchi appearing predominantly during expiration.

General Considerations

Bronchitis is inflammation of the major conducting airways within the lung and is unusual as an isolated entity in children. However, inflammation within this section of the airways commonly occurs in association with disease processes involving other areas of the respiratory tract. In adults, the diagnosis of chronic bronchitis is based on a history of at least 3 months of productive cough occurring for 2 or more years, but no generally acceptable criteria for this diagnosis exist in children. A differential diagnosis for 3–4 weeks of cough and sputum production in a child is given in the text that follows.

Clinical Findings

A. Symptoms and Signs: Acute bronchitis usually begins as a nonproductive cough that may be associated with other features of an upper respiratory illness of viral origin. The longer the cough persists, the more likely it is to become productive. In general, children with uncomplicated acute bronchitis appear nontoxic, and fever, if present, is low-grade. There are diffuse rhonchi predominantly during expiration. In uncomplicated acute bronchitis, mucus production decreases, and the cough disappears over a period of 7–10 days.

B. Laboratory Findings: The white blood count is usually normal and, if elevated, may suggest a viral infection. Pulmonary function tests may reveal variable degrees of airway obstruction.

C. Imaging: X-ray examination of the chest may be normal or may show a mild increase in bronchovascular markings.

Differential Diagnosis

Most attacks of acute bronchitis are caused by viral infections. Certain viral pathogens (eg, adenovirus) can produce a more severe clinical picture that resembles a pertussis-like illness. Bacteria that may produce disease in which bronchitis is a prominent symptom include *Bordetella pertussis, Mycobacterium tuberculosis, Corynebacterium diphtheriae,* and *Mycoplasma pneumoniae.*

Noninfectious diseases need to be considered in the evaluation of acute bronchitis that differs from the clinical picture described above and in cases of chronic or recurrent bronchitis. Asthma may present as a persistent cough with little or no wheezing. Sinus infections may provide a source of persistent irritation to the respiratory tract and lead to a chronic cough. Cystic fibrosis, an immunodeficiency, or primary ciliary dyskinesia must also be considered if the bronchitis persists or recurs and if bronchiectasis is present or suspected. In the younger child, respiratory tract anomalies, foreign bodies, and recurrent aspiration must also be considered. Tobacco or marijuana smoking may contribute to this process in older children. In patients of all ages, the potential role of irritants within the environment must also be evaluated.

Complications

In otherwise healthy children, complications of acute bronchitis secondary to viral infection are few but include otitis media, sinusitis, and pneumonia.

Treatment

When bronchitis is secondary to an uncomplicated acute viral infection, supportive therapy is all that is necessary. Expectorants and cough suppressants, though commonly used, are seldom indicated. Avoidance of irritants during the viral infection may also decrease symptoms and morbidity. When the bronchitic syndrome is due to other underlying problems, treatment must address the primary process.

Loughlin GM: Bronchitis. In: *Disorders of the Respiratory Tract in Children,* 5th ed. Chernick V, Kendig EL Jr (editors). Saunders, 1990.

BRONCHIOLITIS

Bronchiolitis is a common cause of acute hospital admissions in infants under 2 years of age, especially during the winter months. The typical presentation is acute onset of tachypnea, cough, rhinorrhea, and expiratory wheezing. Respiratory syncytial virus (RSV) is by far the most common pathogen; parainfluenza and influenza viruses, adenovirus, *Mycoplasma, Chlamydia, Ureaplasma,* and *Pneumocystis* are less common causes of wheezing-associated respiratory illness during early infancy. Major concerns include not only the acute effects of bronchiolitis but also the possible development of chronic airway hyperreactivity (asthma). Bronchiolitis due to respiratory syncytial virus infection contributes substantially to morbidity and mortality in children with underlying cardiopulmonary disorders, including bronchopulmonary dysplasia, cystic fibrosis, and congenital heart disease, especially when pulmonary hypertension is present.

Clinical Findings

A. Symptoms and Signs: The usual course of RSV bronchiolitis is 1–2 days of fever, rhinorrhea, and cough, followed by wheezing, tachypnea, and respiratory distress. Typically, the breathing pattern is shallow, with rapid respirations. Nasal flaring, cyanosis, retractions, and rales may be present, along with prolongation of the expiratory phase and wheezing, depending on the severity of illness. Some young infants present with apnea and few findings on auscultation but may subsequently develop rales, rhonchi, and expiratory wheezing.

B. Laboratory Findings: The peripheral white blood cell count may be normal or may show a mild lymphocytosis.

C. Imaging: Chest x-ray findings typically include hyperinflation with mild interstitial infiltrates, but segmental atelectasis is common.

Treatment

Susceptibility to RSV in high-risk children can be reduced by giving immune globulin with a high titer of antibodies against RSV. Prevention by new vaccines is also being explored. Although most children with RSV bronchiolitis are readily managed as outpatients by supportive therapy, hospitalization is required in children younger than 2 months of age and in patients with hypoxemia on room air, a history of apnea, moderate tachypnea with feeding difficulties, marked respiratory distress with retractions, or underlying chronic cardiopulmonary disorders. Initial management includes an assessment of oxygenation and ventilation and, if hypoxemia is present, administration of supplemental oxygen. The response to therapy should be checked by oximetry since this provides early warning of impending respiratory failure in infants. In one series, 7% of normal children admitted for viral bronchiolitis subsequently required mechanical ventilation; infants with bronchopulmonary dysplasia and cystic fibrosis hospitalized with RSV bronchiolitis develop respiratory failure at higher rates. Progressive respiratory distress (including progressive hypoxemia and hypercapnia) and apnea are common indications for admission to the intensive care unit and mechanical ventilation.

Intravenous fluids should be given as required, avoiding fluid overload and pulmonary edema. Although β-adrenergic drug therapy and corticosteroids may attenuate airway obstruction, their use remains controversial and empiric, and patients should be assessed individually to determine responsiveness.

The availability of rapid diagnostic testing for RSV infection may permit early intervention with antiviral therapy (ribavirin), especially in children with marked respiratory distress or chronic cardiopulmonary disease. Although ribavirin's efficacy remains unclear, its use may be considered for hospitalized infants with severe disease; for those with congenital heart disease, bronchopulmonary dysplasia, cystic fibrosis, immunodeficiencies, or other chronic lung disorders; and for recent transplant recipients and patients undergoing chemotherapy. Children younger than 6 weeks and those with underlying metabolic, neurologic, or congenital abnormalities should also be considered for ribavirin therapy.

Prognosis

Although the outcome in bronchiolitis is good for healthy children, the mortality rate in patients with cardiopulmonary disease can be high. Recurrent episodes of wheezing may follow acute infection in almost half of the hospitalized infants.

American Academy of Pediatrics, Committee on Infectious Diseases: Reassessment of the indications for ribavirin therapy in respiratory syncytial virus infections. Pediatrics 1996;97:137.

Groothuis JR et al: Prophylactic administration of respiratory syncytial virus immune globulin to high-risk infants and young children. N Engl J Med 1993;329:1524.

Levin MJ: Treatment and prevention options for respiratory syncytial virus infections. J Pediatr 1994;124:S22.

Makela J, Ruuskanen O: RSV in children. Curr Opin Pediatr 1994;6:17.

Zucker AR, Meadows WL: Pediatric critical care physicians' attitudes about guidelines for the use of ribavirin in critically ill children with RSV pneumonia. Crit Care Med 1995;23:767.

BRONCHIECTASIS

Essentials of Diagnosis & Typical Features

- Chronic cough with sputum production.
- Persistent abnormalities on physical examination of the chest.
- Persistent abnormalities on chest x-ray.
- Diagnosis confirmed by high-resolution CT.

General Considerations

"Bronchiectasis" means dilation of bronchi. The dilation may be regular, with the airway continuing to have a smooth outline (cylindric bronchiectasis); irregular, with areas of dilation and constriction (varicose bronchiectasis); or marked, with destruction of structural components of the airway wall (saccular bronchiectasis). Although the incidence in the general population is low (< 0.5%), the morbidity associated with severe forms of bronchiectasis is significant. Medical treatment can halt the progression of a potentially reversible (cylindric) form to an irreversible destructive airway disease (saccular bronchiectasis).

Bronchiectasis results from obstruction of the airway and poor drainage (from such causes as cystic fibrosis, foreign bodies) along with infection. Infection or obstruction occurring alone is unlikely to lead to the more severe forms of bronchiectasis.

Clinical Findings

A. Symptoms and Signs: Manifestations range from chronic cough with early morning sputum production in an overtly healthy child to recurrent pneumonia with or without hemoptysis in a chronically ill one. There may be a history of recurrent respiratory infections, dyspnea on exertion, and a productive cough precipitated by exercise. Some children present with recurrent fevers. Chronic cough, persistent atelectasis, and failure of a chest x-ray to clear after respiratory infection are typical. On physical examination, finger clubbing may be seen, and there may be evidence of sinusitis. Persistent moist rales, rhonchi, and decreased air entry are often noted over the bronchiectatic area when saccular changes are present.

B. Laboratory Findings and Imaging: Cultures from the respiratory tract usually reveal mixed flora; *H influenzae* is a common isolate.

Chest films may be mildly abnormal with slightly increased bronchovascular markings or areas of atelectasis, or they may demonstrate cystic changes in one or more areas of the lung. The extent of bronchiectasis is best defined by high-resolution CT scan of the lung, which often reveals far wider involvement of lung than expected from the plain chest film. Bronchography is not widely used.

Pulmonary function testing often reveals an obstructive pattern even in the absence of asthma, cystic fibrosis, or other disease processes leading to airway obstruction. This obstruction may result from difficulty in clearing secretions. Evaluation of lung function after use of a bronchodilator is helpful in assessing the benefit a patient may have from bronchodilators. Serial assessments of lung function help define the progression or resolution of the disease.

Differential Diagnosis

Bronchiectasis can develop in patients with cystic fibrosis, antibody deficiency, and abnormal mucociliary clearance (primary ciliary dyskinesia). Bronchiectasis has also been described in children with HIV infection. Recurrent aspiration of a foreign body must also be considered, especially when bronchiectatic changes are confined to one area of the lung.

Although congenital causes of bronchiectasis are relatively uncommon compared with the predisposing factors listed above, they must still be considered in the differential diagnosis. Bronchiectasis may result from defective development of bronchial cartilage (Williams-Campbell syndrome) and developmental failure of elastic and muscular tissues of the trachea and bronchi (tracheobronchomegaly, or Mounier-Kuhn syndrome). Bronchial stenosis, either congenital or acquired, also predisposes to bronchiectasis.

Complications

Major concerns are severe pneumonia, hemoptysis, and cor pulmonale. Less frequent complications are abscesses of the lung or central nervous system, empyema, and bronchopleural fistula.

Treatment

Initial management consists of antibiotics as well as pulmonary physiotherapy, consisting of bronchodilators followed by postural drainage and chest percussion to affected areas. Sinusitis must be vigorously treated if present.

Surgical removal of an area of lung affected with severe saccular bronchiectasis is considered when the response to therapy is poor. Other indications for operation include extensive or repeated hemoptysis and recurrent pneumonia in one area of lung. Operation is best performed when the bronchiectatic area is well localized and the rest of the lung appears normal—most likely in a child who has saccular bronchiectasis due to foreign body aspiration or a congenital defect. Children with more serious underlying disorders (cystic fibrosis, hypogammaglobulinemia) are likely to have bronchiectatic changes in several areas of the lung and are not good candidates for surgery.

Prognosis

The prognosis depends on the underlying cause and severity of bronchiectasis, the extent of lung involvement, and the response to medical management. Good pulmonary hygiene and avoidance of infectious complications in the involved areas of lung may reverse cylindric bronchiectasis.

Amorosa JK et al: Bronchiectasis in children with lymphocytic interstitial pneumonia and acquired immune deficiency syndrome: Plain film and CT observations. Pediatr Radiol 1992;22:603.

Brown MA, Lemen RJ: Bronchiectasis. In: *Disorders of the Respiratory Tract in Children,* 5th ed. Chernick V, Kendig EL Jr (editors). Saunders, 1990.

BRONCHIOLITIS OBLITERANS

Bronchiolitis obliterans is characterized by obstruction of bronchi and bronchioles by fibrous tissue. The disorder follows damage to the lower respiratory tract, such as inhalation of toxic gases, infections (adenovirus, influenza virus, rubeola virus, *Bordetella, Mycoplasma*), connective tissue diseases, transplantation, and aspiration. Many cases of bronchiolitis obliterans are idiopathic. Adenovirus-induced bronchiolitis obliterans occurs more frequently in the Native American population in Canada and in Polynesian children in New Zealand.

Clinical Findings

A. Symptoms and Signs: Bronchiolitis obliterans should be considered when there is persistent cough, wheezing, or sputum production after an episode of acute pneumonia. Prolonged rales or wheezing or persistent exercise intolerance following a pulmonary insult should also suggest this disease.

B. Laboratory Findings and Imaging: Chest x-ray abnormalities include evidence of localized or generalized air trapping as well as (in some cases) nodular densities and alveolar opacification. Scattered areas of matched decreases in ventilation and perfusion are seen when the lung is scanned. Pulmonary angiograms reveal decreased vasculature in the area of lung involvement, whereas bronchograms demonstrate marked pruning of the bronchial tree. An assessment of lung function demonstrates an obstructive process that may be combined with evidence of restriction. Inhaled bronchodilators or corticosteroids provide little improvement in lung function.

Differential Diagnosis

Poorly treated asthma, cystic fibrosis, and bronchopulmonary dysplasia must be considered in children with persistent airway obstruction. A trial of medications (including bronchodilators and corticosteroids) may help to determine the reversibility of the process when the primary differential is between asthma and bronchiolitis obliterans. Although the results of imaging and pulmonary function testing are very suggestive, the best way to establish a definitive diagnosis is by lung biopsy.

Complications

Sequelae of bronchiolitis obliterans include persistent airway obstruction, recurrent wheezing, bronchiectasis, chronic atelectasis, recurrent pneumonia, and unilateral hyperlucent lung syndrome.

Treatment

Supplemental oxygen should be given to patients with oxygen desaturation during normal activities or sleep. In addition, early treatment should be directed at preventing ongoing airway damage due to problems such as aspiration, which may be either the primary insult or an acquired problem secondary to marked hyperinflation. The effectiveness of other forms of treatment may be more difficult to evaluate. Oral and inhaled bronchodilators may reverse airway obstruction if there is a reactive component to the disease. Many children also receive at least one course of corticosteroid treatment in an attempt to reverse the obstruction or prevent ongoing damage. Antibiotics should be used as indicated for pneumonia.

Prognosis

Prognosis may depend in part on the underlying cause as well as the age at which the insult occurred. The course varies from mild asthma-like symptoms to rapidly fatal deterioration despite therapy.

Hardy KA: Obliterative bronchiolitis. In: *Pediatric Respiratory Disease*. Hilman BC (editor). Saunders, 1993.

BRONCHOPULMONARY DYSPLASIA

Essentials of Diagnosis & Typical Features

- Acute respiratory distress in first week of life.
- Required oxygen therapy or mechanical ventila-

tion, with persistent oxygen requirement at 1 month.
- Persistent respiratory abnormalities, including physical signs and radiographic findings.

General Considerations

Bronchopulmonary dysplasia remains one of the most significant sequelae of acute respiratory distress in the neonatal intensive care unit, with an incidence between 10% and 40% (depending on the criteria used for definition and the gestational age of the population base). This disease was first characterized in 1967 when Northway and coworkers reported the clinical, radiologic, and pathologic findings in a group of premature newborns who required prolonged mechanical ventilation and oxygen therapy to treat hyaline membrane disease. The progression from acute hyaline membrane disease to chronic lung disease was divided into four stages: acute respiratory distress shortly after birth, usually hyaline membrane disease (stage I); clinical and radiographic worsening of the acute lung disease, often due to increased pulmonary blood flow secondary to a patent ductus arteriosus (stage II); and progressive signs of chronic lung disease (stages III and IV).

The precise definition of bronchopulmonary dysplasia remains unclear. This confusion results from several factors, including our ignorance of the mechanisms causing some children to develop the disorder, the lack of specific diagnostic tests, and the room for subjective variability in the present diagnostic criteria. This is a chronic respiratory disorder of infancy that follows treatment (usually mechanical ventilation) during the first week of life for acute respiratory distress and is subsequently associated with persistent signs of respiratory distress, a requirement for supplemental oxygen, and radiographic abnormalities beyond 30 days of age. This broad definition does not accommodate some key issues, including the following: (1) although most of these children were premature and had hyaline membrane disease, full-term newborns with such disorders as meconium aspiration or persistent pulmonary hypertension can also develop bronchopulmonary dysplasia; (2) some severely preterm newborns require minimal ventilator support yet subsequently develop a prolonged oxygen requirement despite the absence of severe acute manifestations of respiratory failure; (3) newborns dying within the first weeks of life can already have the aggressive, fibroproliferative pathologic lesions that resemble bronchopulmonary dysplasia; and (4) physiologic abnormalities (increased airway resistance) and biochemical markers of lung injury (altered protease and antiprotease ratios, increased inflammatory cells and mediators), which are predictive of bronchopulmonary dysplasia, are already present in the first week of life.

Although the exact mechanisms leading to chronic lung disease are not completely understood, bronchopulmonary dysplasia represents the consequences of lung injury caused by oxygen toxicity, barotrauma, and inflammation superimposed on a susceptible, generally immature lung. The premature lung often makes insufficient functional surfactant; furthermore, the antioxidant defense mechanisms are not sufficiently mature to protect the lung from the toxic oxygen metabolites generated from hyperoxia. The lungs destined to develop bronchopulmonary dysplasia show early inflammation and hypercellularity followed by healing with fibrosis. Thus, abnormal lung mechanics due to structural immaturity, surfactant deficiency, atelectasis, and pulmonary edema—plus lung injury secondary to hyperoxia and mechanical ventilation—lead to further abnormalities of lung function, causing increases in ventilator and oxygen requirements and ending in a vicious circle that compounds the progression of lung injury. Excessive fluid administration, patent ductus arteriosus, pulmonary interstitial emphysema, pneumothorax, infection, pulmonary hypertension, and inflammatory stimuli secondary to lung injury or infection also play important roles in the pathogenesis of the disease.

Differential Diagnosis

The radiologic differential diagnosis includes meconium aspiration syndrome, congenital infection (such as with cytomegalovirus or *Ureaplasma*), cystic adenomatoid malformation, recurrent aspiration, pulmonary lymphangiectasia, total anomalous pulmonary venous return, overhydration, and idiopathic pulmonary fibrosis.

Clinical Course & Treatment

The clinical course of infants with bronchopulmonary dysplasia ranges from a mild increased oxygen requirement that gradually resolves over a few months to more severe disease requiring chronic tracheostomy and mechanical ventilation for the first 2 years of life. In general, patients show slow, steady improvements in oxygen or ventilator requirements but can have frequent respiratory exacerbations leading to frequent or prolonged hospitalizations. Clinical management generally includes careful attention to growth, nutrition (caloric requirements of infants with oxygen dependence and respiratory distress are quite high), metabolic status, developmental and neurologic status, and related problems, along with the various cardiopulmonary abnormalities described below.

Increased airway resistance and bronchial hyperreactivity are common in affected infants, so inhaled corticosteroids or cromolyn sodium together with occasional use of β-adrenergic agonists are commonly part of the treatment plan. Part of the rationale for the use of corticosteroids is to decrease lung inflammation and enhance responsiveness to β-adrenergic drugs, as in the treatment of severe asthma. β-Adrenergic agonists followed by chest physiotherapy are often used for the thick secretions that may contribute to airway obstruction or recurrent atelectasis.

Although bronchial hyperreactivity in affected infants is well recognized, structural lesions (such as subglottic stenosis, vocal cord paralysis, tracheal stenosis, tracheomalacia, bronchial stenosis, and granulomatous bronchial polyps) often contribute to airflow limitation. Children with significant stridor, sleep apnea, chronic wheezing, or excessive respiratory distress need bronchoscopy.

Infants often have recurrent pulmonary edema, which may be due to increased permeability of the injured pulmonary circulation or to increases in hydrostatic pressure if left ventricular dysfunction is present. Salt and water retention secondary to chronic hypoxemia, hypercapnia, or other stimuli may be present. Chronic or intermittent diuretic therapy with furosemide, hydrochlorothiazide, and spironolactone is commonly used if there are rales or signs of persistent pulmonary edema, with acute improvement in lung function demonstrated by clinical studies. Unfortunately, diuretics often have adverse effects, including severe volume contraction, hypokalemia, alkalosis, and hyponatremia. Potassium and arginine chloride supplements are commonly required.

Infants with bronchopulmonary dysplasia often have pulmonary hypertension, and in many children even mild hypoxia can cause significant elevations of pulmonary arterial pressure. To minimize the harmful effects of hypoxia, the PaO_2 should be kept above 55–60 mm Hg. Because even intermittent hypoxia contributes to the development or progression of pulmonary hypertension and cor pulmonale, noninvasive assessments of oxygenation must be made during all activities, including the infant's waking, sleeping, and feeding periods. Serial electrocardiographic and echocardiographic studies monitor the development of right ventricular hypertrophy. If hypertrophy persists or if it develops where it was not previously present, intermittent hypoxia should be considered and further assessments of oxygenation pursued, especially while the infant sleeps. Infants with a history of intubation can develop obstructive sleep apnea secondary to a high-arched palate or subglottic narrowing. Barium swallow, esophageal pH probe studies, bronchoscopy, and cardiac catheterization may reveal unsuspected cardiac or pulmonary lesions—aspiration, tracheomalacia, obstructive sleep apnea, anatomic cardiac lesions, etc—that contribute to the underlying pathophysiology. Long-term care should include monitoring systemic hypertension and the development of left ventricular hypertrophy.

Nutritional problems in infants may be due to increased oxygen consumption, feeding difficulties, gastroesophageal reflux, and chronic hypoxia. Hypercaloric formulas and gastrostomies are often required to ensure adequate intake while avoiding overhydration. Influenza vaccine is recommended.

With the onset of acute wheezing secondary to suspected viral infection, rapid diagnostic testing for RSV infection may facilitate early treatment. The recent development of prophylactic intravenous immune globulin therapy specific for RSV has shown promise in reducing the morbidity of bronchiolitis in infants with bronchopulmonary dysplasia.

For children who remain ventilator-dependent, the authors believe that $PaCO_2$ should be maintained below 60 mm Hg—even when pH is normal—because of the potential adverse effects of hypercapnia on salt and water retention, cardiac function, and perhaps pulmonary vascular tone. Changes in ventilator settings in children with severe lung disease should be slow, because the effects of many of the changes may not be manifested for days. These signs may include poor feeding, irritability, weight loss, vomiting, increased retractions, wheezing, and CO_2 retention. Medical staff should meet frequently with the parents to review progress and changes in treatment plans and thereby ease some of the family stresses involved in caring for a child with severe chronic disease. Patience, continued family support, attention to developmental issues, and speech and physical therapy help to improve the long-term outlook.

Prognosis

Although the mortality rate is high in infants with severe (stage IV) bronchopulmonary dysplasia, the long-term outlook is generally favorable. More time and further study is needed, however, to assess the impact in adolescence and early adulthood of such sequelae as persistent airway hyperreactivity, exercise intolerance, and perhaps abnormal lung growth. Long-term follow-up studies suggest that lung function may be altered for life. Hyperinflation and damage to small airways has been reported in children 10 years out from the first signs of bronchopulmonary dysplasia. Late development of cor pulmonale also influences the prognosis adversely. New therapeutic approaches such as surfactant replacement and high-frequency ventilation have not yet been shown to reduce the incidence of bronchopulmonary dysplasia. Controlled trials using systemic corticosteroids at the time of diagnosis of bronchopulmonary dysplasia have resulted in improvements in respiratory status and inflammatory mediators in lung fluid. However, studies have shown the development of alveolar wall thinning, impairment of alveoli formation, and decreased alveolar surface area in neonatal animals treated with dexamethasone. Long-term effects of dexamethasone in treated humans are unknown. The possible role of antioxidant therapy or specific anti-inflammatory agents must be pursued.

Abman SH, Groothuis JR: Pathophysiology and treatment of bronchopulmonary dysplasia: Current issues. Pediatr Clin North Am 1994;41:277.

Hislop AA: Bronchopulmonary dysplasia: Pre- and postnatal influences and outcome (commentary). Pediatr Pulmonol 1997;23:71.

Holtzman RB, Frank L (editors): *Bronchopulmonary Dysplasia. Clinical Perinatology,* Vol 19. Saunders, 1992.

Northway WH, Rosan RC, Porter DY: Pulmonary disease following respiratory therapy of hyaline membrane disease: Bronchopulmonary dysplasia. N Engl J Med 1967;276:357.

Northway WH et al: Late pulmonary sequelae of bronchopulmonary dysplasia. N Engl J Med 1990;323:1793.

Ozdemir A et al: Markers and mediators of inflammation in neonatal lung disease. Pediatr Pulmonol 1997;23:292.

CYSTIC FIBROSIS

Essentials of Diagnosis & Typical Features

- Sweat chloride > 60 mmol/L.
- Mutated CFTR protein.
- Pulmonary, gastrointestinal, or hepatic dysfunction.

General Considerations

Cystic fibrosis is the most common lethal genetic disease in the United States, with an incidence of 1:3000–1:2000 white births. It is a major cause of pulmonary and gastrointestinal morbidity in children and a leading cause of death in early adulthood. Although cystic fibrosis causes abnormalities in the hepatic, gastrointestinal, and male reproductive systems, lung disease is the major cause of morbidity and mortality. Almost all patients develop obstructive lung disease associated with chronic infection that leads to progressive loss of pulmonary function. The prognosis has improved steadily over the past 20 years, so that the median survival is now 31 years—perhaps because of antibiotics, better treatment of malabsorption, and development of a network of cystic fibrosis care centers. The centers usually emphasize a multidisciplinary approach to patient care.

The cystic fibrosis gene is on the long arm of human chromosome 7 and codes for the cystic fibrosis transmembrane conductance regulator (CFTR) protein. The CFTR is involved in chloride channel activity. Approximately 75% of the mutations in cystic fibrosis patients correspond to a specific deletion of three base pairs, which results in loss of a phenylalanine residue at amino acid position 508 of the CFTR. The remainder of the cystic fibrosis mutant gene pool consists of many different mutations. Part of the variability in clinical course in cystic fibrosis can be explained by differences in genotype.

Clinical Findings & Treatment

A. Clinical Presentations and Diagnosis: Seventeen percent of infants with cystic fibrosis present at birth with a type of intestinal obstruction known as meconium ileus. Abdominal distention and the presence of a thick, sticky meconium throughout the large colon on meglumine diatrizoate enema examination suggest the diagnosis. In the past, surgical removal of the meconium was common and often led to resection of bowel. Improved techniques of enema administration under radiologic observation have reduced the need for surgery.

Roughly 50% of patients with cystic fibrosis present in infancy with failure to thrive, respiratory compromise, or both. The age at presentation, however, can be variable; some patients are not diagnosed until adulthood. Neonatal screening based on elevations of immunoreactive trypsinogen in the blood is an alternative method of case identification.

Whether the clinical suspicion of cystic fibrosis is based on meconium ileus, failure to thrive, recurrent respiratory infections, or elevated immunoreactive trypsinogen in infancy, the diagnosis is made only after a positive sweat test or demonstration of a genotype consistent with cystic fibrosis. The sweat of individuals with cystic fibrosis contains elevated concentrations of chloride and sodium. Although elevated sweat electrolytes are associated with other conditions, a positive sweat test combined with the clinical picture usually confirms the diagnosis. Laboratories routinely performing sweat chloride tests give more reliable results than those that perform them only occasionally. The Gibson-Cooke quantitative technique is the only acceptable method. Measurements of electrical conductivity alone can be unreliable.

B. Gastrointestinal and Nutritional Findings and Treatment: Untreated patients with cystic fibrosis have abdominal distention and discomfort; bulky, greasy stools; and increased flatulence secondary to exocrine pancreatic insufficiency and malabsorption. Some infants present with hypoalbuminemia, anemia, edema, and hepatomegaly. Infants with severe protein-calorie malnutrition have particularly difficult courses, with high morbidity and mortality rates. Children and adults with cystic fibrosis are subject to intestinal blockage from inspissated stool. This "meconium ileus equivalent" is now most often treated with cathartics and enemas and only rarely requires surgery. Patients with cystic fibrosis are more prone to intussusception (especially of the appendix) than are normal individuals.

The cornerstone of gastrointestinal treatment is pancreatic enzyme supplementation. Patients are required to take the enzyme capsules with each meal and with snacks. Newer enzyme preparations contain more lipase per capsule than older preparations; therefore, patients take fewer capsules, making administration easier. Occasionally, enzyme supplementation alone does not control the malabsorption, and antacids are added to the regimen.

Individuals with cystic fibrosis may have fat-soluble vitamin deficiency, hypoalbuminemia, and poor growth with decreased stores of body fat. In the past, fat-restricted diets were recommended. It is now rec-

ognized that patients with cystic fibrosis need all the calories they can take, and unrestricted diets are now the norm in most centers. Moreover, caloric supplements, such as high-calorie commercial supplements or formulas or food modules (including Polycose and medium-chain triglycerides) are often added to the patient's diet. In patients who do not respond to oral supplementation, night-time nasogastric feeding or feeding by means of gastrostomy or jejunostomy has been tried. Although there is general agreement that quality of life is enhanced by improved nutrition, it is not known whether aggressive nutritional treatment increases longevity. The goals of nutritional treatment are to achieve normal height and weight. Patients may require many more calories than predicted because of stool loss of fat and protein and ongoing pulmonary infection and inflammation.

C. Pulmonary Findings and Treatment: Infants with cystic fibrosis frequently have respiratory symptoms severe enough to require hospitalization. Cough, tachypnea, rales, and wheezing are common findings. RSV infection is associated with marked morbidity in early infancy. Some patients develop cough only later in childhood or adolescence, but by adulthood almost all patients with cystic fibrosis have productive coughs. In more advanced disease, hemoptysis due to bronchiectasis, exercise limitation, and cor pulmonale may be present. Rales may be heard on physical examination. Clubbing also develops as the lung disease progresses.

Pulmonary function abnormalities initially show obstructive patterns with diminished flow rates and increased lung volumes. As the disease progresses, vital capacity is also affected. The incidence of airway reactivity in cystic fibrosis has been estimated to be 25–50%, several times the incidence in the general population. Initially, the airway is colonized with *Staphylococcus aureus,* but in most patients *Pseudomonas aeruginosa* becomes predominant at some point. Acquisition of the characteristic mucoid *Pseudomonas* is associated with a more rapid decline in pulmonary function. In addition, infection with *Pseudomonas cepacia* has been associated with rapid deterioration and death. Pathologically, the earliest lesions involve hyperplasia of the mucus glands of the bronchial epithelium and mucosal and submucosal cellular infiltrates. Bronchiolectasis and bronchiectasis throughout all lung fields usually follow.

Treatment of the pulmonary disease in cystic fibrosis includes chest physical therapy, antibiotics, bronchodilators, and (more recently) anti-inflammatory agents. Each of these treatments is controversial. Postural drainage and percussion have demonstrated benefit over a 3-year period in a recent study. Antibiotics play a major role in pulmonary treatment and are used liberally in outpatient treatment (eg, with a change in cough or respiratory symptoms). For patients colonized with *S aureus* or nontypeable *H influenzae,* trimethoprim-sulfamethoxazole and cefalexin are commonly used oral antibiotics. For patients colonized with *P aeruginosa,* oral ciprofloxacin is frequently effective. Pulmonary exacerbations associated with *Pseudomonas* colonization are usually treated with two antibiotics to avoid development of resistance. Ceftazidime and tobramycin are the most commonly used intravenous antibiotics; however, the choice of antibiotic should be guided by sensitivity tests.

Recent studies have indicated a benefit from inhaled antibiotics. The high incidence of airway reactivity suggests that bronchodilators could be useful, but some studies have shown paradoxic responses—which may result in part from earlier airway closure due to increasing compliance of large airways.

Current speculation on the development of lung disease in cystic fibrosis includes not only the effects of the bacterial pathogens but also the host response. If activated neutrophils or immune complexes are important in the genesis of the airway injury, anti-inflammatory agents may be helpful. Although corticosteroids may be beneficial in patients with increased airway reactivity, a multicenter trial has identified glucose intolerance, diabetes, and decreased linear growth as complications of alternate-day prednisone. Human recombinant DNase when used chronically improves pulmonary function and reduces the need for hospitalizations, probably by decreasing the viscosity of mucus and improving clearance of secretions.

A subgroup of patients with cystic fibrosis have frequent pulmonary exacerbations characterized by difficult breathing, increased sputum production, decreased exercise tolerance, and diminished pulmonary function. These patients often benefit from hospital treatment, including intensive physical therapy, intravenous antibiotics, bronchodilators, and concentrated efforts at nutritional rehabilitation. Increasingly, outpatient intravenous therapy is being used to shorten or eliminate the hospital stay.

D. Hepatic Disease: Although most patients with cystic fibrosis have cirrhosis at autopsy, only a small percentage develop portal hypertension. In these individuals, however, the clinical manifestations of the liver disease may be severe, with esophageal varices leading to life-threatening gastrointestinal bleeding and hypersplenism requiring splenic embolization.

E. Reproductive Tract Involvement: Failure of development of the vas deferens leaves more than 95% of males with cystic fibrosis infertile. Cystic fibrosis is occasionally diagnosed through infertility evaluations in men with relatively mild involvement of the respiratory and gastrointestinal tracts. In general, women with cystic fibrosis are fertile, but pregnancy may place considerable stress on patients with limited pulmonary function.

Prognosis

The rate of progression of lung involvement usu-

ally determines survival. Most patients now reach adulthood. Lung transplant for end-stage disease is an accepted treatment. In addition, new treatments, including gene therapy trials, are being developed based on improved understanding of the disease at the cellular and molecular levels.

Aitken ML et al: Recombinant human DNase inhalation in normal subjects and patients with cystic fibrosis: A phase 1 study. JAMA 1992:267:1947.

Kerem B-S et al: Identification of the cystic fibrosis gene: Genetic analysis. Science 1989;245:1073.

Kerem E et al: The relation between genotype and phenotype in cystic fibrosis: Analysis of the most common mutation (delta F508). N Engl J Med 1990;323:1517.

MacLusky I: Cystic fibrosis for the primary care pediatrician. Pediatr Ann 1993;22:541.

Ramsey BW: Management of pulmonary disease in patients with cystic fibrosis. N Engl J Med 1996;335:179.

Stern RC: The primary care physician and the patient with cystic fibrosis. J Pediatr 1989; 114:31.

CONGENITAL MALFORMATIONS OF THE LUNG

What follows is a brief description of selected congenital pulmonary malformations that involve or compromise alveoli.

PULMONARY AGENESIS & HYPOPLASIA

With unilateral pulmonary agenesis (complete absence of one lung), the trachea continues into a main bronchus and often has complete tracheal rings. The left lung is affected more often than the right. With compensatory postnatal growth, the remaining lung often herniates into the contralateral chest. Chest x-ray study shows a mediastinal shift toward the affected side, and vertebral abnormalities may be present. Absent or incomplete lung development may be associated with other congenital abnormalities, such as absence of one or both kidneys or fusion of ribs, and the outcome is primarily related to the severity of associated lesions. About 50% of patients survive; the mortality rate is higher with agenesis of the right lung than of the left lung. This difference is probably not related to the higher incidence of associated anomalies but rather to a greater shift in the mediastinum that leads to tracheal compression and distortion.

Pulmonary hypoplasia is incomplete development of one or both lungs, resulting in reduction of the number of bronchial branchings and their associated alveoli. Pulmonary hypoplasia may be present in up to 10–15% of perinatal autopsies. The hypoplasia can be caused by an intrathoracic mass, resulting in lack of space for the lungs to grow; decreased size of the thorax; decreased fetal breathing movements; decreased blood flow to the lungs; or possibly a primary mesodermal defect affecting multiple organ systems. Congenital diaphragmatic hernia is the most common cause, with an incidence of 1:2200 births. Other causes include extralobar sequestration, diaphragmatic eventration or hypoplasia, thoracic neuroblastoma, fetal hydrops, and fetal hydrochylothorax. Chest cage abnormalities, diaphragmatic elevation, oligohydramnios, chromosomal abnormalities, severe musculoskeletal disorders, and cardiac lesions may also lead to hypoplastic lungs. Postnatal factors may play important roles—eg, infants with advanced bronchopulmonary dysplasia can have pulmonary hypoplasia.

Clinical Findings

A. Symptoms and Signs: The clinical presentation is highly variable and is related to the severity of hypoplasia as well as associated abnormalities. Lung hypoplasia is often associated with pneumothorax. Some newborns present with perinatal stress, severe acute respiratory distress, and persistent pulmonary hypertension of the newborn secondary to primary pulmonary hypoplasia (without associated anomalies). Children with lesser degrees of hypoplasia may present with chronic cough, tachypnea, wheezing, and recurrent pneumonia.

B. Laboratory Findings and Imaging: Chest x-ray findings include variable degrees of volume loss in a small hemithorax with mediastinal shift. Computed tomography is the optimal diagnostic imaging procedure if the chest x-ray is not definitive. Ventilation/perfusion scans, angiography, and bronchoscopy are often helpful in the evaluation, demonstrating decreased pulmonary vascularity or premature blunting of airways associated with the mal-developed lung tissue. The degree of respiratory impairment is defined by analysis of arterial blood gases.

Treatment & Prognosis

Treatment is supportive. The outcome is determined by the severity of underlying medical problems, the extent of the hypoplasia, and the degree of pulmonary hypertension.

Langston C, Thurlbeck WM: Conditions altering normal lung growth and development. In: *Neonatal Pulmonary Care.* Thibeault DW, Gregory GA (editors). Appleton-Century-Crofts, 1986.

Phelan PD, Landau LI, Olinsky A: Congenital malformations of the bronchi, lungs, diaphragm and rib cage. In: *Respiratory Illness in Children,* 3rd ed. Phelan PD, Landou LI, Olinsky A (editors). Blackwell Scientific, 1990.

Schwartz MZ et al: Congenital malformations of the lung and mediastinum: A quarter century of experience from a single institution. J Pediatr Surg 1997;32:44.

PULMONARY SEQUESTRATION

Pulmonary sequestration is abnormal pulmonary tissue that does not communicate with the tracheobronchial tree and receives its blood supply from one or more anomalous systemic arteries. It is classified as either extralobar or intralobar. Extralobar sequestration is a mass of pulmonary parenchyma anatomically separate from the normal lung, with a distinct pleural investment. Its blood supply derives from the systemic circulation (more typical), from pulmonary vessels, or from both. Although it can rarely communicate with the esophagus or stomach, it does not communicate directly with the tracheobronchial tree. Pathologically, extralobar sequestration appears as a solitary thoracic lesion near the diaphragm. Abdominal sites are rare. Size varies from 0.5 to 12 cm. The left side is involved in over 90% of cases. In contrast to intralobar sequestrations, venous drainage is usually through the systemic or portal venous system.

Histologic findings include uniformly dilated bronchioles, alveolar ducts, and alveoli. Occasionally, the bronchial structure appears normal; often, however, the cartilage in the wall is deficient, or no cartilage-containing structures can be found. On occasion, lymphangiectasia is found within the lesion. Extralobar sequestration can be associated with other anomalies, including bronchogenic cysts, heart defects, and diaphragmatic hernia, the latter occurring in over half of cases.

Intralobar sequestration is an isolated segment of lung within the normal pleural investment but without connection to the tracheobronchial tree. The arterial supply is often provided by one or more arteries arising from the aorta or its branches. Intralobar sequestration is usually found within the lower lobes (98%) and is rarely associated with other congenital anomalies (less than 2% versus 50% with extralobar sequestration). It is rarely seen in the newborn period (unlike extralobar sequestration). Some have hypothesized that intralobar sequestration is an acquired lesion secondary to chronic infection. Clinical presentation includes chronic cough, wheezing, or "recurrent pneumonias." Rarely, intralobar sequestration can present with hemoptysis. Diagnosis is often made by angiography, demonstrating large systemic arteries perfusing the lesion. Treatment is by surgical resection.

Katzenstein AA: Pediatric Disorders. In: *Katzenstein and Askin's Surgical Pathology of Non-neoplastic Lung Disease,* 3rd ed. Saunders, 1997.

CONGENITAL LOBAR EMPHYSEMA

Congenital lobar emphysema—also known as infantile lobar emphysema, congenital localized emphysema, unilobar obstructive emphysema, congenital hypertrophic lobar emphysema. or congenital lobar overinflation—presents in most patients as severe neonatal respiratory distress or as progressive respiratory impairment during the first year of life. Rarely, the mild or intermittent nature of the symptoms in older children or young adults results in delayed diagnosis. Most patients are white males. Although the cause of congenital lobar emphysema is not well understood, some lesions exhibit bronchial cartilaginous dysplasia due to abnormal orientation or distribution of the bronchial cartilage. This leads to expiratory collapse, producing obstruction and the symptoms outlined below.

Clinical Findings

A. Symptoms and Signs: Clinical features include tachypnea, cyanosis, wheezing, retractions, and cough. Physical examination reveals decreased breath sounds on the affected side, perhaps with hyperresonance to percussion, mediastinal displacement, and bulging of the chest wall on the affected side.

B. Imaging: Radiologic findings include overdistention of the affected lobe (usually an upper or middle lobe), with wide separation of bronchovascular markings, collapse of adjacent lung, shift of the mediastinum away from the affected side, and a depressed diaphragm on the affected side. The radiographic diagnosis may be confusing in the newborn because of retention of alveolar fluid in the affected lobe causing the appearance of a homogeneous density. Other diagnostic studies include chest x-ray with fluoroscopy, ventilation/perfusion study, and perhaps CT scan followed by bronchoscopy with or without bronchography, angiography, and exploratory thoracotomy.

Differential Diagnosis

The differential diagnosis of congenital lobar emphysema includes pneumothorax, pneumatocele, atelectasis with compensatory hyperinflation, diaphragmatic hernia, and congenital cystic adenomatoid malformation. The most common site of involvement is the left upper lobe (42%) or right middle lobe (35%). Evaluation must differentiate regional obstructive emphysema from lobar hyperinflation secondary to an uncomplicated ball-valve mechanism due to extrinsic compression from a mass (eg, bronchogenic cyst, tumor, lymphadenopathy, foreign body, "pseudotumor" or plasma cell granuloma, vascular compression) or intrinsic obstruction from a mucus plug due to infection and inflammation from various causes.

Treatment

Management generally involves surgery, especially when respiratory distress is marked, with either segmental or complete lobectomy. Conservative management in less symptomatic older children may lead to an outcome not different from those treated surgically with lobectomy.

Azizkhan RG et al: Acquired lobar emphysema (overinflation): Clinical and pathological evaluation of infants requiring lobectomy. J Pediatr Surg 1992; 27:1145.

Katzenstein AA: Pediatric Disorders. In: *Katzenstein and Askin's Surgical Pathology of Non-neoplastic Lung Disease,* 3rd ed. Saunders, 1997.

Kravitz RM: Congenital malformations of the lung. Pediatr Clin North Am 1994; 41:453.

CONGENITAL CYSTIC ADENOMATOID MALFORMATION

Congenital cystic adenomatoid malformations are unilateral hamartomatous lesions that generally present as marked respiratory distress within the first days of life. This disorder accounts for 95% of cases of congenital cystic lung disease.

Right and left lungs are involved with equal frequency. These lesions appear as gland-like space-occupying masses or have an "adenomatoid" increase in terminal respiratory structures, forming intercommunicating cysts of various sizes, lined by cuboidal or ciliated pseudostratified columnar epithelium. They may have polypoid formations of mucosa, with focally increased elastic tissue in the cyst wall beneath the bronchial type of epithelium. Air passages appear malformed and tend to lack cartilage.

There are three types. Type 1 is most common (75%) and consists of single or multiple large cysts (1–5 cm in diameter) with features of mature lung tissue. Type 1 is amenable to surgical resection. A mediastinal shift is evident on examination or chest x-ray film in 80% of patients and can mimic infantile lobar emphysema. Approximately 75% of type 1 lesions are right-sided. A survival rate of 90% is generally reported.

Type 2 lesions (20% of cases) consist of multiple small cysts (0.5–1.5 cm) resembling dilated simple bronchioles and are often (60%) associated with other anomalies, especially renal agenesis or dysgenesis, cardiac malformations, and intestinal atresia. Approximately 60% of type 2 lesions are on the left side. Mediastinal shift is evident less often (10%) than in type 1, and the survival rate is worse (40%).

Type 3 lesions consist of small cysts (< 0.5 cm). They appear as a bulky, firm mass. The reported survival rate is 50%.

Recently, two additional types have been described: type 0, a malformation of the proximal tracheobronchial tree (incompatible with life), and type 4, a malformation of the distal acinus. Both types are extremely uncommon.

Clinical Findings

A. Symptoms and Signs: Clinically, respiratory distress is noted soon after birth. Expansion of the cysts occurs with the onset of breathing and produces compression of normal lung areas with mediastinal herniation. Breath sounds are decreased. With type 3 lesions, dullness to percussion may be present. The disorder can present in older patients as a spontaneous pneumothorax or "pneumonia."

B. Imaging: In type 1, chest x-ray shows an intrapulmonary mass of soft tissue density with scattered radiolucent areas of varying sizes and shapes, usually with a mediastinal shift and pulmonary herniation. Placement of a radiopaque feeding tube into the stomach helps in the differentiation from diaphragmatic hernia. Type 2 lesions appear similar except that the cysts are smaller. Type 3 may appear as a solid homogeneous mass filling the hemithorax and causing a marked mediastinal shift. Differentiation from sequestration is not difficult as there is no systemic blood supply to a congenital cystic adenomatoid malformation.

Treatment

Treatment of types 1 and 3 is surgical removal of the affected lobe. Resection is often indicated because of the risk of infection and air trapping, since the malformation communicates with the tracheobronchial tree but mucous clearance is compromised. Because type 2 is often associated with other severe anomalies, management may be more complex. Segmental resection is not feasible because smaller cysts may expand after removal of the more obviously affected area.

Cloutier MM et al: Congenital cystic adenomatoid malformation. Chest 1993;103:761.

Stocker JT: Congenital and developmental diseases. In: *Pulmonary Pathology,* 2nd ed. Dial AH, Hammar AP (editors). Springer, 1994.

ACQUIRED DISORDERS INVOLVING ALVEOLI

BACTERIAL PNEUMONIA

Essentials of Diagnosis & Typical Features

- Fever cough, dyspnea.
- Abnormal chest examination (rales or decreased breath sounds).
- Abnormal chest radiograph (infiltrates, hilar adenopathy, pleural effusion).

General Considerations

Bacterial pneumonia is inflammation of the lung

classified according to the infecting organism. It usually develops when one or more of the defense mechanisms normally protecting the lung is inadequate. Patients with the following problems are particularly predisposed to this disease: aspiration, immunodeficiency or immunosuppression, congenital anomalies (intrapulmonary sequestration, tracheoesophageal fistula, cleft palate), abnormalities in clearance of mucus (cystic fibrosis, ciliary dysfunction, tracheomalacia, bronchiectasis), congestive heart failure, and perinatal contamination.

Clinical Findings

A. Symptoms and Signs: The bacterial pathogen, severity of the disease, and age of the patient may cause substantial variations in the presentation of acute bacterial pneumonia. Infants may manifest few or nonspecific findings on history and physical examination. Immunocompetent older patients may not be extremely ill. Some patients may present with fever only or only with signs of generalized toxicity. Others may have additional symptoms or signs of (1) lower respiratory tract disease (respiratory distress, cough, sputum production), (2) pneumonia (rales, decreased breath sounds, dullness to percussion, abnormal tactile or vocal fremitus), or (3) pleural involvement (splinting, pain, friction rub, dullness to percussion). Some patients may manifest additional extrapulmonary findings, such as meningismus or abdominal pain, due to pneumonia itself. Others may have evidence of infection at other sites due to the same organism causing their pneumonia: meningitis, otitis media, sinusitis, pericarditis, epiglottitis, or abscesses.

B. Laboratory Findings: Elevated white blood cell counts (> 15,000/μL) frequently accompany bacterial pneumonia. However, a low white blood count (< 5000/μL) can be an ominous finding in this disease.

C. Imaging: Chest radiographic findings (lateral and frontal views) define bacterial pneumonia. Patchy infiltrates, atelectasis, hilar adenopathy, or pleural effusion may be observed. Films should be taken in the lateral decubitus position to identify pleural fluid. Complete lobar consolidation is not a common finding in infants and children. Severity of disease may not correlate with radiographic findings. Clinical resolution precedes resolution by chest x-ray.

D. Special Examinations: Invasive diagnostic procedures (transtracheal aspiration, bronchial brushing or washing, lung puncture, or open biopsy) should be undertaken in critically ill patients when other means do not adequately identify the cause (see Culture of Material From the Respiratory Tract).

Differential Diagnosis

The differential diagnosis of pneumonia varies with the age and immunocompetence of the host. The spectrum of potential pathogens to be considered includes aerobic, anaerobic, and acid-fast bacteria as well as *Chlamydia trachomatis* and *C psittaci*, *Rickettsia quintana* (Q fever), *Pneumocystis carinii*, *Bordetella pertussis*, *Mycoplasma pneumoniae*, *Legionella pneumophila*, and respiratory viruses.

Noninfectious pulmonary disease (including gastric aspiration, foreign body aspiration, atelectasis, congenital malformations, congestive heart failure, malignant growths, tumors such as plasma cell granuloma, chronic interstitial lung diseases, and pulmonary hemosiderosis) should be considered in the differential diagnosis of localized or diffuse infiltrates. When effusions are present, additional noninfectious disorders such as collagen diseases, neoplasm, and pulmonary infarction should also be considered.

Complications

Empyema may occur frequently with staphylococcal and group A β-hemolytic streptococcal disease. Pneumococcal effusions have a more benign course. Distal sites of infection—meningitis, otitis media, sinusitis (especially of the ethmoids), and septicemia—may be present, particularly with disease due to *S pneumoniae* or *H influenzae*. Certain immunocompromised patients, such as those who have undergone splenectomy or who have hemoglobin SS or SC disease or thalassemia, are especially prone to overwhelming sepsis with these organisms. Distal infection of the bones, joints, or other organs (eg, liver abscess) may occur in certain hosts with specific organisms.

Treatment

Appropriate antimicrobial therapy varies according to which organisms are the likely cause. Treatment should be guided by (1) Gram's stain of sputum, tracheobronchial secretions, or pleural fluid if available; (2) radiographic findings; (3) age and known or suspected immunocompetence of the host; and (4) local epidemiologic information.

Reasonable coverage for pneumonia in the sick, immunocompromised, or debilitated patient, pending the results of bronchoalveolar lavage or thoracoscopic biopsy, should include (1) ceftazidime, (2) clindamycin, (3) vancomycin, (4) erythromycin for *Legionella* and *Mycoplasma*, and possibly trimethoprim-sulfamethoxazole for *P carinii*. Depending on the circumstances and the level of illness, empiric antifungal or antiviral therapy may be considered. In specific circumstances such as aspiration due to neurologic impairment or in patients with tracheostomies, clindamycin is indicated, pending culture and sensitivity studies, due to the likely presence of resistant anaerobes.

Children with less severe pneumonias can often be treated with an initial injection of ceftazidime, depending on presentation, followed by oral clarithromycin or azithromycin. However, persistence or worsening of symptoms within 3–5 days suggests the presence of a resistant organism, and agents such as clindamycin or vancomycin may be required. When possible, therapy can be guided by the antibiotic sensitivity pattern of the organisms isolated.

Whether or not a child should be hospitalized depends on its age, the severity of illness, the suspected organism, and the anticipated reliability of compliance at home. Home treatment is adequate for most older children. With febrile pneumonias, infants generally—and toddlers often—require admission. Moderate to severe respiratory distress, apnea, hypoxemia, poor feeding, clinical deterioration on treatment, or associated complications (large effusions, empyema, or abscess) indicate the need for immediate hospitalization. Careful follow-up within 12 hours to 5 days is often indicated in those not admitted.

Therapy is also guided by results of studies for bacterial, fungal, and viral pathogens (see Culture of Material From the Respiratory Tract, above) and is based on other diagnostic studies (see below).

Additional therapeutic considerations include (1) oxygen, (2) humidification of inspired gases, (3) hydration and electrolyte supplementation, (4) oral hygiene, and (5) nutrition. Removal of pleural fluid for diagnostic purposes is indicated initially to guide antimicrobial therapy. Many feel that early chest tube drainage of empyema fluid due to *S aureus* is indicated. Empyema due to group A β-hemolytic streptococci or *H influenzae* can also necessitate chest tube drainage, whereas pleural effusions due to *S pneumoniae* rarely do. Repeat pleural taps should be considered in the patient who has persistent high fever for more than 10 days in association with significant pleural effusions. The persistence of organisms in this fluid or the persistence of toxicity, malaise, anorexia, and wasting in the patient suggests the potential need for pleural decortication, a procedure that can be made less morbid by thoracoscopy in skilled hands.

Endotracheal intubation or mechanical ventilation may be indicated in patients with respiratory failure or those too debilitated or overwhelmed to handle their secretions.

Prognosis

For the immunocompetent host in whom bacterial pneumonia is adequately recognized and treated, the survival rate is high. For example, the mortality rate from uncomplicated pneumococcal pneumonia is less than 1%. If the patient survives the initial illness, persistently abnormal pulmonary function following empyema is surprisingly uncommon, even when treatment has been delayed or inappropriate.

Austrian R: Confronting drug-resistant pathogenic bacteria: A report on the Rockefeller University workshop. N Engl J Med 1994;330:1247.

Brook I: Treatment of aspiration or tracheostomy-associated pneumonia in neurologically impaired children: Effect of antimicrobials effective against anaerobic bacteria. Int J Pediatr Otorhinolaryngol 1996;35:171.

Jadavji T et al: A practical guide for the diagnosis and treatment of pediatric pneumonia. Can Med Assoc J 1997;156:S703.

Scheld WM, Mandell GL: Nosocomial pneumonia: Pathogenesis and recent advances in diagnosis and therapy. Rev Infect Dis 1991;13(Suppl 9):S743.

Schutze GE, Jacobs RF: Management of community-acquired bacterial pneumonia in hospitalized children. Pediatr Infect Dis J 1992;11:160.

Tomasz A: Multiple antibiotic-resistant pathogenic bacteria: A report on the Rockefeller University workshop. N Engl J Med 1994;330:1247.

VIRAL PNEUMONIA

Essentials of Diagnosis & Typical Features

- Upper respiratory infection prodrome (fever, coryza, cough, hoarseness).
- Wheezing or rales.
- Myalgia, malaise, headache (older children).

General Considerations

Viral pneumonia constitutes the majority of pediatric pulmonary infections. Respiratory syncytial virus (RSV), parainfluenza (1, 2, and 3) viruses, and influenza (A and B) viruses are responsible for more than 75% of cases. Severity of disease, height of fever, radiographic findings, and the characteristics of cough or lung sounds do not reliably differentiate viral from bacterial pneumonias. However, substantial pleural effusions, pneumatoceles, abscesses, lobar consolidation with lobar volume expansion, and "round" pneumonias are generally inconsistent with viral disease.

Clinical Findings

A. Symptoms and Signs: An upper respiratory infection frequently precedes the onset of lower respiratory disease due to viruses. Although wheezing or stridor may be prominent in viral disease, cough, signs of respiratory difficulty (retractions, grunting, nasal flaring) and physical findings (rales, decreased breath sounds) may not be distinguishable from those in bacterial pneumonia.

B. Laboratory Findings: The peripheral white blood cell count can be normal or slightly elevated and is not useful in distinguishing viral from bacterial disease. A markedly elevated neutrophil count, however, indicates that viral disease is less likely.

Rapid viral diagnostic methods—such as fluorescent antibody tests or ELISA for RSV—are increasingly available and should be performed on nasopharyngeal secretions to confirm this diagnosis in high-risk patients and for epidemiology or infection control. Rapid diagnosis of RSV infection does not preclude the possibility of concomitant infection with other pathogens.

C. Imaging: Chest radiographs frequently show perihilar streaking, increased interstitial markings, peribronchial cuffing, or patchy bronchopneumonia. Lobar consolidation may occur, however, as in bacterial pneumonia. Patients with adenovirus disease may have severe necrotizing pneumonias, resulting in the development of pneumatoceles. Hyperinflation of the lungs may occur when involvement of the small airways is prominent.

Differential Diagnosis

The differential diagnosis of viral pneumonia is the same as for bacterial pneumonia. In patients in whom wheezing is a prominent feature, the physician should consider asthma, airway obstruction caused by foreign body aspiration, acute bacterial or viral tracheitis, and parasitic disease.

Complications

Bronchiolitis obliterans or severe chronic respiratory failure may follow adenovirus pneumonia. Bronchiolitis or viral pneumonia may contribute to persistent reactive airway disease in some patients. Bronchiectasis, persistent interstitial lung diseases (fibrosis and desquamative interstitial pneumonitis), and unilateral hyperlucent lung (Swyer-James syndrome) may follow measles, adenovirus, and influenzal pneumonias. Viral pneumonia or laryngotracheobronchitis may predispose the patient to subsequent bacterial tracheitis or pneumonia as immediate sequelae. Plasma cell granuloma may develop as a rare sequela of viral or bacterial pneumonia.

Treatment

General supportive care for viral pneumonia does not differ from that for bacterial pneumonia. Patients can be quite ill and should be hospitalized according to the level of their illness. Because bacterial disease often cannot be definitively excluded, antibiotics may be indicated.

Patients at risk for life-threatening RSV infections, eg, those with bronchopulmonary dysplasia or other severe pulmonary conditions, congenital heart disease, or significant immunocompromise, should be hospitalized and treated with ribavirin. Rapid viral diagnostic tests may be a useful guide for such therapy. These high-risk patients should be immunized annually against influenza A and B viruses. Despite immunization, however, influenza can still occur. When available epidemiologic data indicate an active influenza A infection in the community, rimantadine or amantadine hydrochloride should be considered early for high-risk infants and children who appear to be infected.

Children with suspected viral pneumonia should be placed in respiratory isolation.

Prognosis

Although most children with viral pneumonia recover uneventfully, worsening reactive airway disease, abnormal pulmonary function or chest radiographs, persistent respiratory insufficiency, and even death may occur in high-risk patients such as newborns or those with underlying lung, cardiac, or immunodeficiency disease. Patients with adenovirus infection or those concomitantly infected with RSV and second pathogens such as influenza, adenovirus, cytomegalovirus or *P carinii* also have a poorer prognosis.

Heidemann SM: Clinical characteristics of parainfluenza virus infection in hospitalized children. Pediatr Pulmonol 1992;13:86.
Kim PE et al: Association of invasive pneumococcal disease with season, atmospheric conditions, air pollution, and the isolation of respiratory viruses. Clin Infect Dis 1996;22:100.
Stretton M et al: Intensive care course and outcome of patients infected with respiratory syncytial virus. Pediatr Pulmonol 1992;13:143.
Tristram DA et al: Simultaneous infection with respiratory syncytial virus and other respiratory pathogens. Am J Dis Child 1988;142:834.

CHLAMYDIAL PNEUMONIA

Essentials of Diagnosis & Typical Features

- Cough, tachypnea, rales, few wheezes, and no fever.
- Appropriate age: 2–12 weeks.
- Inclusion conjunctivitis, eosinophilia, and elevated immunoglobulins can be seen.

General Considerations

Pulmonary disease due to *C trachomatis* usually evolves gradually as the infection descends the respiratory tract. Infants may appear quite well despite the presence of significant pulmonary illness. Infant infections are now at epidemic proportions in urban environments worldwide. Other sexually transmitted organisms such as *U urealyticum* may also be widespread and contribute to lung disease in infants. Unlike other bacteria, the chlamydiae are unable to synthesize their own ATP and are sometimes called "energy parasites."

Clinical Findings

A. Symptoms and Signs: About 50% of patients with chlamydial pneumonia have active inclusion conjunctivitis or a history of it. Rhinopharyngitis with nasal discharge or otitis media may have occurred or may be currently present. Female patients may have vulvovaginitis.

Cough is usually present. It can have a staccato character and resemble the cough of pertussis. The infant is usually tachypneic. Scattered inspiratory rales are commonly heard, but wheezes rarely. Significant fever suggests a different or additional diagnosis.

B. Laboratory Findings: Although patients may frequently be hypoxemic, CO_2 retention is not common. Peripheral blood eosinophilia (400 cells/μL) has been observed in about 75% of patients. Serum immunoglobulins are usually abnormal. IgM is virtually always elevated, IgG is high in many, and IgA is less frequently abnormal. *C trachomatis* can usually be identified in nasopharyngeal washings using fluorescent antibody or culture techniques.

C. Imaging: Chest radiographs may reveal diffuse interstitial and patchy alveolar infiltrates, peribronchial thickening, or focal consolidation. A small pleural reaction can be present. Despite the usual absence of wheezes, hyperexpansion is commonly present.

Differential Diagnosis

Bacterial, viral, and fungal *(P carinii)* pneumonias should be considered. Premature infants and those with bronchopulmonary dysplasia may also have chlamydial pneumonia.

Treatment

Erythromycin or sulfisoxazole therapy should be administered for 14 days. Hospitalization may be required for infants with significant respiratory distress, coughing paroxysms, or posttussive apnea. Oxygen therapy may be required for prolonged periods in some patients.

Prognosis

An increased incidence of obstructive airway disease and abnormal pulmonary function tests may occur for at least 7–8 years following infection.

Brayden RM et al: Apnea in infants with *Chlamydia trachomatis* pneumonia. Pediatr Infect Dis J 1987;6:423.
Grayston JT et al: A new respiratory pathogen: *Chlamydia pneumoniae,* strain TWAR. J Infect Dis 1990; 161:618.
Hammerschlag MR et al: Persistent infection with *Chlamydia pneumoniae* following acute respiratory infection. Clin Infect Dis 1992;14:178.

MYCOPLASMAL PNEUMONIA

Essentials of Diagnosis & Typical Features

- Fever.
- Cough.
- Appropriate age: over 5 years.

General Considerations

M pneumoniae is a common cause of symptomatic

pneumonia in older children. Endemic and epidemic infection can occur. The incubation period is long (2–3 weeks), and the onset of symptoms is slow. Although the lung is the primary infection site, there are sometimes extrapulmonary complications.

Clinical Findings

A. Symptoms and Signs: Fever, cough, headache, and malaise are common symptoms as the illness evolves. Although cough is usually dry at the onset, sputum production may develop as the illness progresses. Sore throat, otitis media, otitis externa, and bullous myringitis may occur. Rales are frequently present on chest examination; decreased breath sounds or dullness to percussion over the involved area may be present.

B. Laboratory Findings: The total and differential white blood cell counts are usually normal. The cold hemagglutinin titer should be determined, because it may be elevated during the acute presentation. A titer of 1:64 or higher supports the diagnosis. Acute and convalescent titers for *M pneumoniae* demonstrating a fourfold or greater rise in specific antibodies confirm the diagnosis.

C. Imaging: Chest radiographs usually demonstrate interstitial or bronchopneumonic infiltrates, frequently in the middle or lower lobes. Pleural effusions are extremely uncommon.

Complications

Extrapulmonary involvement of the blood, central nervous system, skin, heart, or joints can occur. Direct Coombs-positive autoimmune hemolytic anemia, occasionally a life-threatening disorder, is the most common hematologic abnormality that can accompany *M pneumoniae* infection. Coagulation defects and thrombocytopenia can also occur. Cerebral infarction, meningoencephalitis, Guillain-Barré syndrome, cranial nerve involvement, and psychosis all have been described. A wide variety of skin rashes, including erythema multiforme and Stevens-Johnson syndrome, can occur. Myocarditis, pericarditis, and a rheumatic fever-like illness can also occur.

Treatment

Antibiotic therapy with erythromycin for 7–10 days usually shortens the course of illness. Ciprofloxacin is a possible alternative. Supportive measures, including hydration, antipyretics, and bed rest, are helpful.

Prognosis

In the absence of the less common extrapulmonary complications, the outlook for recovery is excellent. The extent to which *M pneumoniae* can initiate or exacerbate chronic lung disease is not well understood.

Hammerschlag MR: Atypical pneumonias in children. Adv Pediatr Infect Dis 1995; 10:1.

Klein JP: History of macrolide use in pediatrics. Pediatr Infect Dis J 1997;16:427.
Leigh MW, Clyde WA Jr: Chlamydial and mycoplasmal pneumonias. Semin Respir Infect 1987;2:152.
Orlicek SL, Walker MS, Kuhls TL: Severe mycoplasma pneumonia in young children with Down syndrome. Clin Pediatr 1992;31:409.

TUBERCULOSIS

Essentials of Diagnosis & Typical Features
- Positive tuberculin skin test or anergic host.
- Positive culture for *Mycobacterium tuberculosis*.

General Considerations

There is a resurgence of tuberculosis in all age groups, including children. The clinical spectrum of tuberculosis includes a positive tuberculin skin test without evident disease, asymptomatic primary infection, the Ghon complex, bronchial obstruction with secondary collapse or obstructed airways, segmental lesions, calcified nodules, pleural effusions, progressive primary cavitating lesions, contiguous spread into adjacent thoracic structures, acute miliary tuberculosis, adult respiratory distress syndrome (ARDS), overwhelming reactivation infection in the immunocompromised host, occult lymphohematogenous spread, and metastatic extrapulmonary involvement at almost any site. Symptoms of airway obstruction, sometimes with secondary bacterial pneumonia resulting from hilar adenopathy, are common presenting features in children.

Clinical Findings

A. Symptoms and Signs: The most important aspect of the history is contact with an individual with tuberculosis—often an elderly relative, a caretaker, or a person previously residing in a region where tuberculosis is endemic—or a history of travel to or residence in such an area. Homeless and extremely impoverished children are also at high risk, as are those in contact with high-risk adults (AIDS patients, residents or employees of correctional institutions or nursing homes, drug users, and health care workers). Once exposed, pediatric patients at risk for developing active disease include infants and those with malnutrition, AIDS, diabetes mellitus, or immunosuppression (cancer chemotherapy, corticosteroids). In suspected cases, the patient, immediate family, and suspected carriers should be tuberculin-tested. Spread is mainly respiratory, so isolated pulmonary parenchymal tuberculosis constitutes more than 95% of presenting cases. The primary focus, which is usually single, and the nodal involvement may or may not be radiographically visible. Because healing—rather than progression—is the usual course in the uncompromised host, a positive tuberculin test may be the only manifestation. However, for patients born outside the United States, a positive test may indicate only a previous BCG immunization.

The tuberculous complications listed previously most often occur during the first year of infection. Thereafter, infection remains quiescent until adolescence, when reactivation of pulmonary tuberculosis is common. At any stage, chronic cough, anorexia, weight loss or failure to gain weight, and fever are useful clinical signs if present. Except in cases with complications or advanced disease, physical findings are few. Most children with pulmonary tuberculosis are asymptomatic.

B. Laboratory Findings: A positive tuberculin skin test is defined as 10 mm or more of induration 48–72 hours after intradermal injection of 5 tuberculin units of PPD. Tine tests should not be used. Appropriate control skin tests, such as those for hypersensitivity to diphtheria-tetanus, mumps, or *Candida albicans,* should be applied at the same time PPD is applied. If the patient fails to respond to PPD and all of the controls, the possibility of tuberculosis is not excluded.

Anteroposterior and lateral chest radiographs should be obtained in all suspected cases. Culture for *M tuberculosis* is critical for proving the diagnosis and for defining drug susceptibility. Early morning gastric lavage following an overnight fast should be performed on three occasions in infants and children with suspected active pulmonary tuberculosis prior to the onset of drug therapy when the severity of illness allows. Although stains for acid-fast bacilli on this material are of little value, this is the ideal culture site. Despite the increasing importance of isolating organisms because of multiple drug resistance, only 40% of children will yield positive cultures.

Sputum cultures from older children and adolescents are similarly useful. Stains and cultures of bronchial secretions are useful if bronchoscopy is performed as part of the patient's evaluation. When pleural effusions are present, pleural biopsy for cultures and histopathologic examination for granulomas or organisms provide diagnostic information. Meningeal involvement is a real possibility in young children, and lumbar puncture should be considered in their initial evaluation.

Differential Diagnosis

Fungal diseases that affect mainly the lungs, such as histoplasmosis, coccidioidomycosis, cryptococcosis, and North American blastomycosis, may resemble tuberculosis and in doubtful cases should be excluded by appropriate serologic studies. Atypical tuberculous organisms may involve the lungs, especially in the immunocompromised patient. Depending on the presentation, diagnoses such as lymphoreticular and other malignancies, collagen-vascular disorders, or other pulmonary infections may be considered.

Complications

In addition to those listed above, lymphadenitis, meningitis, osteomyelitis, arthritis, enteritis, peritonitis, and renal, ocular, middle ear, and cutaneous disease may occur. The infant born to tuberculous parents is at great risk for developing illness. The possibility of life-threatening airway compromise must always be considered in patients with large mediastinal or hilar lesions.

Treatment

Because the risk of hepatitis due to isoniazid is extremely low in children, this drug is indicated in those with a positive tuberculin skin test. This greatly reduces the risk of subsequent active disease and complications with minimal morbidity. Isoniazid plus rifampin treatment for 6 months, plus pyrazinamide during the first 2 months, is indicated when the chest radiograph is abnormal or when there is extrapulmonary disease. Without pyrazinamide, isoniazid plus rifampin must be given for 9 months. In general, the more severe tuberculous complications are treated with a larger number of drugs. Enforced, directly observed therapy (twice weekly or oftener) is indicated when noncompliance is suspected. Recommendations for antituberculosis chemotherapy, based on disease stage, are continuously being updated. The most current edition of the AAP *Red Book* is a reliable source for these protocols.

Corticosteroids are used to control inflammation in selected patients with (1) potentially life-threatening airway compression by lymph nodes, (2) acute pericardial effusion, (3) massive pleural effusion with mediastinal shift, and, perhaps, (4) miliary tuberculosis with respiratory failure.

Prognosis

In patients with an intact immune system, modern antituberculous therapy offers good potential for recovery. The outlook for patients with immunodeficiencies, organisms resistant to multiple drugs, poor drug compliance, or advanced complications is guarded. Organisms resistant to multiple drugs are increasingly common. Resistance emerges either because the physician prescribes an inadequate regimen or because the patient discontinues medications. When resistance to or intolerance of isoniazid and rifampin prevents their use, cure rates are 50% or less.

American Academy of Pediatrics Committee on Infectious Diseases: Screening for tuberculosis in infants and children. Pediatrics 1994;93:131.

Serwint JR et al: Outcomes of annual tuberculosis screening by Mantoux test in children considered to be at high risk: Results from one urban clinic. Pediatrics 1997; 99:529.

Starke JR, Jacobs RF, Jereb J: Resurgence of tuberculosis in children. J Pediatr 1992;120:839.

StarkE JR: Universal screening for tuberculosis infection: School's out! JAMA 1995;274:652.

Starke JR: Current chemotherapy for tuberculosis in children. Infect Dis Clin North Am 1992;6:215.

Vallejo JG, Starke JR: Intrathoracic tuberculosis in children. Semin Respir Infect 1996;11:184.

ASPIRATION PNEUMONIA

Patients whose anatomic defense mechanisms are impaired are at risk of aspiration pneumonia (Table 17–2). Acute disease is commonly caused by bacteria present in the mouth (especially gram-negative anaerobes). Chronic aspiration often causes recurrent bouts of acute febrile pneumonia. It may also lead to chronic focal infiltrates, atelectasis, or illness resembling asthma or interstitial lung disease.

Clinical Findings

A. Symptoms and Signs: Acute onset of fever, cough, respiratory distress, or hypoxemia in a patient at risk suggests aspiration pneumonia. Chest physical findings, such as rales, rhonchi, or decreased breath sounds, may initially be limited to the lung region into which aspiration occurred. Although any region may be affected, the right side—especially the right upper lobe in the supine patient—is commonly affected. In patients with chronic aspiration, diffuse wheezing may occur. Generalized rales may also be present. Such patients may not develop acute febrile pneumonias.

B. Laboratory Findings and Imaging: Chest radiographs may reveal lobar consolidation or atelectasis and focal or generalized alveolar or interstitial infiltrates. In some patients with chronic aspiration, perihilar infiltrates with or without bilateral air trapping may be seen.

In severely ill patients with acute febrile illnesses, a bacteriologic diagnosis should be made. In addition to blood cultures, cultures of tracheobronchial secretions and bronchoalveolar lavage or lung puncture

Table 17–2. Risk factors for aspiration pneumonia.

Seizures
Depressed sensorium
Recurrent gastroesophageal reflux, emesis, or
   gastrointestinal obstruction
Neuromuscular disorders with suck-swallow dysfunction
Anatomic abnormalities (laryngeal cleft, tracheoesophageal
   fistula, vocal cord paralysis)
Debilitating illnesses
Occult brain stem lesions
Near-drowning
Nasogastric, endotracheal, or tracheostomy tubes
Severe periodontal disease

specimens may be desirable. (See Culture of Material From the Respiratory Tract, above.)

In patients with chronic aspiration pneumonitis, solid documentation of aspiration as the cause of illness may be elusive. Barium contrast studies may provide evidence of suck-swallow dysfunction, laryngeal cleft, occult tracheoesophageal fistula, or gastroesophageal reflux. Overnight or 24-hour esophageal pH probe studies may also help establish the latter. Although radionuclide scans are commonly used, the yield from such studies is disappointingly low. Rigid bronchoscopy in infants or flexible bronchoscopy in older children can be useful in (1) more definitively excluding tracheoesophageal fistula and (2) obtaining bronchoalveolar lavage specimens to search for lipid-laden macrophages as evidence of chronic aspiration.

Differential Diagnosis

In the acutely ill patient, bacterial and viral pneumonias should be considered. In the chronically ill patient, the differential diagnosis may include disorders causing (1) recurrent pneumonia (eg, immunodeficiencies, ciliary dysfunction, foreign body, etc), (2) chronic wheezing, or (3) interstitial lung disorders (see Interstitial Lung Disease), depending on the presentation.

Complications

Empyema or lung abscess may result from acute aspiration pneumonia. Chronic disease may result in bronchiectasis.

Treatment

Antimicrobial therapy for acute aspiration pneumonia includes coverage for gram-negative anaerobic organisms. In general, clindamycin is appropriate initial coverage. However, in some hospital-acquired infections, additional coverage for multiply resistant *P aeruginosa,* streptococci, and other organisms may be required.

Treatment of recurrent and chronic aspiration pneumonia may include the following: (1) surgical correction of anatomic abnormalities; (2) improved oral hygiene; (3) improved hydration; and (4) inhaled bronchodilators, chest physical therapy, and suctioning. In patients with compromise of the central nervous system, exclusive feeding by gastrostomy and (in some) tracheostomy may be required to control airway secretions. Gastroesophageal reflux, often requiring surgical correction, is commonly present in such patients.

Prognosis

The outlook is directly related to the disorder causing aspiration.

Brook I: Treatment of aspiration or tracheostomy-associated pneumonia in neurologically impaired children: Effect of antimicrobials effective against anaerobic bacteria. Int J Pediatr Otorhinolaryngol 1996;35:171.

Colombo JL, Hallberg TK, Sammut PH: Time course of lipid-laden macrophages with acute and recurrent milk aspiration in rabbits. Pediatr Pulmonol 1992;12:95.

Colombo JL, Hallberg TK: Recurrent aspiration in children: Lipid-laden alveolar macrophage quantitation. Pediatr Pulmonol 1987;3:86.

Finegold SM: Aspiration pneumonia. Rev Infect Dis 1991;13(Suppl 9):S737.

Moran JR et al: Lipid-laden alveolar macrophage and lactose assay as markers of aspiration in neonates with lung disease. J Pediatr 1988;112:643.

PNEUMONIA IN THE IMMUNOCOMPROMISED HOST

Pneumonia in an immunocompromised host may be due to any common bacteria (streptococci, staphylococci, *M pneumoniae*) or less common pathogens such as *Toxoplasma gondii, P carinii, Aspergillus* species, *Mucor, Candida* species, *Cryptococcus neoformans,* gram-negative enteric and anaerobic bacteria, *Nocardia, Legionella pneumophila,* mycobacteria, and viruses (cytomegalovirus, varicella-zoster, herpes simplex, influenza virus, respiratory syncytial virus, adenovirus). Multiple organisms are commonly present.

Clinical Findings

A. Symptoms and Signs: Patients often present with subtle signs such as mild cough, tachypnea, or low-grade fever that can rapidly progress to high fever, respiratory distress, and hypoxemia. An obvious portal of infection, such as an intravascular catheter, may predispose to bacterial or fungal infection.

B. Laboratory Findings and Imaging: Fungal, parasitic, or bacterial infection, especially with antibiotic-resistant bacteria, should be suspected in the neutropenic child. Cultures of peripheral blood, sputum, tracheobronchial secretions, urine, nasopharynx or sinuses, bone marrow, pleural fluid, biopsied lymph nodes, or skin lesions or cultures through intravascular catheters should be obtained as soon as infection is suspected.

Invasive methods are commonly required to make a diagnosis. Appropriate samples should be obtained soon after a patient with pneumonia fails to respond to initial treatment. The results of these procedures usually lead to important changes in empiric preoperative therapy. Sputum is frequently unavailable. Bronchoalveolar lavage frequently provides the diagnosis of one or more organisms and should be done early in evaluation. The combined use of a wash, brushing, and lavage has a high yield. In patients with rapidly advancing disease, open lung biopsy becomes more urgent. The morbidity and mortality rates of this procedure can be reduced by a thoracoscopic approach by a skilled operator. Because of the multiplicity of organisms that may cause disease, a comprehensive set of studies should be done on lavage or biopsy material. These consist of (1) rapid diagnostic studies, including fluorescent antibody studies for *Legionella;* rapid culture and antigen detection for viruses; (2) Gram's, acid-fast, and fungal stains; (3) cytologic examination for viral inclusions; (4) cultures for viruses, anaerobic and aerobic bacteria, fungi, mycobacteria, and *Legionella;* and (5) rapid immunofluorescent studies for *P carinii.*

Chest radiographs may be useful. In *P carinii* pneumonia, dyspnea and hypoxemia may be marked despite minimal radiographic abnormalities

Differential Diagnosis

The organisms causing disease vary with the type of immunocompromise present. For example, the splenectomized patient may be overwhelmed by infection with *S pneumoniae* or *H influenzae.* The infant receiving ACTH therapy may be more likely to have *P carinii* infection. The febrile neutropenic child who has been receiving adequate doses of intravenous broad-spectrum antibiotics may have fungal disease, including pneumocystis pneumonia. The key to diagnosis, however, is to consider all possibilities of infection.

Depending on the form of immunocompromise, perhaps only one-half to two-thirds of new pulmonary infiltrates in such patients represent infection. The remainder are caused by (1) pulmonary toxicity of radiation, oxygen, chemotherapy, or other drugs; (2) pulmonary disorders, including hemorrhage, embolism, atelectasis, aspiration, or ARDS; (3) recurrence or extension of primary malignant growths or immunologic disorders; (4) transfusion reactions, leukostasis, or tumor cell lysis; or (5) interstitial lung disease, such as lymphocytic interstitial pneumonitis with HIV infection.

Complications

Respiratory failure, shock, multiple organ damage, disseminated infection, and death commonly occur in the infected immunocompromised host.

Treatment

Broad-spectrum intravenous antibiotics are indicated early in febrile, neutropenic, or immunocompromised children. Trimethoprim-sulfamethoxazole (for *Pneumocystis*) and erythromycin (for *Legionella*) are also indicated early in the treatment of immunocompromised children before an organism is identified. Further therapy should be based on studies of specimens obtained from bronchoalveolar lavage or lung biopsy.

Prognosis

Prognosis is based on the severity of the underlying immunocompromise, appropriate early diagnosis and treatment, and the infecting organisms.

Frankel LR et al: Bronchoalveolar lavage for diagnosis of pneumonia in the immunocompromised child. Pediatrics 1988;81:785.

Glaser JH et al: Cytomegalovirus and *Pneumocystis carinii* pneumonia in children with acquired immunodeficiency syndrome. J Pediatr 1992;120:929.

Grubman S, Simonds RJ: Preventing *Pneumocystis carinii* pneumonia in human immunodeficiency virus-infected children: New guidelines for prophylaxis. Pediatr Infect Dis J 1996;15:165.

Lanino E et al: Fiberoptic bronchoscopy and bronchoalveolar lavage for the evaluation of pulmonary infiltrates after BMT in children. Bone Marrow Transplant 1996; 18(Suppl 2):117.

Martin WJ II: Diagnostic bronchoalveolar lavage in immunosuppressed patients with new pulmonary infiltrates. Mayo Clin Proc 1992;67:296.

McSherry GD: Human immunodeficiency-virus-related pulmonary infections in children. Semin Respir Infect 1996;11:173.

Shaw NJ, Elton R, Eden OB: Pneumonia and pneumonitis in childhood malignancy. Acta Paediatr 1992;81:222.

HYPERSENSITIVITY PNEUMONIA

Essentials of Diagnosis
& Typical Features

- History of exposure (eg, birds, organic dusts or molds).
- Interstitial infiltrates on chest radiograph or diffuse rales.
- Recurrent cough, fever, wheezing, or weight loss can occur.

GENERAL CONSIDERATIONS

Hypersensitivity pneumonitis is a disease involving the peripheral airways, interstitium, and alveoli. Both acute and chronic forms may occur. In children, the most common forms are brought on by exposure to birds or bird droppings (eg, pigeons, parakeets, parrots, doves). Inhalation of almost any organic dust, however (moldy hay, compost, logs or tree bark, sawdust, or aerosols from humidifiers), can cause disease.

Clinical Findings

A. Symptoms and Signs: Episodic cough and fever can occur with acute exposures. Chronic exposure results in weight loss, fatigue, dyspnea, cyanosis, and, ultimately, respiratory failure.

B. Laboratory Findings: Acute exposure may be followed by polymorphonuclear leukocytosis with eosinophilia and evidence of airway obstruction on pulmonary function testing. Chronic disease results in a restrictive picture on lung function tests. Arterial blood gases may reveal hypoxemia with a decreased $PaCO_2$ and normal pH.

The serologic key to diagnosis is the finding of precipitins (precipitating IgG antibodies) to the organic dusts that contain avian proteins or fungal or bacterial antigens. However, exposure may invoke precipitins without causing disease.

Differential Diagnosis

Patients with mainly acute symptoms must be differentiated from those with atopic asthma. Patients with chronic symptoms must be distinguished from those with collagen-vascular, immunologic, or primary interstitial pulmonary disorders.

Complications

Prolonged exposure to offending antigens may result in pulmonary hypertension due to chronic hypoxemia, cor pulmonale, irreversible restrictive lung disease due to pulmonary fibrosis, or respiratory failure.

Treatment

Complete elimination of exposure to the offending antigens is required. Corticosteroids may hasten recovery.

Prognosis

With appropriate diagnosis and avoidance of offending antigens, the prognosis is excellent. A good prognosis, however, is dependent on early diagnosis before pulmonary damage is irreversible.

Carlsen K-H et al: Allergic alveolitis in a 12-year-old boy: Treatment with budesonide nebulizing solution. Pediatr Pulmonol 1992;12:257.

Eisenberg JD, Montanero A, Lee RG: Hypersensitivity pneumonitis in an infant. Pediatr Pulmonol 1992;12:186.

O'Connell EJ et al: Childhood hypersensitivity pneumonitis (farmer's lung): Four cases in siblings with long-term follow-up. J Pediatr 1989;114:995.

Selman M, Chapela R, Raghu G: Hypersensitivity pneumonitis: Clinical manifestations, pathogenesis, diagnosis, and therapeutic strategies. Semin Respir Med 1993;14:353.

INTERSTITIAL LUNG DISEASE

Essentials of Diagnosis
& Typical Features

- Tachypnea, dyspnea, retractions, or hypoxemia.
- Cough or rales.
- Bilateral pulmonary infiltrates.

General Considerations

The presentation of interstitial lung disorders in children is often subtle and gradual in onset. Such disorders in the child are commonly caused by infection, immunodeficiency, aspiration, cardiac disease, or pulmonary vascular disease. Children are less likely than adults to have primary (idiopathic) pulmonary interstitial lung disorders (eg, desquamative, usual, or lymphocytic interstitial pneumonitis), hypersensitivity pneumonitis, or collagen-vascular diseases.

Clinical Findings

A. Symptoms and Signs: Children may present with a chronic dry cough or a history of dyspnea on exertion. The child with more advanced disease may have increased dyspnea, tachypnea, retractions, cyanosis, clubbing, failure to thrive, or weight loss. Physical examination may reveal these findings, and dry ("Velcro") rales may be present on chest auscultation, especially at the lung bases.

B. Laboratory Findings and Imaging: Chest radiographs are normal in up to 10–15% of patients. More commonly, diffuse or perihilar bilateral reticular interstitial infiltrates are present. Nodular and reticulonodular diseases are uncommon in children except in HIV infection. Bilateral disease is the rule except in cases of infection and aspiration-related disorders, which may be unilateral.

On pulmonary function testing, interstitial disorders often show a restrictive pattern of decreased lung volumes, compliance, and diffusing capacity for carbon monoxide, whereas the FEV_1/FVC ratio may be normal or increased. However, exercise-induced hypoxemia is often the earliest detectable abnormality of lung function. Blood gas abnormalities include hypoxemia, a low $PaCO_2$, and normal pH.

Many chronically ill patients can be investigated in a sequence: (1) "serologic," (2) bronchoscopic, and (3) biopsy steps. Although bronchoalveolar lavage may be useful in identifying patients with pulmonary hemosiderosis (hemosiderin-laden macrophages), aspiration (lipid-laden macrophages), and infectious disorders, lung biopsy is the most reliable method for definitive diagnosis.

During the initial phase, the following diagnostic studies may be considered: x-rays, barium swallow, pulmonary function tests, skin tests (see Tuberculosis); complete blood count and ESR; sweat chloride test for cystic fibrosis; ECG or echocardiogram; serum immunoglobulins, and other immunologic evaluations; sputum studies (see Pneumonia in the Immunocompromised Host, above); and studies for Epstein-Barr virus, cytomegalovirus, *M pneumoniae, Chlamydia, Pneumocystis,* and *U urealyticum.*

During the second phase, rigid bronchoscopy should be performed to exclude anatomic abnormalities and obtain multiple bronchial biopsies to examine cilia. At the same procedure, bronchoalveolar lavage should be done, preferably through a flexible bronchoscope and an endotracheal tube if the patient is large enough, for microbiologic and cytologic testing. In patients with static or slowly progressing disease, one can then await results of bronchoscopic studies. In patients with acute, rapidly progressive

disease, this stage should be combined with thoracoscopic or open lung biopsy. Special stains and cultures, immunofluorescence for immune complexes, and electron microscopy should be ordered. Although transbronchial biopsy may be useful in diagnosing a few disorders (eg, sarcoidosis), its overall usefulness in pediatrics is limited.

Differential Diagnosis

Malignant disorders (histiocytosis X, disseminated carcinoma), congenital disorders (Gaucher's disease, neurofibromatosis, tuberous sclerosis, familial interstitial lung disease), pulmonary hemosiderosis, pulmonary telangiectasia or lymphangiectasia, bronchiolitis obliterans, sarcoidosis, and ciliary dyskinesia should be considered in addition to the groups of disorders mentioned above.

Complications

Respiratory failure or pulmonary hypertension with cor pulmonale may occur.

Treatment

Therapy for interstitial lung disease due to infection, aspiration, or cardiac disorders should be directed toward the primary disorder. Most of the primary pulmonary interstitial disorders are treated initially with prednisone (2 mg/kg/d) for 6 weeks to 6 months depending on the severity of disease and the response. Many patients require even more protracted therapy with alternate-day prednisone. Chloroquine (5–10 mg/kg/d) may be useful in selected disorders such as desquamative interstitial pneumonitis. Addition of cytotoxic drugs (azathioprine, cyclophosphamide) has not been shown to be more beneficial than prednisone alone.

Prognosis

The prognosis is guarded in children with interstitial lung disease due to collagen-vascular and primary pulmonary interstitial diseases, immunodeficiency diseases, and cancer.

Bokulic RE, Hilman BC: Interstitial lung disease in children. Pediatr Clin North Am 1994;41:543.

Fan LL et al: Clinical spectrum of chronic interstitial lung disease in children. J Pediatr 1992;121:867.

Fan LL: Evaluation and therapy of chronic interstitial pneumonitis in children. Curr Opin Pediatr 1994;6:248.

Rothenberg SS et al: The safety and efficacy of thoracoscopic lung biopsy in infants and children. J Pediatr Surg 1996;31:100.

EOSINOPHILIC PNEUMONIA

Essentials of Diagnosis & Typical Features

- Pulmonary infiltrates, often migratory, on chest radiograph.

- Persistent cough; wheezes or rales on chest auscultation.
- Increased eosinophils in peripheral blood or in lung biopsy specimens.

General Considerations

A spectrum of diseases should be considered under this heading: (1) transient pulmonary infiltrates with eosinophilia (Löffler's syndrome), (2) tropical eosinophilia, (3) pulmonary eosinophilia with asthma (allergic bronchopulmonary aspergillosis and related disorders), (4) hypereosinophilic mucoid impaction, (5) bronchocentric granulomatosis, and (6) collagen-vascular disorders. Many occur in children with personal or family histories of allergies or asthma. These disorders may be related to hypersensitivity to migratory parasitic nematodes *(Ascaris, Strongyloides, Ancylostoma, Toxocara, Trichuris),* larval forms of filariae *(Wuchereria bancrofti),* or fungi *(Aspergillus, Candida).* Eosinophilic pneumonias can be associated also with drug hypersensitivity, sarcoidosis, Hodgkin's disease or other lymphomas, and bacterial infections, including brucellosis and those caused by *M tuberculosis* and atypical mycobacteria.

Clinical Findings

A. Symptoms and Signs: Cough, wheezing, and dyspnea are common presenting complaints. In Löffler's syndrome, fever, malaise, sputum production, and, rarely, hemoptysis may be present. In allergic bronchopulmonary aspergillosis, patients may present all of these findings and commonly produce brown mucus plugs. Anorexia, weight loss, night sweats, and clubbing can also occur.

B. Laboratory Findings and Imaging: Elevated absolute peripheral blood eosinophil counts (3000/μL and often exceeding 50% of leukocytes) are present in Löffler's syndrome, tropical eosinophilia, and allergic bronchopulmonary aspergillosis. Serum IgE levels as high as 1000–10,000 IU/mL are common. In allergic bronchopulmonary aspergillosis, the serum IgE concentration appears to correlate with activity of the disease. Stools should be examined for ova and parasites—often several times—to clarify the diagnosis. Isohemagglutinin titers are often markedly elevated in Löffler's syndrome.

In allergic bronchopulmonary aspergillosis and related disorders, patients may show central bronchiectasis on chest x-ray ("tramlines") or CT scan. Saccular proximal bronchiectasis of the upper lobes is pathognomonic. Although the chest radiograph may be normal, peribronchial haziness, focal or plate-like atelectasis, or patchy to massive consolidation can occur. Positive immediate skin tests, serum IgG precipitating antibodies, or IgE specific for the offending fungus are present.

Differential Diagnosis

These disorders must be differentiated from exacerbations of asthma, cystic fibrosis, or other underlying lung disorders that cause infiltrates on chest x-ray films. Allergic bronchopulmonary aspergillosis can occur in patients with cystic fibrosis.

Complications

Delayed recognition and treatment of allergic bronchopulmonary aspergillosis may cause progressive lung damage and bronchiectasis. Lesions of the conducting airways in bronchocentric granulomatosis can extend into adjacent lung parenchyma and pulmonary arteries, resulting in secondary vasculitis.

Treatment

Therapy for parasites causing Löffler's syndrome should be given, and corticosteroids may be required when illness is severe. Treatment of disease due to microfilariae is both diagnostic and therapeutic. Allergic bronchopulmonary aspergillosis and related disorders are treated with prolonged courses of oral corticosteroids, bronchodilators, and chest physical therapy.

Buchheit J et al: Acute eosinophilic pneumonia with respiratory failure: A new syndrome? Am Rev Respir Dis 1992;145:716.

Christensen WN, Hutchins GM: Hypereosinophilic mucoid impaction of bronchi in 2 children under 2 years of age. Pediatr Pulmonol 1985;1:278.

Howard WA: Pulmonary infiltrates with eosinophilia (Löffler syndrome). In: *Disorders of the Respiratory Tract in Children,* 5th ed. Chernick V, Kendig EL Jr (editors). Saunders, 1990.

Wilmott RW, Kravitz RM: Allergic bronchopulmonary aspergillosis. In: *Pediatric Respiratory Disease: Diagnosis and Treatment.* Hilman BC (editor). Saunders, 1993.

LUNG ABSCESS

Lung abscesses are most likely to occur in immunocompromised patients, in those with severe infections elsewhere (embolic spread), or in those with recurrent aspiration, malnutrition, or blunt chest trauma. Although organisms such as *S aureus, H influenzae, S pneumoniae,* and viridans streptococci more commonly affect the previously normal host, anaerobic and gram-negative organisms as well as *Nocardia, Legionella* species, and fungi *(Candida, Aspergillus)* should also be considered in the immunocompromised host.

Clinical Findings

A. Symptoms and Signs: High fever, malaise, and weight loss are often present. Symptoms and signs referable to the chest may or may not be present. In infants, evidence of respiratory distress can be present.

B. Laboratory Findings and Imaging: Elevated peripheral white blood cell count with a neutrophil predominance or an elevated erythrocyte sedimentation rate may be present. Blood cultures are rarely positive except in the overwhelmed host.

Chest radiographs usually reveal single or multiple thick-walled lung cavities. Air-fluid levels can be present. Local compressive atelectasis, pleural thickening, or adenopathy may also occur. Chest CT scan may provide better localization of the lesions.

In patients producing sputum, stains and cultures may provide the diagnosis. Direct percutaneous aspiration of material for stains and cultures guided by fluoroscopy or ultrasonography should be considered in the severely compromised or ill.

Differential Diagnosis

Loculated pyopneumothorax, an *Echinococcus* cyst, neoplasms, plasma cell granuloma, and infected congenital cysts and sequestrations should be considered.

Complications

Although complications due to abscesses are now rare, mediastinal shift, tension pneumothorax, and spontaneous rupture can occur. Diagnostic maneuvers such as lung puncture may also cause complications (pneumothorax).

Treatment

Because of the risks of lung puncture, uncomplicated abscesses are frequently treated in the uncompromised host with appropriate broad-spectrum antibiotics directed at *S aureus, H influenzae,* and streptococci. Additional coverage for anaerobic and gram-negative organisms should be provided for others. Prolonged therapy (3 weeks or more) may be required. Attempts to drain abscesses via bronchoscopy have caused life-threatening airway compromise. Surgical drainage or lobectomy is occasionally required, primarily in immunocompromised patients. However, such procedures may themselves cause life-threatening complications.

Prognosis

Although radiographic resolution may be very slow, resolution occurs in most patients without risk factors for lower respiratory tract infections or loss of pulmonary function. In the immunocompromised host, the outlook depends on the underlying disorder.

Bruckheimer E et al: Primary lung abscess in infancy. Pediatr Pulmonol 1995;19:188.

Emanuel B, Shulman ST: Lung abscess in infants and children. Clin Pediatr Pulmonol 1995;19:188.

Lewin S et al: Legionnaire's disease: A cause of severe abscess-forming pneumonia. Am J Med 1979;67:339.

Tan TQ, Seiheimer DK, Kaplan SL: Pediatric lung abscess: Clinical management and outcome. Pediatr Infect Dis J 1995;14:51.

Zuhdi MK et al: Percutaneous catheter drainage of tension pneumatocele, secondarily infected pneumatocele, and lung abscess in children. Crit Care Med 1996;24:330.

PULMONARY TUMORS

Primary tumors of the airway and parenchyma of the lung are unusual in pediatrics. Most intrathoracic tumors occur in or close to the mediastinum (see Mediastinal Masses). Other pulmonary tumors may be classified as benign, malignant, or metastatic. Benign pulmonary tumors include plasma cell granulomas, hamartomas, adenomas, papillomas, angiomas, leiomyomas, lipomas, and neurogenic tumors. The most common malignant tumor in children is a bronchogenic carcinoma, but this is again very rare. Other malignant tumors include fibrosarcomas and leiomyosarcomas. Metastatic tumors in childhood include Wilms' tumor, hepatoblastoma, osteogenic sarcoma, chondrosarcoma, Ewing's tumor, reticulum cell sarcoma, and soft tissue sarcomas. Lung tumors in children are more often metastatic than primary.

Clinical Findings

A. Symptoms and Signs: Symptoms, when they occur, may include pain, fever, cough, wheezing, weight loss, malaise, anemia, anorexia, and hemoptysis. On physical examination, signs of a pleural effusion, volume loss, or consolidation may be present if the tumor has led to significant airway obstruction.

B. Laboratory Findings and Imaging: In addition to frontal and lateral chest x-rays, fluoroscopy, CT scans, and angiography may be helpful in defining and delineating the tumor. Sputum cultures and cytology, as well as tuberculin and fungal skin tests plus fungal serology, may be needed to exclude other conditions.

Differential Diagnosis

The differential diagnosis includes acute, recurrent, or persistent viral and bacterial pneumonia, tuberculosis, and pulmonary infiltrates due to fungal infections. In infants, congenital malformations (pulmonary sequestration, cystic adenomatoid malformation) may also present as mass lesions.

Treatment & Prognosis

Both the appropriate therapy and the response to therapy depend on the type and location of the tumor. Benign lesions may be cured with surgical resection, but the prognosis is more guarded with both primary and metastatic malignant lesions.

Cohen MC, Kaschula ROC: Primary pulmonary tumors in childhood: A review of 31 years' experience and the literature. Pediatr Pulmonol 1992;14:222.

Hammer J et al: Plasma cell granuloma of the lung: Associated laboratory findings and ultrastructural evidence of inflammatory origin. Pediatr Pulmonol 1991;10:299.

Hartman GE, Shochat SJ: Primary pulmonary neoplasms in childhood: A review. Ann Thorac Surg 1983;36:108.

Watterson J et al: Thoracopulmonary neoplasms and lung complications of childhood cancer. In: *Pediatric Respiratory Disease: Diagnosis and Treatment.* Hilman BC (editor). Saunders, 1993.

DISEASES OF THE PULMONARY CIRCULATION

PULMONARY HEMORRHAGE

Pulmonary hemorrhage is caused by a spectrum of disorders affecting the large and small airways and alveoli. It can occur as an acute or chronic process. Hemorrhage involving the alveoli is termed "diffuse alveolar hemorrhage." If pulmonary hemorrhage is subacute or chronic, hemosiderin-laden macrophages are found in the sputum and tracheal or gastric aspirate. Many cases are secondary to infection (bacterial, mycobacterial, parasitic, viral, or fungal), lung abscess, bronchiectasis (cystic fibrosis or other causes), foreign body, coagulopathy (often with overwhelming sepsis), or elevated pulmonary venous pressure (secondary to congestive heart failure or anatomic heart lesions). Other causes include lung contusion from trauma, arteriovenous fistula, multiple telangiectasia, pulmonary sequestration, agenesis of a single pulmonary artery, and esophageal duplication or bronchogenic cyst. Rarer causes are tumors, such as bronchial adenoma or left atrial myxoma, and pulmonary infarction secondary to pulmonary embolus.

Diffuse alveolar hemorrhage may be idiopathic or drug-related or may occur in Goodpasture's syndrome, rapidly progressive glomerulonephritis, and systemic vasculitides (often associated with such collagen-vascular diseases as systemic lupus erythematosus, rheumatoid arthritis, Wegener's granulomatosis, polyarteritis nodosa, Schönlein-Henoch purpura, and Behçet's disease). Idiopathic pulmonary hemosiderosis refers to the accumulation of hemosiderin in the lung, especially the alveolar macrophage, as a result of chronic or recurrent hemorrhage (usually from pulmonary capillaries) that is not associated with the causes listed above. Children and young adults are mainly affected, with the age at onset ranging from 6 months to 20 years. This group of disorders includes milk allergy in young infants (Heiner's syndrome).

Clinical Findings

A. Symptoms and Signs: Pulmonary hemorrhage has as many symptoms as it has causes. Large airway hemorrhage presents with hemoptysis and symptoms of the underlying cause, such as infection, foreign body, or bronchiectasis in cystic fibrosis. Hemoptysis from larger airways is often bright red or contains clots. Idiopathic pulmonary hemosiderosis usually presents with nonspecific respiratory symptoms (cough, tachypnea, retractions) with or without hemoptysis, poor growth, and fatigue. Some children or young adults may present with massive hemoptysis, marked respiratory distress, stridor, or a pneumonia-like syndrome. Fever, abdominal pain, digital clubbing, and chest pain may be reported. Jaundice and hepatosplenomegaly may be present with chronic bleeding. Physical examination often reveals decreased breath sounds, rales, rhonchi, or wheezing.

B. Laboratory Findings and Imaging: Laboratory studies vary depending on the cause of hemorrhage. Following long-standing idiopathic pulmonary hemorrhage there is iron deficiency anemia and heme-positive sputum. Nonspecific findings may include lymphocytosis and an elevated erythrocyte sedimentation rate. Peripheral eosinophilia is present in up to 25% of patients. Chest x-rays demonstrate a range of findings, from transient perihilar infiltrates to large, fluffy alveolar infiltrates with or without atelectasis and mediastinal adenopathy. Pulmonary function testing generally reveals restrictive impairment, with low lung volumes, poor compliance, and an increased diffusion capacity. Hemosiderin-laden macrophages are found in bronchial or gastric aspirates. The diagnostic usefulness of lung biopsy is controversial.

Diffuse alveolar hemorrhage with underlying systemic disease such as systemic lupus erythematosus, Wegener's granulomatosis, and occasionally Goodpasture's syndrome can occur with the histologic entity known as necrotizing pulmonary capillaritis. On lung biopsy the alveolar septa are infiltrated with neutrophils, and alveolar hemorrhage is acute or chronic. The septa can fill with edema or fibrinoid necrosis. It is possible that idiopathic pulmonary hemosiderosis represents a mild form of capillaritis associated with alveolar hemorrhage. It might represent a process that waxes and wanes, and capillaritis may be focal or mild. Likewise, idiopathic pulmonary hemosiderosis may be caused by an immune-mediated process, though no serologic marker has yet been identified. Although capillaritis has been described without evidence of underlying systemic disease, the search for collagen-vascular disease, vasculitis, or pulmonary fibrosis should be exhaustive.

The investigation should include serologic studies such as antineutrophil cytoplasmic antibodies (c-ANCA) for Wegener's granulomatosis, p- or c-ANCA for microscopic polyangiitis, antinuclear antibodies for systemic lupus erythematosus, and anti-basement membrane antibodies for Goodpasture's syndrome. α1-Antitrypsin deficiency has been associated with vasculitides and should be considered.

Suspected cases of cow's milk-induced pulmonary hemosiderosis can be confirmed by laboratory findings that include high titers of serum precipitins to multiple constituents of cow's milk and positive intradermal skin tests to various cow's milk proteins. Improvement after an empiric trial of a diet free of cow's milk also supports the diagnosis.

Differential Diagnosis

The search for the site of respiratory bleeding, underlying systemic illness, and cardiac or vascular abnormalities will help define the diagnosis. When gross hemoptysis is present, large airway bronchiectasis, epistaxis, foreign body, and arteriovenous or pulmonary malformations should be ruled out.

Alveolar bleeding with hemoptysis is often frothy and pink. The differential diagnosis includes the disorders causing diffuse alveolar hemorrhage listed above. In contrast to idiopathic pulmonary hemosiderosis, Goodpasture's syndrome presents in a slightly older age group (15–35 years), tends to have a more aggressive pulmonary course, and has renal involvement (crescentic proliferative glomerulonephritis and circulating anti-glomerular basement membrane antibody). Wegener's granulomatosis also has renal involvement (granulomatous glomerulitis with necrotizing vasculitis, but renal biopsy may be nonspecific) and other systemic manifestations, especially with upper and lower respiratory tract inflammation. Upper tract involvement includes sinusitis, rhinitis, recurrent epistaxis, otitis media, saddle nose deformity, and subglottic stenosis. Wegener's granulomatosis may present without renal involvement early in the course of the disease. The diagnosis can be made by biopsy or an elevated antineutrophil cytoplasmic antibody titer.

Treatment

Therapy should be aimed at direct treatment of the underlying disease. Supportive measures, including iron therapy, supplemental oxygen, and blood transfusions, may be needed. A cow's milk-free diet should be tried in infants. Systemic corticosteroids have been used for various causes of diffuse alveolar hemorrhage and have been particularly successful in those secondary to collagen-vascular disorders and vasculitis. Case reports have been published on the variable effectiveness of steroids, chloroquine, cyclophosphamide, and azathioprine for idiopathic pulmonary hemosiderosis.

Prognosis

The outcome of idiopathic pulmonary hemosiderosis is variable, characterized by a waxing and waning course of intermittent intrapulmonary bleeds and the gradual development of pulmonary fibrosis over time. The severity of the underlying renal disease contributes to the mortality rates associated with Goodpasture's syndrome and Wegener's granulo-matosis. Diffuse alveolar hemorrhage is considered a lethal pulmonary complication of systemic lupus erythematosus.

Bowman CM: Pulmonary hemosiderosis. In: *Respiratory Disease in Children*. Loughlin GM, Eigen H (editors). William & Wilkins, 1994.

Fauci AS et al: Wegener's granulomatosis: Prospective clinical and therapeutic experience with 85 patients for 21 years. Ann Intern Med 1983;98:76.

Jennings CA et al: Diffuse alveolar hemorrhage with underlying isolated pauciimmune pulmonary capillaritis. Am J Respir Crit Care Med 1997;155:1101.

Savage JA et al: Alpha 1-antitrypsin deficiency and anti-proteinase 3 antibodies in anti-neutrophil cytoplasmic antibody (ANCA)-associated systemic vasculitis. Clin Exp Immunol 1995;100:194.

Travis WD et al: A clinicopathologic study of 34 cases of diffuse pulmonary hemorrhage with lung biopsy confirmation. Am J Surg Pathol 1990; 14:1112.

Zamora MR et al: Diffuse alveolar hemorrhage and systemic lupus erythematosus. Medicine 1997:76:192.

PULMONARY EMBOLISM

Although pulmonary embolism is apparently rare in children, the incidence is probably underestimated because it is often not considered in the differential diagnosis of respiratory distress. It occurs most commonly in children with sickle cell anemia as part of the "acute chest syndrome" and with rheumatic fever, infective endocarditis, schistosomiasis, bone fracture, dehydration, polycythemia, nephrotic syndrome, atrial fibrillation, "complicated" pneumonia, and other conditions. Emboli may be single or multiple, large or small, with clinical signs and symptoms dependent on the severity of pulmonary vascular obstruction.

Clinical Findings

A. Symptoms and Signs: Pulmonary embolism usually presents clinically as an acute onset of dyspnea and tachypnea. Heart palpitations or "a sense of impending doom" may be reported.

Pleuritic chest pain and hemoptysis may be present (not common), along with splinting, cyanosis, and tachycardia. Massive emboli may be present with syncope and cardiac arrhythmias. Physical examination is usually normal (except for tachycardia and tachypnea) unless the embolism is associated with an underlying disorder. Mild hypoxemia, rales, focal wheezing, or a pleural friction rub may be found.

B. Laboratory Findings and Imaging: Radiologic findings may be normal, but a peripheral infiltrate, small pleural effusion, or elevated hemidiaphragm can be present. If the emboli are massive, differential blood flow and pulmonary artery enlargement may be appreciated. The ECG is usually normal unless the pulmonary embolus is massive. Ventilation/perfusion scans show localized areas of ventilation without perfusion. If this study is normal, pulmonary embolus is virtually excluded. Further evaluation may include radiofibrinogen leg scanning and impedance plethysmography to search for deep venous thrombosis. Coagulation studies, including assessments of antithrombin III and protein C or S deficiencies or defective fibrinolysis, may be indicated. However, 90% of adult patients with venous thromboembolism have no identified coagulopathy.

Treatment

Acute treatment includes supplemental oxygen, sedation, and anticoagulation. Although controversial, current recommendations include heparin administration to maintain an activated partial thromboplastin time that is one and one-half or more times the control value. Thrombolytic therapy with streptokinase and urokinase may be necessary if the embolus is massive. In patients with identifiable deep venous thrombosis of the lower extremities and significant pulmonary emboli (with hemodynamic compromise despite anticoagulation), inferior vena caval interruption may be necessary. Long-term prospective data regarding this latter therapy are lacking, however.

Evans DA et al: Pulmonary embolism in children. Pediatr Clin North Am 1994; 41:569.

Moser KM: Pulmonary embolism. In: *Textbook of Respiratory Medicine*, 2nd ed. Murray JF, Nadel JA (editors). Saunders, 1994.

PULMONARY EDEMA

Pulmonary edema is excessive accumulation of extravascular fluid in the lung. This occurs when fluid is filtered into the lungs faster than it can be removed, leading to changes in lung mechanics such as decreased lung compliance, worsening hypoxemia from ventilation/perfusion mismatch, bronchial compression, and, if advanced, decreased surfactant function. There are two basic types of pulmonary edema: increased pressure (cardiogenic or hydrostatic) and increased permeability (noncardiogenic or "primary"). Hydrostatic pulmonary edema is usually due to excessive increases in pressure, which is most commonly due to congestive heart failure from multiple causes. In contrast, many lung diseases, especially ARDS (see below), are characterized by the development of pulmonary edema secondary to changes in permeability due to injury to the alveolocapillary barrier. In these settings, pulmonary edema occurs independently of the elevations of pulmonary venous pressure.

Clinical Findings

A. Symptoms and Signs: Cyanosis, tachypnea, tachycardia, and respiratory distress are commonly present. Physical findings include rales, diminished breath sounds, and (in young infants) expiratory wheezing. More severe disease is characterized by progressive respiratory distress with marked retractions, dyspnea, and severe hypoxemia.

B. Imaging: Chest x-ray findings depend on the cause of the edema. Pulmonary vessels are prominent, often with diffuse interstitial or alveolar infiltrates. Heart size is usually normal in permeability edema but enlarged in hydrostatic edema.

Treatment

Although specific therapy depends on the underlying cause, supplemental oxygen therapy and, if needed, ventilator support for respiratory failure are instituted. Diuretics, digoxin, and vasodilators may be indicated for congestive heart failure along with restriction of salt and water. Recommended interventions for permeability edema are reduction of vascular volume and maintenance of the lowest central venous or pulmonary arterial wedge pressure possible without sacrificing cardiac output or causing hypotension (see below). Beta-adrenergic agonists such as terbutaline have been shown to increase alveolar clearance of lung water, perhaps through the action of a sodium-potassium channel pump. Maintaining normal albumin levels in the capillaries maintains the filtration of lung liquid toward the capillaries, avoiding low oncotic pressure.

Cope DK et al: Pulmonary capillary pressure: A review. Crit Care Med 1992;20:1043.

Demling RH et al: Pulmonary edema: Pathophysiology, methods of measurement, and clinical importance in acute respiratory failure. New Horiz 1993;1:371.

Staub NC: Pathogenesis of pulmonary edema. Prog Cardiovasc Dis 1980;23:53.

CONGENITAL PULMONARY LYMPHANGIECTASIA

Structurally, congenital pulmonary lymphangiectasia appears as dilated subpleural and interlobular lymphatic channels and may present as part of a generalized lymphangiectasis (in association with obstructive cardiovascular lesions—especially total anomalous pulmonary venous return) or as an isolated idiopathic lesion. Pathologically, the lung appears firm, bulky, and noncompressible, with prominent cystic lymphatics visible beneath the pleura. On cut section, dilated lymphatics are present near the hilum, along interlobular septa, around bronchovascular bundles, and beneath the pleura. Histologically, dilated lymphatics have a thin endothelial cell lining overlying a delicate network of elastin and collagen.

Clinical Findings

Congenital pulmonary lymphangiectasia is a rare,

usually fatal disease that generally presents as acute or persistent respiratory distress at birth. Although most patients do not survive the newborn period, some survive longer, and there are isolated case reports of its diagnosis later in childhood. It may be associated with features of Noonan's syndrome, asplenia, total anomalous pulmonary venous return, septal defects, atrioventricular canal, hypoplastic left heart, aortic arch malformations, and renal malformations. Chylothorax has been reported. Chest x-ray findings include a "ground glass" appearance, prominent interstitial markings suggesting lymphatic distention, diffuse hyperlucency of the pulmonary parenchyma, and hyperinflation with depression of the diaphragm.

Prognosis

Although the onset of symptoms may be delayed for as long as the first few months of life, prolonged survival is extremely rare. Most deaths occur within weeks after birth. Rapid diagnosis is essential in order to expedite the option of pulmonary transplant.

Huber A et al: Congenital pulmonary lymphangiectasia. Pediatr Pulmonol 1991; 10:310.

Sindel LJ et al: Progressive pulmonary lymphangiectasia. Pediatr Pulmonol 1991; 10:57.

DISORDERS OF THE CHEST WALL

EVENTRATION OF THE DIAPHRAGM

Eventration of the diaphragm occurs when striated muscle is replaced with connective tissue and is demonstrated on x-ray film by elevation of part or all of the diaphragm. This congenital disorder is thought to represent incomplete formation of the diaphragm in utero. When defects are small, there is no paradoxic movement of the diaphragm and little symptomatology. Small eventrations may be detected on a chest x-ray film taken for another reason. When defects are large, there may or may not be paradoxic movement of the diaphragm, depending on the nature of the tissue replacing the normal diaphragm. The degree of respiratory distress depends in large part on the amount of paradoxic motion of the diaphragm. When the diaphragm moves upward during inspiration, instability of the inferior border of the chest wall increases the work of breathing and can lead to respiratory muscle fatigue. Treatment for respiratory distress is surgical plication, which stabilizes the diaphragm.

The differential diagnosis of eventration includes phrenic nerve injury and partial diaphragmatic hernia. The former can result from birth or other trauma and may also be seen following cardiac surgery. In most cases, only one phrenic nerve is involved. An elevated hemidiaphragm is noted on chest x-ray, and paradoxic motion of the diaphragm may be seen by fluoroscopy or ultrasonography. Patients often cannot be extubated or have persistent respiratory compromise, particularly with feeding. If symptoms persist for 2–4 weeks, the diaphragm is surgically plicated as described previously. Function returns to the diaphragm in about 50% of cases of phrenic nerve injury whether or not plication was performed. Recovery periods of up to 100 days have been reported in these cases.

Ribet M, Linder JL: Plication of the diaphragm for unilateral eventration or paralysis. Eur J Cardiothorac Surg 1992;6:357.

SCOLIOSIS

Scoliosis—lateral curvature of the spine—can, if uncorrected, lead to severe restrictive lung disease and death from cor pulmonale. Most cases of idiopathic scoliosis occur in adolescent girls and are corrected before there is significant pulmonary impairment. Congenital scoliosis of severe degree or with other major abnormalities carries a more guarded prognosis. Scoliosis may also occur in patients with progressive neuromuscular disease, such as Duchenne's muscular dystrophy, and can be a major contributor to respiratory failure.

Day GA et al: Pulmonary functions in congenital scoliosis. Spine 1994;19:1027.

Kearon C et al: Factors determining pulmonary function in adolescent idiopathic thoracic scoliosis. Am Rev Respir Dis 1993;148:288.

PECTUS EXCAVATUM

Pectus excavatum is anterior depression of the chest wall that may be symmetric or asymmetric with respect to the midline. Reports of exercise testing and pulmonary function testing in patients with pectus excavatum have not clearly demonstrated any marked abnormalities. Therefore, the decision to repair the deformity is usually based on cosmetic considerations. Care of patients following pectus excavatum repair requires mechanical ventilation and careful respiratory monitoring because of the weak chest wall following surgery.

Morshius W et al: Pulmonary function before surgery for pectus excavatum and at long-term follow-up. Chest 1994;105:1646.

PECTUS CARINATUM

Pectus carinatum is a bowing out of the sternum, usually apparent at birth. The abnormality may be associated with systemic diseases such as the mucopolysaccharidoses. As with pectus excavatum, pulmonary function tests are not usually abnormal in the absence of other disorders. The decision to repair this deformity is based primarily on cosmetic grounds. Postoperative care similarly requires careful monitoring because of chest wall instability produced by the repair.

Kobayashi S et al: Correction of pectus excavatum and pectus carinatum assisted by the endoscope. Plast Reconstr Surg 1997;99:1037.

NEUROMUSCULAR DISORDERS

Weakness of the respiratory and pharyngeal muscles leads to chronic or recurrent pneumonia secondary to aspiration and infection, atelectasis, hypoventilation, and respiratory failure in severe cases. Scoliosis, which frequently accompanies long-standing neuromuscular disorders, may further compromise respiratory function. Typical physical findings are a weak cough, decreased air exchange, rales, wheezing, and dullness to percussion. Signs of cor pulmonale (loud pulmonary component to the second heart sound, hepatomegaly, elevated neck veins) may be evident in advanced cases. Chest films generally show small lung volumes. If chronic aspiration is present, increased interstitial infiltrates and areas of atelectasis or consolidation may be present. Arterial blood gases demonstrate hypoxemia in the early stages and compensated respiratory acidosis in the late stages. Typical pulmonary function abnormalities include low lung volumes and decreased inspiratory force generated against an occluded airway. Treatment is supportive and includes vigorous pulmonary toilet, antibiotics with infection, and oxygen to correct hypoxemia. Unfortunately, despite aggressive medical therapy, many neuromuscular conditions progress to respiratory failure and death. The decision to intubate and ventilate is a difficult one; it should be made only when there is real hope that deterioration, though acute, is potentially reversible or when chronic ventilation is wanted. Chronic mechanical ventilation using either noninvasive or invasive techniques is being used more frequently in patients with chronic respiratory insufficiency.

Fields AI et al: Outcome of home care for technology-dependent children: Success of an independent, community-based care management model. Pediatr Pulmonol 1991;11:310.

Shaffner DH, Gioia FR: Neuromuscular disease and respiratory failure. In: *Textbook of Pediatric Intensive Care*, 2nd ed. Rogers MC (editor). Williams & Wilkins, 1992.

DISORDERS OF THE PLEURA & PLEURAL CAVITY

The visceral pleura covers the outer surface of the lungs, and the inner surface of the chest wall is the parietal pleura. Disease processes can lead to accumulation of air or fluid in the pleural space. Pleural effusions are classified as transudates or exudates. Transudates occur when there is imbalance between hydrostatic and oncotic pressure, so that fluid filtration exceeds reabsorption (eg, congestive heart failure). Exudates form as a result of inflammation of the pleural surface leading to increased capillary permeability (eg, parapneumonic effusions). Other pleural effusions include chylothorax and hemothorax.

Thoracentesis is helpful in characterizing the fluid and providing definitive diagnosis. Recovered fluid is considered an exudate (as opposed to a transudate) if any of the following are found: a pleural fluid to serum protein ratio greater than 0.5, a pleural fluid to serum lactic dehydrogenase (LDH) ratio greater than 0.6, or a pleural fluid LDH greater than 200 units/L. Important additional studies on pleural fluid include cell count; pH and glucose; Gram's, acid-fast, and fungal stains; cultures; counterimmunoelectrophoresis for specific organisms; and, occasionally, amylase concentration. Cytologic examination of pleural fluid should be performed to rule out leukemia or other neoplasm.

PARAPNEUMONIC EFFUSION & EMPYEMA

Bacterial pneumonia is often accompanied by pleural effusion. Some of these effusions harbor infection, and others are inflammatory reactions to pneumonia. The nomenclature in this area is somewhat confusing. Some use the term empyema for grossly purulent fluid and parapneumonic effusion for nonpurulent fluid. It is clear, however, that some nonpurulent effusions will also contain organisms and represent either partially treated or early empyema. It is probably best to refer to all effusions associated with pneumonia as parapneumonic effusions, some of which are infected and some not.

The most common organism associated with empyema is *S pneumoniae*. Other common organisms include *H influenzae* and *S aureus*. Less common causes are group A streptococci, gram-negative organisms, anaerobic organisms, and *Mycoplasma pneumoniae*. Effusions associated with tuberculosis are almost always sterile and constitute an inflammatory reaction.

Clinical Findings

A. Symptoms and Signs: Patients usually present with typical signs of pneumonia, including fever, tachypnea, and cough. They may have chest pain, decreased breath sounds, and dullness to percussion on the affected side and may prefer to lie on the affected side. With large effusions, there may be tracheal deviation to the contralateral side.

B. Laboratory Findings: The white blood count is often elevated, with left shift. Blood cultures are sometimes positive. The tuberculin skin test is positive in most cases of tuberculosis. Thoracentesis reveals findings consistent with an exudate. Cells in the pleural fluid are usually neutrophils in bacterial disease and lymphocytes in tuberculous effusions. In bacterial disease, pleural fluid pH and glucose are often low. pH less than 7.2 suggests active bacterial infection. The pH of the specimen should be determined in a blood gas syringe sent to the laboratory on ice. Extra heparin should not be used in the syringe since it can falsely lower the pH. Although in adults the presence of low pH and glucose necessitates aggressive and thorough drainage procedures, the prognostic significance of these findings in children is not known. Gram's stain, cultures, and counterimmunoelectrophoresis are often positive for the offending organism.

C. Imaging: The presence of pleural fluid is suggested by a homogeneous density on chest x-ray that obscures the underlying lung. Large effusions may cause a shift of the mediastinum to the contralateral side. Small effusions may only blunt the costophrenic angle. Lateral decubitus films may help to detect freely movable fluid by demonstrating a "layering-out" effect. If the fluid is loculated, no such effect is perceived. Ultrasonography can be extremely valuable in localizing the fluid and detecting loculations, especially when thoracentesis is contemplated.

Treatment & Prognosis

After initial thoracentesis and identification of the organism, appropriate intravenous antibiotics and adequate drainage of the fluid remain the mainstay of therapy. Although there is a trend toward managing smaller pneumococcal empyemas without a chest tube, most larger effusions require chest tube drainage. More aggressive procedures such as thoracotomy with open drainage or decortication are rarely indicated except for less common causes of this disorder such as infection with group A streptococci and gram-negative and anaerobic organisms. Early decortication using thoracoscopic techniques may reduce morbidity and the need for prolonged hospitalization.

The prognosis is related to the severity of disease but is generally excellent, with complete or nearly complete recovery expected in most instances.

Alkrinawi S et al: Pleural infection in children. Semin Respir Infect 1996;11:148.

Bouros D et al: Intrapleural streptokinase versus urokinase in the treatment of complicated parapneumonic effusions: A prospective, double blind study. Am J Resp Crit Care Med 1997;155:291.

Bryant RE et al: Pleural empyema. (State of the Art.) Clin Infect Dis 1996;22:747.

Freij B et al: Parapneumonic effusions and empyema in hospitalized children: A retrospective review of 227 cases. Pediatr Infect Dis 1984;3:578.

Redding GJ et al: Lung function in children following empyema. Am J Dis Child 1990;144:1337.

HEMOTHORAX

Accumulation of blood in the pleural space can be caused by surgical or accidental trauma, coagulation defects, and pleural or pulmonary tumors. With blunt trauma, hemopneumothorax may be present. Symptoms are related to blood loss and compression of underlying lung parenchyma. There is some risk of secondary infection, resulting in empyema. Drainage of a hemothorax is required when significant compromise of pulmonary function is present, as with hemopneumothorax. In uncomplicated cases, observation is indicated because blood is readily absorbed spontaneously from the pleural space.

Parry GW et al: Management of haemothorax. Ann R Coll Surg Engl 1996;78:325.

CHYLOTHORAX

The accumulation of chyle in the pleural space usually results from accidental or surgical trauma to the thoracic duct. In the newborn, chylothorax can be congenital or secondary to birth trauma. This condition also occurs as a result of superior vena caval obstruction secondary to central venous lines and following Fontan procedures for tricuspid atresia. Symptoms of chylothorax are related to the amount of fluid accumulation and the degree of compromise of underlying pulmonary parenchyma. Thoracentesis reveals typical milky fluid (unless the patient has been fasting) containing chiefly T lymphocytes.

Treatment should be conservative because many chylothoraces resolve spontaneously. Oral feedings with medium-chain triglycerides reduce lymphatic flow through the thoracic duct. Drainage of chylous effusions should be performed only for respiratory compromise because the fluid often rapidly reaccumulates. Repeated or continuous drainage may lead to protein malnutrition and T cell depletion, rendering the patient relatively immunocompromised. If reaccumulation of fluid persists, surgical ligation of the thoracic duct or sclerosis of the pleural space can be attempted, though the results may be less than satisfactory.

Hillerdal G: Chylothorax and pseudochylothorax. Eur Respir J 1997;10:1157.

Merrigan BA et al: Chylothorax. Br J Surg 1997;84:15.

van Straaten HL, Gerards LJ, Krediet TG: Chylothorax in the neonatal period. Eur J Pediatr 1993;152:2.

PNEUMOTHORAX & RELATED AIR LEAK SYNDROMES

Pneumothorax can occur spontaneously in newborns and in older children or, more commonly, as a result of birth trauma, positive-pressure ventilation, underlying obstructive or restrictive lung disease, and rupture of a congenital or acquired lung cyst. Pneumothorax can also occur as an acute complication of tracheostomy. Air usually dissects from the alveolar spaces into the interstitial spaces of the lung. Migration to the visceral pleura ultimately leads to rupture into the pleural space. Associated conditions - include pneumomediastinum, pneumopericardium, pneumoperitoneum, and subcutaneous emphysema. These conditions are more commonly associated with dissection of air into the interstitial spaces of the lung with retrograde dissection along the bronchovascular bundles toward the hilum.

Clinical Findings

A. Symptoms and Signs: The clinical spectrum can vary from asymptomatic to severe respiratory distress. Associated symptoms include cyanosis, chest pain, and dyspnea. Physical examination may reveal decreased breath sounds and hyperresonance to percussion on the affected side with tracheal deviation to the opposite side. When pneumothorax is under tension, cardiac function may be compromised, resulting in hypotension or narrowing of the pulse pressure. Pneumopericardium is a life-threatening condition that presents with muffled heart tones and shock. Pneumomediastinum rarely causes symptoms by itself.

B. Imaging: Chest films usually demonstrate the presence of free air in the pleural space. If the pneumothorax is large and under tension, compressive atelectasis of the underlying lung and shift of the mediastinum to the opposite side may be demonstrated. Cross-table lateral and lateral decubitus films can aid in the diagnosis of free air. Pneumopericardium is identified by the presence of air completely surrounding the heart, whereas in patients with pneumomediastinum, the heart and mediastinal structures may be outlined with air but the air does not involve the diaphragmatic cardiac border.

Differential Diagnosis

When a patient on a ventilator acutely deteriorates, one must consider not only tension pneumothorax but also obstruction or dislodgment of the endotracheal tube and failure of the mechanical ventilator. Radiographically, pneumothorax must be distinguished from diaphragmatic hernia, lung cysts, congenital lobar emphysema, and cystic adenomatoid malformation, but this task is usually not difficult.

Treatment

Small or asymptomatic pneumothoraces usually do not require treatment and can be managed with close observation. Larger or symptomatic ones usually require drainage, though inhalation of 100% oxygen to wash out blood nitrogen can be tried.

Needle aspiration should be used to relieve tension acutely, followed by chest tube placement. Pneumopericardium requires immediate identification and needle aspiration to prevent death, followed by pericardial tube placement.

In older patients with spontaneous pneumothorax, recurrences are common; sclerosing and surgical procedures are often required.

Bertrand PC et al: Immediate and long term results after surgical treatment of primary spontaneous pneumothorax by VATS. Ann Thorac Surg 1996;61:1641.

Fan LL et al: Giant pulmonary cyst simulating a pneumothorax. Am J Dis Child 1988;142:189.

Warwick WJ: Pneumothorax. In: *Pediatric Respiratory Disease: Diagnosis and Treatment.* Hilman BC (editor). Saunders, 1993.

DISORDERS OF THE CONTROL OF BREATHING

ACUTE LIFE-THREATENING EPISODES IN INFANCY

A substantial number of infants are brought to medical attention following apparently acute life-threatening episodes of cardiorespiratory instability involving cyanosis, pallor, or apnea. In 50% of cases, no cause can be found for the episode. The infants in whom no explanation for the episode can be found are said to have apnea of infancy. There is a weak relationship between apnea of infancy and SIDS, with only a small percentage of patients with apnea of infancy at risk for sudden death. In addition, only a small percentage of infants succumbing to SIDS have prior episodes of apnea.

The following section describes an approach to the patient who has undergone an acute life-threatening episode, taking note of the very broad differential diagnosis and uncertainties in both evaluation and treatment.

Differential Diagnosis

Table 17–3 classifies disorders associated with acute life-threatening events. A careful history is often the most helpful part of the evaluation. It is useful to determine whether the infant has been chronically ill or essentially well. A history of several days of poor feeding, temperature instability, or respiratory or gastrointestinal symptoms suggests an infectious process. Reports of "struggling to breathe" or "trying to breathe" imply airway obstruction. Association of the episodes with feeding implies discoordinated swallowing, gastroesophageal reflux, or airway obstruction. Episodes that typically follow crying may be related to breath-holding. Association of episodes with sleeping may also suggest gastroesophageal reflux or apnea of infancy. Attempts should be made to determine the duration of the episode, but this is often difficult. It is helpful to role-play the episode with the family. Details regarding the measures taken to resuscitate the infant and the infant's recovery from the episode are often useful in determining severity.

The physical examination provides further direction in pursuing the diagnosis. Fever or hypothermia suggests infection. An altered state of consciousness implies a postictal state or drug overdose. Respiratory distress implies cardiac or pulmonary lesions.

Most patients are hospitalized for observation in order to reduce stress on the family and allow prompt completion of the evaluation. Laboratory evaluation includes a complete blood count for evidence of infection. Serum electrolytes are usually obtained. Elevations in serum bicarbonate suggest chronic hypoventilation, whereas decreases suggest acute acidosis, perhaps due to hypoxia during the episode. Chronic acidosis is suggestive of an inherited metabolic disorder. The chest radiograph is examined for infiltrates suggesting acute infection or chronic aspiration and for cardiac size as a clue to intrinsic cardiac disease. Arterial blood gas studies provide an initial assessment of oxygenation and acid-base status, and low PaO_2 or elevated $PaCO_2$ (or both) implies cardiorespiratory disease. A significant base deficit suggests that the episode was accompanied by hypoxia or circulatory impairment. On-line oxygen saturation measurements in the hospital assess oxygenation status during different activities and are more comprehensive than a single blood gas sample.

Because apnea has been associated with respiratory infections, diagnostic studies for infection—with respiratory syncytial virus in particular but also other viruses and pertussis—may contribute to the diagnostic process. The apnea seen with infection often precedes other physical findings. If there is any possibility that the episode involved airway obstruction, the airway should be examined either directly, by fiberoptic bronchoscopy, or radiographically, by CT or barium swallow. If reflux is suspected, it should be documented by esophageal pH monitoring coupled with respiratory pattern recording. Most infants with reflux and apnea can be treated with medical antireflux measures. Infants with reflux and repeated episodes of apnea may benefit from a surgical antireflux procedure.

There are several neurologic causes of acute life-threatening episodes. Apnea as the sole manifestation of a seizure disorder is unusual but may occur. In cases of repeated episodes, 24-hour electroencephalographic monitoring may be helpful in detecting a seizure disorder. Leigh's disease, a brain stem disorder characterized pathologically by neuronal dropout, may present with apneic episodes.

Apneic episodes have been linked to child abuse in several ways. Head injury following nonaccidental trauma may be first brought to medical attention because of apnea. Other signs of abuse are usually immediately apparent in such cases. Drug overdose, either accidental (eg, mistakes in application of anticolic medications containing barbiturates) or intentional, may also present with apnea. Several series document that apneic episodes may be falsely reported by parents seeking attention, ie, Munchausen-by-proxy syndrome. Parents may physically interfere with a child's respiratory efforts, in which case pinch marks on the nares are sometimes found.

Treatment

Therapy is directed at the underlying cause if one

Table 17–3. Differential diagnosis of acute life-threatening episodes.

Infectious	Viral: respiratory syncytial virus and other respiratory viruses Bacterial: sepsis, pertussis
Gastrointestinal	Gastroesophageal reflux with or without obstructive apnea
Respiratory	Airway abnormality; vascular rings, pulmonary slings, tracheomalacia Pneumonia
Neurologic	Seizure disorder CNS infection: meningitis, encephalitis Vasovagal response Leigh's encephalopathy Brain tumor
Cardiovascular	Congenital malformation Dysrhythmias Cardiomyopathy
Nonaccidental trauma	Battering Drug overdose Munchausen-by-proxy syndrome
No definable cause	Apnea of infancy

is found. After blood cultures are taken, antibiotics should be administered to infants who appear toxic. Seizure disorders are treated with anticonvulsants. Vascular rings and pulmonary slings must be corrected surgically because of severe morbidity and high mortality rates in uncorrected cases.

The approach to care in apnea of infancy is controversial. These infants present with acute life-threatening episodes where no cause can be ascertained. Treatment has emphasized the use of electronic monitors for detection of apnea or bradycardia in the home. Parents are then taught cardiopulmonary resuscitation. The rationale for the use of monitors is that infants at risk for subsequent severe episodes can be identified. Attempts to predict which infants are at risk have included hypoxic and hypercapnic challenges and determinations of the frequency of periodic breathing or apnea, usually through the use of pneumograms. None of these techniques are sufficiently specific or selective to be useful. Furthermore, the efficacy of home monitoring has never been demonstrated in controlled trials.

The decision to monitor these infants involves the participation of the family. Infants with severe initial episodes or repeated severe episodes are now thought to be at significant increased risk and should probably be monitored in the home. Episodes in these children are so severe that the parents want to know the infant's condition at all times. Monitoring is not indicated in patients who have isolated episodes of lesser severity unless the parents clearly express a wish for it. Pneumograms can be used to determine whether apnea is occurring. However, pneumograms are not predictive and play no role in the decision to monitor or when to stop monitoring. The decision to discontinue monitoring is usually based on the infant's ability to go several months without triggering the alarm.

Aminophylline has been suggested as treatment for apnea of infancy, but controlled trials are lacking. At this point, this drug is not recommended.

Brooks JG: Apparent life-threatening events and apnea of infancy. Clin Perinatol 1992;19:809.

National Institutes of Health Consensus Development Conference Statement: Infantile apnea and home monitoring. Sept 29 to Oct 1, 1986. Pediatrics 1987;79:292.

SUDDEN INFANT DEATH SYNDROME

Sudden infant death syndrome (SIDS) is a poorly understood disorder encompassing cases of sudden and unexpected death of previously well or nearly well infants that remain unexplained after an adequate postmortem examination. The postmortem examination is an important feature of the definition because approximately 20% of cases of sudden death can be explained by autopsy findings. The incidence of SIDS in the United States (1–2:1000) makes it the

leading cause of death in infancy after the neonatal period. The overall incidence of SIDS has steadily declined over the past few decades.

Epidemiologic and pathologic data constitute most of what is known about SIDS. The number of deaths peaks at age 2 months, and most deaths occur in infants a few weeks to 6 months of age. There is an increase in deaths during the peak respiratory virus season, and most deaths occur between midnight and 8 AM. The syndrome is more common among ethnic and racial minorities and socioeconomically disadvantaged populations. There is a 3:2 male predominance in most series. Other risk factors include low birth weight, teenage or drug-addicted mothers, maternal smoking, and a family history of SIDS. Most of these risk factors are associated with a two- to threefold elevation of incidence but are not specific enough to be useful in predicting which infants will die unexpectedly. Recent immunization is not a risk factor.

The most consistent pathologic findings are intrathoracic petechiae and mild inflammation and congestion of the respiratory tract. Subtler pathologic findings include brain stem gliosis, extramedullary hematopoiesis, and increases in periadrenal brown fat. These latter findings suggest that infants who succumb to SIDS have had intermittent or chronic hypoxia before death.

The mechanism or mechanisms of death in SIDS are unknown. For example, it is not known whether the initiating event at the time of death is cessation of breathing or cardiac arrhythmia or asystole. Suggested hypotheses have included upper airway obstruction, catecholamine excess, brain stem immaturity or injury, and increased fetal hemoglobin. It has been recognized that some infants who presented with apneic episodes subsequently died from SIDS; however, study of these infants and prospective studies of large numbers of newborns have indicated that most infants with apnea do not die from SIDS and that most infants with SIDS have no identifiable episodes of apnea (see Acute Life-Threatening Episodes, above).

A history of mild symptoms of upper respiratory infection before death is not uncommon, and SIDS victims are sometimes seen by physicians a day or so before death. When infants are discovered blue, cold, and motionless by parents or caretakers, they are most commonly taken to the emergency room, where resuscitative efforts are almost uniformly of no avail. Families must then be supported following the death. The National Sudden Infant Death Syndrome Foundation provides information about psychosocial support groups and counseling for families of SIDS victims. The postmortem examination can be of value to the family; when the diagnosis of SIDS is established, lingering questions about other possible causes of death are resolved. For this reason, as well as for ascertaining causes of death in infancy, postmortem examination should always be recommended. Some recent reports have suggested that a death scene investigation may also be important in determining the cause of sudden unexpected deaths in infancy.

Positioning & SIDS

A variety of recent studies from other countries have presented evidence that the incidence of SIDS is significantly higher when infants are put down in the prone position. A Task Force on Infant Positioning and SIDS of the American Academy of Pediatrics has recommended that healthy infants be positioned on the side or back. This statement acknowledges the limitations of many of the studies and that there are valid reasons why certain infants— such as preterm infants with respiratory distress, infants with gastroesophageal reflux, or certain airway anomalies—do better sleeping in the prone position. Nevertheless, the current evidence is compelling for recommending the side or back position for sleeping in healthy term infants.

Berry PJ: Pathological findings in SIDS. J Clin Pathol 1992;45:11.

Goldberg J: The counseling of SIDS parents. Clin Perinatol 1992;19:927.

Freed GE et al: Sudden infant death syndrome prevention and an understanding of selected clinical issues. Pediatr Clin North Am 1994;41:967.

Willinger M, Hoffman HJ, Hartford RB: Infant sleep position and risk for sudden infant death syndrome. Pediatrics 1994;93:814.

II. MEDIASTINUM

MEDIASTINITIS

Acute infection involving the mediastinum in pediatric patients is usually due to perforation of the esophagus secondary to trauma. The trauma may be self-induced (foreign body, puncture injury to the pharynx with a sharp object) or iatrogenic (endoscopy, attempted endotracheal intubation). Spontaneous esophageal perforation leading to mediastinitis can accompany vomiting, but this is rare. In addition, acute suppurative mediastinitis without trauma does occur but is unusual.

Clinical Findings

A. Symptoms and Signs: The early symptoms and signs of acute mediastinitis may be vague and include the gradual onset of fever, chills, and dysphagia with substernal pain. Dyspnea and cough may also be present. Inspiration may be accompanied

by discomfort due to stretching of inflamed mediastinal structures, leading to a pattern of spasmodic or "halting" inspiration. On physical examination, evidence of obstruction of venous return may be present, with substernal pain elicited on palpation of the structures of the thorax. In addition, subcutaneous emphysema may be appreciated in the thoracic and cervical areas.

B. Laboratory Findings and Imaging: The white blood count of the patient with mediastinitis is usually high, with neutrophils and band forms prominent on the differential. The chest x-ray may reveal widening of the upper mediastinum; the lateral view shows anterior displacement of the trachea and the esophagus. Mediastinal emphysema, pleural effusions, and pyopneumothorax may also be present.

Differential Diagnosis

The differential diagnosis includes diseases that lead to the toxic appearance of an infant or child. A primary bacterial pneumonia as well as septicemia must be considered. Retropharyngeal abscesses may also lead to the pattern of respiratory distress seen with a suppurative mediastinitis.

Complications

If not recognized and rapidly treated, mediastinitis can progress rapidly and lead to death from the infection or tracheal obstruction. Mediastinal abscess may also complicate the clinical course of the disease.

Treatment

As soon as the diagnosis is made, parenterally administered broad-spectrum antibiotics must be given. If significant tracheal obstruction is present, an airway must be provided. Drainage of abscesses in the mediastinum may also be indicated.

Templeton JM: Thoracic emergencies. In: *Textbook of Pediatric Emergency Medicine,* 3rd ed. Fleisher GR, Ludwig S (editors). Williams & Wilkins, 1993.

MEDIASTINAL MASSES

Mediastinal masses may present because of symptoms produced by pressure on the esophagus, airways, nerves, or vessels within the mediastinum or may be discovered on a routine chest x-ray. Once the mass is identified, localization to one of four mediastinal compartments aids in the differential diagnosis (Figure 17–1). The superior mediastinum is the area above the pericardium that is bordered inferiorly by an imaginary line from the manubrium to the fourth thoracic vertebra. The anterior mediastinum is bordered by the sternum anteriorly and the pericardium posteriorly, whereas the posterior mediastinum is defined by the pericardium and diaphragm anteriorly and the lower eight thoracic vertebrae pos-

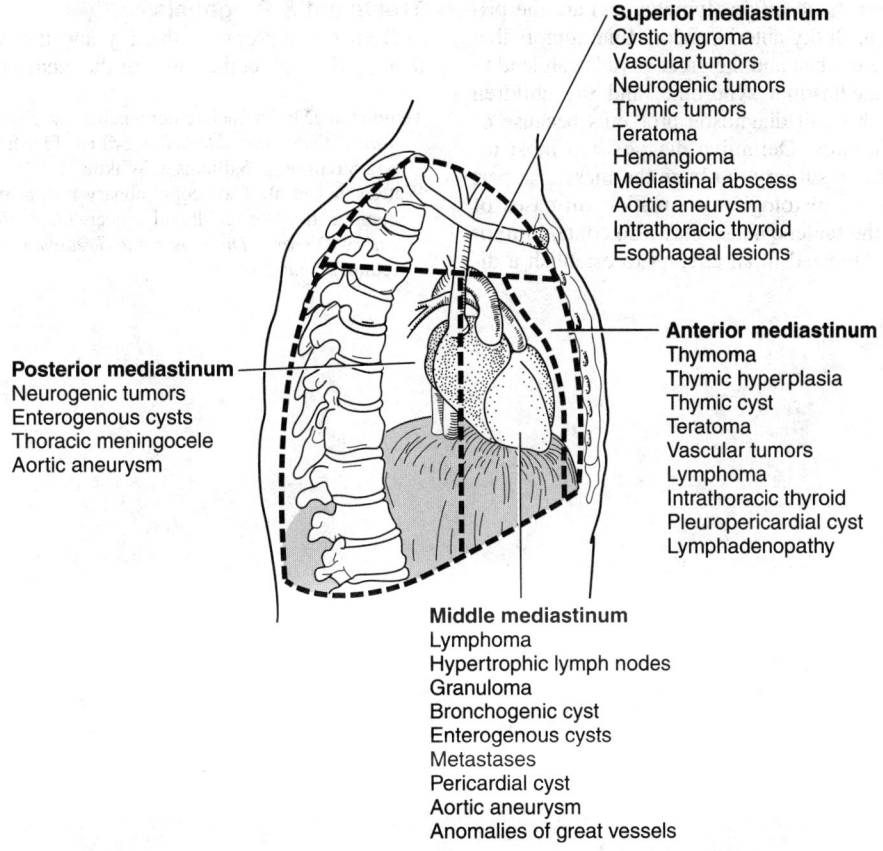

Superior mediastinum
Cystic hygroma
Vascular tumors
Neurogenic tumors
Thymic tumors
Teratoma
Hemangioma
Mediastinal abscess
Aortic aneurysm
Intrathoracic thyroid
Esophageal lesions

Posterior mediastinum
Neurogenic tumors
Enterogenous cysts
Thoracic meningocele
Aortic aneurysm

Anterior mediastinum
Thymoma
Thymic hyperplasia
Thymic cyst
Teratoma
Vascular tumors
Lymphoma
Intrathoracic thyroid
Pleuropericardial cyst
Lymphadenopathy

Middle mediastinum
Lymphoma
Hypertrophic lymph nodes
Granuloma
Bronchogenic cyst
Enterogenous cysts
Metastases
Pericardial cyst
Aortic aneurysm
Anomalies of great vessels

Figure 17–1. Anatomic compartments within the mediastinum. The differential diagnosis of mediastinal masses is based on location within these four compartments.

teriorly. The mid mediastinum is surrounded by these three compartments.

Clinical Findings

A. Symptoms and Signs: Respiratory symptoms, when present, are due to pressure on an airway and may include cough, wheezing, and complaints consistent with an infectious process caused by partial or complete obstruction of an airway (unresolving pneumonia in one area of lung). Hemoptysis can also occur but is an unusual presenting symptom. Dysphagia may occur secondary to compression of the esophagus. Encroachment of the mass on the recurrent laryngeal nerve can cause hoarseness due to paralysis of the left vocal cord. Superior vena caval obstruction can lead to dilation of neck vessels as well as other signs and symptoms of obstruction of venous return from the upper part of the body (superior mediastinal syndrome).

B. Laboratory Findings and Imaging: The mass is initially defined by frontal and lateral chest x-rays together with thoracic CT scans and perhaps

MRI. A barium swallow may also help define the extent of a mass. Other studies that may be required include angiography (to define the blood supply to large tumors), electrocardiography, echocardiography, ultrasound of the thorax, fungal and mycobacterial skin tests, and urinary catecholamine assays. MRI or myelography may be necessary in children suspected of having a neurogenic tumor in the posterior mediastinum.

Differential Diagnosis

The differential diagnosis classified according to the mediastinal compartment housing the mass is set forth in Figure 17–1. Several general points should be kept in mind. In some series, more than 50% of mediastinal tumors occur in the posterior mediastinum and are mainly neurogenic tumors or enterogenous cysts. Most neurogenic tumors in children under 4 years of age are malignant (neuroblastoma, neuroganglioblastoma), whereas a benign ganglioneuroma is the most common histologic type in older children. In the mid and anterior mediastinum, tumors of lymphatic origin (lymphomas) are the primary concern. Bulky anterior mediastinal tumors that compress the trachea and the great vessels can lead to a superior mediastinal syndrome, and the children can present difficult diagnostic problems because of anesthesia hazards. Definitive diagnosis in most instances relies on surgery to obtain the mass or a part of the mass for histologic examination. In cases of lymphoma, the scalene nodes may also contain tumor and may be biopsied in an attempt to establish a diagnosis.

Treatment & Prognosis

Both the appropriate therapy and the response to therapy depend on the cause of the mediastinal mass.

Templeton JM: Thoracic emergencies. In: *Textbook of Pediatric Emergency Medicine,* 3rd ed. Fleisher GR, Ludwig S (editors). Williams & Wilkins, 1993.

Watterson J et al: Thoracopulmonary neoplasms and lung complications of childhood cancer. In: *Pediatric Respiratory Disease: Diagnosis and Treatment.* Hilman BC (editor). Saunders, 1993.

Cardiovascular Diseases 18

Robert R. Wolfe, MD, Mark M. Boucek, MD, Michael S. Schaffer, MD, & James W. Wiggins, Jr., MD

Cardiovascular disease is a significant cause of death and chronic illness in children. In North America, more than 1% of newborn infants have congenital heart disease, usually resulting from multifactorial causes. Preventive medicine is the most important aspect of pediatrics, and it is becoming obvious that the prevention of adult heart disease must begin in childhood (eg, prevention of atherosclerosis by diet modification). But prevention requires an understanding of the causes of disease, and in this there are wide discrepancies, ranging from significant accomplishments in the case of rheumatic fever to the very tentative steps being taken to understand the causes of congenital heart disease, atherosclerosis, and essential hypertension.

DIAGNOSTIC EVALUATION

The most important clues to the presence of heart disease requiring prompt attention are congestive heart failure and cyanosis. These clinical conditions are discussed in more detail in subsequent sections. The presence of a heart murmur may suggest the possibility of heart disease in an infant, or the murmur may be a functional or innocent one. Not all serious cardiovascular disorders are accompanied by an easily detectable murmur.

Sequence of Evaluation
(1) History
(2) Physical examination
(3) Electrocardiogram
(4) Chest x-ray
(5) Echocardiogram
(6) Cardiac catheterization (with angiography)

HISTORY

In obtaining a medical history from the family or the patient, one must keep in perspective the patient's age and activity level relative to age. A history of increasing feeding difficulties and diaphoresis is the most common feature of early congestive heart failure.

Family History
Most cardiac diseases are familial, so the history of heart disease in a first-degree relative should be sought. These details might suggest the need to evaluate the child for hyperlipidemia.

Pregnancy
The history of pregnancy should elicit information regarding first-trimester exposure to illness or medications that place infants at high risk for congenital heart disease. A history of significant problems related to labor and delivery, such as perinatal stress or asphyxia at birth, suggests causes of myocardial dysfunction and pulmonary hypertension in the neonate.

Growth & Development
Major cardiac problems frequently affect a child's ability to grow. There may be a history of poor feeding (early fatigue, vomiting, lethargy) or failure to thrive despite adequate caloric intake. Gross motor development may also be delayed in children with significant congestive heart failure or cyanosis, though other aspects of development are less frequently affected.

Tachypnea
Parents frequently notice rapid breathing in the child. Although infants at rest rarely breathe faster than 40 respirations per minute, infants in congestive heart failure usually have respiratory rates in excess of 60/min (often 80–100/min). Tachypnea may be considered the cardinal sign of left-sided heart failure in the pediatric patient.

Cyanosis
Cyanotic heart disease may go unrecognized because of lack of appreciation of the subtleties of diagnosing cyanosis. The infant with a cyanotic heart lesion may be more gray than blue (and may have no heart murmur).

Hypoxemic Spells

It is important to determine whether the patient with a cyanotic heart lesion such as tetralogy of Fallot is having hypoxemic spells, because prompt surgical intervention may be required. These spells usually occur on morning awakening or after a feeding or bowel movement; the infant begins breathing fast, becomes progressively more gray or blue, and cries as if having severe pain. Such a spell rarely may progress to unconsciousness, paresis, or even death.

Other Clinical Clues

Orthopnea, dyspnea, easy fatigability, growth failure, sweating, squatting, and pneumonia are common clues to the presence of heart disease.

PHYSICAL EXAMINATION

The examination should begin with a careful general inspection to note activity (agitation, lethargy) and skin perfusion and color. Vital signs, including temperature, pulse rate, respiratory rate, and particularly blood pressure (in all four extremities in symptomatic infants), can reflect the overall status of the patient. Auscultation of the heart and lungs should be performed early in the overall examination, because the infant's crying limits the physician's ability to hear even pronounced cardiac sounds. Abdominal examination for position and size of organs is also important. The presence of other congenital abnormalities, particularly chromosomal disorders, increases the probability of congenital heart disease.

1. CARDIOVASCULAR EXAMINATION

Inspection & Palpation

Conformation of the chest can give clues to past or present cardiomegaly. Prominence of the precordial chest wall is frequently seen in infants and children with cardiomegaly. Increased cardiac activity is often noted on inspection.

Palpation may reveal precordial activity, right ventricular lift, or left-sided heave; a diffuse point of maximal impulse; or the presence of a thrill caused by a loud murmur. Thrills are typically located where the murmur is most intense and can sometimes be felt at the point of radiation, as in a suprasternal notch or carotid thrill with aortic stenosis. In patients with severe pulmonary hypertension, palpable pulmonary closure is frequently noted, usually at the mid to upper left sternal border.

Auscultation

A. Normal Heart Sounds: S_1 (the first heart sound) is the sound of atrioventricular valve closure. It is best heard at the lower left sternal border and is usually medium-pitched. Although four components

of S_1 can be detected by phonocardiography, only one or two of these are usually heard with a stethoscope.

S_2 (the second heart sound) is the sound of semilunar valve closure. It has a higher pitch than S_1 and is best heard along the lower and upper left sternal border. S_2 has two component sounds, A_2 and P_2 (aortic and pulmonary valve closure). A_2 is best appreciated at the mid and lower left sternal border, whereas P_2 is best heard at the upper left sternal border and is normally softer than A_2. Splitting of S_2 varies with respirations, widening with inspiration and narrowing with expiration. It is best heard at the second left intercostal space at the sternal border.

S_3 (the third heart sound) is the sound of rapid filling of the left ventricle. It occurs in early diastole and after S_2 and is a medium- to low-pitched thud. When heard in healthy children, the sound diminishes or disappears when the position changes from supine to sitting or standing; it is usually intermittent.

S_4 (the fourth heart sound) is associated with atrial contraction and increased atrial pressure and has a low pitch similar to that of S_3. It occurs just prior to S_1 and is not normally audible.

B. Abnormal Heart Sounds: Abnormalities in splitting or intensity of the component sounds of S_2 can be helpful in the diagnosis of major heart problems. With inspiration, there is a decrease in the intrathoracic pressure; this decrease causes increased filling of the right side of the heart, thereby prolonging the ejection time and delaying closure of the pulmonary valve. Normal intrathoracic pressure changes have little effect on the filling of the left side of the heart. Widening of splitting can be a clue to right-sided volume overload, whereas narrowing may indicate increased pulmonary artery pressure. A single S_2 is often heard in cases of malposition of the great vessels or severe pulmonary hypertension.

Ejection clicks are high-pitched and are usually related to dilated great vessels or valve abnormalities (or both). They can be heard throughout the ventricular systole and are classified as early, mid, or late. Early ejection clicks at the upper left sternal border are usually of pulmonary origin. Aortic clicks are heard in a wider distribution but best at the apex. Widespread clicks originating or loudest at the apex can be mitral or aortic in origin. The mid to late ejection click at the apex is most typically mitral valve prolapse. Early clicks may also be heard in spontaneous closure of ventricular septal defects.

S_3 can be a functional sound in childhood, although it often is associated with cardiac abnormalities.

S_4 is not normally audible; its finding on auscultation is almost always associated with cardiac abnormalities.

Opening snap is a relatively rare sound in pediatrics, occurring early in diastole and usually preceding a diastolic murmur of atrioventricular stenosis. It is medium-pitched in intensity.

C. Murmurs: Murmurs are the most common cardiovascular finding. The presence of a murmur in a child almost always causes alarm in the parents, who associate murmurs with major heart disease. However, most children have functional or innocent murmurs.

1. Characteristics–Murmurs can be evaluated on the basis of the following characteristics:

a. Location and radiation–Where the murmur is best heard and where the sound extends.

b. Relationship to cardiac cycle and duration–Systolic (with the pulse), diastolic, continuous, or to-and-fro.

c. Intensity–Classified as grade I, soft and heard with difficulty; grade II, soft but easily heard; grade III, loud but without a thrill; grade IV, loud and associated with a precordial thrill; grade V, loud, with thrill, and audible with the edge of the stethoscope; or grade VI, very loud and audible with the stethoscope off the chest or with the naked ear.

d. Quality–Harsh, musical, or rough; high, medium, or low in pitch.

e. Variation with position–Audible when the patient is supine, sitting, standing, or squatting.

2. Functional murmurs–The seven most common functional murmurs heard in childhood are as follows:

a. Newborn murmur–As the name implies, this murmur is frequently heard within the first few days of life. Typically, it is located at the lower left sternal border, without significant radiation. Newborn murmur is a soft, short, vibratory grade I–II/VI early systolic murmur that often subsides when mild pressure is applied to the abdomen. Newborn murmur usually disappears by 2–3 weeks of age.

b. Functional murmur of peripheral arterial pulmonary stenosis–This murmur is frequently heard in the premature infant, often after closure of a patent ductus arteriosus. It is secondary to mild narrowing of the branches of the pulmonary artery. Typically, the murmur is heard with equal intensity at the upper left sternal border, at the back, and in both axillas. It is a soft, short, high-pitched, grade I–II/VI systolic ejection murmur and usually disappears by 6 months of life. This murmur must be differentiated from true peripheral arterial pulmonary stenosis (rubella syndrome), coarctation of the thoracic aorta, valvular pulmonary stenosis, and atrial septal defect. These entities should, however, have other findings to suggest their organic nature.

c. Still's murmur–Probably the most common murmur of early childhood, this murmur can be heard in infancy, although it is most typically heard from the age of 2 years until adolescence. Classically, Still's murmur is loudest midway between the apex and the lower left sternal border, and often it may be transmitted (depending on loudness) to the remainder of the precordial area. Still's murmur is a musical or vibratory, short, high-pitched, grade I–III

early systolic ejection murmur. It is loudest when the patient is in the supine position; it diminishes or disappears when the patient sits or stands or during Valsalva's maneuver. Still's murmur may be louder in patients with fever or tachycardia.

d. Pulmonary outflow ejection murmur–This murmur may be heard throughout childhood. It is usually a soft, short, systolic ejection murmur, grade I–II in intensity and well localized to the upper left sternal border. The murmur becomes louder when the patient is in the supine position or when cardiac output is increased and softens with standing or during Valsalva's maneuver. Pulmonary outflow ejection murmur must be differentiated from other murmurs, such as those associated with pulmonary stenosis, coarctation of the aorta, atrial septal defect, and peripheral pulmonary artery stenosis.

e. Venous hum–This very common murmur of childhood is usually heard after 3 years of age. The murmur is located at the upper right and left sternal borders and in the lower neck. It is described as a continuous musical hum of grade I–II intensity, and it may be accentuated in diastole and with inspiration. This murmur always disappears when the patient is placed in a supine position or when the jugular vein is compressed. Venous hum is thought to be produced by turbulence in the subclavian and jugular veins.

f. Innominate or carotid bruit–This murmur is more common in the older child and adolescent. It is heard in the right supraclavicular and neck areas. This is a long systolic ejection murmur, somewhat harsh and of grade II–III intensity. The bruit can be accentuated by light pressure on the carotid artery and must be differentiated from all types of aortic stenosis.

g. Hemic murmur–Hemic murmurs are heard whenever anemia, fever, stress, or any increase in cardiac output is present. Typically, they are heard best in the aortic and pulmonary areas. These systolic ejection murmurs are of grade I–II intensity and are high-pitched. They disappear with normalization of cardiac output.

When functional murmurs are found in a child, the physician should assure the parents that these are normal heart sounds of the developing child and that they represent no abnormality of the heart.

3. Organic murmurs–Organic murmurs are evaluated on the basis of the characteristics outlined above (eg, location, intensity). These murmurs are discussed in relation to specific lesions later in this chapter.

2. NONCARDIAC EXAMINATION

Arterial Pulse

A. Rate and Rhythm: Cardiac rate and rhythm are usually determined by palpation of the radial or brachial pulse. Throughout infancy and childhood, the rate is subject to great variation. Multiple determinations must be made under properly evaluated conditions before conclusions can be drawn about their significance. This cautious approach is particularly important in infants.

Marked variations in heart rate occur with activity; therefore, the resting heart rate may be most accurately determined during sleep. In older children, exercise and emotional factors have a marked effect on the heart rate. All of these factors should be taken into account when examining the child, because many children are apprehensive and may react emotionally to the initial phases of the examination. It is possible for normal infants to have heart rates of 180 or 190 during the activity associated with a physical or electrocardiographic examination. Average resting heart rates range from 120/min in infants to 80/min in older children.

In the pediatric age group, the rhythm may be regular, or there may be a phasic variation in the heart rate (sinus arrhythmia), which is normal. Variations occasionally occur without relation to the respiratory cycle.

B. Quality and Amplitude of Pulse: Examination of the cardiovascular system should always include comparison of the pulses of the upper and lower extremities. A bounding pulse is characteristic of patent ductus arteriosus or aortic regurgitation. Narrow or thready pulses are found in patients with congestive heart failure or severe aortic stenosis.

The suprasternal notch should be examined, where visible pulsation is usually abnormal, although it may be seen in patients who are emotionally excited. A prominent pulsation is found in aortic insufficiency, patent ductus arteriosus, and coarctation of the aorta. A palpable thrill in the suprasternal notch is characteristic of aortic stenosis and is occasionally found with valvular pulmonary stenosis, coarctation of the aorta, and patent ductus arteriosus.

Assessment of the femoral pulse is an essential part of the physical examination of every infant and child. The femoral pulse should be readily palpable and equal in amplitude and time of appearance with the brachial pulse. A femoral pulse that is absent or weak or one that is delayed in comparison with the brachial pulse suggests coarctation of the aorta. An absent or diminished femoral pulse may be the only clue to the cause of a life-threatening problem.

Arterial Blood Pressure

Blood pressures should be obtained in the upper and lower extremities. Systolic pressure in the lower extremities determined by the auscultatory technique is usually higher than that found in the upper extremities in patients *over age 1 year.* In normal infants, the pressure in the arms may be slightly higher. The cuff must cover the same relative area of the arm and leg; for this reason, a larger cuff usually must be used for the leg than for the arm.

A. Procedures: Because of variation of blood pressure with respiration and slower rhythmic variations (Mayer or Traube-Hering waves), pressure obtained by any method should be repeated several times.

1. Auscultatory method–Hearing Korotkoff sounds by stethoscope and sphygmomanometer is the most common measure of blood pressure in children and correlates well with direct intra-arterial measurements. However, many factors affect its accuracy. Among these are the dimensions of the inflatable bag within the cuff. The length of the bag should be 100% and the width 50% of the circumference of the limb. A cuff that is too narrow or too short will produce a blood pressure reading that is higher than the true pressure.

2. Doppler ultrasound or automated blood pressure method–The combination of a small ultrasound transducer and a sphygmomanometer has proved to be especially applicable to the small infant. Considerations of cuff dimensions are still critical, however.

B. Pulse Pressure: Pulse pressure is determined by subtracting the diastolic pressure from the systolic pressure. Normally, the pulse pressure is less than 50 mm Hg or less than half the systolic pressure. A widened pulse pressure (which is associated with a bounding pulse) is present in aorticopulmonary shunt (eg, patent ductus arteriosus), aortic insufficiency, fever, anemia, and complete heart block. A narrow pulse pressure is seen in congestive heart failure, severe aortic stenosis, and pericardial tamponade.

Venous Pressure & Pulse

The level of the distended jugular vein above the suprasternal notch when the patient is at a 45-degree angle is a measure of venous pressure in older children and adults. Normally, one may observe the level of the transition between collapse and distention of the jugular vein approximately 1–2 cm above the notch. In addition to the level of the pulse, the wave pattern should be observed. Two waves can frequently be seen: (1) The *a* wave, because of right atrial contraction, is a rather sharply rising wave and therefore occurs immediately before or with the first heart sound or point of maximum impulse. (2) The *v* wave, caused by filling of the right atrium during ventricular systole, is a more slowly rising wave and occurs toward the end of ventricular systole. The venous pulse is not too helpful in examining infants and young children, however, because their necks are short and fat.

Extremities

Cyanosis of the extremities usually indicates congenital heart disease, but severe pulmonary disease must be excluded. Cyanosis is characterized by a bluish discoloration of the nails and mucous membranes.

A. Clubbing of Fingers and Toes: Clubbing implies fairly severe cyanotic congenital heart disease. It usually does not appear until approximately age 1, although occasionally, in patients with severe cyanosis, it may occur earlier. The first sign of clubbing is softening of the nail beds, followed by rounding of the fingernails and then by thickening and shininess of the terminal phalanx, with loss of creases.

Hypoxemia producing cyanosis is by far the most common cause, but clubbing occurs also in patients with infective endocarditis, severe liver disease, and lung abscess.

B. Edema: Edema of the lower extremities is characteristic of right ventricular heart failure in older children and adults. However, in infants and younger children, peripheral edema is more likely to affect first the face, then the presacral region, and eventually the extremities.

Abdomen

Hepatomegaly is the cardinal sign of right heart failure in the infant and child. Presystolic pulsation of the liver may occur with right atrial hypertension and systolic pulsation with tricuspid insufficiency. Congestive splenomegaly may be present in patients who have had long-standing congestive heart failure. Enlargement of the spleen is one of the characteristic features of subacute infective endocarditis. Ascites is occasionally present in right heart failure.

Payne RM et al: Toward a molecular understanding of congenital heart disease. Circulation 1995;91:494.

Rosner B et al: Blood pressure nomograms for children and adolescents, by height, sex, and age, in the United States. J Pediatr 1993;123:871.

Van Oort A et al: The vibratory innocent heart murmur in schoolchildren: A case-control Doppler echocardiographic study. Pediatr Cardiol 1994;15:275.

ELECTROCARDIOGRAPHY & VECTORCARDIOGRAPHY

The electrocardiogram (ECG) is an essential part of the evaluation of the cardiovascular system. The ECG is the sine qua non for the diagnosis of dysrhythmias and may offer the best clue to the specific diagnosis of congenital lesions (eg, left axis deviation in a blue baby, suggesting tricuspid atresia). Conversely, the ECG may provide little or no help (as in assessing right ventricular hypertrophy in the newborn or left ventricular hypertrophy in the child with congenital aortic stenosis).

It is not possible, within the limitations of this presentation, to teach the interpretation of the ECG, but

a few basic facts and definitions should help to orient the student.

A. Propagation of Electrical Force: As shown in Figure 18–1, a wave of electrical force traveling toward an electrode inscribes a positive (upward) deflection; away from an electrode, a negative deflection; and perpendicular to an electrode, a low-voltage, isodiphasic complex. These forces are inscribed as loops on the vectorcardiogram (VCG), and abnormalities are manifested as alterations in direction and duration of force or as increased or decreased electrical force (amplitude of QRS complex on the ECG or loop on the VCG).

B. Age-Related Variations: The ECG and VCG evolve with the age of the patient. The rate gradually decreases and intervals generally increase with age. There is also progressive change in dominance of ventricles from right ventricular dominance in the young infant to left ventricular dominance in the older infant, child, and adult. The normal ECG of the 1-week-old would be highly abnormal for a 1-year-old, and the ECG of a 5-year-old would not be normal for an adult.

C. Electrocardiographic Interpretation: Figure 18–2 defines the events recorded on the ECG. The sequence of recording the findings of the ECG is usually as follows: rate, rhythm, P wave, PR interval, QRS complex (including axis, amplitude, and duration), QT interval, ST segment, and T wave.

1. Rate–The paper speed at which ECGs are usually taken is 25 mm/s. Each small square is 1 mm, and each large square, 5 mm. Therefore, five large squares represent 1 second, one large square 0.2 s, and one small square 0.04 s. A common method of estimating the ventricular rate is to count the number of large squares between two QRS complexes: If QRS complexes appear at a rate of one per large

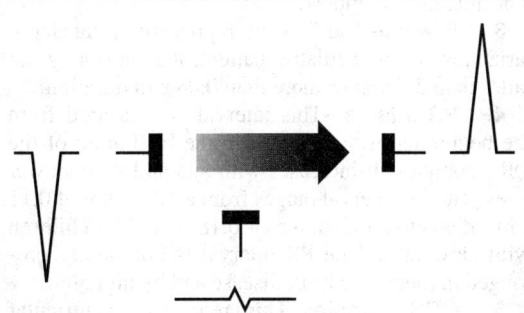

Figure 18–1. Depolarization of the myocardium. The arrow represents the wave of electrical force. As it travels toward the electrode, it inscribes a positive (upward) deflection; away from the electrode, a negative (downward) deflection; and perpendicular to the electrode, a low-voltage, isodiphasic deflection.

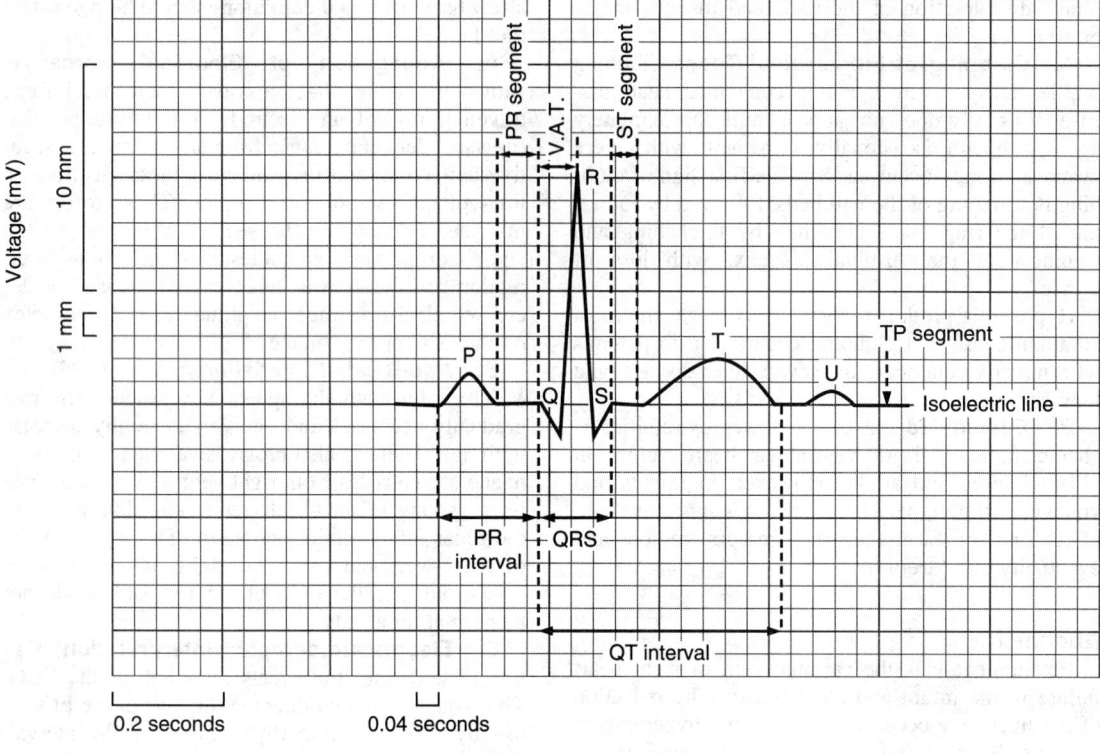

Figure 18–2. Complexes and intervals of the electrocardiogram.

square (5/s), the ventricular rate is 300; if QRS complexes appear every two squares, the ventricular rate is 150, and so on. The formula is to divide the number of large squares between QRS complexes into 300 and roughly interpolate for fractions of large squares.

2. Rhythm–Normal sinus rhythm consists of a normal P wave followed by a normal PR interval and a normal QRS complex.

3. P wave–The P wave represents atrial depolarization. In the pediatric patient, it is normally not taller than 2.5 mm or more than 0.08 s in duration.

4. PR interval–This interval is measured from the beginning of the P wave to the beginning of the QRS complex. It increases with age and with slower rates. The PR interval ranges from a minimum of 0.11 s in infants to a maximum of 0.18 s in older children with slow rates. The PR interval is commonly prolonged in rheumatic heart disease and by digitalis.

5. QRS complex–This represents ventricular depolarization, and its amplitude and direction of force (axis) reveal the relative size of (viable) ventricular mass in hypertrophy, hypoplasia, and infarction. Abnormal ventricular conduction (eg, right bundle branch block, anterior fascicular block) is also revealed. Interpretation of the QRS complex is one of

the most important aspects of cardiologic diagnosis. VAT is the ventricular activation time.

6. QT interval–This interval is measured from the beginning of the QRS complex to the end of the T wave. The QT duration is affected by drugs such as digitalis and electrolyte imbalances such as hypocalcemia and hypokalemia (really QU interval prolongation). The normal duration is rate-related and must be corrected using the following formula:

$$QT_c = \frac{QT\ interval(s)}{\sqrt{R - R\ interval(s)}}$$

The normal QT_c is usually less than 0.44 s.

7. ST segment–This short segment lying between the end of the QRS complex and the beginning of the T wave is affected by drugs and electrolyte imbalances and reflects myocardial injury.

8. T wave–The T wave represents myocardial repolarization and is altered by electrolytes, myocardial hypertrophy, and ischemia.

9. Impression–The ultimate impression of the ECG is derived from a systematic analysis of features such as those described above as compared with expected normal values for the age of the child.

Benson DW Jr: The normal electrocardiogram. In: *Moss and Adams Heart Disease in Infants, Children, and Adolescents,* 5th ed. Emmanouilides GC et al (editors). Williams & Wilkins, 1995.

Gillette PC, Garson A Jr: *Pediatric Arrhythmias: Electrophysiology and Pacing.* Saunders, 1990.

Liebman J, Plonsey R, Gillette PC: Pediatric Electrocardiography. Williams & Wilkins, 1982.

Park MK: Electrocardiography. In: *Pediatric Cardiology for Practitioners.* Mosby, 1996.

CHEST X-RAY

The chest x-ray requires systematic evaluation. Accurate conclusions about the presence or absence of congenital heart defects and bone abnormalities can be drawn only if the proper procedures were followed—eg, the penetration of x-ray was adequate, and the films were obtained on adequate inspiration (distortions resulting from inadequate inspiration may look like cardiomegaly and increased vascular markings). The size of the heart, as seen on the chest x-ray film, must be evaluated in relation to the age and size of the patient. Chest films of the normal newborn show a greater heart size and more pronounced vascular markings than those of the normal older child. These factors must all be taken into consideration in evaluating heart size and configuration and lung fields. The standard posteroanterior and left lateral chest films are usually adequate for this evaluation (Figure 18–3). If there is suspicion of vascular ring or mediastinal mass, multiple-view films with barium swallow are indicated.

Condon V: The heart and great vessels. In: *Caffey's Pediatric X-Ray Diagnosis: An Integrated Imaging Approach.* Silverman FN (editor). Year Book, 1985.

Park MK: Chest radiography. In: *Pediatric Cardiology for Practitioners.* Mosby, 1996.

ECHOCARDIOGRAPHY & DOPPLER ULTRASONOGRAPHY

Echocardiography is now the major noninvasive method for diagnosis of congenital heart defects and is used to define anatomy, function, chamber and vessel size, and valve abnormalities. The use of M-mode and two-dimensional echocardiography will, in most instances, allow accurate diagnosis. These methods, along with doppler ultrasonography (color, pulsed, or continuous-wave ultrasound measurements) can now be used to predict cardiac output, flow direction, valve gradients, and pulmonary artery pressure. New techniques of transesophageal and three-dimensional echocardiography are adding anatomic information that is particularly helpful in the surgical management of patients with congenital heart disease. Interpretation of the results of these studies requires the skill of the pediatric cardiologist. In cases of major heart disease, cardiac catheterization should also be performed.

Park MK: Noninvasive techniques. Echocardiography. In: *Pediatric Cardiology for Practitioners.* Mosby, 1996.

Silverman NH: *Pediatric Echocardiography.* Williams & Wilkins, 1993.

Stümper O, Sutherland GR: *Transesophageal Echocardiography in Congenital Heart Disease.* Arnold, 1994.

NUCLEAR CARDIOLOGY

Use of radionuclide tracers in infants and children includes detection and quantification of left-to-right and right-to-left intracardiac shunting, quantification

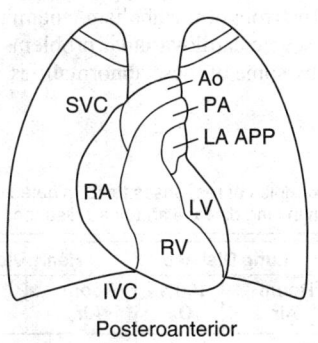

Posteroanterior

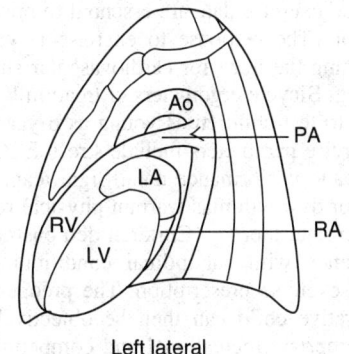

Left lateral

Figure 18–3. Position of cardiovascular structures in principal x-ray views. Ao = aorta, IVC = inferior vena cava, LA = left atrium, LA APP = left atrial appendage, LV = left ventricle, PA = pulmonary artery, RA = right atrium, RV = right ventricle, SVC = superior vena cava.

of cardiac output at rest and during exercise using gated blood pool scintigraphy, and myocardial imaging with thallium 201 (^{201}Tl) and technetium 99m (^{99m}Tc) sestamibi for ischemia or infarction. In the older child, the latter method can be enhanced by exercise stress testing. These tests yield more objective data for evaluation of children with heart disease.

Gibbons RJ: Nuclear cardiology. In: *Mayo Clinical Practice of Cardiology*. Mosby, 1996.

Hurwitz RA: Radionuclide methods. In: *Moss and Adams Heart Disease in Infants, Children, and Adolescents*, 5th ed. Emmanouilides GC et al (editors). Williams & Wilkins, 1995.

Wiles HB: Nuclear cardiology. In: *The Science and Practice of Pediatric Cardiology*. Garson A Jr, Bricker JT, McNamara DG (editors). Lea & Febiger, 1990.

MAGNETIC RESONANCE IMAGING

Magnetic resonance imaging (MRI) is now a valuable tool in the evaluation and noninvasive follow-up of many congenital heart defects. Particularly in the imaging of vascular structures of the thorax, MRI can be matched only by angiography. The addition of "gated" imaging or cine MRI now allows dynamic evaluation of the structure and blood flow patterns within the heart and great vessels. MRI is invaluable in the long-term follow-up of coarctation of the aorta after angioplasty.

Breen JF, Julsrud PR: Cardiac magnetic resonance imaging. In: *Mayo Clinical Practice of Cardiology*. Mosby, 1996.

ERGOMETRY

Pediatric ergometry is a newly evolving technique. It has long been hampered by lack of appreciation of its applications and availability of normal data. Most children with heart disease are capable of normal activity, and exercise data are essential to prevent overprotection. The response to exercise is valuable in determining the need for cardiovascular surgery and its timing. Bicycle ergometers or treadmills can often be used to test children as young as 6 years. Important exercise parameters include stress ECGs, conditioning, and performance data. Significant stress ischemia or dysrhythmias warrant physical restrictions or appropriate therapy. Children demonstrating poor performance with suboptimal conditioning benefit from an exercise prescription. The preoperative and postoperative child can then be objectively guided into appropriate recreational and competitive activities and given prevocational guidance.

Driscoll DJ: Exercise testing. In: *Moss and Adams Heart Disease in Infants, Children, and Adolescents*, 5th ed.
Emmanouilides GC et al (editors). Williams & Wilkins, 1995.

ARTERIAL BLOOD GASES
(Arterial Po$_2$, Systemic O$_2$ Saturation)

Because cyanosis is difficult to measure (and sometimes to recognize) by inspection of the patient, objective laboratory determinations are required. The quantitative response of arterial Po$_2$ or O$_2$ saturation (eg, by pulse oximetry) to administration of 100% oxygen is one of the most useful methods of distinguishing cyanosis produced by heart disease from cyanosis related to lung disease in sick infants. In cyanotic heart disease, PaO$_2$ increases very little from values obtained while breathing ambient room air compared with values during 100% oxygen administration. However, there is usually a very significant increase in PaO$_2$ when oxygen is administered to a patient with lung disease. Continuous noninvasive methods for monitoring arterial Po$_2$ include the transcutaneous O$_2$ monitor and pulse oximetry. Inherent limitations have prevented the general substitution of these noninvasive methods for direct arterial sampling in this evaluation, but they are valuable in overall cardiopulmonary care of the sick infant. Table 18–1 illustrates the sort of response one might expect following at least 10 minutes of 100% oxygen administration to cyanotic infants with heart disease versus lung disease.

OTHER NONINVASIVE LABORATORY STUDIES

In children of all ages, but particularly in the infant and newborn, many metabolic abnormalities can have a major influence on the performance of the cardiovascular system. In evaluating the symptomatic infant, it is important to rule out infection, hypoglycemia, hypocalcemia, hypovolemia, hyperkalemia, inborn errors of metabolism, anemia, and so on. Likewise, severe cardiovascular problems may be accompanied by some of these abnormalities.

Table 18–1. Examples of responses to 10 minutes of 100% oxygen in lung disease and heart disease.

	Lung Disease		Heart Disease	
	Room Air	100% O$_2$	Room Air	100% O$_2$
Color	Blue →	Pink	Blue →	Blue
Oximetry	60% →	99%	60% →	62%
PaO$_2$ (mm Hg)	35 →	120	35 →	38

CARDIAC CATHETERIZATION & ANGIOCARDIOGRAPHY

The definitive anatomic and physiologic study of infants and children with heart disease is cardiac catheterization. It is essential for the primary physician to distinguish those infants and children who require the specialized diagnostic and therapeutic facilities of the pediatric cardiac center from those who may be safely managed without such facilities and consultation. On the basis of the preceding steps of diagnostic evaluation—history, physical examination, ECG, chest x-ray, and other noninvasive laboratory studies—the consulting pediatric cardiologist has a rather precise assessment of the anatomic and physiologic abnormalities in simple malformations and considerable useful information about complex malformations.

Indications & Objectives

A. Infants:

1. Indications–

a. Infants with cyanosis presumed to be cardiovascular in origin should be catheterized as soon as a reasonably stable clinical condition can be achieved. This should be performed for diagnosis of anatomic abnormalities not easily appreciated by echocardiography and for therapeutic interventions such as balloon atrial septostomy or valvuloplasty of a stenotic pulmonary or aortic valve.

b. Infants with severe congestive heart failure that does not respond promptly and satisfactorily to anticongestive measures.

c. Infants in whom early operation for congenital heart disease is contemplated.

d. Infants in whom the anatomic and physiologic abnormality is sufficiently vague that appropriate medical management is not possible.

e. Infants who have evidence of complicating or potentially progressive problems, such as pulmonary hypertension.

2. Objectives–(In descending order of importance.)

a. To perform the study with the lowest possible rate of death or serious complications. Pediatric cardiologists and pediatric cardiac catheterization laboratories with experience in studying infants are required so that these objectives can be met: to gain meaningful information promptly; to care for the critically ill infant with temperature and pH control, fluid management, and all essential pediatric treatment; and to anticipate and handle life-threatening crises.

b. To gain information which is not available by other methods and which will provide the basis for therapeutic decisions (medical or surgical).

c. To provide therapeutic intervention (eg, Rashkind septostomy, balloon valvuloplasty).

d. To obtain sufficient physiologic and anatomic data so that repeat catheterization to complete the study will not be necessary.

B. Children:

1. Indications–

a. All children for whom heart surgery is contemplated (with the exception of children with unequivocal patent ductus arteriosus or atrial septal defect [or both] or other uncomplicated anatomy or physiology).

b. All children in whom there is question about the anatomic or physiologic abnormality which would significantly influence management and which cannot be completely answered by noninvasive methods.

c. Children with progressive lesions that require careful physiologic monitoring (eg, pulmonary hypertension).

d. Children who have had cardiovascular surgery and require assessment of the adequacy of the repair.

e. Children with mild to moderate cardiovascular lesions when important information about the natural history is required. This procedure should be done only in the setting of a well-designed protocol and fully informed consent.

2. Objectives–Conducting the study with the lowest possible risk is the most important objective of cardiac catheterization of the child as well as the infant; and the risk to the child (< 0.2%) is certainly much less than the risk to the sick infant (2%). Complete anatomic and physiologic data are important objectives of catheterization in children and infants. No physician or laboratory should undertake the catheterization of a child unless prepared to obtain a completely informative study and unless physicians and surgeons are available who are capable of proceeding with whatever medical or surgical therapy may be indicated.

Contraindications

Cardiac catheterization is contraindicated in infants and children who present with no clinical urgency and none of the indications listed above. It should not be done if personnel and facilities fail to meet high standards of patient safety and clinical diagnostic and therapeutic expertise.

Cardiac Catheterization Data

Figure 18–4 shows oxygen saturation (in percent) and pressure (in mm Hg) values obtained at cardiac catheterization from the chambers and great arteries of the heart. These values would be within the normal range for a child.

A. Oxygen Content and Saturation; Pulmonary and Systemic Blood Flow (Cardiac Output): In most laboratories, evidence of left-to-right shunt is determined by changes of blood oxygen content or saturation during passage of the catheter through the right side of the heart. A significant in-

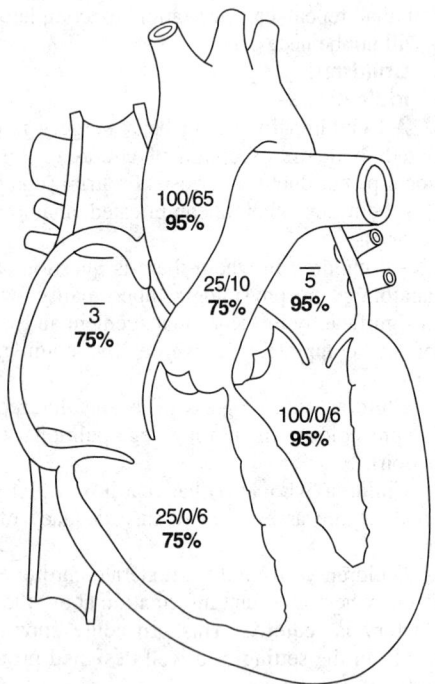

100/65
95%

25/10
75%

5̄
95%

3̄
75%

100/0/6
95%

25/0/6
75%

Figure 18–4. Pressures (in mm Hg) and oxygen saturation (in percent) obtained by cardiac catheterization in a healthy child. 3 = mean pressure of 3 mm Hg in the right atrium, 5 = mean pressure of 5 mm Hg in the left atrium.

crease in oxygen content or oxygen saturation from one chamber to another indicates the presence of a left-to-right shunt at the site of the increase. The oxygen saturation of the peripheral arterial blood should always be determined during cardiac catheterization. Normal arterial oxygen saturation is 91–97%. A decrease (at sea level) below 91% suggests the presence of a right-to-left shunt, underventilation, or pulmonary disease.

The size of a left-to-right shunt is usually expressed as a ratio of the pulmonary to systemic blood flow or as liters per minute as determined by the Fick principle:

$$\frac{\text{Cardiac output}}{(\text{L/min})} = \frac{\text{Oxygen consumption (mL/min)}}{\text{Arteriovenous difference (mL/L)}}$$

B. Pressures: Pressures should be determined in all chambers and vessels entered. Pressures should always be recorded when a catheter is pulled back from a distal chamber or vessel into a more proximal chamber. It is not normal for systolic pressure in the ventricles to exceed systolic pressure in the great arteries or mean diastolic pressure in the atria to exceed end-diastolic pressure in the ventricles. If a "gradient" in pressure does exist, it means that there is ob

struction, and the severity of the gradient is one criterion for the necessity of operative repair. A right ventricular systolic pressure of 100 mm Hg and a pulmonary artery systolic pressure of 20 mm Hg yield a gradient of 80 mm Hg. In this case, the patient would be classified as having severe pulmonary stenosis requiring repair.

C. Pulmonary and Systemic Vascular Resistance: The vascular resistance is calculated from the following formula and reported in units or in dynes $\cdot$ cm^{-5}/m^2:

$$\text{Resistance} = \frac{\text{Pressure}}{\text{Flow}}$$

Pulmonary vascular resistance equals mean pulmonary artery pressure minus the mean pulmonary artery wedge or left atrial pressure divided by pulmonary blood flow per square meter of body surface area. (Pulmonary blood flow is determined from the Fick principle, as noted previously.) **Systemic vascular resistance** equals mean systemic arterial pressure minus the mean central nervous pressure divided by systemic blood flow.

Normally, the pulmonary vascular resistance ranges from 1 to 3 units, or from 80 to 240 dynes $\cdot$ cm^{-5}/m^2. If pulmonary resistance is above 10 units or the pulmonary/systemic resistance ratio is above 0.7, all other diagnostic findings should be reviewed carefully to confirm the presence of pulmonary hypertension that is so severe as to render the patient inoperable.

D. Special Techniques: Special techniques used during cardiac catheterization include the following:

1. Hydrogen electrode catheter–Used to determine the presence of very small left-to-right shunts, this technique enables the operator to detect such shunts even in the absence of any increase in oxygen saturation.

2. Indicator dilution curves–This involves injection of an indicator, such as indocyanine green (Cardio-Green), at specific places in the heart and detection of the dye downstream, usually in a peripheral artery. This technique permits the detection of both right-to-left and left-to-right shunts at the specific points within the cardiovascular system. Cardiac output is frequently determined by this method.

3. Selective angiocardiography and cineangiocardiography–In this technique, contrast material is injected in a specific chamber or vessel and the course of the contrast material is followed by serial large-film x-rays (angiocardiography) or by motion pictures (cineangiocardiography).

4. Contrast echocardiography–Saline or indocyanine green is rapidly injected via the cardiac catheter, and downstream "clouding" is imaged with either M-mode or two-dimensional echocardiogra phy. Dynamic spatial or structural relationships of chambers, valves, and vessels are visualized; this procedure may be done repetitively without the risk of radiation.

5. Interventional catheterization—Specially designed catheters are now used for dilatation of stenotic valves and vascular structures. Balloon valvuloplasty-angioplasty is now the treatment of choice for valve pulmonary stenosis, coarctation of the thoracic aorta, aortic valve stenosis, and pulmonary arterial stenoses. Other valve and vascular dilating techniques, such as intravascular stents, are now in use along with techniques for closure of patent ductus arteriosus and atrial septal defect (under study). Many simple defects are now treated effectively through these and other procedures.

Bridges ND, Freed MD: Cardiac catheterization, angiocardiography. In: *Moss and Adams Heart Disease in Infants, Children, and Adolescents,* 5th ed. Emmanouilides GC et al (editors). Williams & Wilkins, 1995.

Mullins CE, O'Laughlin MP: Therapeutic cardiac catheterization. In: *Moss and Adams Heart Disease in Infants, Children, and Adolescents,* 5th ed. Emmanouilides GC et al (editors). Williams & Wilkins, 1995.

PRENATAL & NEONATAL CIRCULATION

Fetal Circulation

In the fetus, the placenta is the organ of respiration and for exchange of waste products. Oxygenated blood (approximately 80% saturated) passes from the placenta through the umbilical vein to the heart. As it flows toward the heart, it mixes with blood from the inferior vena cava and the portal vein, so that blood entering the right atrium is approximately 65% saturated. A considerable amount of this blood is shunted immediately across the foramen ovale into the left atrium. The venous blood derived from the upper part of the body is much less saturated (approximately 30%), and most of it enters the right ventricle through the tricuspid valve. Thus, the blood in the right ventricle is a mixture of both relatively highly saturated blood from the umbilical vein and desaturated blood from the venae cavae. This mixture results in a blood oxygen saturation of approximately 50% in the right ventricle.

The blood in the left atrium is derived from the blood shunting across the foramen ovale and the blood returning from the pulmonary veins. A great deal of the left ventricular output goes to the head, whereas the lower portion of the body is supplied by blood both from the right ventricle, through the patent ductus arteriosus, and from the left ventricle.

Physiologic Changes at Birth & in the Neonatal Period

At birth, two dramatic events that affect the cardiovascular and pulmonary system occur: (1) the umbilical cord is clamped, removing the placenta from the circulation; and (2) breathing commences. As a result, marked changes in the circulation occur. During fetal life, the placenta offers little resistance to the flow of blood, so that the systemic circuit is a low-resistance one. On the other hand, the pulmonary arterioles are markedly constricted and offer strong resistance to the flow of blood into the lung. Clamping the cord causes a sudden increase in resistance to flow in the systemic circuit. As the lung becomes the organ of respiration, the oxygen tension (PO_2) increases in the vicinity of the small pulmonary arterioles, resulting in a release of the constriction and thus a significant decrease in the pulmonary arteriolar resistance. Indeed, the pulmonary vascular resistance shortly after birth is less than that of the systemic circuit.

Because of the changes in resistance, most of the right ventricular outflow now passes into the lung rather than through the ductus arteriosus into the descending aorta. In fact, functional closure of the ductus arteriosus begins to develop shortly after birth. Recent studies have demonstrated that the ductus arteriosus remains patent for a variable period, usually 24–48 hours. During the first hour after birth, there is a small right-to-left shunt (as in the fetus). However, after 1 hour, bidirectional shunting occurs, with the left-to-right direction predominating. In most cases, right-to-left shunting completely disappears by 8 hours. However, in patients with severe hypoxia (eg, in respiratory distress syndrome), the pulmonary vascular resistance remains elevated, resulting in a continued right-to-left shunt. The cause of the functional closure of the ductus arteriosus is not completely known. However, evidence indicates that the increased PO_2 of the arterial blood causes spasm of the ductus. Anatomically, however, the ductus arteriosus does not close until approximately age 3 months.

In fetal life, the foramen ovale serves as a one-way valve, permitting shunting of blood from the inferior vena cava through the right atrium into the left atrium. At birth, because of the changes in the pulmonary and systemic vascular resistance and the increase in the quantity of blood returning from the pulmonary veins to the left atrium, the left atrial pressure rises above that of the right atrium. This functionally closes the flap of the one-way valve, essentially preventing flow of blood across the septum. It has been shown, however, that a small right-to-left shunt does continue for the first week of life. Although the foramen ovale remains functionally closed throughout life, it remains patent in about 25% of patients.

A clinical syndrome has been recognized that is characterized in term infants by onset of tachypnea, cyanosis, and clinical evidence of pulmonary hypertension during the first 8 hours after delivery. These infants have massive right-to-left ductal or foramen shunting or both for 3–7 days because of the high pulmonary vascular resistance. The clinical course is generally one of progressive cor pulmonale, hypoxia, and acidosis, terminating in early death unless the pulmonary resistance can be lowered. The resistance can usually be reversed by instituting appropriate means to increase alveolar PO_2: high-frequency, low tidal volume hyperventilation (to produce respiratory alkalosis) and intravenous administration of vasoactive drugs. Recently, extracorporeal membrane oxygenation (ECMO) and inhaled nitric oxide have shown promise in selected cases. At postmortem, the findings include increased thickness of the pulmonary arteriolar media, which is believed to represent persistence of the fetal circulation.

Changes in the First Year of Life

The most significant changes occur at birth and within the neonatal period. However, pulmonary vascular resistance and the pulmonary arterial pressure continue to fall during the first year of life. This phenomenon results from the involution of the pulmonary arteriole from a relatively thick-walled, small-lumen vessel to a thin-walled, large-lumen vessel. Adult levels of resistance and pressure are usually achieved by age 6 months to 1 year.

Heymann MA: Fetal and postnatal circulation: Pulmonary circulation. In: *Moss and Adams Heart Disease in Infants, Children, and Adolescents,* 5th ed. Emmanouilides GC et al (editors). Williams & Wilkins, 1995.

Kanto WP Jr: A decade of experience with neonatal extracorporeal membrane oxygenation. J Pediatr 1994;124: 335.

Kinsella JP et al: Clinical responses to prolonged treatment of persistent pulmonary hypertension of the newborn with low doses of inhaled nitric oxide. J Pediatr 1993; 123:103.

MAJOR CLUES TO HEART DISEASE IN INFANTS & CHILDREN

CONGESTIVE HEART FAILURE

Congestive heart failure at the clinical level is the failure of the heart to meet the circulatory and metabolic needs of the body. Congestive heart failure is one of the two major clues to the presence of important heart disease. (The other is cyanosis; see later in this chapter.) It has been estimated that congestive heart failure begins before age 1 year in over 90% of infants and children who ever develop the disorder in the pediatric age period—and most of these patients are less than 6 months of age.

Congestive heart failure beginning in infancy may

persist throughout childhood until operation relieves the underlying malformation (unless surgery is not possible). Other infants with moderately severe heart failure in the first few months of life may gradually compensate (for a variety of reasons) and not require medical intervention after age 12 or 18 months even though their congenital heart lesions are still unrepaired.

Clinical Findings

The three cardinal signs of congestive heart failure in the pediatric patient are cardiomegaly (the sine qua non), tachypnea (left side), and hepatomegaly (right side).

Cardiomegaly represents a homeostatic (compensatory) mechanism that maintains adequate cardiac output by enlarging the capacity of the pump. This mechanism is frequently referred to as Starling's law of the heart. Up to a point, the enlarging heart can deliver a greater stroke volume output, but limits are soon reached (the descending limb of Starling's curve). Figure 18–5 shows a family of ventricular performance curves. The curve at the right depicts a damaged myocardium; the curve in the center, a normal myocardium; and the curve at the left, a myocardium under inotropic stimulation. One should be very cautious about the diagnosis of congestive heart failure in the absence of an enlarged heart (an exception being a condition such as total anomalous venous return below the diaphragm, which will, for a short period of time, be characterized by other signs of congestive heart failure without an enlarged heart). Cardiomegaly without other signs of congestive failure may well be taken as early or homeostatically compensated congestive heart failure.

Tachypnea may be considered the cardinal sign of

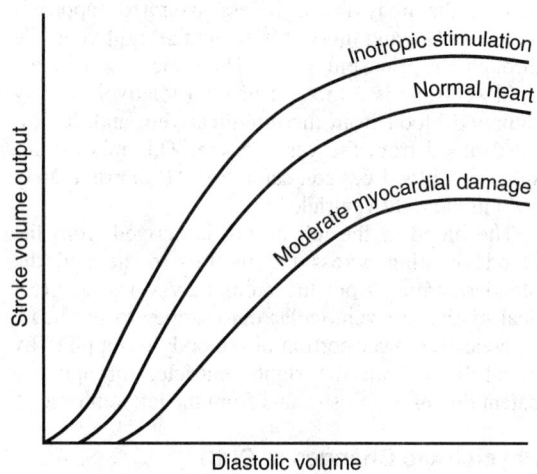

Figure 18–5. Ventricular performance curves.

left-sided heart failure. It may be present for a short time before hepatomegaly occurs, although pure left-sided or pure right-sided heart failure does not commonly exist independently for long.

Hepatomegaly is the cardinal sign of right-sided heart failure. The liver is capable of trapping relatively large amounts of edema fluid in the infant that would be more evident as peripheral edema in the older child and adult. It is therefore common rather than unusual for the infant in moderately severe heart failure to have an enlarged liver with no pretibial or even presacral or facial edema. Peripheral edema is found in infants only in the most severe cases of congestive heart failure.

Additional signs and symptoms of congestive heart failure are feeding difficulties, dyspnea, restlessness, easy fatigability, weak pulses, pallor, rales, peripheral edema, weight gain from fluid accumulation, tachycardia, sweating, pneumonia, orthopnea, and growth failure.

Underlying Causes of Heart Failure in the Pediatric Age Group

By far the most common cause of congestive heart failure in the pediatric patient is congenital heart disease. Causes in infancy and childhood appear in the outline below:

A. Heart Failure in Infancy:

1. Cardiovascular causes–Congenital heart disease (producing volume overload, outflow obstruction, myocardial impairment), congenital vascular disease (eg, coarctation of the aorta, an outflow obstruction disorder; peripheral arteriovenous shunts, a volume overload disorder), acquired myocardial disease (eg, myocarditis), dysrhythmias, rheumatic fever (very rare in infants in the United States).

2. Noncardiovascular causes–Acidosis, respiratory disease, central nervous system disease, anemia, sepsis, hypoglycemia.

B. Heart Failure in Childhood: Cardiovascular causes are potentially the same as in infancy except that rheumatic fever plays a more important role in childhood. Noncardiovascular causes become less important with increasing age—especially such mechanisms as acidosis and hypoglycemia.

Treatment

The physician caring for children must have facility with routine measures and familiarity with some emergency measures for treating congestive heart failure.

A. Routine Measures:

1. Digitalis–Digitalis is the keystone of the treatment of congestive heart failure. The desired effect is improvement in myocardial performance (inotropic effect), shifting the patient to a more efficient ventricular performance in the family of curves shown in Figure 18–5. The preparation most widely used in pediatrics is digoxin, which may be adminis-

tered (in order of rapidity of onset of effect) intravenously, intramuscularly, or orally. The clinical urgency of the individual case dictates how quickly digitalization should be accomplished. Although there are general guidelines, the ultimate dosage (on a milligram-per-kilogram basis) must be individualized for each patient.

a. Protocols for digitalization–

(1) In hospital–

Age	Parenteral	Oral
Premature	0.035 mg/kg	0.04 mg/kg
1 week to 2 years	0.05 mg/kg	0.07 mg/kg
< 1 week or > 2 years	0.04 mg/kg	0.06 mg/kg

Use of the elixir (0.05 mg/mL) is advisable even in older children because the bioavailability of the tablet preparations is unreliable.

The routine schedule consists of giving one-quarter of the digitalizing dose intramuscularly or orally every 6 hours for four doses. For rapid digitalization, give half the digitalizing dose intravenously or intramuscularly and repeat in 4–6 hours. For very rapid digitalization, give the full digitalizing dose intravenously with very close monitoring. For maintenance, give one-quarter to one-third of the oral digitalizing dose daily (divided into morning and evening doses).

(2) Digitalization of outpatients–Give the maintenance dose of digoxin (see above) divided into morning and evening doses. In less than 1 week, adequate digitalization is obtained without running the risk of a parent's inadvertently failing to revert to a maintenance dosage schedule and continuing a high digitalizing dose to the point of toxicity (even death).

b. Digitalis toxicity–Slowing of the heart rate below 100 in infants, below 80 in young children, and below 60 in older children is often taken as a guide to reducing the dosage of digoxin. Any dysrhythmia that occurs during digitalis therapy should be attributed to the drug until proved otherwise, although ventricular bigeminy and various degrees of atrioventricular block are characteristic of digitalis toxicity. Age-specific serum levels suggestive of toxicity during maintenance therapy are as follows: newborn, over 4 ng/mL; 1 month to 1 year, over 3 ng/mL; after 1 year, over 2 ng/mL.

c. Digitalis poisoning–_This is an acute emergency that must be treated without delay._ The sooner the stomach is emptied, the better the prognosis, but even if many hours have passed, the stomach should still be emptied. Attention must then be paid to maintaining an adequate cardiac rate and output and to controlling the dysrhythmia. A useful basic intravenous solution is 10% glucose in water to which KCl (3 mEq/kg/d) and regular insulin (20 units/1000 mL) have been added. KCl must be used with caution in patients with electrocardiographic high-grade block. It should be given in amounts not to exceed the maintenance requirement per 24 hours for the weight or surface area of the patient. To this solution may be added isoproterenol (in the calibrated administration set) titrated in quantities appropriate to maintain adequate heart rate and output in the face of complete heart block. Phenytoin may be administered through the intravenous tubing to treat arrhythmias by beginning with a 1 mg/kg slow intravenous push followed every 5–10 minutes with doubling doses to a maximum total combined dose of 15 mg/kg. In severe cases, digoxin immune Fab (ovine) dosage is determined by total body load (TBL) of digoxin:

$$\text{IV TBL} = \text{C (ng/mL)} \times 5.6 \times \text{body weight (kg)}/1000$$
$$or$$
$$\text{TBL} = \text{mg of digoxin ingested} \times 0.8$$

where C = the postdistribution digoxin concentration (serum digoxin level). The dose of digoxin immune Fab (in mg) = TBL × 66.7. Fab is infused over 15–20 minutes. If this agent is not available, a temporary transvenous pacemaker may be required to control arrhythmias.

2. Diuretics–If digitalis alone is inadequate to achieve satisfactory compensation, diuretics may be required. For rapid inpatient diuresis, give furosemide intravenously or intramuscularly; for maintenance therapy, give thiazides or furosemide orally daily along with spironolactone.

The dosages are as follows:

a. Furosemide–
(1) Intravenously or intramuscularly, 1 mg/kg per dose, given two or three times daily while monitored in the hospital; monitor electrolytes.
(2) Orally, 2–5 mg/kg/d.

b. Thiazides–These drugs should be given daily with spironolactone (which helps to prevent excessive potassium loss). Do not give daily for prolonged periods unless spironolactone is being given also and serum electrolytes are being monitored periodically.
(1) Chlorothiazide suspension (250 mg/tsp), 20 mg/kg/d.
(2) Hydrochlorothiazide tablets, 2 mg/kg/d.

c. Spironolactone–Give 2–4 mg/kg/d in two divided doses.

3. Rest and sedation–The decompensated and mildly distressed patient requires rest; the severely distressed and anxious infant or child requires sedation. Parenteral morphine, 0.1 mg/kg, is useful for sedation as well as for control of acute pulmonary edema, but it should be given only with good airway control.

4. Oxygen–Oxygen will not make a patient with cyanotic heart disease pink, but it will raise the systemic PaO_2 in patients with severe congestive heart failure, overcoming the capillary-alveolar block of pulmonary edema and alleviating the hypoxemic contribution to congestive failure.

5. Salt restriction–Salt restriction must be approached with caution in infants and children. Treatment of the disease entity known as low-salt congestive heart failure is one of the more hazardous undertakings in medical management. Our feeling is that there is no place for salt-free formulas in the treatment of congestive failure in infants. Standard Similac 60/40 has about the same sodium content as human milk and about half the sodium content of cow's milk and other prepared formulas. Most cases of "low-salt failure" are largely the result of overly vigorous salt restriction (sometimes combined with the other major factor, overly vigorous diuretic therapy). Clearly, salty foods such as potato chips and bacon should be avoided, and no salt should be used beyond what is normally used in cooking. It is important that food be palatable enough to eat for a child, who may already be undernourished as a consequence of chronic, poorly compensated heart failure.

B. Emergency and Heroic Measures: The acute emergencies of congestive heart failure are usually related to fluid retention with pulmonary edema and low cardiac output. Some emergency therapeutic measures that may be lifesaving include the following:

1. Morphine–For acute pulmonary edema, give 0.1 mg/kg intravenously or subcutaneously.

2. Diuretics–Furosemide or ethacrynic acid may be given intravenously in an initial dosage of 1 mg/kg to produce a rapid diuresis.

3. Positive-pressure breathing–Pulmonary edema may sometimes be managed by intubation or mask with bag-breathing or a respirator to raise the alveolar pressure above pulmonary capillary pressure.

4. Peritoneal dialysis–Although furosemide has largely met the need for the extremely rapid relief of fluid retention, there are three specific instances in which peritoneal dialysis with a hypertonic solution may be indicated: (1) when fluid retention (especially pulmonary edema) is life-threatening and diuretics are unsuccessful; (2) in low-salt congestive heart failure when both the fluid retention and the electrolyte imbalance require correction; and (3) in the early postoperative care of an infant who may have transient renal failure with both fluid retention and hyperkalemia.

The advantages of hypertonic peritoneal dialysis are that the procedure promptly (within minutes) draws fluid into the peritoneal cavity, where it is subject to immediate removal, while simultaneously correcting the electrolyte imbalance, whether it is low-sodium, high-potassium, or both. For methods of dialysis, see Chapter 21. If the major problem is electrolyte imbalance, such as potassium retention, a hypertonic solution is not required and the usual "isotonic" dialyzing fluid is indicated.

5. Intravenous inotropic support–Use of agents such as dopamine (1–20 mg/kg/min), dobutamine (2–15 mg/kg/min), isoproterenol (0.1–1 mg/kg/min), and amrinone (0.75 mg/kg bolus, then 5–10 mg/kg/min) may help in stabilizing patients with severe myocardial dysfunction, hypotension, or low cardiac output. These agents can be lifesaving in myocarditis and cardiogenic shock.

6. Afterload reduction–A relatively new form of therapy for "pump" failure is to effect afterload reduction by decreasing systemic vascular resistance with an intravenous infusion of vasodilators. Experience in children is limited. The procedure has been used largely in postoperative patients with reduced cardiac output and peripheral vasoconstriction. Agents such as nitroprusside have been lifesaving but must be used in a setting where central venous pressure, arterial pressure, cardiac output, and so on, can be carefully monitored.

Latson L: Captopril in children with cardiomyopathies. Circulation 1991;83:707.

Padbury JF et al: Dopamine pharmacokinetics in newborn infants. J Pediatr 1990;117:472.

Wernovsky G, Chang AC, Wessel DL: Intensive care. In: *Moss and Adams Heart Disease in Infants, Children, and Adolescents,* 5th ed. Emmanouilides GC et al (editors). Williams & Wilkins, 1995.

CYANOSIS

One of the two major clues to the presence of heart disease in the infant and child is cyanosis. (The other is congestive heart failure; see previous section.)

Cyanosis represents an increased concentration (4–5 g/dL) of reduced hemoglobin in the blood. Bluish discoloration is usually, but not always, a sign. Patients with anemia and cyanosis may not appear blue; patients with polycythemia may appear cyanotic, even though inadequate blood oxygen content is not present. Visible cyanosis accompanies low cardiac output, hypothermia, and systemic venous congestion, even in the presence of adequate oxygenation.

In patients with true central cyanosis, the cause of cyanosis (cardiac, pulmonary, hematologic, or central nervous system disorder) must be determined. Most often, the physician is faced with differentiating between cardiac and pulmonary problems. Evaluation of arterial blood gases (see above) is one of the easiest ways to differentiate between lung and heart disease. Cyanosis in heart disease is also related to pulmonary blood flow. In some "cyanotic" congenital heart defects, the decrease in pulmonary blood flow is minimal and results in minimal cyanosis. Presence of pulmonary hypertension also influences pulmonary blood flow, and thus oxygen therapy may cause a partial increase in oxygen saturation; the increase is usually much less in patients with heart disease than in those with pulmonary disease.

Evaluation for methemoglobinemia may be necessary to rule out hematologic causes of cyanosis. If the cause of cyanosis is a disease of the central nervous system, the patient usually responds to oxygen therapy.

Cyanotic heart disease is usually a medical emergency, most often requiring palliative or corrective surgery.

CONGENITAL HEART DISEASE

Congenital heart disease is present in about 1% of studied North American and British populations, making this the most common category of congenital structural malformation. Curative or palliative surgical correction is now available for over 90% of patients with congenital heart disease.

The customary division of congenital heart diseases into noncyanotic and cyanotic types is useful if one understands the basis for it. By convention, patients with right-to-left shunts fall into the cyanotic category whether they have readily recognizable cyanosis or not; patients who do not have right-to-left shunts—even if they are cyanotic for other reasons, such as low cardiac output—are placed in the noncyanotic category.

Etiologic Considerations

Only 8% of all congenital heart defects are known to be associated with single mutant gene or chromosome abnormalities, and the remainder are the result of various other causes. Multiple environmental factors, including diabetes, alcohol consumption, progesterone use, certain viruses, and other teratogens, are now associated with an increased incidence of malformations. These factors probably represent environmental triggers in persons susceptible or predisposed to congenital heart defects. The effect of rubella virus is probably independent of hereditary factors and consequently predisposes the patient to patent ductus arteriosus and pulmonary artery branch stenosis. Acquired heart diseases, such as rheumatic fever, appear to have much stronger environmental influence. Atherosclerosis clearly can have distinct familial patterns but in some circumstances can be influenced by diet, drugs, or lifestyle.

In dealing with families of children with congenital heart disease, the physician must often answer the question of risk to future pregnancies. Table 18–2

Table 18–2. Observed and expected recurrence risks in siblings of 1478 probands with congenital heart lesion.[1]

Anomaly	Probands	Affected Siblings		
		No.	Percent	Exp. ($\sqrt{p}$)
Ventricular septal defect	212	24/543	4.4	5.0
Patent ductus arteriosus	204	17/505	3.4	3.5
Tetralogy of Fallot	157	9/338	2.7	3.2
Atrial septal defect	152	11/342	3.2	3.2
Pulmonary stenosis	146	10/345	2.9	2.9
Aortic stenosis	135	7/317	2.2	2.1
Coarctation of aorta	128	5/272	1.8	2.4
Transpositions of great vessels	103	4/209	1.9	2.2
Atrioventricular canal	73	4/151	2.6	2.0
Tricuspid atresia	51	1/96	1.1	1.4
Ebstein's anomaly	42	1/96	1.1	0.7
Truncus arteriosus	41	1/86	1.2	0.7
Pulmonary atresia	34	1/77	1.3	1.0
Total	1478	95/3377		

[1]Reproduced, with permission, from Nora JJ: Etiologic factors in congenital heart disease. Pediatr Clin North Am 1971;18:1059.

outlines the risk for certain lesions in patients with one affected first-degree relative. Studies indicate that the incidence in children of affected mothers may be as high as 10–15%. With more than one affected first-degree relative, recurrence is also much higher, and some families may have a hereditary predisposition to congenital heart disease.

Ferencz C, Villasenor AC: Epidemiology of cardiovascular malformations: The state of the art. Cardiol Young 1991; 1:264.

Nora JJ, Nora AH: Maternal transmission of congenital heart disease: New recurrence risk figures and the questions of cytoplasmic inheritance and vulnerability to teratogens. Am J Cardiol 1987;59:459.

NONCYANOTIC CONGENITAL HEART DISEASE

ATRIAL SEPTAL DEFECT OF THE OSTIUM SECUNDUM VARIETY

Essentials of Diagnosis & Typical Features

- Right ventricular heave.
- S_2 widely split and usually fixed.
- Grade I–III/VI ejection systolic murmur at the pulmonary area.
- Widely radiating systolic murmur mimicking peripheral pulmonary artery stenosis (common in infancy).

- Diastolic flow murmur at the lower left sternal border (if the shunt is significant in size).
- ECG with rsR′ in lead V_1.

General Considerations

An atrial septal defect is an opening in the atrial septum permitting the shunting of blood between the two atria. There are three major types: (1) The ostium secundum type (discussed here) is the most common and is in an intermediate position. (2) The sinus venosus type is positioned high in the atrial septum, is the least common, and is frequently associated with partial anomalous venous return. (3) The ostium primum type is low in position and is a form of atrioventricular septal defect; it is discussed in that section.

Atrial septal defect of the ostium secundum variety occurs in approximately 10% of patients with congenital heart disease and is twice as common in females as in males. Diagnosis in infancy is becoming more common.

Pulmonary hypertension and growth failure are increasingly recognized in infancy and childhood. After the third decade, an increased pulmonary vascular resistance develops, the left-to-right shunting decreases, and right-to-left shunting begins.

Clinical Findings

A. Symptoms and Signs: Infants may present with congestive heart failure often unresponsive to medical management, necessitating early total corrective surgery. However, children with atrial septal defects often have no cardiovascular symptoms. Some patients remain asymptomatic throughout life; others develop easy fatigability as older children or adults. Cyanosis does not occur until pulmonary hypertension develops. This may never occur; if it does, it is usually not seen until after the third decade of life. Congestive heart failure is uncommon in infants and young children.

The arterial pulses are normal and equal throughout. In the usual case, the heart is hyperactive, with a heaving impulse felt best at the lower left sternal border and over the xiphoid process. There are usually no thrills. S_2 at the pulmonary area is widely split and sometimes fixed. The pulmonary component is normal in intensity. A grade I–III/VI ejection-type systolic murmur is heard best at the left sternal border in the second intercostal space. An additional murmur of relative peripheral pulmonary artery stenosis may be heard, more commonly in infants. A mid-diastolic murmur can often be heard in the fourth intercostal space at the left sternal border. This murmur is caused by increased blood flow across the tricuspid valve during diastole (tricuspid flow murmur). The presence of this murmur suggests a high flow (pulmonary to systemic blood flow ratio greater than 2:1).

B. Imaging: Chest x-ray films usually demonstrate cardiac enlargement. The main pulmonary artery may be dilated. The pulmonary vascular markings are increased as a result of increased pulmonary blood flow. However, occasionally the chest x-ray is unimpressive despite a significant L–R shunt.

C. Electrocardiography and Vectorcardiography: The usual ECG shows right axis deviation with a clockwise loop in the frontal plane. In the right precordial leads, there is usually an rsR′ pattern.

D. Echocardiography: M-mode echocardiography shows (1) paradoxic motion of the ventricular septal wall (moving in the same direction rather than the direction opposite that of the free left ventricular wall) and (2) dilated right ventricular cavity with increased tricuspid valve excursion. Direct visualization of the atrial septal defect by two-dimensional echocardiography, plus demonstration of a left-to-right shunt through the defect by color flow Doppler, confirms the diagnosis and has largely eliminated the need for cardiac catheterization.

E. Cardiac Catheterization: Oximetry reveals evidence of a significant increase in oxygen saturation at the atrial level. The pulmonary artery pressure is usually normal. The right ventricular pressure is occasionally greater than the pulmonary artery pressure, the increased right-sided "flow." Pulmonary vascular resistance is usually normal. The ratio of pulmonary to systemic blood flow may vary from 1.5:1 to 4:1. A catheter can easily be passed across the atrial septum into the left atrium.

Treatment

Surgical closure is generally recommended for ostium secundum-type atrial septal defects in which the ratio of pulmonary to systemic blood flow is greater than 2:1. Operation is usually performed electively in patients between ages 2 and 4 years. The death rate for surgical closure is less than 1%. When surgical intervention is early, late complications of right ventricular dysfunction and significant dysrhythmias may be avoided or diminished. Early surgery is also indicated in infants presenting with congestive heart failure or significant pulmonary hypertension. Devices to close selected atrial septal defects by interventional cardiac catheterization are in clinical trials.

Course & Prognosis

Patients with atrial septal defects usually tolerate them very well in the first 2 decades of life, and an occasional patient may live a completely normal life without symptoms. Frequently, however, pulmonary hypertension and reversal of the shunt develop by the third or fourth decade. Heart failure may also occur at this time. Subacute infective endocarditis is a very rare complication. Spontaneous closure occurs and is sometimes associated with an aneurysm of the atrial septum. Exercise tolerance and oxygen consumption

in surgically corrected children are generally normal, and physical limitations are unnecessary.

Ettedgui J et al: Diagnostic echocardiographic features of the sinus venosus defect. Br Heart J 1990;64:329.

Fukazawa M, Fukushige J, Ueda K: Atrial septal defects in neonates with reference to spontaneous closure. Am Heart J 1988;116:123.

Mahoney LT et al: Atrial septal defects that present in infancy. Am J Dis Child 1986;140:1115.

Pollick C et al: Doppler color flow imaging assessment of shunt size in atrial septal defect. Circulation 1987;78:522.

Reybrouck T et al: Cardiorespiratory exercise capacity after surgical closure of atrial septal defect is influenced by the age at surgery. Am Heart J 1991;122:1073.

Rome JJ et al: Double umbrella closure of atrial defects. Circulation 1990;82:751.

VENTRICULAR SEPTAL DEFECTS

Essentials of Diagnosis & Typical Features

Small- to moderate-sized left-to-right shunt without pulmonary hypertension:
- Acyanotic, relatively asymptomatic.
- Grade II–IV/VI pansystolic murmur, maximal along the lower left sternal border.
- P_2 not accentuated.

Large left-to-right shunt:
- Acyanotic.
- Easy fatigability.
- Congestive heart failure in infancy (often).
- Hyperactive heart; biventricular enlargement.
- Grade II–V/VI pansystolic murmur, maximal at the lower left sternal border.
- P_2 usually accentuated.
- Diastolic flow murmur at the apex.

Insignificant left-to-right shunt or bidirectional shunt with pulmonary hypertension:
- Quiet precordium with right ventricular lift.
- Palpable P_2.
- Short ejection systolic murmur along the left sternal border; single accentuated S_2.
- Systemic arterial oxygen desaturation may be present; pulmonary arterial pressure and systemic arterial pressures are equal; little or no oxygen saturation increase at the right ventricular level by catheterization.

General Considerations

Simple ventricular septal defect (without other lesions) is the single most common congenital heart malformation, accounting for about 25% of all cases of congenital heart disease. Defects in the ventricular septum can occur both in the membranous portion of the septum (most common) and in the muscular portion.

There are five different courses that patients with ventricular septal defect may follow:

A. Spontaneous Closure: Thirty to 50 percent of all ventricular septal defects close spontaneously. The small defects close in 60–70% of cases. Larger defects may occasionally also close spontaneously, and there are many documented examples of spontaneous closure of ventricular septal defects in the second and third decades of life. Half of the defects that do not close become functionally or anatomically smaller.

B. Shunts Too Small to Justify Repair: Asymptomatic patients with hearts normal in size (as seen on x-ray film) and without pulmonary hypertension are generally not subjected to surgical repair. In those who have had cardiac catheterization, the ratio of pulmonary to systemic blood flow is usually found to be less than 2:1, and serial cardiac catheterizations demonstrate that the shunts get progressively smaller.

C. Disease Severe Enough to Require Surgery: The time of surgery depends on the nature of the disease. Patients may require surgery in infancy because of intractable congestive heart failure; surgery before 2 years of age because of progression of pulmonary hypertension; or surgery between 2 and 5 years of age to prevent chronic left ventricular volume overload and progressive pulmonary hypertension.

D. Defect Inoperable Because of Pulmonary Hypertension: The vast majority of patients with inoperable pulmonary hypertension develop this condition progressively. The combined data of the multicenter National History Study indicate that most cases of irreversible pulmonary hypertension can be prevented by surgical repair of a large defect before 2 years of age.

E. Development of Infundibular Pulmonary Stenosis: Approximately 5% of infants with large left-to-right shunts will develop progressive infundibular obstruction effecting an outflow gradient and diminution of the shunt. A small proportion of these infants have precyanotic tetralogy of Fallot, as evidenced by coexistent right aortic arch or abnormal spatial orientation of the infundibulum.

Clinical Findings

A. Symptoms and Signs: Patients with small or moderate left-to-right shunts usually have no cardiovascular symptoms. There may be a history of frequent respiratory infections in infancy and early childhood. Patients with large left-to-right shunts frequently are sick early in infancy. Such patients have frequent respiratory infections, including bouts of pneumonitis. They grow slowly, with very poor weight gain. Dyspnea, exercise intolerance, and fatigue are quite common. Congestive heart failure may develop between 1 and 6 months of age. Patients who survive the first year usually improve, although easy fatigability may persist. With severe pulmonary hypertension (Eisenmenger's syndrome), cyanosis is present.

1. Small left-to-right shunt–There are usually no lifts, heaves, thrills, or shocks. The first sound at the apex is normal, and the second sound at the pulmonary area is split physiologically. The pulmonary component is normal. A grade II–IV/VI, medium- to high-pitched, blowing pansystolic murmur is heard best at the left sternal border in the third and fourth intercostal spaces. There is slight radiation over the entire precordium. No diastolic murmurs are heard.

2. Moderate left-to-right shunt–Slight prominence of the precordium is common. There is a moderate left ventricular thrust. A systolic thrill may be palpable at the lower left sternal border between the third and fourth intercostal spaces. The second sound at the pulmonary area is most often split but may be single. A grade IV/VI, harsh pansystolic murmur is heard best at the lower left sternal border in the fourth intercostal space. A diastolic flow murmur is heard and indicates that the pulmonary venous return across the mitral valve is large and that the pulmonary to systemic blood flow ratio is at least 2:1.

3. Very large ventricular septal defects with pulmonary hypertension–The precordium is prominent, and the sternum bulges. A left ventricular thrust and a right ventricular heave are palpable. A shock of the second sound can be felt at the pulmonary area. A thrill may or may not be present at the lower left sternal border. A second heart sound is usually single or narrowly split, with accentuation of the pulmonary component. The murmur ranges from grade II to grade V/VI and is usually harsh and pansystolic. Occasionally, when the defect is large, very little murmur can be heard. A diastolic flow murmur may or may not be heard, depending on the size of the shunt.

B. Imaging: X-ray findings of the chest vary, depending on the size of the shunt. In patients with small shunts, x-ray findings may be normal. The heart is normal in size, and the pulmonary vascular markings may be just beyond the upper limits of normal. Patients with large shunts usually show significant cardiac enlargement involving both the left and right ventricles and the left atrium. The aorta is usually small to normal in size, and the main pulmonary artery segment is dilated. The pulmonary vascular markings are significantly increased in patients with large shunts.

C. Electrocardiography: There is some correlation between the electrocardiographic and hemodynamic findings. The ECG is normal in patients with small left-to-right shunts and normal pulmonary arterial pressures. Left ventricular hypertrophy is usually found in patients with large left-to-right shunts and normal pulmonary vascular resistance (moderate-sized defects). Combined ventricular hypertrophy (both right and left) is found in patients with pulmonary hypertension caused by increased flow, increased resistance, or both. Pure right ventricular hypertrophy is found in patients with pulmonary hypertension secondary to pulmonary vascular obstruction (Eisenmenger's syndrome).

D. Echocardiography: Two-dimensional echocardiography provides visualization of defects that are 2 mm or larger in about 75% of cases and often can be used to pinpoint the anatomic location. Addition of color flow Doppler, however, allows detection of virtually all defects, including the smaller defects. Multiple defects can be detected by combining two-dimensional and color flow imaging. Conventional Doppler can aid in evaluation of ventricular septal defects by estimating the pressure difference (if any) between the left and right ventricles. A pressure difference greater than 25 mm Hg usually indicates a moderate-sized defect and absence of severe pulmonary hypertension.

E. Cardiac Catheterization and Angiocardiography: Oxygen saturation is increased at the right ventricular level. The pulmonary artery pressure may vary from normal to equal that in the systemic arteries. Left atrial pressure (pulmonary capillary pressure) may be normal to increased. Pulmonary vascular resistance varies from normal to markedly increased. The ratio of pulmonary to systemic blood flow may vary from 1.1:1 to 4:1. Angiocardiographic examination defines the number, size, and location of the defects.

Treatment

A. Medical Management: Patients who develop congestive heart failure should be treated vigorously with anticongestive measures (see Congestive Heart Failure, above). If the patient does not respond to vigorous anticongestive measures or shows signs of progressive pulmonary hypertension, surgery is indicated without delay. Transcatheter closure of selected ventricular septal defects is being evaluated as an experimental procedure.

B. Surgical Treatment: Historically, a pulmonary artery band was placed to protect the pulmonary vascular bed and decrease heart failure when there was a large ventricular defect. Today, a pulmonary artery band is used only when there are multiple defects or other anomalies. Primary closure of the defect with a prosthetic patch is now used for virtually all symptomatic singular defects. The age for elective surgery is becoming progressively younger in most centers, with most defects usually closed in infancy.. Patients with cardiomegaly, poor growth, poor exercise tolerance, or other clinical abnormalities who have cardiac catheterization findings of significant shunt ($\geq$ 2:1) without significant pulmonary hypertension (> 10 units of resistance) are candidates for surgery. In general, patients with mean pulmonary artery pressures equal to systemic pressure who are unresponsive to oxygen administration, with little or no left-to-right shunt or bidirectional shunt-

ing, and pulmonary resistance calculated to be greater than 10 resistance units (or pulmonary/systemic resistance ratios > 0.7) are considered inoperable. There are patients who have pulmonary hypertension of lesser degree who remain operable, but there is a progressively greater operative risk when there is increasing pulmonary hypertension (from 1% risk for patients without pulmonary hypertension to 25% for those at the upper limits of operability).

To prevent pulmonary hypertension from reaching inoperable levels, early surgical intervention is recommended for patients who have increased pulmonary vascular resistance. In centers with the capability of doing total correction on infants with or without deep hypothermia, complete repair before 2 years of age is recommended. The presence of multiple muscular defects in a tiny symptomatic infant is still considered to be an indication for pulmonary artery banding as an initial palliative procedure. Transcatheter closure of selected defects is in clinical trials.

Course & Prognosis

Significant late dysrhythmias are uncommon. Functional exercise capacity and oxygen consumption are usually normal, and physical restrictions are unnecessary. Adults with corrected defects have a normal quality of life. Definite congenital heart disease occurred in approximately 3% of probands of male and female patients with ventricular septal defect.

Driscoll DJ et al: Occurrence risk for congenital heart disease in relatives of patients with aortic stenosis, pulmonary stenosis, or ventricular septal defect. Circulation 1993;87(Suppl):I-121.

Hornberger LK et al: Elucidation of the natural history of ventricular septal defects by serial Doppler color flow mapping studies. J Am Coll Cardiol 1989;13:1111.

Lock JE et al: Transcatheter closure of ventricular septal defects. Circulation 1988;78:361.

Mehta AV et al: Ventricular septal defect in the first year of life. Am J Cardiol 1992;70:364.

Soto B, Ceballos R, Kirklen JW: Ventricular septal defects: A surgical viewpoint. J Am Coll Cardiol 1989;14:1291.

ATRIOVENTRICULAR SEPTAL DEFECT

Essentials of Diagnosis & Typical Features

- Murmur often inaudible in neonates.
- Loud pulmonary component of S_2.
- Common in infants with Down's syndrome.
- ECG with left axis deviation.

General Considerations

An atrioventricular septal defect is a congenital cardiac abnormality that results from incomplete fusion of the embryonic endocardial cushions. The endocardial cushions help to form the lower portion of the atrial septum, the membranous portion of the ventricular septum, and the septal leaflets of the tricuspid and mitral valves. These defects are not very common. They account for about 4% of all cases of congenital heart disease. The incidence of this abnormality is 20% in patients with Down syndrome.

Atrioventricular septal defects may be divided into incomplete and complete forms. The complete form, also known as persistent common atrioventricular canal, consists of a posterior ventricular septal defect, a low atrial septal defect of the ostium primum variety that is continuous with the ventricular septal defect, and a cleft in both the septal leaflet of the tricuspid valve and the anterior leaflet of the mitral valve. In the incomplete form, any one of these components may be present. The most common partial form of atrioventricular septal defect is the ostium primum type of atrial septal defect with a cleft in the mitral valve.

The complete form (persistent common atrioventricular canal) results in large left-to-right shunts at both the ventricular and atrial levels, tricuspid and mitral regurgitation, and marked pulmonary hypertension, usually with some increase in pulmonary vascular resistance. When the latter is present, the shunts may be bidirectional. The hemodynamics in the incomplete form are dependent on the lesions present.

Clinical Findings

A. Symptoms and Signs: The clinical picture varies depending on the severity of the defect. In the incomplete form, these patients may be indistinguishable from patients with the ostium secundum type of atrial septal defect. They are often asymptomatic. On the other hand, patients with atrioventricular canal usually are severely affected. Congestive heart failure often develops in infancy, and recurrent bouts of pneumonitis are common.

In the complete form, the murmur may be inaudible in the neonate. After 4–6 weeks, a nonspecific systolic murmur develops; the murmur is usually not as harsh as that of an isolated ventricular septal defect. The heart is significantly enlarged (both the right and left sides), and a systolic thrill may be palpated at the lower left sternal border. The second heart sound is split, with an accentuated pulmonary component. A pronounced diastolic flow murmur may be heard at the apex and the lower left sternal border.

When severe pulmonary vascular obstruction is present, there is evidence of dominant right ventricular enlargement. A shock of the second sound can be palpated at the pulmonary area. No thrill is felt. The second sound is markedly accentuated and single. A nonspecific short systolic murmur is heard at the lower left sternal border. No diastolic flow murmurs are heard. Cyanosis is detectable in severe cases with predominant right-to-left shunts.

The physical findings in the incomplete form depend on the lesions. In the most common variety (ostium primum atrial septal defect with mitral regurgitation), the findings are similar to those of the ostium secundum type of atrial septal defect with or without findings of mitral regurgitation.

B. Imaging: As indicated on x-ray film, cardiac enlargement is present depending on the degree of specific anatomic defect and the severity. In the complete (canal) form, there is enlargement of all four chambers. The pulmonary vascular markings are increased. In patients with pulmonary vascular obstruction, only the main pulmonary artery segment and its branches are prominent. The peripheral markings are usually decreased.

C. Electrocardiography: In all forms of atrioventricular septal defect, left axis deviation with a counterclockwise loop in the frontal plane is present. The mean axis varies from approximately −30 to −90 degrees. Since left axis deviation is present in all patients with this defect, the ECG is a very important diagnostic tool. Only 5% of isolated ventricular septal defects have this electrocardiographic abnormality. First-degree heart block is present in over 50% of cases. Right, left, or combined ventricular hypertrophy is present depending on the particular type of defect and the presence or absence of pulmonary vascular obstruction.

D. Echocardiography: Echocardiography is the diagnostic technique of choice. On M-mode echocardiography, excursion of the atrioventricular valve through the plane of the interventricular septal defect is characteristic. The anatomy can be directly visualized by two-dimensional echocardiography; the sensitivity of this method is equal to or superior to that of selective cineangiography. Color flow mapping can indicate the location of septal defects and valve regurgitation and the direction of the shunt.

E. Cardiac Catheterization and Angiocardiography: The results of cardiac catheterization vary depending on the type of defect present. When catheterization is performed from the leg, the catheter is easily passed across the atrial septum in its lowest portion and frequently enters the left ventricle directly. This catheter course is a result of the very low atrial septal defect and the cleft in the mitral valve. Increased oxygen saturation in the right ventricle or the right atrium identifies the level of the shunt. Angiocardiography reveals a characteristic "gooseneck" deformity in the complete canal form.

Treatment

Treatment consists of anticongestive measures and eventual surgical correction. In the incomplete form, surgery is associated with a relatively low death rate (2–5%). The complete form is associated with a significantly higher death rate (about 15%), but complete correction in the first year of life, prior to the onset of irreversible pulmonary hypertension, is advisable.

Pulmonary artery banding procedures are rarely used for atrial septal defects. They are less effective in patients with predominantly ventricular level shunts than in patients with simple ventricular septal defect. At corrective surgery, transesophageal echo is useful in assessing the adequacy of repair.

Haworth SG: Pulmonary vascular bed in children with complete atrioventricular septal defect: Relation between structure and hemodynamic abnormalities. Am J Cardiol 1986;57:833.

Marino B et al: Atrioventricular canal in Down syndrome. Am J Dis Child 1990;144:1120.

Moscoso G: Developmental morphology of atrioventricular cushions and atrioventricular septal structures: A clue to understanding atrioventricular septal defects. J Perinatal Med 1991;19:215.

PATENT DUCTUS ARTERIOSUS

Essentials of Diagnosis & Typical Features

- Variable murmur, with active precordium and full pulses, in newborn premature infants.
- Continuous murmur and full pulses in older infants.

General Considerations

Patent ductus arteriosus is the persistence in extrauterine life of the normal fetal vessel that joins the pulmonary artery to the aorta. It closes spontaneously in normal term infants by 4 days of age. It is a common abnormality, accounting for about 12% of all cases of congenital heart disease. It is very common in children born to mothers who had rubella during the first trimester of pregnancy. There is a higher incidence of patent ductus arteriosus in infants born at high altitudes (over 10,000 ft). It is twice as common in females as in males. In preterm infants weighing less than 1500 g, the frequency of patent ductus arteriosus may be as high as 20–60%.

The defect occurs as an isolated abnormality, but associated lesions are not infrequent. Coarctation of the aorta, patent ductus arteriosus, and ventricular septal defect are commonly associated. Even more important to recognize are those patients with murmurs of patent ductus but without readily apparent findings of other associated lesions who are being kept alive by the patent ductus (eg, a patient with patent ductus with unsuspected pulmonary atresia).

Clinical Findings

A. Symptoms and Signs: The clinical findings and the clinical course depend on the size of the shunt and the degree of pulmonary hypertension.

1. Typical patent ductus arteriosus–The pulses are bounding, and pulse pressure is widened (pulse pressure is greater than half of the systolic pressure). The first heart sound is normal. The sec-ond heart sound is usually narrowly split and very rarely (when the shunt is maximal) paradoxically split (ie, the second sound closes on inspiration and splits on expiration). The paradoxic splitting is caused by the maximal overload of the left ventricle and the prolonged ejection of blood from this chamber.

The murmur is quite characteristic. It is a very rough "machinery" murmur that is maximal at the second intercostal space at the left sternal border and inferior to the left clavicle. It begins shortly after the first heart sound, rises to a peak at the second heart sound, and passes through the second heart sound into diastole, where it becomes a decrescendo murmur and fades or disappears before the first heart sound. The murmur tends to radiate fairly well over the lung fields anteriorly but relatively poorly over the lung fields posteriorly. A diastolic flow murmur is often heard at the apex. Depending on the pulmonary artery pressure, the murmur may be only systolic in time. This characteristic should be fully appreciated when trying to reach a diagnosis of patent ductus arteriosus in infants.

2. Patent ductus arteriosus with pulmonary hypertension–The physical findings depend on the cause of the pulmonary hypertension. If pulmonary hypertension is primarily the result of a marked increase in blood flow and only a slight increase in pulmonary vascular resistance, the physical findings are similar to those listed above. The significant difference is the presence of an accentuated pulmonary component of S_2. Bounding pulses and a loud continuous heart murmur are present. In patients with pulmonary vascular resistance and predominant right-to-left shunt, the findings are quite different. There may be evidence of cyanosis. The second heart sound is single and quite accentuated, and there is no significant heart murmur. The pulses are normal rather than bounding.

3. Patent ductus arteriosus in the premature neonate with associated respiratory distress syndrome–A preterm neonate during or after the clinical course of respiratory distress syndrome may have a significant associated patent ductus arteriosus that may be difficult to detect clinically but is often threatening in magnitude. A soft, nonspecific systolic murmur or no murmur is more common than the classic continuous murmur. The peripheral pulse and precordium are often bounding but typically are not characteristic for several days after the onset of a large left-to-right shunt. An early sign indicating the presence of a significant left-to-right shunt with concomitant congestive heart failure is increasing dependence on oxygen and respiratory support. In addition, increasing radiographic cardiomegaly and pulmonary edema plus increasing echocardiographic evidence of a left-to-right shunt differentiate this clinical and laboratory picture from bronchopulmonary dysplasia.

B. Imaging: In simple patent ductus arteriosus,

the x-ray appearance depends on the size of the shunt. If the shunt is relatively small or moderate in size, the heart is not enlarged. If the shunt is large, there is evidence of both left atrial and left ventricular enlargement. In both cases, the aorta is prominent, as is the main pulmonary artery segment.

C. Electrocardiography: The ECG may be normal or may show left ventricular hypertrophy, depending on the size of the shunt. In patients with pulmonary hypertension caused by increased blood flow, there is usually biventricular hypertrophy. In those with pulmonary vascular obstruction, there is pure right ventricular hypertrophy. An anterior ST depression (V_1) of 2 mm suggests subendocardial ischemia as a result of a diastolic "steal" from the coronary arteries via the ductus; this finding indicates the need for closure.

D. Echocardiography: Enlargement of the left atrium as measured by M-mode echocardiography was historically an important clue to the presence of congestive heart failure and is especially useful in diagnosing patent ductus arteriosus in the preterm infant. A left atrial to ascending aorta ratio of greater than 1.2 or 1.3 is considered evidence of a sizable left-to-right ductal shunt. The use of color flow, pulsed doppler ultrasonography, and two-dimensional echocardiography can provide direct visualization of the ductus and confirmation of the direction and degree of shunting and usually eliminates the need for a diagnostic cardiac catheterization. Preterm infants with a suspected patent ductus arteriosus should have a complete echocardiographic evaluation to make a definitive diagnosis, assess the magnitude of the left-to-right shunt, and rule out associated, particularly ductus-dependent lesions.

E. Cardiac Catheterization and Angiocardiography: Cardiac catheterization is rarely indicated in the premature infant with symptomatic ductus. Older children with a patent ductus arteriosus diagnosed by echocardiography need only catheterization if there are plans to close the ductus during catheterization.

Treatment

Treatment consists of surgical correction when the ductus arteriosus is large, except in patients with pulmonary vascular obstruction. Patients with large left-to-right shunts and pulmonary hypertension should be operated on very early (even under the age of 1 year) to prevent the development of progressive pulmonary vascular obstruction. Simple patent ductus arteriosus should be corrected after the child reaches age 1, although the operation may be delayed until later without increasing the risk of death. Transcatheter closure with an occluder device is being evaluated as an experimental technique. Transcatheter closure of small defects with a coil is becoming standard therapy.

Patients with nonreactive pulmonary vascular ob-

struction who have resistance greater than 10 units and a pulmonary/systemic resistance ratio greater than 0.7 despite vasodilator therapy (eg, nitric oxide) should not be operated on. These patients are made worse by closure of the ductus, because the ductus serves as an escape route and limits the degree of pulmonary hypertension.

The preterm infant with symptomatic ductus presents a special and controversial problem. At some institutions, it is customary to operate on virtually all preterm infants weighing under 1200 g. At other institutions, surgery is rarely done, and most infants receive a maximum of three doses of either oral indomethacin (0.1–0.3 mg/kg every 8–24 hours) or parenteral indomethacin (0.1–0.3 mg/kg every 12 hours) if adequate renal, hematologic, and hepatic function is demonstrated. Contraindications to indomethacin treatment include hyperbilirubinemia of 12 mg/dL or greater, renal failure, shock, necrotizing enterocolitis, intracranial hemorrhage, hemorrhagic disease, and evidence of a spontaneously closing ductus. Efficacy and safety of indomethacin use are enhanced by the careful monitoring of serum levels of indomethacin. A serum level of less than 250 ng/mL is associated with treatment failure. Conventional conservative management includes fluid restriction with or without diuretics and ligation only if these fail. Factors to be considered in making a rational decision on the modality of therapy include a high rate of spontaneous ductus closure without therapy and an extremely low surgical risk in experienced centers; the inability of a laboratory to monitor serum levels of indomethacin may influence the decision.

Course & Prognosis

Patients with simple patent ductus arteriosus and small to moderate shunts usually do quite well even without surgery. However, in the third or fourth decade of life, symptoms of easy fatigability, dyspnea on exertion, and exercise intolerance appear, usually as a consequence of the development of pulmonary hypertension or congestive heart failure.

Spontaneous closure of a patent ductus arteriosus may occur within the first 2 years of life or beyond. This is especially true in infants who were born preterm. After age 2, spontaneous closure is less common. Because subacute infective endocarditis is a potential complication, surgical ligation is recommended if the defect persists beyond age 2 years.

Patients with large shunts or pulmonary hypertension do not do as well. Poor growth and development, frequent episodes of pneumonitis, and the development of congestive heart failure are not uncommon in patients with large left-to-right shunts. If these patients do not succumb to congestive heart failure in early infancy, they frequently go on to develop pulmonary vascular obstruction in later childhood or adolescence. Life expectancy is markedly reduced, and these patients often die in their second or third decade. Those rare patients with pulmonary vascular obstruction from very early infancy are actually less symptomatic than those with pulmonary hypertension without obstruction.

Cambier PA et al: Percutaneous closure of the small patent ductus arteriosus using coil embolization. Am J Cardiol 1992;69:815.

Goldberg SJ: Response of the patent ductus arteriosus to indomethacin treatment. Am J Dis Child 1987;141:250.

Rashkind WJ et al: Nonsurgical closure of patent ductus arteriosus. Circulation 1987;75:583.

Reller MD et al: Duration of ductal shunting in healthy preterm infants: An echocardiographic color flow Doppler study. J Pediatr 1988;112:441.

Reller MD et al: The timing of spontaneous closure of the ductus arteriosus in infants with respiratory distress syndrome. Am J Cardiol 1990;66:75.

Valdez-Cruz M et al: Real-time Doppler color flow mapping for detection of patent ductus arteriosus. J Am Coll Cardiol 1986;8:1105.

MALFORMATIONS ASSOCIATED WITH OBSTRUCTION TO BLOOD FLOW ON THE RIGHT SIDE OF THE HEART

1. VALVULAR PULMONARY STENOSIS WITH INTACT VENTRICULAR SEPTUM

Essentials of Diagnosis & Typical Features

- No symptoms with mild and moderately severe cases.
- Cyanosis and a high incidence of right-sided congestive heart failure in very severe cases in infancy.
- Right ventricular lift; systolic ejection click at the pulmonary area in mild to moderately severe cases.
- S_2 widely split with soft to inaudible P_2; grade I–VI/VI obstructive systolic murmur, maximal at the pulmonary area.
- Dilated pulmonary artery on posteroanterior chest x-ray film.

General Considerations

Obstruction of right ventricular outflow at the pulmonary valve level accounts for about 10% of all cases of congenital heart disease. In the usual case, the cusps of the pulmonary valve are fused to form a membrane or diaphragm with a hole in the middle that varies from 2 mm to 1 cm in diameter. Occasionally, there may be a fusion of only two cusps, producing a bicuspid pulmonary valve. Very frequently, especially in the more severe cases, there is secondary infundibular stenosis. The pulmonary valve ring is usually small. There is usually moderate to marked poststenotic dilatation of both the main and left pulmonary arteries. Patent foramen ovale is fairly common.

Obstruction to blood flow across the pulmonary valve results in an increase in pressure developed by the right ventricle to maintain an adequate output across that valve. Pressures greater than systemic are potentially life-threatening and are associated with "critical" obstruction. As a consequence of the increased work required of the right ventricle, severe right ventricular hypertrophy and eventual right ventricular failure can occur. In contrast to patients with right ventricular outflow obstruction, patients with this obstruction who also have a large ventricular septal defect (ie, tetralogy of Fallot) are not at great risk for heart failure; because of the septal defect, there is communication between the ventricles, which limits the amount of pressure developed in the right ventricle (pressure is equal to systemic pressure) and thereby makes heart failure extremely uncommon.

When the obstruction is severe and the ventricular septum is intact, a right-to-left shunt will often occur at the atrial level through a patent foramen ovale. Accordingly, patients with this condition may have a varying degree of cyanosis. The presence of cyanosis indicates a relatively severe degree of valvular obstruction.

Clinical Findings

A. Symptoms and Signs: The history depends on the severity of the obstruction. Patients with a mild or even a moderate degree of valvular pulmonary stenosis are completely asymptomatic throughout infancy, childhood, and adolescence. Patients with a more severe type of valvular obstruction may develop cyanosis and congestive heart failure very early—even in the neonatal period. Hypoxemic spells characterized by a sudden onset of marked cyanosis and dyspnea are much less common than in tetralogy of Fallot.

Patients with mild to moderate obstruction are acyanotic. Patients with severe or critical stenosis usually show evidence of central cyanosis. These patients are usually well developed and well nourished. They often have a round face and widely spaced eyes. The pulses are normal and equal throughout. Clubbing may occur in severe cases in which cyanosis has persisted for a long time. On examination of the heart, there may be prominence of the precordium. A heaving impulse of the right ventricle can frequently be palpated. A systolic thrill is often palpated in the pulmonary area and occasionally in the suprasternal notch. The first heart sound is normal. In patients with mild to moderate stenosis, a prominent ejection click of pulmonary origin is heard best at the second left intercostal space. This click varies with respiration. It is much more prominent during expiration than inspiration. In patients with severe stenosis, the click tends to merge with the first heart sound. The second heart sound also varies with the degree of stenosis. In mild valvular stenosis, the second heart sound is normally split and the pulmonary component is normal in intensity. In moderate degrees of obstruction, the second heart sound is more widely split and the pulmonary component is softer. In severe pulmonary stenosis, the second heart sound is single, since the pulmonary component cannot be heard. An ejection-type, rough, obstructive systolic murmur is best heard at the second interspace at the left sternal border. It radiates very well to the back. With severe obstruction of the valve, the murmur is usually short and peaks in late systole. No diastolic murmurs are audible. In older children, a prominent *a* wave is seen in the jugular venous pulse. If there is congestive heart failure, the liver is enlarged.

B. Imaging: In the mild form of pulmonary stenosis, the heart may be normal in size. Poststenotic dilatation of the main pulmonary artery segment and the left pulmonary artery is often present. In moderate to severe cases, there may be a slight right ventricular enlargement, and there may or may not be poststenotic dilatation of the main pulmonary artery. In patients who are cyanotic, the pulmonary vascular markings are decreased; otherwise, they are normal.

C. Electrocardiography: Electrocardiographic findings are usually normal in patients with mild obstruction. Right ventricular hypertrophy is present in patients with moderate to severe valvular obstruction. In severe obstruction, right ventricular hypertrophy and the right ventricular strain pattern (deep inversion of the T wave) are seen in the right precordial leads. In the most severe form, right atrial hypertrophy is also present. Right axis deviation is also seen in the moderate to severe forms. Occasionally, the axis is greater than +180 degrees.

D. Echocardiography: The pulmonary valve appears to be unusually echo-dense. The pulmonary valve image on two-dimensional echocardiography shows a thickened structure with less than normal excursion. The transvalvular pressure gradient can be noninvasively and accurately estimated by echo Doppler technique.

E. Cardiac Catheterization and Angiocardiography: There is no increase in oxygen saturation or oxygen content in the right side of the heart. In the more severe cases, there is a right-to-left shunt at the atrial level. Pulmonary artery pressure is normal in milder cases and quite low in moderately severe to severe cases. Right ventricular pressure is always higher than pulmonary artery pressure. The gradient across the pulmonary valve varies from 10 to 200 mm Hg. In severe cases, the right atrial pressure is often elevated, with a predominant *a* wave. Cineangiocardiography with injection of contrast material into the right ventricle shows thickening of the pulmonary valve and the very narrow opening of the pulmonary valve. This produces a jet of contrast from the right ventricle into the pulmonary artery. Infundibular hypertrophy may be present. Diagnostic catheterization is usually combined with a balloon pulmonary valvotomy.

Treatment

Elective valvotomy is recommended for children with right ventricular pressures of greater than 50 mm Hg or higher than two-thirds of systemic pressure. Immediate correction is indicated for patients with systemic or greater right ventricular pressure. Percutaneous balloon valvuloplasty has become the procedure of choice in most institutions. It appears to be as effective as surgery in relieving obstruction and causes less valve insufficiency.

The need for additional surgical resection of associated infundibular hypertrophy is controversial. Because additional surgery increases the risk and because the outflow obstruction usually regresses, many centers perform only the balloon valvotomy.

Course & Prognosis

Patients with mild pulmonary stenosis live a normal life and have a normal life span. Those with stenosis of moderate severity rarely are symptomatic. Those with severe valvular obstruction may develop severe cyanosis and congestive heart failure in early life.

Postoperative follow-up suggests that most patients with right ventricular pressure equal to or less than systemic pressure who were treated surgically early in life have good voluntary maximum exercise capacity. If relief of valvular obstruction occurs prior to 20 years of age, longevity is essentially the same as that of the general population. Physical restriction is unwarranted in these patients. The quality of life of adults with pulmonary stenosis is comparable to that of the normal population. The risk of congenital coronary heart disease is 1.7% in the offspring of males and approximately 4% in probands of females.

Driscoll DJ et al: Occurrence risk for congenital heart defects in relatives of patients with aortic stenosis, pulmonary stenosis, or ventricular septal defect. Circulation 1993;87(Suppl):I-121.

Kopecky SL et al: Long term outcome of patients undergoing surgical repair of isolated pulmonary valve stenosis. Circulation 1988;78:1150.

Lloyd T, Donnerstein R: Rapid T-wave normalization after balloon pulmonary valvuloplasty in children. Am J Cardiol 1989;64:399.

Marantz PM et al: Results of balloon valvuloplasty in typical and dysplastic pulmonary valve stenosis: Doppler echocardiographic follow up. J Am Coll Cardiol 1988; 12:476.

McCrindle B, Kan J: Long term results after balloon valvuloplasty. Circulation 1991;83:1915.

Rey C et al: Percutaneous transluminal balloon valvuloplasty of congenital pulmonary valve stenosis, with a special report on infants and neonates. J Am Coll Cardiol 1988;11:815.

2. INFUNDIBULAR PULMONARY STENOSIS WITHOUT VENTRICULAR SEPTAL DEFECT

Pure infundibular pulmonary stenosis is rare. One should suspect infundibular pulmonary stenosis where there is evidence of mild to moderate pulmonary stenosis and intact ventricular septum and (1) no pulmonary ejection click is audible and (2) the murmur is maximal in the third and fourth intercostal spaces rather than in the second intercostal space. The clinical picture is identical.

3. DISTAL PULMONARY STENOSIS

Supravalvular Pulmonary Stenosis

Supravalvular pulmonary stenosis, a relatively rare condition, is caused by coarctation of the body of the main pulmonary artery. The clinical picture may be identical to that of valvular pulmonary stenosis, although the murmur is maximal in the first intercostal space at the left sternal border and in the suprasternal notch. No ejection click is audible. A second heart sound is usually narrowly split, and the pulmonary component is quite loud as a result of closure of the pulmonary valve under high pressure. The murmur radiates extremely well into the neck and over the lung fields.

Peripheral Pulmonary Branch Stenosis

In peripheral pulmonary branch stenosis, there are multiple small coarctations of the branches of the pulmonary artery in the periphery of the lung. Systolic murmurs may be heard over both lung fields, both anteriorly and posteriorly. The transient pulmonary branch stenosis murmurs of infancy (previously described in the section on heart murmurs, under Diagnostic Evaluation) are innocent. Pulmonary artery branch stenosis murmurs may be the most audible murmurs in atrial septal defects in infancy and early childhood. The most common cause of significant pulmonary artery branch stenosis is maternal rubella. Several types of supravalvular aortic stenosis syndromes may be found in association with this condition.

Surgery is often unsuccessful. Transvenous angioplasty is currently being assessed but does not appear to be as efficacious in patients with peripheral pulmonary branch stenosis as in patients with pulmonary valvular stenosis.

Absence of a Pulmonary Artery

Absence of a pulmonary artery may be an isolated malformation or may occur in association with other congenital heart diseases. It is occasionally seen in patients with tetralogy of Fallot.

Dunkle LM, Rowe RD: Transient murmur simulating pulmonary artery stenosis in premature infants. Am J Dis Child 1972;124:666.

Rothma A et al: Early results and follow-up of balloon angioplasty for branch pulmonary artery stenosis. J Am Coll Cardiol 1990;15:1109.

MALFORMATIONS ASSOCIATED WITH OBSTRUCTION TO BLOOD FLOW ON THE LEFT SIDE OF THE HEART

1. COARCTATION OF THE AORTA

Essentials of Diagnosis & Typical Features

- Pulse lag in lower extremities.
- Blood pressure of 20 mm Hg or pressure greater in the upper than in the lower extremities.
- Blowing systolic murmur in the left axilla.

General Considerations

Coarctation is a common cardiac abnormality accounting for about 6% of all cases of congenital heart disease. Three times as many males as females are affected. In the vast majority of cases, coarctation occurs in the thoracic portion of the descending aorta. The abdominal aorta is very rarely involved. Coarctations are usually in the juxtaductal position rather than the preductal or postductal position. The term "coarctation of aorta syndrome" is a useful concept, because most symptomatic infants have associated patent ductus arteriosus, tubular hypoplasia of the aortic isthmus (frequently erroneously termed a coarctation), ventricular septal defect, and bicuspid aortic valve. The tubular hypoplasia of the aortic isthmus is probably related to paucity of blood flow in the fetus and often spontaneously enlarges with postnatal growth.

Clinical Findings

A. Symptoms and Signs: Patients with coarctation may or may not have cardiovascular symptoms in infancy, childhood, and adolescence. Congestive heart failure may develop in early infancy, and symptoms of decreased exercise tolerance and fatigability may appear in childhood.

The important physical finding is diminution or absence of femoral pulses. However, a significant number of infants will initially have equal upper and lower extremity pulses until the coexistent patent ductus arteriosus closes. Normally, the blood pressure in the upper extremities is slightly higher than in the lower extremities during the first few months of life. After 1 year of age, blood pressure higher in the arms than in the legs is suggestive of coarctation of the aorta. The actual level of blood pressure in the arms may be only moderately elevated, even in severe coarctation, or it may be significantly elevated. In the presence of severe congestive heart failure, the differences in pulses in the upper and lower extremities may not be readily apparent, but with compensation, the pulses in the arms are palpably stronger than those of healthy infants; the pulses in the legs remain diminished or absent in affected infants. The left subclavian artery is occasionally involved in the coarctation, in which case the left brachial pulse is weak. If the coarctation is uncomplicated, the heart sounds are normal. The aortic component of the second heart sound is occasionally increased in intensity. An ejection systolic murmur of grade II/VI intensity is often heard at the aortic area and the lower left sternal border. The pathognomonic murmur of coarctation is heard in the left axilla. This murmur is usually systolic in timing but may spill into diastole. If the coarctation is complicated by other malformations, murmurs associated with these other abnormalities will be audible.

B. Imaging: In the older child, x-ray findings may indicate a heart normal in size, although there is usually some evidence of left ventricular enlargement. The ascending aorta is usually normal in size. On barium swallow, the esophagus has a characteristic e shape. The first arc of the e is caused by dilatation of the aorta just proximal to the coarctation. The second arc results from poststenotic dilatation of the aorta. The middle bar of the e is due to the coarctation itself. In older children, notching or scalloping of the ribs caused by marked enlargement of the intercostal collaterals can be seen. MRI has become extremely useful for determining noninvasively the anatomy of the coarctation.

In infants in congestive heart failure, there is evidence of marked cardiac enlargement and pulmonary venous congestion.

C. Electrocardiography: ECGs in children may be normal or may show evidence of slight left ventricular hypertrophy. In infants with or without congestive heart failure, the ECG usually demonstrates right ventricular hypertrophy.

D. Echocardiography: Real-time two-dimensional echocardiography and color flow Doppler may visualize the coarctation directly, and continuous wave doppler may serve as a predictor of severity. However, if the ductus arteriosus is still patent, echocardiography may not detect the coarctation. Associated lesions such as a bicuspid aortic valve or mitral abnormalities may suggest the presence of a coarctation.

E. Cardiac Catheterization and Angiocardiography: These studies demonstrate the position, anatomy, and severity of the coarctation and will assess the adequacy of the collateral circulation.

Treatment

Infants with coarctation of the aorta and congestive heart failure require vigorous anticongestive measures. Dilation of the associated patent ductus arteriosus with a constant infusion of prostaglandin E_1 (PGE_1) at 0.05–0.20 µg/kg/min may stabilize the critically ill infant until operation can be performed. **Many with isolated coarctation and no associated lesions respond well to inotropic therapy and may not require surgery in infancy.** In infants with striking congestive heart failure and without associated cardiovascular abnormalities, severe systemic hypertension is often a contributing factor.

Infants with associated intracardiac defects sometimes need immediate surgery but frequently require revision of the recoarctation later in life. Modification of the surgical technique utilizing a subclavian flap anastomosis or an extended end-to-end anastomosis reduces the likelihood of this late complication.

Percutaneous balloon angioplasty has been used successfully as a palliative procedure to stabilize critically ill infants with coarctation of aorta syndrome and as primary therapy in older children. Percutaneous balloon angioplasty is also being utilized to dilate recoarctations in postoperative patients.

Patients who do not require surgery early in infancy may be corrected electively up to 4 years of age unless significant systemic hypertension develops. Older children should be repaired either with surgery or with angioplasty at the time of diagnosis.

Course & Prognosis

Children who survive the neonatal period without developing congestive heart failure do quite well throughout childhood and adolescence. Fatal complications (eg, hypertensive encephalopathy, intracranial bleeding) occur uncommonly. Subacute infective endocarditis is also rare before adolescence.

Children with coarctation corrected during school age are at significant risk for systemic hypertension and myocardial dysfunction. Careful exercise testing is mandatory prior to their participation in athletic activities.

Balderson S et al: Maximal voluntary exercise variables in children with postoperative coarctation of the aorta. J Am Coll Cardiol 1992;191:154.

Cohen M et al: Coarctation of the aorta: Long-term follow-up and prediction of outcome after surgical correction. Circulation 1989;80:840.

Mendelsohn AM et al: Rapid progression of aortic aneurysms after patch aortoplasty repair of coarctation of the aorta. J Am Coll Cardiol 1992;20:381.

Simpson IA et al: Color flow Doppler flow mapping in patients with coarctation of the aorta: New observations and improved evaluation with color flow diameter and proximal acceleration as predictors of severity. Circulation 1988;77:736.

Ward KE et al: Delayed detection of coarctation in infancy:

Implications for timing newborn follow-up. Pediatrics 1990;86:972.

2. AORTIC STENOSIS

Essentials of Diagnosis & Typical Features

- Systolic ejection murmur at the upper right sternal border.
- Thrill in the carotid arteries.
- Systolic click at the apex.
- Dilatation of the ascending aorta on chest x-ray.

General Considerations

Aortic stenosis may be defined from the anatomic or physiologic point of view. Anatomically, it consists of an obstruction to the outflow from the left ventricle at or near the aortic valve. Physiologically, aortic stenosis may be defined as a condition in which a systolic pressure gradient of more than 10 mm Hg exists between the left ventricle and the aorta. Aortic stenosis accounts for approximately 5% of all cases of congenital heart disease. Anatomically, congenital aortic stenosis may be divided into four types:

A. Valvular Aortic Stenosis (75%): Critical aortic stenosis presenting in infancy usually consists of a unicuspid diaphragm-like structure without well-defined commissures. Preschool and school-age children more commonly present with a bicuspid valve. Teenagers and young adults characteristically present with tricuspid but partially fused leaflets. This lesion is more common in males than in females.

B. Discrete Membranous Subvalvular Aortic Stenosis (20%): This consists of a membranous or fibrous ring just below the aortic valve. The ring forms a diaphragm with a hole in the middle and results in obstruction to left ventricular outflow. The aortic valve itself and the anterior leaflet of the mitral valve are often deformed.

C. Supravalvular Aortic Stenosis: In this variety, there is a constriction of the ascending aorta just above the coronary arteries. This condition is often associated with a family history, abnormal facies, and mental retardation (Williams syndrome).

D. Idiopathic Hypertrophic Subaortic Stenosis (IHSS): In this case, there is a marked hypertrophy of the entire left ventricle and, predominantly, the ventricular septum. With contraction of the ventricle, the hypertrophic portion of the septum, together with the mitral valve, causes obstruction of left ventricular outflow. A family history is often present.

Obstruction to outflow from the left ventricle causes the left ventricle to work harder to maintain an adequate pressure and flow in the systemic arterial circuit, resulting in hypertrophy of the left ventricle and increased oxygen requirement. If the stenosis is severe, the oxygen requirements may exceed the capacity of the coronary arteries to supply oxygen, and relative coronary insufficiency may develop. In critical aortic stenosis, left ventricular failure may occur. The left ventricle is usually able to adapt to the increased pressure load for a considerable period before heart failure or coronary insufficiency develops.

Clinical Findings

A. Symptoms and Signs: Most patients with aortic stenosis have no cardiovascular symptoms. Except in the most severe cases, the patient may do well up until the third to fifth decades of life, although some patients have mild exercise intolerance and easy fatigability. A small percentage of patients have significant symptoms within the first decade, that is, dizziness and syncope. Sudden death, although uncommon, may occur in all forms of aortic stenosis, the greatest risk being IHSS.

Although isolated valvular aortic stenosis seldom causes symptoms in infancy, severe heart failure occasionally occurs when critical obstruction is present. The response to medical management is poor; therefore, an aggressive surgical approach is recommended.

The physical findings vary somewhat depending on the anatomic type of lesion:

1. Valvular aortic stenosis–Affected patients are well developed and well nourished. The pulses are usually normal and equal throughout. If the stenosis is severe and there is a gradient of greater than 80 mm Hg, the pulses are small with a slow upstroke. Examination of the heart reveals a left ventricular thrust at the apex. A systolic thrill at the right base, the suprasternal notch, and both carotid arteries accompanies moderate disease. If only one carotid artery manifests a thrill, it is the right carotid (usually seen in milder disease).

The first heart sound is normal. A prominent aortic-type ejection click or ejection sound is best heard at the apex. In infants, this click can be heard at the lower left sternal border and at the aortic area. It is separated from the first heart sound by a short but appreciable interval. It does not vary with respiration. The second heart sound at the pulmonary area is physiologically split. The aortic component of the second heart sound is of good intensity. There is a grade III–V/VI, rough, medium- to high-pitched ejection-type systolic murmur, loudest at the first and second intercostal spaces, which radiates well into the suprasternal notch and along the carotids. The murmur also radiates fairly well down the lower left sternal border and can be heard at the apex. The murmur transmits to the neck, and its grade correlates roughly with the severity of the stenosis.

2. Discrete membranous subvalvular aortic stenosis–The findings are essentially the same as those of valvular aortic stenosis. Absence of an aortic ejection click is an important differentiating point, and the thrill and murmur are usually somewhat more intense at the left sternal border in the third and fourth intercostal spaces than at the aortic area. Frequently, however, the murmur is equally intense at both areas. A diastolic murmur of aortic insufficiency is commonly heard after 5 years of age.

3. Supravalvular aortic stenosis–Affected patients often have abnormal facies and are mentally retarded. The thrill and murmur are characteristically best heard in the suprasternal notch and along the carotids, although they are well transmitted over the aortic area and near the mid left sternal border. A difference in pulses and blood pressure between the right and left arms may be found, with the more prominent pulse and pressure in the right arm.

4. Idiopathic hypertrophic subaortic stenosis–The murmur in this case is ejection in quality, grade II–III/VI, and heard from the left sternal border toward the apex and sometimes associated with a murmur of mitral insufficiency. There is often an atrial fourth heart sound with a diastolic murmur. No ejection click is audible. The arterial pulse wave has a rapid upstroke and frequently a bisferious quality.

B. Imaging: In most cases, x-ray findings indicate that the heart is not enlarged. The left ventricle, however, is slightly prominent. In valvular and discrete subvalvular aortic stenosis, dilatation of the ascending aorta is frequently seen (more commonly in the former). The ascending aorta is usually normal in IHSS and in supravalvular aortic stenosis.

C. Electrocardiography: There is some correlation between the severity of the obstruction and the ECG. Patients with mild aortic stenosis have normal ECGs. Patients with severe obstruction frequently demonstrate evidence of left ventricular hypertrophy and left ventricular strain, but many do not. In about 25% of severe cases, the ECG is normal. Progressive increase in left ventricular hypertrophy on serial ECGs indicates a significant degree of obstruction. Left ventricular strain is taken as a potential indication for operation.

D. Echocardiography: This has become a reliable noninvasive technique for the initial diagnosis and follow-up evaluation of IHSS. It also provides clues to the progression of other forms of aortic stenosis. Doppler echocardiographic techniques can now predict transvalvular gradients quite accurately.

E. Cardiac Catheterization and Angiocardiography: Left heart catheterization demonstrates the pressure differential between the left ventricle and the aorta and the level at which the gradient exists. Patients with severe aortic stenosis may be asymptomatic and have normal ECGs and chest x-rays. Historically, serial cardiac catheterization was frequently the only reliable guide to the progression and severity of the lesion. Currently, echocardiography has largely replaced the need for serial catheterizations. In the case of valvular aortic stenosis, an asymptomatic patient with a resting gradient of 60–80 mm Hg is considered to require surgery. In the face of symptoms, patients with lesser gradients are surgical candidates. Cineangiocardiography is helpful in demonstrating the level of the obstruction.

Treatment

Because operation offers less than a cure, surgical repair should be considered only in patients with symptoms or a large resting gradient (60–80 mm Hg). In many cases, the gradient can be only moderately to minimally relieved without producing aortic insufficiency (which is potentially more harmful than the lesion for which surgery was undertaken). Percutaneous balloon valvuloplasty is now accepted as standard treatment. Discrete subvalvular aortic stenosis requires a lesser gradient for surgical intervention, because continued trauma to the aortic valve by the subvalvular jet may destroy the valve. Unfortunately, simple resection is followed by recurrence in more than 25% of patients with subvalvular aortic stenosis. Asymmetric septal hypertrophy has even less satisfactory results than muscle resection; therefore, medical management with propranolol should be tried initially.

All patients should have close follow-up, and those over age 6 years should undergo yearly exercise testing. If exercise testing is normal, restriction of physical activity may not be necessary in patients with mild to moderate aortic stenosis; in many cases, these patients may participate in competitive sports.

Course & Prognosis

All forms of left ventricular outflow tract obstruction tend to be progressive diseases. However, regression of the obstruction has been documented in a few patients with supravalvular obstruction. Pediatric patients with left ventricular outflow tract obstruction—with the exception of those with critical aortic stenosis of infancy—are usually asymptomatic. Symptoms accompanying severe unoperated obstruction (angina, syncope, congestive heart failure) are all rare currently because of detection and surgical intervention. The vast majority of children without asymmetric septal hypertrophy not only are asymptomatic but also tend to have the personality and capabilities to compete in sports. There is increasing evidence that preoperative or postoperative children whose obstruction is mild to moderate have above-average oxygen consumption and maximum voluntary working capacity. Children in this category with normal findings on resting and exercising ECG and normal heart size may safely participate in vigorous physical activity, including nonisometric competitive sports. Children with severe aortic stenosis tend to demonstrate ventricular dysrhythmias as adults.

Kasten-Sportas CH et al: Percutaneous balloon valvuloplasty in neonates with critical aortic stenosis. J Am Coll Cardiol 1991;13:1101.

Kennedy KD et al: Natural history of moderate aortic stenosis. J Am Coll Cardiol 1991;17:313.

Oh JK et al: Prediction of the severity of aortic stenosis by Doppler aortic valve area determination. J Am Coll Cardiol 1988;11:1227.

Shaddy RE et al: Gradient reduction aortic valve regurgitation and prolapse after balloon aortic valvuloplasty in 32 consecutive patients with congenital aortic stenosis. J Am Coll Cardiol 1990;16:451.

Witsenburg M et al: Short and midterm results of balloon valvuloplasty for valvar aortic stenosis in children. Am J Cardiol 1992;69:945.

Wolfe RR et al: Arrhythmias in patients with valvar aortic stenosis, valvar pulmonic stenosis, and ventricular septal defect. Circulation 1993;87(Suppl):I-89.

Zeevi B et al: Neonatal critical valvar aortic stenosis. Circulation 1989;80:831.

3. MITRAL VALVE PROLAPSE

Essentials of Diagnosis & Typical Features

- Midsystolic click best heard with the patient in the standing or squatting position.
- Occasional late systolic murmur.

General Considerations

Mitral valve prolapse is the most common entity to present with abnormal auscultatory findings in older pediatric patients. It is secondary to redundant valve tissue or abnormal tissue comprising the mitral valve apparatus. The mitral valve prolapses, moving posteriorly or superiorly into the left atrium during ventricular systole. A systolic click occurs at the time of this movement and is the clinical hallmark of this entity. Mitral insufficiency may occur late in systole, causing an atypical, short, late systolic murmur with variable radiation. It is most commonly found in individuals with the following characteristics: over 6 years of age, female, slender habitus, and bony thoracic abnormalities. Its incidence is estimated to vary from 2% to 20%, with the higher part of the range representing incidence in slender teenage females.

Clinical Findings

A. Symptoms and Signs: The vast majority of patients with mitral valve prolapse are asymptomatic. Chest pain, palpitations, and dizziness are reported, but it is not clear whether or not these symptoms are more common in affected patients than in the normal population. Significant dysrhythmias are uncommon, and true exercise intolerance is rare. The standard approach to auscultation must be modified to diagnose mitral valve prolapse; that is, auscultation should be performed with the patient placed in various positions. Clicks with or without systolic murmur are more commonly elicited in the standing and squatting positions than in the supine and sitting positions. The systolic click occurs earlier in children than in adults; that is, it tends to be midsystolic rather than late systolic. Although it is usually heard at the apex, it may be audible at the left sternal border or even occasionally may be panthoracic. A midsystolic or systolic murmur following the click implies mitral insufficiency and is much less common than isolated prolapse. The murmur tends to be atypical for mitral insufficiency in that it is not pansystolic and radiates to the sternum rather than to the left axilla. A coexistent diastolic murmur of relative or real mitral stenosis is rare. Occasionally, a systolic "honk" is heard.

B. Imaging: In the rare case of significant mitral insufficiency, the left atrium may be enlarged; this is visualized best on lateral film x-ray. Most chest x-rays show normal findings, and their use is therefore largely unwarranted.

C. Electrocardiography: Despite the fact that flat or inverted T waves in precordial lead V6 have been reported, almost all electrocardiographic findings are normal. Disabling chest pain is rare and should be assessed with ergometric electrocardiography.

D. Echocardiography: Significant posterior systolic movement of the anterior mitral valve leaflet is considered diagnostic. Many false-positive results are the result of multiple leaflet images (chevroning) or to the presence of insignificant (small duration and amplitude) posterior systolic valve movement. False-negative results are also common, partly because of performance of the procedure when the patient is in the supine position. If the physical findings are typical for isolated prolapse, echocardiography can assess the degree of myxomatous change of the mitral apparatus.

E. Cardiac Catheterization and Angiography: Invasive procedures are very rarely indicated.

Treatment & Prognosis

Use of oral propranolol may be effective in rare cases of disabling chest pain. Prophylaxis for subacute infectious endocarditis is indicated only in individuals with associated mitral insufficiency.

The natural course of disease is largely unknown. Twenty years of observation indicate, however, that mitral valve prolapse in childhood is a largely benign entity. It merges with a common variation from normal in slender children and is associated with an asthenic body build that presumably results from altered geometry of the left ventricle and mitral valve.

Alpert MA et al: Frequency of isolated panic attacks and panic disorder in patients with mitral valve prolapse syndrome. Am J Cardiol 1992;69:1489.

Arfken CL et al: Mitral valve prolapse: Associations with symptoms and anxiety. Pediatrics 1990;85:311.

Barlow JB, Pocock WA: Billowing, floppy, prolapsed or flail valves? Am J Cardiol 1985;55:501.

Kessler KM: Prolapse paranoia. J Am Coll Cardiol 1988; 11:48.

Levine RA: Reconsideration of echocardiographic standards for mitral valve prolapse: Lack of association between leaf displacement isolated to the apical four-chamber view and independent echocardiographic evidence of abnormality. J Am Coll Cardiol 1988;11:1010.

4. OTHER CONGENITAL VALVULAR LESIONS

Congenital Mitral Stenosis

In this rare disorder, the valve leaflets are thickened and fused to produce a diaphragm-like or funnel-like structure with an opening in the center. Frequent associated malformations include subaortic and aortic stenosis and coarctation of the aorta. This lesion complex is known as Shone syndrome. Most patients develop symptoms early in life. Early symptoms include tachypnea, dyspnea, and severe failure to thrive. Physical examination reveals a first heart sound that is accentuated, and the pulmonary closure sound is loud. No opening snap can be heard. In most cases, a presystolic crescendo murmur is heard at the apex. Occasionally, only a mid-diastolic murmur can be heard. Rarely, no murmur at all is heard. Electrocardiography shows right axis deviation, biatrial enlargement, and right ventricular hypertrophy. X-ray reveals evidence of left atrial enlargement and, frequently, pulmonary venous congestion. Echocardiography shows abnormal valve structures with reduced excursion and left atrial enlargement. Cardiac catheterization reveals an elevated pulmonary capillary pressure and wedge pressure and pulmonary hypertension.

Surgical treatment, including valve replacement with a prosthetic mitral valve, has become possible even in infants weighing 3–5 kg.

Cor Triatriatum

This is an extremely rare abnormality in which the pulmonary veins enter a separate chamber rather than pass directly into the left atrium. The chamber communicates with the left atrium through an opening of variable size. The physiologic consequences of this condition are very similar to those of mitral stenosis. The clinical findings depend on the size of the opening. If the opening is extremely small, symptoms develop very early in life. If the opening is large, patients may be asymptomatic for a considerable period of time. Echocardiography may reveal a dense shadow in the left atrium. Two-dimensional color flow doppler echocardiographic techniques have greatly enhanced the noninvasive accuracy of the diagnosis. Cardiac catheterization may be diagnostic. Finding a high pulmonary capillary pressure (high pulmonary venous pressure) and a low left atrial pressure (if the catheter can be passed through the foramen ovale into the true left atrial chamber) makes the diagnosis certain. Angiocardiographic studies may identify two "left atrial" chambers.

Surgical repair is usually successful.

Congenital Mitral Regurgitation

This is a relatively rare abnormality that is usually associated with other congenital heart lesions, including corrected transposition of the great vessels, endocardial cushion defect, and endocardial fibroelastosis. Uncomplicated congenital mitral regurgitation is very rare. It is sometimes present in patients with Marfan syndrome. Occasionally, there is a congenital dilatation of the valve ring with an otherwise normal valve. In other cases, the chordae tendineae are malformed, resulting in mitral regurgitation.

Congenital Aortic Regurgitation

The most common causes of this disorder are bicuspid aortic valve, either uncomplicated or with coarctation of the aorta; ventricular septal defect and aortic insufficiency; and fenestration of the aortic valve cusp (one or more holes in the cusp).

Absence of the Pulmonary Valve

This rare abnormality is usually associated with ventricular septal defect. In about 50% of cases, pulmonary stenosis is present (tetralogy of Fallot).

Ebstein's Malformation of the Tricuspid Valve

This uncommon abnormality consists of downward displacement of the tricuspid valve such that the greater portion of the valve is attached to the ventricular wall rather than to the fibrous ring. As a result, the upper portion of the right ventricle is functionally within the right atrium. The portion of the ventricle below the apex of the tricuspid valve is very small and represents the true functioning right ventricle. Clinically, there is a wide spectrum of abnormalities ranging from relative absence of symptoms to death in early infancy. The severity depends on the degree of malattachment of the valve and the associated abnormalities. Echocardiography is useful in diagnosis.

Surgical repair consists of an annuloplasty procedure to modify the level of tricuspid orifice and diminish mitral insufficiency. The procedure's rate of success is highly variable. Late arrhythmias are common. Postoperative tolerance of exercise is significantly increased compared to preoperative status but decreased compared to healthy individuals.

Driscoll DJ, Mottram CD, Danielson GK: Spectrum of exercise intolerance in 45 patients with Ebstein's anomaly and observations on exercise tolerance in 11 patients after surgical repair. J Am Coll Cardiol 1988;11:831.

Lang D et al: Pathologic spectrum of malformations of the tricuspid valve in prenatal and neonatal life. J Am Coll Cardiol 1991;17:1161.

Quaegebeur JN et al: Surgery for Ebstein's anomaly. J Am Coll Cardiol 1991;17:722.

Saxena A et al: The left ventricular function in patients 20 years of age with Ebstein's anomaly of the tricuspid valve. Am J Cardiol 1991;67:217.

Spevak PJ et al: Balloon angioplasty for congenital mitral stenosis. Am J Cardiol 1990;66:472.

MYOCARDIAL DISEASES

Myocardial diseases are characterized by significant cardiac enlargement. Murmurs may or may not be present. Electrocardiographic changes include left ventricular hypertrophy, ST depression, and T wave inversion.

1. GLYCOGEN STORAGE DISEASE OF THE HEART

At least 10 types of glycogen storage disease are recognized. The type that primarily involves the heart is known as Pompe's disease. The deficient enzyme (acid maltase) is necessary for hydrolysis of the outer branches of glycogen, and its absence results in marked deposition of glycogen within the myocardium. Cardiac glycogenosis is a rare heritable (autosomal recessive) disorder.

Affected infants are usually normal at birth, but onset commonly begins by the sixth month of life. These children have a history of retardation of growth and development, feeding problems, poor weight gain, and then the findings of heart failure. Physical examination reveals generalized muscular weakness, a large tongue, cardiomegaly, no significant heart murmurs, and, occasionally, evidence of congestive heart failure. Chest x-rays reveal marked cardiomegaly with or without pulmonary venous congestion. The ECG shows a short PR interval with left ventricular hypertrophy and shows ST depression and T wave inversion over the left precordial leads. Echocardiography shows extremely thick ventricular wall structures.

Children with this disease usually die within the first year of life. Death may be sudden or the result of progressive congestive heart failure.

2. ANOMALOUS ORIGIN OF THE LEFT CORONARY ARTERY

In this condition, the left coronary artery arises from the pulmonary artery rather than from the aorta. In the neonatal period, while the pulmonary arterial pressure is relatively high, blood is supplied to the left ventricle from the pulmonary artery. Accordingly, during this period the child is asymptomatic and does well. However, within the first 2 months of life, the pulmonary arterial pressure decreases to normal. This phenomenon results in a marked decrease of flow to the left coronary artery. Infarction of the heart usually occurs. If the patient survives, collateral channels appear that join the peripheral branches of the right with the branches of the left coronary artery.

As a result, the direction of blood flow in the left coronary artery changes. Whereas previously there was some flow from the pulmonary artery into the myocardium through the left coronary, flow now occurs from the right coronary artery through the collateral into the left coronary artery and then into the pulmonary artery. In essence, then, an arteriovenous fistula is formed that further removes blood from the myocardium, resulting in further myocardial infarction and fibrosis. Death occurs eventually as a result of marked dilatation of the heart and congestive heart failure. At autopsy, the left ventricle is found to be markedly fibrosed and thin.

Clinical Findings

A. Symptoms and Signs: Patients appear to be healthy at birth. Growth and development are relatively normal for a few months, although detailed questioning of the parents often discloses a history of intermittent episodes of severe abdominal pain, pallor, and sweating, especially during or after feeding. These episodes are thought to be secondary to "colic," and attacks are similar to anginal attacks in adults.

On physical examination, the patients are usually well developed and well nourished. The pulses are usually weak but equal throughout. The heart is enlarged but not very active. A murmur of mitral regurgitation is frequently present, although no murmur may be heard.

B. Imaging: Chest x-ray films show significant cardiac enlargement with or without pulmonary venous congestion.

C. Electrocardiography: The ECG is usually diagnostic. There are T wave inversions in leads I and aVL. The precordial leads show T wave inversions from V4 to V7. Deep Q waves are often seen in leads I, aVL, and V4 to V6. These findings of myocardial infarction are similar to those in adults.

D. Echocardiography: The diagnosis can be made with two-dimensional techniques by visualizing a single large right coronary artery arising from the aorta.

E. Cardiac Catheterization and Angiocardiography: A small left-to-right shunt (a result of the flow of blood from the right through the left coronary artery into the pulmonary artery) can often be detected at the pulmonary artery level. Frequently, however, the shunt is very small and can be detected only by the most sensitive techniques, for example, by the use of a hydrogen electrode catheter. Cineangiocardiography following injection of contrast material into the root of the aorta shows absence of origin of the left coronary artery from the aorta. A huge right coronary artery fills directly from the aorta, and the contrast material will flow through the right coronary system into the left coronary arteries and finally into the pulmonary artery.

Treatment & Prognosis

Medical management with anticongestives and afterload reduction is advocated by some but fails to correct the anatomic defect. Operations requiring cardiopulmonary bypass to effect two functional coronary arteries from the aorta are preferred. Simple ligation of the left coronary artery or subclavian to coronary artery anastomosis (without cardiopulmonary bypass) should be considered for the most critically ill infants.

The prognosis is guarded. No therapeutic modality has been shown to be superior in follow-up studies of survivors.

Midgley A et al: Repair of anomalous origin of the left coronary artery in the infant and small child. J Am Coll Cardiol 1984;4:1231.

Sauer U et al: Risk factors for perioperative mortality in children with anomalous origin of the left coronary artery from the pulmonary artery. J Thorac Cardiovasc Surg 1991;102:566

3. ENDOCARDIAL FIBROELASTOSIS

The incidence of endocardial fibroelastosis has decreased dramatically over the past 2 decades, and this entity is now uncommon. The cause is not known, although intrauterine infection with mumps or coxsackievirus B has been suggested.

Pathologic examination discloses a marked milky white thickening of the endocardium, the subendocardial layers of the left ventricle, and, usually, the left atrium. The mitral valve is frequently involved also. The myocardial fibers themselves are fibrotic and disorganized, and associated hypervascularization is common. Serial sections often show coexistent evidence of myocarditis. Thus, endocardial fibroelastosis appears to be part of a continuum of primary endomyocardial diseases and may be a sequela to myocarditis.

Clinical Findings

A. Symptoms and Signs: Patients appear normal at birth, and growth and development during early infancy are normal. About half develop symptoms within the first 5 months of life, and most are symptomatic by age 1 year. An occasional patient may have no symptoms until age 5 years.

The symptoms and signs that do develop are associated with left ventricular heart failure. These include dyspnea, easy fatigability, feeding difficulties, and, eventually, findings of left and right heart failure.

On physical examination, these children are often small and undernourished. The heart is usually enlarged, and the heart tones are poor (when there is evidence of decompensation). A murmur of mitral regurgitation may be present.

B. Imaging: Chest x-ray films show generalized cardiac enlargement with or without pulmonary venous congestion.

C. Electrocardiography: The ECG almost always shows evidence of left ventricular hypertrophy and, quite frequently, ST depression and T wave inversion. If there has been pulmonary hypertension secondary to left heart failure, right ventricular hypertrophy may be present. Right atrial hypertrophy is sometimes present. Complete heart block is occasionally seen.

D. Echocardiography: M-mode and two-dimensional techniques reveal dilatation of cardiac chambers and echo-dense endocardial images. Myocardial systolic function is decreased.

E. Cardiac Catheterization and Angiocardiography: Catheterization reveals the absence of left-to-right shunts. Pulmonary hypertension may be present. Cineangiocardiography demonstrates diminished myocardial contractility. Transcatheter endomyocardial biopsy has become a more common technique in infants and children for primary myocardial disease but seldom reveals a cause.

Treatment & Prognosis

Treatment of endocardial fibroelastosis is medical and consists of adequate and prolonged use of digitalis afterload reduction and oral diuretics. If response to the usual dose is not satisfactory, the dosage of both digitalis and diuretics can be increased until a satisfactory response is noted or toxicity occurs. Infants who respond favorably to medical therapy should continue these agents for several years. Infants and children who fail to respond to medical therapy will require cardiac transplantation.

Some children appear to improve initially with treatment but then develop recurrent bouts of heart failure. Complete recovery in such patients is very infrequent, and unless receiving a transplant, most eventually die with intractable congestive heart failure. The prognosis is most favorable in patients who present between 6 months and 3 years of age and respond promptly to treatment.

Chan KY et al: Immunosuppressive therapy in the management of acute myocarditis in children: A clinical trial. J Am Coll Cardiol 1991;17:458.

CYANOTIC CONGENITAL HEART DISEASE

TETRALOGY OF FALLOT

Essentials of Diagnosis & Typical Features

- Cyanosis after the neonatal period.
- Hypoxemic spells during infancy.
- Right-sided aortic arch in 25%.

- Systolic ejection murmur at the upper left sternal border.

General Considerations

In Fallot's tetralogy, there is a ventricular septal defect and severe obstruction to right ventricular outflow such that the intracardiac shunt is predominantly from right to left. This is the most common type of cyanotic heart lesion, accounting for 10–15% of all cases of congenital heart disease. The ventricular defect is usually located in the membranous portion of the septum but may be totally surrounded by muscular tissue and is usually quite large. Obstruction to right ventricular outflow may be solely at the infundibular level (50–75%), at the valvular level alone (rarely), or at both levels (25% or more). The primary embryologic abnormality is in the septation of the conus and truncus arteriosus, resulting in an enlarged overriding aorta and hypoplasia of the pulmonary trunk. Experimental lesions in specific loci of ectodermal (neural crest) tissue which migrate to the conus can reproduce the defects seen in tetralogy of Fallot. The term "tetralogy" has been used to describe this combination of lesions, since there is always associated right ventricular hypertrophy and a varying degree of "overriding of the aorta." The overriding is present because of the position of the ventricular septal defect in relation to a dilated and often dextroposed aorta. These two factors (right ventricular hypertrophy, overriding aorta) plus the major lesions make up the tetralogy. A right-sided aortic arch is present in 25% of cases, and an atrial septal defect in 15%.

Severe obstruction to right ventricular outflow plus a large ventricular septal defect results in a right-to-left shunt at the ventricular level and desaturation of the arterial blood. The degree of desaturation and the extent of cyanosis depend on the size of the shunt. This in turn is dependent on the resistance to outflow from the right ventricle, the size of the ventricular septal defect, and the systemic vascular resistance. The greater the obstruction, the larger the ventricular septal defect, and the lower the systemic vascular resistance, the greater the right-to-left shunt. Although the patient may be deeply cyanotic, the amount of pressure the right ventricle can develop is limited to that of the systemic (aortic) pressure. In other words, right ventricular pressure cannot exceed left ventricular pressure. The right ventricle is usually able to maintain this level of pressure without developing heart failure. A new etiologic consideration is the association of cardiac conotruncal abnormalities with chromosome 22q11 deletion (CATCH 22).

Clinical Findings

A. Symptoms and Signs: The clinical findings vary depending on the degree of right ventricular outflow obstruction. Patients with a mild degree of obstruction are only minimally cyanotic or acyanotic and may even present initially with congestive heart failure. Those with maximal obstruction are deeply cyanotic from birth. However, few children are asymptomatic; most have cyanosis by 4 months of age, and the cyanosis usually is progressive. Growth and development are retarded, and easy fatigability and dyspnea on exertion are common. Squatting is seen when the children become old enough to walk.

Hypoxemic spells (cyanotic spells) are characterized by the following signs and symptoms: (1) sudden onset of cyanosis or deepening of cyanosis; (2) sudden onset of dyspnea; (3) alterations in consciousness, encompassing a spectrum from irritability to syncope; and (4) decrease in intensity or disappearance of the systolic murmur. These episodes may begin in the neonatal period and continue until nearly school age. It is unusual, however, for the initial episode to occur after 2 years of age. Acute treatment of cyanotic spells consists of giving oxygen and placing the patient in the knee-chest position. Acidosis, if present, should be corrected with intravenous sodium bicarbonate. Morphine sulfate should be administered cautiously by a parenteral route in a dosage of 0.1 mg/kg. Propranolol, 0.1–0.2 mg/kg intravenously, has been found to be useful. Chronic (daily) treatment of cyanotic spells with propranolol, 1 mg/kg orally every 4 hours while awake, remains controversial; however, in a significant number of patients, this regimen has prevented subsequent "spells" and made it possible to delay operation until total correction can be performed.

Patients with tetralogy are usually small and thin. The degree of cyanosis is variable. The fingers and toes show varying degrees of clubbing depending on the age of the child and the severity of the cyanosis.

On examination of the heart, a right ventricular lift is palpable. No thrills are present. The first sound is normal; occasionally, there is an ejection click at the apex that is aortic in origin. The second sound is predominantly aortic and single and best heard at the left sternal border between the third and fourth intercostal spaces. The second heart sound at the pulmonary area is soft. There is a grade I–III/VI, rough, ejection-type systolic murmur that is maximal at the left sternal border in the third intercostal space.

B. Laboratory Findings: The hemoglobin, hematocrit, and red blood cell count are usually mildly to markedly elevated, depending on the degree of arterial oxygen desaturation.

C. Imaging: Chest x-rays reveal the overall heart size to be normal, and indeed the x-ray film may sometimes be interpreted as being entirely normal. However, the right ventricle is hypertrophied, and this is often shown in the posteroanterior projection by an upturning of the apex (boot-shaped heart). The main pulmonary artery segment is usually concave, and the aorta in 25% of cases arches to the right. The pulmonary vascular markings are usually decreased.

D. Electrocardiography: The cardiac axis is to the right, ranging from +90 to +180 degrees. The P waves are usually normal, although there may be evidence of slight right atrial hypertrophy. Right ventricular hypertrophy is always present, but right ventricular strain patterns are rare.

E. Echocardiography: Two-dimensional imaging reveals thickening of the free right ventricular wall, with overriding of the aorta and a membranous ventricular septal defect, and is diagnostic. Furthermore, obstruction at the level of the infundibulum and pulmonary valve can be identified, and the size of the proximal pulmonary arteries can be measured. The anatomy of the coronary arteries may be visualized.

F. Cardiac Catheterization and Angiocardiography: Cardiac catheterization reveals the presence of a right-to-left shunt in most cases. There is arterial blood desaturation of varying degree. The right-to-left shunt exists at the ventricular level. The right ventricular pressure is at systemic levels, and the pressure contour in the right ventricle is identical to that of the left ventricle. The pulmonary artery pressure is extremely low (mean ranges of 5–10 mm Hg). The pressure gradients may be noted at the valvular level, the infundibular level, or both. The catheter frequently is passed from the right ventricle into the overriding ascending aorta but may cause a transient right bundle branch block.

Cineangiocardiography is diagnostic. Injection of contrast material into the right ventricle reveals the right ventricular outflow obstruction and the right-to-left shunt at the ventricular level. With improved echocardiographic techniques, the major indications for cardiac catheterization are to establish coronary artery and distal pulmonary artery anatomy. In addition, some patients may be palliated by balloon dilatation of the right ventricular outflow tract.

Treatment

A. Palliative Treatment: Palliative treatment is performed at some centers for very small infants who are markedly symptomatic (severely cyanotic, frequent severe anoxic spells) and in whom complete correction is a higher risk. Medical (chronic oral beta-blocking agents) or, more often, surgical (creation of a systemic arterial to pulmonary arterial anastomosis) palliation can be used.

The most common surgical palliation is the creation of a Gortex shunt from the subclavian artery to a branch pulmonary artery (modified Blalock-Taussig shunt).

B. Total Correction: The timing of total correction ranges from birth to 2 years, varying with the philosophies and results of each treatment center. It involves closing the ventricular septal defect and removing the obstruction to right ventricular outflow.

The surgical death rate varies from 1% to 5%. The major limiting anatomic feature of total correction is the size of the pulmonary artery and its branches.

Course & Prognosis

Infants with the most severe form of the disease are usually deeply cyanotic at birth. Hypoxemic spells may occur during the neonatal period. Death is extremely rare during a severe hypoxemic spell. Many patients who survive the first year of life seem to improve. This may be because of the development of systemic-to-pulmonary collateral vessels. Although hypoxemic spells may decrease in severity, these children remain deeply cyanotic and markedly limited in their activity. They seldom survive the second decade of life without surgical treatment.

Complete repair prior to the school-age years usually results in fair to good function, although patients are occasionally subject to sudden death from dysrhythmias. A competent pulmonary valve without a dilated right ventricle appears to diminish arrhythmias and enhance exercise performance.

Bricker JT: Sudden death and tetralogy of Fallot: Risks, markers, and causes. Circulation 1995;92:158.

Garson A Jr, Gillette PC, McNamara DG: Propranolol: The preferred palliation for tetralogy of Fallot. Am J Cardiol 1981;47:1098.

Gatzoulig MA et al: Right ventricular diastolic function 15 to 35 years after repair of tetralogy of Fallot. Circulation 1995;91:1775.

Kreutzer J et al: Tetralogy of Fallot with diminutive pulmonary arteries. J Am Coll Cardiol 1996;27:1741.

Momma K et al: Tetralogy of Fallot with pulmonary atresia associated with chromosome 22q11 deletion. J Am Coll Cardiol 1996;27:198.

Murphy JG et al: Long-term outcome in patients undergoing surgical repair of tetralogy of Fallot. N Engl J Med 1993;9:593.

Warner KG et al: Restoration of the pulmonary valve reduces right ventricular volume overload after previous repair of tetralogy of Fallot. Circulation 1993; 88(Suppl):II-189.

PULMONARY ATRESIA WITH VENTRICULAR SEPTAL DEFECT

This condition consists of complete atresia of the pulmonary valve in association with ventricular septal defect. Essentially, it is an extreme form of tetralogy of Fallot. Since there is no flow outward from the right ventricle into the pulmonary artery, the pulmonary blood flow must be derived either from a patent ductus arteriosus or from collateral channels.

The clinical picture depends entirely on the size of the ductus or the collateral channels (or both). If they are large, patients may do well and actually do better than those with severe tetralogy of Fallot. If effective pulmonary blood flow is small, death occurs secondary to severe anoxia early in life. This may occur suddenly with postnatal closure of a patent ductus arteriosus.

Echocardiography or cardiac catheterization and angiocardiography are diagnostic. If patent ductus arteriosus dependency is established, a PGE_1 infusion to dilate the patent ductus arteriosus may help stabilize the patient until surgery.

Infants who are severely hypoxemic require urgent systemic-to-pulmonary anastomosis in order to provide sufficient oxygenated blood to the body.

A corrective surgical procedure that has been successful in patients with adequate-sized pulmonary arteries consists of bypassing the obstructed right ventricular outflow and closing the ventricular septal defect. Success may depend on precise definition of pulmonary arterial and collateral blood supply to the lung and prior unifocalization of segments with dual arterial blood supply. More recently, an approach has been adopted to create initially a central connection between the right ventricle or aorta to the central pulmonary artery.

Hoffback KM et al: Analysis of survival in patients with pulmonic valve atresia and ventricular septal defect. Am J Cardiol 1991;67:737.

Marelli AJ et al: Pulmonary atresia with ventricular septal defect in adults. Circulation 1994;89:243.

Redington AN, Sommerville J: Stenting of aortopulmonary collaterals in complex pulmonary atresia. Circulation 1996;94:2479.

PULMONARY ATRESIA WITH INTACT VENTRICULAR SEPTUM

Essentials of Diagnosis & Typical Features

- Cyanosis at birth.
- Chest x-ray film with a concave pulmonary artery segment and the apex tilted upward.

General Considerations

In this uncommon condition, the pulmonary valve is absent and is replaced by a small diaphragm consisting of the fused cusps. The ventricular septum is intact. The main pulmonary artery segment is somewhat hypoplastic but almost always patent. In type 1 deformity (80%), the cavity volume of the right ventricle is extremely small and the wall is thickened and fibrotic. In type 2, the right ventricular cavity is frequently of normal size.

During intrauterine life, if the tricuspid valve is intact and normal, very little blood enters the right ventricle, since there is no outlet for this chamber. Almost all of the blood passes through the foramen ovale directly into the left side of the heart. In type 2 deformity, there is usually an outlet for the right ventricle (tricuspid valve insufficiency), and the right

ventricle receives a sufficient quantity of blood to permit it to develop in a relatively normal fashion.

Following birth, the pulmonary circulation is maintained primarily by a patent ductus arteriosus. Although a bronchial pulmonary collateral network is present, it is usually insufficient to maintain the pulmonary circulation. Accordingly, whether or not the patients live depends on the patency of the ductus arteriosus. The ductus usually remains open for only a short period. As it closes, hypoxia becomes progressively more severe, and death occurs within several hours.

Clinical Findings

A. Symptoms and Signs: Patients may be normal at birth, although they are usually cyanotic. Cyanosis becomes progressively more severe and is associated with severe dyspnea. A blowing systolic murmur resulting from the associated patent ductus arteriosus may be heard at the pulmonary area and under the left clavicle. In type 2 deformity, a loud pansystolic murmur caused by the tricuspid insufficiency is heard at the lower left sternal border. Not infrequently, the liver is pulsatile.

B. Imaging: Chest x-rays vary from a small to a markedly enlarged heart, depending on the presence or degree of tricuspid insufficiency. With striking tricuspid insufficiency, right atrial enlargement may be massive and the cardiac silhouette may virtually fill the chest.

C. Electrocardiography: Electrocardiography reveals an axis that is usually normal in the frontal plane. Evidence for right atrial enlargement is usually striking. Voltage criteria for other chamber enlargement are variable.

D. Echocardiography: M-mode and two-dimensional echocardiography shows absence of the pulmonary valve, with varying degrees of hypoplasia of the right ventricular cavity and tricuspid annulus. The severity of tricuspid regurgitation often correlates positively with right ventricular size.

E. Cardiac Catheterization and Angiocardiography: Right ventricular pressure is very high (greater than systemic). A cineangiocardiogram following injection of contrast material into the right ventricle reveals absence of filling of the pulmonary artery from the right ventricle. It also demonstrates the size of the right ventricular chamber, relative hypoplasia of the components of the tripartite right ventricle (inflow, trabecular, infundibulum), and the presence or absence of tricuspid regurgitation, and right ventricular sinusoids that anastomose with the coronary arteries may fill.

Treatment & Prognosis

As in pulmonary atresia with ventricular septal defect, a PGE_1 infusion is useful in stabilizing the patient and maintaining patency of the ductus until surgery can be performed. Surgery should be undertaken as soon as the diagnosis is made. A Rashkind atrial septostomy is performed, depending on right ventricular size, to open up the communication across the atrial septum. Increasingly, the pulmonary valve plate is being perforated at cardiac catheterization by a variety of means. Subsequent surgical approaches vary widely. In cases of type 1 deformity, it is necessary to immediately establish a surgical aorticopulmonary anastomosis (usually a Blalock-Taussig shunt). Later in infancy, a communication between the right ventricle and pulmonary artery should be created in an attempt to stimulate right ventricular cavity growth. If right ventricular dimensions or function are inadequate for a two-ventricular repair, a one-ventricular systemic venous to pulmonary artery palliation is indicated. In cases of type 2 deformity, a closed valvotomy may be all that is necessary initially, with a more definitive reconstruction of the right ventricular outflow tract accomplished at a later date.

The prognosis is unpredictable for patients with type 1 or type 2 deformity who survive the surgery. In type 1 patients, the dimensions of the right ventricle can increase significantly after the initial procedure. Overall, however, this disorder remains one of the least satisfactory forms of cyanotic congenital heart disease.

Hanley FL et al: Outcomes in neonatal pulmonary atresia with intact ventricular septum: A multiinstitutional study. J Am Coll Cardiol 1993;21:1454.

Wright SB, Radtke WA, Gillette PC: Percutaneous radiofrequency valvotomy using a standard 5Fr electrode catheter for pulmonary atresia in neonates. Am J Cardiol 1996;77:1370.

TRICUSPID ATRESIA

Essentials of Diagnosis & Typical Features

• Marked cyanosis present from birth.
• ECG with left axis deviation, right atrial enlargement, and left ventricular hypertrophy.

General Considerations

This relatively rare condition (< 1% of cases of congenital heart disease) is characterized by complete atresia of the tricuspid valve. As a result, no direct communication exists between the right atrium and the right ventricle.

Tricuspid atresia may be divided into two types, depending on the relationship of the great vessels (Table 18–3).

Because there is no direct communication between the right atrium and the right ventricle, the entire systemic venous return must flow through the atrial septum (either an atrial septal defect or patent foramen ovale) into the left atrium. Accordingly, the left

Table 18–3. Tricuspid atresia.

Type 1: Without transposition of the great arteries	Type 2: With transposition of the great arteries
(a) No ventricular septal defect; hypoplasia or atresia of the pulmonary artery; patent ductus arteriosus (b) Small ventricular septal defect; pulmonary stenosis; hypoplastic pulmonary artery (c) Large ventricular septal defect and no pulmonary stenosis; normal-sized pulmonary artery	(a) With ventricular septal defect and pulmonary stenosis (b) With ventricular septal defect but without pulmonary stenosis

atrium receives both the systemic venous return and the pulmonary venous return. Complete mixing occurs in the left atrium, resulting in a greater or lesser degree of arterial desaturation.

As a result of this lack of direct communication, the development of the ventricle depends on the presence of a left-to-right shunt at the ventricular level. Therefore, severe hypoplasia of the right ventricle occurs in those forms in which there is no ventricular septal defect or in which the ventricular septal defect is very small.

Clinical Findings

A. Symptoms and Signs: In most patients with tricuspid atresia, symptoms develop very early in infancy. Except in patients whose pulmonary blood flow is great, cyanosis is present at birth. Growth and development are very poor, and there is usually easy fatigability on feeding, tachypnea, dyspnea, anoxic spells, and evidence of right heart failure. Patients with marked increase in pulmonary blood flow—types 1(c) and 2(b)—may develop evidence of left heart failure as well.

Clubbing is present if the child is old enough. On examination of the heart, a slight bulge on the right side of the sternum may occasionally be seen. The first heart sound is normal. The second heart sound is most often single (owing to aortic closure). A murmur is usually present, although it is variable. It ranges from grade I to grade III/VI in intensity and usually is a harsh blowing murmur heard best at the lower left sternal border.

B. Imaging: Chest x-ray findings are variable. The heart may be slightly to markedly enlarged. The main pulmonary artery segment is usually small or absent. The size of the right atrium varies from huge to only moderately enlarged, depending on the size of the communication at the atrial level. The pulmonary vascular markings are usually decreased, although in types 1(c) and 2(b) they are increased.

C. Electrocardiography: The ECG is usually helpful. It often shows a left axis deviation with a counterclockwise loop in the frontal plane. The P waves are tall and peaked, indicative of right atrial hypertrophy. The size of the P wave depends on the right atrial pressure, which in turn depends on the size of the interatrial communication (the taller the P wave, the smaller the communication). Left ventricular hypertrophy or left ventricular preponderance is found in almost all cases. Voltage over the right precordium is usually low.

D. Echocardiography: M-mode and two-dimensional methods are diagnostic and show absence of the tricuspid valve, the relationship of the great vessels, and the sources of pulmonary blood flow.

E. Cardiac Catheterization and Angiocardiography: This reveals the marked right-to-left shunt at the atrial level and desaturation of the left atrial blood. Because of the complete mixing in the left atrial chambers, oxygen saturation in the left ventricle, right ventricle, pulmonary artery, and aorta is identical to that in the left atrium. The right atrial pressure is increased. Left ventricular and systemic pressures are normal. The catheter cannot be passed through the tricuspid valve from the right atrium to the right ventricle. The course of the catheter is always from the right atrium into the left atrium and from there into the left ventricle. An atrial balloon septostomy is performed if a restrictive communication is present.

Treatment & Prognosis

In infants with high pulmonary artery flow, conventional anticongestive therapy should be given until the infant begins to outgrow the ventricular septal defect. Occasionally, a pulmonary artery band is needed to protect the pulmonary vascular bed in preparation for a Fontan procedure. A Fontan procedure (connection of the systemic venous return to the right ventricle or pulmonary artery) is performed when increasing cyanosis occurs.

In infants with extremely low pulmonary artery flow, PGE_1 should be infused until an aorticopulmonary shunt can be performed. A Fontan procedure or Glenn procedure is usually performed after 6 months of age.

The prognosis for all patients with tricuspid atresia depends on achieving a balance of pulmonary blood flow that permits adequate oxygenation of the tissues without producing intractable congestive heart failure. For children treated by the Fontan procedure, the prognosis is as yet undefined; initial results are moderately encouraging.

Bradley SM et al: Bidirectional superior cavopulmonary connection in young infants. Circulation 1996;94 (Suppl):II-5.
Franklin RCG et al: Tricuspid atresia presenting in infancy:

Survival and suitability for the Fontan operation. Circulation 1993;87:427.

HYPOPLASTIC LEFT HEART SYNDROME

Essentials of Diagnosis & Typical Features
- Mild cyanosis at birth. Minimal auscultatory findings.
- Rapid onset of shock with ductal closure.

General Considerations

Hypoplastic left heart syndrome includes a number of conditions in which there are either valvular or vascular lesions on the left side of the heart, resulting in hypoplasia of the left ventricle. The syndrome is found in 1.4–3.8% of infants with congenital heart disease.

The lesions that make up this syndrome are mitral atresia, aortic atresia, or both. In all of these conditions, there is severe obstruction to either filling or emptying of the left ventricle. As a result, during intrauterine life, the quantity of blood filling the left ventricle is extremely small, resulting in hypoplasia of this chamber. Following birth, survival depends on a patent ductus arteriosus. there is marked impairment of the circulation because of the very small size of the left ventricle and the presence of obstructing lesions. Congestive heart failure develops rapidly, in most cases within several days to 3 months of life.

Patients with aortic atresia develop congestive heart failure very early, usually within the first week. Death occurs earliest in this group. Patients with mitral atresia who have large atrial and ventricular communications may live longer. Some patients have lived beyond the first decade. Patients with involvement of the aortic arch usually die within 1 month or less.

Clinical Findings

A. Symptoms and Signs: The clinical picture depends on the type of obstructing lesion. Cyanosis is usually present early in life and is usually generalized. Patients with hypoplasia or atresia of the aortic arch may show differential cyanosis. Murmurs may or may not be present and are usually nondiagnostic. Congestive heart failure and shock accompany closure of the ductus arteriosus.

B. Imaging: Chest x-ray findings usually are relatively normal at birth. Rapid and progressive cardiac enlargement then occurs, frequently associated with pulmonary venous congestion. These changes occur earliest in patients with aortic atresia.

C. Electrocardiography: The ECG usually demonstrates right axis deviation, right atrial hypertrophy, and right ventricular hypertrophy with relative paucity of left ventricular forces and absence of a Q wave in V_6.

D. Echocardiography: Echocardiography is usually diagnostic and eliminates the need for cardiac catheterization. A diminutive aorta and left ventricle with a poorly defined mitral valve in the presence of a normal and easily definable tricuspid valve are diagnostic. The systemic circulation is dependent on the patent ductus arteriosus. There is retrograde flow in the aortic arch with color doppler imaging.

Treatment & Prognosis

PGE_1 infusion is essential initial management, since systemic circulation depends on a patent ductus arteriosus. Further management depends on balancing pulmonary and systemic blood flow, because the right ventricle provides both. With increasing postnatal age, the pulmonary resistance falls, favoring pulmonary overcirculation and compromised systemic perfusion. Techniques to increase pulmonary vascular tone—such as hypoxia and hypercapnic ventilation, increased viscosity (hematocrit), and avoidance of pharmacologic pulmonary vasodilators—can improve systemic perfusion.

Palliative therapy at present is creation of single-ventricle physiology operatively, as with the Norwood procedure and its variants. An increasing number of infants are receiving orthotopic cardiac transplantation in infancy to replace the defective cardiac anatomy.

The prognosis for this once uniformly lethal syndrome is improving. Palliative operations can now be performed with survival rates of 50–75%. Many palliated infants may ultimately require transplantation. The 1-year survival rates with primary transplantation are over 80%. Further advances in surgery and immunology are likely to continue to improve the prognosis.

Boucek MM, Bernstein D: Heart transplantation in infancy. Prog Pediatr Cardiol 1993;2:20.

Morris CD, Outcalt J, Menashe VD: Hypoplastic left heart syndrome: Natural history in a geographically defined population. Pediatrics 1990;85:977.

Shaddy RE et al: Outcome of cardiac transplantation in children. Survival in a contemporary multi institutional experience. Circulation 1996;94(Suppl):II-69.

COMPLETE TRANSPOSITION OF THE GREAT ARTERIES

Essentials of Diagnosis & Typical Features

- Cyanotic newborn without respiratory distress.
- More common in males.

General Considerations

Complete transposition of the great vessels is the second most common variety of cyanotic congenital heart disease, accounting for about 16% of all cases. The male/female ratio is 3:1. The disorder is caused by an embryologic abnormality in the spiral division of the truncus arteriosus.

The aorta is located anterior to the pulmonary artery—either directly anterior or to the left or right. The pulmonary artery usually ascends parallel to the aorta rather than crosses it. In most cases, associated intracardiac abnormalities are present. These include ventricular septal defect, atrial septal defect, pulmonary stenosis, and patent ductus arteriosus. Obstructive changes within the pulmonary arteriolar bed are common in patients past infancy.

Transposition of the great vessels can be classified in two types (Table 18–4).

Since the aorta arises directly from the right ventricle, life would not be possible unless there were mixing between the systemic and pulmonary circulations; oxygenated blood from the pulmonary veins must, in some way, reach the systemic arterial circuit. In patients with intact ventricular septum (group 1), mixing occurs at the atrial and also at the ductal levels. However, in most patients, these communications are small, and the ductus arteriosus often closes shortly after birth. These patients are therefore severely cyanotic, and congestive heart failure occurs rapidly as a result of the marked increase in cardiac output. Patients with a ventricular septal defect show greater or lesser degrees of cyanosis, depending on the ratio of the pulmonary to systemic blood flow. Patients with ventricular septal defect and pulmonary stenosis—groups 2(a) and 2(b)—are usually severely cyanotic because of the limited blood flow to the lungs. Patients with ventricular septal defect and pulmonary vascular obstruction (group 2[b]) show a moderate degree of cyanosis. Patients with ventricular septal defect and normal pulmonary vascular resistance (group 2[c]) show the least cyanosis but often develop heart failure very early because of the enormous pulmonary blood flow.

Congestive heart failure develops not only because of the high cardiac output but also because of the poor oxygenation of the myocardium and the presence of systemic pressure in both ventricles.

Table 18–4. Complete transposition of the great arteries.

Group 1: With intact ventricular septum	Group 2: With ventricular septal defect
(a) Without pulmonary stenosis	(a) With pulmonary stenosis
(b) With pulmonary stenosis subvalvular or valvular (or both)	(b) With pulmonary vascular obstruction
	(c) Without pulmonary vascular obstruction (normal pulmonary vascular resistance)

Clinical Findings

A. Symptoms and Signs: Many of the neonates are large, some weighing 4 kg at birth, and most are cyanotic at birth, although cyanosis occasionally does not develop until later. Patients in groups 1 and 2(a) are most cyanotic. Retardation of growth and development after the neonatal period is common. Congestive heart failure occurs in patients in groups 1 and 2(c). Patients in group 2(a) show no evidence of congestive heart failure but often have severe anoxic spells in early life.

Although these infants are usually large at birth, growth and development are retarded before definitive surgery. The findings on cardiovascular examination depend somewhat on the intracardiac defects. Group 1(a) patients have only soft murmurs or none at all. The first heart sound is usually normal. The second heart sound is single and accentuated and is best heard at the lower left sternal border. Patients in group 1(b) have loud obstructive systolic murmurs that are maximal at the second and third intercostal spaces and the left sternal border, radiating well to the first and second intercostal spaces. Group 2(a) patients have a murmur of pulmonary stenosis (obstructive systolic murmur at the base of the heart, best heard to the right of the sternum). Those in group 2(c) have a systolic murmur along the lower sternal border and a mitral diastolic flow murmur at the apex.

B. Imaging: In the sick, blue newborn, at a time when any diagnostic clues are greatly appreciated, the chest x-ray in transposition is often very nonspecific.

C. Electrocardiography: Early in infancy, the ECG is usually of little positive help. It reveals the usual amount of right ventricular hypertrophy expected for age.

D. Echocardiography: Two-dimensional imaging and doppler evaluation can accurately describe the anatomy and physiology in infants with transposition. The abnormal relationship of the great vessels is the hallmark of transposition on echocardiography. Even the balloon septostomy may be performed with echo guidance.

E. Cardiac Catheterization and Angiocardiography: Cardiac catheterization has a dual purpose in this malformation: diagnosis and therapy. As soon as the cardiologist has confidently demonstrated that complete transposition of the great arteries exists and that there are two well-developed ventricles, a Rashkind septostomy may be performed. The coronary anatomy can be delineated by ascending aortography.

Treatment

It has become increasingly apparent at many pediatric cardiology centers throughout the world that survival of patients with transposition of the great arteries depends on early, aggressive management.

Cardiac catheterization is no longer routine for all types of transposition. Complex variations such as 2(a), 2(b), and 2(c) may still require invasive evaluation. PGE_1 infusion may improve mixing of oxygenated blood by opening the ductus arteriosus.

All patients with favorable anatomic and hemodynamic criteria (type 1) should be offered corrective surgery by 2 weeks of age. Surgery traditionally involved insertion of an intra-atrial baffle (by either a Mustard or a Senning operation) to redirect systemic and pulmonary venous blood to the appropriate pulmonary and aortic ventricles. Since 1975, surgical techniques to "switch" the great vessels to their anatomically appropriate locations have undergone a slow evolution. A key feature in the development of techniques has been careful patient selection. The left ventricular musculature in this entity rapidly loses its muscle mass and potential to meet systemic afterload unless a large ventricular septal defect or left ventricular outflow obstruction occurs; consequently, newborns with either of these conditions are appropriate candidates.

The incidence of death from this type of surgery has fallen from 25% to approximately 5% or less. Although the death rate following an intra-atrial baffling procedure may be lower, there is growing concern about the long-term ability of an anatomic right ventricle to function as a systemic circulation pump. During the past several years, most institutions have begun using anatomic correction techniques in almost all patients. As the use of anatomic correction (vessel switch) techniques has spread to more centers, postoperative complications such as supravalvular pulmonary stenosis and stenoses or kinking of coronary arteries have been noted. The long-term exercise capacity of patients after interatrial rerouting operations has, in some studies, turned out to be better than that projected by early studies. Long-term results for anatomic correction are yet to be determined. The intermediate-term results appear to be excellent for the arterial switch procedure.

Bonhoeffer P et al: Coronary artery obstruction after the arterial switch operation for transposition of the great arteries in newborns. J Am Coll Cardiol 1997;29:202.

Gelatt M et al: Arrhythmia and mortality after the Mustard procedure: A 30-year single-center experience. J Am Coll Cardiol 1997;29:194.

ORIGIN OF BOTH GREAT VESSELS FROM THE RIGHT VENTRICLE

In this rare malformation, the aorta is completely transposed, but the pulmonary artery occupies a relatively normal position. Accordingly, both great vessels arise from the right ventricle. Ventricular septal defect is present in all cases and provides the only outlet for the left ventricle.

This malformation may be divided into five types on the basis of the relationship of the ventricular septal defect to the great arteries and the presence or absence of pulmonary stenosis: (1) ventricular septal defect related to the aorta, (2) ventricular septal defect related to the pulmonary artery (Taussig-Bing type), (3) ventricular septal defect committed to both great vessels, (4) ventricular septal defect uncommitted to the great vessels, and (5) ventricular septal defect related to the aorta, with pulmonary stenosis (tetralogy of Fallot type).

The clinical and laboratory features depend on which of the five anatomic types occurs. Two-dimensional echocardiography has proved to be extremely important in the diagnosis and classification of this entity.

Surgical correction is most satisfactory in patients with ventricular septal defect related to the aorta and is effected by closing the defect and creating a tunnel from the left ventricle to the aorta via the patch. Correction of uncommitted defects or defects related to the pulmonary artery requires patch closure and directing the blood to the pulmonary artery, thereby creating a transposition of the great vessels and an associated interatrial rerouting procedure. The use of a valved external conduit may be necessary in the complex varieties.

Roberson DA, Silverman NH: Malaligned outlet septum with subpulmonary ventricular septal defect and abnormal ventriculoarterial connection: A morphologic spectrum defined echocardiographically. J Am Coll Cardiol 1990;16:459.

Tchervenkov CI et al: Institutional experience with a protocol of early primary repair of double outlet right ventricle. Ann Thorac Surg 1995;60(Suppl):610.

TOTAL ANOMALOUS PULMONARY VENOUS RETURN WITH OR WITHOUT OBSTRUCTION

Essentials of Diagnosis & Typical Features

- Cyanosis.
- Systolic ejection murmur with left sternal border flow rumble and accentuated P_2.
- Right atrial and right ventricular hypertrophy.
- Pulmonary venous connection.

General Considerations

This malformation accounts for approximately 2% of all congenital heart lesions. The pulmonary venous blood drains not into the left atrium but either directly or indirectly (via a systemic venous connection) into the right atrium. Thus, the entire venous drainage of the body drains into the right atrium.

This malformation may be classified according to the site of entry of the pulmonary veins into the right side of the heart.

Type 1 (55%): Entry into the left superior vena cava (persistent anterior cardinal vein) or right superior vena cava.

Type 2: Entry into the right atrium or into the coronary sinus.

Type 3: Entry below the diaphragm (usually into the portal vein).

Type 4: Multiple types of entry.

Since the entire venous drainage from the body drains into the right atrium, a right-to-left shunt is always present at the atrial level. This may take the form of either a large atrial septal defect or a patent foramen ovale. Relatively complete mixing of the systemic and pulmonary venous return occurs in the right atrium, so that the left atrial and hence the systemic arterial saturation levels approximately equal that of the right atrial saturation.

The degree of desaturation of the blood (and thus the degree of cyanosis present) is determined by the ratio of the quantity of pulmonary blood flow to that of the systemic blood flow.

Clinical Findings

A. With Normal Pulmonary Vascular Resistance: Most patients in this group have some elevation of the pulmonary artery pressure owing to the marked increase in pulmonary blood flow. In most cases, the pressure does not reach systemic levels.

1. Symptoms and signs–These patients may have a history of mild cyanosis in the neonatal period and during early infancy. Thereafter, they do relatively well except for frequent respiratory infections. They are usually rather small and thin and resemble patients with very large atrial septal defects.

Careful examination discloses duskiness of the nail beds and mucous membranes, but definite cyanosis and clubbing are usually not present. The arterial pulses are normal. The jugular venous pulses usually show a significant v wave. Examination of the heart shows left chest prominence. A right ventricular heaving impulse is palpable.

The pulmonary component of the second sound is usually increased in intensity. A grade II–IV/VI ejection-type systolic murmur is heard at the pulmonary area. It radiates very well over the lung fields anteriorly and posteriorly. An early to mid-diastolic flow murmur is often heard at the lower left sternal border in the third and fourth intercostal spaces (tricuspid flow murmur).

2. Imaging–Chest x-ray reveals evidence of cardiac enlargement primarily involving the right atrium, right ventricle, and pulmonary artery. There is a marked increase in pulmonary vascular markings. There is often a characteristic contour called a "snowman" or "figure of 8," which is seen where the anomalous veins drain into a persistent left superior vena cava.

3. Electrocardiography–Electrocardiography reveals right axis deviation and varying degrees of right atrial and right ventricular hypertrophy. There is often a QR pattern over the right precordial leads.

4. Echocardiography–Demonstration by echocardiography of a chamber posterior to the left atrium is strongly suggestive of the diagnosis. However, echocardiographic discrimination between anomalies of pulmonary venous return and persistence of pulmonary fetal circulation can still be challenging. The availability of two-dimensional echocardiography plus color flow Doppler has increased the diagnostic accuracy.

B. With Increased Pulmonary Vascular Resistance: This group includes patients in whom the pulmonary veins drain into a systemic venous structure below the diaphragm. It also includes a small number of patients in whom the venous drainage is into a systemic vein above the diaphragm.

1. Symptoms and signs–These infants are usually quite sick. Fifty percent die within the first 6 months; most are dead by age 1 year unless treated surgically. Cyanosis is common at birth and is evident by 1 week. Another common early symptom is severe tachypnea. Congestive heart failure develops later.

Cardiac examination discloses a striking right ventricular impulse. A shock of the second sound is palpable. The first heart sound is accentuated. The second heart sound is markedly accentuated and single. A grade I–II/VI ejection-type systolic murmur is frequently heard over the pulmonary area with radiation over the lung fields. Diastolic murmurs are uncommon. In many cases, no murmur is heard at all.

2. Imaging–In the most severe and classic cases, the heart is small and pulmonary venous congestion is marked. In less severe cases, the heart may be slightly enlarged or normal in size, with only slight pulmonary venous congestion.

3. Electrocardiography–The ECG shows right axis deviation, right atrial hypertrophy, and right ventricular hypertrophy.

4. Echocardiography–Echocardiography may demonstrate the combination of a small left atrium and a vessel lying parallel and anterior to the descending aorta and to the left of the inferior vena cava. Color flow Doppler echocardiographic patterns are useful in establishing the diagnosis and are often diagnostic.

5. Cardiac catheterization and angiocardiography–These procedures are diagnostic. Cardiac catheterization demonstrates the presence of total anomalous pulmonary venous return and (usually) the site of entry of the anomalous veins. It also demonstrates the ratio of the pulmonary to systemic blood flow and the degree of pulmonary hypertension and pulmonary vascular resistance.

Cineangiocardiography following injection of contrast material into the right ventricle or pulmonary artery demonstrates the presence of anomalous pulmonary venous return and the site of entry of the anomalous veins.

Treatment

If immediate surgical intervention is not contemplated, atrial balloon septostomy should be performed during the initial diagnostic cardiac catheterization. This procedure, combined with vigorous medical management, may sustain some infants for several months. Most centers have reported excellent surgical results using either cardiopulmonary bypass or deep hypothermia (cooling to 20 °C). A modification of the anastomosis allowing a larger communication has also greatly improved the surgical results. In such centers, the option of immediate surgical correction may be taken.

Course & Prognosis

Patients with normal pulmonary vascular resistance and only modest elevation of pulmonary artery pressures may do well through the first or second decade. Eventually, however, a progressive increase in pulmonary vascular resistance and pulmonary hypertension does occur. Patients with increased pulmonary vascular resistance and pulmonary hypertension do poorly, and most die unless treated before age 1 year.

Bando K et al: Surgical management of total anomalous pulmonary venous connection: 30 year trends. Circulation 1996;94(Suppl):II-12
Wang JK et al: Obstructed total anomalous pulmonary venous connection. Pediatr Cardiol 1993;14:28.

PERSISTENT TRUNCUS ARTERIOSUS

Essentials of Diagnosis & Typical Features
- Neonatal cyanosis.
- Systolic ejection click.

General Considerations

Persistent truncus arteriosus probably accounts for less than 1% of all congenital heart malformations. Only one (huge) great vessel arises from the heart and supplies both the systemic and pulmonary arterial beds. It develops embryologically as a result of complete lack of formation of the spiral ridges that divide the fetal truncus arteriosus into the aorta and the pulmonary artery. A high ventricular septal defect is always present. The number of valve leaflets varies from two to six, and the valve may be sufficient, insufficient, or stenotic.

The classification most commonly used is into four types:

Type 1: One pulmonary artery that arises from the base of the trunk just above the semilunar valve and runs parallel with the ascending aorta (48%).

Type 2: Two pulmonary arteries that arise side by side from the posterior aspect of the truncus (29%).

Type 3: Two pulmonary arteries that arise independently from either side of the trunk (11%).

Type 4: No demonstrable pulmonary artery (12%). Pulmonary circulation is derived from bronchials arising from the descending thoracic aorta. (The existence of this variety of truncus is controversial. Many authorities consider it an extreme form of tetralogy of Fallot with an atretic main pulmonary artery.)

In this condition, blood leaves the heart through a single common exit. Therefore, the saturation of the blood in the pulmonary artery is the same as that in the systemic arteries. The degree of systemic arterial oxygen saturation depends on the ratio of the pulmonary to systemic blood flow. If pulmonary vascular resistance is normal, the pulmonary blood flow is much greater than the systemic blood flow and the saturation is relatively high. If pulmonary vascular resistance is great, owing either to pulmonary vascular obstruction or to very small pulmonary arteries, pulmonary blood flow is reduced and oxygen saturation is low. The systolic pressures in both ventricles are identical to that in the aorta.

Clinical Findings

A. Symptoms and Signs: The clinical picture varies depending on the degree of pulmonary blood flow.

1. Large pulmonary blood flow–Patients with large pulmonary blood flow do well and are usually acyanotic, although the nail beds are commonly dusky. They function similarly to patients with large ventricular septal defects and pulmonary hypertension. Examination of the heart reveals a hyperactive impulse, felt both at the apex and over the xiphoid process. A systolic thrill is common at the lower left sternal border. The first heart sound is normal. A loud early systolic ejection click is commonly heard. The second sound is single and accentuated. A grade IV/VI, completely pansystolic murmur is audible at the lower left sternal border. A diastolic flow murmur can often be heard at the apex (mitral flow murmur).

2. Decreased pulmonary blood flow–Patients with decreased pulmonary blood flow have marked cyanosis early and do very poorly. The most common manifestations include retardation of growth and development, easy fatigability, dyspnea on exertion, and congestive heart failure. The heart is not unduly active. The first and second heart sounds are loud. A systolic grade II–IV/VI murmur is heard at the lower left sternal border. No diastolic flow murmur is heard. A continuous heart murmur is very uncommon except in type 4, in which the continuous murmur is caused by the large bronchial collateral vessels. A very loud systolic ejection click is commonly heard.

B. Imaging: The most common x-ray findings are a boot-shaped heart, absence of the main pulmonary artery segment, and a large aorta that frequently arches to the right. The pulmonary vascular markings vary, depending on the degree of pulmonary blood flow.

C. Electrocardiography: The axis is usually normal, although left axis deviation occurs rarely. Evidence of right ventricular hypertrophy or combined ventricular hypertrophy is commonly present. Left ventricular hypertrophy as an isolated finding is rare.

D. Echocardiography: A characteristic image would exhibit override of a single great artery (similar to tetralogy of Fallot) without a demonstrable right ventricular infundibulum. The origin or the pulmonary arteries and the degree of truncal valve abnormality can be seen. Color flow doppler can aid in the description of pulmonary flow.

E. Angiocardiography: This procedure is usually diagnostic. Injection of contrast material into the right ventricle demonstrates the presence of a ventricular septal defect and the single vessel arising from the heart. The exact type of truncus, however, may be somewhat difficult to determine even from angiocardiograms.

Treatment

Anticongestive measures are indicated for patients with high pulmonary blood flow and congestive failure. Aortic homografting for "total correction" of the truncus has been performed in selected patients. During the past several years, the number of severely symptomatic infants undergoing successful "total correction" in the first 3 months of life has increased. Operative repair requires placement of a conduit from right ventricle to the pulmonary artery, and as the child grows replacement will be necessary.

Course & Prognosis

The outcome depends to a great extent on the status of the pulmonary circulation and the competence of the truncal valve. Patients with a low pulmonary blood flow usually do very poorly and die within 1 year. Those with increased pulmonary blood flow can survive for a variable period. A few cases of survival without surgery into the third decade have been reported. Death is usually the result of congestive heart failure, hypoxia, subacute infective endocarditis, or brain abscess. Surgical repair has dramatically improved the prognosis.

Juanida E, Haworth SG: Pulmonary vascular disease in children with truncus arteriosus. Am J Cardiol 1984; 54:1315.

NaKae S et al: Correction of truncus arteriosus in autologous arterial flap in neonates and small infants. Ann Thorac Surg 1996;62:123.

Samanek M: Children with congenital heart disease: Probability of natural survival. Pediatr Cardiol 1992;13:152.

DEXTROCARDIA

This lesion consists of right-sided heart with or without reversal of position of other organs (situs inversus). If there is no reversal of other organs, the heart usually has other severe defects. With complete situs inversus, the heart is usually normal.

Apical pulse and sounds are heard on the right side of the chest. X-ray film shows the cardiac silhouette on the right side. On electrocardiography, the P waves are usually inverted in lead I; QRS is predominantly down in lead I; and lead II resembles normal lead III and vice versa. Two-dimensional echocardiography is extremely useful in defining the complex anatomy.

With situs inversus and no heart defects, the prognosis is excellent. If severe heart defects are present, definitive diagnosis is imperative, because corrective surgery is frequently beneficial.

Emmanouilides GC, Baylen BG: Dextrocardia and the cardiosplenic syndromes. In: *Neonatal Cardiopulmonary Distress.* Emmanouilides GC, Baylen BG (editors). Year Book, 1988.

Van Praagh R et al: Malposition of the heart. In: *Heart Disease in Infants, Children, and Adolescents,* 4th ed. Adams FH, Emmanouilides GC, Riemenschneider TA (editors). Williams & Wilkins, 1989.

ACQUIRED HEART DISEASE

RHEUMATIC FEVER

Rheumatic fever is a disease in transition. Although it is still an important disease in the United States, its incidence has diminished significantly over the past half-century. Penicillin is largely responsible, but the decrease in rheumatic fever was already apparent before the antibiotic era. In the United States and other developed countries in the temperate zone, improvement in standards of living, general hygiene, and opportunities for medical care have greatly reduced the incidence of this disease. However, there has been a resurgence of acute rheumatic fever in several regions of the United States (the Midwest in 1984 and the intermountain West in 1987). In addition, the character of the illness is more malignant than that seen in the 1970s, with a high incidence of associated carditis and chorea. The reason for these regional epidemics is not as yet known, but it is clear that the disease has returned.

Until the recent epidemic, the symptomatic presentation of the disease had also changed significantly in the United States within the past 2 decades. The frequency with which one encounters severe, disabling carditis has greatly diminished, and the attack rate of acute rheumatic fever is considerably less than the original estimate of 0.3% in untreated children. Current manifestations of carditis are often mild and transient and require serial examinations by a skilled auscultator or echocardiography to confirm or rule out the diagnosis. The combination of chorea and carditis, previously noted to be rare, has been common during the recent epidemic. One can only speculate on the reasons for these changes in the epidemiologic characteristics of the disease in different communities.

Group A β-hemolytic streptococcal infection of the upper respiratory tract is the essential environmental trigger that acts on predisposed individuals. The latest attempts to define host susceptibility implicate immune response (Ir) genes, which are present in approximately 15% of the population. The immune response triggered by colonization of the pharynx with group A streptococci consists of (1) sensitization of B lymphocytes by streptococcal antigens, (2) formation of antistreptococcal antibody, (3) formation of immune complexes that cross-react with cardiac sarcolemma antigens, and (4) myocardial and valvular inflammatory response.

The peak period of risk in the United States is age 5–15 years. The disease is slightly more common in girls and is now more common in blacks, perhaps reflecting socioeconomic factors. The average annual attack rate in the total North American population is less than 1:10,000, and the presence of rheumatic heart disease in the school-age population is less than 1:1000. The annual death rate from rheumatic heart disease in school-age children (whites and nonwhites) recorded in the 1980s was less than 1:100,000.

Jones Criteria (Revised) for Diagnosis of Rheumatic Fever

Major manifestations
Carditis
Polyarthritis
Sydenham's chorea
Erythema marginatum
Subcutaneous nodules

Minor manifestations
Clinical
Previous rheumatic fever or rheumatic heart disease
Polyarthralgia
Fever
Laboratory
Acute phase reaction: elevated erythrocyte sedimentation rate, C-reactive protein, leukocytosis
Prolonged PR interval

Plus

Supporting evidence of preceding streptococcal infection, ie, increased titers of antistreptolysin O or other streptococcal antibodies, positive throat culture for group A *Streptococcus.*

Traditionally, two major or one major and two minor criteria (plus supporting evidence of streptococcal infection) justified the presumptive diagnosis of rheumatic fever. However, the major modern dilemma regarding diagnosis is that the physical findings may be so subtle and transient that the criteria are marginal. Since improper diagnosis has lifelong and serious consequences, it is justified to hospitalize patients with marginal findings so that serial clinical studies of the patient, including multiple examinations by a pediatric cardiologist, can be performed. If rheumatic fever appears likely on the basis of appropriate and careful evaluation but does not fully meet the revised Jones criteria, the diagnosis of suspect acute rheumatic fever is appropriate. This diagnosis mandates anti-infective prophylaxis but attempts to avoid the social and economic sequelae of the full diagnosis.

Major Manifestations of Rheumatic Fever

A. Active Carditis: Any one of the following.

1. A significant *new* murmur that is clearly mitral insufficiency (with or without a transient apical diastolic Carey Coombs murmur) or aortic insufficiency. It should be remembered that mitral insufficiency, while commonly caused by rheumatic fever, has many other causes in childhood.

2. Pericarditis, manifested by a pericardial friction rub or evidence of pericardial effusion.

3. Evidence of congestive heart failure.

B. Polyarthritis: Two or more joints must be involved; involvement of one joint does not constitute a major manifestation. The joints may be involved simultaneously or (more diagnostically) in a migratory fashion. The most commonly involved joints are the ankles, knees, hips, wrists, elbows, and shoulders. Heat, redness, swelling, severe pain, and tenderness are usually all present. Arthralgia alone without the other signs of inflammation is not sufficient to meet the criterion of polyarthritis.

C. Sydenham's Chorea: Sydenham's chorea is characterized by emotional instability and involuntary movements. These findings become progressively more severe and are often followed by the development of ataxia and slurring of speech. Muscular weakness becomes apparent following the onset of the involuntary movements. The individual attack of chorea is self-limiting, although it may last up to 3 months. It is not uncommon to find involvement on only one side. Manifestations may not be apparent for months to years after the acute episode of rheumatic fever.

D. Erythema Marginatum: Although this is a specific and major manifestation of acute rheumatic fever, many physicians fail to distinguish it from other skin lesions. It usually occurs only in severe cases and is rarely an essential diagnostic clue. It consists of a macular erythematous rash with a circinate border and appears primarily on the trunk and the extremities. The face is usually not involved.

E. Subcutaneous Nodules: These are usually seen only in severe cases, and then most commonly over the joints, scalp, and spinal column. They vary from a few millimeters to 2 cm in diameter and are nontender and freely movable under the skin.

Minor Manifestations of Rheumatic Fever

A. Polyarthralgia: Pain in two or more joints without heat, swelling, and tenderness is a minor rather than a major manifestation.

B. Fever: The fever is usually low-grade, although occasionally it reaches 39.4–40 °C.

C. Acute Phase Reaction: The sedimentation rate is accelerated and, more specifically, the C-reactive protein is elevated. Congestive heart failure does not influence the C-reactive protein and usually does not affect the sedimentation rate. Leukocytosis is the rule.

D. Electrocardiographic Changes: Prolongation of the PR interval represents only a minor manifestation and does not qualify as active carditis.

E. History: There is a prior history of acute rheumatic fever or the presence of inactive rheumatic heart disease.

Essential Manifestation

Except in cases of rheumatic fever presenting solely as Sydenham's chorea or long-standing carditis, there should be clear supporting evidence of a streptococcal infection such as scarlet fever, a positive throat culture for group A β-hemolytic *Streptococcus,* and increased antistreptolysin O or other streptococcal antibody titers. The antistreptolysin O titer is significantly higher in rheumatic fever than in uncomplicated streptococcal infections.

Other Manifestations

Associated findings may include erythema multiforme; abdominal, back, and precordial pain; and nontraumatic epistaxis, vomiting, malaise, weight loss, and anemia. The abdominal pain may mimic a "surgical abdomen," and many negative laparotomies have been performed in patients with acute rheumatic fever.

Treatment & Prophylaxis

A. Treatment of the Acute Episode:

1. Anti-infective therapy–Eradication of the streptococcal infection is essential. Benzathine penicillin G is the drug of choice. Depending on the age and weight of the patient, give a single intramuscular injection of 0.6–1.2 million units; alternatively, give penicillin V, 125–250 mg orally four times a day for 10 days. Erythromycin, 250 mg orally four times a day, may be substituted if the patient is allergic to penicillin.

2. Anti-inflammatory agents–

a. Aspirin–Patients with the contemporary form of the disease need significantly less aspirin than in the past. Currently, 30–60 mg/kg/d is given in four divided doses; this dosage is often more than sufficient to effect dramatic relief of the arthritis and fever. In general, higher dosages carry a greater risk of side effects, and there are no proved short-term or long-term benefits of giving high doses to effect salicylate blood levels of 20–30 mg/dL. The duration of therapy must be tailored to meet the needs of the patient, but use of aspirin for 2–6 weeks, with reduction in dosage toward the end of the course, is usually sufficient.

b. Corticosteroids–Corticosteroids are rarely indicated in current therapy. However, in the unusual patient with severe carditis and manifestations of congestive heart failure (as evidenced by radiographic findings of cardiomegaly or by cardiopulmonary symptoms or a gallop rhythm), therapy may be not only effective but lifesaving. Corticosteroid therapy may be given as follows: prednisone, 2 mg/kg/d orally for 2 weeks (or comparable doses of other corticosteroids); reduce prednisone to 1 mg/kg/d the third week, and begin aspirin, 50 mg/kg/d; stop prednisone at the end of 3 weeks, and continue aspirin for 8 weeks or until the C-reactive protein is negative and the sedimentation rate is falling.

3. Therapy of congestive heart failure–See Congestive Heart Failure, above.

4. Bed rest and ambulation–Strict bed rest is not required for patients with arthritis and mild carditis without congestive heart failure. It is preferable to maintain a regimen of bed-to-chair with bathroom privileges and meals at the table for patients who are relatively asymptomatic while on aspirin therapy. Asymptomatic patients can be kept in bed only under duress anyway. Patients with severe carditis (congestive heart failure) have no desire to get out of bed and should be at bed rest at least as long as corticosteroid therapy is required. Gradual indoor ambulation followed by modified outdoor activity may be ordered when symptoms have disappeared but there is still clinical and laboratory evidence of rheumatic activity. Modified bed rest for 2–6 weeks is generally adequate. Children should not return to school while there is clear evidence of rheumatic activity. Most children are now managed on an outpatient basis.

B. Treatment After the Acute Episode:

1. Prevention–The patient who has had rheumatic fever has a greatly increased risk of developing rheumatic fever following the next inadequately treated group A β-hemolytic streptococcal infection. *Prevention is thus the most important therapeutic course for the physician to emphasize.* The purpose of follow-up visits after the acute episode is not so much to evaluate the evolution of mitral insufficiency murmurs as to reinforce the physician's advice about the necessity for antibacterial prophylaxis

with penicillin benzathine G. At such times, the physician should stress that greater protection is afforded by administration via the intramuscular route than via the oral route (penicillin V) and that, in addition, failure to comply with regular oral medication programs increases the risk for recurrence of rheumatic fever. Thus, patients should be informed that the parenteral route will be favored until they are adults, at which time their internists may elect oral medication.

If myocardial or valvular disease persists, antibacterial prophylaxis is a lifelong commitment. More commonly with transient cardiac involvement, 3–5 years of therapy or discontinuance at adolescence is a practical and effective approach.

The following regimens are in current use:

a. Penicillin benzathine G, 1.2 million units intramuscularly every 21–28 days, is the drug of choice.

b. Sulfadiazine, 500 mg daily as a single oral dose for patients weighing over 27 kg, is the drug of second choice. Blood dyscrasias and a lesser effectiveness in reducing streptococcal infections make this drug less satisfactory than penicillin benzathine G.

c. Penicillin V, 250,000 units orally twice daily, offers approximately the same protection afforded by sulfadiazine but is much less effective than intramuscular penicillin benzathine G (5.5 versus 0.4 streptococcal infections per 100 patient-years).

d. Erythromycin, 250 mg orally twice a day, may be given to patients allergic to both penicillin and sulfonamides.

2. Residual valvular damage–Chronic congestive heart failure may follow a single severe episode of acute rheumatic carditis or, more commonly, may follow repeated episodes. In children in the United States, the typical manifestations of residual valvular damage are heart murmurs of mitral and aortic insufficiency; murmurs are not accompanied by congestive heart failure during most of the pediatric age period *as long as repeated attacks are prevented.*

Methods of managing congestive heart failure have been discussed previously. Children with severe valvular damage who cannot be adequately managed on a medical regimen must be considered for valve replacement—and considered before the myocardium is irreversibly damaged.

Ayoub EM: Resurgence of rheumatic fever in the United States: The changing picture of a preventable illness. Postgrad Med 1992;92:139.

Dajani AS et al: Guidelines for the diagnosis of rheumatic fever: Jones criteria, updated 1992. Circulation 1993;87:302.

Loeffler AM et al: Identification of cases of acute rheumatic fever managed on an outpatient basis. Pediatr Infect Dis J 1995;141:975.

Vasan RS et al: Echocardiographic evaluation of patients

with acute rheumatic fever and rheumatic carditis. Circulation 1996;94:73.

RHEUMATIC HEART DISEASE

Mitral Insufficiency

Mitral insufficiency, the most common valvular residual of acute rheumatic carditis, is characterized by a pansystolic murmur that is localized at the apex. In patients with mitral involvement, the murmur appears early in the course of rheumatic carditis, and, depending on the severity of the damage, may disappear over a period of days or months or may persist for life.

Among the many other causes of mitral insufficiency, the most common is the mitral dysfunction syndrome, characterized by a mid to late apical systolic murmur introduced by a click.* Other causes are myocarditis, endocardial fibroelastosis, anomalous left coronary artery, and congenital anomalies of the mitral valve, which occur as isolated lesions or as part of a complex of anomalies (eg, endocardial cushion defects).

Mitral Stenosis

There are murmurs of mitral stenosis that are secondary to structural stenosis of the valve; those that result from relative excess of flow (in large volumes of regurgitation); and those that are present during acute valvulitis (Carey Coombs murmur). Mitral stenosis caused by structural stenosis is rarely encountered in the United States before 5–10 years following the first episode of acute rheumatic carditis and is much more commonly discovered in adults than in children. Early structural mitral stenosis murmurs, flow murmurs, and Carey Coombs murmurs are short and heard in mid diastole. Progressively more severe mitral stenosis murmurs become longer in duration until they attain the classic crescendo, presystolic configuration. Interventional cardiovascular balloon dilation of significant mitral stenosis is now being evaluated.

Aortic Insufficiency

This early decrescendo diastolic murmur is not commonly encountered as the sole valvular involvement of rheumatic carditis. It is the second most common valve affected in polyvalvular as well as in single valvular disease. It appears that the aortic valve is involved more often in males and in blacks. A short aortic systolic murmur resulting from excess

---

*A word of caution about diagnosing the mitral dysfunction syndrome: The echocardiographic finding of prolapse (redundancy) of the mitral valve, which characterizes mitral dysfunction, may also be found in patients with acute rheumatic fever and recently acquired rheumatic heart disease.

flow may accompany the aortic insufficiency murmur.

Aortic Stenosis

Dominant aortic stenosis of rheumatic origin does not occur in pediatric patients. Aortic stenosis in children is congenital. In one large series, the shortest length of time observed for a patient to develop dominant aortic stenosis secondary to rheumatic heart disease was 20 years.

Edwards BS, Edwards JE: Congestive heart failure in rheumatic carditis: Valvular or myocardial origin? J Am Coll Cardiol 1993;22:830.
Shrivastava S et al: Mitral valvotomy with the Inoue balloon in juvenile rheumatic mitral stenosis. Am J Cardiol 1995;76:404.

MYOCARDITIS

In most cases, the cause of myocarditis is not determined. Coxsackievirus B is the most common infectious agent isolated. Coxsackievirus A, rubella virus, cytomegalovirus, mumps virus, herpesvirus, adenovirus, and many other viral agents have been implicated. Virtually every other infectious agent, including bacteria, fungi, rickettsiae, chlamydiae, spirochetes, parasites, and HIV, has been suggested as a cause of myocarditis, but laboratory confirmation is seldom possible. It is important to emphasize that myocarditis is part of a spectrum of primary endomyocardial diseases and may be one of the causes of endocardial fibroelastosis.

Clinical Findings

A. Symptoms and Signs: The clinical picture usually falls into two separate patterns: (1) Onset of congestive heart failure is sudden in a newborn who has been in relatively good health 12–24 hours previously. This is a malignant form of the disease and is thought to be solely secondary to overwhelming viremia and tissue invasion of multiple organ systems, including the heart. (2) In the older child, the onset of cardiac findings tends to be much more gradual. There is often a history of an upper respiratory tract infection or gastroenteritis within the month prior to the development of cardiac findings. This is a more insidious form of the disease and may have a late postinfectious or autoimmune component. Recovery from the initial infection is followed by gradual and progressive development of easy fatigability, dyspnea on exertion, and malaise.

In the newborn infant, the signs of congestive heart failure are usually apparent. The skin is pale and gray, and peripheral cyanosis may be present. The pulses are rapid, weak, and thready. Edema of the face and extremities may be seen. Significant cardiomegaly is present, and the left and right ventricular impulses are weak. On auscultation, the heart sounds may be muffled and distant. Third and fourth heart sounds are common, resulting in a gallop rhythm. Murmurs are usually absent, although a murmur of tricuspid or mitral insufficiency can occasionally be heard. Moist rales are usually present at both lung bases. The liver is enlarged and frequently tender. The level of the jugular venous pulse is elevated.

B. Imaging: Generalized cardiomegaly can be seen on x-ray. There is evidence of moderate to marked pulmonary venous congestion. Pneumonitis is commonly present.

C. Electrocardiography: The ECG is variable. Classically, there is evidence of low voltage of the QRS throughout all frontal and precordial leads and depression of the ST segment and inversion of the T waves in leads I, III, and aVF and in the left precordial leads during the acute malignant stage. Dysrhythmias are common, and atrioventricular and intraventricular conduction disturbances may be present. With the more benign form—or during the recovery phase of the malignant form—high-voltage QRS complexes are commonly seen and are indicative of left ventricular hypertrophy.

D. Echocardiography: Echocardiography demonstrates four-chamber dilation with poor ventricular function and atrioventricular valve regurgitation.

Treatment

A. Digitalis: The use of digitalis in a rapidly deteriorating child with myocarditis is dangerous and should be undertaken with great caution. Because the inflamed myocardium is markedly sensitive to digitalis, only about two-thirds of the usual total digitalizing dose should be used. During the initial phase of therapy, ECGs should be taken frequently. If serious dysrhythmias or other evidence of digitalis intoxication develops, the drug should be stopped and not reinstituted until all evidence of digitalis toxicity has disappeared. If toxicity is not evident and there is no clinical response, digitalis doses should be increased until one or the other is noted.

B. Diuretics: Diuretics should be administered with caution, since they may potentiate digitalis toxicity.

C. Corticosteroids: The administration of corticosteroids is controversial but seems more rational when used in the treatment of the more benign postinfectious autoimmune cases. If the patient's condition continues to deteriorate despite anticongestive measures, corticosteroids are commonly used.

D. Systemic Vasodilators: The use of systemic vasodilators such as nitroprusside in a hypotensive deteriorating critically ill patient is risky but may be lifesaving. Initial results using ACE inhibitors such as captopril are promising.

Prognosis

The prognosis for a patient with myocarditis is related to the age at onset, the response to therapy, and the presence or absence of recurrences. If the patient is less than 6 months of age or older than 3 years, responds poorly to therapy, and manifests multiple recurrences of congestive heart failure, the prognosis is poor. Many patients recover clinically but have persistent cardiomegaly. It is possible that subclinical myocarditis in childhood is the pathophysiologic basis for some of the idiopathic myocardiopathies seen later in life.

Chan KY et al: Immunosuppressive therapy in the management of acute myocarditis in children. J Am Coll Cardiol 1991;17:458.
Rezkalla SH et al: Treatment of viral myocarditis with focus on captopril. Am J Cardiol 1996;77:634.

INFECTIVE ENDOCARDITIS

Essentials of Diagnosis & Typical Features
- Preexisting organic heart murmur.
- Persistent fever.
- Increasing symptoms of heart disease (ranging from easy fatigability to heart failure).
- Splenomegaly (70%).
- Embolic phenomena (50%).
- Leukocytosis, elevated erythrocyte sedimentation rate, hematuria, positive blood culture.

General Considerations

Bacterial infection of the endocardial surface of the heart or the intimal surface of certain arterial vessels (coarcted segment of aorta and ductus arteriosus) is a rare condition that usually occurs when an abnormality of the heart or great vessels exists. It may develop in a normal heart during the course of septicemia.

The incidence of infective endocarditis appears to be increasing owing to many factors, including (1) increased survival rates for children with congenital heart disease, (2) greater long-term use of central venous catheters, and (3) increased use of prosthetic material and valves. Pediatric patients without preexisting heart disease also are at increased risk for infective endocarditis owing to (1) increased survival rates for children with immune deficiencies, (2) greater long-term use of indwelling lines in critically ill newborns, and (3) increased incidence of intravenous drug abuse.

Patients at greatest risk include those with aorticopulmonary shunts, left-sided outflow obstruction, and ventricular septal defects. Predisposing factors can be identified approximately 30% of the time and include dental procedures, nonsterile surgical procedures, and cardiovascular surgery.

Organisms causing endocarditis include viridans

streptococci (about 50% of cases), *Staphylococcus aureus* (about 30%), and fungal agents (about 10%).

Clinical Findings

A. History: Almost all patients with infective endocarditis have a history of heart disease. There may or may not be a history of infection or a surgical procedure (tooth extraction, tonsillectomy).

B. Symptoms, Signs, and Laboratory Findings: In one large study, the following symptoms, signs, and laboratory findings were reported (in order of decreasing frequency): changing murmurs, fever, positive blood culture, weight loss, cardiomegaly, elevated sedimentation rate, splenomegaly, petechiae, embolism, and leukocytosis. Other findings are hematuria, signs of congestive heart failure, clubbing, joint pains, and hepatomegaly. Echocardiography has become a valuable tool in diagnosing large vegetations.

Prevention

It is recommended that patients at risk for infective endocarditis be given appropriate antibiotics before any type of dental work (tooth extraction, cleaning) and before operations within the oropharynx, gastrointestinal tract, and genitourinary tract. Continuous antibiotic prophylaxis (as in the treatment of rheumatic fever) is *not* recommended in patients with congenital heart disease.

The following schedule is recommended: under 15 kg, 750 mg of oral amoxicillin; 15–30 kg, 1500 mg; over 30 kg, 3000 mg. This dose is to be given 1 hour prior to dental procedures.

Treatment

In a patient with known heart disease, the presence of an otherwise unexplained fever should alert the physician to the possibility of infective endocarditis. A positive blood culture or other major findings of infective endocarditis confirm the diagnosis. If a positive blood culture is obtained and the organism is identified, specific treatment should be begun immediately. Even if blood cultures are negative after 48 hours, it is advisable to begin penicillin therapy (if there is other evidence of infective endocarditis), because most positive cultures are obtained within the first 48 hours. Nafcillin parenterally or dicloxacillin enterally are the drugs of choice in most cases. Other antibiotics may be added (see Chapter 33). If congestive heart failure occurs and progresses unremittingly in the face of adequate antibiotic therapy, surgical excision of the infected area and prosthetic valve replacement should be considered.

Course & Prognosis

The prognosis depends on how early in the course of the infectious process treatment is instituted. The prognosis is better in patients in whom blood culture is positive. If congestive heart failure develops, the prognosis is usually poor.

Even though bacteriologic cure of the infectious process is achieved, death may occur as a result of congestive heart failure secondary to severe valvular destruction. Intractable congestive heart failure may occur weeks or months following bacteriologic cure. Embolization may occur following bacteriologic cure when vegetations tear off from the involved area.

The death rate for infective endocarditis is still about 20%.

Biancaniello TM, Romero JR: Bacterial endocarditis after adjustment of orthodontic appliances. J Pediatr 1991; 118:248.

Dajani AS et al: Prevention of bacterial endocarditis: Recommendations by the American Heart Association. JAMA 1997;277:1794.

Mansur AJ et al: Determinants of prognosis in 300 episodes of infective endocarditis. Thorac Cardiovasc Surg 1996; 44:22.

Saiman L, Prince A, Gerony WM: Pediatric infective endocarditis in the modern era. J Pediatr 1993;122:847.

PERICARDITIS

Essentials of Diagnosis
& Typical Features

- Retrosternal pain made worse by deep inspiration and decreased by leaning forward.
- Fever.
- Shortness of breath and grunting respirations are common.
- Pericardial friction rub.
- Tachycardia.
- Hepatomegaly and distention of the jugular veins.
- ECG with elevated ST segment.

General Considerations

Involvement of the pericardium rarely occurs as an isolated event. In most cases, pericardial disease occurs in association with a more generalized process. Important causes include rheumatic fever, viral pericarditis, purulent pericarditis, rheumatoid arthritis, uremia, and tuberculosis.

In the pediatric age group, pericardial disease usually takes the form of acute pericarditis. In most cases, there is effusion of fluid into the pericardial cavity. The consequences of such effusion depend on the amount, type, and speed of fluid accumulation. Under certain circumstances, serious compression of the heart occurs. The direct compression and the body's attempt to correct it result in cardiac tamponade. Unless the pericardial fluid is evacuated, death occurs very rapidly.

Clinical Findings

A. Symptoms and Signs: The symptoms depend to a great extent on the cause of the pericarditis. Pain is common. It is usually sharp and stabbing, located in the mid chest and in the shoulder and neck, made worse by deep inspiration, and considerably decreased by sitting up and leaning forward. Shortness of breath and grunting respirations are common findings in all patients.

The physical findings depend on whether or not a significant amount of effusion is present: (1) In the absence of significant accumulation of fluid, the pulses are normal and the level of the jugular venous pulse is normal. On examination of the heart, a characteristic scratchy, high-pitched friction rub may be heard. It is often systolic and diastolic and can be located at any point between the apex and the left sternal border. The location and timing vary considerably from time to time. The heart sounds are usually normal, and the heart is not enlarged to percussion. (2) If there is a considerable accumulation of pericardial fluid, the cardiovascular findings are different. The heart is enlarged to percussion, but on inspection of the precordium, it seems to be very quiet. Auscultation reveals distant and muffled heart tones. Friction rub is usually not present. In the absence of cardiac tamponade, the peripheral, venous, and arterial pulses are normal.

Cardiac tamponade is characterized by distention of the jugular veins, tachycardia, enlargement of the liver, peripheral edema, and "paradoxic pulse,"* in which the systolic pressure drops by more than 10 mm Hg during inspiration. (Normally, the systolic pressure drops by no more than 5 mm Hg.) This finding is best determined with the use of a blood pressure cuff. At this point, the patient is critically ill and has all the symptoms and signs suggestive of right-sided congestive heart failure.

Not all patients with marked cardiac compression demonstrate all the findings listed above. If the patient appears critically ill and has evidence of pericarditis and effusion, treatment should be instituted even though all the clinical signs of cardiac tamponade are not present.

B. Imaging: In pericarditis without effusion, chest x-ray findings are normal. With pericardial effusion, the cardiac silhouette is enlarged, often in the shape of a water bottle, with blunting of the cardiodiaphragmatic borders. When there is evidence of cardiac tamponade, the lung fields are clear. This is in contrast to patients with myocardial dilatation, who show evidence of pulmonary congestion.

C. Electrocardiography: A number of electrocardiographic abnormalities occur in patients with pericarditis. Low voltage is commonly seen in patients with significant pericardial effusion, although the voltage may be normal. The ST segment is commonly elevated during the first week of involvement. The T wave is usually upright during this time. Following this, the ST segment is normal and the T

wave becomes flattened. After about 2 weeks, the T wave inverts and remains inverted for several weeks or months. In contrast to findings in patients with myocardial infarction, there is no reciprocal relationship between the findings in lead I and lead III in the frontal plane and the right and left precordial leads.

D. Echocardiography: Echocardiography has become a most reliable form of noninvasive diagnosis of pericardial effusion. The results must be considered in light of the clinical picture in deciding whether or not to remove the fluid.

Treatment

Treatment depends on the cause of pericarditis. Cardiac tamponade resulting from any cause must be treated by evacuation of the fluid. It is usually desirable to perform wide resection of the pericardium through a surgical incision. However, insertion of a needle into the pericardial sac may be lifesaving in an emergency situation.

Prognosis

The prognosis depends to a great extent on the cause of the pericardial disease. Cardiac tamponade from any cause results in death unless the fluid is evacuated.

SPECIFIC DISEASES INVOLVING THE PERICARDIUM

Acute Rheumatic Fever

When pericarditis occurs during the course of acute rheumatic fever, it is almost always associated with involvement of the myocardium and the endocardium (pancarditis). Thus, heart murmurs are almost always present. The pericarditis is usually of the serofibrinous variety and usually not associated with significant pericardial effusion.

Patients with acute rheumatic fever and pericarditis are usually very ill, with severe cardiac involvement. They respond extremely well to corticosteroid therapy. Pericarditis usually disappears rapidly (1 week) after corticosteroid therapy is started. Constrictive pericarditis almost never occurs secondary to this disease.

Viral Pericarditis

Viral pericarditis is uncommon in children and young adults. The most common cause is coxsackievirus B4. Influenza virus has also been implicated. There is usually a history of a protracted upper respiratory tract infection.

The pericardial effusion usually lasts for several weeks. Cardiac tamponade is rare. Recurrences of pericardial effusion are common even months or years after the initial episode. Constrictive pericarditis has been reported in this disease.

---

*"Paradoxic pulse" is a misnomer, since the drop is only an accentuation of a normal event.

Purulent Pericarditis

The most common causes of purulent pericarditis are pneumococci, streptococci, staphylococci, *Escherichia coli,* and *Haemophilus influenzae.* This disorder is always secondary to infection elsewhere, although occasionally the primary site is not obvious. In addition to demonstrating signs of cardiac compression, patients are septic and run extremely high fevers. The purulent fluid accumulating within the pericardial sac is usually quite thick and filled with polymorphonuclear leukocytes. Although antibiotics will sterilize the pericardial fluid, pericardial tamponade commonly develops, and evacuation of the pericardial sac is usually necessary. Wide resection of the pericardium through a surgical incision performed in the operating room is most desirable, but pericardiocentesis is often dramatically effective and lifesaving. Drainage of the purulent fluid is followed by marked improvement of symptoms.

Postpericardiotomy Syndrome

Postpericardiotomy syndrome is characterized by fever, chest pain, friction rub, and elevation of ST segment noted on ECG 1–2 weeks after open heart surgery. It appears to be an autoimmune disease with high titers of antiheart antibody and with detectable evidence of fresh or reactivated viral illness. The syndrome is often self-limited and responds well to short courses of aspirin or corticosteroid therapy. Occasionally, it lasts for months to years and may require pericardiocentesis or pericardiectomy.

Dupuis C et al: Bacterial pericarditis in infancy and childhood. Am J Cardiol 1994;74:807.
Friedland IR et al: Cardiac complications in children with staphylococcus bacteremia. J Pediatr 1995;127:746.
Guindo J et al: Recurrent pericarditis: Relief with colchicine. Circulation 1990;82:1117.

HYPERTENSION*

Blood pressure determinations are being more routinely obtained in the examination of infants and children; as a result, systemic hypertension has become more widely recognized as a pediatric problem. Pediatric standards for blood pressure have been published, but the studies from which these standards were derived suffered from three methodologic problems. The first and most important is that the widest cuff that would fit between the axilla and the antecubital fossa was not routinely used. The use of a wide cuff either has no effect on blood pressure or decreases blood pressure by a maximum of 5 mm Hg. Use of a narrow cuff, however, routinely increases blood pressure by

10–50 mm Hg. The second methodologic problem was lack of an ethnic cross section. Third, the fact that systemic blood pressure decreases with increasing altitude of residence was not taken into consideration.

These three problems were addressed in a study of a triracial population at sea level and at an altitude of 3100 m. The widest cuff that would fit between the axilla and the antecubital fossa was used in each case. Most children 10–11 years of age needed a standard adult-size cuff (bladder width of 12 cm), and many high school students needed a large adult-size cuff (width of 16 cm) or leg cuff (width of 18 cm). Results of the study are shown in Table 18–5. The 95th percentile value for blood pressure was similar for both sexes and all three ethnic groups. Blood pressure varied more with altitude and body weight than with sex or ethnic origin. If the blood pressure taken in a quiet atmosphere and sitting position exceeds the 95th percentile for systolic, diastolic muffle, or diastolic disappearance pressures, it should be repeated twice in 1- to 2-week intervals. If it is abnormal all three times, a pediatric hypertension diagnostic center should be consulted.

Essential hypertension is the most common form of pediatric hypertension. Coarctation of the thoracic or abdominal aorta, renal artery stenosis, renal disease, and pheochromocytoma should be ruled out.

Patients with essential hypertension often show improvement with reduction of obesity, reduction of excessive salt intake, institution of an exercise program, avoidance of cigarette smoking, and avoidance of oral contraceptives.

Badenhop RF, Wang XL, Wilcken DEL: Angiotensin-converting enzyme genotype in children and coronary events in their grandparents. Circulation 1995;91:1655.

Table 18–5. The 95th percentile value for blood pressure (mm Hg) taken in the sitting position.[1]

Age (years)	Sea Level			10,000 ft		
	S	Dm	Dd	S	Dm	Dd
5				92	72	62
6	106	64	60	96	74	66
7	108	72	66	98	76	70
8	110	76	70	104	80	70
9	114	80	76	106	80	70
10	118	82	76	108	80	70
11	124	82	78	108	80	72
12	128	84	78	108	80	72
13	132	84	80	116	84	76
14	136	86	80	120	84	76
15	140	88	80	120	84	80
16	140	90	80	120	84	80
17	140	92	80	122	84	80
18	140	92	80	130	84	80

[1]Blood pressures: S = systolic (Korotkoff's sound 1; onset of tapping), Dm = diastolic muffling (Korotkoff's sound 4), Dd = diastolic disappearance (Korotkoff's sound 5).

*The diagnostic evaluation of renal hypertension and the treatment of hypertensive emergencies, as well as the ambulatory treatment of chronic hypertension, are discussed in Chapter 21.

Gifford RW et al: The fifth report of the Joint National Committee on detection, evaluation, and treatment of high blood pressure. Arch Intern Med 1993;153:154.

Gillman MW et al: Identifying children at high risk for the development of essential hypertension. J Pediatr 1993;122:837.

Hegyi T et al: Blood pressure ranges in premature infants. J Pediatr 1994124:627.

Steinfeld L et al: Sphygmomanometry in pediatric patients. J Pediatr 1978;92:934.

Update on 1987 Task Force report on high blood pressure in children and adolescents. Pediatrics 1996;98:649.

ATHEROSCLEROSIS AS A PEDIATRIC PROBLEM

Awareness of the importance of coronary artery risk factors in general—and atherosclerosis in particular—has risen dramatically in the general population during the past 25 years. In adults, the incidence of death from ischemic heart disease has been decreasing over the last decade, presumably as a result of modifying the diet or lifestyle to avoid known risks for heart disease. During this same decade, a large number of serum samples from the pediatric population have been collected and analyzed for lipids, and epidemiologic studies have been performed to determine the relationship of lipid levels to coronary heart disease. The level of serum lipids in childhood usually remains the same through adolescence. Biochemical abnormalities in the lipid profile appear early in childhood and correlate with higher risk for coronary artery disease in adulthood. High-density lipoprotein has been identified as an antiatherogenic agent through these studies.

The concept of pediatric screening for hyperlipidemia has been evaluated carefully. Currently, only children at high risk—that is, children with a family history of early myocardial infarction (prior to 50–55 years) in parents or grandparents or with known familial hyperlipidemia or adopted children—are screened routinely. In addition, some researchers consider adolescents with total cholesterol levels of greater than 180 mg/dL or low-density lipoprotein levels of greater than 110 mg/dL to be at risk for coronary artery disease in adulthood.

In most cases, treatment consists of dietary restrictions, exercise, abstinence from smoking, and avoidance of other ischemic heart disease risk factors. In patients with life-threatening familial hyperlipidemia, pharmacologic and surgical intervention (ileal bypass, portacaval shunt) may be considered.

Lauer RM, Clark WR: Use of cholesterol measurements in childhood for the prediction of adult hypercholesterolemia: The Muscatine Study. JAMA 1990;264:3034.

Lauer RM et al: National cholesterol education program (NCEP): Highlights of report. Pediatrics 1992;89:495.

Muhonen LE et al: Coronary risk factors in adolescents related to their knowledge of familial coronary heart disease and hypercholesterolemia: The Muscatine Study. Pediatrics 1994;93:444.

MUCOCUTANEOUS LYMPH NODE SYNDROME

Mucocutaneous lymph node syndrome, also known as Kawasaki disease, was first described in Japan in 1967. The acute illness is characterized by (1) prolonged fever (over 5 days) that is unresponsive to antibiotics; (2) conjunctivitis; (3) cracking and fissuring of the lips, with inflammation of mucous membranes; (4) cervical lymphadenopathy; (5) rash involving the trunk and the extremities, with reddened palms and soles of the hands and feet and subsequent desquamation of tips of the toes and fingers; and (6) edema. Patients may also have associated arthritis. Thrombocytosis and increased sedimentation rate are seen on laboratory examination.

Cardiovascular complications during the acute illness include myocarditis, pericarditis, and arteritis that predisposes the patient to aneurysm formation in the coronary arteries in approximately 20% of patients. Aneurysm formation may occur 7–45 days after the onset of illness. Acute myocardial infarction may occur during the acute illness secondary to thrombosis of these aneurysms. Death occurs in 1–2% of patients during this phase of the illness. Long-term follow-up of patients with aneurysms shows some resolution of aneurysms in 50% of those affected; the remainder may continue to have aneurysms, may develop stenosis, and, possibly later, may develop myocardial ischemia.

During the acute illness and for 2–3 months after, patients should be monitored closely by serial electrocardiography, chest x-ray, and M-mode and two-dimensional echocardiography. Selective coronary angiography is recommended in those patients with coronary abnormalities detected by echocardiography.

The acute illness is now treated with high doses of intravenous immune globulin (IVIG), 2 g/kg as a single dose given over 10–12 hours. If fever recurs within 48–72 hours and no other source of the fever is detected, a repeat dose is recommended, and high doses of aspirin, 20 mg/kg per dose given four times a day until day 14 of illness, then 3–5 mg/kg/d for 2–3 months from the onset of illness if the echocardiogram is normal or indefinitely if coronary abnormalities are present. Evidence of myocardial ischemia or infarction warrants early cardiac catheterization and bypass surgery if obstruction exists.

American Heart Association Committee on Rheumatic Fever, Endocarditis, Kawasaki Disease: Guidelines for long term management of patients with Kawasaki disease. Circulation 1994;89:916.

Gersony WM: Diagnosis and management of Kawasaki disease. JAMA 1991;265:2699.

Shulman, ST et al: Kawasaki disease. Pediatr Clin North Am 1995;42:1205.

DISORDERS OF RATE & RHYTHM & OF ELECTROLYTE IMBALANCE

The recognition and treatment of cardiac arrhythmias have markedly increased in the recent past. Better monitoring (electrocardiography, bedside monitors, Holter monitors, etc) has increased the awareness and detection of rhythm disturbances. There is also a true rise in the incidence of arrhythmias. More children are now surviving cardiac surgery and acute carditis and live chronically with altered hemodynamics, physiology, and structural changes. These changes over time will create altered conduction and new arrhythmias.

The advent of invasive electrophysiology with recordings from the endocardium has greatly improved our understanding of the conduction system. And now, with cardiac ablation techniques, we can offer these children a "cure" rather than lifelong antiarrhythmia treatment.

Sinus Arrhythmia

It is normal to have phasic variation in the heart rate (sinus arrhythmia). Typically, the sinus rate varies with the respiratory cycle, while P-QRS-T intervals remain normal. "Marked" sinus arrhythmia is defined as a greater than 100% variation in heart rate. It may be found in association with respiratory distress or increased intracranial pressure, or it may be present in normal children. It alone virtually never requires treatment. However, it may be associated with sinus node dysfunction (see below).

Sinus Bradycardia

Depending on the age of the patient, sinus bradycardia is defined as either (1) a heart rate below the normal limit for age (neonates to 6 years, 60 beats/min; 7–11 years, 45 beats/min; > 12 years, 40 beats/min) or (2) a heart rate inappropriately slow for the functional status of the patient (chronotropic incompetence). In critically ill patients, common causes of sinus bradycardia include hypoxia, central nervous system damage, and iatrogenic medication side effects. Only symptomatic bradycardia (syncope, low cardiac output, or exercise intolerance) requires treatment (atropine or artificial cardiac pacing).

Sinus Tachycardia

The heart rate normally accelerates in response to stress (eg, fever, hypovolemia, anemia, congestive heart failure). Tachycardia with decreased cardiac output is more ominous and warrants evaluation for shock or tachyarrhythmia. Treatment may be indicated for correction of the underlying cause of tachycardia (eg, transfusion for anemia, correction of hypovolemia or fever).

Wren C, Campbell RWF: *Paediatric Cardiac Arrhythmias.* Oxford Univ Press, 1996.

PREMATURE ATRIAL CONTRACTIONS

Premature atrial contractions are triggered by an ectopic focus in the atrium. They are one of the most common premature beats seen in the pediatric population, particularly during the fetal and newborn periods. They may be conducted (with associated QRS) or nonconducted (without associated QRS) (Figure 18–6). There is usually some delay until the next normal sinus beat. Depending on the ectopic focus of the premature contraction, the frontal plane vector of the P wave may be normal (+30–90 degrees) or abnormal. As an isolated finding, premature atrial contractions are benign and require no treatment. They may need to be suppressed with antiarrhythmic agents when they trigger tachyarrhythmias or produce bradycardia secondary to nonconduction.

PREMATURE JUNCTIONAL CONTRACTIONS

Premature junctional contractions arise within the atrioventricular node or the bundle of His. Most often, they induce a normal QRS complex with no preceding P wave. When conducted aberrantly to the ventricles, they cannot be distinguished from premature ventricular contractions except by invasive electrophysiologic study. Premature junctional contractions are usually benign and require no specific therapy.

PREMATURE VENTRICULAR CONTRACTIONS

Premature ventricular contractions may originate in either ventricle and are characterized by a bizarre QRS of over 80 ms duration in newborns and 120 ms in children (Figure 18–7). Premature ventricular contractions originating from a single ectopic focus all have the same configuration; those of multifocal origin show varying configurations. The consecutive occurrence of more than one beat can result in cou-

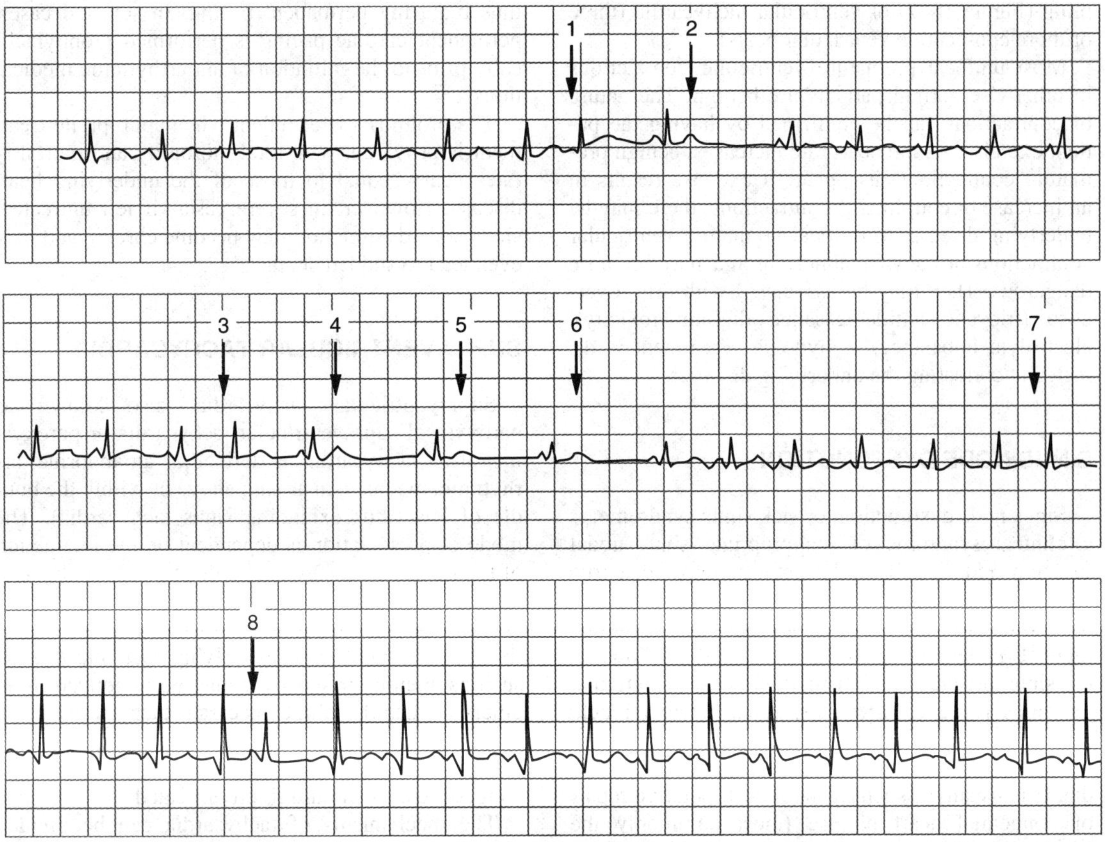

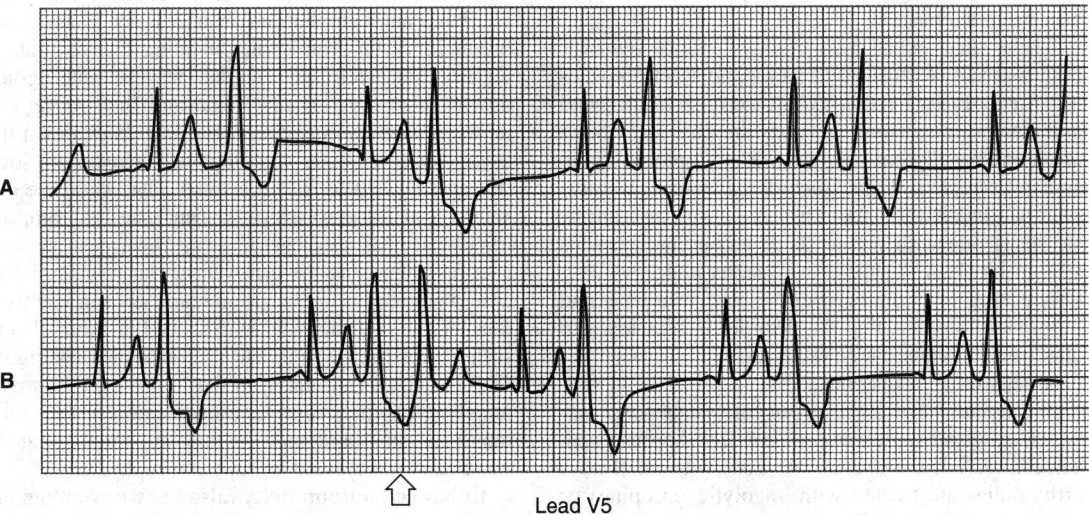

Figure 18–6. Lead II rhythm strip with premature atrial contractions. Beats 1, 3, 7, and 8 are conducted to the ventricles, whereas beats 2, 4, 5, and 6 are not.

Figure 18–7. Lead V5 rhythm strip with unifocal premature ventricular contractions in a bigeminy pattern. The arrow shows a ventricular couplet.

pling (Figure 18–7) or ventricular tachycardia (three or more consecutive ventricular beats).

Most unifocal premature ventricular contractions in otherwise normal patients are benign. The nature of contractions can be confirmed by having the patient exercise. As the heart rate increases, benign premature contractions disappear. If exercise results in an increase or coupling of contractions, there may be underlying disease. Multifocal premature ventricular contractions are always abnormal and may be more dangerous. They may be associated with drug overdose (tricyclic antidepressants, digoxin toxicity), electrolyte imbalance, or hypoxia. Treatment is directed at correcting the underlying disorder.

SINUS NODE DYSFUNCTION

Sinus node dysfunction, or sick sinus syndrome, is a clinical syndrome of inappropriate sinus nodal function and rate. The abnormality may be a true anatomic defect of the sinus node or its surrounding tissue, or it may be an abnormality of autonomic input. It is defined as one or more of the following: (1) sinus bradycardia, (2) marked sinus arrhythmia, (3) sinus pause or arrest, (4) sinoatrial exit block, (5) combined brady- and tachyarrhythmias, (6) sinus node reentry, and (7) atrial muscle reentry tachycardia. It is usually associated with postoperative repair of congenital heart disease (most commonly the Mustard or Senning repair for transposition of the great arteries or the Fontan procedure), but it is also seen in unoperated congenital heart disease, in acquired heart diseases, and in normal hearts. In some cases the disorder is inherited. Symptoms usually manifest between 2 and 17 years and consist of episodes of syncope, presyncope, or disorientation. Some patients may experience palpitations, pallor, or exercise intolerance.

The evaluation of sinus node dysfunction involves both external electrocardiography and electrophysiologic recordings. Resting ECGs, exercise testing, and ambulatory monitoring help define the arrhythmia and correlate rhythm changes with symptoms. Invasive electrophysiologic recordings measure sinus node automaticity, sinoatrial conduction, and intrinsic heart rate with and without autonomic nervous system blockade. Correction of sinus node dysfunction during autonomic blockade with atropine and propranolol implies that the disorder is secondary to abnormal autonomic tone rather than an anatomic abnormality of the sinus node.

Treatment is usually reserved for symptomatic patients. Asymptomatic patients can just be observed, since there is little chance of sudden death. Bradyarrhythmias are treated with vagolytic (atropine) or adrenergic (aminophylline) agents or permanent cardiac pacemakers. Antiarrhythmic treatment of tachyarrhythmias often produces or enhances bradycardia, thus requiring permanent pacing. In selected cases, permanent cardiac pacing is performed prophylactically prior to the initiation of antiarrhythmic medications.

The prognosis is excellent when appropriate treatment is provided, with total morbidity and mortality rates nearly equal to those of the underlying heart disease. However, in severe cases, if left untreated, sinus node dysfunction may become chronic and may even lead to sudden death.

SUPRAVENTRICULAR TACHYCARDIA

Supraventricular tachycardia, also known as paroxysmal supraventricular tachycardia or paroxysmal atrial tachycardia, is defined as an abnormal arrhythmia mechanism arising above or within the bundle of His (thus excluding sinus tachycardia). The mode of presentation is dependent on the interaction of the rate of the tachycardia, the cardiovascular system, and the patient in general. A tachycardia may be poorly tolerated in a child with preexisting congestive heart failure or an underlying systemic disease such as anemia or sepsis or may go unnoticed in an otherwise healthy child. Incessant tachycardia in an otherwise healthy individual, albeit slow (120–150 beats/min), may cause myocardial dysfunction and congestive heart failure if left untreated.

The mechanisms of tachycardia can be divided into three groups: reentry, enhanced automaticity, and triggered dysrhythmias.

Reentry is conduction through two or more pathways, creating a sustained repetitive circular loop. The circuit can be confined to the atrium (intra-atrial reentry, a form of atrial flutter) (Figure 18–8). It may be confined within the atrioventricular node (atrioventricular nodal reentrant tachycardia) or it may encompass an atrioventricular accessory connection, producing orthodromic reciprocating tachycardia, in which the electrical impulse travels anterograde down the atrioventricular node and then retrograde up the accessory connection and then back down the atrioventricular node to complete the reentrant loop (Figure 18–9). Wolff-Parkinson-White syndrome is a subclass of these in which, during sinus rhythm, the impulse travels anterograde down the accessory connection, bypassing the atrioventricular node and creating ventricular preexcitation (early eccentric activation of the ventricle with a short PR interval and slurred upstroke of the QRS, a delta wave (Figure 18–10). Reentrant tachycardia represents approximately 80% of pediatric arrhythmias, has a wide range of rates, and may or may not demonstrate P waves and initiate and terminate abruptly.

Enhanced automaticity (also known as automatic or ectopic tachycardia) is created when a focus of cardiac tissue develops an abnormally fast spontaneous rate of depolarization. These arrhythmias rep-

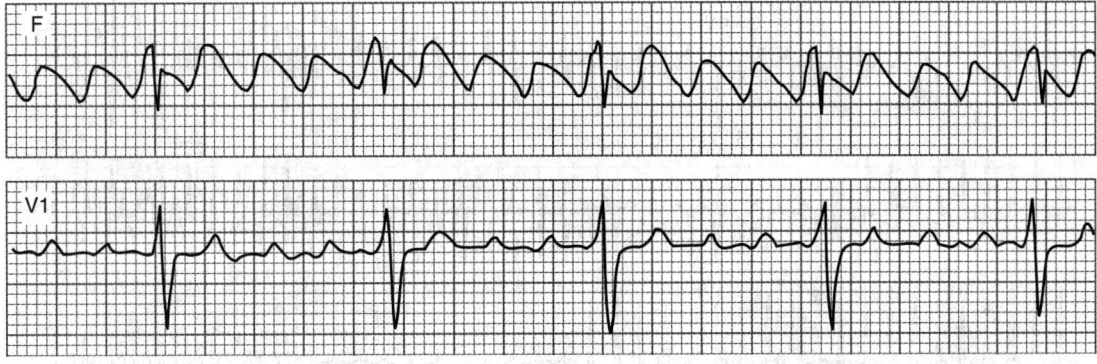

Figure 18–8. Leads aVF (F) and V1, showing atrial flutter with "sawtooth" atrial flutter waves.

resent approximately 20% of childhood arrhythmias and are usually under autonomic influence. Electrocardiography demonstrates a normal QRS complex preceded by an abnormal P wave (Figure 18–11). Junctional ectopic tachycardia may show atrioventricular dissociation or 1:1 retrograde conduction (Figure 18–12). These tachycardias demonstrate a gradual onset and offset and may be paroxysmal or incessant. When they are incessant, they usually present with congestive heart failure and a clinical picture of dilated cardiomyopathy.

Triggered dysrhythmia is extremely rare. It is caused by enhanced afterdepolarizations of the action potential that reach the takeoff potential. It is one of the side effects of digitalis toxicity.

Clinical Findings

A. Symptoms and Signs: Clinical presentation varies with the age of the patient. Infants tend to turn pale and mottled with onset of tachycardia and may become irritable. With long duration of tachycardia, symptoms of congestive heart failure develop. Heart rates can be from 240 to 300 beats/min. Older children may complain of dizziness, palpitations, fatigue, and chest pain. Heart rates usually range from 240/min in the younger child to 150–180/min in the teenager. Congestive heart failure is less common in children than in infants. Tachycardia may be associated with either congenital heart defects such as Ebstein's anomaly or acquired conditions such as cardiomyopathies and myocarditis.

B. Imaging: Findings on chest x-ray are normal during the early course of tachycardia. If congestive heart failure is present, the heart is enlarged and there is evidence of pulmonary venous congestion.

C. Electrocardiography: Electrocardiography is the most important tool in the diagnosis of supraventricular tachycardia.

1. The heart rate is rapid and out of proportion to the patient's physical status (ie, a rate of 140/min with an abnormal P wave while quiet and asleep).

2. The rhythm is extremely regular. There is little variation in the rate throughout the entire tracing.

3. P waves may or may not be present. If they are present, there is no variation in the appearance or in the PR interval. P waves may be difficult to find because they are superimposed on the preceding T wave. Furthermore, if the abnormal focus is located within the atrioventricular node, the P waves will not be seen (Figure 18–9).

4. The QRS complex is usually the same as during normal sinus rhythm. However, the QRS complex is occasionally widened (supraventricular tachycardia with aberrant ventricular conduction), in which case the condition may be difficult to differentiate from ventricular tachycardia.

Treatment

A. Acute Treatment: During initial episodes of supraventricular tachycardia, patients require close monitoring. Correction of acidosis and electrolyte abnormalities is also indicated.

1. Vagal maneuvers–The "diving reflex," an icebag placed on the nasal bridge for 20 seconds (for infants) or facial immersion in ice water (for children or adolescents), will increase parasympathetic tone and terminate some tachycardias. The Valsalva maneuver, which can be performed by older compliant children, may also terminate supraventricular tachycardia.

2. Adenosine–Adenosine transiently blocks atrioventricular conduction and terminates tachycardias that incorporate the atrioventricular node.

Adenosine does not convert tachycardias whose mechanism is confined to the atria (atrial ectopic tachycardia, intra-atrial reentry). However, it serves as a diagnostic tool in these arrhythmias by demonstrating continuation of the tachycardia during atri-

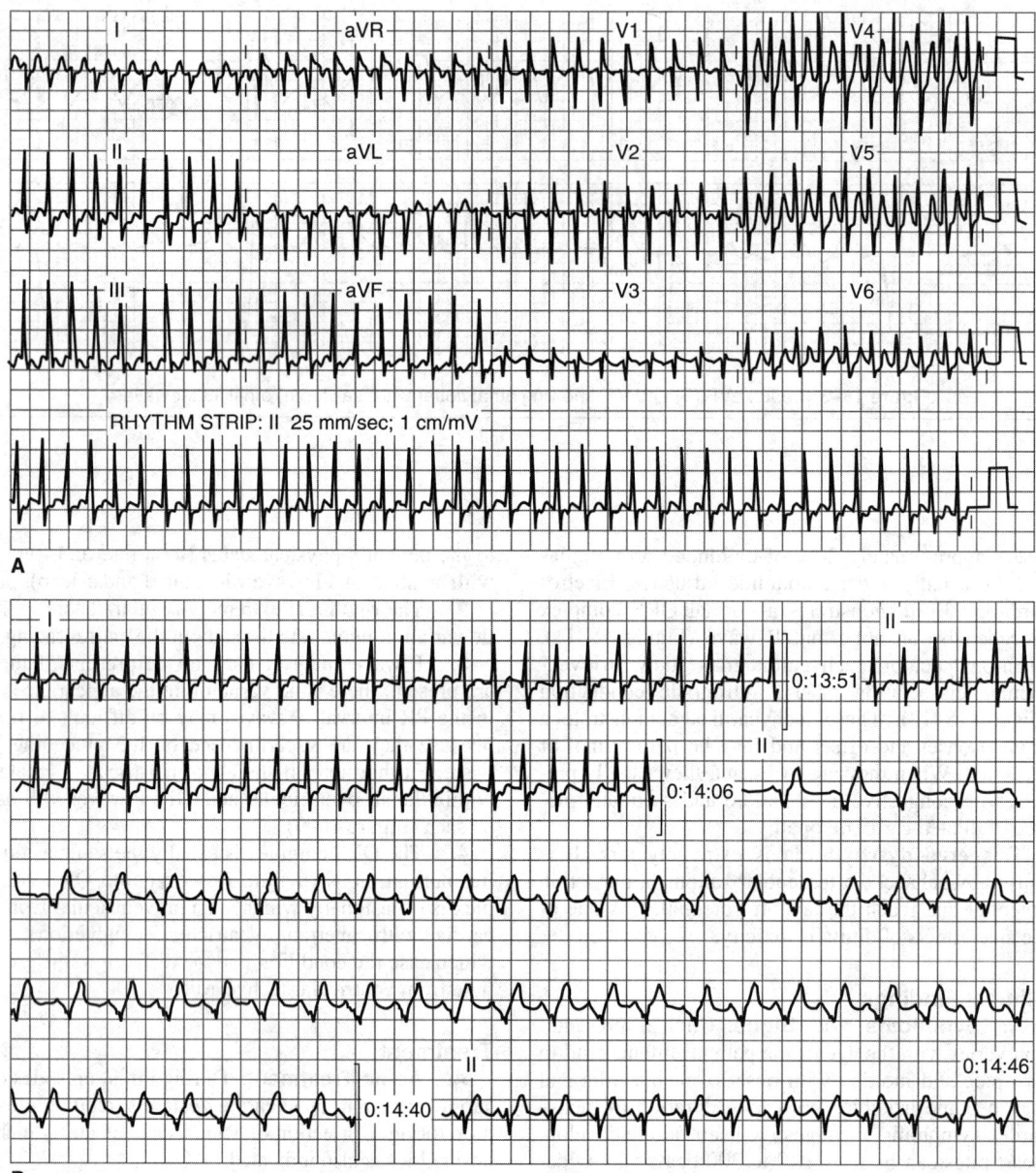

Figure 18–9. Supraventricular tachycardia. **A:** Twelve-lead ECG showing orthodromic reciprocating tachycardia (see text). **B:** Lead II rhythm strip showing spontaneous conversion to normal sinus rhythm with ventricular preexcitation (Wolff-Parkinson-White syndrome) and then spontaneous resolution with loss of the delta wave and a normal PR interval at the end of the tracing.

oventricular block, implying that atrioventricular node conduction is not a crucial element of the tachycardia circuit. The dose is 50–250 mcg/kg by rapid intravenous bolus. It is antagonized by aminophylline and should be used with caution in patients with asthma.

3. Transesophageal atrial pacing–Atrial overdrive pacing and termination can be performed from a bipolar electrode-tipped catheter positioned in the esophagus adjacent to the left atrium. Overdrive pacing at rates approximately 30% faster than the tachycardia rate will interrupt the tachycardia circuit and restore sinus rhythm.

4. DC cardioversion–Direct current (DC) car-

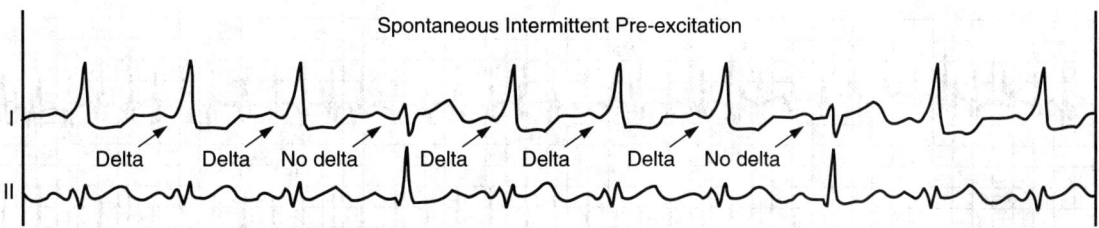

Figure 18–10. Leads I and II with spontaneous intermittent ventricular preexcitation (Wolff-Parkinson-White syndrome).

dioversion (0.5–2 synchronized J/kg) should be used immediately when a patient presents in cardiovascular collapse.

B. Chronic Treatment:

1. Digitalis–Digitalis is the drug of choice for long-term therapy. Conversion should be accomplished within 8–12 hours. Doses used are the same as those for congestive heart failure.

2. Beta-adrenergic blocking agents–Propranolol decreases sinus heart rate and atrioventricular nodal conduction. It is effective in the treatment of both reentrant and ectopic arrhythmias in doses ranging from 1 to 4 mg/kg/d. Newer beta-blockers such as atenolol and nadolol have recently become popular because they have fewer central nervous system side effects than propranolol and may be given only once or twice a day.

3. Calcium channel antagonists–Verapamil and other calcium channel blockers markedly prolong conduction through the atrioventricular node and are effective in interrupting and preventing reentrant tachycardias that incorporate the atrioventricular node. They are ineffective in terminating atrial tachycardias but may be useful to control the ventricular response by producing atrioventricular blockade. Verapamil comes in short- and long-acting preparations; the dose is 3–5 mg/kg/d. It may cause myocardial dysfunction and is contraindicated in infants.

4. Other drugs–Recently introduced antiarrhythmic medications (eg, flecainide, propafenone, sotalol, amiodarone) have increased pharmacologic actions and are extremely effective. However, these drugs also have serious side effects, including proarrhythmia (production of arrhythmias) and sudden

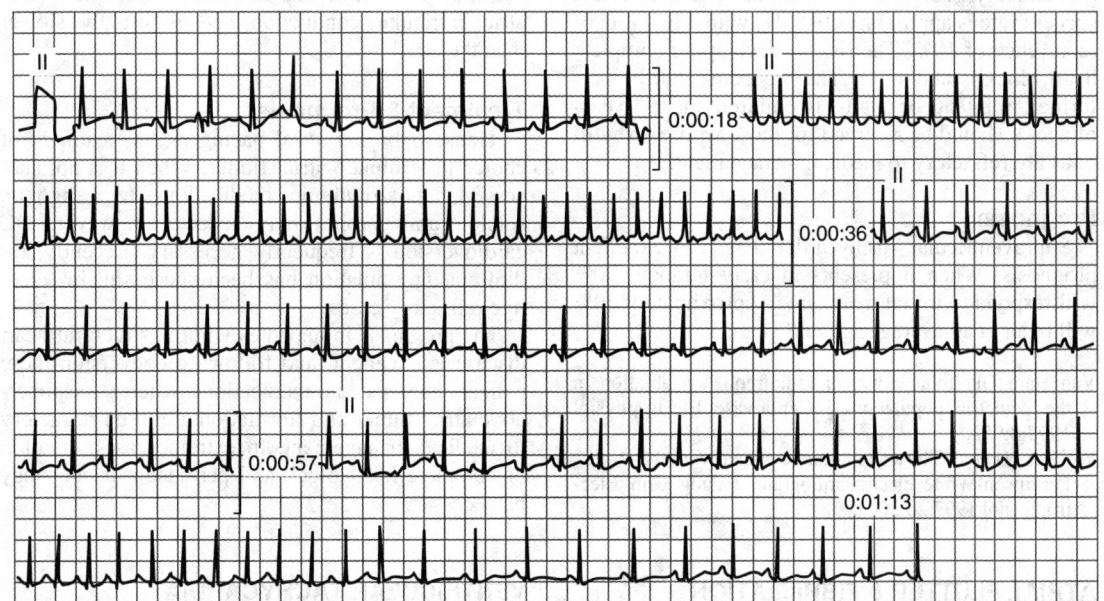

Figure 18–11. Lead II rhythm strip of ectopic atrial tachycardia. The tracing demonstrates a variable rate with a maximum of 260 beats/min, an abnormal P wave, and a gradual termination.

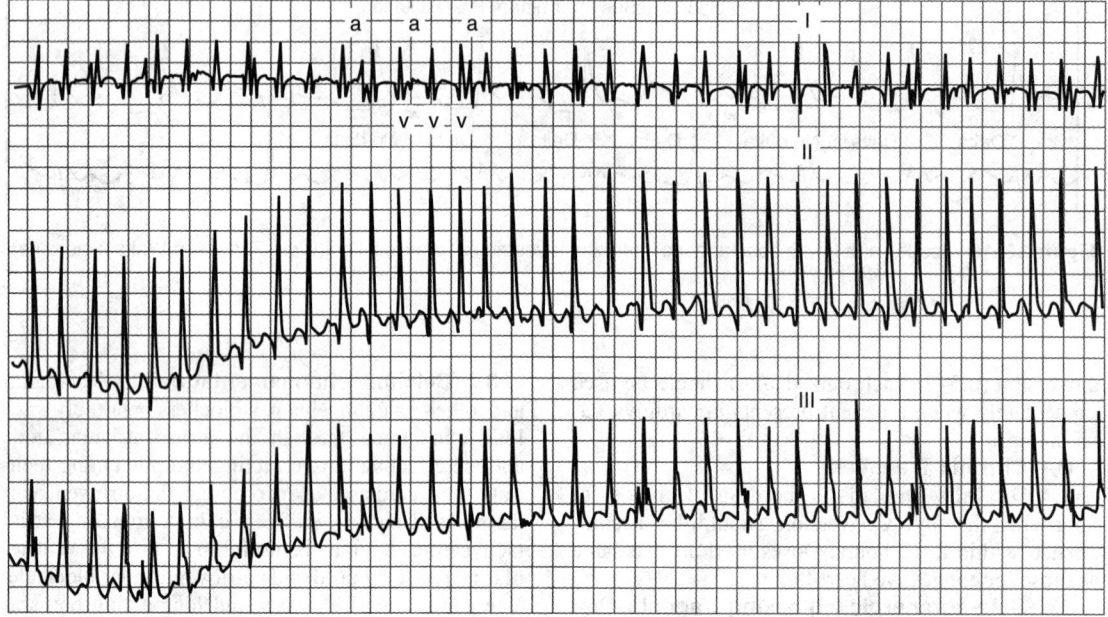

Figure 18–12. Three-lead rhythm strip of junctional ectopic tachycardia. Lead I is an atrial electrogram showing atrial (a)–ventricular (v) dissociation.

death, and should be used only under the direction of a pediatric cardiologist.

5. Radiofrequency ablation–This is a nonsurgical transvenous catheter technique that will desiccate an arrhythmia focus or accessory pathway and permanently "cure" an arrhythmia. The immediate success rate is approximately 85%, with a low rate of recurrence of 10%. The risk of developing complete heart block is about 1%. The procedure can be performed in infants or adults. In children under 4 years of age, it should be reserved for those whose arrhythmias are refractory to medical management.

Prognosis

Supraventricular tachycardia has an excellent prognosis. When it presents in early infancy, 90% will respond to initial treatment. Approximately 30% will recur at an average age of 8 years.

Van Hare GF: Indications for radiofrequency ablation in the pediatric population. J Cardiovasc Electrophysiol 1997;8:952.

Wellens HJ et al: The asymptomatic patient with the Wolff-Parkinson-White electrocardiogram. Pacing Clin Electrophysiol 1997;20:2082.

ATRIAL FLUTTER & FIBRILLATION

Atrial flutter and fibrillation are rare in children and are most often associated with organic heart dis-

ease—particularly postoperative congenital heart disease and sinus node dysfunction. Atrial flutter (Figure 18–8) can present in infancy and can mimic supraventricular tachycardia. The atrial rate is usually greater than 240/min and often more than 300/min. The ventricular rate depends on the rate of atrioventricular conduction and is usually slower than the atrial rate.

Treatment & Prognosis

Transesophageal atrial pacing is the treatment of choice to terminate atrial flutter. When it is not successful, antiarrhythmic medications (eg, digoxin, sotalol, amiodarone) may succeed; however, DC cardioversion is frequently necessary. Recently, radiofrequency ablation has been successful in selective refractory cases.

The prognosis in neonates without structural heart disease is excellent, and following conversion these patients may need no medications, whereas postoperative atrial flutter and fibrillation are often refractory to medical management. In extreme cases, creation of complete heart block and permanent pacing may be necessary.

VENTRICULAR TACHYCARDIA

Ventricular tachycardia is uncommon in childhood (Figure 18–13). It is usually associated with underly-

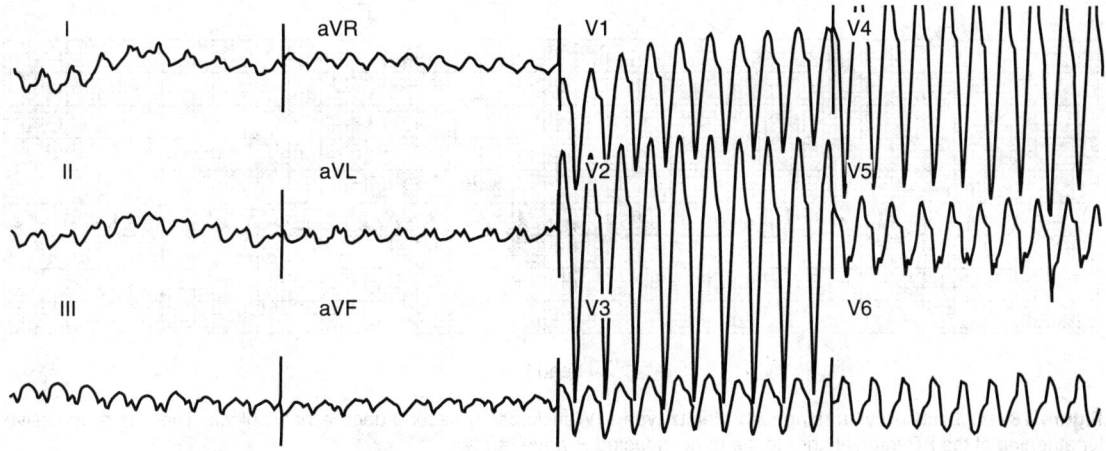

Figure 18–13. Twelve-lead ECG from a child with imipramine toxicity and ventricular tachycardia.

ing abnormalities of the myocardium (myocarditis, cardiomyopathy, myocardial tumors, postoperative congenital heart disease) or toxicity (hypoxia, electrolyte imbalance, drug toxicity). Sustained tachycardia is generally an unstable situation and, if left untreated, will usually degenerate into ventricular fibrillation.

Accelerated idioventricular rhythm is a sustained ventricular tachycardia seen in neonates with normal hearts. The rate is within 10% of the preceding sinus rate, and it is a self-limiting arrhythmia that requires no treatment.

Acute termination of ventricular tachycardia involves restoration of the normal myocardium when possible (correct electrolyte imbalance, drug toxicity, etc) and DC cardioversion (1–4 J/kg), cardioversion with lidocaine (1 mg/kg), or both. Chronic suppression of ventricular arrhythmias with antiarrhythmic drugs has many side effects (including proarrhythmia and death), and it must be initiated in the hospital under the direction of a pediatric cardiologist.

Davis AM et al: Clinical spectrum, therapeutic management and follow-up of ventricular tachycardia in infants and young children. Am Heart J 1996;131:186.

LONG QT SYNDROME

The long QT syndrome in children is an arrhythmic disorder in which ventricular repolarization is irregular and prolonged ($QT_c > 0.44$ s). It presents as syncope or seizures in response to exercise or sudden death, and if untreated it has a very high mortality rate (5% per year). It is transmitted genetically in an autosomal dominant or recessive pattern (the latter associated with congenital deafness), or it may be sporadic. Treatment is with beta blockade and exercise limitation and is only partially successful.

Moss AJ: Clinical management of patients with long QT syndrome: Drugs, devices, and gene-specific therapy. Pacing Clin Electrophysiol 1997;20:2058.

HEART BLOCK

1. FIRST-DEGREE HEART BLOCK

First-degree heart block is an electrocardiographic diagnosis of prolongation of the PR interval. The block does not in itself cause problems, but it is frequently seen in association with such congenital heart defects as atrial septal defect and with diseases such as rheumatic carditis. The PR interval may also be prolonged as a result of digoxin therapy.

2. SECOND-DEGREE HEART BLOCK

Mobitz type I (Wenckebach) heart block is recognized by progressive prolongation of the PR interval until there is no QRS following a P wave (Figure 18–14). Mobitz type I heart block occurs in normal hearts at rest and is usually benign. In **Mobitz type II** heart block, there is no progressive lengthening of the PR interval before the dropped beat (Figure 18–15). Mobitz type II heart block is frequently associated with organic heart disease, and a complete evaluation is necessary.

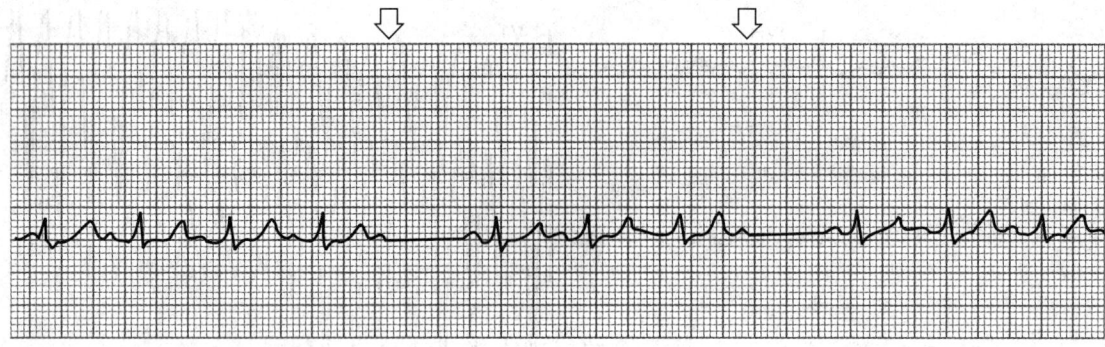

Lead I

Figure 18–14. Lead I rhythm strip with Mobitz type I (Wenckebach) second-degree heart block. There is progressive lengthening of the PR interval prior to the nonconducted P wave (arrow).

3. COMPLETE HEART BLOCK

In complete heart block, the atria and ventricles beat independently. Ventricular rates can range from 40 to 80 beats/min, whereas atrial rates may be faster (Figure 18–16).

Congenital complete heart block, the most common form of complete heart block, has a very high association with maternal systemic lupus erythematosus. Serologic screening should be performed in the mother of an infant with complete heart block even if she has no symptoms of collagen vascular disease. Congenital complete heart block is also associated with congenitally corrected transposition of the great vessels and endocardial cushion defect. Acquired complete heart block may be secondary to acute myocarditis, drug toxicity, electrolyte imbalance, hypoxia, and cardiac surgery.

Clinical Findings

Prenatal bradycardia is frequently noted in infants with congenital complete heart block, and emergent delivery is required if hydrops fetalis develops. Postnatal adaptation is largely dependent on the heart rate; infants with heart rates lower than 55 beats/min are at significantly greater risk for low cardiac output, congestive heart failure, and death. Wide QRS complexes and a rapid atrial rate are also poor prognostic signs. Most patients have an innocent flow murmur from increased stroke volume. In symptomatic patients, the heart can be quite enlarged and pulmonary edema may be present. In older patients, Stokes-Adams syncope can be the presenting symptom, or heart block may be found unexpectedly on routine physical examination. Complete cardiac evaluation, including echocardiography and Holter monitoring, is necessary to assess the patient for ventricu-

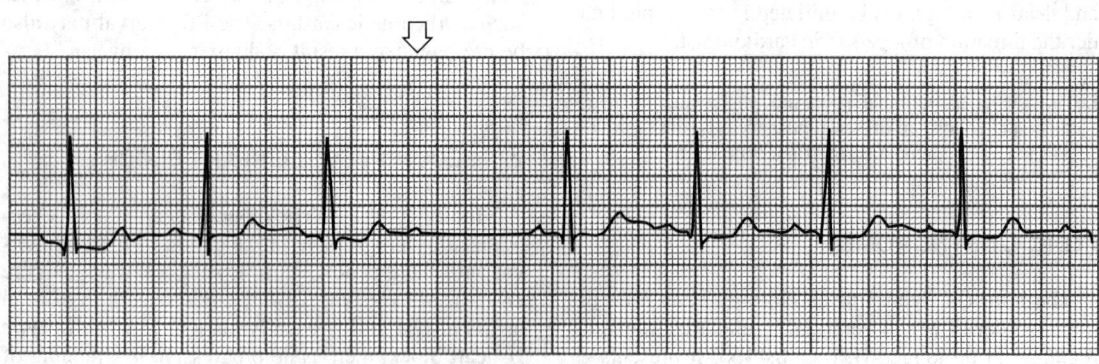

Lead III

Figure 18–15. Lead III rhythm strip with Mobitz type II second-degree heart block. There is a consistent PR interval with occasional loss of atrioventricular conduction (arrow).

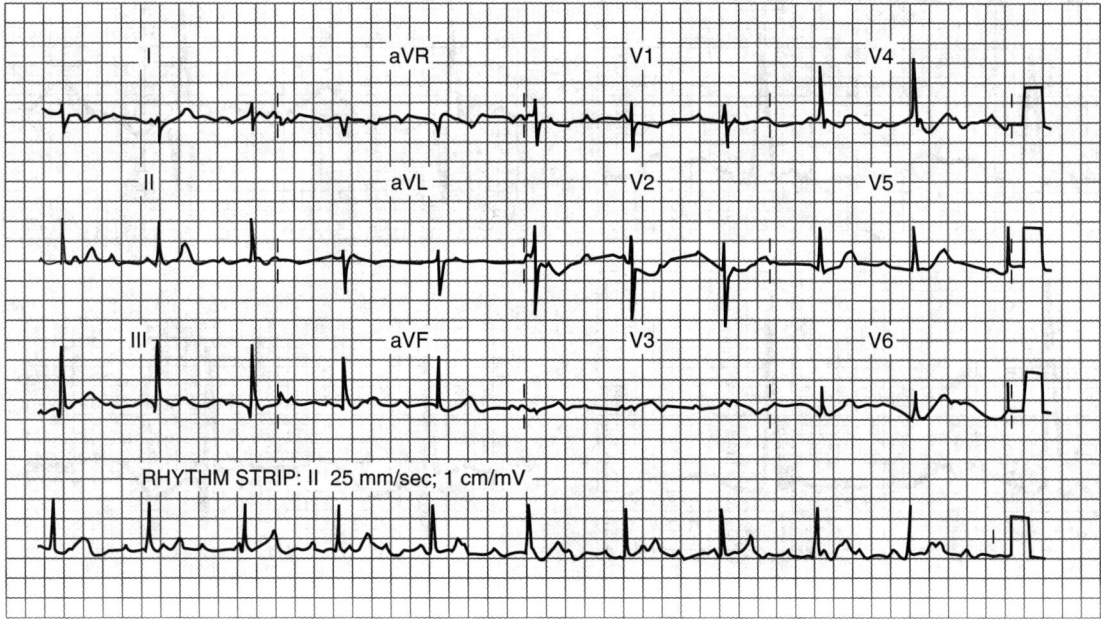

Figure 18–16. Twelve-lead ECG and lead II rhythm strip of complete heart block. The atrial rate is 150/min and the ventricular rate is 60/min.

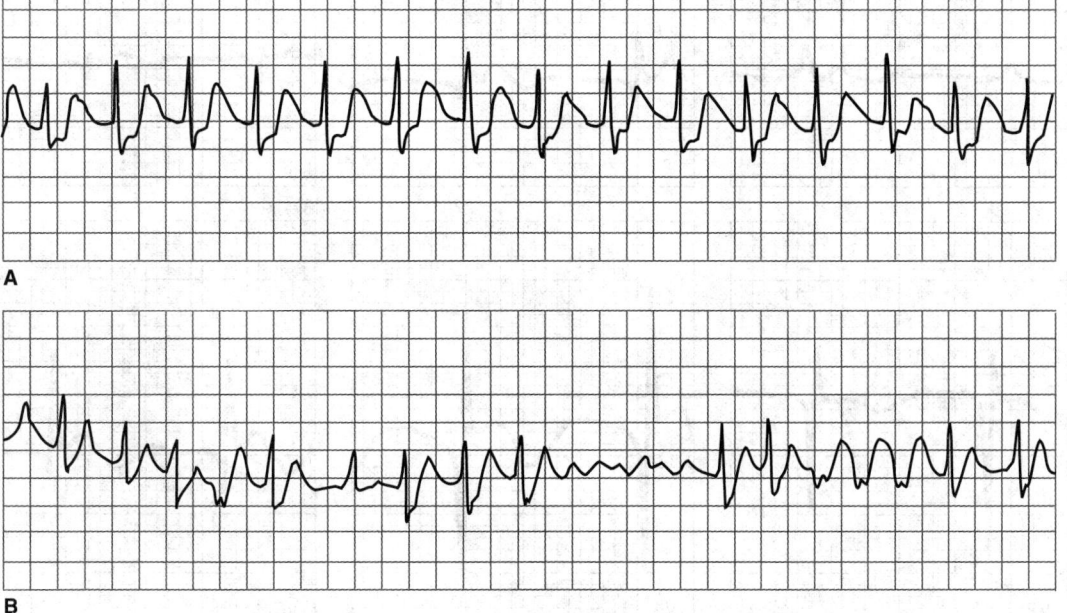

Figure 18–17. Rhythm strips of hyperkalemia, beginning with tall, peaked T waves and progressing to sinusoidal ventricular tachycardia.

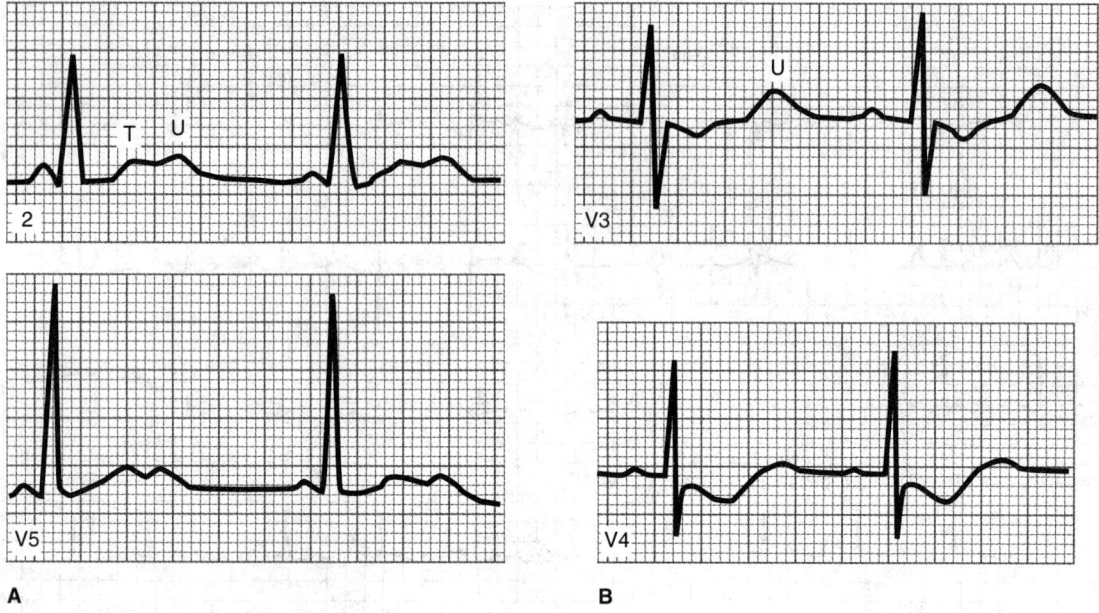

Figure 18–18. ECGs of hypokalemia, showing ST-segment depression and prominent U waves.

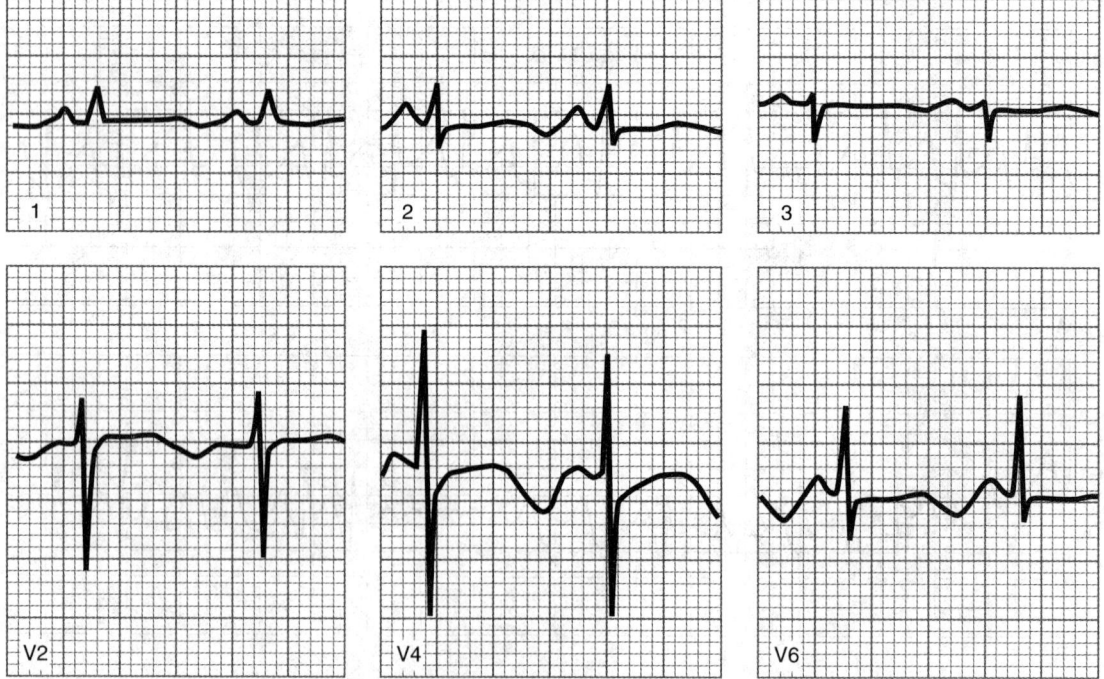

Figure 18–19. ECGs of hypocalcemia, demonstrating QT interval prolongation and T wave inversion.

lar dysfunction and to relate any symptoms to concurrent arrhythmias.

Treatment

In patients thought to be at risk for Stokes-Adams attacks or congestive heart failure, the treatment of choice for complete heart block is surgical insertion of a permanent pacemaker. Until permanent pacing can be instituted, patients can be temporarily assisted by infusions of isoproterenol or by temporary transcutaneous pacemakers.

Michaelson M: Congenital complete atrioventricular block. Progr Pediatr Cardiol 1995;4:1.

SYNCOPE
(Fainting)

Syncope is a sudden transient loss of consciousness that resolves spontaneously. The common form of syncope (simple fainting) occurs in 15% of children and is a disorder of control of heart rate and blood pressure by the autonomic nervous system that causes hypotension or bradycardia. It is often associated with rapid rising and postural hypotension, prolonged standing, or hypovolemia. Patients exhibit "vagal" symptoms such as pallor, nausea, or diaphoresis. Syncope, also known as autonomic dysfunction, can be evaluated with head-up tilt table testing. The patient is placed supine on a tilt table, and then—under constant heart rate and blood pressure monitoring—is tilted to the upright position. If symptoms develop, they can be classified as vasode-

pressor (hypotension), cardioinhibitory (bradycardia), or mixed. Treatment can then be directed accordingly. Syncope is usually self-limited and can be controlled with dietary salt and volume loading to prevent hypovolemia. Syncope that occurs during exercise or stress or is associated with a positive family history is a warning sign that there may be a serious underlying dysrhythmia calling for further investigation.

Balaji S et al: Neurocardiogenic syncope in children with a normal heart. J Am Coll Cardiol 1994;23:779.

ELECTROLYTE IMBALANCE

Potassium, calcium, and, to a lesser extent, magnesium imbalances are reflected in the ECG. Electrolyte disturbances resulting from potassium and calcium excess or deficiency are of greatest concern to the pediatrician, and some familiarity with these abnormal tracings is essential. In hyperkalemia (Figure 18–17), there is gradual progression from tall, peaked T waves (5–7 mEq/L) through widening of the QRS complex (8–9 mEq/L) to a broad, almost sinusoidal ventricular tachycardia configuration (> 10 mEq/L). Hypokalemia (Figure 18–18) is characterized by progressive prominence of the U wave and prolongation of the QT interval with ST segment depression. In hypocalcemia (Figure 18–19), there is prolongation of the QT interval, and in extreme cases T wave inversion occurs.

Judith M. Sondheimer, MD

EVALUATION OF THE CHILD WITH VOMITING (Table 19–1)

Assessment of the child with vomiting should start with a complete history, physical examination, and description of the vomitus. Emesis of gastric contents is characteristic of gastric outlet obstruction, central nervous system masses or infection, peptic disease, urinary tract infection, otitis or sinusitis, metabolic diseases (especially those causing acidosis), rumination, and psychogenic vomiting. Gastroesophageal reflux should be suspected in a healthy child with effortless postprandial spitting. An upper gastrointestinal series is essential to rule out anatomic causes. Further evaluations may include serum electrolytes, calcium, magnesium, urea nitrogen, urinalysis, and urine culture. The decision to obtain x-rays and scans of the central nervous system, chest, or sinuses is based on a specific indication from the history or physical examination.

The child who vomits bile-stained material may have small intestinal obstruction and should be investigated urgently. Bile staining may be gold or green in color. The history and physical examination are the essential starting points and should include duration of vomiting, the presence of blood in the vomitus, the presence of abdominal pain or distention, the character of the stools, and the presence of fever. Pain localized to the right lower quadrant suggests appendicitis. Midline or diffuse abdominal pain suggests pancreatitis or generalized peritonitis. Abdominal distention suggests intestinal obstruction. Viral and bacterial gastroenteritis associated with diarrhea and may produce generalized ileus with bilious vomiting. Gallbladder disease is uncommon in childhood but should be suspected in children with a positive family history or primary medical conditions promoting gallstones. The presence of mucus and blood in the stool should arouse suspicion of intestinal intussusception or bacterial or toxic colitis. Three-way radiographs of the abdomen are a first diagnostic step in localizing the site of intestinal obstruction.

The evaluation of bloody vomitus should start with confirmation that the material vomited is indeed blood. Numerous causes must be considered, including swallowed maternal blood in newborns, oropharyngeal lesions, nosebleed, peptic disease, bleeding disorders, foreign bodies, and esophageal varices. Mallory-Weiss tear of the gastroesophageal junction is common after prolonged vomiting. Careful assessment of the cardiovascular stability of the child is essential before extensive evaluation is initiated. Passage of a nasogastric tube will help determine whether bleeding is ongoing. Hematocrit should be measured. The history and physical examination will provide specific clues to diagnosis that may make further testing unnecessary. If further diagnostic investigation is desired, the most productive test is upper intestinal endoscopy.

GASTROESOPHAGEAL REFLUX

Postprandial regurgitation is the most common symptom of gastroesophageal reflux in young infants. Regurgitation ranges from effortless spitting to forceful vomiting. Although usually harmless, severe gastroesophageal reflux may cause failure to thrive, esophagitis with hematemesis, occult blood loss, anemia, esophageal stricture, and inflammatory esophageal polyps. Aspiration pneumonia, chronic cough, wheezing, and asthma-like attacks are reported. Dysphagia, colic after feedings, and neck contortions (Sandifer's syndrome) may occur. Ruminative behavior is sometimes a symptom. Apneic spells in young infants, especially occurring with position change after feeding, may be caused by gastroesophageal reflux. Gastroesophageal reflux is common in neurologically impaired children.

Gastroesophageal reflux is usually diagnosed clinically in thriving infants under 6 months of age. It can be diagnosed on barium swallow by observing free regurgitation of barium from stomach to esophagus. However, both false-positive and false-negative tests are common. An upper GI series is important to rule out anatomic causes of vomiting. Prolonged monitoring of esophageal pH is a more sensitive test.

Table 19–1. Causes of vomiting and regurgitation.

GASTROINTESTINAL TRACT DISORDERS

Esophagus
- Achalasia
- Gastroesophageal reflux (chalasia)
- Hiatal hernia
- Esophagitis
- Atresia with or without fistula
- Congenital vascular or mucosal rings, webs
- Stenosis
- Duplication and diverticulum
- Foreign body
- Periesophageal mass

Stomach
- Hypertrophic pyloric stenosis
- Pylorospasm
- Diaphragmatic hernia
- Peptic disease and gastritis
- Antral web

Duodenum
- Annular pancreas
- Duodenitis and ulcer
- Malrotation
- Mesenteric bands
- Superior mesenteric artery syndrome

Intestine and colon
- Atresia and stenosis
- Meconium ileus
- Malrotation, volvulus
- Duplication
- Intussusception
- Foreign body
- Polyposis
- Soy or cow's milk protein intolerance
- Gluten enteropathy
- Food allergy
- Hirschsprung's disease
- Chronic intestinal pseudo-obstruction
- Appendicitis
- Inflammatory bowel disease
- Gastroenteritis, infections

Other abdominal organs
- Hepatitis
- Gallstones
- Pancreatitis
- Peritonitis

EXTRA-GASTROINTESTINAL TRACT DISORDERS

- Sepsis
- Pneumonia
- Otitis media
- Urinary tract infection
- Meningitis
- Subdural effusion
- Hydrocephalus
- Brain tumor
- Reye's syndrome
- Rumination
- Intoxications
  - Alcohol
  - Aspirin
  - Acetaminophen
- Adrenal insufficiency
- Renal tubular acidosis
- Inborn errors
  - Urea cycle disorders
  - Phenylketonuria
  - Maple syrup urine disease
  - Organic acidemia
  - Galactosemia
  - Fructose intolerance
  - Tyrosinosis
- Scleroderma
- Epidermolysis bullosa

Esophageal and gastric scintiscanning is sometimes helpful in identifying pulmonary aspiration. Esophagoscopy is not diagnostic, but esophagitis can be identified.

Treatment & Prognosis

In 85% of patients, gastroesophageal reflux is self-limited, disappearing between 6 and 12 months, often coincident with assumption of erect posture and initiation of solid feedings. Regurgitation is reduced by conservative measures such as frequent small feedings thickened with rice cereal (2–3 tsp/oz of formula) and placing the child in a prone position. H-2–receptor antagonists (ranitidine, 5 mg/kg/d in two

doses) and proton pump inhibitors (eg, omeprazole) are effective in controlling esophagitis. Use of the latter agents promotes hypergastrinemia, whose long-term effects in infants are not defined. Prokinetic agents such as metoclopramide (0.1 mg/kg before meals) or cisapride (0.2 mg/kg/dose three or four times daily) hasten gastric emptying and improve esophageal motor function. Their impact on the symptoms of typical GE reflux of infants is not well documented by controlled studies. Recently there has been concern about prolongation of QT interval and cardiac arrythmia during treatment with cisapride. This is most likely to occur in patients simultaneously receiving erythromycin or other macrolides, in premature infants, in patients with antecedent heart disease or multi-organ system failure.

Surgery is indicated if reflux causes (1) persistent vomiting with failure to thrive (2) esophagitis or esophageal stricture and (3) apneic spells or chronic pulmonary disease unresponsive to 2–3 months of medical therapy. Children over 18 months, children with large hiatus hernias, and neurologically handicapped children respond less well to medical therapy.

Laneau S et al: Proarrythmia associated with cisapride in children. Pediatrics 1998; 101:1053.
Nelson SP et al: Prevalence of symptoms of gastroesophageal reflux during infancy. Arch Pediatr Adolesc Med 1997;151:569.
Scott RB et al: Cisapride in pediatric gastroesophageal reflux. J Pediatr Gastroenterol Nutr 1997;25:499.
Sondheimer JM: Gastroesophageal reflux in children: Clinical presentation and diagnostic evaluation. Gastrointest Endosc Clin North Am 1994;4:55.

ACHALASIA OF THE ESOPHAGUS

Esophageal achalasia is characterized by failure of relaxation of the lower esophageal sphincter and lack of propulsive peristalsis in the esophageal body.

Clinical Findings

A. Symptoms and Signs: Achalasia occurs at any age but is uncommon under age 5 years. Typical symptoms include retrosternal pain and episodes of food "sticking" in the throat or upper chest. Patients eat slowly and often drink large amounts of fluid with meals. Dysphagia is relieved by repeated forceful swallowing or by vomiting. Familial cases have been described. Chronic cough, wheezing, recurrent pneumonitis, anemia, and weight loss may occur.

B. Imaging and Manometric Studies: The barium swallow shows a dilated esophagus with a short, tapered "beak" at the distal end. In infants, esophageal dilation may not be present. Cinefluoroscopy may show absence of normal peristalsis. Esophageal manometry may show high resting pressure in the lower esophageal sphincter, failure of the sphincter to relax with swallowing, and abnormal or absent peristalsis. The cause is unknown. Decrease in tissue nitric oxide in the area of the lower esophageal sphincter may be a secondary phenomenon or may be primary to the motor abnormalities preventing sphincter relaxation.

Differential Diagnosis

Congenital esophageal stricture, esophageal webs, peptic stricture secondary to chronic reflux, and esophageal masses may mimic esophageal achalasia.

Treatment & Prognosis

Pneumatic dilation of the lower esophageal sphincter is of value in most cases and can be repeated if symptoms recur. Botulinum toxin injected into the lower esophageal sphincter has been effective temporarily in adults. More definitive results can be achieved by surgically splitting the lower esophageal sphincter muscle (Heller myotomy), a procedure that can now be performed laparoscopically. Because of the shorter duration of the illness, the prognosis for return of the esophagus to normal caliber after surgical treatment is better in pediatric patients than in adults.

Lelli JL, Drongowski RA, Coran AG: Efficacy of the transthoracic modified Heller myotomy in children with achalasia. J Pediatr Surg 1997;32:338.

Pasricha PJ, Kalloo AN: Recent advances in the treatment of achalasia. Gastrointest Endosc Clin North Am 1997;7:191.

CAUSTIC BURNS OF THE ESOPHAGUS

Ingestion of caustic solids or liquids (pH > 12.0) may produce esophageal lesions ranging from superficial inflammation to coagulative necrosis with ulceration, perforation, and mediastinitis (or peritonitis if the stomach is involved). The severity of the accompanying oral or laryngeal lesions does not correlate well with the degree of esophageal injury. Esophageal or laryngeal obstruction secondary to edema and exudate formation occurs within 24 hours. Pain may be severe. Strictures of the esophagus may develop quickly, or gradually over several months. Esophageal strictures develop in areas of anatomic narrowing such as the cervical region, at the point at which the left bronchus crosses the esophagus, and at the gastroesophageal junction. Stricture occurs only with full-thickness esophageal necrosis. Short circumferential strictures may occur, or the entire esophagus may become twisted and narrowed. Shortening of the esophagus may lead to hiatal hernia.

The child with a history of alkali ingestion should have a careful examination of the lips and mouth and of the airway. Drooling is common. Oral lesions are especially common with solid agents. Vomiting

should not be induced. Intravenous corticosteroids (eg, methylprednisolone, 1–2 mg/kg/d), are started immediately if oral cavity swelling is severe and laryngeal edema is suspected. Intravenous fluids may be necessary if dysphagia is present. Esophagoscopy should be done within 24–48 hours after ingestion.

Treatment may be stopped if there are only first-degree burns. Corticosteroids may be beneficial in first- and second-degree burns but are not likely to prevent stricture formation from third-degree burns. Repeated esophageal dilations may be necessary as a stricture develops but are not performed acutely. When x-rays show erosion into the mediastinum or peritoneum, antibiotics are mandatory. Intraluminal esophageal stenting may be beneficial during early management. Surgical replacement of the esophagus with a segment of colon may be necessary if dilation fails to control stricture.

Although other ingestants may cause esophageal irritation (eg, bleach, detergents, or acids), it is rare for any but the strongest acids and detergents to result in full-thickness necrosis and stricture.

Byrne W: Foreign bodies, bezoars and caustic ingestion. Gastrointest Endosc Clin North Am 1994;4:99.

HIATAL HERNIA

Hiatal hernias are classified as (1) paraesophageal, in which the esophagus and gastroesophageal junction are normally placed with the gastric cardia, herniated beside the esophagus through the esophageal hiatus; and (2) sliding, in which the gastroesophageal junction and a portion of the proximal stomach are herniated through the esophageal hiatus. Paraesophageal hernia is rare in childhood and presents with pain, esophageal obstruction, or respiratory compromise. Sliding hernia is common in children. Gastroesophageal reflux may accompany sliding hiatal hernia, though many—even those of large size—cause no symptoms.

Surgical correction of paraesophageal or hiatus hernia is indicated only if symptoms persist in spite of medical treatment.

PYLORIC STENOSIS

The cause of postnatal pyloric circular muscle hypertrophy leading to gastric outlet obstruction is not known. The incidence is 1–8:1000 births, with a 4:1 male predominance and a positive family history in 13%.

Clinical Findings

A. Symptoms and Signs: Vomiting usually begins between 2 and 4 weeks of age and rapidly becomes projectile after every feeding; it starts at birth in about 10% of cases. Onset of symptoms may be delayed in premature infants. The vomitus is rarely bilious but may be blood-streaked. The infant is hungry and nurses avidly. Constipation, dehydration, weight loss, fretfulness, and finally apathy occur. The upper abdomen may be distended after feeding, and prominent gastric peristaltic waves from left to right may be seen. An olive-sized mass can often be felt on deep palpation in the right upper abdomen, especially after the child has vomited.

B. Laboratory Findings: There is hypochloremic alkalosis with potassium depletion. Hemoconcentration is reflected by elevated hemoglobin and hematocrit values. Elevated unconjugated bilirubin occurs in 2–5% of cases.

C. Imaging: An upper gastrointestinal series reveals delay in gastric emptying and an elongated narrowed pyloric channel with a double tract of barium. The enlarged pyloric muscle causes characteristic semilunar impressions on the gastric antrum. Ultrasonography shows a hypoechoic ring with a hyperdense center. Thickness of circular muscle is greater than 4 mm in pyloric stenosis.

Differential Diagnosis

Other causes of vomiting must be ruled out (Table 19–1). In esophageal stenosis or achalasia, the vomitus contains no gastric contents, and metabolic alkalosis is rare. With annular pancreas, malrotation, volvulus, and lesions causing small bowel obstruction, the vomitus is bilious. The absence of virilization and hyperkalemia generally rules out congenital adrenal hyperplasia with adrenal insufficiency. Seizures, irritability, and metabolic acidosis are often associated with other metabolic disorders. Sepsis and urinary tract infections should be checked by culture. Pylorospasm during barium x-ray may cause delay in gastric emptying, but the elongated narrow pyloric canal is not seen and no mass is palpable. Antral webs or diaphragms, duplications, cysts, and ulcers of the pyloric canal are rare causes of gastric outlet obstruction.

Treatment & Prognosis

Pyloromyotomy is the treatment of choice and consists of incision down to the mucosa along the pyloric length. Prior to surgery, it is imperative to repair dehydration and electrolyte abnormalities even if it takes 24–48 hours.

The outlook is excellent following surgery. Sometimes there is vomiting postoperatively in cases with a long preoperative history. The postoperative barium x-ray remains abnormal despite relief of symptoms.

Moazam F, Kolts BE, Rodgers B: In pursuit of the etiology of congenital hypertrophic pyloric stenosis. J Pediatr Gastroenterol Nutr 1982;1:97.

Stunden RJ, LeQuense GW, Little KET: The improved ultrasound diagnosis of pyloric stenosis. Pediatr Radiol 1986;16:200.

PEPTIC DISEASE

Peptic ulcers may occur at any age but are more common between 12 and 18 years. Boys are affected more frequently than girls. Most ulcers in childhood are secondary to an underlying illness, toxin, or drug. Secondary peptic disease is caused by breakdown in the normal mucosal defense, which permits acid peptic digestion of gastric or duodenal mucosa. Causes include (1) reduced mucous protective layer (aspirin, nonsteroidal anti-inflammatory drugs, hypoxia); (2) reduced metabolic activity of the mucosal cell, which allows for diffusion of hydrogen ions into the cell (hypoxia, hypotension); (3) increased secretion of acid or pepsin (increased parietal cell mass, increased postprandial secretion of gastrin, increased vagal tone); (4) reflux of bile from duodenum to stomach; and (5) decreased neutralizing activity in duodenal secretions. The most common causes of secondary ulcer are toxins (alcohol, aspirin, and nonsteroidal anti-inflammatory medications), sepsis, hypotension, burns, and injury of the central nervous system.

There is a close association between *Helicobacter pylori* infection of the gastric antrum and the primary peptic conditions—antral gastritis, duodenal ulcer, and gastric ulcer. The incidence of *H pylori* infection is low in North American children but increases with age. Antibody positivity is found in 10–20% of healthy North American children. There is no evidence that *H pylori* infection causes recurrent abdominal pain of childhood or dyspepsia without gastritis. The prevalence of *H pylori* varies. It is often higher in areas with poor sanitation and water supply.

Clinical Findings

A. Symptoms and Signs: In children under 6 years of age, vomiting and upper gastrointestinal bleeding are the most common manifestations of peptic ulcer disease. Older children are more likely to complain of abdominal pain, with occult gastrointestinal bleeding and emesis occurring in less than 50%. Large ulcers in the pyloric channel may cause gastric outlet obstruction. Acute illnesses responsible for secondary ulcers include central nervous system disease, burns, sepsis, and multiple organ system failure. Chronic conditions such as pulmonary insufficiency, Crohn's disease, hepatic cirrhosis, and rheumatoid arthritis are associated with peptic disease. Gross upper gastrointestinal bleeding requiring transfusion is more commonly seen in secondary ulcers, particularly following ingestion of aspirin, alcohol and nonsteroidal anti-inflammatory drugs, than in primary ulcer disease. Ulcers may occur throughout the upper gastrointestinal tract secondary to nonsteroidal anti-inflammatory medications.

B. Imaging and Endoscopy: An upper gastrointestinal x-ray may show an ulcer crater. Such soft signs of peptic disease as duodenal spasticity and irregularity, which are suggestive of ulcer in adults, are often found in normal infants and are unreliable. Upper intestinal endoscopy is the most accurate diagnostic test for peptic disease. If the purpose of endoscopy is to identify the site of acute upper gastrointestinal bleeding, it should be performed within 48 hours after the episode. Endoscopy is necessary for the identification of *H pylori* (by culture of tissue, urease testing, or histologic identification of organisms). It also allows for identification of other causes of peptic symptoms such as esophagitis, eosinophilic enteropathy, and celiac disease.

Differential Diagnosis

Secondary ulcers should be suspected in any child with a severe underlying disease who suddenly presents with hematemesis or melena. The differential diagnosis of primary peptic ulcer includes recurrent abdominal pain, irritable bowel syndrome, esophagitis, pancreatitis, cholelithiasis, and recurrent midgut volvulus. Suspicion should increase when there is a family history of primary peptic ulcer disease or *H pylori* infection.

Treatment

Peptic ulcer disease may be treated with liquid antacids, but these are poorly tolerated by children. H-2–receptor antagonists such as cimetidine (5 mg/kg/dose given orally before meals and at bedtime) or ranitidine (2.5 mg/kg/dose given orally every 12 hours) produce healing in 4–8 weeks. Proton pump inhibitors (omeprazole and lansoprazole) are powerful inhibitors of gastric acid secretion but pediatric dosages have not been determined and the effects of prolonged hypergastrinemia seen with these agents are not known.

Strict "ulcer diets" are not indicated. Foods that cause pain should be avoided. Caffeine should be avoided because it increases gastric secretion. Three regular meals are recommended, and snacks are to be avoided especially at bedtime. Aspirin and nonsteroidal anti-inflammatory drugs should not be used.

Cure of peptic disease associated with *H pylori* infection requires eradication of the organism. The optimal therapeutic regimen is still undetermined. A recent National Institutes of Health consensus conference recommends "triple therapy" with amoxicillin, metronidazole, and bismuth subsalicylate for 10–14 days. Double therapy with omeprazole and amoxicillin may be equally effective.

George DE, Glassman M: Peptic ulcer disease in children. Gastrointest Endosc Clin North Am 1994;4:23.

MacArthur C, Saunders M, Feldman W: *H pylori*, gastroduodenal disease and recurrent abdominal pain in children. JAMA 1995;273:729.

CONGENITAL DIAPHRAGMATIC HERNIA

Diaphragmatic hernia may be secondary to a posterolateral defect in the diaphragm (foramen of Bochdalek) or, in about 5% of cases, to a retrosternal defect (foramen of Morgagni). It represents failure of division of the thoracic and abdominal cavities at the eighth to tenth weeks of fetal life. All degrees of protrusion of the abdominal viscera through the diaphragmatic opening may occur. Eighty percent of posterolateral defects involve the left diaphragm. In eventration of the diaphragm, a leaf of the diaphragm with hypoplastic muscular elements balloons into the chest and leads to similar but milder symptoms.

Mild to severe respiratory distress is usually present at birth. The abdomen may be scaphoid because of displacement of the viscera. Breath sounds in the affected hemithorax are absent, with displacement of the point of maximal cardiac impulse. Occasionally, a diaphragmatic hernia may be found on incidental chest x-ray. Thirty percent of infants with diaphragmatic hernia die, mostly mfrom pulmonary insufficiency. The lung on the affected side is hypoplastic, with decreased generations of airways and pulmonary arteries, and there is pulmonary hypertension. Other complications include mediastinal shift with vascular kinking, pulmonary infection, prematurity, cardiac anomalies, and intestinal malrotation. Extracorporeal membrane oxygenation may decrease the early postoperative mortality rate in patients with poor lung compliance. Inhaled nitric oxide reduces pulmonary vascular hypertension, and it was hoped that its use might improve the outcome in patients with diaphragmatic hernia. Results in controlled trials have thus far been disappointing.

Inhaled nitric oxide and hypoxic respiratory failure in infants with congenital diaphragmatic hernia. The Neonatal Inhaled Nitric Oxide Study Group. Pediatrics 1997;99:838.

Wilson JM et al: Congenital diaphragmatic hernia: A tale of two cities, the Boston experience. J Pediatr Surg 1997;32:401.

CONGENITAL DUODENAL OBSTRUCTION

Extrinsic duodenal obstruction is usually due to congenital peritoneal bands associated with intestinal malrotation, annular pancreas, or duodenal duplication. Intrinsic obstruction is a result of stenosis, mucosal diaphragm ("wind sock" deformity), or duodenal atresia. The duodenal lumen may be obliterated by a membrane or completely interrupted with a fibrous cord between the two segments. Atresia may be proximal or distal to the ampulla of Vater.

Clinical Findings

A. Atresia: A history of polyhydramnios is common. Vomiting (usually bile-stained) begins within a few hours after birth, with epigastric distention. Meconium may be normally passed. Duodenal atresia is commonly associated with other congenital anomalies (30%), including esophageal atresia, other intestinal atresias, and cardiac and renal anomalies. Prematurity (25–50%) and Down's syndrome (20–30%) are associated conditions. Abdominal x-rays show distention of the stomach and proximal duodenum with air ("double bubble"). With protracted vomiting, there may be less air in the stomach. Absence of gas distal to the obstruction suggests atresia or an extrinsic obstruction severe enough to completely occlude the lumen, whereas air scattered over the lower abdomen may indicate a partial duodenal obstruction. A barium enema may be helpful in determining the presence of malrotation or atresia lower in the gastrointestinal tract.

B. Duodenal Stenosis: Obvious symptoms of duodenal obstruction may be delayed for weeks or years. Although the stenotic area is usually postampullary, the vomitus does not always contain bile.

Treatment & Prognosis

Duodenoduodenostomy is performed to bypass stenosis or atresia. Thorough exploration is necessary to ensure that no additional anomalies are present lower in the gastrointestinal tract. The mortality rate (35–40%) is significantly affected by prematurity, Down's syndrome, and associated congenital anomalies. Postoperative duodenal dilation and hypomotility may cause continued symptoms.

CONGENITAL INTESTINAL ATRESIAS & STENOSES

Excluding anal anomalies, intestinal atresia and stenosis account for one-third of all cases of neonatal intestinal obstruction. Polyhydramnios occurs in most affected infants and can be diagnosed before birth by ultrasonography. Neonates present with a clinical triad of abdominal distention, bilious vomiting, and obstipation or failure to pass meconium. Prematurity and other congenital anomalies may be present. The localization and relative incidence of atresias and stenoses are listed in Table 19–2.

Bile-stained vomiting with abdominal distention usually begins in the first 48 hours of life. Atresias, stenoses, and obstructing membranes may affect multiple sites. The small intestine may be significantly shortened. X-ray features include dilated loops of small bowel and absence of colonic gas. Barium enema reveals narrow-caliber microcolon if the atresia is in the lower small bowel. In over 10% of cases of intestinal atresia, there is absence of the mesentery, and the superior mesenteric artery cannot be

Table 19–2. Localization and relative frequency of congenital gastrointestinal atresias and stenoses.

	Area Involved	Type of Lesion	Relative Frequency
Pylorus		Atresia; web or diaphragm	1%
Duodenum	80% are distal to the ampulla of Vater	Atresia, stenosis; web or diaphragm	45%
Jejunoileal	Proximal jejunum and distal ileum	Atresia (multiple in 6–29%); stenosis	50%
Colon	Left colon and rectum	Atresia (usually associated with atresias of the small bowel)	5–9%

identified beyond the origin of the right colic and ileocolic arteries. The ileum coils around one of these two arteries, giving rise to the "Christmas tree" deformity. The tenuous blood supply often compromises surgical anastomoses. Multiple intestinal atresias may be associated with immunodeficiency. The differential diagnosis includes Hirschsprung's disease, paralytic ileus secondary to sepsis, gastroenteritis or pneumonia, midgut volvulus, and meconium ileus. Surgery is mandatory in newborn infants with small bowel atresia. Postoperative complications include short bowel syndrome and hypomotility.

Walker MW et al: Multiple areas of intestinal atresia associated with immunodeficiency and post transfusion graft versus host disease. J Pediatr 1993;123:93.

ANNULAR PANCREAS

Annular pancreas is a result of incomplete rotation and fusion of the dorsal and ventral pancreatic anlagen. The symptoms are those of partial or complete duodenal obstruction. Down's syndrome and congenital anomalies of the gastrointestinal tract occur frequently. Polyhydramnios is common. Clinical manifestations can develop late in childhood.

Treatment consists of duodenoduodenostomy or duodenojejunostomy without operative dissection or division of the pancreatic annulus.

INTESTINAL MALROTATION WITH OR WITHOUT VOLVULUS

Normally, the midgut, extending from the duodenojejunal junction to the mid transverse colon and supplied by the superior mesenteric artery, returns to the intra-abdominal position during the tenth week of embryonic life. The root of the mesentery rotates in a counterclockwise direction during retraction. This causes the colon to cross ventrally; the cecum moves from the left to the right lower quadrant, and the duodenum crosses dorsally to become partly retroperitoneal. When this rotation is incomplete, the posterior fixation of the mesentery is defective, so that the bowel from the ligament of Treitz to the mid transverse colon may twist, causing a volvulus around the narrow mesenteric root.

Clinical Findings

A. Symptoms and Signs: Malrotation accounts for 10% of neonatal intestinal obstructions. Most infants present with recurrent bile-stained vomiting or acute small bowel obstruction in the first 3 weeks of life. The first signs may occur later in life, with symptoms of intermittent intestinal obstruction or, rarely, with malabsorption, protein-losing enteropathy, or diarrhea. Associated congenital anomalies, especially cardiac, occur in over 25% of symptomatic cases.

B. Imaging: An upper gastrointestinal series may show partial or complete small bowel obstruction. The duodenojejunal junction may lie to the right of the spine along with the jejunal loops. The diagnosis of malrotation can be further confirmed by barium enema, which may demonstrate a mobile cecum located in the midline, right upper quadrant, or left abdomen.

Treatment & Prognosis

Midgut volvulus is a surgical emergency. Bowel necrosis results from occlusion of the superior mesenteric artery. When necrosis is extensive, it is recommended that a first operation include only reduction of the volvulus with lysis of mesenteric bands. Intestinal resection should be delayed if possible until a second-look operation 24–48 hours later can be undertaken in the hope that some bowel can be salvaged. The prognosis is guarded if there is perforation, peritonitis, or extensive intestinal necrosis.

Janik JS, Ein SH: Normal intestinal rotation with nonfixation: A cause of chronic abdominal pain. J Pediatr Surg 1979;14:670.

Millar AJW et al: The deadly vomit: Malrotation and midgut volvulus. Pediatr Surg Int 1987;2:172.

Stewart DR et al: Malrotation of the bowel in infants and children: A 15 year experience. Surgery 1976;79:716.

MECKEL'S DIVERTICULUM & OMPHALO-MESENTERIC DUCT REMNANTS

1. MECKEL'S DIVERTICULUM

Meckel's diverticulum is the most common of the omphalomesenteric duct remnants. It is usually found on the antimesenteric border of the mid to distal ileum. It is present in 1.5% of the population but rarely causes symptoms. In addition to the ileal mucosa, diverticula may contain gastric, pancreatic, jejunal, or colonic mucosa. Familial cases have been reported. Complications occur three times more frequently in males than in females and in 50–60% of cases within the first 2 years of life. Acid secreted by heterotopic gastric tissue causes ulceration and bleeding from adjacent ileal mucosa.

Clinical Findings

A. Symptoms and Signs: In 40–60% of symptomatic cases, painless passage of maroon or melanotic blood per rectum occurs. Acute bleeding may cause shock. Occult bleeding is less common. Intestinal obstruction occurs in 25% of symptomatic cases as a result of ileocolonic intussusception. Intestinal volvulus may occur around a fibrous remnant of the vitelline duct extending from the tip of the diverticulum to the abdominal wall. In some cases, entrapment of a bowel loop under a band running between the diverticulum and the base of the mesentery occurs. The diverticulum may be trapped in an inguinal hernia (Littre's hernia). Diverticulitis occurs in 10–20% of symptomatic cases and is clinically indistinguishable from acute appendicitis. Perforation and generalized peritonitis may occur. There may be chronic recurrent abdominal pain.

B. Imaging: Diagnosis of Meckel's diverticulum is seldom made on barium x-ray. Radionuclide imaging utilizes ^{99m}Tc pertechnetate, which is taken up by the diverticulum lined with heterotopic gastric mucosa. Stimulation of ^{99m}Tc pertechnetate uptake by pentagastrin or cimetidine can reduce the number of false-negative results. Angiography may be useful when bleeding is brisk.

Treatment

Treatment is surgical. At laparoscopy or laparotomy, the ileum proximal and distal to the diverticulum may reveal ulcerations and heterotopic tissue adjacent to the neck of the diverticulum.

Prognosis

The prognosis for Meckel's diverticulum is good. Marked hemorrhage may occur but is rarely exsanguinating.

2. OTHER REMNANTS OF THE OMPHALOMESENTERIC DUCT

Fecal discharge from the umbilicus is evidence of a patent omphalomesenteric duct. The duct may be completely closed, causing a fibrous cord joining ileum and umbilicus and potentially the origin of a volvulus. A mucoid umbilical discharge may be indicative of a mucocele, which can protrude through the umbilicus and be mistaken for an umbilical granuloma, since it is firm and bright red. In all cases, surgical excision of the omphalomesenteric remnant is indicated.

Moore TC: Omphalomesenteric duct malformations. Semin Pediatr Surg 1996;5:116.

DUPLICATIONS OF THE GASTROINTESTINAL TRACT

Duplications are congenital anomalies of the gastrointestinal tract. They are fluid-filled, spherical, or tubular structures found anywhere along the gastrointestinal tract, most commonly in the ileum. Duplications usually contain fluid and sometimes blood if necrosis has taken place. Most duplications do not communicate with the intestinal lumen but are attached to the mesenteric side of the gut and share a common muscular coat. The epithelial lining of the duplication is usually of the same type as that from which it originates. Some duplications (neuroenteric cysts) are attached to the spinal cord and are associated with hemivertebrae and anterior or posterior spina bifida.

Symptoms of vomiting, abdominal distention, colicky pain, rectal bleeding, partial or total intestinal obstruction, or an abdominal mass may start in infancy. Diarrhea and malabsorption may result from bacterial overgrowth in communicating duplications. Physical examination reveals a rounded, smooth, freely movable mass, and x-ray films of the abdomen show a noncalcified mass displacing the intestines or stomach. Scanning with ^{99m}Tc pertechnetate is useful in duplications containing gastric mucosa. Involvement of the terminal small bowel can give rise to an intussusception. Prompt surgical treatment is indicated.

Bissler JJ, Klein RL: Alimentary tract duplications in children. Clin Pediatr 1988;27:152.

CONGENITAL AGANGLIONIC MEGACOLON
(Hirschsprung's Disease)

Hirschsprung's disease results from an absence of ganglion cells in the mucosal and muscular layers of the colon. There is a failure of neural crest cells to migrate to the mesodermal layers, possibly mediated by abnormalities in end-organ cell surface receptors or local deficiency of nitric oxide synthesis. The rectum alone (30%) or the rectosigmoid (44%) is usually affected. The entire colon is aganglionic in 8% of cases. Segmental aganglionosis is very rare and may be an acquired lesion. The aganglionic segment is narrowed, with dilation of the proximal normal colon. The mucosa of the dilated colonic segment may become thin and inflamed (enterocolitis), resulting in diarrhea, bleeding, and protein loss.

A familial pattern has been described, particularly in total colonic aganglionosis. The disease is four times more common in boys than in girls, and 10–15% of patients have Down's syndrome.

Clinical Findings

A. Symptoms and Signs: Failure of the newborn to pass meconium—followed by vomiting, abdominal distention, and reluctance to feed—suggests the diagnosis of Hirschsprung's disease. In some cases, symptoms of distention and vomiting appear later. Bouts of enterocolitis manifested by fever, explosive diarrhea, and prostration are reported in about 50% of newborns with this disease. These episodes may lead to acute inflammatory and ischemic changes in the colon, with perforation (especially cecal) and sepsis. In later infancy, alternating obstipation and diarrhea predominate. The older child is more likely to present with constipation. The stools are offensive and ribbon-like, the abdomen enlarged, and the veins prominent; peristaltic patterns are readily visible, and fecal masses are palpable. Intermittent bouts of intestinal obstruction due to fecal impaction, hypochromic anemia, hypoproteinemia, and failure to thrive are common. Encopresis is rarely seen.

On digital examination, the anal canal and rectum are devoid of fecal material despite fecal impaction obvious on abdominal examination or x-ray. If the aganglionic segment is short, there may be a gush of flatus and stool as the finger is withdrawn.

B. Laboratory Findings: Ganglion cells are absent in both the submucosal and muscular layers of the involved bowel. Special stains may show nerve trunk hypertrophy and increased acetylcholinesterase activity.

C. Imaging: X-ray examination of the abdomen may reveal dilated proximal colon and absence of gas in the pelvic colon. A barium enema using a catheter with the tip inserted barely beyond the anal sphincter usually demonstrates the narrowed segment distally with a sharp transition to proximal dilated colon. However, a "transition zone" may not be seen in neonates. Retention of barium for 24–48 hours is not diagnostic of Hirschsprung's disease but can be seen in retentive constipation as well.

D. Special Examinations: Failure of reflex relaxation of the internal sphincter muscle after balloon distention of the rectum is seen in all patients with Hirschsprung's disease regardless of the length of the aganglionic segment.

Differential Diagnosis

Hirschsprung's disease accounts for 15–20% of cases of neonatal intestinal obstruction. In childhood, this disease must be differentiated from retentive constipation. It can also be confused with celiac disease because of the striking abdominal distention and failure to thrive.

Treatment

Treatment is surgical. Initially, diverting colostomy (or ileostomy) is performed proximal to the aganglionic segment. Resection of the aganglionic segment is usually delayed until the infant is at least 6 months of age. During operation, the transition zone between ganglionated and nonganglionated bowel is identified. Aganglionic bowel is resected, and a surgical pull-through of ganglionated bowel to the preanal remnant is made.

Prognosis

Complications following surgery include chronic constipation, fecal incontinence, anastomotic breakdown, or stricture. Postoperative obstruction may result from inadvertent retention of a distal aganglionic segment or postoperative destruction of ganglion cells secondary to vascular impairment. Neuronal dysplasia of the remaining bowel may result in a pseudo-obstruction syndrome. Enterocolitis may occur postoperatively in 15% of procedures.

Kubota M, Kamimura T, Suita S: External anal sphincter dysfunction and postoperative bowel habits in patients with Hirschsprung's disease. J Pediatr Surg 1997;32:22.

Shimotake T et al: Germline mutations of the RET proto-oncogene in children with total aganglionosis. J Pediatr Surg 1997;32:498.

Wilcox DT et al: One-stage neonatal pull-through to treat Hirschsprung's disease. J Pediatr Surg 1997;32:243.

CHYLOUS ASCITES

Chylous ascites due to congenital infection or developmental abnormality of the lymphatic system may be observed at birth. If the thoracic duct is involved, chylothorax may be present. Later in life, chylous ascites may result from congenital lymphatic abnormality, tumors, peritoneal bands, or trauma to major lymphatics.

Clinical Findings

A. Symptoms and Signs: In both congenital and acquired forms, diarrhea and failure to thrive are noted. The abdomen is distended, with a fluid wave and shifting dullness. Unilateral or generalized peripheral edema may be present.

B. Laboratory Findings: Laboratory findings include hypoalbuminemia, hypogammaglobulinemia, and lymphopenia. Ascitic fluid contains lymphocytes and has the biochemical composition of chyle if the patient has just been fed; otherwise, it is indistinguishable from ascites secondary to cirrhosis.

Differential Diagnosis

Chylous ascites must be differentiated from ascites

due to liver failure and, in the older child, from constrictive pericarditis and neoplastic, infectious, or inflammatory diseases causing lymphatic obstruction.

Complications & Sequelae

Severe chylous ascites can be fatal. Chronic loss of albumin and gamma globulin through the gastrointestinal tract may lead to edema and increase the risk of infection. Rapidly accumulating chylous ascites may cause respiratory complications.

Treatment & Prognosis

If there is a congenital abnormality due to hypoplasia, aplasia, or ectasia of the lymphatics, little can be done for the patient. Shunting of peritoneal fluid into the venous system is sometimes effective. A fat-free diet supplemented with medium-chain triglycerides decreases the formation of chylous ascitic fluid. Total parenteral nutrition may be necessary. The congenital form of chylous ascites may spontaneously disappear following paracentesis and a medium-chain triglyceride diet. The prognosis is guarded, though spontaneous cures have been reported.

Chye JK, Lim CT, Vander Heuvel M: Neonatal chylosis ascites: Report of 3 cases and review of the literature. Pediatr Surg Int 1997;12:296-298.

Cochran WJ et al: Chylous ascites in infants and children: A case report and literature review. J Pediatr Gastroenterol Nutr 1985;4:668.

CONGENITAL ANORECTAL ANOMALIES

Anorectal anomalies occur once in every 3000–4000 births, and most types are more common in males. Inspection of the perianal area is essential in all newborns.

Classification & Presentation

A. Anterior Displacement of the Anus: This anomaly is more common in girls than in boys. It may be associated with a posterior rectal shelf and usually is characterized by constipation that responds poorly to medical management.

B. Anal Stenosis: In anal stenosis, the anal aperture is very small and filled with a dot of meconium. Defecation is difficult, and there may be ribbon-like stools, fecal impaction, and abdominal distention. This malformation accounts for about 10% of cases of anorectal anomalies.

C. Imperforate Anal Membrane: In imperforate anal membrane, the infant fails to pass meconium, and a greenish bulging membrane is seen. After excision, bowel and sphincter function are normal.

D. Anal Agenesis: In the child with anal agenesis, an anal dimple is present, and stimulation of the perianal area leads to puckering indicative of the presence of the external sphincter. If there is no associated rectoperineal fistula, intestinal obstruction occurs. Fistulas may also be vulvar in the female and urethral in the male.

E. Anorectal Agenesis: Anorectal agenesis accounts for 75% of total anorectal anomalies. Fistulas are almost invariably present. In the female, they may be vaginal or may enter a urogenital sinus, which is a common passageway for the urethra and vagina. In the male, fistulas are rectovesical or rectourethral. Associated major congenital malformations are common. Sacral defects and absence of internal and external anal sphincters are common.

Radiologic Findings

Careful radiologic evaluation is indicated immediately so that the anal anomaly and the extent of associated anomalies of the bowel and the urogenital tract can be fully appraised.

Treatment & Prognosis

Dilation of the anus should be undertaken in cases of anal stenosis. Treatment for imperforate anal membrane consists of excision of the membrane and dilation. Colostomy is advocated for all cases of anorectal agenesis. In patients with anal agenesis and a visible fistula of sufficient size to pass meconium, surgery can be deferred. Males without a visible fistula may have a urethral fistula; therefore, colostomy is recommended.

Of the patients with "low" defects, 80–90% are continent after surgery; with "high" defects, only 30% achieve continence. Gracilis muscle transplants may improve continence. Levatorplasty may also be used as a secondary operation following surgery for anorectal agenesis. Antegrade continence enema procedures may allow for continence in children without anal sphincter function.

Bar-Maor JA, Eiten A: Determination of the normal location of the anus. J Pediatr Gastroenterol Nutr 1987;6:559.

Koyle MA et al: The Malone antegrade continence enema for neurogenic and structural fecal incontinence and constipation. J Urol 1995;154:759.

Smith ED: The bathwater needs changing, but don't throw out the baby: An overview of anorectal anomalies. J Pediatr Surg 1987;22:335.

ACUTE ABDOMEN

Many disorders must be considered in the differential diagnosis of acute abdomen. Emergency surgery should not be considered until the differential diagnosis has been completed. The patient may be too young to describe symptoms, and the parent's description is a subjective interpretation of what he or she thinks is wrong. A classification of acute abdomen is shown in Table 19–3. Some of the specific entities are discussed in subsequent sections. Reaching a speedy and accurate diagnosis in the patient with an acute abdomen is critical and requires skill in physical diagnosis, intimate acquaintance with the characteristic symptoms of a large number of conditions, and the judicious selection of laboratory and radiologic tests.

PERITONITIS

Primary bacterial peritonitis is rare. The most common organisms responsible include *Escherichia coli* and other enteric organisms, hemolytic streptococci, and pneumococci. Primary peritonitis occurs in patients with splenectomy, splenic dysfunction, or ascites (nephrotic syndrome, advanced liver dis-

Table 19–3. Etiologic classification of acute abdomen.[1]

Mechanical Obstruction		Inflammatory Diseases and Infections			
Intraluminal Obstruction	Extraluminal Obstruction	Gastrointestinal Disease	Paralytic Ileus	Blunt Trauma	Miscellaneous
Foreign body	Hernia	Appendicitis	Sepsis	Accident	Lead poisoning
Bezoar	Intussusception	Crohn's disease	Pneumonia	Battered child syndrome	Sickle cell crisis
Fecalith	Volvulus	Ulcerative colitis	Pyelonephritis		Familial Mediterranean fever
Gallstone	Duplication	Henoch-Schönlein purpura and other causes of vasculitis	Peritonitis		Porphyria
Parasites	Stenosis		Pancreatitis		Diabetic acidosis
Meconium ileus equivalent	Tumor	Peptic ulcer	Cholecystitis		Addisonian crisis
Tumor	Mesenteric cyst	Meckel's diverticulitis	Renal and gallbladder stones		Torsion of testis
Fecaloma	Superior mesenteric artery syndrome	Acute gastroenteritis	Pelvic inflammation		Torsion of ovarian pedicle
	Pyloric stenosis	Pseudomembranous enterocolitis	Lymphadenitis due to viral or bacterial infection		

[1]Reproduced, with permission, from Roy CC, Morin CL, Weber AM: Gastrointestinal emergency problems in paediatric practice. Clin Gastroenterol 1981;10:225.

ease, kwashiorkor). It occurs also in infants with pyelonephritis or pneumonia. Secondary peritonitis is associated with peritoneal dialysis, penetrating abdominal trauma, or a ruptured viscus. Organisms not commonly pathogenic such as *Staphylococcus epidermidis* and *Candida* may cause secondary peritonitis, especially if foreign bodies are present. Intraabdominal abscesses may form in pelvic, subhepatic, or subphrenic areas, but localization of infection is less common in young infants than in adults.

Symptoms include severe abdominal pain, fever, nausea, and vomiting. Respirations are shallow. The abdomen is tender, rigid, and distended, with involuntary guarding. Bowel sounds may be absent. Diarrhea is fairly common in primary peritonitis and less so in secondary peritonitis.

The leukocyte count is high initially (> 20,000/μL), with a predominance of immature forms, and later may fall to neutropenic levels, especially in primary peritonitis. Bacterial peritonitis should be suspected if paracentesis fluid contains more than 500 leukocytes/μL or more than 32 mg/dL of lactate; if it has a pH less than 7.34; or if the pH of ascites fluid is more than 0.1 pH unit less than arterial blood pH. Etiologic diagnosis is made by Gram's stain and culture, preferably of 5–10 mL of fluid for optimal yield. The blood culture is often positive in primary peritonitis.

Antibiotic treatment and supportive therapy for dehydration, shock, and acidosis are indicated. Surgical treatment of the underlying cause of secondary peritonitis is critical. Removal of infected catheters in patients with secondary peritonitis is recommended, and is mandatory if *Candida* infection is present.

Bell MJ: Peritonitis in the newborn: Current concepts. Pediatr Clin North Am 1985;32:1181.
Kimber CP, Hutson JM: Primary peritonitis in children. Aust N Z J Surg 1996;66:169.

ACUTE APPENDICITIS

Acute appendicitis is the most common indication for emergency abdominal surgery in childhood. The frequency increases with age and peaks between 15 and 30 years. Obstruction of the appendix by fecaliths (25%) or parasites is a predisposing factor.

The incidence of perforation is high (40%) in infants and children. In order to avoid delay in diagnosis, it is important to maintain close communication with parents, perform a thorough physical examination and sequential examinations of the abdomen over several hours, and interpret correctly the evolving symptoms and signs.

Clinical Findings

A. Symptoms and Signs: The typical child with appendicitis has low-grade fever and periumbili-

cal abdominal pain, which then localizes to the right lower quadrant, accompanied by signs of peritoneal irritation. Anorexia, vomiting, constipation, and diarrhea also occur. The clinical picture is often atypical and includes generalized pain, tenderness around the umbilicus, and no leukocytosis. Rectal examination should always be done and may reveal localized mass or tenderness. Because many conditions give rise to symptoms mimicking appendicitis and because physical findings are often inconclusive, it is important to repeat examinations of the abdomen. In children under 2 years of age, the pain of appendicitis is poorly localized, and perforation before surgery is common.

B. Laboratory Findings: White blood cell counts are seldom higher than 15,000/μL. Pyuria, fecal leukocytes, and guaiac-positive stool are occasionally found.

C. Imaging: A radiopaque fecalith is reportedly present in two-thirds of cases of ruptured appendix. A positive diagnosis of nonperforated appendicitis cannot be made by barium enema. Ultrasonography of the acutely inflamed appendix shows a noncompressible, thickened appendix in 93% of cases. A localized fluid collection adjacent to or surrounding the appendix may also be seen. Indium-labeled white blood cell scan may localize to an inflamed appendix. Enlarged mesenteric lymph nodes are a nondiagnostic finding.

Differential Diagnosis

The presence of intrathoracic infection (eg, pneumonia) or urinary tract infection should be kept in mind, along with other medical and surgical conditions leading to acute abdomen (see previous section).

Treatment & Prognosis

Exploratory laparotomy or laparoscopy is indicated whenever the diagnosis of appendicitis cannot be ruled out after a period of close observation. Postoperative antibiotic therapy directed to the treatment of anaerobes and coliforms is reserved for cases with gangrenous or perforated appendix. A single intraoperative dose of cefoxitin or cefotetan is recommended for all cases to prevent postoperative complications. The mortality rate is less than 1% during childhood despite the high incidence of perforation. Laparoscopic removal of a nonruptured appendix is associated with a shortened hospital stay.

Mason JD: The evaluation of acute abdominal pain in children. Emerg Med Clin North Am 1996;14:629.
Ramachandran P et al: Ultrasonography as an adjunct in the diagnosis of acute appendicitis: A 4-year experience. J Pediatr Surg 1996;31:164.

INTUSSUSCEPTION

Intussusception is the most frequent cause of intestinal obstruction in the first 2 years of life. It is three times more common in males than in females. In most cases (85%) the cause is not apparent, though polyps, Meckel's diverticulum, Schönlein-Henoch purpura, lymphomas, lipomas, parasites, foreign bodies, or adenovirus or rotavirus infections with hypertrophy of Peyer's patches are predisposing factors. Intussusception of the small intestine occurs in patients with celiac disease and cystic fibrosis—related to the bulk of stool in the terminal ileum. In children over 6 years of age, lymphoma is the most common lesion. Intermittent small bowel intussusception is a rare cause of recurrent abdominal pain.

The intussusception usually starts just proximal to the ileocecal valve, so that invagination is ileocolic. Other forms include ileoileal and colocolic. Swelling, hemorrhage, incarceration with necrosis of the intussuscepted bowel, and eventual perforation and peritonitis occur as a result of impairment of venous return.

Clinical Findings

Characteristically, a thriving infant 3–12 months of age develops paroxysmal abdominal pain with screaming and drawing up of the knees. Vomiting and diarrhea occur soon afterward (90% of cases), and bloody bowel movements with mucus appear within the next 12 hours (50%). Prostration and fever supervene. The abdomen is tender and becomes distended. On palpation, a sausage-shaped mass may be found usually in the upper mid abdomen. Some patients show signs of altered consciousness—particularly lethargy between spasms of pain—or have seizures.

The intussusception can persist for several days when obstruction is not complete, and such cases may present as separate attacks of enterocolitis. In older children, sudden attacks of abdominal pain may be related to chronic recurrent intussusception with spontaneous reduction.

Treatment

A. Conservative Measures: Barium enema or pneumatic enema is both diagnostic and therapeutic. However, neither pneumatic nor hydrostatic reduction should be attempted if there are signs of strangulated bowel, perforation, or severe toxicity.

The barium solution should be allowed to drip by gravity through a Foley catheter inserted in the rectum from a height not more than 1 m above the fluoroscopy table.

There should be no manipulation of the abdomen during hydrostatic reduction under fluoroscopic examination, because this may increase intraluminal pressure and thus the risk of perforation.

Upon reduction, there should be free reflux of barium for a distance of 24–30 cm into the ileum; this is best demonstrated in a postevacuation film.

Careful air insufflation is a simple, safe, and effective alternative to hydrostatic reduction.

B. Surgical Measures: For patients not suitable for hydrostatic or pneumatic reduction or in whom these procedures are unsuccessful (25%), surgery is required. This has the advantages of demonstrating any lead point (such as Meckel's diverticulum) and of a lower recurrence rate.

Prognosis

The prognosis relates directly to the duration of the intussusception before reduction. The mortality rate with treatment is 1–2%. The patient should be observed carefully after hydrostatic or pneumatic reduction because intussusception recurs within 24 hours in 3–4% of patients.

Eshel G et al: Intussusception: A nine year survey. J Pediatr Gastroenterol Nutr 1997;24:253.

FOREIGN BODIES IN THE ALIMENTARY TRACT

Most foreign bodies pass through the gastrointestinal tract without difficulty, though objects longer than 5 cm may have difficulty negotiating the ligament of Treitz. Ingested foreign bodies tend to lodge in areas of natural constriction—valleculae, thoracic inlet, gastroesophageal junction, pylorus, ligament of Treitz, and ileocecal junction. Foreign bodies lodged in the esophagus for more than 24 hours require removal. Smooth foreign bodies in the stomach, such as buttons or coins, may be watched without attempting removal for up to several months if the child is free of symptoms. Straight pins, screws, and nails generally pass without incident. Removal of open safety pins or wooden toothpicks is recommended. Button batteries lodged in the esophagus should be removed immediately. Button batteries in the stomach will generally pass uneventfully. The use of balanced electrolyte lavage solutions containing polyethylene glycol (eg, GoLYTELY) may help the passage of small, smooth foreign bodies lodged in the stomach or intestine. Lavage is especially useful in hastening the passage of button batteries or ingested tablets that may be toxic. Failure of a smooth foreign body to exit the stomach suggests the possibility of gastric outlet obstruction.

Esophagogastroscopy will permit the removal of most foreign bodies lodged in the esophagus and stomach. A Foley catheter may be used to dislodge smooth, round esophageal foreign bodies in healthy children with no previous esophageal disease. It is introduced into the esophagus, and the balloon at the distal end is inflated below the foreign body. Careful withdrawal of the catheter under fluoroscopic observation will bring the foreign body into the mouth, where it can be extracted. Only an experienced radiologist should attempt this maneuver.

Campbell JB, Foley LC: A safe alternative to endoscopic removal of blunt esophageal foreign bodies. Arch Otolaryngol 1983;109:323.

Litovitz T, Schmitz BF: Ingestion of cylindrical and button batteries: An analysis of 2382 cases. Pediatrics 1992;89:747.

Paul RI et al: Foreign body ingestions in children: Risk of complication varies with site of initial health care contact. Pediatrics 1993;91:121.

ANAL FISSURE

Anal fissure is a slit-like tear in the anal canal, usually secondary to the passage of large, hard, fecal masses. Anal stenosis, anal crypt abscess, and trauma can be contributory factors. Sexual abuse must be considered in any child with large, irregular, or multiple anal fissures. Anal fissures may be the presenting symptoms of Crohn's disease in older children.

The infant or child with anal fissure typically cries with defecation and will try to hold back stools. Sparse, bright red bleeding is seen on the outside of the stool or on the toilet tissue following defecation. The fissure can often be seen if the patient is examined in a knee-chest position with the buttocks spread apart. When a fissure cannot be identified, it is essential to rule out other causes of rectal bleeding such as juvenile polyp, perianal inflammation (due to group A streptococcal infection), or inflammatory bowel disease. Anal fissures should be treated promptly to break the constipation → fissure → retention → constipation cycle. A stool softener should be given. Anal dilation relieves sphincter spasm. Warm sitz baths after defecation may be helpful. In rare cases, silver nitrate cauterization or surgery is indicated. Anal surgery should be avoided in Crohn's disease.

INGUINAL HERNIA

A peritoneal sac precedes the testicle as it descends from the genital ridge to the scrotum. The lower portion of this sac envelops the testis to form the tunica vaginalis, and the remainder normally atrophies by the time of birth. In some cases, peritoneal fluid may become trapped in the tunica vaginalis of the testis (noncommunicating hydrocele). If the processus vaginalis remains open, peritoneal fluid or an abdominal structure may be forced into it (indirect inguinal hernia).

Most inguinal hernias are of the indirect type and occur much more frequently (9:1) in boys than in girls. Hernias may be present at birth or may appear at any age thereafter. The incidence in premature infants is close to 5%. In those weighing 1000 g or less, inguinal hernia is reported in 30%.

Clinical Findings

There are no symptoms associated with an empty processus vaginalis. In most cases, a hernia is a painless inguinal swelling of variable size. There may be a history of inguinal fullness associated with coughing or long periods of standing; or there may be a firm, globular, and tender swelling, sometimes associated with vomiting and abdominal distention.

Spontaneous reduction frequently occurs during sleep or with slight external pressure. In some instances, a herniated loop of intestine may become partially obstructed, leading to pain and partial intestinal obstruction. Rarely, bowel becomes trapped in the hernia sac and complete intestinal obstruction occurs. Gangrene of the hernia contents or testis may occur; in the female, the ovary may prolapse into the hernial sac.

Inspection of the two inguinal areas may reveal a characteristic bulging or mass. Infants should be observed for evidence of swelling after crying and older children after bearing down.

A suggestive history is often the only criterion for diagnosis, along with the "silk glove" feel of the rubbing together of the two walls of the empty hernial sac.

Differential Diagnosis

An inguinal mass may represent lymph nodes. They are usually multiple and more discrete. Hydrocele of the cord transilluminates. An undescended testis may be moved along the canal and is associated with absence of the gonad in the scrotum.

Treatment

Manual reduction of incarcerated inguinal hernia can be attempted after the sedated infant is placed in the Trendelenburg position with an ice bag on the affected side. This is contraindicated if incarceration has been present for more than 12 hours or if bloody stools are noted. Surgery is usually indicated if a hernia has once incarcerated. Hydroceles frequently resolve by the age of 2 years. There is still controversy about exploring the opposite side. Exploration of the unaffected groin can document the patency of the processus vaginalis, but patency does not always mean that herniation will occur, especially in patients over 1 year of age, in whom the risk of contralateral hernia is about 10%.

Incarcerated inguinal hernias occur most often in the first 10 months of life and are more common in girls than in boys.

Pellegrin K et al: Laparoscopic evaluation of the contralateral patent processus vaginalis in children. Am J Surg 1996;172:602.

Gahukamble DB, Khamage AS: Early vs delayed repair of reduced incarcerated inguinal hernias in the pediatric population. J Pediatr Surg 1996;31:1218.

UMBILICAL HERNIA

Umbilical hernias are more common in premature than in full-term infants and more common in black than in white infants.

Small bowel may incarcerate in small-diameter umbilical hernias. Most umbilical hernias regress spontaneously if the fascial defect has a diameter of less than 1 cm. Large defects and smaller hernias persisting after 4 years of age should be treated surgically. Reducing the hernia and strapping the skin does not accelerate the healing process.

TUMORS OF THE GASTROINTESTINAL TRACT

1. JUVENILE POLYPS

Juvenile polyps are usually pedunculated and solitary. The head of the polyp is composed of hyperplastic glandular and vascular elements, often with cystic transformation. Juvenile polyps are benign, and 80% occur in the rectosigmoid. Their incidence is highest between 3 and 5 years of age, and they are rare before age 1 and, because of autoamputation, after age 15 years. They are more frequent in boys. The painless passage of small amounts of bright red blood on a normal or constipated stool is the most frequent manifestation. Abdominal pain is infrequent, but a juvenile polyp can be the lead point for an intussusception. Low-lying polyps may prolapse during defecation.

Rarely, there are many juvenile polyps in the colon, causing anemia, diarrhea, and protein loss. A few cases of generalized juvenile polyposis involving the stomach and the small and large bowel have been reported. These cases are associated with a slightly increased risk of cancer.

Colonoscopy is both diagnostic and therapeutic when polyps are suspected. After removal of the polyp by electrocautery, nothing further should be done if histologic findings confirm the diagnosis. There is a slight risk of developing further juvenile polyps.

Other polyposis syndromes are summarized in Table 19–4.

Coburn MC et al: Malignant potential in intestinal juvenile polyposis syndromes. Ann Surg Oncol 1995;2:386.
Rustgi A: Hereditary gastrointestinal polyposis and non-polyposis syndromes. N Engl J Med 1994;31:1694.

2. CANCERS OF THE ESOPHAGUS, SMALL INTESTINE, & COLON

Esophageal cancer is rare in childhood. Cysts, leiomyomas, and hamartomas predominate. Caustic injury of the esophagus increases the risk of squamous cell carcinoma, and chronic peptic esophagitis is associated with Barrett's esophagus, a precancerous lesion.

The most common gastric or small bowel cancer in children is lymphoma or lymphosarcoma. Intermittent abdominal pain, abdominal mass, intussusception, or a celiac-like picture may be present. Carcinoid tumors are usually benign, discovered incidentally following appendectomy. Metastasis is rare, as are symptoms associated with serotonin secretion.

Adenocarcinoma of the colon is rare in the pediatric age group. The transverse colon and rectosigmoid are the two most commonly affected sites. The low 5-year survival relates to the nonspecificity of presenting complaints and the large percentage of undifferentiated types. Children with a family history of colon cancer, chronic ulcerative colitis, or familial polyposis syndromes are at greater risk.

Aiges HW et al: Adenocarcinoma of the colon in an adolescent with the family cancer syndrome. J Pediatr 1979;94:632.
Hassall E: Barrett's esophagus: New definitions and approaches in children. J Pediatr Gastroenterol Nutr 1993;16:345.

3. MESENTERIC CYSTS

These rare tumors may be small or large and single or multiloculated. Invariably thin-walled, they contain either serous, chylous, or hemorrhagic fluid. They are commonly located in the mesentery of the small intestine but may also be seen in the mesocolon. Most mesenteric cysts are asymptomatic. Traction on the mesentery eventually leads to colicky abdominal pain, which can be mild and recurrent but may present acutely with vomiting. Volvulus is reported, as is hemorrhage into the cyst. A rounded mass can occasionally be palpated or seen on x-ray film to displace adjacent intestine. Abdominal ultrasonography is usually diagnostic. Surgical removal is indicated.

4. INTESTINAL HEMANGIOMA

Hemangiomas of the bowel may cause acute or chronic blood loss. They may also cause intestinal obstruction via intussusception, local stricture, or intramural hematoma formation. Thrombocytopenia and consumptive coagulopathy are occasional complications. Some lesions are telangiectasias (Rendu-Osler-Weber syndrome), and others are capillary hemangiomas. However, the largest group consists of cavernous hemangiomas, which are composed of large, thin-walled vessels arising from the submucosal vascular plexus. They may protrude into the lumen as polypoid lesions or may invade the intestine from mucosa to serosa.

Abrahamson J, Shandling B: Intestinal hemangiomata in childhood and a syndrome for diagnosis: A collective review. J Pediatr Surg 1973;8:487.

Table 19–4. Gastrointestinal polyposis syndromes.

	Location	Number	Histology	Extraintestinal Findings	Malignant Potential	Recommended Therapy
Juvenile polyps	Colon	Single (70%) Several (30%)	Hyperplastic, hamartomatous	None	None	Remove polyp for continuous bleeding or prolapse.
Familial juvenile polyposis coli[1]	Colon	More than ten	Hyperplastic with focal adenomatous change	None	10–25%; higher if familial	Remove all polyps. Consider colectomy if very numerous or adenomatous.
Generalized juvenile polyposis[1]	Stomach, small bowel, colon	Multiple	Hyperplastic with focal adenomatous change	Hydrocephaly, cardiac lesions, mesenteric lymphangioma, malrotation	10–25%	Colectomy and close surveillance.
Familial adenomatous polyposis[1]	Colon; less commonly, stomach and small bowel	Multiple	Adenomatous	None	95–100%	Colectomy by age 18.
Peutz–Jeghers syndrome[1]	Small bowel, stomach, colon	Multiple	Hamartomatous	Pigmented cutaneous and oral macules; ovarian cysts and tumors; bony exostoses	2–3%	Remove accessible polyps or those causing obstruction or bleeding.
Gardner's syndrome	Colon; less commonly, stomach and small bowel	Multiple	Adenomatous	Cysts, tumors, and desmoids of skin and bone; ampullary tumors; other tumors, retinal pigmentations can be a screening tool in families	95–100%	Colectomy by age 18. Upper tract surveillance.
Cronkhite-Canada syndrome	Stomach, colon; less commonly, esophagus and small bowel	Multiple	Hamartomatous	Alopecia; onychodystrophy; hyperpigmentation	Rare	None
Turcot's syndrome[2]	Colon	Multiple	Adenomatous	Thyroid and brain tumors are the usual presentation	Possible	CNS screening most important

[1]Autosomal dominant.
[2]Autosomal recessive.

Mestre JR, Andres JM: Hereditary hemorrhagic telangiectasia causing hematemesis in an infant. J Pediatr 1982;101:577.

ACUTE INFECTIOUS DIARRHEA
(Gastroenteritis)

Viruses are the most common cause of acute gastroenteritis in developing and developed countries. Bacterial and parasitic enteric infections are discussed in Chapters 36 and 37. Of the viral agents proved to cause enteric infection, rotavirus, a 67-nm double-stranded RNA virus with at least eight serotypic variants, is the most common. As with most viral pathogens, rotavirus affects the small intestine, causing voluminous watery diarrhea without leukocytes or blood. In the United States, rotavirus affects mainly infants between 3 and 15 months of age. Peak incidence in the United States is in the winter months. Sporadic cases occur at other times. The virus is transmitted via the fecal-oral route and survives for hours on hands and for days on environmental fomites.

Diagnosis & Treatment
of Rotavirus Infections

The incubation period for rotavirus is 24–48 hours. Vomiting is the first symptom in 80–90% of cases, followed within 24 hours by low-grade fever and profuse watery diarrhea. Diarrhea usually lasts 4–8 days but may last longer in young infants or immunocompromised patients. The white blood cell count is rarely elevated. The stool sodium is usually less than 40 mEq/L. Thus, as patients become dehydrated from unreplaced stool losses, they may become hypernatremic. The stool does not contain blood or white cells. Metabolic acidosis results from bicarbonate loss in the stool, ketosis from poor intake, and lactic acidemia from hypotension and hypoperfusion.

Replacement of fluid and electrolyte deficits and ongoing losses is critical, especially in small infants. (Oral and intravenous therapy are discussed in Chapter 39.) The use of oral rehydration fluid is appropriate in most cases, but clear liquid and hypocaloric (dilute formula) diets for more than 48 hours are not advisable in uncomplicated viral gastroenteritis because starvation depresses digestive function and prolongs diarrhea.

Intestinal lactase levels are reduced during rotavirus infection. Brief use of a lactose-free diet is associated with a shorter period of diarrhea but is not critical to successful recovery in most healthy infants. Reduced fat intake during recovery may reduce nausea and vomiting.

Antidiarrheal medications are ineffective (kaolin-pectin combinations) or even dangerous (loperamide, tincture of opium, diphenoxylate with atropine). Bismuth subsalicylate preparations may reduce stool volume but are not critical to recovery. Oral immunoglobulin has occasionally been useful in limiting duration of disease in immunocompromised patients.

Specific identification of rotavirus is not required in every case, especially in epidemic outbreaks. Rotavirus antigens can be identified in stool. False-positives (which may actually be nonpathogenic rotavirus) are seen in neonates. Electron microscopy of the stool will also reveal the virus but is less sensitive.

Some immunity is imparted by the first episode of rotavirus infection. Serum antibodies are present, but their role in prevention of subsequent attacks is not clear. Repeat infections occur, but are usually less severe. Prevention of rotavirus is mainly by good hygiene and prevention of fecal-oral contamination. A quadrivalent oral vaccine that incorporates attenuated viruses of the four major pathogenic serotypes is under investigation, with protection ranging from 57–77%.

Diagnosis & Treatment
of Other Viral Infections

Other viral pathogens in stool have been identified by electron microscopy, special viral cultures, or enzyme-linked immunoassays in infants with diarrhea. Enteric adenoviruses (serotypes 40 and 41) are the second most common viral pathogens in infants. The symptoms of enteric adenovirus infection are similar to those produced from rotavirus, but infection is not seasonal and duration of illness may be longer. The Norwalk agent is a small RNA virus that causes chiefly vomiting but also some diarrhea in older children and adults, usually in common source outbreaks (perhaps water-borne). The duration of symptoms is short, usually 24–48 hours. Other potentially pathogenic viruses include astroviruses, caliciviruses, corona-like viruses, and other small round viruses. Cytomegalovirus (CMV) and herpesvirus rarely cause diarrhea but may cause colitis or enteritis in immunocompromised hosts. CMV enteritis is particularly common after bone marrow transplantation and in late stages of HIV infection.

Kapikian AZ: Viral gastroenteritis. JAMA 1993;269:627.
Leiberman JM: Rotavirus and other viral causes of gastroenteritis. Pediatr Ann 1994;23:529.

CHRONIC DIARRHEA

It is difficult to define chronic diarrhea because there are wide variations in normal bowel habits. Some infants pass one firm stool every second to third day, whereas others may have 5–8 soft small stools daily. A gradual or sudden increase in the number and volume of stools (> 15 g/kg/d) combined with an increase in fluidity should raise a suspicion that an organic cause of chronic diarrhea is present.

Diarrhea may result from any of the following pathogenetic mechanisms: (1) interruption of normal cell transport processes for water, electrolytes, or nutrients; (2) decrease in the surface area available for absorption, which may be due to shortening of the bowel or mucosal disease; (3) increase in intestinal motility; (4) increase in unabsorbable osmotically active molecules in the intestinal lumen; and (5) increase in intestinal permeability, leading to increased loss of water and electrolytes.

The differential diagnosis of chronic diarrhea is lengthy. Table 19–5 lists some disease categories and specific conditions in which diarrhea is a prominent feature.

Noninfectious Causes of Diarrhea

A. Antibiotic Therapy: Diarrhea accompanies antibiotic therapy in up to 60% of cases. Some antibiotics decrease carbohydrate transport and intestinal lactase levels. Eradication of normal gut flora and overgrowth of other organisms may cause diarrhea. Most antibiotic-associated diarrhea is watery in nature, unassociated with systemic symptoms, and decreases when antibiotic therapy is stopped. Pseudomembranous colitis, caused by the toxins produced by *Clostridium difficile,* occurs in 0.2–10% of patients treated with antibiotics, especially clindamycin, cephalosporins, and amoxicillin. Patients develop fever, tenesmus, and abdominal pain with diarrhea, which contains leukocytes and sometimes gross blood up to 8 weeks after antibiotic exposure. Treatment with oral vancomycin (30–50 mg/kg/d) or metronidazole (30 mg/kg/d) for 7 days is recommended. Relapse occurs after treatment in 10–50% of cases.

B. Extraintestinal Infections: Infections of the urinary tract and upper respiratory tract (especially otitis media) are at times associated with diarrhea. The mechanism remains obscure. Antibiotic treatment of the primary infection, toxins released by infective agents, and local irritation of the rectum (in patients with bladder infections) may play a role.

C. Malnutrition: Malnutrition is associated with an increased frequency of enteral infections; decreased bile acid synthesis, pancreatic enzyme output, and disaccharidase activity; altered motility; and changes in the intestinal flora—all of which may cause diarrhea.

D. Diet: Overfeeding may cause diarrhea, especially in young infants. Relative deficiency of pancreatic amylase in young infants may produce diarrhea after starchy foods. Fruit juices, especially those high in fructose or sorbitol, produce osmotic diarrhea. Intestinal irritants (spices and foods high in roughage) and histamine-containing or histamine-releasing foods (eg, citrus fruits, tomatoes, certain cheeses, red wines, and fish) also cause diarrhea.

E. Allergic Diarrhea: Diarrhea caused by allergy to dietary proteins is a frequently entertained but rarely authenticated diagnostic entity. Protein allergy is more common in infants under 12 months of age, who may experience mild to severe colitis. A personal or family history of atopy is common in infants with protein allergy. Older children may develop a celiac-like syndrome with flattening of mucosal villi, steatorrhea, hypoproteinemia, and occult blood loss. Skin testing is not reliable. Double-blind oral challenge with the suspected food under careful observation is necessary to confirm intestinal protein allergy. In infants, the condition usually disappears after 12 months. Allergies to fish, peanuts, and eggs are more likely to be lifelong. Multiple food allergy (more than three) is rare.

F. Chronic Nonspecific Diarrhea: Chronic nonspecific diarrhea is the most common cause of loose stools in thriving children. The typical patient is a healthy child 6–20 months of age who was a colicky baby and who has three to six loose mucoid stools per day during the waking hours. The diarrhea worsens with a low-residue, low-fat, or high-carbohydrate diet and during periods of stress and infection. It clears spontaneously at about 3½ years of age (usually coincident with toilet training). No organic disease is discoverable. Possible causes include abnormalities of bile acid absorption in the terminal ileum, incomplete carbohydrate absorption (excessive fruit juice ingestion seems to worsen the condition), and abnormal motor function. A high familial incidence of functional bowel disease is observed. Stool tests for blood, white cells, fat, parasites, and bacterial pathogens are negative.

The following measures are helpful: institution of a high-fat (about 40% of total calories), low-carbohydrate, high-fiber diet; avoidance of between-meal snacks; and avoidance of chilled fluids, especially fruit juices. It may be helpful to give loperamide, 0.1–0.2 mg/kg/d in two or three divided doses; cholestyramine, 2–4 g in divided doses; or psyllium agents, 1–2 tsp twice daily.

Hoekstra JH et al: Apple juice malabsorption: Fructose or sorbitol? J Pediatr Gastroenterol Nutr 1993;16:39.
Hyams JS et al: Carbohydrate malabsorption following fruit juice ingestion in young children. Pediatrics 1988;82:64.
Kelly CP et al: *Clostridium difficile* colitis. N Engl J Med 1994;330:257.
Leung AK, Robson WL: Evaluating the child with chronic diarrhea. Am Fam Physician 1996;53:635.

THE MALABSORPTION SYNDROMES

Malabsorption of ingested food has many causes. Shortening of the small bowel (usually via surgical resection) or mucosal damage (celiac disease) both reduce surface area. Impaired motility of the small

Table 19–5. Guide to differential diagnosis of chronic diarrhea.

Disease	Age	Type of Diarrhea	Associated Features
Bacterial infections	Any age	Mucoid, bloody stool with poly-morphonuclear leukocytes.	Rarely chronic except in immunocompromised hosts; *Salmonella, Yersinia, Campylobacter* most likely.
Viral infections	Any age	Watery.	Rarely chronic except in immunocompromised hosts; cytomegalovirus, adenovirus, rotavirus.
Parasitic infections	Any age	Depends on organism.	*Entamoeba, Giardia, Cryptosporidium, Cyclospora, Isospora*
Dietary factors Overfeeding (especially starches)	< 6 months	Watery.	Colicky behavior without weight loss.
Protein allergy	< 2 months	Watery with or without malabsorption of fat; at times, blood and mucus.	Colic, vomiting, anemia, hypoproteinemia.
Acrodermatitis enteropathica	< 12 months	Voluminous with steatorrhea.	Malnutrition, skin rash; low serum zinc; usually genetic; sometimes secondary to severe dietary zinc deficiency.
Primary bile acid malabsorption	< 1 month	Voluminous with steatorrhea.	Malnutrition; defective ileal transport of bile acids.
Irritable colon or chronic, non-specific diarrhea	6–36 months	Watery, frequent, with mucus, undigested food; no steatorrhea.	Healthy child; often starts with bout of gastroenteritis.
Toxic diarrhea (antibiotics, cancer chemotherapy, radiation)	Any age	Loose; sometimes steatorrhea, with occult blood or pus.	Vomiting; anorexia.
Functional tumors (neuroblastoma, carcinoid, pancreatic cholera, Zollinger-Ellison syndrome)	Any age	Secretory diarrhea, watery; persists when patient fasts.	Hypokalemia; other symptoms depend upon tumor.
Carbohydrate malabsorption Congenital deficiencies Sucrase-isomaltase	< 6 months	Watery; low pH; reducing substance-positive after acid hydrolysis; volume varies with sucrose intake.	Abdominal distention; poor growth; deficiency present in 0.8% of United States Caucasians, 10% of Alaskan natives.
Glucose-galactose malabsorption	< 1 month	Intractable diarrhea with feeding; stool pH low; watery; reducing substances present.	Poor growth; defect in glucose sodium cotransporter; gene locus 22g.
Genetic deficiencies Lactase	> 4 years	Watery diarrhea with lactose; low pH; reducing substances present.	Deficiency develops in 100% of Asians, 80% of African-Americans, 15% of American whites.
Acquired deficiencies Lactase and sucrase	Any age	Watery; low pH; reducing substances present.	Follows intestinal injury or infection.
Monosaccharide intolerance	< 6 months	Watery; low pH; reducing substances present.	Rare; follows infection, made worse by malnutrition.
Pancreatic disorders Cystic fibrosis	< 6 months	Steatorrhea; bulky, foul, pale.	Respiratory infection; poor weight gain.
Shwachman syndrome	< 2 years	Steatorrhea; bulky, foul, pale.	Neutropenia; short stature, bacterial infections; metaphysial dysostosis.
Chronic pancreatitis	Any age	Steatorrhea; bulky, foul, pale.	Rare in children; usually associated with alcoholism.
Celiac disease	> 12 months	Steatorrhea; bulky, foul, pale.	Vomiting, distention, irritability, anorexia.

(continued)

Table 19–5. Guide to differential diagnosis of chronic diarrhea. (continued)

Disease	Age	Type of Diarrhea	Associated Features
Intestinal lymphangiectasia	3 months	Voluminous; steatorrhea.	Lymphedema, lymphopenia, hypoalbuminemia.
Immune defects Hypogammaglobulinemia; IgA deficiency	Any age	Watery; sometimes steatorrhea.	Recurrent cutaneous and respiratory infection.
Combined immunodeficiency	< 1 month	Severe; watery.	Stomatitis, skin rash, recurrent infection, opportunistic infection.
HIV infection	Any age	Steatorrhea.	Other opportunistic infections.
Defective cellular immunity	< 2 years		
Genetic-metabolic disorders Chloride-losing diarrhea	< 1 month	Watery.	Alkalosis; growth failure.
Abeta- and hypobetalipoproteinenemia	< 3 months	Profuse; steatorrhea.	Progressive neurologic symptoms; low serum cholesterol; acanthocytosis.
Wolman's disease	< 1 month	Profuse; steatorrhea.	Vomiting; severe growth failure; adrenal calcification; hypercholesterolemia.
Folate malabsorption	< 1 month	Watery.	Megaloblastic anemia, stomatitis, seizures, retardation.
Anatomic abnormalities Blind (stagnant) loop or bacterial overgrowth	Any age	Watery; fat and carbohydrate malabsorption.	Caused by surgical adhesions, intestinal duplication, abnormal gastrointestinal motility, partial obstruction.
Short bowel	Any age	Watery; malabsorption of all nutrients.	Rarely congenital; usually secondary to surgical resection.
Intestinal pseudo-obstruction	Any age	Watery; malabsorption of all nutrients.	Distention; may be acquired or congenital; diarrhea secondary to bacterial overgrowth.
Inflammatory bowel disease Crohn's disease	Usually > 10 years	Loose with or without steatorrhea. failure; joint pain, perianal disease.	Pain, fever, abdominal mass, growth
Ulcerative colitis	Usually > 10 years	Bloody stools with polymorphonuclear leukocytes.	Tenesmus, anemia, abdominal pain, fever, joint pain; less severe growth failure.
Eosinophilic gastroenteritis	Any age	Watery or bloody, depending upon site of disease.	Intestinal or gastric obstruction, eczema, asthma.
Hirschsprung's disease with enterocolitis	< 1 year	Foul, liquid with white and red blood cells.	Abdominal distention, fever, history of constipation.
Malnutrition	< 1 year	Loose, steatorrhea; sometimes with carbohydrate malabsorption.	Becomes temporarily worse with refeeding.
Endocrine disorders Hyperthyroidism	Any age	Frequent, loose stool without malabsorption.	Other signs of hyperthyroidism.

intestine may interfere with normal propulsive movements and mixing of food with pancreatic and biliary secretions. Anaerobic bacteria proliferate under these conditions and impair fat absorption by deconjugation of bile acids (intestinal pseudo-obstruction, postoperative blind loop syndrome). Impaired intestinal lymphatic (congenital lymphangiectasis) or venous drainage also causes malabsorption. Diseases reducing pancreatic exocrine function (cystic fibrosis,

Shwachman syndrome) or the production and flow of biliary secretions cause nutrient malabsorption. Malabsorption may be genetically determined (disaccharidase deficiency, glucose-galactose malabsorption, and abetalipoproteinemia).

Clinical Findings

Gastrointestinal symptoms such as diarrhea, vomiting, anorexia, abdominal pain, and bloating are common. Certain physical features such as potbelly and wasted buttocks may indicate celiac disease. Observation of the stools for abnormal color, consistency, bulkiness, odor, mucus, and blood is important. Microscopic examination of stools for neutral fat and fatty acids is helpful because most malabsorption syndromes involve some fat malabsorption. Pancreatic insufficiency is associated with neutral fat in the stool. Fatty acids are the major fatty material found in the stool of patients with mucosal disease (celiac disease) and liver disease.

Quantitative assessment of fat absorption requires measurement of fat excreted in the feces as a proportion of fat intake for a defined period. Five percent excretion of ingested fat is normal for an infant over 1 year of age; 10–15% in a younger infant. Prothrombin time, serum carotene, vitamin E, and vitamin D levels may be depressed by fat malabsorption. Accurate assessment of protein absorption is difficult and requires isotopic labeling of amino acids. Loss of serum proteins across the intestinal mucosa can be estimated by measurement of fecal α_1-antitrypsin. Malabsorption of complex carbohydrate is rarely measured. Disaccharide or monosaccharide malabsorption is estimated by reduction in stool pH, increased breath hydrogen, or decreased intestinal mucosal disaccharidase activity.

Other tests that may be helpful in suggesting a cause in a child with malabsorption include sweat chloride concentration (cystic fibrosis), intestinal mucosal biopsy (eg, celiac disease, intestinal lymphangiectasia, giardiasis, inflammatory bowel disease), liver function tests, and pancreatic secretion of enzymes after stimulation with secretin and cholecystokinin.

Differential Diagnosis

The pathophysiologic classification in Table 19–6 may be helpful in view of the variety of disorders giving rise to malabsorption.

Treatment & Prognosis

See specific syndromes (eg, celiac disease, disaccharidase deficiency).

Branski D, Lerner A, Lebenthal E: Chronic diarrhea and malabsorption. Pediatr Clin North Am 1996;43:307.
Talusan-Soriano K, Lake AM: Malabsorption in childhood. Pediatr Rev 1996;17:135.

CONSTIPATION

Constipation is passage of bulky or hard stool at infrequent intervals. Retention of feces in the rectum results in encopresis (involuntary fecal leakage) in 60% of affected children. Organic causes of constipation are listed in Table 19–7. Most constipation in childhood is not organic but a result of voluntary or involuntary retentive behavior.

Clinical Findings

Normal infants under 3 months of age often grunt, strain, and turn red in the face while passing normal stools. This pattern may be erroneously viewed as constipation. Failure to appreciate this normal developmental pattern may lead to the unwise use of laxatives or enemas. Infants and children may gradually develop the ability to ignore the sensation of rectal fullness and retain stool. Many factors promote and reinforce this behavior, which finally results in impaction of the rectum and overflow incontinence or encopresis: painful defecation; skeletal muscle weakness; psychologic issues, especially those relating to control and authority; modesty and distaste for school bathrooms; medications; and others listed in Table 19–7. The dilated rectum becomes less sensitive to dilation, thus perpetuating the problem, regardless of the original cause. As many as 1–2% of healthy primary school children have retentive constipation. The ratio of males to females is 4:1 in some studies.

Differential Diagnosis

Features distinguishing retentive constipation from Hirschsprung's disease are summarized in Table 19–8.

Treatment of Retentive Constipation

Increased intake of fluids and high-residue foods such as bran, whole wheat, fruits, and vegetables may be sufficient therapy in mild constipation. The use of a barley malt extract (Maltsupex) 1–2 tsp added to feedings two or three times daily, is helpful in small infants. Stool softeners such as dioctyl sodium sulfosuccinate, 5–10 mg/kg/d, prevent excessive drying of the stool and are effective unless there is voluntary stool retention. Cathartics such as standardized extract of senna fruit (eg, Senokot syrup), 1–2 tsp twice daily depending on age, can be used for short periods.

If encopresis is present, treatment should start with relieving fecal impaction. Then, an effective stool softener should be given in amounts sufficient to induce three or four loose stools per day (2–5 mL/kg/d of mineral oil in two doses). After several weeks to months of regular loose stools, the dosage of mineral oil can be tapered and stopped. Mineral oil should not be given to nonambulatory infants, retarded children, or those with gastroesophageal reflux. Aspiration of mineral oil may cause lipid pneumonia.

The prevention of stool holding and the establishment of a regular bowel habit are accomplished by toileting the child at regular times each day and by the daily administration of mineral oil over several months. Recurrence of encopresis should be treated promptly with a short course of laxatives or enemas. A multiple vitamin is recommended while mineral oil is administered.

Table 19–6. Malabsorption syndromes.

Intraluminal phase abnormalities	Intestinal phase abnormalities (cont'd)
Acid hypersecretion; Zollinger-Ellison syndrome	Circulatory disturbances
Gastric resection	Cirrhosis
Exocrine pancreatic insufficiency	Congestive heart failure
Cystic fibrosis	Abnormal structure of gastrointestinal tract
Chronic pancreatitis	Dumping syndrome after gastrectomy
Pancreatic pseudocysts	Malrotation
Schwachman syndrome	Stenosis of jejunum or ileum
Enterokinase deficiency	Small bowel resection; short bowel syndrome
Lipase and colipase deficiency	Polyposis
Malnutrition	Selective inborn absorptive defects
Decreased conjugated bile acids	Congenital malabsorption of folic acid
Liver production and excretion	Selective malabsorption of vitamin B_{12}
Neonatal hepatitis	Cystinuria, methionine malabsorption
Biliary atresia: intrahepatic and extrahepatic	Hartnup disease, blue diaper syndrome
Acute and chronic active hepatitis	Glucose-galactose malabsorption
Disease of the biliary tract	Primary disaccharidase deficiency
Cirrhosis	Acrodermatitis enteropathica
Fat malabsorption in the premature infant	Abetalipoproteinemia
Intestinal malabsorption of bile acids	Congenital chloridorrhea
Short bowel syndrome	Primary hypomagnesemia
Bacterial growth	Hereditary fructose intolerance
Blind loop	Familial hypophosphatemic rickets
Fistula	Endocrine diseases
Strictures, regional enteritis	Diabetes mellitus
Scleroderma, intestinal pseudo-obstruction	Addison's disease
Intestinal phase abnormalities	Hyperthyroidism
Mucosal diseases	Hypoparathyroidism, pseudohypoparathyroidism
Infections, bacterial or viral	Neuroblastoma, ganglioneuroma
Infections, parasitic	**Vascular and lymphatic disorders**
Giardia lamblia	Whipple's disease
Fish tapeworm	Intestinal lymphangiectasis
Hookworm	Congestive heart failure
Cryptosporidium	Regional enteritis with lymphangiectasis
Malnutrition	Lymphoma
Marasmus	Abetalipoproteinemia
Kwashiorkor	**Miscellaneous**
Dermatitis herpetiformis	Renal insufficiency
Folic acid deficiency	Carcinoid, mastocytosis
Drugs: methotrexate, antibiotics	Immune deficiency disorders
Crohn's disease	Familial dysautonomia
Cow's milk and soy protein intolerance	Collagen-vascular disease
Secondary disaccharidase deficiency	Wolman's disease
Secondary monosaccharide intolerance	Histiocytosis X
Hirschsprung's disease with enterocolitis	
Tropical sprue	
Celiac disease	
Radiation enteritis	
Lymphoma	

Psychiatric consultation may be indicated for patients with resistant symptoms or severe emotional disturbances.

Loening-Baucke V: Chronic constipation in children. Gastroenterology 1993;105:1557.

GASTROINTESTINAL BLEEDING

Vomiting blood and passing blood per rectum are alarming symptoms. The history is the key to identifying the bleeding source. The following questions should be answered:

(1) Is it really blood, and is it coming from the gastrointestinal tract? A number of substances simulate hematochezia or melena (Table 19–9). The presence of blood should be confirmed chemically. A history of genitourinary problems, coughing, tonsillitis, lost teeth, or epistaxis may identify an extraintestinal bleeding source.

(2) How much blood is there and what is its color and character? Table 19–10 lists the sites of gastrointestinal bleeding predicted by the appearance of the blood in the stools. Table 19–11 lists causes of rectal bleeding.

(3) Is the child acutely or chronically ill? The physical examination should be thorough. Physical

Table 19–7. Causes of constipation.[1]

Functional or retentive causes	Abnormalities of myenteric ganglion cells
Dietary causes	Hirschsprung's disease
Undernutrition, dehydration	Waardenburg's syndrome
Excessive milk intake	Multiple endocrine neoplasia IIA
Lack of bulk	Hypo- and hyperganglionosis
Cathartic abuse	von Recklinghausen's disease
Drugs	Multiple endocrine neoplasia IIB
Narcotics	Intestinal neuronal dysplasia
Antihistamines	Chronic intestinal pseudo-obstruction
Some antidepressants	Spinal cord defects
Vincristine	Metabolic and endocrine disorders
Structural defects of gastrointestinal tract	Hypothyroidism
Anus and rectum	Hyperparathyroidism
Fissure, hemorrhoids, abscess	Renal tubular acidosis
Anterior ectopic anus	Diabetes insipidus (dehydration)
Anal and rectal stenosis	Vitamin D intoxication (hypercalcemia)
Presacral teratoma	Idiopathic hypercalcemia
Small bowel and colon	Skeletal muscle weakness or incoordination
Tumor, stricture	Cerebral palsy
Chronic volvulus	Muscular dystrophy/myotonia
Intussusception	
Smooth muscle diseases	
Scleroderma and dermatomyositis	
Systemic lupus erythematosus	
Chronic intestinal pseudo-obstruction	

[1]Modified and reproduced, with permission, from Silverman A, Roy CC: *Pediatric Clinical Gastroenterology,* 3rd ed. Mosby, 1983.

Table 19–8. Differentiation of retentive constipation and Hirschsprung's disease.

	Retentive Constipation	Hirschsprung's Disease
Onset	2–3 years	At birth
Abdominal distention	Rare	Present
Nutrition and growth	Normal	Poor
Soiling and retentive behavior	Intermittent or constant	Rare
Rectal examination	Ampulla full	Ampulla may be empty
Rectal biopsy	Ganglion cells present	Ganglion cells absent
Rectal manometry	Normal rectoanal reflex	Nonrelaxation of internal anal sphincter after rectal distention
Barium enema	Distended rectum	Narrow distal segment with proximal megacolon

Table 19–9. Pitfalls in the diagnosis of gastrointestinal bleeding in children.[1]

Exogenous blood
Maternal blood[2]
Epistaxis
Uncooked meat
Pseudoblood
Medications in red syrup
Red Kool-Aid, fruit punch, red gelatin
Tomato skin
Tomato juice
Cranberry juice
Beets
Peach skin
Red diaper syndrome[3]
Red cherries
Black stools
Iron preparations[4,5]
Pepto-Bismol
Grape juice
Purple grapes
Spinach
Chocolate

[1]Modified and reproduced, with permission, from Treem WR: Gastrointestinal bleeding in children. Gastrointest Endosc Clin North Am 1994;4:75.
[2]From cracked nipples in a breast-fed baby.
[3]Red pigmentation of soiled diapers due to *Serratia marcescens* in stool.
[4]Ferrous sulfate and ferrous gluconate with guaiac and ortho-tolidine-based tests.
[5]High false-positive rate with orthotolidine-based tests.

Table 19–10. Identification of sites of gastrointestinal bleeding.

Symptom or Sign	Location of Bleeding Lesion
Effortless bright red blood from the mouth	Nasopharyngeal or oral lesions; tonsillitis; esophageal varices; lacerations of esophageal or gastric mucosa (Mallory-Weiss syndrome)
Vomiting of bright red blood or of "coffee grounds"	Lesion proximal to ligament of Treitz
Melanotic stool	Lesion proximal to ligament of Treitz, upper small bowel. Blood loss in excess of 50–100 mL/24 h
Bright red or dark red blood in stools	Lesion in the ileum or colon. (Massive upper gastrointestinal bleeding may also be associated with bright red blood in stool.)
Streak of blood on outside of a stool	Lesion in the rectal ampulla or anal canal

signs of portal hypertension, intestinal obstruction, or coagulopathy are particularly important. The nasal passages should be inspected for signs of recent epistaxis, the vagina for menstrual blood, and the anus for fissures and hemorrhoids.

A systolic blood pressure below 100 mm Hg and a pulse rate above 100/min in an older child suggest at least a 20% reduction of blood volume. A pulse rate increase of 20/min or a drop in systolic blood pressure greater than 10 mm Hg when the patient sits up is also a sensitive index of significant volume depletion.

(4) Is the child still bleeding? Serial determinations of vital signs and hematocrit are essential to assess ongoing bleeding. Detection of blood in the gastric aspirate confirms a bleeding site proximal to the ligament of Treitz. However, its absence does not rule out the duodenum as the source.

Treatment

If a hemorrhagic diathesis is detected, vitamin K should be given intravenously. In severe bleeding, the need for volume replacement is monitored by measurement of central venous pressure. In less severe cases, vital signs, serial hematocrits, and gastric aspirates are sufficient.

If blood is recovered from the gastric aspirate, gastric lavage with saline should be performed for 30–60 minutes until only a blood-tinged return is obtained. Panendoscopy is then done to identify the bleeding site. Endoscopy is superior to barium contrast study for lesions such as esophageal varices,

stress ulcers, and gastritis. Colonoscopy may identify the source of bright red rectal bleeding and should be performed if the extent of bleeding warrants immediate investigation and if plain x-ray films show no signs of intestinal obstruction.

Small or large bowel lesions that bleed briskly (> 0.5 mL/min) may be localized by angiography or radionuclide scanning following injection of labeled red cells.

Persistent vascular bleeding (varices, vascular anomalies) may be temporarily relieved using vasopressin (20 units/1.73 m^2 intravenously over a 20-minute period). Thereafter, it may be necessary to sustain the infusion for 24 hours at a rate of 0.2–0.4 units/1.73 m^2/min. Bleeding from esophageal varices may be stopped by temporary compression with a pediatric Sengstaken-Blakemore tube. Sclerotherapy or banding of uncontrolled bleeding varices is the treatment of choice.

If gastric decompression, antacid therapy, and transfusion are ineffective in stopping ulcer bleeding, laser therapy, local injection of epinephrine, electrocautery, or emergency surgery may be necessary.

Treem WR: Gastrointestinal bleeding in children. Gastrointest Endosc Clin North Am 1994;4:75.

RECURRENT ABDOMINAL PAIN

About 10% of healthy school children between 5 and 15 years of age will at some time experience recurrent episodes of abdominal pain severe enough to interfere with normal activities. An organic cause can be found in fewer than 10% of cases.

Clinical Findings

A. Symptoms and Signs: Attacks of abdominal pain are characteristically of variable duration and intensity. Although the pain is usually located in the periumbilical area, location far from the umbilicus does not rule out recurrent abdominal pain. Pain may occur both day and night. Weight loss is rare. Pain may be associated with dramatic reactions; patients may clutch the abdomen, double over, or even throw themselves to the ground. School attendance may suffer. Indeed, reluctance to attend school (school phobia) may be an important etiologic factor. The pain may be associated with pallor, nausea, vomiting, and slight temperature elevation.

The pain usually bears little relationship to bowel habits and physical activity. However, some patients have a constellation of symptoms strongly suggesting irritable bowel syndrome—bloating, postprandial pain, lower abdominal discomfort, and erratic stool habits with a sensation of obstipation or incomplete evacuation of stool. A precipitating or stressful situation in the child's life at the time the pains began can sometimes be elicited. A history of functional gas-

Table 19–11. Differential diagnosis of gastrointestinal bleeding in children by symptoms and age at presentation.[1]

	Infant	Child (2–12)	Adolescent (> 12)
Hematemesis	Swallowed maternal blood Peptic esophagitis Mallory-Weiss tear Gastritis Gastric ulcer Duodenal ulcer Gastric, duodenal ulcer	Epistaxis Peptic esophagitis Caustic ingestion Mallory-Weiss tear Esophageal varices Gastritis Gastric ulcer Duodenal ulcer Hereditary hemorrhagic telangiectasia Hemobilia Henoch-Schönlein purpura	Esophageal ulcer Peptic esophagitis Mallory-Weiss tear Esophageal varices Gastric ulcer Gastritis Duodenal ulcer Hereditary hemorrhagic telangiectasia Hemobilia Henoch-Schönlein purpura
Painless melana	Duodenal ulcer Duodenal duplication Ileal duplication Meckel's diverticulum Gastric heterotopia[2]	Duodenal ulcer Duodenal duplication Ileal duplication Meckel's diverticulum Gastric heterotopia[2]	Duodenal ulcer Leiomyoma (sarcoma)
Melena with pain, obstruction, peritonitis, perforation	Necrotizing enterocolitis Intussusception[3] Volvulus	Duodenal ulcer Hemobilia[4] Intussusception[3] Volvulus Ileal ulcer (isolated)	Duodenal ulcer Hemobilia[4] Crohn's disease (ileal ulcer)
Hematochezia with diarrhea, crampy abdominal pain	Infectious colitis Pseudomembranous colitis Eosinophilic colitis Hirschspring's enterocolitis	Infectious colitis Pseudomembranous colitis Granulomatous (Crohn's) colitis Hemolytic-uremic syndrome Henoch-Schönlein purpura Lymphonodular hyperplasia	Infectious colitis Pseudomembranous colitis Granulomatous (Crohn's) colitis Hemolytic-uremic syndrome Henoch-Schönlein purpura
Hematochezia without diarrhea or abdominal pain	Anal fissure Eosinophilic colitis Rectal gastric mucosa heterotopia Colonic hemangiomas	Anal fissure Solitary rectal ulcer Juvenile polyp Lymphonodular hyperplasia	Anal fissure Hemorrhoid Solitary rectal ulcer Colonic arteriovenous malformation

[1]Reproduced, with permission, from Treem WR: Gastrointestinal bleeding in children. Gastrointest Endosc Clin North Am 1994;4:75.
[2]Ectopic gastric tissue in jejunum or ileum without Meckel's diverticulum.
[3]Classically, "currant jelly" stool.
[4]Hemobilia often accompanied by vomiting, right upper quadrant pain.

trointestinal complaints is often found in family members.

A thorough physical examination is essential and usually normal. Complaints of abdominal tenderness elicited during palpation sometimes seem out of proportion to visible signs of distress.

B. Laboratory Findings: Complete blood count, sedimentation rate, urinalysis, and stool test for occult blood usually suffice. If the pain is atypical, further testing suggested by symptoms should be done.

Differential Diagnosis

Abdominal pain secondary to disorders of the urinary tract and extra-abdominal sources are listed in Table 19–3. Pinworms, mesenteric lymphadenitis, and chronic appendicitis are improbable causes of recurrent abdominal pain. Lactose intolerance usually causes pain, gas, and diarrhea. At times, however, abdominal discomfort may be the only symptom. Abdominal migraine and abdominal epilepsy are rare conditions. The incidence of peptic gastritis, esophagitis, duodenitis, and ulcer disease is probably underappreciated. Upper intestinal endoscopy may be useful.

Treatment & Prognosis

Treatment consists of reassurance based on a thorough physical appraisal and a sympathetic explanation of the functional nature of the complaint. Therapy for emotional problems is sometimes required, but drugs should be avoided. The prognosis is good.

Antonson DL: Abdominal pain. Gastrointest Endosc Clin North Am 1994;4:1.

Hyams J: Recurrent abdominal pain in children. Curr Opin Pediatr 1995;7:529.

PROTEIN-LOSING ENTEROPATHIES

Excessive loss of plasma proteins into the gastrointestinal tract occurs in association with a number of disorders.

Clinical Findings

Signs and symptoms include edema, chylous ascites, poor weight gain, and sometimes deficiencies of fat-soluble vitamins and anemia. Serum albumin is usually less than 2.5 g/dL. Serum globulins may also be decreased. Fecal α_1-antitrypsin, a marker for protein loss, is elevated (> 3 mg/g dry weight stool; slightly higher in breast-fed infants).

Disorders associated with protein-losing enteropathy are listed in Table 19–12.

Differential Diagnosis

Hypoalbuminemia may be due to an increased catabolic rate or may be associated with poor protein intake, impaired hepatic protein synthesis, or congenital malformations of lymphatics outside the gastrointestinal tract. It is important to rule out proteinuria from such conditions as urinary infection, nephritis, and nephrotic syndrome as causes of protein loss.

Treatment

Albumin infusions in conjunction with diuretics

Table 19–12. Disorders associated with protein-losing enteropathy.

Vascular obstruction
  Congestive heart failure
  Constrictive pericarditis
  Atrial septal defect
  Primary myocardial disease
  Increased right atrial pressure[1]
Stomach
  Giant hypertrophic gastritis (Ménétrier's disease), often
    secondary to CMV infection
  Polyps
  Gastritis secondary to H pylori infection
Small intestine
  Celiac disease
  Intestinal lymphangiectasia
  Blind loop syndrome
  Abetalipoproteinemia
  Chronic mucosal ischemia (eg, from chronic volvulus or
    radiation enteritis)
  Allergic enteropathy
  Malrotation
  Inflammatory bowel disease
Colon
  Ulcerative colitis
  Hirschsprung's disease
  Pseudomembranous colitis
  Polyposis syndromes
  Villous adenoma
  Solitary rectal ulcer

[1]Children who undergo Fontan procedure for tricuspid atresia are especially prone.

may relieve symptoms temporarily. Treatment must be directed toward the primary underlying cause.

CELIAC DISEASE
(Gluten Enteropathy)

Celiac disease results from intestinal sensitivity to the gliadin fraction of gluten from wheat, rye, barley, and oats. Most pediatric cases present during the second year of life, but the age at onset and the severity are both variable. The disease is more common in Europe and Canada than in the United States and is uncommon in blacks and Asians.

It is thought that intestinal damage and villous atrophy result from a cell-mediated immune response to gliadin, the alcohol-soluble fraction of gluten. Ten percent of first-degree relatives may be affected. The inheritance is probably polygenic, but it might result from a single gene in combination with an environmental precipitant such as intestinal adenovirus infection. The increased incidence of celiac disease in children with type I diabetes mellitus, IgA deficiency, and Down's syndrome is consistent with possible immunologic factors in the development of celiac disease. Individuals with HLA-DR3 and -DR4 tissue type are at higher risk.

Clinical Findings
A. Symptoms and Signs:
1. Diarrhea–Affected children present with a history of digestive disturbances starting at 6–12 months of age—the age at which wheat, rye, or oat glutens are first fed. Initially, the diarrhea may be intermittent; subsequently it is continuous, with bulky, pale, frothy, greasy, foul-smelling stools. During celiac crises, dehydration, shock, and acidosis are seen. In cases in which anorexia is severe (about 10%), diarrhea is absent.

2. Constipation, vomiting, and abdominal pain–This triad of symptoms may in a small number of cases dominate the clinical picture and suggest a diagnosis of intestinal obstruction. Constipation generally results from a combination of anorexia, dehydration, muscle weakness, and bulky, fatty stools.

3. Failure to thrive–The onset of diarrhea is usually accompanied by loss of appetite, failure to gain weight, and irritability. Weight loss is most marked in the limbs and buttocks. The abdomen becomes distended secondary to gas and fluid in the intestinal tract. Short stature and delayed puberty are characteristic in older children.

4. Anemia and vitamin deficiencies–Anemia usually responds to iron supplementation and is rarely megaloblastic. Deficiencies in fat-soluble vitamins are common. Rickets can be seen when growth has not been completely halted by the disease. Osteomalacia is more common, however, and pathologic fractures may occur. Hypoprothrombinemia secondary to vitamin K malabsorption can cause easy bleeding.

B. Laboratory Findings:

1. Fat content of stools–A 3-day collection of stools usually reveals excessive fecal fat. A normal child will excrete 5–10% of ingested fats. The untreated celiac patient will excrete more than 15% of daily fat intake. Anorexia may be so severe that steatorrhea may not be present in 10–25% of cases until normal intake is established.

2. Impaired carbohydrate absorption–A low oral glucose tolerance curve is seen. Absorption of D-xylose is impaired, with blood levels lower than 20 mg/dL 60 minutes after ingestion.

3. Hypoproteinemia–Hypoalbuminemia can be severe enough to lead to edema. There is evidence of increased protein loss in the gut lumen and poor hepatic synthesis secondary to malnutrition.

C. Imaging: A small bowel series shows a malabsorptive pattern characterized by segmentation, clumping of the barium column, and hypersecretion. These changes are nonspecific and can be found in other malabsorption states (Table 19–6).

D. Biopsy Findings: Intestinal biopsy is the most reliable test for celiac disease. It is a safe and simple procedure even in infants. Under the dissecting microscope, the jejunal mucosa lacks the slender, finger-like projections that characterize normal villi. Under the light microscope, the celiac mucosa has shortened or absent villi, lengthened crypts of Lieberkühn, and intense plasma cell infiltration of the lamina propria.

E. Serologic Tests: Antigliadin, antireticulin, and antiendomysial antibodies are useful screening tests. IgG antibodies to gliadin are present in 10% of normal children. Antiendomysial antibodies are the most sensitive and specific screening test for celiac disease if the patient is not IgA-deficient.

Differential Diagnosis

The differential diagnosis includes disorders that cause malabsorption. Strict adherence to two diagnostic criteria is essential—the characteristic small bowel microscopic changes and clinical improvement on a gluten-free diet. Repeated mucosal biopsies to prove histologic recovery on gluten-free diet and relapse on gluten challenge are not critical to the diagnosis in typical patients. Endomysial antibody titers may decrease on a gluten-free diet.

Treatment

A. Diet: Treatment consists of dietary gluten restriction for life. All sources of wheat, rye, barley, and oat gluten must be eliminated during the initial treatment. Some patients may be able to tolerate oats in the diet, but this should be tested only after recovery has occurred. Lactose is poorly tolerated in the acute stage because the extensive mucosal damage causes disaccharidase deficiency. Normal amounts of

fat are advisable. Supplemental calories, vitamins, and minerals are indicated in the acute phase. Clinical improvement is usually evident within a week, and histologic repair is complete after 3–12 months.

B. Corticosteroids: Corticosteroids can hasten clinical improvement but are indicated only in very ill patients with signs and symptoms of celiac crisis (profound malnutrition, diarrhea, edema, abdominal distention, and hypokalemia).

Prognosis

Clinical and histologic recovery is the rule but may be slow. Malignant lymphoma of the small bowel occurs with increased frequency in adults with long-standing disease. Dietary treatment seems to decrease the risk of this complication.

Taminiau JA: Celiac disease. Curr Opin Pediatr 1996;8:483.

DISACCHARIDASE DEFICIENCY

Starches and the disaccharides sucrose and lactose are quantitatively the most important dietary carbohydrates. The dietary disaccharides and oligosaccharide products of pancreatic amylase action on starch require hydrolysis by intestinal brush border disaccharidases before significant absorption can take place. Disaccharidase levels are higher in the jejunum and in the proximal ileum than in the distal ileum and duodenum.

In primary disaccharidase deficiency, a single enzyme is affected, disaccharide intolerance is likely to persist, intestinal histologic findings are normal, and a family history is common.

Because disaccharidases are confined to the outer cell layer of the intestinal epithelium, they are susceptible to mucosal damage. Many conditions cause secondary disaccharidase deficiency, with lactase usually most severely depressed. Histologic examination reveals changes compatible with the underlying disorder.

Clinical Findings

A. Primary (Congenital):

1. Lactase deficiency–Congenital lactase deficiency is a rare condition leading to diarrhea after lactose is ingested. The stools are frothy and acid; their pH may fall below 4.5 owing to the presence of organic acids. Vomiting is common. Severe malnutrition may occur. Reducing substances are present in the stools, and lactosuria may occur. Infants with lactosuria, aminoaciduria, proteinuria, acidosis, and elevated blood urea nitrogen have been described. Blood glucose fails to rise more than 10 mg/dL after ingestion of 1 g/kg of lactose. A rise in breath hydrogen after oral administration of lactose (from hydrogen produced by normal colon flora during fermentation of unabsorbed carbohydrate) is also diagnostic.

Patients respond to reduction of dietary lactose. Tolerance for dietary starch and sucrose is normal. Lactase extracted from *Aspergillus* and *Kluyvera* species can be added to milk products or taken with meals to enhance lactose hydrolysis (Lactaid).

2. Sucrase and isomaltase deficiency–This is a combined defect that is inherited as an autosomal recessive trait. Ten percent of Alaskan natives are affected. The condition is rare in other groups. Abdominal distention, failure to thrive, and chronic diarrhea may be the presenting symptoms. Distaste for and avoidance of sucrose occurs even in young infants.

Because sucrose is not a reducing sugar, tests for reducing substances in the stool will be negative unless the sucrose in the stool is hydrolyzed. A sucrose tolerance test (1 g/kg) is likely to be abnormal. Breath hydrogen will be elevated after ingestion of sucrose. Treatment of primary sucrase-isomaltase deficiency requires elimination of most sucrose. A preparation of yeast sucrase taken with meals is also effective.

B. Secondary (Acquired):
1. Secondary lactase deficiency–Diarrhea may be produced in normal individuals if a large dose of lactose is ingested. The threshold for lactose tolerance is much lower than that for sucrose. There is a high prevalence of genetically determined lactase deficiency in certain racial groups (70% in North American blacks and nearly 100% in Asian populations) after 3–5 years of age. It is estimated that 30–60% of Caucasians become lactase-deficient after 3–5 years. Neomycin and kanamycin administration can reduce lactase activity. Celiac disease, giardiasis, malnutrition, viral or bacterial gastroenteritis, abetalipoproteinemia, immunoglobulin deficiencies, and intestinal mucosal injury secondary to radiation and cancer chemotherapy all can decrease intestinal lactase activity.

2. Secondary sucrase deficiency–Intestinal mucosal damage tends to lower the levels of all disaccharidases. Signs of sucrose intolerance are usually masked by the more striking symptoms of lactose intolerance. Infectious diarrhea is the most common cause of secondary sucrose intolerance.

Prognosis

Primary disaccharidase deficiency is a lifelong defect. However, in both lactase and sucrase deficiencies, tolerance for the disaccharide may increase with age. The prognosis in the secondary or acquired forms of disaccharidase deficiency depends on the underlying illness. Normal tolerance for lactose may not be regained for many months after an acute mucosal injury.

Baudon JJ et al: Sucrase-isomaltase deficiency: Changing pattern over 2 decades. J Pediatr Gastroenterol Nutr 1996;22:284.

Rings EH, Grand RJ, Buller HA: Lactose intolerance and lactase deficiency in children. Curr Opin Pediatr 1994;6:562.

GLUCOSE-GALACTOSE MALABSORPTION

Glucose-galactose malabsorption is a rare disorder in which the Na glucose transport protein is defective. The gene has been localized to the long arm of chromosome 22. Severe diarrhea begins with the first feedings. Small bowel histologic findings are normal. Glycosuria and aminoaciduria may occur. The glucose tolerance test is flat. Fructose is well tolerated. The diarrhea promptly subsides on withdrawal of glucose and galactose from the diet. Reducing substances are consistently found in the stool. The acquired form of glucose-galactose malabsorption is mainly seen in infants under 6 months of age, usually following acute viral or bacterial enteritis. Both disaccharides and monosaccharides, including fructose, are malabsorbed.

In the congenital disease, exclusion of glucose and galactose from the diet is mandatory. A satisfactory formula is one with a carbohydrate-free base plus added fructose. The prognosis is good if the disease is diagnosed early, because tolerance for glucose and galactose improves with age. In the secondary form, prolonged parenteral nutrition may be required until intestinal transport mechanisms for monosaccharides return.

Elsas LJ, Longo N: Glucose transporters. Ann Rev Med 1992;43:377.

Nichols VN et al: Acquired monosaccharide intolerance in infants. J Pediatr Gastroenterol Nutr 1989;8:51.

INTESTINAL LYMPHANGIECTASIA

This form of protein-losing enteropathy results from a congenital abnormality of the bowel lymphatic system, often associated with abnormalities of the lymphatics in the extremities. Obstruction of lymphatic drainage of the intestine leads to rupture of the intestinal lacteals with leakage of lymph into the lumen of the bowel. Fat loss may be significant and lead to steatorrhea. Chronic loss of lymphocytes and immunoglobulins increases the susceptibility to infections.

Clinical Findings

Peripheral edema, diarrhea, abdominal distention, lymphedematous extremities, chylous effusions, and repeated infections are common. Laboratory findings are low serum albumin, decreased immunoglobulin levels, lymphocytopenia, and anemia. Serum calcium is frequently depressed, and stool fat may be elevated. Lymphocytes may be seen in large numbers on a stool smear. Fecal α_1-antitrypsin is elevated. X-ray studies reveal an edematous small bowel mucosal pattern, and biopsy reveals dilated lacteals in the villi and lamina propria. If only the lymphatics of the deeper layers of bowel or intestinal mesenterics are involved, laparotomy may be necessary to establish the diagnosis.

Differential Diagnosis

Other causes of protein-losing enteropathy must be considered, though an associated lymphedematous extremity strongly favors this diagnosis.

Treatment & Prognosis

Medium chain triglycerides as a fat source are effective only in mucosal lymphangiectasia. Vitamin and calcium supplements should be given. Antibiotics are used for specific infections. Total parenteral nutrition is helpful on a temporary basis. Surgery is needed when the lesion is localized to a small area of the bowel or in cases of constrictive pericarditis or obstructing tumors. Intravenous albumin and immune globulin may also be used to control symptoms. The prognosis is not favorable, though there may be remission with age.

Mehta MN et al: Intestinal lymphangiectasia. Indian Pediatr 1996;33:866.

COW'S MILK PROTEIN INTOLERANCE

Milk protein intolerance is more common in males and in young infants with a family history of atopy. The estimated prevalence is 0.5–1%. Colic, vomiting, and diarrhea are the major symptoms. Stools often contain blood and mucus. Sigmoidoscopic examination reveals a superficial colitis, often with an eosinophilic infiltrate. Pneumatosis intestinalis may be present on x-ray. Viral gastroenteritis sometimes precedes the onset of symptoms. Less commonly, milk protein may induce eosinophilic gastroenteritis with protein-losing enteropathy, hypoalbuminemia, and hypogammaglobulinemia. A celiac-like syndrome with villous atrophy, malabsorption, hypoalbuminemia, occult blood in the stool, and anemia can occur in older children. IgE-mediated anaphylactic shock is a rare manifestation of milk protein sensitivity in infancy.

Breast-fed infants under 6 months of age can also develop blood-streaked stools and a sigmoidoscopic picture similar to that of infants with milk protein sensitivity. Tiny amounts of intact allergen passed in breast milk may be the cause. Elimination of whole cow's milk from the mother's diet sometimes causes resolution of bloody diarrhea. A switch to semielemental diet (in which the protein source has been partially or completely hydrolyzed) almost always results in improvement. Because the blood loss and diarrhea in these breast-fed infants are rarely severe, it is not essential that breast feeding be stopped. If symptoms are severe or prolonged, however, a trial of semielemental formula is recommended. The colitic pattern of milk protein sensitivity and colitis in breast-fed infants usually clears spontaneously by 6–12 months of age.

Patients with milk protein allergy have a 30% incidence of sensitivity to soy protein, with similar symptoms. It is therefore best to use a partially or completely hydrolyzed formula as an elimination diet.

Host A: Cow's milk protein allergy and intolerance in infancy. Some clinical, epidemiological, and immunologic aspects. Pediatr Allergy Immunol 1994;5(Suppl 5):5.

Moon A, Kleinman RE: Allergic gastroenteropathy in children. Ann Allergy Asthma Immunol 1995;74:5.

IMMUNOLOGIC DEFICIENCY STATES WITH DIARRHEA OR MALABSORPTION

Diarrhea is common in immune deficiency states, but the cause is often obscure. Fifty to 60 percent of patients with idiopathic acquired hypogammaglobulinemia have steatorrhea and intestinal villous atrophy. Lymphonodular hyperplasia is a common feature in this group of patients. Patients with congenital or Bruton type agammaglobulinemia uniformly have diarrhea and abnormal intestinal morphology. Patients with isolated IgA deficiency may also present with chronic diarrhea, a celiac-like picture, lymphoid nodular hyperplasia, and giardiasis. Patients with isolated cellular immunity defects, combined cellular and humoral immune incompetence, and HIV infection may have severe chronic diarrhea leading to malnutrition. The cause of diarrhea may be common bacterial, viral, fungal, or parasitic pathogens, organisms usually considered nonpathogenic (*Blastocystis hominis, Candida*), or unusual organisms (cytomegalovirus, *Cryptosporidium, Isospora belli, Mycobacterium* species, microsporidia, and algal organisms such as Cyanobacteria). Often the cause is not found. There is a high incidence of disaccharidase deficiency. Chronic granulomatous disease may be associated with intestinal symptoms suggestive of chronic inflammatory bowel disease. A rectal biopsy may reveal the presence of typical macrophages.

Treatment must be directed toward correction of the immunologic defect. Specific treatments are available or are being developed for many of the unusual pathogens causing diarrhea in the immunocompromised host. Thus, a vigorous diagnostic search for specific pathogens is warranted in these individuals.

Deveikis A: Gastrointestinal disease in immunocompromised children. Pediatr Ann 1994;23:562.

INFLAMMATORY BOWEL DISEASE

Crohn's disease and ulcerative colitis are the two major idiopathic inflammatory bowel diseases of children. They share many features resulting from bowel inflammation, such as diarrhea, pain, fever, and blood loss, but they differ in important aspects, such as distribution of disease, histologic findings, incidence and type of extraintestinal symptoms, response to medications and surgery, and prognosis. A comparison of these two conditions is shown in Table 19–13. The cause is unknown but is probably an abnormal or uncontrolled, genetically determined immunologic or inflammatory response to an environmental antigenic trigger, possibly a virus or bacterium. There is no indication that emotional factors are a primary cause of these diseases.

Differential Diagnosis

A. Crohn's Disease: When extraintestinal

Table 19–13. Features of Crohn's disease and ulcerative colitis.[1]

	Crohn's Disease	Ulcerative Colitis
Age at onset	10–20 years	10–20 years
Incidence	4–6 per 100,000	3–15 per 100,000
Area of bowel affected	Oropharynx, esophagus, and stomach, rare; small bowel only, 25–30%, colon and anus only, 25%; ileocolitis, 40%; diffuse disease, 5%	Total colon, 90%; proctitis, 10%
Distribution	Segmental; disease-free skip areas common.	Continuous; distal to proximal
Pathology	Full-thickness, acute, and chronic inflammation; noncaseating granulomas (50%), extraintestinal fistulas, abscesses, stricture, and fibrosis may be present	Superficial, acute inflammation of mucosa with microscopic crypt abscess
X-ray findings	Segmental lesions; thickened, circular folds, cobblestone appearance of bowel wall secondary to longitudinal ulcers and transverse fissures; fixation and separation of loops; narrowed lumen; "string sign"; fistulas	Superficial colitis; loss of haustra; shortened colon and pseudopolyps (islands of normal tissue surrounded by denuded mucosa) are late findings
Intestinal symptoms	Abdominal pain, diarrhea (usually loose with blood if colon involved), perianal disease, enteroenteric or enterocutaneous fistula, abscess, anorexia	Abdominal pain, bloody diarrhea, urgency, and tenesmus
Extraintestinal symptoms Arthritis/arthralgia	15%	9%
Fever	40–50%	40–50%
Stomatitis	9%	2%
Weight loss	90% (mean 5.7 kg)	68% (mean 4.1 kg)
Delayed growth and sexual development	30%	5–10%
Uveitis, conjunctivitis	15% (in Crohn's colitis)	4%
Sclerosing cholangitis	—	4%
Renal stones	6% (oxalate)	6% (urate)
Pyoderma gangrenosum	1–3%	5%
Erythema nodosum	8–15%	4%
Laboratory findings	High erythrocyte sedimentation rate; microcytic anemia; low serum iron and total iron-binding capacity; increased fecal protein loss; low serum albumin; antineutrophil cytoplasmic antibodies present in 10–20%; Saccharomyces cerevisiae antibodies positive in 60%.	High erythrocyte sedimentation rate; microcytic anemia, high white blood cell count with left shift; antineutrophil cytoplasmic antibodies present in 80%

Reproduced, with permission, from Kirschner BS: Inflammatory bowel disease in children. Pediatr Clin North Am 1988;35:189.

symptoms predominate, Crohn's disease can be mistaken for rheumatoid arthritis, systemic lupus erythematosus, or hypopituitarism. Frequently, the acute onset of ileocolitis is mistaken for acute appendicitis. Symptoms sometimes suggest celiac disease, peptic ulcer, intestinal obstruction, or intestinal lymphoma.

B. Ulcerative Colitis: In the acute stage, bacterial pathogens and toxins causing colitis must be ruled out. These include *Shigella, Salmonella, Yersinia, Campylobacter, Entamoeba histolytica,* invasive *Escherichia coli, Aeromonas hydrophila,* and the toxin-producing pathogens *E coli* and *Clostridium difficile.* Mild ulcerative colitis sometimes mimics irritable bowel symptoms. Crohn's disease of the colon is an important differential possibility.

Complications
(See Table 19–13.)

A. Crohn's Disease: Intestinal obstruction, fistula, and abscess formation are common. Perforation and hemorrhage are rare. Malnutrition is caused by anorexia and compounded by malabsorption, protein-losing enteropathy, disaccharidase deficiency, and diarrhea induced by bile salts. Systemic complications include perianal disease, pyoderma gangrenosum, arthritis, amyloidosis, and growth retardation. The risk of colon cancer is increased in patients with Crohn's colitis, though probably not to the extent seen in ulcerative colitis.

B. Ulcerative Colitis: Arthritis, uveitis, pyoderma gangrenosum, and malnutrition all occur. Growth failure and delayed puberty are less common than in Crohn's disease. Liver disease (chronic active hepatitis, sclerosing cholangitis) is more common. In patients with pancolitis, carcinoma of the colon occurs with an incidence of 1–2% per year after the first 10 years of disease. Cancer risk is a function of disease duration and not age at onset. The mortality rate from colon cancer is high because the usual signs (occult blood in stool, pain, and abnormal x-ray findings) are not specific and may be ignored in a patient with colitis. Routine cancer screening via colonoscopy, with multiple biopsies and evaluation of specimens by histology for metaplasia and by flow cytometry for aneuploidy, is recommended in pediatric patients after 10 years of pancolitis. Dysplasia that persists in absence of inflammation is an indication for colectomy, as is aneuploidy in multiple biopsies.

Treatment

A. Medical Treatment: Medical treatment for Crohn's disease and ulcerative colitis is similar and includes anti-inflammatory, antidiarrheal, and antibiotic medication. No medical therapy has proved uniformly effective.

1. Diet–A high-protein, high-carbohydrate diet with normal amounts of fat is recommended. Decreased amounts of roughage may help decrease symptoms in those with colitis or with partial intestinal obstruction. Lactose is poorly tolerated when disease is active. The main concern should be ensuring adequate caloric intake. Restrictive or "bland" diets are counterproductive because they usually result in poor intake. Vitamin and iron supplements are recommended. Zinc levels are often low in patients with Crohn's disease and should be repleted. Supplemental calories in the form of liquid diets are well tolerated. Total parenteral nutrition for periods of 4–6 weeks may induce remission of symptoms and stimulate linear growth and sexual development. Enteral administration of low-residue or elemental liquid diets may also be associated with rapid nutritional repletion and temporary remission of symptoms, perhaps because of a reduced enteral antigen load. Home programs of both enteral and parenteral nutritional support have been used in patients with intractable symptoms or growth failure.

2. Nonabsorbable salicylate derivatives–Sulfasalazine is effective in mild cases of ulcerative colitis and perhaps in cases of Crohn's disease of the colon. It prevents relapse of ulcerative colitis once remission is induced. The drug is not absorbed in the small intestine. It is hydrolyzed by colon flora into sulfapyridine and 5-aminosalicylate. The sulfonamide moiety is probably inactive but is responsible for the allergic side effects of the drug. The salicylate moiety probably has local anti-inflammatory activity in the colon. Side effects are common, including skin rash, nausea, headache, and abdominal pain. More rarely, serum sickness, hemolytic anemia, aplastic anemia, and pancreatitis occur. Response to therapy may be slow. Sulfasalazine inhibits folic acid absorption, and supplemental folic acid is recommended.

Two to 3 grams per day in three divided doses are recommended for children over age 10, or 50 mg/kg/d for younger children. Half of this dose is used as a maintenance medication for well-controlled ulcerative colitis. Salicylate polymers for both oral and rectal use (olsalazine, mesalamine) are available. They are no more effective than sulfasalazine but can be tolerated by sulfonamide-sensitive patients and have fewer side effects.

3. Corticosteroids–With more severe inflammatory bowel disease, corticosteroids are used. Methylprednisolone, 2 mg/kg/d, or hydrocortisone, 10 mg/kg/d, may be given intravenously when disease is severe. Prednisone, 1–2 mg/kg/d orally in two or three divided doses, is given for 6–8 weeks, followed by a gradual tapering. Alternate-day steroids are associated with fewer side effects as the dosage of drug is tapered. There is no evidence that corticosteroids prevent relapses. Prednisone is often given in conjunction with sulfasalazine. The patient's varicella immunity should be confirmed by history or antibody screen and the parents appropriately counseled as to risk and therapy after varicella exposure. Serum titers against *Entamoeba histolytica* and stool examination for that parasite must be checked before starting therapy with corticosteroids, since amebic colitis may become generalized with steroid therapy. Hydrocortisone in the form of enema or foam can be instilled into the rectum in patients with tenesmus or ulcerative proctitis.

4. Azathioprine–Azathioprine, 1–2 mg/kg/d orally, is used only when a high maintenance dose of corticosteroids is necessary to keep the disease under control and there are serious risks of steroid-induced complications. Positive results of this therapy may be delayed weeks to months. Similarly, mercaptopurine is now under evaluation as a steroid-sparing maintenance medication for severe Crohn's disease in childhood.

5. Metronidazole–This drug is now used routinely in Crohn's disease patients with perianal disease. Disease tends to recur when the drug is discontinued. It may also be effective in Crohn's disease of the colon. The dosage of metronidazole is 15–30 mg/kg/d in three divided doses. Peripheral neuropathy may be a side effect with prolonged use. Ciprofloxacin may have similar therapeutic effects.

6. Cyclosporine–This powerful immunosuppressant is effective in severe, steroid-resistant ulcerative colitis, but because of side effects and rapid relapse after discontinuation, it is usually used to "buy time" in severely affected patients for whom surgical treatment is planned.

7. Anticytokines–Still in clinical trials in children. Anti-TNFα will soon be released for use in adults with severe Crohn's disease.

B. Surgical Treatment:

1. Crohn's disease–Crohn's disease is not cured by surgery. However, 70% of patients eventually require surgery to relieve obstruction, drain abscess, relieve intractable symptoms, or encourage growth and sexual maturation. The relapse rate 6 years after surgery is 60%. Recurrence usually occurs at the site of anastomosis, most likely within 2 years. The rate of recurrence may be less in disease limited to the colon. Surgery performed to correct growth retardation must be performed before puberty.

2. Ulcerative colitis–Surgery is curative and is recommended for those with uncontrolled hemorrhage, toxic megacolon, unrelenting pain and diarrhea, growth failure, high-grade mucosal dysplasia, or malignant tumors. There are now several surgical approaches (ileoanal anastomosis, Koch-type continent ileostomy) that allow a near-normal lifestyle after colectomy. Liver disease may not be improved by colectomy.

Prognosis

A. Crohn's Disease: Although the mortality rate is low (2% in the first 7 years), morbidity is high. The disease is progressive in most cases, and its course is interspersed with acute and chronic complications, leading to variable degrees of disability. Over 50% of patients experience symptoms that affect the quality of life. About 20% have severe disabling disease, and 20% have so few symptoms that they describe themselves as healthy.

B. Ulcerative Colitis: The prognosis is good. About 5% of patients present with toxic megacolon—massive colonic dilation secondary to full-thickness enterocolitis accompanied by shock and fever—and require immediate colectomy. Seventy-five percent have a relapsing and remitting course. Twenty-five to 40 percent require colectomy—especially those with pancolitis, anemia, and hypoalbuminemia at the time of presentation.

Griffiths AM, Sherman PM: Colonoscopic surveillance for cancer in ulcerative colitis: A critical review. J Pediatr Gastroenterol Nutr 1997;24:202.

Hyams JS: Extraintestinal manifestations of inflammatory bowel disease in children. J Pediatr Gastroenterol Nutr 1994;19:7.

Justinich C, Hyams JS: Inflammatory bowel disease in children and adolescents. Gastrointest Endosc Clin North Am 1994;4:39.

Noel RA, Ferry GD: Pediatric inflammatory bowel disease. Curr Opin Gastroenterol 1992;8:676.

REFERENCES

Silverman A, Roy CC: *Pediatric Clinical Gastroenterology,* 4th ed. Mosby, 1995.

Suchy FJ (editor): *Liver Disease in Children.* Mosby, 1994.

Walker WA et al (editors): *Pediatric Gastrointestinal Disease.* BC Decker, 1995.

Wyllie R, Hyams JS (editors): *Pediatric Gastrointestinal Disease.* Saunders, 1993.

Liver & Pancreas 20

Ronald J. Sokol, MD, & Michael R. Narkewicz, MD

LIVER

PROLONGED NEONATAL CHOLESTATIC JAUNDICE

The main clinical features of disorders causing prolonged neonatal cholestasis are (1) elevated direct-reacting bilirubin fraction (> 2 mg/dL or > 20% of total bilirubin), (2) elevated serum bile acids (> 10 mmol/L), (3) variably acholic stools, (4) dark urine, and (5) hepatomegaly.

Prolonged neonatal cholestasis (decreased bile flow) may be the result of intrahepatic or extrahepatic causes. Attention to specific clinical clues distinguishes these two major categories of jaundice in 85% of cases. Histologic examination of tissue obtained by percutaneous liver biopsy increases the accuracy of differentiation to 95% (Table 20–1).

INTRAHEPATIC CHOLESTASIS

Essentials of Diagnosis & Typical Features
- Elevated total and direct bilirubin.
- Hepatomegaly and dark urine.
- Patency of extrahepatic biliary tree.

General Considerations

Intrahepatic cholestasis is characterized by patency of the extrahepatic biliary system—despite cholestasis—and abnormalities of liver function tests. A specific cause can be identified in about 25% of cases. Patency of the extrahepatic biliary tract is suggested by pigmented stools and can least invasively be confirmed by hepatobiliary scintigraphy using ^{99m}Tc-diethyliminodiacetic acid (diethyl-IDA, DIDA). Radioactivity in the bowel within 4–24 hours is evidence of patency. Patency of the extrahepatic biliary system can also be determined by cholangiography carried out intraoperatively, percutaneously by transhepatic cholecystography, or by utilizing the newly designed pediatric-sized side-viewing endoscope.

1. PERINATAL OR NEONATAL HEPATITIS RESULTING FROM INFECTION

This diagnosis is considered in infants with jaundice, hepatomegaly, vomiting, lethargy, fever and petechiae. A perinatally acquired viral, bacterial, or protozoal infection must be identified. Infection may occur by transplacental spread, via the ascending route from vaginal or cervical structures into amniotic fluid; from swallowed contaminated fluids (maternal blood, urine) during delivery; or from breast milk, contaminated hands, etc. Infectious agents often associated with neonatal intrahepatic cholestasis include herpes simplex virus, varicella virus, coxsackieviruses, cytomegalovirus, rubella virus, echoviruses, adenovirus, parvovirus, HHV type 6, hepatitis B virus, human immunodeficiency virus, *Treponema pallidum,* and *Toxoplasma gondii.* Although hepatitis C may be transmitted vertically, it rarely causes neonatal cholestasis. The degree of liver cell injury caused by these agents is variable, ranging from massive hepatic necrosis (herpes simplex) to focal necrosis and mild inflammation (cytomegalovirus, hepatitis B virus). Serum bilirubin, bile acids, ALT, AST, and alkaline phosphatase are elevated. The infant is jaundiced and generally appears ill.

Clinical Findings

A. Symptoms and Signs: Clinical symptoms usually appear in the first 2 weeks of life but may appear as late as 2–3 months. Jaundice may be noted in the first 24 hours or may develop later. Loss of appetite, poor sucking reflex, lethargy, and vomiting are frequent. Stools may be normal to pale in color but are seldom acholic. Dark urine stains the diaper.

Table 20–1. Differentiating clinical and histologic features of intrahepatic and extrahepatic neonatal cholestasis.

	Intrahepatic	Extrahepatic
Clinical features	Preterm, small for gestational age, appears ill; hepatosplenomegaly, other organ or system involvement; incomplete cholestasis (stools with some color); associated cause identified (infections, metabolic, familial, etc)	Full-term, seems well; hepatomegaly (firm to hard); complete cholestasis (acholic stools); polysplenia syndrome, equal right and left hepatic lobes
Histologic features	Cholestasis, lobular disarray, giant cells, portal inflammation, minimal fibrosis, rare neoductular formation, steatosis, extramedullary hematopoiesis	Cholestasis, neoductular proliferation, portal fibrosis, bile lakes, normal lobular architecture, rare giant cells

Hepatomegaly is present, and the liver has a uniform firm consistency. Splenomegaly is variably present. Macular, papular, or petechial rashes may occur. In less severe cases, failure to thrive may be the major complaint. Unusual presentations include liver failure, hypoproteinemia, and anasarca (nonhemolytic hydrops) and hemorrhagic disease of the newborn.

B. Laboratory Findings: The blood count often shows neutropenia, thrombocytopenia, and signs of mild hemolysis. Mixed hyperbilirubinemia, elevated aminotransferases with near-normal alkaline phosphatase, prolongation of clotting studies, mild acidosis, and elevated cord serum IgM suggest congenital infection. Nasopharyngeal washings, urine, stool, and cerebrospinal fluid should be cultured for virus. Specific serologic tests may be useful, as are long-bone x-rays to determine the presence of "celery stalking" in the metaphysial regions of the humeri, femurs, and tibias. When indicated, CT and MRI can identify intracranial calcifications. Nuclear hepatobiliary imaging shows decreased hepatic clearance of the circulating isotope with excretion into the gut.

A percutaneous liver biopsy is performed to distinguish intrahepatic from extrahepatic cholestasis, rather than to identify a specific infectious agent within the liver tissue. Nevertheless, the presence of intracytoplasmic and intranuclear inclusions of cytomegalovirus in hepatocytes or bile duct epithelial cells, or the presence of intranuclear acidophilic inclusions of herpes simplex can be diagnostic. Variable degrees of lobular disarray characterized by focal necrosis, multinucleated giant cell transformation, and ballooned pale hepatocytes with loss of cord-like arrangement of liver cells are usual. Intrahepatocytic and canalicular cholestasis may be prominent. Portal changes are not striking, but modest neoductular pro-

liferation and mild fibrosis may occur. Special stains, in situ hybridization or viral cultures of biopsy material may be helpful.

Differential Diagnosis

Great care must be taken to distinguish infectious causes of intrahepatic cholestasis from genetic or metabolic causes (inborn errors), because the clinical presentations are very similar. Galactosemia, congenital fructose intolerance, and tyrosinemia must be investigated promptly, because specific dietary therapy is available. Alpha$_1$-antitrypsin deficiency, cystic fibrosis, and neonatal iron storage disease must also be considered. Specific physical features may be helpful when considering Alagille's or Zellweger's syndrome.

Unless the extrahepatic bile duct has spontaneously perforated, infants with extrahepatic cholestasis do not appear ill; stools are usually completely acholic, and the liver is enlarged and firm. Histologic findings are shown in Table 20–1.

Treatment

Most forms of viral neonatal hepatitis are treated symptomatically. Infants with herpes simplex or varicella infections are treated with acyclovir. Fluids and adequate calories are encouraged. Intravenous dextrose is needed if feedings are not well tolerated. The consequences of cholestasis are treated as indicated (Table 20–2). Vitamin K orally or by injection and vitamins D and E orally should be provided. Choleretics (cholestyramine, phenobarbital, ursodeoxycholic acid) are used if cholestasis persists. Corticosteroids are contraindicated. Penicillin for suspected syphilis or antibiotics for bacterial hepatitis need to be administered promptly.

Prognosis

Multiple organ involvement is commonly associated with neonatal infectious hepatitis and has a poor outcome. Death from hepatic or cardiac failure, intractable acidosis, or intracranial hemorrhage is seen, especially in herpesvirus or echovirus infection and occasionally in cytomegalovirus or rubella infection. Hepatitis B virus may rarely cause fulminant neonatal viral hepatitis; most infected infants become asymptomatic carriers of hepatitis B. Persistent liver disease results in mild chronic hepatitis, portal fibrosis, or cirrhosis. Chronic cholestasis, although rare following infections, may lead to dental enamel hypoplasia, failure to thrive, biliary rickets, severe pruritus, and xanthoma.

Specific Infectious Agents

A. Neonatal Hepatitis B Virus Disease: Infection with hepatitis B virus (HBV) may occur at any time during perinatal life, but the risk is higher when acute maternal disease occurs during the last trimester of pregnancy. However, most cases of

Table 20–2. Treatment of complications of chronic cholestatic liver disease.

Indication	Treatment	Dose	Toxicity
Intrahepatic cholestasis	Phenobarbital	3–10 mg/kg/d	Drowsiness, irritability, interference with vitamin D metabolism
	Cholestyramine/colestipol hydrochloride	250–500 mg/kg/d	Constipation, acidosis, binding of drugs, increased steatorrhea
	Ursodeoxycholic acid	15–20 mg/kg/d	Transient increase in pruritus
Pruritus	Phenobarbital or cholestyramine/colestipol (or both)	Same as above	
	Antihistamines: Diphenhydramine hydrochloride Hydroxyzine	5–10 mg/kg/d 2–5 mg/kg/d	Drowsiness
	Ultraviolet light B	Exposure as needed	Skin burn
	Carbamazepine	20–40 mg/kg/d	Hepatotoxicity, marrow suppression, fluid retention
	Rifampin	10 mg/kg/d	Hepatotoxicity, marrow suppression
	Ursodeoxycholic acid	15–20 mg/kg/d	Transient increase in pruritus
Steatorrhea	Formula containing medium-chain triglycerides (eg, Pregestimil)	120–150 calories/kg/d for infants	Expensive
	Oil supplement containing medium-chain triglycerides	1–2 mL/kg/d	Diarrhea, aspiration
Malabsorption of fat-soluble vitamins	Vitamin A	10,000–25,000 units/d	Hepatitis, pseudotumor cerebri, bone lesions
	Vitamin D	800–5000 units/d	Hypercalcemia, hypercalciuria
	25-Hydroxycholecalciferol (vitamin D)	3–5 μg/kg/d	Hypercalcemia, hypercalciuria
	1,25-Dihydroxycholecalciferol (vitamin D)	0.05–0.2 μg/kg/d	Hypercalcemia, hypercalciuria
	Vitamin E (oral)	25–200 IU/kg/d TPGS,[1] 15–25 IU/kg/d	Potentiation of vitamin K deficiency
	Vitamin E (intramuscular)	1–2 mg/kg/d	Muscle calcifications
	Vitamin K (oral)	2.5 mg twice per week to 5 mg/d	
	Vitamin K (intramuscular)	2–5 mg each 4 wk	
Malabsorption of other nutrients	Multiple vitamin	1–2 times the standard dose	
	Calcium	25–100 mg/kg/d	Hypercalcemia, hypercalciuria
	Phosphorus	25–50 mg/kg/d	Gastrointestinal intolerance
	Zinc	1 mg/kg/d	Interference with copper absorption

[1]Tocopheryl polyethylene glycol-1000 succinate (water-soluble vitamin E).

neonatal disease are acquired from mothers who are asymptomatic carriers of hepatitis B. HBV has been found in most body fluids, including breast milk, but it is not present in feces. In chronic HBsAg carrier mothers, fetal and infant acquisition risk is greatest if the mother (1) is also HBeAg-positive and HBeAb-negative, (2) has detectable levels of serum-specific hepatitis B DNA polymerase, or (3) has high serum levels of HBcAb. These findings are markers of high infectivity; however, hepatitis B can be transmitted even if HBsAg is the only marker present.

Neonatal liver disease resulting from HBV is extremely variable. The infant has a 70–90% chance of acquiring HBV at birth from HBsAg-positive mothers if nothing is done to prevent infection (ie, administration of hepatitis B immune globulin [HBIG] or vaccine). Most infected infants become asymptomatic carriers of HBV, usually for life. Fulminant hepatic necrosis has rarely been reported, especially in association with intrapartum or postpartum transfusions of infected blood. However, it also can occur from maternally transmitted virus. In such cases, progressive jaundice, stupor, shrinking liver size, and coagulation abnormalities dominate the clinical picture. Respiratory, circulatory, and renal failure usually follow. Histologically, the liver shows massive hepatocyte necrosis, collapse of the reticulum framework, minimal inflammation, and occasional pseudoacinar structures. Rare survivors are reported with reasonable restitution of liver architecture toward normal.

In less severe cases, focal hepatocyte necrosis is seen with a mild portal inflammatory response. Cholestasis is intracellular and canalicular. Chronic persistent and chronic active hepatitis may be present for many years, with serologic evidence of persisting antigenemia (HBsAg) and mildly elevated serum aminotransferases. Chronic active hepatitis may rarely progress to cirrhosis within 1–2 years.

To prevent perinatal transmission, all infants of mothers who are HBsAg-positive (regardless of HBeAg status) should receive HBIG and hepatitis B vaccine within the first 24 hours after birth and vaccine again at 1 and 6 months of age (see Chapter 10).

B. Neonatal Bacterial Hepatitis: Most bacterial liver infections in newborns are acquired by transplacental invasion from amnionitis with ascending spread from maternal vaginal or cervical infection. Onset is abrupt, usually within 48–72 hours after delivery, with signs of sepsis and often shock. Jaundice, seen in less than 25% of cases, appears early and is of the mixed type. The liver enlarges rapidly, and the histologic picture is that of diffuse hepatitis with or without micro- or macroabscess. The most common organisms are *Escherichia coli, Listeria monocytogenes,* and group B streptococci and, rarely, *Mycobacterium tuberculosis.* Isolated neonatal liver abscess caused by *E coli* or *Staphylococcus aureus* is often associated with omphalitis or umbilical vein catheterization. Bacterial hepatitis and neonatal liver abscesses require specific antibiotics in large doses and, rarely, surgical drainage. Deaths are common, but survivors show no long-term consequences of liver disease.

C. Neonatal Jaundice With Urinary Tract Infection: Jaundice in affected infants—usually males—typically appears between the second and fourth weeks of life. The manifestations of this disorder are lethargy, fever, poor appetite, jaundice, and hepatomegaly. Except for mixed hyperbilirubinemia, other liver function tests are not remarkable. Leuko-

cytosis is present, and infection is confirmed by culture techniques. The mechanism for the liver impairment is unknown, although toxic action of bacterial products (endotoxins) and the inflammatory response have been incriminated.

Treatment of the infection leads to prompt resolution of the cholestasis without hepatic sequelae. Metabolic liver diseases may present with gram-negative bacterial urinary tract infection and must be considered.

Kim SC et al: Universal hepatitis B immunization. Pediatrics 1995;95:764.
Krugman S: Viral hepatitis: A, B, C, D, and E: Prevention. Pediatr Rev 1992;13:245.
Pickering LK: Management of the infant of a mother with viral hepatitis. Pediatr Rev 1988;9:315.
Rosenthal P: Neonatal hepatitis and congenital infections. In: *Liver Disease in Children.* Suchy FJ (editor). Mosby-Year Book, 1994.
Stevens CE et al: Perinatal hepatitis B virus transmission in the United States. JAMA 1985;253:1740.
Zuccotti GV et al: Hepatitis B vaccination in infants of mothers infected with human immunodeficiency virus. J Pediatr 1994;125:70.

2. INTRAHEPATIC CHOLESTASIS RESULTING FROM INBORN ERRORS OF METABOLISM, FAMILIAL CAUSES, & "TOXIC" CAUSES

These cholestatic syndromes are caused by specific enzyme deficiencies or other inherited disorders; a positive history of certain precipitants associated with neonatal liver disease; and features of intrahepatic cholestasis—ie, jaundice, hepatomegaly, and normal to completely acholic stools. Some of the specific clinical conditions have characteristic clinical signs.

Enzyme Deficiencies & Other Inherited Disorders

Early specific diagnosis is important because dietary or pharmacologic treatment may be available (Table 20–3). Reversal of liver disease and clinical symptoms is prompt and permanent in several disorders as long as the diet is maintained. As with other inborn errors of metabolism, parents of the affected infant should be offered genetic counseling.

Cholestasis caused by metabolic diseases such as galactosemia, fructose intolerance, and tyrosinemia may be accompanied by vomiting, lethargy, poor feeding, and irritability. Hepatomegaly is a constant finding. The infants often appear septic; gram-negative bacteria can be cultured from blood in 25–50% of cases, especially in patients with galactosemia. Other inherited conditions that present with neonatal intrahepatic cholestasis are outlined in Table 20–3. Treatment of these disorders is outlined in Chapter 30.

Table 20–3. Metabolic and genetic causes of neonatal cholestasis.[1]

Disease	Inborn Error	Hepatic Pathology	Diagnostic Studies
Galactosemia	Galactose-1-phosphate uridylyltransferase	Cholestasis, steatosis, necrosis, pseudoacini, fibrosis	Galactose-1-phosphate uridylyltransferase assay of red blood cells
Fructose intolerance	Fructose-1-phosphate aldolase	Steatosis, necrosis, pseudoacini, fibrosis	Liver fructose-1-phosphate aldolase assay or leukocyte DNA analysis
Tyrosinemia	Fumarylacetoacetase	Necrosis, steatosis, pseudoacini, portal fibrosis	Urinary succinylacetone, fumarylacetoacetase assay of red blood cells
Cystic fibrosis	Cystic fibrosis transmembrane regular gene abnormality	Cholestasis, neoductular proliferation, excess bile duct mucus, portal fibrosis	Sweat test and leukocyte DNA analysis
Hypopituitarism	Deficient production of pituitary hormones	Cholestasis, giant cells	Thyroxine, TSH, cortisol levels
α_1-Antitrypsin deficiency	Abnormal α_1-antitrypsin molecule (Pi ZZ phenotype)	Giant cells, cholestasis, steatosis, neoductular proliferation, fibrosis, PAS-diastase-resistant cytoplasmic granules	Serum α_1-antitrypsin phenotype
Gaucher's disease	β-Glucosidase	Cholestasis, cytoplasmic inclusions in Kupffer's cells (foam cells)	β-Glucosidase assay in leukocytes
Niemann-Pick disease	Lysosomal sphingomyelinase	Cholestasis, cytoplasmic inclusions in Kupffer's cells	Sphingomyelinase assay of leukocytes or liver
Glycogen storage disease type IV	Branching enzyme	Fibrosis, cirrhosis, PAS-diastase-resistant cytoplasmic inclusions	Brancher enzyme analysis of leukocytes or liver
Neonatal hemochromatosis	Unknown	Giant cells, portal fibrosis, hemosiderosis, cirrhosis	Histology, iron stains
Peroxisomal disorders (eg, Zellweger's syndrome)	Deficient peroxisomal enzymes or assembly	Cholestasis, necrosis, fibrosis, cirrhosis, hemosiderosis	Plasma very long chain fatty acids, qualitative bile acids, plasmalogen, pipecolic acid, liver electron microscopy
Abnormalities in bile acid metabolism	Several enzyme deficiencies defined	Cholestasis, necrosis, giant cells	Urine, serum, duodenal fluid analyzed for bile acids by fast atom bombardment-mass spectroscopy
Byler's disease (familial progressive intrahepatic cholestasis)	FIC-1 and spgp genes	Cholestasis, necrosis, giant cells, fibrosis	Histology, family history, normal cholesterol, low or normal γ-glutamyl transpeptidase
Alagille's syndrome (syndromic paucity of interlobular bile ducts)	Jagged 1 gene mutations	Cholestasis, paucity of interlobular bile ducts, increased copper levels	Three or more clinical features, liver histology

[1]TSH = thyroid-stimulating hormone, PAS = periodic acid-Schiff.

"Toxic" Causes of Neonatal Cholestasis

A. Neonatal Ischemic-Hypoxic Conditions: Perinatal events that result in hypoperfusion of the gastrointestinal system are sometimes followed in 1–2 weeks by cholestasis. This is seen in premature infants with respiratory distress, severe hypoxia, hypoglycemia, shock, and acidosis. When these perinatal conditions develop in association with gastrointestinal lesions such as ruptured omphalocele, gastroschisis, or necrotizing enterocolitis, a subsequent cholestatic picture is common (25–50% of cases). Liver function studies reveal mixed hyperbilirubinemia, elevated alkaline phosphatase and γ-glutamyl transpeptidase values, and variable elevation of the aminotransferases. Stools are seldom persistently acholic.

Choleretics (cholestyramine, phenobarbital, ursodeoxycholic acid), introduction of enteral feedings as soon as possible, and nutritional support are the mainstays of treatment until the cholestasis resolves (see Table 20–2). In some cases, this resolution may take 3–6 months. Complete resolution of the hepatic abnormalities is the rule, but portal fibrosis with periportal scarring is occasionally seen on follow-up biopsy.

B. Prolonged Parenteral Nutrition: Cholestasis may develop after 1–2 weeks in premature newborns receiving total parenteral nutrition. Contributing factors include possible toxicity of intravenous amino acids, diminished stimulation of bile flow from prolonged absence of feedings, translocation of intestinal bacteria and their cell wall products, missing nutrients or antioxidants, photo-oxidation of amino acids, and the "physiologic cholestatic" propensity of the premature infant. Histology of the liver may resemble that of extrahepatic biliary atresia. Early introduction of feedings has reduced the frequency of this disorder. The prognosis is generally good. Rare cases of portal fibrosis, cirrhosis, and hepatoma may develop, particularly in infants with intestinal resections or anomalies.

C. "Inspissated Bile Syndrome": This is the result of accumulation of bile in canaliculi and in the small and medium-sized bile ducts in hemolytic disease of the newborn (Rh, ABO) and in some infants receiving total parenteral nutrition. The same mechanisms may cause intrinsic obstruction of the common duct. An ischemia-reperfusion injury may also contribute to cholestasis in Rh incompatibility. In extreme hemolysis, the cholestasis may be seemingly complete, with acholic stools. Levels of bilirubin may reach 40 mg/dL, primarily direct-reacting. If inspissation of bile occurs within the extrahepatic biliary tree, differentiation from biliary atresia may be difficult. A trial of choleretics is indicated. Once stools show a return to normal color or ^{99m}Tc-DIDA scanning shows biliary excretion into the duodenum, patency of the extrahepatic biliary tree is ensured. Small bile-colored plugs in the stools are sometimes reported by parents at the time stool color becomes normal. Although most cases slowly improve over 2–6 months, persistence of complete cholestasis for more than 2 weeks requires further studies (ultrasonography, DIDA scanning, liver biopsy) with possible examination of the extrahepatic biliary tree. Irrigation of the common bile duct is sometimes necessary to dislodge the obstructing inspissated biliary material.

Balistreri WF, Bove KE: Hepatobiliary consequences of parenteral alimentation. Prog Liver Dis 1990;9:567.

Bhatia J et al: Total parenteral nutrition-associated alterations in hepatobiliary function and histology in rats: Is light exposure a clue? Pediatr Res 1993;33:487.

Dunn L et al: Beneficial effects of early hypocaloric enteral feedings on neonatal gastrointestinal function: Preliminary report of a randomized trial. J Pediatr 1988; 112:622.

Roy CC, Silverman A, Alagille D (editors): Inborn errors of metabolism. In: *Pediatric Clinical Gastroenterology*, Mosby, 1995.

Sokol RJ et al: Hepatic oxidant injury associated with glutathione depletion during total parenteral nutrition in weanling rats. Am J Physiol 1995;270:G691.

3. IDIOPATHIC NEONATAL HEPATITIS (Giant Cell Hepatitis)

This type of cholestatic jaundice of unknown cause presents with features of cholestasis and a typical liver biopsy appearance; it accounts for up to 50% of cases of neonatal intrahepatic cholestasis. The degree of cholestasis is variable, and the disorder may be indistinguishable from extrahepatic causes in 10% of cases. Alpha$_1$-antitrypsin deficiency, Alagille's syndrome, and Byler's disease and bile acid synthesis defects may present in a similar clinical and histologic manner. However, in Byler's disease and bile acid synthesis defects the γ-glutamyl transpeptidase levels are normal or low.

Intrauterine growth retardation, prematurity, poor feeding, emesis, poor growth, and partially or intermittently acholic stools are characteristic of intrahepatic cholestasis. Neonatal lupus erythematosus may present with giant cell hepatitis; however, thrombocytopenia, skin rash, or congenital heart block is usually also present.

In cases of suspected idiopathic neonatal hepatitis (absence of infectious, metabolic, and toxic causes), patency of the biliary tree should be verified to exclude extrahepatic "surgical" disorders. DIDA scanning and ultrasonography may be helpful in this regard. Some have used the enteral string test during DIDA scanning to confirm bile duct patency. Liver biopsy findings are usually diagnostic after 6–8 weeks of age (see Table 20–1) but may be misleading before 4 weeks of age. Failure to detect patency of the biliary tree, nondiagnostic liver biopsy findings, or persisting complete cholestasis (acholic stools) are indications for minilaparotomy and intraoperative cholangiography by an experienced surgeon. Occasionally, a small but patent (hypoplastic) extrahepatic biliary tree is demonstrated and is probably the result rather than the cause of diminished bile flow; surgical reconstruction of hypoplastic biliary trees should not be attempted.

Once a patent extrahepatic tree is confirmed, therapy should include choleretics, a special formula with medium-chain triglycerides (Pregestimil, Alimentum), and supplemental fat-soluble vitamins in water-miscible form. (See Table 20–2.) These are continued as long as significant cholestasis remains (conjugated bilirubin > 1 mg/dL). Fat-soluble vitamin levels should be monitored while supplements are given.

Eighty percent of patients recover without significant hepatic fibrosis. However, if a relative previously had neonatal hepatitis, there is a 70–80% probability of progression to cirrhosis (Byler's disease). Long-term consequences correlate best with the duration of the cholestasis. In general, failure to resolve the cholestatic picture by 6–12 months is associated with progressive liver disease and evolving cirrhosis. This may occur either with normal or diminished numbers of interlobular bile ducts (paucity of interlobular ducts). Perilobular and intralobular fibrosis both progress, and portal hypertension eventually ensues, with splenomegaly and esophageal varices. Finally, ascites with rising bilirubin levels heralds the onset of hepatic failure. Liver transplantation has been successful when signs of hepatic decompensation are noted (rising bilirubin, intractable ascites).

Dick MC, Mowat AP: Hepatitis syndrome in infancy: An epidemiological survey with 10 year follow-up. Arch Dis Child 1985;60:512.

Laim W et al: Differential diagnosis of extrahepatic biliary atresia from neonatal hepatitis: A prospective study. J Pediatr Gastroenterol Nutr 1994;18:121.

Odievre M et al: Long-term prognosis for infants with intrahepatic cholestasis and patent extrahepatic biliary tract. Arch Dis Child 1981;56:373.

Ramirez RO, Sokol RJ: Medical management of cholestasis. In: *Liver Disease in Children.* Suchy FJ (editor). Mosby-Year Book, 1994.

4. PAUCITY OF INTERLOBULAR BILE DUCTS

Forms of intrahepatic cholestasis caused by decreased numbers of interlobular bile ducts may be classified according to whether or not they are associated with other malformations. The gene for the syndromic form, Alagille's syndrome is located on chromosome 20p, and codes for a ligand of the "notch" receptor, though the pathogenesis is not understood. Alagille's syndrome (arteriohepatic dysplasia), is sometimes recognized by identification of the characteristic facies, which becomes more obvious with age. The forehead is prominent, as is the nasal bridge. The eyes are set deep and sometimes widely apart (hypertelorism). Often the chin is small and slightly pointed and projects forward. Ears are prominent. The severity of cholestasis is variable; thus, stool color varies. Pruritus begins by 3–6 months of age. Firm, smooth hepatomegaly is present, and cardiac murmurs are frequent. Xanthomas develop later in the disease. Occasionally, early cholestasis is mild and not recognized.

Direct hyperbilirubinemia may be mild to severe (2–15 mg/dL). Serum alkaline phosphatase, γ-glutamyl transpeptidase, and cholesterol are markedly elevated, especially early in life. Serum bile acids are always elevated. Aminotransferases are slightly increased, but clotting factors and other liver proteins are usually normal.

The cardiovascular abnormalities include peripheral and valvular pulmonary stenoses (most common), atrial septal defect, coarctation of the aorta, and tetralogy of Fallot.

Vertebral arch defects are common, including incomplete fusion of the vertebral body or anterior arch (butterfly deformity) and diminished interpedicle distance in the thoracolumbar spine. Eye abnormalities (posterior embryotoxon) and renal abnormalities (dysplastic kidneys, renal tubular ectasia, single kidney, hematuria) are also associated with this disorder. Growth retardation with normal to increased levels of growth hormone is common. Although variable, the IQ is frequently low. Hypogonadism with micropenis may be present. A weak, high-pitched voice may develop. Neurologic disorders resulting from vitamin E deficiency (areflexia, ataxia, ophthalmoplegia) eventually develop in many children.

In the nonsyndromic form, paucity of interlobular bile ducts is seen in the absence of the extrahepatic malformations. Paucity may also be seen in α_1-antitrypsin deficiency, in Zellweger's syndrome and in association with lymphedema (Aagenaes' syndrome), in Byler's disease, in cystic fibrosis, in cytomegalovirus or rubella infection, and in inborn errors of bile acid metabolism.

High doses (250 mg/kg/d) of cholestyramine may control pruritus, lower cholesterol, and clear xanthomas. Phenobarbital may lower serum bilirubin. Ursodeoxycholic therapy (10–20 mg/kg/d) appears to be more effective and less toxic than cholestyramine or phenobarbital. Nutritional therapy to prevent wasting and deficiencies of fat-soluble vitamins is of particular importance because of the severity of cholestasis (see Table 20–2).

Prognosis is more favorable in the syndromic than in the nonsyndromic varieties. In the former, only 30–40% of patients have severe complications of disease, whereas over 70% of patients suffering from the latter progress to cirrhosis. In Alagille's syndrome, cholestasis may improve by age 2–4 years, with minimal residual hepatic fibrosis. Survival into adulthood despite raised serum bile acids, aminotransferases, and alkaline phosphatase is common. Several patients have developed hepatocellular carcinoma. Hypogonadism has been noted; however, fertility is not obviously affected. Cardiovascular anomalies may shorten life expectancy. Some patients have persistent, severe cholestasis, rendering their quality of life poor; liver transplantation has been performed under these circumstances.

Alagille D et al: Syndromic paucity of interlobular bile ducts (Alagille syndrome or arteriohepatic dysplasia): Review of 80 cases. J Pediatr 1987;110:195.

Hoffenberg EJ et al: Outcome of syndromic paucity of interlobular bile ducts (Alagille syndrome) with onset of cholestasis in infancy. J Pediatr 1995;127:220.

Li L et al: Alagille syndrome is caused by mutations in human Jagged 1, which encodes a ligand for notch 1. Nat Genet 1997;16:243.

Schwarzenberg SJ et al: Long-term complications of arteriohepatic dysplasia. Am J Med 1992;93:171.

Sokol RJ et al: Multicenter trial of *d*-alpha tocopheryl polyethylene glycol-1000 succinate for treatment of vitamin E deficiency in children with chronic cholestasis. Gastroenterology 1993;104:1727.

EXTRAHEPATIC NEONATAL CHOLESTASIS

Extrahepatic neonatal cholestasis is characterized by complete and persistent cholestasis (acholic stools) in the first 2 months of life, lack of patency of the extrahepatic biliary tree proved by intraoperative, percutaneous, or endoscopic cholangiography, firm to hard hepatomegaly, and typical features on histologic examination of liver biopsy tissue. (See Table 20–1.) Causes include extrahepatic biliary atresia, choledochal cyst, intrinsic obstruction of the common duct, and spontaneous perforation of the extrahepatic ducts.

1. EXTRAHEPATIC BILIARY ATRESIA

In whites, extrahepatic biliary atresia occurs in 1:13,000–1:8000 births, and the incidence in both sexes is equal. In Asians, the incidence is higher, and the disorder is twice as common in girls. The abnormality found most commonly is complete atresia of all extrahepatic biliary structures. The specific cause is not known, although evidence supports an insult to the biliary structures in the perinatal period that progresses in postnatal life. Extrahepatic atresia has not been found in stillborn fetuses and is rarely seen in premature infants. Meconium and first-passed stools are usually normal in color, suggesting early patency of the ducts. Evidence obtained from surgically removed remnants of the extrahepatic biliary tree suggests an inflammatory or sclerosing cholangiopathy. Although an infectious cause seems reasonable, no agent has been consistently found in such cases. A role for reovirus type 3 and rotavirus group C in biliary atresia has been suggested but recently disputed. Although other congenital malformations, especially vascular ones, occur in 20–30% of cases of extrahepatic biliary atresia, only polysplenia syndrome (situs inversus, preduodenal portal vein, interruption of the inferior vena cava, polysplenia, midline liver) is consistently associated with extrahepatic biliary atresia. Thus, it is felt that 2 forms exist: the perinatal (infectious) type (about 80% of cases), and the fetal-embryonic type (about 20%).

Jaundice may be noted in the newborn period but is more often delayed until 2–3 weeks of age. The urine stains the diaper, and the stools are often pale yellow, buff-colored, gray, or acholic. Seepage of bilirubin products across the intestinal mucosa gives some yellow coloration to the stools. Hepatomegaly is common, and the liver may feel firm to hard; splenomegaly develops later. Pruritus, digital clubbing, xanthomas, and a rachitic rosary may be noted in older patients. Murmurs reflecting increasing cardiovascular output or shunting through bronchial arteries may be heard over the entire precordium and back. By 2–6 months, the growth curves reveal poor weight gain. Late in the course, ascites and bleeding complications occur.

No single laboratory test will consistently differentiate this entity from other causes of "complete" obstructive jaundice. A DIDA excretion study performed early in the course of disease and after pretreatment with phenobarbital (3–5 mg/kg/d for 5–7 days) helps to distinguish intrahepatic from extrahepatic causes of cholestasis, but is not diagnostic. Although biliary atresia is suggested by persistent elevation of serum γ-glutamyl transpeptidase or alkaline phosphatase levels, high cholesterol levels, and prolonged prothrombin times, these findings have also been reported in severe neonatal hepatitis, α_1-antitrypsin deficiency, and bile duct paucity. Furthermore, these tests will not differentiate the location of the obstruction within the extrahepatic system. Generally, the aminotransferases are only modestly elevated in biliary atresia. Serum proteins and blood clotting factors are not affected early in the disease. Routine chest x-ray may reveal abnormalities suggestive of polysplenia syndrome. Ultrasonography of the biliary system should be performed to ascertain the presence of choledochal cyst and intra-abdominal anomalies. Liver biopsy specimens can differentiate intrahepatic causes of cholestasis from biliary atresia in over 90% of cases.

The major diagnostic dilemma is between this entity and neonatal hepatitis, bile duct paucity, choledochal cyst, or intrinsic bile duct obstruction (stones, bile plugs). Although spontaneous perforation of extrahepatic bile ducts leads to jaundice and acholic stools, the infants are usually quite ill with chemical peritonitis from biliary ascites, and hepatomegaly is not found.

If the diagnosis of biliary atresia cannot be excluded by the diagnostic evaluation before 60 days of life, surgical exploration is necessary. Laparotomy must include liver biopsy and an operative cholangiogram if a gallbladder is present. The presence of yellow bile in the gallbladder implies patency of the proximal extrahepatic duct system. Radiographic visualization of dye in the duodenum excludes obstruction to the distal extrahepatic ducts.

In the absence of surgical correction, the following eventually develop: failure to thrive, marked pruritus, portal hypertension, hypersplenism, bleeding diathesis, rickets, ascites, and cyanosis. Bronchitis and pneumonia are common. Eventually, hepatic failure and death occur, almost always by age 18–24 months.

Except for the occasional example of "correctable" biliary atresia where choledochojejunostomy is feasible, the standard procedure is hepatoportoenterostomy (Kasai procedure). Occasionally, portocholecystostomy (gallbladder Kasai procedure) may be performed if the gallbladder is present and the passage from it to the duodenum is patent. These procedures are best done in specialized centers where experienced surgical, pediatric, and nursing personnel are available. It is recommended that surgery be performed as early as possible (age 6–10 weeks); the Kasai procedure should generally not be undertaken in infants over 4 months of age, because the likelihood of bile drainage at this age is very low. Orthotopic liver transplantation is now indicated for patients who fail to drain bile after the Kasai procedure or who progress to end-stage biliary cirrhosis despite surgical treatment. The 5-year survival rate following transplantation is 60–80%.

Whether or not the Kasai procedure is performed, supportive medical treatment measures consist of vitamin and caloric support (using water-miscible forms of vitamins A, D, K, and E and formulas containing medium-chain triglycerides [Pregestimil or Alimentum]). (See Table 20–2.) Bacterial infections (eg, ascending cholangitis) should be treated promptly with broad-spectrum antibiotics, and signs of bleeding tendency should be corrected with intramuscular vitamin K. Ascites can be managed with reduced sodium intake and spironolactone. Choleretics and bile acid-binding products (cholestyramine, aluminum hydroxide gel) are of little use. The value of ursodeoxycholic acid remains to be determined.

When bile flow is sustained, the 5-year survival rate is 35–50%. Complete surgical failures have the same outcome as nonoperated cases, but patients die sooner (age 8–15 months versus age 18–36 months). Death is usually caused by liver failure, sepsis, acidosis, or respiratory failure secondary to intractable ascites. Surprisingly, terminal hemorrhage is unusual. Liver transplantation has dramatically changed the outlook for these patients.

Butler SN, Smith D: Living with chronic pediatric liver disease: The parent's experience. Pediatr Nurs 1992; 18:453.

Karrer FM et al: Biliary atresia registry, 1976 to 1989. J Pediatr Surg 1990;25:1076.

Karrer FM et al: Long term results with Kasai's operation for biliary atresia. Arch Surg 1996;131:493.

Lilly JR et al: The surgery of biliary atresia. Ann Surg 1989;210:289.

Ramirez RO, Sokol RJ: Medical management of cholestasis. In: *Liver Disease in Children.* Suchy FJ (editor). Mosby-Year Book, 1994

Riepenhoff-Talty M et al: Group A rotaviruses produce ex-

trahepatic biliary obstruction in orally inoculated newborn mice. Pediatr Res 1993;33:394.

Ryckman F et al: Improved survival in biliary atresia patients in the present era of liver transplantation. J Pediatr Surg 1993;28:382.

Silveira TR et al: Association between HLA and extrahepatic biliary atresia. J Pediatr Gastroenterol Nutr 1993;16:114.

Yoon PW et al: Epidemiology of biliary atresia: A population-based study. Pediatrics 1997;99:376.

2. CHOLEDOCHAL CYST

Choledochal cysts cause 2–5% of cases of extrahepatic neonatal cholestasis; the incidence is fourfold higher in girls and higher in Asians. In most cases, the clinical manifestations, basic laboratory findings, and histopathologic features on liver biopsy are indistinguishable from those seen in biliary atresia. Neonatal symptomatic cysts are usually associated with atresia of the distal common duct—accounting for the diagnostic dilemma—and may simply be part of the spectrum of biliary atresia. However, a palpable subhepatic mass, positive ultrasound scan, or pressure deformity on the first and second portions of duodenum seen on upper gastrointestinal series promptly resolves the question. Immediate operation is indicated once abnormalities in clotting factors have been corrected and bacterial cholangitis, if present, has been treated with intravenous antibiotics. Discovery of such a mass eliminates the need for other studies. In older children, choledochal cyst presents as recurrent episodes of obstructive jaundice or abdominal pain or as a right abdominal mass.

Excision of the cyst and choledochojejunal anastomosis are recommended. In some cases, because of technical problems, only the mucosa of the cyst can be removed with jejunal anastomosis to the proximal bile duct. Anastomosis of cyst to jejunum or duodenum is not recommended.

The prognosis depends on the presence or absence of associated evidence of atresia and the appearance of the intrahepatic ducts. If atresia is found, the prognosis is similar to that described above. If an isolated extrahepatic cyst is encountered, the outcome is generally excellent, with resolution of the jaundice and return to normal liver cellular architecture the rule. However, bouts of ascending cholangitis, particularly if intrahepatic cysts are present, or obstruction of the anastomotic site may occur. The risk of biliary carcinoma developing within the cyst is about 5–15% at adulthood; therefore, cystectomy should be done whenever possible.

Bancroft JD et al: Antenatal diagnosis of choledochal cyst. J Pediatr Gastroenterol Nutr 1994;18:142.

Lilly JR et al: Forme fruste choledochal cyst. J Pediatr Surg 1985;20:449.

Stein JE, Vacanti JP: Biliary atresia and other disorders of the extrahepatic biliary tree. In: *Liver Disease in Children.* Suchy FJ (editor). Mosby-Year Book, 1994.

Voyles CR et al: Carcinoma in choledochal cysts: Age-related incidence. Arch Surg 1983;118:986.

3. SPONTANEOUS PERFORATION OF THE EXTRAHEPATIC DUCTS

The sudden appearance of obstructive jaundice, acholic stools, and abdominal enlargement with ascites in a sick newborn is suggestive of this condition. The liver is usually normal in size, and a yellow-green discoloration can often be discerned under the umbilicus or in the scrotum. In 24% of cases, stones or sludge is found obstructing the common bile duct. DIDA scan shows leakage from the biliary tree, and ultrasonography confirms ascites or fluid around the bile duct.

Treatment is surgical. Simple drainage, without attempt at oversewing the perforation, is sufficient in primary perforations. A diversion anastomosis is constructed in cases associated with choledochal cyst or stenosis. The prognosis is generally good.

Haller JO et al: Spontaneous perforation of the common bile duct in children. Radiology 1989;172:621.

Megison SM et al: Management of common bile duct obstruction associated with spontaneous perforation of the biliary tree. Surgery 1992;111:237.

OTHER NEONATAL HYPERBILIRUBINEMIC CONDITIONS (Noncholestatic Nonhemolytic)

This group of disorders associated with hyperbilirubinemia is of two types: (1) unconjugated hyperbilirubinemia, consisting of breast milk jaundice, Lucey-Driscoll syndrome, congenital hypothyroidism, upper intestinal obstruction, Gilbert's syndrome, Crigler-Najjar syndrome, and drug-induced hyperbilirubinemia; and (2) conjugated noncholestatic hyperbilirubinemia, consisting of Dubin-Johnson syndrome and Rotor's syndrome.

1. UNCONJUGATED HYPERBILIRUBINEMIA

Breast Milk Jaundice

Persistent elevation of the indirect bilirubin fraction may occur in up to 36% of breast-fed infants. Recent studies implicate an enhancer of intestinal absorption of unconjugated bilirubin in jaundice-causing human milk rather than an inhibitor of bilirubin conjugation acting on hepatocytes. The increased enterohepatic shunting of unconjugated bilirubin exceeds the normal conjugating capacity in the liver of these infants.

Hyperbilirubinemia does not usually exceed 20 mg/dL, with most in the range of 10–15 mg/dL. In those whose bilirubin levels are above 4–5 mg/dL, the jaundice is noticeable by the fifth to seventh days of breast feeding. It may accentuate the underlying physiologic jaundice—especially early, when total fluid intake may be less than optimal. Except for jaundice, the physical examination is usually normal; urine does not stain the diaper, and the stools are golden yellow.

The jaundice peaks by the third week and clears before 3 months in almost all infants, even when breast feedings are continued. All infants who remain jaundiced past 2 weeks should have measurements of direct bilirubin to exclude hepatobiliary disease.

Kernicterus has never been reported in this condition. In special situations, breast feeding may be temporarily discontinued and replaced by formula feedings for 2–3 days until serum bilirubin decreases by 2–8 mg/dL. Cow's milk formulas inhibit the intestinal reabsorption of unconjugated bilirubin. When breast-feeding is reinstituted, the serum bilirubin may increase slightly but not to the previous level. Phototherapy is not indicated in the healthy term infant with this condition.

Alonso EM et al: Enterohepatic circulation of nonconjugated bilirubin in rats fed with human milk. J Pediatr 1991;118:425.

Gourley GR, Aren RA: β-Glucuronidase and hyperbilirubinemia in breast-fed and formula-fed babies. Lancet 1986;1:644.

Gourley GR: Bilirubin metabolism and neonatal jaundice. In: *Liver Disease in Children.* Suchy FJ (editor). Mosby-Year Book, 1994.

Newman TB, Maisels MJ: Evaluation and treatment of jaundice in the term newborn: A kinder, gentler approach. Pediatrics 1992;89:809.

Congenital Hypothyroidism

Although the differential diagnosis should always include consideration of congenital hypothyroidism as a cause of indirect hyperbilirubinemia, the diagnosis may be obvious from other clinical and physical clues or from the newborn screening results. The jaundice quickly clears with replacement thyroid hormone therapy, although the mechanism is unclear.

Labrune P et al: Bilirubin uridine diphosphate glucuronosyltransferase hepatic activity in jaundice associated with congenital hypothyroidism. J Pediatr Gastroenterol Nutr 1992;14:79.

Upper Intestinal Obstruction

The association of indirect hyperbilirubinemia with high intestinal obstruction—eg, duodenal atresia, annular pancreas, pyloric stenosis—in the newborn has been observed repeatedly; the mechanism is unknown. Diminished levels of hepatic glucuronyl transferase have been found on liver biopsy in pyloric stenosis.

Treatment is that of the underlying obstructive condition (usually surgical). Jaundice disappears once adequate nutrition is achieved.

Wolley MM et al: Jaundice, hypertrophic pyloric stenosis and hepatic glucuronyl transferase. J Pediatr Surg 1974;9:359.

Gilbert's Syndrome

This is a common form (3–7% of the population) of familial hyperbilirubinemia associated with a partial reduction of hepatic bilirubin uridine diphosphate glucuronyl transferase activity and perhaps an abnormality in the function or amount of one or more hepatocyte membrane protein carriers. Mild fluctuating jaundice, especially with illness, and vague constitutional symptoms are common. Jaundice is first recognized after puberty. Shortened red blood cell survival time in some patients is thought to be caused by reduced activity of enzymes involved in heme biosynthesis (protoporphyrinogen oxidase). Subsidence of hyperbilirubinemia has been achieved in patients by administration of phenobarbital (5–8 mg/kg/d), though this therapy is not justified.

The disease is actually inherited as an autosomal recessive abnormality of the promoter region of UDP-glucuronyl transferase-1; however, another factor is necessary for disease expression. The homozygous (16%) and heterozygous states (40%) are very common. Males are affected more often than females (4:1). Serum unconjugated bilirubin is less than 3–6 mg/dL. The findings on liver biopsy and most other liver function tests are normal except for prolonged indocyanine green and sulfobromophthalein (BSP) retention. An increase of 1.4 mg/dL or more in the level of unconjugated bilirubin after a 2-day fast (300 kcal/d) is consistent with the diagnosis of Gilbert's syndrome. The nicotinic acid provocation test is seldom used in pediatric patients.

Bosma PJ et al: The genetic basis of the reduced expression of bilirubin UDP-glucuronyl transferase 1 in Gilbert's syndrome. N Engl J Med 1995;333:1171.
Gentile S et al: Dose dependence of nicotinic acid-induced hyperbilirubinemia and its dissociation from hemolysis in Gilbert's syndrome. J Lab Clin Med 1986;107:166.

Crigler-Najjar Syndrome

Patients with type I disease usually develop rapid severe elevation of unconjugated bilirubin (> 30–40 mg/dL), with neurologic consequences (kernicterus). Consanguinity is often present. Prompt recognition of this entity and treatment with exchange transfusions are required, followed by phototherapy. Some survive without neurologic signs until adolescence or early adulthood, at which time deterioration may suddenly occur. For diagnosis, a duodenal bile specimen should be obtained. It is colorless and contains a predominance of unconjugated bilirubin, small amounts of monoconjugates, and only traces of conjugated bilirubin. Phenobarbital administration in these patients does not significantly alter these findings, nor does it lower serum bilirubin levels. The glucuronyl transferase deficiency is inherited in an autosomal recessive pattern. A combination of phototherapy and cholestyramine may keep bilirubin levels below 25 mg/dL. The use of tin protoporphyrin or tin mesoporphyrin remains experimental. Liver transplantation is curative and may prevent kernicterus if performed early. An auxiliary orthotopic transplantation also relieves the jaundice while the patient retains native liver.

A milder form (type II) with both autosomal dominant and recessive inheritance is rarely associated with neurologic complications. Hyperbilirubinemia is less severe, and the bile is pigmented and contains bilirubin mono- and diglucuronide. Patients with this form respond to phenobarbital with lowering of serum bilirubin levels. An increased proportion of monoconjugated and diconjugated bilirubin in the bile follows phenobarbital treatment.

Liver biopsy findings and liver function tests are consistently normal in both types.

Berg CL: The physiology of jaundice: Molecular and functional characterization of the Crigler-Najjar syndromes. Hepatology 1995;22:1338.
Galbraith RA et al: Suppression of bilirubin production in the Crigler-Najjar type I syndrome: Studies with the heme oxygenase inhibitor tin mesoporphyrin. Pediatrics 1992;89:175.
Rubaltelli FF et al: Serum and bile bilirubin pigments in the differential diagnosis of Crigler-Najjar disease. Pediatrics 1994;94:553.
Shevell MI et al: Crigler-Najjar syndrome type I: Treatment by home phototherapy followed by orthotopic liver transplantation. J Pediatr 1987;110:429.
Whitington PF et al: Orthotopic auxiliary liver transplantation for Crigler-Najjar syndrome type I. Lancet 1993;342:779.

Drug-Induced Hyperbilirubinemia

Vitamin K_3 (menadiol) may elevate indirect bilirubin levels by causing hemolysis. Vitamin K_1 (phytonadione) can be safely used in neonates. Rifampin may cause unconjugated hyperbilirubinemia. Other drugs (eg, ceftriaxone, sulfonamides) may displace bilirubin from albumin, potentially increasing the risk of kernicterus–especially in the sick premature infant.

Fink S, Karp W, Robertson A: Ceftriaxone effect on bilirubin-albumin binding. Pediatrics 1987;80:873.

2. CONJUGATED NONCHOLESTATIC HYPERBILIRUBINEMIA (Dubin-Johnson Syndrome & Rotor's Syndrome)

These diagnoses are suspected with persistent or recurrent conjugated hyperbilirubinemia and jaundice with normal liver blood tests. The basic defect in Dubin-Johnson syndrome affects the multiple organic anion transport (MOAT) protein of the bile canaliculus, causing impaired hepatocyte excretion of conjugated bilirubin into bile, with a variable degree of impairment in uptake and conjugation complicating the picture. Transmission is autosomal recessive, so a positive family history is occasionally obtained. In Rotor's syndrome, the defect lies in hepatic uptake and storage of bilirubin. Bile acids are normally handled, so that cholestasis does not occur. Bilirubin values range from 2 to 5 mg/dL, and other liver function tests are normal. In Rotor's syndrome, the liver is normal; in Dubin-Johnson syndrome, it is darkly pigmented on gross inspection. Microscopic examination reveals numerous dark-brown pigment granules consisting of polymers of epinephrine metabolites, especially in the centrilobular regions. However, the amount of pigment varies within families, and some jaundiced members may have no demonstrable pigmentation in the liver. Otherwise, the liver is histologically normal. Oral cholecystography fails to visualize the gallbladder in Dubin-Johnson syndrome but is normal in Rotor's syndrome. Differences in the excretion patterns of sulfobromophthalein, in results of DIDA cholescintigraphy, in urinary coproporphyrin I and III levels, and in the serum pattern of monoglucuronide and diglucuronide conjugates of bilirubin can help distinguish between these two conditions.

The prognosis is excellent, and no treatment is needed.

Crawford JM, Gollan JL: Bilirubin metabolism and the pathophysiology of jaundice. In: *Diseases of the Liver,* 7th ed. Schiff L, Schiff ER (editors). Lippincott, 1993.
Paulusma CC et al: A mutation in the human canalicular multispecific organic anion transporter gene causes the Dubin-Johnson syndrome. Hepatology 1997;25:1539.
Rosenthal P et al: The distribution of serum bilirubin conjugates in pediatric hepatobiliary diseases. J Pediatr 1987;110:201.
Shieh CC et al: Dubin-Johnson syndrome presenting with neonatal cholestasis. Arch Dis Child 1990;65:898.

HEPATITIS A

Essentials of Diagnosis & Typical Features

- Gastrointestinal upset (anorexia, vomiting, diarrhea).
- Jaundice.
- Liver tenderness and enlargement.
- Abnormal liver function tests.
- Local epidemic of the disease.
- Anti-HAV IgM elevation.

General Considerations
(See Table 20–4.)

Hepatitis A virus (HAV) infection occurs in both epidemic and sporadic fashion. Transmission by the fecal-oral route explains epidemic outbreaks from contaminated food or water supplies, particularly by food handlers. Particles 27 nm in diameter have been found in stools during the acute phase of type A hepatitis and are similar in appearance to the enteroviruses. Sporadic cases usually result from contact with an affected individual. Transmission through blood products obtained during the viremic phase has occurred, though very rarely. The overt form of the disease is easily recognized by the clinical manifestations, but two-thirds of affected individuals have an anicteric and unrecognized form of the disease. This has been especially true in outbreaks of hepatitis A reported in day care centers accepting children younger than 3 years of age. Lifelong immunity to HAV follows infection. In developing coun-

Table 20–4. Hepatitis viruses.

	HAV	HBV	HCV	HDV	HEV
Type of virus	Enterovirus (RNA)	Hepadnavirus (DNA)	Flavivirus (RNA)	Incomplete (RNA)	Calicivirus (RNA)
Transmission routes	Fecal-oral	Parenteral, sexual, vertical	Parenteral, sexual	Parenteral, sexual	Fecal-oral
Incubation period	15–40 days	50–150 days	1–5 months	20–90 days	2–9 weeks
Diagnostic test	Anti-HAV IgM	HBsAg, anti-HBc IgM	Anti-HCV, PCR-RNA test	Anti-HDV	Anti-HEV
Mortality rate (acute)	0.1–0.2%	0.5–2%	1–2%	2–20%	1–2% (in pregnant women, 20%)
Carrier state	No	Yes	Yes	Yes	No
Vaccine available	Yes	Yes	No	Yes (HBV)	No
Treatment	None	Interferon-alfa	Interferon-alfa	Interferon-alfa	None

HEPATITIS VIRUS ABBREVIATIONS	
HAV	Hepatitis A virus
Anti-HAV IgM	IgM antibody to HAV
HBV	Hepatitis B virus
HBsAg	HBV surface antigen
HBcAg	HBV core antigen
HBeAg	HBV e antigen
Anti-HBs	Antibody to HBsAg
Anti-HBc	Antibody to HBcAg
Anti-HBc IgM	IgM antibody to HBcAg
Anti-HBe	Antibody to HBeAg
HCV	Hepatitis C virus
Anti-HCV	Antibody to HCV
HDV	Hepatitis D (delta) virus
Anti-HDV	Antibody to HDV
HEV	Hepatitis E virus
Anti-HEV	Antibody to HEV
NANBNC	Non-A, non-B, non-C hepatitis virus

tries, most children are exposed to HAV by age 10 years, whereas only 20% are exposed by age 20 years in developed countries.

Antibody to HAV appears within 1–4 weeks of clinical symptoms. While the great majority of children with infectious hepatitis are asymptomatic or have mild disease and recover completely, some will develop fulminant hepatitis. Children who die during the initial attack of the disease do so from massive hepatic necrosis secondary to overwhelming viremia, an immunologic deficiency state, or perhaps exposure to a mutant strain of virus.

Clinical Findings

A. History: A history of direct exposure to a previously jaundiced individual or of eating seafood or drinking contaminated water in the recent past should be sought. Following an incubation period of 15–40 days, the initial nonspecific symptoms usually precede the development of jaundice by 5–10 days.

B. Symptoms and Signs: Fever, anorexia, vomiting, headache, and abdominal pain are the usual symptoms. Darkening of the urine precedes jaundice, which peaks in 1–2 weeks and then begins to subside. The stools may become light or clay-colored during this time. Clinical improvement can be noted as jaundice develops. Tender hepatomegaly and jaundice are typically present; splenomegaly is variable.

C. Laboratory Findings: Aminotransferases and conjugated and unconjugated bilirubin levels are elevated. The leukocyte count is normal to low; the sedimentation rate is elevated. Serum proteins are generally normal, but an elevation of the gamma globulin fraction (> 2.5 g/dL) can occur and indicates a worse prognosis. Hypoalbuminemia, hypoglycemia, and marked prolongation of prothrombin time are serious prognostic findings. Urine bile and urobilinogen are increased. Diagnosis is made by serology. A positive anti-HAV IgM indicates acute

disease, whereas IgG anti-HAV persists after recovery.

Percutaneous liver biopsy is rarely indicated but may be safely performed in most children—provided the partial thromboplastin time, platelet count, and bleeding time are normal and the prothrombin time is prolonged no more than 4–5 seconds. The presence of ascites may increase the risk of percutaneous liver biopsy. "Balloon cells" and acidophilic bodies are characteristic histologic findings. Liver cell necrosis may be diffuse or focal, with accompanying infiltration of inflammatory cells containing polymorphonuclear leukocytes, lymphocytes, macrophages, and plasma cells, particularly in portal areas. Some bile duct proliferation may be seen in the perilobular portal areas alongside areas of bile stasis. Regenerative liver cells and proliferation of reticuloendothelial cells are present. Occasionally, massive hepatocyte necrosis is seen, portending a bad prognosis.

Differential Diagnosis

Before jaundice appears, the symptoms are those of a nonspecific viral enteritis. Other diseases with somewhat similar onset include pancreatitis, infectious mononucleosis, leptospirosis, drug-induced hepatitis, Wilson's disease, autoimmune hepatitis, and, most often, type B, C, E, or NANBNC hepatitis. Acquired cytomegalovirus disease may also mimic HAV, although lymphadenopathy is usually present in the former.

Prevention

Some attempt at isolation of the patient during initial phases of illness is indicated, although most patients with type A hepatitis are noninfectious by the time the disease becomes overt. Stool, diapers, and other fecally stained clothing should be handled with care for 1 month after the appearance of jaundice.

Passive-active immunization of exposed susceptibles can be achieved by giving standard immune globulin, 0.02–0.04 mL/kg intramuscularly. Illness is prevented in 80–90% of individuals if immune globulin is given within 1–2 weeks of exposure. Individuals traveling to endemic disease areas should receive HAV vaccine or 0.02–0.06 mL/kg of immune globulin as prophylaxis if there is insufficient time for vaccination.

Treatment

There are no specific measures. Sedatives and corticosteroids should be avoided.

At the start of the illness, a light diet is preferable. During the icteric phase, lower-fat foods may diminish gastrointestinal symptoms but do not affect overall outcome. Drugs and elective surgery should be avoided.

Prognosis

Ninety-five percent of children recover without sequelae. In rare cases of fulminant hepatitis, the patient may die in 5 days or may survive as long as 1–2 months. The prognosis is poor if the signs and symptoms of hepatic coma develop, with deepening of jaundice and development of ascites; orthotopic liver transplantation is indicated under these circumstances. Incomplete resolution leads to prolonged hepatitis or chronic cholestatic hepatitis but not to cirrhosis. Rare cases of aplastic anemia following acute infectious hepatitis have also been reported. A benign relapse of symptoms may occur in 10–15% of cases after 6–10 weeks of apparent resolution.

Balistreri WF: Acute and chronic viral hepatitis. In: *Liver Disease in Children.* Suchy FJ (editor). Mosby-Year Book, 1994.

Hoofnagle JH, DiBisceglie AM: Serologic diagnosis of acute and chronic viral hepatitis. Semin Liver Dis 1991;11:73.

Katkov WN, Dienstag JL: Hepatitis vaccines. Gastroenterol Clin North Am 1995;24:147.

Noble RC et al: Post transfusion hepatitis A in a neonatal intensive care unit. JAMA 1984;252:2711.

Werzberger A et al: A controlled trial of a formalin-inactivated hepatitis A vaccine in healthy children. N Engl J Med 1992;327:453.

HEPATITIS B

Essentials of Diagnosis
& Typical Features

- Gastrointestinal upset, anorexia, vomiting, diarrhea.
- Jaundice, tender hepatomegaly, abnormal liver function tests.
- Serologic evidence of hepatitis B disease: HBsAg, HBeAg, anti-HBc IgM.
- History of parenteral, sexual, or household exposure or maternal HBsAg carriage.

General Considerations
(See Table 20–4.)

In contrast to hepatitis A, hepatitis B has a later onset with an incubation period of 21–135 days. The disease is caused by a DNA virus (42-nm Dane particle) that is usually acquired perinatally from a carrier mother; from blood products, shared needles, needle sticks, skin piercing, or tattoos; or through sexual transmission. Breast milk, urine, and saliva have been shown to contain viral antigen. Transmission via blood products has been almost eliminated by HBsAg donor-screening protocols. Mutant viruses may predispose the patient to fulminant hepatitis.

The complete Dane particle is composed of a core (28-nm particle) that is found in the nucleus of infected liver cells and a double outer shell (surface antigen). The Dane particle is found in the cytoplasm where the completed virus particle is synthesized. The surface antigen in blood is termed HBsAg. This is found as a 22-nm spherical particle in the serum but occasionally occurs as a filamentous structure as well. The antibody to it is anti-HBs. The core antigen is termed HBcAg and its antibody is anti-HBc. A specific anti-HBc IgM occurs during primary viral replication.

Another important antigen-antibody system associated with HBV disease is the "e" (envelope) antigen system. HBeAg, a truncated soluble form of HBcAg, appears in the serum of infected patients early and correlates with active virus replication. Persistence of HBeAg is a marker of infectivity, whereas the appearance of anti-HBe generally implies termination of viral replication. Other serologic markers indicating viral replication include the presence of DNA polymerase and circulating HBV DNA.

Clinical Findings

A. Symptoms and Signs: The symptoms are nonspecific, consisting only of slight fever (which may be absent) and mild gastrointestinal upset. Visible jaundice is usually the first significant finding. It is accompanied by darkening of the urine and pale or clay-colored stools. Hepatomegaly is present. Occasionally, a symptom complex of macular rash, urticarial lesions, and arthritis antedates the appearance of icterus. When acquired vertically at birth, chronic disease is frequently asymptomatic despite ongoing liver injury.

B. Laboratory Findings: To diagnose acute HBV infection, the HBsAg and anti-HBc IgM are the only tests needed. To document recovery, immunity, or response to the HBV vaccine, the anti-HBs is useful. If HBsAg persists after 8 weeks in acute infections, it may signify a chronic infection. Vertical transmission to newborns is documented by positive HBsAg.

Liver function test results are similar to those discussed previously for hepatitis A. Liver biopsy seldom differentiates HAV and HBV disease, although specific stains may detect HBcAg or HBsAg in the liver.

Renal involvement may be suspected on the basis of urinary findings suggesting glomerulonephritis.

Differential Diagnosis

The differentiation between HAV and HBV disease is made easier by a history of parenteral exposure, a parent who is HBsAg-positive, and an unusually long period of incubation. HBV and hepatitis C infection are differentiated serologically. The history may suggest a drug-induced hepatitis, especially if a serum sickness prodrome is reported. Autoimmune hepatitis, Wilson's disease and alpha$_1$-antitrypsin deficiency should also be considered.

NANBNC hepatitis is diagnosed in the absence of serologic markers of hepatitis type A, B, or C, a history of drug exposure, autoimmune markers, abnormal ceruloplasmin, iron indices, or α_1-antitrypsin concentration.

Prevention

Control of hepatitis B in the population is based on screening of blood donors and pregnant women, use of properly sterilized needles and surgical equipment, avoidance of sexual contact with carriers, and vaccination of household contacts, sexual partners, medical personnel, and those at high risk. Universal immunization of all infants born in the United States and of adolescents is now recommended. When acquired vertically at birth, chronic disease is frequently asymptomatic despite ongoing liver injury. The vaccine is highly effective for pre-exposure prophylaxis (see Chapter 9). Postexposure administration of hepatitis B immune globulin (0.06 mL/kg intramuscularly, given as soon as possible after exposure, up to 7 days) and initiation of vaccination are also effective.

Treatment

Supportive measures such as bed rest and a nutritious diet are used during the active stage of disease. Corticosteroids are contraindicated. No other treatment is needed for acute HBV infection. For patients with progressive disease (chronic active hepatitis), treatment with interferon alfa (5–6 million units/m^2 body surface area three times a week for 4–6 months) inhibits viral replication in 30–40% of patients, normalizes ALT, and converts HBeAg to Anti-HBe. Side effects are common. Younger children may respond better. Asymptomatic HBsAg carriers (normal serum ALT, no hepatomegaly) do not respond. Liver transplantation is successful in acute fulminant hepatitis B; however, reinfection is common following liver transplantation performed as treatment for chronic hepatitis B. Chronic HBIG therapy or lamivudine therapy reduces recurrence after transplantation.

Prognosis

The prognosis is good, although fulminant hepatitis, chronic persistent hepatitis, or chronic active hepatitis and cirrhosis may supervene in 10% of patients. The course of the disease is variable, but jaundice seldom persists for more than 2 weeks. HBsAg disappears in 95% of cases at the time of clinical recovery. Persistent asymptomatic antigenemia may occur, particularly in children with Down's syndrome or leukemia and those undergoing chronic hemodialysis. Persistence of neonatally acquired HBsAg occurs in 70–90% of infants, and the presence of e antigen in the HBsAg carrier patient seems to imply a poorer prognosis. Chronic hepatitis B disease predisposes the patient to development of hepatocellular carcinoma. After 8–10 years of HBV infection, surveillance for development of hepatocellular carcinoma with hepatic ultrasonography and serum alpha-fetoprotein is performed annually.

Bortolotti F et al: Long-term outcome of chronic hepatitis type B in patients who acquired hepatitis B infection in childhood. Gastroenterology 1990;99:805.

Chang MH et al: Factors affecting clearance of hepatitis B e antigen in hepatitis B surface antigen carrier children. J Pediatr 1989;115:385.

Hepatitis B virus: A comprehensive strategy for eliminating transmission in the United States through universal childhood vaccination. Recommendations of the Immunization Practices Advisory Committee. MMWR Morb Mortal Wkly Rep 1991;40:1.

Narkewicz MR et al: Clearance of chronic hepatitis B virus infection in young children after alpha interferon treatment. J Pediatr 1995;127:815.

Ruiz-Moreno M et al: Prospective, randomized controlled trial of interferon-a in children with chronic hepatitis B. Hepatology 1991;13:1035.

Shapiro CN et al: Hepatitis B virus transmission between children in day care. Pediatr Infect Dis J 1989;8:870.

Xu Z-Y et al: Prevention of perinatal acquisition of hepatitis B virus carriage using vaccine: Preliminary report of a randomized, double-blind placebo-controlled and comparative trial. Pediatrics 1985;76:713.

HEPATITIS C

Hepatitis C virus (HCV) causes the chronic form of non-A, non-B hepatitis (90% of posttransfusion hepatitis cases). Risk factors include illicit use of intravenous drugs (40%), occupational or sexual exposure (10%), and transfusions (10%); 30% of cases are associated with no known risk factors. Children with hemophilia or on chronic hemodialysis are particularly at risk. The risk from transfused blood products has greatly diminished (from 1–2:100 to 1:1000 units of blood) since the advent of blood testing for ALT and anti-HCV. Cases have been caused by contaminated immune serum globulin preparations. Vertical transmission from HCV-infected mothers appears to occur more commonly in mothers who are HIV-positive (10–20%) compared with HIV-negative (0–6%); infected infants have raised ALT, but outcome is unknown at present. Transmission from breast milk is probably quite rare. HCV rarely causes fulminant hepatitis in children or adults in Western countries, but different serotypes do so in Asia.

HCV is a single-stranded RNA virus in the flavivirus family. At least seven genotypes of HCV exist. Several well-defined HCV antigens are the basis for serologic antibody tests. The second-generation ELISA test for anti-HCV is highly accurate; anti-HCV is generally present when symptoms occur. HCV RNA, which can be detected in serum by polymerase chain reaction and the new branched-DNA test, indicates active infection.

Clinical Findings

A. Symptoms and Signs: The incubation period is 1–5 months, but the onset of symptoms is insidious. Many childhood cases are asymptomatic despite development of chronic hepatitis. More typical flu-like prodromal symptoms and jaundice occur in less than 25% of cases. Hepatosplenomegaly is evident in chronic hepatitis. Ascites, clubbing, palmar erythema, or spider angiomas indicate progression to cirrhosis.

B. Laboratory Findings: Fluctuating mild to moderate elevations of aminotransferases over long periods are characteristic of chronic HCV infection. Diagnosis is established by the presence of anti-HCV (second-generation ELISA) confirmed by the radioimmunoblot assay (RIBA) or HCV RNA by polymerase chain reaction. Anti-HCV is acquired passively at birth and does not indicate disease for the first 6–12 months. HCV RNA testing should be performed in suspicious cases.

Percutaneous liver biopsy is indicated in chronic cases. Histologic examination shows portal triaditis with chronic inflammatory cells, occasional lymphocyte nodules in portal tracts, mild macrovesicular steatosis, and variable bridging necrosis, fibrosis, and cirrhosis.

Differential Diagnosis

HCV hepatitis should be distinguished from HAV, HBV, and NANBNC cases by serologic testing. Other causes of childhood cirrhosis should be considered in chronic cases (eg, Wilson's disease, α_1-antitrypsin deficiency), or chronic hepatitis may be caused by drug or autoimmune reactions.

Treatment

Treatment of acute hepatitis is supportive. Chronic HCV infection responds to interferon-alfa (3 million units/m^2 three times a week for 6–12 months) in 40–50% of cases. Relapses are common and appear to depend on genotype of the virus. Treatment for 12–15 months appears to be more durable. End-stage liver disease secondary to HCV responds well to liver transplantation, although reinfection is common and gradually progressive. There appears to be no benefit from using immune globulin in infants born to infected mothers.

Prognosis

In adults, 85% of HCV cases develop chronic hepatitis, and cirrhosis develops in 20% of those with chronic disease in 10 to more than 30 years. A strong association exists between chronic HCV disease and the development of hepatocellular carcinoma as little as 15 years after infection. The outcome of infected children is less well defined, though cirrhosis may develop rapidly or after decades. Infants infected at birth generally have concomitant HIV infection; their outcome is unknown at present. In adults, chronic HCV infection has been associated with mixed cryoglobulinemia, polyarteritis nodosa, a sicca-like syndrome, and membranoproliferative glomerulonephritis.

Bortolotti F et al: Hepatitis C virus infection and related liver disease in children of mother with antibodies to the virus. J Pediatr 1997;130:990.

Choo Q-L et al: Isolation of a cDNA clone derived from a blood-borne non-A, non-B hepatitis genome. Science 1989;244:359.

Clemente MG et al: Effect of iron overload on the response to recombinant interferon-alfa treatment in transfusion-dependent patients with thalassemia major and chronic hepatitis C. J Pediatr 1994;125:123.

Jonas MM: Interferon-alpha for viral hepatitis. J Pediatr Gastroenterol Nutr 1996;23:93.

Nowicki MJ, Balistreri WF: The hepatitis C virus: Identification, epidemiology, and clinical controversies. J Pediatr Gastroenterol Nutr 1995;20:248.

Ohto H et al: Transmission of hepatitis C virus from mothers to infants. N Engl J Med 1994;330:744.

HEPATITIS D (Delta Agent)

The hepatitis D virus (HDV) is a 35-nm defective virus that requires a coat of HBsAg to be infectious. HDV infection thus can occur only in the presence of HBV infection. In developing countries, transmission is by intimate contact; in Western countries, by parenteral exposure. HDV is rare in North America. HDV can coinfect simultaneously with HBV, causing acute hepatitis, or can superinfect a patient with chronic HBV infection, predisposing the individual to chronic hepatitis or fulminant hepatitis. In children, there is a strong association between chronic HDV coinfection with HBV and chronic active hepatitis and cirrhosis. Vertical HDV transmission is rare. The diagnosis of HDV is made by anti-HDV IgM. Treatment is directed at therapy for HBV infection (eg, interferon-alfa) or for fulminant hepatic failure.

Bortolotti F et al: Long-term evaluation of chronic delta hepatitis in children. J Pediatr 1993;122:736.

HEPATITIS E

Hepatitis E virus (HEV) is the cause of enterically transmitted, epidemic non-A, non-B hepatitis. It is rare in the United States. HEV is a calicivirus-like agent that is transmitted via the fecal-oral route. It occurs predominantly in developing countries, is associated with water-borne epidemics, and has only a 3% secondary attack rate in household contacts. Areas reporting epidemics include southeast Asia, China, the Indian subcontinent, the Middle East, northern and western Africa, Mexico, and Central America. Its clinical manifestations are similar to those of HAV except that symptomatic disease is rare in children but more common in adolescents and adults and is associated with a high mortality rate

(10–20%) in pregnant women, particularly in the third trimester of pregnancy. Diagnosis is established by anti-HEV. The outcome in nonpregnant individuals is benign, with no chronic hepatitis or chronic carrier state reported. There is no effective treatment or vaccine.

Hyams KC et al: Acute sporadic hepatitis E in Sudanese children: Analysis based on a new Western blot assay. J Infect Dis 1992;165:1001.
Krawczynski K: Hepatitis E. Hepatology 1993;17:932.

OTHER HEPATITIS VIRUSES

The recently discovered hepatitis G virus (HGV), also called the GB virus, is relatively common and parenterally and vertically transmitted, but has not been shown to produce acute or chronic liver disease. Its clinical importance is unknown.

Another NANBNC virus causes the majority of cases of fulminant hepatitis in children. Infection with this uncharacterized agent is associated with the development of aplastic anemia in a small proportion of patients recovering from hepatitis and in 15–20% of those undergoing liver transplantation for fulminant hepatitis.

Other cases of acute hepatitis are not associated with any of the known hepatitis viruses. Epstein-Barr virus, cytomegalovirus, adenovirus, and leptospirosis may cause acute hepatitis.

Chen H-L et al: Hepatitis G virus infection in normal and prospectively followed posttransfusion children. Pediatr Res 1997;42:784.
Hibbs JR et al: Aplastic anemia and viral hepatitis. Non-A, Non-B, Non-C? JAMA 1992;267:2051.

FULMINANT HEPATITIS
(Acute Massive Hepatic Necrosis, Acute Yellow Atrophy)

Essentials of Diagnosis & Typical Features
- Acute hepatitis with deepening jaundice.
- Extreme evaluation of AST and ALT.
- Prolonged prothrombin time.
- Encephalopathy and cerebral edema.
- Asterixis and fetor hepaticus.

General Considerations
Fulminant hepatitis is defined as acute hepatitis resulting in hepatic coma and coagulopathy within 6 weeks after onset and has a mortality rate of 80–90% in children (without liver transplantation). An unusually virulent infectious agent or peculiar host susceptibility is postulated in these cases. In the first few weeks of life, fulminant hepatic necrosis can be caused by herpes simplex, echovirus, or adenovirus.

Metabolic diseases that may be responsible include galactosemia, fructose intolerance, tyrosinemia, neonatal iron storage disease, respiratory chain defects, bile acid synthesis defects, and peroxisomal diseases. Later, HBV, NANBNC hepatitis viruses, and HEV are sometimes causative. HAV rarely is responsible. Patients with immunologic deficiency diseases and those receiving immunosuppressive drugs are especially vulnerable. In the older child, Wilson's disease, autoimmune hepatitis, and drugs (eg, acetaminophen, anesthetic agents) or toxins (eg, poisonous mushrooms) and leukemia must also be considered.

Clinical Findings
In a number of patients, the disease proceeds in a rapidly fulminant course with deepening jaundice, coagulopathy, hyperammonemia, ascites, a rapidly shrinking liver, and progressive coma. Terminally, AST and ALT, which were greatly elevated (2000–10,000 units/L), may improve at the time when the liver is getting smaller and undergoing massive necrosis and collapse. Another group of patients start with a course typical of "benign" hepatitis and then suddenly become ill once again during the second week of the disease. Fever, anorexia, vomiting, and abdominal pain may be noted, and worsening of liver function tests parallels changes in sensorium or impending coma. Hyperreflexia and a positive extensor plantar response are seen. A characteristic breath odor (fetor hepaticus) is present. A generalized bleeding tendency occurs at this time. Impairment of renal function, manifested by either oliguria or anuria, is an ominous sign. The striking laboratory findings include elevated serum bilirubin levels (usually > 20 mg/dL), high AST and ALT (> 5000 units/L) that may decrease terminally, low serum albumin, hypoglycemia, and prolonged prothrombin time. Blood ammonia levels may be elevated, whereas blood urea nitrogen is often very low. Hyperpnea is frequent, and mixed respiratory alkalosis and metabolic acidosis is present. A rise in the polymorphonuclear white blood cell count often presages acute liver failure.

Differential Diagnosis
Other known causes of fulminant hepatitis, such as drugs and other chemical poisons or naturally occurring plant toxins, may be difficult to exclude. Patients with Reye's syndrome or urea cycle defects are typically anicteric. A liver biopsy may be helpful. Wilson's disease, autoimmune chronic active hepatitis, acute leukemia, cardiomyopathy, and Budd-Chiari syndrome should be considered.

Complications
The development and depth of hepatic coma determine the prognosis. Patients in grade 3 or 4 coma (combativeness, unresponsiveness to verbal stimuli,

decorticate function) rarely survive without transplantation. Cerebral edema, which usually accompanies coma, is frequently the cause of death. Sepsis, hemorrhage, renal failure, or cardiorespiratory arrest is a common terminal event. Thus, when patients enter grade 3 coma, liver transplantation should be performed. The rare survivor without transplantation may have degrees of residual fibrosis or even cirrhosis.

Treatment

Many regimens have been tried, but controlled evaluation of therapy remains difficult. Exchange transfusion (with fresh heparinized blood) temporarily repairs both the chemical and hematologic abnormalities. Response may be delayed, and repeated exchange transfusions may become necessary. Plasmapheresis with plasma exchange, total body washout, charcoal hemoperfusion, and hemodialysis using a special high-permeability membrane have been used in the treatment of fulminant hepatic failure. Removal of circulating toxins may be of greater benefit to extrahepatic organ function (brain) than to the liver itself. Reversal of hepatic encephalopathy may follow any of these therapeutic modalities but without improvement in the final prognosis. Orthotopic liver transplantation has met with success in approximately 60–85% of cases; however, patients in grade 4 coma may not always recover cerebral function. Therefore, patients in hepatic failure should be transferred early to centers where liver transplantation can be performed. Criteria for deciding when to perform transplantation on these patients are not firmly established; however, serum bilirubin over 20 mg/dL, prothrombin time over 30 seconds, and factor V levels less than 20% indicate a poor prognosis. The prognosis is better for acetaminophen ingestion, particularly when *N*-acetylcysteine treatment is given.

Corticosteroids may actually be harmful. Sterilization of the colon with oral antibiotics such as metronidazole, neomycin, or gentamicin is recommended. An alternative is acidification of the colon with lactulose, 1–2 mL/kg three or four times daily, which reduces blood ammonia levels and traps ammonia in the colon. Intravenous infusions of prostaglandin E are of questionable benefit.

Close monitoring of fluid and electrolytes is mandatory and requires a central venous line. Ten percent dextrose solutions should be infused (6–8 mg/kg/min) to maintain normal blood glucose. Diuretics, sedatives, and tranquilizers are to be used sparingly. Early signs of cerebral edema are treated with infusions of mannitol (0.5–1 g/kg).

Comatose patients are intubated, given mechanical ventilatory support, and monitored for signs of infection. Coagulopathy is treated with fresh-frozen plasma, other clotting factor concentrates, platelet infusions, or exchange transfusion. Plasmapheresis and

hemodialysis may help maintain a patient while awaiting liver transplantation. Epidural monitoring for increased intracranial pressure in patients awaiting liver transplantation is advocated. Artificial hepatic support devices are being developed and tested to "bridge" patients to transplantation. Prophylactic immune globulin, 0.02 mL/kg intramuscularly, should be given to close contacts of the patient with HAV and, perhaps, NANBNC hepatitis.

Prognosis

The overall prognosis remains grave. Exchange transfusions or other modes of heroic therapy do not improve survival figures. The presence of nests of liver cells seen on liver biopsy amounting to more than 25% of the total cells and rising levels of clotting factors V and VII coupled with rising levels of serum alpha-fetoprotein may signify a more favorable prognosis for early survival. Only the rare survivor escapes postnecrotic cirrhosis. Results of liver transplantation (60–85% survival) exceed survival in nontransplanted patients (20–25%).

Alonso E et al: Fulminant hepatitis associated with centrilobular necrosis in young children. J Pediatr 1995;127:888.

Devictor D et al: Emergency liver transplantation for fulminant liver failure in infants and children. Hepatology 1992;16:1156.

O'Grady JG et al: Early indicators of prognosis in fulminant hepatic failure. Gastroenterology 1989;97:439.

Psacharopoulos HT et al: Fulminant hepatic failure in childhood. Arch Dis Child 1980;55:252.

Riordan SM, Williams R: Treatment of hepatic encephalopathy. N Engl J Med 1997;337:473.

Sokol RJ et al: Outcome of acute hepatic failure in children. J Pediatr Gastroenterol Nutr 1997;24:480.

Sokol RJ: Fulminant hepatic failure and hepatic coma. In: *Pediatric Clinical Gastroenterology*, 4th ed. Roy CC, Silverman A, Alagille D (editors). Mosby-Year Book, 1995.

AUTOIMMUNE HEPATITIS (Lupoid Hepatitis)

Autoimmune hepatitis is most common in teenage girls, although it occurs at all ages and in either sex. Chronic active hepatitis may also follow HBV, HCV, and delta hepatitis infections. Rarely, chronic active hepatitis evolves from drug-induced hepatitis (eg, pemoline) or may develop in conjunction with such diseases as ulcerative colitis, Sjögren's syndrome, or autoimmune hemolytic anemia. Wilson's disease and α_1-antitrypsin deficiency may also present as chronic active hepatitis. A positive HBsAg test indicates chronic active hepatitis caused by HBV, and anti-HCV and anti-HDV indicate HCV and delta hepatitis, respectively. Positive antinuclear antibodies, smooth muscle antibodies or liver-kidney microsomal antibodies, and systemic manifestations (eg, arthralgia, acne, amenorrhea) are characteristic of autoimmune hepatitis.

A genetic susceptibility to development of this entity is suggested by the increased incidence of the histocompatibility antigens HLA-A1 and HLA-B8. These histocompatibility antigens may be related to a defect in suppressor T cell function noted in patients with chronic active hepatitis. Increased autoimmune disease in families of patients and a high prevalence of seroimmunologic abnormalities in relatives have been noted.

Clinical Findings

Fever, malaise, recurrent or persistent jaundice, skin rash, arthritis, amenorrhea, gynecomastia, acne, pleurisy, pericarditis, or ulcerative colitis may be found in the history of these patients, or asymptomatic hepatomegaly or splenomegaly may be found on examination. Occasional patients present in acute liver failure. Cutaneous signs of chronic liver disease may be noted (eg, spider angiomas, liver palms, digital clubbing). Hepatosplenomegaly is frequently present.

Liver function tests reveal moderate elevations of serum bilirubin, AST, ALT, and serum alkaline phosphatase. Serum albumin may be low. Serum IgG levels are strikingly elevated (in the range of 2–6 g/dL), with reports of values as high as 11 g/dL. Low levels of C3 complement have been seen. Three subtypes have been described based on autoantibodies present: anti-smooth muscle (anti-actin), anti-liver-kidney microsome, and anti-soluble liver antigen.

Histologic examination of liver biopsy specimens shows loss of the lobular limiting plate, "piecemeal" necrosis, portal fibrosis, an inflammatory reaction of lymphocytes and plasma cells in the portal areas and perivascularly, and some bile duct and Kupffer cell proliferation and pseudolobule formation. Cirrhosis may be present at diagnosis in up to 50% of patients.

Differential Diagnosis

Laboratory and histologic findings differentiate other types of chronic hepatitis (eg, HBV, HCV, and HDV infection; Wilson's disease; chronic persistent hepatitis; α_1-antitrypsin disease; primary sclerosing cholangitis). Wilson's disease and α_1-antitrypsin deficiency must be excluded if HBV and HCV studies are negative. Drug-induced (isoniazid, methyldopa, pemoline) chronic active hepatitis should be ruled out. In acute, severe viral hepatitis, histologic examination may also show an "aggressive" lesion early in the disease (< 3 months).

Complications

Untreated disease that continues for months to years eventually results in postnecrotic cirrhosis. Persistent malaise, fatigue, and anorexia parallel disease activity. Bleeding from esophageal varices and development of ascites usually usher in hepatic failure.

Treatment

Corticosteroids (prednisone, 2 mg/kg/d) decrease the mortality rate during the early active phase of the disease. Azathioprine, 1–2 mg/kg/d, is of value in decreasing the side effects of long-term corticosteroid therapy but should not be used alone during the "induction" phase of treatment. Steroids are reduced over a 6- to 12-month period, and azathioprine is continued for 1–2 years. Relapses are treated similarly. Many patients require chronic azathioprine therapy. Ursodeoxycholic acid or cyclosporine may be helpful in poorly responsive cases. Liver transplantation is indicated when disease progresses to decompensated cirrhosis despite therapy.

Prognosis

The overall prognosis for chronic active hepatitis has been significantly improved by early therapy. Some report cures (normal histologic findings) in 15–20% of cases. Relapses (seen clinically and histologically) occur in 40–50% of cases after cessation of therapy; remissions follow repeat treatment. Survival for 10 years is common despite residual cirrhosis. Progressive portal hypertension is seen, and complications (bleeding varices, ascites) require specific therapy. Liver transplantation is successful 70–90% of the time. Disease recurrence after transplantation is rare.

Johnson PJ et al: Meeting report: International Autoimmune Hepatitis Group. Hepatology 1993;18:998.

Maddrey WC: Subdivisions of idiopathic autoimmune chronic active hepatitis. Hepatology 1987;7:1372.

Maggiore G et al: Liver disease associated with anti-liver-kidney microsome antibody in children. J Pediatr 1986;108:399.

Maggiore G et al: Treatment of autoimmune chronic active hepatitis in childhood. J Pediatr 1984;104:839.

Roy CC, Silverman A, Alagille D: Chronic hepatitis. In: *Pediatric Clinical Gastroenterology.* Mosby, 1994.

STEATOHEPATITIS

Steatohepatitis presents as asymptomatic soft hepatomegaly or the finding of mild to moderately elevated aminotransferases (two to ten times the upper limit of normal). Serum bilirubin, alkaline phosphatase, and γ-glutamyl transpeptidase are normal. Liver biopsy shows macrovesicular steatosis, mild portal tract inflammation, normal bile ducts, and variable degrees of portal fibrosis to cirrhosis. Ultrasonography or CT scanning indicates fat density in the liver. Most cases are associated with obesity or type II diabetes mellitus. Steatohepatitis is also seen in Wilson's disease, hereditary fructose intolerance, tyrosinemia, HCV hepatitis, cystic fibrosis, fatty acid oxidation defects, kwashiorkor, Reye's syndrome, respiratory chain defects, and toxic hepatopathy (ethanol and others). Treatment is weight reduction for obesity or treatment for the other causes. A similar entity called non-alcoholic steatohepatitis is seen in adults.

Vajro P: Persistent hyperaminotransferasemia resolving after weight reduction in obese children. J Pediatr 1994;125:239.

CIRRHOSIS

Cirrhosis is a histologically defined condition of the liver characterized by diffuse hepatocyte injury and regeneration, an increase in connective tissue (fibrosis), and disorganization of the lobular and vascular architecture. It may be micronodular or macronodular in appearance and may vary from one area of the liver to the next, but the entire liver is typically involved. It is the vasculature distortion that leads to increased resistance to blood flow, producing portal hypertension and its consequences.

Many liver diseases may progress to cirrhosis. In children, the two most common forms of cirrhosis are postnecrotic and biliary—with different causes, symptomatology, and treatment requirements. Both forms can eventually lead to liver failure and death.

In the pediatric population, postnecrotic cirrhosis is often a result of acute or chronic liver disease (eg, idiopathic neonatal giant cell hepatitis; viral HBV, HCV, or NANBNC; autoimmune hepatitis, drug-induced hepatitis) or certain inborn errors of metabolism (Table 20–3). Cirrhosis is an exceptional outcome of HAV infection and only follows massive hepatic necrosis. The evolution to cirrhosis may be insidious, with no recognized icteric phase, as in some cases of hepatitis B or C, Wilson's disease, hemochromatosis, or α_1-antitrypsin deficiency. At the time of diagnosis of cirrhosis, the underlying liver disease may be active, with abnormal liver function test results; or it may be quiescent, with normal liver tests. Most cases of biliary cirrhosis result from congenital abnormalities of the bile ducts (biliary atresia, choledochal cyst, common duct stenosis), tumors of the bile duct, Caroli's disease, Byler's disease, primary sclerosing cholangitis, hypoplasia of the intrahepatic bile ducts, and cystic fibrosis.

Occasionally, cirrhosis may follow a hypersensitivity reaction to certain drugs, such as phenytoin. Parasites *(Clonorchis sinensis, Fasciola, Ascaris)* may be causative in children living in endemic areas.

Clinical Findings

A. Symptoms and Signs: General malaise, loss of appetite, failure to thrive, and nausea are frequent complaints, especially in anicteric varieties. Easy bruising may be reported. Jaundice may or may not be present. The first indication of underlying liver disease may be ascites, gastrointestinal hemorrhage, or hepatic encephalopathy. There may be variable hepatosplenomegaly, spider angiomas, warm skin, and palmar erythema. A small, shrunken liver may be detected by percussion over the right chest wall that reveals resonance rather than expected dullness. Most often, the liver is slightly enlarged, especially in the subxiphoid region, where it has a firm to hard quality and an irregular edge. Ascites may be detected as shifting dullness or a fluid wave. Gynecomastia may be noted in males. Digital clubbing is found in 10–15% of cases. Pretibial edema is often seen, reflecting underlying hypoproteinemia. In adolescent girls, irregularities of menstruation and amenorrhea may be early complaints.

In biliary cirrhosis, patients often have jaundice, dark urine, pruritus, hepatomegaly, and sometimes xanthoma in addition to the above clinical findings. Undernutrition and failure to thrive because of steatorrhea may be more apparent in this form of cirrhosis.

B. Laboratory Findings: Mild abnormalities of aminotransferases (AST, ALT) are often present, with a decreased level of albumin and a variable increase in the level of gamma globulins. Prothrombin time is prolonged and may be unresponsive to vitamin K administration. Burr and target red cells may be noted on the peripheral blood smear. Anemia, thrombocytopenia, and leukopenia are present if hypersplenism exists.

In biliary cirrhosis, elevated conjugated bilirubin, bile acids, γ-glutamyl transpeptidase, alkaline phosphatase, and cholesterol are common.

C. Imaging: Hepatic ultrasound or CT examination may demonstrate abnormal hepatic texture and nodules. In biliary cirrhosis, abnormalities of the biliary tree may be apparent by ultrasonography, CT, hepatobiliary scintigraphy, or cholangiography.

D. Pathologic Findings: Liver biopsy findings of regenerating nodules and surrounding fibrosis are hallmarks of cirrhosis. Pathologic features of biliary cirrhosis also include canalicular and hepatocyte cholestasis, as well as plugging of bile ducts. The interlobular bile ducts may be increased or decreased, depending on the cause and the stage of the disease process.

Complications & Treatment

Major complications of cirrhosis in childhood include progressive nutritional disturbances, hormonal disturbances, the evolution of portal hypertension and its complications. Hepatocarcinoma occurs with increased frequency in the cirrhotic liver, especially in patients with the chronic form of hereditary tyrosinemia or after long-standing HBV or HCV disease. At present, there is no proven medical treatment for cirrhosis, but wherever a treatable condition is identified (eg, Wilson's disease, galactosemia, congenital fructose intolerance) or an offending agent eliminated (drugs, toxins), disease progression can be altered; in occasional cases, regression of fibrosis has been noted. Immunosuppressive treatment in autoimmune hepatitis can halt the progression of cirrhosis. Surgical correction of biliary tree abnormalities can stabilize the disease process or lead to a reversal in some situations. Liver transplantation may be appropriate in patients with cirrhosis whose disease is continuing to progress or in whom the complications of cirrhosis are no longer manageable.

Prognosis

Postnecrotic cirrhosis has an unpredictable course. Without transplantation, affected patients may die from liver failure within 15 years. Patients with a rising bilirubin or a vitamin K-resistant coagulopathy along with diuretic refractory ascites usually survive less than 1 year. The terminal event in some patients may be generalized hemorrhage, sepsis, or cardiorespiratory arrest. For patients with biliary cirrhosis, the prognosis is similar, except for those with surgically corrected lesions that result in regression or stabilization of the underlying liver condition. With liver transplantation, survival is 70–80%.

Conn HO, Atterbury CE: Cirrhosis. In: *Diseases of the Liver,* 7th ed. Schiff L, Schiff ER (editors). Lippincott, 1993.

Hardy SC, Kleinman RE: Cirrhosis and chronic liver failure. In: *Liver Disease in Children.* Suchy FJ (editor). Mosby-Year Book, 1994.

ALPHA$_1$-ANTITRYPSIN DEFICIENCY LIVER DISEASE

Essentials of Diagnosis & Typical Features

- Serum α_1-antitrypsin level less than 50–80 mg/dL.
- Identification of a specific phenotype (Pi ZZ, SZ).
- Detection of diastase-resistant glycoprotein deposits in periportal hepatocytes.
- Histologic evidence of liver disease.
- Family history of early-onset pulmonary disease or liver disease.

General Considerations

The disease is caused by a deficiency in the protease inhibitor system (Pi), predisposing patients to chronic liver disease and an early onset of pulmonary emphysema. It is most often associated with the Pi phenotype ZZ. With the intermediate serum levels of α_1-antitrypsin present in the heterozygote phenotype (MZ), the incidence of liver disease in adults is only slightly greater than that in the general population, despite the presence of glycoprotein deposits in hepatocytes. The exact relationship between low levels of serum α_1-antitrypsin and the development of liver disease is unclear. Emphysema develops because of a lack of inhibition of elastase, which destroys pulmonary connective tissue. Although all patients with the ZZ genotype have antitrypsin inclusions in hepatocytes, that may be the only histologic evidence of

liver disease. An associated abnormality in the microsomal disposal of accumulated aggregates may be necessary for the liver disease phenotype.

About 20% of affected individuals present with neonatal cholestasis. At 18 years of age, about 10% of individuals with α_1-antitrypsin deficiency have or have had clinically significant liver injury. Very few children have pulmonary involvement. Most children are asymptomatic, with no laboratory or clinical evidence of liver disease.

Clinical Findings

A. Symptoms and Signs: α_1-Antitrypsin deficiency should be suspected in all small-for-gestational-age newborns with neonatal cholestasis. Poor appetite, lethargy, slight irritability, and jaundice suggest neonatal hepatitis but are not pathognomonic of any one cause. Hepatosplenomegaly is present. The family history may be positive for emphysema or cirrhosis.

In the older child, hepatomegaly or physical findings suggestive of cirrhosis, especially in the face of a negative history of liver disease, should always lead one to suspect α_1-antitrypsin deficiency. Recurrent pulmonary disease (bronchitis, pneumonia) may be present in a few children.

B. Laboratory Findings: Low levels ($<$ 0.2 mg/dL) of the α_1-globulin fraction may be noted on serum protein fractionation. Specific quantitation of α_1-antitrypsin reveals levels of less than 50–80 mg/dL in homozygotes (ZZ) deficient in this glycoprotein. Specific Pi phenotyping should be done to confirm the diagnosis. Liver function tests often reflect underlying hepatic pathologic changes. Hyperbilirubinemia (mixed) and elevated aminotransferases, alkaline phosphatase, and γ-glutamyl transpeptidase are present early. Hyperbilirubinemia generally resolves, while aminotransferase elevation may persist. Signs of cirrhosis and portal hypertension may develop.

Liver biopsy after 2–6 months of age shows diastase-resistant intracellular granules positive to periodic acid-Schiff staining, with hyaline masses, particularly in periportal zones.

Differential Diagnosis

In the newborn, other specific causes of neonatal cholestasis need to be considered. In the older child, other causes of insidious cirrhosis (eg, viral hepatitis type B or C, autoimmune hepatitis, Wilson's disease, cystic fibrosis, glycogen storage disease) should be considered.

Complications

Of all infants with Pi ZZ α_1-antitrypsin deficiency, only 20% develop liver disease in childhood. The complications of portal hypertension, cirrhosis, and chronic cholestasis predominate in affected children.

Early-onset pulmonary emphysema occurs in young adults (aged 30–40 years), particularly in smokers. An increased susceptibility to hepatocarcinoma has been noted in cirrhosis with α_1-antitrypsin deficiency.

Treatment

There is no specific treatment for the liver disease of this disorder. Affected infants who are breast-fed may have less severe liver disease. Replacement of the protein by transfusion therapy is successful in preventing pulmonary disease in affected adults. The neonatal cholestatic condition is treated with choleretics, medium-chain triglyceride-containing formula, and water-miscible vitamins (see Table 20–2). Ursodeoxycholic acid may reduce AST, ALT and γ-glutamyl transpeptidase, but its effect on outcome is unknown. Portal hypertension, esophageal bleeding, ascites, and other complications are treated as described elsewhere. Genetic counseling is indicated whenever the diagnosis is made. Diagnosis by prenatal screening is possible. Liver transplantation has been shown to cure the deficiency.

Prognosis

Thirty to 50 percent of patients with liver injury either die from progressive liver disease or develop cirrhosis. A correlation between histologic patterns and clinical course has been documented in the infantile form of the disease. Liver failure can be expected 5–15 years after development of cirrhosis. Recurrence or persistence of hyperbilirubinemia along with worsening coagulation studies indicates the need for evaluation for possible liver transplantation. Decompensated cirrhosis caused by this disease is an excellent indication for liver transplantation; the survival rate is 70–90%.

Perlmutter DH: Alpha-1-antitrypsin deficiency: Biochemical and clinical manifestations. Ann Med 1996;28:385.

Sveger T, Eriksson S: The liver in adolescents with α_1-antitrypsin deficiency. Hepatology 1995;22:514.

Sveger T: Prospective study of children with alpha$_1$-antitrypsin deficiency: Eight-year-old follow-up. J Pediatr 1984;104:91.

Teckman JH et al: Molecular pathogenesis of liver disease in alpha-1-antitrypsin deficiency. Hepatology 1996;24:1504.

Wewers MD et al: Replacement therapy for alpha$_1$-antitrypsin deficiency associated with emphysema. N Engl J Med 1987;316:1055.

BILIARY TRACT DISEASE

1. CHOLELITHIASIS

Essentials of Diagnosis & Typical Features

- Episodic right upper quadrant abdominal pain.
- Elevated bilirubin, alkaline phosphatase, and γ-glutamyl transpeptidase.
- Stones or sludge seen on abdominal ultrasound.

General Considerations

Gallstones may develop at all ages in the pediatric population and in utero. Gallstones may be divided into cholesterol stones, which contain more than 50% cholesterol, and pigment stones, black (sterile bile) and brown (infected bile). Pigment stones predominate in the first decade of life, while cholesterol stones account for up to 90% of gallstones in adolescence. For some patients, gallbladder dysfunction is associated with biliary sludge formation, which may evolve into "sludge balls" or tumefaction bile and thence into gallstones. The process is reversible in many patients.

Clinical Findings

A. History: Most symptomatic gallstones present with acute and recurrent episodes of moderate to severe, sharp right upper quadrant or epigastric pain. The pain may radiate substernally or to the right shoulder. On rare occasions, the presentation may include a history of jaundice, back pain, or generalized abdominal discomfort, where it is associated with pancreatitis, suggesting stone impaction in the common duct or ampulla hepatopancreatica. Nausea and vomiting may occur during attacks. Pain episodes often occur postprandially, especially with ingestion of fatty foods. The groups at risk for gallstones include the following: patients with known or suspected hemolytic disease; females; teenagers with prior pregnancy; obese individuals; certain racial or ethnic groups, particularly Native Americans (Pima Indians); Hispanics; and infants and children with ileal disease (Crohn's disease) or prior ileal resection. Fasting premature infants on prolonged parenteral hyperalimentation (with or without chronic furosemide therapy) are at particular risk for gallstone formation. Patients with cystic fibrosis or Wilson's disease also have an increased incidence of gallstones. Other, less certain risk factors include a positive family history, use of birth control pills, and diabetes mellitus.

B. Symptoms and Signs: During acute episodes of pain, tenderness is present in the right upper quadrant or epigastrium, with a positive inspiratory arrest (Murphy's sign) but usually without peritoneal signs. If present, scleral icterus is helpful. Evidence of underlying hemolytic disease in addition to icterus may include pallor (anemia), splenomegaly, tachycardia, and high-output cardiac murmur. Fever is unusual in uncomplicated cases.

C. Laboratory Findings: Laboratory tests are usually normal unless calculi have lodged in the extrahepatic biliary system, in which case the serum bilirubin and γ-glutamyl transpeptidase (or alkaline phosphatase) may be elevated. Amylase and lipase may be increased if stone obstruction occurs at the ampulla hepatopancreatica.

D. Imaging: Ultrasound evaluation is the best imaging technique, showing abnormal intraluminal contents (stones, sludge) as well as anatomic alterations of the gallbladder or dilation of the biliary ductal system. The presence of an anechoic acoustic shadow differentiates calculi from intraluminal sludge or sludge balls. Plain abdominal x-rays will show calculi with a high calcium content in the region of the gallbladder in up to 15% of cases. Lack of visualization of the gallbladder with hepatobiliary scintigraphy may suggest chronic cholecystitis. In selected cases, endoscopic retrograde cholangiopancreatography (ERCP) may be helpful in defining subtle abnormalities of the bile ducts and locating intraductal stones.

Differential Diagnosis

Other abnormal conditions of the biliary system with similar presentation are summarized in Table 20–5. Liver disease (hepatitis, abscess, tumor) can cause similar symptoms or signs. Peptic disease, reflux esophagitis, paraesophageal hiatal hernia, cardiac disease, and pneumomediastinum must be considered when the pain is epigastric or substernal in location. Renal or pancreatic disease is a possible explanation if the pain is localized to the right flank or mid back. Subcapsular or supracapsular lesions of the liver (abscess, tumor, hematoma) or right lower lobe infiltrate may also be a cause of nontraumatic right shoulder pain.

Complications

Major problems are related to stone impaction in either the cystic or common duct and lead to stricture formation or perforation. Acute distention and subsequent perforation of the gallbladder may occur when gallstones cause obstruction of the cystic duct. Stones impacted at the level of the ampulla hepatopancreatica often cause "gallstone pancreatitis."

Treatment

Symptomatic cholelithiasis is best treated by either open or laparoscopic cholecystectomy. Intraoperative cholangiography via the cystic duct is required so that the physician can be certain the ductal system is free of retained stones. Calculi in the extrahepatic bile ducts may be removed by ERCP, sphincterotomy, and balloon extraction or by surgical exploration and removal, often with T tube drainage. There is an increased risk of cholangitis and bile duct stricture with the latter procedure.

Gallstones developing in premature infants on total parenteral nutrition can be followed by ultrasound examination. Most of the infants are asymptomatic, and the stones will resolve in 3–12 months. Gallstone dissolution using cholelitholytics (ursodeoxycholic acid) or mechanical means (lithotripsy) has not been approved for use in children. Asymptomatic gallstones do not usually require treatment, as only 20% will eventually cause problems.

Prognosis

The prognosis is excellent in uncomplicated cases that come to surgery not requiring exploration and T tube drainage of the common bile duct. Cystic duct "stump pain" is not reported in children.

Bowen JC et al: Gallstone disease: Pathophysiology, epidemiology, natural history, and treatment options. Med Clin North Am 1992;76:1143.

Debray D et al: Cholelithiasis in infancy: A study of 40 cases. J Pediatr 1993;122:385.

Schwesinger WH, Diehl AK: Changing indications for laparoscopic cholecystectomy: Stones without symptoms and symptoms without stones. Surg Clin North Am 1996;76:493.

2. OTHER BILIARY TRACT DISORDERS

For a schematic representation of the various types of choledochal cysts, see Figure 20–1. For acute hydrops, choledochal cyst, acalculous cholecystitis, primary sclerosing cholangitis, Caroli's disease, and congenital hepatic fibrosis, see Table 20–5.

PYOGENIC & AMEBIC LIVER ABSCESS

Pyogenic liver abscesses are caused by intestinal bacteria seeded via the portal vein from infected viscera and occasionally from ascending cholangitis or gangrenous cholecystitis. Blood cultures are positive in up to 60% of cases. The resulting lesion tends to be solitary and located in the right hepatic lobe. Bacterial seeding may also occur from infected burns, pyodermas, and osteomyelitis. Unusual causes include omphalitis, subacute infective endocarditis, pyelonephritis, Crohn's disease, and perinephric abscess. Multiple pyogenic liver abscesses are associated with severe sepsis. Children receiving anti-inflammatory and immunosuppressive agents and children with defects in white blood cell function (chronic granulomatous disease) are more prone to pyogenic hepatic abscesses, especially those caused by *Staphylococcus aureus*.

Amebic liver abscess is rare in children. An increased risk is associated with travel through endemic areas (Mexico, Southeast Asia). *Entamoeba histolytica* invasion occurs via the large bowel, although a history of diarrhea (colitis-like picture) is not always obtained.

Clinical Findings

With pyogenic liver abscess, nonspecific complaints of fever, chills, malaise, and abdominal pain are frequent. Weight loss is very common, especially in delayed diagnosis. A few patients have shaking chills and jaundice. The dominant complaint is a constant dull pain over an enlarged liver that is tender to palpation. An elevated hemidiaphragm with reduced

Table 20–5. Biliary tract abnormalities.

	Acute Hydrops Transient Dilatation of Gallbladder[1,2]	Choledochal Cyst[3,4] (See Figure 20–1.)	Acalculous Cholecystitis[5]	Primary Sclerosing Cholangitis[6-8]	Caroli's Disease[9] (Idiopathic Intrahepatic Bile Duct Dilation)	Congenital Hepatic Fibrosis[10]
Predisposing or associated conditions	Premature infants with prolonged fasting or systemic illness. Hepatitis. Abnormalities of cystic duct. Kawasaki disease. Bacterial sepsis, EBV.	Congenital lesion. Female sex. Asians. Rarely with Caroli's disease or congenital hepatic fibrosis.	Systemic illness, sepsis (Streptococcus, Salmonella, Kiebsiella, etc), HIV infection. Gallbladder stasis, obstruction of cystic duct (stones, nodes, tumor).	Most have chronic ulcerative colitis (70%); 75% are males. Increased incidence of HLA-B8. Sicca syndrome, fibroinflammatory conditions, immunodeficiency syndromes, histiocytosis.	Congenital lesion. Also found in congenital hepatic fibrosis or with choledochal cyst. Female sex. Autosomal recessive polycystic kidney disease.	Familial (autosomal recessive) 25% with autosomal recessive polycystic kidney disease. Choledochal cyst. Caroli's disease. Meckel-Gruber, Ivemark's, or Jeune's syndrome.
Symptoms	Absent in premature infants. Vomiting, abdominal pain in older children.	Abdominal pain, vomiting, jaundice	Acute severe abdominal pain, vomiting, fever	Pruritus, jaundice, abdominal pain, fatigue	Recurrent abdominal pain, vomiting. Fever, jaundice when cholangitis occurs.	Hematemesis, melena from bleeding esophageal varices
Signs	Right upper quadrant abdominal mass. Tenderness in some.	Icterus, acholic stools, dark urine in neonatal period. Right upper quadrant abdominal mass or tenderness in older child.	Tenderness in mid and right upper abdomen. Occasional palpable mass in right upper quadrant.	Icterus, hepatomegaly, splenomegaly	Icterus, hepatomegaly	Hepatosplenomegaly
Laboratory abnormalities	Most are normal. Increased WBC count in sepsis (may be decreased in premature infants). Abnormal LFTs in hepatitis.	Conjugated hyperbilirubinemia, elevated GGTP, slightly increased AST. Elevated pancreatic serum amylase if ampulla hepatopancreatica is involved.	Elevated WBC count, normal or slight abnormality of LFTs	Elevated serum bile acids, bilirubin, GGTP. Slight elevation of AST. Perinuclear antineuclear cytoplasmic antibodies (pANCA) often positive.	Abnormal LFTs. Increased WBC count with cholangitis. Urine abnormalities if associated with CHF.	Low platelet and WBC count (hypersplenism), slight elevation of AST, GGTP. Inability to concentrate urine.
Diagnostic studies most useful	Gallbladder ultrasonography	Gallbladder ultrasonography hepatobiliary scintigraphy, and ERCP, or MRCP	Scintigraphy to confirm nonfunction of gallbladder. Ultrasonography or abdominal CT scan to rule out other neighboring disease.	Ultrasonography of the biliary tree, ERCP, hepatobiliary scintigraphy	Transhepatic cholangiography, ERCP, MRCP, scintigraphy, ultrasonography, intravenous pyelography	Liver biopsy. Ultrasonography of the liver and kidneys. Upper endoscopy, splenoportography.
Treatment	Treatment of associated condition. Needle or tube cystostomy rarely required. Cholecystectomy seldom indicated.	Surgical resection and choledochoenterostomy	Broad-spectrum antibiotic coverage, then cholecystectomy or cholecystostomy drainage and definitive surgery 3–4 weeks later	Ursodeoxycholic acid, cholestyramine. Liver transplantation. Balloon dilation, stenting of extrahepatic bile ducts.	Antibiotics and surgical or endoscopic drainage for cholangitis. Liver transplantation for some. Lobectomy for localized disease.	Treatment of portal hypertension. Liver kidney transplantation for some.

Complications	Perforation with bile peritonitis rare	Progressive biliary cirrhosis. Increased incidence of cholangiocarcinoma. Cholangitis in some.	Perforation and bile peritonitis, sepsis, abscess or fistula formation. Pancreatitis.	Progressive biliary cirrhosis, portal hypertension, fat malabsorption, vitamin deficiencies, cholangiocarcinoma, liver failure	Sepsis with episodes of cholangitis, biliary cirrhosis, portal hypertension. Intraductal stones. Cholangiocarcinoma.	Bleeding from varices. Splenic rupture, severe thrombocytopenia. Progressive renal failure.
Prognosis	Excellent with resolution of underlying condition. Consider cystic duct obstruction if disorder fails to resolve.	Depends on anatomic type of cyst, associated condition, and success of surgery. Liver transplantation required in some.	Good with early diagnosis and treatment	Guarded; disease progression is expected even with medical treatment. Course not changed by colectomy.	Poor, with gradual deterioration of liver function. Multiple surgical drainage procedures expected. Liver transplantation should alter long-term prognosis.	Good in absence of serious renal involvement and with control of portal hypertension. Slightly increased risk of cholangiocarcinoma.

Ultrasonography = liver and biliary tract scanning; scintigraphy = hepatobiliary scan using radiolabeled [99mtechnetium]; AST = aspartate aminotransferase (SGOT); CHF = congenital hepatic fibrosis; CT = computed tomography; ERCP = endoscopic retrograde cholangiopancreatography; LFT = liver function tests; GGTP = γ-glutamyl transpeptidase; WBC = white blood count; MRCP = magnetic resonance cholangiopancreatography

[1]Crankson S et al: Acute hydrops of the gallbladder in childhood. Eur J Pediatr 1992;151:318.
[2]Suddleson E et al: Hydrops of the gallbladder associated with Kawasaki syndrome. J Pediatr Surg 1987;22:956.
[3]Shian WJ et al: Choledochal cysts: A nine year review. Acta Paediatr 1993;82:383.
[4]Altman RP: Choledochal cyst. Semin Pediatr Surg 1992;1:130.
[5]Barie PS, Fischer E: Acute acalculous cholecystitis. J Am Coll Surg 1995;180:232.
[6]El-Shabrawi M et al: Primary sclerosing cholangitis in childhood. Gastroenterology 1987;92:1226.
[7]Lee YM, Kaplan MM: Primary sclerosing cholangitis N Engl J Med 1995;332:924.
[8]Beuers U et al: Ursodeoxycholic acid for treatment of primary sclerosing cholangitis: A placebo-controlled trial. Hepatology 1992;16:707.
[9]Inui A et al: A case of Caroli's disease with special reference to hepatic CT and US finding. J Pediatr Gastroenterol Nutr 1992;14:463.
[10]Perisic VN: Long term studies on congenital hepatic fibrosis in children. Acta Paediatr 1995;85:695.

TYPE | FINDINGS

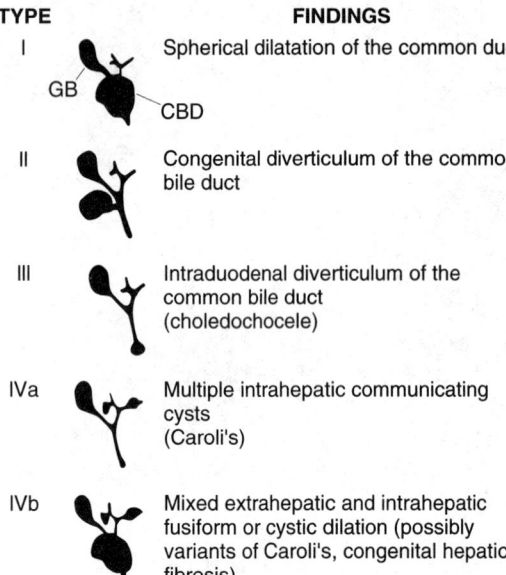

I — Spherical dilatation of the common duct

GB — CBD

II — Congenital diverticulum of the common bile duct

III — Intraduodenal diverticulum of the common bile duct (choledochocele)

IVa — Multiple intrahepatic communicating cysts (Caroli's)

IVb — Mixed extrahepatic and intrahepatic fusiform or cystic dilation (possibly variants of Caroli's, congenital hepatic fibrosis)

Figure 20–1. Classification of cystic dilation of the bile ducts. Types I, II, and III are extrahepatic. Type IVa is solely intrahepatic, and type IVb is both intrahepatic and extrahepatic.

or absent respiratory excursion may be demonstrated on physical examination and confirmed by fluoroscopy. Laboratory studies show leukocytosis and, at times, anemia. Liver function tests may be normal or reveal mild elevation of transaminases and alkaline phosphatase. Elevated vitamin B_{12} levels are reported. Amebic liver abscesses are usually heralded by an acute illness with high fever, chills, and leukocytosis. Early in the course, liver tests may suggest mild hepatitis. An occasional prodrome may include cough, dyspnea, and shoulder pain as rupture of the abscess into the right chest occurs. Consolidation of the right lower lobe is common (30%).

Ultrasound liver scan is the most useful diagnostic aid in evaluating pyogenic and amebic abscesses, detecting lesions as small as 1–2 cm. Nuclear scanning with gallium or technetium sulfur colloid or CT imaging may be useful to differentiate tumor or hydatid cyst.

The distinction between pyogenic and amebic abscesses is best made by indirect hemagglutination test (which is positive in more than 95% of patients with amebic liver disease) and the prompt response of the latter to antiamebic therapy (metronidazole). Examination of material obtained by needle aspiration of the abscess using ultrasound guidance is often diagnostic.

Differential Diagnosis

Hepatitis, hepatoma, hydatid cyst, gallbladder dis-

ease, or biliary tract infections can mimic liver abscess. Subphrenic abscesses, empyema, and pneumonia may give a similar picture. Inflammatory disease of the intestines or of the biliary system may be complicated by liver abscess.

Complications

Spontaneous rupture of the abscess may occur with extension of infection into the subphrenic space, thorax, peritoneal cavity, and, occasionally, the pericardium. Bronchopleural fistula with large sputum production and hemoptysis can develop in severe cases. Simultaneously, the amebic liver abscess may be secondarily infected with bacteria (10–20% of cases). Metastatic hematogenous spread to the lungs and the brain has been reported.

Treatment

Ultrasound- or CT-guided percutaneous needle aspiration for aerobic and anaerobic culture with simultaneous placement of a catheter for drainage, combined with appropriate antibiotic therapy, is the treatment of choice for solitary pyogenic liver abscess. Multiple liver abscesses may also be treated successfully by this method. Surgical intervention may be indicated if there is rupture outside the capsule of the liver or if enterohepatic fistulae are suspected.

Amebic abscesses should be treated promptly. Only those that are sufficiently large and threaten to rupture need to be aspirated. Uncomplicated cases can be treated with oral metronidazole, 35–50 mg/kg/d in three divided doses for 10 days. Intravenous metronidazole can be used in patients unable to take oral medication. In severe cases, give dehydroemetine, 1–1.5 mg/kg/d intramuscularly for 5 days, and chloroquine, 10 mg/kg/d in one or two divided doses for 21 days. Failure to improve after 72 hours of drug therapy indicates superimposed bacterial infection or an incorrect diagnosis. At this point, needle aspiration or surgical drainage is indicated. Once oral feedings can be tolerated, a 20-day course of iodoquinol (30 mg/kg/d in three doses) is started as a luminal amebicide. Resolution of the abscess cavity occurs over 3–6 months.

Prognosis

An unrecognized and untreated pyogenic liver abscess is universally fatal. With drainage and antibiotics, the cure rate is about 90%. Most amebic abscesses are cured with conservative medical management; the mortality rate is less than 3%. If extrahepatic complications occur (empyema, bronchopleural fistula, pericardial complications), 10–15% of patients will succumb.

Moore SW et al: Conservative initial treatment for liver abscesses in children. Br J Surg 1994;81:872.

Nazir Z, Moazam F: Amebic liver abscess in children. Pediatr Infect Dis J 1993;12:929.

Novak DA, Dolson DJ: Bacterial, parasitic and fungal infections of the liver. In: *Liver Disease in Children.* Suchy FJ (editor). Mosby-Year Book, 1994.

PORTAL HYPERTENSION

Essentials of Diagnosis & Typical Features

- Splenomegaly.
- Recurrent ascites.
- Variceal hemorrhage.
- Hypersplenism.

General Considerations

Portal hypertension is defined as an increase in the portal venous pressure to more than 5 mm Hg greater than the inferior vena caval pressure. Portal hypertension is most commonly a result of cirrhosis. However, portal hypertension without cirrhosis may be divided into prehepatic, suprahepatic, and intrahepatic causes. Although the specific lesions vary somewhat in clinical signs and symptoms, the end result of portal hypertension is common to all.

A. Prehepatic Portal Hypertension: Prehepatic portal hypertension from acquired abnormalities of the portal and splenic veins accounts for 5–8% of cases of gastrointestinal bleeding in children. A history of neonatal omphalitis, sepsis, dehydration, and umbilical vein catheterization is present in 30–50% of cases. Less common causes in older children include local trauma, peritonitis (pylephlebitis), hypercoagulable states, and pancreatitis. Symptoms may occur before 1 year of age, but in most cases the diagnosis is not made until 3–5 years of age. Those with a positive neonatal history tend to be symptomatic earlier.

A variety of portal or splenic vein malformations, some of which may be congenital, have been described, including valves and atretic segments. "Cavernous" transformation is probably the result of attempted collateralization around the thrombosed portal vein rather than a congenital malformation. The site of the venous obstruction may be anywhere from the hilum of the liver to the hilum of the spleen.

B. Suprahepatic Vein Occlusion or Thrombosis (Budd-Chiari Syndrome): In most instances, no cause can be demonstrated. Endothelial injury to hepatic veins by bacterial endotoxins has been demonstrated experimentally. The occasional association of hepatic vein thrombosis in inflammatory bowel disease favors the presence of endogenous toxins traversing the liver. Allergic vasculitis leading to endophlebitis of the hepatic veins has been described occasionally. In addition, hepatic vein obstruction may be secondary to tumor, abdominal trauma, hyperthermia, or sepsis, or it may occur fol-

lowing the repair of an omphalocele or gastroschisis. Congenital vena caval bands, webs, a membrane, or strictures above the hepatic veins are sometimes causative. Hepatic vein thrombosis may be a complication of oral contraceptive medications. Underlying thrombotic conditions (antithrombin III, protein C, factor V Leiden, phospholipid antibodies, or protein S deficiency) should be evaluated.

C. Intrahepatic:

1. Cirrhosis (see above).

2. Veno-occlusive disease (acute stage)–This entity now occurs most frequently in bone marrow transplant patients. It may also develop after chemotherapy for acute leukemia, particularly with thioguanine. Additional causes include the ingestion of pyrrolizidine alkaloids ("bush tea") or other herbal teas and a familial form of the disease seen in congenital immunodeficiency states.

The acute form of the disease generally occurs in the first month after bone marrow transplantation and is heralded by the triad of weight gain (ascites), tender hepatomegaly, and jaundice. The disease may be rapidly fatal, although about 50% of patients recover. Subacute and chronic forms also exist.

3. Congenital hepatic fibrosis–This is a rare autosomal recessive cause of intrahepatic presinusoidal portal hypertension (Table 20–5). Liver biopsy is generally diagnostic, demonstrating von Meyenberg complexes. On angiography, the intrahepatic branches of the portal vein may be duplicated. Renal abnormalities (microcystic disease) are often associated with the hepatic lesion; therefore, renal ultrasonography and urography should be routinely performed.

4. Other rare causes–Hepatoportal sclerosis (idiopathic portal hypertension, noncirrhotic portal fibrosis), noncirrhotic nodular transformation of the liver, and schistosomal hepatic fibrosis are also rare causes of intrahepatic presinusoidal portal hypertension.

Clinical Findings

A. Symptoms and Signs: Splenomegaly in an otherwise well child is the most constant physical sign. Recurrent episodes of abdominal distention resulting from ascites may also be noted. The usual presenting symptoms are hematemesis and melena.

The presence of prehepatic portal hypertension is suggested by the following: (1) an episode of severe infection in the newborn period or early infancy—especially omphalitis, sepsis, gastroenteritis, severe dehydration, or prolonged or difficult umbilical vein catheterizations; (2) no previous evidence of liver disease; (3) a history of well-being prior to onset or recognition of symptoms; and (4) normal liver size and tests with splenomegaly.

Most patients with suprahepatic portal hypertension present with hepatomegaly of acute onset and abdominal enlargement caused by ascites. Abdominal pain and tender hepatosplenomegaly are frequent, whereas jaundice is present in only 25% of cases. Vomiting, hematemesis, and diarrhea are less common. Cutaneous signs of chronic liver disease are often absent, as the obstruction is usually acute. The presence of distended superficial veins on the back and the anterior abdomen, along with dependent edema, is seen with inferior vena cava obstruction affecting hepatic vein outflow. Absence of hepatojugular reflux (jugular distention when pressure is applied to the liver) is a helpful clinical sign.

The symptoms and signs of intrahepatic portal hypertension are generally those of cirrhosis (see above).

B. Laboratory Findings and Imaging: Most other common causes of splenomegaly or hepatosplenomegaly may be excluded by proper laboratory tests. Cultures, Epstein-Barr virus titers, hepatitis serologies, blood smear examination, bone marrow studies, and liver function tests may be necessary. In prehepatic portal hypertension, liver function tests are generally normal. In Budd-Chiari syndrome and veno-occlusive disease, mild to moderate hyperbilirubinemia with modest elevations of aminotransferases and prothrombin time are often present. Hypersplenism with mild leukopenia and thrombocytopenia is often present. Upper endoscopy will reveal varices in symptomatic patients. When possible, confirmation of a normal liver is best obtained by liver biopsy.

Doppler-assisted ultrasound scanning of the liver, portal vein, splenic vein, inferior vena cava, and hepatic veins may assist in defining the vascular anatomy. In prehepatic portal hypertension, abnormalities of the portal or splenic vein may be apparent, whereas the hepatic veins are normal. When noncirrhotic portal hypertension is suspected, angiography often is diagnostic. Selective arteriography of the superior mesenteric artery is recommended prior to surgical shunting to determine the patency of the superior mesenteric vein.

For suprahepatic portal hypertension, an inferior venacavogram using catheters from above or below the suspected obstruction may reveal an intrinsic filling defect, an infiltrating tumor, or extrinsic compression of the inferior vena cava by an adjacent lesion. A large caudate lobe of the liver suggests Budd-Chiari syndrome. Care must be taken in interpreting extrinsic pressure defects of the subdiaphragmatic inferior vena cava if ascites is significant.

Simultaneous wedge hepatic vein pressure and hepatic venography are useful to demonstrate obstruction to major hepatic vein ostia and smaller vessels. In the absence of obstruction, reflux across the sinusoids into the portal vein branches can be accomplished. Pressures should also be taken from the right heart and supradiaphragmatic portion of the inferior vena cava to eliminate constrictive pericarditis and pulmonary hypertension from the differential diagnosis.

Differential Diagnosis

All causes of splenomegaly must be included in the differential diagnosis, the most common ones being infections, immune thrombocytopenic purpura, blood dyscrasias, lipidosis, reticuloendotheliosis, cirrhosis of the liver, and cysts or hemangiomas of the spleen. When hematemesis or melena occurs, other causes of gastrointestinal bleeding are possible, that is, gastric or duodenal ulcers, tumors, duplications, or inflammatory bowel disease.

As ascites is almost always present in suprahepatic portal hypertension, cirrhosis resulting from any cause must be excluded. Other suprahepatic (cardiac, pulmonary) causes of portal hypertension must also be ruled out. Although ascites may occur in prehepatic portal hypertension, it is uncommon.

Complications

The major manifestation and complication of portal hypertension is bleeding esophageal varices. Fatal exsanguination is uncommon, but hypovolemic shock or resulting anemia may require prompt treatment. Congestive splenomegaly with granulocytopenia and thrombocytopenia occurs but seldom causes major symptoms. Rupture of the enlarged spleen secondary to trauma is always a threat. Retroperitoneal edema has been reported (Clatworthy's sign).

Without treatment, complete and persistent hepatic vein obstruction leads to liver failure, coma, and death. A nonportal type of cirrhosis may develop in the chronic form of hepatic veno-occlusive disease in which small and medium-sized hepatic veins are affected. Death from renal failure may occur in rare cases of congenital hepatic fibrosis.

Treatment

Definitive treatment of noncirrhotic portal hypertension is generally lacking. In prehepatic portal hypertension, the experience with surgical portosystemic shunts is complicated by a lack of sustained patency in most children less than 10 years old. Therefore, aggressive medical treatment of the complications of prehepatic portal hypertension is the preferred option. However, some centers have reported good results with shunting procedures, and the new meso-rex shunt may offer improved outcome. Veno-occlusive disease may be prevented somewhat by the prophylactic use of ursodeoxycholic acid prior to conditioning for bone marrow transplantation. Withdrawal of the suspected offending agent, if possible, may increase the chance of recovery. For suprahepatic portal hypertension, efforts should be directed at determining the underlying cause and correction, if possible. Either surgical or angiographic relief of obstruction should be attempted if a defined obstruction of the vessels is apparent. Liver transplantation should be considered early in the course if direct correction is not possible.

However, in most cases, management of portal hypertension is directed at management of the complications (Table 20–6).

Prognosis

For prehepatic portal hypertension, the prognosis depends on the site of the block, the effectiveness of variceal eradication, the availability of suitable vessels for shunting procedures, and the experience of the surgeon. Each unsuccessful surgical procedure worsens the prognosis. In patients managed by medical means, bleeding episodes seem to diminish with adolescence.

The prognosis in patients managed by medical and supportive therapy may be better than in the surgically treated group, especially when surgery is performed at an early age. Portacaval encephalopathy is unusual in the post-shunted child except when protein intake is excessive.

The mortality rate of hepatic vein obstruction is very high—95%. In veno-occlusive disease, the prognosis is better, with complete recovery possible in 50% of acute forms and 5–10% of subacute forms.

Brown RS Jr, Lake JR: Transjugular intrahepatic portosystemic shunt as a form of treatment for portal hypertension: indications and contraindications. Adv Intern Med 1997;42:485.

Carreras E et al: Hepatic veno-occlusive disease after bone marrow transplant. Blood Rev 1993;7:43.

Dilawari JB et al: Hepatic outflow obstruction (Budd-Chiari syndrome). Experience with 177 patients and a review of the literature. Medicine 1994;73:21.

Gentil-Kocher S et al: Budd-Chiari syndrome in children: Report of 22 cases. J Pediatr 1988;113:30.

Hassall E: Nonsurgical treatments for portal hypertension in children. Gastrointest Endosc Clin North Am 1994;4:223.

Price MR et al: Management of esophageal varices in children by endoscopic variceal ligation. J Pediatr Surg 1996;31:1056.

HEPATOMA

Essentials of Diagnosis & Typical Features

- Abdominal enlargement and pain, weight loss, anemia.
- Hepatomegaly with or without a definable mass.
- Laparotomy and tissue biopsy.

General Considerations

Primary epithelial neoplasms of the liver represent 0.2–5.8% of all malignant conditions in children. After Wilms' tumor and neuroblastoma, hepatomas are the third most common intra-abdominal cancer. The incidence is higher in Southeast Asia, where childhood cirrhosis is more common. There are two basic morphologic types with certain clinical and prognostic differences. Hepatoblastoma predominates in male infants and children, with most cases appearing before age 3. Most lesions are found in the right lobe of the liver. Pathologic differentiation from hepatocarcinoma may be difficult. Hepatocarcinoma, the other major malignant tumor of the liver, occurs more frequently after age 3. This type of neoplasm carries a poorer prognosis than hepatoblastoma and causes more abdominal discomfort. Patients with chronic hepatitis B, cirrhosis, glycogen storage disease type I, tyrosinemia, or α_1-antitrypsin deficiency have an increased risk for hepatic adenoma and carcinoma. The late development of hepatoma in patients treated with androgens for de Toni-Fanconi

Table 20–6. Treatment of complications of portal hypertension.

Complication	Diagnosis	Treatment[1]
Bleeding esophageal varices	Endoscopic verification of variceal bleeding	Endosclerosis or variceal ligation. Octreotide, 30 µg/m^2/h IV Pediatric Sengstaken-Blakemore tube. Surgical variceal ligation, selective venous embolization, TIPS, OLT. Propranolol may be useful to prevent recurrent bleeding.
Ascites	Clinical examination (fluid wave, shifting dullness), abdominal ultrasonography	Sodium restriction (1–2 mEq/kg/d), spironolactone (3–5 mg/kg/d), furosemide (1–2 mg/kg/d), IV albumin (0.5–1 g/kg per dose), paracentesis, peritoneovenous (LeVeen) shunt, TIPS, surgical portosystemic shunt, OLT.[2]
Hepatic encephalopathy	Abnormal neurologic examination, elevated plasma ammonia	Protein restriction (0.5–1 g/kg/d), IV glucose (6–8 mg/kg/min), neomycin (2–4 g/m^2 BSA PO in 4 doses), lactulose (1 mL/kg per dose [up to 30 mL] every 4–6 h PO), plasmapheresis, hemodialysis, OLT.[2]
Hypersplenism	Low WBC count, platelets, and/or hemoglobin. Splenomegaly.	No intervention, partial splenic embolization, TIPS, surgical portosystemic shunt, OLT. Splenectomy may worsen variceal bleeding.

[1]TIPS = transjugular intrahepatic portosystemic shunt, OLT = orthotopic liver transplantation, BSA = body surface area.
[2]In order of sequential management.

syndrome and aplastic anemia must also be kept in mind. The increased use of anabolic steroids by body-conscious adolescents poses a risk of hepatic neoplasia. An interesting aspect of primary epithelial neoplasms of the liver has been the increased incidence of associated anomalies and unusual conditions found in these children. Virilization has been reported as a consequence of gonadotropin activity of the tumor. Feminization with bilateral gynecomastia may occur in association with high estradiol levels in blood, the latter a consequence of increased aromatization of circulating androgens by the liver. Leydig cell hyperplasia without spermatogenesis is found on testicular biopsy. Hemihypertrophy, congenital absence of the kidney, macroglossia, and Meckel's diverticulum have been found in association with hepatocarcinoma.

Clinical Findings

A noticeable increase in abdominal girth with or without pain is the most constant feature of the history. A parent may note a "bulge" in the upper abdomen or report feeling a hard mass. Constitutional symptoms (anorexia, fatigue, fever, chills, etc) may be present. A teenage male may complain of gynecomastia.

A. Symptoms and Signs: Weight loss, pallor, and abdominal pain associated with a large abdomen are common. Physical examination reveals hepatomegaly with or without a definite tumor mass, usually to the right of the midline. In the absence of cirrhosis, signs of chronic liver disease are usually absent. However, evidence of virilization or feminization in prepubertal children may be noted.

B. Laboratory Findings: Normal liver function tests are the rule. Anemia is frequently seen, especially in cases of hepatoblastoma. Cystathioninuria has been reported. Alpha-fetoprotein levels are often elevated, especially in hepatoblastoma. Elevated estradiol levels are sometimes seen. Final tissue diagnosis is best obtained at laparotomy, although ultrasound- or CT-guided needle biopsy of the liver mass can be used.

C. Imaging: Ultrasonography, CT, and MRI are useful for diagnosis and for following tumor response to therapy. A scintigraphic study of bone and lung and selective angiography are generally part of the preoperative workup to evaluate metastatic disease.

Differential Diagnosis

In the absence of a palpable mass, the differential diagnosis is that of hepatomegaly with or without anemia or jaundice. Hematologic and nutritional conditions should be ruled out, as well as HBV and HCV infection, α_1-antitrypsin deficiency disease, lipid storage diseases, histiocytosis X, glycogen storage disease, tyrosinemia, congenital hepatic fibrosis, hepatic abscess (pyogenic or amebic), cysts, adenoma, focal nodular hyperplasia, inflammatory pseudotumor, and hemangiomas. If fever is present, hepatic abscess (pyogenic or amebic) must be considered. Veno-occlusive disease and hepatic vein thrombosis are rare possibilities. Tumors in the left lobe may be mistaken for pancreatic pseudocysts.

Complications

Progressive enlargement of the tumor, abdominal discomfort, ascites, respiratory difficulty, and widespread metastases (especially to the lungs and the abdominal lymph nodes) are the rule. Rupture of the neoplastic liver and intraperitoneal hemorrhage have been reported. Progressive anemia and emaciation predispose the patient to an early septic death.

Treatment

An aggressive surgical approach has resulted in the only long-term survivals. Complete resection of the lesion offers the only chance for cure. It appears that every isolated lung metastasis should also be surgically resected. Radiotherapy and chemotherapy have been disappointing in the treatment of primary liver neoplasms, although new combinations of drugs are continually being evaluated. These modalities are also used for initial cytoreduction of tumors found to be unresectable at the time of primary surgery. Second-look celiotomy has, in some cases, allowed resection of the tumor, resulting in a reduced mortality rate. Organ transplantation has been disappointing but continues to be performed in selected patients. The survival rate may be better for those patients in whom the tumor is incidental to another disorder (tyrosinemia, biliary atresia, cirrhosis). In HBV-endemic areas, childhood HBV vaccination has reduced the incidence of hepatocellular carcinoma.

Prognosis

The survival rate if the tumor is completely removed is 90% for hepatoblastoma and 33% for hepatocellular carcinoma. Fibrolamellar oncocytic hepatocarcinoma has a more favorable prognosis. The overall survival and cure rate is less than 20%.

Chang MH et al: Universal hepatitis B vaccination in Taiwan and the incidence of hepatocellular carcinoma in children. N Engl J Med 1997;336:1855.

Newman KD: Hepatic tumors in children. Semin Pediatr Surg 1997;6:38.

Raney B: Hepatoblastoma in children: A review. J Pediatr Hematol Oncol 1997;19:418.

Stocker JT: Hepatic tumors in children. In: *Liver Disease in Children.* Suchy FJ (editor). Mosby-Year Book, 1994.

WILSON'S DISEASE (Hepatolenticular Degeneration)

Essentials of Diagnosis & Typical Features

- Acute or chronic liver disease.
- Deteriorating neurologic status.

- Kayser-Fleischer rings.
- Elevated liver copper.
- Abnormalities in levels of ceruloplasmin and serum and urine copper.

General Considerations

In Wilson's disease, the increased hepatic copper is caused by a mutation in the gene on chromosome 13 coding for a specific P-type ATPase involved in copper transport. This results in impaired bile excretion of copper and incorporation of copper into ceruloplasmin by the liver. The accumulated copper causes oxidant (free radical) damage to the liver. The disease should be considered in all children with evidence of liver disease or with suggestive neurologic signs. A family history is often present, and 25% of cases are identified by screening asymptomatic homozygous family members. The disease is autosomal recessive and occurs in 1:30,000 live births in all populations.

Clinical Findings

A. Symptoms and Signs: Hepatic involvement may be fulminant, may masquerade as chronic active liver disease, or may progress insidiously to postnecrotic cirrhosis. Findings include jaundice, hepatomegaly early in childhood, splenomegaly, Kayser-Fleischer rings, and neurologic manifestations such as tremor, dysarthria, and drooling beginning after 10 years of age. Deterioration in school performance is often the earliest neurologic expression of disease. Psychiatric symptoms may also occur. The Kayser-Fleischer rings can sometimes be detected by unaided visual inspection as a brown band at the junction of the iris and cornea, but slit-lamp examination is always necessary. Absence of Kayser-Fleischer rings does not exclude this diagnosis unless neurologic signs are present.

B. Laboratory Findings: The laboratory diagnosis is sometimes difficult. Serum ceruloplasmin levels (measured by the oxidase method) are usually less than 20 mg/dL. (Normal values are 23–43 mg/dL.) Low values, however, are seen normally in infants under 3 months of age, and in 3–5% of homozygotes the levels may be toward the lower end of the normal range (20–30 mg/dL). Serum copper levels are low, but the overlap with normal is too great for satisfactory discrimination. In acute fulminant Wilson's disease, serum copper levels are markedly elevated owing to hepatic necrosis and release of copper. The presence of anemia, hemolysis, very high serum bilirubin (> 20–30 mg/dL), and low alkaline phosphatase are characteristic of acute Wilson's disease. Urine copper excretion in children over 3 years of age is normally less than 30 mg/d; in Wilson's disease, it is greater than 190 mg/d. Finally, the tissue content of copper from a liver biopsy, normally less than 20 mg/g wet tissue, is greater than 250 mg/g in Wilson's disease.

Glycosuria, aminoaciduria, and depressed serum uric acid levels have been reported. Hemolysis and gallstones may be present; bone lesions simulating those of osteochondritis dissecans have also been found.

The coarse nodular cirrhosis and glycogen nuclei seen on liver biopsy may distinguish Wilson's disease from other types of cirrhosis. Early in the disease, vacuolation of liver cells, steatosis, and lipofuscin granules can be seen, as well as Mallory bodies. The presence of the latter in a child is strongly suggestive of Wilson's disease. Stains for copper may sometimes be negative despite high copper content in the liver. Therefore, liver copper levels must be determined on biopsy specimens.

Differential Diagnosis

During the icteric phase, acute viral hepatitis, α_1-antitrypsin deficiency, chronic active hepatitis, Indian childhood cirrhosis, and drug-induced hepatitis are the usual diagnostic possibilities. Later, other causes of cirrhosis and portal hypertension require consideration. Laboratory testing for serum ceruloplasmin, urine copper excretion, and liver copper concentration will differentiate Wilson's disease from the others. The radiocopper ceruloplasmin incorporation test is sometimes needed to differentiate Wilson's disease with a normal ceruloplasmin level from other liver disease with increased liver and urine copper values. Urinary copper excretion during penicillamine challenge may help differentiate Wilson's disease from other causes. Genetic testing may be necessary in confusing cases.

Complications

Progressive liver disease, postnecrotic cirrhosis, hepatic coma, and death are common in the untreated patient. The complications of portal hypertension (variceal hemorrhage, ascites) are poorly tolerated by these patients. Progressive degenerating central nervous system disease and terminal aspiration pneumonia are common in untreated older people. Acute hemolytic disease may result in renal impairment and profound jaundice as part of the presentation of fulminant hepatitis.

Treatment

Penicillamine, 1000–2000 mg/d orally, is the drug of choice in all cases, whether or not the patient is symptomatic. It is best to begin with 250 mg/d and increase the dose weekly by 250 mg increments. The target dose is 20 mg/kg/d. Dietary restriction of copper intake is not practical. Supplementation with zinc sulfate may reduce copper absorption. Penicillamine is continued for life, although doses may be transiently reduced at the time of surgery or early in pregnancy. Vitamin B_6 (25 mg) is given daily while on penicillamine to prevent optic neuritis. For patients who cannot tolerate penicillamine, trientine hydrochloride is effective at a dose of 1–1.5 g/d. Non-compliance with the drug regimen can lead to fulminant liver failure and death.

General treatment measures for acute hepatitis are as outlined for infectious hepatitis. Liver transplantation is indicated for all cases of acute fulminant disease, progressive hepatic decompensation despite several months of penicillamine, and severe progressive hepatic insufficiency in patients who unadvisably discontinue penicillamine therapy.

Prognosis

The prognosis of untreated Wilson's disease is poor. Without transplantation, all patients with the fulminant presentation succumb. Copper chelation reduces hepatic copper content and reverses many of the liver lesions, but it does not have a profound effect on established cirrhosis. Neurologic symptoms generally respond to therapy. All siblings should be immediately screened and homozygotes treated with copper chelation even if asymptomatic. Genetic testing is now available for family members.

DaCosta CM et al: Value of urinary copper excretion after penicillamine challenge in the diagnosis of Wilson's disease. Hepatology 1992;15:609.

Scheinberg IH, Sternlieb I: *Wilson's Disease.* Saunders, 1984.

Sokol RJ: Wilson's disease and Indian childhood cirrhosis. In: *Liver Disease in Children.* Suchy FJ (editor). Mosby-Year Book, 1994.

Sternlieb I: Perspectives on Wilson's disease. Hepatology 1990;12:1234.

Tanzi RE et al: The Wilson disease gene is a copper transporting ATPase with homology to the Menkes disease gene. Nature Genet 1993;5:344.

REYE'S SYNDROME (Encephalopathy With Fatty Degeneration of the Viscera)

Essentials of Diagnosis & Typical Features

- Prodromal upper respiratory tract infection, influenza A or B illness, or chickenpox.
- Vomiting.
- Lethargy, drowsiness progressing to semicoma.
- Elevated AST, hyperammonemia, normal or slightly elevated bilirubin, prolonged prothrombin time.
- Variable hypoglycemia.
- Microvesicular steatosis of the liver, kidneys, brain, etc.

General Considerations

The number of reported cases of Reye's syndrome is decreasing, perhaps because of a decline in the use of salicylates among younger children, who seem to be at greater risk. Varicella, influenzas A and B, echovirus 2, coxsackievirus A, and Epstein-Barr virus have been isolated from some patients. Epidemics of Reye's syndrome seem to cluster during influenza B epidemics. Salicylate use is associated with Reye's syndrome. Many apparent cases are actually caused by defects in fatty acid oxidation. The mode of onset may lead to confusion with other causes of coma, particularly toxic encephalopathy and hepatic coma.

The mechanism is thought to be damage to mitochondria caused by salicylate metabolites or some other toxin or chemical in the milieu of a viral infection. Mitochondrial dysfunction leads to elevated short-chain fatty acids and hyperammonemia as well as directly to cerebral edema.

Clinical Findings

A. Symptoms and Signs: Chickenpox or minor upper respiratory tract illness precedes the development of vomiting, irrational behavior, progressive stupor, and coma. Restlessness and convulsions may also occur. Striking physical findings are hyperpnea, irregular respirations, and dilated, sluggishly reacting pupils. Jaundice is minimal or absent. The liver may be normal or slightly enlarged. Splenomegaly is absent. A positive Babinski sign, hyperreflexia, and decorticate and decerebrate posturing are consistent with cerebral edema.

B. Laboratory Findings: Cerebrospinal fluid is acellular, and cerebrospinal fluid glucose may be low in younger patients. Cerebrospinal fluid pressure is variably elevated. The serum glucose is proportionately decreased. Moderate to severe elevations of AST, ALT, and lactate dehydrogenase are found. Serum bilirubin and alkaline phosphatase values are normal to slightly elevated. The prothrombin time is usually prolonged, and the blood ammonia is usually elevated. A mixed respiratory alkalosis and metabolic acidosis is seen. In a few cases, the blood urea nitrogen has been elevated. Hyperaminoacidemia (glutamine, alanine, lysine) and hypocitrullinemia are present.

Histopathologic changes in Reye's syndrome are most striking in the brain, liver, and kidneys, less so in the heart and pancreas. The brain shows gross cerebral edema, occasionally with evidence of herniation. Histologically, loss of neurons and fatty vacuolation around small vessels have been noted. The liver shows diffuse microvesicular steatosis with minimal inflammatory changes. Glycogen is virtually absent from the hepatocytes in biopsy specimens taken before administration of hypertonic glucose. Ultrastructural changes are mitochondrial.

The kidney changes include swelling and fatty degeneration of the proximal lobules.

C. Electroencephalography: The EEG shows diffuse slow wave activity.

Differential Diagnosis

Differentiation of Reye's syndrome from en-

LIVER & PANCREAS / 591

cephalitis, acute toxic encephalopathy, hepatic coma, or fulminant hepatitis can be made on clinical and laboratory grounds. A negative history and urine screen for ingestion of poisons and drugs, absence of cells in the cerebrospinal fluid, and absence of jaundice favor a diagnosis of Reye's syndrome. The fatty acid oxidation defects (eg, medium-chain acyl-CoA dehydrogenase deficiency) and other metabolic disorders may resemble Reye's syndrome; urine gas chromatographic analysis will help differentiate them. Liver biopsy and electron microscopy can be diagnostic and are indicated in atypical cases.

Complications

Aspiration pneumonitis and respiratory failure are common, as with any comatose patient. Most patients die of cerebral edema rather than hepatic or renal failure. Cardiac dysrhythmias may develop, as may inappropriate vasopressin excretion, diabetes insipidus, and acute pancreatitis.

Treatment

Treatment is supportive. A nasogastric tube, Foley catheter, and arterial and central venous pressure lines should be inserted immediately. Mechanical ventilation may become necessary if the patient reaches grade 3 coma (agitated delirium, combativeness). Intracranial pressure should be monitored directly and kept below 15–20 mm Hg, and systemic blood pressure should be kept high enough to maintain cerebral perfusion pressure above 45–50 mm Hg. Hyperventilation, mannitol infusions (0.5–1 g/kg every 4 hours), barbiturates, or ventricular drainage is used to lower intracranial pressure. Maintenance fluids using 10% glucose should be given at a rate sufficient to produce a urine flow of 1–1.5 mL/kg/h. Careful attention to central venous pressure is needed when using hyperosmolar agents. Vitamin K_1, 3–5 mg intramuscularly, should be administered. Hypothermia (30–33 °C) and pharmacologic doses of intravenous pentobarbital (1–3 mg/kg/h) to maintain a serum level of 2.5–4 mg/dL have been used to decrease body (brain) metabolic needs during the period of uncontrolled intracranial pressure.

Prognosis

At least 70% of these patients survive. The prognosis is related to the depth of coma and the peak ammonia level on admission. Because Reye's syndrome is less common now, many patients are diagnosed only when comatose. Severe neurologic residuals are common in younger children (< 2 years) who recover from prolonged grade 3–4 coma (Lovejoy). All patients should be screened for fatty acid oxidation and other metabolic defects.

Heubi JE et al: Grade I Reye's syndrome: Outcome and predictors of progression to deeper coma grades. N Engl J Med 1984;311:1539.

Heubi JE et al: Reye's syndrome: Current concepts. Hepatology 1987;7:155.
Partin JC: Reye's syndrome. In: Liver Disease in Children. Suchy FJ (editor). Mosby-Year Book, 1994.
Shaywitz BA, Rothstein P, Venes JL: Monitoring and management of increased intracranial pressure in Reye's syndrome: Results in 29 patients. Pediatrics 1980; 66:198.

LIVER TRANSPLANTATION

Orthotopic liver transplantation is no longer experimental. Children with end-stage liver disease, acute fulminant hepatic failure, or complications from metabolic liver disorders should be considered for liver transplantation. Recent advances in immunosuppression (eg, introduction of cyclosporine and tacrolimus, use of monoclonal antibodies against T cells), better candidate selection, improvements in surgical techniques, and experience in postoperative management have contributed to improved results.

The major indications for childhood transplantation are (1) a failed Kasai operation or decompensated cirrhosis caused by extrahepatic biliary atresia, (2) α_1-antitrypsin deficiency, (3) posthepatitic (autoimmune chronic active hepatitis, hepatitis B or C disease) cirrhosis, (4) tyrosinemia, (5) Crigler-Najjar syndrome type I, (6) Wilson's disease, (7) acute fulminant hepatic failure when recovery is unlikely, (8) primary sclerosing cholangitis, and (9) cases in which the consequences of chronic cholestasis severely impair the patient's quality of life. Children should be referred early for evaluation because the limiting factor for success is the small donor pool. Pared-down adult livers and organs from living related donors are being used in children in many centers. In general, 75–85% of children survive at least 2–5 years after transplantation, with long-term survival expected to be comparable. Lifetime immunosuppression therapy using combinations of cyclosporine, tacrolimus, prednisone, or azathioprine, with its incumbent risks, appears necessary to prevent rejection. The overall quality of life for children with a transplanted liver appears to be excellent. The lifelong risk of Epstein-Barr virus-induced lymphoproliferative disease is increased.

Broelsch CE et al: Application of reduced-size liver transplants as split grafts, auxiliary orthotopic grafts, and living related segmental transplants. Ann Surg 1990; 212:368.
de Ville de Goyet J: Split liver transplantation in Europe—1988 to 1993. Transplantation 1995;59:1371.
Emond JC et al: Improved results of living-related liver transplantation with routine application in a pediatric program. Transplantation 1993;55:835.
Rand EB et al: Measles vaccination after orthotopic liver transplantation. J Pediatr 1993;123:87.
Ryckman FC et al: Liver transplantation in children. In:

Liver Disease in Children. Suchy FJ (editor). Mosby-Year Book, 1994.

Whitington PF, Balistreri WF: Liver transplantation in pediatrics: Indications, contraindications, and pretransplant management. J Pediatr 1991;118:169.

Zitelli BJ et al: Changes in life-style after liver transplantation. Pediatrics 1988;82:173.

PANCREAS

ACUTE PANCREATITIS

Essentials of Diagnosis & Typical Features

- Epigastric abdominal pain radiating to the back.
- Nausea and vomiting.
- Elevated serum amylase and lipase.
- Evidence of pancreatic inflammation by CT or ultrasound.

General Considerations

Most cases of acute pancreatitis are the result of drugs, viral infections, systemic diseases, or abdominal trauma; more than 20% are idiopathic. Other causes of obstruction of pancreatic flow include stones, choledochal cyst, tumors of the duodenum, pancreas divisum, and ascariasis. Acute pancreatitis has been seen sulfasalazine, thiazides, valproic acid, azathioprine, mercaptopurine, asparaginase, antiretroviral drugs (especially ddI), high-dose corticosteroids, and other drugs. It may also occur in cystic fibrosis, systemic lupus erythematosus, α_1-antitrypsin deficiency, diabetes, Crohn's disease, glycogen storage disease type I, hyperlipidemia types I and V, hyperparathyroidism, Schönlein-Henoch purpura, Reye's syndrome, organic acidopathies, Kawasaki disease, or chronic renal failure; during rapid refeeding in cases of malnutrition; and in familial cases. Alcohol-induced pancreatitis should be considered in the teenage patient.

Clinical Findings

A. Symptoms and Signs: An acute onset of persistent (hours to days), moderate to severe upper abdominal and midabdominal pain occasionally referred to the back, with vomiting and fever, is the common presenting picture. The abdomen is tender but not rigid, and bowel sounds are diminished, suggesting peritoneal irritation. Abdominal distention is common in infants and younger children. Jaundice is unusual. Ascites may be noted, and a left-sided pleural effusion is present in some. Periumbilical and flank bruising indicate hemorrhagic pancreatitis.

B. Laboratory Findings: Leukocytosis and an elevated serum amylase ($> 1\frac{1}{2}$–2 times normal) should be expected early, except in infants under 6 months of age who may have hypoamylasemia. Serum lipase is elevated and persists longer than serum amylase. The immunoreactive trypsinogen test may also be of value. Pancreatic amylase isoenzyme determination can help differentiate nonpancreatic causes (salivary, intestinal, tubo-ovarian, etc) of serum amylase elevation. Hyperglycemia (serum glucose > 300 mg/dL), hypocalcemia, falling hematocrit, rising blood urea nitrogen, hypoxemia, and acidosis may all occur in severe cases and imply a poor prognosis.

C. Imaging: Plain x-ray films of the abdomen may show a localized ileus (sentinel loop). Ultrasonography shows decreased echodensity of the gland in comparison to the left lobe of the liver. Pseudocyst formation can also be seen early in the course. CT scanning is better for detecting pancreatic phlegmon or abscess formation. Endoscopic retrograde or perhaps magnetic resonance pancreatography may be useful in confirming patency of the main pancreatic duct in cases of abdominal trauma, in recurrent acute pancreatitis, or in revealing stones, ductal strictures, and pancreas divisum.

Differential Diagnosis

Other causes of acute upper abdominal pain include lesions of the stomach, duodenum, liver, and biliary system; acute gastroenteritis or atypical appendicitis; pneumonia; volvulus; intussusception; and nonaccidental trauma.

Complications

Complications early in the disease include shock caused by fluid and electrolyte disturbances, ileus, acute respiratory distress syndrome, and hypocalcemic tetany. Hypervolemia is seen between the third and fifth days, at which time renal tubular necrosis may occur. The gastrointestinal, neurologic, musculoskeletal, hepatobiliary, dermatologic, and hematologic systems may also be involved.

Later, 5–20% of patients develop a pseudocyst heralded by recurrence of abdominal pain and rise in the serum amylase. Up to 60–70% of these will resolve spontaneously. Infection, hemorrhage, rupture, fistulization, or obstruction may occur. Phlegmon formation is frequently seen (30–50%) and may extend from the gland into the retroperitoneum or into the lesser sac. Most regress, but some require drainage. Infection in this inflammatory mass is a constant threat. Pancreatic abscess formation is rare (3–5%) and develops 2–3 weeks after the initial insult. Fever, leukocytosis, and pain occur; diagnosis is by ultrasound or CT scanning.

Chronic pancreatitis, exocrine or endocrine pancreatic insufficiency, and pancreatic lithiasis are rare sequelae of acute pancreatitis.

Treatment

Medical management includes rest, gastric suction, fluids, electrolyte replacement, and blood or colloid as needed. Pain should be controlled with opioids. Oxygen may be required if desaturation occurs. An H_2 blocker helps to maintain gastric neutrality at a pH greater than 4.5. Nutrition is provided by the parenteral route. Broad-spectrum antibiotic coverage is used only in severe hemorrhagic pancreatitis. Drugs known to produce acute pancreatitis should be discontinued. Recurrence of pain after oral feedings may be prevented by giving pancreatic enzymes with the meal.

Surgical treatment is reserved for traumatic disruption of the gland, intraductal stone, other anatomic obstructive lesions, and unresolved or infected pseudocysts or abscesses. Early endoscopic decompression of the biliary system reduces the morbidity associated with biliary pancreatitis.

Prognosis

In the pediatric age group, the prognosis is surprisingly good with conservative management. The mortality rate is 5–10% in patients treated by operation and 1% in those treated medically. The morbidity rate is high with surgery as a result of fistula formation.

Steinberg W, Tenner S: Acute pancreatitis. N Engl J Med 1994;330:1198.

Young CY et al: Pancreatitis in children: Experience with 43 cases. Eur J Pediatr 1996;155:458.

Weizman Z, Durie PR: Acute pancreatitis in childhood. J Pediatr 1988;113:24.

CHRONIC PANCREATITIS

Chronic pancreatitis is differentiated from acute pancreatitis in that the pancreas is structurally or functionally abnormal before and after an attack.

The causes include stenotic lesions of the ampulla hepatopancreatica, strictures of the pancreatic ducts, intraductal stones, or persisting pseudocyst following acute pancreatitis. The role of pancreas divisum in chronic pancreatitis remains controversial. Chronic disease rarely follows acute nontraumatic pancreatitis. Choledochal and duplication cysts can be an unrecognized cause of chronic pancreatitis. Hyperlipidemias (types I and V), hyperparathyroidism, familial chronic relapsing pancreatitis, and cystic fibrosis should be considered. Alcohol abuse is the leading cause in adults in the United States.

Clinical Findings

The diagnosis often is delayed by the nonspecific symptoms and the lack of persistent laboratory abnormalities.

A. Symptoms and Signs: There is usually a history of recurrent upper abdominal pain of variable severity but prolonged (1–6 days) duration. Radiation of the pain into the back is a frequent complaint. Fever and vomiting are not common in the chronic form. Steatorrhea and symptoms of diabetes may develop later in the course of this disease, and malnutrition secondary to failure of pancreatic exocrine secretions may also occur.

B. Laboratory Findings: The serum amylase and lipase are usually elevated during early acute attacks but are often normal later. Pancreatic insufficiency and reduced volume and bicarbonate response may be found at duodenal intubation after intravenous administration of synthetic cholecystokinin (0.02 mg/kg) and secretin (2 U/kg). A threefold increase above normal serum amylase is considered a positive test for obstruction.

Blood lipids and urinary amino acids are elevated in familial forms of the disease associated with hyperlipoproteinemia and should be studied in all cases. A mutation of the cationic trypsinogen gene is the cause of hereditary pancreatitis. Elevated blood glucose and glycohemoglobin levels and glycosuria are frequently found in protracted disease. Sweat chloride should be checked for cystic fibrosis and serum calcium for hyperparathyroidism.

C. Imaging: X-rays of the abdomen may show pancreatic calcifications in up to 30%. Ultrasound or CT examination demonstrates pancreatic enlargement, ductal dilation, and calculi in up to 80%. ERCP is the procedure of choice to establish the diagnosis. Pancreatograms show ductal dilation, stones, strictures, or stenotic segments.

Differential Diagnosis

Other causes of recurrent abdominal pain must be considered. Specific causes of pancreatitis such as hyperparathyroidism, systemic lupus erythematosus, infectious disease, and ductal obstruction by tumors, stones, or helminths must be excluded by appropriate tests.

Complications

Disabling abdominal pain, steatorrhea, nutritional deprivation, pancreatic pseudocysts, and diabetes are the most frequent long-term complications. Pancreatic carcinoma occurs in 4% of patients within 20 years of their diagnosis.

Treatment

Medical management of acute attacks is indicated (see Acute Pancreatitis, above). If ductal obstruction is strongly suspected, endoscopic therapy (balloon dilation, stenting, stone removal, sphincterotomy) should be pursued. Biliary sphincterotomy and biopsy are recommended even when obvious obstruction is not found. Relapses seem to occur in most patients. Orally ingested pancreatic enzymes at mealtime may reduce pain episodes in some patients.

The daily injection of a somatostatin analogue (octreotide acetate) has shown promise in relieving pain episodes and decreasing the serum amylase of some patients. Antioxidant therapy is being investigated. Pseudocysts may be marsupialized to the surface or drained into the stomach or into a loop of jejunum in those failing to regress spontaneously. Experience in pediatric patients indicates that lateral pancreaticojejunostomy can reduce pain in patients with a dilated pancreatic duct and may prevent or delay progression of functional pancreatic impairment.

Prognosis

In the absence of a correctable lesion, the prognosis is not good. Disabling episodes of pain, pancreatic insufficiency, and diabetes may ensue. Narcotic addiction and suicide are risks in teenagers with disabling disease.

Crombleholme TM et al: The modified Puestow procedure for chronic relapsing pancreatitis in childhood. J Pediatr Surg 1990;25:749.
Little JM et al: Chronic pancreatitis beginning in childhood and adolescence. Arch Surg 1992;127:90.
Steer ML et al: Chronic pancreatitis. N Engl J Med 1995;332:1482.

GASTROINTESTINAL & HEPATOBILIARY MANIFESTATIONS OF CYSTIC FIBROSIS

Cystic fibrosis is a disease with protean manifestations. Although pulmonary and pancreatic involvement dominates the clinical picture for most patients (see Chapter 19), a variety of other organs can be involved. Table 20–7 lists the important gastrointestinal, pancreatic, and hepatobiliary conditions that may affect cystic fibrosis patients along with their clinical findings, incidence, most useful diagnostic studies, and preferred treatment.

Colombo C et al: Hepatobiliary disease in cystic fibrosis. Semin Liver Dis 1994;14:259.
Dodge JA, Macpherson C: Colonic strictures in cystic fibrosis. J R Soc Med 1995;88(Suppl 25):3.
Littlewood JM: Cystic fibrosis: Gastrointestinal complications. Br Med Bull 1992;48:847.

SYNDROMES WITH PANCREATIC EXOCRINE INSUFFICIENCY

Several syndromes are associated with exocrine pancreatic insufficiency. Clinically, the patients present with a history of failure to thrive, diarrhea, fatty stools, and an absence of respiratory symptoms. Laboratory findings include a normal sweat chloride, with low to absent pancreatic lipase, amylase, and trypsin on duodenal intubation. Each disorder has several associated clinical features that aid in the dif-

ferential diagnosis. In Schwachman's syndrome, pancreatic exocrine hypoplasia with widespread fatty replacement of the glandular acinar tissue is associated with neutropenia because of maturational arrest of the granulocyte series. Metaphysial dysostosis and an elevated fetal hemoglobin are common, while immunoglobulin deficiency and hepatic dysfunction are also reported. CT examination of the pancreas demonstrates the widespread fatty replacement. Serum immunoreactive trypsinogen levels are extremely low.

Other causes of exocrine pancreatic insufficiency include (1) exocrine pancreatic insufficiency with aplastic alae, aplasia cutis, deafness (Johanson-Blizzard syndrome); (2) exocrine pancreatic insufficiency with sideroblastic anemia, developmental delay, seizures, and liver dysfunction (Pearson bone marrow pancreas syndrome); (3) exocrine pancreatic insufficiency associated with duodenal atresia or stenosis; (4) exocrine pancreatic insufficiency associated with malnutrition; and (5) exocrine pancreatic insufficiency associated with pancreatic hypoplasia or agenesis.

The complications and sequelae of deficient pancreatic enzyme secretion are malnutrition, diarrhea, and growth failure. The degree of steatorrhea may lessen with age. Intragastric lipolysis primarily caused by lingual lipase may compensate in patients with low or absent pancreatic function. In Schwachman's syndrome, the major sequela seems to be short stature. Increased numbers of infections may be the result of chronic neutropenia. Neutrophil mobility is also impaired in many patients. In addition, an increased incidence of leukemia has been noted in these patients.

Pancreatic enzyme replacement therapy and fat-soluble vitamin replacement are required in most patients. The prognosis appears to be good for those able to survive the increased number of bacterial infections early in life and those patients without severe associated defects.

Cleghorn GJ et al: Exocrine pancreatic dysfunction in malnourished Australian aboriginal children. Med J Aust 1991;154:45.
Lerner A et al: Pancreatic diseases in children. Pediatr Clin North Am 1996;43:125.
Mack DR et al: Shwachman syndrome: Exocrine pancreatic dysfunction and variable phenotypic expression. Gastroenterolgy 1996;111:1593.
McShane MA et al: Pearson syndrome and mitochondrial encephalomyopathy in a patient with a deletion of mtDNA. Am J Hum Genet 1991;48:39.
Sarles J, Guys JM, Sauniere JF: Pancreatic function and congenital duodenal abnormalities. J Pediatr Gastroenterol Nutr 1993;16:284.
Wright NM et al: Permanent neonatal diabetes mellitus and pancreatic exocrine insufficiency resulting from congenital pancreatic agenesis. Am J Dis Child 1993;47:607.

Table 20–7. Gastrointestinal and hepatobiliary manifestations of cystic fibrosis.

Organ	Condition	Symptoms	Age at Presentation	Incidence	Diagnostic Evaluation	Management
Esophagus	Gastroesophageal reflux, esophagitis	Pyrosis, dysphagia, epigastric pain, hematemesis	All ages	10–20%	Endoscopy and biopsy, overnight pH study	H_2 blockers, antacids, carafate, omeprazole, cisapride, surgical antireflux procedure
	Varices	Hematemesis, melena	Childhood and adolescents	3–10%	Endoscopy, barium swallow	Endosclerosis, drugs (see text), portacaval shunt, liver transplantation
Stomach	Gastritis	Upper abdominal pain, vomiting, hematemesis	School age and older	10–25%	Endoscopy and biopsy	H_2 blockers, antacids, carafate, omeprazole, cisapride
	Hiatal hernia	Reflux symptoms (see above), epigastric pain	School age and older	3–5%	Endoscopy: barium swallow	As above. Surgery in some.
Intestine	Meconium ileus	Abdominal distention, bilious emesis	Neonate	10–15%	X-ray studies, plain abdominal films; contrast enema shows microcolon	Dislodgement of obstruction with Gastrografin enema. Surgery if unsuccessful or if case complicated by atresia, perforation, or volvulus.
	Distal intestinal obstruction syndrome	Abdominal pain, acute and recurrent; distention; occasional vomiting	Any age, usually school age through adolescence	10–15%	Palpable mass in right lower quadrant, x-ray studies	Gastrografin enema, intestinal lavage solution, diet, bulk laxatives, adjustment of pancreatic enzyme intake
	Fibrosing colonopathy	As above. History of high enzyme dosage.	≥3 years	< 1%	Barium enema or UGI/SBFT, abdominal ultrasound, or CT	Reduce pancreatic enzyme dose to < 2000 units of lipase/kg per dose if indicated. Surgical resection may be necessary.
	Intussusception	Acute, intermittent abdominal pain; distention; emesis	Infants through adolescence	1–3%	X-ray studies, barium enema	Reduction by barium or air enema or surgery if needed, diet, bulk laxatives. Adjustment of pancreatic enzyme intake.
	Rectal prolapse	Anal discomfort, rectal bleeding	Infants and children to age 4–5 years	15–25%	Visual mass protruding from anus	Manual reduction, adjustment of pancreatic enzyme dosage, reassurance as problem resolves by age 3–5 years
	Carbohydrate intolerance	Abdominal pain, flatulence, continued diarrhea with adequate enzyme replacement therapy	Any age	10–25%	Intestinal mucosal biopsy and disaccharidase analysis. Breath hydrogen after lactose load.	Reduce lactose intake; reduction of gastric hyperacidity if mucosa shows partial villous atrophy. Beware concurrent celiac disease or *Giardia* infection.
Pancreas	Total exocrine insufficiency	Diarrhea, steatorrhea, malnutrition, failure to thrive. Specific fat-soluble vitamin deficiency states.	Neonate through infancy	85–90%	72-hour fecal fat evaluation	Pancreatic enzyme replacement, may need elemental formula, fat-soluble vitamin and vitamin E supplements

(continued)

Table 20–7. Gastrointestinal and hepatobiliary manifestations of cystic fibrosis. (continued)

Organ	Condition	Symptoms	Age at Presentation	Incidence	Diagnostic Evaluation	Management
Pancreas (cont'd)	Pancreatic sufficiency (partial exocrine insufficiency)	Occasional diarrhea, mild growth delay	Any age	10–15%	72-hours fecal fat evaluation, direct pancreatic function tests	Pancreatic enzyme replacement in selected patients. Fat-soluble vitamin supplements as indicated by biochemical evaluation.
	Pancreatitis	Recurrent abdominal pain, vomiting	Older children through adolescence. Primarily in patients with pancreatic sufficiency.	0.1%	Increased serum lipase and amylase, pancreatic provocative test, endoscopic pancreatogram	Addition of pancreatic enzymes to feeds, endoscopic removal of sludge or stones if present, endoscopic papillotomy
	Diabetes	Weight loss, polyuria, polydipsia	Older children through adolescence	5–7%	Glucose tolerance test and insulin levels	Diet, insulin
Liver	Steatosis	Hepatomegaly	Neonates and infants, but can be seen at all ages	20–60%	Liver biopsy	Improved nutrition, replacement of pancreatic enzymes and vitamins
	Focal biliary cirrhosis	Hepatomegaly	Infants and older patients Prevalence increases with age.	20–70%	Liver biopsy	As above. Taurine supplements (still experimental), ursodeoxycholic acid (unproved benefit).
	Multilobular biliary cirrhosis	Hepatosplenomegaly, hematemesis from esophageal varices; hypersplenism; jaundice, ascites late in course	School age through adolescence	7–13%	Liver biopsy, endoscopy	Improved nutrition, ursodeoxycholic acid (unproved benefit), endosclerosis of varices, splenic embolization, liver transplantation
	Neonatal jaundice	Cholestatic jaundice hepatomegaly; often seen with meconium ileus	Neonates	0.1–1%	Sweat chloride test, liver biopsy	Nutritional support, special formula with medium-chain triglyceride-containing oil, pancreatic enzyme replacement
Gallbladder	Microgallbladder	None	Congenital—present at any age	30%	Ultrasound or hepatobiliary scintigraphy	None needed
	Cholelithiasis	Recurrent abdominal pain, rarely jaundice	School age through adolescence	1%	Ultrasound	Surgery if symptomatic and low risk, trial of cholelitholytics in others
Extrahepatic bile ducts	Intraluminal obstruction (sludge, stones, tumor)	Jaundice, hepatomegaly, abdominal pain	Neonates, then older children through adolescence	Rare in neonates (< 0.1%)	Ultrasound and hepatobiliary scintigraphy, endoscopic cholangiography	Surgery in neonates, endoscopic intervention in older patients or surgery
	Extraluminal obstruction (intrapancreatic compression, tumor)	As above	As above	Rare (< 1%)	As above	Surgical biliary drainage procedure or biliary stent placement endoscopically
	Stenosis	As above	As above	1–40%	As above	Endoscopic balloon dilation, surgical drainage

ISOLATED EXOCRINE PANCREATIC ENZYME DEFECT

Normal premature infants and most newborns produce little, if any, pancreatic amylase following meals or exogenous hormonal stimulation. This temporary physiologic insufficiency may persist for the first 3–6 months of life and be responsible for diarrhea when complex carbohydrates (cereals) are introduced into their diet.

Congenital pancreatic lipase deficiency and congenital colipase deficiency are extremely rare disorders, causing diarrhea and variable malnutrition with malabsorption of dietary fat and fat-soluble vitamins. The sweat chloride is normal, and neutropenia is absent. Treatment is oral replacement of pancreatic enzymes and a low-fat diet or formula containing medium-chain triglycerides.

Exocrine pancreatic insufficiency of proteolytic enzymes (trypsinogen, trypsin, chymotrypsin, etc) is caused by enterokinase deficiency, a duodenal mucosal enzyme required for activation of the pancreatic proenzymes. These patients present with malnutrition associated with hypoproteinemia and edema but are free of respiratory symptoms and have a normal sweat test. They respond to pancreatic enzyme replacement therapy and feeding formulas that contain a casein hydrolysate (eg, Nutramigen, Pregestimil).

Gaskin KJ: Hereditary disorders of the pancreas. In: *Pediatric Gastrointestinal Disease: Pathophysiology, Diagnosis, Management,* 2nd ed. Walker WA et al (editors). Mosby-Year Book, 1996.

Mann NS, Mann SK: Enterokinase. Proc Soc Exp Biol Med 1994;206:114.

PANCREATIC TUMORS

Pancreatic tumors, whether benign or malignant, are rare lesions. They most often arise from ductal or acinar epithelium (malignant adenocarcinoma) or from islet (endocrine) components within the gland, such as the benign insulinoma (adenoma) derived from B cells. Other pancreatic tumors also originate from these pluripotential endocrine cells (gastrinoma, VIPoma, glucagonoma). These malignant lesions produce diverse symptoms, because they release biologically active polypeptides from this ectopic location. The clinical features of these tumors are summarized in Table 20–8. The differential diagnosis of these abdominal tumors includes Wilms' tumor, neuroblastoma, and malignant lymphoma. In older children, endoscopic ultrasonography can aid in localizing these tumors.

Jaksic T et al: A 20-year review of pediatric pancreatic tumors. J Pediatr Surg 1992;27:1315.

Weber HC et al: Diagnosis and management of Zollinger-Ellison syndrome. Semin Gastrointest Dis 1995;6:79.

Wynick D, Williams SJ, Bloom SR: Symptomatic secondary hormone syndromes in patients with established malignant pancreatic endocrine tumors. N Engl J Med 1988;319:605.

Table 20–8. Pancreatic tumors.

	Age	Major Findings	Diagnosis[1]	Treatment	Associated Conditions
Insulinoma	Any age	Hypoglycemia, seizures; high serum insulin; abdominal pain and mass infrequent	Ultrasound, CT scan, MRI	Surgery	
Adenocarcinoma	Any age	Epigastric pain, mass weight loss, anemia, biliary obstruction	Ultrasound, CT scan, MRI	Surgery	Hereditary (calcific) pancreatitis
Gastrinoma	Over age 5–8 years	Male sex, gastric hypersecretion, peptic symptoms, multiple ulcers, gastrointestinal bleeding, anemia, diarrhea	Elevated fasting gastrin and postsecretin suppression test (> 300 pg/mL), CT scan, MRI, laparotomy	H$_2$ blockers, omeprazole, surgical resection, total gastrectomy	Zollinger-Ellison syndrome, multiple endocrine neoplasia syndrome type I, neurofibromatosis
VIPoma	Any age	Secretory diarrhea, hypokalemia, weight loss	Elevated vasoactive intestinal polypeptide (VIP) levels; sometimes, elevated serum gastrin and pancreatic polypeptide	Surgery, octreotide	
Glucagonoma	Older patients	Necrolytic rash, diarrhea, anemia, thrombotic events	Elevated glucagon, gastrin, VIP	Surgery	

[1]CT = computed tomography, MRI = magnetic resonance imaging.

REFERENCES

Lebenthal E (editor): Pediatric gastroenterology. (Two parts.) Pediatr Clin North Am 1996;43:1.

Roy CC, Silverman A, Alagille D (editors): *Pediatric Clinical Gastroenterology,* 4th ed. Mosby-Year Book, 1995.

Suchy FJ (editor): *Liver Disease in Children.* Mosby-Year Book, 1994.

Walker WA et al (editors): *Pediatric Gastrointestinal Disease: Pathophysiology, Diagnosis, Management,* 2nd ed. Mosby-Year Book, 1996.

Kidney & Urinary Tract

21

Gary M. Lum, MD

EVALUATION OF THE KIDNEY & URINARY TRACT

HISTORY

When renal disease is suspected, the history should include (1) family history of cystic disease, hereditary nephritis, deafness, dialysis, or renal transplantation; (2) preceding acute or chronic illnesses (eg, urinary tract infection, pharyngitis, impetigo, or endocarditis); (3) rashes or joint pains; (4) growth delay or failure to thrive; (5) polyuria, polydipsia, enuresis, urinary frequency, or dysuria; (6) hematuria or discolored urine; (7) pain (abdominal, costovertebral angle, or flank) or trauma; (8) sudden weight gain or edema; and (9) drug or toxin exposure. In the newborn or small infant, obtain birth history and information regarding prenatal ultrasonographic studies, birth asphyxia, Apgar scores, oligohydramnios, dysmorphic features, abdominal masses, voiding patterns, anomalous development, and umbilical artery catheterization.

PHYSICAL EXAMINATION

Important aspects of the physical examination include the height, weight, skin lesions (café-au-lait or ash leaf spots), pallor, edema, or skeletal deformities. Anomalies of the ears, eyes, or external genitalia may be associated with renal disease. The blood pressure should be measured in a quiet setting. The cuff should cover two-thirds of the child's upper arm, and peripheral pulses should be noted. An ultrasonic device is useful for measurements in infants. The abdomen should be palpated, with attention to the kidneys, abdominal masses, musculature, and the presence of ascites.

LABORATORY EVALUATION OF RENAL FUNCTION

Urinalysis

Commercially available dipsticks can be used to screen for the presence of red blood cells, hemoglobin, leukocytes, nitrites, and protein and to approximate pH. Positive results should be checked by microscopy, as should any suspicion of crystalluria. Significant proteinuria (> 150 mg/d) detected by dipstick should be quantitated in the laboratory.

Serum Analysis

The standard indicators of renal function are serum levels of urea nitrogen and creatinine; their ratio is normally about 10:1. The ratio may increase in cases where renal perfusion or urine flow is decreased (as in urinary tract obstruction), because serum urea nitrogen levels are more affected by these and other factors (eg, nitrogen intake, catabolism, use of corticosteroids) than are creatinine levels. The most reliable indicator of glomerular function is the serum level of creatinine. For example, serum creatinine increasing from 0.5 mg/dL to 1 mg/dL represents a 50% decrease in glomerular filtration rate. Small children should have serum creatinine levels well under 0.8 mg/dL, and only the larger adolescents should have levels exceeding 1 mg/dL. Laboratory results should be compared with age-matched control values. Less precise but nonetheless important indicators of the presence of renal disease are abnormalities of serum electrolytes, pH, calcium, phosphorus, magnesium, albumin, or complement.

Measurement of Glomerular Filtration Rate (GFR)

The determination of GFR is of paramount importance in the evaluation of suspected renal disease or in the serial follow-up of the child with established renal insufficiency.

The endogenous creatinine clearance (C_{cr}) in milliliters per minute gives an estimate of the GFR. A 24-hour urine collection is usually obtained; however, in small children from whom collection is difficult, a 12-hour daytime specimen, collected when urine flow rate is greatest, is acceptable. The procedure for collecting a quantitative urine specimen should be carefully explained so that the parent or patient understands fully the rationale of (1) first emptying the bladder (discarding that urine) and noting the time; and (2) putting all urine subsequently voided into the collection receptacle, including the last void, 12 or 24 hours later. Reliability of the 24-hour collection can be approximated by measurement of the total 24-hour creatinine excretion in the specimen. Total daily creatinine excretion (creatinine index) should be in the range of 14–20 mg/kg. If the creatinine index does not fall within this range, collections may be either inadequate or excessive. Calculation by the following formula requires measurements of plasma creatinine (P_{cr}) in mg/mL, urine creatinine (U_{cr}) in mg/mL, and urine volume (V) expressed as mL/min.

$$C_{Cr} = \frac{U_{Cr}\ V}{P_{Cr}}$$

Creatinine is a reflection of body muscle mass. Because accepted ranges of normal creatinine clearance are based on adult parameters, "correction" for size is needed to determine normal ranges in children. Clearance is "corrected" to a standard body surface area of 1.73 m^2 in the formula:

$$\text{"Corrected" } C_{Cr} = \frac{\text{Patient's } C_{Cr} \times 1.73 \text{ m}^2}{\text{Patient's body surface area}}$$

Although 80–125 mL/min/1.73 m^2 is the normal range for creatinine clearance, estimates at the lower end of this range may indicate problems.

A simple and tested formula for quick approximation of creatinine clearance incorporates use of the plasma creatinine level and the child's length in centimeters:

$$C_{Cr}\ (\text{mL/min/1.73 m}^2) = \frac{0.55 \times \text{Height in cm}}{P_{Cr} \text{ in mg/dL}}$$

Note: This formula takes the body surface area into account, so further correction is not necessary. Use 0.45 × length in centimeters in newborns less than 1 year old. This method of calculation is not meant to detract from the importance of clearance determinations but is useful when a suspicious plasma creatinine needs to be checked.

Urine Concentrating Ability

Inability to concentrate urine is associated with polyuria, polydipsia, or enuresis and is often the first sign of chronic renal failure. The first morning void should be concentrated. Evaluation of other abnor-

malities of urinary concentration or dilution is discussed under specific disease entities, such as diabetes insipidus.

Microhematuria or Isolated Proteinuria

In children with asymptomatic hematuria or proteinuria, the search for renal origins will yield the most results. Isolated proteinuria may reflect urologic abnormalities, benign excretion or glomerular alterations. The presence of red cell casts supports a diagnosis of glomerulonephritis, but the absence of casts does not rule out the disease. Anatomic abnormalities such as cystic disease may be a source of hematuria.

Benign hematuria, including benign familial hematuria, is diagnosed by exclusion. In this group are children whose hematuria is caused by asymptomatic hypercalciuria. Figure 21–1 suggests an approach to the renal workup of hematuria. Further discussion of glomerulonephritis follows.

The association of proteinuria with hematuria is characteristic of more significant glomerular disease. A spot urine sample that reveals a protein:creatinine ratio of more than 0.2 is abnormal. A timed (usually 24-hour) urine collection is useful, especially to demonstrate orthostatic or "postural" proteinuria. Urine voided upon arising in the morning is collected in one container, and urine formed in the upright position during the rest of the day is collected in a separate container, finishing with a void just before going to bed. The two quantities can then be used to calculate total protein excretion, and the amount of protein can be compared in upright versus recumbent specimens to determine an orthostatic component. If the upright collection contains 80–100% of the measured protein and does not exceed a total of 1.5 g, the diagnosis of orthostatic (benign) proteinuria is acceptable. Measuring the creatinine in the specimen and calculating the creatinine index confirms specimen reliability.

An approach to the workup of isolated proteinuria is shown in Figure 21–2. Note that corticosteroid therapy is indicated in the algorithm because this may be initiated prior to referral. Discussion of other renal lesions with proteinuric presentations follows.

Special Tests of Renal Function

Measurements of urinary sodium, creatinine, and osmolality are useful in differentiating prerenal causes of renal insufficiency from renal causes when the possibility of acute tubular necrosis is raised.

The physiologic response to decreased renal perfusion is an increase in urine concentration (osmolality usually > 800 mOsm/L), a rise in urinary solutes, and a decrease in urinary sodium (usually < 20 mEq/L). Therefore, when an increase in serum creatinine or blood urea nitrogen concentration or a decrease in urinary output suggests the possibility of renal failure, appropriate steps can be taken to assess the sta-

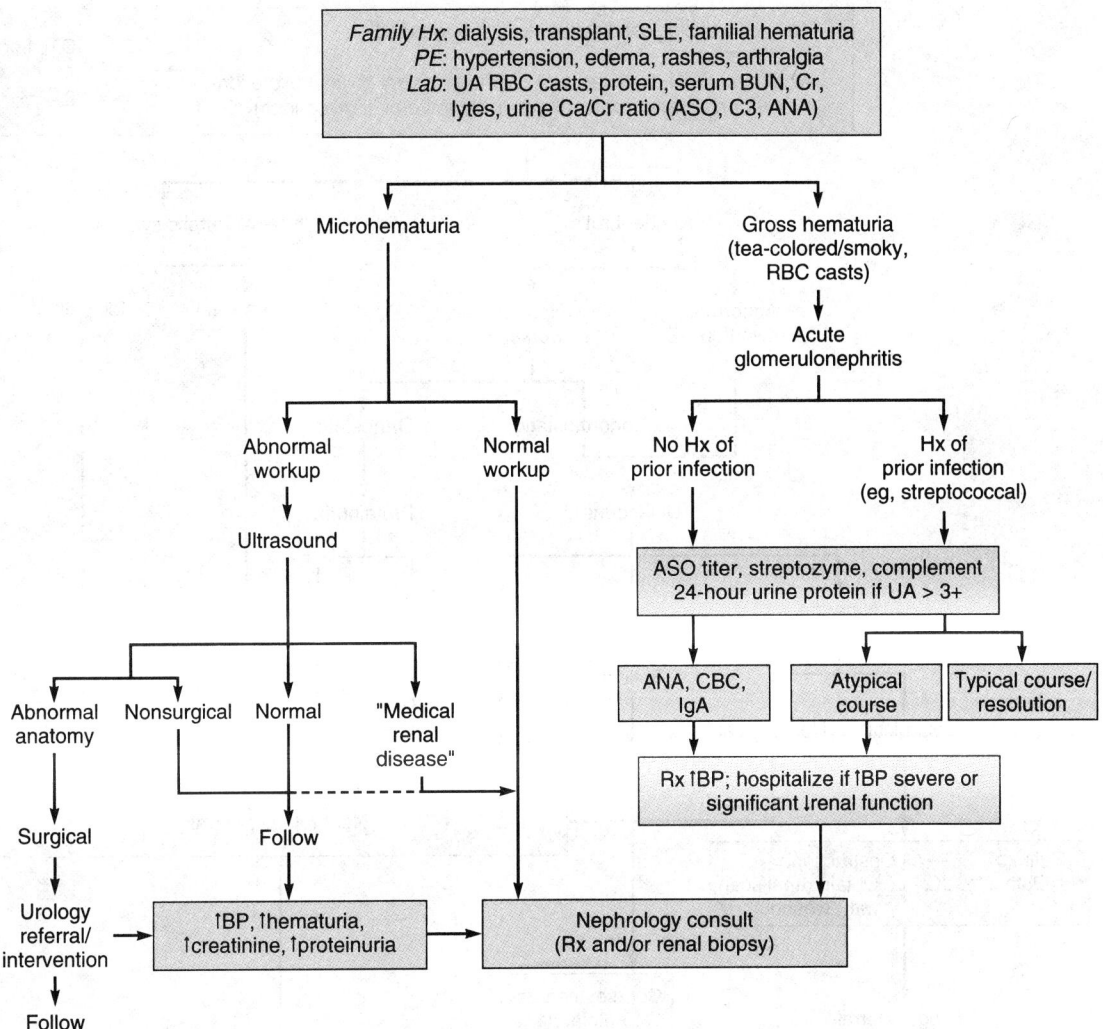

Figure 21–1. Approach to the renal workup of hematuria. (Exclude urinary tract infection, lithiasis, trauma, bleeding disorders, sickle cell disease.)

tus of renal function by qualitative and quantitative urinalysis. (See Acute Renal Failure.)

The presence of some substances in urine suggests tubular dysfunction. For example, urine glucose should be less than 5 mg/dL. Hyperphosphaturia occurs with significant tubular abnormalities (eg, Fanconi's syndrome). Measurement of the phosphate concentration of a 24-hour urine specimen and evaluation of tubular reabsorption of phosphorus (TRP) will help document renal tubular diseases as well as hyperparathyroid states. TRP (expressed as percentage of reabsorption) is calculated as follows:

$$TRP = 100\left[1 - \frac{S_{Cr} \times U_{PO4}}{S_{PO4} \times U_{Cr}}\right]$$

where S_{Cr} = serum creatinine; U_{cr} = urine creatinine; S_{PO4} = serum phosphate; and U_{PO4} = urine phosphate. All values for creatinine and phosphate are expressed in milligrams per deciliter for purposes of calculation. A TRP value of 80% or more is considered normal, though it depends somewhat on the S_{PO4}.

The urinary excretion of amino acids in generalized tubular disease reflects a quantitative increase rather than a qualitative change.

The ability of the proximal tubule to reabsorb bicarbonate is affected in several disease states—including isolated renal tubular acidosis, Fanconi's syndrome (which is present in such diseases as cystinosis), and chronic renal failure—and is discussed later under specific entities.

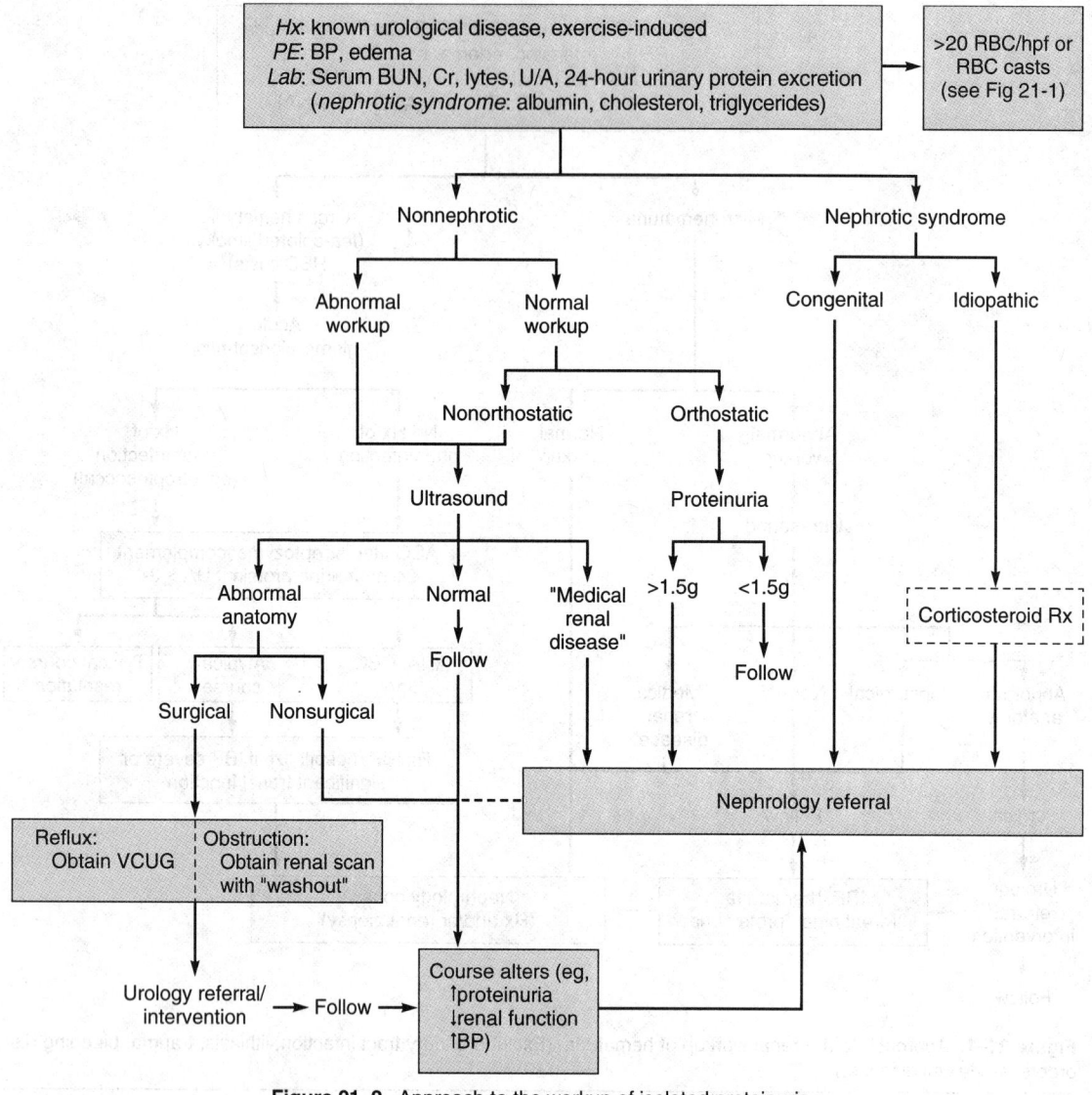

Figure 21–2. Approach to the workup of isolated proteinuria.

LABORATORY EVALUATION OF IMMUNOLOGIC FUNCTION

Much of parenchymal renal disease is mediated by immune mechanisms, many of which are not well defined or known. Examples of mechanisms in the kidney include (1) deposition of circulating antigen-antibody complexes that are themselves injurious or incite injurious responses and (2) formation of antibody directed against the glomerular basement membrane itself (rare in children).

Total serum complement, the C3 and C4 complement components, and serum immunoglobulins should be measured when immune-mediated renal injury or chronic glomerulonephritis is suspected. Abnormal serum protein levels are often associated with immune complex deposition; in such cases, tests should be performed to detect antinuclear antibodies, hepatitis-associated antigen, rheumatoid factor, and cold-precipitable proteins (cryoglobulins). Where indicated, special studies to measure circulating immune complexes, C3 "nephritic" factor, and anti-glomerular basement membrane (anti-GBM) antibody may be performed. Very often, the diagnosis rests on the description of renal histology.

RADIOGRAPHIC EVALUATION

Renal ultrasonography is a useful noninvasive tool in the evaluation of renal parenchymal disease, urinary tract abnormalities, or renal blood flow. Excretory urography is useful in assessing the anatomy and function of the kidney, collecting system, and bladder. Radioisotope studies provide valuable information concerning renal anatomy, blood flow, and glomerular, tubular, and collecting system function.

Evaluation of the lower urinary tract (voiding cystourethrography or cystoscopy) is indicated when vesicoureteral reflux or bladder outlet obstruction is suspected. Cystoscopy is rarely useful in the evaluation of asymptomatic hematuria or proteinuria in children.

Renal arteriography or venography is indicated in children to define vascular abnormalities (eg, renal artery stenosis) prior to surgical intervention. Less invasive measures such as ultrasonography and Doppler studies can demonstrate renal blood flow or thromboses.

RENAL BIOPSY

Histologic information is valuable for diagnosis, treatment, and prognosis. Satisfactory evaluation of renal tissue requires examination by light microscopy, immunofluorescence microscopy, and electron microscopy.

When a biopsy is anticipated, a pediatric nephrologist should be consulted. In children, percutaneous renal biopsy is an acceptable low-risk procedure—avoiding the risks of general anesthesia—when performed by an experienced physician. A surgeon should perform the biopsy procedure if operative exposure of the kidney is necessary, if an increased risk factor (eg, bleeding disorder) is present, or if a wedge biopsy is preferred.

CONGENITAL ANOMALIES OF THE URINARY TRACT

RENAL PARENCHYMAL ANOMALIES

About 10% of children have congenital anomalies of the genitourinary tract. Severity ranges from abnormalities that remain asymptomatic through adult life to malformations incompatible with intrauterine or extrauterine life.

Some asymptomatic abnormalities have significant complications. For example, patients with horseshoe kidney (kidneys fused in their lower poles) have a higher incidence of renal calculi. Unilateral agenesis is usually accompanied by compensatory hypertrophy of the contralateral kidney and thus should be compatible with normal renal function. Supernumerary and ectopic kidneys are usually of no significance. Abnormal genitourinary development can result in varying degrees of renal maldevelopment and function, of which complete renal agenesis is the most severe. When the agenesis is bilateral it causes early death. Oligohydramnios is present and can result in pulmonary hypoplasia and peculiar (Potter) facies.

Renal Dysgenesis

Renal dysgenesis represents a spectrum of anomalies. In simple hypoplasia, which may be unilateral or bilateral, the affected organs are smaller than normal. In the various forms of dysplasia, immature, undifferentiated renal tissue persists. In some of the dysplasias, the number of normal nephrons is insufficient to sustain life once the child reaches a critical body size. Such lack of renal tissue may not be readily discernible in the newborn period because the infant's urine production, though poor in concentration, may be adequate in volume. Often, the search for renal insufficiency is initiated only when growth fails or chronic renal failure develops.

Other forms of renal dysplasia include oligomeganephronia (characterized by the presence of only a few large glomeruli) and the cystic dysplasias (characterized by the presence of renal cysts). This group includes microcystic disease (congenital nephrosis). A simple cyst within a kidney may be clinically unimportant because it does not predispose to progressive polycystic development. An entire kidney lost to multicystic development with concomitant hypertrophy and normal function of the contralateral side may also be of little clinical consequence. Nonetheless, even a simple cyst could pose problems if it becomes a site for lithiasis, infection, or hematuria.

Polycystic Kidney Disease

The autosomal recessive form of polycystic kidney disease ("infantile" polycystic kidney disease) is characterized by large cystic kidneys, often accompanied by cystic malformations in multiple organ systems. Some children with this type die in the newborn period, but because of improvements in medical management many progress over an undetermined number of months or years to end-stage renal failure. When autosomal recessive polycystic kidney disease is diagnosed at a later age, it may be manifested chiefly by liver rather than renal involvement. Autosomal dominant disease ("adult" form), though rarely of clinical significance (if at all) before the fourth decade, may also be detected in the newborn period and, depending on severity, could be fatal. Although renal insufficiency and hypertension usually occur late in this type, there are exceptions. Careful documentation (usually by ultrasonography), close monitoring and management of the complications of renal insufficiency, and strict attention to hypertension control—as well as genetic counseling—are suggested. Management of end-stage renal failure is by dialysis or renal transplantation.

Medullary Cystic Disease (Juvenile Nephronophthisis)

Medullary cystic disease is characterized by varying sizes of cysts in the renal medulla and is associated with tubular and interstitial nephritis. Children present with renal failure and signs of tubular dysfunction (decreased concentrating ability, Fanconi's syndrome). This lesion should not be confused with medullary sponge kidney (renal tubular ectasia), a frequently asymptomatic disease seen in adults.

Gabow PA: Autosomal dominant polycystic kidney disease. N Engl J Med 1993;329:332.
Kissane JM: Renal cysts in pediatric patients. Pediatr Nephrol 1990;4:69.

DISTAL URINARY TRACT ANOMALIES

Obstruction at the ureteropelvic junction may be the result of intrinsic muscle abnormalities, aberrant vessels, or fibrous bands. The lesion can cause hydronephrosis and usually presents as an abdominal mass in the newborn. Obstruction can occur in other parts of the ureter, especially at its entrance into the bladder, with resulting proximal hydroureter and hydronephrosis. Whether impediments to normal flow of urine are intrinsic or extrinsic, steps should be taken immediately to rectify the problem and minimize damage to the renal parenchyma.

Severe bladder malformations such as exstrophy are clinically obvious and provide a surgical challenge. More subtle—but urgent in terms of diagnosis—is obstruction of urine flow from aberrant posterior urethral valves. This anomaly, which occurs almost exclusively in males, usually presents as anuria or a poor voiding stream in the newborn period, with severe obstruction of urine flow. Ascites may occur, and the kidneys and bladder may be easily palpable. Provided that severe, irreversible damage to renal development has not occurred in utero, timely intervention must be taken to avert further renal damage. The same can be said of many such complex genitourinary anomalies, including those of the external genitalia.

Complex Anomalies

Prune belly syndrome is an association of urinary tract anomalies with cryptorchidism and absent abdominal musculature. Although complex anomalies, especially renal dysplasia, usually cause early death or the need for dialysis or transplantation, some patients have lived into the third decade with varying degrees of renal insufficiency. Early urinary diversion is essential to sustain renal function. A renal biopsy at the time of this surgery may predict subsequent renal function.

Other complex malformations and such external genitalia anomalies as hypospadias are beyond the scope of this text. Overall, urologic abnormalities resulting in severe compromise and destruction of renal tissue provide therapeutic and management challenges aimed at preserving all remaining function and treating the complications of progressive chronic renal failure.

Fernbach SK: The dilated urinary tract in children. Urol Radiol 1992;14:34.
Gordon I: Vesico-ureteric reflux, urinary-tract infection, and renal damage in children. Lancet 1995;346:489.
Noe HN: The current status of screening for vesicoureteral reflux. Pediatr Nephrol 1995;9:638.
Peters CA: Urinary tract obstruction in children. J Urol 1995;154:1874.
Tripp BM, Honsy YL: Neonatal hydronephrosis: The controversy and the management. Pediatr Nephrol 1995; 9:503.

HEMATURIA & GLOMERULAR DISEASE

Children with painful hematuria should be investigated for causes of direct injury to the urinary tract whether the pain is dysuria, associated with cystitis or urethritis; back pain secondary to pyelonephritis; or colicky flank pain accompanying the passage of a stone. "Bright red" blood or clots in the urine occur with bleeding disorders, trauma, and arteriovenous malformations. Abdominal masses suggest the presence of urinary tract obstruction, cystic disease, or tumors involving the renal or perirenal structures.

Asymptomatic hematuria is a challenge because clinical and diagnostic data must be obtained to determine whether the problem is transient or whether the child should be referred to a nephrologist. Figure 21–1 delineates the outpatient approach to renal hematuria. The concern regarding the differential diagnosis is the possible presence of glomerular disease.

GLOMERULONEPHRITIS

Acute poststreptococcal glomerulonephritis is the most common form of postinfectious glomerulonephritis. The epidemiologic relationship between certain strains of streptococci and glomerulonephritis is well recognized. Antigen-antibody complexes are formed in the bloodstream and deposited in the glomeruli. These deposited complexes may incite glomerular inflammation and activate the complement system.

The diagnosis of poststreptococcal disease may be supported by a recent history (7–14 days previously) of group A β-hemolytic streptococcal infection. If a positive culture is not available, recent infection may be supported by an elevated antistreptolysin titer or by elevation of one or more antibody titers in the streptozyme panel. Other infections have been shown to cause similar glomerular injury; thus, "postinfection glomerulonephritis" is a better term for this type of acute glomerulonephritis. Patients whose renal function deteriorates rapidly should undergo renal biopsy.

The clinical presentation of glomerulonephritis is usually with gross hematuria ("coffee-colored" or "tea-colored" urine), with or without some (eg, periorbital) edema. Symptoms are usually nonspecific; in cases of severe hypertension, there may be headache. Fever is not expected. Severe glomerular injury (which usually occurs in severe, acute presentations of the more chronic or destructive forms of glomerulonephritis) may be accompanied by massive proteinuria (nephrotic syndrome), anasarca or ascites, and severe compromise of renal function.

There is no specific treatment for typical poststreptococcal glomerulonephritis. Appropriate antibiotic therapy is indicated for infection if still present. The disturbances in renal function and resulting hypertension may require dietary management, diuretics, or antihypertensive drugs. In severe cases, hemodialysis or peritoneal dialysis may be necessary; corticosteroids may also be administered in an attempt to influence the course.

The acute abnormalities generally resolve in 2–3 weeks; serum complement may be normal as early as 3 days or as late as 30 days after onset. Although microscopic hematuria may persist for as long as a year, most children recover completely. Persistent deterioration in renal function, urinary abnormalities beyond 18 months, persistent hypocomplementemia, and nephrotic syndrome are ominous signs and are indications for renal biopsy.

The various types of glomerulonephritis present similarly. The most commonly encountered entities in childhood and their clinical and histopathologic descriptions are listed in Table 21–1. Severe glomerular histopathologic and clinical entities, such as anti-GBM antibody disease (Goodpasture's syndrome) and idiopathic, rapidly progressive glomerulonephritis, may be considered in the differential diagnosis of acute glomerulonephritis, but these disorders are exceedingly rare in children.

Andreoli SP: Chronic glomerulonephritis in childhood: Membranoproliferative glomerulonephritis, Henoch-Schönlein purpura nephritis, and IgA nephropathy. Pediatr Clin North Am 1995;42:1487.

Cameron JS: Lupus nephritis in childhood and adolescence. Pediatr Nephrol 1994;8:230.

Stapleton FB: Hematuria associated with hypercalciuria and hyperuricosuria: A practical approach. Pediatr Nephrol 1995;9:671.

Yadin O: Hematuria in children. Pediatr Ann 1994;23:474.

ACUTE INTERSTITIAL NEPHRITIS

Acute interstitial nephritis is characterized by diffuse or focal inflammation and edema of the renal interstitium and secondary involvement of the tubules. It seems to be related most often to drugs (eg, antibiotics, especially methicillin).

Fever, rigor, abdominal or flank pain, and rashes may occur in drug-associated cases. Urinalysis should reveal leukocyturia and hematuria. Hansel's staining of the urinary sediment is helpful in demonstrating the presence of eosinophils. The inflammation can be severe enough to cause significant deterioration of renal function. Histologic demonstration of tubular and interstitial inflammation of the kidneys is helpful for diagnosis. Immediate identification and removal of the causative agent is imperative. A relentless course with progressive renal insufficiency or nephrotic syndrome may require supportive dialysis and treatment with corticosteroids.

Dhillon S, Higgins RM: Interstitial nephritis. Postgrad Med J 1997;73:151.

PROTEINURIA & RENAL DISEASE

Urine is not normally completely protein-free, but the average excretion is well below 150 mg/24 h. Small increases in urinary protein can accompany febrile illnesses or exertion and in some cases are produced while in the upright posture.

An algorithm for investigation of isolated proteinuria is presented in Figure 21–2. In idiopathic nephrotic syndrome without associated features of glomerulonephritis, treatment with corticosteroids may be initiated as described below. Nephrologic advice or follow-up should be sought, especially in difficult or frequently relapsing cases.

CONGENITAL NEPHROSIS

Congenital nephrosis is a rare autosomal recessive disorder. The kidneys are pale and large and may show microcystic dilations (microcystic disease) of the proximal tubules and glomerular changes. The

Table 21–1. Glomerular diseases encountered in childhood.

Entity	Clinical Course	Prognosis
Postinfection glomerulonephritis (GN). Onset occurs 10–14 days after acute illness, commonly streptococcal. Characteristics include acute onset, tea-colored urine, mild to severe renal insufficiency and edema.	Acute phase is usually over in 2 weeks. There is complete resolution in 95% of cases. Severity of renal failure and hypertension varies. Microhematuria may persist to 18 months. Hypocomplementemia resolves in 1–30 days.	Excellent. Chronic disease is rare. Severe proteinuria, atypical presentation/course, or persistent hypocomplementemia suggest another entity is likely.
Membranoproliferative glomerulonephritis. Presentation ranges from mild microhematuria to acute GN syndrome. Diagnosis is made by renal biopsy. Etiologic origin is unknown. Type I and Type II are most common. Lesion is chronic.	Course can be mild to severe (rapid deterioration in renal function); may mimic postinfection GN. Proteinuria can be severe. Complement depression is intermittent to persistent. Hypertension is usually significant.	Type I may respond to corticosteroids. Type II (dense deposit disease) is less treatable; functions decrease immediately to as long as 15 years later in 30–50% of untreated cases.
IgA Nephropathy. Classic presentation consists of asymptomatic gross hematuria during acute unrelated illness, with microhematuria between episodes. There are occasional instances of acute GN syndrome. Etiologic origin is unknown. Diagnosis is made by biopsy.	90% of cases resolve in 1–5 years. Gross hematuric episodes resolve with recovery from acute illness. Severity of renal insufficiency and hypertension varies. Proteinuria occurs in more severe, atypical cases.	Generally good. Small percentage develops chronic renal failure. Proteinuria in the nephrotic range is a poor sign. There is no universally accepted medication. (Corticosteroids may be useful in severe cases.)
Schönlein-Henoch purpura glomerulonephritis. Degree of renal involvement varies. Asymptomatic microhematuria is most common, but GN syndrome can occur. Renal biopsy is recommended in severe cases; it can provide prognostic information.	Presentation varies with severity of renal lesion. In rare cases, course may progress rapidly to serious renal failure. Hypertension varies. Proteinuria in the nephrotic range and severe decline in function can occur.	Overall, prognosis is good. Cases presenting with greater than 50% reduction in function or proteinuria exceeding 1 g/24 h may develop chronic renal failure. Severity of renal biopsy picture can best guide approach in such cases. There is no universally accepted medication.
Glomerulonephritis of systemic lupus erythematosus (SLE). Microhematuria and proteinuria are rarely first signs of this systemic disease. Renal involvement varies. GN often causes the most concern.	Renal involvement is mild to severe. Clinical complexity depends on degree of renal insufficiency and other systems involved. Hypertension is significant. Manifestations of the severity of the renal lesion guide therapeutic intervention.	Renal involvement accounts for most of significant morbidity in SLE. Control of hypertension affects renal prognosis. Medication is guided by symptoms, serology, and renal lesion. End-stage renal failure can occur.
Hereditary glomerulonephritis (eg, Alport's syndrome). Transmission is autosomal dominant/X-linked, with family history marked by end-stage renal failure, especially in young males. Deafness and eye abnormalities are associated.	There is no acute syndrome. Females are generally less affected but are carriers. Hypertension and increasing proteinuria occur with advancing renal failure. There is no known treatment.	Progressive proteinuria and hypertension occur early, with gradual decline in renal function in those most severely affected. Disease progresses to end-stage renal failure in most males.

latter consist of proliferation, crescent formation, and thickening of capillary walls. The pathogenesis is not well understood.

Infants with congenital nephrosis commonly have low birth weight, a large placenta, wide cranial sutures, delayed ossification, and mild edema. The edema may become apparent after the first few weeks or months of life. Anasarca follows, and the abdomen can become greatly distended by ascites. Massive proteinuria associated with typical-appearing nephrotic syndrome and hyperlipidemia is the rule. Hematuria is common. If the patient lives long enough, progressive renal failure occurs. Most affected infants succumb to infections at the age of a few months.

Treatment has little to offer other than nutrition support and management of the chronic renal failure, including dialysis and transplantation.

Ettenger RB: The evaluation of the child with proteinuria. Pediatr Ann 1994;23:486.
Roy S III: Proteinuria. Pediatr Ann 1996;25:277.

IDIOPATHIC NEPHROTIC SYNDROME OF CHILDHOOD
("Nil" Disease, Lipoid Nephrosis, Minimal Change Disease)

Nephrotic syndrome is characterized by proteinuria, hypoproteinemia, edema, and hyperlipidemia. It may occur as a result of any form of glomerular disease and may be associated with a variety of extrarenal conditions. In children under 5 years of age, the disease usually takes the form of idiopathic nephrotic syndrome of childhood ("nil" disease, lipoid nephrosis), which has characteristic clinical and laboratory findings.

Clinical Findings

Affected patients are generally under 5 years of age at the time of their first episode. Often following an influenza-like syndrome, the child is noted to have periorbital swelling and perhaps oliguria. Within a few days, increasing edema—even anasarca—becomes evident. Other than vague malaise and occasionally abdominal pain, complaints are few. With significant "third spacing" of plasma volume, however, some children may present with hypotension. With marked edema, there may also be dyspnea due to pleural effusions.

Despite heavy proteinuria, the urine sediment is usually normal. Microscopic hematuria (< 20 RBCs/hpf) may be present. Plasma albumin is low and lipids are raised. Humoral immunity does not appear to cause this nephrotic syndrome. When azotemia occurs, it is usually secondary to intravascular volume depletion rather than to impairment of function.

Glomerular morphology is unremarkable except for fusion of foot processes of the visceral epithelium of the glomerular basement membrane. This finding, however, is nonspecific and is seen in many proteinuric states. There may be "minimal changes" in the glomerular mesangium, with unremarkable findings on immunofluorescence and electron microscopic examination.

Complications

Infectious complications (eg, peritonitis) are occasionally encountered, and pneumococci are frequently responsible. Immunization with pneumococcal vaccine is helpful. Hypercoagulability may be present, and thromboembolic phenomena are commonly reported.

Treatment & Prognosis

As soon as the diagnosis of idiopathic nephrotic syndrome is made, corticosteroid treatment should be started. Prednisone, 2 mg/kg/d (maximum, 60 mg/d), is given as a single daily dose until the urine protein falls to "trace" or "negative" for a maximum of 8 weeks. The same dose is then administered on an alternate-day schedule for 1 month; thereafter, the dose is very gradually tapered and discontinued over the ensuing 2 months. If remission is achieved only to be followed by another relapse, the treatment course may be repeated. If at any time the nephrosis becomes refractory to treatment or if there are three relapses within a year's time, renal biopsy may be

considered. If the histologic findings are consistent with "minimal change disease," cytotoxic agents can be considered; however, these agents are generally most helpful when there is corticosteroid dependence and not resistance. If corticosteroid treatment gives little or no response, one should suspect a more significant glomerular lesion.

Other therapeutic measures may be directed toward the complications of the nephrotic syndrome itself. Unless the edema is symptomatic (eg, respiratory compromise due to ascites), diuretics should be used with extreme care; the patients are expected to have a decreased circulating volume and are also at risk for intravenous thrombosis. However, careful restoration of compromised circulating volume with intravenous albumin infusion and administration of diuretics is helpful in mobilizing edema. Immediate attention to infections (eg, acute peritonitis) is important to reduce morbidity.

Prognosis is often suggested by the initial response to corticosteroids. A prompt remission lasting for over a year is almost always permanent. Failure to respond or early relapse usually heralds a prolonged series of relapses, which may indicate the presence of more serious nephropathy. Chlorambucil or other cytotoxic drug therapy is predictably successful only in children who respond to corticosteroids. Patients who do not respond to corticosteroids or who relapse frequently should be referred to a pediatric nephrologist.

Mendoza SA, Tune BM: Management of the difficult nephrotic patient. Pediatr Clin North Am 1995;42:1459.

Salcedo JR et al: Nephrosis in childhood. Nephron 1995; 71:373.

Schnaper HW: Primary nephrotic syndrome of childhood. Curr Opin Pediatr 1996;8:141.

FOCAL GLOMERULAR SCLEROSIS

Focal glomerular sclerosis is one cause of corticosteroid-resistant or frequent relapsing nephrotic syndrome. The etiology is unknown. The diagnosis is made by renal biopsy, which shows normal-appearing glomeruli as well as some partially or completely sclerosed glomeruli. The lesion has serious prognostic implications; as many as 15–20% of cases can progress to end-stage renal failure. The clinical response to corticosteroid treatment is variable. Experience with cyclosporine is accumulating, and significant improvement is being reported.

Gregory MJ et al: Long-term cyclosporine therapy for pediatric nephrotic syndrome: a clinical and histologic analysis. J Am Soc Nephrol 1996;7:543.

Ingulli E et al: Aggressive long-term cyclosporine therapy for steroid-resistant focal segmental glomerulosclerosis. J Am Soc Nephrol 1995;5:1820.

Niaudet P et al: Cyclosporine in the therapy of steroid-resistant idiopathic nephrotic syndrome. Kidney Int Suppl 1997;58:S85.

MESANGIAL NEPHROPATHY
(Mesangial Glomerulonephritis)

Mesangial nephropathy is another cause of corticosteroid-resistant nephrotic syndrome. The renal biopsy shows a distinct increase in the mesangial matrix of the glomeruli. Very often the expanded mesangium contains deposits of IgM demonstrated on immunofluorescent staining. The origin is unknown. Corticosteroid therapy may induce remission, but relapses are common. Treatment with cyclosporine may be helpful.

Faedda R et al: Immunosuppressive treatment of the nephrotic syndrome due to mesangial lesions. Clin Nephrol 1996;46:237.

MEMBRANOUS NEPHROPATHY
(Membranous Glomerulonephritis)

Although largely idiopathic in nature, membranous nephropathy can be found in association with diseases such as hepatitis B antigenemia, systemic lupus erythematosus, congenital and secondary syphilis, and renal vein thrombosis; with immunologic disorders such as autoimmune thyroiditis; and with administration of drugs such as penicillamine. The pathogenesis is unknown, but it is thought that the glomerular lesion is the result of prolonged deposition of circulating antigen-antibody complexes.

The onset of membranous nephropathy may be insidious or may resemble that of idiopathic nephrotic syndrome of childhood (see previous text). It occurs more often in older children. The proteinuria of membranous nephropathy responds little if at all to corticosteroid therapy. Low-dose corticosteroid therapy, however, has been shown to reduce or delay development of chronic renal insufficiency. The diagnosis is made by renal biopsy.

Cameron JS: Membranous nephropathy in childhood and its treatment. Pediatr Nephrol 1990;4:193.

DISEASES OF THE RENAL VESSELS

RENAL VEIN THROMBOSIS

In the newborn period, renal vein thrombosis may suddenly complicate sepsis or dehydration. It may be observed in an infant of a diabetic mother, or it may be the result of umbilical vein catheterization. Renal vein thrombosis is less common in older children and adolescents; it may develop following trauma or without any apparent predisposing factors. Nephrotic syndrome may either cause or result from renal vein thrombosis. Spontaneous renal vein thrombosis has been associated with membranous glomerulonephropathy.

Clinical Findings

Renal vein thrombosis in newborns generally presents with the sudden development of an abdominal mass. If the thrombosis is bilateral, oliguria may be present; urine output may be normal with a unilateral thrombus. In older children, flank pain, sometimes with a palpable mass, is a common presentation.

No single laboratory test is diagnostic of renal vein thrombosis. Hematuria usually is present. Proteinuria is less constant. In the newborn, thrombocytopenia may be found; this is rare in older children. The diagnosis is made by ultrasonography and Doppler flow studies.

Treatment

Anticoagulation with heparin is the treatment of choice both in newborns and in older children. In the newborn, a course of heparin combined with treatment of the underlying problem is usually all that is required. Management in other cases is less straightforward. The tendency for recurrence and embolization has led some workers in this field to recommend long-term anticoagulation. If an underlying membranous glomerulonephritis is suspected, biopsy should be performed.

Course & Prognosis

The mortality rate in newborns from renal vein thrombosis depends on the underlying cause. With unilateral thromboses, the prognosis for adequate renal function is good. Renal vein thrombosis may rarely recur in the same kidney or occur in the other kidney years after the original episode of thrombus formation. Extension into the vena cava, with pulmonary emboli, is possible.

Kothari SS, Varma S, Wasir HS: Thrombolytic therapy in infants and children. Am Heart J 1994;127:651.

RENAL ARTERIAL DISEASE

Children may develop renovascular hypertension due to fibromuscular hyperplasia, congenital stenosis, or other renal arterial lesions. The proportion of children whose hypertension is due to these lesions is small. Unfortunately, there are few clinical clues to underlying arterial lesions. Nonetheless, arterial lesions should be suspected in children whose hypertension is severe, with onset at or below 10 years, or associated with delayed visualization with nuclear medicine scan. The diagnosis is established by renal arteriography with selective renal vein renin measurements. Some of these lesions may be approached by transluminal angioplasty or surgery (see Hypertension in the following text), but repair may be technically impossible in many small children. Although thrombosis of renal arteries is rare, it should be considered in a patient with acute onset of hypertension and hematuria in an appropriate setting (eg, in association with hyperviscosity or umbilical artery catheterization). Early diagnosis and treatment (eg, heparin) provides the best chance of reestablishing renal blood flow.

Textor SC, Canzanello VJ: Radiographic evaluation of the renal vasculature. Curr Opinion Nephrol Hypertens 1996;5:541.

HEMOLYTIC-UREMIC SYNDROME

Hemolytic-uremic syndrome is the commonest single cause of renal failure due to glomerular vascular injury in childhood. The glomerular damage is exacerbated by severe fluid imbalances during the gastrointestinal prodrome. Epidemiologic studies suggest genetic and infectious or immunologic etiologic components. The primary lesion seems to be in the arteriolar endothelium, especially in the kidney, with formation of platelet thrombi and resulting microangiopathic hemolysis. Recent data suggest that hemolytic-uremic syndrome involves a disorder of immunoregulation and that a unique class of anti-endothelial cell antibodies is produced which may play a role in pathogenesis of the vascular injury. However, the epidemic form of the disease in most cases is precipitated by E coli O157. It may also be seen in association with pneumococcal infections, where neuraminidase plays a role.

Clinical Findings

Hemolytic-uremic syndrome is most common under 2 years of age but is more severe in older children. The epidemic form begins with a prodromal phase characterized by gastrointestinal symptoms, including abdominal pain, diarrhea, and vomiting. Oliguria, pallor, and bleeding manifestations, principally gastrointestinal, occur next. Hypertension and seizures develop in some children—especially those who develop severe renal failure and fluid overload—but there may be significant involvement of the CNS.

The triad of anemia, thrombocytopenia, and renal failure characterizes the syndrome. Anemia is profound and is associated with red blood cell fragments on smear. A high reticulocyte count confirms the hemolytic nature of the anemia. The platelet count is almost invariably below 100,000/μL. Other coagulation abnormalities are less consistent. Serum fibrin split products are often present, but fulminant disseminated intravascular coagulation is rare. Hematuria is often present. The serum complement level is normal.

Complications

The complications of hemolytic-uremic syndrome usually result from renal failure. Neurologic problems, particularly seizures, may result from electrolyte abnormalities such as hyponatremia, hypertension, or central nervous system vascular disease. Severe bleeding, transfusion requirements, and complicating infections must be anticipated.

Treatment

Meticulous attention to fluid and electrolyte status is crucial. Early dialysis improves the prognosis; the size of the patient will usually dictate peritoneal dialysis as the technique of choice. Seizures usually respond to control of hypertension and electrolyte abnormalities. It has been suggested that the plasma in some cases lacks a prostacyclin-stimulating factor that is a potent inhibitor of platelet aggregation. Therefore, plasma infusion or plasmapheresis has been advocated in severe cases. Platelet inhibitors have also been tried, but the results have not been impressive, especially late in the disease. Nonetheless, it appears that using a platelet inhibitor early in the disease may obviate the need for platelet transfusion and in some cases reduce the progression of renal failure. Red cell and platelet transfusions may be necessary; although the risk of volume overload is significant, it can be minimized by dialysis. Erythropoietin (epoetin alfa) treatment may reduce red cell transfusion needs. While there is no universally accepted therapy for patients with this syndrome, the strict control of hypertension and nutrition and the timely use of dialysis reduces morbidity and mortality.

Education regarding ingestion of undercooked meats or unpasteurized products may reduce the incidence. Investigative studies for prevention are currently under way.

Course & Prognosis

Geographic factors may determine the severity of hemolytic-uremic syndrome. Most commonly, children recover from the acute episode within 2–3 weeks, and follow-up reveals no residual renal insufficiency. However, some patients who recover from the acute episode have severe and occasionally progressive renal dysfunction or hypertension. Thus, follow-up of children recovering from hemolytic-uremic syndrome should include serial determinations of renal function for 1–2 years and meticulous attention to blood pressure for 5 years. Mortality is of greatest concern in the early phase from the complications of central nervous system disease.

Siegler RI: The hemolytic uremic syndrome. Pediatr Clin North Am 1995;42:1505.

RENAL FAILURE

ACUTE RENAL FAILURE

Acute renal failure is the sudden inability to excrete urine of sufficient quantity or adequate composition to maintain body fluid homeostasis. Causes include impaired renal perfusion, acute renal disease, renal ischemia, renal vascular compromise, or obstructive uropathy. Prerenal, renal, and postrenal causes are listed in Table 21–2.

Clinical Findings

The hallmark of early renal failure is oliguria. Al-

Table 21–2. Classifications of renal failure.

Prerenal
  Dehydration due to gastroenteritis, malnutrition, or diarrhea
  Hemorrhage, aortic or renal vessel injury, trauma, surgery, cardiac surgery, renal arterial thrombosis
  Diabetic acidosis
  Hypovolemia associated with capillary leak or nephrotic syndrome
  Shock
  Heart failure
Renal
  Hemolytic-uremic syndrome
  Acute glomerulonephritis
  Extension of prerenal hypoperfusion
  Nephrotoxins
  Acute tubular necrosis or vascular nephropathy
  Renal (cortical) necrosis
  Intravascular coagulation—septic shock, hemorrhage
  Diseases of the kidney and vessels
  Iatrogenic disorders
  Severe infections
  Drowning, especially fresh water
  Hyperuricacidemia from cancer treatment
  Hepatic failure
Postrenal
  Obstruction due to tumor, hematoma, or the presence of posterior urethral valves or ureteropelvic junction stricture, ureterovesical junction stricture, ureterocele
  Crystalluria: sulfonamide or uric acid
  Stones
  Trauma to a solitary kidney or collecting system
  Renal vein thrombosis

though an exact etiologic diagnosis may not be clear at the onset, classifying the oliguria as outlined in Table 21–2 is helpful before starting treatment.

If the cause of renal failure or oliguria is not clear, entities that can be treated (eg, volume depletion) should be considered first. After treatable problems or glomerular diseases are ruled out, a diagnosis of acute tubular necrosis (eg, vasomotor nephropathy, ischemic injury) may be entertained.

A. Postrenal Causes: Postrenal failure is found in newborns with anatomic abnormalities. Obstruction of the bladder outlet should be relieved by insertion of a urethral catheter followed by surgical correction. Timely intervention may prevent irreversible renal injury and chronic renal failure. Delayed voiding in the newborn period, anuria, or poor urinary stream usually suggests obstruction. Ureteropelvic junctional obstruction usually presents as an abdominal mass. Obstructive uropathy is accompanied by variable degrees of renal insufficiency.

B. Prerenal Causes: The commonest cause of decreased renal function in children is compromised renal perfusion. It is usually secondary to dehydration, though abnormalities of renal vasculature and poor cardiac performance may also be considered. Possible secondary causes should be addressed and, if possible, eliminated in order to determine if true renal functional disturbances are present.

C. Renal Causes: The various acute glomerulonephritides, hemolytic-uremic syndrome, acute interstitial nephritis, and nephrotoxic injury are examples of "renal" entities that produce varying degrees of acute renal failure. The diagnosis of acute tubular necrosis or vasomotor nephropathy is considered in clinical situations where—with no evidence of specific renal parenchymal diseases—the elimination of any prerenal or postrenal factors produces no improvement in renal performance.

Table 21–3 lists the urinary indices that are helpful in distinguishing prerenal conditions from acute tubular necrosis.

Complications

The clinical severity of the complications depends

Table 21–3. Urine studies.

Prerenal Failure	Acute Tubular Necrosis
Urine osmolality 50 mOsm/kg greater than plasma osmolality	Urine osmolality equal to or less than plasma osmolality
Urine sodium < 10 mEq/L	Urinary sodium > 20 mEq/L
Ratio of urine creatinine to plasma creatinine > 14:1	Ratio of urine creatinine to plasma creatinine < 14:1
Specific gravity > 1.020	Specific gravity 1.012–1.018

on the degree of renal functional impairment and oliguria. Common complications include (1) fluid overload (hypertension, congestive heart failure, pulmonary edema), (2) electrolyte disturbances (hyperkalemia), (3) metabolic acidosis, (4) hyperphosphatemia, and (5) uremia.

Treatment

An indwelling catheter is inserted to monitor urine output. If urine volume is insignificant and renal failure is established, the catheter should be removed to minimize infection risks. Prerenal or postrenal factors should be excluded or rectified and the circulating volume maintained with appropriate fluids. The patient's response is assessed by physical examination and observed urinary output. Measurement of central venous pressure may be indicated. If diuresis does not occur in response to the above measures, give furosemide, 1–5 mg/kg intravenously, the dose being higher with greater functional compromise. Allow 1 hour for a response to occur. If the urine output remains low (< 0.5 mL/kg/h), increase the furosemide (up to 5 mg/kg). If no diuresis occurs with maximum dosing, the further administration of diuretics will not be helpful.

If these maneuvers stimulate some urine flow but biochemical evidence of acute renal failure persists, the resulting "nonoliguric" acute renal failure should be more manageable. Fluid overload and dialysis may be averted. However, if the medications and nutrients required exceed the urinary output, dialysis is indicated. Institution of dialysis before the early complications of acute renal failure develop is likely to improve clinical management and outcome. It is important to adjust medication dosage according to degree of renal function.

Acute Dialysis

A. Indications for Dialysis: The need for dialysis is determined on the basis of clinical findings. Immediate indications for dialysis are (1) severe hyperkalemia; (2) unrelenting metabolic acidosis (usually in a situation where fluid overload prevents sodium bicarbonate administration); (3) fluid overload with or without severe hypertension or congestive heart failure (a situation that would seriously compromise nutrition or drug administration); and (4) symptoms of uremia, usually manifested in children by central nervous system depression. The rate of rise of both urea nitrogen and creatinine levels may indicate the need for dialysis; it is generally accepted that the urea nitrogen level should not be allowed to exceed 100 mg/dL in small children.

B. Methods of Dialysis: The choice between peritoneal dialysis and hemodialysis may be dictated by their availability. Peritoneal dialysis is generally preferred in children because of the ease of performance and patient tolerance. Although peritoneal dialysis is technically less efficient than hemodialysis, hemodynamic stability and metabolic control can be better sustained because this technique can be applied on a relatively continuous basis. However, hemodialysis should be considered (1) if rapid removal of toxins is desired, (2) if the size of the patient makes hemodialysis less technically cumbersome and hemodynamically well-tolerated, or (3) if impediments to efficient peritoneal dialysis are present (eg, ileus).

C. Complications of Dialysis: Complications of peritoneal dialysis include peritonitis, volume depletion, and such technical complications as dialysate leakage or respiratory compromise from intraabdominal dialysate fluid. Peritonitis can be avoided by strict observance of aseptic technique. Peritoneal fluid cultures are obtained as clinically indicated. Dialysate can leak around the dialysis catheter or through tissue planes, causing dissection. Leakage is reduced by good catheter placement technique and appropriate intra-abdominal dialysate volumes. Any technical problems that result in abnormal flow of dialysate in and out of the peritoneal cavity require the attention of the nephrology consultant. Dialysis is useful in maintaining electrolyte balance; because potassium is absent from standard dialysate solutions, potassium may be added to the dialysate as clinically indicated. Phosphate is also absent because hyperphosphatemia is an expected problem in renal failure. Nonetheless, if phosphate intake is inadequate, hypophosphatemia must be addressed. High dextrose concentrations (maximum 4.25%) can correct fluid overload rapidly at the risk of causing hyperglycemia. Fluid removal may be increased with more frequent exchanges of the dialysate, but rapid osmotic transfer of water may result in hypernatremia.

Even in small infants, hemodialysis can rapidly correct major metabolic and electrolyte disturbances, as well as volume overload. The process is highly efficient, but the speed of the changes can cause such problems as hemodynamic instability. Anticoagulation is usually required but may entail minimal exposure to the risks of heparin administration. Careful monitoring of the appropriate biochemical parameters is important. Note that during or immediately following the procedure, blood sampling will produce misleading results because equilibration between extravascular compartments and the blood will not yet have been completed. Vascular access must be obtained and carefully monitored.

Course & Prognosis

The period of severe oliguria, if it occurs, usually lasts about 10 days. Oliguria lasting longer than 3 weeks, or anuria, makes a diagnosis of acute tubular necrosis very unlikely; vascular injury, severe ischemia (cortical necrosis), glomerulonephritis, or obstruction is more probable. The diuretic phase begins with an increase in urinary output to passage of large volumes of isosthenuric urine containing sodium levels of 80–150 mEq/L. During the recovery phase, signs and symptoms subside rapidly, although polyuria may persist for several days or weeks. Urinary abnormalities usually disappear completely within a few months. If renal recovery does not ensue, arrangements are made for chronic dialysis and eventual renal transplantation.

Sehic A, Chesney RW: Acute renal failure: Therapy. Pediatr Rev 1995;16:137.

CHRONIC RENAL FAILURE

Chronic renal failure in children most commonly results from developmental abnormalities of the kidneys or urinary tract. The kidneys may develop poorly (dysgenesis) or not at all (agenesis). Cystic development may result in immediate or progressive insufficiency. Abnormal development of the urinary tract may not permit normal renal development. Depending, however, on the degree of interference with normal renal parenchymal development, timely surgery may minimize parenchymal injury and perhaps even achieve completely normal function. In older children, the chronic glomerulonephritides and nephropathies, irreversible nephrotoxic injury, or hemolytic-uremic syndrome may also result in chronic renal failure.

When chronic renal failure is the result of an inadequate amount of normally functioning renal tissue, the inability to concentrate urine results in polyuria, polydipsia, or enuresis. Depending on the degree of renal insufficiency, failure to thrive may be the chief concern. Renal failure due to abnormalities of the collecting system may follow unrecognized urinary tract infection. Progressive deterioration of renal function may occur in the absence of infection. Without appropriate health maintenance, children may present with overt complications of long-standing chronic renal failure such as rickets or growth delay.

Chronic renal failure resulting from glomerulonephritis may be expected after an acute presentation. In unsuspected chronic glomerulonephritis, presentations range from hypertension to overt uremic symptoms. Growth failure depends on age at presentation and the rapidity of functional decline. Some of the chronic glomerulonephritides (eg, membranoproliferative glomerulonephritis) can progress unnoticed if subtle abnormalities of the urinary sediment are undetected or ignored. Any child with a history of chronic glomerulonephritis or significant renal injury needs close follow-up and monitoring of renal function. The use of angiotensin-converting enzyme (ACE) inhibitors has been shown to be useful in decreasing the glomerulosclerosis that occurs after glomerular injury and thus is commonly used in the treatment of associated hypertension.

Complications

Despite the kidney's ability to compensate for gradual loss of functioning nephrons in progressive chronic renal, there are early complications as well as those that occur toward end-stage renal disease (GFR < 15 mL/min/1.73 m^2); at this point, the compensatory capability is exhausted. In children who have developmentally reduced function but are unable to concentrate the urine, polyuria and thus dehydration is more likely to be a problem than fluid overload. As renal homeostatic capability approaches end stage, there may be a reduction in output; however, many such children can continue to produce generous quantities of urine (but not of "good quality") even when renal replacement therapies are initiated. Moreover, a "salt-wasting" state can occur. On the other hand, children who develop chronic renal failure due to the glomerular disease will characteristically have difficulty with sodium and water retention and hypertension relatively early in the course.

Other early manifestations of chronic renal failure include metabolic acidosis and growth retardation. Disturbances in calcium, phosphorus, and vitamin D metabolism leading to renal osteodystrophy require prompt attention. Although renal compensation and increased parathyroid hormone can maintain a normal serum phosphate early in the course, this will result in secondary hyperparathyroidism with resulting skeletal abnormalities. This can be reflected early by an increase in serum alkaline phosphatase.

Overt uremic symptoms are late manifestations of chronic renal failure. If left unchecked, chronic renal failure eventually affects every organ system adversely. The subjective symptoms of uremia are anorexia, nausea, and malaise. Children fail to thrive. Central nervous system manifestations occur late in the course and range from subtle changes to confusion, apathy, and lethargy. With advancing uremia, stupor and coma may be present. Associated electrolyte abnormalities may precipitate seizures (more commonly, a result of untreated hypertension). Anemia is the rule in chronic renal failure. It is usually normochromic and normocytic and results from decreased renal erythropoietin synthesis. Platelet dysfunction and other abnormalities of the coagulation system may be present. Bleeding phenomena—especially gastrointestinal bleeding—may be a problem. Cardiovascular manifestations may be life-threatening. Uremic pericarditis may develop. Congestive heart failure or hypertension may be seen.

Treatment

The aims of treatment in chronic renal failure prior to dialysis are to preserve any remaining renal function and to avoid complications. Controlling hypertension (see Treatment of Hypertension), hyperphosphatemia, and urinary tract infection contribute toward this endeavor. Acidosis may be treated with sodium citrate solutions provided the added sodium will not aggravate hypertension. Hyperphosphatemia is controlled by dietary restriction and the use of dietary phosphate binders (eg, calcium carbonate). Vitamin D should be administered to maintain normal serum calcium. When the blood urea nitrogen exceeds approximately 50 mg/dL, or if the child is lethargic or anorexic, dietary protein restriction should be initiated. Sodium restriction is advisable when hypertension is present. Potassium restriction will be necessary as the GFR falls to a level where urinary output decreases sharply. Meanwhile, the diet must continue to provide the child's specific daily requirements.

Renal function must be regularly monitored (creatinine and blood urea nitrogen) as well as serum electrolytes, calcium, phosphorus, alkaline phosphatase, and hemoglobin and hematocrit. Results guide changes in fluid and dietary management as well as dosages of phosphate binder, citrate buffer, vitamin D, and blood pressure medications. Anemia may be treated with epoetin alfa. All of these areas require careful monitoring to minimize symptoms while continuing to assess the need for chronic dialysis and transplantation.

Care must be taken to avoid medications that aggravate hypertension, increase the body burden of sodium, potassium, or phosphate, or increase production of blood urea nitrogen. Successful management relies greatly upon education of the patient and family.

Attention must also be directed toward the psychosocial needs of the patient and family during adjustment to chronic illness. The strategy for patient management—and the need for family education and adjustment—changes when a plan for chronic dialysis and possible renal transplantation is initiated. These changes may include a reduction in medications or dietary limitations, with the potential for improving growth. Some uremic children will grow significantly when given human recombinant growth hormone.

Dialysis & Transplantation

The best-tolerated treatment of end-stage renal disease in a child is a successful and uncomplicated renal transplant. The North American Pediatric Renal Transplant Collaborative Study reports a 1-year graft survival rate of living-related kidney transplants of 90%, with 85% at 2 years and 75% at 5 years. With cadaveric transplantation, percentages of graft survivals are 76%, 71%, and 62%, respectively. Overall, the mortality rate is 4% for recipients of living-related donors and 6.8% for recipients of cadaver donors. These percentages are affected by the increased mortality rate—reported to be as high as 75%—in infants under 1 year of age. Most transplantation centers are waiting until infants reach a body weight of about 15 kg. This appears to be associated with a significantly improved survival rate. Adequate

growth and well-being are directly related to acceptance of the graft, the degree of normal function, and the side effects of medications.

Great advances have also been made in peritoneal dialysis and hemodialysis, both in technique and in our understanding of the specialized approach required. Hemodialysis is now performed in major centers that devote their entire effort to the management of pediatric patients and is regarded as a reasonable long-range method of treating the older child with end-stage renal disease. The demonstrated feasibility of chronic peritoneal dialysis in children, however, has made it the primary choice of dialysis therapy, especially for small children. It is well accepted and can be performed in the home.

The best measure of the success of chronic dialysis in children is the level of physical and psychosocial rehabilitation achieved. Patients continue to participate in day-to-day activities and attend school. Although catch-up growth rarely occurs, patients can grow at an acceptable rate even though they may remain in the lower percentiles. Use of epoetin alfa, growth hormone, and better control of renal osteodystrophy contribute to improved outcome.

Fine RN et al: Recombinant human growth hormone in infants and young children with chronic renal insufficiency. Pediatr Nephrol 1995;9:451.

Maschio G et al: Effect of the angiotensin-converting enzyme of chronic renal insufficiency. N Engl J Med 1996;334:939.

McEnery PT et al: Renal transplantation in children: A report of the North American Pediatric Renal Transplant Cooperative study. N Engl J Med 1992;326:1721.

Nakano M et al: Protein intake and renal function in children. Am J Dis Child 1989;143:160.

RENAL HYPERTENSION

Hypertension in children is commonly of renal origin. It is anticipated as a complication of known renal parenchymal disease, but it may be found on routine physical examination in an otherwise normal child. Increased understanding of the roles of water and salt retention on the one hand and overactivity of the renin-angiotensin system on the other has done much to guide therapy; it is nevertheless clear that not all forms of hypertension can be explained by these two mechanisms.

The causes of hypertension in the newborn period include (1) congenital anomalies of the kidneys or renal vasculature; (2) obstruction of the urinary tract; (3) thrombosis of renal vasculature or kidneys; and (4) volume overload. There are also reported instances of apparent paradoxic elevations of blood pressure in clinical situations in which chronic diuretic therapy is used, such as in bronchopulmonary dysplasia. Hypertensive infants should also be examined for renal, vascular, or aortic abnormalities (eg, thrombosis, neurofibromatosis, coarctation), as well as some endocrine disorders.

Diagnosis

A child is normotensive if the average recorded systolic and diastolic blood pressures are lower than the 90th percentile for age and sex. The 90th percentile in the newborn period is approximately 85–90/55–65 mm Hg for both sexes. In the first year of life, the acceptable levels are 90–100/60–67 mm Hg. Incremental increases with growth occur, gradually approaching young adult ranges of 100–120/65–75 mm Hg in the late teens. Careful measurement of blood pressure includes ensuring correct cuff size and reliable equipment. The cuff should be wide enough to cover two-thirds of the upper arm and should encircle the arm completely without causing an overlap in the inflatable bladder. Although an anxious child may have an elevation in blood pressure, abnormal readings must not be too hastily attributed to this cause. Repeat measurement is helpful, especially after the child has been consoled.

Routine laboratory studies include a complete blood count, urinalysis, and urine culture. Radiography and ultrasonography are used to study the anatomy of the urinary tract, the blood flow to the kidneys, and their function. A renal biopsy (which rarely reveals the cause of hypertension unless there is clinical evidence of renal disease) should always be undertaken with special care in the hypertensive patient and preferably after pressures have been controlled by therapy. A suggested approach to the outpatient workup is presented in Figure 21–3.

Treatment

A. Treatment of Acute Emergent Hypertension: A hypertensive emergency exists when central nervous system signs of hypertension appear, such as papilledema or encephalopathy. Retinal hemorrhages or exudates indicate a need for prompt and effective control. It is common in children, however, to see no end-organ abnormalities secondary to hypertension. Treatment varies with the clinical presentation. The primary classes of useful antihypertensive drugs are (1) diuretics, (2) alpha- and beta-adrenergic blockers, (3) ACE inhibitors, (4) calcium channel blockers, and (5) vasodilators.

Whatever method is used to control emergent hypertension, medications for sustained control should also be initiated so that the effect will be maintained when the emergent measures are discontinued (Table 21–4).

Acute elevations of blood pressure not exceeding the 95th percentile for age may be approached with oral medication, and measures should be aimed at progressive improvement and control within 48 hours.

1. Sublingual nifedipine, a calcium channel blocker, is rapid-acting and in appropriate doses should not result in hypotensive blood pressure levels. The liquid from a 10-mg capsule can be withdrawn with a syringe and the dosage approximated. The exact dosage for children who weigh less than 10–30 kg is difficult to ascertain by this method, but 5 mg is a safe starting point. Because the treatment is given for rising blood pressure, it is unlikely that the effects will be greater than desired. Larger children with malignant hypertension require 10 mg. In such cases, the capsule may simply be pierced and the medication squeezed under the patient's tongue.

2. Intravenous hydralazine can be effective in some cases. Dosage varies according to the severity of the hypertension and should begin at about 0.15 mg/kg.

3. Sodium nitroprusside is also effective in an intensive care setting for reducing severely elevated blood pressure. Intravenous administration of 0.5–10 mg/kg/min will reduce blood pressure in seconds, but the dose must be carefully monitored.

4. Furosemide, 1–5 mg/kg intravenously, will reduce blood volume and enhance the effectiveness of antihypertensive drugs.

B. Treatment of Sustained Hypertension: There are several choices (Table 21–5). A single drug such as a beta blocker (unless contraindicated—eg, in reactive airway disease) may be adequate in mild hypertension. Diuretics are useful in renal insufficiency, but disadvantages of possible electrolyte imbalance must be considered. Single-drug therapy with an ACE inhibitor is useful, especially since most hypertension in children has renal causes. The use of the vasodilator type of antihypertensive drug requires concomitant administration of a diuretic to counter the effect of vasodilation on increasing renal sodium and water retention and a beta-blocker to counter reflex tachycardia. Minoxidil, considered the most powerful of the orally administered vasodilators, can be extremely efficacious in the treatment of severe, sustained hypertension, but its effect is greatly offset by the other effects described. Hirsutism is a significant side effect. Hydralazine hydrochloride may still be the most common vasodilator in pediatric use—but, again, the necessity of using two additional drugs for maximum benefit keeps vasodilators in reserve for those severe situations calling for management with three or four drugs. The advice of a pediatric nephrologist should be sought.

Bandel-Stenzel M, Najarian JS, Sinaiko AR: Renal artery stenosis in infants: Long-term medical treatment before surgery. Pediatr Nephrol 1996;10:147.

Hanna JD, Chan JCM, Gill JR Jr: Hypertension and the kidney. J Pediatr 1991;118:327.

Hohn AR: Diagnosis and management of hypertension in childhood. Pediatr Ann 1997;26:105.

Sinaido AR: Treatment of hypertension in children. Pediatr Nephrol 1994;8:603.

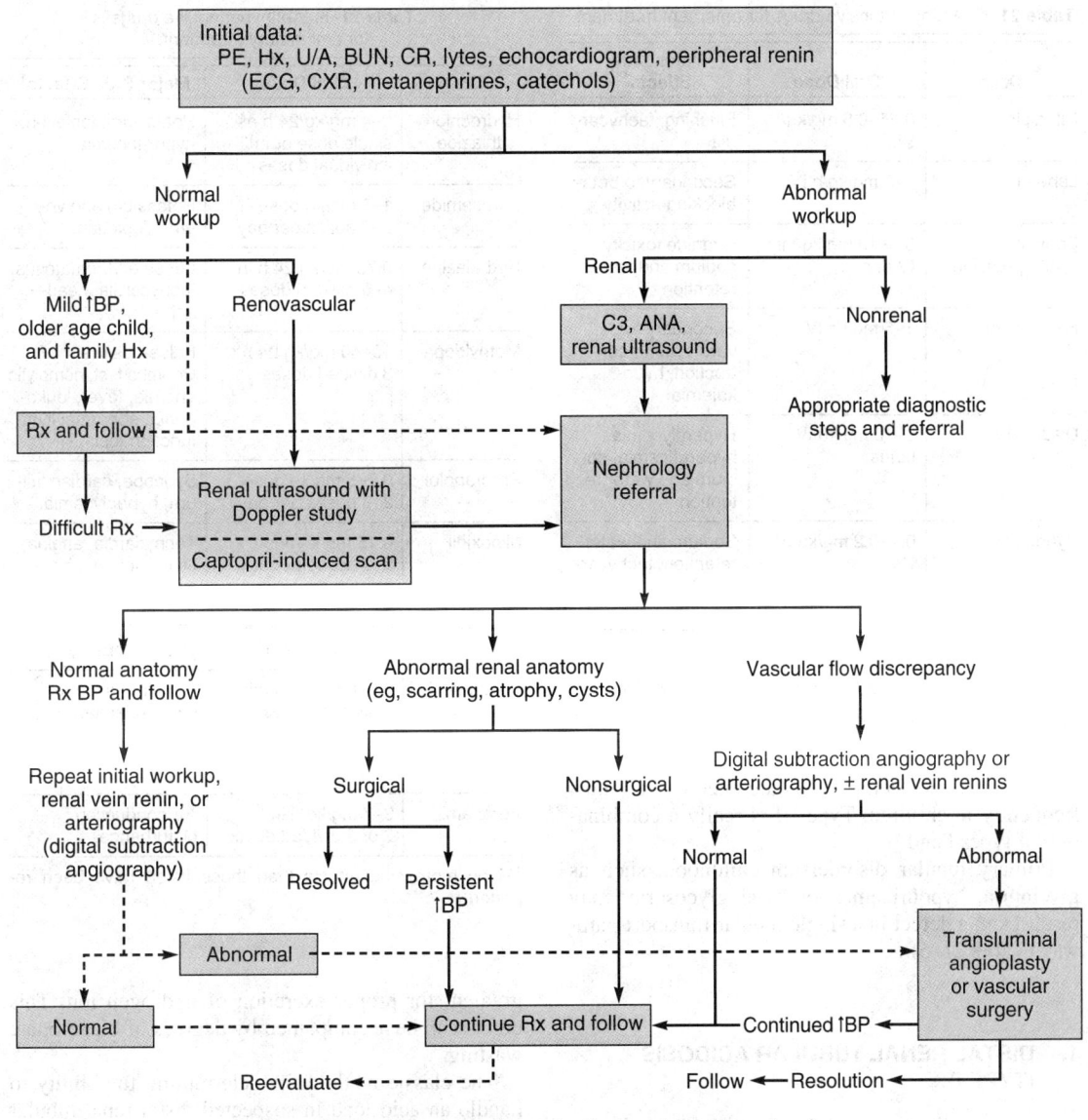

Figure 21–3. Approach to the outpatient workup of hypertension.

INHERITED OR DEVELOPMENTAL DEFECTS OF THE URINARY TRACT

There are many developmental, hereditary, or metabolic defects of the kidneys and collecting system. The clinical consequences include metabolic abnormalities, failure to thrive, nephrolithiasis, renal glomerular or tubular dysfunction, and chronic renal failure. Table 21–6 lists some of the major entities;

discussion of the rarer conditions is beyond the scope of this book.

DISORDERS OF THE RENAL TUBULES

Three subtypes of renal tubular acidosis are well recognized: (1) the "classic" form, called type I or distal renal tubular acidosis; (2) the bicarbonate "wasting" form, called type II or proximal renal tubular acidosis; and (3) type IV, or hyperkalemic renal tubular acidosis (rare in children), which is asso-

Table 21–4. Antihypertensive drugs for emergent treatment.

Drug	Oral Dose	Major Side Effects[1]
Nifedipine	0.25–0.5 mg/kg/ SL	Flushing, tachycardia
Labetalol	1–3 mg/kg/h IV	Secondary to beta-blocking activity
Sodium nitroprusside	0.5–10 mg/kg/min IV drip	Cyanide toxicity, sodium and water retention
Furosemide	1–5 mg/kg IV	Secondary to severe volume contraction, hypokalemia
Diazoxide	2–10 mg/kg IV bolus	Hyperglycemia, hyperuricemia, sodium and water retention
Hydralazine	0.1–0.2 mg/kg IV	Sodium and water retention, tachycardia, flushing

[1]Many more side effects than those listed have been reported.

Table 21–5. Antihypertensive drugs for ambulatory treatment.

Drug	Oral Dose	Major Side Effects[1]
Hydrochloro-thiazide	2–4 mg/kg/24 h as single dose or in 2 individual doses	Potassium depletion, hyperuricemia.
Furosemide	1–5 mg/kg/dose, 2–3 doses per day	Potassium and volume depletion.
Hydralazine	0.75 mg/kg/24 h in 4–6 divided doses	Lupus erythematosus, tachycardia, headache.
Methyldopa	10–40 mg/kg/24 h in 3 divided doses	False-positive Coombs test, hemolytic anemia, fever, leukopenia, abnormal liver function tests.
Propranolol	0.2–5 mg/kg/dose, 2–3 doses per day	Syncope, cardiac failure, hypoglycemia.
Minoxidil	0.15 mg/kg/dose, 2–3 doses per day	Tachycardia, angina, fluid retention, hirsutism.
Captopril	0.3–2 mg/kg/dose, 2–3 doses per day	Rash, hyperkalemia, glomerulopathy.
Enalapril	0.2–0.5 mg/kg/d in 2 divided doses	Proteinuria, cough, hyperkalemia.
Nifedipine	0.5–1 mg/kg/d, 3 doses per day	Flushing, tachycardia.
Verapamil	3–7 mg/kg/d in 2 or 3 divided doses	AV conduction disturbance.

[1]Many more side effects than those listed have been reported.

ciated with hyporeninemic hypoaldosteronism. Type I and type II and their variants are encountered most frequently in children. Type III is really a combination of types I and II.

Primary tubular disorders in childhood, such as glycinuria, hypouricemia, or renal glycosuria, may result from a defect in a single tubular transport pathway (Table 21–6).

1. DISTAL RENAL TUBULAR ACIDOSIS (TYPE I)

The most common form of distal renal tubular acidosis in childhood is the hereditary form. The clinical presentation is one of failure to thrive, anorexia, vomiting, and dehydration. Hyperchloremic metabolic acidosis occurs, with hypokalemia and a urinary pH exceeding 6.5. The acidosis is more severe in the presence of a bicarbonate "leak." This variant of distal renal tubular acidosis with bicarbonate wasting has been called type III but for clinical purposes need not be considered as a distinct entity. Concomitant hypercalciuria may lead to rickets, nephrocalcinosis, nephrolithiasis, and renal failure.

Other situations that may be responsible for distal renal tubular acidosis are found in some of the entities listed in Table 21–6.

Distal renal tubular acidosis results from a defect in the distal nephron, in the tubular transport of hydrogen ion, or in the maintenance of a steep enough gradient for proper excretion of hydrogen ion. This defect can be accompanied by degrees of bicarbonate wasting.

The classic method for determining the ability to handle an acid load in suspected distal renal tubular acidosis is the administration of NH_4Cl. The acid load testing is cumbersome to perform and can produce severe acidosis. A clinical trial of alkali administration should be used to rule out proximal (type II) renal tubular acidosis. The dose of alkali required to achieve a normal plasma HCO_3^- concentration in patients with distal renal tubular acidosis is low (seldom exceeds 2–3 meq/kg/24 h)—in contrast to that required in proximal renal tubular acidosis (> 10 meq/kg/24 h). Higher doses are needed, however, if distal renal tubular acidosis is accompanied by bicarbonate wasting. Correction of acidosis can result in reduced complications and improved growth.

Distal renal tubular acidosis is usually a permanent disorder, though it sometimes occurs as a secondary complication. If the defect does not represent a greater tubular disorder and renal damage is prevented, the prognosis is good.

Table 21–6. Inherited or developmental defects of the urinary tract.

Cystic diseases of genetic origin
  Polycystic disease
    Autosomal recessive form (infantile)
    Autosomal dominant form (adult)
    Other syndromes that include either form
  Cortical cysts
    Several syndromes are known to have various renal
      cystic manifestations, including "simple" cysts; may
      not have significant effect on renal functional status
      nor be associated with progressive disease
  Medullary cysts
    Medullary sponge kidney
    Medullary cystic disease (nephronophthisis)
  Hereditary and familial cystic dysplasia
    Congenital nephrosis
    "Finnish" disease
Dysplastic renal diseases
  Renal aplasia (unilateral, bilateral)
  Renal hypoplasia (unilateral, bilateral, total, segmental)
  Multicystic renal dysplasia (eg, unilateral, bilateral,multilocular,
    postobstructive)
  Familial and hereditary renal dysplasias
  Oligomeganephronia
Hereditary diseases associated with nephritis
  Hereditary nephritis with deafness and ocular defects (Alport's
    syndrome)
  Nail-patella syndrome
  Familial hyperprolinemia
  Hereditary nephrotic syndrome
  Hereditary osteolysis with nephropathy
  Hereditary nephritis with thoracic asphyxiant dystrophy
    syndrome
Hereditary diseases associated with intrarenal
    deposition of metabolites
  Angiokeratoma corporis diffusum (Fabry's disease)
  Heredopathia atactica polyneuritiformis (Refsum's disease)
  Various storage diseases (eg, G_{M1} monosialogangliosido-
    sis, Hurler's syndrome, Niemann-Pick disease, familial
    metachromatic leukodystrophy, glycogenosis type I [von
    Gierke's disease], glycogenosis type II [Pompe's disease])
  Hereditary amyloidosis (familial Mediterranean fever; heredofa-
    milial urticaria with deafness and neuropathy; primary famil-
    ial amyloidosis with polyneuropathy)
Hereditary renal diseases associated with tubular
    transport defects
  Hartnup disease
  Immunoglycinuria
  Fanconi's syndrome
  Oculocerebrorenal syndrome of Lowe
  Cystinosis (infantile, adolescent, adult types)
  Wilson's disease
  Galactosemia
  Hereditary fructose intolerance
  Renal tubular acidosis (many types)
  Hereditary tyrosinemia
  Renal glycosuria
  Vitamin D-resistant rickets
  Pseudohypoparathyroidism
  Vasopressin-resistant diabetes insipidus
  Hypouricemia
Hereditary diseases associated with lithiasis
  Hyperoxaluria
  L-Glyceric aciduria
  Xanthinuria
  Lesch-Nyhan syndrome and variants, gout
  Nephropathy due to familial hyperparathyroidism
  Cystinuria (types I, II, III)
  Glycinuria
Miscellaneous
  Hereditary intestinal vitamin B_{12} malabsorption
  Total and partial lipodystrophy
  Sickle cell anemia
  Bartter's syndrome

2. PROXIMAL RENAL TUBULAR ACIDOSIS (TYPE II)

Proximal renal tubular acidosis is characterized by an alkaline urine pH, loss of bicarbonate in the urine, and mildly reduced serum bicarbonate concentrations. About 85–90% of bicarbonate reabsorption occurs in the proximal tubules. The lesion in proximal renal tubular acidosis is a lowering of the renal bicarbonate threshold, ie, the concentration of serum bicarbonate above which bicarbonate appears in the urine. With more severe acidosis, the concentration of serum bicarbonate drops and bicarbonate disappears from the urine; this reflects normal distal tubular acidification.

The proximal type is the most common type of renal tubular acidosis encountered in children. It is often an isolated defect, and in the newborn infant it can be considered an aspect of renal immaturity. Onset in infants is accompanied by failure to thrive, hyperchloremic acidosis, hypokalemia, and, rarely, nephrocalcinosis. Secondary forms result from reflux or obstructive uropathy and are seen in association with other tubular disorders (Table 21–6).

As previously described, the amount of alkali required to correct acidosis may aid in distinguishing the proximal (requires > 3 mEq/kg of alkali per day) from the distal type. Serum bicarbonate should be monitored weekly until a level of at least 20 mEq/L is attained.

The available forms of bicarbonate therapy that are somewhat more easily tolerated than sodium bicarbonate are the citrate solutions (eg, Bicitra, Polycitra). Bicitra contains 1 mEq of Na^+ and citrate per milliliter. Polycitra contains 2 mEq per milliliter of citrate and 1 mEq each of Na^+ and K^+. The required daily dosage is given in three divided doses. Potassium supplementation may be required, because the added sodium load presented to the distal tubule may exaggerate potassium losses.

In cases of isolated defects, especially where the problem is related to renal immaturity, the prognosis is excellent. Alkali therapy can usually be discontinued after several months to 2 years. Growth should be normal, and the gradual increase in the serum bicarbonate level to above 22 mEq/L heralds the presence of a raised bicarbonate threshold in the tubules. If the defect is part of a more complex tubular abnormality (Fanconi's syndrome with attendant phosphaturia, glycosuria, and amino aciduria), the prognosis depends on the underlying disorder or syndrome.

Rodriguez-Soriano J, Vallo A: Renal tubular acidosis. Pediatr Nephrol 1990;4:268.

OCULOCEREBRORENAL SYNDROME (Lowe's Syndrome)

Lowe's syndrome has been described in males only and is therefore thought to be transmitted as an X-linked recessive gene leading to anomalies involving the eyes, brain, and kidneys. The physical stigmas and the degree of mental retardation are variable. In addition to congenital cataracts and buphthalmos, the typical facies includes prominent epicanthal folds, frontal prominence, and a tendency to scaphocephaly. Muscle hypotonia is a prominent finding. The incidence of hypophosphatemic rickets is variable; it is characterized by low serum phosphorus levels, low to normal serum calcium levels, elevated serum alkaline phosphatase levels, renal tubular acidosis, and aminoaciduria. Treatment includes alkali therapy, phosphate replacement, and vitamin D. Mothers of affected males have punctate lens opacities.

CONGENITAL HYPOKALEMIC ALKALOSIS (Bartter's Syndrome)

Bartter's syndrome is characterized by severe hypokalemic, hypochloremic metabolic alkalosis; extremely high levels of circulating renin and aldosterone; and a paradoxic absence of hypertension. On renal biopsy, there is a striking juxtaglomerular hyperplasia. Most patients present in early infancy with severe failure to thrive.

The cause and pathogenesis are not known. The pathogenesis is thought to be related to sodium reabsorption defects in the proximal or distal tubule. Studies have associated elevated levels of prostaglandins with the syndrome, and treatment with inhibitors of prostaglandins (eg, indomethacin) has been advocated. A prostaglandin-independent chloride-reabsorptive defect has been proposed.

Treatment with prostaglandin inhibitors and potassium-conserving diuretics (eg, amiloride combined with magnesium supplements) and potassium is beneficial. Although the prognosis is guarded, a few patients seem to have less severe forms of the disease that are compatible with long survival times.

CYSTINOSIS

Three types of cystinosis have been identified: adult, adolescent, and infantile. The adult type is a relatively benign condition characterized by cystine deposition in the corneas, granulocytes, and fibroblasts but no renal disease. The adolescent type is also characterized by cystine deposition but is accompanied by the development of mild renal failure with Fanconi's syndrome during adolescence; growth is normal. The infantile type is both the most common and the most severe. Characteristically, children present in the first or second year of life with Fanconi's syndrome.

Cystinosis is an autosomal recessive condition.

The exact biochemical nature of the disease remains obscure. Cystine is stored in cellular lysosomes in virtually all tissues—the consequence of a now-recognized lysosomal cystine afflux transport system. Eventually, cystine accumulation results in cell damage and cell death, particularly in the renal tubules. Renal failure between ages 6 and 12 is common.

Whenever the diagnosis of cystinosis is suspected, slitlamp examination of the corneas by an ophthalmologist should be performed, since cystine crystal deposition causes an almost pathognomonic ground-glass "dazzle" appearance. Increased white cell cystine levels are diagnostic. Hypothyroidism is common.

Phosphocysteamine therapy is giving good results in the treatment of cystinosis. Depending on the progression of chronic renal failure, management is directed toward all side effects of renal failure, with particular attention being paid to the control of renal osteodystrophy. Dialysis and transplantation may be needed.

Markello TC, Bernadini IM, Gahl WA: Improved renal function in children with cystinosis treated with cysteamine. N Engl J Med 1993;328:1157.

PHOSPHATE-LOSING RENAL TUBULAR SYNDROMES & OTHER FORMS OF RICKETS

Recent investigation of the metabolic products of vitamin D_3 has done much to clarify the causes of various forms of rickets. Those forms due primarily to a lack of available calcium are described in Chapter 10. They include idiopathic hypercalciuria, in which there is low calcium intake or excessive urinary calcium loss; lack of vitamin D_3 because of low dietary intake or from steatorrhea; and vitamin D dependency and azotemic rickets. In vitamin D_3 dependency, there is an inborn or acquired inability to synthesize 1,25-dihydroxycholecalciferol (the calcium transport stimulating factor, type I), or there may be end-organ insensitivity to this factor (type II). Treatment consists of giving supplementary calcium or vitamin D in appropriate doses.

Diseases associated with decreased availability of phosphorus also cause rickets. Excessive use of antacids may be responsible. Most commonly, the defect is an inherited or acquired one in which a defect of phosphorus reabsorption is variably associated with other transport defects (eg, Fanconi's syndrome). Certain generalized metabolic diseases—notably Wilson's disease, galactosemia, fructose intolerance, and cystinosis—may cause similar tubular damage. Treatment of the primary type is to give extra phosphorus. Treatment of the acquired forms is that of the basic disease.

Familial hypophosphatemic vitamin D-resistant

rickets is an example of a tubular nephropathy in which only phosphorus transport is affected. Most patients present during the second year of life, but some conditions have onset in the first 6 months.

Clinical features vary. Changes may be only biochemical, with a strikingly low serum phosphorus and an elevated alkaline phosphatase level. Muscle hypotonia may be severe; growth failure, bowing of the legs, and enlargement of the wrists, knees, and costochondral junctions are often associated with spinal deformities. Craniosynostosis has been described in infants with this disease. Pathologic fractures may be seen on x-ray as well as certain unique findings consisting of an irregular mosaic formation of the haversian system and trabecular "halos" of low-density bone.

In most cases, the serum phosphorus level is less than 2 mg/dL. The urinary calcium level is low, and the serum calcium level may be normal or slightly low. Serum levels of 1,25-dihydroxycholecalciferol are low, probably because high levels of phosphate in the tubule cell shut off the 1α-hydroxylase activity. Aminoaciduria is rare.

Treatment consists of giving 1–3 g of phosphorus daily, either as a buffered monosodium and disodium hydrogen phosphate solution at pH 7.4 or as Fleet's Phospho-Soda. Magnesium oxide, 10–15 mg/kg/d by mouth, may be of value. Supplementary calcitriol, up to 40 mg/kg/d, should be given if the serum calcium levels remain below normal.

Normal growth is never achieved unless every effort is made to keep the serum phosphorus level over 3 mg/dL.

NEPHROLITHIASIS

Renal calculi in children may result from certain inborn errors of metabolism, such as cystine in cystinosis, glycine in hyperglycinuria, urates in Lesch-Nyhan syndrome, and oxalates in oxalosis. Stones may occur secondary to hypercalciuria in distal tubular acidosis, and large stones are quite often seen in children with spina bifida who have paralyzed lower limbs. Treatment is limited to that of the primary condition, if possible. Surgical removal of stones should be considered only for obstruction, intractable severe pain, and chronic infection.

Cystinuria

Cystinuria, like Hartnup disease and a number of other disorders, is primarily an abnormality of amino acid transport across both the enteric and proximal renal tubular epithelium. There appear to be at least three biochemical types. In the first type, the bowel transport of basic amino acids and cystine is impaired, but transport of cysteine is not impaired. In the renal tubule, basic amino acids are again rejected by the tubule, but cystine absorption appears to be normal. The reasons for the cystinuria are, therefore, still obscure. Heterozygotes have no aminoaciduria. The second type is similar to the first except that the heterozygotes excrete excess cystine and lysine in the urine, and cystine transport in the bowel is normal. In the third type, only the nephron is involved. The only clinical manifestations are related to stone formation—ureteral colic, dysuria, hematuria, proteinuria, and secondary urinary tract infection. Urinary excretion of cystine, lysine, arginine, and ornithine is increased.

The most reliable way to prevent stone formation is to maintain a constantly high free water clearance. This involves generous fluid intake. Alkalinization of the urine is helpful. If these measures do not prevent significant renal lithiasis, the use of tiopronin is recommended.

Primary Hyperoxaluria

Oxalate production in humans is derived from the oxidative deamination of glycine to glyoxalate (about 40%), from the serine-glycolate pathway (about 50%), and from ascorbic acid. At least two enzymatic blocks have been described. Type 1 is a deficiency of liver-specific peroxisomal alanine:glyoxylate aminotransferase. Type 2 is glyoxalate reductase deficiency.

Excess oxalate combines with calcium to form insoluble deposits in the kidneys, lungs, and other tissues. The onset is during childhood. The joints are occasionally involved, but the main impact is on the kidneys, where progressive oxalate deposition leads to fibrosis and eventual renal failure.

Pyridoxine supplementation and a low-oxalate diet have been tried as therapy, but the overall prognosis is poor, and most patients succumb to uremia by early adulthood. Renal transplantation is not very successful because of destruction of the transplant kidney. However, there are encouraging results with concomitant liver transplantation, correcting the metabolic defect.

Hyperoxaluria may also occur secondary to ileal disease or after ileal resection.

Coe FL, Parks JH, Asplin JR: The pathogenesis and treatment of kidney stones. N Engl J Med 1992;327:1721.

Leumann E, Hoppe B, Neuhaus T: Management of primary hyperoxaluria: Efficacy of oral citrate administration. Pediatr Nephrol 1993;7:207.

NEPHROGENIC DIABETES INSIPIDUS

In the normal kidney, the interstitial fluid of the papilla is hyperosmolar to the fluid in the collecting duct. The luminal cells have a specific receptor for antidiuretic hormone (ADH), which, acting via cAMP, permits water to move across the cell membrane in response to the osmotic gradient. In the common X-linked recessive form (type I) of nephro-genic diabetes insipidus, there is a disorder of the ADH:adenylyl cyclase receptor, and urinary adenylyl cyclase is not increased after administration of vaso-pressin. In the type II variety, cAMP is formed by ADH action but has no effect on water transport. There are probably many variants of this complex mechanism, which is also influenced by prostaglan-din E_1 and by its inhibitor, indomethacin.

The symptoms are limited to polyuria, polydipsia, and failure to thrive. In some children, particularly if the solute intake is unrestricted, some adjustment to an elevated serum osmolality may develop. How-ever, these children are particularly liable to episodes of dehydration, fever, vomiting, and convulsions.

Clinically, the diagnosis can be made on the basis of a history of polydipsia and polyuria that are not sensitive to the administration of vasopressin, desmo-pressin acetate (DDAVP), or lypressin. It is wise to confirm this in all cases by performing a vasopressin test. Carefully monitored water restriction does not increase the tubular reabsorption of water (T^cH_2O) to above 3 mL/min/m^2. Urine osmolality will remain lower than 450 mOsm/kg, whereas serum osmolality rises and total body weight falls. Before weight re-duction greater than 5% occurs or before serum os-molality exceeds 320 mOsm/kg, administer vaso-pressin. Urine concentrating ability is impaired in a number of conditions—sickle cell anemia, pyelonephritis, potassium depletion, hypercalcemia, cystinosis and other renal tubular disorders and ob-structive uropathy—and as a result of nephrotoxic drugs.

In infants, it is usually best to allow water as de-manded and to restrict salt. Serum sodium levels should be evaluated at intervals to avoid hyperosmo-lality from inadvertent water restriction. In later childhood, sodium intake should continue to be re-stricted to 2–2.5 mEq/kg/24 h.

Treatment with hydrochlorothiazide is helpful, and many individuals show improvement with adminis-tration of prostaglandin inhibition with drugs such as indomethacin or tolmetin.

URINARY TRACT INFECTIONS

Urinary tract infections occur in approximately 1% of premature infants and newborns. Many of these infections are hematogenously spread; how-ever, outside the clinical setting of perinatal acute ill-ness and prematurity, urinary tract infections raise the possibility of urinary tract abnormalities. During the first year of life, males are more likely to have an anatomic basis for developing urinary tract infection;

nevertheless, the initial infection in a small child should alert the physician to the possibility of abnor-mal anatomy regardless of the patient's sex.

Older boys with a first infection should be exam-ined for urinary tract abnormalities, whereas a more conservative, watchful approach may be taken with older girls, especially if sexual activity or poor per-sonal hygiene is a possible cause. Such an approach, of course, assumes there are no other clinical abnor-malities present that arouse suspicion of significant urinary tract disease (eg, enuresis or short stature).

The most common causes of urinary tract infec-tions are *Escherichia coli, Klebsiella, Staphylococ-cus,* and the enteric streptococci—all present in nor-mal rectal and perineal flora. Unless there is reason to suspect that bacteremia is responsible, bacteria usually are presumed to gain access to the urinary tract via the urethra. The problem is greatly aggra-vated by poor hygiene, perineal infection (eg, pin-worms), sexual activity, and instrumentation. Despite the fact that voiding provides some safeguard against such contamination developing into infection, abnor-malities of the collecting system contribute to clinical infection and may lead to upper tract disease and re-nal parenchymal damage.

Clinical Findings

A. Symptoms and Signs: Newborns may pre-sent with fever, hypothermia, poor feeding, jaundice, failure to thrive, or sepsis. Infants may have strong-smelling urine and irritability. Preschool children may have abdominal pain, vomiting, strong-smelling urine, fever, enuresis, increased frequency of urina-tion, dysuria, or urgency. School-age children may develop the "classic" signs of urinary tract infection, including enuresis, increased frequency of urination, dysuria, urgency, fever, and costovertebral angle ten-derness (flank pain). Occasionally, children with bac-terial urinary tract infection present with hemor-rhagic cystitis.

Not all symptoms suggestive of urinary tract infec-tion actually prove to be related to bacterial infection. Anatomic abnormalities producing voiding discom-fort, irritation of the external genitalia, or viral hem-orrhagic cystitis are examples of such problems. On the other hand, some infections may actually be rela-tively asymptomatic. In either case, the presence of a urinary tract infection should be documented by urinalysis and urine culture.

B. Laboratory Tests: The clean-catch, mid-stream method may be satisfactory for children who can void upon request and who can be assisted in ob-taining a proper specimen or be relied upon to obtain one unassisted. Bladder catheterization or suprapubic bladder tap may be performed when necessary (eg, highly suspicious clinical picture but inability to ob-tain a satisfactory clean-catch specimen). Any proce-dure, however, carries the risk of contamination, and for this reason the more invasive procedures should be used only upon appropriate indication and with proper technique.

After the specimen is obtained, care must be taken to decant an aliquot for urinalysis prior to sending the specimen for culture and sensitivity testing. The aliquot is then spun and prepared for microscopic analysis. The presence of bacteria in the specimen is highly suggestive of urinary tract infection provided that the specimen is clean-catch and midstream. The presence of pyuria (> 5 WBCs/hpf) is also consistent with infection—but, again, specimen reliability is important because the perineal region, vagina, or external genitalia may be the source of blood cells in urine specimens. Nonetheless, such findings plus highly suspicious symptoms warrant initiation of antibiotic treatment until culture results are reported.

The presence of multiple organisms suggests specimen contamination; however, this possibility must be evaluated in light of the method used in obtaining the specimen as well as the level of confidence in the technical performance of the procedure used. If the child is not already receiving the appropriate antibiotic as indicated by the sensitivity test results, a change should be made accordingly.

Nonculture methods such as nitrite sticks for early detection of urinary tract infection may be useful in following the child with recurrent infection or being treated prophylactically with antibiotic suppression therapy.

Treatment

A. Initial Treatment: After urinary tract infection is confirmed, initial therapy should be based on the patient's history of antibiotic use, the location of the infection, and the subsequent drug sensitivities of the organism.

For uncomplicated cases of urethritis or cystitis, a single oral antibiotic that the patient has not used recently (eg, ampicillin, a sulfonamide, nitrofurantoin) can be administered for 10 days. The choice of antibiotic therapy must be verified by prior culture and sensitivity testing. A patient with suspected pyelonephritis need not always be admitted to the hospital, but antibiotic coverage should be broad (ampicillin, a sulfonamide, or a cephalosporin plus gentamicin). This regimen ensures adequate coverage until the patient improves and the results of antibiotic sensitivity tests are available, allowing selection of a single effective oral antibiotic. Antibiotic dosages (depending on choice of drug) are appropriately modified in patients with acute or chronic renal failure.

Most urinary tract infections can be successfully treated with inexpensive drugs given orally. Follow-up urinalysis or use of nitrite sticks within 2–3 days can confirm therapeutic success. If symptoms persist, reexamination and repeat urine culture are necessary.

B. Treatment of Refractory Infection: Persistent bacteriuria indicates superinfection with a different organism or with the same organism due to obstruction, the presence of a foreign body, or conversion of the organism to a variant form.

C. Urologic Intervention: Voiding cystourethrography should be obtained with proved infection. Renal ultrasonography is a helpful noninvasive tool for evaluating the anatomy of the urinary tract.

Obvious structural ureteral reflux or obstructive anomalies require referral to a urologist experienced in dealing with children. Vesicoureteral reflux is common in younger children. Mild reflux does not cause renal damage and will disappear in time if repeated infections can be prevented. Severe reflux generally requires ureteral reimplantation.

In patients without structural or functional urinary tract abnormalities, possible causes of recurrent infection include infrequent or incomplete voiding, poor perineal hygiene, pinworms, constipation, and the use of bubble bath. If attempts to deal with these problems are unsuccessful, single-dose prophylaxis at bedtime with agents such as nitrofurantoin or trimethoprim-sulfamethoxazole may be useful in combination with a program of frequent voiding.

D. Follow-Up of Patients With Urinary Tract Infection: All patients with urinary tract infection should be checked for recurrence every 1–2 months until they have remained free of infection for 1 year. Home testing of first morning concentrated urine specimens by nitrite stick may reduce the cost of follow-up without compromising accuracy.

Prognosis

As long as urinary tract infections can be confined to the lower urinary tract (bladder and below), the prognosis is excellent. Once an infectious process has entered the kidney, the prognosis becomes more guarded. Therefore, every diagnostic and therapeutic effort should be made to prevent recurrences.

Chandra M: Reflux nephropathy, urinary tract infection, and voiding disorders. Curr Opin Pediatr 1995;7:164.

Hellerstein S: Urinary tract infections: Old and new concepts. Pediatr Clin North Am 1995;42:1433.

Nash MA, Seigle RL: Urinary tract infections in infants and children. Adv Pediatr Infect Dis 1996;11:403.

REFERENCES

Edelmann CM Jr et al (editors): *Pediatric Kidney Disease,* 2nd ed. Little, Brown, 1992.

Holliday MA, Barratt TM, Avner ED: *Pediatric Nephrology,* 4th ed. Williams & Wilkins, 1994.

Neurologic & Muscular Disorders

Paul G. Moe, MD, & Alan R. Seay, MD

NEUROLOGIC ASSESSMENT & NEURODIAGNOSTIC PROCEDURES

NEUROLOGIC HISTORY & EXAMINATION

The history is usually taken with the child and parents together. Questions can be addressed directly to the older child with further details supplemented by the parent. If time permits, a teenager should be interviewed alone. If strong psychosocial factors become evident by the end of the joint interview, the parent may be asked to leave. Sensitive issues (eg, drug use, sexual activity) can then be reexplored with the older child.

A patient data form filled out by the parent in advance of the visit or in the physician's waiting room is helpful. The form should include the chief complaint, the patient's strengths and talents, birth and family history, medical history, and school and behavioral history. A checklist of behavioral issues such as hyperactivity, depression, short attention span, and so on, can bring attention to areas that need to be more carefully explored during the interview. Developmental delays suspected in the infant or older child can also be addressed in a checklist. A physician interviewing a child aged 5–7 can begin with neutral questions regarding age and birthday. It is often informative to see whether these children know their birthday or even year of birth.

The core of the history is the present illness. What the parent or child sees as important should be the initial focus. In recurrent conditions (eg, seizures or headaches), it is important to find out what happened during the first as well as the most recent episode. Details of recurrent episodes should be thoroughly discussed, including frequency, duration, change in character over time, and precipitating and alleviating factors. The effect of emotions, medications, and environmental manipulations such as diet change should be reviewed. The physician should ascertain, if possible, whether the disease is congenital or age-acquired and whether it is progressive.

As the interview progresses, the clinician begins to form ideas about a possible diagnosis; these can be explored with searching questions. Occasionally, the patient and parent see things from different viewpoints. The child, for instance, may consider the headaches a trivial matter that does not interfere with activity; the mother may feel differently. It may be helpful to observe the emotional interchange between parent and child and to note each one's opinions regarding the severity of disease, the degree of interference with peer group and school activities, side effects and efficacy of medications, and the like.

Depending on the nature of the complaint, the past medical history may or may not be extremely detailed. For example, in the case of a teenager with headaches, the mother's history of pregnancy and birth is of little importance. In the case of a 2-month-old child with hypotonia, detailed information about these events is essential. The family and genetic history may be important. A strong family history of migraine or a history of myotonic dystrophy in an uncle might be the key to diagnosis in the examples cited. The parents may have to do some searching with inquiries to relatives or hospitals to assemble family history details.

Available health records, roentgenograms, electroencephalograms (EEGs), and school records may complement the interview. Developmental history is essential in the assessment of any infant. The Denver Developmental Screening Test (DDST) is one helpful tool for reviewing each major area of behavior in infancy, that is, gross motor, fine motor, personal/social, and language. Some developmental expectations and landmarks are listed in Table 22–1.

In the older child, the developmental history can be explored with questions concerning school progress. The clinician should ask how the patient is getting along with the peer group, in physical activities, and in the family setting. Open-ended questions (eg, "What is she like? What is an average day in her

Table 22–1. Neurologic developmental landmarks.

	Birth	3 Months	6 Months	9 Months	12–15 Months	24 Months
Motor	Flexor posture, lifts head prone, hands grasped	Sits: head forward, bobbing, lifts head supine, hands open, retains briefly	Rolls both ways, begins to sit alone, supports (erect), bounces	Creeps, pulls up standing, pincer grasp, sits well	Walks with one or both hands held, stands alone briefly, releases on command	Walks and runs well, walks downstairs, turns pages singly
Special senses	Regards (vision), may follow 45 degrees	Looks at hands, follows 90–180 degrees	Discriminates voices, localizes sounds	Picks up raisin, "bye-bye"	Localizes noises, localizes pain	Towers six or seven cubes, imitates scribble
Adaptive	Startles to sound, delayed nociceptive response	Smiles socially, vocalizes socially, follows vertically	Holds cube, palmar grasp, retrieves toy, transfers and rakes raisin	Bangs toys together, pat-a-cake	Assists in dressing, attempts spoon feeding, tries two-cube tower	Asks for toilet, pulls on garments, spoon-feeds well, parallel play
Language	Throaty noises	Coos, chuckles, vocal social response	Babbles (polysyllables), "mmm-mmm"	"Ma-ma, Da-da," one other "word"	Understands simple command, speaks one to three words	Speaks in phrases, names three to five pictures, pronouns: "I, me, you"
Reflex	Tonic neck, palmar grasp	Disappearing tonic neck, Moro reflex	Begins voluntary stepping	Parachute response		
Automatisms	Moro reflex, sucks, roots, stepping, supporting, traction: head lag	Landau response, traction: no head lag	Neck righting, blinks to threat			

life? What does she do?") can help the clinician assess the child's social functioning.

During examination, the infant or toddler is often held in the mother's lap. Much information can be obtained by observing a child carefully and noting spontaneous movements, curiosity, ability to understand directions, and alertness to visual and auditory cues (eg, a tinkling bell).

Part of the neurologic examination includes a brief general physical examination with emphasis on the skin (birth marks), spine, neck, and skull (including palpation of the fontanelle and measurement of head circumference). At some point in the examination, the baby should be inspected virtually unclothed. In an older child, asking about birthmarks and inspecting the spine with the shirt pulled up and the child bent over for evaluation of scoliosis may be sufficient.

Developmental assessment should be included in the neurologic examination of the infant. At an appropriate age (eg, 6–18 months), the physician may start with handing blocks to the baby, offering a raisin, and evaluating reach and type of grasp. A younger baby often enjoys a bell, the older child a reflex hammer. Using the block and the raisin, the clinician can assess the items on the DDST that have not been elucidated by the history.

Having the child run around the room and retrieve a ball allows testing of his or her **station and gait.** Children usually enjoy having their **reflexes** tested. Be sure reflexes are present proximally and distally, such as knee jerk, ankle jerk, triceps, brachial radialis. Sometimes, a subtle case of hemiparesis can be suggested by a unilateral absence of abdominal or cremasteric cutaneous reflexes. Occasionally, tapping one's finger over a hamstring or biceps reflex can show an absent reflex or asymmetry in a lumbosacral plexus or brachial plexus injury.

Infantile automatisms—their presence, absence, or asymmetry—are important in examination of the newborn and very young infant (Table 22–1).

Running around the room, squatting, jumping, etc, are tests of the child's **motor functions.** In infants, tone—the examiner's subjective feeling while manipulating the limb—is important. (See the section on hypotonic infants.) Occasionally, formal muscle testing is necessary, such as abduction at the shoulder and hand grasp, rising from a squat, and dorsiflexion of the foot to test proximal and distal strength. **Sensory testing** is rarely contributory, but touch, tickle, and pinprick testing can be used in small children.

At this point, the infant's **cranial nerves** have usually been satisfactorily assessed by observation (eg, extraocular movements, vision, and hearing). If there is concern about swallowing or tongue size or function, these areas can be examined with a flashlight and tongue blade. Lastly, the fundi should be assessed by having the infant look at a distant object or by having the parent attract the child's attention with a pinwheel or bell. The physician can approach from the side to observe the disk before light on the macula causes miosis. Sometimes, mydriatics to dilate the pupil are necessary.

In the older child, formal examination of **mental status** is rarely necessary. Simple assessment of cognition can be achieved by having the child obey right-and-left commands (eg, "Put your right hand on your left ear"), do simple arithmetic problems, and read paragraphs appropriate for grade level (Table 22–2).

In the older child, the **Romberg test** (standing with eyes closed, feet together, and hands straight out), tandem walking, and standing and hopping on each foot are tests of station and gait. Limb coordination can be tested by finger pursuit, that is, having children touch the clinician's moving finger with their own. Finger-nose alternating movements and patting the palm and the back of the hand alternately on the lap are other tests of lateral coordination. In the older child, tests for sense of position, vibration, and even cortical sensory status (eg, position of the limb in space and finger writing) are occasionally important.

Because children can be uncooperative and findings uncertain, serial examinations are sometimes necessary. Reasons for a follow-up examination should be explained in detail to the parent. No neurologic examination is a complete failure. The clinician has the opportunity to observe the child during the interview and during play; these observations may give a reasonable assessment of neurologic function.

Finally, it must be emphasized that a complete examination should be performed and results told to the parents in plain language, even when the complaint seems trivial.

Table 22–2. Mental status examination for school-age children.

Orientation: Time, place, situation, name, date, year.
Memory: Recent and remote, eg, "What did you have for lunch?" "What did you do on your birthday?" Remember (for 10 minutes): "Red flag, Washington's birthday, Christmas presents."
Calculation: Depends on educational background. Example: Subtract serial sevens.
Proverbs: Interpret: "Too many cooks spoil the broth." "A rolling stone gathers no moss."
Situation: "What would you do if you saw a fire?"
Aphasia: "What's this?" (chalk). "Stick out your tongue." "Put your right finger on your left ear." Sample speech, reading, and writing.

Johnson CP, Blasco PA: Infant growth and development. Pediatr Rev 1997;18:224.

LUMBAR PUNCTURE

The principal purpose of lumbar puncture is to obtain an aliquot of cerebrospinal fluid (CSF) for the diagnosis of infectious and inflammatory conditions of the central nervous system (Table 22–3). The uses of CSF specimens in cytologic studies, bioassays of enzymes and neurotransmitters, and specific rapid tests for viruses are widening the clinical (and research) applicability of lumbar puncture. Polymerase chain reaction (PCR) testing can amplify tiny amounts of virus or bacterial DNA to diagnose meningoencephalitis. Examples are encephalitis due to herpesvirus, enterovirus, and *Mycobacterium tuberculosis.*

Therapeutically, lumbar puncture may be used to drain CSF to reduce its hematotoxic effects in hemorrhagic conditions (eg, intraventricular hemorrhage in newborns, ruptured berry aneurysm) and to lower intracranial pressure in pseudotumor cerebri. Symptoms may be improved in viral meningitis.

Lumbar puncture is usually performed with the patient in the lateral recumbent or decubitus position. Entry is at the level of the iliac crest or the L3–L4 interspace, with the patient's head initially flexed and then extended. In small infants—especially premature infants and neonates in the first months of life—lumbar puncture is more safely and satisfactorily performed with the infant in the sitting position and the head only slightly flexed or supported with a pillow propped between the outstretched arms and legs resting against the infant's chest and abdomen. The wrists and ankles should be held by an assisting nurse, and the needle should be pointed slightly cephalad.

Note: Before lumbar puncture is performed, the fundi should always be checked for papilledema. Lumbar puncture is contraindicated in the presence of elevated intracranial pressure, especially when there are focal neurologic deficits, because of the risk of tentorial or tonsillar herniation. This risk is less likely when there is diffuse cerebral swelling than when elevated pressure is due to a mass lesion. Therefore, if equipment for computed tomographic (CT) brain scanning is readily available, lumbar puncture should usually be delayed until a scan can be done; it should not be delayed, however, if examination of cerebrospinal fluid is indispensable for diagnosis and vital therapeutic intervention.

Lumbar puncture must be performed promptly when a diffuse central nervous system infection (meningitis, meningoencephalitis, encephalitis, cerebritis) is suspected. Only a small-gauge needle should be used, and only enough fluid should be withdrawn to permit cell count, protein and glucose

Table 22–3. Characteristics of cerebrospinal fluid (CSF) in the normal child and in central nervous system infections and inflammatory conditions.

Condition	Initial Pressure (mm H₂O)	Appearance	Cells/μL	Protein (mg/dL)	Glucose (mg/dL)	Other Tests	Comments
Normal	< 60	Clear	0–5 lymphocytes. First 3 mos, 1–3 PMNs. Neonates, up to 30 lymphocytes, 20–50 RBCs.	15–35 (lumbar), 5–15 (ventricular). Up to 150 (lumbar) for short time after birth; to 6 months, up to 65.	50–80 (two-thirds of blood glucose); may be increased after seizure	CSF-IgG index < 0.7[1] LDH 2–27 units/L	CSF protein in first month may be up to 170 mg/dL in small-for-dates or premature infants. No increase in WBCs due to seizure.
Bloody tap	Normal or low	Bloody (sometimes with clot)	One additional WBC/700 RBCs.[2] RBCs not crenated.	One additional milligram per 800 RBCs[2]	Normal	RBC number should fall between first and third tubes; wait 5 minutes between tubes	Spin down fluid; supernatant will be clear and colorless.
Bacterial meningitis, acute	200–750+	Opalescent to purulent	Up to thousands, mostly PMNs. Early, few cells.	Up to hundreds	Decreased; may be none	Smear and culture mandatory. LDH > 24 units/L. Bacterial antigen tests if Gram stain and culture are negative.	Very early, glucose may be normal. Latex agglutination for *S pneumoniae* and group B *Streptococcus*.
Bacterial meningitis, partially treated	Usually increased	Clear or opalescent	Usually increased. PMNs usually predominate.	Elevated	Normal or decreased	LDH usually > 24 units/L. Bacterial antigen tests.	Smear and culture may be negative if antibiotics have been in use.
Tuberculous meningitis	150–750+	Opalescent; fibrin web or pellicle	250–500, mostly lymphocytes. Early, more PMNs.	45–500; parallels cell count; increases over time	Decreased; may be none	Smear for acid-fast organism: CSF culture and inoculation; PCR	Consider AIDS.
Fungal meningitis	Increased	Variable; often clear	10–500. Early, more PMNs; then mostly lymphocytes.	Elevated and increasing	Decreased	India ink preparations, cryptococcal antigen, culture, inoculations, immunofluorescence tests	Often superimposed in patients who are debilitated or on immunosuppressive therapy.
Aseptic meningoencephalitis (viral meningitis, or parameningeal disease)	Normal or slightly increased	Clear unless cell count > 300/μL	None to a few hundred, mostly lymphocytes; PMNs predominate early.	20–125	Normal; may be low in mumps, herpes, or other viral infections	CSF, stool, blood, throat washings for viral cultures. LDH < 28 units/L PCR for HSV, CMV, EBV, enterovirus, etc.	Acute and convalescent antibody titers for some viruses. In mumps, up to 1000 lymphocytes; serum amylase often elevated. Rarely, several thousand cells present in enteroviral infection.
Neurosyphilis	Normal to 400	Clear unless protein is very high	10–100, mostly lymphocytes	25–150; higher in meningitis	Normal	Positive CSF serology CSF-IgG index increased	Serology positive in untreated cases; *Treponema pallidum* immobilization test positive.
Parainfectious encephalomyelitis	80–450, usually increased	Usually clear	0–50, mostly lymphocytes.	15–75	Normal	CSF-IgG index may be increased. Oligoclonal bands variable.	No organisms. Fulminant cases resemble bacterial meningitis.
Polyneuritis	Normal and occasionally increased	Early: normal; late: xanthochromic if protein high	Normal; occasionally slight increase	Early: normal; late: 45–1500	Normal	CSF-IgG index may be increased. Oligoclonal bands variable.	Try to find cause (viral infections, toxins, lupus, diabetes, etc)
Meningeal carcinomatosis	Often elevated	Clear to opalescent	Cytologic identification of tumor cells	Often mildly to moderately elevated	Often depressed	Cytology	Seen with leukemia, medulloblastoma, meningeal melanosis, histiocytosis X. *Note:* May mimic meningitis.
Brain abscess	Normal or increased	Usually clear	5–500 in 80%; mostly PMNs	Usually slightly increased	Normal; occasionally decreased	Imaging study of brain (MRI)	Cell count related to proximity to meninges; findings as in purulent meningitis if abscess perforates.

[1] CSF-IgG index = CSF IgG/serum IgG ÷ CSF albumin/serum albumin.

[2] Many studies document pitfalls in using these ratios due to WBC lysis. Clinical judgment and repeat taps may be necessary to rule out meningitis in this situation.

Key: PMN = polymorphonuclear neutrophil; CSF = cerebrospinal fluid; WBC = white blood cell; RBC = red blood cell; LDH = lactate dehydrogenase; AIDS = acquired immunodeficiency syndrome; PCR = polymerase chain reaction; HSV = herpes simplex virus; CMV = cytomegalovirus; EBV = Epstein Barr virus determination, and such stains and cultures (bacterial, fungal, and viral) and other studies as may be needed. A specimen of 2–3 mL is usually adequate for microchemical determinations.

It is occasionally important to obtain opening and closing CSF pressures. To obtain valid pressure readings, the child's head, neck, and legs should be gently brought into a straight line. Pressure in the sitting position should be measured with the level of the foramen magnum as "zero"; the length of the fluid column above that level is the pressure in millimeters of water.

Carraccio C, Blotny K, Fisher MC: CSF analysis in systemically ill children without CNS disease. Pediatrics 1995;96:48.

Jaffe M et al: The ameliorating effect of lumbar puncture in viral meningitis. Am J Dis Child 1989;143:682.

Markowitz H, Kokmen E: Neurologic diseases and the cerebrospinal fluid immunoglobin profile. Mayo Clin Proc 1983;58:273.

Novak RW: Lack of validity of standard corrections for white blood cell counts of blood-contaminated cerebrospinal fluid in infants. Am J Clin Pathol 1984;82:95.

Portnoy J, Olson L: Normal cerebrospinal fluid values in children: Another look. Pediatrics 1985;75:484.

Ricevuti G: Meningeal leukemia diagnosed by cytocentrifuge study of cerebrospinal fluid. Arch Neurol 1986;43:466.

Rubenstein S, Yager R: What represents pleocytosis in blood-contaminated ("traumatic tap") CSF in childhood? J Pediatr 1985;107:249.

Ward EM, Gushurst D: Uses and techniques of pediatric lumbar puncture. Am J Dis Child 1992;196:1160.

ELECTROENCEPHALOGRAPHY

This widely used noninvasive electrophysiologic method for recording cerebral activity has its greatest clinical applicability in the study of seizure disorders. "Activation" techniques to accentuate abnormalities or disclose latent abnormalities include photic stimulation, well-sustained hyperventilation for 3 minutes, and depriving the patient of sleep from about midnight until after breakfast, at which time the EEG is recorded. The latter is an excellent though less widely used "activation" method.

Electroencephalography is also used in the evaluation of tumors, cerebrovascular accidents, neurodegenerative diseases, and other neurologic disorders causing brain dysfunction; but with some notable exceptions, it is nonspecific. Recordings over a 24-hour period or all-night recordings are invaluable in the diagnosis of sleep disturbances and narcolepsy. Electroencephalography with telemetry or simultaneous monitoring of behavior on videotape, has great usefulness in selected cases. The EEG can be helpful in determining a possible cause or mechanism of coma and is frequently used to help determine whether coma is irreversible and brain death has occurred.

The limitations of electroencephalography are considerable: In most cases, the duration of the actual tracing is about 45 minutes and reflects only surface cortical function. Many drugs—especially barbiturates and benzodiazepines—have considerable effects on the EEG and may confuse interpretation. Moreover, about 15% of nonepileptic individuals, especially children, may have an abnormal EEG. Electroencephalographic findings such as those seen in migraine, learning disabilities, or behavior disorders do not reflect permanent "brain damage." A major usefulness of EEG is to show epileptiform activity in children with seizure disorders; sometimes the findings are virtually diagnostic, as in the hypsarrhythmia EEG of infantile spasms or the prolonged 3-second spike wave of absence seizures.

At present, use of CT scans, evoked potentials, positron emission tomography, regional cerebral blood flow studies, single-photon emission computed tomography (SPECT), and magnetic resonance imaging (MRI) supplements the use of EEGs as a diagnostic and prognostic tool.

EVOKED POTENTIALS

Cortical auditory, visual, or somatosensory evoked potentials (evoked responses) may be recorded from the scalp surface over the temporal, occipital, or frontoparietal cortex after repetitive stimulation of the retina by light flashes, of the cochlea by sounds, or of a nerve by galvanic stimuli of varying frequency and intensity, respectively. Computer averaging is used to recognize and enhance these responses while subtracting or suppressing the asynchronous background electroencephalographic activity. The presence or absence of evoked potential waves and their latencies (time from stimulus to wave peak or time between peaks) figure in the clinical interpretation.

The reproducible and quantifiable results obtained from brain stem auditory, pattern-shift visual, and short-latency somatosensory evoked potentials (see below) indicate the level of function of the relevant sensory pathway or system and identify the site of anatomic disruption. Although results of these tests alone are usually not diagnostic, the tests are noninvasive, sensitive, objective, and relatively inexpensive extensions of the clinical neurologic examination. Because the auditory and somatosensory tests and one type of visual test are completely passive, requiring only that the patient remain still, they are particularly useful in the evaluation of neonates and small children as well as in patients unable to cooperate (eg, as a result of mental retardation, degenerative disorder, anesthesia, or coma). Knowledge of normal values and experience in testing of the applicable patient group are mandatory.

Brain Stem Auditory Evoked Potentials

A brief auditory stimulus (click) of varying intensity and frequency is delivered to the ear to activate the auditory nerve (nerve VIII) and sequentially activate the cochlear nucleus, tracts and nuclei of the lateral lemniscus, and inferior colliculus. Thus, this technique assesses hearing and function of the brain stem auditory tracts.

Hearing in the neonate or uncooperative (but sedated) patient can be objectively assessed, making the technique particularly useful in high-risk infants—especially those in intensive care nurseries— and in retarded and autistic patients. Brain stem auditory evoked potentials are used to judge brain stem dysfunction in sleep apnea, in Arnold-Chiari malformation, and achondroplasia. Because high doses of anesthetic agents or barbiturates do not seriously affect results, the test is used to assess and monitor brain stem function of surgical patients (in the operating room) and those in hypoxic-ischemic coma or coma following head injury. Absence of evoked potential waves beyond the first wave from the auditory nerve usually signifies brain death. Brain stem auditory evoked potentials are also useful in the early evaluation of diseases affecting myelin—the various leukodystrophies and multiple sclerosis (although auditory evoked potentials are less valuable than visual evoked potentials in the latter)—and in intrinsic brain stem gliomas. They are sometimes useful in evaluation of hereditary ataxias, Wilson's disease (hepatolenticular degeneration), and other degenerative disorders affecting the brain stem.

Pattern-Shift Visual Evoked Potentials

The preferred stimulus is a shift (reversal) of a checkerboard pattern, and the response is a single wave (called P100) generated in the striate and parastriate visual cortex. The absolute latency of P100 (time from stimulus to wave peak) and the difference in latency between the two eyes are sensitive indicators of disease. The amplitude of response is affected by any process resulting in poor fixation on the stimulus screen or affecting visual acuity. Ability to focus on a checkerboard pattern is necessary. An LED (light-emitting diode), goggles, or bright flash stimulus can be used in younger and uncooperative children, but the norms are less standardized. Evoked potentials suggest that visual acuity may be 20/20 in infants by 6–7 months of age.

Clinical application of the test includes detection and monitoring of strabismus (ie, in amblyopia ex anopsia), optic neuritis, and lesions near the optic nerve and chiasm such as optic gliomas and craniopharyngiomas. Degenerative and immunologic diseases that affect visual transmission may be detected early and followed by serial evaluations by this technique, including adrenoleukodystrophy, Pelizaeus-

Merzbacher disease, some spinocerebellar degenerations, sarcoidosis, and even multiple sclerosis. Flash visual evoked potentials are used to monitor function during surgery involving the eyes and optic nerve; to assess cortical or hysterical blindness; and to evaluate patients with photosensitive epilepsy, who may have exaggerated responses.

Short-Latency Somatosensory Evoked Potentials

Responses are commonly produced by electrical stimulation of peripheral sensory nerves, since this evokes potentials of greatest amplitude and clarity; finger tapping and muscle stretching may also be used. The function of this test is similar to that of the auditory test in closely correlating wave forms with function of the sensory pathways and permitting localization of conduction defects.

Short-latency somatosensory evoked potentials are used in the assessment of a wide variety of lesions of the peripheral nerve, root, spinal cord, and central nervous system following trauma, neuropathies (eg, in diabetes mellitus or Guillain-Barré syndrome), myelodysplasias, cerebral palsy, and many other disorders. The procedure is often performed on an outpatient basis. One method is stimulation of the median nerve at the wrist with small (nonpainful) electrical shocks and recording of responses from the brachial plexus above the clavicle, the neck (cervical cord), and the opposite scalp area overlying the sensorimotor cortex. After stimulation from the knee (peroneal nerve) or ankle (tibial nerve), impulses are recorded from the lower lumbar spinal cord, cervical cord, and sensorimotor cortex. Such potentials are used to monitor spinal cord sensory functioning during surgery for disorders including scoliosis, myelodysplasias, and tumors and other lesions of the spinal cord or blood vessels supplying the cord. The technique is also used in leukodystrophies involving peripheral nerves, in multiple sclerosis, and in the differential diagnosis of hysteria and malingering (anesthetic limbs). In the diagnosis of coma and brain death, somatosensory evoked potentials supplement the results of auditory evoked potentials.

Aldrich MS, Jahnke B: Diagnostic value of video EEG polysomnography. Neurology 1991;41:1060.

Cohen BA, Schenk VA, Sweeney DB: Meningitis-related hearing loss evaluated with evoked potentials. Pediatr Neurol 1988;4:18.

DeMeirleir LJ, Taylor MJ: Prognostic utility of SEPs in comatose children. Pediatr Neurol 1987;3:78.

Eyre JA (editor): The neurophysiologic examination of the newborn infant. *Clinics in Developmental Medicine,* No. 120. MacKeith Press, 1992.

Fagan ER, Taylor MJ, Logan WJ: Somatosensory evoked potentials. A review of the clinical applications in pediatric neurology. Pediatr Neurol 1987;3:189.

Kamimura N et al: Spinal somatosensory evoked potentials in infants and children with spinal cord lesions. Brain Dev 1988;10:355.

Taylor MJ, McCullough D: Prognostic value of VEPs in young children with acute-onset cortical blindness. Pediatr Neurol 1992;7:111.

Whyte HE et al: Prognostic utility of visual evoked potentials in term asphyxiated neonates. Pediatr Neurol 1986;2:220.

BRAIN ELECTRICAL ACTIVITY MAPPING (BEAM)

Brain electrical activity mapping is a relatively new technique in which electroencephalographic and evoked potential data recorded from multiple scalp electrodes are graphically displayed in color on a computer-driven video screen. Values between electrodes are obtained by interpolation. Learning-disabled, dyslexic, and epileptic children are being studied in research protocols. Expense, lack of normative data, and lack of numbers of homogeneous clinical patients preclude current use of this modality in pediatric practice.

Duffy FH: The BEAM method for neurophysiological diagnosis. Ann N Y Acad Sci 1985;457:19.

Nuwer M: Quantitative EEG. 1. Techniques and problems of frequency, analysis, and topographic mapping. Neurol Clin 1988;5:1.

Nuwer M, Sharbrough F: American EEG Society statement on clinical use of quantitative EEG. Neurology 1987;37:28A.

PEDIATRIC NEURORADIOLOGIC PROCEDURES

Sedation for Procedures

Radiologic procedures in infants and children are usually performed by pediatric radiologists, but sedation for these procedures remains largely the responsibility of the physician caring for the child. The choice of sedation must take into account the patient's age and physical condition, the type of neurologic disorder, the effect and duration of the procedure, and whether immediate neurosurgery is anticipated. The prescribing physician should be familiar with the agent used.

Oral or rectal chloral hydrate, 30–60 mg/kg/dose, is safest. Many radiology departments, however, use only nonoral administration because of the risks of vomiting and aspiration. One favorite is pentobarbital, 6 mg/kg for children weighing less than 15 kg and 5 mg/kg for larger children (up to a maximum of 200 mg) given intramuscularly or rectally (at least 20 minutes before a procedure) or 2–4 mg/kg given intravenously. Equipment to support blood pressure and respiration must be available. This dosage usually achieves sedation for up to 2 hours. If, however, sedation is inadequate 30 minutes after injection— and if the condition of the child permits—a second dose of pentobarbital, 2 mg/kg, is given. General anesthesia may be indicated, especially if the child is to undergo surgery immediately on completion of a radiologic examination.

Computed Tomography (CT Scanning)

CT scanning consists of a series of cross-sectional (axial) roentgenograms and can be performed on an outpatient basis. Radiation exposure is approximately the same as that from a skull roentgenogram series. The images can be viewed on an oscilloscope as the scan is being done and later examined on printed-out films; both oscilloscope views and films record variations in tissue densities. CT scanning is of high sensitivity (88–96% of lesions larger than 1–2 cm can be seen) but low specificity (a tumor, focus of infection, or infarct may have the same appearance).

The CT scan is often repeated after intravenous injection of iodized contrast for enhancement, which reflects the vascularity of a lesion or its surrounding tissues. Precautions should be taken to ensure that the patient is not hypersensitive to iodinated dyes and that allergic reactions can be managed promptly. Sufficient information is often obtained from a nonenhanced scan; in these cases, cost and risk are minimized.

Sedation may be required for CT scanning. For positioning the head of children up to 8 years of age, a specially shaped headrest may be needed. The indications for CT scanning and the findings in specific conditions are discussed below in the sections on specific disorders.

Magnetic Resonance Imaging

MRI is a noninvasive technique that uses the magnetic properties of certain nuclei to produce diagnostically useful signals. Currently, the technique is based on detecting the response (resonance) of hydrogen proton nuclei to applied radiofrequency electromagnetic radiation; these nuclei are abundant in the body and more sensitive to MRI than other nuclei. The strength of MRI signals varies with the relationship of water to protein and the amount of lipids present. The image displayed, which is made up of a mixture of signals and is similar to the CT film, provides high-resolution contrast of soft tissues. MRI can, in fact, provide information about the histologic, physiologic, and biochemical status of tissues in addition to gross anatomic data.

MRI has been used to delineate brain tumors, edema, ischemic and hemorrhagic lesions, hydrocephalus, vascular disorders, inflammatory and infectious lesions, and degenerative processes. MRI can be used to study myelination and demyelination and, through the demonstration of changes in relaxation time, metabolic disorders of the brain, muscles, and glands. Because bone causes no artifact in the images, the posterior fossa and its contents can be studied far better using MRI than with CT scans; even blood vessels and the cranial nerves can be imaged. On the other hand, the inability of MRI to detect calcification limits its usefulness in the investigation of calcified lesions such as craniopharyngioma or leptomeningeal angiomatosis.

It is believed that the strong magnetic fields used in this procedure do not cause molecular or cellular damage. Work is progressing on imaging from nuclei other than hydrogen, such as phosphorus and sodium.

The cost of MRI is two or three times that of a contrast-enhanced CT scan. The procedure can be frightening and requires sedated sleep or light anesthesia for the child to ensure complete immobility. Magnetic resonance angiography (MRA) is a noninvasive (no arterial or venous puncture or dye injection) technique to show large extra- and intracranial blood vessels; it often now replaces the more hazardous intra-arterial injection angiogram.

Positron Emission Tomography

Positron emission tomography (PET) is an imaging technique that measures the metabolic rate at a given site by CT scanning to detect positron (proton) emission. For measurement of local cerebral metabolism, the radiolabeled substrate most frequently used has been fluorodeoxyglucose ^{18}F by injection. Gray matter and white matter are clearly distinguishable; the skull and air- or fluid-filled cavities are least active metabolically.

PET has been used to study the cerebral metabolism of neonates and brain activation by visual or auditory stimuli. Pathologic states that have been studied include epilepsy (during and between seizures), brain infarcts and tumors, and dementias. This functional test of brain metabolism is clinically useful in preoperative evaluation for epilepsy surgery. The "epileptogenic zone" will often be hypermetabolic during ictal events and hypoactive during the time between seizures. The information complements electrical (EEG) and imaging (MRI) findings to aid in the decision about tissue removal.

With PET, infants with infantile spasms have occasionally been found to have a focal lesion, sometimes leading to successful surgical removal.

Clinical application is limited by the cost of the procedure and the clinician's need for access to a nearby cyclotron for preparation of the radiopharmaceuticals.

Ultrasonography

Ultrasonography offers a pictorial display (eg, echoencephalogram, echocardiogram) of the varying densities of tissues in a given anatomic region or structure by recording the echoes of ultrasonic waves reflected from it. These waves, modulated by pulsations, are introduced into the tissue by means of a piezoelectric transducer. The many advantages of ultrasonography include the ability to assess a structure and its positioning quickly by means of portable equipment, without ionizing radiation and at about one fourth the cost of CT scanning. Sedation is usually not necessary, and the procedure can be repeated as often as indicated. In brain imaging, B-mode and real-time sector scanners are usually used, permitting excellent detail in the coronal and sagittal planes. Contiguous structures can be studied by a continuous sweep and reviewed on videotape.

Ultrasonography has been used for in utero diagnosis of hydrocephalus and other anomalies. In neonates, the thin skull and the open anterior fontanelle have facilitated imaging of the brain, and ultrasonography is now used in many nurseries to screen and follow all infants of less than 32 weeks' gestation or under 1500 g for intracranial hemorrhage. Other uses in neonates include detection of hydrocephalus, major brain and spine malformations, and even calcifications from intrauterine infection with cytomegalovirus or *Toxoplasma*.

Cerebral Angiography

Arteriography remains a useful procedure in the diagnosis of many cerebrovascular disorders, particularly in cerebrovascular accidents or in potentially operable vascular malformations. In some instances of brain tumor, arteriography may be necessary to define the precise location or vascular bed, to differentiate among tumors, or to distinguish tumor from abscess or infarction. Noninvasive CTs, MRIs, and MRAs are often satisfactory in cases of static or flowing blood disorders (eg, sinus thromboses). Thus, invasive arteriography is usually done via femoral artery-aorta catheterization.

Myelography

X-ray examination of the spine following injection of a dye, water-soluble contrast medium, or air into the subarachnoid space via the lumbar or, rarely, the cervical route may be indicated in cases of spinal cord tumors or various forms of spinal dysraphism and in rare instances of herniated disks in children. However, in most institutions, MRI or CT metrizamide myelography is employed instead.

Adams C et al: Comparison of SPECT, EEG, CT, MRI, and pathology in partial epilepsy. Pediatr Neurol 1992;8:97.

Barkovich AJ: Pediatric Neuroimaging. Raven Press, 1995.

Chugani K: The role of positron emission tomography in childhood epilepsy. Int Pediatr 1992;7:260.

Edelman RR, Warach S: Magnetic resonance imaging. (Two parts.) N Engl J Med 1993;11:708, 785.

Faerber EN (editor): CNS magnetic resonance imaging in infants and children. *Clinics in Developmental Medicine*. No. 134. MacKeith Press, 1995.

Harvey AS: Functional neuro-imaging with SPECT and PET in childhood developmental disabilities. Int Pediatr 1995;10:177.

Koelfen W et al: Magnetic resonance angiography in 140 patients. Pediatr Neurol 1995;12:31.

Morris MC et al: Neurodiagnostic techniques. Pediatr Rev 1997;18:192.

Shields WD: Anatomic & functional imaging in epilepsy. Int Pediatr 1995;10:72.

DISORDERS AFFECTING THE NERVOUS SYSTEM IN INFANTS & CHILDREN

ALTERED STATES OF CONSCIOUSNESS

Essentials of Diagnosis & Typical Features

- Reduction or alteration in cognitive and affective mental functioning and in arousability or attentiveness.
- Acute onset.

General Considerations

Coma and other states of unconsciousness are imprecisely defined. Many terms are used to describe the continuum from full alertness and attentiveness to complete unresponsiveness and deep coma, including clouding, obtundation, somnolence or stupor, semicoma or light coma, and deep coma. Several scales have been used to grade the depth of unconsciousness (Tables 22–4 and 22–5). Physicians should use one of these tables and provide further descriptions in case narratives. These descriptions help subsequent observers quantify unconsciousness and evaluate changes in the patient's condition.

The neurologic substrate for consciousness is the reticular activating system in the brain stem, up to and including the thalamus and paraventricular hypothalamus. Large lesions of the cortex, especially of the left hemisphere, can also cause coma. **"Locked-in syndrome"** is a term used for patients who are conscious but have no access to motor or verbal expression because of massive loss of motor function of the brain stem. **"Coma vigil"** is the term used for patients who seem to be comatose but have some spontaneous motor behavior, such as eye opening or eye tracking, almost always at a reflex level. **"Persistent vegetative state"** denotes a chronic condition in which there is preservation of the sleep-wake cycle but no awareness and no recovery of mental function; this has been documented in infants.

Emergency Measures

The clinician's first response is to ensure that the patient will survive the initial examination. The "ABCs" of resuscitation are pertinent: *A*irway must be kept open with positioning or even endotracheal intubation. *B*reathing and adequate air exchange can be assessed by auscultation; hand bag respiratory assistance with oxygen may be needed. *C*irculation must be ensured by assessing pulse and blood pressure. *An intravenous line is always necessary.* Fluids, plasma, blood, or even a dopamine drip (5–20 μg/kg/min) may be required in cases of hypotension. An extremely hypothermic or febrile child may require vigorous cooling or warming to save life. The assessment of vital signs may signal the diagnosis. Slow, insufficient respirations suggest poisoning by hypnotic drugs; apnea may indicate diphenoxylate hydrochloride poisoning. Rapid, deep respirations suggest acidosis, possibly metabolic, as with diabetic coma; toxic, such as that due to aspirin; or neurogenic, as in Reye's syndrome. Hyperthermia may in-

Table 22–4. Gradation of coma.

	"Deep Coma"		"Light Coma"		
	Grade 4	Grade 3	Grade 2	Grade 1	Stupor
Response to pain	0	+	Avoidance	Avoidance	Arousal unsustained
Tone/posture	Flaccid	Decerebrate	Variable	Variable	Normal
Tendon reflexes	0	+/–	+	+	+
Pupil response	0	+	+	+	+
Response to verbal stimuli	0	0	0	0	+
Other corneal reflex	0	+	+	+	+
Gag reflex	0	+	+	+	+

Table 22–5. "Glasgow Coma Scale" for recording assessment of consciousness.[1,2]

		Date				
		Time	**Time**	**Time**	**Time**	**Etc**
Best motor response	6 Obeys commands 5 Localizes pain 4 Withdraws 3 Abnormal flexing 2 Extensor response 1 None					
Best verbal response	5 Oriented 4 Confused conversation (words) 3 Inappropriate words (vocal sounds) 2 Incomprehensible sounds (cries) 1 None					
Eye opening	4 Spontaneous 3 To speech 2 To pain 1 None					
	Total Score					

[1]Modified and reproduced, with permission, from Jennett B, Teasdale G: Aspects of coma after severe head injury. Lancet 1977;1:878.
[2]The scale can also be modified for infants. The sections regarding motor response and eye opening remain unchanged; items in parentheses in verbal response section are to be applied to infants. Under 6 months of age, the best verbal response is a cry (score 2) and the best motor response is usually flexion (score 3), for a total maximal score of 9. Adjusted maximal scores are as follows:

Birth–6 months:	9	2–5 years:	13
6–12 months:	11	Over 5 years:	14–15
1–2 years:	12		

dicate infection or heat stroke; hypothermia may indicate cold exposure, ethanol poisoning, or hypoglycemia (especially in infancy).

The signs of impending brain herniation are another priority of the initial assessment. Bradycardia, high blood pressure, irregular breathing, increased extensor tone, and third nerve palsy with the eye deviated outward and the pupil dilated are possible signs of impending temporal lobe or brain stem herniation. These signs suggest a need for hyperventilation, reducing cerebral edema, prompt neurosurgical consultation, and possibly, in an infant with a bulging fontanelle, subdural or ventricular tap (or both).

Initial intravenous fluids should contain glucose until further assessment disproves hypoglycemia as a cause.

A history obtained from parents or witnesses is desirable. Sometimes the only history will be obtained from ambulance attendants. An important point is whether the child is known to have a chronic illness, such as diabetes, hemophilia, epilepsy, or cystic fibrosis. Recent acute illness raises the possibility of coma caused by Reye's syndrome, viral or bacterial meningitis, or the much rarer hemolytic-uremic syndrome. A combination of viral illness with 1–3 days of sudden and intractable vomiting invariably precedes the coma of Reye's syndrome. (The illness is usually respiratory, sometimes varicella.)

Trauma is a common cause of coma. Lack of a history of trauma, especially in infants, does not rule it out; nonaccidental trauma or a fall unwitnessed by caretakers may have occurred.

In coma of unknown cause, poisoning is always a possibility. Absence of a history of ingestion of a toxic substance or of medication in the home does not rule out poisoning as a cause.

Often the history is obtained concurrently with a brief pediatric and neurologic screening examination. After the assessment of vital signs and their meaning, the general examination proceeds with a trauma assessment. Palpation of the head and fontanelle, inspection of the ears for infection or hemorrhage, and a careful examination for neck stiffness are indicated. If circumstances suggest head or neck trauma, the head and neck must be immobilized so that any fracture or dislocation will not be aggravated. The skin must be inspected for petechiae or purpura that might suggest bacteremia, infection, bleeding disorder, or traumatic bruising. Examination of the chest, abdomen, and limbs is important to exclude enclosed hemorrhage, traumatic fractures, and the like.

Neurologic examination quantifies the stimulus response and depth of coma, such as responsiveness to verbal or painful stimuli. Examination of the eyes in reference to pupils, fundi, and eye movements is important. Are the eye movements spontaneous, or is it necessary to do the doll's-eye maneuver (rotating the head rapidly to see whether the eyes follow)? Motor and sensory examinations assess reflex asymmetries, Babinski's sign, and evidence of spontaneous posturing or posturing induced by noxious stimuli (eg, decorticate or decerebrate posturing).

If the cause of the coma is not obvious, emergency laboratory tests must be obtained. Table 22–6 lists some of the causes of coma in children and mnemon-

ics for its investigation. An immediate blood glucose (or Dextrostix), complete blood count, urine obtained by catheterization if necessary, pH and electrolytes (including bicarbonate), serum urea nitrogen, and AST are initial screens. Urine, blood, and even gastric contents must be saved for toxin screen if the underlying cause is not obvious. Spinal tap is often necessary to rule out central nervous system infection. Papilledema is a relative contraindication to lumbar

Table 22–6. Some causes of coma in childhood.[1]

Mechanism of Coma	Likely Cause	
	Newborn Infant	Older Child

Anoxia
  Asphyxia
  Respiratory
    obstruction
  Severe anemia
	Birth asphyxia
	Meconium aspiration, infection (especially respiratory syncytial virus)
	Hydrops fetalis
		CO poisoning
		Croup, epiglottitis
		
		Hemolysis, blood loss

Ischemia
  Cardiac
  Shock
	Shunting lesions, hypoplastic left heart
	Asphyxia (cardiac), sepsis
		Shunting lesions, aortic stenosis
		Blood loss, infection

Head trauma	Birth contusion, hemorrhage, nonaccidental trauma	Falls, auto accidents
Infection	Gram-negative meningitis, herpes encephalitis, postimmunization encephalitis	Bacterial meningitis, viral encephalitis, postinfectious encephalitis
Vascular	Intraventricular hemorrhage (premature), sinus thrombosis	Arterial or venous occlusion with congenital heart disease
Neoplasm	Medulloblastoma	Brain stem glioma, increased pressure with posterior fossa tumors
Drugs	Maternal sedatives, injected analgesics	Overdose, many drugs
Epilepsy	Constant minor motor seizures	Constant minor motor seizures, petit mal status, postictal state
Toxins	Lead	Arsenic, alcohol, drugs, pesticides
Hypoglycemia	Birth injury, diabetic progeny, toxemic progeny	Diabetes, "prediabetes," "idiopathic," hypoglycemic agents
Increased intracranial pressure	Anoxic brain damage, hydrocephalus, metabolic disorders (urea cycle; amino-, organic acidurias)	Toxic encephalopathy, Reye's syndrome, head trauma, tumor of posterior fossa
Hepatic causes	Hepatic failure, inborn metabolic errors in bilirubin conjugation	Hepatic failure, chronic aggressive hepatitis
Renal causes	Hypoplastic kidneys	Nephritis, acute and chronic
Hypertensive encephalopathy		Acute nephritis, vasculitis
Hypercapnia	Congenital lung anomalies, bronchopulmonary dysplasia	Cystic fibrosis

Electrolyte abnormalities
  Hypernatremia
  Hyponatremia
 	
  Severe acidosis
  Hyperkalemia
	Iatrogenic ($NaHCO_3$ use), salt poisoning
	Inappropriate antidiuretic hormone, adrenogenital syndrome, dialysis (iatrogenic)
	Septicemia, cold injury, metabolic errors
	Renal failure, adrenogenital syndrome
		Diarrhea, dehydration
		Diarrhea, dehydration, gastroenteritis
		
		Infection, diabetic coma, poisoning (eg, aspirin)
		Poisoning (aspirin)

Purpuric	Disseminated intravascular coagulation, hemolytic-uremic syndrome	Disseminated intravascular coagulation, leukemia, thrombotic purpura (rare)

[1]Modified and reproduced, with permission, from Lewis J, Moe PG: The unconscious child. In: *Current Diagnosis,* 5th ed. Conn H, Conn R (editors). WB Saunders, 1977.

puncture. Occasionally, blood culture is obtained, antibiotics started, and imaging study of the brain done prior to a diagnostic spinal tap. If meningitis is suspected and a tap is believed to be hazardous, antibiotics should be started and the diagnostic spinal puncture done later. Tests that are less readily available but helpful in obscure cases of coma include PO_2, PCO_2, ammonia levels, serum and urine osmolality, porphyrins, lead levels, and, in the newborn, urine and serum amino acids and urine organic acids.

If there is any suspicion of head trauma or increased pressure, an emergency CT scan or MRI is necessary. Bone windows on the former study or skull x-rays can be done at the same sitting. The absence of skull fracture, of course, does not rule out coma caused by life-threatening closed head trauma; injury that results from shaking a child is one example. In a child with an open fontanelle, a real-time ultrasound may be substituted for the other, more definitive imaging studies if there is good local expertise.

Rarely, an emergency EEG aids in diagnosing the cause of coma. A nonconvulsive status epilepticus or focal finding seen with herpes encephalitis (periodic lateralized epileptiform discharges) or focal slowing as seen with stroke or cerebritis are cases in which the EEG might be helpful. The EEG also may correlate with the stage of coma (eg, in Reye's syndrome) and add prognostic information. An improving (or deteriorating) EEG may herald clinical improvement, aid in predicting outcome, and suggest the need for more (or less) heroic therapy.

Treatment

A. General Measures: Vital signs must be monitored and maintained. Most emergency rooms and intensive care units have flow sheets that provide space for repeated monitoring of the coma; one of the coma scales can be a useful tool for this purpose. The patient's response to vocal or painful stimuli and orientation to time, place, and situation when coming out of the coma are monitored. Posture and movements of the limbs, either spontaneously or in response to pain, are serially noted. Pupillary size, equality, and reaction to light and movement of the eyes to the doll's-eye maneuver or ice-water calorics should be recorded. Intravenous fluids can be tailored to the situation, as for treatment of acidosis, shock, or hypovolemia. Nasogastric suction is initially important; when the coma is prolonged, nasogastric feedings are sometimes part of treatment. The patient needs to be catheterized for monitoring urine output and for urinalysis. The child should be protected from decubiti with frequent turning and, if necessary, by providing a foam mattress. The eyes should be protected with pads and artificial tears.

B. Seizures: An EEG should be ordered if there is a question of ongoing seizures. If there are obvious motor seizures, treatment for status epilepticus is given with intravenous drugs (see below). If there is suggestion of brain stem herniation or increased pressure, an intracranial monitor may be necessary. This procedure is described in more detail in Chapter 12. Initial treatment of this possible complication includes keeping the patient's head up (15–30 degrees) and hyperventilation. Mannitol, diuretics, corticosteroids, and drainage of CSF are more heroic measures covered in detail elsewhere.

Prognosis

About 50% of children with nontraumatic causes of coma have a good outcome. In studies of adults assessed on admission or within the first days after the onset of coma, an analysis of multiple variables was most helpful in assessing prognosis. Abnormal neuro-ophthalmologic signs (eg, the absence of pupillary reaction or of eye movement in response to the doll's-eye maneuver or ice water calorics and the absence of corneal responses) were unfavorable. Delay in the return of motor responses, tone, or eye opening was also unfavorable. In children, the assessment done on admission is about as predictive as one done in succeeding days. Approximately two thirds of outcomes can be successfully predicted at an early stage on the basis of coma severity, extraocular movements, pupillary reactions, motor patterns, blood pressure, temperature, and seizure type. Other characteristics, such as the need for assisted respiration, the presence of increased intracranial pressure, and the duration of coma, were not significantly predictive.

Published reports suggest that an anoxic (in contrast to traumatic, metabolic, toxic, and so on) cause of coma, such as that caused by near drowning, has a much grimmer outlook.

BRAIN DEATH

Many medical and law associations have endorsed the following definition of death: "An individual who has sustained either (1) irreversible cessation of circulatory and respiratory functions, or (2) irreversible cessation of all functions of the entire brain, including the brain stem, is dead. A determination of death must be made in accordance with accepted medical standards." Representatives from several pediatric and neurologic associations have endorsed the Guidelines for the Determination of Brain Death in Children. The criteria in term infants (older than 38 weeks) were applicable 1 week after the neurologic insult. Difficulties in assessing premature infants and term infants shortly after birth were acknowledged.

Prerequisites

In assessment of brain death, the history is important. The physician must determine proximate causes to make sure there are no remediable or reversible conditions. Examples of such causes are metabolic conditions, toxic agents, sedative-hypnotic drugs, surgically remediable conditions, hypothermia, and paralytic agents.

Physical Examination Criteria (Chapter 12)

The following criteria are those established by the Task Force on Brain Death in Children.

1. Coexistence of coma and apnea–The patient must exhibit complete loss of consciousness, vocalization, and volitional activity.

2. Absence of brain stem function–As defined by the following: (a) Midposition or fully dilated pupils that do not respond to light. Drugs may influence and invalidate pupillary assessment. (b) Absence of spontaneous eye movements and those induced by oculocephalic and caloric (oculovestibular) testing. (c) Absence of movement of bulbar musculature, including facial and oropharyngeal muscles. The corneal, gag, cough, sucking, and rooting reflexes are absent. (d) Absence of respiratory movements when the patient is off the respirator. Apnea testing using standardized methods can be performed but is done after other criteria are met.

3. Temperature and blood pressure–The patient must not be significantly hypothermic or hypotensive for age.

4. Tone is flaccid, and spontaneous or induced movements, excluding spinal cord events such as reflex withdrawal or spinal myoclonus, are absent.

5. The examination should remain consistent with brain death throughout the observation and testing period.

Confirmation

Details of apnea testing suggest documentation of a PCO_2 level greater than 60 mm Hg, with oxygenation maintained throughout; this level may be reached 3–15 minutes after taking the patient off the respirator. The recommended observation period to confirm brain death (repeated examinations) is 12–24 hours (longer in infants); *reversible causes must be ruled out.*

If an irreversible cause is documented, laboratory testing is not essential. Helpful tests to support the clinical assertion of brain death include electroencephalography and angiography:

(1) Electrocerebral silence on EEG should persist for 30 minutes, and drug concentrations must be insufficient to suppress EEG activity. (2) Failure of arterial intracerebral blood flow on angiography confirms brain death. Carotid arteriography and cerebral radionuclide angiography are two methods. Dural sinus flow may persist and does not invalidate the diagnosis of brain death.

Other laboratory studies have not been sufficiently well documented to be considered definitive; cerebral evoked potentials and ultrasound blood pulsa-

tions are two common examples. Xenon-enhanced computed tomography is a more elaborate method.

In rare cases, preserved intracranial perfusion in the presence of electroencephalographic silence has been documented, and the converse has also been reported. Controversy attends the definition and criteria of brain death in the newborn. This debate inevitably acknowledges the issue of withdrawing support from the infant with a hopeless prognosis who is not brain dead.

Alfonso I et al: Evaluation of the comatose fullterm neonate. Int Pediatr 1997;12:74.

Ashwal S, Schneider S, Thompson J: Xenon computed tomography measuring cerebral blood flow in the determination of brain death in children. Ann Neurol 1989;25:539.

Fishman MA: Validity of brain death criteria in infants. Pediatrics 1995;96:513.

Jones KM, Barnes PD: MR diagnosis of brain death. AJNR Am J Neuroradiol 1992;13:65.

Lang CJG: Apnea testing by artificial CO_2 augmentation. Neurology 1995;45:966.

Mizrahi EM, Pollack MA, Kellaway P: Neocortical death in infants: Behavioral, neurologic, and electroencephalographic characteristics. Pediatr Neurol 1985;1:302.

Shewmon DA: Commentary on guidelines for the determination of brain death in children. Ann Neurol 1988; 24:789.

Task Force on Brain Death in Children: Guidelines for the determination of brain death in children. Ann Neurol 1987;21:616. [Also available in Arch Neurol 1987;44:587, Neurology 1987;37:1077, Pediatr Neurol 1987;3:242, and Pediatrics 1987;80:298.]

Vegetative state: Report of the American Neurological Association Committee on Ethical Affairs. Ann Neurol 1993;33:386.

Yager JY, Johnston B, Seshia SS: Coma scales in pediatric practice. Am J Dis Child 1990;144:1088.

SEIZURE DISORDERS (Epilepsies)

Essentials of Diagnosis & Typical Features

- Recurrent nonfebrile seizures.
- Often, interictal electroencephalographic changes.

General Considerations

A seizure is a sudden, transient disturbance of brain function, manifested by involuntary motor, sensory, autonomic, or psychic phenomena, alone or in any combination, often accompanied by alteration or loss of consciousness. A seizure may occur after a transient metabolic, traumatic, anoxic, or infectious insult to the brain.

Repeated seizures without evident time-limited cause justify the label of **epilepsy.** Seizures and epilepsy occur most commonly at the extremes of life. The incidence is highest in the newborn and higher in childhood than in later life. Epilepsy in childhood often remits. Prevalence flattens out after age 10–15. The chance of having a second seizure after an initial unprovoked episode is 30%. The chance of remission from epilepsy in childhood is 50%. The recurrence rate after the withdrawal of drugs is about 30%. Factors adversely influencing recurrence include (1) difficulty in getting the seizures under control (ie, the number of seizures occurring before control is achieved); (2) neurologic dysfunction or mental retardation; (3) age at onset under 2 years; and (4) abnormal EEG at the time of discontinuing medication. The type of seizures also often determines prognosis.

Seizures are caused by any factor that can disturb brain function. Seizures and epilepsy are often classified as **symptomatic** (the cause is strongly identified or presumed) or **idiopathic** (the cause is unknown, or genetic influences are strongly etiologic). The younger the infant or child, the more likely that the cause can be identified. Idiopathic or genetic epilepsy most often appears between ages 4 and 16. A seizure disorder or epilepsy should not be considered idiopathic unless a searching history, examination, and appropriate laboratory tests have turned up no apparent cause.

Clinical Findings

A. Symptoms and Signs: The key to the diagnosis of epilepsy is the history. The initial symptom often identifies the aura to the seizure itself. A feeling of fear, numbness or tingling in the fingers, or bright lights in one visual field might be examples of an aura (really the onset of the seizure). Sometimes the patient recalls nothing because there has been no aura or warning. The parent might report that the patient's eyes went off to one side or that extreme pallor, trismus, or overall body stiffening occurred first. Occasionally there is a prodrome; for example, a feeling of "unwellness," of something about to happen, or a recurrent thought over minutes or hours prior to the aura and seizure itself.

Minute details of the seizure can help determine the site of onset and aid in classification. Did the patient become extremely pale before falling? Was the patient able to respond to queries during the episode? Did the patient become completely unconscious? Did the patient fall stiffly or gradually slump to the floor? Was there an injury? How long did the stiffening or jerking last? Where were the sites of jerking?

Events after the seizure can be helpful in diagnosis. Was there loss of speech? Was the patient able to respond accurately before going to sleep?

All these events prior to, during, and after the seizure can help to classify the seizure and, indeed, may help to determine if the event actually was a probable epileptic seizure or a pseudoseizure (a nonepileptic phenomenon mimicking a seizure). Classifying the seizure may aid in diagnosis or prognosis and suggest desirable or necessary laboratory tests and medications (Tables 22–7 and 22–8).

B. Status Epilepticus: Status epilepticus is a clinical or electrical seizure lasting at least 30 minutes, or a series of seizures without complete recovery over the same period of time. After 30 minutes, the brain begins to suffer from hypoxia and acidosis, with depletion of local energy stores, cerebral edema, and structural damage. Eventually, high fever, hypotension, respiratory depression, and even death may occur. Thus, *status epilepticus is a relative medical emergency.*

Status epilepticus is classified as (1) convulsive—the common tonic-clonic, or "grand mal" status epilepticus; or (2) nonconvulsive, such as simple motor status without loss of consciousness. Other nonconvulsive types include absence status, or "spike-

Table 22–7. Clinical seizure correlation with electroencephalographic patterns.[1]

Clinical Seizure Type	EEG Ictal	EEG Interictal
Focal (partial) Simple partial Motor, sensory	Persistent long-standing local contralateral discharge (eg, spike, slow wave)	Transient contralateral spike, slow wave discharge
Complex partial (psychomotor)	Focal or bilateral frontal, temporal discharge	Temporofrontal local discharge, or normal
Partial seizures with generalization	Above discharges become generalized (all leads)	
Generalized Absence (petit mal) Simple[2] Complex[3]	Generalized (all leads) 3/s spike-wave lasting > 1–2 seconds	Brief generalized 3/s spike-wave lasting < 1–2 seconds. Normal background.
Atypical absence	Irregular 1–4/s spike-wave	Abnormal; often slow spike-wave, asymmetric
Myoclonic seizures	Multiple spike-wave	Multiple spike-wave
Tonic-clonic (grand mal)	10/s spike/slowing, then spike/slow wave	Multiple spikes, spike wave sharp, slow
Atonic (astatic, akinetic)	Multiple spike-wave	Multiple spike-wave

[1]According to the International Classification of Epileptic Seizures. Some subtypes are not listed. Some age-limited syndromes occurring in childhood are not easily incorporated into this scheme.
[2]Impairment of consciousness only.
[3]With tonic, clonic, autonomic component.

Table 22–8. Seizures by age at onset, pattern, and preferred treatment.

Age Group and Seizure Type	Age at Onset	Clinical Manifestations	Causative Factors	Electroencephalographic Pattern	Other Diagnostic Studies	Treatment and Comments (Anticonvulsants by Order of Choice)
Neonatal seizures	Birth to 2 weeks	Often "atypical"; sudden limpness or tonic posturing, brief apnea, and cyanosis; odd cry; eyes "rolling up"; blinking or mouthing or chewing movements; nystagmus, twitchiness or clonic movements—focal, multifocal, or generalized. Some seizures are nonepileptic-decerebrate, or other posturings; release from forebrain inhibition; poor response to drugs.	Neurologic insults (hypoxia/ischemia; intracranial hemorrhage) present more in first 3 days or after eighth day; metabolic disturbances alone between third and eighth days; hypoglycemia, hypocalcemia, hyper- and hyponatremia. Drug withdrawal. Pyridoxine deficiency and other metabolic causes. CNS infections and structural abnormalities.	May correlate poorly with clinical seizures. Focal spikes or slow rhythms; multifocal discharges. "Electroclinical dissociation" may occur; EEG-electrical seizure without clinical manifestations and vice versa.	Lumbar puncture; serum Ca^{2+}, PO_4^{3-}, glucose, Mg^{2+}; BUN, amino acid screen, blood ammonia, organic acid screen, TORCHES[1] screen. Ultrasound or CT scan for suspected intracranial hemorrhage and structural abnormalities.	Phenobarbital, IV or IM; if seizures not controlled, add phenytoin IV (loading dose 20 mg/kg each). Diazepam 0.3 mg/kg. Treat underlying disorder. Seizures due to brain damage often resistant to anticonvulsants. When cause in doubt, stop protein feedings until enzyme deficiencies of urea cycle or amino acid metabolism ruled out.
West's syndrome "infantile spasms." (See also Lennox-Gastaut syndrome, below.)	3–18 months; occasionally up to 4 years	Sudden, usually symmetric adduction and flexion of limbs with concomitant flexion of head and trunk; also abduction and extensor movements like Moro reflex. Tendency for spasms to occur in clusters, on waking or falling asleep, or may be noted particularly when the infant is being handled, is ill, or is otherwise irritable. Tendency for each patient to have own stereotyped pattern.	Pre- or perinatal brain damage or malformation in approximately one-third; biochemical, infectious, degenerative causes in approximately one-third; unknown in approximately one-third. With early onset, pyridoxine deficiency, amino- or organic aciduria. Tuberous sclerosis in 5–10%. Chronic inflammatory disease and toxoplasmosis. Aicardi syndrome (females with mental retardation, agenesis of corpus callosum, ocular and vertebral anomalies).	Hypsarrhythmia; chaotic high-voltage slow waves, random spikes, all leads (90%); other abnormalities in rest. Rarely "normal." EEG normalization usually correlates with reduction of seizures; not helpful prognostically regarding mental development.	Funduscopic and skin examination, trial of pyridoxine. Amino and organic acid screen. Chronic inflammatory disease. TORCHES[1] screen, CT or MRI scan should be done to (1) establish definite diagnosis, (2) aid in genetic counseling. SPECT or PET scan may identify focal lesion.	ACTH preferred (2–4 units/kg/d IM Acthar gel once daily, then slow withdrawal). Some prefer oral corticosteroids. Clonazepam, valproic acid. In resistant cases, ketogenic or medium-chain triglyceride diet (see text). Retardation of varying degree in approximately 90% of cases. Occasionally, surgical extirpation of focal lesion may be curative.
Febrile convulsions	3 months to 5 years (maximum 6–18 months)	Usually generalized seizures, less than 15 minutes; rarely focal in onset. May lead to status epilepticus. Latter usually benign. Recurrence risk of second febrile seizure 30%; 50% if under 1 year of age.	Nonneurologic febrile illness (temperature rises to 39°C or higher); family history frequently positive for febrile convulsions.	Normal interictal EEG, especially when obtained 8–10 days after seizure. In older infants, 3/s spikes often seen.	Lumbar puncture in infants or whenever suspicion of meningitis exists.	Treat underlying illness, fever. Diazepam orally or rectally as needed, 0.3–0.5 mg/kg three times daily during illness. Prophylaxis with phenobarbital (valproic acid if phenobarbital not tolerated), with neurologic deficits, prolonged seizure, family history of epilepsy.
Myoclonic-astatic (akinetic, atonic) seizures, formerly atypical absence. When mental retardation is presented, this is called Lennox-Gastaut syndrome.	Any time in childhood; normally 2–7 years	Shock-like violent contractions of one or more muscle groups, singly or irregularly repetitive; may fling patient suddenly to side, forward, or backward. Usually no or only brief loss of consciousness. Half of patients or more also have generalized grand mal seizures.	Multiple causes, usually resulting in diffuse neuronal damage. History of West's syndrome; prenatal or perinatal brain damage; viral meningoencephalitis; subacute sclerosing panencephalitis; CNS degenerative disorders; lead or other encephalopathies; structural cerebral abnormalities, eg, porencephaly.	Atypical slow (1–2.5 Hz) spike-wave complexes ("petit mal variant") and bursts of high-voltage generalized spikes, often with diffusely slow background frequencies. See text.	As dictated by index of suspicion. Lumbar puncture with measles antibody titer and CSF-IgG index. Nerve conduction studies. Skin biopsy for electron microscopy, MRI scan, WBC lysosomal enzymes if metabolic degenerative disease suspected.	Difficult to treat. Valproic acid, clonazepam, or ethosuximide. Felbamate. Diazepam. Ketogenic or medium-chain triglyceride diet. ACTH or corticosteroids as in West's syndrome. Perhaps lamotrigine, vigabatrin. Protect head with helmet and chin padding.
Absence ("petit mal"). Also juvenile and myoclonic absence.	3–15 years	Lapses of consciousness or vacant stares, lasting about 10 seconds, often in "clusters." Automatisms of face and hands; clonic activity in 30–45%. Often confused with complex partial seizures but no aura or postictal confusion.	Unknown. Genetic component: probably an autosomal dominant gene.	3/s bilaterally synchronous, symmetric, high-voltage spikes and waves. EEG "normalization" correlates closely with control of seizures.	Hyperventilation when patient on inadequate or no medication often provokes attacks. CT scan is rarely of value.	Valproic acid or ethosuximide; with latter, add phenobarbital or valproate if major motor seizures. In resistant cases, ketogenic or medium-chain triglyceride diet. Also, in resistant cases, valproic acid and ethosuximide together.

Seizure type	Age	Clinical features	EEG	Diagnostic studies	Treatment
Simple partial or focal seizures (motor/sensory/ jacksonian). (Complex partial or psychomotor seizures, below.)	Any age	Seizure may involve any part of body; may spread in fixed pattern (jacksonian march), becoming generalized. In children, epileptogenic focus often "shifts," and epileptic manifestations may change concomitantly.	Focal spikes or slow waves in appropriate cortical region; sometimes diffusely abnormal or even normal.	Often secondary to birth trauma, inflammatory process, vascular accidents, meningoencephalitis, etc. If seizures are coupled with new or progressive neurologic deficits, a structural lesion (eg, brain tumor) is likely	If seizures are difficult to control or progressive deficits occur, neuroradiodiagnostic studies, particularly CT brain scan, imperative (see text).	Carbamazepine, phenytoin, phenobarbital, or primidone. Valproic acid useful adjunct.
Complex partial seizures (psychomotor, temporal lobe, or limbic seizures)	Any age	Aura may be a sensation of fear, epigastric discomfort, odd smell or taste (usually unpleasant), visual or auditory hallucination (either vague and "unformed" or well-formed image, words, music). Aura and seizure stereotyped for each patient. Seizure may consist of vague stare; facial, tongue, or swallowing movements and throaty sounds; or various complex automatisms. Unlike absences, complex partial seizures tend not to occur in clusters but singly and to last longer (1 minute or more), followed by confusion. History of aura (or child running to adult from "vague fear") and of automatisms involving more than face and hands establish diagnosis.	As above, but occurring in temporal lobe and its connections, eg, frontotemporal, temporoparietal, temporo-occipital regions.	As above. Temporal lobes especially sensitive to hypoxia; thus, this seizure type may be a sequela of birth trauma, febrile convulsions, etc. Also especially vulnerable to certain viral infections, especially herpes simplex. Remediable other causes are small cryptic tumors or vascular malformations.	MRI when structural lesions suspected. PCR of cerebrospinal fluid in acute febrile situation for herpes; rarely, temporal lobe biopsy. Carotid amobarbital injection when lateralization of speech dominance in question and surgical extirpation of epileptogenic area is contemplated.	Carbamazepine, phenytoin, phenobarbital, or primidone. More than one drug may be necessary. Valproic acid may be useful. In cases uncontrolled by drugs and where a primary epileptogenic focus is identifiable, excision of anterior third of temporal lobe. Adjunctive psychotherapy required frequently. Gabapentin, topiramate, lamotrigine, and tiagabine (for > 16-year-olds).
"Benign epilepsy of childhood" (with "centrotemporal" or "rolandic" foci)	5–16 years	Partial motor or generalized seizures. Similar seizure patterns may be observed in patients with focal cortical lesions.	Centrotemporal spikes or sharp waves ("rolandic discharges") appearing paroxysmally against a normal EEG background.	Seizure history of abnormal EEG findings in relatives of 40% of affected probands and 18–20% of parents and siblings, suggesting transmission by a single autosomal dominant gene, possibly with age-dependent penetrance.	Seldom need CT or MRI scan.	Carbamazepine or phenytoin. Primidone or phenobarbital.
Juvenile myoclonic epilepsy (of Janz)	Late childhood and adolescence, peaking at 13 years	Mild myoclonic jerks of neck and shoulder flexor muscles after awakening. Intelligence usually normal.	Interictal EEG shows fast variety of spike-and-wave sequences or 4- to 6-Hz multispike and wave complexes.	40% of relatives have myoclonias, especially in females; 15% have the abnormal EEG pattern with clinical attacks.	Differentiate from progressive myoclonic encephalopathy of Unverricht-Lafora and other degenerative disorders by appropriate biopsies (muscle, liver, etc).	Valproic acid. Phenobarbital. Primidone.
Generalized tonic-clonic seizures (grand mal)	Any age	Loss of consciousness; tonic-clonic movements, often preceded by vague aura or cry. Bladder and bowel incontinence in approximately 15%. Postictal confusion; sleep. Often mixed with or masking other seizure patterns.	Bilaterally synchronous, symmetric multiple high-voltage spikes, spikes and waves, mixed patterns. Often normal under age 4.	Often unknown. Genetic component. May be seen with metabolic disturbances, trauma, infection, intoxication, degenerative disorders, brain tumors.	As above.	Phenobarbital in first 12 months; carbamazepine or valproic acid; phenytoin; primidone. Combinations may be necessary.

637

[1]TORCHES is a mnemonic formula for toxoplasmosis, rubella, cytomegalovirus, herpes simplex, and syphilis.

wave stupor," and (very rare) partial complex status epilepticus.

An EEG may be necessary to aid in diagnosing the less common variants, such as a patient with known absence who now is in a partially-in-contact, stuporous state.

A child with status epilepticus often has a high fever with or without intracranial infection, such as viral encephalitis or bacterial meningitis. Status epilepticus may be the initial seizure; various studies show that 25–75% of children experience status epilepticus as the initial seizure. Often, it is a reflection of a remote insult (eg, anoxic or traumatic). Tumor, vascular disease (strokes), or head trauma, which are common causes of status epilepticus in adults, are uncommon causes in childhood. Fifty percent of cases are symptomatic of acute (25%) or chronic (25%) CNS disorders. Infection or metabolic disorders are the most common symptomatic causes in children. The cause is unknown in 50% of cases, but many of these will be febrile.

Status epilepticus is more common in children under 1 year of age, with 37% of cases occurring under that age and 85% under age 5. Thus, the pediatrician sees status epilepticus most commonly in infants and preschoolers. For treatment, see Table 22–9.

C. Febrile Seizures: Criteria for febrile seizures are (1) age of 3 months to 5 years (most occur between the ages of 6–18 months), (2) fever of 38.8 °C, and (3) non-central nervous system infection. Most (greater than 90%) are generalized and brief (less than 5 minutes) and occur early in an OMPA (otitis media, pharyngitis, adenitis) illness. Febrile seizures occur in 2–3% of children. Gastroenteritis, especially when caused by *Shigella* or *Campylobacter,* and urinary tract infections are less common causes. Roseola infantum is a rare but classic cause. One study implicated viral causes in 86% of cases. Immunizations may be a cause.

Rarely, status epilepticus may occur; fever is a common cause of status epilepticus in early childhood. Febrile seizures rarely (2–4%) lead to epilepsy or recurrent nonfebrile seizures in later childhood and adult life. The chance of later epilepsy is higher if the febrile seizures have complex features, such as a duration of over 15 minutes, more than one seizure in the same day, or focal features. Other adverse factors are an abnormal neurologic status preceding the seizures (eg, cerebral palsy or mental retardation); early onset of febrile seizure (before 1 year of age); and a family history of epilepsy. Even with adverse factors, the risk of epilepsy in later life is low, in the range of 15–20%.

Recurrent febrile seizures occur in 20–40% of cases but, in general, do not worsen the long-term outlook.

The child with a febrile seizure must be examined. Routine studies such as serum electrolytes, glucose, calcium, skull x-rays, or brain imaging studies are

Table 22–9. Status epilepticus treatment.

1. ABCs
   a. Airway: Maintain oral airway; intubation may be necessary.
   b. Breathing: Oxygen by mouth (if available).
   c. Circulation: Assess pulse, blood pressure; support with IV fluids, drugs. Monitor vital signs.
2. Start glucose-containing IV; evaluate serum glucose; electrolytes, HCO_3^-, CBC, BUN, anticonvulsant levels.
3. May need arterial blood gases, pH.
4. Give 50% glucose if dextrose low (1–2 mL/kg).
5. Begin IV drug therapy; goal is to control status epilepticus in 20–60 minutes.
   a. Diazepam 0.3–0.5 mg/kg over 1–5 minutes (20 mg maximum); may repeat in 5–20 minutes (short action: 20 minutes; watch for respiratory depression); or, lorazepam 0.05–0.2 mg/kg (less effective with repeated doses, longer-acting than diazepam). Midazolam IM or IV: 0.1–0.3 mg/kg; intranasally, 0.2 mg/kg.
   b. Phenytoin 10–20 mg/kg IV (not IM) over 5–20 minutes; 1000 mg maximum); monitor with blood pressure and ECG. Fosphenytoin may be given more rapidly—even IM—in the same dosage; order 10–20 mg/kg of "phenytoin equivalent."
   c. Phenobarbital 5–20 mg/kg (sometimes higher in newborns or refractory status in intubated patients).
6. Correct metabolic perturbations (eg, low-sodium, acidosis).
7. Other drug approaches in refractory status:
   a. Repeat phenytoin, phenobarbital (5–10 mg/kg). Monitor blood levels. Support respiration, blood pressure as necessary.
   b. Valproic acid suspension, 50 mg/mL diluted 1:1, 30–60 mg/kg orally (nasogastric tube) or rectally. Valproate sodium (Depacon), available as 100 mg/mL for IV use; give 15–60 mg/kg/d over 1 hour or more.
   c. General anesthetic.
8. Consider underlying causes:
   a. Structural disorders or trauma. Consider CT scan.
   b. Infection: Spinal tap, blood culture, antibiotics.
   c. Metabolic disorders: Lactic acidosis, toxins, uremia. May need HCO_3^-, medication, toxin screen, judicious fluid administration.
9. Give maintenance drug (if diazepam only was sufficient to halt status epilepticus): phenytoin 10 mg/kg, phenobarbital 5 mg/kg, daily dose IV (or by mouth) divided every 12 hours.

seldom helpful. A white count above 20,000/μL or with an extreme left shift may correlate with bacteremia; complete blood count and blood cultures may be appropriate studies. Serum sodium is often slightly low but not low enough to require treatment or to cause the seizure. *Meningitis must be ruled out.* Bacterial meningitis can present with a fever and seizure. Signs of meningitis (eg, bulging fontanelle, stiff neck, stupor, and irritability) may all be absent, especially in a child under 18 months of age.

After controlling the fever and stopping an ongoing seizure, the physician must decide whether to do a spinal tap. The fact that the child has had a previous febrile seizure does not rule out meningitis as the cause of the current episode. The younger the child, the more important the tap, because physical findings are less reliable in diagnosing meningitis. Although the yield is low, a tap should probably be done if the child is under age 2, if recovery is slow, if no other cause for the fever is found, or if close follow-up will not be possible. Occasionally, observation in the emergency room for several hours obviates the need for a tap. A negative tap does not rule out the emergence of meningitis during the same febrile illness; sometimes a second tap needs to be done.

Treatment after the seizure is problematic. Many clinicians choose to treat the child with maintenance dosage of anticonvulsant medication during the course of that febrile illness. Diazepam, 0.5 mg/kg two or three times a day orally or rectally, has been used in Europe and Japan with success both for prophylaxis and for prevention of subsequent seizures. (Suppositories are not currently available in the United States.) Phenobarbital and valproate sodium are other choices; however, the somnolence due to the phenobarbital load (about 5–10 mg/kg) is often disquieting to both the doctor and parent and sometimes confuses follow-up assessments. Valproic acid imposes greater risks and should not be given if there is vomiting or acidosis.

Most clinicians choose to follow up the patient without administering anticonvulsant medication. Measures to control fever (sponging, antipyretics, and appropriate antibiotics if a bacterial illness is suspected or found) are the mainstays of treatment. The family can be reassured that simple febrile seizures are not thought to have any long-term adverse consequences. An EEG should be ordered if the febrile seizure is complicated or unusual; in the uncomplicated febrile seizure, the EEG is most often normal. About 10% will have slowing or other occipital abnormalities. Ideally, the study should be done at least a week after the illness to avoid transient findings due to the fever or seizure itself. In older children, 3 per second spike-wave discharge, suggestive of a genetic propensity to epilepsy, may occur. In the young infant, electroencephalographic findings seldom aid in assessing the chance of recurrence of febrile or nonfebrile seizures.

Prophylactic anticonvulsants are not indicated in the uncomplicated febrile seizure patient. If febrile seizures are complicated or prolonged, or if medical reassurance fails to relieve family anxiety, anticonvulsant prophylaxis may be indicated and can reduce the incidence of recurrent febrile or nonfebrile seizures. One remedy is to use diazepam at the first onset of fever for the duration of the febrile illness as noted above. Phenobarbital, 3–5 mg/kg/d as a single bedtime dose, is an inexpensive and safe alternative. Often, increasing the dose gradually (eg, starting with 2 mg/kg/d the first week and increasing to 3 mg/kg/d the second week, and so on) decreases side effects and noncompliance. A plasma phenobarbital level in the range of 15–40 mg/mL is desirable.

Valproate sodium is more hazardous. In infants, the liquid suspension must often be used but has a short half-life and causes more gastrointestinal upset than the coated capsules used in older children. The dose is 15–60 mg/kg/d in three or four divided doses. Precautionary laboratory studies are necessary.

Phenytoin and carbamazepine have not shown effectiveness in the prophylaxis of febrile seizures.

D. Laboratory Findings and Imaging: Ordering of laboratory tests depends on the age of the child, the severity and type of the seizure, whether the child is ill or injured, and the clinician's suspicion about the underlying cause. *Every case of suspected seizure disorder warrants an EEG.* Other studies are used selectively. Seizures in early infancy are often symptomatic. Therefore, the younger the child, the more careful must be the laboratory assessment (Table 22–10).

Table 22–10. Laboratory studies in first seizure of epilepsy (nonneonatal).

Well infant	EEG, calcium, BUN, or urinalysis, and perhaps CT or MRI. (Abnormal examination or focally abnormal EEG may prompt an imaging study.)
Well older child	EEG; consider CT or MRI
Ill infant	Calcium, magnesium, CBC, BUN, electrolytes, blood culture, lumbar puncture, EEG, possibly CT or MRI
Ill older child	CBC, BUN, lumbar puncture, EEG, CT or MRI
Generalized tonic-clonic seizure	As above
Generalized absence	EEG only
Atypical absence	EEG, CT, MRI: Consider studies for mental retardation: serum and urine amino and organic acids and chromosomes, including fragile X. If there is progressive worsening, consider lysosomal enzymes, lumbar puncture (protein, enzymes, IgG), long-chain fatty acids, skin or conjunctival biopsies.
Infantile spasms	See Atypical absence
Myoclonic progressive seizure with mental retardation	See Atypical absence
Focal	EEG. In cases of mental retardation, positive neurologic examination, EEG focal slow wave, or poorly controlled seizures, do CT or MRI. In refractory cases, consider surgical evaluation.

Metabolic abnormalities are seldom found in the well child with seizures; unless there is a high clinical suspicion of uremia, hyponatremia, or other serious condition, laboratory tests are not necessary. Special studies may be necessary in unusual circumstances, as when hemolytic-uremic syndrome or lead poisoning is a suspected cause. CT scans are overused in patients with seizures. The youngster with a routine febrile seizure, a nonfebrile generalized seizure with normal examination and normal EEG, or an absence seizure does not need a CT or MRI scan. The yield in a child with normal neurologic examination and EEG is less than 5%. Conversely, in children with symptomatic epileptic syndromes, the yield of positive results is as high as 60–80%. Examples include infantile spasms, Lennox-Gastaut syndrome, and progressive myoclonic epilepsy.

In focal seizures, children with benign rolandic epilepsy do not need a CT scan; it will invariably be normal. The yield with other focal seizures is 15–30%, with most of the findings unimportant in relation to diagnosis and prognosis (eg, a mildly dilated single ventricle, superficial atrophy). Nonetheless, an imaging study eases anxiety and rules out the remote possibility of tumor or vascular malformation. Other indications for CT or MRI scan include difficulty in controlling seizures, progressive neurologic findings on serial examinations, worsening focal findings on the EEG, suspicion of increased pressure, and, of course, any case in which surgery is being considered. A previous normal scan does not rule out an emerging tumor; if the course is unsatisfactory, repeating the scan may be necessary. A neoplasm or other unexpected treatable lesion is found in a small number, perhaps 2–3%, of CT scans.

E. Electroencephalography: The limitations of electroencephalography—even in epilepsy, where it is most useful—are considerable. *A seizure is a clinical phenomenon;* an EEG showing epileptiform activity may confirm and even extend the clinical diagnosis, but it cannot make the diagnosis.

The EEG need not be abnormal in the presence of a definite seizure disorder. Normal EEGs are seen following a first generalized seizure in one third of children under 4 years of age; the initial EEG is normal in about 20% of older epileptic children and in about 10% of adults with epilepsy. These percentages are reduced when serial tracings are obtained. On the other hand, various grades of "arrhythmias" are frequently observed in children; focal spikes and generalized spike-wave discharges are seen in 30% of close nonepileptic relatives of patients with centrencephalic epilepsy.

1. Diagnostic value–The greatest value of the EEG in convulsive disorders is to help classify seizure types and thus to select appropriate therapy (Table 22–7). Petit mal absences and partial complex or psychomotor seizures are sometimes difficult to distinguish, especially when the physician must rely

on the history and cannot observe one; their differing electroencephalographic patterns will then prove most helpful. Another frequent illustration of the role of the EEG in guiding therapy is the finding of mixed seizure patterns in a child who clinically has only grand mal or only petit mal absences, since some anticonvulsants efficacious for one seizure type may provoke the other. The EEG may often help in diagnosing neonatal seizures with minimal and "atypical" clinical manifestations; it may show "hypsarrhythmia" in infantile spasms or the pattern associated with the Lennox-Gastaut syndrome, both expressions of diffuse brain dysfunctioning of multiple causes and generally of grave significance. The EEG may help differentiate "convulsive equivalents" from somatic complaints of psychogenic origin.

The EEG may show focal slowing that, if constant—particularly when there are corresponding focal seizure manifestations and abnormal neurologic findings—will alert the physician to the presence of a structural lesion, in which case brain imaging may establish the cause and help determine further investigation and treatment.

2. Prognostic value–A normal EEG following a first convulsion suggests (but does not guarantee) a favorable prognosis. Markedly abnormal EEGs may become normal with treatment (1) immediately following intravenous injection of 50 mg of vitamin B_6 in pyridoxine dependency or deficiency; (2) in infantile spasms and sometimes the Lennox-Gastaut syndrome (ACTH or corticosteroids); (3) in petit mal absences (anticonvulsants); and (4) in petit mal and other minor motor seizures, including the Lennox-Gastaut syndrome (ketogenic diet). If so, it is likely that seizure control will be achieved (though this offers no clues to the mental status of the patient).

Electroencephalography should be repeated when there is an increase in the severity and frequency of seizures despite exhaustive and adequate anticonvulsant therapy; when there is a significant change in the clinical seizure pattern; or when there are progressive neurologic deficits. Focal or diffuse slowing may indicate a progressive lesion.

The EEG may be helpful in determining when to discontinue anticonvulsant therapy. The presence or absence of epileptiform activity on the EEG prior to withdrawal of anticonvulsants after a seizure-free period of several years on the medications has been shown to be correlated with the degree of risk of recurrence of seizures.

Differential Diagnosis

It is extremely important that a nonepileptic condition be accurately labeled. To the layperson, epilepsy often has connotations of brain damage and limitation of activity; a person so diagnosed may be precluded from certain occupations in later life. It is often very difficult to change an inaccurate diagnosis of many years' standing.

Some of the common nonepileptic events that mimic seizure disorder are listed in Table 22–11.

Complications

Emotional disturbances—notably anxiety, depression, anger, feelings of guilt and inadequacy—often occur in the parents of the affected child as a reaction to the seizures, as well as in the child old enough to understand. The seizures, particularly the hallucinatory auras and psychomotor attacks, frequently set off in the prepubescent and adolescent patient fantasies (and sometimes obsessive ruminations) about dying and death that may become so strong that they lead to suicidal behavior and attempts. The limitations many school systems place on epileptic children add to the problem. Commonly, the child expresses painful feelings by "acting out."

Pseudoretardation may occur in poorly controlled epileptic children because their seizures (or the subclinical paroxysms sustained) may interfere with their learning ability. Anticonvulsants are less likely to "slow the child down" but may do so when given in toxic amounts; phenobarbital is particularly implicated.

True mental retardation is most commonly part of the same pathologic process that causes the seizures but may occasionally occur when seizures are frequent, prolonged, and accompanied by hypoxia.

Physical injuries, especially lacerations of the forehead and chin, are frequent in astatic or akinetic seizures ("drop attacks"). In all other seizure disorders in childhood, injuries as a direct result of an attack are impressively rare.

Treatment

The ideal treatment of seizures is the correction of specific causes. However, even when a biochemical disorder (eg, leucine hypoglycemia), a tumor, or septic meningitis is being treated, anticonvulsant drugs are often still required.

A. Precautionary Management of Individual Brief Seizures: Protect the patient against self-injury and aspiration of vomitus. Beyond that, no specific therapy is necessary. The less done to the patient during a relatively brief seizure (up to 10 or 15 minutes), the better. Thrusting a spoon handle or tongue depressor into the clenched mouth of a convulsing patient or trying to restrain tonic-clonic movements may cause worse injuries than a bitten tongue or bruised limb. Mouth-to-mouth resuscitation is rarely necessary.

B. General Management of the Young Epileptic:

1. Education–The patient and parents must be helped to understand the problem of seizures and their management. Many children—some even as young as 3 years of age—are capable of cooperating with the physician in problems of seizure control.

All bottles containing antiepileptic drugs should bear a label. The parents should know the names and dosage of the anticonvulsants being administered.

Materials on epilepsy—including pamphlets (some in Spanish), monographs, films, and videotapes suitable for children and teenagers, parents, teachers, and medical professionals—may be purchased through the Epilepsy Foundation of America, Materials Service Center, 4351 Garden City Drive, Landover, MD 20785. The Foundation's local chapter and other community organizations are eager to provide guidance and other services. In many cities, there are support groups for older children and adolescents and for their parents and others concerned.

2. Privileges and precautions in daily life–Encourage normal living within reasonable bounds. Children should engage in physical activities appropriate to their age and social group. After seizure control is established, swimming is generally permissible with a "buddy system" or adequate lifeguard coverage. High diving and high climbing should not be permitted. Physical training and sports (other than contact sports) are usually to be welcomed rather than restricted. Driving is discussed below.

Loss of sleep should be avoided. Emotional disturbances may need to be treated. Alcohol intake—a serious problem usually beginning in adolescence—should be avoided because it may precipitate seizures. Prompt attention should be given to infections. Further neurologic disturbances should be brought to the physician's attention promptly.

Although every effort should be made to control seizures, this must not interfere with a child's ability to function. Sometimes a child is better off having an occasional mild seizure than being so heavily sedated that function at home, in school, or at play is impaired. Therapy and medication adjustment often require much art and fortitude on the physician's part. Indeed, some pediatricians and pediatric neurologists, after discussion with the parents, are now not instituting anticonvulsant therapy after up to three nonfebrile convulsions in an otherwise neurologically intact child.

3. Driving–Driving becomes important to most young people at age 15 or 16. Restrictions vary from state to state; in most, a learner's permit or driver's license will be issued if the patient has been under a physician's care and free of seizures for at least 2 years, provided that the treatment or basic neurologic problem does not interfere with the ability to drive. A guide to this and other legal matters pertaining to persons with epilepsy is published by the Epilepsy Foundation of America, whose legal department may be able to provide additional information (see reference below).

4. Pregnancy–In the pregnant teenager with epilepsy, the possibility of teratogenic effects of anticonvulsants, such as facial clefts (about 5%), must be weighed against the risks from seizures. Such mal-

Table 22–11. Nonepileptic paroxysmal events.

Breath-holding attacks

Age 6 months to 3 years. Always precipitated by trauma and fright. Cyanosis; sometimes stiffening, tonic (or jerking-clonic) convulsion (anoxic seizure). Patient may sleep following attack. Family history positive in 30%. EEG normal. Treatment is interpretation and reassurance.

Infantile syncope (pallid breath holding)

No external precipitant (perhaps internal pain, cramp, or fear?). Pallor may be followed by seizure (anoxic-ischemic). Vagally (heart-slowing) mediated, like adult syncope. EEG normal; may see cardiac slowing with vagal stimulation (eyeball pressure, cold cloth on face) during EEG.

Tics or Tourette's syndrome

Simple or complex stereotyped (the same time after time) jerks or movements, coughs, grunts, sniffs. Worse at repose or with stress. May be suppressed during physician visit. Family history often positive. EEG negative. Nonanticonvulsant drugs may benefit.

Night terrors, sleep talking, walking, "sit-ups"

Age 3–10. Usually occur in first sleep cycle (30–90 minutes after going to sleep), with crying, screaming, and "autonomic discharge" (pupils dilatated, perspiring, etc). Lasts minutes. Child goes back to sleep and has no recall of event next day. Sleep studies (polysomnogram and EEG) are normal. Disappears with maturation. Sleep talking and walking and short "sit-ups" in bed are fragmentary arousals. If a spell is recorded, EEG shows arousal from deep sleep, but the behavior seems wakeful. The youngster needs to be protected from injury and gradually settled down and taken back to bed.

Nightmares

Nightmares or vivid dreams occur in subsequent cycles of sleep, often in the early morning hours, and generally are partially recalled the next day. The bizarre and frightening behavior may sometimes be confused with complex partial seizures. These occur during REM (rapid eye movement) sleep; epilepsy usually does not occur during that phase of sleep. In extreme or difficult cases, an all-night sleep EEG may help to differentiate seizures from nightmares.

Migraine

One variant of migraine can be associated with an acute confusional state. There may be the usual migraine prodrome with spots before the eyes, dizziness, visual field defects, and then agitated confusion. A history of other, more typical migraine with severe headache and vomiting but without confusion may aid in the diagnosis. The severe headache with vomiting as the youngster comes out of the migraine may aid in distinguishing the attack from epilepsy. Other seizure manifestations are practically never seen, eg, tonic-clonic movements, falling, and complete loss of consciousness. The EEG in migraine is usually normal and seldom has epileptiform abnormalities often seen in patients with epilepsy. Lastly, migraine and epilepsy are sometimes linked: migraine-caused ischemia on the brain surface sometimes leads to later epilepsy.

Benign nocturnal myoclonus

Common in infants and may last even up to school age. Focal or generalized jerks (the latter also called "hypnic" or "sleep jerks") may persist from onset of sleep on and off all night. A video record for physician review can aid in diagnosis. EEG taken during jerks is normal, proving that these jerks are not epilepsy. Treatment is by reassurance.

Shuddering

Shuddering or shivering attacks can occur in infancy and be a forerunner of essential tremor in later life. Often, the family history is positive for tremor. The shivering may be very frequent. EEG is normal. There is no clouding or loss of consciousness.

Gastroesophageal reflux

Seen more commonly in children with cerebral palsy or brain damage, reflux of acid gastric contents may cause pain that cannot be described by the child. At times, there may be unusual posturings (dystonic or other) of the head and neck or trunk, an apparent attempt to stretch the esophagus or close the opening. There is no loss of consciousness, but there may be eye rolling, apnea, occasional vomiting that may simulate a seizure. An upper GI series, cine of swallowing, sometimes even an EEG (which is always normal) may be necessary to distinguish this from seizures.

Masturbation

Rarely in infants, repetitive rocking or rubbing motions may simulate seizures. The youngster may look out of contact, be poorly responsive to the environment, and have autonomic expressions (eg, perspiration, dilated pupils) that may be confused with seizures. Observation by a skilled individual, sometimes even in a hospital situation, may be necessary to distinguish this from seizures. EEG is of course normal between or during attacks. Interpretation and reassurance are the only necessary treatment.

Conversion reaction/pseudoseizures

As many as 50% of patients with pseudoseizures have epilepsy. Episodes may be writhing, intercourse-like movements, tonic episodes, bizarre jerking and thrashing around, or even apparently sudden unresponsiveness. Often, there is ongoing psychological trauma. Often, but not invariably, the patients are developmentally delayed. The spells must often be seen or recorded on videotape in a controlled situation to distinguish them from epilepsy. A normal EEG during a spell is a key diagnostic feature. Often, the spells are so bizarre that they are easily distinguished. Sometimes, pseudoseizures can be precipitated by suggestion with injection of normal saline in a controlled situation. Combativeness is common; self-injury and incontinence rare.

Temper tantrums and rage attacks

These are sometimes confused with epilepsy. The youngster is often amnesic or at least claims amnesia for events during the spell. The attacks are usually precipitated by frustration or anger and are often directed either verbally or physically and subside with behavior modification and isolation. EEGs are generally normal but unfortunately seldom obtained during an attack. Anterior temporal leads may be helpful in ruling out temporal or lateral frontal abnormalities, the latter sometimes seen in partial complex seizures. Improvement of the attacks with psychotherapy, milieu therapy, or behavioral modification helps rule out epilepsy.

Benign paroxysmal vertigo

These are brief attacks of vertigo in which the youngster often appears frightened and pale and clutches the parent. The attacks last 5–30 seconds. Sometimes, nystagmus is identified. There is no loss of consciousness. Usually, the child is well and returns to play immediately afterward. The attacks may occur in clusters, then disappear for months. Attacks are usually seen in infants and preschoolers aged 2–5. EEG is normal. If caloric tests can be obtained (often very difficult in this age group), abnormalities with hypofunction of one side are sometimes seen. Medications are usually not desirable or necessary.

Staring spells

Teachers often make referral for absence or petit mal seizures in youngsters who stare or seem preoccupied at school. Helpful in the history is the lack of these spells at home, eg, in the early morning hours prior to breakfast, as might be seen with absence seizures. A lack of other epilepsy in the child or family history often is helpful. Sometimes, these children have difficulties with school and a cognitive or learning disability. The child can generally be brought out of this spell by a firm command. An EEG is sometimes necessary to confirm that absence seizures are not occurring. A 24-hour ambulatory EEG to record attacks during the child's everyday school activities is occasionally necessary.

formations occur in the infants of about 2.5% of untreated epileptic mothers.

C. Principles of Anticonvulsant Therapy:

1. Treat with the drug appropriate to the clinical situation, as outlined in Table 22–12.

2. Start with one drug in conventional dosage, and increase the dosage until seizures are controlled. If seizures are not controlled on the tolerated maximal dosage of one major anticonvulsant, gradually switch over to another before adding a second anticonvulsant. The dosages and usually effective blood levels listed in Table 22–12 are guides. Individual variations must be expected. The "therapeutic range" may also vary somewhat with the method used to determine levels.

3. Advise the parents and the patient that the prolonged use of anticonvulsant drugs will not produce significant or permanent "mental slowing" (although the underlying cause of the seizures might) and that prevention of seizures for 2–4 years substantially reduces the chances of recurrence. Advise them also that anticonvulsants are given to prevent further seizures and that they should be taken as prescribed. Changes in medications or dosages should not be made without the physician's knowledge. Unsupervised sudden withdrawal of anticonvulsant drugs may precipitate severe seizures or even status epilepticus.

Anticonvulsants must be kept where they cannot be ingested by small children or suicidal patients.

4. Check the patient at intervals, depending on the underlying cause of the seizures, the degree of control, and the toxic properties of the anticonvulsant drug or drugs used. Blood counts, urinalyses, and liver function or other biologic tests must be obtained periodically in the case of some anticonvulsants, as indicated in Table 22–12.

Periodic neurologic reevaluation is important. CT scanning may be indicated. Repeat EEGs are not needed to achieve seizure control. Indications for repeat EEGs are discussed above.

5. Continue anticonvulsant treatment until the patient is free of seizures for 2 or more years or, in some cases, through adolescence. In about 75% of cases, seizures may not recur. Such variables as younger age at onset, normal EEG, and ease of controlling seizures carry a favorable prognosis, whereas later onset, slowing or spikes on EEG, a history of atypical febrile convulsions, and possibly an abnormal neurologic examination carry a higher risk of recurrence.

6. In general, there is no need to withdraw anticonvulsants before taking an EEG.

7. Discontinue anticonvulsants gradually. If it becomes necessary to withdraw anticonvulsants abruptly, the patient should be under close medical surveillance. If seizures recur during or after withdrawal, anticonvulsant therapy should be reinstituted and again maintained for at least 2 or more years.

D. Blood Levels of Antiepileptic Drugs:

1. General comments–Most anticonvulsants take two or three times the length of their half-life to reach the "steady states" indicated in Table 22–12. This must be considered when blood levels are assessed after anticonvulsants are started or dosages are changed.

Individuals vary in their metabolism and their particular pharmacokinetic characteristics. These and external factors, including, for example, food intake or illness, also affect the blood level. Thus, the level reached on a milligram per kilogram or surface area basis varies among patients.

Experience and clinical research in the determination of antiepileptic blood levels have shown that there is some correlation between (1) drug dose and blood level, (2) blood level and therapeutic effect, and (3) blood level and some toxic effects.

2. Effective levels–The ranges given in Table 22–12 are those within which seizure control without toxicity will be achieved in most patients. The level for any given individual will vary not only with metabolic makeup (including biochemical defects) but also with the nature and severity of the seizures and their underlying cause, with other medications being taken, and other factors. Seizure control may be achieved at lower levels in some, and higher levels may be reached without toxicity in others. When control is achieved at a lower level, the dose should not be increased merely to get the level into the "therapeutic range." Likewise, toxic side effects will be experienced at different levels even within the "therapeutic range"; lowering the dose usually resolves the problem, but sometimes the drug must be withdrawn or another added (or both). Some serious toxic effects, including allergic reactions, LE phenomenon, and bone marrow or liver toxicity, are independent of dosage; liver toxicity especially may be the effect not just of a particular drug but also of its use in a patient who is or has been on several—and often a whole gamut—of other drugs.

3. Interaction of antiepileptic drugs–Blood levels of anticonvulsants may be affected by other drugs. Individual variations occur; adjustment of doses may be required.

4. Indications for determination of blood levels–Drug blood levels should be measured in a new patient or after a new drug is introduced and seizure control without toxicity is achieved to determine the effective level for that patient. Blood level monitoring is useful also when expected control on a "usual" dosage has not been achieved, either with a single drug or after adding another; when seizures recur in a previously well-controlled patient; or when control is poor in a patient taking anticonvulsants being seen for the first time. A low level may indicate inadequate dosage, drug interaction, or noncompliance with the prescribed regimen. A high level may indicate slowed metabolism or excretion or drug interaction.

Table 22–12. Guide to pediatric anticonvulsant drug therapy.[1]

Drug	Average Total Dosage (mg/kg/d)	Steady State	Effective Blood Levels[2]	Side Effects and Precautions	Directions and Remarks
Primary anticonvulsant					
Carbamazepine (Tegretol)	15–25 mg/kg/d in 2–4 divided doses	3–6 days	4–12 µg/mL (> 15)	Dizziness, ataxia, diplopia, thrombocytopenia leukopenia, rash. *Rare:* hepatotoxicity, bone marrow depression, dystonia, inappropriate priate ADH secretion, bizarre behaviors, tics.	Monitor CBC, platelet count, liver function tests closely for first 6 months, then periodically. Blood effects usually early and transient. *Drug interactions:* ↑ by fluoxetine, propoxyphene, erythromycin, cimetidine; ↓ by felbamate, phenobarbital, phenytoin.
Valproic acid (Depakene, Depakote)	15–60 mg/kg/d in 2–4 divided doses	2–4 days	50–120 µg/mL (> 140)	Weight gain, occasional gastric discomfort, constipation. Tremor, hair loss in 5%. *Rare:* hepatotoxicity, hyperammonemia, leukopenia.	For prophylaxis in febrile convulsions, see text. Monitor CBC, platelets, liver function tests closely in forst 6 months, then periodically. Can be given rectally (suspension: 250 mg/5 mL). Depacon is a new IV preparation, 100 mg/mL. Drug interactions: ↑ by cimetidine and lamotrigine; ↓ by phenobarbital, phenytoin, carbamazepine, lamotrigine.
Phenytoin (Dilantin)	5–10 mg/kg/d in 1 or 2 doses	5–10 days	5–20 µg/mL (>25)	Gum hypertrophy, hirsutism, ataxia, nystagmus, diplopia, rash, anorexia, nausea, osteomalacia. *Rare:* macrocytic anemia, lymph node involvement, exfoliative dermatitis, peripheral neuropathy.	Generally very effective and safe. Good dental hygiene reduces gum hyperplasia. May aggravate absence andmyoclonic seizures. Consider supplemental vitamin D. Poorly absorbed by neonatal gut. Use 50 mg Infantabs in infants (may be crushed to adjust dosage). Suspension not recommended. *Drug interactions:* ↑ by felbamate, phenobarbital; ↓ by carbamazepine, phenobarbital, antacids.
Phenobarbital	3–8 mg/kg/d as single daily dose	10–21 days	15–40 µg/mL (> 45)	Irritability and overactivity in many children; sedative effects in others. Mild ataxia, nystagmus, skin rash. May interfere with learning.	Overall, the safest drug. Bitter taste. Higher blood levels sometimes required and tolerated in severe chronic epileptics. Useful in neonatal seizures and status epilepticus.
Primidone (Mysoline)	10–25 mg/kg/d in 3 or 4 divided doses	1–5 days	4–12 µg/mL (> 15)	Drowsiness, ataxia, vertigo, anorexia, nausea, vomiting, rash.	Start slowly with 25–35% of expected maintenance dose; increase every other day until full dose reached.
Ethosuximide (Zarontin)	10–40 mg/kg/d in 1 or 2 doses	5–6 days	40–100 µg/mL (> 150)	Nausea, gastric discomfort, hiccups, blood dyscrasias.	May aggravate generalized seizures. Combine with valproic acid in refractory abscence seizures.
Clonazepam (Klonopin)	0.1–0.2 mg/kg/d in 2 or 3 divided doses	5–10 days	15–80 ng/mL (> 80)	Drowsiness (> 50%): soporific effects greatest drawback. Behavior problems in 25%. Slurred speech, ataxia, salivation.	Start slowly with 25% of expected maintenance dosage; increase every 2 or 3 days. Useful with refractory minor motor seizures (astatic, myoclonic, infantile spasms; absences). Tolerance may occur.

Table 22–12. Guide to pediatric anticonvulsant drug therapy.[1] (continued)

Drug	Average Total Dosage (mg/kg/d)	Steady State	Effective Blood Levels[2]	Side Effects and Precautions	Directions and Remarks
Adjunctive or secondary drug					
Acetazolamide (Diamox)	5–20 mg/kg/d in 2 or 3 divided doses	1–2 days	10–14 µg/mL	Anorexia; numbness and tingling. Urinary frequency, so do not give in evening. Renal stones.	Supplement to other medications, especially in absence and complex partial seizures. Also in females 4 days prior to and in the first 2 or 3 days of menstrual period for catamenial seizures.
Methsuximide (Celontin)	15–30 mg/kg/d in 2–4 divided doses	Not known (? 14 days)	10–40 µg/mL (normethsuximide)	Drowsiness, ataxia, headache, diplopia. Skin rash in 15%.	Useful in complex partial and myoclonic-astatic seizures.
Clorazepate (Tranxene)	0.3–1 mg/kg/d in 2 or 3 divided doses	Not known (? 21 days)	0.2–1.5 µg/mL (> 2)	Lethargy.	May be useful adjunct in generalized tonic-clonic, partial, and astatic seizures. Not for children under age 9 years.
Felbamate (Felbatol)	15–45 mg/kg/d in 3 or 4 divided doses	5–7 days	22–137 µg/mL	Anorexia, vomiting, insomnia, headache, somnolence. Rash in 1%. Aplastic anemia and hepatic failure are significant hazards.	A dangerous drug. Used in children with Lennox-Gastaut syndrome; in adults with complex partial seizures. Obtain informed consent. *Drug interactions:* ↑ by phenytoin, carbamazepine. ↓ by valproic acid.
Phenacemide (phenurone)	25–50 mg/kg/d in 2–4 divided doses	Not known	. . .	Rash, anorexia, nausea: *Caution:* hepatitis, psychosis, blood dyscrasias.	Especially effective in complex partial seizures when all other drugs fail. Monitor CBC and liver function tests frequently in first 3–4 months, then 2–4 times a year.
Gabapentin (Neurontin) > 12 years	30–60 mg/kg/d in 3 divided doses (900–1800 mg total per day)	1–2 days	. . .	Drowsiness, dizziness, ataxia.	Add-on drug for partial seizures; no effect on other anticonvulsant drug levels.
Topiramate (Topamax)	10 mg/kg/d rarely 20 mg/kg/d) in 2 divided doses (maximum, 400 mg/d)	Not known	Not known	Somnolence, slowed mentation, dizziness, language problems (word finding), rarely kidney stones	Adjunctive drug for complex partial seizures. Minimal effect on other drug levels.
Trimethadione (Tridione)	20–50 mg/kg/d in 3 or 4 divided doses	Not known	470–1200 µg/mL (dimethadione)	Rash, photophobia, irritability. *Caution:* Leukopenia, agranulocytosis. LE phenomenon.	Useful primary drug in absence seizures if ethoxuximide and valproic acid fail. May aggravate generalized seizures; if so, add phenobarbital. CBC and urinalysis once a month.
Mephobarbital (Mebaral)	4–10 mg/kg/d in 1 or 2 doses	As with phenobarbital	15–40 µg/mL (phenobarbital)	As with phenobarbital.	Twice the quantity of phenobarbital required for comparable effect.
Lamotrigine (Lamictal) > 16 years	5–15 mg/kg/d in 2–4 divided doses (1–5 mg if taking valproic acid); 50–300 mg/d total	8–15 days	. . .	Dizziness, headaches, diplopia, ataxia, nausea. Rash in 5–10%.	Add-on drug for children over age 16 with complex partial seizures. Increase dose slowly over 2 months (see package insert).

Table 22–12. Guide to pediatric anticonvulsant drug therapy.[1] (continued)

Drug	Average Total Dosage (mg/kg/d)	Steady State	Effective Blood Levels[2]	Side Effects and Precautions	Directions and Remarks
Treatment of status epilepticus[3]					
Diazepam (Valium)	0.3 mg/kg IV. Repeat dose: 0.1–0.3 mg/kg IV.			Administer slowly. Monitor pulse and blood pressure. May cause respiratory depression in presence of phenobarbital.	May need to be repeated every 3–4 hours. Follow with phenytoin or phenobarbital for long-range control. ***Note:*** Intramuscular administration for status epilepticus is ineffective.
Phenobarbital	5–20 mg/kg IV initially: Repeat dose 5–10 mg/kg IV.			See above.	Rule out pyridoxine deficiency. In neonatral seizures, load with 15–20 mg/kg IV.
Phenytoin (Dilantin)	10–20 mg/kg IV initially: Repeat dose: 5–10 mg/kg IV.			Administer IV over a 5-minute period. Absorption after IM administration uncertain. Monitor blood levels.	Adjunct in neonatal seizures (20 mg/kg IV) if phenobarbital alone fails. Fos-phenytoin, new safe preparation. Same dose. May give rapidly IV.
Lorazepam (Ativan)	0.05–0.2 mg/kg IV. May repeat.			Mild respiratory depression.	May be more effective than diazepam. Longer-acting.
Midazolam (Versed)	0.1–0.3 mg/kg IM or IV; 0.2 mg/kg as nasal spray			See other benzodiapines.	Short-acting.
Lidocaine (Xylocaine)	2 mg/kg IV			Administer slowly.	Useful especially when reluctant to give more diazepam, or barbiturates. Effect brief (about 30 minutes).

[1]Treatment of infantile spasms: See text regarding use of corticotropin or corticosteroids. See also clonazepam or valproic acid, especially with recurrences.
[2]In parentheses are shown the levels at which clinical toxicity becomes manifest in monotherapy.
[3]General anesthesia if other measures fail.

Blood levels are mandatory when there are signs and symptoms of toxicity—particularly where there is polydrug therapy, the dosage of a drug has been raised, or another drug has been added. Blood levels may be the only means of detecting intoxication in a comatose patient or very young child. Toxic levels also occur with drug abuse or liver disease.

Finally, when the patient is well controlled (or is controlled as well as one may hope for in a patient refractory to antiepileptics or one with difficult-to-control seizures) and free of toxic signs, blood levels are unnecessary.

E. Side Effects of Antiepileptic Drugs: (See also Table 22–12.)

1. Serious allergic reactions usually necessitate discontinuance of a drug. However, not every rash in a child receiving an anticonvulsant is due to the drug. If a useful antiepileptic drug is discontinued for this reason and the rash disappears, restarting the drug in a smaller dosage is often warranted to see if the reaction recurs.

2. Signs of drug toxicity often disappear when the daily dosage is reduced by 25–30%.

3. The sedative effect of many of the anticonvulsants may be forestalled by slowly working up to the usual therapeutic dose, eg, over 3–4 weeks for phenobarbital.

4. Gingival hyperplasia secondary to phenytoin is best minimized through good dental hygiene but occasionally requires gingivectomy. This condition (but not hypertrichosis) usually disappears within about 6 months after the drug is discontinued.

F. ACTH and Corticosteroids:

1. Indications–These drugs are indicated for infantile spasms not due to causes amenable to specific therapy and in the Lennox-Gastaut syndrome which cannot be controlled by anticonvulsant drugs.

Duration of therapy is guided by cessation of clinical seizures and normalization of the EEG. ACTH or oral corticosteroids are usually continued in full doses for 2 weeks and then, if seizures have ceased, tapered over 1 week. Others use a total treatment period of about 2 months. If seizures recur, the dosage is increased to the last effective level and repeated for 2–4 weeks, or switching to or from prednisone is tried. Some clinicians maintain the patient for up to 6 months on this dosage before attempting withdrawal. There is no strong evidence, however, that longer courses of treatment are more beneficial.

2. Dosages–

a. ACTH gel, starting with 2–4 units/kg/d intramuscularly in a single morning dose. Parents can be taught to give injections.

b. Prednisone, starting with 2–4 mg/kg/d orally in two or three divided doses.

3. Precautions–Give additional potassium, guard against infections, and discuss the cushingoid appearance and its disappearance. Do not withdraw oral corticosteroids suddenly. Side effects in some series occur in up to 40% of cases, especially with higher doses than those listed here (used by some authorities).

G. Ketogenic or Medium-Chain Triglyceride Diet in Treatment of Epilepsy: A ketogenic diet should be recommended in astatic and myoclonic seizures and absence seizures not responsive to drug therapy; it is occasionally recommended for infantile spasms that do not respond to corticotropin or the corticosteroids. Ketosis is induced by a diet high in fats and very limited in carbohydrates with sufficient protein for body maintenance and growth; by the feeding of medium-chain triglycerides (MCT); or by a combination of these methods. The MCT diet induces ketosis more readily than does a high level of dietary fats and thus requires less carbohydrate restriction. The mechanism for the anticonvulsant action of the ketogenic diet is not understood. It is, however, the ketosis, not the acidosis, that raises the seizure threshold.

The diet is usually most effective in young children under the age of 8 years, but when all other measures fail, it should be tried even in adolescents.

As ketosis is achieved, a repeat EEG may be helpful; seizure control by the diet is more likely to occur if the EEG shows improvement.

The ketogenic diet is difficult and expensive, tends to be monotonous, and depends on the caregiver's ability to weigh out the foods as well as on absolute adherence to the diet prescribed. Whether the ketosis is achieved by high-fat meals or an MCT diet is often a matter of the physician's, the dietitian's, or the patient's preference. The result may also depend on which form of the diet is better tolerated. Full cooperation of all family members is required, including the patient if old enough. However, when seizure control is achieved by this method, the child is alert, often needs no anticonvulsants or only small amounts, and parental and patient satisfaction is most gratifying.

H. Surgery: In seizure disorders intractable to anticonvulsant therapy and primarily of focal origin, neurosurgery should be considered. Useful procedures, depending on the lesion, include corticectomy, hemispherectomy, anterior temporal lobectomy (for complex partial seizures), callosotomy (or commissurotomy), and stereotactic ablation.

Arroyo S, Freeman JM: Epilepsy surgery in children: State of the art. Adv Pediatr 1994;41:53.

Bobele GB, Bodensteiner JB: Infantile spasms. Neurol Clin 1990;8:633.

Brodie MJ, Dichter MA: Antiepileptic drugs. (Drug Therapy.) N Engl J Med 1996;334:168.

Camfield CS, Camfield PR: Febrile seizures: An Rx for parent fears and anxieties. Contemp Pediatr 1993;10:26.

Committee on Drugs, American Academy of Pediatrics: Behavioral and cognitive effects of anticonvulsant therapy. Pediatrics 1985;76:644.

Coulter DL: Comprehensive management of epilepsy in persons with mental retardation. Epilepsia 1997;38 (Suppl 4):S524.

Dieckmann RA: Rectal diazepam for prehospital pediatric status epilepticus. Ann Emerg Med 1994;24:216.

Duchowny MS et al: Surgical treatment of epilepsy in childhood. Int Pediatr 1997;12:106.

Dulac O, Chugani M, Dalla Bernardina B: *Infantile Spasms and West Syndrome.* Saunders, 1994.

Evans OB: Breath-holding spells. Pediatr Ann 1997; 26:410.

Farwell JR et al: Phenobarbital for febrile seizures: Effects on intelligence and on seizure recurrence. N Engl J Med 1990;322:364.

Feit LR: Syncope in the pediatric patient: Diagnosis, pathophysiology, and treatment. Adv Pediatr 1996;43:469.

Gilman J et al: Intractable epilepsy: Are the new antiepileptic agents beneficial? Int Pediatr 1997;12:48.

Haslam RHA: Nonfebrile Seizures. Pediatr Rev 1997; 18:39.

Hirtz DG: Febrile Seizures. Pediatr Rev 1997;18:5.

Jayakar P: The role of EEG in management of childhood epilepsy. Int Pediatr 1993;8:253.

Kaplan PW: Nonconvulsive status in the ER. Epilepsia 1996;37:643.

Marson A et al: New antiepileptic drugs: A systematic review of their efficacy and tolerability. BMJ 1996;313: 1169.

Maytal J, Shinnar S: Febrile status epilepticus. Pediatrics 1990;86:611.

McBride MC: Status epilepticus. Pediatr Rev 1995;16:386.

Nordli DR, DeVivo DC: The ketogenic diet revisited: Back to the future. Epilepsia 1997;38:743.

Painter MJ, Gaines L: Neonatal seizures: Diagnosis and treatment. J Child Neurol 1991;6:101.

Pellock JM: The classification of childhood seizures and epilepsy syndromes. Neurol Clin 1990;8:619.

Resnick TJ et al: Epilepsy and the ketogenic diet. Int Pediatr 1997;12:102.

Rosman NP et al: A controlled trial of diazepam administered during febrile illnesses to prevent recurrence of febrile seizures. N Engl J Med 1993;328:79.

Stafstrom CE: Neonatal Seizures. Pediatr Rev 1995;16:248.

Wolf SM et al: Infantile spasms: Current therapy and progress. Pediatr Rev 1996;17:356.

Wyllie E: Temporal lobe epilepsy in children. Int Pediatr 1993;8:267.

Zupanc ML: Update on epilepsy in pediatric patients. Mayo Clin Proc 1996;71:899.

SYNCOPE & FAINTING

Fainting is transient loss of consciousness and postural tone due to a cerebral ischemia or anoxia. Up to

20–50% of children (0–20 years) will faint. There may be a prodrome of dizziness, light-headedness, nausea, "gray-out," sweating, and pallor. After falling, many children stiffen or have jerking motions when unconscious, a tonic-clonic, anoxic-ischemic seizure mimicking epilepsy.

Watching or undergoing a venipuncture is a common precipitant of fainting, as is prolonged standing, fatigue, illness, overheating and sweating, dehydration, hunger, and athleticism with slow baseline pulse. The family history is positive for similar episodes in 90% of cases.

Classification

Ninety-five percent of cases of syncope are of the **vasovagal-vasodepressive** or **neurocardiogenic** type. Vasodilation, cardiac slowing, and hypotension cause transient (1–2 minutes) cerebral ischemia and "passing out." The patient arouses in 1–2 minutes, but full recovery may take an hour or more. Besides those listed above, rare precipitants include hair grooming, cough, micturition, neck stretching, and emotional stress.

More ominous is **cardiac syncope,** which often occurs during exercise; angina or palpitations may occur. An obstructive lesion (stenosis), cardiomyopathy, coronary disease, or dysrhythmia may be the cause (Table 22–13).

Other spells that may mimic syncope are listed in Table 22–13.

Clinical Findings

A. Symptoms and Signs: The workup includes, as well as the history, a physical examination with emphasis on blood pressure, cardiac, and neurologic features. A blood pressure drop of more than 30 mm Hg after standing for 5–10 minutes (adolescent) or a baseline systolic pressure of less than 80 mm Hg suggests orthostasis.

Table 22–13. Classification of syncope in childhood.

Vasovagal, neurocardiogenic (neurally mediated)
  Orthostatic
  Athleticism
  Pallid breath-holding
  Situational (stress, blood drawing)
Cardiac
  Obstructive
  Arrhythmia
  Prolonged QT_c
  Hypercyanotic (eg, in tetralogy of Fallot)
Nonsyncope mimicker
  Migraine with confusion or stupor
  Seizure
  Hypoglycemia
  Hysteria
  Hyperventilation
  Vertigo

B. Laboratory Findings and Imaging: Hemoglobin should be checked if anemia is suggested by the history. Electrocardiography should be done. Consider Holter monitoring, cardiac referral, and echocardiography if cardiac causes seem likely. Tilt testing (though norms are vague) may have a role in frequent recurrent syncope to confirm a vasodepressive cause and avoid more expensive methods of investigation.

Treatment

Treatment consists mostly of giving advice about the benign nature of "fainting" and about avoiding precipitating situations. The patient should be cautioned to lie down if there are prodromal symptoms. Good hydration and reasonable salt intake are advisable. In some cases beta blockers and rarely fludrocortisone may have a role.

Braden DS, Gaymes CH: The diagnosis and management of syncope in children and adolescents. Pediatr Ann 1997;26:422.

Feit LR: Syncope in the pediatric patient: Diagnosis, pathophysiology, and treatment. Adv Paediatr 1996;43:469.

Kaufman H: Neurally mediated syncope and syncope due to autonomic failure: Differences and similarities. J Clin Neurophysiol 1997;14:183.

HEADACHES

Headache is not usually a psychosomatic symptom in very young children, whereas it is more apt to be so in older children and adolescents. Headaches occur in 37% and migraine in 2.7% of children by 7 years of age; by 14 years, the rates are 69% and 10.9%, respectively. A careful description of the headaches, associated circumstances, and other neurologic and systemic symptoms should be obtained. The family history and emotional problems should be discussed in detail. Systemic and neurologic examination, including blood pressure, ophthalmoscopic examination, and station and gait, will usually distinguish organic from psychogenic headaches. Differential features are given in Table 22–14.

If there is evidence of a specific intracranial cause or systemic disorder (eg, renal disease), diagnosis and treatment should be directed at the primary disorder.

The most common headache with onset in adolescence is tension headache. Unlike vascular headache of migraine, the typical tension headache is variable in location, frontal, generalized ("hatband-like"), or occipital, not accompanied by visual, gastrointestinal, neurologic (eg, dizziness) symptoms. Unless accompanied by depression (a linkage common in adults, less common in children), markedly decreased school attendance or diminished athletic prowess seldom occurs. Adolescents with tension

Table 22–14. Differential features of headaches in children.

	Muscle Contraction (Tension/Psychogenic)	Vascular (Migraine)	Traction and Inflammatory (Increased Intracranial Pressure)
Time course	Chronic, recurrent	Acute, paroxysmal, recurrent	Chronic or intermittent but increasingly frequent; progressive severity
Prodromes	No	Yes	No
Description	Diffuse, band-like, tight	Intense, pulsatile, unilateral in older child (70%)	Diffuse; more occipital with infratentorial mass, more frontal with supratentorial mass
Characteristic findings	Feelings of inadequacy, depression, or anxiety	Neurologic symptoms and signs usually transient	Positive neurologic signs, especially papilledema
Predisposing factors	Problems at home or school or socially (sexually)	Positive family history (75%); trivial head trauma may precipitate	No

headaches usually, in spite of head pain, continue to function well. If there is fall-off in peer group or family relationships or schoolwork, more extensive interviewing in reference to adverse events or stress in those areas is needed.

Physical and neurologic examination in tension headaches is normal. Underlying depression must be ruled out. Laboratory studies are unnecessary. Treatment includes searching out and avoiding precipitants (eg, stress, noise) and use of minor analgesics, relaxation techniques, even biofeedback. Prophylactic medication (eg, amitriptyline) may be helpful.

The prognosis is guarded. Minor morbidity and decreased school and work efficiency may persist. Psychogenic etiology or enmeshment may be sought out in the especially difficult headache patient; psychiatric consultation may be needed.

A chronic progressive headache may represent brain tumor causing headache because of its midline location, obstructing spinal fluid flow, resulting in a painful, progressive hydrocephalus. Or, the tumor mass may distort pain-sensitive structures, such as blood vessels, meninges, or dura.

Although brain tumor headache may initially mimic migraine, tension, or sinus headaches, certain history and physical findings alert the clinician.

Headache of recent onset in a child in the age group from 3 to 10, the peak age for brain tumors, is worrisome. A progressive headache with worsening frequency (eg, from weekly to daily) and severity (eg, from mild to prostrating) suggests tumor.

Headache in the morning, perhaps due to change of position and change in intracranial dynamics, with vomiting (often without nausea) is ominous.

A child with headache who is deteriorating in social, school, and athletic (coordination) prowess causes concern.

Even more important are positive neurologic findings. *The typical headache patient has a normal physical and neurologic examination.* Strabismus,

weakness of extraocular muscles, visual loss, poor pupillary response, and papilledema or optic atrophy must be ruled out. Coordination and gait must be assessed with finger-nose-finger pursuit, balancing on each leg, hopping, and tandem walking forward and backward on a straight line.

If suspicion remains high in spite of a normal neurologic examination, a follow-up examination is essential. An imaging study should be strongly considered.

The preferred study is MRI, which is superior to CT scan for posterior fossa tumors and for visualization around bony structures such as the sella and foramen magnum. However, if suspicion for tumor is low, the more available and less expensive CT scan is a sensible alternative.

To summarize, a history with the key points listed above and a good physical and neurological examination usually picks up the rare headache with brain tumor. A recent study of 104 children with onset of headaches prior to 7 years of age, seen by age 9, found mostly (75%) migraines. A pertinent quote from that article: "No child who presented for evaluation of headaches with a normal neurologic exam was found to have a brain tumor."

Migraine attacks are usually paroxysmal, throbbing, pulsating, or pounding in character (initial vasoconstriction of intracranial vessels followed by vasodilation of extracranial vessels). The pain in children is as often bilateral as unilateral, frontal or retro-orbital as hemicranial. Between attacks, the child is asymptomatic. Migraine in children is associated (in order of frequency) with nausea, gastric discomfort, or vomiting; dizziness or vertigo; photophobia, visual auras, and, less frequently, visual loss; sensory and motor disturbances, especially involving the face and arms; speech disturbances; and, occasionally, hemiplegia (sometimes alternating), acute confusional states, or impairment of space, time, and body image perceptions (termed the "Alice-in-Wonderland syndrome"). The child frequently seeks rest in a dark, quiet room.

Migraine of varying severity may occur in up to 6.6% of children between 7 and 14 years of age. Onset by age 4 is not uncommon. After 10 years of age, it is twice as common in girls as in boys. The family history is positive for migraine in up to 75% of patients and not infrequently also for epilepsy. School stresses (headache often occurs after school) and foods occasionally precipitate migraine. Head trauma may precipitate onset. In most instances, the migraine attack is brief (hours, not days), and sleep gives relief. Motion sickness is an associated feature in 45% of cases.

EEG may be abnormally slow to mildly or moderately dysrhythmic in up to 80% of patients soon after an attack of complicated migraine (emphasizing the relationship between migraine and epilepsy). Neuroradiologic studies, such as CT scanning, are usually not warranted unless there are definite neurologic or progressive abnormalities.

Acetaminophen or ibuprofen is often effective in children. The patient should be allowed to remain quiet in a darkened room. In children over 12 years of age, severe migraine may often be controlled by Fiorinal, Fioricet, or Midrin, one or two capsules or tablets every 4 hours. If these measures are ineffective, especially in the older child, and when anxiety and nausea are prominent symptoms, Cafergot is often useful.*

In the prevention of severe, frequent, and disabling migraine—especially in children too young to alert an adult to their symptoms or to follow the above regimen—prophylaxis is recommended as follows: propranolol, 10–40 mg three times daily depending on weight (contraindications are respiratory and cardiac disorders); cyproheptadine, 2–4 mg every 8–12 hours; or calcium channel blockers (in varying forms and dosages; they may be anticonvulsant action as well). Antidepressants such as imipramine or amitriptyline may be useful (25–50 mg at bedtime). Methysergide maleate is not recommended in children.

Operant conditioning and biofeedback are lengthy and expensive options, studied almost exclusively in children in conjunction with vascular, not tension, headaches. Biofeedback was studied and reported in a position paper of the American College of Physicians in 1985 and was thought unproved. A recent pediatric study suggested utility of these therapies in vascular headaches in children.

---

*One capsule of Fiorinal or Lanorinal contains butalbital, 50 mg; aspirin, 325 mg; and caffeine, 40 mg. One tablet of Fioricet contains butalbital, 50 mg; acetaminophen, 325 mg; and caffeine, 40 mg. One capsule of Midrin contains isometheptene mucate, 65 mg; dichloralphenazone, 100 mg; and acetaminophen, 325 mg. Cafergot tablets contain ergotamine tartrate, 1 mg, and caffeine, 100 mg.

Chu ML, Shinnar S: Headaches in children younger than 7 years of age. Arch Neurol 1992;49:79.

Hääläinen ML et al: Ibuprofen or acetaminophen for the acute treatment of migraine in children: A double-blind, randomized, placebo-controlled, crossover study. Neurology 1997;48:103.

Hääläinen ML et al: Sumatriptan for migraine attacks in children: A randomized placebo-controlled study. Neurology 1997;48:1100.

Jensen R, Brinck T, Olesen J: Sodium valproate has a prophylactic effect in migraine without aura: A triple-blind, placebo-controlled crossover study. Neurology 1994; 44:647.

Maytal J et al: The value of brain imaging in children with headaches. Pediatrics 1995;96:413.

Parker C: Complicated migraine syndromes and migraine variants. Pediatr Ann 1997;26:417.

Rothner AD: Classification, pathogenesis, evaluation, and management of headaches in children and adolescents. Curr Opin Pediatr 1992;4:949.

Singer HS et al: Chronic recurrent headaches in children. Pediatr Ann 1992;21:369.

Singer HS: Migraine headaches in children. Pediatr Rev 1994;15:94.

Visser WH et al: Sumatriptan in clinical practice: A 2-year review of 453 migraine patients. Neurology 1996;47:46.

SLEEP DISORDERS

1. SLEEP APNEA SYNDROME IN OLDER CHILDREN

Sleep apnea syndrome should be considered if there is a history of restless sleep with snoring or respiratory noise during sleep and frequent awakenings in an older child who shows poor school performance associated with excessive daytime sleepiness or irritability and hyperactivity. Children with these problems frequently have hypertrophied tonsils or adenoids, causing partial airway obstruction. Occasionally, they have facial dysmorphism; neuromuscular disorders with muscle hypotonia and poor pharyngeal muscle control; and hyperplastic tissues, as seen in myxedema, Hodgkin's disease, or pickwickian syndrome. Evaluation includes soft tissue x-rays of the lateral neck; chest x-ray; electrocardiography to rule out cardiomegaly, sinus dysrhythmias, and incipient or actual right-sided heart failure; arterial blood gas determinations while awake and during sleep; and polysomnography. Therapy is generally surgical, ranging from tonsillectomy and adenoidectomy when appropriate, to tracheostomy when medical measures fail.

2. NARCOLEPSY

Narcolepsy, a primary disorder of sleep and wakefulness, is characterized by chronic, excessive daytime sleeping that occurs regardless of activity or surroundings and is not relieved by increased sleep at night. Onset occurs as early as 3 years of age; about 18% of patients are 10 years or younger. Sixty percent are between puberty and their late teens. Narcolepsy usually interferes severely with normal living. Often months to years after onset, there may also be cataplexy (transient partial or total loss of muscle tone, often triggered by laughter, anger, or other emotional upsurge); hypnagogic hallucinations (visual or auditory); and sensations of paralysis on falling asleep. Studies have shown that rapid eye movement (REM) sleep, with loss of muscle tone and an electroencephalographic low-amplitude mixed frequency pattern, occurs soon after sleep onset in patients with cataplexy, whereas normal subjects experience 80–100 minutes or longer of non-REM (NREM) sleep before the initial REM period.

Narcolepsy is treated with a CNS stimulant (dextroamphetamine or long-acting methylphenidate is preferred); occasionally, a tricyclic antidepressant, in low doses titrated to the need of the patient, is added to the treatment regimen. The condition persists throughout life.

3. SOMNAMBULISM

Somnambulism has been assigned to a group of sleep disturbances known as disorders of arousal. It is characterized by abrupt onset early in the night of an episode of veiled consciousness and coordinated activity (eg, walking, sometimes moving objects without seeming purpose). The episode is relatively brief and ceases spontaneously. There is poor recall of the event on waking in the morning. Somnambulism may be related to mental activities occurring in stages 3 and 4 of NREM sleep. Incidence has been estimated at only 2–3%, but up to 15% of cases are reported in children 6–16 years of age, with boys affected more often than girls and many having recurrent episodes. No psychopathologic features can usually be demonstrated, but a strong association (30%) between childhood migraine and somnambulism has been noted. Episodes of somnambulism may be triggered in predisposed children by stresses, including febrile illnesses. No treatment of somnambulism is required, and it is not necessary to seek psychiatric consultation.

4. NIGHT TERRORS

Night terrors (pavor nocturnus) are a disorder of arousal from NREM sleep. Most cases occur in children 3–8 years of age, and the disorder rarely occurs after adolescence. It is characterized by sudden (but only partial) waking, with the severely frightened child unable to be fully roused or comforted. Concomitant autonomic symptoms include rapid breathing, tachycardia, and perspiring. The next morning, the child has no recall of any nightmare. Psychopathologic mechanisms are unclear, but falling asleep after watching scenes of violence on television or hearing frightening stories may play a role. Elimination of such causes and administration of a mild antianxiety agent such as chlordiazepoxide may be helpful. It is important to differentiate these episodes from complex partial (psychomotor) seizures. (See also Chapter 3.)

Blum NJ, Carey WB: Sleep problems among infants and young children. Pediatr Rev 1996;17:87.

Kotagal S, Hartse KM, Walsh JK: Characteristics of narcolepsy in preteenaged children. Pediatrics 1990;85:205.

Sheldon S, Spire JP, Levy H: *Pediatric Sleep Medicine.* Saunders, 1992.

Wise MS: Parasomnias in children. Pediatr Ann 1997; 26:427.

HEAD & SPINAL INJURIES

Serious accidental injury constitutes one of the most common causes of childhood hospitalization and death in the United States. (See also Chapter 11.)

Injury of the brain can result from sudden acceleration-deceleration movements or from sudden rotational or torsional movements of the head. Direct impact of the brain against the inner table of the skull, together with blood vessel rupture and dural tears, leads to parenchymal damage.

Closed head injury includes injuries in which the skull remains intact or in which there is only a small linear fracture. **Open head injury** consists of injuries involving major scalp lacerations and compound or depressed skull fractures. Brain parenchymal injury can occur in either closed or open head injuries but is more frequent and often more severe with open head injury.

The clinical severity of head injury is classified as mild, moderate, or severe, depending on the type and extent of brain damage, the presence of brain edema, and the presence or absence of intracranial hemorrhage. Intracranial hemorrhages can occupy a variety of potential spaces within the cranial vault, including epidural, subdural, and subarachnoid spaces. Cerebral contusions consist of a localized region of petechial hemorrhage and edema. Intraparenchymal hemorrhages can be small or massive, rapidly expanding to produce markedly elevated intracranial pressure and cerebral herniation.

Clinical Findings

A. Symptoms and Signs: In mild head injuries, loss of consciousness may not occur or may be only momentary. Frequently, patients experience mild to moderate headache, nausea, vomiting, vertigo, and lightheadedness. Although tachycardia may be present, blood pressure and other vital signs are normal. There is rapid resolution of all symptoms. Occasionally, a brief, generalized clonic seizure may occur shortly after the head injury, but posttraumatic epilepsy is rare.

Moderately severe head injuries are associated with loss of consciousness for several minutes to 1 hour. Headache may be severe, and the patient may experience severe irritability, drowsiness, emotional lability, and signs of mild to moderate delirium. Nausea and vomiting can be prominent. Vertigo, tinnitus, and lightheadedness may be moderately severe for a short period. Symptoms resolve in 1–2 days, though vertigo and some alteration in behavior, mood, and concentration persist for several days. Some children also experience relatively protracted problems regarding attention, concentration, and school performance after seemingly mild or moderate head injury.

Severe head injury is associated with prolonged loss of consciousness, usually longer than 1 hour. Headache, nausea, vomiting, and tinnitus are severe and at times incapacitating. Marked behavioral changes and seizures can develop immediately after the head injury. Posttraumatic epilepsy occurs in approximately 10% of children. Symptoms usually persist for several days or weeks, in some patients for months.

When intracranial hemorrhages occur, symptoms of progressively increasing intracranial pressure may develop. Patients have progressive loss of consciousness and severe nausea and vomiting. Seizures occur in about 50–70% of children with subdural hematomas. Fever and nuchal rigidity are often present with subdural hematomas, and meningitis may be suspected. Epidural and acute subdural hematomas may be acute and require emergency surgical drainage. These forms of intracranial hemorrhage can rapidly lead to death, particularly if they occur in the posterior fossa. Subarachnoid hemorrhages are unusual in childhood unless they are associated with an underlying cerebrovascular malformation. Intracerebral hematomas, particularly in the frontal and temporal regions, can occur after either a closed or open head injury. When intracerebral hemorrhages occur, an underlying bleeding diathesis should be excluded by appropriate laboratory testing.

B. Physical Examination: Initial assessment of patients who have suffered head injury includes frequent monitoring of heart rate, blood pressure, and temperature. Sudden changes in blood pressure, particularly hypotension, may be an indication of intrathoracic, intra-abdominal, or other systemic injury associated with bleeding.

Head circumference should be measured in infants after head injury; size and tension of the fontanelle should be carefully documented. Evaluation of the head and neck region is important in the search for signs of CSF leakage from the ear and nose. Care should be taken to move the head as little as possible because injury to the spinal cord and cervical vertebrae may not be initially apparent. The patient should be examined thoroughly for signs of injury to extremities, abdomen, back, and chest. The skin should also be carefully examined for evidence of recent or remote injury. The possibility of nonaccidental trauma should be suspected when multiple sites of injury or injuries of different ages are present.

Neurologic examination includes assessment of pupillary size, symmetry, and light reflexes. Evidence of ocular and orbital injury may be associated with basilar skull fracture. Funduscopic examination may disclose retinal flame-shaped hemorrhages that can be indicative of subdural or subarachnoid hemorrhages. Increased intracranial pressure related to intracranial hemorrhages or cerebral edema may result in dilated, nonpulsating retinal veins and swelling of the optic disk. Assessment of muscle tone, strength, and reflexes may provide evidence of focal or lateralized neurologic dysfunction.

C. Laboratory Studies and Imaging: A sudden or progressive decrease in hematocrit may suggest rapidly evolving acute subdural hematoma. Injury may result in fluid and electrolyte abnormalities as a consequence of inappropriate secretion of antidiuretic hormone or diabetes insipidus.

Radiographic studies, particularly CT scanning, should be conducted to search for skull fracture, intracranial hemorrhage, and intracranial foreign bodies. Skull films in general are not as helpful as CT scanning; however, in certain situations when CT scanning is not available, skull films may demonstrate clinically significant depressed or comminuted skull fractures. In addition, plain radiographs of the neck, chest, abdomen, and extremities are important in searching for more generalized evidence of injury. X-ray films of the neck should be obtained on all patients with head injury because unsuspected spinal injury can be present and require immediate stabilization. MRI can also demonstrate intracranial hemorrhage and some types of foreign bodies. MRI is not, however, as helpful as CT scanning at defining bony abnormalities. Cerebral angiography may be required at times when major vascular damage is suspected or when the patient develops clinical signs suggesting arterial dissection.

Lumbar puncture is rarely needed in the evaluation of patients with head injury and in most instances is contraindicated. Infants with tense fontanelles and fever may be suspected initially of having bacterial meningitis; in this situation lumbar puncture may be necessary.

Subdural tap is an important immediate diagnostic as well as therapeutic maneuver in acute and rapidly progressing subdural or epidural hematomas. When an acute subdural hematoma is suspected and the patient is deteriorating rapidly, a subdural tap should be performed as an emergency procedure. *The tap should not be delayed in order to obtain a CT scan.*

With posterior fossa subdural and epidural hematomas, a cisternal tap can also be life-saving.

EEGs after acute head injury are frequently abnormal but nonspecific, and their role is quite limited in initial evaluation and management of head injury. EEGs may be useful in monitoring seizure activity and may complement serial neurologic examinations and assessments of a patient's progress after head injury.

Differential Diagnosis

Whenever the cause for the head injury is not readily apparent, nonaccidental trauma should be suspected. Intracranial hemorrhage may occur with relatively minor injuries in patients with bleeding diatheses. Some metabolic disorders, such as scurvy, rickets, and Menkes' disease, may predispose the patient to pathologic fractures and intracranial hemorrhage.

Complications

Seizures, either focal or generalized, have been reported in 5–15% of children with head injury. Usually the seizures are brief, but a few patients experience status epilepticus. Chronic posttraumatic epilepsy develops in 10% of children who have suffered brain lacerations or who have experienced prolonged loss of consciousness immediately after head injury. When posttraumatic seizures develop, approximately 50% occur in the first 6 months after the injury, and 80% will have developed within 2 years. Antiepileptic medications may be started when patients have one or more immediate posttraumatic seizures and continued for up to 6 months. If seizures develop later, chronic antiepileptic medication is continued for 2–4 years.

Massive cerebral swelling, cerebral edema, and intracranial hematomas may lead to herniation of the temporal lobe through the tentorial notch with subsequent brain stem compression and rapid deterioration of the patient's mental status and neurologic function. Cerebellar tonsillar herniation results from posterior fossa hematomas and leads to clinical evidence of lower brain stem dysfunction, progressive loss of consciousness, and impaired cardiorespiratory functions.

Cerebrospinal fluid leakage through basilar skull fractures predisposes the patient to chronic, recurrent bacterial meningitis with organisms that normally inhabit the upper airway, such as *Streptococcus pneumoniae* and *Haemophilus influenzae*. Most CSF leaks stop spontaneously, but chronic leaks require surgical closure. If the patient develops signs of fever, nuchal rigidity, or other evidence of possible meningitis, antibiotics are necessary.

Hydrocephalus can develop after head injury, particularly when subarachnoid hemorrhage leads to basilar arachnoiditis or impairment of the cerebrospinal fluid absorption through the arachnoid villi.

Some patients develop pseudotumor cerebri shortly after head injury. The mechanism is not clear.

Patients with diastatic linear fractures develop leptomeningeal cysts. This type of cyst develops when a tear in the dura and arachnoid is followed by entrapment of the arachnoid between the margins of the diastatic fracture. CSF accumulates within the cyst and produces a progressively enlarging, fluid-filled mass over the fracture line. Removal of the cyst and closure of the dural tear requires surgical repair.

Postconcussion syndrome is seen in children, adolescents, and adults, but its pathogenesis is not clear. Principal manifestations are changes in behavior, personality, and sleep pattern, headache, vertigo, tinnitus, and various head and neck pains. School or job performance deteriorates, and the ability to concentrate is impaired. Hyperactivity can impair the child's normal daily function. Treatment is symptomatic, and postconcussion syndrome usually abates gradually over a period of days to weeks.

Treatment

Immediate treatment of a patient with serious head injury consists of securing the airway and supporting the cardiovascular system. Seizures, particularly status epilepticus, may require acute anticonvulsant medication. Subdural or cisternal taps are required if the patient is rapidly deteriorating because of an acute subdural or epidural hematoma.

After initial assessment, the patient must be observed carefully for several hours after head injury, whether in the emergency room, in an ambulatory clinic setting, or at home. The patient's arousability, pupillary light reflexes, extraocular movements, and extremity movements must be serially documented. Hospitalization of patients after head injury is necessary when the patient has focal or asymmetric neurologic deficits that do not rapidly resolve or when loss of consciousness is prolonged. It is important to admit and monitor carefully patients who show signs of deterioration and to initiate rapid treatment to relieve intracranial pressure.

Severe headache, nausea, vomiting, and restlessness can usually be treated symptomatically. Tetanus prophylaxis (0.5 mL tetanus toxoid) may be required for patients with scalp lacerations or open head injuries. Most patients do not require antibiotics. However, patients with CSF leakage from the nose or ears should be monitored carefully and antibiotics started if meningitis is suspected. Cerebral edema may be treated with diuretics, osmotic agents, or glucocorticoids or by lowering the patient's PCO_2. If acute obstructive hydrocephalus occurs, a ventricular drain aids in controlling increased intracranial pressure.

Patients with depressed or displaced fractures, epidural hematomas, progressive acute subdural hematomas, and some chronic subdural hematomas require operation. Evacuation of intracerebral hematomas is usually not indicated, though superficial intracerebral hematomas occasionally may be evacuated in an attempt to relieve severe and rapidly increasing mass effect.

Prognosis

Ninety percent or more of children who suffer from mild to moderate head injuries become free of symptoms and do not develop serious, long-term complications. Severe head injury is associated with a mortality rate of 5–10%. Three to 5 percent of children with severe head injury have severe, long-term neurologic deficits, and another 5–6% have moderate long-term deficits. Over 80% of children with severe head injury, however, enjoy good functional recovery.

SPINAL CORD INJURY

Spinal cord injury can occur at any age and often coexists with head injury. A high degree of suspicion is required to promptly diagnose and treat spinal injuries in infants and children. In neonates, spinal cord injury results from traction and hyperextension during difficult delivery. Generalized flaccidity and respiratory failure are frequently the predominant acute clinical manifestations, with spasticity and hyperreflexia developing later. In older children, the clinical signs of spinal cord injury depend on the level at which the injury occurs. Cervical cord injury results in respiratory weakness, flaccid weakness, and areflexia in the upper extremities; loss of bowel and bladder control; and spasticity and hyperreflexia in the lower extremities. A sensory level may be detectable in older children with low cervical, thoracic, and lumbosacral cord injury.

Diagnosis is based on the clinical history, pattern of neurologic deficits, and MRI. Plain films can be useful in the initial evaluation if fractures and bone displacements are present, but a normal plain x-ray of the spinal column does not exclude spinal cord injury or replace the need for MRI if a spinal cord injury is suspected. Initial management of suspected spinal cord injury involves stabilizing the neck, minimizing movement of the patient, and supporting respiratory and cardiovascular functions. Additional measures include use of osmotic agents and corticosteroids to reduce edema, surgery to remove epidural or subdural hematoma, and surgery to stabilize bone fractures and displacements. Long-term management of residual neurologic dysfunction requires intensive rehabilitation; bowel and bladder care; treatment of spasticity with baclofen, diazepam, or dantrolene sodium; and psychologic counseling.

The prognosis varies with the severity of the injury. Children with complete cord transections have a poor prognosis for recovery. Late complications include progressive spinal deformity, contractures, dysesthetic pain syndromes, recurrent infections, and decubitus ulcers.

Cogen PH: Craniospinal trauma in children. In: *Principles of Child Neurology.* Berg BO (editor). McGraw-Hill, 1996.
Davis PC et al: Spinal injuries in children: Role of MR. AJNR Am J Neuroradiol 1993;14:607.

PERINATAL HEAD INJURY

Injury to the scalp and skull occurs during the perinatal period in association with prolonged pressure on the infant's skull, breech presentation, shoulder dystocia, or malpositioned forceps. Several types of head and scalp injury may be visibly apparent at the time of birth. **Caput succedaneum** is characterized by hemorrhagic edema of the scalp skin and muscles. **Cephalhematoma** is a localized subperiosteal hemorrhage; this type of hemorrhage is limited in extent by the periosteum that attaches at suture margins. Caput and cephalhematomas resolve spontaneously and require no specific treatment. Cephalhematomas occasionally prolong neonatal jaundice, and approximately 25% of them overlie linear skull fractures. **Subgaleal hemorrhage** represents the most dangerous extracranial hemorrhage in the neonate. The blood of this hemorrhage dissects underneath the fascia of muscles of the head and neck. Blood may dissect and extend into the face, down the neck, and over the chest and back. Massive blood loss can take place, and subgaleal hemorrhage can result in exsanguination. Subgaleal hemorrhage usually occurs in association with an underlying bleeding disorder or after severe head trauma that results in tears of the dura that form the dural sinuses.

Skull fractures in the perinatal period involving the skull base and occipital region can be associated with dural tears and massive intracranial hemorrhage. Hemorrhage secondary to dural tear often results in catastrophic, rapid clinical deterioration and death.

Intracranial hemorrhage is the most serious consequence of head injury during the perinatal period. Epidural hematomas are usually associated with depressed skull fractures. *Emergency surgical removal is mandatory.* Subarachnoid hemorrhage is relatively frequent in the perinatal period and is often asymptomatic. However, hydrocephalus may develop after subarachnoid hemorrhage and may require ventriculoperitoneal shunting. Subdural hematomas are occasionally seen in the perinatal period and are often associated with cerebral laceration or contusion. Acute subdural hematomas may progress rapidly, and the patient may require emergency surgery for evacuation of the hematoma. Chronic subdural hematomas are manifested by increasing head circumference and the gradual appearance of neurologic deficits, anemia, poor weight gain, irritability, and somnolence.

Intracerebral hematomas usually indicate severe head trauma in the perinatal period and are frequently associated with dural lacerations or with bleeding disorders.

Intracranial Hemorrhage in the Premature

Approximately 25–40% of all newborns weighing less than 2000 g develop periventricular-interventricular hemorrhage. This type of hemorrhage originates in the germinal matrix and is related to immature blood vessel structure, poor blood vessel support by the germinal matrix, and the unusual tortuous course of veins in the region of the germinal matrix in the premature brain. Germinal matrix hemorrhages are classified as grade I, II, or III. Grade I indicates a hemorrhage limited to the subependymal, germinal matrix region with little or no intraventricular extension. Grade II represents the germinal matrix hemorrhage with moderate extension into the ventricular system. Grade III represents germinal matrix hemorrhage with massive intraventricular extension and usually ventriculomegaly. Furthermore, intraventricular hemorrhage may be associated with hemorrhagic infarction of the white matter dorsal and lateral to the anterior lateral ventricle.

Clinical symptoms of intraventricular-periventricular hemorrhage are related to the size of the hemorrhage and its degree of extension into the ventricular system. In addition, symptoms are modified by the degree of the infant's systemic illness. Small grade I hemorrhages limited to the germinal matrix can be asymptomatic and are often diagnosed by ultrasonography but not suspected clinically. Some patients develop a waxing and waning course with a gradual, stuttering evolution of neurologic deficits. The most dramatic presentation of intraventricular-periventricular hemorrhage, however, is the sudden catastrophic onset of seizures, anemia, and cardiovascular instability. Acute grade III hemorrhages combined with periventricular hemorrhagic infarction are associated with a mortality rate of more than 60% (Table 22–15).

Laboratory evaluation of infants with periventricular-intraventricular hemorrhage includes assessment of the hematocrit, electrolytes, calcium, magnesium, blood glucose concentration, coagulation system, and acid-base status. Examination of CSF after intraventricular hemorrhage is usually not necessary but reveals grossly bloody spinal fluid with elevated protein and decreased glucose concentration.

The primary diagnostic test in neonates suspected of having periventricular-intraventricular hemorrhage is cranial ultrasonography. This test is excellent for displaying germinal matrix hemorrhage with or without intraventricular extension and can be used for serial monitoring of ventricular size. However, ultrasonography is not an adequate method for evaluating cerebral hemispheres or structures of the posterior fossa. CT or MRI scanning is necessary for full evaluation of the cerebral parenchyma, the posterior fossa, and the subarachnoid, subdural, and epidural spaces.

Treatment

Treatment of infants with periventricular-intraventricular hemorrhage is directed at stabilizing and supporting the cardiovascular system. Abnormalities of the cardiovascular, renal, gastrointestinal, and other organ systems require specific monitoring and management. Fluid, electrolyte, and acid-base disturbances should be identified and corrected. Secondary infections and seizures should be treated with antibiotics and anticonvulsant medications. Any underlying bleeding diathesis should be corrected, and vitamin K_1 should be given to infants to ensure that a bleeding diathesis secondary to vitamin K deficiency does not contribute to the patient's problems.

For patients with progressive ventriculomegaly and hydrocephalus, ventricular drains and subsequent ventriculoperitoneal shunting are often required. The value of serial lumbar punctures is controversial, but this procedure can be useful in some patients if ventriculostomy is not readily available to relieve acute posthemorrhagic ventriculomegaly.

Prognosis

The outcome of intracranial hemorrhage is related to the extent of underlying brain injury. Brain lacerations and contusions predispose to the development of posttraumatic epilepsy and focal or multifocal areas of cerebral atrophy.

The outcome of neonatal intraventricular-periventricular hemorrhage is related to the size and extent of the hemorrhage and associated factors such as the presence of hemorrhagic infarction and systemic complications secondary to cardiovascular, renal, gastrointestinal, and other systemic abnormalities. Table 22–15 displays the mortality and morbidity rates with regard to neurologic deficits and hydrocephalus.

Table 22–15. Prognosis of periventricular-intraventricular hemorrhage (IVH) in premature infants.

	Acute		Long-Term
	Mortality (%)	Hydrocephalus (%)	Neurologic Impairment (%)
Grade I	5	5	5
Grade II	10	25	15
Grade III	20	55	40
IVH and periventricular hemorrhagic infarction (grade IV)	50	80	90

Lescohier I, DiScala C: Blunt trauma in children: Causes and outcomes of head versus extracranial injury. Pediatrics 1993;91:721.

Volpe JJ: Intraventricular hemorrhage in the premature infant: Current concepts. (Two parts.) Ann Neurol 1989;25:3, 109.

NEOPLASMS OF THE CENTRAL NERVOUS SYSTEM

1. INTRACRANIAL TUMORS

Neoplasms of the central nervous system (CNS) account for approximately 20% of all malignant neoplasms of childhood and are second only to leukemia in frequency. The incidence of primary CNS tumors in people under 20 years of age is 20–25 per million per year, or about one-third to one-half of the incidence of childhood leukemia. The incidence of CNS tumors in children under age 2 is approximately 10% of that in older children, or approximately 2–2.5 per million per year. Approximately 1500 new cases of brain tumor occur each year in the United States, including 150–200 cases in children under 2 years old. The peak incidence of brain tumors occurs between the ages of 5 and 10 years, and the male:female ratio is approximately 1.2:1. Primary brain tumors can be classified generally by their cell of origin (Table 22–16). In children over the age of 2, approximately 65% of brain tumors are infratentorial and 35% supratentorial. Secondary involvement of the nervous system is common in the early stages of acute leukemia, and the brain may be invaded directly by tumors that involve extraneural tissue in the head and neck region. Hematogenous metastatic spread from solid malignant tumors outside the nervous system is rare in childhood, but the true incidence of this phe-

nomenon is unknown. Some highly aggressive and malignant intracranial tumors in childhood, such as medulloblastoma, commonly spread throughout the subarachnoid spaces within the central nervous system. Rarely, primary CNS tumors may metastasize to extraneural sites such as bone marrow, lung, and viscera.

Clinical Manifestations

Manifestations of intracranial tumors consist of nonspecific signs due to increased intracranial pressure (Table 22–17). Infratentorial tumors, regardless of histologic type, frequently present with gait disturbance, incoordination, multiple and often asymmetric cranial nerve deficits, and nystagmus. The patient may tilt the head in an attempt to relieve discomfort at the base of the skull due to cerebellar tonsillar herniation, or head tilt may be a compensatory adjustment to correct double vision.

Specific neurologic manifestations of supratentorial tumors are dictated by the location of the tumor. Focal motor and sensory abnormalities and focal seizures occur frequently in the more common types of hemispheric tumors. Abnormalities of eye movements and vision are also common. Endocrine and autonomic disturbances may indicate the presence of a hypothalamic or thalamic tumor.

Diagnosis

When the clinical history and the findings of physical examination suggest the presence of an intracranial mass, a CT or MRI scan of the head should be obtained to define the precise anatomic site and extent of the tumor. Skull x-rays may show scalloping of the inner table of the skull, truncation of the sella turcica, or widening of the suture lines as evidence of increased intracranial pressure. Electroencephalographic findings in brain tumors are nonspecific, and EEGs are rarely necessary in the initial diagnostic evaluation of brain tumor. However, EEGs done on

Table 22–16. Classification of primary brain tumors of childhood.

Tumor Type	Incidence (%)	Common Examples
Glial cell tumors	50–60	Astrocytoma Optic nerve glioma Brain stem glioma Ependymoma
Neuroectodermal tumors	25–35	Medulloblastoma Pinealoblastoma
Craniopharyngioma	5–10	
Germ cell tumors	< 10	Teratoma Dermoid Germinoma
Meningeal tumors	< 5	Meningioma Meningeal sarcoma
Lymphoma (non-Hodgkin's)	< 1	

Table 22–17. Signs of increased intracranial pressure.

Acute
  Macrocephaly
  Excessive rate of head growth
  Altered behavior
  Decreased level of consciousness
  Vomiting
  Blurred vision
  Double vision
  Optic disk swelling
  Abducens nerve paresis
Chronic
  Macrocephaly
  Growth impairment
  Developmental delay
  Optic atrophy
  Visual field loss

patients who have focal or generalized seizures as a manifestation of their tumor may show localized epileptiform discharges. An EEG done before initiation of treatment for the brain tumor may provide a useful baseline assessment of electrocerebral activity for future reference. Examination of CSF is usually not necessary in the diagnosis of localized mass lesions within the nervous system. However, examination of spinal fluid, particularly cytopathologic examination, may be helpful when tumors are disseminated throughout the subarachnoid space.

Treatment

Some tumors, such as cerebellar astrocytomas, may be completely removed by surgery and require no additional treatment. Most primary CNS tumors, however, are currently treated by a combination of surgery, radiation, and chemotherapy. Surgery is frequently used to reduce the mass of tumor and is followed by localized radiation to the tumor bed. Some tumors with a propensity for subarachnoid seeding and spread (eg, medulloblastoma) are also treated with prophylactic total craniocerebral radiation. Given the many chemotherapeutic agents available, it is recommended that children with brain tumors be enrolled in multicenter protocols that use combinations of surgery, radiation, and chemotherapy.

2. PSEUDOTUMOR CEREBRI

Pseudotumor cerebri is a condition characterized by increased intracranial pressure in the absence of an identifiable intracranial mass or hydrocephalus. Clinical manifestations of pseudotumor cerebri are those of increased intracranial pressure as outlined in Table 22–17. The precise cause is usually not known, but pseudotumor cerebri has been described in association with a variety of inflammatory, metabolic, toxic, and connective tissue disorders (Table 22–18). The diagnosis of pseudotumor cerebri is one of exclusion. CT or MRI scans of the head are needed to exclude hydrocephalus and intracranial masses; these studies demonstrate ventricles of small or normal size but no other structural abnormalities. Lumbar puncture should be performed to document elevated CSF pressure. Examination of cerebrospinal fluid reveals a normal cell count, a normal glucose concentration, and a normal or low protein concentration. In some inflammatory and connective tissue diseases, however, the CSF protein may be increased.

Specific treatment of pseudotumor cerebri is aimed at correcting any identifiable underlying predisposing condition. In addition, some patients may benefit from the use of furosemide or acetazolamide to decrease the volume and pressure of cerebrospinal fluid within the central nervous system. These drugs may be used in combination with repeated lumbar punctures to remove CSF. If a program of repeated

Table 22–18. Conditions associated with pseudotumor cerebri.

Metabolic-toxic disorders
Hypervitaminosis A
Hypovitaminosis A
Prolonged steroid therapy
Steroid withdrawal
Tetracycline therapy
Nalidixic acid therapy
Iron deficiency
Plumbism
Hypocalcemia
Hyperparathyroidism
Adrenal insufficiency
Lupus erythematosus
Chronic CO_2 retention
Infectious and parainfectious disorders
Chronic otitis media
Poliomyelitis
Guillain-Barré syndrome
Dural sinus thrombosis
Minor head injury

spinal fluid removal and medical management is not successful or if visual field loss is detected despite these measures, lumboperitoneal shunt or another surgical decompression procedure may be necessary to prevent irreparable visual loss and damage to the optic nerves.

3. SPINAL CORD TUMORS

The incidence of tumors within the spinal canal is one sixth to one fifth that of tumors within the intracranial compartment. The peak age at occurrence is approximately 4 years. Spinal tumors can be classified as intradural or extradural. Intradural tumors within the substance of the spinal cord are referred to as intramedullary and those outside as extramedullary. Recent reports suggest that approximately one-third of intraspinal tumors are intramedullary, approximately one-third are intradural extramedullary, and approximately one-third are extradural. About 10% of intraspinal tumors arise in the sacral region, and the remainder are distributed equally in the cervical, thoracic, and lumbar regions. Neurofibromas, meningiomas, dermoid cysts, teratomas, and metastatic tumors constitute the most frequent tumors that are extradural or intradural extramedullary. Astrocytomas and ependymomas are the most common intramedullary tumors.

Clinical manifestations of spinal cord tumors result from direct invasion of the tumor into neural tissue as well as from compression of neural tissue. Symptoms of gait disturbance, pain, and bowel and bladder dysfunction occur in association with abnormal muscle stretch reflexes, weakness, and sensory loss. The specific patterns of neurologic deficits are determined by the location and size of tumor mass.

When the clinical course and physical examination suggest the presence of an intraspinal mass, neuroimaging procedures are required. Spinal CT scan, metrizamide myelography, and spinal MRI scans are used to define tumors. The use of gadolinium with MRI scanning enhances the definition of tumors within the spinal cord and within the spinal subarachnoid and extradural spaces. Although examination of CSF may demonstrate the presence of neoplastic cells and markedly elevated protein concentrations, this test is not required for the diagnosis of intraspinal tumors and is contraindicated when significant cord compression is suspected clinically.

Primary intraspinal tumors may be totally removed by surgery, but many intramedullary tumors require a combination of surgery, radiation, and chemotherapy similar to the treatment of intracranial tumors discussed in the preceding section.

In addition to primary intraspinal tumors, the spinal cord and intraspinal compartment may be the site of direct invasion or hematogenous metastatic spread of tumors that arise outside the nervous system. Important examples include spinal neuroblastoma that may be an extension of paraspinous retroperitoneal neuroblastoma. Lymphoma, sarcoma, and leukemia may involve paraspinous tissue and spread to the intraspinal compartment through neural foramina. Treatment of these secondary neoplasms usually requires some combination of surgical excision, radiation, and chemotherapy.

Allen ED et al: The clinical and radiological evaluation of primary brain tumors in children. Part I: Clinical evaluation. J Natl Med Assoc 1993;85:445.

Babikian P, Corbett J, Bell W: Idiopathic intracranial hypertension in children. The Iowa experience. J Child Neurol 1994;9:144.

Fort DW, Rushing EJ: Congenital central nervous system tumors. J Child Neurol 1997;12:157.

Murovic J, Sundaresen N: Pediatric spinal axis tumors. Neurosurg Clin North Am 1992;3:947.

Packer RJ: Brain tumors in children. Curr Opin Pediatr 1995;7:64.

Schoeman JF: Childhood pseudotumor cerebri: Clinical and intracranial pressure response to acetazolamide and furosemide treatment in a case series. J Child Neurol 1994;9:130.

CEREBROVASCULAR DISEASE

Cerebrovascular disease, or stroke, occurs with an incidence in the pediatric population of approximately 1.2–2.5:100,000 per year. Although stroke occurs most frequently between the ages of 1 and 5 years, it may occur at any age during infancy and childhood. Congenital cyanotic heart disease is the most common underlying systemic disorder predisposing to stroke.

The initial approach to the patient should take into account the patient's age and any underlying systemic or neurologic illness. A systematic search for evidence of cardiac, vascular, or hematologic disease and intracranial disorders should be undertaken (Table 22–19).

Clinical Findings

A. Symptoms and Signs: Clinical manifestations of stroke in childhood vary according to the vascular distribution to the brain that is involved. Because many conditions leading to childhood stroke result in emboli, multifocal neurologic involvement is common. Children may present with acute hemi-

Table 22–19. Etiologic risk factors for stroke in children.

Cardiac disorders
  Cyanotic heart disease
  Valvular disease
    Rheumatic
    Endocarditis
  Cardiomyopathy
  Cardiac dysrhythmia
Vascular occlusive disorders
  Arterial trauma (carotid dissections)
  Homocystinuria
  Mitochondrial encephalomyopathy
  Vasculitis
    Meningitis
    Polyarteritis nodosa
    Systemic lupus erythematosus
    Drug abuse (amphetamines)
  Fibromuscular dysplasia
  Moyamoya disease
  Diabetes
  Nephrotic syndrome
  Systemic hypertension
  Dural sinus and cerebral venous thrombosis
    Meningitis
    Hyperviscosity
    Hypovolemia
  Cortical venous thrombosis
  Carotid-cavernous fistula
Hematologic disorders
  Polycythemia
  Thrombotic thrombocytopenia
  Thrombocytopenic purpura
  Thrombocythemia
  Hemoglobinopathies
    Sickle cell disease
    S-C disease
  Coagulation defects
    Hemophilia
    Vitamin K deficiency
  Hypercoagulable states
    Pregnancy
    Systemic lupus erythematosus
    Use of oral contraceptives
    Antithrombin III deficiency
    Protein C and S deficiencies
  Leukemia
Intracranial vascular anomalies
  Arteriovenous malformation
  Arterial aneurysm
  Carotid-cavernous fistula

plegia similar to stroke in adults. Symptoms of unilateral weakness, sensory disturbance, dysarthria, and dysphasia may develop over a period of minutes, but at times progressive worsening of symptoms may evolve over several hours. Bilateral hemispheric involvement may lead to a depressed level of consciousness. The patient may also demonstrate disturbances of mood and behavior and experience focal or multifocal seizures. Physical examination of the patient is aimed not only at identifying the specific deficits related to impaired cerebral blood flow but also at seeking evidence for any predisposing disorder. Retinal hemorrhages, splinter hemorrhages in the nail beds, cardiac murmurs, and signs of trauma are especially important findings.

When stroke is ushered in by a focal hemiconvulsion followed by hemiplegia, a chronic epilepsy syndrome may persist for years in association with hemiplegia. This combination of hemiconvulsion, hemiplegia, and chronic epilepsy has been referred to as the **HHE syndrome.**

B. Laboratory Findings: Laboratory investigation can be carried out systemically, with particular attention to disorders involving the heart, blood vessels, platelets, red cells, hemoglobin, and coagulation proteins. Additional laboratory tests for systemic disorders such as systemic lupus erythematosus and polyarteritis nodosa are usually indicated.

Examination of spinal fluid is indicated in patients with fever, nuchal rigidity, or marked obtundation when the diagnosis of intracranial infection requires exclusion. Lumbar puncture, however, may be deferred until a neuroimage excluding brain abscess or a space-occupying lesion that might contraindicate lumbar puncture has been obtained. In the absence of infection and frank intracranial subarachnoid hemorrhage, CSF examination is rarely helpful in defining the cause of the cerebrovascular disorder.

C. Imaging: CT and MRI scans of the brain are often helpful in defining the extent of cerebral involvement with ischemia or hemorrhage. CT scans, however, may be normal within the first few hours of an ischemic stroke and may need to be repeated several hours later. A CT scan early after the onset of neurologic deficits is valuable in excluding significant intracranial hemorrhage. This information may be helpful in the early stages of management and in the decision to treat with anticoagulants.

Cerebral angiography is usually not urgently needed but may be needed to confirm such disorders as fibromuscular dysplasia and cerebral arteritis. If angiography is done, all major vessels should be studied. If evidence of fibromuscular dysplasia is present in the intracranial or extracranial vessels, renal arteriography is indicated. With additional technical advances, MRA will soon replace conventional contrast angiography for most cases of childhood stroke.

When seizures are prominent, an EEG may be used as an adjunct in the patient's evaluation. An EEG and sequential electroencephalographic monitoring may help in patients with severely depressed consciousness.

Electrocardiography and echocardiography are useful both in the diagnostic approach to the patient and in ongoing monitoring and management, particularly when hypotension or cardiac arrhythmias complicate the clinical course.

Differential Diagnosis

Patients with an acute onset of neurologic deficits must be evaluated not only for cerebrovascular disease but also for other disorders that can cause focal neurologic deficits. Hypoglycemia, prolonged focal seizures, a prolonged postictal paresis (Todd's paralysis), meningitis, encephalitis, and brain abscess should all be considered. Migraine with focal neurologic deficits may be difficult to differentiate initially from ischemic stroke. Occasionally, the onset of a neurodegenerative disorder (eg, adrenoleukodystrophy) may begin with the abrupt onset of seizures and focal neurologic deficits. The possibility of drug abuse (particularly cocaine) and other toxic exposures must be investigated diligently.

Treatment

The initial management of children with stroke is aimed at providing support for pulmonary, cardiovascular, and renal function. Appropriate fluid and electrolyte infusions should be started, and careful monitoring of heart rate and rhythm and blood pressure are required. Specific treatment of stroke depends in part upon the underlying pathogenesis and the specific predisposing disorder. In some situations, heparinization for emboli and consumption coagulopathies is indicated. In other disorders, such as fibromuscular dysplasia, treatment to decrease platelet adhesiveness may be an acceptable alternative to anticoagulation.

Long-term management requires intensive rehabilitation efforts, anticonvulsant treatment, and therapy aimed at improving the child's language, educational, and psychologic performance.

Prognosis

The outcome of stroke in infants and children is variable. Underlying predisposing conditions and the vascular territory involved all play a role in dictating the outcome for an individual patient. When the stroke involves extremely large portions of one hemisphere or large portions of both hemispheres and cerebral edema develops, the patient's level of consciousness may deteriorate rapidly, and death may occur within the first few days. Some patients may achieve almost complete recovery of neurologic function within several days if the cerebral territory is small. Seizures, either focal or generalized, may occur in 30–50% of patients at some point in the course of their cerebrovascular disorder. Chronic problems with learning, behavior, and activity are common.

Broderick J et al: Stroke in children within a major metropolitan area: The surprising importance of intracerebral hemorrhage. J Child Neurol 1993;8:250.

Kerr LM et al: Ischemic stroke in the young: Evaluation and age comparison of patients six months to thirty-nine years. J Child Neurol 1993;8:266.

Reila AR, Roach ES: Etiology of stroke in children. J Child Neurol 1993;8:201.

Roach ES, Riela AR: *Pediatric Cerebrovascular Disorders,* 2nd ed. Futura, 1995.

Yang JS, Park YD, Hartlage PL: Seizures associated with stroke in childhood. Pediatr Neurol 1995;12:136.

CONGENITAL MALFORMATIONS OF THE NERVOUS SYSTEM

Malformations of the nervous system occur in 1–3% of living neonates and are present in 40% of infants who die. Developmental anomalies of the central nervous system may result from a variety of causes, including infectious, toxic, metabolic, and vascular insults that affect the fetus. The specific type of malformation that results from such insults, however, may depend more upon the gestational period during which the insult occurs than on the specific cause. The period of induction, days 0–28 of gestation, is the period during which the neural plate appears and the neural tube forms and closes. Insults during this phase can result in a major absence of neural structures, such as anencephaly, or in a defect of neural tube closure, such as spina bifida, meningomyelocele, or encephalocele. Cellular proliferation and migration characterize neural development that occurs after 28 days of gestation. Lissencephaly, pachygyria, agyria, and agenesis of the corpus callosum are caused by insults that occur during the period of cellular proliferation and migration.

1. ABNORMALITIES OF NEURAL TUBE CLOSURE

Defects of neural tube closure constitute some of the most common congenital malformations affecting the nervous system. Spina bifida with associated meningomyelocele or meningocele is commonly found in the lumbosacral region. Depending on the extent and severity of the involvement of the spinal cord and peripheral nerves, clinical findings include lower extremity weakness, bowel and bladder dysfunction, and hip dislocation. Operation to close meningoceles and meningomyeloceles is usually indicated. Additional treatment is necessary to manage chronic abnormalities of the urinary tract, orthopedic

abnormalities such as kyphosis and scoliosis, and paresis of the lower extremities. Hydrocephalus associated with meningomyelocele usually requires ventriculoperitoneal shunting.

Arnold-Chiari Malformations

Arnold-Chiari malformation type I consists of elongation and displacement of the caudal end of the brain stem into the spinal canal with protrusion of the cerebellar tonsils through the foramen magnum. In association with this hindbrain malformation, there are often minor to moderate abnormalities of the base of the skull, including basilar impression (platybasia) and small foramen magnum. Arnold-Chiari malformation type I may remain asymptomatic for years, but in older children and young adults it may cause progressive ataxia, paresis of the lower cranial nerves, and progressive vertigo. Posterior cervical laminectomy may be necessary to provide relief from cervical cord compression. Ventriculoperitoneal shunting is required for hydrocephalus.

Arnold-Chiari malformation type II consists of the malformations found in Arnold-Chiari type I plus an associated lumbosacral meningomyelocele. Hydrocephalus is present in approximately 90% of children with Arnold-Chiari type II. These patients may also have aqueductal stenosis, hydromyelia, or syringomyelia. The clinical manifestations of Arnold-Chiari type II are most commonly caused by the associated hydrocephalus and meningomyelocele. In addition, dysfunction of the lower cranial nerves may be present.

Arnold-Chiari malformation type III is characterized by occipital encephalocele, a closure defect of the rostral end of the neural tube. Hydrocephalus is extremely common with this malformation.

In general, the diagnosis of neural tube defects is obvious at the time of birth. Diagnosis may be strongly suspected prenatally on the basis of ultrasonographic findings and the presence of elevated alpha-fetoprotein in the amniotic fluid. Folate deficiency in pregnant women has been associated with an increased incidence of neural tube defects in their infants.

2. DISORDERS OF CELLULAR PROLIFERATION AND MIGRATION

Lissencephaly

Lissencephaly is a severe malformation of the brain characterized by an extremely smooth cortical surface with minimal sulcal and gyral development. Such a smooth surface is characteristic of fetal brain at the end of the first trimester. In addition, many lissencephalic brains have a primitive cytoarchitectural construction with a four-layered cerebral mantle instead of the mature six-layered mantle. **Pachygyria** (thick gyri) and **agyria** (absence of gyri) are closely associated with lissencephaly but represent more restricted forms of migrational abnormalities. Patients with lissencephaly usually suffer from severe neurodevelopmental delay, microcephaly, and seizures (including infantile spasms) and frequently have additional associated malformations and dysmorphic features. Walker-Warburg syndrome or Miller-Dieker syndrome can often be identified in some of these patients. Walker-Warburg syndrome is an autosomal recessive disorder, and Miller-Dieker syndrome is associated with defects of chromosome 17; it is particularly important to identify these syndromes because of their genetic importance. In addition to these two syndromes, lissencephaly may be a component of Zellweger's syndrome, a metabolic peroxisomal abnormality associated with the presence of elevated concentrations of very long-chain fatty acids in plasma. A peroxisomal defect in fatty acid degradation in cultured skin fibroblasts confirms the diagnosis. No specific treatment for lissencephaly is available. Seizures may be controlled by the use of phenobarbital, phenytoin, or clonazepam.

MRI scans have helped to define a number of presumed migrational defects that are similar to but anatomically more restricted than lissencephaly. A distinctive example is bilateral perisylvian cortical dysplasia. Patients with this disorder have pseudobulbar palsy, variable cognitive deficits, facial diplegia, dysarthria, developmental delay, and epilepsy. Seizures are often difficult to control with antiepileptic drugs; some patients have benefited from corpus callosotomy. The cause of this syndrome is as yet unknown, though intrauterine cerebral ischemic injury has been postulated. Therapy is aimed at improving speech and oromotor functions and controlling seizures.

Agenesis of the Corpus Callosum

Agenesis of the corpus callosum, once thought to be a relatively rare cerebral malformation, has been seen frequently with modern neuroimaging techniques such as CT and MRI. The cause of this malformation is unknown. Occasionally, it appears to be inherited in an autosomal dominant or autosomal recessive pattern. X-linked recessive patterns have also been described. Agenesis of the corpus callosum has been found in some patients with pyruvate dehydrogenase deficiency and in others with nonketotic hyperglycinemia. Most cases, however, are sporadic. Maldevelopment of the corpus callosum may be partial or complete. No specific syndrome is typical of agenesis of the corpus callosum, although many patients have seizures, developmental delay, microcephaly, or mental retardation. Neurologic abnormalities may be related to microscopic cytoarchitectural abnormalities of the brain that occur in association with agenesis of the corpus callosum. The malformation may be found coincidentally by neuroimaging studies in otherwise normal patients, and has been described as a coincidental finding at autopsy in neurologically normal individuals. A special form of agenesis of the corpus callosum occurs in Aicardi's syndrome. In this X-linked disorder, agenesis of the corpus callosum is associated with infantile spasms, mental retardation, lacunar chorioretinopathy, and vertebral body abnormalities.

Dandy-Walker Malformation

Dandy-Walker malformation is characterized by aplasia of the vermis, cystic enlargement of the fourth ventricle, rostral displacement of the tentorium, and absence or atresia of the foramina of Magendie and Luschka. Although hydrocephalus is usually not present congenitally, it develops within the first few months of life; 90% of patients who develop hydrocephalus do so by the age of 1 year. On physical examination, there is often a rounded protuberance or exaggeration of the cranial occiput. In the absence of hydrocephalus and increased intracranial pressure, there may be few physical findings to suggest neurologic dysfunction. An ataxic syndrome occurs in fewer than 20% of patients and is usually late in appearing. Many long-term neurologic deficits result directly from hydrocephalus. Diagnosis of Dandy-Walker malformation is confirmed by CT or MRI scanning of the head. Treatment is directed at the management of hydrocephalus.

3. CRANIOSYNOSTOSIS

Craniosynostosis, or premature closure of cranial sutures, is usually sporadic and idiopathic. However, some patients have hereditary disorders, such as Apert's syndrome and Crouzon's disease, that are associated with abnormalities of the digits, extremities, and heart. Occasionally, craniosynostosis may be associated with an underlying metabolic disturbance such as hyperthyroidism and hypophosphatasia. The most common form of craniosynostosis involves the sagittal suture and results in scaphocephaly, an elongation of the head in the anterior to posterior direction. Premature closure of the coronal sutures causes brachycephaly, an increase in cranial diameter from left to right. Unless many or all cranial sutures close prematurely, intracranial volume will not be compromised, and the brain's growth will not be impaired. Closure of only one or a few sutures will not cause impaired brain growth or neurologic dysfunction. Management of craniosynostosis is directed at preserving normal skull shape and consists of excising the fused suture and applying material to the edge of the craniectomy to prevent reossification of the bone edges. The best cosmetic effect on the skull is achieved when surgery is done during the first 6 months of life.

4. HYDROCEPHALUS

Hydrocephalus is characterized by an increased volume of cerebrospinal fluid in association with progressive ventricular dilation. In communicating hydrocephalus, CSF circulates through the ventricular system and into the subarachnoid space without obstruction. In noncommunicating hydrocephalus, an obstruction blocks the flow of spinal fluid within the ventricular system or blocks the egress of spinal fluid from the ventricular system into the subarachnoid space. A wide variety of disorders, such as hemorrhage, infection, tumors, and congenital malformations, may play an etiologic role in development of hydrocephalus.

Clinical features of hydrocephalus include macrocephaly, an excessive rate of head growth, irritability, vomiting, loss of appetite, impaired upgaze, impaired extraocular movements, hypertonia of the lower extremities, and generalized hyperreflexia. Without treatment, optic atrophy may occur. In infants, papilledema may not be present, whereas older children with closed cranial sutures can eventually develop swelling of the optic disk. Hydrocephalus can be diagnosed on the basis of the clinical course, findings on physical examination, and CT or MRI scan.

Treatment of hydrocephalus is directed at providing an alternative outlet for CSF from the intracranial compartment. The most common method is ventriculoperitoneal shunting. Other treatment should be directed, if possible, at the underlying cause of the hydrocephalus.

Dobyns WB, Trumit CL: Lissencephaly and other malformations of cortical development: 1995 update. Neuropediatrics 1995;26:132.

Hirsch JF et al: The Dandy-Walker malformation. J Neurosurg 1984;61:515.

Kuzniecky R et al: Congenital bilateral perisylvian syndrome: Study of 31 patients. Lancet 1993;341:608.

ABNORMAL HEAD SIZE

Bone plates of the skull have almost no intrinsic capacity to enlarge or grow, unlike long bones. They depend on extrinsic forces to stimulate new bone formation at the suture lines. Although gravity and traction on bone by muscle and scalp probably stimulate some growth, the single most important stimulus for head growth during infancy and childhood is brain growth. Therefore, accurate assessment of head growth is one of the most important aspects of the neurologic examination of young children. A head circumference that is 2 SD above or below the mean for age requires investigation and explanation.

1. MICROCEPHALY

A head circumference more than 2 SD below the mean for age and sex is by definition microcephaly. More important, however, than a single head circumference measurement is the rate or pattern of head growth through time. Head circumference measurements that progressively drop to lower percentiles with increasing age are indicative of a process or condition that has impaired the brain's capacity to grow. The causes of microcephaly are numerous. Some examples are listed in Table 22–20.

Clinical Findings

A. Symptoms and Signs: Microcephaly may be suspected in the full-term newborn and in infants up to 6 months of age whose chest circumference exceeds the head circumference (unless the child is very obese). Microcephaly may be discovered when the child is examined because of delayed developmental milestones or neurologic problems, such as seizures or spasticity. There may be a marked backward slope of the forehead (as in familial microcephaly) with narrowing of the bitemporal diameter.

Table 22–20. Microcephaly.

Causes	Examples
Chromosomal	Trisomy 13, 18, 21
Malformation	Lissencephaly, schizencephaly
Syndromes	Rubenstein-Taybi, Cornelia de Lange
Toxins	Alcohol, anticonvulsants (?), maternal phenylketonuria
Infections (intrauterine)	TORCHES[1]
Radiation	Maternal pelvis, first and second trimester
Placental insufficiency	Toxemia, infection
Familial	Autosomal dominant, autosomal recessive
Perinatal hypoxia, trauma	Birth asphyxia, injury
Infections (perinatal)	Bacterial meningitis (especially group B streptococci) Viral encephalitis (coxsackie B, herpes simplex)
Metabolic	Hypoglycemia, phenylketonuria, maple syrup urine disease
Degenerative disease	Tay-Sachs, Krabbe's

[1]A mnemonic formula for *to*xoplasmosis, *r*ubella, *c*ytomegalovirus, *h*erpes simplex, and *s*yphilis.

The fontanelle may close earlier than expected, and sutures may be prominent.

B. Laboratory Findings: These vary with the cause. Abnormal dermatoglyphics may be present when the injury occurred before the 19th week of gestation. In the newborn, IgM, antibody titers for toxoplasmosis, rubella, cytomegalovirus, herpes simplex virus, and syphilis must be assessed. Elevated specific IgM titer is indicative of congenital infection. The urine culture for cytomegalovirus (CMV) will be positive at birth when this virus is the cause of microcephaly. Eye, cardiac, and bone abnormalities may also be clues to congenital infection. The child's serum and urine amino and organic acid determination are occasionally diagnostic. The mother may require screening for phenylketonuria. Karyotyping, including fragile X, should be considered.

C. Imaging: CT or MRI scans may aid in diagnosis and prognosis. These studies may demonstrate calcifications, malformations, or atrophic patterns that suggest specific congenital infections or genetic syndromes. Plain skull x-rays may show closed sutures, but these studies are of limited value in diagnosis and have been replaced by more sensitive and more informative scanning procedures. Genetic counseling should be done in any infant with significant microcephaly.

Differential Diagnosis

Congenital craniosynostosis involving multiple sutures is easily differentiated by inspection (head shape), history, identification of syndromes, hereditary pattern, and sometimes signs and symptoms of increased intracranial pressure. Common forms of craniosynostosis involving sagittal, coronal, and lambdoidal sutures are associated with abnormally shaped heads but do not cause microcephaly. Treatable undergrowth of the brain due to hypopituitarism, hypothyroidism, or severe protein-calorie undernutrition is recognized by the history and clinical findings.

Treatment & Prognosis

Except for the treatable disorders noted above, treatment is usually supportive and directed at the multiple neurologic and sensory deficits, endocrine disturbances (eg, diabetes insipidus) and seizures. Many children with head circumferences more than 2 SD below the mean show variable degrees of mental retardation. The notable exceptions are found in cases of hypopituitarism (rare) or familial autosomal dominant microcephaly.

Ishihara T et al: Growth and achievement of large and small headed children in a normal population. Brain Dev 1988;10:295.

Rios A: Microcephaly. Pediatr Rev 1996;17:386.

2. MACROCEPHALY

A head circumference more than 2 SD above the mean for age and sex denotes macrocephaly. Excessive head growth rate through time suggests increased intracranial pressure most likely caused by hydrocephalus, extra-axial fluid collections, or neoplasms. Macrocephaly with normal head growth rate suggests familial macrocephaly or true megalencephaly, as might occur in neurofibromatosis. Other example of causes of macrocephaly are listed in Table 22–21.

Clinical Findings

Clinical and laboratory findings vary with the underlying process. In infants, transillumination of the skull with an intensely bright light in a completely darkened room may disclose subdural effusions, hydrocephalus, hydranencephaly, and cystic defects.

A surgically or medically treatable condition must be ruled out. Thus, the first decision is whether and when to perform an imaging study.

A. Imaging Study Deferred:

1. "Catch-up growth," as in the thriving, neurologically intact premature infant whose rapid head

Table 22–21. Macrocephaly.

Causes	Examples
Pseudomacrocephaly, pseudohydrocephalus, catch-up growth crossing percentiles	Growing premature infant; recovery from malnutrition, congenital heart disease

Increased intracranial pressure
  With dilated ventricles
  With other mass
	
	Progressive hydrocephalus, subdural effusion
	Arachnoid cyst, porencephalic cyst, brain tumor

Benign familial macrocephaly (idiopathic external hydrocephalus)	External hydrocephalus, benign enlargement of the subarachnoid spaces, congenital communicating hydrocephalus, benign subdural collections of infancy

Megalencephaly (large brain)
  With neurocutaneous disorder
  With gigantism
  With dwarfism
  Metabolic
  Lysosomal
  Other leukodystrophy
	Benign familial (see above).
	Neurofibromatosis, tuberous sclerosis, etc.
	Soto's syndrome.
	Achondroplasia.
	Mucopolysaccharidoses.
	Metachromatic leukodystrophy.
	Canavan's spongy degeneration.

Thickened skull	Fibrous dysplasia (bone), hemolytic anemia (marrow), sicklemia, thalassemia

enlargement is most marked in the first weeks of life, or the infant in the early phase of recovery from deprivation dwarfism. As the expected "normal" is reached, head growth slows down, then resumes a normal growth pattern. If the fontanelle is open, cranial ultrasonography can assess ventricular size and diagnose or exclude hydrocephalus.

2. Familial macrocephaly, in which another family member may have an unusually large head with no signs or symptoms referable to such disorders as neurocutaneous dysplasias (especially neurofibromatosis) or cerebral gigantism (Soto's syndrome) nor significant mental or neurologic abnormalities in the child.

B. Imaging Study: CT or MRI scans (or ultrasonography, if the anterior fontanelle is open) are used to define any structural cause of macrocephaly and to determine an operable disorder. Even when the condition is not treatable (or is benign), the information gained may permit more accurate diagnosis and prognosis, guide management and genetic counseling, and serve as a basis for comparison should future abnormal cranial growth or neurologic changes necessitate a repeat study. An imaging study is necessary if there are any signs or symptoms of increased intracranial pressure (Table 22–17).

Gooskens RHJM et al: Megalencephaly: Definition and classification. Brain Dev 1988;10:1.

Wilms G et al: CT and MR in infants with pericerebral collections and macrocephaly: Benign enlargement of the subarachnoid spaces versus subdural collections. AJNR Am J Neuroradiol 1993;14:855.

NEUROCUTANEOUS DYSPLASIAS

Neurocutaneous dysplasias are diseases of the neuroectoderm and sometimes involve endoderm and mesoderm. Birthmarks and skin growths appearing later often suggest a need to look for brain, spinal cord, and eye disease. **Hamartomas** (histologically normal tissue growing abnormally rapidly or in aberrant sites) are common. The most common dysplasias are dominantly inherited. Benign and even malignant tumors may develop.

1. NEUROFIBROMATOSIS
(Recklinghausen's Disease)

Essentials of Diagnosis & Typical Features

- More than six café au lait spots 5 mm in greatest diameter in prepubertal individuals and over 15 mm in greatest diameter in postpubertal individuals.
- Two or more neurofibromas of any type or one plexiform neurofibroma.
- Freckling in the axillary or inguinal regions.
- Optic glioma.
- Two or more Lisch nodules (iris hamartomas).
- Distinctive osseous lesions, such as sphenoid dysplasia or thinning of long bone with or without pseudarthroses.
- First-degree relative (parent, sibling, offspring) with neurofibromatosis type 1 by above criteria.

General Considerations

Neurofibromatosis is a multisystem disorder with a prevalence of 1:4000. Fifty percent of cases are due to new mutations in the *NF1* gene. Forty percent of patients will develop medical complications of the disorder in their lifetime.

Clinical Findings

A. Symptoms and Signs: The most common presenting symptoms are cognitive or psychomotor problems such as school difficulties; 40% of patients have learning disabilities, and mental retardation is seen in 8%. The family history is important in identifying dominant gene manifestations in parents; they should be examined in detail. The history should focus on lumps or masses causing disfigurement, functional problems, or pain. The clinician should ask about visual problems; strabismus or amblyopia dictates a search for optic glioma, a common tumor in neurofibromatosis. Any progressive neurologic deficit might call for studies to rule out tumor of the spinal cord or central nervous system. Tumors of the eighth nerve are virtually never seen in common neurofibromatosis type 1.

The physician should check blood pressure and examine the spine for scoliosis and the limbs for pseudarthroses. Head measurement often shows macrocephaly. Hearing and vision need to be assessed. The eye examination should include a check for proptosis and iris Lisch nodules; the optic disk should be examined for atrophy or papilledema. Short stature and precocious puberty are occasional findings. An examination for neurologic manifestations of tumors (eg, asymmetric reflexes, spasticity) is important.

B. Laboratory Findings: Laboratory tests are not likely to be of any value in asymptomatic patients. Selected patients require brain MRI or CT scans with special cuts through the optic nerves to rule out optic glioma. Hypertension necessitates a look at renal arteries for dysplasia and stenosis as a cause. Cognitive and school achievement testing may be indicated. Scoliosis or limb abnormalities should be studied by appropriate roentgenograms such as an MRI scan of the spinal cord and roots.

Differential Diagnosis

Patients with Albright's syndrome often have larger café au lait spots with precocious puberty. Many normal individuals have one or two café au lait spots.

Treatment

Genetic counseling is important. The risk to siblings is up to 50%. The disease may be progressive, with serious complications rarely seen. Patients sometimes worsen during puberty or pregnancy. Family members need to be evaluated for the presence of the gene. Annual or semiannual visits are important in the early detection of school problems or bony or neurologic abnormalities.

Multidisciplinary clinics at medical centers around the United States are often an excellent resource. Prenatal diagnosis is probably on the horizon, but the variability of manifestations (trivial to severe) will make therapeutic abortion an unlikely option. Chromosomal linkage studies are under way (chromosome 17q11.2).

Information for lay people and physicians is available from the National Neurofibromatosis Foundation, Inc., 70 West 40th Street, New York, NY 10018.

Committee on Genetics: Health supervision for children with neurofibromatosis. Pediatrics 1995;96:368.

Goldberg Y et al:Neurofibromatosis type 1:an update and review for the primary pediatrician. Clin Pediatr 1996;35:545.

Gutmann DH et al: The diagnostic evaluation and multidisciplinary management of neurofibromatosis 1 and neurofibromatosis 2. JAMA 1997;278:51.

North K: *Neurofibromatosis Type 1 in Childhood.* MacKeith Press, 1997.

Sevick RJ et al: Evolution of white matter lesions in neurofibromatosis type I: MR findings. AJR Am J Roentgenol 1992;159:171.

2. TUBEROUS SCLEROSIS (Bourneville's Disease)

Essentials of Diagnosis & Typical Features

- Facial angiofibromas or subungual fibromas.
- Often hypomelanotic macules, gingival fibromas.
- Retinal hamartomas.
- Cortical tubers or subependymal glial nodules, often calcified.
- Renal angiomyolipomas.

General Considerations

Tuberous sclerosis, a disease of unknown cause, is of autosomal dominant inheritance. A triad of seizures, mental retardation, and adenoma sebaceum is seen in only 33% of patients. The disease was earlier thought to have a high rate of mutation. As a result of more sophisticated techniques such as MRI, parents formerly thought not to harbor the gene are now being diagnosed as asymptomatic carriers.

Like neurofibromatosis, tuberous sclerosis may present with a wide variety of symptoms. The patient may be asymptomatic but for skin findings or may be devastated by severe infantile spasms in early infancy, by continuing epilepsy, and by mental retardation. Seizures in early infancy correlate with later mental retardation.

Clinical Findings

A. Symptoms and Signs:

1. Dermatologic features–Skin findings bring most cases to the physician's attention. Ninety-six percent have one or more hypomelanotic macules, facial angiofibromas, ungual fibromas, or shagreen patches. Adenoma sebaceum, the facial skin hamartomas, may first appear in early childhood, often on the cheek, chin, and dry sites of the skin where acne is not usually seen. They often have a reddish hue. The off-white hypomelanotic macules are more easily seen in tanned or dark-skinned individuals. They often are oval or "ash leaf" in shape and follow dermatomes. A Wood lamp (ultraviolet light) shows the macules more clearly—a great help in the light-skinned patient. In the scalp, poliosis (whitened hair) is the equivalent. In infancy, the presence of these macules accompanied by seizures is virtually diagnostic of the disease. Subungual or periungual fibromas are more common in the toes. Leathery, orange peel-like shagreen patches support the diagnosis. Café au lait spots are occasionally seen. Fibrous or raised plaques may resemble coalescent angiofibromas.

2. Neurologic features–Seizures are the most common presenting symptom. Five percent of cases of infantile spasm (a serious epileptic syndrome) occur in patients with tuberous sclerosis. Thus, any patient presenting with infantile spasms (and the parents as well) should be carefully examined for this disorder. An imaging study of the central nervous system, such as a CT scan, may show calcified subependymal nodules; MRI may show dysmyelinating white matter lesions or cortical tubers. Virtually any kind of symptomatic seizure (eg, atypical absence, partial complex, and generalized tonic-clonic seizures) may occur.

3. Mental retardation–Mental retardation is seen in up to 50% of patients referred to centers; the incidence is probably much lower in randomly selected patients. Patients with seizures are more prone to retardation or learning disabilities.

4. Renal lesions–Renal cysts or angiomyolipomas may be asymptomatic. Hematuria or obstruction of urine flow sometimes occurs; the latter requires operation. Ultrasonography of the kidneys should be done in any patient suspected of tuberous sclerosis, both to aid in diagnosis if lesions are found and to rule out renal obstructive disease.

5. Cardiopulmonary involvement–Rarely, cystic lung disease may occur. Rhabdomyomas of the heart may be asymptomatic but can lead to outflow obstruction, conduction difficulties, and death. Chest x-rays and echocardiograms can detect these rare manifestations.

6. Eye involvement–Retinal hamartomas are often near the disk.

7. Skeletal involvement–Findings sometimes helpful in diagnosis are cystic rarefactions of the bones of the fingers or toes.

B. Diagnostic Studies: Plain radiographs may detect areas of thickening within the skull, spine, and pelvis; and cystic lesions in the hands and feet. Chest x-rays may show lung honeycombing. More helpful is CT scanning, which can show the virtually pathognomonic subependymal nodular calcifications and sometimes widened gyri or tubers and brain tumors. Contrast material may show the often classically located tumors near the foramen interventriculare. Hypomyelinated lesions may be seen with magnetic resonance imaging.

EEG is helpful in delineating the presence of seizure discharges.

Treatment

Therapy is as indicated by underlying disease (eg, seizures and tumors of the brain, kidney, and heart). Skin lesions on the face may need dermabrasion or laser treatment. Genetic counseling emphasizes identification of the carrier. There is a 50% risk of appearance in offspring if either parent is a carrier. The patient should be seen annually for counseling and reexamination in childhood. Identification of the chromosomes (9,16; *TSCI* and *TSC2* genes) may in the future make intrauterine diagnosis possible.

Aicardi J: Tuberous sclerosis. Int Pediatr 1993;8:171.

Martin N et al: Gadolinium-DTPA enhanced MR imaging in tuberous sclerosis. Neuroradiology 1990;31:492.

Oppenheimer EY et al: Late appearance of hypopigmented maculae in tuberous sclerosis. Am J Dis Child 1985;139:408.

Valenzuela JR, Duarte AM: Neurocutaneous syndromes. Int Pediatr 1997;12:113.

3. ENCEPHALOFACIAL ANGIOMATOSIS (Sturge-Weber Disease)

Sturge-Weber disease consists of a facial port wine nevus involving the upper part of the face (in the first division of the fifth nerve), a venous angioma of the meninges in the occipitoparietal regions, and choroidal angioma. The syndrome has been described without the facial nevus.

Clinical Findings

In infancy, the eye may show congenital glaucoma, or buphthalmos, with a cloudy, enlarged cornea. In early stages, the facial nevus may be the only indication, with no findings in the brain even on radiologic studies. The characteristic atrophy and calcifications of the cortex and meningoangiomatosis may appear with time, solidifying the diagnosis.

Physical examination may show focal seizures or hemiparesis on the side opposite the cerebral lesion. The facial nevus may be much more extensive than the first division of the fifth nerve; it can involve the lower face, mouth, lip, neck, and even torso. Hemiatrophy of the opposite limbs may occur. Mental handicap may result from poorly controlled seizures. Late-appearing glaucoma and, rarely, CNS hemorrhage occur.

Radiologic studies may show calcification of the cortex; CT scanning may show this much earlier than plain film studies. MRI scans often show underlying brain involvement.

The EEG often shows depression of voltage over the involved area in early stages; later, epileptiform abnormalities may be present focally.

Treatment

Sturge-Weber disease is sporadic. Early control of seizures is important to avoid consequent developmental setback. If seizures do not occur, normal development can be anticipated. Careful examination of the newborn, with ophthalmologic assessment to detect early glaucoma, is indicated. Rarely, surgical removal of the involved meninges and the involved portion of the brain may be indicated, even hemispherectomy.

Strauss RP, Resnick SD: Pulsed dye laser therapy for port-wine stains in children: Psychosocial and ethical issues. J Pediatr 1993;122:505.

Sujansky E, Conradi S: Sturge-Weber syndrome: Age of onset of seizures and glaucoma and the prognosis for affected children. J Child Neurol 1995;10:49.

Tallman B et al: Location of port-wine stains and the likelihood of ophthalmic and/or central nervous system complications. Pediatrics 1991;87:322.

4. VON HIPPEL-LINDAU DISEASE (Retinocerebellar Angiomatosis)

Von Hippel-Lindau disease is a rare, dominantly inherited condition with retinal and cerebellar hemangioblastomas; cysts of the kidneys, pancreas, and epididymis; and sometimes renal cancers. The patient may present with ataxia, slurred speech, and nystagmus due to a hemangioblastoma of the cerebellum or with a medullary spinal cord cystic hemangioblastoma. Retinal detachment may occur from hemorrhage or exudate in the retinal vascular malformation. Rarely, a pancreatic cyst or renal tumor may be the presenting symptom.

The diagnostic criteria for the disease are a retinal or cerebellar hemangioblastoma with or without a positive family history, intra-abdominal cyst, or renal cancer.

Choyke PL et al: von Hippel-Lindau disease: Genetic, clinical, and imaging features. Radiology 1995;194:629.

CENTRAL NERVOUS SYSTEM DEGENERATIVE DISORDERS OF INFANCY & CHILDHOOD

The CNS degenerative disorders of infancy and childhood are characterized by arrest of psychomotor development and loss, usually progressive but at variable rates, of mental and motor functioning and often of vision as well. Seizures are common in some disorders. Symptoms and signs vary with age at onset and primary sites of involvement of specific types.

These disorders are fortunately rare. An early clinical pattern of decline often follows normal early development. Referral for sophisticated biochemical testing is usually necessary before definitive diagnosis can be made. (See Tables 22–22 and 22–23.)

Aubourg P et al: Brain MRI and electrophysiologic abnormalities in preclinical and clinical adrenomyeloneuropathy. Neurology 1992;42:85.

Brown FR et al: Peroxisomal disorders: Neurodevelopmental and biochemical aspects. Am J Dis Child 1993;147:617.

Goebel HH: Neuronal ceroid-lipofuscinoses: The current status. Brain Dev 1992;14:203.

Jaeken J, Carchon H: The carbohydrate-deficient glycoprotein syndromes: Recent developments. Int Pediatr 1993;8:60.

Vadasz AG, Epstein LG: Degenerative central nervous system disease. Pediatr Rev 1995;16:426.

ATAXIAS OF CHILDHOOD

1. ACUTE CEREBELLAR ATAXIA

Acute cerebellar ataxia occurs most commonly in children 2–6 years of age. The onset is abrupt, and the evolution of symptoms is rapid. In about 50% of cases, there is a prodromal illness with fever, respiratory or gastrointestinal symptoms, or an exanthem within 3 weeks of onset. Associated viral infections include varicella, rubeola, mumps, rubella, echovirus infections, poliomyelitis, infectious mononucleosis, and influenza. Bacterial infections such as scarlet fever and salmonellosis have also been incriminated.

Clinical Findings

A. Symptoms and Signs: Ataxia of the trunk and extremities may be severe, so that the child exhibits a staggering, reeling gait and inability to sit without support or to reach for objects; or there may be only mild unsteadiness. Hypotonia, tremor of the extremities, and horizontal nystagmus may be present. Speech may be slurred. The child is frequently irritable, and vomiting may occur.

There are no clinical signs of increased intracranial pressure. Sensory and reflex testing usually shows no abnormalities.

B. Laboratory Findings: CSF pressure and protein and glucose levels are normal; slight lymphocytosis (up to about 30/mL) may be present. Attempts should be made to identify the etiologic viral agent.

C. Imaging: CT scans are normal; MRI may show cerebellar postinfectious demyelinating lesions. The EEG may be normal or may show nonspecific slowing.

Differential Diagnosis

Acute cerebellar ataxia must be differentiated from acute cerebellar syndromes due to phenytoin, phenobarbital, primidone, or lead intoxication. For phenytoin, the toxic level in serum is usually above 25 µg/mL; for phenobarbital, above 50 µg/mL; for primidone, above 14 µg/mL. (See Seizure Disorders.) With lead intoxication, papilledema, anemia, basophilic stippling of erythrocytes, proteinuria, typical x-rays, and elevated CSF protein are clinical clues, confirmed by serum, urine, or hair lead levels. An occult neuroblastoma, usually seen with the polymyoclonus-opsoclonus syndrome (see below) occasionally begins as acute cerebellar ataxia.

In rare cases, acute cerebellar ataxia may be the presenting sign of acute bacterial meningitis or may be mimicked by corticosteroid withdrawal, vasculitides such as in polyarteritis nodosa, trauma, the first attack of ataxia in a metabolic disorder such as Hartnup disease, or the onset of acute disseminated encephalomyelitis or of multiple sclerosis. The history and physical findings may differentiate these disturbances, but appropriate laboratory studies are often necessary. For ataxias with more chronic onset and course, see the sections on spinocerebellar degeneration (below) and the other degenerative disorders.

Treatment & Prognosis

Treatment is supportive. The use of corticosteroids has no rational justification.

Eighty to 90 percent of children with acute cerebellar ataxia not secondary to drug toxicity recover without sequelae within 6–8 weeks. In the remainder, neurologic disturbances, including disorders of behavior and of learning, ataxia, abnormal eye movements, and speech impairment, may persist for months or years, and recovery may remain incomplete.

Cohen HA et al: Mumps-associated acute cerebellar ataxia. Am J Dis Child 1992;146:930.

DeAngelis C: Ataxia. Pediatr Rev 1995;16:114

2. POLYMYOCLONIA-OPSOCLONUS SYNDROME OF CHILDHOOD (Infantile Myoclonic Encephalopathy, "Dancing Eyes—Dancing Feet" Syndrome)

The symptoms and signs of this syndrome are at first similar to those of acute cerebellar ataxia. Often

Table 22–22. Central nervous system degenerative disorders of infancy.

Disease	Enzyme Defect and Genetics	Onset	Early Manifestations	Vision and Hearing	Somatic Findings	Motor System	Seizures	Laboratory and Tissue Studies	Course
WHITE MATTER									
Globoid (Krabbe's) leukodystrophy	Recessive. Galactocerebrosidase and lactosylceramidase 1 deficiency.	First 6 months; "late-onset forms"	Feeding difficulties. Shrill cry. Irritability. Arching of back.	Optic atrophy, mid-course to late. Hyperacusis occasionally.	Head often small. Often underweight.	Early spasticity, occasionally preceded by hypotonia. Prolonged nerve condition.	Early. Myoclonic, and generalized, decerebrate posturing	CSF protein elevated; usually normal in late-onset forms. Sural nerve; nonspecific myelin breakdown. Enzyme deficiency in leukocytes, cultured skin fibroblasts. Demyelination, gliosis; low-signal CT scan, high-signal T$_2$-weighted MRI.	Rapid. Death usually by 1½–2 years. Late-onset cases may live 5–10 years.
Metachromatic leukodystrophy	Recessive. Arylsulfatase A deficiency.	Second year. Less often, later in childhood, or adult.	Incoordination, especially gait disturbance; then general regression. Reverse in juveniles.	Optic atrophy, usually late. Hearing normal.	Head enlarged late. None in juvenile form.	Combined upper and lower motor neuron signs. Prolonged nerve conduction.	Infrequent, usually late and generalized	Metachromatic cells in urine: negative sulfatase A test. CSF protein elevated: occasionally normal early. Sural nerve biopsy: metachromasia. Enzyme deficiency in leukocytes, cultured skin fibroblasts. Imaging: Same as globoid leukodystrophy.	Moderately slow. Death in infantile form by 3–8 years, in "juvenile" form by 10–15 years.
Neuroaxonal degeneration (Seitelberger's disease). Same as, or resembling, Hallervorden-Spatz disease.	Familial, (?) recessive. More common in girls than boys; defect unknown.	1–3 years	Arrest of development and dementia. Loss of motor functions. Occasionally hypesthesia over trunk and legs.	Nystagmus frequent; optic atrophy, hearing impairment	Early, may lie in	Combined upper and lower motor neuron lesions. Prominent feature "frog" position.	Variable, but usually not a prominent tion counter probes over the temples.	Denervation on EMG; elevated serum LDH and aminotransferase. Increased iron uptake in region of basal ganglia by scintillation. Brain and sural nerve: axonal swellings or "spheroids." Iron deposition in globus pallidus.	Very slowly progressive, with death early in second decade or earlier.
Pelizaeus-Merzbacher disease	X-linked recessive; rare female. Proteolipid protein (myelin).	(?) Birth to 2 years	"Eye rolling" often shortly after birth. Head bobbing. Slow loss of intellect.	Slowly developing optic atrophy. Hearing normal. Nystagmus.	Head and body normal	Cerebellar signs early, hyperactive deep reflexes. Spasticity.	Usually only late	None specific. Brain biopsy: extensive demyelination with small perivascular islands of intact myelin. Exon imitations in PLP gene in 10–25%.	Very slow, often seemingly stationary.
DIFFUSE, BUT PRIMARILY GRAY MATTER									
Poliodystrophy (Alpers') disease	Occasionally familial, recessive. Possibly viral. Metabolic forms.	Infancy to adolescence	Variable: loss of intellect, seizures, incoordination. Vomiting, hepatic failure.	"Cortical blindness and deafness	Head normal initially; may fail to grow	Variable: incoordination, spasticity	Often initial manifestation: myoclonic, akinetic, and generalized	Nonspecific. CSF protein normal or slightly elevated. Extensive neuronal loss in cortex: may occur very late. Variably increased serum pyruvate, lactate; liver steatosis, cirrhosis late. Increased serum pyruvate, lactate.	Usually rapid, with death within 1–3 years after onset.
Tay-Sachs disease and G$_{M2}$ gangliosidosis variants: Sandhoff disease; juvenile; chronic-adult	Recessive. Hexosaminidase deficiencies. Tay-Sachs 93% East European Jewish, hexosaminidase A deficiency. Others panethnic. Sandhoff hexosaminidase A and B deficiency.	Tay-Sachs, Sandhoff similar: 3–6 months. Others 2–6 years or later. Juvenile-partial hexosaminidase A.	Variable: shrill cry, loss of vision, infantile spasms, arrest of development. In juvenile and chronic forms: motor difficulties; later, mental difficulties.	Cherry-red macula, early blindness. Hyperacusis early. Strabismus in juvenile form, blindness late.	Head enlarged late. Liver occasionally enlarged. None in juvenile chronic forms.	Initially floppy. Eventual decerebrate rigidity. In juvenile and chronic forms: dysarthria, ataxia, spasticity.	Frequent, in mid-course and late. Infantile spasms and generalized	Blood smears: vacuolated lymphocytes; basophilic hypergranulation. Enzyme deficiencies in serum. leukocytes, culture skin fibroblasts. High-density thalami on CT scan, low-density white matter.	Moderately rapid. Death usually by 2–5 years. In juvenile form, 5–15 years.

668

Disease	Genetics / Enzyme defect	Age at onset	Early signs	Eyes	Head and organs	Tone / neurologic	Seizures	Laboratory	Course
Niemann-Pick disease and variants	50% Jewish. Recessive. Sphingomyelinase deficiency in types A and C involving the CNS.	First 6 months. In variants, later onset: often non-Jewish.	Slow development. Protruding belly.	Cherry-red macula in 35–50%. Blindness late. Deafness occasionally.	Head usually normal. Spleen enlarged more than liver. Occasional xanthomas of skin.	Initially floppy. Eventually spastic. Occasionally extrapyramidal signs.	Rare and late	Blood: vacuolated lymphocytes; increased lipids. X-rays: "mottled" lungs, decalcified bones. "Foam cells" in bone marrow, spleen, lymph nodes.	Moderately slow. Death usually by 3–5 years.
Infantile Gaucher's disease (glucosyl ceramide lipidosis)	Recessive. Glucocerebrosidase deficiency.	First 6 months; rarely, late infancy	Stridor or hoarse cry; retraction; feeding difficulties	Occasional cherry-red macula. Convergent squint. Deafness occasionally.	Head usually normal. Liver and spleen equally enlarged.	Opisthotonos early, followed rapidly by decerebrate rigidity	Rare and late	Anemia. Increased acid phosphatase. X-rays: thinned cortex, trabeculation of bones. "Gaucher cells" in bone marrow, spleen. Enzyme deficiency in leukocytes or cultured skin fibroblasts.	Very rapid
Lipogranulomatosis (Farber's disease)	Ceramidase deficiency	Early in infancy	Hoarseness, irritability, restricted joint movements	Usually normal	Painful nodular swelling of joints; subcutaneous nodules	Psychomotor retardation and progressive paralysis	Usually none	Chest x-rays may show pulmonary infiltrates. Nodules: granulomatous lesions, resembling those in reticuloendotheliosis. Multiple infarcts on CNS imaging.	Rapid: death usually in 1–2 years.
Generalized gangliosidosis and juvenile type (G_{M1} gangliosidoses)	Recessive; β-galactosidase deficiency	First year; less often, second year	Arrest of development. Protruding belly. Coarse facies in infantile (generalized) form.	50% "cherry-red spot." Hearing usually normal. In juvenile type, occasionally retinitis pigmentosa.	Head enlarged early: liver enlarged more than spleen	Initially floppy, eventually spastic	Usually late	Blood: vacuolated lymphocytes. X-rays: dorsolumbar kyphosis, "beaking" of vertebrae. "Foam cells" similar to those in Niemann-Pick disease.	Very rapid. Death within a few years. Slower in juvenile type (to 10 years).
Subacute necrotizing encephalomyelopathy (Leigh's disease)	Recessive or variable. May have deficiency of pyruvate carboxylase, pyruvate dehydrogenase, cytochrome enzymes.	Infancy to late childhood	Difficulties in feeding; feeble or absent cry; floppiness	Optic atrophy, often early. Roving eye movements. Ophthalmoplegia.	Head usually normal, occasionally small; cardiac and renal tubular dysfunction occasionally	Flaccid and immobile; may become spastic. Spinocerebellar forms; ataxia.	Rare and late	Increased CSF and blood lactate and pyruvate. High-signal MRI T_2 foci in thalami; globus pallidus, subthalamic nuclei.	Usually rapid in infants, but may be slow with death after several years. Central hypoventilation a frequent cause of death.
"Steel wool," or kinky hair," disease (Menkes')	X-linked recessive; defect in copper absorption	Infancy	Peculiar facies; secondary hair white, twisted, split; hypothermia	May show optic disk pallor and microcysts of pigment epithelium	Normal to small	Variable: floppy to spastic	Myoclonic infantile spasms; status epilepticus	Defective absorption of copper. Cerebral angiography shows elongated arteries. Hair shows pili torti; split shafts. CT scan may show diffuse multifocal areas of low density.	Moderately rapid. Death usually by 3–4 years.
Carbohydrate-deficient glycoprotein syndrome	Recessive glycoprotein abnormality	Infancy	Failure to thrive, retardation	Strabismus		Variable	Rare	Transferrin decreased. Liver steatosis. Cerebellar hypoplasia.	Cardiomyopathy, thrombosis
Bassen-Kornzweig disease	Recessive; primary defect unknown	Early childhood	Diarrhea in infancy	Retinitis pigmentosa; late ophthalmoplegia	None	Ataxia, late extrapyramidal movement disorder	None	Abetalipoproteinemia: acanthocytosis, low serum vitamin E; cerebellar atrophy on imaging.	Progression arrested with vitamin E

Table 22–23. Central nervous system degenerative disorders of childhood.[1]

Disease	Enzyme Defect and Genetics	Onset	Early Manifestations	Vision and Hearing	Motor System	Seizures	Laboratory and Tissue Studies	Course
Adrenoleukodystrophy and variants	X-linked recessive. Neonatal form recessive. Acyl-CoA synthetase deficiency.	5–10 years. Newborn.	Impaired intellect, behavioral problems	"Cortical blindness and deafness"	Ataxia, spasticity. Motor deficits may be asymmetric, or one-sided initially.	Occasionally	Hyperpigmentation and adrenocortical insufficiency. ACTH elevated. Accumulation of very long chain fatty acids. Plasma test available for long-chain fatty acids.	Fairly rapid. Death usually within 2–3 years after onset.
Neuronal ceroid lipofuscinosis (NCL) (cerebromacular degeneration, Batten's disease)	Recessive; Defect unknown	8–18 months INCL: 4–8 years JNCL	Ataxia. Visual difficulties. Arrested intellectual development.	Pigmentary degeneration of macula. Optic atrophy. Hearing may be impaired.	Ataxia, spasticity progressing to decerebrate rigidity	Often early: myoclonus and later generalized; difficult to control	Blood: vacuolated lymphocytes, azurophilic dispersed hypergranulation of polymorphonuclear cells. Electrotretinography helpful. In skin, skeletal muscle, peripheral nerves, brain: "curvilinear bodies" and "fingerprint profiles" autofluorescent lipopigments.	Moderately slow. Death in 3–8 years.
Subacute sclerosing panencephalitis (SSPE Dawson's disease)	None. Measles "slow virus" infection. Also reported as result of rubella.	3–22 years; rarely earlier or later	Impaired intellect, emotional lability, incoordination	Occasionally chorioretinitis or optic atrophy. Hearing normal.	Ataxia, slurred speech, occasionally involuntary movements, spasticity progressing to decerebrate rigidity	Myoclonic and akinetic seizures relatively early; later, focal and generalized	CSF protein normal to moderately elevated. High CSF IgG;[2] oligoclonal bands. Elevated CSF and serum measles (or rubella) antibody titers. Characteristic EEG. Brain biopsy: inclusion body encephalitis; culturing of measles virus, perhaps rubella virus.	Variable, death in months to years. Remissions of variable duration may occur.
Multiple sclerosis	None. Diagnosis difficult in childhood.	Adolescent; rare in childhood	Highly variable. May strike one or more sites of CNS. Paresthesias common.	Optic neuritis; diplopia, nystagmus at some time. Vestibulocochlear nerves occasionally affected.	Motor weakness, spasticity, ataxia, sphincter disturbances, slurred speech, mental difficulties	Rare: focal or generalized	CSF may show slight pleocytosis, elevation of protein and gamma globulin;[2] oligoclonal bands present. CT scan may show areas of demyelination. Auditory, visual, and somatosensory evoked responses often show lesions in respective pathways. Changes in T cell subsets.	Variable: complete remission possible. Recurrent attacks and involvement of multiple sites are prerequisites for diagnosis.
Cerebrotendinous xanthomatosis	?Recessive. Abnormal accumulation of cholesterol.	Late childhood to adolescence	Xanthomas in tendons. Mental deterioration.	Cataracts; xanthelasma	Cerebellar defects; bulbar paralysis late	Myoclonus	Xanthomas may appear in lungs. Xanthomas in tendons (especially Achilles).	Very slowly progressive into middle life. Replace deficient bile acid.
Huntington's disease	Dominant. Chromosome 4p CAG repeat.	10% childhood onset	Rigidity, dementia	Ophthalmoplegia late	Rigidity; chorea frequently absent in children	50% with major motor seizures	CT scan may show "butterfly" atrophy of caudate and putamen	Moderately rapid with death in 15 years
Refsum's disease	Recessive. Phytanic acid oxidase deficiency.	5–10 years	Ataxia, ichthyosis, cardiomyopathy	Retinitis pigmentosa	Ataxia	None	Serum phytanic acid elevated. Slow nerve conduction velocity. Elevated CSF protein. Peroxisomal disease.	Treat with low phytanic acid diet

[1]For late infantile metachromatic leukodystrophy, Pelizaeus-Merzbacher disease, poliodystrophy, Gaucher's disease of later onset, and subacute necrotizing encephalomyelopathy, see Table 22–22.
[2]CSF gamma globulin (IgG) is considered elevated in children when > 9% of total protein (possibly even > 8.3%); definitively elevated when > 14%.

of sudden onset, polymyoclonia-opsoclonus syndrome is characterized by severe incoordination of the trunk and extremities with lightning-like jerking or flinging movements of a group of muscles, causing the child to be in constant motion while awake. Extraocular muscle involvement results in sudden irregular eye movements (opsoclonus). Irritability and vomiting are often present, but there is no depression of level of consciousness. This syndrome occurs in association with viral infections, tumors of neural crest origin, and many other disorders. Immunologic mechanisms have been postulated. There are usually no signs of increased intracranial pressure. Cerebrospinal fluid may show normal or mildly increased protein levels. Special techniques show increased CSF levels of plasmacytes and abnormal immunoglobulins. The EEG may be slightly slow, but when performed together with electromyography, it shows no evidence of association between cortical discharges and the muscle movements. An assiduous search must be made to rule out tumor of neural crest origin by x-rays of the chest and CT scan or ultrasound (or both) of the adrenal area as well as by assays of urinary catecholamine metabolites (vanillylmandelic acid, etc) and cystathionine.

The symptoms respond (often dramatically) to large doses of corticotropin. Otherwise, treatment is as for specific entities. When a neural crest (or other) tumor is found, surgical excision should be followed by irradiation and chemotherapy. Life span is determined by the biologic behavior of the tumor.

The syndrome is usually self-limited but may be characterized by exacerbations and remissions. However, even after removal of a neural crest tumor and without other evidence of its recurrence, symptoms may reappear. Mild mental retardation may be a sequela.

Mitchell WG, Snodgrass SR: Opsoclonus-ataxia due to childhood neural crest tumors: A chronic neurologic syndrome. J Child Neurol 1990;5:153.

Pranzatelli MR: The neurobiology of the opsoclonus-myoclonus syndrome. Clin Neuropharmacol 1992;15:186.

3. SPINOCEREBELLAR DEGENERATION DISORDERS

Spinocerebellar degeneration disorders may be hereditary or may occur in sporadic distribution. Hereditary disorders include Friedreich's ataxia, dominant hereditary ataxia, and a group of miscellaneous diseases.

Friedreich's Ataxia

This is a recessive disorder characterized by onset of gait ataxia or scoliosis before puberty, becoming progressively worse. Reflexes, light touch, and position sensation are reduced. Dysarthria becomes progressively more severe. Cardiomyopathy usually develops, and diabetes mellitus is found in 40% of patients, with half of these requiring insulin. Pes cavus typically is found. The GAA trinucleotide repeats on chromosome 9 can be utilized for laboratory diagnosis.

Treatment includes surgery for scoliosis and intervention as needed for cardiac disease and diabetes. Patients are usually confined to a wheelchair after age 20 years. Death occurs, usually from heart failure or dysrhythmias, in the third or fourth decade; some patients survive longer.

Dominant Ataxia

This disease (also known as olivopontocerebellar atrophy, Holmes's ataxia, Marie's ataxia, etc) occurs with varying manifestations, even among members of the same family. Ataxia occurs at onset, and progression continues with ophthalmoplegias, extrapyramidal tract and motor neuron degeneration, and later dementia. One type has been found to be caused by a CAG trinucleotide repeat. Levodopa may ameliorate rigidity and bradykinesia, but no other therapy is available. Only 10% of cases have onset in childhood, and their course is often more rapid.

Miscellaneous Hereditary Ataxias

Associated findings permit identification of these recessive disorders. These include ataxia-telangiectasia (telangiectasia, immune defects; see below), Wilson's disease (Kayser-Fleischer rings), Refsum's disease (ichthyosis, cardiomyopathy, retinitis pigmentosa, large nerves), Rett's syndrome (regression to autism at 7–18 months in girls, loss of use of hands, progressive failure of brain growth), and abetalipoproteinemia (infantile diarrhea, acanthocytosis, retinitis pigmentosa). Patients with juvenile and chronic gangliosidoses and some hemolytic anemias and long-term survivors of Chédiak-Higashi disease may develop spinocerebellar degeneration. Idiopathic familial ataxia is called Behr's syndrome. Neuropathies such as Charcot-Marie-Tooth disease produce ataxia.

Dubourg O et al: Analysis of the SCA1 CAG repeat in a large number of families with dominant ataxia: Clinical and molecular correlations. Ann Neurol 1995;37:176.

Haas R, Rapin I, Moser H: Rett syndrome and autism. J Child Neurol 1988;3(Suppl):52.

Montermini L et al: Phenotypic variability in Friedreich ataxia: Role of the associated GAA triplet repeat expansion. Ann Neurol 1997;41:675.

Sheu KFR et al: Mitochondrial enzymes in hereditary ataxias. Metab Brain Dis 1988;3:151.

Stumpf DA: The inherited ataxias. Neurol Clin 1985;3:47.

ATAXIA-TELANGIECTASIA (Louis-Bar Syndrome)

Ataxia-telangiectasia is a multisystem disorder inherited as an autosomal recessive trait. It is characterized by progressive ataxia; telangiectasia of the bulbar conjunctiva, external ears, nares, and (later) other body surfaces, appearing in the third to sixth year; and recurrent respiratory, sinus, and ear infections. Ocular dyspraxia, slurred speech, choreoathetosis, hypotonia and areflexia, and psychomotor and growth retardation may be present. Endocrinopathies are common. Nerve conduction velocities may be reduced. The entire nervous system may be affected in late stages of the disease. A spectrum of involvement may be seen in the same family. Immunodeficiencies of IgA and IgE are common (see Chapter 27), and the incidence of certain cancers is high.

Gatti RA: Ataxia-telangiectasia. Dermatol Clin 1995;13:1.

Lavin MF, Shiloh Y: Ataxia-telangiectasia: A multifaceted genetic disorder associated with defective signal transduction. Curr Opin Immunol 1996; 8:459.

Swift M et al: Incidence of cancer in 161 families affected by ataxia-telangiectasia. N Engl J Med 1991;325:1831.

EXTRAPYRAMIDAL DISORDERS

Extrapyramidal disorders are characterized by the presence in the waking state of one or more of the following features: dyskinesias, athetosis, ballismus, tremors, rigidity, and dystonias.

For the most part, precise pathologic and anatomic localization is not understood. Motor pathways synapsing in the striatum (putamen and caudate nucleus), globus pallidus, red nucleus, substantia nigra, and the body of Luys are involved; this "system" is modulated by pathways originating in the thalamus, cerebellum, and reticular formation.

1. SYDENHAM'S POSTRHEUMATIC CHOREA

Sydenham's chorea is characterized by an acute onset of choreiform movements and variable degrees of psychologic disturbance. It is frequently associated with rheumatic endocarditis and arthritis. Although the disorder follows infections with group A β-hemolytic streptococci, the interval between infection and chorea may be greatly prolonged; throat cultures and antistreptolysin O (ASO) titers may therefore be negative. Chorea has also been associated with hypocalcemia; with vascular lupus erythematosus; and with toxic, viral, infectious and parainfectious, and degenerative encephalopathies.

Clinical Findings

A. Symptoms and Signs: Chorea, or rapid involuntary movements of the limbs and face, is the hallmark physical finding. In addition to the jerky incoordinate movements, the following are noted: emotional lability, waxing and waning ("milkmaid's")

grip, darting tongue, "spooning" of the extended hands and their tendency to pronate, and knee jerks slow to return from the extended to their prestimulus position ("hung up"). Seizures, while uncommon, may be masked by choreic jerks.

B. Laboratory Findings: Anemia, leukocytosis, and an increased erythrocyte sedimentation rate (ESR) may be present. The ASO titer may be elevated and C-reactive protein (CRP) present. Throat culture is sometimes positive for group A β-hemolytic streptococci.

Electrocardiography and echocardiography are often essential to detect cardiac involvement. Antineuronal antibodies are present in most patients but are not specific. Electroencephalography may show nonspecific slowing or seizure activity.

Differential Diagnosis

The diagnosis of Sydenham's chorea is usually not difficult. Tics, drug-induced extrapyramidal syndromes, Huntington's chorea, and hepatolenticular degeneration (Wilson's disease), as well as other rare movement disorders, can usually be ruled out on historical and clinical grounds.

Other causes of chorea can be ruled out by laboratory tests, such as ANA (antinuclear antibody) for lupus, TSH, T_4 for thyroid disease, serum calcium for hypocalcemia, Monospot for mononucleosis.

Treatment

There is no specific treatment. Dopaminergic blockers such as haloperidol, 0.5 mg to 3–6 mg/d, or pimozide, 4–12 mg/d, have been used. Parkinsonian side effects such as rigidity and masked facies and, with high doses, tardive dyskinesia rarely occur in childhood. A variety of other drugs have been used with success in individual cases, such as the anticonvulsant sodium valproate, 50–60 mg/kg/d in divided doses; or prednisone, 0.5–2 mg/kg/d in divided doses. Emotional lability and depression sometimes warrant administration of antidepressants such as amitriptyline.

All patients should be given antistreptococcal rheumatic fever prophylaxis.

Prognosis

Sydenham's chorea is a self-limiting disease that may last from a few weeks to months. Two-thirds of patients relapse one or more times, but the ultimate outcome does not appear to be worse in those with recurrences. Valvular heart disease occurs in about one third of patients, particularly if other rheumatic manifestations appear. Psychoneurotic disturbances, if not already present at the onset of illness, occur in a significant percentage of patients.

Kiessling LS, Marcotte AC, Culpepper L: Antineuronal antibodies in movement disorders. Pediatrics 1993;92:39.

Pranzatelli MR: Movement disorders in childhood. Pediatr Rev 1996;17:388.

Swedo SE et al: Sydenham's chorea: Physical and psychological symptoms of St. Vitus' dance. Pediatrics 1993;91:706.

Swedo SE: Sydenham's chorea. JAMA 1994;272:1788.

Vedanarayanan VV: Paroxysmal movement disorders. Pediatr Ann 1997;26:402.

2. TICS
(Habit Spasms)

Tics, or habit spasms, are quick repetitive but irregular movements, often stereotyped, and briefly suppressible. Coordination and muscle tone are not affected. A psychogenic basis is seldom discernible.

Transient tics of childhood (12–24% incidence in school-age children) last from 1 month to 1 year and seldom need treatment. Many children with tics have a history of encephalopathic past events, "soft signs" on neurologic examination, and school problems.

Facial tics such as grimaces, twitches, and blinking predominate, but the trunk and extremities are often involved and there are twisting or flinging movements. Vocal tics are less common.

Gilles de la Tourette's syndrome is a chronic disorder of multiple fluctuating motor and vocal tics, with onset in childhood, lasting more than a year, with absence of other recognizable causes for tics. Tics evolve slowly, new ones being added to or replacing old ones. Coprolalia and echolalia are relatively infrequent. Partial forms are common. The usual age at onset is 2–15 years, and the familial incidence is 35–50%; the disorder is now reported in almost all ethnic groups. Gilles de la Tourette's syndrome may be triggered by stimulants such as methylphenidate and dextroamphetamine. An imbalance of neurotransmitters, especially dopamine and serotonin, has been hypothesized.

In relatively mild cases, tics are self-limited and, when disregarded, disappear. When attention is paid to one tic, it may disappear only to be replaced by another that is often worse. If the tic and its underlying anxiety or compulsive neurosis are severe, psychiatric evaluation and treatment are needed.

Important comorbidities are attention deficit hyperactivity disorder (ADHD) and obsessive-compulsive disorder (OCD). Medications such as methylphenidate and dextroamphetamine should be carefully titrated to treat ADHD and avoid worsening tics. Fluoxetine and clomipramine may be useful for OCD in patients with tics.

When medication is required to treat Tourette's syndrome, the most effective agents are dopamine blockers. However, many pediatric patients can manage without drug treatment. Generally, medications are reserved for patients with disabling symptoms; treatment may be relaxed or discontinued when the symptoms abate (Table 22–24).

Table 22–24. Medications for Tourette's syndrome and tics.

Dopamine blockers (many are antipsychotics)
Haloperidol (Haldol)
Pimozide (Orap)
Fluphenazine (Prolixin)
Trifluperazine (Stelazine)
Risperidone (Resperdal)
Serotonergic drugs[1]
Fluoxetine (Prozac)
Paroxetine (Sertraline)
Paxil (Paroxetine)
Luvox (Fluvoxamine)
Anafranil (Clomipramine)
Clonazepam (Klonopin)
Noradrenergic drugs[2]
Clonidine (Catapres)
Guanfacine (Tenex)

[1]Useful for obsessive-compulsive disorder.
[2]Useful for attention deficit hyperactivity disorder.

Nonpharmacologic treatment of Tourette's syndrome includes education of patients, family members, and school personnel. In some cases, restructuring the school environment to prevent tension and teasing may be necessary; supportive counseling, either at or outside school, should be provided.

Usually, medications will not eradicate the tics. Accordingly, the goal of treatment should be to reduce the tics to tolerable levels without inducing undesirable side effects. Dosage should be increased at weekly intervals until a satisfactory response is obtained. Often, a single dose at bedtime is sufficient. The two neuroleptic agents used most often are haloperidol and fluphenazine; side effects to be avoided include akathisia and tardive dyskinesia. The newest neuroleptic agent in use is pimozide; motor side effects of this drug are the same as those encountered with the use of other dopamine blockers.

Clonidine, clonazepam, and calcium channel blockers have been used in individual patients with some success; sometimes these agents are used for combined therapy (eg, haloperidol with nifedipine).

Calderone-Gonzales R, Calderone-Sepulveda R: Tourette syndrome: Current concepts. Int Pediatr 1993;8:176.

Freeman RD: Attention deficit hyperactivity disorder in the presence of Tourette syndrome. Neurol Clin 1997;15:411.

Kurlan R: Tourette syndrome. Treatment of tics. Neurol Clin 1997;15:403.

Singer H: Neurobiological issues in Tourette syndrome. Brain Develop 1994;16:353.

Singer H: Tic disorders. Pediatr Ann 1993;33:33.

INFECTIONS & INFLAMMATORY DISORDERS OF THE CENTRAL NERVOUS SYSTEM

Infections of the central nervous system are among the most common neurologic disorders encountered by pediatricians. Although infections are among the CNS disorders most amenable to treatment, they also have a very high potential for causing catastrophic destruction of the nervous system. It is imperative for the clinician to recognize such infections early, in order to treat as early as possible to prevent massive tissue destruction.

Clinical Manifestations

Patients with central nervous system infections, whether caused by bacteria, viruses, or other microorganisms, present with similar manifestations. Systemic signs of infection include fever, generalized malaise, or impaired heart, lung, liver, or kidney function. General features suggesting CNS infection include headache, stiff neck, fever or hypothermia, changes in mental status (including hyperirritability evolving into lethargy and coma), seizures, and focal sensory and motor deficits. On examination, meningeal irritation is manifested by the presence of Kernig's and Brudzinski's signs. In very young infants, signs of meningeal irritation may be absent, and temperature instability and hypothermia are often more prominent than fever. In young infants, a bulging fontanelle and an increased head circumference are common. Papilledema may eventually develop, particularly in older children and adolescents. Cranial nerve palsies may develop acutely or gradually during the course of neurologic infections. No specific clinical sign or symptom is reliable in distinguishing bacterial infections from infections caused by other microbes.

During the initial clinical assessment, conditions that predispose the patient to infection of the central nervous system should be sought. Infections involving the sinuses or other structures in the head and neck region can result in direct extension of infection into the intracranial compartment. Open head injuries, recent neurosurgical procedures, immunodeficiencies, and the presence of a mechanical shunt may predispose to intracranial infection.

Laboratory Investigation

When CNS infections are suspected, blood should be obtained for a complete blood count, general chemistry panel, and culture. Most important, however, is obtaining cerebrospinal fluid. In the absence of focal neurologic deficits or signs of increased intracranial pressure, CSF should be obtained immediately from any patient in whom serious CNS infec-

tion is suspected. When papilledema or focal motor signs are present, a lumbar puncture may be delayed until a neuroimaging procedure has been done to exclude brain abscess or other space-occupying lesion. It is generally safe to obtain spinal fluid from infants with nonfocal neurologic examination even if the fontanelle is bulging. Spinal fluid should be examined for the presence of red and white blood cells, protein concentration, glucose concentration, bacteria and other microorganisms; a sample should be cultured. In addition, serologic, immunologic, and nucleic acid detection (PCR) tests may be performed on the spinal fluid in an attempt to identify the specific organism. As a general rule, spinal fluid that contains a high proportion of polymorphonuclear leukocytes, a high protein concentration, and a low glucose concentration strongly suggests bacterial infection. CSF containing predominantly lymphocytes, a high protein concentration, and a low glucose concentration suggests infection with mycobacteria, fungi, uncommon bacteria, and some viruses such as lymphocytic choriomeningitis virus, herpes simplex virus, mumps virus, and arboviruses. Cerebrospinal fluid that contains a high proportion of lymphocytes, normal or only slightly elevated protein concentration, and a normal glucose concentration is most suggestive of viral infections, although partially treated bacterial meningitis and parameningeal infections may also result in this type of CSF formula. Typical spinal fluid findings in a variety of infectious and inflammatory disorders are shown in Table 22–3.

Neuroimaging with CT and MRI scans may be helpful in demonstrating the presence of brain abscess, meningeal inflammation, or secondary problems such as venous and arterial infarctions, hemorrhages, and subdural effusions when these are expected. In addition, these procedures may identify sinus or other focal infections in the head or neck region that are related to the central nervous system infection. CT scanning may demonstrate bony abnormalities, such as basilar fractures.

EEGs may be helpful in the assessment of patients who have had seizures at the time of presentation. The changes are often nonspecific and characterized by generalized slowing. In some instances, such as herpes simplex virus infection, focal electronegative activity may be seen early in the course and may be one of the earliest laboratory abnormalities to suggest the diagnosis. EEGs may also show focal slowing over regions of abscesses. Unusual but characteristic electroencephalographic patterns are seen in some patients with subacute sclerosing panencephalitis.

In some cases, brain biopsy may be needed to identify the presence of specific organisms and clarify the diagnosis. Herpes simplex virus infections can be confirmed using the PCR to assay for herpes DNA in spinal fluid. This test has a 95% sensitivity and 99% specificity.

Brain biopsy may be needed to detect the rare PCR-negative case of herpes simplex and various parasitic infections, brain tumors, and other structural abnormalities.

BACTERIAL MENINGITIS

Bacterial infections of the central nervous system may present acutely (symptoms evolving rapidly over 1–24 hours), subacutely (symptoms evolving over 1–7 days), or chronically (symptoms evolving over more than 1 week). Diffuse bacterial infections involve the leptomeninges, superficial cortical structures, and blood vessels. Although the term "meningitis" is used to describe these infections, it should not be forgotten that the brain parenchyma is also inflamed and that blood vessel walls may be infiltrated by inflammatory cells that result in endothelial cell injury, vessel stenosis, and secondary ischemia and infarction.

Pathologically, the inflammatory process involves all intracranial structures to some degree. Acutely, this inflammatory process may result in cerebral edema or impaired cerebrospinal fluid flow through and out of the ventricular system resulting in hydrocephalus.

Treatment

A. Specific Measures: (See also Chapter 36, *Haemophilus influenzae* type B infections; and Chapter 33.)

While awaiting the results of diagnostic tests, the physician should start broad-spectrum antibiotic coverage as noted below. After specific organisms are identified, antibiotic therapy can be tailored based on antibiotic sensitivity patterns. Children under 3 months of age are treated initially with cefotaxime (or ceftriaxone if over 1 month of age) and ampicillin; the latter agent is used to treat *Listeria* and enterococci, agents that rarely affect older children. Children older than 3 months are treated with ceftriaxone, cefotaxime, or ampicillin plus chloramphenicol. If *S pneumoniae* cannot be ruled out by the initial Gram's stain, vancomycin or rifampin are added until cultures are reported, since penicillin-resistant pneumococci are common in the United States. Therapy may be narrowed when organism sensitivity allows. Duration of therapy is 7 days for meningococcal infections, 10 days for *H influenzae* or pneumococcal infection, and 14–21 days for other organisms. Slow clinical response or the occurrence of complications may prolong the need for therapy. Although therapy for 7 days has proved successful in many children with *Haemophilus* infection, it cannot be recommended if steroids are also used (see below) without further study.

B. General and Supportive Measures: Children with bacterial meningitis are often systemically ill. The following complications should be looked for and treated aggressively: hypovolemia, hypoglycemia, hyponatremia, acidosis, septic shock, increased intracranial pressure, seizures, disseminated intravascular coagulation, and metastatic infection (eg, pericarditis, arthritis, and pneumonia). Children should initially be monitored closely (cardiorespiratory monitor, strict fluid balance and frequent urine specific gravity assessment, daily weights, neurologic assessment every few hours), not fed until neurologically very stable, isolated until the organism is known, rehydrated with isotonic solutions until euvolemic, and then given intravenous fluids containing dextrose and sodium at no more than maintenance rate (assuming no unusual losses occur).

Complications

Abnormalities of water and electrolyte balance result from either excessive or insufficient production of antidiuretic hormone and require careful monitoring and appropriate adjustments in fluid administration. Monitoring serum sodium every 8–12 hours during the first 1 or 2 days, and urine sodium if the inappropriate secretion of antidiuretic hormone is suspected, usually uncovers significant problems.

Seizures occur in up to 30% of children with bacterial meningitis. Seizures tend to be most common in neonates and less common in older children. Persistent focal seizures or focal seizures associated with focal neurologic deficits strongly suggest subdural effusion, abscess, or vascular lesions such as arterial infarct, cortical venous infarcts, or dural sinus thrombosis. Because generalized seizures in a metabolically compromised child may have severe sequelae, early recognition and therapy are critical; some practitioners prefer phenytoin for acute management because it is less sedating than phenobarbital.

Subdural effusions occur in as many as 50% of young children with *H influenzae* meningitis. Subdural effusions are often seen on CT scans of the head during the course of meningitis. They do not require treatment unless they are producing increased intracranial pressure or progressive mass effect. Although subdural effusions may be detected in children with persistent fever, such effusions do not usually have to be sampled or drained if the infecting organism is *Haemophilus,* meningococcus, or pneumococcus. These are usually sterilized with the standard treatment duration, and slowly waning fever during an otherwise uncomplicated recovery may be followed clinically. Under any other circumstance, however, aspiration of the fluid for documentation of sterilization or relief of pressure should be considered.

Cerebral edema can participate in the production of increased intracranial pressure, requiring treatment with dexamethasone, osmotic agents, diuretics, or hyperventilation; continuous pressure monitoring may be needed.

Long-term sequelae of meningitis result from direct inflammatory destruction of brain cells, vascular injuries, or secondary gliosis. Focal motor and sensory deficits, visual impairment, hearing loss, seizures, hydrocephalus, and a variety of cranial nerve deficits can result from meningitis. Sensorineural hearing loss in *H influenzae* meningitis occurs in approximately 5–10% of cases during long-term follow-up. Recent studies have suggested that early addition of dexamethasone to the antibiotic regimen may modestly decrease the risk of hearing loss in some children with *H influenzae* meningitis (Chapter 36).

In addition to the variety of disorders mentioned above, some patients with meningitis suffer from mental retardation and severe behavioral disorders that limit their function at school and later performance in life. Table 22–25 lists the overall mortality and morbidity figures for the most common organisms associated with acute bacterial meningitis in childhood.

BRAIN ABSCESS

Patients with brain abscess often appear to have systemic illness similar to patients with bacterial meningitis, but in addition they show signs of focal neurologic deficits, papilledema, and other evidence of increased intracranial pressure or a mass lesion. Symptoms may be present for a week or more; children with bacterial meningitis usually present within a few days. Conditions predisposing to development of brain abscess include penetrating head trauma; chronic infection of the middle ear, mastoid, or sinuses (especially the frontal sinus); chronic dental or pulmonary infection; cardiovascular lesions allowing right-to-left shunting of blood (including arteriovenous malformations); and endocarditis.

When brain abscess is strongly suspected, a neuroimaging procedure such as CT or MRI scans should be done prior to lumbar puncture. If a brain abscess is identified, lumbar puncture may be dangerous and rarely alters the choice of antibiotic or clinical management since the CSF abnormalities usually reflect only parameningeal inflammation. With spread from contagious septic foci, streptococci

and anaerobic bacteria are most common. Staphylococci most often enter from trauma or from infections. Enteric organisms may form an abscess from chronic otitis. Unfortunately, cultures from a large number of brain abscesses remain negative.

The diagnosis of brain abscess is based primarily on a strong clinical suspicion and confirmed by a neuroimaging procedure. Electroencephalographic changes are nonspecific but frequently demonstrate focal slowing in the region of brain abscess. Initial therapy for infection from presumed contagious foci uses penicillin and metronidazole. Cefotaxime is a good alternative to penicillin, especially if enteric organisms are suspected. Enteric organisms are also often susceptible to trimethoprim-sulfamethoxazole. Suspicion of staphylococci, or their recovery from an aspirate, should be treated with nafcillin or vancomycin. Treatment may include neurologic consultation and anticonvulsant and edema therapy if necessary. In their early stages, brain abscesses are areas of focal cerebritis and can be "cured" with antibiotic treatment alone. Well-developed abscesses require surgical drainage.

Differential diagnosis of brain abscess includes any condition that produces focal neurologic deficits and increased intracranial pressure, such as neoplasms, subdural effusions, cerebral infarctions, and certain infections (herpes simplex, cysticercosis, and toxocariasis).

The surgical mortality rate in the treatment of brain abscess is lower than 5%. Untreated cerebral abscesses lead to irreversible tissue destruction and may rupture into the ventricle, producing catastrophic deterioration in neurologic function and death. Because brain abscesses are often associated with systemic illness and systemic infections, the death rate is frequently high in these patients.

VIRAL INFECTIONS

Viral infections of the central nervous system can involve primarily meninges (meningitis) (see Chapter

Table 22–25. Outcome of acute bacterial meningitis by organism.

Organism	Mortality (%)	Motor Handicap (%)		Intellect (%)	
		None	Severe	Normal	Severe Mental Retardation
Escherichia coli, other coliforms	20–50	62	25	75	25
Haemophilus influenzae	5–10	87	3	82	5
Streptococcus pneumoniae	10–30	96	0	83	0
Neisseria meningitidis	5–10	100	0	93	0
Group B streptococci	20	85	10–15	100	0
Overall total	10–25	85	5	82	6

34) or cerebral parenchyma (encephalitis). All patients, however, have some degree of involvement of both the meninges and cerebral parenchyma (meningoencephalitis). Many viral infections are generalized and diffuse, but some viruses, notably herpes simplex and some arboviruses, characteristically cause prominent focal disease. Focal cerebral involvement is clearly evident on neuroimaging procedures. Some viruses have an affinity for specific CNS cell populations. Poliovirus and other enteroviruses can selectively infect anterior horn cells (poliomyelitis) and some intracranial motor neurons.

Although most viral infections of the nervous system present with an acute or subacute course in childhood, chronic infections can occur. Subacute sclerosing panencephalitis, for example, represents a chronic indolent infection caused by measles virus and is characterized clinically by progressive neurodegeneration and seizures.

Inflammatory reactions within the nervous system may occur during the convalescent stage of systemic viral infections. Parainfectious or postinfectious inflammation of the central nervous system results in several well-recognized disorders: acute disseminated encephalomyelitis, transverse myelitis, optic neuritis, polyneuritis, and Guillain-Barré syndrome.

Congenital viral infections can also affect the central nervous system. Cytomegalovirus, herpes simplex virus, and rubella virus are the most notable causes of viral brain injury in utero.

Treatment of CNS viral infections is usually limited to symptomatic and supportive measures, except for herpes simplex virus. Acyclovir is the treatment in suspected or proved cases of herpes simplex virus encephalitis. Acyclovir is also useful in some patients with varicella-zoster virus infections of the central nervous system.

Encephalopathy of HIV Infection

Neurologic syndromes associated directly with HIV infection include subacute encephalitis, meningitis, myelopathy, polyneuropathy, and myositis. In addition, secondary opportunistic infections of the central nervous system occur in patients with HIV-induced immunosuppression; toxoplasmal and cytomegaloviral infections are particularly common. Progressive multifocal leukoencephalopathy, a secondary papillomavirus infection, herpes simplex virus, and herpes zoster virus infections also occur frequently in patients with HIV infection. A variety of fungal (especially cryptococcal), mycobacterial, and bacterial infections have been described.

Neurologic abnormalities in these patients can also be the result of noninfectious neoplastic disorders. Primary CNS lymphoma and metastatic lymphoma to the nervous system are the most frequent neoplasms involving the nervous system in these patients. See Chapters 27 and 34 for diagnosis and management of HIV infection.

OTHER INFECTIONS

A wide variety of other microorganisms, including *Toxoplasma,* mycobacteria, spirochetes, rickettsiae, amebas, and mycoplasmas, can cause CNS infections. Central nervous system involvement in these infections is usually secondary to systemic infection or other predisposing factors. Appropriate cultures and serologic testing are required to confirm infections by these organisms. Parenteral antimicrobial treatment for these infections is discussed elsewhere in this text.

NONINFECTIOUS INFLAMMATORY DISORDERS OF THE CENTRAL NERVOUS SYSTEM

The differential diagnosis of bacterial, viral, and other microbial infections of the central nervous system includes disorders that cause inflammation but for which no specific etiologic organism has been identified. Sarcoidosis, Behçet's syndrome, systemic lupus erythematosus (SLE), other collagen-vascular disorders, and Kawasaki disease are examples. In these disorders, CNS inflammation usually occurs in association with characteristic systemic manifestations that allow proper diagnosis. Management of central nervous system involvement in these disorders is the same as the treatment of the systemic illness.

OTHER PARAINFECTIOUS ENCEPHALOPATHIES

In association with systemic infections or other illnesses, CNS dysfunction may occur in the absence of direct central nervous system inflammation or infection. **Reye's syndrome** is a prominent example of this type of encephalopathy that often occurs in association with varicella virus or other respiratory or systemic viral infections. In Reye's syndrome, cerebral edema and cerebral dysfunction occur, but there is no evidence of any direct involvement of the nervous system by the associated microorganism or inflammation. Cerebral edema in Reye's syndrome is accompanied by liver dysfunction and fatty infiltration of the liver. As a result of efforts to discourage use of aspirin in childhood febrile illnesses, there has been a marked decrease in the number of patients with Reye's syndrome. The precise relationship, however, between aspirin and Reye's syndrome is not clear.

Ashwal S et al: Bacterial meningitis in children. Neurology 1992;42:739.

Brook I: Brain abscess in children: Microbiology and management. J Child Neurol 1995;10:283.

Burns D: The neuropathology of pediatric acquired immunodeficiency syndrome. J Child Neurol 1992;7:332.

Chamberlain MC: Pediatric AIDS: Longitudinal comparative MRI and CT brain imaging study. J Child Neurol 1993;8:175.

Epstein LG, Gendelman HE: Human immunodeficiency virus type 1 infection of the nervous system: Pathogenetic mechanisms. Ann Neurol 1993;33:429.

Quagliarello V, Scheld WM: Drug therapy: Treatment of bacterial meningitis. N Engl J Med 1997;336:708.

Schaad UB et al: Dexamethasone therapy for bacterial meningitis in children. Lancet 1993;342:457.

SYNDROMES PRESENTING AS ACUTE FLACCID PARALYSIS

Flaccid paralysis evolving over hours or a few days suggests involvement of the lower motor neuron complex (see Floppy Infant Syndrome). **Anterior horn cells** (spinal cord) may be involved by viral infection (paralytic poliomyelitis) or by paraviral or postviral immunologically mediated disease (acute transverse myelitis). The **nerve trunks** (polyneuritis) may be diseased as in Guillain-Barré syndrome or affected by toxins (diphtheria, porphyria). The **neuromuscular junction** may be blocked by tick toxin or botulinum toxin. The paralysis rarely will be due to metabolic (periodic paralysis) or inflammatory muscle disease (myositis). *A lesion compressing the spinal cord must be ruled out.*

Clinical Findings

A. Symptoms and Signs: (Table 22–26.) Features assisting diagnosis are age, a history of preceding or waning illness, the presence (at time of paralysis) of fever, rapidity of progression, cranial nerve findings, and sensory findings. The examination may show "long tract" findings (pyramidal tract), causing increased reflexes and positive Babinski sign. The spinothalamic tract may be interrupted, causing loss of pain and temperature. Back pain, even tenderness to percussion, may occur, as well as bowel and bladder incontinence. Often, the paralysis is ascending, symmetric, and painful (muscle tenderness or myalgia). Laboratory findings occasionally are diagnostic.

B. Laboratory Findings: (Table 22–26.) The examination of spinal fluid is most helpful. Imaging studies of the spinal column (plain films) and spinal cord (MRI, myelogram) are occasionally essential. Viral cultures (spinal fluid, throat, stool) and titers aid in diagnosing poliomyelitis. A high sedimentation rate may suggest tumor or abscess; ANA may suggest lupus arteritis.

Electromyography and nerve conduction velocity can be helpful in diagnosing polyneuropathy. Nerve conduction is usually slowed after 7–10 days. Findings in botulism and tick-bite paralysis can be specific and diagnostic. Rarely, elevation of muscle enzymes—or even myoglobinuria—may aid in diagnosis of myopathic paralysis. Porphyrin urine studies and heavy metal assays (arsenic, thallium, lead) can reveal those rare toxic causes of polyneuropathic paralysis.

Differential Diagnosis

The child who has been well and becomes paralyzed often has polyneuritis. Acute transverse myelitis sometimes occurs in an afebrile child. The child who is ill and febrile at the time of paralysis often has acute transverse myelitis (or poliomyelitis); *acute* epidural spinal cord abscess (or other compressive lesion) must be ruled out. Poliomyelitis is very rare in our immunized population. Paralysis due to tick bites occurs seasonally (spring and summer). The tick is usually found in the occipital hair. Removal is curative.

Paralysis due to botulism occurs most commonly under age 1; food-borne and wound botulism are very rare. An investigative history and laboratory studies are diagnostic. Intravenous drug abuse can lead to myelitis and paralysis. Furthermore, *chronic* myelopathy occurs with two human immunodeficiency virus infections, HTLV-I and HTLV-III (now called HIV-1).

Complications

A. Respiratory Paralysis: Early and careful attention to oxygenation is essential; administration of oxygen, intubation, mechanical respiratory assistance, and careful suctioning of secretions may be required. Increasing anxiety and a rise in diastolic and systolic blood pressures are early signs of hypoxia. Cyanosis is a late sign. Deteriorating spirometric findings (forced expiratory volume in 1 second [FEV_1] and total vital capacity) may indicate the need for controlled intubation and respiratory support.

B. Infections: Pneumonia is common, especially in cases of respiratory paralysis. Prophylactic antibiotic administration is generally contraindicated. Antibiotic therapy is best guided by results of cultures. Bladder infections occur when an indwelling catheter is required because of bladder paralysis. Recovery from myelitis may be delayed by urinary tract infection.

C. Autonomic Crisis: This may be a cause of death in Guillain-Barré syndrome; strict attention to vital signs to detect and treat hypotension or hypertension and cardiac arrhythmias in an intensive care setting is advisable, at least early in the course in severely ill patients.

Treatment

There is no specific treatment in most of these syndromes; however, ticks causing paralysis must be removed. Other therapies include the use of erythromycin in *Mycoplasma* infections and botulism equine antitoxin in wound botulism. Recognized associated disorders (eg, endocrine, neoplastic, toxic) should be treated by appropriate means. Supportive care also involves pulmonary toilet, adequate fluids and nutrition, bladder and bowel care, prevention of decubiti, and, in many cases, psychiatric support.

A. Corticosteroids: These agents are believed by most to be of no benefit in Guillain-Barré syndrome. Autonomic symptoms (eg, hypertension) in polyneuritis may require treatment.

Table 22–26. Acute flaccid paralysis in children.

	Poliomyelitis (Paralytic, Spinal, and Bulbar), With or Without Encephalitis	Landry-Guillain-Barré Syndrome ("Acute Idiopathic Polyneuritis")	Botulism	Tick-Bite Paralysis	Transverse Myelitis and Neuromyelitis Optica
Etiology	Poliovirus types I, II, and III; other enteroviruses; vaccine strain poliovirus (rare)	Likely delayed hypersensitivity-immunologic. Mycoplasmal and viral infections (including infectious mononucleosis) and various systemic or toxic disorders may be underlying cause. *Campylobacter* enteritis. Hepatitis B.	*Clostridium botulinum* toxin. Block at neuromuscular junction. Under age 1, toxin forms in bowel from ingested dust or honey in formula. At older ages, contaminated food (preformed toxin). Rarely from wound infection.	Probable interference with transmission of nerve impulse caused by toxin in tick saliva	Usually unknown; multiple viruses (herpes, EBV, varicella, hepatitis A) often postviral (see Guillain-Barré syndrome)
History	None, or inadequate polio immunization. Upper respiratory or gastrointestinal symptoms followed by brief respite. Bulbar paralysis more frequent after tonsillectomy. Often in epidemics, in summer and early fall.	Nonspecific respiratory or gastrointestinal symptoms in preceding 5–14 days common. Any season, though slightly lower incidence in summer.	Infancy: dusty environment (eg, construction area), suburbs; honey. Older: "food poisoning." Multiple cases hours to days after ingesting contaminated food.	Exposure to ticks (dog tick in eastern United States; wood ticks). Irritability 12–24 hours before onset of a rapidly progressive ascending paralysis.	Rarely symptoms compatible with multiple sclerosis or optic neuritis. Progression from onset to paraplegia often rapid, usually without a history of bacterial infection.
Presenting complaints	Febrile at time of paralysis. Meningeal signs, muscle tenderness, and spasm. Asymmetric weakness widespread or segmental (cervical, thoracic, lumbar). Bulbar symptoms early or before extremity weakness; anxiety; delirium.	Symmetric weakness of lower extremities, which may ascend rapidly to arms, trunk, and face. Verbal child may complain of paresthesias. Fever uncommon. Facial weakness early. Miller-Fisher variant presents as ataxia and ophthalmoplegia.	Infancy: constipation, poor suck and cry. "Floppy." Apnea. Lethargy. Choking (cause of SIDS?). Older: blurred vision, diplopia, ptosis, choking, weakness.	Rapid onset and progression of ascending flaccid paralysis; often accompanied by pain and paresthesias. Paralysis of upper extremities usually occurs on second day after onset.	Root and back pain in about one-third to one-half of cases. Sensory loss below level of lesion accompanying rapidly developing paralysis. Sphincter difficulties common.
Findings	Flaccid weakness, usually asymmetric. Cord level: Lumbar: legs, lower abdomen Cervical: shoulder, arm, neck, diaphragm Thoracic: intercostals, spine, upper abdomen Bulbar: respiratory lower cranial nerves Fever in first days	Flaccid weakness, symmetric, usually greater proximally, but may be more distal or equal in distribution. Facial diplegia in about 85%, rarely IX–XI, III–VI. Bulbar involvement may occur. Slight distal impairment of position, vibration, touch; difficult to assess in young children.	Infants: flaccid weakness. Alert. Eye, pupil, facial weakness. Deep tendon reflexes decreased to 0? Absent suck, gag. Constipation. Older: paralysis accommodation, eye movements. Weak swallow. Respiratory paralysis.	Flaccid, symmetric paralysis. Cranial nerve and bulbar (respiratory) paralysis, ataxia, sphincter disturbances, and sensory deficits may occur. Some fever. Diagnosis rests on finding tick, which is especially likely to be on occipital scalp.	Paraplegia with areflexia below level of lesion early; later, may have hyperreflexia. Sensory loss below and hyperesthesia or normal sensation above level of lesion. Paralysis of bladder and rectum. Optic neuritis rarely may be present.
CSF	Pleocytosis (20–500+ cells) with PMN predominance in first few days, followed by rapid decrease and monocytic preponderance. Glucose normal. Protein frequently elevated (50–150 mg/dL).	Cytoalbuminologic dissociation; ten or fewer mononuclear cells with high protein after first week. Normal glucose. IgG may be elevated.	Normal	Normal	Usually no manometric block; CSF may show increased protein, pleocytosis with predominantly mononuclear cells, increased IgG

(continued)

Table 22–26. Acute flaccid paralysis in children. (continued)

	Poliomyelitis (Paralytic, Spinal, and Bulbar), With or Without Encephalitis	Landry-Guillain-Barré Syndrome ("Acute Idiopathic Polyneuritis")	Botulism	Tick-Bite Paralysis	Transverse Myelitis and Neuromyelitis Optica
EMG	Denervation after 10–21 days. Nerve conduction normal.	Nerve conduction velocities markedly decreased; may be normal early, or axon only damage.	EMG distinctive: BSAP ("brief small abundant potentials").	Nerve conduction slowed; returns rapidly to normal after removal of tick	Normal early. Denervation at level of lesion after 10–21 days.
Other studies	Initially, leukocytosis. Virus in stool and throat. Serologic titers.	Search for specific cause such as infection, intoxication, metabolic or endocrine disease, allergic phenomena, neoplasm. Lymphocyte transformation demonstrated. *Mycoplasma pneumoniae* implicated in some cases.	Infancy: stool culture, toxin. Rare serum toxin positive, Older: serum (or wound) toxin.	Leukocytosis, often with moderate eosinophilia	Normal spine x-rays do not exclude spinal epidural abscess. MRI has largely replaced myelography to rule out cord-compressive lesions. Cord may be swollen myelitis.
Course and prognosis	Paralysis usually maximal 3–5 days after onset. Transient bladder paralysis may occur. Outlook varies with extent and severity of involvement. *Note:* Mortality greatest from respiratory failure and superinfection. Early muscle atrophy common.	Course progressive over a few days to about 2 weeks. Transient bladder paralysis may occur. *Note:* Threat greatest from respiratory failure, autonomic crises (eg, widely variable BP, arrhythmia), and superinfection. Majority recover completely. Plasmapheresis may have a role. Intravenous IgG (IGIV) relapses occasionally occur.	Infancy: supportive. Penicillin. Purge stool. Antitoxin unnecessary. Respiratory support (prolonged often), gavage feeding. Avoid aminoglycosides. Older: penicillin, antitoxin, prolonged respiratory support. Prognosis: excellent with good quality intensive care. Fatality 3%.	Total removal of tick is followed by rapid improvement and recovery. Otherwise, mortality rate due to respiratory paralysis is very high.	Large degree of functional recovery possible. Corticosteroids are of controversial benefit in shortening duration of acute attack or altering the overall course.

B. Plasmapheresis: Plasma exchange or intravenous immunoglobulin G (IgG) has been beneficial in severe cases of Guillain-Barré syndrome.

C. Physical Therapy: Rehabilitative measures are best instituted when acute symptoms have subsided and the patient is stable.

D. Antibiotics: Appropriate antibiotics and drainage are required for epidermal abscess.

Prognosis

Prognosis varies greatly with the extent of involvement, duration of the inflammatory process, complications, and other factors.

Bleck TP: IVIG for GBS: Potential problems in the alphabet soup. Neurology 1993;43:857.

Bolton CF: The changing concepts of Guillain-Barré syndrome. (Editorial.) N Engl J Med 1995;333:1415.

Evans OB, Vedanarayanan V: Guillain-Barré syndrome. Pediatr Rev 1997;18:10.

Irani DN et al: Relapse in Guillain-Barré syndrome after treatment with human immune globulin. Neurology 1993;43:872.

Johnson RT, McArthur J: Myelopathic and retrovirus infections. Ann Neurol 1987;21:113.

Khatri BO et al: Plasmapheresis with acute inflammatory polyneuropathy. Pediatr Neurol 1990;6:17.

Plasma Exchange/Sandoglobulin GBS Trial Group: Randomized trial of plasma exchange, intravenous immunoglobulin, and combined treatments in Guillain-Barré syndrome. Lancet 1997;349:225.

Ropper AH, Wijdicks EFM, Truax BT: *Guillain-Barré Syndrome.* Davis, 1993.

Vriesendorp FJ et al: Serum antibodies to GM_1, GD_{1b}, peripheral nerve myelin, and *Campylobacter jejuni* in patients with Guillain-Barré syndrome and controls: Correlation and prognosis. Ann Neurol 1993;34:130.

DISORDERS OF CHILDHOOD AFFECTING MUSCLES

This section is concerned with specific muscle and neuromuscular disorders, including the muscular dystrophies, myasthenia gravis, and miscellaneous congenital neuromuscular disorders (Table 22–27).

Certain studies that are commonly used in the diagnosis of muscle diseases merit special consideration.

Serum Enzymes

CK (creatine kinase) reflects muscle damage or "leak" from muscle into plasma. Blood should be drawn before electromyography or muscle biopsy, which may lead to release of the enzyme. Corticosteroids may suppress levels despite very active muscle disease.

Muscle Imaging

MRI scans are used in research studies to assist the diagnosis and assessment of muscular dystrophies, congenital myopathies and myotonias, and spinal muscular atrophies.

Electromyography (EMG)

Electromyography is often helpful in grossly differentiating **myopathic** from **neurogenic** processes. Fibrillations occur in both. In the myopathies, very low spikes are more typical, and the motor unit action potentials seen during contraction characteristically are of short duration, polyphasic, and increased in number for the strength of the contraction (increased interference pattern). Neurogenic findings include decreased numbers of motor units, which may be polyphasic, larger than normal, or both. The interference pattern is decreased. In myotonic dystrophy, the EMG is characterized by prolonged discharge of electrical activity on movement of the probing needle ("dive bomber" sound).

Muscle Biopsy

Properly executed (by "open" biopsy or by using the Bergstrom muscle biopsy needle), this procedure is usually most helpful. Histochemical techniques, histogram analysis of muscle fiber types and sizes, and electron microscopy are offering new classifications of the myopathies. Findings common to the dystrophies include variation in the size and shape of muscle fibers, increase in connective tissue, interstitial infiltration of fatty tissue, degenerative changes in muscle fibers, and central location of nuclei.

Dystrophin is a normal intracellular plasma membrane protein in muscle, the gene product missing in Duchenne's (and Becker's) dystrophy. Staining the muscle for dystrophin aids in differentiating Duchenne's from Becker's dystrophy; dystrophin is absent in Duchenne's, reduced in Becker's dystrophy. Electrophoresis can confirm whether the dystrophin is absent or present in small amounts and whether there is a qualitative difference from normal dystrophin, the latter two patterns being characteristic of Becker's dystrophy.

Genetic Testing
& Carrier Detection

To date, detection of carriers for Duchenne's dys-

trophy (mothers and sisters of affected boys) has rested on CK elevations (two-thirds will have this finding); physical findings of mild dystrophy (large calves, muscle weakness); abnormal muscle EMGs; or biopsy results. All are unreliable for diagnostic purposes.

DNA probes are now available for carrier detection and prenatal diagnosis of Duchenne's and Becker's dystrophy. Deletions are often found on the short arm of the X chromosome; it is postulated that all patients and most mothers will show deletions when sufficient probes are developed to search the whole Duchenne genome (perhaps 4000 kb in length).

Amplification of DNA by the polymerase chain reactions (PCR) can detect the deletion. Moreover, this technique plus Southern blot analysis can detect abnormal DNA base repeats. For example, in myotonic dystrophy, a GCT triplet excess is currently the most sensitive test for that disease. The tests can be used for intrauterine diagnosis and prediction of whether the triplet is within the normal or mutant range. Thus, in many cases, the greater the number of repeats, the more severely involved the fetus or patient.

Mutations (especially deletions) of survivor motor neuron (SMN) and neuronal apoptosis inhibitory protein (NAIP) gene on chromosome 5q13 are present in 95% of patients with spinal muscular atrophy.

Lastly, Kearns-Sayer progressive external ophthalmoplegia with retinopathy is inherited via maternal cytoplasmic mitochondria. Assay of mutations and deletions from blood or muscle samples are now commercially available.

Therapy for Duchenne's muscular dystrophy continues to be frustrating. Prednisone in low doses has increased muscle strength and prolonged ambulation. Research emphasis is on gene therapy, but there is great difficulty in finding viral vectors able to carry the very large dystrophin gene into muscle cells.

Connolly AM et al: Congenital muscular dystrophy syndromes distinguished by alkaline and acid phosphatase, merosin, and dystrophin staining. Neurology 1996; 46:810.

Engel A: Gene therapy for Duchenne dystrophy. Ann Neurol 1993;34:3.

Fidzianska A: Spinal muscular atrophy in childhood. Semin Pediatr Neurol 1996;3:53.

Hilton T et al: End of life care in Duchenne muscular dystrophy. Pediatr Neurol 1993;9:165.

Hoffman EP: Characterization of dystrophin in muscle biopsy specimens from patients with Duchenne's or Becker's muscular dystrophy. N Engl J Med 1988; 318:1363.

Holt IF et al: Mitochondrial myopathies: Clinical and biochemical features of 30 patients with major deletions of muscle mitochondrial DNA. Ann Neurol 1989;26:699.

Karpati G et al: Myoblast transfer in muscular dystrophy. Ann Neurol 1993;34:8.

Mendell JR, Sahenk Z, Prior TW: The childhood muscular dystrophies: Diseases sharing a common pathogenesis of membrane instability. J Child Neurol 1995;10:150.

Table 22–27. Muscular dystrophies and myotonias of childhood.

Disease	Genetic Pattern	Age at Onset	Early Manifestations	Involved Muscles	Reflexes
Muscular dystrophies Duchenne's muscular dystrophy (pseudohypertrophic infantile)	X-linked recessive; autosomal recessive unusual. 30–50% have no family history.	2–6 years; rarely in infancy	Clumsiness, easy fatigability on walking, running, and climbing stairs. Walking on toes; waddling gait. Lordosis. (Climbing up on legs rising from supine position—Gower's maneuver.)	Axial and proximal before distal. Pelvic girdle; pseudohypertrophy of gastrocnemius (90%), triceps brachii, and vastus lateralis. Shoulder girdle usually later, also articulation difficulties. Eventually cardiomyopathy (50%).	Knee jerks ± or 0; ankle jerks + to ++
Becker's muscular dystrophy (late onset)	X-linked recessive. (Allele at Xp21)	Childhood (usually later than in Duchenne's)	Similar to Duchenne's	Similar to Duchenne's	Similar to Duchenne's
Limb-girdle muscular dystrophy A. Pelvifemoral (Leyden-Möbius) B. Scapulohumeral (Erb's juvenile) (Chromosome 15)	Autosomal recessive in 60%; high sporadic incidence. A. Relatively common B. Rare	Variable; early childhood to adulthood	Weakness, with distribution according to type. Waddling gait, difficulty climbing stairs. Lordosis.	A. Pelvic girdle usually involved first and to greater extent. B. Shoulder girdle often asymmetric. Quadriceps and hamstrings may be weakest. Pseudohypertrophy of calves uncommon.	Usually present
Facioscapulohumeral muscular dystrophy (Landouzy-Déjérine) scapuloperoneal variant	Autosomal dominant; sporadic cases not uncommon: Linkage to 4q35	Usually late in childhood and adolescence; rare in infancy; not uncommon in 20s	Diminished facial movements with inability to close eyes, smile, or whistle. Face may be flat; unlined. Difficulty in raising arms over head. Lordosis. Tripping in scapuloperoneal type.	Facial muscles followed by shoulder girdle, with occasional spread to hips or distal legs (scapuloperoneal variant)	Present
Spinal muscular atrophy (SMA) Infantile SMA (Werdnig-Hoffman disease)	Autosomal recessive	0–2 years	Floppy infant	"Big" muscles: shoulder, hip. Tongue. Intercostals. Fingerstoes spared.	0 or nearly so
Juvenile SMA (Kugelburg-Welander disease)	Autosomal recessive	Onset after age 2 usually (age 5–15 typical)	Weakness. "Fasciculations" 50%. Rarely a cause of "floppy infant."	Same	Same
Metabolic myopathies Carnitine deficiency (lipid storage myopathy) Primary (rare) Secondary: multiple forms	Genetics variable	Infancy to adolescence	Fasting hypoglycemia and coma; less ketosis than expected. Myopathy. Cardiomyopathy. Fatty liver. Don't confuse with Reye's, SIDS.	Weakness variable; may be precipitated by exercise (with resultant myoglobinuria) or fasting	Normal to decreased
"Oculocraniosomatic syndrome" (ophthalmoplegia and "ragged reds"; progressive external ophthalmoplegia) Kearns-Sayer	(?) Acquired; 80% female; other hereditary neurologic disorders may be found in patient or family	Variable; from infancy to adult life; most at about 10 years of age	Ptosis and limitation of eye movements; hearing and visual loss (retinitis pigmentosa); intellectual loss; cerebellular disturbance (ataxia)	Extraocular muscles, often asymmetric. Variable involvement of axial muscles; cardiac muscles, with conduction defect.	Depressed to ± or 0
Myasthenia gravis Transient neonatal	Variable	At birth	Difficulty sucking, swallowing; trouble with secretions	Somatic and cranial muscles	Normal to decreased

(continued)

Table 22–27. Muscular dystrophies and myotonias of childhood. (continued)

Muscle Biopsy Findings	Other Diagnostic Tests	Treatment	Prognosis
Degeneration and variation in fiber size; proliferation of connective tissue. Basophilia, phagocytosis. Poor differentiation of fiber types on ATPase reaction; deficiency of type 2B fibers. Dystrophin absent.	EMG myopathic. CK (4000–5000 IU) very high with decrease toward normal over the years. ECG. Chest x-ray. Cloned dystrophin cDNA probes to detect deletions on Xp21 chromosome from blood, amniotic fluid, chorionic villi. Sixty percent show deletion.	Physical therapy, braces, wheelchair eventually, weight control	Ten percent show nonprogressive mental retardation. Death from pneumonia 10–15 years after diagnosis with 75% of patients dead by age 20.
Similar to above, except type 2B fibers present. Reduced or abnormal size dystrophin.	Similar to above, although muscle enzymes may not be as elevated	As above. Wheelchair in late childhood or early adult life.	Slower progression than Duchenne's, with death usually in adulthood
Variation in muscle fiber size with many very large fibers. Fiber splitting and internal nuclei common. Many "moth-eaten" whorled fibers. Dystrophin normal.	EMG myopathic. CK variable; often normal but may be elevated ECG.	Physical therapy, weight control	Mildly progressive: spread from lower to upper limbs may take 15–20 years. Life expectancy mid to late adulthood.
Predominantly large fibers with scattered tiny atrophic fibers, "moth-eaten" and whorled fibers. Inflammatory response. Little or no fiber splitting, fibrosis, or type 1 fiber predominance.	EMG myopathic. Muscle enzymes usually normal.	Physical therapy where indicated. Wheelchair in 20%. Forty percent of biopsies show inflammation; steroids ineffective, however.	Very slowly progressive, often with plateaus, except in infantile form where there may be difficulties in walking by adolescence. Usually normal life span.
Small, group atrophy. Twin peak fiber size. Fiber type grouping. Minimal fibrosis.	EMG "neuropathic." Nerve conduction, CSF, muscle enzymes normal. Ninety to 95 percent have deletions or abnormalities in SMN ("survival motor neuron") or other genes at band 5q13.	Supportive: respiratory care, positioning, secretion management. Genetic counseling.	80–95% of patients 0–4 years die of pneumonia and respiratory failure.
Same		Physical therapy, wheelchair positioning to avoid scoliosis. May walk, usually later lose this.	Fairly normal life expectancy. 4–40+ years.
Normal or lipid droplets ("Ragged red" fibers with lipid stain, eg, oil red O).	Muscle biochemistry (carnitine, CPT enzyme). Urine organic acids (at time of illness). Plasma carnitine. WBC, fibroblast enzyme studies.	Avoid fasting and mitochondrial toxins, eg, ASA, valproic acid. Carbohydrate. Treat acidosis. Carnitine orally.	Variable: occasionally fatal in infants. Progressive weakness, developmental delay, cardiomyopathy may occur.
Mitochondrial abnormalities. "Ragged red" fibers. Changes in fiber size, usually due to type 2 fiber atrophy.	CK usually normal. ECG with conduction block. CSF protein elevated. Nerve conduction slowed. CT, brain scan, and brain stem auditory evoked response may be abnormal. Mitochondrial deletions.	Plastic retraction of eyelids. Cardiac support. Anticipate diabetes mellitus. Coenzyme Q?	Dysphagia may develop (50%) as well as generalized muscle weakness. Prognosis fail if disease is confined to ocular muscles. In severe cases, spongy vacuolization of brain and brain stem.
Unnecessary	Edrophonium or neostigmine tests. Acetylcholine receptor (AChR) antibodies. Repetitive nerve stimulation, EMG.	Supportive. Anticholinergic drugs.	Usually transient (< 2 months)

Table 22–27. Muscular dystrophies and myotonias of childhood. (continued)

Disease	Genetic Pattern	Age at Onset	Early Manifestations	Involved Muscles	Reflexes
Persistent neonatal	Variable	Variable: birth, neonatal, infancy	Same	Same	Same
Congenital myopathies Myotonic dystrophy (Neonatal onset)	Autosomal dominant	At birth	Same as myasthenia. Ptosis. Facial diplegia. Arthrogyposis, club feet, thin ribs.	Cranial and somatic, pharyngeal.	Decreased to 0
"Other" Central core Nemaline (rod body) Myotubular (centronuclear) Congenital fiber type disproportion	Variable, often autosomal recessive	Severe variants present at birth; milder variants (more common) infancy, childhood	Severe variant, as in myasthenia, myotonic dystrophy. Later presentation—facial weakness, mild to moderate weakness, even "toe walking" only.	Similar to myotonic dystrophy	Decreased to 0
Congenital muscular dystrophy (Fukayama)	Genetic Chromosome 9dq31–33. Autosomal recessive.	Birth	Hypotonia. Facial weakness, joint contractures, mental retardation. Ocular abnormalities.	Heterogenous. Facial (cranial) and somatic. Contracture common.	Variable
Congenital muscular dystrophy ("occidental")	Unknown; usually not familial	Birth (or early infancy)	As above. Normal IQ.	Same	Same
Benign congenital hypotonia (Oppenheim)	Variable	Variable	Hypotonia only. Deep tendon reflexes positive. Laboratory tests, biopsy normal.	Somatic muscles (respiratory muscles spared)	Normal to decreased
Myotonias Myotonia congenita (Thomsen)	Autosomal dominant (autosomal recessive cases reported)	Early infancy to late childhood	Difficulty in relaxing muscles after contracting them, especially after sleep; aggravated by cold, excitement.	Hands especially; muscles may be diffusely enlarged, giving patient herculean appearance.	Normal
Myotonic dystrophy (Steinert) (childhood and adult form)	Autosomal dominant	Late childhood to adolescence; neonatal and infantile forms increasingly recognized (see above)	Myotonia of grasp, tongue; worsened by cold, emotions. "Hatchet-face." Nasal voice. Weakness and easy fatigability. Mild to moderate mental retardation noted.	Wasting, weakness of facial muscles, (mastication); sternocleidomastoids, hands. Myotonic phenomena: "bunching up" of muscles of tongue, thenar eminance, finger extensors after tapping with percussion hammer.	In infantile form, marked hyporeflexia

(continued)

Miller G, Wessel HB: Diagnosis of dystrophinopathies: Review for the clinician. Pediatr Neurol 1993;9:3.

Miller RG, Hoffman EP: Molecular diagnosis and modern management of Duchenne muscular dystrophy. Neurol Clin 1994;12:699.

Milu JM, Gilbert-Barnes E: Type I spinal muscular atrophy (Werdnig-Hoffman disease). Am J Dis Child 1993;147:908.

Parano E et al: Congenital muscular dystrophy: Clinical review and proposed classification. Pediatr Neurol 1995;13:97.

Pegoraro E et al: Congenital muscular dystrophy with pri-

Table 22–27. Muscular dystrophies and myotonias of childhood. (continued)

Muscle Biopsy Findings	Other Diagnostic Tests	Treatment	Prognosis
Sophisticated end plate, nerve terminal ultrastructural studies may be necessary	May be similar to above. AChR antibodies negative.	May not respond to ACh-ase drugs, steroids, or immunosuppressants	Variable, may have long-term severe course
Generalized fiber hypertrophy, delay in maturation. Type I atrophy. Internal nuclei.	EMG "myotonic" in some (waning amplitude and pitch). Test mother. CK often normal. DNA testing (chromosome 19) for GCT repeat.	Supportive, even respiratory support. Genetic counseling.	Severely involved infant may improve dramatically over months; expect mental retardation in this same variant
Distinctive diagnostic histochemistry, eg, "central cores," "nemaline rods," myotubes type II–I fibers of unequal size	Myopathic EMG	Supportive. Genetic counseling.	Variable. May shorten life. Death in infancy or severe handicap. Scoliosis prominent.
"Dystrophic" changes. Fibrosis. Necrotic fibers. Internal nuclei. ? regenerative fibers.	Myopathic EMG. CK increased or normal. Positive CT, MRI scans: white matter low density, polymicrogyria, lissencephaly, etc.	Supportive	Physical and mental handicap lifelong
Same	As above, CT, MRI variably low density; may have absent dystrophin-associated protein (DAP), merosin deficiency		May improve, walk. Scoliosis.
Normal with sophisticated studies (histochemistry, electron microscopy, even metabolic studies)	Use of this diagnosis is shrinking with increasingly sophisticated biochemical (eg, cytochrome oxidase) studies	Supportive	Good (by definition). (Few documented long-term studies.)
Nonspecific and minor changes; type 2B fibers may be absent	EMG "myotonic"	Usually none. Phenytoin, especially in cold weather, may improve muscle functioning.	Normal life expectancy, with only mild disability
Type I fiber atrophy, type 2 hypertrophy, sarcoplasmic masses, internal nuclei, phagocytosis, fibrosis, and cellular reaction.	EMG markedly "myotonic." Glucose tolerance test, thyroid tests. ECG. Chest x-ray and pulmonary function tests. Immunoglobulins. PCR amplification of GCT repeat on chromosome 19q13 to distinguish normal from mutant alleles.	Procainamide, 250 mg 3 times daily orally, increased to tolerance; phenytoin 5–7 mg/kg/d orally. (Drugs usually little role.)	Frontal baldness, cataracts (85%), gonadal atrophy (85% of males), thyroid dysfunction, diabetes mellitus (20%). Cardiac conduction defects; impaired pulmonary function. Low IgG. Life expectancy decreased.

mary laminin (merosin) deficiency presenting as inflammatory myopathy. Ann Neurol 1996;40:782.

Redman JB et al: Relationship between parental trinucleotide GTC repeat length and severity of myotonic dystrophy in offspring. JAMA 1993;269:1960.

Roland EM: Neuromuscular diseases in childhood. Curr Opin Pediatr 1994;6:636.

Russman BS, Schwartz RC: Neuromuscular diseases of childhood. Curr Opin Pediatr 1993;5:669.

Russman BS: Rehabilitation of the pediatric patient with a neuromuscular disease. Neurol Clin 1990;8:727.

Spiro AJ: Muscular dystrophy. Pediatr Rev 1995;16:437.

Tawil R et al: A pilot trial of prednisone in facioscapulohumeral muscular dystrophy. Neurology 1997;48:46.

Tritschler HJ, Medori R: Mitochondrial DNA alterations as a source of human disorders. Neurology 1993;43:280.

Van der Knaap MS et al: Magnetic resonance imaging in classification of congenital muscular dystrophies with brain abnormalities. Ann Neurol 1997;42:50.

Voskova-Goldman A et al: DMD-specific FISH probes are diagnostically useful in the detection of female carriers of DMD gene deletions. Neurology 1997;48:1633.

Wang CH et al: Extensive DNA deletion associated with severe disease alleles on spinal muscular atrophy homologues. Ann Neurol 1997;42:41.

Wolff JA: Gene therapy for neuromuscular disorders. Int Pediatr 1993;8:14.

BENIGN ACUTE CHILDHOOD MYOSITIS

Benign acute childhood myositis (myalgia cruris epidemica) is characterized by transient severe muscle pain and weakness affecting mainly the calves and occurring 1–2 days following an upper respiratory tract infection. Though symptoms involve mainly the gastrocnemius muscles, all skeletal muscles appear to be invaded directly by virus; recurrent episodes are due to different viral types. By seroconversion or isolation of the virus, acute myositis has been shown to be largely due to influenza types B and A and occasionally due to parainfluenza and adenovirus.

MYASTHENIA GRAVIS

Essentials of Diagnosis & Typical Features

- Weakness, chiefly of muscles innervated by the brain stem, usually coming on or increasing with use (fatigue).
- Positive response to neostigmine and edrophonium.
- Acetylcholine receptor antibodies in serum (except in congenital form).

General Considerations

Myasthenia gravis is characterized by easy fatigability of muscles, particularly the extraocular muscles and those of mastication, swallowing, and respiration. In the neonatal period, however, or in early infancy, the weakness may be so constant and general that an affected infant may present nonspecifically as a "floppy infant." Girls are affected more frequently than boys. The age at onset is over 10 years in 75% of cases, often shortly after menarche. If diagnosed before age 10, congenital myasthenia should be considered in retrospect. Thyrotoxicosis is found in almost 10% of affected female patients. The essential abnormality is a circulating antibody that binds to the acetylcholine receptor protein and thus reduces the number of motor end plates for binding by acetylcholine.

Clinical Findings

A. Symptoms and Signs:

1. Neonatal (transient) myasthenia gravis– This disorder occurs in 12% of infants born to myasthenic mothers. The condition is due to maternal acetylcholine receptor antibody transferred across the placenta; a thymic factor in the infant may also be involved. A sibling may have died in the neonatal period with similar symptoms and nondiagnostic autopsy.

2. Congenital (persistent) myasthenia gravis– In this form of the disease, the mothers of the affected infants rarely have myasthenia gravis, but other relatives may. Sex distribution is equal. Symptoms are often subtle and not recognized initially. Differential diagnosis includes many other causes of the "floppy infant" syndrome, such as infant botulism, ocular myopathy, congenital ptosis, and Möbius' syndrome (facial nuclear aplasia and other anomalies). Congenital myasthenia gravis is not caused by receptor antibodies and often responds poorly to therapy. It may result from a genetic abnormality of the acetylcholine receptor protein or other neurotransmitter vagaries.

3. Juvenile myasthenia gravis– In this autoimmune form, the symptoms and signs are similar to those in adults. Receptor antibodies are usually present. The patient may be first seen by an otolaryngologist or psychiatrist. The more prominent signs are difficulty in chewing, dysphagia, a nasal voice, ptosis, and ophthalmoplegia. Pathologic fatigability of limbs, chiefly involving the proximal limb and neck muscles, may be more prominent than the bulbar signs and may lead to an initial diagnosis of conversion hysteria, muscular dystrophy, or polymyositis. Weakness may be limited to ocular muscles only. Associated disorders include autoimmune conditions, especially thyroid disease.

An acute fulminant form of myasthenia gravis has been reported in children of age 2–10 years and presents with rapidly progressive respiratory difficulties. Bulbar paralysis may evolve within 24 hours. There is no history of myasthenia. The differential diagnosis includes Guillain-Barré syndrome and bulbar poliomyelitis. Administration of anticholinesterase agents establishes the diagnosis and is lifesaving.

B. Laboratory Findings:

1. Neostigmine test– In newborns and very young infants, the neostigmine test may be preferable to the edrophonium (Tensilon) test because the longer duration of its response permits better observation, especially of sucking and swallowing movements. The test dose of neostigmine is 0.02 mg/kg subcutaneously, usually given with atropine, 0.01 mg/kg subcutaneously. There is a delay of about 10 minutes before the effect may be manifest. The physician should be prepared to suction secretions.

2. Edrophonium test– Testing with edrophonium is used in older children who are capable of cooperating in certain tasks, such as raising and lowering their eyelids and squeezing a sphygmomanometer bulb or the examiner's hands. The test dose is 0.1–1 mL intravenously, depending on the size of the child. Maximum improvement occurs within 2 minutes.

3. Other laboratory tests–Serum acetylcholine receptor antibodies are often found in the neonatal and juvenile forms. Ophthalmologic tests of ocular motility with edrophonium are often positive in patients able to cooperate. In juveniles, thyroid studies are appropriate.

C. Electrical Studies of Muscle: Repetitive stimulation of a motor nerve at slow rates (3/s) with recording over the appropriate muscle reveals a progressive fall in amplitude of the muscle potential in myasthenic patients. A maximal stimulus must be given. At higher rates of stimulation (50/s), there may be a transient repair of this defect before the progressive decline is seen.

If this study is negative, single-fiber electromyography is now employed to determine if "mean jitter" exceeds the normal rate.

D. Imaging: Chest x-ray and CT scanning in older children may disclose benign thymus enlargement. Thymus tumors are rare in children.

Treatment

A. General and Supportive Care: In the newborn or in a child in myasthenic or cholinergic crisis (see following text), suctioning of secretions is essential. Respiratory assistance may be required.

Treatment should be conducted by physicians with experience in this disorder.

B. Anticholinesterase Drug Therapy:

1. Pyridostigmine bromide–The dose must be adjusted for each patient. A frequent starting dose is 15–30 mg orally every 6 hours.

2. Neostigmine–Fifteen milligrams of neostigmine are roughly equivalent to 60 mg of pyridostigmine bromide. Neostigmine often causes gastric hypermotility with diarrhea, but it is the drug of choice in newborns, in whom prompt treatment may be lifesaving. It may be given parenterally.

3. Atropine–Atropine may be added on a maintenance basis to control mild cholinergic side effects such as hypersecretion, abdominal cramps, and nausea and vomiting.

4. Immunologic intervention–This is primarily with prednisone. Plasmapheresis is effective in removing acetylcholine receptor antibody in severely affected patients.

5. Myasthenic crisis–Relatively sudden difficulties in swallowing and respiration may be observed in myasthenic patients. Edrophonium results in dramatic but brief improvement; this may make evaluation of the condition of the small child difficult. Suctioning, tracheostomy, respiratory assistance, and fluid and electrolyte maintenance may be required.

6. Cholinergic crisis–Cholinergic crisis may result from overdosage of anticholinesterase drugs. The resulting weakness may be similar to that of myasthenia, and the muscarinic effects (diarrhea, sweating, lacrimation, miosis, bradycardia, hypotension) are often absent or difficult to evaluate. The edrophonium test may help to determine whether the patient is receiving too little of the drug or is manifesting toxic symptoms due to overdosage. Improvement after the drugs are withdrawn suggests cholinergic crisis. A respirator should be available. The patient may require atropine and tracheostomy.

C. Surgical Measures: Early thymectomy is beneficial in many patients whose disease is not confined to ocular symptoms; the effects may be delayed. Experienced surgical and postsurgical care are prerequisites.

Prognosis

Neonatal (transient) myasthenia presents a great threat to life, primarily due to aspiration of secretions. With proper treatment, the symptoms usually begin to disappear within a few days to 2–3 weeks, after which the child usually requires no further treatment.

In the congenital (persistent) form, the symptoms may initially be as acute as in the transient variety; more commonly, however, they are relatively benign and constant, with gradual worsening as the child grows older. Fatal cases occur.

In the juvenile form, patients may become resistant or unresponsive to anticholinesterase compounds and require corticosteroids or treatment in a hospital, where respiratory assistance can be given. The overall prognosis for survival, for remission, and for improvement after therapy with prednisone and thymectomy is favorable.

Death in myasthenic or cholinergic crisis may occur unless prompt treatment is given.

Engel AG: Myasthenia gravis and myasthenic syndromes: Neurologic progress. Ann Neurol 1984;16:519.

Gordon N: Congenital myasthenia. Dev Med Child Neurol 1986;28:810.

Lefvert AK, Osterman PO: Newborn infants to myasthenic mothers: A clinical study and investigation of acetylcholine receptor antibodies in 17 children. Neurology 1983;33:133.

Morel E et al: Neonatal myasthenia gravis: A new clinical and immunologic appraisal in 30 cases. Neurology 1988;38:138.

Pascuzzi RM, Coslett HB, Johns TR: Long-term corticosteroid treatment of myasthenia gravis: Report of 116 patients. Ann Neurol 1984;15:291.

PERIPHERAL NERVE PALSIES

1. FACIAL WEAKNESS

Facial asymmetry may be present at birth or may develop later, either suddenly or gradually, unilaterally or bilaterally. Nuclear or peripheral involvement of the facial nerves results in sagging or drooping of the mouth and inability to close one or both eyes, particularly when newborns and infants cry. Inability to wrinkle the forehead may be demonstrated in infants and young children by getting them to follow an object (light) moved vertically above the forehead. Loss of taste of the anterior two-thirds of the tongue on the involved side may be demonstrated in intelligent, cooperative children by age 4 or 5; playing with a younger child and the judicious use of a tongue blade may enable the physician to note whether the child's face puckers up when something sour (eg, lemon juice) is applied with a swab to the anterior tongue. Ability to wrinkle the forehead is preserved, owing to bilateral innervation, in supranuclear facial paralysis.

Injuries to the facial nerve at birth occur in 0.25–6.5% of consecutive live births. Forceps delivery is the cause in some cases; in others, the side of the face affected may have abutted in utero against the sacral prominence. Often, no cause can be established.

Acquired peripheral facial weakness (Bell's palsy) of sudden onset and unknown cause is common in children. It often follows a viral illness (postinfectious) or physical trauma (eg, cold). It may be a presenting sign of a disorder such as tumor, hypertension, infectious mononucleosis, herpes simplex, or Guillain-Barré syndrome, usually diagnosable by the history, physical examination, and appropriate laboratory tests.

Bilateral facial weakness in early life may be due to agenesis of the affected muscles or to nuclear causes (part of Möbius' syndrome) or may even be familial. Myasthenia gravis, polyneuritis, and myotonic dystrophy must be considered.

"Asymmetric crying facies," in which one side of the lower lip depresses with crying (this is the normal side) and the other does not, is a common innocent congenital malformation inherited as an autosomal dominant. The defect in the parent (the asymmetry often improves with age) may be almost inapparent. Electromyography suggests congenital absence of the depressor anguli oris muscle of the lower lip. Forceps pressure is often erroneously incriminated as a cause of this innocent congenital anomaly. Occasionally, other major (eg, cardiac septal) congenital defects accompany the palsy.

In the vast majority of cases of isolated peripheral facial palsy—both those present at birth and those acquired later—improvement begins within 1–2 weeks, and near or total recovery of function is observed within 2 months. Methylcellulose drops, 1%, should be instilled into the eyes to protect the cornea during the day; at night, the lid should be taped down with cellophane tape. Upward massage of the face for 5–10 minutes three or four times a day may help maintain muscle tone. Prednisone therapy reduces the pain of Bell's palsy and promotes recovery of facial strength. Acyclovir (herpes antiviral agent) therapy may have a role.

In the few children with permanent and cosmetically disfiguring facial weakness, plastic surgical intervention at 6 years of age or older may be of benefit. New procedures, such as attachment of facial muscles to the temporal muscle or transplantation of cranial nerve XI, are being developed.

Murakami S et al: Bell palsy and herpes simplex virus: Identification of viral DNA in endoneurial fluid and muscle. Ann Intern Med 1996;124:27.

Painter ML, Bergman I: Obstetrical trauma to the neonatal central and peripheral nervous system. Semin Perinatol 1982;6:89.

Sudarshan A, Goldie WD: The spectrum of congenital facial diplegia (Moebius syndrome). Pediatr Neurol 1985; 1:180.

Wilson Chris, Grant CC: Facial nerve palsy secondary to Epstein-Barr virus infection. Arch Pediatr Adolesc Med 1997;151:739.

CHRONIC POLYNEUROPATHY

Polyneuropathy, usually insidious in onset and slowly progressive, occurs in children of any age. The presenting complaints are chiefly disturbances of gait and easy fatigability in walking or running and, slightly less often, weakness or clumsiness of the hands. Pain, tenderness, or paresthesias are less frequently mentioned. Neurologic examination discloses muscular weakness, greatest in the distal portions of the extremities, with steppage gait and depressed or absent deep tendon reflexes. Cranial nerves are sometimes affected. Sensory deficits (difficult to demonstrate in fearful children or those under 5 years of age) occur in a stocking and glove distribution. The muscles may be tender, and trophic changes such as glassy or "parchment" skin and absent sweating may occur. Thickening of the ulnar and peroneal nerves may be felt. Pure sensory neuropathies show up as chronic trauma; that is, the patient does not feel minor trauma and burns to the fingers and toes.

Known causes include (1) toxins (lead, arsenic, mercurials, vincristine, and benzene); (2) systemic disorders (diabetes mellitus, chronic uremia, recurrent hypoglycemia, porphyria, polyarteritis nodosa, and lupus erythematosus); (3) "inflammatory" states (chronic or recurrent Guillain-Barré syndrome and neuritis associated with mumps or diphtheria); (4) hereditary, often degenerative conditions, which in some classifications include certain storage diseases, leukodystrophies, spinocerebellar degenerations with neurogenic components, and Bassen-Kornzweig syndrome (Table 22–27); and (5) hereditary sensory or combined motor and sensory neuropathies. Polyneuropathies associated with carcinomas, beriberi or other vitamin deficiencies, or excessive vitamin B_6 intake are not reported or are exceedingly rare in children.

The most common chronic neuropathy of insidious onset often has no identifiable cause. This "chronic idiopathic neuropathy" is assumed to be immunologically mediated and may have a relapsing course. Sometimes there is facial weakness. Spinal fluid protein is elevated. Nerve conduction is slowed, and nerve biopsies are abnormal. Immunologic abnormalities are seldom demonstrated, although nerve biopsies may show round cell infiltration. Corticosteroids and other immunosuppressants may give long-term benefit.

Of the four defined hereditary sensory neuropathies, the prototype is **familial dysautonomia,** also called Riley-Day syndrome and hereditary sensory neuropathy type III. Transmitted as an autosomal recessive trait and seen mostly in Jewish children, this disorder has its onset in infancy. It is characterized by vomiting and difficulties in feeding that are due to abnormal esophageal motility, pulmonary infections, decreased or absent tearing, indifference to pain, diminished or absent tendon reflexes, absence of fungiform papillae of the tongue, emotional lability, abnormal temperature control with excessive sweating, labile blood pressure, abnormal intradermal histamine responses, and other evidences of autonomic dysfunction.

A careful genetic history (pedigree) and examination and electrical testing (motor and sensory nerve conduction, electromyography) of relatives are keys to diagnosis of hereditary neuropathy. This is the most common cause of chronic neuropathy in children.

Other hereditary neuropathies may have ataxia as a prominent finding often overshadowing the neuropathy. Examples are Friedreich's ataxia, dominant cerebellar ataxia, and Marinesco-Sjögren syndrome. Finally, some hereditary neuropathies are associated with identifiable and occasionally treatable metabolic errors (Table 22–28). These disorders are described in more detail in other sections.

Laboratory diagnosis of chronic polyneuropathy is made by measurement of motor and sensory nerve conduction velocities; electromyography may show a neurogenic polyphasic pattern. Cerebrospinal fluid protein levels are often elevated, sometimes with an increased IgG index as well. Nerve biopsy, with teasing of the fibers as well as staining for metachromasia, may demonstrate loss of myelin and (to a lesser degree) loss of axons and increased connective tissue or concentric lamellas ("onion skin" appearance) around the nerve fiber. Muscle biopsy may show the pattern associated with denervation. Other laboratory studies directed toward specific causes mentioned above include screening for heavy metals and for metabolic, renal, or vascular disorders. Chronic lead intoxication, which rarely causes neuropathy in childhood, may escape detection until the child is given edetate calcium disodium (EDTA) and lead levels are determined in timed urines.

Therapy is directed at specific disorders whenever possible. Occasionally, the weakness is profound and involves bulbar nerves, in which case tracheostomy and respiratory assistance are required. Corticosteroid therapy may be of considerable benefit in cases where the cause is unknown or neuropathy is considered to be due to "chronic inflammation" (this is not the case in acute Guillain-Barré syndrome). Prednisone, 1–2.5 mg/kg/d orally, with tapering to the lowest effective dose—discontinued if the process seems to be arresting and reinstituted when symptoms recur—is recommended. Prednisone should probably not be used for treatment of hereditary neuropathy. In all cases considered for corticosteroid therapy, the risks and benefits should be carefully weighed. When treatment is available, symptoms regress and may disappear altogether over a period of months.

The long-term prognosis varies with the cause and the ability to offer specific therapy. In the "corticosteroid-dependent" group, residual deficits and deaths within a few years are more frequent.

Axelrod FB, Pearson J: Congenital sensory neuropathies: Diagnostic distinction from familial dysautonomia. Am J Dis Child 1984;138:947.

Bird SJ, Slodky JT: Corticosteroid responsive dominant neuropathy in childhood. Neurology 1991;41:437.

Chance PF, Pleasure D: Charcot-Marie-Tooth syndrome. Arch Neurol 1993;50:1180.

Chutorian AM: Chronic polyneuropathy in childhood. Int Pediatr 1988;3:125.

Dyck PJ et al: The 10 P's: A mnemonic helpful in characterization and differential diagnosis of peripheral neuropathy. Neurology 1992;42:14.

Hagberg B: Polyneuropathies in paediatrics. Eur J Pediatr 1990;149:296.

MISCELLANEOUS NEUROMUSCULAR DISORDERS

FLOPPY INFANT SYNDROME

Essentials of Diagnosis & Typical Features

- In early infancy, decreased muscular activity, both spontaneous and in response to postural reflex testing and to passive motion.
- In young infants, "frog posture" or other unusual positions at rest.
- In older infants, delay in motor milestones.

General Considerations

In the young infant, ventral suspension, ie, supporting the infant with a hand under the chest, normally results in the infant's holding its head slightly

Table 22–28. Hereditary motor and sensory neuropathies (HMSN); metabolic error unknown.

Name	Prototype Unknown	Inheritance	Clinical Features	Nerve Biopsy
Sensory and autonomic neuropathy	Familial dysautonomia	Autosomal recessive	See text	Decreased unmyelinated fibers posterior column and cord
	Other	Autosomal recessive, ?autosomal dominant	Rare (see references)	Variable (see references)
HMSN I (if tremor is present, Roussy-Lévy syndrome) (60–90% of HMSN are type I)	"Classic" Charcot-Marie-Tooth (CMT) disease (1) CMT 1A (2) CMT 1B (3) CMT 1C	Autosomal dominant (1) Chromosome 17p11.2–12 duplication (2) Rare. Chromosome 1—linkage to Duffy blood group (3) No linkage yet	Onset 0–15 years. Weakness, atrophy of feet, calves (pes cavus, "stork legs"), hands. Sensory loss 0 or variable. Deep tendon reflexes 0. Motor nerve conduction velocities slowed. Often hypertrophic (palpable) nerves. Linked to Duffy blood group.	Segmental demyelination
HMSN II (10–30% of cases)	Neuronal, axonal Charcot-Marie-Tooth disease	Autosomal dominant	Less severe; onset 10–20. Leg cramps, numbness, motor nerve conduction velocities normal or slightly slow. CSF protein often normal.	Axonal loss, secondary demyelination
HMSN III	Hypertrophic Charcot-Marie-Tooth disease; Déjérine-Sottas disease	Autosomal recessive	Onset in infancy. Severe. CSF protein increased. Very slow MNCV. Slowly progressive.	Hypertrophic ("onion bulb") interstitial changes
HMSN IV	Refsum's disease		Severe sensory, mild motor. Thick nerves. CSF protein elevated. Ichthyosis, retinitis pigmentosa, ataxia, deafness. Urine phytanic acid.	See HMSN III
HMSN V	Charcot-Marie-Tooth disease with spastic paraparesis		Abnormal pyramidal tract findings. Rule out adrenomyelopathy.	Defined in pedigrees. Rule out adrenomyelopathy with long chain fatty acids.
HMSN VI, VII	Optic atrophy, retinitis pigmentosa, etc		Poorly defined. Multiple systems involved.	See HMSN V

up (45 degrees or less), the back straight or nearly so, the arms flexed at the elbows and slightly abducted, and the knees partly flexed. The "floppy" infant droops over the hand like an inverted U. The normal newborn attempts to keep the head in the same plane as the body when pulled up from supine to sitting by the hands (traction response). Marked head lag is characteristic of the floppy infant. Hyperextensibility of the joints is not a dependable criterion.

The usual reasons for seeking medical evaluation in older infants are delays in walking, running, or climbing stairs or motor difficulties and lack of endurance.

Hypotonia or decreased motor activity is a frequent presenting complaint in neuromuscular disorders but may also accompany a variety of systemic conditions or may be due to certain disorders of connective tissue.

Clinical Types

A. Paralytic Group: There is significant lack of movement against gravity (eg, failure to kick the legs, hold up the arms, or attempt to stand when held) or in response to stimuli such as tickling or slight pain.

B. Nonparalytic Group: There is floppiness without significant paralysis.

Note: Deep tendon reflexes may be depressed or absent in the nonparalytic group also. Brisk reflexes with hypotonia point to suprasegmental or general cerebral dysfunction.

1. PARALYTIC GROUP

The hypotonic infant who is weak ("paralyzed") usually has a lesion of the lower motor neuron complex (Table 22–29). Infantile progressive spinal muscular atrophy (Werdnig-Hoffman disease) is the most common cause. Neuropathy is rare. Botulism and myasthenia gravis (rare) are neuromuscular junction causes. Myotonic dystrophy and rare myopathies (eg, central core myopathy) are muscle disease entities.

In anterior horn cell or muscle disease, weakness is proximal (shoulder and hips); finger movement is preserved. Tendon reflexes are absent or depressed; strength (to noxious stimuli) is decreased (paralytic). Intelligence is preserved. Fine motor, personal/social, and language milestones are normal, such as on a Denver Developmental Screening Test (DDST).

Myopathies

The congenital, relatively nonprogressive myopathies, muscular dystrophy, myotonic dystrophy, polymyositis, and periodic paralysis are discussed elsewhere. Most cases of congenital or early infantile muscular dystrophy reported in the past probably represented congenital myopathies (Table 22–27). Congenital muscular dystrophy, diagnosed by muscle biopsy, occurs in two forms: (1) a benign form, with gradual improvement in strength; and (2) a severe form, in which there is either rapid progression of weakness and death in the first months or year of life or severe disability with little or no progression but lifelong marked limitation of activity.

Glycogenosis With Muscle Involvement

Glycogen storage diseases are described in Chapter 30. Patients with type II (Pompe's disease, due to a deficiency of acid maltase) are most likely to present as floppy infants. The weakness in type III (limit dextrinosis) is less marked than in type II, while the rare instances of type IV (amylopectinosis) are severely hypotonic. Muscle cramps on exertion or easy fatigability, rather than floppiness in infancy, is the presenting complaint in type V (McArdle's phosphorylase deficiency) or the glycogenosis due to phosphofructokinase deficiency or phosphohexose isomerase inhibition.

Myasthenia Gravis

Neonatal transient and congenital persistent myasthenia gravis, with patients presenting as "paralytic" floppy infants, is described elsewhere in this chapter.

Arthrogryposis Multiplex (Congenital Deformities About Multiple Joints)

This symptom complex, sometimes associated with hypotonia, may be of "neurogenic" or "myopathic" origin (or both) and may be associated with a wide variety of other anomalies. Orthopedic aspects are discussed in Chapter 23.

Spinal Cord Lesions

Severe limpness in newborns following breech ex-

Table 22–29. Floppy infant: paralytic causes.

Disease	Genetic	Early Manifestations
IPSMA (Infantile Progressive Spinal Muscular Atrophy) "Malignant" form	Autosomal recessive (AR)	In utero movements decreased by one-third. Gradual weakness, delay in gross motor milestones. Weak cry. Abdominal breathing. Poor limb motion ("no kicking"). Deep tendon reflexes (DTR)—0. Fasciculations of tongue. Normal personal-social behavior.
"Intermediate" form	AR	Onset under age 1 usual. *Progression slower:* may be impossible to predict early course of IPSMA. Hand tremors common.
Infantile botulism	Acquired under age 1 (mostly under 6 months); botulism spore in stool makes toxin	Poor feeding. Constipation. Weak cry. Failure to thrive. Lethargy. Facial weakness, ptosis, ocular muscle palsy. Inability to suck, swallow. Apnea. Source: soil dust (outdoor construction workers may bring it home on clothes), honey.
Myasthenia gravis Neonatal transient	12% of infants born from a myasthenia mother	Floppiness. Poor sucking and feeding; choking. Respiratory distress. Weak cry.
Congenital persistent	Mother normal. Rare AR (AD)	As above; may improve and later exacerbate.
Myotonic dystrophy	Autosomal dominant (AD) (almost always *mother* transmits gene in neonatal/infant severe form)	Polyhydramnios; failure of suck, respirations. Facial diplegia. Ptosis. Arthrogryposis. Thin ribs. Later, developmental delay.
Neonatal "rare myopathy," severe variant Nemaline, central core, "minimal change," myotubular (centronuclear), reducing body	AR, AD	Virtually all of the rare myopathies may have a severe (even fatal) neonatal or early infant form. Clinical features similar in infancy to infantile myotonic dystrophy.
Congenital muscular dystrophy Fukayama	? Genetic ? infectious	Early onset. Facial weakness. Joint contractures. Severe mental retardation. Ill-defined.
Other		Severe or benign (improve). No mental retardation.
Essential hypotonia ("benign congenital hypotonia")	Unknown cause	Diagnosis of exclusion. Family history variable. Mild to moderate hypotonia with weakness.

traction with stretching or actual tearing of the lower cervical to upper thoracic spinal cord is rarely seen today, owing to improved obstetric delivery. Klumpke's lower brachial plexus paralysis may be present; the abdomen is usually exceedingly soft, and the lower extremities are flaccid. Urinary retention is present initially; later, the bladder may function autonomously. Myelography or MRI scanning may define the lesion. After a few weeks, spasticity of the lower limbs becomes obvious. Treatment is symptomatic and consists of bladder and skin care and eventual mobilization on crutches or in a wheelchair.

2. NONPARALYTIC GROUP

The nonparalytic group often has "brain damage" (Table 22– 29). Intrauterine or perinatal insults to brain or spinal cord, while sometimes difficult to document, are major causes. (Occasionally, severe congenital myopathies presenting in the newborn period cause confusion.) Persisting severe hypotonia is ominous. Tone will often vary. Spasticity and other forms of cerebral palsy may emerge; hypertonia and hypotonia may occur at varying times in the same in-

fant. Choreoathetoid or ataxic movements and developmental delay can clarify the diagnosis. Reflexes are often increased; pathologic reflexes (Babinski, tonic neck) may persist or worsen.

The creatine kinase level and the EMG are usually normal. Prolonged nerve conduction velocities point to polyneuritis or leukodystrophy. Muscle biopsies, utilizing special stains and histographic analysis, often show a remarkable reduction in size of type II fibers associated with decreased voluntary motor activity.

Limpness in the neonatal period and early infancy and subsequent delay in achieving motor milestones are the presenting features in a large number of children with a variety of CNS disorders, including mental retardation, as in trisomy 21. In many such cases, no specific diagnosis can be made. Close observation and scoring of motor patterns and adaptive behavior, as by the DDST, are most helpful.

Burlet P et al: Large scale deletions of the 5q13 region are specific to Werdnig-Hoffmann disease. J Med Genet 1996;33:281.
Crawford TO: Clinical evaluation of the floppy infant. Pediatr Ann 1992;21:348.

Table 22–29. Floppy infant: nonparalytic causes.

	Causes	Manifestations
Central nervous system disorders Atonic diplegia ("prespastic diplegia")	Intrauterine, perinatal asphyxia, cord injury	Limpness, stupor; poor suck, cry, Moro reflex, grasp; later, irritability, increased tone and reflexes
Choreoathetosis	As above; kernicterus	Hypotonic early; movement disorder emerges later (6–18 months)
Ataxic cerebral palsy	Same as choreoathetosis	Same as choreoathetosis
Syndromes with hypotonia (CNS origin) Trisomy 21	Genetic	All have hypotonia early
Prader-Willi syndrome	Genetic deletion 15q11	Hypotonia, hypomentia, hypogonadism, obesity
Marfan syndrome	Autosomal dominant	Arachnodactyly
Dysautonomia	Autosomal recessive	Respiratory, corneal anesthesia
Turner's syndrome	45X, or mosaic	Somatic stigmata (Chapter 31)
Degenerative disorders Tay-Sachs	Autosomal recessive	Cherry-red spot on macula
Metachromatic leukodystrophy	Autosomal recessive	Deep tendon reflexes increased early, polyneuropathy late; mental retardation
Systemic diseases[1] Malnutrition	Deprivation, cystic fibrosis, celiac disease	
Chronic illness	Congenital heart disease; chronic pulmonary disease (eg, bronchopulmonary dysplasia); uremic, renal acidosis	
Metabolic disease	Hypercalcemia, Lowe's disease	
Endocrinopathy	Hypothyroid	

[1]See elsewhere in text for manifestations.

Crawford TO: From enigmatic to problematic:the new molecular genetics of childhood spinal muscular atrophy. Neurology 1996;46:335.

Dobyns WB: Classification of the cerebro-oculo-muscular syndrome(s). Brain Dev 1993;15:242.

Gay CT, Bodensteiner JB: The floppy infant: Recent advances in the understanding of disorders affecting the neuromuscular junction. Neurol Clin 1990;8:715.

Glatman-Freedman A: Infant botulism. Pediatr Rev 1996;17:185.

Sarnat HB: Congenital myopathies. Int Pediatr 1997;12:87.

Stiefel L: Hypotonia in infants. Pediatr Rev 1996;17:104.

CEREBRAL PALSY

Essentials of Diagnosis & Typical Features

- Impairment of movement and posture since birth or early infancy.
- Nonprogressive and nonhereditary.

General Considerations

Cerebral palsy is a term of clinical convenience for disorders of impaired motor functioning and posture with onset before or at birth or during the first year of life, basically nonprogressive, and varying widely in their causes, manifestations, and prognosis. The most obvious manifestation is impaired function of voluntary muscles. In the United States, cerebral palsy affects about 0.2% of neonatal survivors.

Classification

Classification is commonly based on the predominant motor deficit.

A. Spastic Forms: About 75% of cases. Often associated with other forms.

1. Quadriplegia (tetraplegia)–The four extremities may be involved about equally, or upper limbs may show more severe involvement. The main lesion is in the cerebral white matter. Quadriplegia due to perinatal damage often shows symptoms earlier than that due to fetal undernutrition or prematurity. Nearly 90% of patients are profoundly retarded.

2. Diplegia–Legs involved more than arms.

3. Hemiplegia–One side involved primarily.

4. Paraplegia–Legs only involved.

5. Monoplegia–One extremity only involved.

6. Triplegia–Three extremities involved.

B. Ataxia: About 15% of cases. Pure and in combination with other forms.

C. Dyskinesia (Choreoathetosis): About 5% of cases. Often associated with rigidity or spastic quadriplegia or diplegia.

D. Hypotonic Form: Fewer than 1% of cases. Persistent hypotonia with variable degrees of weakness.

Etiology

The cause is often obscure or multifactorial. No definite etiologic diagnosis is possible in over one-third of cases. The incidence is high among infants small for gestational age. Intrauterine hypoxia is a frequent cause. Other known causes are intrauterine bleeding, infections, toxins, congenital malformations, obstetric complications (including birth hypoxia), neonatal infections, kernicterus, neonatal hypoglycemia, acidosis, and a small number of genetic syndromes (about 2%).

Associated Deficits

A. Seizures: Seizures afflict about 50% of all children with cerebral palsy and are more prevalent in those with severe involvement.

B. Mental Retardation: Mild to moderate retardation is seen in 26% of patients and profound retardation in 27%. The incidence is correlated with the severity of cerebral palsy.

C. Sensory and Speech Deficits: Impairment of speech, vision, hearing, and perceptual functions is found often in varying degrees and combinations.

Clinical Findings

A. Symptoms and Signs: The typical spastic child exhibits muscular hypertonicity of the clasp-knife type that may eventually end in contractures. In the limb or limbs involved, tendon reflexes, if sufficient muscle relaxation can be achieved, are hyperactive; clonus may be present, and the plantar responses are often extensor. Although voluntary control, especially of fine movements, is decreased, there is spread or overflow of associated movements. In extreme cases, the child may lie with elbows flexed and fists clenched ("straphanger's posture") and legs crossed or scissored. In early infancy, the child may appear floppy, although tendon jerks are abnormally increased (hypotonic, atonic, or prespastic diplegia). Rigidity often accompanies cerebral palsy.

Ataxia may be difficult to delineate in the presence of spasticity or hyperkinetic movements.

Microcephaly (head circumference 2 SD below the mean for age and sex and decreasing) is present in about 25% of spastic quadriplegics and diplegics. Partial atrophy of the cranium on the involved side or of involved extremities is observed frequently.

A smaller hand or foot, when combined with mild weakness on muscle testing or hyperreflexia, often justifies a diagnosis of mild cerebral palsy of which the patient or the family may not even have been aware. Occasionally, multiple minor malformations suggest an intrauterine origin.

B. Laboratory and Other Findings: No routine workup can be outlined. The clinical findings, the presence or absence of seizures, and the overall outlook for the child—particularly with respect to intelligence and the ability to carry on activities of daily living—determine what studies should be performed. Hip films in abduction are indicated to rule out dislocations secondary to spasticity. Electroencephalography is indicated when seizures are present or suspected. MRI scans may be helpful in determining timing of insult or malformation, eg, prenatal-intrauterine or perinatal.

Urine screening tests for amino and organic acidurias are indicated. In choreoathetosis with self-injury, serum uric acid determinations should be considered to rule out Lesch-Nyhan syndrome. Macrocephaly and dystonia suggest glutaricaciduria (organic acid).

Differential Diagnosis

The diagnosis is usually not difficult. Progressive deterioration in the first 3 months is more likely to denote a metabolic disorder; subsequently, it denotes one of the CNS degenerative disorders (Tables 22–22 and 22–23). In the ataxic form, cerebellar dysgenesis (sometimes familial) or a spinocerebellar degeneration may have to be ruled out.

Prevention

Obstetric advances in late third-trimester management and delivery have resulted in less cerebral palsy. Much more needs to be done in prenatal care, especially during the second and early third trimester. Examples are maternal counseling to avoid cocaine and alcohol abuse and earlier detection of hypertensive disorders of pregnancy. The number of cases in which cerebral palsy is associated with aggressive efforts to salvage premature infants has decreased as a result of advances in neonatal care.

Treatment

Realistically, a child with cerebral palsy should be helped to achieve maximum potential rather than "normality." Special educational programming depends on the physical and mental potential of the child. The degree of improvement with physical therapy correlates positively with better intelligence. Treat seizures in the same way as those occurring in other children. The orthopedic aspects of cerebral palsy are discussed in Chapter 23.

Spasticity occasionally is reduced by diazepam or baclofen. Optimal doses vary according to the degree of spasticity, the size and age of the child, and other medications taken. Surgical amelioration of moderate to severe spasticity in cerebral palsy has been attempted by various procedures over many years; dorsal rhizotomy is the newest procedure.

Management of "hyperactivity" is dealt with in Chapter 5 in connection with attention deficit hyperactivity disorder.

Psychologic counseling and support of the child and family are of paramount importance.

Prognosis

In patients with severe cerebral palsy, especially spastics with profound retardation and seizures that are difficult to control, death due to intercurrent infections is not uncommon; nearly 50% die by 10 years of age. In nearly 30% of patients—chiefly in those with mild involvement—motor deficits resolve by the seventh birthday. Many children with cerebral palsy and average or near-average intelligence lead fairly normal, satisfying, and productive lives.

Coorssen EA, Msall ME, Duffy LC: Multiple minor malformations as a marker for prenatal etiology of cerebral palsy. Dev Med Child Neurol 1991;33:730.

Hendricks-Ferguson VL, Ortman MR: Selective dorsal rhizotomy to decrease spasticity in cerebral palsy. AORN J 1995;61:514.

Hughes I, Newton R: Genetic aspects of cerebral palsy. Dev Med Child Neurol 1992;34:80.

Kuban KCK, Leviton A: Cerebral palsy. N Engl J Med 1994;330:1888.

Nelson KB et al: Uncertain value of electronic fetal monitoring in predicting cerebral palsy. N Engl J Med 1996;334:613.

Nelson KB: Magnesium sulfate and risk of cerebral palsy in very low-birth-weight infants. JAMA 1996;276:1843.

Perlman JM: Intrapartum hypoxic-ischemic cerebral injury and subsequent cerebral palsy: Medicolegal issues. Pediatrics 1997;99:851.

Rosenbloom L: Diagnosis and management of cerebral palsy. Arch Dis Childhood 1995;72:350.

Scheuerle AE et al: Arginase deficiency presenting as cerebral palsy. Pediatrics 1993;91:995.

Tuft LT: Cerebral palsy. Pediatr Rev 1995;16:411.

Volpe JJ: Value of MR in definition of the neuropathology of cerebral palsy in vivo. AJNR Am J Neuroradiol 1992;13:79.

REFERENCES

Aicardi J: *Diseases of the Nervous System in Childhood.* MacKeith Press, 1992.

Aicardi J: *Epilepsy in Children.* Raven Press, 1994.

Dodson WE, Pellock JM: *Pediatric Epilepsy: Diagnosis and Therapy.* Demos, 1993.

Fenichel GM: *Clinical Pediatric Neurology.* Saunders, 1997.

Freeman JM et al: *Seizures and Epilepsy in Childhood: A Guide for Parents.* Johns Hopkins Univ Press, 1997.

Guilleminault C: *Sleep and Its Disorders in Children.* Raven Press, 1987.

Illingworth RS: *The Development of the Infant and Young Child: Normal and Abnormal,* 8th ed. Churchill Livingstone, 1983.

Menkes JH: *Textbook of Child Neurology,* 5th ed. Williams & Wilkins, 1995.

Plum F, Posner J: *The Diagnosis of Stupor and Coma,* 3rd ed. Davis, 1980.

Shinnar S, Amir N, Branski D: *Childhood Seizures: Pediatric and Adolescent Medicine,* vol. 6. S Karger, 1995.

Swaiman KF: *Pediatric Neurology: Principles and Practice,* vols 1 and 2. Mosby, 1994.

Volpe JJ: *Neurology of the Newborn,* 3rd ed. Saunders, 1995.

Orthopedics

23

Robert E. Eilert, MD, & Gaia Georgopoulos, MD

Orthopedics is the medical discipline that deals with disorders of the neuromuscular and skeletal systems. Patients with orthopedic problems usually present with pain, loss of function, or deformity. Their symptoms must be considered not only in terms of the anatomy of the bones and joints, particularly of the extremities, but also in relationship to the blood vessels, skin, nerves, tendons, and muscles. The physical examination is the most important feature of orthopedic diagnosis and depends upon an intimate knowledge of human anatomy.

DISTURBANCES OF PRENATAL ORIGIN

CONGENITAL AMPUTATIONS

Congenital amputations may be due to teratogens (eg, drugs or viruses), amniotic bands, or metabolic diseases (eg, diabetes in the mother). Rarely, they are genetically determined. The history of the pregnancy must be reviewed for possible teratogenic factors. There is a 30% incidence of multiple limb involvement, and children with congenital limb deficiencies also have a high incidence of associated congenital anomalies, including genitourinary and cardiac defects and cleft palates. According to the currently accepted international classification, amputations are either terminal or longitudinal. In terminal amputation, all parts are missing distal to the level of involvement—such as absence of the forearm, wrist, and hand in the case of a terminal below-the-elbow amputation. A longitudinal amputation consists of partial absence of structures in the extremity along one side or the other. In radial clubhand, the entire radius is absent, but the thumb may be either hy-poplastic or completely absent; that is, the effect on structures distal to the amputation may vary. Complex tissue defects are nearly always associated with longitudinal bone deficiency in that the associated nerves and muscles are not completely represented when a bone is absent.

Terminal amputations are treated by prosthesis, such as to compensate for shortness of one leg. With longitudinal deficiencies, reconstructive surgery may reduce deformity and stabilize joints. In certain types of severe anomalies, operative treatment is indicated to remove a portion of the malformed foot so that a prosthesis can be fitted early. This applies to such anomalies as congenital absence of the fibula, which is the most common congenital long bone deficiency. In cases where limb deficiency is treated by amputation, all possible length should be preserved in children.

Lower extremity prostheses are best fitted between 12 and 15 months of age when walking starts. They are consistently well accepted, since they are necessary for balancing and walking. Upper extremity prostheses are not as well accepted. Fitting the child with a dummy-type prosthesis as early as 6 months of age has the advantage of instilling an accustomed pattern of proper length and bimanual manipulation. Children fitted later than age 2 years nearly always reject upper extremity prostheses.

Children quickly learn how to function with their prostheses and can lead active lives, participating in sports with peers.

Alman BA, Krajbich JI, Hubbard S: Proximal femoral focal deficiency; Results of rotationplasty and Syme amputation. J Bone Joint Surg Am 1995;77:1876.

Choi DH, Kumar SJ, Bowen JR: Amputation or limb lengthening for partial or total absence of the fibula. J Bone Joint Surg Am 1990;72:1391.

van der Windt D et al: Energy expenditure during walking in subjects with tibial rotation-plasty, above-knee amputation, or hip dislocation. Arch Phys Med Rehabil 1992;73:1174.

DEFORMITIES OF THE EXTREMITIES

1. METATARSUS VARUS

Metatarsus varus is a common congenital foot deformity characterized by inward deviation of the forepart of the foot. The longitudinal arch is often creased vertically when the deformity is more rigid. The lateral border of the foot demonstrates sharp angulation at the level of the base of the fifth metatarsal, and this bone will be especially prominent. The deformity varies from flexible to rigid. Most flexible deformities are secondary to intrauterine posture and usually resolve spontaneously. Several investigators have noticed that 10–15% of children with metatarsus varus have hip dysplasia. The hips in these children should be very carefully checked.

If the deformity is rigid and cannot be manipulated past the midline, it is worthwhile to use a cast changed at intervals of 2 weeks to correct the deformity. "Corrective" shoes do not live up to their name, although they can be used to maintain correction obtained by casting.

The prognosis for this common deformity of the foot is excellent. If the deformity persists, the child will exhibit an in-toed gait and may have some problems with shoe wear secondary to the prominence of the base of the fifth metatarsal.

Rushforth GF: The natural history of the hooked forefoot. J Bone Joint Surg Br 1978;60:530.
Smith JT et al: Simple method of documenting metatarsus adductus. J Pediatr Orthop 1991;11:679.

2. CLUBFOOT
(Talipes Equinovarus)

The diagnosis of classic talipes equinovarus, or clubfoot, requires three features: (1) equinus or plantar flexion of the foot at the ankle joint, (2) varus or inversion deformity of the heel, and (3) forefoot varus. The incidence of talipes equinovarus is approximately 1:1000 live births. There are three major categories of clubfoot: (1) idiopathic; (2) neurogenic; and (3) those associated with syndromes, such as arthrogryposis and Larsen's syndrome. Any infant with a clubfoot should be examined carefully for associated anomalies, especially of the spine. Idiopathic clubfeet may be hereditary.

Treatment consists of manipulation of the foot to stretch the contracted tissues on the medial and posterior aspects, followed by splinting to hold the correction. When this treatment is instituted shortly after birth, correction is rapid. When treatment is delayed, the foot tends to become more rigid within a matter of days. Treatment in the nursery by strapping and splinting is often effective until formal casting can be started. The casts are applied sequentially, correcting first the forefoot adduction, then the inversion of the heel, and finally the equinus of the ankle. After full correction is obtained, a night brace is often prescribed for long-term maintenance of correction. Treatment by means of casting requires patience and experience; if it is not done properly in sequence, iatrogenic deformities of the foot may result, such as rocker-bottom foot.

About 50% of children with clubfoot eventually need an operative procedure to lengthen the tightened structures about the foot. A supple foot that is easily corrected by strapping and casting has a more favorable prognosis. If the foot is rigid and resistant to cast treatment, surgical release and correction are appropriate.

Johnston CE II et al: Three-dimensional analysis of clubfoot deformity by computed tomography. J Pediatr Orthop B 1995;4:39.
Ponseti IV: Treatment of congenital clubfoot. J Bone Joint Surg Am 1992;74:448.

3. CONGENITAL DYSPLASIA
OF THE HIP JOINT

Dysplasia means abnormal growth or development. Dysplasia of the hip encompasses a spectrum of conditions in which there is an abnormal relationship between the proximal femur and the acetabulum. In the most severe condition, the femoral head is not in contact with the acetabulum and is classified as a dislocated hip. A dislocatable hip is one in which the hip is within the acetabulum but can be dislocated with a provocative (Barlow) maneuver. A subluxatable hip is one in which the femoral head comes partially out of the joint with a provocative maneuver. Acetabular dysplasia is the term used to denote insufficient acetabular development on x-ray.

Congenital dislocation of the hip occurs in approximately 1:1000 live births. At birth, there is lack of the development of both the acetabulum and the femur. The dysplasia becomes progressive with growth unless the dislocation is corrected. If the dislocation is corrected in the first few days or weeks of life, the dysplasia is completely reversible and a normal hip will develop. As the child becomes older and the dislocation or subluxation persists, the deformity will worsen to the point where it will not be completely reversible, especially after the walking age. For this reason, it is important to diagnose the deformity in the nursery or, at the latest, the 6-week checkup.

Clinical Findings
The diagnosis of hip dislocation in the newborn depends upon demonstrating instability of the joint by placing the infant on the back and obtaining complete relaxation by feeding with a bottle if necessary.

The examiner's long finger is then placed over the greater trochanter and the thumb over the inner side of the thigh. Both hips are flexed 90 degrees and then slowly abducted from the midline, one hip at a time. With gentle pressure, an attempt is made to lift the greater trochanter forward. A feeling of slipping as the head relocates is a sign of instability. In other infants, the joint is more stable, and the deformity must be provoked by applying slight pressure with the thumb on the medial side of the thigh as the thigh is adducted, thus slipping the hip posteriorly and eliciting a jerk as the hip dislocates. The signs of instability are more reliable than x-ray for diagnosing congenital dislocation of the hip in the newborn. X-rays of the pelvis are notoriously unreliable until about 6 weeks of age. Ultrasonography can be used but tends to result in overdiagnosis in the newborn. Asymmetric skinfolds are present in about 40% of newborns and therefore are not particularly helpful.

After the first month of life, the signs of instability become less evident. Contractures begin to develop about the hip joint, limiting abduction. The hip should abduct fully to 90 degrees on either side during the first few months of life. It is important to hold the pelvis level to detect asymmetry of abduction. When the hips and knees are flexed, the knees are at unequal heights, with the dislocated side lower. After the first 6 weeks of life, x-ray examination becomes more valuable, with lateral displacement of the femoral head being the most reliable sign. In mild cases, the only abnormality may be increased steepness of acetabular alignment, so that the acetabular angle is greater than 35 degrees.

If dysplasia of the hip has not been diagnosed during the first year of life and the child begins to walk, there will be a painless limp and a lurch to the affected side. When the child stands on the affected leg, there is a dip of the pelvis on the opposite side owing to weakness of the gluteus medius muscle. This is called Trendelenburg's sign and accounts for the unusual swaying gait. In children with bilateral dislocations, the loss of abduction is almost symmetric and may be deceiving. Abduction is never complete in a dislocation. X-ray of the pelvis is indicated in children with incomplete abduction in the first few months of life. As a child with bilateral dislocation of the hips begins to walk, the gait is waddling. The perineum is widened as a result of lateral displacement of the hips, and there is flexion contracture as a result of posterior displacement of the hips. This flexion contracture contributes to marked lumbar lordosis, and the greater trochanters are easily palpable in their elevated position. Treatment is still possible in the first 2 years of life, but the results are not nearly as effective as in children treated in the nursery.

Treatment

Dislocation or dysplasia diagnosed in the first few weeks or months of life can easily be treated by splinting, with the hip maintained in flexion and abduction. Forced abduction is contraindicated, since this often leads to avascular necrosis of the femoral head. The use of double or triple diapers is never indicated because diapers are not adequate to obtain proper positioning of the hip. Treatment of children requiring splints is best supervised by an orthopedic surgeon with a special interest in the problem.

In the first 4 months of life, reduction can be obtained by simply flexing and abducting the hip; no other manipulation is usually necessary. If force is used to reduce the hip, the excessive pressure may cause avascular necrosis. In such cases, preoperative traction for 2–3 weeks is important to relax soft tissues about the hip. Following traction in which the femur is brought down opposite the acetabulum, reduction can be easily achieved without force under general anesthesia. It is then necessary to place the child in a plaster cast for approximately 6 months. If the reduction is not stable within a reasonable range following closed reduction, open reduction, combined with tightening of the lax capsule in order to maintain reduction, may be necessary.

If reduction is done at an older age, operations to correct the deformities of the acetabulum and femur may be necessary during growth.

Beoree NR, Clarke NM: Ultrasound imaging and secondary screening for congenital dislocation of the hip. J Bone Joint Surg Br 1994;76:525.

Bialik V et al: Clinical assessment of hip instability in the newborn by an orthopaedic surgeon and a pediatrician. J Pediatr Orthop 1986;6:703.

Hernandez RJ, Cornell RG, Hensinger RN: Ultrasound diagnosis of neonatal congenital dislocation of the hip: A decision analysis assessment. J Bone Joint Surg Br 1994;76:539.

Viere RG, Birch JG, Herring JA: Use of the Pavlik harness in congenital dislocation of the hip: An analysis of failure of treatment. J Bone Joint Surg Am 1990;72:238.

4. TORTICOLLIS

Wryneck deformities in infancy may be due either to injury to the sternocleidomastoid muscle during delivery or to disease affecting the cervical spine. In the case of muscular deformity, the chin is rotated to the side opposite to the affected sternocleidomastoid muscle contracture, and the head is tilted toward the side of the contracture. A mass felt in the midportion of the sternocleidomastoid muscle is not a true tumor, but fibrous transformation within the muscle.

In mild cases, passive stretching is usually effective. If the deformity has not been corrected by passive stretching within the first year of life, surgical division of the muscle will correct it. It is not necessary to excise the "tumor" of the sternocleidomastoid muscle, because this tends to resolve spontaneously.

If the deformity is left untreated, an unsightly facial asymmetry will result.

Torticollis is occasionally associated with congenital deformities of the cervical spine, and x-rays of the spine are indicated in all cases. In addition, there is a 20% incidence of hip dysplasia.

Acute torticollis may follow upper respiratory infection or mild trauma in children. Rotatory subluxation of the upper cervical spine should be sought by appropriate x-ray views. Traction or a cervical collar usually results in resolution of the symptoms within 1 or 2 days. Other causes of torticollis include spinal cord or cerebellar tumors, syringomyelia, and rheumatoid arthritis.

Davids JR, Wenger DR, Mubarek SJ: Congenital muscular torticollis: Sequela of intrauterine or perinatal compartment syndrome. J Pediatr Orthop 1993;13:141.
Phillips WA, Hensiger RN: The management of rotary atlanto-axial subluxation in children. J Bone Joint Surg Am 1989;71:664.

GENERALIZED AFFECTIONS OF SKELETAL OR MESODERMAL TISSUES

1. ARTHROGRYPOSIS MULTIPLEX CONGENITA (Amyoplasia Congenita)

Arthrogryposis multiplex congenita consists of incomplete fibrous ankylosis (usually symmetric) of many or all joints of the body. There may be contractures either in flexion or extension. Upper extremity deformities usually consist of adduction of the shoulders, extension of the elbows, flexion of the wrists, and stiff, straight fingers with poor muscle control of the thumbs. In the lower extremities, common deformities are dislocation of the hips, extension of the knees, and severe clubfoot. The joints are fusiform and the joint capsules decreased in volume, producing contractures. Various investigations have attributed the basic defect to an abnormality of muscle or the lower motor neuron. Muscle development is poor, and muscles may be represented only by fibrous bands. The joint deformities appear to be secondary to a lack of active motion during intrauterine development.

Passive mobilization of joints should be done early. Because of poor muscle control, however, joint mobility cannot be maintained by active motion. Prolonged casting for correction of deformities is contraindicated in these children because further stiffness is often produced. Use of removable splints combined with vigorous therapy is the most effective conservative treatment. Surgical release of the affected joints is often necessary. The clubfoot associated with arthrogryposis is very stiff and nearly always requires an operation. Surgery about the knees, including capsulotomy, osteotomy, and tendon lengthening, is used to correct deformity. In the young child, a dislocated hip may be reduced operatively by the medial approach. Multiple operative procedures about the hip are contraindicated because further stiffness may be produced with consequent impairment of motion. The dislocation of the hip that occurs in arthrogryposis is associated with severe dysplasia of the bones and does not respond to treatment as ordinary congenital hip dislocation does. Affected children are often able to walk with bilateral dislocation of the hips, and in cases of severe rigidity it is better to leave the hips out of joint. The long-term disability is not worse than with incomplete surgical reduction of the hips.

The long-term prognosis for physical and vocational independence is poor. Patients usually have normal intelligence, but they have such severe physical restrictions that gainful employment is hard to find.

Mennen U: Early corrective surgery of the wrist and elbow in arthrogryposis multiplex congenita. J Hand Surg Br 1993;18:304.
Sodergard J, Ryoppy S: Knee in arthrogryposis multiplex congenita. J Pediatr Orthop 1990;10:177.

2. MARFAN'S SYNDROME

Marfan's syndrome is a connective tissue disorder characterized by unusually long fingers and toes (arachnodactyly); hypermobility of the joints; subluxation of the ocular lenses; other eye abnormalities including cataract, coloboma, megalocornea, strabismus, and nystagmus; a high-arched palate; a strong tendency to scoliosis; pectus carinatum; and thoracic aortic aneurysms due to weakness of the media of the vessels (see Chapter 31). Serum mucoproteins may be decreased and urinary excretion of hydroxyproline increased. The condition is easily confused with homocystinuria, since the phenotypic presentation is identical. The two diseases are differentiated by the presence of homocystine in the urine in homocystinuria.

Treatment is usually supportive for associated problems such as flatfoot. Scoliosis may involve more vigorous treatment by bracing or spine fusion. The long-term prognosis has improved for patients because better treatment for their aortic aneurysms has been devised.

Joseph KN et al: Orthopaedic aspects of the Marfan phenotype. Clin Orthop 1992;277:251.

3. KLIPPEL-FEIL SYNDROME

Klippel-Feil syndrome is characterized by fusion of some or all of the cervical vertebrae. Multiple spinal anomalies may be present, with hemivertebrae and scoliosis. The neck is short and stiff, the hairline is low, and the ears are often low-set. Common associated defects include congenital scoliosis, cervical rib, spina bifida, torticollis, web neck, high scapula, renal anomalies, and deafness. Examination of the urinary tract by urinalysis and renal ultrasound is indicated as well as a hearing test. Scoliotic deformities, if progressive, are an indication for spinal arthrodesis.

Guilde JT et al: The natural history of Klippel-Feil syndrome: Clinical roentgenographic and magnetic resonance imaging findings at adulthood. J Pediatr Orthop 1995;15:617.

4. SPRENGEL'S DEFORMITY

Sprengel's deformity is a congenital condition in which one or both scapulas are elevated and small. The child cannot raise the arm completely on the affected side, and torticollis may be present. The deformity occurs alone or may be associated with Klippel-Feil syndrome.

If the deformity is functionally limiting, the scapula may be surgically relocated lower in the thorax. Excision of the upper portion of the scapula improves cosmetic appearance but has little effect on function.

Leibovic SJ et al: Sprengel deformity. J Bone Joint Surg Am 1990;72:192.

5. OSTEOGENESIS IMPERFECTA

Osteogenesis imperfecta is a rare, mainly dominantly inherited connective tissue disease characterized by multiple and recurrent fractures. The severe fetal type (osteogenesis imperfecta congenita) is characterized by multiple intrauterine or perinatal fractures. Affected children continue to have fractures and are dwarfed as a result of bony deformities and growth retardation. Intelligence is not affected. The shafts of the long bones are reduced in cortical thickness, and wormian bones are present in the skull. Other features include blue scleras, thin skin, hyperextensibility of ligaments, "otosclerosis" with significant hearing loss, and hypoplastic and deformed teeth. In the tarda type, fractures begin to occur at variable times after the perinatal period, resulting in relatively fewer fractures and deformities in these cases. Affected patients are sometimes suspected of having suffered induced fractures, and the condition should be ruled out in any case of nonaccidental trauma.

Metabolic defects include elevated serum pyrophosphate, decreased platelet aggregation, and decreased incorporation of sulfate into acid mucopolysaccharides by skin fibroblasts. Normal parents can be counseled that the likelihood of a second affected child is negligible.

There is no effective medical treatment. Surgical treatment involves correction of deformity of the long bones. Multiple intramedullary rods have been used to prevent deformity from poor healing of fractures.

The overall prognosis is poor, and patients are often confined to wheelchairs during adulthood.

Binder HT al: Comprehensive rehabilitation of the child with osteogenesis imperfecta. Am J Med Genet 1993; 45:265.
Dent JA, Patterson CR: Fractures in early childhood: Osteogenesis imperfecta or child abuse. J Pediatr Orthop 1991;11:184.
Hanscom DA et al: Osteogenesis imperfecta. J Bone Joint Surg Am 1992;74:598.

6. OSTEOPETROSIS
(Osteitis Condensans Generalisata; Marble Bone Disease; Albers-Schönberg Disease)

Osteopetrosis is a rare disorder of osteoclastic resorption of bone resulting in abnormally dense bones. The marrow spaces are reduced, resulting in anemia. There are two types—a milder autosomal dominant type and a more malignant autosomal recessive type. The findings may appear at any age. On x-ray examination, the bones show increased density, transverse bands in the shafts, clubbing of ends, and vertical striations of long bones. There is thickening about the cranial foramina, and there may be heterotopic calcification of soft tissues.

The autosomal recessive form of osteopetrosis can be successfully treated by allogeneic bone marrow transplantation. The failure rate is high, however, as is the complication rate.

Kaplan FS, August CS, Fallon MD: Successful treatment of infantile malignant osteopetrosis by bone marrow transplantation: A case report. J Bone Joint Surg Am 1988; 70:617.

7. ACHONDROPLASIA
(Classic Chondrodystrophy)

Achondroplasia is the most common form of short-limbed dwarfism. The upper arms and thighs are proportionately shorter than the forearms and legs. Findings frequently include bowing of the extremities, a waddling gait, limitation of motion of major joints, relaxation of the ligaments, short stubby fingers of almost equal length, frontal bossing, moderate hydrocephalus, depressed nasal bridge, and lumbar lordosis. Intelligence and sexual function are normal. The disorder is transmitted as an autosomal dominant trait, but 80% of cases result from a random mutation. X-rays demonstrate short, thick tubular bones and irregular epiphysial plates. The ends of the bones are thick, with broadening and cupping. Epiphysial ossification may be delayed. The spinal canal is narrowed, so that herniated disk in adulthood may lead to acute paraplegia.

Osteotomies of the long bones are occasionally necessary if deformities are severe.

Beals RK, Horton W: Skeletal dysplasias: An approach to diagnosis. J Am Acad Orthop Surg 1995;3:174.

8. OSTEOCHONDRODYSTROPHY (Morquio's Disease)

Morquio's disease is an autosomal recessive disorder of mucopolysaccharide storage. Skeletal abnormalities include shortening of the spine, kyphosis, scoliosis, shortened extremities, pectus carinatum, genu valgum, and a hypoplastic odontoid with atlantoaxial instability. The child generally appears normal at birth and begins to develop deformities between 1 and 4 years of age as a result of abnormal deposition of mucopolysaccharides.

X-rays demonstrate wedge-shaped flattened vertebrae and irregular, malformed epiphyses. The ribs are broad and have been likened to canoe paddles. The lower extremities are more severely involved than the upper ones.

There is no treatment, and the prognosis is poor, although many individuals survive into adulthood. Progressive clouding of the cornea leads to increasing visual impairment. Bone marrow transplantation has been successful in alleviating some of the symptoms.

GROWTH DISTURBANCES OF THE MUSCULOSKELETAL SYSTEM

SCOLIOSIS

Lateral curvature of the spine (scoliosis) is always associated with some rotation of the involved vertebrae. Scoliosis is classified by its anatomic location, in either the thoracic or lumbar spine, with rare involvement of the cervical spine. The convexity of the curve is designated right or left. Thus, a right thoracic scoliosis would denote a thoracic curve in which the convexity is to the right; this is the most common type of idiopathic curve. Posterior curvature

of the spine (kyphosis) is normal in the thoracic area, although excessive curvature may become pathologic. Anterior curvature is called lordosis and is normal in the lumbar and cervical spines. Idiopathic scoliosis generally begins at 8 or 10 years of age and progresses during growth. In rare instances, infantile scoliosis may be seen in children 2 years of age or less.

Idiopathic scoliosis is about four or five times more common in girls. The disorder is usually asymptomatic in the adolescent years, but severe curvature may lead to impairment of pulmonary function in later years. It is important to examine the back of any adolescent during a routine physical examination in order to identify scoliosis early. The examination is performed by having the patient bend forward 90 degrees with the hands joined in the midline. An abnormal finding consists of asymmetry of the height of the ribs or paravertebral muscles on one side, indicating rotation of the trunk associated with lateral curvature.

Diseases that may be associated with scoliosis include neurofibromatosis, Marfan's syndrome, cerebral palsy, muscular dystrophy, poliomyelitis, and myelodysplasia. Neurologic examination should be performed in all children with scoliosis to determine whether some of these disorders are present.

Five to 7 percent of cases of scoliosis are due to congenital vertebral anomalies such as a hemivertebra or unilateral vertebral bridge. These curves are more rigid than the more common idiopathic curve (see below) and will often increase with growth, especially during adolescence. Eighty percent of cases of scoliosis are idiopathic. Since 30% of family members are also affected, siblings of an affected child should be examined.

Idiopathic infantile scoliosis, occurring in children 2–4 years of age, is uncommon in the United States but more common in Great Britain. If the rib-vertebral angle of Mehta is less than 20 degrees, the curve will resolve spontaneously. If the angle is greater, the curve will progress. Postural compensation of the spine may lead to lateral curvature from such causes as unequal length of the lower extremities. Sciatic scoliosis may result from pressure on the spinal cord or roots by infectious processes or herniation of the nucleus pulposus; the underlying cause must be sought. The curvature will resolve as the primary problem is treated.

Clinical Findings

A. Symptoms and Signs: Scoliosis in adolescents is classically asymptomatic. It is imperative to seek the underlying cause in any case where there is pain, since in these instances the scoliosis is almost always secondary to some other disorder such as a bone or spinal cord tumor. Deformity of the rib cage and asymmetry of the waistline are evident with curvatures of 30 degrees or more. A lesser curvature may be detected by the forward bending test described above, which is designed to detect early abnormalities of rotation that are not apparent when the patient is standing erect.

B. Imaging: The most valuable x-rays are those taken of the entire spine in the standing position in both the anteroposterior and lateral planes. Usually, there is one primary curvature with a compensatory curvature that develops to balance the body. At times there may be two primary curvatures, usually in the right thoracic and left lumbar regions. Any left thoracic curvature should be suspected of being secondary to neurologic or muscular disease, prompting a more meticulous neurologic examination. If the curvatures of the spine are balanced (compensated), the head is centered over the center of the pelvis and the patient is "in balance." If the spinal alignment is uncompensated, the head will be displaced to one side, which produces an unsightly deformity. Rotation of the spine may be measured by scoliometer as described by Bunnell (1984). This rotation is associated with a marked rib hump as the lateral curvature increases in severity. Deformity of the rib cage causes long-term problems when lung volumes are reduced.

Treatment

Treatment of scoliosis depends on curve magnitude, skeletal maturity, and risk of progression. Curvatures of less than 20 degrees usually do not require treatment unless they show progression. Bracing is indicated for curvature of 20–40 degrees in a skeletally immature child. Treatment is indicated for any curvature that demonstrates progression on serial x-ray examination. Curvatures greater than 40 degrees are resistant to treatment by bracing. Thoracic curvatures greater than 60 degrees have been correlated with poor pulmonary function in adult life. Curvatures of such severity are an indication for surgical correction and posterior spinal fusion to maintain the correction. Curvatures between 40 and 60 degrees may also require spinal fusion if they are progressive, are causing decompensation of the spine, or are cosmetically unacceptable.

Surgical fusion involves decortication of the bone over the laminas and spinous processes, with the addition of autogenous bone graft from the iliac crest. Postoperative correction is usually maintained by rods and hooks, with activity restriction for several months until the fusion is solid. Treatment is prolonged and difficult and is best done in centers where full support facilities are available.

Prognosis

Compensated small curves that do not progress may be well tolerated throughout life, with very little cosmetic concern. The patients should be counseled regarding the genetic transmission of scoliosis and cautioned that their children should be examined at regular intervals. Large thoracic curvatures greater than 60 degrees are associated with shortened life span and may progress during adult life. Large lumbar curvatures may lead to subluxation of the vertebrae and premature arthritic degeneration of the spine, producing disabling pain in adulthood. Early detection allows for simple brace treatment. In patients so treated, the long-term prognosis is excellent, and surgery is not necessary. For this reason, school screening programs for scoliosis have gained popular support.

Bunnell WP: An objective criterion for scoliosis screening. J Bone Joint Surg Am 1984;66:1381.

Nachemson AL et al: Effectiveness of treatment with a brace in girls who have adolescent idiopathic scoliosis. J Bone Joint Surg Am 1995;77:815.

Peterson LE et al: Prediction of progression of the curve in girls who have adolescent idiopathic scoliosis of moderate severity. J Bone Joint Surg Am 1995;77:823.

Weinstein SL: Idiopathic scoliosis: Natural history. Spine 1986;11:780.

SLIPPED CAPITAL FEMORAL EPIPHYSIS

Slipped capital femoral epiphysis is separation of the proximal femoral epiphysis through the growth plate. The head of the femur is usually displaced medially and posteriorly relative to the femoral neck. The condition occurs in adolescence and is most common in obese males. The cause is not clear, although some authorities have shown experimentally that the strength of the perichondrial ring stabilizing the epiphysial area is sufficiently weakened by hormonal changes during adolescence that the overload of excessive body weight can produce a pathologic fracture through the growth plate. Hormonal studies in these children are normal. The histology of the area of separation is identical with that seen with traumatic separation.

The condition occasionally occurs acutely following a fall or direct trauma to the hip. More commonly, there are vague symptoms over a protracted period in an otherwise healthy child who presents with pain and limp. The pain is often referred into the thigh or the medial side of the knee. It is important to examine the hip joint in any child complaining of knee pain. The consistent finding on physical examination is limitation of internal rotation of the hip. There usually is also an associated hip flexion contracture as well as local tenderness about the hip. X-rays should be taken in both the anteroposterior and lateral planes as the diagnosis may be apparent only in the lateral view.

Treatment is based on the same principles that govern treatment of fracture of the femoral neck in adults in that the head of the femur is fixed to the neck of the femur and the fracture line allowed to heal. Unfortunately, the severe complication of avascular necrosis occurs in 30% of these patients. There is a positive correlation between forceful reduction of the slip and avascular necrosis. In cases of acute slip, as evidenced by the absence of any callus formation about the growth plate, it may be possible to reduce the hip by gentle traction. In more chronic cases, a more expeditious procedure is to pin the slip as it lies. Remodeling of the fracture site often improves the position of the hip without further surgery.

The long-term prognosis is guarded because most of these patients continue to be overweight and overstress their hip joints. Follow-up studies have shown a high incidence of premature degenerative arthritis in this disease—even in those who do not develop avascular necrosis. The development of avascular necrosis almost always guarantees a poor prognosis, because new bone does not replace the femoral head at this late stage of skeletal growth.

About 30% of patients have bilateral involvement, which may occur as late as 1 or 2 years after the primary episode.

Aronson DD, Carlson WE: Slipped capital femoral epiphysis: A prospective study of fixation with a single screw. J Bone Joint Surg Am 1992;74:810.

Loder RT et al: Slipped capital femoral epiphysis associated with endocrine disorders. J Pediatr Orthop 1995; 15:349.

Stanitski CL: Acute slipped capital femoral epiphysis: Treatment alternatives. J Am Acad Orthop Surg 1994; 2:96.

GENU VARUM & GENU VALGUM

Genu varum (bowleg) is normal from infancy through 2 years of life. The alignment then changes to **genu valgum** (knock-knee) until about 8 years of age, at which time adult alignment is attained. Criteria for referral to an orthopedist include persistent bowing beyond age 2, bowing that is increasing rather than decreasing, bowing of one leg only, and knock-knee associated with short stature.

Bracing may be appropriate. Rarely, an osteotomy is necessary for a severe problem such as Blount's disease (proximal tibial epiphysial dysplasia).

Health CH, Staheli LT: Normal limits of knee angle in white children: Genu varum and genu valgum. J Pediatr Orthop 1993;13:259.

Stricker SJ et al: Langenskïold classification of tibia vara: An assessment of interobserver variability. J Pediatr Orthop 1994;14:152.

TIBIAL TORSION

The physician is often asked about "toeing in" in small children. Tibial torsion is rotation of the leg between the knee and the ankle. Internal rotation amounts to about 20 degrees at birth but decreases to neutral rotation by 16 months of age. The deformity is sometimes accentuated by laxity of the knee ligaments, allowing excessive internal rotation of the leg in small children. In children who have a persistent internal rotation of the tibia beyond 16–18 months of age, the condition is often due to sleeping with feet turned in and can be reversed with an external rotation splint worn only at night.

FEMORAL ANTEVERSION

"Toeing in" beyond 2 or 3 years of age is usually secondary to femoral anteversion, which produces excessive internal rotation of the femur rather than external rotation. This femoral alignment follows a natural history of progressive decrease toward neutral up to 8 years of age, with slower change to 16 years of age. Studies comparing the results of treatment with shoes or braces to the natural history have shown that little is gained by active treatment. Active external rotation exercises such as ballet, skating, or bicycle riding may be worthwhile. Osteotomy for rotational correction is rarely required. Refer those who have no external rotation of hip in extension.

Staheli LT et al: Lower-extremity rotational problems in children: Normal values to guide management. J Bone Joint Surg Am 1985;67:39.

Staheli LT: Rotational problems in children. In: *Instructional Course Lectures,* vol 43. American Academy of Orthopaedic Surgeons, 1993.

COMMON FOOT PROBLEMS

When a child begins to stand and walk, the long arch of the foot is flat with a medial bulge over the inner border of the foot. The forefeet are mildly pronated or rotated inward, with a slight valgus alignment of the knees. As the child grows and joint laxity decreases, the long arch is better supported and more normal relationships occur in the lower extremities. (See also Metatarsus Varus and Talipes Equinovarus.)

1. FLATFOOT

Flatfoot is a normal condition in infants. Children presenting for examination should be checked to determine that the heel cord is of normal length when the heel is aligned in the neutral position, allowing complete dorsiflexion and plantar flexion. As long as the foot is supple and a longitudinal arch is noted when the child is sitting in a non-weight-bearing position, the parents can be assured that a normal arch will probably develop. There is usually a familial incidence of relaxed flatfeet in children who have no apparent arch. In any child with a shortened heel cord or stiffness of the foot, other causes of flatfoot such as tarsal coalition or vertical talus should be ruled out by a complete orthopedic examination and x-ray.

In the child with an ordinary relaxed flatfoot, no active treatment is indicated unless there is calf or leg pain. In children who have leg pains attributable to flatfoot, a supportive shoe with scaphoid pad, such as a good-quality sports shoe, is useful. An orthotic that holds the heel in neutral and supports the arch may relieve discomfort if more is needed. An arch insert should not be prescribed unless passive correction of the arch is easily accomplished; otherwise, there will be irritation of the skin over the medial side of the foot.

Any child with a painful or rigid flatfoot should be referred to an orthopedist.

Rao UB, Joseph B: The influence of footwear on the prevalence of flat foot: A survey of 2,300 children. J Bone Joint Surg Br 1992;74:525.
Wenger DR et al: Corrective shoes and inserts as treatment for a flexible flatfoot in infants and children. J Bone Joint Surg Am 1989;71:800.

2. TALIPES CALCANEOVALGUS

Talipes calcaneovalgus is characterized by excessive dorsiflexion at the ankle and eversion of the foot. It is often present at birth and is due to intrauterine position. Treatment consists of passive exercises by the mother, stretching the foot into plantar flexion. In rare instances, it may be necessary to use plaster casts to help with manipulation and positioning. Complete correction is the rule.

3. CAVUS FOOT

This deformity consists of an unusually high longitudinal arch of the foot. It may be hereditary or associated with neurologic conditions such as poliomyelitis, Charcot-Marie-Tooth disease, Friedreich's ataxia, or diastematomyelia. There is usually an associated contracture of the toe extensor, producing a claw toe deformity in which the metatarsal phalangeal joints are hyperextended and the interphalangeal joints acutely flexed. Any child presenting with cavus feet should have a careful neurologic examination and x-rays of the spine.

Conservative therapy is ineffective. In symptomatic cases, operation may be necessary to lengthen the contracted extensor and flexor tendons and to release the plantar fascia and other tight plantar structures. Arthrodesis of the foot may be necessary later. The associated varus heel deformity causes more problems with gait than the high arch.

4. BUNIONS (Hallux Valgus)

Girls may present in adolescence with lateral deviation of the great toe associated with a prominence over the head of the first metatarsal. This deformity is painful only with shoe wear and almost always can be relieved by fitting shoes that are wide enough. Surgery should be avoided in the adolescent age group, because further growth tends to cause recurrence of the deformity.

Groiso J: Juvenile hallux: A conservative approach to treatment. J Bone Joint Surg Am 1992;74:1375.
Peterson HA et al: Adolescent bunion deformity treated with double osteotomy and longitudinal pin fixation of the first ray. J Pediatr Orthop 1993;13:80.

DEGENERATIVE PROBLEMS (Arthritis, Bursitis, & Tenosynovitis)

Degenerative arthritis may follow childhood skeletal problems such as infection, slipped capital femoral epiphysis, avascular necrosis, or trauma or may occur in association with hemophilia. Early effective treatment of these disorders will prevent arthritis. Late treatment is often unsatisfactory.

Degenerative changes in the soft tissues around joints may occur as a result of overuse syndrome in adolescent athletes. Young boys throwing excessive numbers of pitches, especially curve balls, may develop "little leaguer's elbow," consisting of degenerative changes around the humeral condyles associated with pain, swelling, and limitation of motion. In order to enforce the rest necessary for healing, a plaster cast may be necessary. A more reasonable preventive measure is to limit the number of pitches thrown by children.

Acute bursitis is uncommon in childhood, and other causes should be ruled out before this diagnosis is accepted.

Tenosynovitis is most common in the region of the knees and feet. Children taking dancing lessons, particularly toe dancing, may have pain around the flexor tendon sheaths in the toes or ankles. Rest is effective treatment. At the knee level, there may be irritation of the patellar ligament, with associated swelling in the infrapatellar fat pad. Synovitis in this area is usually due to overuse and is treated by rest. Corticosteroid injections are contraindicated.

Kunnamo I et al: Clinical signs and laboratory tests in the differential diagnosis of arthritis in children. Am J Dis Child 1987;141:34.
Pugh MT, Southwood TR, Gaston JS: The role of infection

in juvenile chronic arthritis. Br J Rheumatol 1993; 32:838.

TRAUMA

SOFT TISSUE TRAUMA
(Sprains, Strains, & Contusions)

A sprain is the stretching of a ligament, and a strain is a stretch of a muscle or tendon. In either of these injuries, there may be some degree of tissue tearing. Contusions are generally due to tissue compression, with damage to blood vessels within the tissue and the formation of hematoma.

A severe sprain is one in which the ligament is completely disrupted, resulting in instability of the joint. A mild or moderate sprain is one in which incomplete tearing of the ligament occurs, but in which there is associated local pain and swelling.

Mild or moderate sprains are treated by rest of the affected joint, with ice and elevation to prevent prolonged symptoms. By definition, mild or moderate sprain is not associated with instability of the joint.

If there is more severe trauma resulting in tearing of a ligament, instability of the joint may be demonstrated by gross examination or by stress testing with x-ray documentation. Such deformity of the joint may cause persistent instability resulting from inaccurate apposition of the ligament ends during healing. If instability is evident, surgical repair of the torn ligament may be indicated. If a muscle is torn at its tendinous insertion, it should be repaired.

The initial treatment of any sprain consists of ice, compression, and elevation. The purpose of the treatment is to decrease local edema and residual stiffness resulting from gelling of blood proteins in the interstitial space. Splinting of the affected joint protects against further injury and relieves swelling and pain. Ibuprofen or other nonsteroidal anti-inflammatory agents are useful for pain.

1. ANKLE SPRAINS

The history will indicate that the injury was by either forceful inversion or eversion. The more common inversion injury results in tearing or injury to the lateral ligaments, whereas an eversion injury will injure the medial ligaments of the ankle. The injured ligaments may be identified by means of careful palpation for point tenderness around the ankle. The joint should be supported or immobilized at a right angle, which is the functional position. Adhesive taping may be effective to maintain this position but should be applied by one skilled in the use of tape and changed frequently to prevent the formation of blisters and skin damage. A posterior plaster splint is more easily applied and gives good joint rest if the extremity is protected by using crutches for weight bearing. Prolonged use of a plaster cast is usually not necessary, but the sprained ankle should be rested sufficiently to allow complete healing. This may take 3–6 weeks. Rehabilitation to include strengthening and restitution of kinesthetic sensation can prevent long-term disability.

2. KNEE SPRAINS

Sprains of the collateral and cruciate ligaments are uncommon in children. These ligaments are so strong that it is more common to injure the epiphysial growth plates, which are the weakest structures in the region of the knees of children. In adolescence, however, the physes have started to close, and the knee joint is more like that of an adult, so that rupture of the anterior cruciate ligament can result from a twisting injury. If the injury produces avulsion of the tibial spine, open anatomic reduction is often required.

Effusion of the knee after trauma deserves referral to an orthopedic specialist. The differential diagnosis includes torn ligament, torn meniscus, and osteochondral fracture. Nontraumatic effusion should be evaluated for inflammatory conditions (such as juvenile rheumatoid arthritis) or patellar malalignment.

3. INTERNAL DERANGEMENTS OF THE KNEE

Meniscal injuries are uncommon under age 12. Clicking or locking of the knee may occur in young children as a result of a discoid lateral meniscus, which is a rare congenital anomaly. As the child approaches adolescence, internal damage to the knee from a torsion weight-bearing injury may result in locking of the knee if tearing and displacement of the meniscus occur. Osteochondral fractures secondary to osteochondritis dissecans may also present as internal derangements of the knee in adolescence. Posttraumatic synovitis may mimic a meniscal lesion. In any severe injury to the knee, epiphysial injury should be suspected; stress films will sometimes demonstrate separation of the distal femoral epiphysis in such cases. Epiphysial injury should be suspected whenever there is tenderness on both sides of the metaphysis of the femur after injury.

Cahill B: Osteochondritis dissecans of the knee: Treatment of juvenile and adult forms. J Am Acad Orthop Surg 1995;3:237.

Stanitski CL et al: Observations on acute knee hemarthrosis in children and adolescents. J Pediatr Orthop 1993; 13:506.

4. BACK SPRAINS

Sprains of the ligaments and muscles of the back are unusual in children but may occur as a result of violent trauma from automobile accidents or athletic injuries. Back pain in a child warrants clinical investigation because the complaint is more significant than in an adult. Inflammation, infection, and tumors are more common causes of back pain in children than sprains.

5. CONTUSIONS

Contusion of muscle with hematoma formation produces the familiar "charley horse" injury. Treatment of such injuries is by application of ice, compression, and rest. Exercise should be avoided for 5–7 days. Local heat may hasten healing once the acute phase of tenderness and swelling is past.

6. MYOSITIS OSSIFICANS

Ossification within muscle occurs when there is sufficient trauma to cause a hematoma that later heals in the manner of a fracture. The injury is usually a contusion and occurs most commonly in the quadriceps of the thigh or the triceps of the arm. When a severe injury with hematoma is recognized, it is important to splint the extremity and avoid activity. If further trauma causes recurrent injury, ossification may reach spectacular proportions and resemble an osteosarcoma.

Disability is great, with local swelling and heat and extreme pain upon the slightest motion of the adjacent joint. The limb should be rested, with the knee in extension or the elbow in 90 degrees of flexion, until the local reaction has subsided. After local heat and tenderness have decreased, gentle active exercises may be initiated. Passive stretching exercises are not indicated, because they may stimulate the ossification reaction. It is occasionally necessary to excise excessive bony tissue if it interferes with muscle function once the reaction is mature. Surgery should not be attempted before 9 months to 1 year after injury, because it may restart the process and lead to an even more severe reaction.

Micheli LJ (editor): Injuries in the young athlete. Clin Sports Med 1988;7:459.

TRAUMATIC SUBLUXATIONS & DISLOCATIONS

Dislocation of a joint is always associated with severe damage to the ligaments and joint capsule. In contrast to fracture treatment, which may be safely postponed, dislocations must be reduced immediately. Dislocations can usually be reduced by gentle sustained traction. It often happens that no anesthetic is necessary for several hours after the injury, because of the protective anesthesia produced by the injury. Following reduction, the joint should be splinted for transportation of the patient.

The dislocated joint should be treated by immobilization for at least 3 weeks, followed by graduated active exercises through a full range of motion. Physical therapy is usually not indicated for children with injuries. As a matter of fact, vigorous manipulation of the joint by a therapist may be harmful. The child should be permitted to exercise actively. No passive stretching should be permitted.

1. SUBLUXATION OF THE RADIAL HEAD (Nursemaid's Elbow)

Infants frequently sustain subluxation of the radial head as a result of being lifted or pulled by the hand. The child appears with the elbow fully pronated and painful. The usual complaint is that the child's elbow will not bend. X-ray findings are normal, but there is point tenderness over the radial head. When the elbow is placed in full supination and slowly moved from full flexion to full extension, a click may be palpated at the level of the radial head. The relief of pain is remarkable, as the child usually stops crying immediately. The elbow may be immobilized in a sling for comfort for a day. Occasionally, symptoms last for several days, requiring more prolonged immobilization.

Pulled elbow may be a clue to battering. This should be considered during examination, especially if the problem is recurrent.

2. RECURRENT DISLOCATION OF THE PATELLA

Recurrent dislocation of the patella is more common in loose-jointed individuals, especially adolescent girls. If the patella completely dislocates, it nearly always goes laterally. Pain is severe, and the patient is brought to the doctor with the knee slightly flexed and an obvious bony mass lateral to the knee joint and a flat area over the usual location of the patella. X-ray examination confirms the diagnosis. The patella may be reduced by extending the knee and placing slight pressure on the patella while gentle traction is exerted on the leg. In subluxation of the patella, the symptoms may be more subtle, and the patient may say that the knee "gives out" or "jumps out of place."

In the case of complete dislocation, the knee should be immobilized for 3–4 weeks, followed by a physical therapy program for strengthening the quadriceps muscle. Operation may be necessary to tighten the knee joint capsule if dislocation or subluxation is recurrent. In such instances, if the patella is not stabilized, repeated dislocation produces damage to the articular cartilage of the patellofemoral joint and premature degenerative arthritis.

Vähäsarja V et al: Operative realignment of patellar malalignment in children. J Pediatr Orthop 1995;15:281.

EPIPHYSIAL SEPARATIONS

In children, epiphysial separations and fractures are more common than ligamentous injuries. This finding is based on the fact that the ligaments of the joints are generally stronger than the associated growth plates. In instances in which dislocation is suspected, an x-ray should be taken in order to rule out epiphysial fracture. Films of the opposite extremity, especially for injuries around the elbow, may be valuable for comparison. Reduction of a fractured epiphysis should be done under anesthesia to align the growth plate with the least amount of force. Fractures across the growth plate may produce bony bridges that will cause premature cessation of growth or angular deformities of the extremity. Epiphysial fractures around the shoulder, wrist, and fingers can usually be treated by closed reduction, but fractures of the epiphyses around the elbow often require open reduction. In the lower extremity, accurate reduction of the epiphysial plate is necessary to prevent joint deformity if a joint surface is involved. If angular deformities result, corrective osteotomy may be necessary.

Mosely CF: General features of fractures in children. In: *Instructional Course Lectures,* 41:337–346. Eilert RE (editor). American Academy of Orthopaedic Surgeons, 1992.

TORUS FRACTURES

Torus fractures consist of "buckling" of the cortex due to compression of the bone.They usually occur in the distal radius or ulna. Alignment is usually satisfactory, and simple immobilization for 3 weeks is sufficient.

GREENSTICK FRACTURES

With greenstick fractures there is frank disruption of the cortex on one side of the bone but no discernible cleavage plane on the opposite side. These fractures are angulated but not displaced, since the bone ends are not separated. Reduction is achieved by straightening the arm into normal alignment, and reduction is maintained by a snugly fitting plaster cast. It is necessary to x-ray children with greenstick

fractures again in a week to 10 days to make certain that the reduction has been maintained in plaster. A slight angular deformity can be corrected by remodeling of the bone. The farther the fracture is from the growing end of the bone, the longer the time required for remodeling. The fracture can be considered healed when there is no tenderness or local heat and when adequate bony callus is seen on x-ray.

FRACTURE OF THE CLAVICLE

Clavicular fractures are very common injuries in infants and children. They can be immobilized in a sling for comfort. The healing callus will be apparent when the fracture has consolidated, but this unsightly lump will generally resolve over a period of months to a year.

SUPRACONDYLAR FRACTURES OF THE HUMERUS

Supracondylar fractures tend to occur in the age group from 3 to 6 years and are potentially dangerous because of the proximity to the brachial artery in the distal arm. They are usually associated with a significant amount of trauma, so that swelling may be severe. **Volkmann's ischemic contracture** of the forearm may occur as a result of vascular embarrassment. When severe swelling is present, the safest course is to place the arm in traction and carefully observe nerve function and the vascular supply to the hand. In these cases, the children should be hospitalized and followed up carefully by experienced nurses. If the blood supply is compromised, exposure of the brachial artery may be necessary, although this is rarely needed when satisfactory reduction and traction are employed. Most often, these fractures are treated by closed reduction and percutaneous pinning. Complications associated with supracondylar fractures also include a resultant cubitus varus (decreased carrying angle) secondary to poor reduction. Such a "gunstock" deformity of the elbow may be somewhat unsightly but does not usually interfere with joint function.

Kurer MH, Regan MW: Completely displaced supracondylar fracture of the humerus in children: A review of 1708 comparable cases. Clin Orthop 1990;256:205.
Topping RE et al: Clinical evaluation of crossed pin versus lateral pin fixation in displaced supracondylar humerus fractures. J Pediatr Orthop 1995;15:435.

GENERAL COMMENTS ON OTHER FRACTURES IN CHILDREN

Reduction of fractures in children is usually accomplished by simple traction and manipulation;

open reduction is rarely indicated. Remodeling of the fracture callus usually produces an almost normal appearance of the bone over a matter of months. The younger the child, the more remodeling is possible. Angular deformities remodel with ease. Rotatory deformities do not remodel, and this produces the cubitus varus deformity sometimes seen after supracondylar fractures.

The physician should be suspicious of child abuse whenever the age of a fracture does not match the history given or when the severity of the injury is more than the alleged accident would have produced. In suspected cases of battering where no fracture is present on the initial x-ray film, a repeat film 10 days later is in order. Bleeding beneath the periosteum will be calcified by 7–10 days, and the x-ray appearance is almost diagnostic of severe closed trauma characteristic of a battered child.

Dent JA, Patterson CR: Fractures in early childhood: Osteogenesis imperfecta or child abuse? J Pediatr Orthop 1991;11:184.

Ogden JA: *Skeletal Injury in the Child.* Lea & Febiger, 1982.

Rang M: *Children's Fractures,* 2nd ed. Lippincott, 1983.

Rockwood CA Jr, Wilkins K, Beaty JH (editors): *Fractures in Children,* 4th ed. Lippincott-Raven, 1996.

Weber BG, Brunner C, Freuler F (editors): *Treatment of Fractures in Children and Adolescents.* Springer, 1980.

INFECTIONS OF THE BONES & JOINTS

OSTEOMYELITIS

Osteomyelitis is an infectious process that usually starts in the spongy or medullary bone and then extends to involve compact or cortical bone. The lower extremities are most often affected, and there is commonly a history of trauma. Osteomyelitis may occur as a result of direct invasion from the outside through a penetrating wound (nail) or open fracture, but hematogenous spread of infection (eg, pyoderma or upper respiratory tract infection) from other infected areas is much more common. The most common infecting organism is *Staphylococcus aureus,* which has a tendency to infect the metaphyses of growing bones. Anatomically, circulation in the long bones is such that the arterial supply to the metaphysis just below the growth plate is by end arteries, which turn sharply to end in venous sinusoids, causing a relative stasis. In the infant under 1 year of age, there is direct vascular communication with the epiphysis across the growth plate, so that direct spread may occur from the metaphysis to the epiphysis and subse-

quently into the joint. In the older child, the growth plate provides an effective barrier and the epiphysis is usually not involved, although the infection spreads retrograde from the metaphysis into the diaphysis and, by rupture through the cortical bone, down along the diaphysis beneath the periosteum.

1. EXOGENOUS OSTEOMYELITIS

To avoid osteomyelitis by direct extension, all wounds must be carefully examined and cleansed. Puncture wounds are especially liable to lead to osteomyelitis if not carefully debrided. Cultures of the wound made at the time of exploration and debridement may be useful if signs of infection develop subsequently. Copious irrigation is necessary, and all nonviable skin, subcutaneous tissue, fascia, and muscle must be excised. In extensive or contaminated wounds, antibiotic coverage is indicated. Contaminated wounds should be left open and secondary closure performed 3–5 days later. If at the time of delayed closure further necrotic tissue is present, it should be excised. Leaving the wound open allows the infection to stay at the surface rather than extend inward to the bone.

Initially, broad-spectrum antibiotics should be used. After cultures have been read, an appropriate antibiotic can be chosen if there is lingering inflammation. A tetanus toxoid booster may be indicated. Gas gangrene is best prevented by adequate debridement.

After exogenous osteomyelitis has become established, treatment becomes more complicated, requiring extensive surgical debridement and drainage in hospital with intravenous antibiotics.

2. HEMATOGENOUS OSTEOMYELITIS

Hematogenous osteomyelitis is usually caused by pyogenic bacteria; 85% of cases are due to staphylococci. Streptococci are a less common cause of osteomyelitis. *Pseudomonas* organisms are common in cases of nail puncture wounds. Children with sickle cell anemia are especially prone to osteomyelitis caused by salmonellae.

Clinical Findings

A. Symptoms and Signs: In infants, the manifestations of osteomyelitis may be subtle, presenting as irritability, diarrhea, or failure to feed properly; the temperature may be normal or slightly low; and the white blood count may be normal or only slightly elevated. There may be pseudoparalysis of the involved limb. In older children, the manifestations are more striking, with severe local tenderness and pain, high fever, rapid pulse, and elevated white blood count and sedimentation rate. Osteomyelitis of a lower extremity often presents around the knee in a child 7–10 years of age. Tenderness is most marked over the metaphysis of the bone where the process has its origin. The child may limp or refuse to bear weight.

B. Laboratory Findings: Blood cultures are often positive early. The most significant test in infancy is the aspiration of pus when suspicion arises because of lack of movement in a painful extremity. It is useful to needle the bone in the area of suspected infection and aspirate any fluid present. This fluid should be stained for organisms as well as cultured. Even edema fluid may be useful for determining the causative organism. The white blood cell count is usually elevated, as is the sedimentation rate.

C. Imaging: Nonspecific local swelling is the first x-ray finding. This is followed by elevation of the periosteum, with formation of new bone from the cambium layer of the periosteum occurring after 3–6 days. As the infection becomes chronic, areas of cortical bone are isolated by pus spreading down the medullary canal, causing rarefaction and demineralization of the bone. Such isolated pieces of cortex become ischemic and form sequestra (dead bone fragments). These x-ray findings are late but specific. Osteomyelitis should be diagnosed clinically before significant x-ray findings are present. Bone scan is sensitive but nonspecific in suspected cases before x-ray findings become positive. MRI can demonstrate edema early or soft tissue thickening later.

Treatment

A. Specific Measures: Oral antibiotics are appropriate when tenderness, fever, the white cell count, and the erythrocyte sedimentation rate are all decreasing and the culture is positive. Serum bactericidal levels should exceed 1:8. Antibiotics should be started intravenously as soon as the diagnosis of osteomyelitis is made. Agents that cover *Staphylococcus aureus* and *Streptococcus pyogenes* (eg, oxacillin, nafcillin, or cefazolin) are appropriate for most cases. For specific recommendations and for possible *Pseudomonas* infection, see Chapter 36.

Chronic infections are treated for months. Following surgical debridement, *Pseudomonas* foot infections usually respond to 1–2 weeks of treatment.

B. General Measures: Splinting of the limb minimizes pain and decreases spread of the infection by lymphatic channels through the soft tissue. The splint should be removed periodically to allow active use of adjacent joints and prevent stiffening and muscle atrophy. In chronic osteomyelitis, splinting may be necessary to guard against fracture of the weakened bone.

C. Surgical Measures: Aspiration of the metaphysis for culture and Gram stain is the most useful diagnostic measure in any case of suspected osteomyelitis. In the first 23–72 hours, it may be possible to treat osteomyelitis by antibiotics alone. If frank pus

is aspirated from the bone, however, surgical drainage is indicated. If the infection has not shown a dramatic response within 24 hours, surgical drainage is also indicated. It is important that all devitalized soft tissue be removed and adequate exposure of the bone obtained to permit free drainage. Excessive amounts of bone should not be removed when draining acute osteomyelitis, because they may not be completely replaced by the normal healing process. Little damage is done by surgical drainage, but failure to drain the pus in acute cases may lead to more severe damage.

Prognosis

When osteomyelitis is diagnosed in the early clinical stages and prompt antibiotic therapy is begun, the prognosis is excellent. If the process has been unattended for a week to 10 days, there is almost always some permanent loss of bone structure, as well as the possibility of growth abnormality.

Dormans JP, Drummond DS: Pediatric hematogenous osteomyelitis: New trends in presentation, diagnosis and treatment. J Am Acad Orthop Surg 1994;2:333.
Jacobs RF et al: Management of *Pseudomonas* osteochondritis complicating puncture wounds of the foot. Pediatrics 1982;69:432.
Mazur JM et al: Usefulness of magnetic resonance imaging for diagnosis of acute musculoskeletal infections in children. J Pediatr Orthop 1995;15:144.

PYOGENIC ARTHRITIS

The source of pyogenic arthritis varies according to the age of the child. In the infant, pyogenic arthritis often develops by spread from adjacent osteomyelitis. In the older child, it presents as an isolated infection, usually without bony involvement. In teenagers with pyogenic arthritis, an underlying systemic disease is usually the cause, such as an obvious generalized infection or an organism (eg, the gonococcus) that has an affinity for joints.

The infecting organism varies with age: group B streptococcus and *Staphylococcus aureus* in those under 4 months; *Haemophilus influenzae* and *Staphylococcus* in those 4 months to 4 years old; and *Staphylococcus* and *Streptococcus pyogenes* in older children and adolescents. *Haemophilus influenzae* is now uncommon because of effective immunization.

The initial effusion of the joint rapidly becomes purulent. An effusion of the joint may accompany osteomyelitis in the adjacent bone. A white cell count exceeding 100,000/μL in the joint fluid indicates a definite purulent infection. Generally, spread of infection is from the bone into the joint, but unattended pyogenic arthritis may also affect adjacent bone. The sedimentation rate is often above 50 mm/h.

Clinical Findings

A. Symptoms and Signs: In older children,

the signs are striking, with fever, malaise, vomiting, and restriction of motion. In infants, paralysis of the limb due to inflammatory neuritis may be evident. Infection of the hip joint in infants can be diagnosed if suspicion is aroused by decreased abduction of the hip in an infant who is irritable or feeding poorly. A history of umbilical catheter treatment in the newborn nursery should alert the physician to the possibility of pyogenic arthritis of the hip.

B. Imaging: Early distention of the joint capsule is nonspecific and difficult to measure by x-ray. In the infant with unrecognized pyogenic arthritis, dislocation of the joint may follow within a few days as a result of distention of the capsule by pus. Later changes include destruction of the joint space, resorption of epiphysial cartilage, and erosion of the adjacent bone of the metaphysis. The bone scan shows increased flow and increased uptake about the joint.

Treatment

Diagnosis may be made by aspiration of the joint. In the hip joint, pyogenic arthritis is most easily treated by surgical drainage because the joint is deep and difficult to aspirate as well as being inaccessible to thorough cleaning through needle aspiration. More recently, arthroscopic irrigation and debridement have been successful in treating pyogenic arthritis of the knee. If fever and clinical symptoms do not subside within 24 hours after treatment is begun, open surgical drainage is indicated. Antibiotics can be selected based on age, Gram's stain, and culture of the aspirated pus. Reasonable empiric therapy in infants is nafcillin or oxacillin plus a third-generation cephalosporin. An antistaphylococcal agent alone is usually adequate for children over 5 years. For staphylococcal infections, 3 weeks of therapy is recommended; for other organisms, 2 weeks is usually sufficient. Oral therapy may be begun when clinical signs have markedly improved. It is not necessary to give intra-articular antibiotics, since good levels are achieved in the synovial fluid.

Prognosis

The prognosis for the patient with pyogenic arthritis is excellent if the joint is drained early, before damage to the articular cartilage has occurred. If infection is present for more than 24 hours, there is dissolution of the proteoglycans in the articular cartilage, with subsequent arthrosis and fibrosis of the joint. Damage to the growth plate may also occur, especially within the hip joint, where the epiphysial plate is intracapsular.

Betz RR et al: Late sequelae of septic arthritis of the hip in infancy and childhood. J Pediatr Orthop 1990;10:365.

Shaw BA, Kasser JR: Acute septic arthritis in infancy and childhood. Clin Orthop 1990;257:212.

TUBERCULOUS ARTHRITIS

Tuberculous arthritis is now a rare disease in the United States. It must be considered, however, in children with resistant infections of the joints, especially those with a history of tuberculosis in family members. Generally, the infection may be ruled out by skin testing. The joints most commonly affected in children are the intervertebral disks, resulting in gibbus or dorsal angular deformity at the site of involvement.

Treatment is by local drainage of the "cold abscess," followed by antituberculous therapy. Prolonged immobilization in a plaster cast or prolonged bed rest is necessary to promote healing. Spinal fusion may be required to preserve stability of the vertebral column.

DISKITIS

Results of a study of 47 patients support the view that so-called diskitis is pyogenic infectious spondylitis in children and that specific treatment and intravenous antibiotics are more likely to lead to rapid relief of symptoms and signs without recurrence.

TRANSIENT SYNOVITIS OF THE HIP

The most common cause of limping and pain in the hip of children in the United States is transitory synovitis, an acute inflammatory reaction that often follows an upper respiratory infection and is generally self-limited. In questionable cases, aspiration of the hip yields only yellowish fluid, ruling out pyogenic arthritis. Generally, however, toxic synovitis of the hip is not associated with elevation of the erythrocyte sedimentation rate, the white blood count or a temperature above 38.3 °C. It classically affects children 3–10 years of age and is more common in boys. There is limitation of motion of the hip joint, particularly internal rotation, and x-ray changes are nonspecific, with some swelling apparent in the soft tissues around the joint.

Treatment consists of bed rest and the use of traction with slight flexion of the hip. Nonsteroidal antiinflammatory medications may shorten the course of the disease, though even with no treatment duration of the disease usually is limited to days. It is important to maintain x-ray follow-up because toxic synovitis may be the precursor of avascular necrosis of the femoral head (next section) in a small percentage of patients. X-ray films can be obtained at 1 month and 3 months, or earlier if there is persistent limp or pain.

Hodges DL, McGuire TJ: Hip pain in children: An anatomic approach. Orthop Rev 1988;17:251.

Terjesen T, Osthus P: Ultrasound in the diagnosis and follow-up of transient synovitis of the hip. J Pediatr Orthop
1991;11:608.

VASCULAR LESIONS & AVASCULAR NECROSIS (Osteochondroses)

AVASCULAR NECROSIS OF THE PROXIMAL FEMUR (Legg-Calvé-Perthes Disease)

The vascular supply of bone is generally precari-
ous, and when it is interrupted, necrosis results. In
contrast to other body tissues that undergo infarction,
bone removes necrotic tissue and replaces it with living bone in a process called "creeping substitution."
This replacement of necrotic bone may be so complete and so perfect that a completely normal bone
results. Adequacy of replacement depends on the age
of the patient, the presence or absence of associated
infection, the congruity of the involved joint, and
other physiologic and mechanical factors.

Because of their rapid growth in relation to their
blood supply, the secondary ossification centers in
the epiphyses are subject to avascular necrosis. Despite the number of different names referring to avascular necrosis of the epiphyses, the process is identical, necrosis of bone followed by replacement (Table
23–1).

Even though the pathologic and radiologic features of avascular necrosis of the epiphyses are well
known, the cause is not generally agreed upon.
Necrosis may follow known causes such as trauma or
infection, but idiopathic lesions usually develop during periods of rapid growth of the epiphyses. Thus,

Table 23–1. The osteochondroses.

Ossification Center	Eponym	Typical Age
Capital femoral	Legg-Calvé-Perthes disease	3–5
Tarsal navicular	Köhler's bone disease	6
Second metatarsal head	Freiberg's disease	12–14
Vertebral ring	Scheuemann's disease	13–16
Capitellum	Panner's disease	9–11
Tibial tubercle	Osgood-Schlatter disease	11–13
Calcaneus	Sever's disease	8–9

the highest incidence of Legg-Calvé-Perthes disease
is between 4 and 8 years of age.

Clinical Findings

A. Symptoms and Signs: Persistent pain is
the most common symptom, and the patient may present with limp or limitation of motion.

B. Laboratory Findings: Laboratory findings,
including studies of joint aspirates, are normal.

C. Imaging: X-ray findings correlate with the
progression of the process and the extent of necrosis.
The early finding is effusion of the joint associated
with slight widening of the joint space and periarticu-
lar swelling. Decreased bone density in and around
the joint is apparent after a few weeks. The necrotic
ossification center appears more dense than the surrounding viable structures, and there is collapse or
narrowing of the femoral head.

As replacement of the necrotic ossification center
occurs, there is rarefaction of the bone in a patchwork
fashion, producing alternating areas of rarefaction and
relative density or "fragmentation" of the epiphysis.

In the hip, there may be widening of the femoral
head associated with flattening, giving rise to the
term **coxa plana.** If infarction has extended across
the growth plate, there will be a radiolucent lesion
within the metaphysis. If the growth center of the
femoral head has been damaged so that normal
growth does not occur, varus deformity of the
femoral neck will occur as a result of overgrowth of
the greater trochanteric apophysis.

Eventually, complete replacement of the epiphysis
will become apparent as new bone replaces necrotic
bone. The final shape of the head depends on the extent of the necrosis and collapse that has been allowed to occur.

Differential Diagnosis

Differential diagnosis must include inflammatory
and infectious lesions of the joints or apophyses.
Transient synovitis of the hip may be distinguished
from Legg-Calvé-Perthes disease by serial x-rays.

Treatment

Treatment consists simply of protection of the
joint. If the joint is deeply seated within the acetabulum and normal joint motion is maintained, a reasonably good result can be expected. Bracing is no
longer believed to be of benefit.

Prognosis

The prognosis for complete replacement of the
necrotic femoral head in a child is excellent, but the
functional result depends on the amount of deformity
that develops during the time the softened structure exists. In Legg-Calvé-Perthes disease, the prognosis depends on the completeness of involvement of the epiphysial center. In general, patients with metaphysial
defects, those in whom the disease develops late in

childhood, and those who have more complete involvement of the femoral head have a poorer prognosis.

Osteochondrosis due to vascular lesions may affect various growth centers. Table 23–1 indicates the common sites and the typical ages at presentation.

Fulford GE et al: A prospective study of non-operative and operative management for Perthes disease. J Pediatr Orthop 1993;13:281.

Martinez AG, Weinstein SL, Dietz FR: Weight bearing abduction brace treatment of Legg-Calvé-Perthes disease. J Bone Joint Surg Am 1992;74:12.

McAndrew MP, Weinstein SL: A long-term follow-up of Legg-Calvé-Perthes disease. J Bone Joint Surg Am 1984;66:860.

OSTEOCHONDRITIS DISSECANS

In osteochondritis dissecans, a wedge-shaped necrotic area of bone and cartilage develops adjacent to the articular surface. The fragment of bone may be broken off from the host bone and displaced into the joint as a loose body. If it remains attached, the necrotic fragment may be completely replaced by creeping substitution.

The pathologic process is the same as that described previously for avascular necrosing lesions of ossification centers. Because these lesions are adjacent to articular cartilage, however, there may be joint damage.

The most common sites of these lesions are the knee (medial femoral condyle), the elbow joint (capitellum), and the talus (superior lateral dome).

Joint pain is the usual presenting complaint. However, local swelling or locking may be present, particularly if there is a fragment free in the joint. Laboratory studies are normal.

Treatment consists of protection of the involved area from mechanical damage. If there is a fragment free within the joint as a loose body, it must be arthroscopically removed. For some marginal lesions, it may be worthwhile to drill the necrotic fragment to encourage more rapid vascular ingrowth and replacement. If large areas of a weight-bearing joint are involved, secondary degenerative arthritis may result.

NEUROLOGIC DISORDERS INVOLVING THE MUSCULOSKELETAL SYSTEM

ORTHOPEDIC ASPECTS OF CEREBRAL PALSY

Early physical therapy to encourage completion of the normal developmental patterns may be of benefit in patients with cerebral palsy. The greatest gains from this therapy are obtained during the first few years of life, and therapy should not be continued when no improvement is apparent.

Bracing and splinting are of questionable benefit, although night splints may be useful in preventing equinus deformity of the feet or adduction contractures of the hips. Orthopedic surgery is useful for treating joint contractures that interfere with function. In general, muscle transfers are unpredictable in cerebral palsy, and most orthopedic procedures are directed at tendon lengthening or bony stabilization by osteotomy or arthrodesis. Recently, selective dorsal rhizotomy has been used in selected cases.

Flexion and adduction of the hip due to hyperactivity of the adductors and flexors may produce a progressive paralytic dislocation of the hip, which can lead to pain and dysfunction. Treatment of this dislocation is difficult and unsatisfactory. The principal preventive measure is abduction bracing, but this must often be supplemented by release of the adductors and hip flexors in order to prevent dislocation. In severe cases, osteotomy of the femur may also be necessary to correct the bony deformities of femoral anteversion and coxa valga that are invariably present. Patients with a predominantly athetotic pattern are poor candidates for any surgical procedure or bracing.

Because it is difficult to predict the outcome of surgical procedures in cerebral palsy, the surgeon must examine patients on several occasions before any operative procedure is undertaken. Follow-up care by a physical therapist to maximize the anticipated long-term gains should be arranged before the operation.

Bleck EE: Orthopaedic Management of Cerebral Palsy. MacKeith, 1987.

Boscarino LF et al: Effects of selective dorsal rhizotomy on gait in children with cerebral palsy. J Pediatr Orthop 1993;13:174.

Little DG et al: Late hip subluxation in spastic diplegia associated with unrecognized hydrocephalus. J Pediatr Orthop 1995;15:368.

Moreau M et al: Adductor and psoas release for subluxation of the hip in children with spastic cerebral palsy. J Pediatr Orthop 1995;15:672.

ORTHOPEDIC ASPECTS OF MYELODYSPLASIA

Patients born with spina bifida cystica (aperta) should be examined early by an orthopedic surgeon. The level of neurologic involvement determines the muscle imbalance that will be present and apt to produce deformity with growth. The involvement is often asymmetric and tends to change during the first 12–18 months of life. Early closure of the sac is the rule, although there has been some hesitancy to treat all of these patients because of the extremely poor prognosis associated with congenital hydrocephalus, high levels of paralysis, and associated congenital anomalies. A high percentage of these children have hydrocephalus, which may be evident at birth or shortly thereafter, requiring shunting. Associated musculoskeletal problems may include clubfoot, congenital dislocation of the hip, arthrogryposis type changes of the lower extremities, and congenital scoliosis, among others. The most common lesions are at the level of L3–4 and tend to affect the hip joint, with progressive dislocation occurring during growth. Foot deformities may be in any direction and are complicated by the fact that sensation is generally absent. Spinal deformities develop in a high percentage of these children, with scoliosis present in approximately 40%. Ambulation may require long leg braces. Careful urologic follow-up must be obtained to prevent complications from bladder dysfunction.

In children who have a reasonable likelihood of walking, operative treatment consists of reduction of the hip and alignment of the feet in the weight-bearing position as well as stabilization of the scoliosis. In children who lack active quadriceps function and extensor power of the knee, the likelihood of ambulation is greatly decreased. In such patients, aggressive surgery in the hip region may result in stiffening of the joints, thus preventing sitting. Multiple foot operations are also contraindicated in these children.

The overall management of the child with spina bifida should be coordinated in a multidiscipline clinic where all doctors can also work with therapists, social workers, and teachers to provide the best possible care.

Beaty JH, Canale ST: Orthopaedic aspects of myelomeningocele. J Bone Joint Surg Am 1990;72:626.

Swank M, Dias LS: Walking ability in spina bifida patients: A model for predicting future ambulatory status based on sitting balance and motor level. J Pediatr Orthop 1994;14:715.

NEOPLASIA OF THE MUSCULOSKELETAL SYSTEM

Neoplastic diseases of the musculoskeletal system are a serious problem because of the poor prognosis of malignant tumors arising in bone or other tissues derived from mesoderm. Fortunately, few of the benign lesions undergo malignant transformation. Accurate diagnosis depends upon correlation of the clinical, x-ray, and microscopic findings. A child with complaints about the knee should be investigated for tumor, though the usual causes of knee pain are traumatic, infectious, or developmental in origin.

Osteochondroma

Osteochondroma is the most common bone tumor in children. It usually presents as a pain-free mass. Any pain that may be present is due to adventitious bursitis or tendinitis due to irritation by the tumor. The lesion may be single or multiple. Pathologically, the lesion is a bone mass capped with cartilage. These masses tend to grow during childhood and adolescence in proportion to the child's growth.

On x-ray the tumors tend to be in the metaphysial region of long bones and may be pedunculated or sessile. The cortex of the underlying bone "flows" into the base of the tumor.

An osteochondroma should be excised if it interferes with function, is frequently traumatized, or is large enough to be deforming. The prognosis is excellent. Malignant transformation is very rare.

Osteoid Osteoma

Osteoid osteoma classically produces night pain that can be relieved by aspirin. On physical examination there usually is tenderness over the lesion. An osteoid osteoma in the upper femur may cause pain referred to the knee.

On x-ray the lesion is a radiolucent nidus surrounded by dense osteosclerosis that may obscure the nidus. Bone scan shows intense uptake in the lesion.

Surgical incision of the nidus is curative and may be done using computed tomography imaging and minimally invasive technique. The prognosis is excellent, with no known cases of malignant transformation, though the lesion has a tendency to recur.

Enchondroma

Enchondroma is usually a silent lesion unless it produces a pathologic fracture. On x-ray it is radiolucent, usually in a long bone. There may be speckled calcification. The classic lesion looks as though someone dragged his fingernails through clay, making streaks in the bones. Enchondroma is treated by surgical curettage and bone grafting. The prognosis is excellent. Malignant transformation may occur but is very rare in childhood.

Chondroblastoma

Chondroblastoma presents with pain around a joint and may produce a pathologic fracture. On x-ray the lesion is radiolucent and can perforate the epiphysial cartilage. Calcification is unusual, with little or no reactive bone. The lesion is treated by surgical curettage and bone grafting. The prognosis is excellent if complete curettage is performed. There is no known malignant transformation.

Nonossifying Fibroma

Nonossifying fibroma is also called "benign cortical defect" and is nearly always an incidental finding on an incidental x-ray. The most frequent sites are the distal femur and proximal tibia. Nonossifying fibroma is a radiolucent lesion eccentrically located in the bone. Usually there is a thin sclerotic border. Multiple lesions may be present. No treatment is needed since these lesions heal as they ossify with maturation of the bone and growth. The prognosis is excellent.

Osteosarcoma

Osteosarcoma usually presents as pain in a long bone, though functional loss, the mass of the tumor, or limp may be the presenting complaint. Pathologic fracture is common. The malignant osseous tumor produces a destructive expanding and invasive lesion. There may be a triangle adjacent to the tumor produced by elevated periosteum and subsequent tumor ossification. The lesion may contain calcification and violates the cortex of the bone. Femur, tibia, humerus, and other long bones are the sites usually affected.

Surgical excision (limb salvage) or amputation is indicated based on the extent of the tumor. The lesion is radioresistant and does not respond to chemotherapy. Adjuvant chemotherapy is routinely used prior to surgical excision. The prognosis is improving, with 30% 5-year survival rates being reported in modern series. Death usually occurs due to lung metastasis.

Ewing's Sarcoma

The presenting complaint is usually pain and tenderness. Fever and leukocytosis may also be present, which makes osteomyelitis part of the differential diagnosis. The lesion may be multicentric. Ewing's sarcoma is radiolucent and destroys the cortex, frequently in the diaphysial region. There may be reactive bone formation about the lesion, seen as successive layers of so-called "onion skin layering."

Treatment is with multiagent chemotherapy, radiation, and surgical resection. The prognosis is poor with large tumor size, pelvic lesions, and poor response to chemotherapy. Metastasis occurs to multiple organs.

Cara JA, Canadell J: Limb salvage for malignant bone tumors in young children. J Pediatr Orthop 1994;14:112.

Gebhardt MC, Ready JE, Mankin JH: Tumors about the knee in children. Clin Orthop 1990;255:86.

Meyer WH, Malawer MM: Osteosarcoma: Clinical features and evolving surgical and chemotherapeutic strategies. Pediatr Clin North Am 1991;38:317.

O'Connor MI, Pritchard DJ: Ewing's sarcoma: Prognostic factors, disease control, and the reemerging role of surgical treatment. Clin Orthop 1991;262:78.

Simon MA, Finn HA: Diagnostic strategy for bone and soft-tissue tumors. J Bone Joint Surg Am 1993;75:622.

MISCELLANEOUS DISEASES OF BONE

FIBROUS DYSPLASIA

Dysplastic fibrous tissue replacement of the medullary canal is accompanied by the formation of metaplastic bone in fibrous dysplasia. Three forms of the disease are recognized: monostotic, polyostotic, and polyostotic with endocrine disturbances (precocious puberty in females, hyperthyroidism, and hyperadrenalism [Albright's syndrome]).

Clinical Findings

A. Symptoms and Signs: The lesion or lesions may be asymptomatic. Pain, if present, is probably due to pathologic fractures. In females, endocrine disturbances may be present in the polyostotic variety and associated with café au lait spots.

B. Laboratory Findings: Laboratory findings are normal unless endocrine disturbances are present, in which case there may be increased secretion of gonadotropic, thyroid, or adrenal hormones.

C. Imaging: The lesion begins centrally within the medullary canal, usually of a long bone, and expands slowly. Pathologic fracture may occur. If metaplastic bone predominates, the contents of the lesion will be of the density of bone. Marked deformity of the bone may result, and a shepherd's crook deformity of the upper femur is a classic feature of the disease. The disease is often asymmetric, and limb length disturbances may occur as a result of stimulation of epiphysial cartilage growth.

Differential Diagnosis

The differential diagnosis includes other fibrous lesions of bone as well as destructive lesions such as unicameral bone cyst, eosinophilic granuloma, aneurysmal bone cyst, nonossifying fibroma, enchondroma, and chondromyxoid fibroma.

Treatment

If the lesion is small and asymptomatic, no treatment is needed. If the lesion is large and produces or threatens pathologic fracture, curettage and bone grafting are indicated.

Prognosis

Unless the lesions impair epiphysial growth, the prognosis for patients with fibrous dysplasia is good. Lesions tend to enlarge during the growth period but are stable during adult life. Malignant transformation is rare.

UNICAMERAL BONE CYST

Unicameral bone cyst occurs in the metaphysis of a long bone, usually in the femur or humerus. It begins within the medullary canal adjacent to the epiphysial cartilage. It probably results from some fault in enchondral ossification. The cyst is "active" as long as it abuts onto the metaphysial side of the epiphysial cartilage and "inactive" when a border of normal bone exists between the cyst and the epiphysial cartilage. The lesion is usually identified when a pathologic fracture occurs, producing pain. Laboratory findings are normal. On x-ray films, the cyst is identified centrally within the medullary canal, producing expansion of the cortex and thinning over the widest portion of the cyst.

Treatment consists of injection with corticosteroid. Several injections may be required. If injection fails, then curettage and bone grafting may be required. The cyst may heal after a fracture and not require treatment. The prognosis is good.

ANEURYSMAL BONE CYST

Aneurysmal bone cyst is similar to unicameral bone cyst, but it contains blood rather than clear fluid. It usually occurs in a slightly eccentric position in the long bone, expanding the cortex of the bone but not breaking the cortex, although some extraosseous mass may be produced. On x-ray films, the lesion appears somewhat larger than the width of the epiphysial cartilage, and this feature distinguishes it from unicameral bone cyst.

The aneurysmal bone cyst is filled by large vascular lakes, and the stoma of the cyst contains fibrous tissue and areas of metaplastic ossification.

The lesion may appear aggressive histologically, and it is important to differentiate it from osteosarcoma or hemangioma. Treatment is by curettage and bone grafting, and the prognosis is good.

INFANTILE CORTICAL HYPEROSTOSIS
(Caffey's Syndrome)

Infantile cortical hyperostosis is a benign disease of unknown cause that has its onset before 6 months of age and is characterized by irritability, fever, and nonsuppurating, tender, painful swellings. Swellings may involve almost any bone of the body and are frequently widespread. Classically, there are swellings of the mandible and clavicle in 50% of cases as well as of the ulna, humerus, and ribs. The disease is limited to the shafts of bones and does not involve subcutaneous tissues or joints. It is self-limited but may persist for weeks or months. Anemia, leukocytosis, an increased sedimentation rate, and elevation of the serum alkaline phosphatase are usually present. Cortical hyperostosis is demonstrable by a typical x-ray appearance and may be diagnosed on physical examination by an experienced pediatrician.

Fortunately, the disease appears to be decreasing in frequency. Corticosteroids are effective in severe cases. The prognosis is good, and the disease usually terminates without deformity.

GANGLION

A ganglion is a smooth, small cystic mass connected by a pedicle to the joint capsule, usually on the dorsum of the wrist. It may also be seen in the tendon sheath over the flexor surfaces of the fingers. These ganglia can be excised if they interfere with function or cause persistent pain.

BAKER'S CYST

Baker's cyst is a herniation of the synovium in the knee joint into the popliteal region. In children, the diagnosis may be made by aspiration of mucinous fluid, but the cyst nearly always disappears with time. Whereas Baker's cysts may be indicative of intra-articular disease in the adult, they usually are of no clinical significance in children and rarely require excision.

Dinham JM: Popliteal cysts in children: The case against surgery. J Bone Joint Surg Br 1975;57:69.

Rheumatic Diseases

24

J. Roger Hollister, MD

JUVENILE RHEUMATOID ARTHRITIS
(Juvenile Chronic Arthritis)

Essentials of Diagnosis
& Typical Features

- Nonmigratory monarticular or polyarticular arthropathy, with a tendency to involve large joints or proximal interphalangeal joints and lasting more than 3 months.
- Systemic manifestations with fever, erythematous rashes, nodules, leukocytosis, and, occasionally, iridocyclitis, pleuritis, pericarditis, anemia, fatigue, and growth failure.

General Considerations

Juvenile rheumatoid arthritis (JRA) patients exhibit different immunogenetic traits from adult rheumatoid arthritis patients. In juvenile rheumatoid arthritis, HLA-DR5 is associated with iritis and the production of antinuclear antibodies, whereas HLA-DR4 is found in seropositive, polyarticular disease. These traits may be important in the formation of anti-suppressor cell antibodies, immune complex generation, and consequent chronic inflammatory disease. Tumor necrosis factor may be the final common cytokine that perpetuates the inflammation.

Clinical Findings

A. Symptoms and Signs: There are three major patterns of presentation in JRA that provide clues to the prognosis and possible sequelae of the disease. In the **acute febrile form,** an evanescent salmon-pink macular rash, arthritis, hepatosplenomegaly, leukocytosis, and polyserositis characterize the constellation described by George Still. These patients have episodic illness, and remission of the systemic features can be expected within 1 year. They do not develop iridocyclitis.

The **polyarticular pattern** resembles the adult disease, with chronic pain and swelling of many joints in a symmetric fashion. Both large and small joints are usually involved. Systemic features are less prominent, although low-grade fever, fatigue, rheumatoid nodules, and anemia may be present.

These patients tend to have long-standing arthritis, although the disease may wax and wane. Iridocyclitis is occasionally seen in this group. Older children may have a positive rheumatoid factor test.

The third pattern consists of **pauciarticular disease,** characterized by chronic arthritis of a few joints—often the large weight-bearing joints—in an asymmetric distribution. The synovitis is usually mild and may be painless. Systemic features are uncommon, but there is severe extra-articular involvement with inflammation in the eye. Up to 30% of children with pauciarticular juvenile rheumatoid arthritis develop insidious, asymptomatic iridocyclitis, which may cause blindness if untreated. The activity of the eye disease does not correlate with that of the arthritis. Therefore, routine ophthalmologic screening with slit-lamp examination must be performed every 6 months for 4 years, after which the risk is much lower.

B. Laboratory Findings: There is no diagnostic test for JRA. Rheumatoid factor is positive by the latex fixation test in about 15% of cases, usually when onset of polyarticular disease occurs after age 8 years. Antinuclear antibodies are most often present in pauciarticular disease with iridocyclitis and may serve as an indication of this complication; they are also fairly common in the late-onset rheumatoid factor-positive group. A normal erythrocyte sedimentation rate does not exclude the diagnosis.

In Table 24–1 are listed the general characteristics of joint fluid in various conditions. A positive Gram stain or culture is the only definitive test for infection. A leukocyte count over 2000/μL suggests inflammation; this may be due to infection, any of the collagen-vascular diseases, leukemia, or reactive arthritis. A very low glucose concentration (< 40 mg/dL) or very high polymorphonuclear leukocyte count (> 60,000/μL) is highly suggestive of bacterial arthritis in a child. Chemical analysis of synovial fluid is otherwise of little diagnostic benefit.

C. Imaging: In the early stages of the disease, only soft tissue swelling and regional osteoporosis are seen. MRI of involved joints may show joint damage earlier in the course of the disease than with other imaging modalities.

Table 24–1. Joint fluid analysis.

Disorder	Cells/μL	Glucose[1]
Trauma	More red cells than white cells; usually < 2000 white cells	Normal
Reactive arthritis	3000–10,000 white cells, mostly mono-nuclears	Normal
Juvenile rheumatoid arthritis and other inflammatory arthritides	5000–60,000 white cells, mostly neutrophils	Usually normal or slightly low
Septic arthritis	> 60,000 white cells, > 90% neutrophils	Low to normal

[1]Normal value is 75% or more of serum glucose value.

Differential Diagnosis

Table 24–2 lists the most common causes of limb pain in childhood. A few points of information may indicate the most likely diagnosis. For instance, orthopedic causes are due to increased physical activity, not major trauma. Reactive arthritides are suggested by a preceding viral infection, strep throat, or purpuric rash, and their course is waxing and waning over several days.

Monarticular arthritis is the most important differential disorder to establish. Pain in the hip or lower extremity is a frequent symptom with childhood cancer, especially leukemia, neuroblastoma, and rhabdomyosarcoma. Infiltration of bone by tumor and actual joint effusion may be seen. X-rays of the affected site and a careful examination of the blood smear for unusual cells and thrombocytopenia are necessary. In doubtful cases, bone marrow examination is indicated.

Bacterial arthritis is usually acute and monarticular except for arthritis associated with *Haemophilus influenzae* infection and gonorrhea, both of which may be associated with a migratory pattern. Fever, leukocytosis, and increased sedimentation rate with an acute process in a single joint demand synovial fluid examination and culture to identify the pathogen.

The arthritis of rheumatic fever is migratory, transient, and often more painful than that of juvenile rheumatoid arthritis. Rheumatic fever is very rare under the age of 5 years. Evidence of rheumatic carditis should be carefully sought. Evidence of recent streptococcal infection is essential to the diagnosis. The fever pattern in rheumatic fever is low grade and persistent compared with the intermittent fever in the systemic form of JRA. Lyme arthritis resembles pauciarticular juvenile rheumatoid arthritis, but it occurs as discrete, recurrent episodes of arthritis lasting 2–6 weeks. A negative test for antibodies to *Borrelia burgdorferi* argues strongly against this diagnosis.

Table 24–2. Differential diagnosis of limb pain in children.

Orthopedic
  Stress fracture
  Overuse syndrome
  Chondromalacia patellae
  Osgood-Schlatter disease
  Slipped capital femoral epiphysis
  Legg-Calvé-Perthes disease
  Hypermobility syndrome
Reactive arthritis
  Schönlein-Henoch purpura
  Reactive arthritis following diarrhea
  Toxic synovitis of the hip
  Transient synovitis following viral infection
  Rheumatic fever
Infections
  Bacterial
    Lyme arthritis
    Osteomyelitis
    Septic arthritis
    Discitis
  Viral
    Parvovirus (in adolescents)
    Rubella
    Hepatitis B arthritis
Collagen-vascular
  Juvenile rheumatoid arthritis
  Spondyloarthropathy
  Systemic lupus erythematosus
  Dermatomyositis
Neoplastic
  Leukemia
  Lymphoma
  Neuroblastoma
  Reticuloendotheliosis
  Osteoid osteoma
  Bone tumors (benign or malignant)
Syndromes of psycho-organic origin
  Growing pains
  Fibromyalgia
  Reflex neurovascular dystrophy

Treatment

The objectives of therapy are to restore function, relieve pain, and maintain joint motion. In recent years, other nonsteroidal anti-inflammatory drugs (NSAIDs) have replaced salicylates in the medical treatment of juvenile rheumatoid arthritis. Although their anti-inflammatory potency is not different from that of aspirin, their liquid form, decreased frequency of dosing, and diminished side effects appear to enhance compliance, cause fewer side effects, and justify their increased cost. Naproxen, 7.5 mg/kg twice daily; ibuprofen, 10 mg/kg four times daily; and tolmetin sodium, 10 mg/kg three times daily, may be used. If benefit occurs in the first 2 days, there will be continued improvement, with the maximum effect at 6 weeks. Aspirin, 75–100 mg/kg/d in three divided doses, is equally effective. Salicylates are withheld if the patient is exposed to chickenpox or Asian flu. Range-of-motion and muscle-strengthening exercises should be taught and supervised by a therapist, and a home program should be instituted. Bed rest is to be avoided except in the most acute stages. Joint casting is almost never indicated.

In JRA patients who fail to respond to aspirin, there are a number of alternatives. Methotrexate has replaced injectable gold salt therapy as a second-line medication. Symptomatic response usually occurs within 3–4 weeks. The low doses used (5–10 mg/m^2/wk as a single dose) have been associated with few side effects. Stomatitis usually resolves with continued administration. Nausea may be prevented by splitting the dose. Hepatotoxicity, including fibrosis, is a concern. A CBC and liver function tests should be obtained at 2-month intervals. Liver biopsy may be performed if there are recurrent elevations of aminotransferases. Injectable gold salts are an alternative in refractory cases.

Iridocyclitis should be treated by an ophthalmologist, and methotrexate may be used in difficult cases. Local corticosteroid injections into joints, synovectomy, or joint replacement may be indicated in selected patients.

Prognosis

In the primarily articular forms of JRA, disease activity progressively diminishes with age and ceases in about 95% of cases by puberty. In a few instances, this will persist into adult life. Problems after puberty therefore relate primarily to residual joint damage. Cases presenting in the teen years usually presage adult disease. The children most liable to be permanently handicapped are those with unremitting synovitis, hip involvement, or positive rheumatoid factor tests.

Dana MR et al: Visual outcomes prognosticators in juvenile rheumatoid arthritis-associated uveitis. Ophthalmology 1997;104:236.

Feldman BM et al: Seasonal onset of systemic-onset juvenile rheumatoid arthritis. J Pediatr 1996;129:513.

Grom AA et al: Patterns of expression of tumor necrosis factor α, tumor necrosis factor β, and their receptors in synovia of patients with juvenile rheumatoid arthritis and juvenile spondylarthropathy. Arthritis Rheum 1996; 39:1703.

Huppertz et al: Intraarticular corticosteroids for chronic arthritis in children: Efficacy and effects on cartilage and growth. J Pediatr 1995;127:317.

Kugathasan S et al: Liver biopsy findings in patients with juvenile rheumatoid arthritis receiving long-term weekly methotrexate therapy. J Pediatr 1996;128:149.

Rosenberg AM: Treatment of juvenile rheumatoid arthritis: Approach to patients who fail standard therapy. J Rheumatol 1996;23:9.

Tibbits G. Juvenile rheumatoid arthritis: Old challenges, new insights. Postgrad Med 1994;96:75.

Wallace CA et al: Increased risk of facial scars in children taking nonsteroidal anti-inflammatory drugs. J Pediatr 1994;125:819.

Wallendal M et al: The discriminating value of serum lactate dehydrogenase levels in children with malignant neoplasms presenting as joint pain. Arch Pediatr Adolesc Med 1996;150:70.

SPONDYLOARTHROPATHY

Lower extremity arthritis, particularly in males over 10 years of age, suggests a form of spondyloarthropathy. Inflammation of tendinous insertions (enthesopathy) such as the tibial tubercle or the heel occurs in these diseases and not in juvenile rheumatoid arthritis. Low back pain and sacroiliitis are quite specific for this form of arthritis. Carriage of HLA-B27 antigen occurs in 80% of these individuals. Specific syndromes of Reiter's disease, inflammatory bowel disease, psoriasis, or postdiarrheal reactive arthritis are suggested by the associated clinical findings and epidemiology. No autoantibodies are found, but inflammatory indicators such as an elevated erythrocyte sedimentation rate or C-reactive protein are usually present. The episodes are usually intermittent, in contrast to the more chronic symptoms of juvenile rheumatoid arthritis. Acute, not chronic, uveitis may occur.

The nonsteroidal medications, particularly indomethacin (2–4 mg/kg/d) and naproxen (15 mg/kg/d), are more effective than salicylates in the spondyloarthropathies. Refractory cases may respond to sulfasalazine. Local corticosteroid injections are contraindicated in Achilles tendinitis.

The arthritis is usually episodic. Unlike adults, children do not frequently progress to joint destruction or ankylosis.

Cabral DA et al: Spondyloarthropathies of childhood. Pediatr Clin North Am 1995;42:1051.

SYSTEMIC LUPUS ERYTHEMATOSUS

Essentials of Diagnosis & Typical Features

- Multisystem inflammatory disease of joints, serous linings, skin, kidneys, and central nervous system.
- Antinuclear antibodies must be present in active, untreated disease.

General Considerations

Systemic lupus erythematosus (SLE) is the prototype of immune complex diseases; its pathogenesis is related to deposition in the tissue of soluble immune complexes existing in the circulation. The spectrum of symptoms appears to be due not to tissue-specific autoantibodies but rather to damage to the tissue by lymphocytes, neutrophils, and complement evoked by the deposition of antigen-antibody complexes. Many such antigen-antibody systems are present in this disorder, but the best correlation exists between DNA–anti-DNA complexes and the activity of the disease. Laboratory tests of these antibodies and complement components give an objective assessment of disease pathogenesis and response to therapy. Autoreactive T lymphocytes that have escaped clonal deletion and unregulated B lymphocyte production of autoantibodies may initiate the disease.

Clinical Findings

A. Symptoms and Signs: The onset of systemic lupus erythematosus is most common in girls (8:1) between the ages of 9 and 15 years. The symptoms depend on what organ is involved with immune complex deposition.

1. Joint symptoms are the most common presenting feature. Nondeforming arthritis may involve any joint, often in a symmetric manner. Myositis may also occur and is more painful than the inflammation in dermatomyositis.

2. Systemic manifestations of SLE include weakness, anorexia, fever, fatigue, and loss of weight.

3. Skin lesions include butterfly erythema and induration, small ulcerations in skin and mucous membranes, purpura, alopecia, and Raynaud's phenomenon. The sun sensitivity of the dermal lesions may be striking.

4. Polyserositis may include pleurisy with effusions, peritonitis, and pericarditis. Libman-Sacks endocarditis may be seen in patients with anti-phospholipid antibodies.

5. Hepatosplenomegaly and lymphadenopathy may occur.

6. Renal systemic lupus erythematosus produces few symptoms at onset but is often progressive and is the leading cause of death. Renal biopsy is indicated in patients who do not respond to corticosteroids or who cannot have corticosteroids tapered to a less toxic alternate-day regimen. The histologic pattern of diffuse proliferative nephritis requires the most aggressive treatment. Late complications are nephrosis and uremia.

7. Central nervous system involvement produces a variety of symptoms such as seizures, coma, hemiplegia, focal neuropathies, chorea, and behavior disturbances, including psychosis.

B. Laboratory Findings: Leukopenia and anemia are frequently found with a low incidence of Coombs positivity. Thrombocytopenia and purpura may be early manifestations even in the absence of other organ involvement. The erythrocyte sedimentation rate (ESR) is elevated, and hypergammaglobulinemia is often present. Renal involvement is indicated by the presence in the urine of red cells, white cells, red cell casts, and proteinuria.

The antinuclear antibody (ANA) test is invariably positive in patients with active untreated SLE, and a negative ANA test effectively excludes the diagnosis. For patients with a positive antinuclear antibody test, a profile identifying individual disease-specific antibodies should be ordered. Anticardiolipin antibody and the lupus anticoagulant are two recently described autoantibodies that identify lupus patients at risk for thrombotic events.

In managing the disease, elevated titers of anti-DNA antibody and depressed levels of serum complement (hemolytic, C3, or C4) accurately reflect active disease, especially renal, central nervous system, and skin disease. A CT or MRI scan may identify pathologic conditions of the brain in lupus cerebritis, such as infarction, vasculitis, or atrophy.

Differential Diagnosis

Systemic lupus erythematosus may simulate many inflammatory diseases such as rheumatic fever, rheumatoid arthritis, and viral infections. It is essential to review all organ systems carefully to establish a clinical pattern. Renal and central nervous system involvement is unique to SLE. A negative ANA test excludes the diagnosis of systemic lupus erythematosus. Tests yielding false-positive results are usually of low titer (< 1:320).

An overlap syndrome known as mixed connective tissue disease, with features of several collagen-vascular diseases, has recently been described in adults and children. The symptom complex is diverse and does not readily fit previous classifications. Arthritis, fever, skin tightening, Raynaud's phenomenon, muscle weakness, and rashes are most commonly present. Important factors in recognition of this disease entity are the relative infrequency of renal disease, which implies a better prognosis than systemic lupus erythematosus, and the corticosteroid responsiveness of symptoms, which distinguishes mixed connective tissue disease from scleroderma. The definition of the disease includes the presence of serum antibody to a ribonuclear protein (RNP). The initial antinuclear antibody test is positive in very high titers. The ANA profile demonstrates the antibody to RNP. Pulmonary disease in childhood produces major morbidity.

Treatment

The treatment of systemic lupus erythematosus should be tailored to the organ system involved so that toxicities may be minimized. Prednisone, 0.5–1 mg/kg/d orally, has significantly lowered the mortality rate in SLE and should be used in all cases with renal, cardiac, or central nervous system involvement. The dose should be varied using clinical and laboratory parameters of disease activity, and the minimum amount of corticosteroid to control the disease should be used. Alternate-day regimens of corticosteroid are frequently possible. Skin manifestations may frequently be treated with antimalarials such as hydroxychloroquine, 5–7 mg/kg/d orally. Pleuritic pain or arthritis can often be managed with nonsteroidal anti-inflammatory medications.

If disease control is inadequate with prednisone or if the dose required produces intolerable side effects, an immunosuppressant should be added. Either azathioprine, 2–3 mg/kg/d orally, or cyclophosphamide, 0.5–1 g/m^2, administered intravenously once a month, has been most widely used. These drugs are ineffective during acute crises such as seizures.

The toxicities of the regimens must be carefully considered. In life-threatening disease, the choices are easier. Growth failure, osteoporosis, Cushing's syndrome, adrenal suppression, and aseptic necrosis are serious side effects of chronic use of prednisone. When high doses of corticosteroids are used (> 2 mg/kg/d), the risk of sepsis is very real. Cyclophosphamide causes bladder epithelial dysplasia, hemorrhagic cystitis, and sterility. Azathioprine has been associated with liver damage and bone marrow suppression. Immunosuppressant treatment should be withheld if the total white count falls below 3000/μL or the neutrophil count below 1000/μL. Retinal damage from chloroquine derivatives has not been observed with recommended dosages. Intravenous pulse steroid therapy and plasmapheresis are treatments that may be useful in selected cases.

Amenorrhea may result from uncontrolled systemic lupus erythematosus but may also be a consequence of prednisone, cyclophosphamide, or azathioprine administration.

Course & Prognosis

The prognosis in SLE relates to the presence of renal involvement or infectious complications of treatment. With improved diagnosis, milder cases are now identified. Nonetheless, the survival rate has improved from 51% at 5 years in 1954 to 90% today. The disease has a natural waxing and waning cycle, and periods of complete remission are not unusual.

Drenkard C et al: Remission of systemic lupus erythematosus. Medicine 1996;75:88.

Khamashta MA et al: The management of thrombosis in the antiphospholipid-antibody syndrome. N Engl J Med 1995;332:993.

Lang BA, Silverman ED: A clinical overview of systemic lupus erythematosus in childhood. Pediatr Rev 1993; 14:194.

Thomas C, Robinson JA: The antinuclear antibody test: When is a positive test clinically relevant. Postgrad Med 1993;94:191.

Tiddens HAWM et al: Juvenile-onset mixed connective tissue disease: Longitudinal follow-up. J Pediatr 1993; 94:55.

West SG et al: Neuropsychiatric lupus erythematosus: A 10-year prospective study on the value of diagnostic tests. Am J Med 1995;99:153.

DERMATOMYOSITIS (Polymyositis)

Essentials of Diagnosis & Typical Features
- Pathognomonic skin rash.
- Weakness of proximal muscles and occasionally of pharyngeal and laryngeal groups.
- Pathogenesis related to vasculitis.

General Considerations

Dermatomyositis, a rare inflammatory disease of muscle and skin in childhood, is uniquely responsive to corticosteroid treatment. The vasculitis observed in childhood dermatomyositis differs pathologically from the adult disease. Small arteries and veins are involved, with an exudate of neutrophils, lymphocytes, plasma cells, and histiocytes. The lesion progresses to intimal proliferation and thrombus formation. These vascular changes are found in the skin, muscle, kidney, retina, and gastrointestinal tract. Postinflammatory calcinosis is frequent.

The autoimmune pathogenesis of dermatomyositis has been difficult to prove. Recent studies have shown that both cellular and humoral mechanisms may be involved. Lymphocytes from patients are stimulated to undergo blastogenesis in the presence of muscle tissue and will release lymphotoxin, which destroys cultured fetal muscle cells. Biopsies studied with immunofluorescence techniques demonstrate immunoglobulin and complement in perivascular distribution. The putative antigen has not been identified and results of viral studies have been negative.

Clinical Findings

A. Symptoms and Signs: The predominant symptom is muscular weakness in proximal distribution affecting pelvic and shoulder girdles. Tenderness, stiffness, and swelling may be found but are not striking. Neurologic findings such as absence of tendon reflexes are not seen until late in the disease. Pharyngeal and respiratory involvement can be life-threatening. Flexion contractures and muscle atrophy produce significant residual deformities. Calcinosis may follow the inflammation in muscle and skin.

The rash of dermatomyositis is very helpful in the diagnosis of unknown muscle disease. Characteristically, the rash involves the upper eyelids and extensor surfaces of the knuckles, elbows, and knees with a distinctive heliotrope color that progresses to a scaling and atrophic appearance. Periorbital edema is not uncommon. Nail-fold capillary abnormalities may identify patients with a poorer prognosis. None of the rashes associated with other childhood rheumatic diseases have these features of distribution. The activity of the rash frequently does not parallel the muscle disease.

B. Laboratory Findings: Determination of muscle enzyme levels is the most helpful tool in diagnosis and treatment. All enzymes, including serum aldolase, should be screened to detect an abnormality that reflects activity of the disease. In later years of the illness, magnetic resonance imaging (MRI) of weak muscles may show disease activity when the enzymes are normal. No autoantibodies are found. Electromyography is useful to distinguish myopathic from neuropathic causes of muscle weakness. Muscle biopsy is indicated in doubtful cases of myositis without the pathognomonic rash.

Treatment

Prednisone in high doses (1–2 mg/kg/d orally) has been shown to speed recovery. The dose should be maintained or increased until muscle enzymes have returned to normal. Functional recovery will lag somewhat behind laboratory improvement. With improvement, the dose may be cut to that level which maintains disease control and normal muscle enzymes. Treatment must be continued for an average of 2 years. Immunosuppressant agents are occasionally required in childhood dermatomyositis. Intravenous immune globulin or cyclosporine therapy may be tried in refractory cases. Physical therapy is critical to prevent or allay contractures.

Course & Prognosis

Most children will recover and discontinue medications in 1–3 years. Relapses may occur. Functional ability is very good in most patients. Myositis in childhood is not associated with an increased risk of cancer.

Basta M, Dalakas MC: High-dose intravenous immunoglobulin exerts its beneficial effect in patients with dermatomyositis by blocking endomysial deposition of activated complement fragments. J Clin Invest 1994; 94:1729.

Lang B, Dooley J: Failure of pulse intravenous methylprednisolone treatment in juvenile dermatomyositis. J Pediatr 1996;128:429.

Miller LC et al: Methotrexate treatment of recalcitrant childhood dermatomyositis. Arthritis Rheum 1992;35: 1143.

Pachman L: Juvenile dermatomyositis: pathophysiology and disease expression. Pediatr Clin North Am 1995;42: 1071.

Zeller V et al: Cyclosporin A therapy in refractory juvenile dermatomyositis. J Rheumatol 1996;23:1424.

POLYARTERITIS NODOSA

Polyarteritis nodosa is a rare disease, but a significant number of cases have been reported in childhood and infancy. No single cause has been found, but evidence of a streptococcal trigger and poorly controlled parvovirus infection have been found in some series.

Pathologically, the disease is a vasculitis of medium-sized arteries with fibrinoid degeneration in the media extending to the intima and adventitia. Neutrophils and eosinophils comprise the inflammatory reaction. Aneurysms may be palpated or seen radiographically. Thrombosis of diseased arteries may cause infarction in many organs. Fibrosis of vessels and surrounding tissues accompanies the healing stages.

Symptomatology involves many tissues, and diagnosis is difficult. In childhood, unexplained fever, conjunctivitis, central nervous system involvement, and cardiac disease are more prominent than is the case in adult disease. Many cases appear as acute myocarditis, and the peripheral neuropathy so common in the adult is unusual. Diagnosis depends on biopsy-proved vasculitis or characteristic aneurysms on angiography.

The mortality rate is high, especially with cardiac involvement. Treatment consists of prednisone, 1–1.5 mg/kg/d orally, immunosuppressants, and intravenous immune globulin, but controlled studies of the efficacy of therapy of this rare disease are not yet available.

Athreya BH: Vasculitis in children. Pediatr Clin North Am 1995;42:1239.

Finkel TH et al: Chronic parvovirus B19 infection and systemic necrotizing vasculitides: Opportunistic pathogen or etiologic agent. Lancet 1994;343:1255.

Ozen S et al: Diagnostic criteria for polyarteritis nodosa in childhood. J Pediatr 1992;120:206.

DIFFUSE SCLERODERMA (Progressive Systemic Sclerosis)

Scleroderma is a rare disease in childhood. Both the generalized systemic type and **morphea** (the more localized benign form) have been described. The diagnosis is made on a clinical basis with the finding of a skin disease that progresses from an edematous phase to an atrophic, taut, immobile dermis involving some or all of the skin. Systemic involvement may include Raynaud's phenomenon, arthralgias, pulmonary fibrosis, and renal disease. Involvement of the lungs and kidneys leads to rapid demise. Histologically, the diagnosis may not be specific but includes dermal atrophy with increased fibrosis and collagen content. The pathogenesis remains obscure, but studies indicate an increased synthesis of immature collagen by cultured scleroderma fibroblasts.

Effective therapy still awaits a better understanding of disease pathogenesis. Physical therapy is sometimes helpful in reducing debilitation from contractures and muscle wasting.

Birdi N et al: Localized scleroderma progressing to systemic disease. Arthritis Rheum 1993;36:410.

Nelson AM: Localized scleroderma including morphea, linear scleroderma, and eosinophilic fasciitis. Curr Probl Pediatr 1996;26:318.

NONRHEUMATIC PAIN SYNDROMES

1. REFLEX SYMPATHETIC DYSTROPHY

Reflex sympathetic dystrophy is a painful condition that is frequently confused with arthritis. There appears to be both an increased prevalence and an increased recognition of the condition. Severe extremity pain leading to nearly complete loss of function is the hall-mark of the condition. Evidence of autonomic dysfunction is demonstrated by color changes, temperature differences, and dyshidrosis in the affected extremity. Foot involvement is more common than hand involvement. A puffy swelling of the entire hand or foot is common. On examination, there is marked cutaneous hyperesthesia to even the slightest touch. Results of laboratory tests are negative. X-ray findings are normal except for late development of osteoporosis. Bone scans are very helpful and demonstrate either increased or decreased blood supply to the painful extremity.

The cause of this condition remains elusive. Unlike adults, children only occasionally have a history of significant physical trauma at onset. How the autonomic dysfunction causes severe somatic pain is not known, but the feedback cycle does provide the basis for treatment. In mild cases, a program of rehabilitative physical therapy in combination with desensitization techniques will restore function and relieve pain. Refractory cases need family counseling and may respond to steroids or ganglionic blocks by local anesthesia. Long-term prognosis is good if recovery is rapid; recurrent episodes imply a less favorable prognosis.

Veldman P et al: Signs and symptoms of reflex sympathetic dystrophy: Prospective study of 829 patients. Lancet 1993;342:1012.

2. FIBROMYALGIA

Fibromyalgia is a diffuse pain syndrome in which patients experience pain all over their bodies without objective swelling. Weather changes and fatigue exacerbate symptoms. A sleep disturbance, such as insomnia or prolonged waking periods in the night, is an almost universal symptom; therefore, patients should be carefully questioned in this regard. On examination, patients are normal except for characteristic trigger points at the insertion of muscles, especially along the neck, spine, and pelvis.

Treatment consists of physical therapy and relieving the sleep disorder. Low-dose antidepressant medication (amitriptyline, 25 mg) taken before sleep may produce remarkable benefit in reduction of pain. Physical therapy should emphasize a graded rehabilitative approach to stretching and exercise. Analgesic medications provide poor pain relief and should be avoided because their use leads to escalation of medication, including narcotics.

The prognosis for young patients is not clear, and long-term strategies may be necessary to enable them to cope with the condition.

Bennett RM: Fibromyalgia: The commonest cause of widespread pain. Comprehensive Ther 1995;21:269.
Wilke WS: Treatment of "resistant" fibromyalgia. Rheum Dis Clin North Am 1995;21:247.

3. CHRONIC FATIGUE SYNDROME

Since 1985, chronic fatigue syndrome has become an increasingly common diagnosis. The distinction between this apparent organic fatigue and emotional causes of fatigue is not easily made. Criteria have been developed by NIH to assist in classification. The fatigue should have a defined date of onset, and there is a long list of excludable diagnoses. Other clinical manifestations include low-grade fevers, sore throat, painful lymph nodes, and neuropsychiatric problems. Epstein-Barr virus (EBV) infection does not account for all the patients described. Treatment is symptomatic and somewhat unsatisfactory.

Buchwald D: Fibromyalgia and chronic fatigue syndrome: similarities and differences. Rheum Dis Clin North Am 1996;22:219.
Wessely S et al: Postinfectious fatigue: Prospective cohort study in primary care. Lancet 1995;345:1333.
Wilson A et al: The treatment of chronic fatigue syndrome: Science and speculation. Am J Med 1994;96:544.

HYPERMOBILITY SYNDROME

Ligamentous laxity, which previously was thought to occur only in Ehlers-Danlos syndrome or Down's syndrome, is now recognized as a common cause of joint pain in our physically competitive society.

Children are now participating in a wide range of physically demanding sports and activities. Patients with hypermobility present with episodic joint pain and occasionally with swelling that lasts a few days after increased physical activity. Depending on the activity, almost any joint may be affected.

Physical examination may reveal joint swelling and tenderness, but the key to diagnosis is the demonstration of ligamentous laxity. Five criteria have been established: (1) passive opposition of the thumb to the flexor surface of the forearm; (2) passive hyperextension of the fingers so that they are parallel to the extensor surface of the forearm; (3) hyperextension of the elbow; (4) hyperextension of the knee (genu recurvatum); and (5) palms on floor with knees extended. Results of laboratory tests are normal. The pain associated with the syndrome is produced by improper joint alignment caused by the laxity during exercise.

Treatment consists of a graded conditioning program designed to provide muscular support of the joints to compensate for the loose ligaments. The prognosis is good provided conditioning before activities is adequate.

Gedalia A, Press J: Articular symptoms in hypermobile schoolchildren: A prospective study. J Pediatr 1991; 119:944.

REFERENCES

Cassidy JT, Petty RE: *Textbook of Pediatric Rheumatology,* 3rd ed. Saunders, 1995.

Jacobs JC: *Pediatric Rheumatology for the Practitioner,* 2nd ed. Springer, 1993.

Pediatric rheumatology. Pediatr Clin North Am 1995;42:5. (Entire issue.)

Hematologic Disorders

25

Peter A. Lane, MD, Rachelle Nuss, MD, & Daniel R. Ambruso, MD

NORMAL HEMATOLOGIC VALUES

The normal ranges for peripheral blood counts vary significantly with age. Normal neonates show a relative polycythemia with a hematocrit of 45–65%. The reticulocyte count at birth is relatively high at 2–8%. Within the first few days of life, erythrocyte production decreases, and the levels of hemoglobin and hematocrit fall to a nadir at about 2–3 months. During this period, known as **physiologic anemia of infancy,** normal infants have hemoglobins as low as 10 g/dL and hematocrits as low as 30%. (Premature infants can reach a nadir hemoglobin of 7–8 g/dL at 8–10 weeks.) Thereafter, the normal values for hemoglobin and hematocrit gradually increase until adult values are reached after puberty.

Newborns have larger red cells than children and adults, with a mean corpuscular volume (MCV) at birth of more than 94 fL. The MCV subsequently falls to a nadir of 70–84 fL at about 6 months of age. Thereafter, the MCV gradually increases until it reaches adult normal values after puberty.

The normal number of white blood cells is higher in infancy and early childhood than later in life. Neutrophils predominate in the differential white count at birth and in the older child. There is a predominance of lymphocytes (up to 80%) between about 1 month and 6 years of age.

Normal values for the platelet count are 150,000–400,000/μL and vary little with age.

BONE MARROW FAILURE

Failure of the marrow to produce adequate numbers of circulating blood cells may be congenital or acquired and may cause pancytopenia (aplastic anemia) or involve only one cell line (single cytopenia). Constitutional and acquired aplastic anemia will be discussed in detail here, whereas the more common single cytopenias (Table 25–1) will be dealt with in subsequent sections. Bone marrow failure caused by malignancy or other infiltrative disease is discussed in Chapter 26. It is also important to remember that many drugs and toxins may affect the marrow and cause single or multiple cytopenias.

Suspicion of bone marrow failure should be high in children with pancytopenia and in children with single cytopenias and without evidence of peripheral red cell, white cell, or platelet destruction. Macrocytosis often accompanies bone marrow failure, and many of the constitutional bone marrow disorders are associated with a variety of congenital anomalies.

Alter BP, Young NS: The bone marrow failure syndromes. In: *Hematology of Infancy and Childhood,* 5th ed. Nathan DG, Orkin SH (editors). Saunders, 1998.
Young NS, Alter BP: *Aplastic Anemia: Acquired and Inherited.* Saunders, 1994.

CONSTITUTIONAL APLASTIC ANEMIA (Fanconi's Anemia)

Essentials of Diagnosis & Typical Features
- Thrombocytopenia or neutropenia progressing to pancytopenia.
- Macrocytosis.
- Multiple congenital anomalies.
- Increased chromosome breakage in peripheral blood lymphocytes.

General Considerations
Fanconi's anemia is a syndrome characterized by defective DNA repair and caused by a variety of different genetic mutations. Inheritance is autosomal recessive, and the disease occurs in all ethnic groups. Hematologic manifestations usually begin with thrombocytopenia or neutropenia and subsequently progress over the course of months or years to pancytopenia. Typically, the diagnosis is made between the ages of 2 and 15 years.

Table 25–1. Important single cytopenias.

Red cell aplasia
  Congenital hypoplastic anemia (Diamond-Blackfan
    anemia)
  Transient erythroblastopenia of childhood
  Transient aplasia with chronic hemolysis
Neutropenia
  Kostmann's syndrome
  Shwachman-Diamond syndrome
  Cyclic neutropenia
Thrombocytopenia
  Thrombocytopenia with absent radii
  Amegakaryocytic thrombocytopenia

Clinical Findings

A. Symptoms and Signs: Symptoms are due principally to the degree of hematologic abnormality. Thrombocytopenia may cause purpura, petechiae, and bleeding; neutropenia may cause severe or recurrent infections; and anemia may cause weakness, fatigue, and pallor. Congenital anomalies are present in at least 50% of patients. The most common include abnormal pigmentation of the skin (generalized hyperpigmentation, café au lait or hypopigmented spots), short stature with delicate features, and skeletal malformations (hypoplasia, anomalies, or absence of the thumb and radius). More subtle anomalies include hypoplasia of thenar eminence or weakness of the radial pulse. Associated renal anomalies include aplasia, horseshoe kidney, and duplication of the collecting system. Other anomalies are microcephaly, microphthalmia, strabismus, ear anomalies, and hypogenitalism.

B. Laboratory Findings: Thrombocytopenia or leukopenia typically occur first, followed over the course of months to years by anemia and progression to severe aplastic anemia. Macrocytosis is virtually always present, is usually associated with anisocytosis and an elevation in fetal hemoglobin, and is an important diagnostic clue. The bone marrow reveals hypoplasia or aplasia consistent with the degree of peripheral cytopenias. The diagnosis is confirmed by the demonstration of an increased number of chromosome breaks and rearrangements in peripheral blood lymphocytes. The use of diepoxybutane to stimulate these breaks and rearrangements provides for a sensitive assay that is virtually always positive in children with Fanconi's anemia, even before the onset of hematologic abnormalities. Such testing is sometimes used for prenatal diagnosis as well.

Differential Diagnosis

Because patients with Fanconi's anemia frequently present with thrombocytopenia, the disorder must be differentiated from idiopathic thrombocytopenic purpura (ITP) and other more common causes of decreased platelets. In contrast to those with ITP, patients with thrombocytopenia of Fanconi's anemia usually present with a gradual fall in the platelet count, and counts less than 20,000/μL are often accompanied by neutropenia or anemia. Furthermore, children with ITP do not have macrocytosis and would not typically have short stature, microcephaly, or other congenital anomalies. Fanconi's anemia may also present initially with pancytopenia and must be differentiated from acquired aplastic anemia and from diseases associated with bone marrow infiltration such as acute leukemia. Examination of the bone marrow in conjunction with chromosome studies of peripheral blood lymphocytes will usually distinguish between these disorders.

Complications

The most important complications of Fanconi's anemia are those related to thrombocytopenia and neutropenia. In addition, persons with Fanconi's anemia have a significantly increased risk of developing malignancies, especially acute nonlymphocytic leukemia and solid tumors, and myelodysplastic syndromes. Death is usually the result of thrombocytopenic hemorrhage, overwhelming infection, or malignancy.

Treatment

Attentive supportive care is a critical feature of management. Patients with neutropenia who develop fever require prompt evaluation and parenteral broad-spectrum antibiotics. Transfusions are important but should be used judiciously, especially in the management of thrombocytopenic patients, who frequently become refractory to platelet transfusions as a consequence of alloimmunization. Transfusions from family members should be discouraged because of the negative impact on the outcome of bone marrow transplantation. At least 50% of patients with Fanconi's aplastic anemia respond, albeit incompletely, to androgen therapy with or without corticosteroids, and many recommend institution of androgens before transfusions are needed. However, such treatments are associated with hepatotoxicity, and masculinization is particularly troublesome in females.

Successful bone marrow transplantation cures the aplastic anemia and this is an important treatment option for children with Fanconi's anemia who are fortunate enough to have an HLA-identical sibling donor. First, it is important to exclude the possibility of Fanconi's anemia in the donor by testing lymphocytes for chromosome breakage.

Prognosis

Many patients succumb to bleeding, infection, or malignancy in adolescence or early adulthood. The long-term outlook for those undergoing successful bone marrow transplantation is uncertain, particularly with regard to the risk of subsequently developing malignancies.

Alter BP: Clinical features of Fanconi's anemia. In: *Aplastic Anemia: Acquired and Inherited.* Young NS, Alter BP (editors). Saunders, 1994.

Butturini A et al: Hematologic abnormalities in Fanconi anemia: An international Fanconi anemia registry study. Blood 1994;84:1650.

Gluckman E et al: Bone marrow transplantation for Fanconi anemia. Blood 1995;86:2856.

ACQUIRED APLASTIC ANEMIA

Essentials of Diagnosis & Typical Features

- Weakness and pallor.
- Petechiae, purpura, and bleeding.
- Frequent or severe infections.
- Pancytopenia with empty bone marrow.

General Considerations

Acquired aplastic anemia is characterized by peripheral pancytopenia with a hypocellular bone marrow. Approximately 50% of the cases in childhood are idiopathic, without evidence of any etiologic agent or associated abnormality. Other cases appear to be secondary to idiosyncratic reactions to drugs such as chloramphenicol, phenylbutazone, sulfonamides, nonsteroidal anti-inflammatory drugs, and anticonvulsants. Toxic causes include exposure to benzene, insecticides, and heavy metals. Infectious causes include viral hepatitis (usually non-A, non-B, non-C), infectious mononucleosis, and HIV. In immunocompromised children, aplastic anemia has been associated with human parvovirus.

Clinical Findings

A. Symptoms and Signs: Weakness, fatigue, and pallor are the result of anemia; petechiae, purpura, and bleeding occur because of thrombocytopenia; and fevers due to generalized or localized infections are the result of neutropenia. Hepatosplenomegaly and significant lymphadenopathy are unusual.

B. Laboratory Findings: Anemia is usually normocytic, with a low reticulocyte count. The white blood cell count is low, with a marked neutropenia. The platelet count is typically below 50,000/µL and frequently below 20,000/µL. Bone marrow aspiration and biopsy are essential to the diagnosis and show hypocellularity, often marked, with the marrow space replaced with fat.

Differential Diagnosis

Examination of the bone marrow usually excludes pancytopenia caused by peripheral destruction of blood cells or by infiltrative processes such as acute leukemia, storage diseases, and myelofibrosis. Many of these other conditions are associated with hepatosplenomegaly. Occasionally, children with pancytopenia and hypocellular bone marrows ultimately prove to have preleukemic conditions. In this regard, cytogenetic analysis of the marrow is helpful, since the presence of a clonal abnormality may predict the subsequent development of leukemia. Some children with Fanconi's anemia do not have congenital anomalies, and for that reason all children with newly diagnosed aplastic anemia should be studied for the presence of chromosome breaks and rearrangements in peripheral blood lymphocytes.

Complications

Acquired aplastic anemia is characteristically complicated by overwhelming infection and severe hemorrhage, and these two complications are the leading causes of death. Other complications are those associated with therapy.

Treatment

Comprehensive supportive care is most important in the management of children with acute acquired aplastic anemia. All febrile illnesses require prompt evaluation and usually parenteral antibiotics. Packed red blood cells should be transfused to alleviate symptoms of anemia. Platelet transfusions may be lifesaving, but they should be used sparingly since many patients eventually develop platelet alloantibodies.

Bone marrow transplantation is the treatment of choice for patients with severe aplastic anemia when an HLA-compatible sibling donor is available. Because the likelihood of success with transplantation is adversely influenced by multiple transfusions, HLA typing of family members should be undertaken as soon as the diagnosis of aplastic anemia is made. An increasing number of patients who lack HLA-matched siblings are able to find unrelated but matched donors through the National Bone Marrow Registry.

The best alternative to bone marrow transplantation for patients without an HLA-identical sibling is immunosuppression, usually with antithymocyte globulin (ATG), cyclosporine, and corticosteroids. Responses are somewhat variable, but most patients show hematologic improvement and become transfusion-independent.

Prognosis

The prognosis for patients with severe aplastic anemia is extremely poor if bone marrow transplantation is not available and if immunosuppression is not effective. In such cases, patients often die of infection or hemorrhage within 6–12 months after diagnosis. Children treated early with bone marrow transplantation from an HLA-identical sibling have a long-term survival rate of greater than 80%. Many treated with immunosuppressive therapy enjoy sustained complete remissions. However, recent studies demonstrate that both therapies are associated with a significantly increased risk of myelodysplastic syndromes, acute leukemia, and other malignancies in long-term survivors.

Brown KE et al: Hepatitis-associated aplastic anemia. N Engl J Med 1997;336:1059.
Lawlor ER et al: Immunosuppressive therapy: A potential alternative to bone marrow transplantation as initial therapy for acquired severe aplastic anemia of childhood. J Pediatr Hematol Oncol 1997;19:115.
Ohara A et al: Myelodysplastic syndrome and acute myelogenous leukemia as a late clonal complication in children with aplastic anemia. Blood 1997;90:1009.
Rosenfeld SJ et al: Intensive immunosuppression with antithymocyte globulin and cyclosporine as treatment for severe aplastic anemia. Blood 1995;85:3058.
Sanders JE et al: Marrow transplant experience for children with severe aplastic anemia. Am J Pediatr Hematol Oncol 1994;16:43.
Young NS, Barrett AJ: The treatment of severe acquired aplastic anemia. Blood 1995;85:3367.

ANEMIAS

APPROACH TO THE CHILD WITH ANEMIA

Anemia is a relatively common finding, and finding the cause is always important. Even though anemia in childhood has many causes, the correct diagnosis can usually be established with relatively little laboratory cost.

Frequently, the cause is suggested by a careful history. The possibility of nutritional causes should be addressed by inquiry about dietary intake, growth and development, and symptoms of chronic disease, malabsorption, or blood loss. Hemolytic disease may be suggested by a history of jaundice (including neonatal jaundice) or by a family history of anemia, jaundice, gallbladder disease, splenomegaly, or splenectomy. The child's ethnic background may suggest the possibility of certain hemoglobinopathies or of deficiencies of red cell enzymes such as glucose-6-phosphate dehydrogenase (G6PD). The review of systems may reveal clues to a previously unsuspected systemic disease with which anemia may be associated. The age of the patient is important because some causes of anemia are age-related. For example, iron deficiency anemia and β-globin disorders present more commonly between 6 and 36 months of age than at other times in life.

The physical examination may also reveal clues to the cause of anemia. Poor growth may suggest chronic disease or hypothyroidism. Congenital

anomalies may be associated with constitutional aplastic anemia (Fanconi's anemia) or with congenital hypoplastic anemia (Diamond-Blackfan anemia). Other disorders may be suggested by the findings of petechiae or purpura (leukemia, aplastic anemia, hemolytic uremic syndrome), jaundice (hemolysis or liver disease), generalized lymphadenopathy (leukemia, juvenile rheumatoid arthritis, HIV infection), splenomegaly (leukemia, sickle syndromes, hereditary spherocytosis, liver disease, hypersplenism), or evidence of chronic or recurrent infections.

The initial laboratory evaluation of the anemic child generally consists of a complete blood count (CBC) with differential and platelet count, review of the peripheral blood smear, and usually a reticulocyte count. The algorithm in Figure 25–1 shows how this limited laboratory information, together with the history and physical examination, may lead to a specific diagnosis or focus additional laboratory investigations to a limited diagnostic category (eg, microcytic anemia, bone marrow failure, pure red cell aplasia, or hemolytic disease). This diagnostic scheme depends principally on the MCV to determine whether the anemia is microcytic, normocytic, or macrocytic, according to the percentile curves of Dallman and Siimes (Figure 25–2).

With regard to microcytic anemias, the incidence of iron deficiency in the United States has decreased significantly with improvements in infant nutrition. Still, iron deficiency is an important cause of microcytic anemia, especially between 6 and 24 months of age. A trial of therapeutic iron is appropriate in such children, provided the dietary history is compatible with the development of iron deficiency and the physical examination or CBC results do not suggest an alternative cause for the anemia. If this is not the case—or if a trial of therapeutic iron fails to correct the anemia and microcytosis—then further laboratory evaluation is warranted.

Another key element of Figure 25–1 is the use of both the reticulocyte count and the peripheral blood smear to determine whether a normocytic or macrocytic anemia is due to hemolysis. Typically, hemolytic disease is associated with an elevated reticulocyte count, but some children with chronic hemolysis initially present during a period of virus-induced aplasia when the reticulocyte count is not elevated. Thus, review of the peripheral smear for evidence of hemolysis (eg, spherocytes, red cell fragmentation, sickle forms) is important in the evaluation of children with normocytic anemias and low reticulocyte counts. When hemolysis is suggested, the correct diagnosis may be suspected by specific abnormalities of red cell morphology or by clues from the history or physical examination. Autoimmune hemolysis can be excluded by Coombs testing. Review of blood counts and the peripheral smears of the mother and father may suggest congenital disorders such as hereditary spherocytosis. Children with

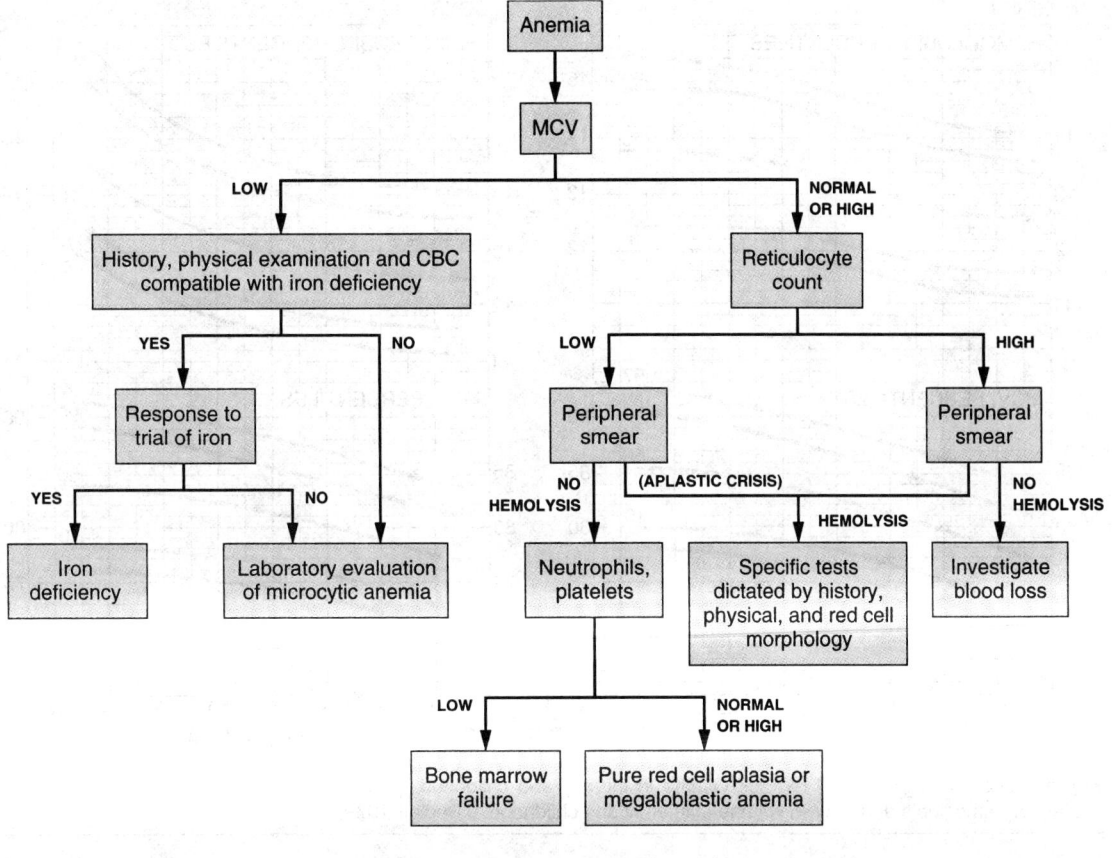

Figure 25–1. Investigation of anemia.

normocytic or macrocytic anemias, with relatively low reticulocyte counts and no evidence of hemolysis on the blood smear, usually have anemias caused by inadequate erythropoiesis in the bone marrow. The presence of neutropenia or thrombocytopenia in such children suggests bone marrow failure and the possibility of aplastic anemia or malignancy and usually dictates examination of the bone marrow. Pure red cell aplasia may be congenital (Diamond-Blackfan anemia), acquired and transient (transient erythroblastopenia of childhood), a manifestation of a systemic disease such as renal disease or hypothyroidism, or due to malnutrition or deficiencies of folate or cobalamin.

Dallman PR et al: Percentile curves for hemoglobin and red cell volume in infancy and childhood. J Pediatr 1979;94:26.

Oski FA, Brugnara C, Nathan DG: A diagnostic approach to the anemic patient. In: *Hematology of Infancy and Childhood,* 5th ed. Nathan DG, Orkin SH (editors). Saunders, 1998.

PURE RED CELL APLASIA

Infants and children with normocytic or macrocytic anemia, a low reticulocyte count, and normal or elevated numbers of neutrophils and platelets should be suspected of having pure red cell aplasia. Examination of the peripheral smear in such cases is important because signs of hemolytic disease suggest the possibility of chronic hemolysis complicated by an aplastic crisis due to parvovirus infection. Appreciation of this phenomenon is important because children with chronic hemolytic disease may not be diagnosed until the anemia is exacerbated by an episode of red cell aplasia that results in a rapidly falling hemoglobin. In such cases, cardiovascular compromise and congestive heart failure are imminent threats.

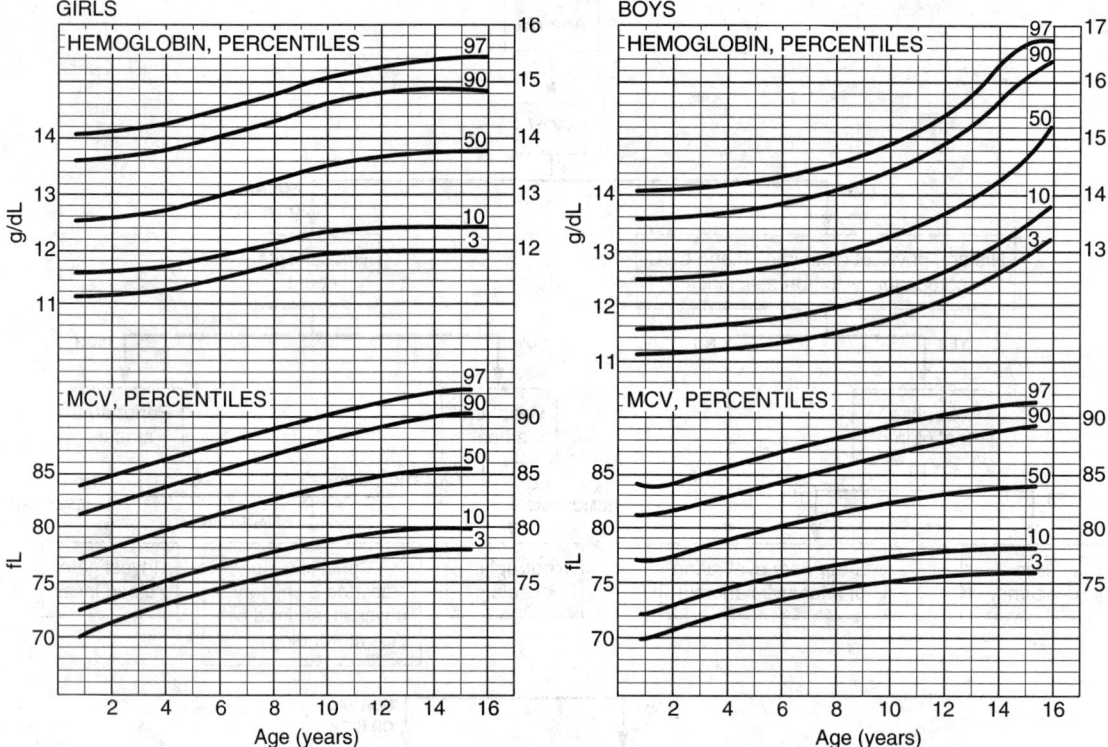

Figure 25–2. Hemoglobin and red cell volume in infancy and childhood. (From Dallman PR, Siimes MA: Percentile curves for hemoglobin and red cell volume in infancy and childhood. J Pediatr 1979;94:26.)

1. CONGENITAL HYPOPLASTIC ANEMIA (Diamond-Blackfan Anemia)

Essentials of Diagnosis & Typical Features

- Age: birth to 1 year.
- Macrocytic anemia with reticulocytopenia.
- Bone marrow with erythroid hypoplasia.
- Short stature or congenital anomalies in one-third.

General Considerations

Diamond-Blackfan anemia is a relatively rare cause of anemia that usually presents in infancy or early childhood. Early diagnosis is important because prompt treatment with corticosteroids results in increased erythropoiesis in about two-thirds of patients, thus avoiding the difficulties and complications of long-term chronic transfusion therapy. The cause of the disorder is unclear, and both autosomal dominant and autosomal recessive modes of inheritance have been suggested.

Clinical Findings

A. Symptoms and Signs: Signs and symptoms are generally those of chronic anemia, such as pallor, and congestive heart failure sometimes follows. Jaundice, splenomegaly, or other evidence of hemolysis is usually absent. Short stature or other congenital anomalies are present in one-third of patients. A wide variety of anomalies have been described, and those affecting the head, face, and thumbs are probably the most common.

B. Laboratory Findings: Diamond-Blackfan anemia is characterized by severe anemia and marked reticulocytopenia. The neutrophil count is usually normal or slightly decreased, and the platelet count is normal or elevated. The bone marrow usually shows a marked decrease in erythroid precursors but is otherwise normal. In older children, levels of fetal hemoglobin are usually increased and there is evidence of persistent fetal erythropoiesis such as the presence of the i antigen on erythrocytes. In addition, the level of adenosine deaminase in erythrocytes is elevated.

Differential Diagnosis

The principal disorder from which Diamond-Blackfan anemia must be differentiated is transient erythroblastopenia of childhood. In contrast to that condition, patients with Diamond-Blackfan anemia generally present at an earlier age, often have macrocytosis, and have evidence of fetal erythropoiesis and an elevated level of red cell adenosine deaminase. In addition, short stature and congenital anomalies, which occur in one-third of patients with Diamond-Blackfan anemia, are not associated with transient erythroblastopenia. Lastly, transient erythroblastopenia of childhood usually resolves within 6–8 weeks of diagnosis, whereas Diamond-Blackfan anemia is generally a lifelong affliction. Other disorders associated with decreased red cell production such as renal failure, hypothyroidism, and the anemia of chronic disease need to be considered.

Treatment

Oral corticosteroids should be initiated as soon as the diagnosis of Diamond-Blackfan anemia is made. Two-thirds of patients will respond to prednisone, 2 mg/kg/d, and many of those who respond subsequently tolerate significant tapering of the dose. Patients who are unresponsive to conventional doses of prednisone may respond to high-dose intravenous methylprednisolone or may require chronic red cell transfusion therapy, which inevitably causes transfusion-induced hemosiderosis and the need for chelation with parenteral deferoxamine. Bone marrow transplantation is an alternative therapy that should be considered for transfusion-dependent patients who have HLA-matched siblings. Hematopoietic growth factors have been used in some cases with limited success. Unpredictable, spontaneous remissions occasionally occur.

Prognosis

The prognosis for patients responsive to corticosteroids is generally good, particularly if remission is maintained with low doses of alternate-day prednisone. Patients dependent upon transfusion are at risk for the complications of hemosiderosis, including death from congestive heart failure, cardiac arrhythmias, or hepatic failure. This remains a significant threat, particularly during adolescence, when compliance with nightly subcutaneous infusions of deferoxamine is often a difficult issue.

Alter BP: Diamond-Blackfan anemia. In: *Aplastic Anemia: Acquired and Inherited.* Young NS, Alter BP. Saunders, 1994.

Bernini JC, Carrillo JM, Buchanan GR: High-dose intravenous methylprednisolone therapy for patients with Diamond-Blackfan anemia refractory to conventional doses of prednisone. J Pediatr 1995;127:654.

Greinix HT et al: Long-term survival and cure after marrow transplantation for congenital hypoplastic anaemia (Diamond-Blackfan syndrome). Br J Haematol 1993;84:515.

Olivieri NF et al: Failure of recombinant human interleukin-3 therapy to induce erythropoiesis in patients with refractory Diamond-Blackfan anemia. Blood 1994;83:2444.

2. TRANSIENT ERYTHROBLASTOPENIA OF CHILDHOOD

Essentials of Diagnosis & Typical Features

- Age: 6 months to 4 years.
- Normocytic anemia with reticulocytopenia.
- Absence of hepatosplenomegaly or lymphadenopathy.
- Erythroid precursors initially absent from bone marrow.

General Considerations

Transient erythroblastopenia of childhood is a relatively common cause of acquired anemia in early childhood. The disorder is generally suspected when a normocytic anemia is discovered during evaluation of pallor or when a CBC is obtained for another reason. Because the anemia is due to decreased red cell production and thus develops slowly, the cardiovascular system has time to compensate. Therefore, children with hemoglobins as low as 4 or 5 g/dL may look remarkably well. The disorder is thought to be autoimmune in most cases, since IgG from some patients has been shown to suppress erythropoiesis in vitro.

Clinical Findings

Pallor is the most common sign, and hepatosplenomegaly and lymphadenopathy are absent. The anemia is normocytic, and the smear shows no evidence of hemolysis. The platelet count is normal or elevated, and the neutrophil count is normal or, in some cases, somewhat decreased. The Coombs test is negative, and there is no evidence of chronic renal disease, hypothyroidism, or other systemic disorder. Bone marrow examination shows severe erythroid hypoplasia initially; subsequently, erythroid hyperplasia develops along with reticulocytosis and the anemia resolves.

Differential Diagnosis

Transient erythroblastopenia of childhood must be differentiated from Diamond-Blackfan anemia, particularly in infants less than 1 year of age. In contrast to Diamond-Blackfan anemia, transient erythroblastopenia is not associated with macrocytosis, short stature, or congenital anomalies, or with evidence of fetal erythropoiesis prior to the phase of recovery. Also in contrast to Diamond-Blackfan anemia, levels of red cell adenosine deaminase are normal. Transient erythroblastopenia of childhood must also be differentiated from chronic disorders associated with decreased red cell production, such as renal failure, hypothyroidism, and other chronic states of infection or inflammation. As with other single cytopenias, the possibility of malignancy (ie, leukemia) should always be considered, particularly if fever, bone pain, hepatosplenomegaly, or lymphadenopathy is present.

In such cases, examination of the bone marrow is generally diagnostic. Confusion may sometimes arise when the anemia of transient erythroblastopenia is first identified during the early phase of recovery when the reticulocyte count is high. In such cases, the disorder may be confused with the anemia of acute blood loss or with hemolytic disease. In contrast to hemolytic disorders, however, there is no jaundice and no evidence of hemolysis on the blood smear.

Treatment & Prognosis

By definition, transient erythroblastopenia of childhood is a transient disorder. Some children require red cell transfusions if signs of cardiovascular compromise are present. Resolution of the anemia is heralded by an increase in the reticulocyte count, which generally occurs within 4–8 weeks of diagnosis. In contrast to other autoimmune disorders of childhood (eg, ITP, autoimmune hemolytic anemia), the use of corticosteroids is of no proven benefit and is not indicated.

Alter BP: Transient erythroblastopenia of childhood. In: Aplastic Anemia: Acquired and Inherited. Young NS, Alter BP. Saunders, 1994.

Cherrick I, Karayalcin G, Lanzkowsky P: Transient erythroblastopenia of childhood: Prospective study of fifty patients. Am J Pediatr Hematol Oncol 1994;16:320.

Miller R, Berman B: Transient erythroblastopenia of childhood in infants < 6 months of age. Am J Pediatr Hematol Oncol 1994;16:246.

NUTRITIONAL ANEMIAS

1. IRON DEFICIENCY ANEMIA

Essentials of Diagnosis & Typical Features

- Pallor and fatigue.
- Poor dietary intake of iron (age 6–24 months).
- Chronic blood loss (age > 2 years).
- Microcytic hypochromic anemia.

General Considerations

Long considered the most common cause of anemia in pediatrics, iron deficiency has seen a dramatic decrease in incidence during the past two decades. This is the direct result of improved nutrition and the increased availability of iron-fortified infant formulas and cereals. Thus, the current approach to anemia in childhood must take into consideration a relatively greater chance of other causes than was formerly the case.

Normal term infants are born with sufficient iron stores to prevent iron deficiency for the first 4 months of life. Thereafter, enough iron needs to be absorbed to keep pace with the needs of rapid growth. For this reason, nutritional iron deficiency is most common between 6 and 24 months of life. A deficiency earlier than 6 months of age may occur if iron stores at birth are reduced by prematurity, small birth weight, neonatal anemia, or perinatal blood loss or if there is subsequent iron loss due to hemorrhage. Iron-deficient children older than 24 months of age should be investigated for blood loss.

A significant body of evidence indicates that iron deficiency, in addition to causing anemia, has adverse effects on behavior and cognitive function. Thus, the importance of the identification of iron deficiency and of its treatment extends past the resolution of any symptoms directly attributable to a lowered hemoglobin concentration.

Clinical Findings

A. Symptoms and Signs: Symptoms and signs vary with the severity of the deficiency. Mild iron deficiency is usually asymptomatic. In infants with more severe iron deficiency, pallor, fatigue, irritability, and delayed motor development are common. Children whose iron deficiency is due in part to ingestion of unfortified cow's milk may be fat and flabby, with poor muscle tone. A history of pica is common.

B. Laboratory Findings: The severity of anemia depends on the degree of iron deficiency, and the hemoglobin may be as low as 3–4 g/dL in severe cases. Red cells are microcytic and hypochromic, with a low MCV and low MCH. The red blood cell distribution width (RDW) is typically elevated, even with mild iron deficiency. The reticulocyte count is usually normal but may be slightly elevated in severe cases. Iron studies show a decreased serum ferritin as well as a low serum iron, elevated total iron-binding capacity, and decreased transferrin saturation. Free erythrocyte protoporphyrin is elevated. All of these laboratory abnormalities are usually present with moderate to severe iron deficiency, but mild cases may show variable laboratory results.

The bone marrow examination is not helpful in the diagnosis of iron deficiency in infants and small children because little or no iron is stored as marrow hemosiderin at these ages.

Differential Diagnosis

The differential diagnosis is that of microcytic, hypochromic anemia. The possibility of thalassemia (α-thalassemia, β-thalassemia, hemoglobin E disorders) should be considered, especially in infants of African, Mediterranean, or Asian ethnic background. In contrast to those with iron deficiency, infants with thalassemia generally have an elevated number of erythrocytes (the index of the MCV divided by the red cell number is usually < 13) and are less likely, in mild cases, to have an elevated RDW. Thalassemias are associated with normal or increased levels of serum iron and ferritin and with normal iron-binding capacity and free erythrocyte protoporphyrin levels.

The hemoglobin electrophoresis in β-thalassemia trait typically shows an elevation of hemoglobin A_2, but coexistent iron deficiency may lower the percentage of hemoglobin A_2 into the normal range. Hemoglobin electrophoresis will also identify children with hemoglobin E, a cause of microcytosis common in Southeast Asians. In contrast, the hemoglobin electrophoresis in α-thalassemia trait is normal. Lead poisoning has also been associated with microcytic anemia, but anemia with lead levels less than 40 μg/dL is usually due to coexistent iron deficiency.

The anemia of chronic inflammation or infection may also be microcytic. This anemia is usually suspected because of the presence of a chronic systemic disorder. The level of serum iron is low, but serum ferritin is elevated. Finally, it should be appreciated that relatively mild infections, particularly during infancy, may cause transient anemia. For this reason, caution should be exercised when the diagnosis of mild iron deficiency is entertained in infants and young children who have had recent viral or bacterial infections. Ideally, screening tests for anemia should not be obtained within 3–4 weeks of such infections.

Treatment

The recommended oral dose of elemental iron is 4–6 mg/kg/d in three divided daily doses. Mild cases may be treated with 3 mg/kg/d given once daily before breakfast. Parenteral administration of iron is rarely necessary. Iron therapy results in an increased reticulocyte count within 3–5 days, which is maximal between 5 and 7 days. The hemoglobin level begins to increase thereafter. The rate of hemoglobin rise is inversely related to the hemoglobin level at diagnosis. In moderate to severe cases, an elevated reticulocyte count 1 week after initiation of therapy confirms the diagnosis and documents compliance and response to therapy. When iron deficiency is the only cause of anemia, adequate treatment usually results in a resolution of the anemia within 4–6 weeks. Treatment is generally continued for a few additional months to replenish iron stores.

Lozoff B: Iron deficiency and infant development. J Pediatr 1994;125:577.

Lozoff B, Wolf AW, Jimenez E: Iron-deficiency anemia and infant development: Effects of extended oral iron therapy. J Pediatr 1996;129:382.

Moffatt MEK et al: Prevention of iron deficiency and psychomotor decline in high-risk infants through use of iron-fortified infant formula: A randomized clinical trial. J Pediatr 1994;125:527.

Oski FA: Iron deficiency in infancy and childhood. N Engl J Med 1993;329:190.

Piscane A et al: Iron status of breast-fed infants. J Pediatr 1995;127:429.

2. MEGALOBLASTIC ANEMIAS

Essentials of Diagnosis & Typical Features

- Pallor and fatigue.
- Nutritional deficiency or intestinal malabsorption.
- Macrocytic anemia.
- Megaloblastic bone marrow changes.

General Considerations

Megaloblastic anemia is a macrocytic anemia caused by deficiency of cobalamin (vitamin B_{12}), folic acid, or both. Cobalamin deficiency due to dietary insufficiency may occur in infants who are breast fed by mothers who are strict vegetarians or who have pernicious anemia. Intestinal malabsorption is the usual cause of cobalamin deficiency in pediatrics and occurs with Crohn's disease, chronic pancreatitis, bacterial overgrowth of the small bowel, infection with the fish tapeworm (Diphyllobothrium latum), or after surgical resection of the terminal ileum. Deficiencies due to inborn errors of metabolism (transcobalamin II deficiency, methylmalonic aciduria) have also been described. Malabsorption of cobalamin due to deficiency of intrinsic factor (pernicious anemia) is rare in childhood.

Folic acid deficiency may be caused by inadequate dietary intake, malabsorption, increased folate requirements, or some combination of the three. Folate deficiency due to dietary deficiency alone is rare but occurs in severely malnourished infants and has been reported in infants fed goat's milk not fortified with folic acid. Folic acid is absorbed in the proximal small bowel, and deficiencies are encountered in malabsorptive syndromes such as celiac disease. Anticonvulsant medications (eg, phenytoin and phenobarbital) and cytotoxic drugs (eg, methotrexate) have also been associated with folate deficiency, caused by interference with folate absorption or metabolism. Finally, folic acid deficiency is more likely to develop in infants and children with increased requirements. This occurs during infancy because of rapid growth and also in children with chronic hemolytic anemia. Premature infants are particularly susceptible to the development of the deficiency because of low body stores of folate.

Clinical Findings

A. Symptoms and Signs: Infants with megaloblastic anemia may show pallor and mild jaundice due to ineffective erythropoiesis. Classically, the tongue is smooth and beefy red. Infants with cobalamin deficiency may be irritable and may be poor feeders. Older children with cobalamin deficiency may complain of paresthesias, weakness, or an unsteady gait and may show decreased vibratory sensation and proprioception on neurologic examination.

B. Laboratory Findings: The laboratory findings of megaloblastic anemia include an elevated

MCV and mean corpuscular hemoglobin (MCH). The blood smear shows numerous macro-ovalocytes with anisocytosis and poikilocytosis. Neutrophils are large and have hypersegmented nuclei. The white cell count and the platelet count are normal with mild deficiencies, but may be decreased in more severe cases. Examination of the bone marrow typically shows erythroid hyperplasia with large erythroid and myeloid precursors. There is nuclear-cytoplasmic dissociation and ineffective erythropoiesis. The serum indirect bilirubin concentration may be slightly elevated.

Children with cobalamin deficiency have a low serum vitamin B_{12} level, but decreased levels of serum vitamin B_{12} may also be seen in about 30% of patients with folic acid deficiency. Serum levels of metabolic intermediates—methylmalonic acid and homocysteine—may help establish the correct diagnosis. Assessment of folate stores is best done by measuring the level of red cell folate rather than the serum folic acid.

Differential Diagnosis

It is important to recognize that most macrocytic anemias in pediatrics are not megaloblastic. Other causes of an increased MCV include an elevated reticulocyte count (hemolytic anemias), bone marrow failure syndromes (Fanconi's anemia, Diamond-Blackfan anemia), liver disease, and hypothyroidism.

Treatment

Treatment of cobalamin deficiency due to inadequate dietary intake is readily accomplished with oral supplementation. Most cases, however, are due to intestinal malabsorption and require parenteral treatment. In severe cases, parenteral therapy may induce life-threatening hypokalemia and require supplemental potassium. Folic acid deficiency is effectively treated with oral folic acid in most cases. Children at risk for the development of folic acid deficiencies such as premature infants and those with chronic hemolysis are usually given supplementary folic acid prophylactically.

Graham SM et al: Long-term neurologic consequences of nutritional vitamin B_{12} deficiency in infants. J Pediatr 1992;121:710.
Pappo AS, Fields BW, Buchanan GR: Etiology of red blood cell macrocytosis during childhood: Impact of new diseases and therapies. Pediatrics 1992;89:1063.

ANEMIA OF CHRONIC DISORDERS

Anemia is a common manifestation of many chronic illnesses in children. In some instances, causes may be mixed. For example, children with chronic disorders involving intestinal malabsorption or blood loss may have anemia of chronic inflamma-tion in combination with nutritional deficiencies of iron, folate, or cobalamin. In other settings, the anemia is due to dysfunction of a single organ (eg, renal failure, hypothyroidism), and correction of the underlying abnormality causes resolution of the anemia.

1. ANEMIA OF CHRONIC INFLAMMATION

Anemia is frequently associated with chronic illness, particularly those with a significant inflammatory component. The anemia is usually mild to moderate in severity, with a hemoglobin of 8–12 g/dL. In general, the severity of the anemia corresponds to the severity of the underlying disorder. The reticulocyte count is low, and the anemia is thought to be due to inflammatory cytokines that inhibit erythropoiesis and impair iron release by reticuloendothelial cells. The serum iron concentration is low, but in contrast to iron deficiency, the iron-binding capacity is not elevated and the serum ferritin is elevated. Treatment consists of correction of the underlying disorder, which, if controlled, generally results in improvement in hemoglobin level.

Abshire TC: The anemia of inflammation: A common cause of childhood anemia. Pediatr Clin North Am 1996;43:623.
Means RT Jr, Krantz SB: Progress in understanding the pathogenesis of the anemia of chronic disease. Blood 1992;80:1639.

2. ANEMIA OF CHRONIC RENAL FAILURE

Severe normocytic anemia occurs in most forms of renal disease that have progressed to renal insufficiency. Although white cell and platelet production remain normal, the bone marrow shows significant hypoplasia of the erythroid series and the reticulocyte count is low. The principal mechanism responsible for this anemia is deficiency of erythropoietin, a hormone normally produced in the kidney. In the presence of significant uremia, there may also be a component of hemolysis. In the past, treatment of the anemia of chronic renal failure depended on transfusions of packed red blood cells. However, recombinant human erythropoietin (epoetin alfa) has been shown to correct the anemia, and its use has largely eliminated the need for transfusions.

Montini G et al: Pharmacokinetics and hematologic response to subcutaneous administration of recombinant human erythropoietin in children undergoing long-term peritoneal dialysis: A multicenter study. J Pediatr 1993;122:297.
Morris KP et al: Non-cardiac benefits of human recombinant erythropoietin in end stage renal failure and anaemia. Arch Dis Child 1993;69:580.
Siimes MA et al: Factors limiting the erythropoietin re-

sponse in rapidly growing infants with congenital nephrosis on a peritoneal dialysis regimen after nephrectomy. J Pediatr 1992;120:44.

3. ANEMIA OF HYPOTHYROIDISM

Some patients with hypothyroidism develop significant anemia. Occasionally, anemia is detected before the diagnosis of the underlying disorder. A decreased growth velocity in an anemic child suggests hypothyroidism. The anemia is usually normocytic or macrocytic, but it is not megaloblastic and hence not due to deficiencies of cobalamin or folate. Replacement therapy with thyroid hormone is usually effective in correcting the anemia.

Cheu J-Y et al: Anemia in children and adolescents with hypothyroidism. Clin Pediatr 1981;20:696.

CONGENITAL HEMOLYTIC ANEMIAS: RED CELL MEMBRANE DEFECTS

The congenital hemolytic anemias are usually divided into three categories: defects of the red cell membrane, hemoglobinopathies, and disorders of red cell metabolism. Hereditary spherocytosis and elliptocytosis are the most common red cell membrane disorders and are described here. The diagnosis is suggested by the peripheral blood smear, which shows characteristic red cell morphology (eg, spherocytes, elliptocytes). These disorders usually have an autosomal dominant inheritance, and the diagnosis may be suggested by a family history. The hemolysis is due to the deleterious effect of the membrane abnormality on red cell deformability. Decreased cell deformability leads to entrapment of the abnormally shaped red cells in the spleen. Many patients have splenomegaly, and splenectomy usually alleviates the hemolysis.

Clark MR, Wagner GM: Disorders of the erythrocyte membrane. In: *The Hereditary Hemolytic Anemias.* Mentzer WC, Wagner GM (editors). Churchill Livingstone, 1989.
Gallagher PG, Forget BG, Lux SE: Disorders of the erythrocyte membrane. In: *Hematology of Infancy and Childhood,* 5th ed. Nathan DG, Orkin SH (editors). Saunders, 1998.

1. HEREDITARY SPHEROCYTOSIS

Essentials of Diagnosis & Typical Features
- Anemia and jaundice.
- Splenomegaly.
- Positive family history of anemia, jaundice, or gallstones.

- Spherocytosis with increased reticulocytes.
- Increased osmotic fragility.
- Negative Coombs test.

General Considerations
Hereditary spherocytosis is a relatively common inherited hemolytic anemia that occurs in all ethnic groups but is most common in persons of Northern European ancestry, in whom the incidence is about 1:5000. The disorder is a heterogeneous one, marked by variable degrees of anemia, jaundice, and splenomegaly. In some persons, the disorder is mild and there is no anemia because erythroid hyperplasia fully compensates for hemolysis. Severe cases are transfusion-dependent prior to splenectomy. The hallmark of hereditary spherocytosis is the presence of microspherocytes in the peripheral blood. The disease is inherited in an autosomal dominant fashion in about 80% of cases; the remainder are thought to be autosomal recessive or to be caused by new mutations.

Hereditary spherocytosis is the result of a partial deficiency of **spectrin,** an important structural protein of the red cell membrane skeleton. Spectrin deficiency weakens the attachment of the cell membrane to the underlying membrane skeleton and causes the red cell to lose membrane surface area. This process creates spherocytes that are poorly deformable and have a shortened life span because they are trapped in the microcirculation of the spleen and engulfed by splenic macrophages. The extreme heterogeneity of hereditary spherocytosis is directly related to variable degrees of spectrin deficiency. In general, children who inherit hereditary spherocytosis in an autosomal dominant fashion have lesser degrees of spectrin deficiency and mild or moderate hemolysis. In contrast, those with nondominant forms of spherocytosis tend to have greater deficiencies of spectrin and a more severe anemia.

Clinical Findings
A. Symptoms and Signs: Symptoms and signs of hereditary spherocytosis are those related to hemolytic anemia. Fifty percent of affected children have significant hyperbilirubinemia in the newborn period. Splenomegaly subsequently develops in the majority and is usually present by the age of 5 years. Jaundice is variably present and in many patients may only be noted during infection. Patients with significant chronic anemia may complain of pallor, fatigue, or malaise. Intermittent exacerbations of the anemia are caused by increased hemolysis or by aplastic crises and may be associated with severe weakness, fatigue, fever, abdominal pain, or even congestive heart failure.

B. Laboratory Findings: Most patients have mild chronic hemolysis with hemoglobin values between 9 and 12 g/dL. In some cases, the hemolysis is fully compensated and the hemoglobin is in the normal range. Rare cases of severe disease require frequent transfusions. The anemia is usually normocytic and hyperchromic, and many patients have an elevated MCHC. The blood smear shows numerous microspherocytes and polychromasia. The reticulocyte count is elevated and is often higher than might be expected for the degree of anemia. White blood cells and platelets are usually normal. The osmotic fragility is increased, particularly after incubation at 37 °C for 24 hours. Serum bilirubin usually shows an elevation in the unconjugated fraction. Coombs testing is negative.

Differential Diagnosis

Spherocytes are frequently present in persons with immune hemolysis. Thus, in the newborn, hereditary spherocytosis must be distinguished from hemolytic disease caused by ABO or Rh incompatibilities. In older patients, autoimmune hemolytic anemia frequently presents with jaundice and splenomegaly and with spherocytes on the blood smear. The direct Coombs test is positive in most cases of immune hemolysis and negative in hereditary spherocytosis. Occasionally, the diagnosis is confused in patients with splenomegaly from other causes, especially when hypersplenism increases red cell destruction and when some spherocytes are noted on the blood smear. In such cases, the true cause of the splenomegaly is frequently suggested by signs or symptoms of portal hypertension or by laboratory evidence of chronic liver disease. In contrast to children with hereditary spherocytosis, those with hypersplenism typically have some degree of thrombocytopenia or neutropenia.

Complications

Severe jaundice may occur in the neonatal period and, if not controlled by phototherapy, may occasionally require exchange transfusion. Splenectomy is associated with an increased risk of overwhelming bacterial infections, particularly with pneumococci. Gallstones occur in 60–70% of adults who have not undergone splenectomy and may form as early as 8–10 years of age.

Treatment

Supportive measures include the administration of folic acid to prevent the development of red cell hypoplasia due to folate deficiency. Acute exacerbations of anemia due to increased rates of hemolysis or to aplastic crises due to infection with human parvovirus may be severe enough to require red cell transfusions. Splenectomy is performed in many cases and always results in significant improvement. The procedure increases the survival of the spherocytic red cells and leads to complete correction of the anemia in most cases. Patients with more severe disease may show some degree of hemolysis after splenectomy. Except in unusually severe cases, the procedure should be postponed until the child is at

least 5 or 6 years of age because of the greater risk of postsplenectomy sepsis prior to this age. Alternatively, partial splenectomy may be considered for young children with severe hemolysis. All patients scheduled for splenectomy should be immunized with pneumococcal vaccine prior to the procedure, and some recommend prophylactic penicillin afterward. The need for splenectomy in mild cases is somewhat controversial. Splenectomy in the middle childhood years prevents the subsequent development of cholelithiasis and eliminates the need for the activity restrictions recommended for children with splenomegaly. However, these benefits must be weighed against the risks of the surgical procedure and the subsequent lifelong risk of postsplenectomy sepsis.

Prognosis

Splenectomy eliminates signs and symptoms in all but the most severe cases and prevents the development of cholelithiasis. The abnormal red cell morphology and increased osmotic fragility persist without clinical consequence.

Eber SW et al: Variable clinical severity of hereditary spherocytosis: Relation to erythrocytic spectrin concentration, osmotic fragility, and autohemolysis. J Pediatr 1990;117:409.

Hassoun H et al: Characterization of the underlying molecular defect in hereditary spherocytosis associated with spectrin deficiency. Blood 1997;90:398.

Manno CS et al: Splenectomy in mild hereditary spherocytosis: Is it worth the risk? Am J Pediatr Hematol Oncol 1989;11:300.

Tchernia G et al: Initial assessment of the beneficial effect of partial splenectomy in hereditary spherocytosis. Blood 1993;81:2014.

2. HEREDITARY ELLIPTOCYTOSIS

Hereditary elliptocytosis is a heterogeneous disorder whose severity ranges from an asymptomatic carrier state with normal red cell morphology to severe hemolytic anemia. Most affected persons have numerous elliptocytes on the blood smear but mild or no hemolysis. Those with hemolysis have an elevated reticulocyte count and may have jaundice and splenomegaly. These disorders are caused by mutations of red cell membrane skeletal proteins, and most have an autosomal dominant inheritance. Because most cases are asymptomatic, no treatment is indicated. Patients with significant degrees of hemolytic anemia may benefit from folate supplementation or from splenectomy.

Some infants with hereditary elliptocytosis present in the neonatal period with moderate to marked hemolysis and significant hyperbilirubinemia. This disorder has been termed **transient infantile poikilocytosis** because such infants exhibit bizarre erythrocyte morphology with elliptocytes, budding red cells, and small misshapen cells that defy description. The MCV is low, and the anemia may be severe enough to require red cell transfusions. Typically, one parent has hereditary elliptocytosis, usually mild or asymptomatic. The infant's hemolysis gradually abates during the first year of life, and the erythrocyte morphology subsequently becomes more typical of hereditary elliptocytosis.

Mentzer WC et al: Modulation of erythrocyte membrane mechanical stability by 2,3-diphosphoglycerate in the neonatal poikilocytosis/elliptocytosis syndrome. J Clin Invest 1987;79:943.
Palek J, Sahr KE: Mutations of the red cell membrane proteins: From clinical evaluation to detection of the underlying genetic defect. Blood 1992;8:308.

CONGENITAL HEMOLYTIC ANEMIAS: HEMOGLOBINOPATHIES

The hemoglobinopathies are an extremely heterogeneous group of congenital disorders that occur in many different ethnic groups. The relatively high frequency of these genetic variants is thought to be related to the protection afforded heterozygotes from malaria. The hemoglobinopathies are generally classified into two major groups. The first, the thalassemias, are caused by quantitative deficiencies in the production of globin chains. These quantitative defects in globin synthesis result in a microcytic and hypochromic anemia. The second group of hemoglobinopathies are those caused by structural abnormalities of globin chains. The most important of these, hemoglobins S, C, and E, are all the result of point mutations and single amino acid substitutions in the β globin.

Figure 25–3 shows the normal developmental changes that occur in globin-chain production during gestation and the first year of life. At birth, the predominant hemoglobin is fetal hemoglobin, which is composed of two α-globin chains and two γ-globin chains. Subsequently, the production of γ-globin decreases and the production of β globin increases so that adult hemoglobin (two α chains and two β chains) predominates after 4–6 months. Because α-globin chains are present in both fetal and adult hemoglobin, disorders of α-globin synthesis (α-thalassemia) are clinically manifest in the newborn as well as later in life. In contrast, β-globin disorders such as β-thalassemia and sickle cell disease are generally asymptomatic during the first 3–4 months of age and present clinically after γ-chain production—and therefore fetal hemoglobin levels—have decreased substantially.

1. ALPHA-THALASSEMIA

Essentials of Diagnosis & Typical Features

- African, Mediterranean, Middle Eastern, Chinese, or Southeast Asian ancestry.
- Microcytic, hypochromic anemia of variable severity.

General Considerations

Most of the α-thalassemia syndromes are the result of deletions of one or more of the α-globin genes on chromosome 16. Normal diploid cells have four α-globin genes, and thus the variable severity of the α-thalassemia syndromes is related to the number of

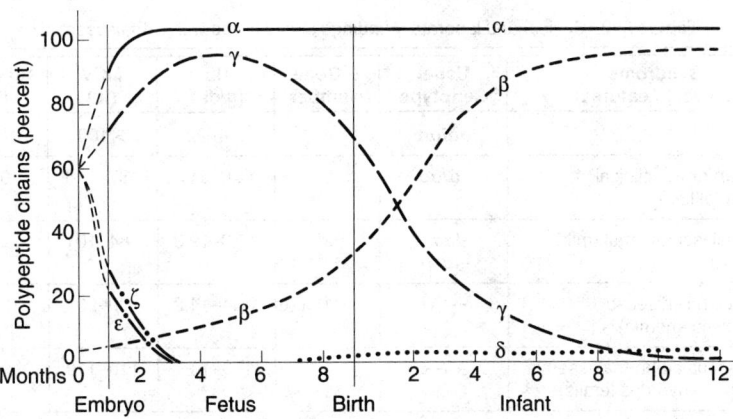

Figure 25–3. Changes in hemoglobin polypeptide chains during human development. (From Miller DR, Baehner RL: *Blood Diseases of Infancy and Childhood,* 6th ed. Mosby, 1989.)

gene deletions. Persons with one α-globin gene deletion (silent carrier) are asymptomatic and have normal blood findings. Persons with two α-globin gene deletions (α-thalassemia trait) have microcytosis and hypochromia with a normal or slightly decreased hemoglobin level. Persons with three α-globin gene deletions (hemoglobin H disease) have a moderately severe anemia. The deletion of all four α-globin genes results in fetal demise due to hydrops fetalis.

The severity of the α-thalassemia syndromes varies among affected ethnic groups, depending on the genetic abnormalities prevalent in the population. In persons of African descent, α-thalassemia is usually caused by the deletion of only one of the two α-globin genes on each chromosome. Thus, heterozygotes in the African population are silent carriers, and homozygotes have α-thalassemia trait. In Asians, however, deletions of one or of both α-globin genes on the same chromosome are common. Thus, heterozygotes are either silent carriers or have α-thalassemia trait and homozygotes or compound heterozygotes have α-thalassemia trait, hemoglobin H disease, or hydrops fetalis. Thus, the presence of α-thalassemia in a child of Asian ancestry may have important implications for genetic counseling, whereas this is not usually the case in families of African ancestry.

Clinical Findings

The clinical findings depend upon the number of α-globin genes deleted. The thalassemia syndromes and associated laboratory findings in newborns are shown in Table 25–2.

Persons with three α-globin genes (one-gene deletion) are asymptomatic and have no hematologic abnormalities. Hemoglobin levels and MCV are normal. Hemoglobin electrophoresis in the neonatal period shows 1–3% Barts hemoglobin, a variant hemoglobin composed of four γ-globin chains. Hemoglobin electrophoresis after the first few months of life is normal. Thus, this condition is usually suspected only in the context of family studies or when a small amount of Barts hemoglobin is detected by neonatal screening for hemoglobinopathies.

Persons with two α-globin genes (two-gene deletion) are typically asymptomatic. The MCV is usually less than 100 fL at birth. Hematologic studies in older infants and children show a normal or slightly decreased hemoglobin level with a low MCV and a slightly hypochromic blood smear with some target cells. The hemoglobin electrophoresis typically shows 5–10% Barts hemoglobin in the neonatal period but is normal in older children and adults.

Persons with one α-globin gene (three-gene deletion) have a moderately severe microcytic hemolytic anemia (Hb 7–10 g/dL), which is often accompanied by hepatosplenomegaly and some bony abnormalities caused by the expanded medullary space. The reticulocyte count is elevated, and the red cells show marked hypochromia and microcytosis with significant poikilocytosis and some basophilic stippling. Hemoglobin electrophoresis in the neonatal period typically shows 15–25% Barts hemoglobin. Later in life, hemoglobin H (composed of four β-globin chains) is detected and may make up as much as 20–30% of the hemoglobin. Incubation of red cells with brilliant cresyl blue (hemoglobin H preparation) shows inclusion bodies formed by denatured hemoglobin H.

The deletion of all four α-globin genes causes severe intrauterine anemia and asphyxia and results in hydrops fetalis and fetal demise or neonatal death shortly following delivery. There is extreme pallor and massive hepatosplenomegaly. Hemoglobin electrophoresis reveals a predominance of Barts hemoglobin with a complete absence of normal fetal or adult hemoglobin.

Table 25–2. Clinical and laboratory findings in newborns with α-thalassemia.[1]

Syndrome (Clinical Features)	Usual Genotype	α Gene Number	Hb (g/dL)	MCV (fL)	Hb Barts (%)
Normal	αα/αα	4	14–22	> 100	None
Silent carrier (no clinical abnormalities)	–α/αα	3	13.6–21	87–116	0–5.8
Alpha-thalassemia trait (mild anemia)	- -/αα or –α/–α	2	14.3–19.3	84–101	2–10
Hemoglobin H disease (hemolytic anemia)	- -/–α	1	12.4–14.2	80–93	19–27
Homozygous alpha-thalassemia (stillborn—hydrops fetalis)	- -/- -	0	3–10	110–119	> 75

[1]From Embury SH, Mentzer WC: The thalassemia syndromes. In: *The Hereditary Hemolytic Anemias*. Mentzer WC, Wagner GM (editors). Churchill Livingstone, 1989.
MCV = mean corpuscular volume.

Differential Diagnosis

α-Thalassemia trait (two-gene deletion) must be differentiated from other mild microcytic anemias including iron deficiency and β-thalassemia trait. In contrast to children with iron deficiency, those with α-thalassemia trait show normal or increased levels of ferritin and serum iron, and the free erythrocyte protoporphyrin is not elevated. In contrast to children with β-thalassemia trait, those with α-thalassemia trait have a normal hemoglobin electrophoresis after 4–6 months of age. Finally, the history of a low MCV (96 fL) at birth or the presence of Barts hemoglobin on the neonatal hemoglobinopathy screening test suggests α-thalassemia.

Children with hemoglobin H disease may have jaundice and splenomegaly, and the disorder must be differentiated from other hemolytic anemias. The key to the diagnosis is the decreased MCV and the marked hypochromia on the blood smear. With the exception of β-thalassemia, most other significant hemolytic disorders have a normal or elevated MCV and are not hypochromic. Infants with hydrops fetalis due to severe α-thalassemia must be distinguished from those with hydrops due to other causes of anemia such as isoimmunization.

Complications

The principal complication of α-thalassemia trait is the needless administration of iron, given in the belief that a mild microcytic anemia is due to iron deficiency. Persons with hemoglobin H disease may have intermittent exacerbations of their anemia, which require blood transfusions. Splenomegaly may become a significant problem, may exacerbate the anemia, and may require splenectomy. Women pregnant with hydropic α-thalassemia infants are subject to increased complications of pregnancy, particularly toxemia and postpartum hemorrhage.

Treatment

Persons with α-thalassemia trait require no treatment. Those with hemoglobin H disease should receive supplemental folic acid and avoid the same oxidant drugs that cause hemolysis in persons with G6PD deficiency, because exposure to these drugs may exacerbate their anemia. The anemia may also be exacerbated during periods of infection, and transfusions may be required. Occasionally, infants with hemoglobin H disease may show failure-to-thrive without red cell transfusions. Hypersplenism may develop later in childhood and require surgical splenectomy. Genetic counseling and prenatal diagnosis should be offered to families at risk for hydropic fetuses.

Embury SH et al: The thalassemia syndromes. In: *The Hereditary Hemolytic Anemias.* Mentzer WC, Wagner GM (editors). Churchill Livingstone, 1989.
Giardina P, Hilgartner MW: Update on thalassemia. Pediatr Rev 1992;13:55.

2. BETA-THALASSEMIA

Essentials of Diagnosis & Typical Features

Beta-thalassemia minor:
- African, Mediterranean, Middle Eastern, or Asian ancestry.
- Mild microcytic, hypochromic anemia.
- No response to iron therapy.
- Elevated level of hemoglobin A_2.

Beta-thalassemia major:
- Mediterranean, Middle Eastern, or Asian ancestry.
- Moderate to very severe microcytic, hypochromic anemia with marked hepatosplenomegaly.
- Elevated fetal and A_2 hemoglobin.

General Considerations

In contrast to the four α-globin genes, only two β-globin genes are present in diploid cells, one on each chromosome 11. Some β-thalassemia genes produce no β-globin chains and are termed β^0-thalassemia. Other β-globin genes produce some β-globin but in diminished quantities and are termed β^+-thalassemia. Persons affected by β-thalassemia may be heterozygous or homozygous. Heterozygotes for most β-thalassemia genes have β-thalassemia minor. Most homozygotes have β-thalassemia major (Cooley's anemia), which is a severe transfusion-dependent anemia. Other homozygotes have a condition known as **thalassemia intermedia** that is more severe than thalassemia minor but not generally transfusion-dependent.

The worldwide importance of β-thalassemia cannot be overstated. β-Thalassemia major is the most common cause of transfusion-dependent anemia in childhood. In addition, β-thalassemia genes interact with genes for structural β-globin variants such as hemoglobin S and hemoglobin E to cause serious disease in compound heterozygotes. These disorders are discussed further in the sections dealing with sickle hemoglobinopathies and with hemoglobin E disorders.

Clinical Findings

A. Symptoms and Signs: Persons with β-thalassemia minor are usually asymptomatic with a normal physical examination. Those with β-thalassemia major are normal at birth but develop a significant anemia during the first year of life as fetal hemoglobin production decreases. If the disorder is not identified and treated with blood transfusions, such children develop massive hepatosplenomegaly and enlargement of the medullary space with thinning of the bony cortex. The skeletal changes cause characteristic facial deformities (prominent forehead and maxilla) and predispose the child to pathologic fractures. Inadequate treatment causes poor growth and development in these children.

B. Laboratory Findings: Laboratory findings

in β-thalassemia minor include a normal or modestly decreased hemoglobin level. The MCV is almost always decreased. The blood smear typically shows hypochromia, target cells, and sometimes basophilic stippling. Hemoglobin electrophoresis is usually diagnostic when hemoglobin A_2 or hemoglobin F or both is elevated. Infants with β-thalassemia major are hematologically normal at birth but develop severe anemia after the first few months of life. The blood smear typically shows a severe hypochromic, microcytic anemia with marked anisocytosis and poikilocytosis. Target cells are prominent, and nucleated red blood cells often exceed the number of circulating white blood cells. The hemoglobin usually falls to 5–6 g/dL or less, and the reticulocyte count is significantly elevated. Platelet and white blood cell counts may be increased, and the serum bilirubin is elevated. The bone marrow shows marked erythroid hyperplasia but is rarely needed for diagnosis. Hemoglobin electrophoresis shows only fetal and A_2 hemoglobin in children with homozygous $β^0$-thalassemia. Those with $β^+$-thalassemia genes make some hemoglobin A but have a marked increase in fetal and in A_2 hemoglobin. The diagnosis of homozygous β-thalassemia may also be suggested by the finding of β-thalassemia minor in both parents.

Differential Diagnosis

β-Thalassemia minor must be differentiated from other causes of mild microcytic, hypochromic anemias, principally iron deficiency and α-thalassemia. In contrast to those with iron deficiency anemia, persons with β-thalassemia minor typically have an elevated number of red blood cells, and the index of the MCV divided by the red cell count is under 13. Generally, the finding of an elevated hemoglobin A_2 is diagnostic; however, the A_2 level is lowered by coexistent iron deficiency, and this may lead to some confusion. Thus, in children thought to be iron-deficient, hemoglobin electrophoresis with quantitation of hemoglobin A_2 is best performed after a course of iron therapy.

β-Thalassemia major is rarely confused with other disorders. Hemoglobin electrophoresis and family studies readily distinguish it from hemoglobin E-β-thalassemia, which is the other important cause of transfusion-dependent thalassemia.

Complications

The principal complication of β-thalassemia minor is the unnecessary use of iron therapy in a futile attempt to correct the microcytic anemia. Children with β-thalassemia major who are inadequately transfused suffer from poor growth and recurrent infections and may have massive hepatosplenomegaly, thinning of the cortical bone, and pathologic fractures. Without treatment, most children die within the first decade of life. The principal complications of β-thalassemia major in transfused children are hemosiderosis, splenomegaly and hypersplenism, and viral infections (especially hepatitis). Transfusional hemosiderosis requires chelation therapy with deferoxamine to prevent cardiac, hepatic, and endocrine dysfunction. Noncompliance with chelation in adolescents and young adults may lead to death from congestive heart failure, cardiac arrhythmias, or hepatic failure. Even with adequate transfusions, most patients develop splenomegaly and some degree of hypersplenism. This necessitates splenectomy because of the increasing transfusion requirements, usually between ages 5 and 10 years. Unfortunately, this procedure leaves the child at risk for overwhelming septicemia.

Treatment

β-Thalassemia minor requires no specific therapy but has important implications for genetic counseling. For those with β-thalassemia major, two approaches to treatment are now available: chronic transfusion with iron chelation or bone marrow transplantation. Programs of blood transfusion are generally targeted to maintain a nadir hemoglobin level above 9–10 g/dL. This gives increased vigor and well-being, improved growth, and fewer overall complications. However, maintenance of good health currently requires iron chelation with nightly subcutaneous infusion of deferoxamine. Small doses of supplemental ascorbic acid may enhance the efficacy of iron chelation. Newly developed oral iron chelators are under study. Patients on chronic transfusion programs generally develop hypersplenism and require splenectomy when their yearly transfusion requirement of packed red cells exceeds 200–250 mL/kg. Splenectomy results in a decrease in the transfusion requirement and hence a lesser rate of iron loading but is associated with a high risk of postsplenectomy sepsis. For this reason, thalassemic patients should receive pneumococcal vaccine prior to the procedure and prophylactic penicillin afterward.

Bone marrow transplantation is an important therapeutic option for children with β-thalassemia major who have an HLA-identical sibling donor. In a large series from Italy, the probability of 3-year event-free survival was 94% when transplantation was performed prior to the development of hepatomegaly or portal fibrosis.

Lucarelli G et al: Marrow transplantation in patients with thalassemia responsive to iron chelation therapy. N Engl J Med 1993;329:840.

Olivieri NF et al: Survival in medically treated patients with homozygous β-thalassemia. N Engl J Med 1994;331:574.

Weatherall DJ: The treatment of thalassemia: Slow progress and new dilemmas. N Engl J Med 1993; 329:877.

3. SICKLE CELL DISEASE

Essentials of Diagnosis & Typical Features

- African, Mediterranean, Middle Eastern, or Indian ancestry.
- Anemia, elevated reticulocyte count, jaundice.
- Recurrent episodes of musculoskeletal or abdominal pain.
- Hemoglobin electrophoresis with hemoglobins S and F, hemoglobins S and C, or hemoglobins S, F, and A with S > A.
- Splenomegaly in early childhood with later disappearance.
- High risk of overwhelming bacterial sepsis.

General Considerations

A high incidence of sickle hemoglobin is found in persons of central African origin. It also occurs in other ethnic groups in Sicily, Italy, Greece, Turkey, Saudi Arabia, and India. Sickle cell anemia is caused by homozygosity for the sickle gene and is the most common form of sickle cell disease. Other clinically important sickling disorders are compound heterozygous conditions in which the sickle gene interacts with genes for hemoglobin C, D_{Punjab}, O_{Arab}, C_{Harlem}, or β-thalassemia.

Overall, sickle cell disease occurs in about one of every 400 African-American infants. Eight percent of African-Americans are heterozygous carriers of the sickle gene and are said to have sickle cell trait.

The protean clinical manifestations of sickle hemoglobinopathies all can be linked directly or indirectly to the propensity of deoxygenated hemoglobin S to polymerize. Polymerization of sickle hemoglobin distorts erythrocyte morphology, decreases red cell deformability, causes a marked reduction in red cell life span, increases blood viscosity, and predisposes to episodes of vaso-occlusion.

Neonatal screening for sickle hemoglobinopathies is now routine in most of the United States. The identification of affected infants at birth, when combined with follow-up programs of parental education, comprehensive medical care, and prophylactic penicillin, markedly reduces the morbidity and mortality rate in early childhood.

Clinical Findings

A. Symptoms and Signs: The symptoms and signs of sickle cell disease are related to the hemolytic anemia and to tissue ischemia and organ dysfunction caused by vaso-occlusion. Children are normal at birth, and onset of symptoms is unusual before 3–4 months of age because high levels of fetal hemoglobin inhibit sickling. A moderately severe hemolytic anemia is often present by 1 year of age, causes pallor, fatigue, and jaundice, and predisposes to the development of gallstones during childhood and adolescence. Intense congestion of the spleen with sickled cells may cause splenomegaly in early childhood and results in functional asplenia as early as 3 months of age. This places children at great risk for overwhelming infection with encapsulated bacteria, particularly pneumococci. Up to 30% of patients experience one or more episodes of acute splenic sequestration, characterized by sudden enlargement of the spleen with pooling of red cells, acute exacerbation of anemia, and, in severe cases, shock and death. Acute exacerbation of anemia also occurs with aplastic crises, usually caused by infection with human parvovirus.

Recurrent episodes of vaso-occlusion and tissue ischemia cause a myriad of acute and chronic problems. Dactylitis, or hand-and-foot syndrome, is the most common initial symptom of the disease and occurs in up to 50% of children before the age of 3 years. Recurrent episodes of ischemic pain—particularly abdominal and musculoskeletal pain—may occur throughout life. Strokes occur in about 8% of children and tend to be recurrent. The acute chest syndrome, characterized by fever, pleuritic chest pain, and acute pulmonary infiltrates with hypoxemia, is caused by pulmonary infection, infarction, or fat embolism from ischemic bone marrow. All tissues are susceptible to damage from vaso-occlusion, and multiple organ dysfunction is common by adulthood. Table 25–3 lists the common manifestations of sickle cell disease in children and adults.

B. Laboratory Findings: Children with sickle cell anemia (Hb SS) generally show a baseline hemo-

Table 25–3. Common clinical manifestations of sickle cell disease.

	Acute	Chronic
Children	Bacterial sepsis or meningitis[1] Splenic sequestration[1] Aplastic crisis Vaso-occlusive events Dactylitis Bone infarction Acute chest syndrome[1] Stroke[1] Priapism	Functional asplenia Delayed growth and development Avasular necrosis of the hip Hyposthenuria Cholelithiasis
Adults	Bacterial sepsis[1] Aplastic crisis Vaso-occlusive events Bone infarction Acute chest syndrome[1] Stroke[1] Priapism Acute multi-organ failure syndrome[1]	Leg ulcers Proliferative retinopathy Avasular necrosis of the hip Cholecystitis Chronic organ failure[1] Liver Lung Kidney Decreased fertility

[1]Associated with significant mortality rate.

globin level between 7 and 10 g/dL. This value may fall to life-threatening levels at the time of a sequestration or aplastic crisis. The baseline reticulocyte count is markedly elevated. The anemia is normocytic or macrocytic, and the blood smear typically shows the characteristic sickle cells as well as numerous target cells. Patients with sickle β-thalassemia generally have a low MCV and hypochromia as well. Those with sickle β^+-thalassemia tend to have lesser degrees of hemolysis and anemia. Persons with sickle hemoglobin C (Hb SC) disease have fewer sickle forms and more target cells, and the hemoglobin level may be normal or only slightly decreased as the rate of hemolysis is much less than in sickle cell anemia.

Most infants with sickle hemoglobinopathies born in the United States are now identified by neonatal screening. Results indicative of possible sickle cell disease require prompt confirmation with hemoglobin electrophoresis. Children with sickle cell anemia and with sickle β^0-thalassemia have only hemoglobins S and F. Persons with sickle β^+-thalassemia have a preponderance of hemoglobin S with a lesser amount of hemoglobin A. Persons with sickle hemoglobin C disease have equal amounts of hemoglobin S and hemoglobin C. The use of solubility tests to screen for the presence of sickle hemoglobin should be avoided because a negative result is frequently encountered in infants with sickle cell disease, and because a positive result an older child does not differentiate sickle cell trait from sickle cell disease. Thus, hemoglobin electrophoresis is always necessary to accurately identify a sickle disorder.

Serum chemistries are often abnormal, depending on the severity of the hemolysis and on the presence of hepatic or renal dysfunction. X-rays of the skull and spine reveal cortical thinning, enlargement of the marrow spaces, and increased trabecular markings.

Differential Diagnosis

Hemoglobin electrophoresis and sometimes hematologic studies of the parents are usually sufficient to confirm the correct diagnosis of a sickle cell disorder. Infants whose neonatal screening test shows only hemoglobin S and F occasionally have disorders other than sickle cell anemia or sickle β^0-thalassemia. The most important of these is a compound heterozygous condition of sickle hemoglobin and pancellular hereditary persistence of fetal hemoglobin. Such children, when older, typically have 30% fetal hemoglobin and 70% hemoglobin S, but they do not have significant anemia nor are they subject to vaso-occlusive episodes.

Complications

Repeated tissue ischemia and infarction causes damage to virtually every organ system. The most important complications are listed in Table 25-3. Patients who require multiple transfusions are at risk for transfusional hemosiderosis and the development of red cell alloantibodies, as well as transmission of infectious agents.

Treatment

The cornerstone of treatment is enrollment in a program that provides for patient and family education, comprehensive outpatient care, and appropriate treatment of acute complications. Important to the success of such a program are psychosocial services, blood bank services, and the ready availability of baseline patient information in the setting where acute problems are handled. Treatment of children with sickle cell anemia and sickle β^0-thalassemia includes prophylactic penicillin, which should be initiated by 2 months of age and continued at least until 5 years of age. The routine use of penicillin prophylaxis in hemoglobin SC disease and sickle β^+-thalassemia is controversial. Pneumococcal vaccine should be administered to all children with sickle cell disease at 2 years of age and again 3 years later. Other routine immunizations, including yearly vaccination against influenza, should be provided. All illnesses associated with fever greater than 38.5 °C should be evaluated promptly with bacterial cultures, administration of parenteral broad-spectrum antibiotics, and careful inpatient or outpatient observation.

Treatment of painful vaso-occlusive episodes includes the maintenance of adequate hydration (with avoidance of overhydration), correction of acidosis if present, administration of adequate analgesia, maintenance of normal oxygen saturation, and the treatment of any associated infections.

Red cell transfusions play an important role in management. Transfusions are indicated to improve oxygen-carrying capacity during acute exacerbations of anemia, as occurs during episodes of splenic sequestration or aplastic crisis. Red cell transfusions are not indicated for the treatment of chronic steady-state anemia, which is usually well tolerated, or for uncomplicated episodes of vaso-occlusive pain. Partial exchange transfusion to reduce the percentage of circulating sickle cells is indicated for a number of severe acute vaso-occlusive events and may be lifesaving. These events include stroke, severe acute chest syndrome, and acute life-threatening failure of other organs. Transfusions may also be used prior to high-risk procedures such as surgery with general anesthesia or arteriograms with ionic contrast materials. A subset of patients are treated with chronic transfusion programs. The most common indication for this type of transfusion is stroke. Without transfusions, children with stroke have a 70–80% chance of recurrent stroke within a 2-year period. This risk of recurrent neurologic events is markedly reduced by the transfusion therapy.

Successful bone marrow transplantation cures sickle cell disease, but to date its use has been limited because of the risks associated with the procedure, the inability to predict in young children the severity of future complications, and the paucity of HLA-identical sibling donors. Therapy using chemotherapeutic agents such as hydroxyurea to ameliorate the disease by increasing levels of fetal hemoglobin is promising but still experimental in children.

Prognosis

Early identification by neonatal screening of infants with sickle cell disease, combined with comprehensive care that includes prophylactic penicillin, has markedly reduced mortality in childhood. Most patients are now expected to live well into adulthood, but they eventually succumb to complications.

Emre U et al: Effect of transfusion in acute chest syndrome of sickle cell disease. J Pediatr 1995;127:901.

Gill FM et al: Clinical events in the first decade in a cohort of infants with sickle cell disease. Blood 1995;86:776.

Lane PA: Sickle cell disease. Pediatr Clin North Am 1996;43:639.

Ohene-Frempong K et al: Cerebrovascular accidents in sickle cell disease: Rates and risk factors. Blood 1998;91:288.

Styles LA, Vichinsky E: Effects of long-term transfusion regimen on sickle cell-related illness. J Pediatr 1994;125:909.

Walters MC et al: Bone marrow transplantation for sickle cell disease. N Engl J Med 1996;335:369.

4. SICKLE CELL TRAIT

Individuals who are heterozygous for the sickle gene are said to have sickle cell trait. This genetic carrier state occurs in 8% of African-Americans and is even more common in some areas of Africa and the Middle East. Accurate identification of persons with sickle cell trait depends on hemoglobin electrophoresis, which typically shows about 60% hemoglobin A and about 40% hemoglobin S with normal levels of hemoglobin A_2 and F. There is no anemia or hemolysis, and the physical examination is normal. Persons with sickle cell trait are generally healthy, and most experience no illness attributable to the presence of sickle hemoglobin in their red cells. Life expectancy is normal.

Sickle trait erythrocytes are capable of sickling, particularly under conditions of significant hypoxemia, and a number of clinical abnormalities have been linked to this genetic carrier state. Exposure to environmental hypoxia (altitude > 3100 m [10,000 ft] above sea level) may precipitate splenic infarction or splenic sequestration. However, most persons with sickle cell trait who choose to visit such altitudes for skiing, hiking, or climbing do so without difficulty. Many develop some degree of hyposthenuria, and about 4% experience painless hematuria, usually microscopic but occasionally macroscopic. For the most part, these renal abnormalities are subclinical, and they do not progress to significant renal dysfunction. The incidence of bacteriuria and pyelonephritis may be increased during pregnancy, but overall rates of maternal and infant morbidity and mortality are not affected by the presence of sickle cell trait in the pregnant woman.

An epidemiologic study of army recruits in military basic training found a higher risk of sudden unexplained death following strenuous exertion in recruits with sickle cell trait than in those with normal hemoglobin. This study has raised concerns about exercise and exertion for persons with the trait. However, considerable evidence suggests that exercise is generally safe and that athletic performance is not adversely affected by sickle cell trait. Exercise tolerance is normal, and the incidence of sickle cell trait in black professional football players is similar to that of the general African-American population, suggesting no barrier to achievement in such a physically demanding profession. Thus, restrictions on athletic competition for children with sickle cell trait are not warranted. Sickle cell trait continues to be most significant for its implications regarding genetic counseling, not for any associated health risks.

Committee on Sports Medicine, American Academy of Pediatrics: Recommendations for participation in competitive sports. Pediatrics 1988;81:737.

Kark JA et al: Sickle cell trait as a risk factor for sudden death in physical training. N Engl J Med 1987;317:781.

Nuss R et al: Cardiopulmonary function in men with sickle cell disease who reside at moderately high altitude. J Lab Clin Med 1993;122:382.

Pearson HA: Sickle cell trait in competitive athletics: Is there a risk? Pediatrics 1989;83:613.

5. HEMOGLOBIN C DISORDERS

Two percent of African-Americans are heterozygous for hemoglobin C and are said to have hemoglobin C trait. Such individuals have no symptoms, anemia, or hemolysis, but the blood smear may show some target cells. Identification of persons with hemoglobin C trait is important for genetic counseling, particularly with regard to the possibility of hemoglobin SC disease in offspring.

Persons with homozygous hemoglobin C have a mild microcytic hemolytic anemia and may develop splenomegaly. The blood smear shows prominent target cells. As with other hemolytic anemias, complications of homozygous hemoglobin C include gallstones and aplastic crises.

Olson JF et al: Hemoglobin C disease in infancy and childhood. J Pediatr 1994;125:745.

6. HEMOGLOBIN E DISORDERS

Hemoglobin E is the second most common hemoglobin variant worldwide, with a gene frequency greater than 10% in some areas of Thailand and Cambodia. In Southeast Asia, an estimated 30 million people have hemoglobin E trait. Persons heterozygous for hemoglobin E are asymptomatic and usually not anemic but there may be mild microcytosis. Persons homozygous for hemoglobin E are also asymptomatic but may have mild anemia; the blood smear shows microcytosis and some target cells.

Hemoglobin E is most important because of its interaction with β-thalassemia. Compound heterozygotes for hemoglobin E and β^0-thalassemia are normal at birth but subsequently develop a moderate to severe microcytic hypochromic anemia. Such children may show jaundice, hepatosplenomegaly, and poor growth if the disorder is not recognized and treated appropriately. In some cases, the anemia becomes severe enough to require lifelong transfusion therapy. In certain areas of the United States, hemoglobin E-β^0-thalassemia has become a more common cause of transfusion-dependent anemia than homozygous β-thalassemia.

Glader BE, Look KA: Hematologic disorders in children from Southeast Asia. Pediatr Clin North Am 1996;43:665.
Johnson JP et al: Differentiation of homozygous hemoglobin E from compound heterozygous hemoglobin E-β-thalassemia by hemoglobin E mutation analysis. J Pediatr 1992;120:775.

7. UNSTABLE HEMOGLOBIN DISORDERS (Congenital Heinz Body Anemias)

Unstable hemoglobin disorders differ from most other structural hemoglobin variants because heterozygotes have hemolytic anemia and often jaundice. The anemia may be exacerbated during hemolytic crises precipitated by fever or by the ingestion of oxidant drugs. Splenomegaly is variably present, and patients are susceptible to the development of gallstones later in life. Patients with more severe hemolysis may have dark brown urine.

Laboratory findings include a variable hemolytic anemia with elevated reticulocyte count. The blood smear may show basophilic stippling. Inclusion bodies of precipitated denatured hemoglobin called Heinz bodies are demonstrated by special stains. Some unstable hemoglobins may be detected by hemoglobin electrophoresis, but many are electrophoretically silent. Thus, the diagnosis depends on the demonstration of hemoglobin instability, usually with the isopropanol precipitation test.

The differential diagnosis includes most other causes of congenital hemolytic anemias. The autosomal dominant genetic transmission may arouse suspicion of a red cell membrane defect, but abnormalities on the peripheral smear are not typical of either spherocytosis or elliptocytosis. The exacerbation of he-

molysis during infection or with ingestion of oxidant drugs and the presence of Heinz bodies may suggest a G6PD deficiency, but normal or elevated levels of G6PD and the increased hemoglobin precipitation with isopropanol are usually sufficient to differentiate unstable hemoglobin disorders from G6PD deficiency.

Treatment of children with unstable hemoglobin disorders generally depends on the severity of the hemolysis. Folic acid may prevent the development of a folate deficiency. The avoidance of oxidant drugs is important for some of these disorders, since their use may precipitate hemolytic crises. The role of splenectomy is unclear.

Vichinsky EP, Lubin PH: Unstable hemoglobins, hemoglobins with altered oxygen affinity, and M-hemoglobins. Pediatr Clin North Am 1980;27:421.
Wagner GM et al: Sickling syndromes and unstable hemoglobin disease. In: *The Hereditary Hemolytic Anemias.* Mentzer WC, Wagner GM (editors). Churchill Livingstone, 1989.

8. OTHER HEMOGLOBINOPATHIES

Hundreds of other human globin-chain variants have been identified and described. Some, such as hemoglobins D and G, are relatively common. Heterozygotes, who are frequently detected during the course of neonatal screening programs for hemoglobinopathies, are generally asymptomatic and usually have no anemia or hemolysis. The principal significance of most hemoglobin variants is the potential for disease in compound heterozygotes who also inherit a gene for β-thalassemia or sickle hemoglobin. For example, children compound heterozygous for hemoglobins S and D_{Punjab} ($D_{Los\ Angeles}$) have a severe hemolytic anemia with a peripheral blood smear and clinical problems virtually identical with those of children with sickle cell anemia.

CONGENITAL HEMOLYTIC ANEMIAS: DISORDERS OF RED CELL METABOLISM

Erythrocytes are dependent on the anaerobic metabolism of glucose for the maintenance of adenosine triphosphate (ATP) levels sufficient for normal homeostasis. Glycolysis also produces the 2,3-DPG levels needed to modulate the oxygen affinity of adult hemoglobin. In addition, glucose metabolism via the hexosemonophosphate shunt is necessary to generate sufficient reduced nicotinamide adenine dinucleotide phosphate (NADPH) and reduced glutathione to protect the red cell against oxidant damage. Congenital deficiencies of many (not all) glycolytic pathway enzymes have been associated with hemolytic anemias. In general, the morphologic abnormalities present on the blood smear are nonspecific, and the inheritance of these disorders is autosomal recessive or X-linked. Thus, the possibility of a red cell enzyme defect should be considered during the evaluation of a congenital hemolytic anemia when the blood smear does not show red cell morphology typical of membrane or hemoglobin defects (eg, spherocytes, sickle forms, target cells), when hemoglobin disorders are excluded by hemoglobin electrophoresis and by isopropanol precipitation tests, and when family studies do not suggest an autosomal dominant disorder. The diagnosis is confirmed by finding a low level of the deficient enzyme.

The following section focuses on the two most common disorders of erythrocyte metabolism: G6PD deficiency and pyruvate kinase deficiency.

1. GLUCOSE-6-PHOSPHATE DEHYDROGENASE (G6PD) DEFICIENCY

Essentials of Diagnosis & Typical Features
- African, Mediterranean, or Asian ancestry.
- Neonatal hyperbilirubinemia.
- Sporadic hemolysis associated with infection or with ingestion of oxidant drugs or fava beans.
- X-linked inheritance.

General Considerations

Deficiency of G6PD is easily the most common red cell enzyme defect that causes hemolytic anemia. The disorder has X-linked recessive inheritance and occurs with high frequency among persons of African, Mediterranean, and Asian ancestry. Hundreds of different G6PD variants have now been identified and characterized. In most instances, enzyme deficiency is due to the instability of the abnormal enzyme, and older red cells are thus more deficient than younger ones. The consequence of the deficiency is the inability of erythrocytes to generate sufficient amounts of NADPH to maintain the levels of reduced glutathione necessary to protect the red cell against oxidant stress. Thus, most persons with G6PD deficiency do not have a chronic hemolytic anemia, but they do have episodic hemolysis at times of exposure to the oxidant stress of infection or of certain drugs or food substances. The severity of the disorder varies among ethnic groups; G6PD deficiency in persons of African ancestry usually is less severe than in other ethnic groups.

Clinical Findings

A. Symptoms and Signs: Infants with G6PD deficiency may have significant hyperbilirubinemia and may require the use of phototherapy or exchange transfusion to prevent kernicterus. The deficiency is an important cause of neonatal hyperbilirubinemia in Mediterranean and Chinese infants but less so in black infants. Older children with G6PD deficiency are asymptomatic and appear normal between episodes of hemolysis. Hemolytic episodes are often triggered by infection or by the ingestion of oxidant drugs, most importantly antimalarial compounds and sulfonamide antibiotics (Table 25–4). Ingestion of fava beans may trigger hemolysis in Mediterranean and Asian children but not in African children. Episodes of hemolysis are associated with pallor, jaundice, hemoglobinuria, and sometimes cardiovascular compromise.

B. Laboratory Findings: The hemoglobin, reticulocyte count, and blood smear are usually normal in the absence of oxidant-induced hemolysis. Episodes of hemolysis are associated with a variable fall in hemoglobin. "Bite" cells or blister cells may be seen, along with a few spherocytes. Hemoglobinuria is common, and the reticulocyte count increases within a few days. Heinz bodies may be demonstrated with appropriate stains. The diagnosis is confirmed by the finding of reduced levels of G6PD in erythrocytes. Because this enzyme is present in increased quantities in reticulocytes, the test is best performed at a time when the reticulocyte count is normal or near normal.

Complications

Kernicterus is a risk for infants with significant neonatal hyperbilirubinemia. Episodes of acute hemolysis in older children may be life-threatening if severe enough to cause cardiovascular collapse. Rare G6PD variants that are associated with chronic hemolytic anemia may be complicated by splenomegaly and by the formation of gallstones.

Treatment

The most important issue is avoidance of drugs known to be associated with hemolysis (see Table 25–4). For some Mediterranean and Asian patients, the consumption of fava beans must also be avoided. Infections should be treated promptly and antibiotics given when appropriate. Most episodes of hemolysis are self-limiting, but red cell transfusions may be lifesaving when signs and symptoms indicate cardiovascular compromise.

Table 25–4. Some common drugs and chemicals that can induce hemolytic anemia in persons with G6PD deficiency.[1]

Acetanilid	Niridazole
Doxorubicin	Nitrofurantoin
Furazolidone	Phenazopyridine
Methylene blue	Primaquine
Nalidixic acid	Sulfamethoxazole

[1]From Beutler E: Glucose-6-phosphate dehydrogenase deficiency. N Engl J Med 1991;324:171.

Beutler E: G6PD deficiency. Blood 1994;84:3613.

Kaplan M et al: Conjugated bilirubin in neonates with glucose-6-phosphate dehydrogenase deficiency. J Pediatr 1996;128:695.

Seidman DS et al: Role of hemolysis in neonatal jaundice associated with glucose-6-phosphate dehydrogenase deficiency. J Pediatr 1995;127:804.

2. PYRUVATE KINASE DEFICIENCY

Pyruvate kinase deficiency is an autosomal recessive disorder that has been described in all ethnic groups but is most common in northern Europeans. The deficiency is associated with a chronic hemolytic anemia of varying severity. Approximately one-third of those affected present in the neonatal period with jaundice and hemolysis that require phototherapy or exchange transfusion. Occasionally, the disorder causes hydrops fetalis and neonatal death. In older children, the hemolysis may require intermittent support with red cell transfusions or may be mild enough to go unnoticed for many years. Jaundice and splenomegaly are frequently present in the more severe cases. The diagnosis of pyruvate kinase deficiency may occasionally be suggested by the presence of echinocytes on the blood smear, but these may be absent prior to splenectomy. Measurement of 2,3-DPG and ATP levels in red cells may suggest the diagnosis of pyruvate kinase deficiency if 2,3-DPG levels are elevated and ATP levels are reduced. The diagnosis depends on the demonstration of low levels of pyruvate kinase activity in red cells.

Treatment of pyruvate kinase depends on the severity of the hemolysis. Blood transfusions may be required for significant anemia, and splenectomy may be beneficial. The procedure does not cure the disorder but does ameliorate the anemia and its symptoms. Characteristically, the reticulocyte count *increases* after splenectomy, despite the decreased hemolysis and increased hemoglobin level. In addition, echinocytes frequently become more prevalent.

Gilsanz F et al: Fetal anaemia due to pyruvate kinase deficiency. Arch Dis Child 1993;69:523.

Mentzer WC Jr: Pyruvate kinase deficiency and disorders of glycolysis. In: *Hematology of Infancy and Childhood,* 4th ed. Nathan DG, Oski FA (editors). Saunders, 1993.

ACQUIRED HEMOLYTIC ANEMIA

1. AUTOIMMUNE HEMOLYTIC ANEMIA

Essentials of Diagnosis & Typical Features

- Pallor, fatigue, jaundice, and dark urine.
- Splenomegaly common.
- Positive Coombs test.
- Reticulocytosis and spherocytosis.

General Considerations

Acquired autoimmune hemolytic anemia is rare during the first 4 months of life but is one of the more common causes of acute anemia after the first year. It may arise as an isolated problem or may complicate an infection (hepatitis, upper respiratory tract infections, mononucleosis, cytomegalovirus infection), systemic lupus erythematosus and other autoimmune syndromes, immunodeficiency states, or malignancies.

Clinical Findings

A. Symptoms and Signs: The disease usually has an acute onset, presenting with weakness, pallor, dark urine, and fatigue. Jaundice is a prominent finding, and splenomegaly is often present. Some cases are chronic and insidious in onset. Clinical evidence of the underlying disease may be present.

B. Laboratory Findings: The anemia is normochromic and normocytic and may vary from mild to severe (hemoglobin concentration < 5 g/dL). The reticulocyte count is usually increased but occasionally may be normal or low. Spherocytes and nucleated red cells may be seen on the peripheral smear. Although leukocytosis and elevated platelet counts are a common finding, thrombocytopenia is occasionally seen. Other laboratory data consistent with hemolysis are present such as increased indirect and total bilirubin, lactic dehydrogenase (LDH), aspartate aminotransferase (AST), and urinary urobilinogen. The hemolysis is intravascular if there is hemoglobinemia or hemoglobinuria. Examination of bone marrow shows marked erythroid hyperplasia and occasionally hemophagocytosis.

Serologic studies provide important information about the disease, which is helpful in defining the pathophysiology, planning therapeutic strategies, and assessing prognosis (Table 25–5). In almost all cases, the direct and indirect antiglobulin (Coombs) tests are positive. Further evaluation allows distinction of three syndromes. The presence of IgG, maximal in vitro activity at 37 °C, and either no antigen specificity or an Rh-like specificity constitute warm autoimmune hemolytic anemia with extravascular destruction by the reticuloendothelial system. In contrast, the detection of complement alone and optimal reactivity in vitro at 4 °C with I or i antigen specificity are diagnostic of cold autoimmune hemolytic anemia with intravascular hemolysis. Paroxysmal cold hemoglobinuria appears identical with cold autoimmune hemolytic anemia but has a different antigen specificity and exhibits hemolysis as well as agglutination in vitro.

Differential Diagnosis

Autoimmune hemolytic anemia must be differentiated from other forms of congenital or acquired hemolytic anemias. The Coombs test discriminates antibody-mediated hemolysis from other causes such as hereditary spherocytosis.

Table 25–5. Classification of autoimmune hemolytic anemia (AIHA) in children.

Syndrome	Warm AIHA	Cold AIHA	Paroxysmal Cold Hematuria

Specific antiglobulin test
  IgG
  Complement
	Strongly positive
	Negative or mildly positive
		Negative
		Strongly positive
			Negative
			Strongly positive

Temperature at maximal reactivity	37 °C	4 °C	4 °C
Antigen specificity	May be panagglutinin or may have an Rh-like specificity	I or i	P
Other	...	...	Positive biphasic hemolysin test
Pathophysiology	Extravascular hemolysis, destruction by the RES (eg, spleen)	Intravascular hemolysis	Intravascular hemolysis
Prognosis	May be more chronic (>3 months) with significant morbidity and mortality. May be associated with a primary disorder (lupus, immunodeficiency, etc)	Generally acute (<3 months). Good outlook: Often associated with infection.	Acute, self-limited. Associated with infection.
Therapy	Respond to RES blockade, including steroids (prednisone, 2 mg/kg/d), IGIV (1 g/kg/d for up to 5 days), or splenectomy	May not respond to RES blockade. Severe cases may benefit from plasmapheresis.	Usually self-limited. Symptomatic management.

RES = reticuloendothelial system.

Complications

The anemia may be very severe and result in cardiovascular collapse requiring emergency management. The complications of the underlying disease such as disseminated lupus erythematosus or lymphoma may be present.

Treatment

Medical management of the underlying disease is important in symptomatic cases. Defining the clinical syndrome provides a useful guide to treatment. Most patients with warm autoimmune hemolytic anemia (in which hemolysis is extravascular) respond to prednisone. After the initial treatment, the dose of corticosteroids may be decreased slowly. Patients may respond to 1 g of intravenous immune globulin (IGIV) per kilogram per day for 1–5 days, but fewer patients respond to IGIV than to prednisone. Although the rate of remission with splenectomy may be as high as 50%, particularly in warm autoimmune hemolytic anemia, this approach should be withheld until other treatments have been tried. In severe cases unresponsive to more conventional therapy, immunosuppressive agents such as cyclophosphamide, azathioprine, or busulfan may be tried alone or in combination with corticosteroids.

Patients with cold autoimmune hemolytic anemia and paroxysmal cold hemoglobinuria are less likely to respond to corticosteroids or IGIV. Since both of these syndromes are most apt to be associated with infections and have an acute, self-limited course,

supportive care may be all that is required. Plasma exchange is effective in cold autoimmune (IgM) hemolytic anemia (and may be helpful in severe cases) because the offending antibody has only an intravascular distribution.

Supportive therapy is crucial. Patients with cold-reacting antibodies, particularly paroxysmal cold hemoglobinuria, should be kept in a warm environment. Transfusion may be necessary because of the complications of severe anemia but should be used only when there is no alternative. In most patients, cross-match-compatible blood will not be found, and the least incompatible unit should be identified. Transfusion must be conducted carefully, beginning with a test dose (see Transfusion Medicine later in this chapter). Identification of the patient's phenotype for minor red cell alloantigens may be helpful in avoiding alloimmunization or providing appropriate transfusions if alloantibodies arise after initial transfusions during the period of supportive care. Patients with severe intravascular hemolysis may have associated disseminated intravascular coagulation (DIC), and heparin therapy should be considered in such cases.

Prognosis

The outlook for autoimmune hemolytic anemia in childhood is usually good unless there are associated diseases (congenital immunodeficiency, AIDS, lupus erythematosus, malignancy), in which case the hemolysis is likely to run a chronic course. In general, children with warm autoimmune hemolytic anemia are at greater risk for more severe and chronic disease with higher morbidity and mortality rates. Hemolysis and positive antiglobulin tests may continue for months or years. Patients with cold autoimmune hemolytic anemia or paroxysmal cold hemoglobinuria are more likely to have acute, self-limited disease (< 3 months). Paroxysmal cold hemoglobinuria is almost always associated with infection (eg, with *Mycoplasma* infection, cytomegalovirus, Epstein-Barr virus).

Hilgartner MW, Bussel J: Use of intravenous gamma globulin for treatment of autoimmune neutropenia of childhood and autoimmune hemolytic anemia. Am J Med 1987;83:25.

Petz LD, Garratty G: Unusual problems regarding autoimmune hemolytic anemias. In: *Acquired Immune Hemolytic Anemias.* Churchill Livingstone, 1980.

Sabio H, Jones D, McKie VC: Biphasic hemolysin hemolytic anemia: Reappraisal of an acute hemolytic anemia of infancy and childhood. Am J Hematol 1992;39:220.

Salama A, Mueller-Eckhardt C: Autoimmune haemolytic anaemia in childhood associated with noncomplement binding IgM autoantibodies. Br J Haematol 1987;65:67.

2. NONIMMUNE ACQUIRED HEMOLYTIC ANEMIA

Hepatic disease may alter the lipid composition of the red cell membrane. This usually results in the formation of target cells and is not associated with significant hemolysis. Occasionally, however, severe hepatocellular damage is associated with the formation of "spur" cells and brisk hemolytic anemia. Renal disease may also be associated with significant hemolysis; hemolytic uremic syndrome is the best-known example. In this disorder, hemolysis is associated with the presence on the blood smear of echinocytes, fragmented red cells, and spherocytes.

A microangiopathic hemolytic anemia with fragmented red cells and some spherocytes may be observed in a number of conditions associated with intravascular coagulation and fibrin deposition within vessels. This occurs with DIC such as may complicate overwhelming infection, but it may also occur when the intravascular coagulation is localized, as with giant cavernous hemangiomas (Kasabach-Merritt syndrome).

POLYCYTHEMIA & METHEMOGLOBINEMIA

CONGENITAL ERYTHROCYTOSIS (Familial Polycythemia)

In pediatrics, polycythemia is usually secondary to some hypoxemic disorder. However, a number of families with congenital erythrocytosis have been described. The disorder differs from polycythemia vera in that it affects only the erythroid series; the white cell count and platelet count are normal. It frequently occurs as an autosomal dominant, although it can also occur as an autosomal recessive. There are usually no physical findings except for plethora and splenomegaly. The hemoglobin may be as high as 27 g/dL, with a hematocrit of 80% and a red cell count of 10 million/μL. There are usually no symptoms other than headache and lethargy. Studies in a number of families have revealed (1) an abnormal hemoglobin with increased oxygen affinity, (2) reduced red cell diphosphoglycerate, (3) autonomous increase in erythropoietin production, or (4) hypersensitivity of erythroid precursors to erythropoietin.

Treatment is not indicated unless symptoms are marked. Phlebotomy is the treatment of choice.

Juvonen E et al: Autosomal dominant erythrocytosis caused by increased sensitivity to erythropoietin. Blood 1991; 78:3066.

Sokol L et al: Primary familial polycythemia: A frameshift mutation in the erythropoietin receptor gene and increased sensitivity of erythroid progenitors to erythropoietin. Blood 1995;86:15.

SECONDARY POLYCYTHEMIA

Secondary polycythemia occurs in response to hypoxemia. The most common cause of secondary polycythemia in children is cyanotic congenital heart disease. It also occurs in chronic pulmonary disease such as cystic fibrosis and in pulmonary arteriovenous shunts. Persons living at extremely high altitudes, as well as some with methemoglobinemia, develop polycythemia. It has on rare occasions been described without hypoxemia in association with renal tumors, brain tumors, Cushing's disease, or hydronephrosis.

Polycythemia occurs normally in the neonatal period; it is particularly exaggerated in infants who are preterm or small for gestational age. In these infants, polycythemia is sometimes associated with other symptoms. It may occur in infants of diabetic mothers, and it has been described as a manifestation of

Down's syndrome in the newborn and as a complication of congenital adrenal hyperplasia.

Iron deficiency may complicate polycythemia and aggravate the hyperviscosity. This complication should always be suspected when the MCV falls below the normal range. Multiple coagulation and bleeding abnormalities have also been described in severely polycythemic cardiac patients, including thrombocytopenia, mild consumption coagulopathy, and elevated fibrinolytic activity. Bleeding at surgery may be severe.

The ideal treatment of secondary polycythemia is correction of the underlying disorder. When this cannot be done, phlebotomy is often necessary to control the symptoms. Iron sufficiency should be maintained. Adequate hydration of the patient and phlebotomy with plasma replacement may be indicated prior to major surgical procedures; these measures prevent the complications of thrombosis and hemorrhage. Isovolumetric exchange transfusion is the treatment of choice in severe cases.

Balcerzak SP, Bromberg PA: Secondary polycythemia. Semin Hematol 1975;12:353.

METHEMOGLOBINEMIA

Methemoglobin is continuously formed at a slow rate by the oxidation of heme iron to the ferric state. Normally, it is enzymatically reduced back to hemoglobin. Methemoglobin is unable to transport oxygen and causes a shift in the dissociation curve of the residual oxyhemoglobin. Cyanosis is produced with methemoglobin levels of approximately 15% or greater. There are several mechanisms for the excess production of methemoglobin, which occurs as a congenital or acquired disorder.

1. HEMOGLOBIN M

The designation M is given to several abnormal hemoglobins associated with methemoglobinemia. Affected individuals are heterozygous for the gene, and it is transmitted as an autosomal dominant. The different types of hemoglobin M result from different amino acid substitutions in the α-globin or β-globin. Hemoglobin electrophoresis at the usual pH will not always demonstrate the abnormal hemoglobin, and isoelectric focusing may be needed. The patient has cyanosis but is otherwise usually asymptomatic. Exercise tolerance may be normal, and life expectancy is not affected. This type of methemoglobinemia does not respond to any form of therapy.

Vichinsky EP, Lubin BH: Unstable hemoglobins, hemoglobins with altered oxygen affinity, and M-hemoglobins. Pediatr Clin North Am 1980;27:421.

2. CONGENITAL METHEMOGLOBINEMIA DUE TO ENZYME DEFICIENCIES

Congenital methemoglobinemia is most frequently caused by congenital deficiency of the reducing enzyme diaphorase I (coenzyme factor I). It is transmitted as an autosomal recessive trait. Affected patients may have as high as 40% methemoglobin but usually have no symptoms, although a mild compensatory polycythemia may be present. Patients with methemoglobinemia associated with a deficiency of diaphorase I respond readily to treatment with ascorbic acid and with methylene blue (see below). However, treatment is not usually indicated.

3. ACQUIRED METHEMOGLOBINEMIA

A number of compounds activate the oxidation of hemoglobin from the ferrous to the ferric state, forming methemoglobin. These include the nitrites and nitrates (contaminated water), chlorates, and quinones. Drugs in this group are the aniline dyes, sulfonamides, acetanilid, phenacetin, bismuth subnitrate, and potassium chlorate. Poisoning with a drug or chemical containing one of these substances should be suspected in any infant or child who presents with sudden cyanosis. Methemoglobin levels in such cases may be extremely high and can produce severe anoxia and dyspnea with unconsciousness, circulatory failure, and death. Young infants and newborns are more susceptible to poisoning because their red cells have difficulty reducing hemoglobin, probably because their NADH methemoglobin reductase is transiently deficient. Infants with metabolic acidosis from diarrhea and dehydration or other causes may also develop methemoglobinemia.

Patients with the acquired form of methemoglobinemia respond dramatically to methylene blue in a dosage of 1–2 mg/kg intravenously. For infants and young children, a smaller dose (1–1.5 mg/kg) is recommended. Ascorbic acid administered orally or intravenously also reduces methemoglobin, but it acts more slowly.

Mansouri A, Lurie AA: Concise review: Methemoglobinemia. Am J Hematol 1993;42:7.

Murray KF, Christie DL: Dietary protein intolerance in infants with transient methemoglobinemia and diarrhea. J Pediatr 1993;122:90.

Osterhoudt KC et al: Rebound severe methemoglobinemia from ingestion of a nitroethane artificial-fingernail remover. J Pediatr 1995;126:819.

Sager S et al: Methemoglobinemia associated with acidosis of probable renal origin. J Pediatr 1995;126:59.

DISORDERS OF LEUKOCYTES

NEUTROPENIA

Essentials of Diagnosis & Typical Features
- Increased frequency of infections.
- Ulceration of oral mucosa and gingivitis.
- Normal numbers of red cells and platelets.

General Considerations

Neutropenia is an absolute neutrophil (granulocyte) count of less than 1500/μL in infancy and childhood, or below 1000/μL between 1 week and 2 years of age. During the first few days of life, an absolute neutrophil count of less than 3500 cells/μL may be considered neutropenia. Neutropenias result from absent or defective granulocyte stem cells, ineffective or suppressed myeloid maturation, decreased production of hematopoietic cytokines (eg, granulocyte colony-stimulating factor [G-CSF], granulocyte-macrophage colony-stimulating factor [GM-CSF]), decreased marrow release, increased neutrophil destruction or consumption, or, in pseudoneutropenia, from an increased neutrophil "marginating pool" (Table 25–6).

The most severe types of congenital neutropenias include reticular dysgenesis (congenital aleukocytosis), Kostmann's syndrome (severe neutropenia with maturation defect in the marrow progenitor cells), Shwachman's syndrome (neutropenia with pancreatic insufficiency), neutropenia with immune deficiency states, cyclic neutropenia, and myelocathexis or dysgranulopoiesis. Neutropenia may also be associated with storage and metabolic diseases and immunodeficiency states. The most common causes of neutropenia are viral infection or drugs resulting either in decreased production in the marrow or increased destruction. Severe bacterial infections may be associated with neutropenia. Although rare, neonatal alloimmune neutropenia can be severe and associated with increased risk for infection. Autoimmune neutropenia in the mother can result in passive transfer of antibody and neutropenia in the neonate. Malignancies, osteopetrosis, marrow failure syndromes, and hypersplenism are not usually associated with isolated neutropenia.

Clinical Findings

A. Symptoms and Signs: Acute severe bacterial or fungal infection is the most significant complication of neutropenia. Although the risk is increased when the absolute neutrophil count is less than 500/μL, the actual susceptibility is variable and depends on the cause of neutropenia, marrow reserves, and other factors. The most common types of infection include septicemia, cellulitis, skin abscesses, pneumonia, and perirectal abscesses. Aphthous ulcers, gingivitis, and periodontal disease also cause

---

Table 25–6. Classification of neutropenia of childhood.

Congenital neutropenia with stem cell abnormalities
    Reticular dysgenesis
    Cyclic neutropenia
Congenital neutropenia with abnormalities of committed myeloid progenitor cells
    Neutropenia with immunodeficiency disorders (T cells and B cells)
    Severe congenital neutropenia (Kostmann)
    Chronic neutropenia of childhood
    Myelokathexis of dysmyelopoiesis
    Shwachman's syndrome
    Cartilage-hair hypoplasia
    Dyskeratosis congenita
    Fanconi's syndrome
    Hyperglycinemia and isovaleric, propionic, and methylmalonic acidemia
    Glycogenosis Ib
    Osteopetrosis
Acquired neutropenias affecting stem cells
    Malignancies (leukemia, lymphoma) and preleukemic disorders
    Drugs or toxic substances
    Ionizing radiation
    Aplastic anemia
Acquired neutropenias affecting committed myeloid progenitors or survival of mature neutrophils
    Ineffective granulopoiesis (vitamin B_{12}, folate, and copper deficiency)
    Infection
    Immune (neonatal alloimmune or autoimmune; autoimmune or chronic benign neutropenia of childhood)
    Hypersplenism

significant problems for these patients. In addition to local signs and symptoms, patients may have chills, fever, and malaise. In most cases, the spleen and liver are not enlarged. *Staphylococcus aureus* and gram-negative bacteria are the most significant causes of infections.

B. Laboratory Findings: Neutrophils are absent or markedly reduced in the peripheral blood. In most forms of neutropenia or agranulocytosis, the monocytes and lymphocytes are normal and the red cells and platelets are not affected. The bone marrow usually shows a normal erythroid series, with adequate megakaryocytes but a marked reduction in the myeloid cells or a significant delay in maturation of this series.

In the evaluation of neutropenia, careful attention should be paid to the duration and pattern of neutropenia, the types of infections and their frequency, and phenotypic abnormalities on physical examination. A careful family history as well as blood counts from the parents is useful. If there is no obvious acquired cause such as viral infection or drug ingestion and no other primary disease, white blood cell counts should be done once or twice weekly for 4–6 weeks to evaluate the possibility of cyclic neutropenia. Bone marrow aspiration and biopsy are most important to characterize the morphologic features of myelopoiesis. Measuring the neutrophil counts in response to steroid infusion will document the marrow reserves. Elevated urinary muramidase levels and elevated serum lactoferrin may be found if increased neutrophil destruction is the cause of neutropenia. Tests for specific causes of neutropenia include measurement of neutrophil antibodies, immunoglobulin levels, antinuclear antibodies, and lymphocyte phenotyping. Cultures of bone marrow are important for defining the numbers of stem cells and progenitors committed to the myeloid series or the presence of cytotoxic lymphocytes or humoral inhibitory factors. Cytokine levels in plasma or by mononuclear cells can be measured directly.

Treatment

Identifiable toxic agents should be eliminated, or associated diseases (such as infections) treated. Prophylactic antimicrobial therapy is not indicated. Recombinant G-CSF and GM-CSF will increase neutrophil counts in most patients. Patients may be started on 5 μg/kg/d of G-CSF (filgrastim) given subcutaneously or intravenously once a day. Depending on the response, the dose may be escalated to 10 μg/kg. For patients with congenital neutropenia, the dose should be regulated to keep the absolute neutrophil count less than 10,000/μL. Some patients maintain adequate counts with G-CSF given on alternate days.

Prognosis

The prognosis varies greatly with the cause and severity of the neutropenia. In severe cases with persistent agranulocytosis, the prognosis is poor in spite of antibiotic therapy; in mild or cyclic forms of neutropenia, symptoms may be minimal and the prognosis for normal life expectancy excellent. Recombinant hematopoietic hormones hold hope in the future for treatment of the more severe syndromes. However, recent studies in Kostmann's syndrome raises the question of malignant potential secondary to cytokine-induced proliferation of progenitor cells.

Ambruso DR et al: Infectious and bleeding complications in patents with glycogenesis Ib. Am J Dis Child 1985;139:691.

Bernini JC: Diagnosis and management of chronic neutropenia during childhood. Pediatr Clin North Am 1996;43:773.

Dale DC et al: A randomized controlled phase III trial of recombinant human granulocyte colony-stimulating factor (filgrastim) for treatment of severe chronic neutropenia. Blood 1993;81:2496.

Guba SC et al: Granulocyte colony stimulating factor (G-CSF) production and G-CSF receptor structure in patients with congenital neutropenia. Blood 1994;83:1468.

Kalra R et al: Monosomy 7 and activating RAS mutations accompany malignant transformation in patients with congenital neutropenia. Blood 1995;86:4579.

McClain K et al: Chronic neutropenia of childhood: Frequent association with parvovirus infection and correlations with bone marrow culture studies. Br J Haematol 1993;85:57.

Neglia JP et al: Autoimmune neutropenia of infancy and early childhood. Am J Pediatr Hematol Oncol 1993; 10:369.

Wright DG et al: Contrasting effects of recombinant human granulocyte-macrophage colony-stimulating activity (CSF) and granulocyte CSF treatment on the cycling of blood elements in childhood-onset cyclic neutropenia. Blood 1994;84:1257.

NEUTROPHILIA

Neutrophilia is an increase in the peripheral blood absolute neutrophil count greater than 7500–8500 cells/μL for infants, children, and adults. To support the increased peripheral count, neutrophils may be mobilized from bone marrow storage or peripheral marginating pools. Acutely, neutrophilia is seen with bacterial or viral infections, inflammatory diseases (eg, juvenile rheumatoid arthritis, inflammatory bowel disease, Kawasaki disease), surgical or functional asplenia, liver failure, diabetic ketoacidosis, azotemia, and patients with congenital disorders of neutrophil function (eg, chronic granulomatous disease and leukocyte adherence deficiency) and hemolysis. Drugs such as corticosteroids, lithium, and epinephrine increase the blood neutrophil count. Corticosteroids cause release of neutrophils from the marrow pool and inhibit egress from capillary beds and postpone apoptotic cell death. Epinephrine causes release of the marginating pool. Acute neutrophilia has been reported after stress such as electric shock, trauma, burns, surgery, and emotional upset. Tumors involving the bone marrow such as lymphomas, neuroblastomas, and rhabdomyosarcoma may be associated with leukocytosis and the presence of immature myeloid cells in the peripheral blood. Infants with Down's syndrome have defective regulation of proliferation and maturation of the myeloid series and may develop neutrophilia. At times this process may affect other cell lines and mimic myeloproliferative disorders or acute myelogenous leukemia.

The neutrophilias must be distinguished from myeloproliferative disorders such as chronic myelogenous leukemia and juvenile chronic myelogenous leukemia. In general, abnormalities involving other cell lines, the appearance of immature cells on the blood smear, and the presence of hepatosplenomegaly are important differentiating characteristics.

DISORDERS OF NEUTROPHIL FUNCTION

Neutrophils play a key role in host defenses. Circulating in capillary beds, they adhere to the vascular endothelium adjacent to sites of infection and inflammation. Moving between endothelial cells, the neutrophil migrates toward the offending agent. Contact with a microbe that is properly opsonized with complement or antibodies triggers ingestion, a process in which cytoplasmic streaming results in the formation of pseudopods that fuse around the invader, encasing it in a phagosome. During the ingestion phase, there is assembly and activation of the oxidase enzyme system, which takes oxygen from the surrounding medium and reduces it to form toxic oxygen metabolites critical to microbicidal activity. Concurrently, granules from the two main classes (azurophil and specific) fuse and release their contents into the phagolysosome. The concentration of toxic oxygen metabolites (hydrogen peroxide, hypochlorous acid, hydroxyl radical, and others) as well as other compounds (proteases, cationic proteins, cathepsins, defensins, and others) increases dramatically, resulting in the death and dissolution of the microbe. Complex physiologic and biochemical processes subserve and control these functions. Defects in any of these may lead to inadequate cell function and an increased risk of infection.

Classification

Congenital defects in neutrophil function are summarized in Table 25–7. Other congenital or acquired causes of mild to moderate neutrophil dysfunction include metabolic defects (glycogen storage disease, diabetes mellitus, renal disease, hypophosphatemia), viral infections and certain drugs. Neutrophils from newborn infants have abnormal adherence, chemotaxis, and bactericidal activity due to maturation-dependent differences in regulation of adhesion glycoproteins, oxidative metabolism, and a deficiency of specific granules and their contents. Cells from patients with thermal injury, trauma, and overwhelming infection have defects in cell motility and bactericidal activity and exhibit similar biochemical abnormalities with neutrophils from newborn infants.

Clinical Findings

Recurrent bacterial or fungal infections are the hallmark of neutrophil dysfunction. Although many patients will have infection-free periods, episodes of pneumonia, sinusitis, cellulitis, cutaneous and mucosal infections (including perianal or peritonsillar abscesses), and lymphadenitis are frequent. As with neutropenia, aphthous ulcers of mucous membranes, severe gingivitis, and periodontal disease are also major complications. In general, S aureus, along with gram-negative organisms, are commonly isolated from infected sites; other organisms may be specifically associated with a defined neutrophil function defect. In some disorders, fungi account for an increasing number of infections. Deep or generalized infections such as osteomyelitis, liver abscesses, sepsis, meningitis, and necrotic or even gangrenous soft tissue lesions occur in specific syndromes (eg, leukocyte adherence deficiency or chronic granulomatous disease). Patients with severe neutrophil dysfunction may die in childhood from severe infections or associated complications. Pertinent laboratory findings are summarized in Table 25–7.

Treatment

The mainstays of management of these patients remain the anticipation of infections and aggressive attempts to identify the foci and the causative agents. Surgical procedures to achieve these goals may be both diagnostic and therapeutic. Broad-spectrum antibiotics covering the range of possible organisms should be initiated without delay, switching to specific antimicrobial agents when the appropriate microbiologic diagnosis is made. When infections are unresponsive or when they recur, granulocyte transfusions may be helpful.

Chronic management includes prophylactic antibiotics. Trimethoprim-sulfamethoxazole and other antibiotic compounds enhance the bactericidal activity of neutrophils from patients with chronic granulomatous disease. Some patients with Chédiak-Higashi syndrome improve clinically when given ascorbic acid. Recombinant γ-interferon has been shown to decrease the number and severity of infections in patients with chronic granulomatous disease. Demonstration of this activity with one patient group raises the possibility that cytokines, growth factors, and other biologic response modifiers may be helpful in other conditions in preventing recurrent infections.

Table 25–7. Classification of congenital neutrophil function deficits.

Disorder	Clinical Manifestations	Functional Defect	Biochemical Defect	Inheritance
Chédiak-Higashi syndrome	Oculocutaneous albinism, photophobia, nystagmus, ataxia. Recurrent infections of skin, respiratory tract, and mucous membranes caused by gram-positive and gram-negative organisms. Many die from lymphoproliferative phase with hepatomegaly, fever. This may be a viral associated hemophagocytic syndrome secondary to Epstein-Barr virus infection.	Neutropenia. Neutrophils, monocytes, lymphocytes, platelets, and all granule-containing cells have giant granules. Most significant defect is in chemotaxis. Also milder defects in microbicidal activity and degranulation.	Unknown. Alterations in membrane fusion with formation of giant granules. Other biochemical abnormalities in cAMP and cGMP, microtubule assembly.	Autosomal recessive
Leukocyte adherence deficiency I	Recurrent soft tissue infections, including gingivitis, otitis, mucositis, periodontitis, skin infections. Delayed separation of the cord in newborn and problems with wound healing.	Neutrophilia. Diminished adherence to surfaces, leading to decreased chemotaxis.	Absence or partial deficiency of CD11/CD18 cell surface adhesive glycoproteins.	Autosomal recessive
Leukocyte adherence deficiency II	Recurrent infections, mental retardation, craniofacial abnormalities, short stature. Red cells have Bombay phenotype.	Neutrophilia. Deficient "rolling" interaction with endothelial cells.	Deficient fucosyl transferase results in deficient sialyl Lewis X antigen, which interacts with P selection on endothelial cell to establish neutrophil rolling, a prerequisite for adherence and diapedesis.	Autosomal recessive
Chronic granulomatous disease	Recurrent purulent infections with catalase-positive bacteria and fungi. May involve skin, mucous membranes. Also develop deep infections (lymph nodes, liver, bones).	Neutrophilia. Neutrophils demonstrate deficient bactericidal activity but normal chemotaxis and ingestion. Defect in the oxidase, resulting in absence or diminished production of toxic oxygen metabolites.	A number of molecular defects in oxidase components. Absent cytochrome b558 with decreased mRNA for either (1) or (2): (1) gp91-phox (2) p22-phox Absent p47-phox or p67-phox (cytosolic components).	(1) X-linked (60–65% of cases). (2) Autosomal recessive (< 5% of cases). Autosomal recessive (30% of cases).
Myeloperoxidase deficiency	Generally healthy	Diminished capacity to enhance hydrogen peroxide-mediated microbicidal activity	Diminished or absent myeloperoxidase; posttranslational defect in processing protein	Autosomal recessive
Specific granule deficiency	Recurrent skin and deep tissue infections	Decreased chemotaxis and bactericidal activity	Failure to produce specific granules or their contents during myelopoiesis	Autosomal recessive

Bone marrow transplantation has been attempted in most major congenital neutrophil dysfunction syndromes, and reconstitution with normal cells and cell function has been documented. Combining genetic engineering with autologous bone marrow transplantation may provide a future strategy for curing these disorders.

Prognosis

For mild to moderate defects, anticipation and conservative medical management ensure a reasonable outlook. For severe defects, excessive morbidity and significant mortality still exist. In some diseases, the development of noninfectious complications, such as the lymphoproliferative phase of Chédiak-Higashi syndrome, may be of significant prognostic importance.

Ambruso DR, Johnston RB Jr: Chronic granulomatous disease of children. In: *Kendig's Disorders of the Respira-*

tory Tract in Children. Chernick V, Boat TF (editors). Saunders, 1998.

Curnutte JT, Orkin SH, Dinauer MC: Genetic disorders of phagocyte function. In: *The Molecular Basis of Blood Diseases.* Stamatoyannopoulos G et al (editors). Saunders, 1994.

Etzioni A et al: Brief report: Recurrent severe infections caused by a novel leukocyte adhesion deficiency. N Engl J Med 1992;327:1789.

Roos D et al: Mutations in the X-linked and autosomal recessive forms of chronic granulomatous disease. Blood 1996;87:1663.

LYMPHOCYTOSIS

From the first week up to the fifth year of life, lymphocytes are the most numerous leukocytes in blood. The ratio then reverses gradually to reach the adult pattern of neutrophil predominance. An absolute lymphocytosis in childhood is seen with acute or chronic viral infections, pertussis, syphilis, tuberculosis, and hyperthyroidism. Other noninfectious conditions, drugs, and hypersensitivity and serum sickness-like reactions cause lymphocytosis.

Clinical features, including fever, upper respiratory symptoms, gastrointestinal complaints, and rashes, are clues in distinguishing infectious from noninfectious causes. The presence of enlarged liver, spleen, or lymph nodes is crucial to the differential diagnosis, which includes acute leukemia and lymphoma. Most cases of infectious mononucleosis present with hepatosplenomegaly or adenopathy. The absence of anemia and thrombocytopenia helps to differentiate these disorders. Evaluation of the morphology of lymphocytes on peripheral blood smear is also crucial. Infectious causes—particularly infectious mononucleosis—are associated with atypical features in the lymphocytes such as basophilic cytoplasm, vacuoles, finer and less dense chromatin, and an indented nucleus. These features are distinct from the characteristic morphology seen in lymphoblastic leukemia. Lymphocytosis in childhood is most commonly associated with infections and resolves with recovery from the primary disease.

EOSINOPHILIA

Eosinophilia in infants and children is an absolute eosinophil count greater than 300/µL. Marrow eosinophil production is stimulated by the cytokine interleukin-5 (IL-5). In children, allergies, and particularly eczema, are the most common primary causes of eosinophilia. Eosinophilia also occurs in drug reactions, with tumors (Hodgkin's and non-Hodgkin's lymphomas and brain tumors), with immunodeficiency and histiocytosis syndromes. Increased eosinophil counts are a prominent feature of parasitic infections. Gastrointestinal disorders such as chronic hepatitis, ulcerative colitis, Crohn's disease, and milk precipitin disease may have eosinophilia. Increased blood eosinophil counts have been identified in several families without association with any specific illness. Rare causes of eosinophilia include the hypereosinophilic syndrome, characterized by counts greater than 1500/µL and organ involvement and damage (hepatosplenomegaly, cardiopathy, pulmonary fibrosis, and central nervous system injury). This is a disorder of middle-aged adults and is rare in children.

Eosinophils are sometimes the last type of mature myeloid cell to disappear after marrow ablative chemotherapy. Increased eosinophil counts are seen with graft versus host disease after bone marrow transplantation, and elevations are sometimes documented during rejection episodes in patients who have solid organ grafts.

Eosinophilic leukemia has been described, but its existence as a distinct entity is controversial.

BLEEDING DISORDERS

Bleeding disorders may occur as a result of (1) quantitative or qualitative abnormalities of platelets, (2) quantitative or qualitative abnormalities in plasma coagulation factors, or (3) vascular abnormalities. The coagulation cascade is shown in Figure 25–4.

Screening tests to investigate patients for possible bleeding disorders should include the following:

(1) Prothrombin time (PT) to screen the clotting activity of factors VII, X, II, V, and fibrinogen.
(2) Activated partial thromboplastin time (aPTT) to screen clotting activity of the following factors: high-molecular-weight kininogen (HMWK), prekallikrein (PK), XII, XI, IX, VIII, X, V, II, and fibrinogen.
(3) Platelet count.
(4) Bleeding time to screen small vessel integrity, von Willebrand and platelet function.
(5) Thrombin time (TT) to measure the generation of fibrin following conversion of prothrombin to thrombin as well as the antithrombin effect of fibrin-split products or heparin.
(6) Fibrinogen level.

Hathaway W, Goodnight Jr S: *Disorders of Hemostasis and Thrombosis.* McGraw-Hill 1993:50.

Sham R, Francis C: Evaluation of mild bleeding disorders and easy bruising. Blood Rev 1994;8:98.

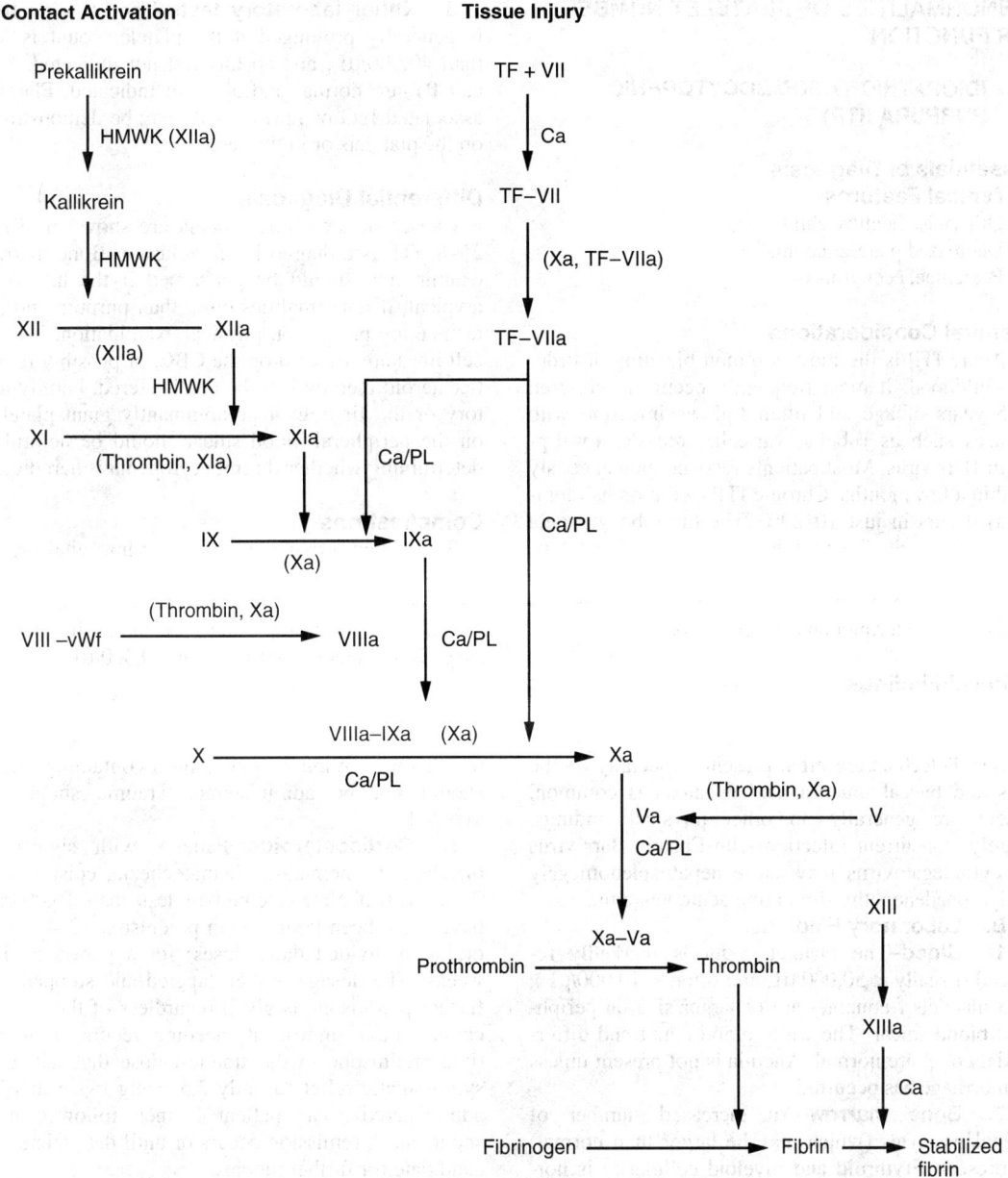

Figure 25–4. Blood coagulation results from a series of reactions involving clotting proteins, calcium, and phospholipids. In the tissue injury pathway, which is the most physiologically active, tissue factor initiates the cascade after it is released from injured cells and forms a complex with factor VIIa. The TF VIIa complex activates factors IX and X. This activation of factor X theoretically bypasses the need to activate factor IX; however, its activation and complexing with factor VIIIa probably amplify the coagulation response. The factor Xa-Va complex catalyzes the conversion of prothrombin to thrombin, which converts fibrinogen to fibrin. Factor XIIIa catalyzes the formation of a stable, cross-linked fibrin clot. Less important physiologically, the contact activation pathway refers to the observation that factor XII can be activated in the presence of a negatively charged surface, such as glass or fatty acids. Prekallikrein and factor XI also bind to such a surface indirectly through their cofactor HMWK. Although the mechanism of factor XII activation is unknown, factor XIIa activates both prekallikrein and factor XI, which in turn activate factor IX. Once factor IX is activated, the cascade proceeds as described previously. A number of steps feature positive feedback by factors shown in parentheses, especially factor Xa and thrombin. Proenzyme forms of clotting factors appear as roman numerals (eg, "VIII"); active clotting factors are designated by "a" (eg, "VIIIa "). (Ca, calcium; HMWK, high-molecular-weight kininogen; PL, phospholipid; TF, tissue factor; vWf, von Willebrand factor. (Adapted from Jesty and Nemerson, 1995.)

ABNORMALITIES OF PLATELET NUMBER OR FUNCTION

1. IDIOPATHIC THROMBOCYTOPENIC PURPURA (ITP)

Essentials of Diagnosis & Typical Features
- Otherwise healthy child.
- Decreased platelet count.
- Petechiae, ecchymoses.

General Considerations
Acute ITP is the most common bleeding disorder of childhood. It most frequently occurs in children 2–5 years of age and often follows infection with viruses such as rubella, varicella, measles, or Epstein-Barr virus. Most patients recover spontaneously within a few months. Chronic ITP (> 6 months' duration) occurs in just 10–20%. The thrombocytopenia generally results from immune clearance of platelets, which generally have IgM or IgG on their surface. The spleen plays a major role by forming antibodies and by sequestering damaged platelets.

Clinical Findings
A. Symptoms and Signs: Onset of ITP is usually acute, with the appearance of multiple ecchymoses. Petechiae are often present, especially on the lips and buccal mucosa, and epistaxis is common. There are generally no other physical findings. Rarely, concurrent infection with Epstein-Barr virus or cytomegalovirus may cause hepatosplenomegaly or lymphadenopathy simulating acute leukemia.

B. Laboratory Findings:

1. Blood–The platelet count is markedly reduced (usually < 50,000/μL and often < 10,000/μL), and platelets frequently are of larger size on peripheral blood smear. The white blood count and differential count are normal. Anemia is not present unless hemorrhage has occurred.

2. Bone marrow–An increased number of megakaryocytes (which may be larger than normal) is present. Erythroid and myeloid cellularity is normal.

3. Other laboratory tests–The bleeding time is generally prolonged if the platelet count is less than 40,000/μL, and so this test not indicated. PTT and PT are normal and also not indicated. Platelet-associated IgG or IgM or both may be demonstrated on the platelets or in the serum.

Differential Diagnosis
Causes of thrombocytopenia are shown in Table 25–8. ITP is a diagnosis of exclusion. Bone marrow examination should be performed if the history is atypical, if abnormalities other than purpura and petechiae are present on physical examination, if other cell lines are affected on the CBC, or possibly if corticosteroid therapy is to be administered. Family history or the finding of predominantly giant platelets on the peripheral blood smear should be helpful in determining whether thrombocytopenia is hereditary.

Complications
Severe hemorrhage and bleeding into vital organs are the feared complications of ITP. Intracranial hemorrhage is the most serious but rarely seen complication. The most important risk factor for hemorrhage is a platelet count less than 20,000/μL.

Treatment
A. General Measures: Many children require no therapy. Aspirin and aspirin-containing drugs should not be administered. Trauma should be avoided.

B. Corticosteroids: Patients with significant bleeding (ie, hematuria, hematochezia, epistaxis) or those with a platelet count of less than 10,000/μL have often been treated with prednisone (2–4 mg/kg orally in divided daily doses) for a period of 1–4 weeks. The dosage is then tapered and stopped. No further prednisone is given regardless of the platelet count unless significant bleeding recurs, at which time prednisone in the smallest dose that will give symptomatic relief (usually 2.5–5 mg twice daily is administered). The patient is then followed until spontaneous remission occurs or until the patient is a candidate for further therapy.

C. Immune Globulin Intravenous (IGIV): As

Table 25–8. Common causes of thrombocytopenia.

Destruction			Decreased Production	
Antibody-Mediated	Coagulopathy	Other	Congenital	Acquired
Idiopathic thrombocytic purpura Infection Immunologic diseases	Disseminated intravascular coagulopathy Sepsis Necrotizing enterocolitis Thrombosis Cavernous hemangioma	Hemolytic uremic syndrome Thrombotic thrombocytopenic purpura Hypersplenism Respiratory distress syndrome	Falconi's syndrome Wiskott-Aldrich syndrome Thrombocytopenia with absent radii Metabolic disorders Osteopetrosis	Aplastic anemia Leukemia and other malignancies Vitamin B_{12} and folate deficiencies

an alternative or adjunct to corticosteroid treatment, IGIV may be given to raise the platelet count in both acute and chronic ITP of childhood. IGIV may be effective even when the patient is resistant to corticosteroids; responses are prompt and may last for several weeks. Most patients respond to 1 g/kg/d for 1–3 days. IGIV is the treatment of choice for severe, life-threatening bleeding. Platelets may be given simultaneously but are rapidly destroyed. IGIV is also appropriate if children with platelet counts < 10,000/μL and minor purpura are to be treated or for children with platelet counts less than 20,000/μL and mucosal membrane bleeding.

D. Rh$_o$(D) Immune Globulin: This agent is as safe as but somewhat less effective than IGIV. The time required for platelet increase is slightly longer than with steroids or IGIV. However, approximately 80% of children with acute or chronic ITP respond well. The drug can only be given to Rh-positive patients, and even so Coombs-positive hemolysis may occur transiently with subsequent anemia. Rho(D) immune globulin is substantially less expensive than IGIV.

E. Splenectomy: Most children with chronic ITP have platelet counts greater than 30,000/μL. Up to 80% of them recover to a platelet count greater than 100,000/μL without therapy over months to years. For those who do not do so, corticosteroids, IGIV, and Rh$_o$(D) immune globulin are treatment options. Splenectomy produces permanent remission in 70–90% but should only be considered after persistence of significant thrombocytopenia for at least 1 year. Preoperative treatment with IGIV or Rh$_o$(D) immune globulin is indicated if the platelet count is significantly decreased. If the patient has been receiving corticosteroid therapy, the dose should be appropriately increased during and after surgery. Anticoagulant therapy is not indicated postoperatively even though the platelet count may rise to 1 million/μL.

The risk of overwhelming infection is increased after splenectomy, particularly in the young child. Therefore, the procedure should be postponed, if possible, until the child is at least 5 years of age. Administration of pneumococcal, meningococcal, and Haemophilus influenzae b vaccines prior to splenectomy is recommended. Prophylactic penicillin following splenectomy should be considered.

Prognosis

Ninety percent of children with ITP will have a spontaneous remission. Features associated with the development of chronic ITP include female sex, age over 10 years at presentation, a more insidious onset of bruising, and the presence of other autoantibodies.

George J et al: Idiopathic thrombocytopenic purpura: A practice guideline developed by explicit methods for The American Society of Hematology. Blood 1996; 88:3.

Medeiros D, Buchanan G: Current controversies in the management of idiopathic thrombocytopenia purpura during childhood. Pediatr Clin North Am 1996;757.

2. THROMBOCYTOPENIA IN THE NEWBORN

Thrombocytopenia is one of the most common causes of purpura in the newborn and should be considered and investigated in any newborn with petechiae or a significant bleeding tendency. A platelet count less than 150,000/μL establishes a diagnosis of thrombocytopenia. A number of specific entities may be responsible (Table 25–8). Infection and intravascular coagulation syndromes are the most common causes of thrombocytopenia in both sick term and preterm newborns. In the well-appearing newborn, antibody-mediated thrombocytopenia (alloimmune or maternal autoimmune), viral syndrome, hyperviscosity, or major vessel thrombosis are important causes. Management is directed toward alleviation of the specific cause.

Thrombocytopenia Associated With Platelet Alloimmunization

Platelet alloimmunization occurs in one out of approximately 550 pregnancies. Unlike Rh incompatibility, it often occurs in first pregnancies. Alloimmunization occurs when a platelet antigen of the infant differs from that of the mother and when the mother is sensitized by platelets that cross from the fetal to the maternal circulation. In whites, sensitization of a mother homozygous for human platelet antigen 1b against paternally acquired fetal HPA-1a antigen results in clinically apparent disease in one per 2–3 thousand births. Severe intracranial bleeding occurs in 10–30% of affected neonates as early as 20 weeks' gestation to after delivery. Petechiae or other bleeding manifestations are usually present shortly after birth. The disease is self-limited with the platelet count normalizing within 4 weeks.

If severe alloimmunization occurs, platelet concentrate from the mother will be more effective in raising the platelet count than random donor platelets. Maternal platelets should be washed and irradiated. IGIV infusions have also been used successfully to raise the platelet count. If less severe, observation alone may be all that is required.

Intracranial hemorrhage in a previous child secondary to alloimmune thrombocytopenia is the worst risk factor for severe fetal thrombocytopenia in a subsequent pregnancy. If alloimmunization has occurred with a previous pregnancy, ultrasound examination of the fetal brain to detect hemorrhage should be obtained at 20 weeks' gestation and repeated regularly. Percutaneous umbilical blood sampling should be performed at mid gestation with concentrated washed maternal platelets transfused to protect against fetal hemorrhage. If the fetal platelet count is low, IGIV should be administered to the mother weekly. Delivery by elective cesarean section is recommended if the fetal platelet count is less than 50,000/μL.

Thrombocytopenia Associated With Idiopathic Thrombocytopenic Purpura in the Mother

Infants born to mothers with ITP or antiphospholipid antibodies may develop thrombocytopenia as a result of transfer of antibody from the mother to the infant. Unfortunately, maternal platelet count, maternal antiplatelet antibody levels, and fetal scalp platelet counts are unreliable predictors of bleeding risk. Antenatal administration of prednisone and IGIV to the mother has been advocated but not shown to be effective.

Most neonates with thrombocytopenia secondary to passive transfer of maternal antibody do not bleed, and thus no specific treatment is indicated. The risk for intracranial hemorrhage is 0.2–2%. If petechiae or puncture wound bleeding ensues, a 1- to 2-week course of oral prednisone, 2 mg/kg/d, may be administered. If the platelet count remains consistently less than 20,000/μL or if severe hemorrhage is present, IGIV should be given. Platelet transfusions may not be helpful without prior removal of antibody by exchange transfusion. The platelet nadir is usually the second day of life. For those with severe thrombocytopenia, it may be 2–4 months before full recovery occurs.

Neonatal Thrombocytopenia Associated With Infections

Thrombocytopenia is commonly associated with severe generalized infections during the newborn period. Fifty to seventy-five percent of neonates with bacterial sepsis are thrombocytopenic. Intrauterine infections such as rubella, syphilis, toxoplasmosis, cytomegalic inclusion disease, herpes simplex, and parvovirus are often associated with thrombocytopenia.

In addition to specific treatment for the underlying disease, platelet transfusions may be indicated in severe cases. Platelet concentrates in doses of 10 mL/kg will raise the platelet count by about 75,000/μL.

Thrombocytopenia Associated With Giant Hemangiomas (Kasabach-Merritt Syndrome)

A rare but important cause of thrombocytopenic purpura in the newborn is giant hemangioma. Platelet sequestration in the lesion results in peripheral depletion of platelets. The bone marrow usually shows megakaryocytic hyperplasia. In the presence of massive hemangiomas, the thrombocytopenia may be associated with DIC and result in fatal hemorrhage. Treatment is indicated if a serious coagulopathy is present or if the lesion exerts pressure on a vital structure or is cosmetically unacceptable.

Surgery is usually contraindicated because of the risk of hemorrhage. Prednisone therapy has been associated with marked regression. If DIC is present, heparin or aminocaproic acid may be useful. Interferon alfa has also been shown to be efficacious but its use has been associated with the development of spastic diplegia.

Bussel J et al: Fetal alloimmune thrombocytopenia. N Engl J Med 1997 337:22.

George D, Bussel J: Neonatal thrombocytopenia. Semin Thromb Hemost 1995;21:276.

Homans A: Thrombocytopenia in the neonate. Pediatr Clin North Am 1996;43:737.

White CW et al: Treatment of childhood angiomatous diseases with recombinant interferon alfa-2a. J Pediatr 1991;118:59.

3. DISORDERS OF PLATELET FUNCTION

Platelet function is studied by assessing aggregation of platelets with agonists such as adenosine diphosphate, collagen, arachidonic acid, and ristocetin. Persons with platelet function defects have skin and mucosal bleeding similar to that seen in persons with thrombocytopenia.

The **hereditary disorders** of platelet function are characterized by a bleeding diathesis, usually associated with a prolonged bleeding time in spite of usually normal numbers of platelets. The findings in these diseases are summarized in Table 25–9.

Acquired disorders of platelet function may occur secondary to uremia, cirrhosis, sepsis, myeloproliferative disorders, acyanotic congenital heart disease, and viral infections. Many pharmacologic agents decrease platelet function. The most common agents are aspirin, nonsteroidal anti-inflammatory agents, and synthetic penicillins.

Treatment

Many individuals with hereditary and acquired platelet function defects will respond to therapy with desmopressin acetate (DDAVP) at a dose of 0.3 μg/kg body weight intravenously or 150–300 μg intranasally depending on body weight. If this is not effective, treatment with random donor platelets at a dose of one bag per 6 kg is indicated. Alternatively, calculations may be based on surface area, where one unit of platelet concentrate per meter squared is expected to raise the platelet count by 20,000/μL.

Hathaway W, Goodnight S: *Disorders of Hemostasis and Thrombosis.* McGraw-Hill, 1993.

Table 25–9. Hereditary platelet function disorders.[1]

Category	Heredity	Morphology	Platelet-Rich Plasma Aggregation to:				Specific Defects
			ADP	Colla-gen	AA	Risto-cetin	
Glanzmann's thrombasthenia[2]	AR	Normal	–	–	–	+	Decreased membrane glycoprotein IIb-IIIa; platelet fibrogen and abnormal adhesion to subendothelium
Bernard-Soulier syndrome[2]	AR	Giant platelets	+	+	+	–	Decreased membrane glycoprotein Ib IX complex
Storage pool deficiency syndromes:[2] Dense body deficiency, Hermansky-Pudlak syndrome	AR	Electron micros-copy: de-creased to absent dense bodies	±	–	±	±	Decreased ADP-ATP, Ca^{2+}, serotonin storage and release
Dense body with α-granule deficiency[2]	AD	Electron micros-copy: de-creased dense bodies and α-granules	±	–	±	±	Decreased ADP, Ca^{2+}, serotonin, PF_4, fibrino-gen, βTG storage and release, decreased PDGF
α-Granule deficiency, gray platelet syndrome[2]	AR	Light gray plate-lets. Electron microscopy: de-creased α-granules	±	±	+	+	Decreased PF_4, βTG, fi-brinogen, decreased PDGF storage and re-lease
Wiskott-Aldrich syndrome[2]	X-linked	Tiny platelets; decreased or-ganelles	±	–	+	+	Abnormal expression of two glycosyltransferases
Failure to release (aspirin-like defect)	Variable	Normal	±	–	–	±	Deficiency of cyclooxygenase or thromboxane synthetase
Platelet factor V Quebec	AD	Normal	?	?	?	?	Decreased platelet fac-tor V function
Pseudo-von Willebrand's disease[2]	AD	Normal	+	+	+	Incr	Intrinsic platelet abnor-mality of increased reac-tion of GPIb with vWF

[1]Modified and reproduced, with permission, from Hathaway WE, Bonnar J: *Hemostatic Disorders of the Pregnant Woman and Newborn Infant.* Elsevier, 1987. © 1987 by Elsevier Science Publishing Co., Inc.
[2]Thrombocytopenia may be seen.
+ = yes; – = no; ± = partial or slight.
AA = arachidonic acid; AD = autosomal dominant; AR = autosomal recessive; PF_4 = platelet factor 4; βTG = β-thromboglobulin; PDGF = platelet-derived growth factor; GPIb = glycoprotein/b.

INHERITED BLEEDING DISORDERS

Normal values for coagulation factors are shown in Table 25–10. The more common factor deficien-cies are discussed here. All persons with bleeding disorders should avoid exposure to medications that inhibit platelet function. Participation in contact sports such as football and ice hockey should be con-sidered in the context of the severity of the bleeding disorder.

1. FACTOR VIII DEFICIENCY (Hemophilia A, Classic Hemophilia)

Essentials of Diagnosis & Typical Features
- Bruising, bleeding, and hemarthroses.
- Prolonged PTT.
- Reduced factor VIII activity.

Table 25–10. Coagulation factor values.[1,2]

	Fetus (20 wk)	Preterm (25–32 wk)	Term Infant	Infant (6 mo)	Normal Adult
Fibrinogen (mg/dL)	96 (40)	250 (100)	240 (150)	251 (160)	278 (61)
II	16 (10)	32 (18)	52 (25)	88 (60)	100 (70)
V	70 (40)	80 (43)	100 (54)	91 (55)	100 (60)
VII	21 (12)	37 (24)	57 (35)	87 (50)	100 (60)
VIII	50 (23)	75 (40)	150 (55)	90 (50)	100 (60)
vWF	65 (40)	150 (90)	160 (84)	107 (60)	100 (60)
IX	10 (5)	22 (17)	35 (15)	86 (36)	100 (50)
X	19 (15)	38 (20)	45 (30)	78 (38)	100 (60)
XI	–	20 (12)	42 (20)	86 (38)	100 (60)
XII	30	22 (9)	44 (16)	77 (39)	100 (60)

[1]Expressed as mean % activity unless otherwise indicated. Values in parentheses are –2SD.
[2]Modified and reproduced, with permission, from Hathaway W, Goodnight S Jr: *Disorders of Hemostasis and Thrombosis.* McGraw-Hill, 1993:31.

General Considerations

Factor VIII deficiency is a bleeding disorder characterized by decreased activity of factor VIII. Factor VIII activity is reported in units per milliliter, with 1 unit/mL equal to 100% of the factor activity found in 1 mL of normal plasma. The normal range for factor VIII activity is 50–150%. The disease occurs predominantly in males and is either inherited in an X-linked manner or is the result of a new mutation. One-third of cases are due to a new mutation. The incidence of factor VIII deficiency is 1:5000 male births.

Clinical Findings

A. Symptoms and Signs: Patients with severe factor VIII deficiency, characterized by frequent spontaneous bleeding episodes involving skin, mucous membranes, joints, muscles, and viscera, have less than 1% circulating factor VIII activity. In contrast, patients with mild factor VIII deficiency, 5–40% factor VIII activity, bleed only at times of trauma or surgery. Those with moderate factor VIII deficiency, 1% to < 5% factor VIII activity, have intermediate bleeding manifestations. The most crippling aspect of factor VIII deficiency is the tendency

to develop recurrent hemarthroses, which incite joint destruction.

B. Laboratory Findings: Persons with factor VIII deficiency have a prolonged PTT. The bleeding time and PT are usually normal. The diagnosis is confirmed by finding decreased factor VIII activity with normal von Willebrand factor (vWF) activity. Cord blood can be accurately assayed to determine factor VIII activity.

In two-thirds of families, the females are carriers and some are mildly symptomatic. Carriers of hemophilia can be detected by determination of the ratio of factor VIII activity to vWF antigen and by molecular genetic techniques.

Complications

Intracranial hemorrhage is the leading disease-related cause of death among those with hemophilia. Up to 50% of intracranial hemorrhages appear to be spontaneous. Hemarthroses begin early in childhood and if recurrent result in joint destruction. Large intramuscular hematomas can lead to a compartment syndrome with resultant muscle and nerve death. Each of these complications is more common in persons with severe hemophilia but may be experienced as well by persons with moderate or mild disease. A serious complication of hemophilia is the development of an acquired circulating antibody to factor VIII after treatment with factor VIII concentrate. Inhibitors or antibodies to factor VIII develop in 15–25% of factor VIII-deficient persons with hemophilia. The inhibitor is an antibody that may be amenable to immunosuppressive therapy. Factor IX concentrate or activated prothrombin complex concentrates may be of help in stopping hemorrhage. Recombinant factor VIIa concentrate is an alternative.

Therapy-related complications have included infection with HIV and hepatitis B (until about 1985 in the United States) and hepatitis C (removed from most United States preparations by 1990). By selecting donors seronegative for these infections and by heat- or chemically treating the factor concentrates to inactivate viruses, the risks of these infections seem to have been eliminated. Safe concentrates are expensive and unobtainable in many parts of the world. Transmission of parvovirus and hepatitis A remains a problem, even with concentrates that have had viral inactivation. Immunization with the killed hepatitis A vaccine may help. Recombinant factor VIII concentrates are available but do contain pooled plasma-derived human albumin.

Treatment

The aim is to normalize the factor VIII activity. Some mild factor VIII-deficient persons may respond to desmopressin; however, most patients require administration of factor VIII concentrates to achieve hemostasis. Factor VIII is available as concentrates from human plasma or as a recombinant protein. The in vivo half-life of factor VIII is generally 8–12 hours. There is no standard vial size for factor VIII concentrates. Factor VIII must be prescribed in units rather than vials. Non-life-threatening hemorrhages are treated with about 20 units/kg body weight factor VIII concentrate. This will increase factor VIII activity to 40%. Life-threatening hemorrhage is initially treated with approximately 50 units/kg factor VIII concentrate; this will increase factor VIII activity by 100%. Subsequent doses are determined according to the situation. The dose given should be as close as possible to the desired dose as determined by vial size. Excess factor VIII concentrate should always be infused rather than discarded. Monitoring the factor VIII activity achieved may be warranted, depending on the situation. The majority of moderately to severely affected persons with hemophilia treat themselves at home with factor concentrate intravenously for routine bleeding episodes.

Hemarthroses are common in persons with hemophilia. Initial therapy is with 20–40 units/kg factor VIII concentrate with subsequent doses in accordance with joint status. Prophylaxis with every other day infusions is likely to prevent the development of arthropathy. A prospective study of this is underway.

Prognosis

When care is coordinated through a hemophilia center where attention is given to the physical, emotional, social, and educational status of the child, the prognosis for a normal life is good.

Bell B et al: Hemophilia: An updated review. Pediatr Rev 1995;16:290.
DiMichele D: Hemophilia 1996. Pediatr Clin North Am 1996;43:709.

2. FACTOR IX DEFICIENCY (Hemophilia B, Christmas Disease)

The mode of inheritance and clinical manifestations of factor IX deficiency are the same as those of factor VIII deficiency. Factor IX deficiency is 15–20% as prevalent as factor VIII deficiency. As in factor VIII deficiency, the PTT in factor IX deficiency is prolonged, but PT and thrombin time are normal. Diagnosis is made by assaying factor IX activity.

Factor IX concentrate is the treatment product. Unlike factor VIII, about 50% of the administered dose of factor IX diffuses into the extravascular space. One unit of factor IX per kilogram is expected to increase the factor IX level by 1%. Factor IX has a half-life of 20–22 hours in vivo. Cryoprecipitates and factor VIII concentrates do *not* contain factor IX. Virus-inactivating techniques for factor IX concentrates appear effective in eradicating HIV and hepatitis C. As with factor VIII, a recombinant concentrate is commercially available. If recombinant factor IX concentrate is administered, the dose must be increased since 1 unit/kg achieves only a 0.6–0.8% rise. Only 1–3% of persons with factor IX deficiency form an inhibitor, but those who do may develop anaphylaxis when treated with factor IX concentrate. The prognosis for persons with factor IX deficiency is comparable to those with factor VIII deficiency.

Warrier I et al: Factor IX inhibitors and anaphylaxis in hemophilia B. J Pediatr Hematol Oncol 1997;19:23.

3. FACTOR XI DEFICIENCY (Hemophilia C)

Factor XI deficiency is a bleeding diathesis of mild to moderate severity. Affected persons may bleed at surgery or following severe trauma but rarely have spontaneous hemarthroses. Factor XI deficiency accounts for less than 5% of all hemophilia diseases.

The defect may be mild, and a sensitive aPTT is required to identify the deficiency. The level of factor XI activity is *not* predictive of risk for bleeding. Intervention is usually only at the time of surgery or trauma. Treatment is with desmopressin or fresh frozen plasma (FFP) to the extent volume expansion is tolerated, or with platelets. Factor XI concentrate is not available in the United States.

The prognosis for an average life span is excellent.

Bolton-Maggs PHB et al: Definition of the bleeding tendency in factor XI-deficient kindreds: A clinical and laboratory study. Thromb Haemost 1995;73:194.

4. OTHER INHERITED BLEEDING DISORDERS

Other hereditary single clotting factor deficiencies are rare. Transmission is generally autosomal. Homozygous individuals with a deficiency or structural abnormality of prothrombin, factor V, factor VII, or factor X have excessive bleeding.

Persons with dysfibrinogenemia (abnormal fibrinogen) are usually asymptomatic but may develop recurrent venous thromboembolic episodes or have a bleeding tendency. Immunologic determinations of fibrinogen are normal, but the thrombin time and PT are often prolonged. Treatment is similar to that outlined for afibrinogenemia.

Afibrinogenemia resembles hemophilia clinically but has an autosomal recessive inheritance. The patients have persistent bleeding from small injuries, hematomas, ecchymoses, and hemarthroses. Fatal bleeding from the umbilical cord has been reported. The principal laboratory finding in afibrinogenemia is complete absence of a fibrin clot by any of the usual clotting tests. Hypofibrinogenemia (fibrinogen level less than 100 mg/dL) is also rarely seen.

Treatment of rare single clotting factor deficient persons is usually with fresh frozen plasma. Cryoprecipitate generally controls the acute bleeding episodes in persons with fibrinogen abnormalities.

Galanakis KK: Fibrinogen anomalies and disease: A clinical update. Hematol Oncol Clin North Am 1992;5:1171.

VON WILLEBRAND'S DISEASE

Essentials of Diagnosis & Typical Features

- Easy bruising and epistaxis from early childhood.
- Bleeding time usually prolonged, with a normal platelet count.
- Reduced activity or abnormal structure of von Willebrand factor.

General Considerations

Von Willebrand's disease and its variants are due to abnormalities of vWF, a plasma protein which forms a multimeric complex that carries factor VIII and also is a cofactor for platelet adhesion. In classic von Willebrand's disease (type I), there is a partial quantitative deficiency of vWF. In von Willebrand's disease type II, there is a qualitative abnormality of vWF. Persons with type III disease have virtually complete deficiency of vWF. Von Willebrand's disease is the most common inherited bleeding disorder; 1% of persons are affected, but only 10% of those affected are symptomatic. It is usually transmitted as an autosomal dominant trait. Acquired von Willebrand's disease may develop in persons with hypothyroidism, Wilms' tumor, cardiac disease, or systemic lupus erythematosus and in those receiving valproic acid.

Clinical Findings

A. Symptoms and Signs: There is usually a history of increased bruising and excessive epistaxis. Increased bleeding will also occur with lacerations or at surgery. Menorrhagia is often a problem.

B. Laboratory Findings: The PTT is usually prolonged but may be normal. The PT is normal. A prolonged bleeding time is often present because vWF is involved in platelet binding to the blood vessel. Platelet number is normal. Factor VIII and vWF antigen are decreased in types I and III but may be normal in type II von Willebrand's disease. Von Willebrand factor activity (ristocetin activity) is decreased in all types.

Treatment

The treatment to prevent or halt bleeding for most persons with types I and II von Willebrand disease is 0.3 μg/kg of desmopressin acetate intravenously in at least 20–30 mL of normal saline given over 20–30 minutes. A twofold to threefold rise in vWF is expected. Efficacy is variable from patient to patient; bleeding time should be measured before and 30 minutes after infusion to assess response. A high concentration nasal desmopressin is an alternative, but the effect varies and response to intravenous desmopressin does not predict response to the nasal preparation. Since stored vWF release is limited, tachyphylaxis is often seen with desmopressin. Children under the age of 2 years are at increased risk for seizures secondary to desmopressin-induced hyponatremia. If further therapy is indicated, vWF-rich concentrate is recommended.

For persons with type IIB and III disease, the usual treatment is with vWF-enriched concentrate. Desmopressin is ineffective in patients with type III von Willebrand's disease. It may benefit those with type IIB disease but may also evoke thrombocytopenia.

Antifibrinolytic drugs (eg, aminocaproic acid) may be useful for control of oral, nasal, or vaginal bleeding.

Prognosis

Life expectancy is normal.

Werner E: Von Willebrand disease in children and adolescents. Pediatr Clin North Am 1996;43:683.

ACQUIRED BLEEDING DISORDERS

1. DISSEMINATED INTRAVASCULAR COAGULATION

Essentials of Diagnosis & Typical Features

- Presence of disorder known to trigger disseminated intravascular coagulation.
- Evidence for activation of coagulation (prolonged PTT, PT, or thrombin time; decreased fibrinogen or platelets).

General Considerations

Disseminated intravascular coagulation (DIC) is an acquired pathologic process characterized by activation of the coagulation system. It may lead to thrombin generation, intravascular fibrin deposition, and platelet consumption. Microthrombi, composed of fibrin and platelets, may produce ischemic tissue damage. The fibrinolytic system is also frequently activated, producing plasmin-mediated destruction of fibrin, fibrinogen, and other clotting factors (factor V, factor VIII). Degradation or split products of fibrin-fibrinogen are formed and function as anticoagulants and inhibitors of platelet function. DIC commonly accompanies disorders seen in critically ill infants and children. Conditions known to trigger DIC include endothelial cell damage (endotoxin, virus), tissue destruction (necrosis, physical injuries), hypoxia (acidosis), ischemic and vascular changes (shock, hemangiomas), and release of tissue procoagulants (cancer, placental disorders).

Clinical Findings

A. Symptoms and Signs: Physical signs of DIC may include (1) diffuse bleeding tendency (hematuria, melena, purpura, petechiae, persistent oozing from needle punctures or other invasive procedures); (2) circulatory collapse, poor skin perfusion, early ischemic changes; and (3) evidence of thrombotic lesions (major vessel thrombosis, gangrene, purpura fulminans).

B. Laboratory Findings: Tests that are most sensitive, easiest to perform, and best reflect the hemostatic capacity of the patient are the PT, PTT, platelet count, fibrinogen level, and a test for fibrin-fibrinogen split products. A test that measures the cross-linked fibrin degradation by-products called d-dimers may also be helpful in demonstrating activation of both coagulation and fibrinolysis. Often, the PT and PTT are prolonged and the platelet count and fibrinogen level are decreased. Levels of fibrin-fibrinogen split products and d-dimers are elevated.

The abnormalities associated with DIC may vary depending on the triggering event. Patients with infections may have primarily thrombocytopenia, with only slight prolongation of the PTT and PT and mild elevation of fibrin-fibrinogen split products; only platelets may be consumed in bacterial sepsis without any other evidence of activated coagulation. In contrast, asphyxia may produce significant consumption of fibrinogen and elevated fibrin-fibrinogen split products without depression of platelets.

Differential Diagnosis

Bleeding with liver disease, vitamin K deficiency, or uremia can mimic DIC. Patients with fulminant hepatitis or advanced cirrhosis often have evidence of both decreased production of liver-dependent coagulation factors and increased consumption of platelets and fibrinogen. Generally, factor VII activity is markedly decreased in liver disease compared with mild to moderate decreases in DIC. Factor VIII activity may be normal or even increased in liver disease compared with decreased activity in DIC.

Treatment

A. Therapy for Underlying Disorder: The most important aspect of therapy is identification and treatment of the triggering event. If this can be treated (eg, hypoxia, shock), often no other therapy is needed for the coagulopathy. Serial coagulation tests help in determining whether specific hemostatic therapy is indicated.

B. Replacement Therapy: Replacement of depleted coagulation factors and platelets may be necessary in severe DIC. FFP replaces depleted coagulation factors; 10–15 mL/kg will raise clotting factor

activities by about 10–15%. Fibrinogen (and factor VIII) can be given as cryoprecipitate also; one bag of cryoprecipitate per 3 kg in infants or one bag of cryoprecipitate per 6 kg in older children will raise the fibrinogen level by 75–100 mg/dL. Platelets are replaced with platelet concentrate; in the neonate, 10 mL of platelet concentrate per kilogram will raise the platelet count by 75,000–100,000/μL. In older children, one bag of platelet concentrate per 5–6 kg is the usual dose. An alternative formula is as follows: 1 unit/m^2 of platelet concentrate will increase the platelet count by about 20,000/μL. The minimal hemostatic goals are a platelet count greater than 40,000/μL, PT of less than 16 seconds, and fibrinogen over 100 mg/dL.

C. Anticoagulant Therapy: Heparin is often given in hopes of interrupting the clotting process. The rationale for heparin therapy is to allow for more effective replacement therapy while the primary disease is being specifically treated, but there is no formal trial to show that heparin is beneficial. The most effective and safest method of giving unfractionated heparin is by continuous intravenous administration. A loading dose of 50–100 units/kg is followed by 15–25 units/kg/h by continuous intravenous infusion. Heparin should be administered to achieve a therapeutic level between 0.4 and 0.7 unit/mL. Low-molecular-weight heparin is an alternative therapy that can be given subcutaneously twice a day; the therapeutic range is 0.5–1 unit/mL.

D. Management of DIC in Neonates: Premature and full-term neonates frequently develop generalized bleeding tendencies associated with illnesses such as respiratory distress syndrome, cyanotic congenital heart disease, cerebral anoxia, and severe sepsis. Often present are hypoxia, acidosis, vascular fragility, decreased platelet number and function, and increased fibrinolytic activity. The pathophysiologic mechanisms of the secondary bleeding syndromes are related to increased consumption or decreased production of clotting factors and platelets. Laboratory tests of bleeding and coagulation are difficult to interpret because results in affected patients overlap with those in normal infants. The values for these tests seen in "normal" full-term and premature neonates are shown in Table 25–10. The pathophysiologic mechanisms of these secondary bleeding syndromes are related to increased consumption or decreased production of clotting factors and platelets.

Treatment consists of eradicating the underlying illnesses and replacing clotting factors, platelets, and red blood cells. Occasionally, exchange transfusion or heparinization is indicated.

2. LIVER DISEASE

The liver is the major synthetic site of HMWK, XIII, XII, XI, X, IX, VII, V, prothrombin, and fibrinogen. It also produces plasminogen and three physiologic anticoagulants, antithrombin III, protein C, and protein S. α_2-Antiplasmin, which regulates fibrinolysis, is produced in the liver. Deficiency of factor V and the vitamin K-dependent factors (II, VII, IX, and X) is most often a problem as a result of decreased hepatic synthesis and is manifested as prolongation of the PT. The PTT may also be prolonged. Extravascular loss and increased consumption of clotting factors may contribute to prolongation of the PT and PTT. The amount of fibrinogen may be decreased, or an abnormal fibrinogen (dysfibrinogen) containing excess sialic acid residues may be synthesized. Dysfibrinogenemia is associated with prolongation of thrombin time and reptilase time. Fibrin-fibrinogen degradation products and d-dimers may be present due to increased fibrinolysis. Thrombocytopenia secondary to hypersplenism and platelet aggregation abnormalities may be seen. Treatment consists of replacement with FFP and platelets as needed. In cases in which liver disease is associated with fat malabsorption, vitamin K (1–5 mg) should be given. Desmopressin may shorten the bleeding time and PTT in patients with chronic liver disease.

3. VITAMIN K DEFICIENCY

All newborns have physiologically depressed activity of the vitamin K-dependent factors (II, VII, IX, and X). If vitamin K is not administered at birth, a bleeding diathesis called **hemorrhagic disease of the newborn** may develop. One of three patterns is seen:

(1) Early hemorrhagic disease of the newborn occurs within 24 hours of birth and is most often manifested by cephalhematoma, intracranial hemorrhage, or intra-abdominal bleeding. Although occasionally idiopathic, it is most often associated with maternal ingestion of drugs that interfere with vitamin K metabolism, eg, warfarin, phenytoin, isoniazid, and rifampin. This is often life-threatening.

(2) Classic hemorrhagic disease of the newborn occurs at 24 hours to 7 days of age and usually is manifested as gastrointestinal, skin, or mucosal bleeding. Bleeding after circumcision may occur. Although occasionally associated with maternal drug usage, it most often occurs in well babies that do not receive vitamin K at birth and are solely breast fed.

(3) Late hemorrhagic disease occurs in infants 1–6 months of age. Manifestations are intracranial, gastrointestinal, or skin bleeding. Usually, it is secondary to chronic diarrhea, malabsorption syndromes, obstructive jaundice, or prolonged antibiotic therapy.

The diagnosis of vitamin K deficiency is based on the history, physical examination, and laboratory results. The PT is markedly prolonged. The PTT may be prolonged. The thrombin time does not prolong until late in the course. Platelet counts are normal. The diagnosis is confirmed by a demonstration of noncarboxlyated proteins in vitamin K's absence (PIVKA) in the plasma and by improvement following treatment with vitamin K. Treatment with vitamin K should be given immediately and not withheld awaiting test results.

4. UREMIA

Qualitative and quantitative platelet abnormalities are the primary hemostatic defect. Decreased activity of factors XII, XI, IX, and prothrombin secondary to increased urinary losses can result in prolongation of the PTT. Bleeding occurs in approximately 50% of patients with chronic renal failure. It is most often manifested as purpura, menorrhagia, or gastrointestinal bleeding. Bleeding may be managed with infusion of desmopressin, red blood cells, and FFP.

Bell B: Bleeding associated with hepatocellular disease. Int J Pediatr Hematol Oncol 1994;1:53.

Huysman M, Sauer P: The vitamin K controversy. Curr Opin Pediatr 1994;6:129.

Manco-Johnson M: Disseminated intravascular coagulation and other hypercoagulable syndromes. Int J Pediatr Hematol Oncol 1994;1:1.

Sagripanti A et al: Bleeding and thrombosis in chronic uremia. Nephron 1997;75:125.

VASCULAR ABNORMALITIES ASSOCIATED WITH BLEEDING

1. HENOCH-SCHÖNLEIN PURPURA (Anaphylactoid Purpura)

Essentials of Diagnosis & Typical Features
- Purpuric cutaneous rash.
- Migratory polyarthritis or polyarthralgias.
- Colicky abdominal pain.
- Nephritis.

General Considerations

Henoch-Schönlein purpura, which is the most common small vessel vasculitis syndrome in children, occurs primarily in males 2–7 years of age. Occurrence is highest in the spring and fall. Two-thirds of affected children have a history of upper respiratory infection in the preceding 1–3 weeks.

Henoch-Schönlein purpura is characterized by vasculitis of the small vessels, particularly those of the skin, gastrointestinal tract, and kidney. Immune complexes are found in the kidney, intestine, and skin. Suspected though not proved inciting antigens include group A β-hemolytic streptococci and other bacteria, viruses, drugs, foods, and insect bites.

Clinical Findings

A. Symptoms and Signs: The skin rash is often urticarial initially and progresses to a macular-papular appearance, which transforms into a diagnostic symmetric purpuric rash distributed on the ankles, buttocks, and elbows. Purpuric areas of a few millimeters in diameter are present and may progress to form larger hemorrhages (palpable purpura). Petechial lesions may occur, but most hemorrhages are slightly larger. The rash usually begins on the lower extremities, but the entire body may be involved. New lesions can continue to appear for 2–4 weeks. Approximately two-thirds of patients develop migratory polyarthralgias or polyarthritis, primarily of the ankles and knees. Edema of the hands, feet, scalp, and periorbital regions may occur. Abdominal colic—due to hemorrhage and edema primarily of the small intestine—occurs in about 50% of those affected. Twenty-five to fifty percent of those affected develop renal involvement, with hematuria, proteinuria, or nephrotic syndrome. Hematuria alone is never the presenting complaint for Henoch-Schönlein purpura, but usually manifests in the second to third week of illness. Renal involvement occurs more commonly in males and in older patients. Testicular torsion may occur. Neurologic symptoms are possible.

B. Laboratory Findings: The platelet count, platelet function tests, and bleeding time are usually normal, although the platelet count may even be elevated. Blood coagulation studies are normal. Urinalysis frequently reveals hematuria. Proteinuria may also be noted, but casts are uncommon. Stool analysis may be positive for blood even though melena is not observed. The ASO titer is frequently elevated and the throat culture positive for group A β-hemolytic streptococci. Serum IgA may be elevated.

Differential Diagnosis

Henoch-Schönlein purpura, in contrast with thrombocytopenic purpura, causes a palpable rash but the platelet count is normal. The rash of septicemia (especially meningococcemia) may be similar to that of Henoch-Schönlein purpura, though the distribution tends to be more generalized with meningococcemia. The possibility of child abuse should be considered in any child presenting with purpura.

Complications

Intussusception of the small bowel may occur. About 15% of patients develop renal failure as a result of advancing proliferative glomerulonephritis with an associated mortality rate of 3%.

Treatment

Generally, treatment is unwarranted. Corticosteroid therapy may provide symptomatic relief for severe gastrointestinal or joint manifestations but does not alter skin or renal manifestations. Aspirin is useful for the pain associated with arthritis. If culture for group A β-hemolytic streptococci is positive or if the ASO titer is elevated, penicillin should be given in full therapeutic doses for 10 days.

Prognosis

The prognosis for recovery is generally good, although symptoms frequently (25–50%) recur over a period of several months. In patients who develop renal manifestations, microscopic hematuria may persist for years. Progressive renal failure occurs in less than 5% of patients with Henoch-Schönlein purpura.

Lanzkowsky S, Lanzkowsky L, Lanzkowsky P: Henoch-Schönlein purpura. Pediatr Rev 1992;13:130.

2. OTHER VASCULAR DISORDERS

Mild to life-threatening bleeding occurs with some types of Ehlers-Danlos syndrome—the most common collagen disorder. Easy bruising is common. Coagulation findings are variable. Spontaneous rupture and dissection of aortic aneurysms have been reported in persons with type IV.

Hausser I, Anton-Lamprecht I: Differential ultrastructural aberrations of collagen fibrils in Ehlers-Danlos syndrome types I–IV as a means of diagnostics and classification. Hum Genet 1994;3:394.

THROMBOTIC DISORDERS

Thrombotic disorders are uncommon in children but are being recognized with increasing frequency. Multiple risk factors, both inherited and acquired, are often present in children who develop a thromboembolic event. Conditions commonly associated with thrombosis during childhood are venous access devices and other implanted foreign bodies, malignancy, infection, trauma, collagen-vascular disease, surgery, renal disease, sickle cell anemia, cardiac disease, and immobilization.

Initial evaluation of the child with a thrombosis must include a family history and definitive imaging study to delineate the type (venous versus arterial) and extent of the thrombosis. Laboratory evaluation is indicated to determine the presence of an underlying congenital or acquired hemostatic abnormality. A deficiency of the anticoagulant proteins, protein C, protein S, or antithrombin III may be congenital or acquired. Activated protein C resistance due to the factor V Leiden mutation is the most common inherited hypercoagulable condition. An acquired condition of activated protein C resistance may occur.

Thrombotic events are generally treated with heparin. Local instillation of a fibrinolytic agent or systemic administration of a fibrinolytic agent are other treatment options. Lifelong warfarin is generally prescribed for individuals with inherited disorders who have a second episode of thrombosis.

INHERITED DISORDERS

1. PROTEIN C DEFICIENCY

Protein C is a vitamin K-dependent protein that is normally activated by thrombin bound to thrombomodulin and inactivates activated factors V and VIII. In addition, it stimulates fibrinolysis. Two phenotypes of hereditary protein C deficiency are seen. Heterozygotes with autosomal dominant protein C deficiency typically present with venous thromboembolism as young adults but may manifest during childhood.

Homozygous or doubly heterozygous individuals generally present within the first 12 hours of life with purpura fulminans. Associated findings may include cerebral or retinal thrombosis resulting in blindness. Immediate treatment with fresh frozen plasma every 6–12 hours should be given. Heparin is generally administered simultaneously. Subsequent management requires chronic anticoagulation with warfarin compounds or infusion of protein C concentrate (not yet available in the United States). The long-term outlook is unknown.

2. PROTEIN S DEFICIENCY

Protein S is a cofactor for protein C. Persons with protein S deficiency have a course similar to those with protein C deficiency. Management for acute thrombotic events is with anticoagulation or fibrinolytic therapy or both. Lifelong warfarin therapy is indicated for those with recurrent thrombotic events.

3. ANTITHROMBIN III DEFICIENCY

Antithrombin III is the most important physiologic inhibitor of thrombin. In addition, it inhibits activated factors IX, X, XI, and XII. Antithrombin III deficiency is transmitted in an autosomal dominant pattern and is associated with venous thromboembolism. Symptoms before puberty are rare.

Initial management of a patient with thrombosis is with anticoagulant therapy. Antithrombin III concentrate is available for replacement. Patients with recurrent venous thrombosis are maintained lifelong on oral anticoagulants. Asymptomatic persons are gen-

erally not anticoagulated except at times of increased risk for thrombosis.

4. FACTOR V LEIDEN MUTATION

An amino acid substitution in the gene coding for factor V results in the production of factor V Leiden, a factor V variant that is resistant to inactivation by activated protein C. About 20% of unselected consecutive adults with deep vein thrombosis and 40–60% of adults from families with unexplained thrombophilia have been identified with this mutation. Venous thrombosis has been reported in children both heterozygous and homozygous for this mutation. Screening is with an assay for activated protein C resistance, which is based on the APTT. Confirmation is by molecular analysis.

5. OTHER INHERITED DISORDERS

Qualitative abnormalities of fibrinogen (dysfibrinogenemias) are usually inherited in an autosomal dominant manner. Most individuals with dysfibrinogenemia are asymptomatic. Some have problems with bleeding, and others develop venous or arterial thrombosis. This diagnosis is suggested by a prolonged thrombin time with a normal fibrinogen level. Dysfunction of the fibrinolytic system may play a role in the development of thrombosis, but the association between defects in this system and thrombosis is less well documented than that between deficiencies of the physiologic anticoagulants and thrombosis.

Hyperhomocysteinemia can be either an inherited or an acquired condition and is associated with an increased risk for both arterial and venous thromboses in adults. Whether or not it is a risk factor for thrombophilia in children has yet to be determined.

Elevated lipoprotein(a), a lipoprotein with homology to plasminogen, has been reported as an important etiologic agent in childhood thrombosis. Lipoprotein(a) levels are genetically transmitted as an autosomal dominant trait.

ACQUIRED DISORDERS

1. ANTIPHOSPHOLIPID ANTIBODIES

Antiphospholipid antibodies include both the lupus anticoagulant and the anticardiolipin antibody. The lupus anticoagulant is an immunoglobulin that inhibits in vitro phospholipid-dependent coagulation assays such as the aPTT and dilute Russell viper venom time. Anticardiolipin antibodies are detected by ELISA assays. Both antibodies are associated with thrombosis. Although common in persons with collagen-vascular disorders, such as systemic lupus erythematosus, they occur following drug exposure, infection, and lymphoproliferative diseases. They are also present in some well individuals.

Treatment for a person with a thrombosis who is found to have an antiphospholipid antibody is generally with heparin anticoagulation. Alternatives are local instillation of a fibrinolytic agent or systemic fibrinolysis. Anticoagulation with warfarin should be continued until the antiphospholipid antibody has resolved. The risk for recurrent thrombosis is very high if anticoagulation is discontinued sooner.

Andrew M et al: Venous thromboembolic complications (VTE) in children: First analyses of the Canadian Registry of VTE. Blood 1994;83:1251.

Dahlback B: Inherited thrombophilia: Resistance to activated protein C as a pathogenic factor of venous thromboembolism. Blood 1995;85:607.

Manco-Johnson M, Nuss R: Lupus anticoagulant in children with thrombosis. Am J Hematol 1995;48:243.

Nuss R, Hays T, Manco-Johnson M: Childhood thrombosis. Pediatrics 1995;96:291.

THE SPLEEN

SPLENOMEGALY & HYPERSPLENISM

The differential diagnosis of splenomegaly in children includes the general categories of congestive splenomegaly, chronic infections, leukemia and lymphomas, hemolytic anemias, reticuloendothelioses, and storage diseases (Table 25–11).

Splenomegaly due to any cause may be associated with hypersplenism and the excessive destruction of circulating red cells, white cells, and platelets. The

Table 25–11. Causes of chronic splenomegaly in children.

Cause	Associated Clinical Findings	Diagnostic Investigation
Congestive splenomegaly	History of umbilical vein catheter or neonatal omphalitis. Signs of portal hypertension (varices, hemorrhoids, dilated abdominal wall veins); pancytopenia, history of hepatitis or jaundice	Complete blood count, platelet count, liver function tests, ultrasonography.
Chronic infections	History of exposure to tuberculosis, histoplasmosis, coccidioidomycosis, other fungal disease; chonic sepsis (foreign body in bloodstream; subacute infective endocarditis)	Appropriate cultures and skin tests, ie, blood cultures; PPD, histoplasmin, coccidioidin skin tests; chest film; HIV serology
Infectious mononucleosis	Fever, fatigue, pharyngitis, rash, adenopathy, hepatomegaly	EBV antibody titers
Leukemia, lymphoma, Hodgkin's disease	Evidence of systemic involvement with fever, bleeding tendencies, hepatomegaly, and lymphadenopathy; pancytopenia	Blood smear, bone marrow examination, chest film, gallium scan, LDH, uric acid
Hemolytic anemias	Anemia, jaundice; family history of anemia, jaundice, and gallbladder disease in young adults	Reticulocyte count, Coombs' test, blood smear, osmotic fragility test, hemoglobin electrophoresis
Reticuloendothelioses (histiocytosis X)	Chronic otitis media, seborrheic or petechial skin rashes, anemia, infections, lymphadenopathy, hepatomegaly, bone lesions	Skeletal x-rays for bone lesions; biopsy of bone, liver, bone marrow, or lymph node
Storage diseases	Family history of similar disorders, neurologic involvement, evidence of macular degeneration, hepatomegaly	Biopsy of liver or bone marrow in search for storage cells
Splenic cyst	Evidence of other infections (postinfectious cyst) or congenital anomalies; peculiar shape of spleen	Radionuclide scan, ultrasonography
Splenic hemangioma	Other hemangiomas, consumptive coagulopathy	Radionuclide scan, arteriography, platelet count, coagulation screen

LDH = lactic dehydrogenase; PPD = purified protein derivative; EBV = Epstein-Barr virus.

degree of cytopenias is variable and, when mild, requires no specific therapy. In other cases, the thrombocytopenia may cause life-threatening bleeding, particularly when the splenomegaly is secondary to portal hypertension and associated with esophageal varices or the consequence of a storage disease. In such cases, treatment with surgical splenectomy or with splenic embolization may be warranted.

Israel DM et al: Partial splenic embolization in children with hypersplenism. J Pediatr 1994;124:95.

ASPLENIA & SPLENECTOMY

There is overwhelming evidence that children who lack normal splenic function are at risk for sepsis, meningitis, and pneumonia due to encapsulated bacteria such as pneumococci and *Haemophilus influenzae*. Such infections are often fulminant and fatal because of inadequate antibody production and impaired phagocytosis of hematogenous bacteria.

Congenital asplenia is usually suspected in an infant born with abnormalities of abdominal viscera and complex cyanotic congenital heart disease. Howell-Jolly bodies are usually present on the peripheral blood smear, and the absence of splenic tissue is confirmed by technetium radionuclide scanning. The prognosis depends on the underlying cardiac lesions, and many children die during the first few months. Prophylactic antibiotics, usually penicillin, and pneumococcal vaccine are recommended for those who survive.

The risk of overwhelming sepsis following surgical splenectomy is related to the child's age and to the underlying disorder. The risk is highest when the procedure is performed earlier in life, so splenectomy is usually postponed until after 5 years. The risk of postsplenectomy sepsis is also greater in children with malignancies, thalassemias, and reticuloendothelioses than in children whose splenectomy is performed for ITP, hereditary spherocytosis, or trauma.

Children with sickle cell anemia develop functional asplenia during the first year of life, and overwhelming sepsis is the leading cause of early deaths in this disease. Prophylactic penicillin has been shown to reduce the incidence of sepsis by 84%.

Lortan JE: Clinical annotation: Management of asplenic patients. Br J Haematol 1993;84:566.

Phoon CK, Neill CA: Asplenia syndrome: Insight into embryology through an analysis of cardiac and extracardiac anomalies. Am J Cardiol 1994;73:581.

TRANSFUSION MEDICINE

DONOR SCREENING & BLOOD PROCESSING: RISK MANAGEMENT

Minimizing the risks of transfusion begins with the donor interview. Questions are asked that will protect the recipient from transmission of infectious agents as well as other risks of transfusions. In addition, information defining high-risk groups whose behavior increases the possible transmission of AIDS, hepatitis, and other diseases is provided, with the request that persons in these groups not donate blood. After completion of the phlebotomy, the donor is given a final opportunity to acknowledge previously undisclosed risk factors by confidentially indicating that his or her blood should not be used for transfusion.

Before blood components can be released for transfusion, donor blood is screened for antibodies to hepatitis B, hepatitis C, HIV-1 and HIV-2 (AIDS), and human T-cell lymphotropic virus (HTLV) I and II; and a serologic test for syphilis is performed. Testing for hepatitis B surface antigen and HIV p24 antigen is also performed. The aminotransferases are measured as surrogate tests for hepatitis (Table 25–12). Positive tests are repeated, and upon their confirmation the unit in question is destroyed and the donor placed in a deferral category. Many of the screening tests used are very sensitive and have a high rate of false-positive results. Because of this, confirmatory tests have been developed to check the initial screening results and separate the false-positives from the true-positives. For special clinical conditions, serologic screening for cytomegalovirus may also be done to identify seronegative units for transfusion.

With these techniques, the risk of an infectious complication from blood components has been minimized (Table 25–12), with the greatest risk being posttransfusion hepatitis (see sections on hepatitis C virus and non-A, non-B, non-C hepatitis elsewhere in this book). Because there is no way to completely eliminate the risk of infection from homologous blood, the safest blood is obtained by autologous donation. Issues of donor size make the techniques of autologous donation difficult to apply to the pediatric population. Whenever possible, however, autologous donation should be considered.

Primary cytomegalovirus infections are important complications of blood transfusion in transplant recipients, neonates, and those with immunodeficiency. Transmission of cytomegalovirus can be avoided by using seronegative donors, apheresis platelet concentrates collected by techniques ensuring low numbers of residual white cells, or red cell or platelet products

Table 25–12. Transmission risks of infectious agents for which screening of blood products is routinely performed.

Disease Entity	Transmission	Screening and Processing Procedures	Approximate Risk of Transmission
Syphilis	Low risk that fresh blood drawn during spirochetemia can transmit infection. Organism not able to survive behond 72 hours during storage at 4 °C.	Donor history. RPR or VDRL.	< 1:100,000
Hepatitis A	Units drawn during prodrome could transmit virus. Because of brief viremia during acute phase, absence of asymptomatic carrier phase, and failure to detect transmission in multiple transfused individuals, infection by this agent is unlikely.	Donor history	< 1:1,000,000
Hepatitis B	Prolonged viremia during various phases of the disease and asymptomatic carrier state make HBV infection a significant risk of transfusion. Incidence has markedly decreased with screening strategies.	Donor history, education, and self-exclusion. Hepatitis B surface antigen (HBsAg). Surrogate tests for non-A, non-B hepatitis and screen for hepatitis C and retroviruses have helped screen out population at risk for transmitting hepatitis B virus.	1:150,000–1:60,000
Hepatitis C	Over two-thirds of cases of non-A, non-B posttransfusion hepatitis may be due to this cause. The agent has characteristics similar to those of HBV which are responsible for the risk from transfusion. Infection may lead to a significant incidence of cirrhosis and end-stage liver disease.	Donor history. Surrogate tests: ALT and hepatitis B core antibody (anti-HBc), anti-HCV.	1:100,000
Non-A, non-B, non-C hepatitis	Not a specific cause but a classification of agents other than HAV, HBV, HCV, Epstein-Barr virus, and cytomegalovirus, which can cause posttransfusion hepatitis.	Donor history. Surrogate tests: ALT and anti-HBc.	Undefined, 1:100,000
Human immunodeficiency virus (HIV-1, HIV-2) infection	Cytotoxic retrovirus spread by sexual contact, parenteral (including transfusion) and vertical routes. Resultant destruction of CD4-positive cells leads to in clinical manifestations of AIDS.	Donor history, education, and self-exclusion. Anti-HIV by EIA, screening test. Western blot confirmatory.	1:500,000
Human T-cell lymphotropic virus I and II (HTLV-I and -II) infection	Transforming retroviruses spread by sexual contact, parenteral (including transfusion) and vertical. Over years to decades, infection with HTLV-I may cause lymphoid malignancies or myelopathy.	Donor history. Anti-HTLV-I and -II by enzyme immunoassay screening test. Western blot confirmatory.	1:600,000

ALT = alanine transaminase; HAV, HBV, HCV = hepatitis A virus, hepatitis B virus, hepatitis C virus; HTLV = human T-cell lymphotropic virus; RPR = rapid plasma reagin; VDRL = syphilis test.

leukodepleted by filtering (white blood cell counts < 5 million per packed red cell unit or apheresis platelet concentrate equivalent).

STORAGE & PRESERVATION OF BLOOD & BLOOD COMPONENTS

Whole blood is routinely fractionated into packed red cells, platelets, and fresh frozen plasma or cryo-precipitate for most efficient use of all blood components. The storage conditions and biologic characteristics of the fractions are summarized in Table 25–13. The conditions provide the optimal environment to maintain appropriate recovery, survival, and function and are different for each blood component. For example, red cells undergo dramatic metabolic changes during their 35-day storage, with a decrease in 2,3-diphosphoglycerate (2,3-DPG) during the second week of storage, a decrease in ATP, and a grad-

Table 25–13. Characteristic of blood and blood components.

Component	Storage Conditions	Composition and Transfusion Characteristics	Indications	Risks and Precautions	Administration
Whole blood	4 °C for 35 days. RBC characteristics. **Survival:** Recovery decreases during storage but is always > 70%. Cells that circulate approximate normal survival. **Function:** 2,3-DPG levels fall to undetectable after second week of storage. This defect repaired within 24 hours of transfusion. **Electrolytes:** With storage, potassium increases in plasma. This rises to high levels after 2 weeks of storage.	Contains RBCs and many plasma compounds of whole blood. Leukocytes and platelets lose activity or viability after a few days under these conditions. Procoagulant clotting factors (particularly VIII and V) deteriorate rapidly during storage. Each unit has about 500 mL volume and Hct 36–40%.	Oxygen carrying capacity (anemia). Volume replacement for blood loss (> 15–20%) or severe shock.	Must be ABO-identical and crossmatch-compatible. Infectious diseases (see Table 28–12). Febrile or hemolytic transfusion reactions. Alloimmunization to red cell, white cell, or platelet antigens.	During acute blood loss, as rapidly as tolerated. In other settings, 2–4 hours. 10 mL/kg will raise Hct by 5% and support volume.
Packed red cells	Same as for whole blood	Contains RBCs; plasma removed in preparation. Status of leukocytes, clotting factors, and platelets same as for whole blood. Hct about 70%, volume 200–250 mL. May request tighter pack to give Hct 80–90%.	Oxygen carrying capacity. Acute trauma or bleeding, or situations requiring intensive cardiopulmonary support (Hct < 25–30%). Chronic anemia (Hct < 20%).	Same as for whole blood	May be given as patient will tolerate based on cardiovascular status over 2–4 hours. Dose of 3 mL packed RBC/kg will raise the Hct by 3%. If cardiovascular status stable, give 10 mL/kg over 2–4 hours. If unstable, use smaller volume or do packed RBC exchange.
Washed or filtered red cells	When cells are washed, there is a 24-hour outdate. Up to that time, they have the same characteristics as packed red cells.	Same as packed red cells	Same as packed red cells. Depending on technique used and extent of reduction of white blood cells, washed red cells may achieve the following: • Avoid febrile reactions. • Decreased the transmission of CMV. • Decreased the incidence of alloimmunization to white cell antigens.	Same as whole blood. Removal of white cells dimishes the risk of febrile reactions. Filtration with white cell filters may decrease rate of alloimmunization to white cell antigens and transmission of CMV.	Same as packed red cells
Frozen red cells	Packed red cells frozen in 40% glycerol solution at under –65 °C. Can be stored 3 years. Retain the same biochemical characteristics, function, and capacity for survival as the day in storage they were frozen; when thawed, 24-hour outdate.	Same as packed red cells	Same as packed red cells. Useful for avoiding febrile reactions, decreasing transmission of CMV, autologous blood donation, and developing an inventory of rare red cell blood groups.	Same as for whole blood. Risk of CMV transmission is at same level as using seronegative components.	Same as packed red cells

(continued)

Table 25–13. Characteristic of blood and blood components. *(continued)*

Component	Storage Conditions	Composition and Transfusion Characteristics	Indications	Risks and Precautions	Administration
Fresh frozen plasma	Plasma from whole blood stored at under –18 °C for up to 1 year	Contains > 80% of all procoagulant and anticoagulant plasma proteins	Replacement of plasma procoagulant and anticoagulant plasma proteins. May provide "other" factors, eg, treatment of TTP.	Need not be crossmatched; should be type-compatible. Volume overload, infectious diseases, allergic reactions.	As rapidly as tolerated by patient but not > 4 hours. Dose: 10–15 mL/kg will increase level of all clotting factors by 10–20%.
Cryoprecipitate	Produced by freezing fresh plasma to under –65 °C, then allowing to thaw 18 hours at 4 °C. After centrifugation, cryoprecipitable proteins are separated. May be stored at under –18 °C for up to 1 year.	Contains factor VIII, fibrinogen, and fibronectin at concentrations greater than those of plasma. Also contains factor XIII. VIII > 80 IU/pack, fibrinogen 100–350 mg/pack.	Treatment of acquired or congenital deficiencies of VIII, von Willebrand factor, and fibrinogen. Useful in making biologic glues that contain fibrinogen. Commercial clotting factor concentrates are the treatment of choice for factor VIII deficiency and von Willebrand disease because sterilization procedures further reduce the risk of viral transmission.	Same as for fresh frozen plasma. ABO agglutinogens may also be concentrated and can give positive direct agglutination test if not type-specific.	Cryoprecipitate can be given as a rapid infusion. Dose: ½ pack per kg body weight will increase factor VIII level by 80–100% and fibrinogen by 200–250 mg/dL.
Platelet concentrates from whole blood donation	Separated from platelet-rich plasma and stored with gentle agitation at 22 °C for 3–5 days. Containers currently in use are plastic and allow for gas exchange, diffusion of CO_2 helps keep pH > 6.00, a major factor in keeping platelets viable and functional.	Each unit contains about 5 $\times 10^{10}$ platelets. Survival: Although there may be some loss with storage, 60–70% recovery should be achieved, with stored platelets correcting the bleeding time in proportion to the peak counts reached.	Treatment of thrombocytopenia or platelet function defects	No crossmatch necessary. Should be ABO type-specific. Other risks as for whole blood.	Can be given as rapid transfusion or as defined by cardiovascular status, not more than 4 hours. Dose: 10 mL/kg should increase platelet count by at least 50,000/μL.
Platelet concentrates by aphersis techniques	Same as random donor units	Platelet content is equivalent to 6–10 units of random donor concentrates. Depending on technique used, these may be relatively free of leukocytes, a product useful in avoiding alloimmunization.	As above, particularly useful in treating patients who have insufficient production in whom alloisoimmunization is a potential problem	Same as above	As above
Granulocytes	Although they may be stored stationary at 20–24 °C, transfuse as soon as possible after collection	Contains at least 1 $\times 10^{10}$ granulocytes but also platelets and red cells	Severely neutropenic individuals (< 500/μL) with poor marrow reserves and suspected bacterial or fungal infections not responding to 48–72 hours of parenteral antibiotics. Also in patients with neutrophil dysfunction.	Same as for platelets. Pulmonary leukostasis reactions. Severe febrile reactions.	Given in an infusion over 2–4 hours. Dose: 1 unit daily for newborns and infants, 1 $\times 10^9$ granulocytes per kg.

CMV = cytomegalovirus.

ual loss of intracellular potassium into the plasma. Fortunately, these changes are readily reversed within hours to days after the red cells are transfused. However, in certain clinical conditions, these effects may define the type of components used. For example, blood less than 7–10 days old would be preferred for exchange transfusion or replacement of red cells in persons with cardiopulmonary disease to ensure adequate oxygen carrying capacity. However, storage time is not an issue when administering transfusions to those with chronic anemia.

Under certain conditions, where excessive potassium load is a problem, one has the option of using blood less than 10 days old, making packed cells out of an older unit of whole blood, or washing blood stored as packed cells. No matter what the age of the blood, over 70% of the red cells will circulate after transfusion and approximate normal survival in the circulation.

Platelets can be stored at 22 °C for a maximum of 3–5 days. At the extremes of storage, there should be at least a 60% recovery, a survival time that approximates turnover of fresh autologous platelets, and normalization of the bleeding time in proportion to the peak platelet count. Frozen components, red cells, fresh frozen plasma, and cryoprecipitate are outdated at 3 years, 1 year, and 1 year, respectively. Frozen red cells retain the same biochemical and functional characteristics as the day they were frozen. Fresh frozen plasma contains 80% or more of all of the clotting factors of fresh plasma. Factor VIII and fibrinogen are concentrated in cryoprecipitate.

PRETRANSFUSION TESTING

Both the donated blood and the recipient are tested for ABO and Rh(D) antigens and for autoantibodies or alloantibodies. The cross-match is required on any component that contains red cells. In the major cross-match, washed donor red cells are incubated with the serum from the patient, and agglutination is detected and graded. The antiglobulin phase of the test is then performed; Coombs reagent, which will detect the presence of IgG or complement on the surface of the red cells, is added to the mixture, and any possible reaction is evaluated. In the presence of a negative antibody screen in the recipient, a negative antiglobulin phase or immediate spin cross-match test confirms the compatibility of the blood. Further testing is required if the antibody screen or the cross-match is positive, and blood should not be given until the nature of the reactivity is delineated. An incompatible cross-match is evaluated first with a direct antiglobulin or Coombs test to detect IgG or complement on the surfaces of the recipient's red cells. The indirect antiglobulin test is also used to determine the presence of antibodies that will coat or activate complement on the surfaces of normal red cells.

TRANSFUSION PRACTICE

General Rules

Several rules should be observed in administering any blood component.

(1) In final preparation of the component, no solutions should be added to the bag or tubing set except for normal saline (0.9% sodium chloride for injection, USP), ABO-compatible plasma, or other specifically approved expanders. Hypotonic solutions cause hemolysis of red cells and, if transfused, result in a severe reaction in the recipient.

(2) Transfusion products should be protected from contact with any calcium-containing solution (such as lactated Ringer's); recalcification and reversal of the citrate effect cause clotting of the blood component.

(3) Blood components should not be warmed to a temperature greater than 37 °C. If a component is incubated in a water bath, it should be enclosed in a watertight bag to prevent contamination of entry ports.

(4) Whenever a blood bag is entered, the sterile integrity of the system is violated, and that unit should be discarded within 4 hours if left at room temperature or within 24 hours if the temperature is between 1 °C and 4 °C.

(5) Transfusions of products containing red cells should not exceed 4 hours. Blood components in excess of what can be infused during this time period should be stored in the blood bank until needed.

(6) Before transfusion, the blood component should be visually inspected for any unusual characteristics—such as the presence of flocculent material, hemolysis, or clumping of cells—and mixed thoroughly.

(7) The unit and the recipient should be properly identified.

(8) The administration set includes a standard 170–260 μm clot filter. Under certain clinical circumstances, an additional microaggregate filter may be used to eliminate small aggregates of fibrin, white cells, and platelets that will not be removed by the standard filter.

(9) The patient should be observed during the entire transfusion but especially during the first 15 minutes. Any adverse symptoms or signs should be evaluated immediately and reactions to the transfusion reported promptly to the transfusion service.

(10) When cross-match-incompatible red cells or whole blood must be given to the patient (as with autoimmune hemolytic anemia), a test dose of 10% of the total volume (not to exceed 75 mL) should be administered over 15–20 minutes; the transfusion is then stopped and the patient evaluated for reaction. If no adverse effects are noted, the remainder of the volume can be carefully infused.

(11) Blood for exchange transfusion in the newborn period may be cross-matched with either in-

fant's or mother's serum. If the exchange is for hemolysis, 500 mL of whole blood stored for less than 7 days will be adequate. If replacement of clotting factors is a key issue, packed red cells (7 days old) reconstituted with fresh frozen plasma may be considered. Based on posttransfusion platelet counts, platelet transfusion may be considered. Other problems to be anticipated are acid-base derangements, hyponatremia, hyperkalemia, hypocalcemia, hypoglycemia, hypothermia, and hypervolemia or hypovolemia.

Choice of Blood Component

In deciding on the need for blood transfusion, several principles should be considered. Indications for blood or blood components must be well defined, and the patient's medical condition and not just the laboratory numbers should be the basis for the decision. Specific deficiencies exhibited by the patient (eg, oxygen carrying capacity, thrombocytopenia) should be treated with appropriate blood components and the use of whole blood minimized. Information about specific blood components is summarized in Table 25–13.

A. Whole Blood: Whole blood may be used in patients who require replacement of oxygen-carrying capacity and volume. More specifically, it should be considered when more than 15% of blood volume is lost. Doses vary depending on volume considerations (Table 25–13). In acute situations, the transfusion may be completed rapidly to support blood volume.

B. Packed Red Cells: Packed red cells (which include leukocyte-poor, filtered, or frozen deglycerolized products) prepared from whole blood by centrifugal techniques are the appropriate choice for almost all patients with deficient oxygen carrying capacity. Exact indications will be defined by the clinical setting, the severity of the anemia, the acuity of the condition, and any other factors affecting oxygen transport.

C. Platelets: The decision to transfuse platelets depends on the clinical condition of the patient, the status of plasma phase coagulation, the platelet count, the cause of the thrombocytopenia, and the functional capacity of the patient's own platelets. With platelet counts less than 10,000–20,000/μL, the risk of severe, spontaneous bleeding is markedly increased, and—in the absence of antibody-mediated thrombocytopenia—transfusion should be considered. Under certain circumstances, especially with platelet dysfunction or treatment that inhibits the procoagulant system, transfusions at higher platelet counts may be necessary.

Transfused platelets are temporarily sequestered in the lungs and spleen before reaching their peak concentrations, 45–60 minutes after transfusion. A significant proportion of the transfused platelets never circulate but remain sequestered in the spleen. This phenomenon results in reduced recovery; only 60–70% of the transfused platelets are accounted for when peripheral platelet count increments are used as a measure of response.

In addition to cessation of bleeding, two variables indicate the effectiveness of platelet transfusions. The first is platelet recovery, the measure of the maximum number of platelets circulating in response to transfusion. The practical measure is the platelet count at 1 hour after transfusion. In the absence of immune or drastic nonimmune factors that markedly decrease platelet recovery, one would expect a 7000/μL increment for each random donor unit and a 40,000–70,000/μL increment for each single-donor apheresis unit in a large child or adolescent. For infants and small children, 10 mL/kg will increase the platelet count by at least 50,000/μL. The second variable is the survival of transfused platelets. Normally, transfused platelets have a half-life of 3–5 days. In the presence of immune or nonimmune destruction, the life span may be shortened to a few days or a few hours. Frequent platelet transfusions may be required to maintain adequate hemostasis.

A particularly troublesome outcome in patients receiving long-term platelet transfusions is the development of a refractory state characterized by poor (< 30%) recovery or no response to platelet transfusion (as measured at 1 hour). Most (70–90%) of these refractory states result from the development of alloantibodies directed against HLA antigens on the platelet. Platelets have class I HLA antigens and the antibodies are primarily against HLA A or B determinants. A smaller proportion of these alloantibodies (10–30%) are directed against platelet-specific alloantigens. The most effective approach is probably to prevent HLA sensitization by using leukocyte-depleted components (< 5 million leukocytes per unit of packed red cells or per apheresis or 6–10 random donor unit concentrates). For the alloimmunized patient, the best approach is to provide HLA A- and HLA B-matched platelets for transfusion. Reports have suggested that platelet cross-matching procedures using HLA-matched or unmatched donors may be helpful in quickly identifying platelet concentrates with the highest probability of resulting in a successful transfusion.

D. Fresh Frozen Plasma (FFP): The indication for FFP is replacement of plasma coagulation factors in clinical situations in which a deficiency of one or more clotting factors exists and there are associated bleeding manifestations. In some hereditary factor deficiencies such as factor VIII deficiency, commercially prepared concentrates contain these factors in higher concentrations and, because of viral inactivation, impose less infectious risk and are more appropriate than plasma.

E. Cryoprecipitate: This component may be used for acquired or congenital disorders of hypofibrinogenemia or afibrinogenemia. The dose given depends on the protein to be replaced. Cryoprecipi-

Table 25–14. Adverse event following transfusions.

Event	Pathophysiology	Signs and Symptoms	Management
Acute hemolytic transfusion reaction	Preformed alloantibodies (most commonly to ABO) and occasionally autoantibodies cause rapid intravascular hemolysis of transfused cells with activation of clotting (DIC), activation of inflammatory mediators, and acute renal failure	Fever, chills, nausea, chest pain, back pain, pain at transfusion site, hypotension, dyspnea, oliguria, dark urine	The risk of this type of reaction overall is low (1:30,000), but the mortality rate is high (up to 40%). Stop the transfusion; maintain renal output with intravenous fluids and diuretics (furosemide or mannitol); treat DIC with heparin; and institute other appropriate supportive measures.
Delayed hemolytic transfusion reaction	Formation of alloantibodies after transfusion and resultant destruction of transfused red cells, usually by extravascular hemolysis	Fever, jaundice, anemia. A small percentage may develop chronic hemolysis.	Detection, definition, and documentation (for future transfusions). Supportive care. Risk, 1:2500.
Bacterial contamination	Contamination of units results in growth of bacteria or production of clinically significant levels of endotoxin	Chills, high fever, hypotension, other symptoms of sepsis or endotoxemia	Stop transfusion; make aggressive attempts to identify organism; provide vigorous supportive medical care
Graft-versus-host disease	Lymphocytes from donor transfused in an immunoincompetent host	Syndrome can present with a variety of organs involved, usually skin, liver, gastrointestinal tract, and bone marrow	Preventive management: Irradiation (> 1500 cGy) of cellular blood components transfused to individuals with congenital or acquired immunodeficiency syndromes, intrauterine transfusion, very premature infants, and when donors are relatives of the recipient
Febrile reactions	Usually caused by leukoagglutinins in recipient cytokines or other biologically active compounds	Fever. May also have chills.	Supportive. Consider leukocyte-poor products for future. Risk per transfusion, 1:200.
Allergic reactions	Most causes not identified. In IgA-deficient individuals, reaction occurs as a result of antibodies to IgA.	Itching, hives, occasionally chills and fever. In severe reactions, may see signs of anaphylaxis: dyspnea, pulmonary edema.	Mild to moderate reactions: diphenhydramine. More severe reactions: epinephrine SC and steroids IV. Risk for mild to moderate allergic reactions, 1:1000; severe anaphylactic reactions, 1:150,000.
Iron overload	There is no physiologic mechanism to excrete excess iron. Target organs include liver, heart, and endocrine organs. In patients receiving red cell transfusions over long periods of time, there is an increase in iron burden.	Signs and symptoms of dysfunctional organs affected by the iron	Chronic administration of iron chelator such as deferoxamine
Dilutional coagulopathy	Massive blood loss and transfusion with replacement with fluids or blood components and deficient clotting factors	Bleeding	Replacement of clotting factors or platelets with appropriate blood components
Transfusion-related acute lung injury	Acute lung injury occurring within 4 hours after transfusion. Two sets of factors interact to produce the syndrome. Patient factors: infection, surgery, cytokine therapy. Blood component factors: lipids, antibodies, cytokines. Two groups of factors interact during transfusion to result in lung injury indistinguishable from ARDS.	Tachypnea, dyspnea, hypoxia. Diffuse interstitial markings. Cardiac evaluation normal.	May consider younger products packed red blood cells ≤ 2 weeks, platelets ≤ 3 days), washing components to prevent syndrome. Management: supportive care.

tate can be given in a rapid transfusion over 30–60 minutes.

F. Granulocytes: With better supportive care over the past 10 years, the need for granulocytes in neutropenic patients with severe bacterial infections has decreased. Indications still remain for severe bacterial infections unresponsive to vigorous medical therapy in either newborns or older children with the presence of bone marrow failure.

G. Apheresis Products and Procedures: Apheresis equipment allows one or more blood components to be collected from a donor while the rest are returned. Apheresis platelet concentrates which have as many platelets as 6–10 units of platelet concentrates from whole blood donations are one example; granulocytes another. Apheresis techniques can also be used to collect hematopoietic stem cells that have been mobilized into the blood by cytokines (G-CSF or GM-CSF) given alone or after chemotherapy. These stem cells are used for autologous bone marrow transplantation. Blood cell separators can be used for the collection of single source plasma or removal of a blood component that is causing disease.

Examples include red cell exchange in sickle cell disease and plasmapheresis in Goodpasture's syndrome or in myasthenia gravis.

Adverse Effects

The noninfectious complications of blood transfusions are outlined in Table 25–14. Most present a small but still significant risk to the recipient.

National Institutes of Health Consensus Conference: Fresh frozen plasma: Indications and risks. JAMA 1985;253: 551.

National Institutes of Health Consensus Conference: Platelet transfusion therapy. JAMA 1987;257:1777.

Rossi EC, Simon TL, Moss GS (editors): *Principles of Transfusion Medicine.* Williams & Wilkins, 1996.

Silliman CC et al: The association of biologically active lipids with the development of transfusion-related acute lung injury: A retrospective study. Transfusion 1997; 37:719.

Stehling L et al: Guidelines for blood utilization review. Transfusion 1994;34:438.

Walker RH (editor): *Technical Manual of the American Association of Blood Banks.*, 12th ed. American Association of Blood Banks, 1996.

REFERENCES

Buchanan GR (editor): Pediatric hematology. Pediatr Clin North Am 1996.

Bunn HF, Forget BG: *Hemoglobin: Molecular, Genetic and Clinical Aspects.* Saunders, 1986.

Embury SH et al: (editors): *Sickle Cell Disease: Basic Principles and Clinical Practice.* Raven Press, 1994.

Hathaway WE, Bonnar J: *Hemostatic Disorders of the Pregnant Woman and Newborn Infant.* Elsevier, 1987.

Hathaway WE, Goodnight SH: *Disorders of Hemostasis and Thrombosis: A Clinical Guide.* McGraw-Hill, 1993.

Mentzer WC, Wagner GM: *The Hereditary Hemolytic Anemias.* Churchill Livingstone, 1989.

Miller DR, Baehner RL: *Blood Diseases of Infancy and Childhood,* 6th ed. Mosby, 1989.

Nathan DG, Orkin SH: *Hematology of Infancy and Childhood,* 5th ed. Saunders, 1998.

Oski FA, Naiman JL: *Hematologic Problems in the Newborn,* 3rd ed. Saunders, 1982.

Petz LD, Garratty G: *Acquired Immune Hemolytic Anemias.* Churchill Livingstone, 1980.

Rossi EC, Simon TL, Moss GS: *Principles of Transfusion Medicine,* 2nd ed. Williams & Wilkins, 1996.

Serjeant GR: *Sickle Cell Disease,* 2nd ed. Oxford Univ Press, 1993.

Stamatoyannopoulos G et al: (editors): *The Molecular Basis of Blood Diseases.* Saunders, 1994.

Young NS, Alter BP: *Aplastic Anemia: Acquired and Inherited.* Saunders, 1994.

26

Neoplastic Disease

*Edythe A. Albano, MD, Linda C. Stork, MD, Brian S. Greffe, MD, CM,
Lorrie F. Odom, MD, & Nicholas K. Foreman, MD*

Cure of cancer in children is being achieved with increasing success. Combined modality therapy (surgery, chemotherapy, radiation therapy) has improved survival dramatically, with the result that the overall cure rate of pediatric malignancies is now 70%. It is estimated that by the year 2000, one in 1000 adults will be a survivor of childhood cancer.

Because pediatric malignancies are rare, the cooperative clinical trial has become the mainstay of treatment planning and therapeutic advances. The Children's Cancer Group (CCG) and the Pediatric Oncology Group (POG) offer the most current therapeutic options and protocols and are able to answer important treatment questions in a timely manner. A newly diagnosed child with cancer should be enrolled in a cooperative clinical trial whenever possible. Because many protocols are associated with significant toxicities, morbidity, and potential mortality, management of pediatric patients should be supervised by a pediatric oncologist familiar with the hazards of treatment.

Advances in molecular genetics, cell biology, and tumor immunology contribute to our understanding of pediatric malignancies and their treatment. It is important that biopsies of suspected malignancies be examined by a pathologist familiar with the role of special ancillary studies. In addition to formalin-fixed tissue, fresh unfixed tissue is essential for metaphase chromosome analysis as well as molecular genetic analysis. The applicability of these procedures can be seen in patients with chronic myeloid leukemia, most of whom have a t(9;22) on cytogenetic analysis. However, not all patients have an obvious karyotype abnormality. In this smaller group, molecular techniques can detect the aberrant gene product that results from the translocation, ensuring greater diagnostic accuracy and leading to appropriate therapy. The polymerase chain reaction (PCR), which amplifies minute DNA fragments in an exponential fashion to yield easily detectable and manipulated amounts of DNA, has wide applicability in the diagnosis of minimal residual disease.

Similar techniques can be used to determine whether a pathologic process is monoclonal (arising from a single cell and generally considered malignant) or polyclonal (arising from multiple cells and usually nonmalignant). Detecting rearrangements of DNA in antigen receptor genes as a clonal marker for the diagnosis of lymphoma is one example. Cells in a benign process have diverse rearrangements of antigen receptor genes, whereas clonal cells that make up a neoplasm have uniform rearrangements.

Similar molecular techniques have led also to the characterization of oncogenes and tumor suppressor genes in human malignancies. An oncogene is one that causes malignant transformation or deregulated cell growth. For example, the proto-oncogene C-*myc* plays an important role in hematopoietic cell proliferation. It has been recognized at the site of three different translocations in Burkitt's lymphomas: t(8;14), t(8;22), and t(2;8). A tumor suppressor gene (anti-oncogene) constrains cell proliferation; its absence can lead to unchecked cell growth. The retinoblastoma gene is the prototypical tumor suppressor gene. Inactivation of both copies of this gene in a cell leads to tumor formation, first recognized in children with retinoblastoma.

Research in supportive care areas such as management of pain, emesis, and infection has improved the survival and quality of life for children undergoing cancer treatment. Long-term follow-up of childhood cancer survivors is yielding information that will provide a rationale for modifying future treatment regimens to decrease morbidity.

MAJOR PEDIATRIC NEOPLASTIC DISEASES

ACUTE LYMPHOBLASTIC LEUKEMIA

Essentials of Diagnosis & Typical Features

- Pallor, petechiae, purpura (50%), bone pain (25%).

- Hepatosplenomegaly (60%), lymphadenopathy (50%).
- Single or multiple cytopenias: neutropenia, thrombocytopenia, anemia.
- Leukopenia or leukocytosis, often with leukemic leukocytes identifiable on blood smear.
- Diagnosis confirmed by bone marrow examination.

General Considerations

Acute lymphoblastic leukemia (ALL) is the most common malignancy of childhood, accounting for about 25% of all cancer diagnoses in patients under the age of 15 years. The worldwide incidence of ALL is about 1:25,000 children per year, including 2500 children per year in the United States. The peak age at onset is 4 years, with 85% of patients diagnosed between the ages of 2 and 10 years. Before the advent of chemotherapy, this disease was fatal, usually within 3–4 months, with virtually no survivors 1 year after diagnosis.

ALL results from uncontrolled proliferation of immature lymphocytes; its cause is unknown, and genetic factors may play a role. Leukemia is defined by the presence of more than 25% malignant hematopoietic cells (blasts) on bone marrow aspirate. Leukemic blasts from the majority of cases of childhood ALL have an antigen on the cell surface called the common ALL antigen (CALLA). These blasts derive from B cell precursors early in their development. Less commonly, lymphoblasts are of T cell origin or of mature B cell origin. Over 70% of children receiving aggressive combination chemotherapy and early presymptomatic treatment to the central nervous system are now cured of ALL.

Clinical Findings

A. Symptoms and Signs: Presenting complaints of patients with ALL include those related to decreased bone marrow production of red cells, white cells, or platelets and to leukemic infiltration of extramedullary (outside bone marrow) sites. Intermittent fevers are common, either as a result of cytokines induced by the leukemia itself or of infections secondary to leukopenia. About 25% of patients experience bone pain, especially in the pelvis, vertebral bodies, and legs. Physical examination at diagnosis ranges from virtually normal to highly abnormal. Signs related to bone marrow infiltration by leukemia include pallor, petechiae, and purpura. Hepatomegaly or splenomegaly occurs in over 60% of cases. Lymphadenopathy is common, either localized or generalized to cervical, axillary, and inguinal regions. The testes may be unilaterally or bilaterally enlarged secondary to leukemic infiltration. Superior vena cava syndrome is caused by mediastinal adenopathy compressing the superior vena cava. A prominent venous pattern develops over the upper chest from collateral vein enlargement. The neck may feel full from venous engorgement. The face may appear plethoric, and the periorbital area may be edematous.

Tachypnea, orthopnea, and respiratory distress from a mediastinal mass may be apparent. Leukemic infiltration of cranial nerves may cause cranial nerve palsies along with mild nuchal rigidity. The optic fundi may show exudates of leukemic infiltration and hemorrhage from thrombocytopenia. The cardiac examination often reveals a flow murmur and tachycardia due to anemia; rarely, signs of congestive heart failure are present. Bone and joint pain may be appreciated on examination, particularly in the pelvis, lower spine, and femurs. There may also be signs of infection.

B. Laboratory Findings: A complete blood count (CBC) with differential is the most useful initial test because 95% of patients with ALL have a decrease in at least one cell type (single cytopenia): neutropenia, thrombocytopenia, or anemia. Most patients have decreases in at least two blood cell lines. The white count is low or normal ($< 10,000/\mu L$) in 50% of patients, but the differential shows neutropenia (absolute neutrophil count $< 1000/\mu L$) along with a small percentage of blasts amid normal lymphocytes. In 30% of patients, the white count is between 10,000 and 50,000/μL, and in 20% of cases it is over 50,000/μL, occasionally higher than 300,000/μL. Blasts are usually readily identifiable on peripheral smears in patients with elevated white counts. Most patients with ALL have decreased platelet counts ($< 150,000/\mu L$) and decreased hemoglobin (< 11 g/dL) at diagnosis. Less than 1% of patients diagnosed with ALL have entirely normal CBCs and blood smears but have bone pain that leads to bone marrow examination. Serum chemistries, particularly uric acid and lactate dehydrogenase (LDH), are often elevated at diagnosis as a result of cell breakdown. Serum phosphorus is occasionally elevated at diagnosis as well.

The diagnosis of ALL is established by bone marrow examination, which shows a homogeneous infiltration of leukemic blasts replacing normal marrow elements. The morphology of blasts on bone marrow aspirate can usually distinguish ALL from acute nonlymphocytic leukemia (ANLL). Lymphoblasts are typically small, with cell diameters of approximately two erythrocytes. Lymphoblasts have scant cytoplasm, usually without granules. The nucleus typically contains no nucleoli or one small, indistinct nucleolus. Immunophenotyping of ALL blasts helps distinguish precursor B cell ALL from T cell ALL. Histochemical stains specific for myeloblastic and monoblastic leukemias (myeloperoxidase and nonspecific esterase) distinguish ALL from acute nonlymphocytic leukemia (ANLL). Between 5% and 10% of patients present with central nervous system leukemia, which is defined as a cerebrospinal fluid white cell count $\geq 5/\mu L$ with blasts apparent on cytocentrifuged specimen.

C. Imaging: Chest x-ray may show mediastinal widening or an anterior mediastinal mass and tracheal compression secondary to lymphadenopathy. Abdominal ultrasound may show kidney enlargement from leukemic infiltration or uric acid nephropathy as well as intra-abdominal adenopathy. Plain films of the long bones and spine may show demineralization, periosteal elevation, or compression of vertebral bodies.

Differential Diagnosis

The differential diagnosis, based on the history and physical examination, includes chronic infections by Epstein-Barr virus and cytomegalovirus, causing lymphadenopathy, hepatosplenomegaly, fevers, and anemia. Prominent petechiae and purpura suggest a diagnosis of immune thrombocytopenic purpura, while significant pallor could be caused by transient erythroblastopenia of childhood, autoimmune hemolytic anemias, or aplastic anemia. Fevers and joint pains, with or without hepatosplenomegaly and lymphadenopathy, suggest juvenile rheumatoid arthritis. The diagnosis of leukemia usually becomes straightforward once the CBC reveals multiple cytopenias and leukemic blasts. Serum LDH levels may help distinguish juvenile rheumatoid arthritis (JRA) from leukemia. LDH is usually normal in JRA but often elevated in ALL patients presenting with bone pain. An elevated white count with lymphocytosis is typical of pertussis; however, in pertussis the lymphocytes are mature, and neutropenia is rarely associated.

Treatment

A. Specific Therapy: Specific treatment is determined by prognostic features present at diagnosis. The first month of therapy consists of induction, at the end of which over 95% of patients exhibit remission on bone marrow aspirates. The drugs most commonly used in induction include oral prednisone, intravenous vincristine and daunorubicin, intramuscular asparaginase, and intrathecal methotrexate. For T cell ALL, intravenous cyclophosphamide has been given during induction as well.

Consolidation is the second phase of treatment, during which intrathecal chemotherapy and sometimes cranial radiation therapy are given to kill lymphoblasts that may be present in the meninges.

Maintenance therapy includes daily oral mercaptopurine, weekly oral or intramuscular methotrexate, and, often, monthly pulses of intravenous vincristine and oral prednisone. Intrathecal chemotherapy, either with methotrexate alone or combined with cytarabine and hydrocortisone, is usually administered every 2–3 months. Several months of intensive chemotherapy, termed delayed intensification, may be interposed within the maintenance chemotherapy phase of treatment.

All these drugs have significant potential side effects. Patients need to be closely monitored to prevent drug toxicities and to ensure early treatment of complications. Most patients are treated on protocols designed by the Children's Cancer Group or Pediatric Oncology Group. The duration of treatment is between 2¼ and 3¼ years.

Treatment for ALL is tailored to prognostic groups. A child 1–9 years of age with a white count under 50,000/μL at diagnosis and without t(9;22) or t(4;11) would be treated with less intensive therapy than a patient who has a white count at diagnosis over 50,000/μL or is older than age 10 years. This treatment approach has significantly increased the cure rate among patients with less favorable prognostic features while minimizing treatment-related toxicities in those with favorable features. Bone marrow relapse is usually heralded by an abnormal CBC. After a patient has completed the entire course of chemotherapy, the chance of relapse is about 10% during the subsequent 4 years.

The CNS and testes are sanctuary sites of extramedullary leukemia. Systemic chemotherapy does not penetrate these tissues as well as it penetrates other organs. "Presymptomatic" intrathecal chemotherapy is a critical part of ALL treatment in preventing CNS relapse. Before the institution of such therapy in the 1970s, the CNS was a major site of initial leukemic relapse. Relapses isolated to the central nervous system now occur in only 5–8% of patients. Symptoms suggestive of CNS disease include headache, nausea and vomiting, irritability, nuchal rigidity, photophobia, and cranial nerve palsies. Previously, up to 15% of boys have testicular relapse following completion of chemotherapy. The presentation of testicular relapse is usually unilateral painless testicular enlargement. The incidence of testicular relapse has decreased significantly as treatment for ALL has intensified. Routine follow-up of boys both on and off treatment includes examination of the testes.

Bone marrow transplantation is rarely used as initial treatment for ALL, as most patients are cured with chemotherapy alone. However, patients whose blasts contain certain chromosomal abnormalities, such as t(9;22) and t(4;11), appear to have a better cure rate with early bone marrow transplant from an HLA-DR-matched sibling donor than with intensive chemotherapy alone. Bone marrow transplantation has cured about 50% of patients who have a relapse of ALL provided a second remission was achieved with chemotherapy before transplant. Children who relapse more than 1 year after completion of chemotherapy (late relapse) may be cured with intensive chemotherapy without bone marrow transplantation.

B. Supportive Care: Tumor lysis syndrome should be anticipated when treatment is started. Hydration, alkalinization of urine with intravenous sodium bicarbonate, and oral allopurinol should be given. If superior vena caval or superior mediastinal syndrome is present, general anesthesia is temporarily contraindicated. If hyperleukocytosis (WBC > 100,000/μL) is accompanied by hyperviscosity and mental status changes, leukapheresis may be indicated to rapidly reduce the number of circulating blasts and minimize the potential thrombotic or hemorrhagic CNS complications. Severe anemia at diagnosis can usually be corrected with a number of small red blood cell transfusions and intravenous furosemide. Throughout the course of treatment, all transfused blood and platelet products should be irradiated in order to prevent graft-versus-host disease from the transfused lymphocytes. Whenever possible, blood products should be leukodepleted to minimize cytomegalovirus (CMV) transmission, transfusion reactions, and sensitization to platelets.

During the course of treatment, fever (temperature > 38.3 °C) and neutropenia (absolute neutrophil count < 500/μL) require treatment with empiric broad-spectrum antibiotics. Patients receiving ALL treatment must receive prophylaxis against *Pneumocystis carinii*. Trimethoprim-sulfamethoxazole is the drug of choice, currently recommended to be given twice each day on 2 or 3 consecutive days per week. Patients nonimmune to varicella are at risk for very serious—even fatal—infection. Such patients should receive varicella-zoster immune globulin (VZIG) within 72 hours after exposure and treatment with intravenous acyclovir for active infection.

The management of a patient on chemotherapy for ALL is very complex because of the infectious complications and potential toxicities of chemotherapy. Treatment of ALL should be guided by physicians and nurses who are specifically trained in pediatric oncology.

Prognosis

Cure rates depend on specific prognostic features present at diagnosis. The two most important features are white count and age. Children aged 2–9 years whose diagnostic white count is < 50,000/μL have a higher rate of cure than other patients. Certain chromosomal abnormalities present in the leukemic blasts at diagnosis influence prognosis. Patients with t(9;22) have a very poor chance of cure even with intensive therapy. Infants t(4;11) have a poor chance of cure. On the other hand, patients whose blasts are hyperdiploid (containing over 50 chromosomes instead of the normal 46) have a greater chance of cure than children without hyperdiploidy. About 25% of children with ALL have blasts that contain a gene rearrangement called TEL-AML1. This rearrangement of genetic material involves chromosomes 12 and 21 and is detected by molecular but not by cytogenetic

techniques. Children with the TEL-AML1 rearrangement appear to have an excellent prognosis as well.

Ablin AR (editor): *Supportive Care of Children With Cancer.* Johns Hopkins Univ Press, 1997.

Pui CH: Childhood leukemia. N Engl J Med 1995; 332:1618.

Rubnitz JE et al: Case-control study suggests a favorable impact of TEL rearrangement in patients with B-lineage ALL treated with antimetabolite therapy: A Pediatric Oncology Group study. Blood 1997;89:1143.

Smith M et al: Uniform approach to risk classification and treatment assignment for children with ALL. J Clin Oncol 1996;14:18.

ACUTE MYELOID LEUKEMIA

Acute myeloid leukemia (AML) is one-fifth as common in childhood as acute lymphoblastic leukemia (ALL). There are 500 new cases per year in the United States. Ionizing radiation, cytotoxic chemotherapeutic agents, benzene exposure, Down's syndrome, and chromosomal instability syndromes are known to be predisposing factors, but most children have no identifiable risk factors. Cytogenetic clonal abnormalities occur in 80% of patients with AML and are often predictive of outcome.

AML is subdivided primarily by morphology and histochemical staining of the leukemic cells (French-American-British [FAB] classification). These subsets have different cytogenetic abnormalities, clinical features, and responses to treatment (Table 26–1).

Clinical presentation is usually with anemia (44%), thrombocytopenia (33%), and neutropenia (69%). Symptoms can be few and innocuous or may be life-threatening. The median hemoglobin at diagnosis is 7 g/dL; platelets are usually < 50,000/μL; and the absolute neutrophil count is under 1000/μL. The total white blood cell count is over 100,000/μL in 25% of children diagnosed with AML. Hyperleukocytosis is associated with life-threatening complications from venous stasis and sludging of blasts in small vessels causing hypoxia, hemorrhage, and infarction, most notably in the lung and CNS. *This is a medical emergency requiring rapid intervention to decrease the leukocyte count.* CNS leukemia is present in 5 to 15% of patients at diagnosis, which is a much higher rate of involvement than in ALL.

Treatment is more difficult than in ALL and requires more intensive chemotherapy, particularly anthracyclines and cytarabine. Toxicities from therapy are common and likely to be life-threatening. Only 70–85% of children achieve remission (versus 98% in ALL); the long-term disease-free survival is 35–50%. Retinoic acid (all-*trans*) can cause differentiation of promyelocytic leukemia cells and induce remission, but cure requires conventional chemother-

Table 26–1. FAB subtypes of ANLL.

FAB Classification	Common Name	Distribution in Childhood		Cytogenetic Associations	Clinical Features
		< 2 Years	> 2 Years		
M$_1$	Acute myeloblastic leukemia without maturation	17%	25%	16q abnormalities	
M$_2$	Acute myeloblastic leukemia with maturation		26%	(18;21)	Myeloblastomas
M$_3$	Acute promyelocytic leukemia		4%	t(15;17)	DIC
M$_4$	Acute myelomonoblastic leukemia	30%	26%	t(3;3) inv 3, inv 16, del 16q, t11/del 11q	Hyperleukocytosis, CNS involvement, skin and gum infiltration
M$_5$	Acute monoblastic leukemia	52%	16%	t(9;11)	Hyperleukocytosis, CNS involvement, skin and gum infiltration
M$_6$	Erythroleukemia		2%		
M$_7$	Acute megakaryoblastic leukemia		5%	t(1;21), t(3;3), inv 3	Down syndrome

apy as well. Allogeneic bone marrow transplantation during first remission may offer a survival advantage over chemotherapy alone. Published results from various centers show a 55–70% survival rate at 5 years. For patients relapsing following conventional chemotherapy, bone marrow transplantation is a potentially curative option.

Grier HE et al: Acute myelogenous leukemia. In: *Principles and Practice of Pediatric Oncology.* Pizzo PA, Poplack DG (editors). Lippincott, 1997.

Smith FO et al: Cellular biology of acute myelogenous leukemia. J Pediatr Hematol Oncol 1995;17:113.

Tallman MS et al: All-*trans*-retinoic acid in acute promyelocytic leukemia. N Engl J Med 1997;337:1021.

CHRONIC MYELOGENOUS LEUKEMIA

Chronic myelogenous leukemia (CML) accounts for less than 5% of the childhood leukemias. Two childhood variants are recognized: the Philadelphia chromosome t(9;22)-positive form, which is essentially identical with that occurring in adults, and the juvenile form (Table 26–2).

Adult CML can be palliated with single-drug chemotherapy such as hydroxyurea. The disease inexorably progresses from the chronic phase, usually within 3 years, to an accelerated phase and then to a blast crisis. The accelerated and blast phases are refractory to therapy. Bone marrow transplantation (BMT) is the only known cure. The 4-year survival rate for patients under 20 years of age transplanted in the chronic phase is 75%. Unfortunately, only one-third of patients have related matched donors available. Consequently, related mismatched, unrelated

matched, cord blood, autologous, and peripheral stem cell bone marrow transplantations are being investigated. BMT is ideally undertaken within a year of diagnosis. Alpha interferon has shown promising results in clinical trials by reducing or eliminating the Philadelphia chromosome-positive malignant clone. The long-term results are not yet known.

Juvenile CML, now called juvenile myelomonocytic leukemia (JMML), accounts for one-third of chronic leukemias in childhood. Compared with the adult form, it is a much more fulminant disease that occurs in infants and very young children. Survival is

Table 26–2. Comparison of juvenile and adult chronic myelogenous leukemia.

	JMML	Adult CML
Age at onset	< 2 years old	> 3 years old
Clinical presentation	Abrupt onset; eczematoid skin rash, markedly lymphadenopathy, bleeding tendency, moderate hepatosplenomegaly.	Nonspecific constitutional complaints, massive splenomegaly, variable hepatomegaly.
Chromosomal alterations	Absent.	t(9;22) present in 90% of cases.
Laboratory features	Moderate leukocytosis (< 100,000/μL), thrombocytopenia, monocytosis, elevated fetal hemoglobin, normal to diminished leukocyte alkaline phosphatase, elevated muramidase, elevated immunoglobulins.	Marked leukocytosis (> 100,000/μL), normal to elevated platelet count, decreased to absent leukocyte alkaline phosphatase, usually normal muramidase.

less than 9 months. Bone marrow transplant has been used successfully.

Enright H, McGlave PB: Biology and treatment of chronic myelogenous leukemia. Oncology 1997;11:1295.

The Italian Cooperative Study Group on Chronic Myeloid Leukemia: Interferon alfa-2a as compared with conventional chemotherapy for the treatment of chronic myeloid leukemia. N Engl J Med 1994;330:820.

Kantarjian HM et al: Treatment of chronic myelogenous leukemia: Current status and investigational options. Blood 1996;87:3069.

BRAIN TUMORS

Essentials of Diagnosis & Typical Features

- Classic triad: morning headache, vomiting, and papilledema.
- Increasing head circumference, cranial nerve palsies, dysarthria, ataxia, hemiplegia, papilledema, hyperreflexia, macrocephaly, cracked pot sign.
- Seizures, personality change, blurred vision, diplopia, weakness, decreased coordination, precocious puberty.

General Considerations

The classic triad of morning headache, vomiting, and papilledema is present in < 30% of children at presentation. School failure and personality changes are common in the older child. Irritability, failure to thrive, and delayed development are common in the very young. Recent-onset head tilt can result from a posterior fossa tumor.

Brain tumors are the most common solid tumors of childhood, accounting for 1500–2000 new malignancies in children each year in the United States and for 25–30% of all childhood cancers. In general, children with brain tumors have a better prognosis than adults. Favorable outcome occurs most commonly with low-grade and fully resectable tumors. Unfortunately, cranial irradiation in young children can have significant neuropsychologic, intellectual, and endocrinologic sequelae.

Brain tumors in childhood are biologically and histologically heterogeneous, ranging from low-grade localized lesions to high-grade tumors with neuraxis dissemination. High-dose systemic chemotherapy is being used more frequently, especially in young children with high-grade tumors, in an effort to delay, decrease, or completely avoid cranial irradiation. Such intensive treatment may be accompanied by autologous bone marrow transplantation or peripheral stem cell reconstitution.

The causes of pediatric brain tumors are unknown. The risk of developing astrocytomas is increased in children with neurofibromatosis or tuberous sclerosis. Several studies show that some childhood brain tumors occur in families with increased genetic susceptibility to childhood cancers in general, brain tumors, or leukemia and lymphoma. An excess of seizures has been observed in relatives of children with astrocytoma. Certain pediatric brain tumors such as ependymoma have been linked to polyomavirus, but the exact relationship remains to be elucidated. The risk of developing a brain tumor is increased in children who received cranial irradiation for treatment of meningeal leukemia.

Because pediatric brain tumors are rare, they are often misdiagnosed or diagnosed late; most pediatricians see no more than two children with brain tumors during their careers.

Clinical Findings

A. Symptoms and Signs: Clinical findings at presentation vary depending on the age of the child and the location of the tumor. Children under 2 years of age more commonly have infratentorial tumors. They usually present with nonspecific symptoms such as vomiting, unsteadiness, lethargy, and irritability. Signs may be surprisingly few or may include macrocephaly, ataxia, hyperreflexia, and cranial nerve palsies. Because the head can expand in young children, papilledema is usually absent. Measuring head circumference and observing gait are essential in evaluating a child for possible brain tumor. Eye findings and apparent visual disturbances such as difficulty tracking can be seen in optic pathway tumors such as optic glioma. Optic glioma occurring in a young child is often associated with neurofibromatosis.

Older children more commonly have supratentorial tumors, which present with headache, visual symptoms, seizures, and focal neurologic deficits. Initial presenting features are often nonspecific. School failure and personality changes are common. Vaguely described visual disturbance is often present, but the child must be directly asked. Headaches are common, but they often will not be predominantly in the morning. The headaches may be confused with migraine.

Infratentorial tumors in older children characteristically present with symptoms and signs of hydrocephalus, which include progressively worsening morning headache and vomiting, gait unsteadiness, double vision, and papilledema. Cerebellar astrocytomas enlarge slowly, and symptoms may worsen over several months. Morning vomiting may be the only symptom of posterior fossa ependymomas, which originate in the floor of the fourth ventricle near the vomiting center. Brain stem tumors may present with facial and extraocular muscle palsies, ataxia, and hemiparesis; hydrocephalus occurs in approximately 25% of these patients at diagnosis.

B. Imaging and Staging: In addition to the tumor biopsy, neuraxis imaging studies are obtained to determine whether dissemination has occurred. It is unusual for brain tumors in children and adolescents to disseminate outside of the CNS. Bone marrow aspirates and biopsies should be considered in children with newly diagnosed medulloblastoma or primitive neuroectodermal tumor, whose tumors are widely disseminated in the neuraxis at diagnosis.

MRI has become the preferred diagnostic study for pediatric brain tumors. MRI provides better definition of the tumor and delineates indolent gliomas that may not be seen on CT scan. On the other hand, a CT scan can be done in 15 minutes as opposed to 45 minutes for MRI and is still useful if an urgent diagnostic study is necessary or to detect calcification of a tumor. Both scans are generally done with and without contrast enhancement. Contrast enhances regions where the blood-brain barrier is disrupted. Postoperative scans to document the extent of tumor resection should be obtained within 48 hours after surgery to avoid postsurgical enhancement.

Imaging of the entire neuraxis and cerebrospinal fluid cytologic examination should be part of the diagnostic evaluation for patients with tumors such as medulloblastoma, ependymoma, and pineal region tumors. Diagnosis of neuraxis "drop metastases" can be accomplished by conventional myelography or, more recently and less invasively, by gadolinium-enhanced MRI incorporating sagittal and axial views. Cerebrospinal fluid should be obtained during the diagnostic surgery. Lumbar CSF is preferred over ventricular CSF for cytologic examination. Levels of biomarkers in the blood and cerebrospinal fluid, such as human chorionic gonadotropin (hCG) and alpha-fetoprotein (AFP), may be helpful at diagnosis and in follow-up. hCG and AFP should be obtained from the blood preoperatively for all pineal and suprasellar tumors.

The neurosurgeon should discuss staging and sample collection with an oncologist before surgery in a newly presenting child with a scan suggestive of brain tumor.

C. Classification: About 50% of the common pediatric brain tumors occur above the tentorium and 50% in the posterior fossa. In the very young child, posterior fossa tumors are more common. Most childhood brain tumors can be divided by the cell of origin into glial tumors (astrocytomas and ependymomas) or nonglial tumors such as medulloblastoma and other primitive neuroectodermal tumors. Some tumors contain both glial and neural elements (eg, ganglioglioma). There are also a group of less common CNS tumors that do not fit into this classification (craniopharyngiomas, germ cell tumors, choroid plexus tumors, and meningiomas). Low-grade and high-grade tumors are found in most categories. Table 26–3 sets forth the location and frequency of the common pediatric brain tumors.

Astrocytoma is the most common brain tumor of childhood. Most are low-grade tumors found in the posterior fossa with a bland cellular morphology and

Table 26–3. Location and frequency of common pediatric brain tumors.

Location	Frequency of Occurrence
Hemispheric	**37%**
Low-grade astrocytoma	23%
High-grade astrocytoma	11%
Other	3%
Posterior fossa	**49%**
Medulloblastoma	15%
Cerebellar astrocytoma	15%
Brain stem glioma	15%
Ependymoma	4%
Midline	**14%**
Craniopharyngioma	8%
Chiasmal glioma	4%
Pineal region tumor	2%

few or no mitotic figures. Low-grade astrocytomas are in many cases curable by complete surgical excision alone. The utility of chemotherapy, however, is increasingly being recognized in low-grade astrocytomas.

Medulloblastoma and related primitive neuroectodermal tumors are the most common high-grade brain tumors in children. These tumors usually occur in the first decade of life, with a peak incidence between 5 and 10 years of age and a 2.1:1.3 female-to-male ratio. These tumors typically arise in the midline cerebellar vermis, with variable extension into the fourth ventricle. Reports of neuraxis dissemination at diagnosis range from 10% to 46% of patients. Prognostic factors are outlined in Table 26–4.

Brain stem tumors are third in frequency of occurrence in children. They are frequently of astrocytic origin and often are high-grade. The tumors that diffusely infiltrate the brain stem and involve primarily the pons have a long-term survival rate of less than 15%. Brain stem tumors that occur above or below the pons and grow in an eccentric or cystic manner

Table 26–4. Prognostic factors in children with medulloblastoma.

Factor	Favorable	Unfavorable
Extent of disease	Nondisseminated	Disseminated
Size of primary tumor after surgery	≤ 3 cm (completely resected)	> 3 cm
Histologic features	Undifferentiated	Foci of glial, ependymal, or neuronal differentiation
Age	≥ 4 years	< 4 years

have a somewhat better outcome. Exophytic tumors in this location may be amenable to surgery. Generally, brain stem tumors are treated without a tissue diagnosis.

Other brain tumors such as ependymomas, germ cell tumors, choroid plexus tumors, and craniopharyngiomas are less common, and each is associated with unique diagnostic and therapeutic challenges.

Treatment

A. Supportive Care: Dexamethasone should be started prior to initial surgery (0.5–1 mg/kg initially, then 0.25–0.5 mg/kg/d in four divided doses). Anticonvulsants (usually phenytoin, 4–8 mg/kg/d) should be started if the child has had a seizure or if the surgical approach is likely to induce seizures. As postoperative treatment of young children with high-grade brain tumors incorporates increasingly more intensive systemic chemotherapy, consideration should also be given to the use of prophylaxis for prevention of oral candidiasis and *Pneumocystis* infection.

Optimum care for the pediatric brain tumor patient requires a multidisciplinary team including subspecialists in pediatric neurosurgery, neuro-oncology, neurology, endocrinology, neuropsychology, radiation therapy, and rehabilitation medicine as well as highly specialized nurses, social workers, and staff in physical therapy, occupational therapy, and speech and language science.

B. Specific Therapy: The goal of treatment is to eradicate the tumor with the least short- and long-term morbidity. Long-term neuropsychologic morbidity becomes an especially important issue related to deficits caused by the tumor itself and the sequelae of treatment. Meticulous surgical removal of as much tumor as possible is generally the preferred initial approach. Technologic advances in the operating microscope, the ultrasonic tissue aspirator, the CO_2 laser (the latter less commonly used in pediatric brain tumor surgery), the accuracy of computerized stereotactic resection, and intraoperative monitoring techniques such as evoked potentials and electrocorticography have increased the feasibility and safety of surgical resection of many pediatric brain tumors. Second-look surgery after chemotherapy is increasingly being used when tumors are incompletely resected at initial surgery.

Radiation therapy for pediatric brain tumors is in a state of evolution. For tumors (such as medulloblastoma) with a high probability of neuraxis dissemination, craniospinal radiation is still standard therapy in children over 3 years of age. In others, such as ependymoma, craniospinal radiation has been abandoned because neuraxis dissemination at first relapse is rare. Approaches to the delivery of radiation to minimize the adverse effects on normal brain are being explored and include hyperfractionation, stereo-

tactic radiation such as the "gamma knife," implantation of interstitial seeds, and use of three-dimensional treatment planning.

Chemotherapy is effective in treating malignant astrocytomas, medulloblastomas, and ependymomas. A series of brain tumor protocols for children under age 3 years involved administering intensive chemotherapy after tumor resection and delaying or omitting radiation therapy. The results of these trials have generally been disappointing. Future trials may give shorter courses of chemotherapy followed by conformal radiotherapy. Conformal techniques allow the delivery of radiation to strictly defined fields and may limit side effects.

In the older child with malignant glioma, the present approach would be surgical resection of the tumor and combined modality treatment with irradiation and intensive chemotherapy. In patients with glioblastoma, the use of high-dose chemotherapy and autologous bone marrow or peripheral stem cell reconstitution is being studied. Surgery is not indicated for diffuse brain stem gliomas. Traditional treatment of these tumors has been local irradiation. Hyperfractionation to increase the dose from the conventional 54 Gy to 72–78 Gy unfortunately showed no apparent benefit in a recent Children's Cancer Group study. New approaches are needed for this prognostically poor tumor.

The treatment of low-grade astrocytomas is also undergoing a process of evolution. Increasing numbers of young children are treated with antitumor chemotherapeutic agents such as carboplatin and vincristine after incomplete resection of these tumors. The role of irradiation after subtotal resection even in the older child is being questioned. A combined CCG/POG study is currently evaluating two different chemotherapy regimens in the treatment of progressive low grade astrocytomas.

Prognosis

Despite improvements in surgery and radiation therapy, the outlook for cure remains poor for children with high-grade brain tumors. For children with high-grade gliomas, an early CCG study showed a 45% progression-free survival rate for children who received radiation therapy and chemotherapy. A follow-up CCG study in which all patients had chemotherapy and radiation therapy showed a 5-year progression-free survival rate of 36%. There is a possibility of effective salvage therapy with high-dose chemotherapy for children who relapse. In addition, the extent of resection appeared to correlate positively with prognosis, with a 3-year progression-free survival rate of 17% for biopsy-only patients, 29–32% for partially or subtotally resected patients, and 54% for those with 90% resections.

The 5- and even 10-year survival rate for low-grade astrocytomas of childhood is 60–90%. However, prognosis depends on both site and grade. A child with a pilocytic astrocytoma of the cerebellum has a considerably better prognosis than a child with a fibrillary astrocytoma of the cerebral cortex. For recurrent or progressive low-grade astrocytoma of childhood, relatively moderate chemotherapy may improve survival.

Conventional craniospinal irradiation for children with low-stage medulloblastoma results in survival rates of 60–90%. Ten-year survival rates are lower (40–60%). Chemotherapy may allow a reduction in the craniospinal radiation dose while preserving survival rates. Five-year survival rates for "poor-risk" medulloblastoma have been 25–40%, but a recent publication reported an 87% survival rate for those treated with chemotherapy and radiation therapy. Children with supratentorial primitive neuroectodermal tumors may also benefit from the addition of chemotherapy to craniospinal radiation.

Finlay JL et al: A pilot study of high-dose thiotepa and etoposide with autologous bone marrow rescue in children and young adults with recurrent central nervous system tumors. J Clin Oncol 1996;14:2495.

Foremen NK et al: Second-look surgery for incompletely resected fourth ventricle ependymomas. Neurosurgery 1997;40;856.

Goldwein JW et al: Update results of a pilot study for low dose craniospinal irradiation plus chemotherapy for children under five with cerebellar primitive neuroectodermal tumors (medulloblastoma). Int J Radiat Oncol Biol Phys 1996;34:899.

LYMPHOMAS

1. HODGKIN'S DISEASE

Essentials of Diagnosis & Typical Features

- Painless cervical (70–80%) or supraclavicular (25%) adenopathy; mediastinal mass (50%).
- Fatigue, anorexia, weight loss, fever, night sweats, pruritus, cough.

General Considerations

Children with Hodgkin's disease have a better response to treatment than do adults, with a 75% overall survival at more than 20 years follow-up. While "adult" therapies are applicable, the management of Hodgkin's disease in children under 16 years of age frequently differs. Because excellent disease control can result from several different therapeutic approaches, selection of staging procedures and treatment are often based on the potential long-term toxicity associated with the intervention.

Although Hodgkin's disease represents 50% of the lymphomas of childhood, only 15% of all cases occur in children 16 years of age or younger. Children less than 5 years of age account for 3% of childhood cases, while 60% occur in the age group from 10 to

16 years of age. There is a 4:1 male predominance in the first decade.

Hodgkin's disease is a histologic diagnosis requiring the presence of the Reed-Sternberg cell or its variants. The histopathology of Hodgkin's disease is unique in that the bulk of the tumor is composed of normal cells, while the malignant Reed-Sternberg cells are relatively scanty. The origin of the malignant cell remains elusive.

Hodgkin's disease is subdivided into four histologic groups, and the distribution parallels that of adults: lymphocyte-predominant (10–20%); nodular sclerosing (40–60%) (increases with age); mixed cellularity (20–40%); and lymphocyte-depleted (5–10%). Prognosis is independent of subclassification, with appropriate therapy based on stage.

Clinical Findings

A. Symptoms and Signs: Painless cervical adenopathy is the usual presentation of Hodgkin's disease. The lymph nodes often feel firmer than inflammatory nodes and have a rubbery texture. They may be discrete or matted together and are not fixed to surrounding tissue. The growth rate is variable, and involved nodes may wax and wane in size over weeks to months.

As Hodgkin's disease nearly always arises in lymph nodes and spreads to contiguous nodal groups, a detailed examination of all nodal sites is mandatory. Lymphadenopathy is common in children, so the decision to perform biopsy is often difficult or delayed for a prolonged period. Indications for early lymph node biopsy include lack of identifiable infection in the region drained by the enlarged node, a node greater than 2 cm in size, supraclavicular adenopathy or abnormal chest x-ray, and lymphadenopathy increasing in size after 2 weeks or failing to resolve within 4–8 weeks.

Constitutional symptoms occur in about one-third of children at presentation. Symptoms of fever > 38 °C, weight loss of 10%, and drenching night sweats are defined by the Ann Arbor staging criteria as "B" symptoms. The "A" designation refers to the absence of these symptoms. "B" symptoms are of prognostic value, and more aggressive therapy is usually required for cure. Generalized pruritus and pain with alcohol ingestion may also occur.

Half of patients have asymptomatic mediastinal disease (adenopathy or anterior mediastinal mass), though symptoms due to compression of vital structures in the thorax may occur. A chest radiograph should be obtained when Hodgkin's disease is being considered. Airway competency must be thoroughly evaluated before any surgical procedure is undertaken to avoid airway obstruction during anesthesia and possible death. Splenomegaly and hepatomegaly (either or both) are generally associated with advanced disease.

B. Laboratory Findings: The blood count is

usually normal, though anemia, neutrophilia, eosinophilia, and thrombocytosis may be present. The erythrocyte sedimentation rate and other acute-phase reactants are often elevated and can serve as markers of disease activity. Immunologic abnormalities occur, particularly in cell-mediated immunity, and anergy is common in advanced-stage disease at diagnosis. Autoantibody phenomena such as hemolytic anemia and an idiopathic thrombocytopenic purpura-like picture have been reported.

C. Staging: A systematic search for thoracic disease includes chest radiography and computed tomography. Assessment of abdominal and pelvic disease is usually accomplished by CT, though lymphangiography may be more accurate. The lack of retroperitoneal fat in young children compromises the adequacy of CT imaging. Lymphangiography in children is variably successful depending on the skill and tenacity of the examiner.

Bilateral bone marrow aspirates and biopsies are performed. Technetium bone scanning may show bony involvement and is usually reserved for patients with bone pain, since bone involvement is rare. Gallium scanning defines gallium-avid tumors and is most useful in evaluating residual mediastinal disease at the completion of treatment.

The staging laparotomy in pediatrics is less important now than previously because almost all patients are given systemic chemotherapy. It is performed only if radiation therapy were the preferred treatment and the detection of abdominal disease would alter therapy. Excellent disease control with radiation therapy can be achieved in laparotomy-staged children, but this option must be weighed against the toxicities of high-dose, extended-field radiation in prepubertal children and the complications of laparotomy, including postsplenectomy sepsis. Reports linking splenectomy with secondary acute myelogenous leukemia following Hodgkin's disease therapy are particularly disturbing.

Treatment & Prognosis

To achieve long-term disease-free survival while minimizing treatment toxicity, Hodgkin's disease is increasingly treated by chemotherapy even in stage I and stage II disease—and less by radiation therapy.

Several combinations of chemotherapeutic agents are effective, but the most commonly used are MOPP (mechlorethamine, Oncovin [vincristine], procarbazine, and prednisone) and ABVD (Adriamycin [doxorubicin], bleomycin, vinblastine, and dacarbazine). These regimens are non-cross-resistant. When these schedules are alternated, exposure to an individual drug is decreased, and the toxicities associated with cumulative doses are minimized. Cyclophosphamide and cytarabine are also being used more.

Radiation continues to play a role in the treatment of childhood Hodgkin's disease, particularly in the control of residual disease following chemotherapy. Combined modality therapy appears to increase the cure rate. The role of radiation therapy at the end of chemotherapy when no residual disease is present is currently being evaluated in a randomized, cooperative, multicenter trial.

With current therapeutic approaches, it is expected that children with stage I and stage II Hodgkin's disease will have at least a 90% disease-free survival 5 years from diagnosis. Since two-thirds of all relapses occur within 2 years after diagnosis and since relapse rarely occurs beyond 4 years, 5-year disease-free survival generally equates with cure. In more advanced disease (stage III and stage IV), 5-year event-free survival ranges from over 60% to 90%.

Treatment of relapsed Hodgkin's disease involves radiation therapy in combination with chemotherapy. An alternative is autologous, stem cell, or allogeneic bone marrow transplantation. Although salvage therapy for Hodgkin's disease is relatively successful, this should not be a consideration in planning primary treatment.

Bierman PJ et al: Autologous transplantation for Hodgkin's disease: Coming of age? Blood 1994;83:1161.

Leventhal BG et al: Hodgkin's disease. In: *Principles and Practice of Pediatric Oncology.* Pizzo PA, Poplack DG (editors). Lippincott, 1997.

Mauch PM: Controversies in the management of early stage Hodgkin's disease. Blood 1994;83:318.

Shankar AG et al: Does histology influence outcome in childhood Hodgkin's disease? Results from the United Kingdom Children's Cancer Study Group. J Clin Oncol 1997;15:2622.

2. NON-HODGKIN'S LYMPHOMA

Essentials of Diagnosis & Typical Features

- Cough, dyspnea, swelling of the face; abdominal pain, abdominal distention, vomiting, constipation.
- Lymphadenopathy, mediastinal mass, pleural effusion, abdominal mass, ascites, hepatosplenomegaly.

General Considerations

Non-Hodgkin's lymphomas are a diverse group accounting for 7–13% of malignancies in children less than 15 years of age (about 390 new cases per year in the United States). In equatorial Africa, non-Hodgkin's lymphoma causes almost 50% of pediatric malignancies. The incidence of non-Hodgkin's lymphoma increases with age. Children 15 years of age or younger account for only 3% of all cases of non-Hodgkin's lymphoma; it is uncommon before 5 years of age. There is a male predominance of approximately 3:1.

Children with congenital or acquired immune deficiencies (eg, Wiskott-Aldrich syndrome, severe combined immunodeficiency syndrome, X-linked lymphoproliferative syndrome, HIV infection, immunosuppressive therapy following solid organ or marrow transplantation) have an increased risk of developing non-Hodgkin's lymphoma. It has been estimated that the risk is 100–10,000 times that of age-matched controls.

Most children who develop non-Hodgkin's lymphoma have no underlying immune defect. Animal models support a viral contribution to pathogenesis. In equatorial Africa, 95% of Burkitt's lymphomas contain Epstein-Barr viral (EBV) DNA. But in North America, less than 20% of Burkitt's tumors contain the EBV genome. Disturbances in host immunologic defenses, perhaps as a consequence of viral infection, chronic immunostimulation, and specific chromosomal rearrangements, are all under investigation as potential triggers in the development of non-Hodgkin's lymphoma.

Pediatric non-Hodgkin's lymphomas are classified by histology into three main groups: lymphoblastic lymphoma, small non-cleaved cell lymphoma (endemic or sporadic Burkitt's lymphoma), and large cell lymphoma (Table 26–5). Malignant lymphoma cells retain features similar to those of the lymphoid lineage cell from which they are derived. Cell membrane markers can therefore help clarify the origins of these cancers and serve as an adjunct to histologic classification. Typically, lymphoblastic lymphoma is associated with T cell surface markers, whereas small non-cleaved cell lymphomas have a B cell phenotype such as surface immunoglobulins. The large cell lymphomas, which make up less than 15% of pediatric non-Hodgkin's lymphomas, may show T cell, B cell, or histiocytic lineage.

Unlike adult non-Hodgkin's lymphoma, virtually all childhood non-Hodgkin's lymphomas are rapidly proliferating, diffuse malignancies arising from nodal or extranodal tissue. These tumors exhibit aggressive behavior but are usually very responsive to treatment.

Clinical Findings

A. Symptoms and Signs: Childhood non-Hodgkin's lymphomas can arise in any site of lymphoid tissue, including lymph nodes, Waldeyer's ring, Peyer's patches, thymus, liver, and spleen. Common extralymphatic sites include bone, bone marrow, CNS, skin, and testes. Signs and symptoms at presentation are determined by the location of lesions and the degree of dissemination. Because non-Hodgkin's lymphoma usually progresses very rapidly, the duration of symptoms is quite brief, from days to a few weeks. Nevertheless, children present with a limited number of syndromes, most of which correlate well with cell type.

Lymphoblastic lymphoma typically presents with symptoms of airway compression (cough, dyspnea, orthopnea) or superior venal caval obstruction (facial edema, chemosis, plethora, venous engorgement) which are a result of mediastinal disease. *These symptoms are a true emergency necessitating rapid diagnosis and treatment.* Pleural and/or pericardia effusions may further compromise the patient's respi-

Table 26–5. Comparison of pediatric non-Hodgkin's lymphomas.

	Lymphoblastic Lymphoma	Small Non-Cleaved Cell Lymphoma	Large Cell Lymphoma
Incidence	30–40%	40–50%	≤ 15%
Histopathologic features	Indistinguishable from ALL lymphoblasts.	Large nucleus with prominent nucleoli surrounded by very basophilic cytoplasm that contains lipid vacuoles.	Large cells with cleaved or noncleaved nuclei.
Immunophenotype	Immature T cell	B cell	B cell, T cell, or histiocyte
Cytogenetic markers	Translocations involving chromosome 14q11 and chromosome 7; interstitial deletions of chromosome 1.	t(8;14), t(8;22), t(2;8)	t(2;5)
Clinical presentation	Intrathoracic tumor, mediastinal mass (50–70%), lymphadenopathy above diaphragm (50–80%).	Intra-abdominal tumor (90%), jaw involvement (10–20% sporadic Burkitt's, 70% epidemic Burkitt's). Bone marrow involvement.	Abdominal tumor most common; unusual sites: lung, face, brain, skin, testes, muscle.
Treatment	Similar to therapy for ALL; 15–18 months' duration	Intensive administration of alkylating agents and intermediate- to high-dose methotrexate; intensive CNS prophylaxis; 6–9 months' duration.	Similar to therapy for small non-cleaved cell lymphomas.

ALL = acute lymphoblastic leukemia.

ratory status. CNS and bone marrow involvement are not common at diagnosis. When bone marrow contains more than 25% lymphoblasts, patients are considered to have acute lymphoblastic leukemia.

Ninety percent of small non-cleaved cell lymphomas present with abdominal disease. Abdominal pain, distention, a right lower quadrant mass, or intussusception in a child older than 5 years of age all suggest the diagnosis of small non-cleaved cell lymphoma (Burkitt's lymphoma). Bone marrow involvement is common (up to 65% of patients). Burkitt's lymphoma is the most rapidly proliferating tumor known and has a high rate of spontaneous cell death as it outgrows its blood supply. Consequently, children with massive abdominal disease frequently have metabolic abnormalities at presentation (hyperuricemia, hyperphosphatemia, and hyperkalemia). Impaired renal function because of tumor infiltration, urinary obstruction by tumor, or urate nephropathy further worsen the biochemical derangements of this life-threatening syndrome of acute tumor lysis. Although similar histologically, there are numerous differences between cases of Burkitt's lymphoma occurring in endemic areas of equatorial Africa and the sporadic cases of North America (Table 26–6).

Large cell lymphomas are similar clinically to the small non-cleaved cell lymphomas, though unusual sites of involvement are more common.

B. Diagnostic Evaluation: Diagnosis is by biopsy with histology, immunophenotyping, and cytogenetic studies. If mediastinal disease is present, anesthesia must be avoided if the airway or vena cava is compromised by tumor. Samples of pleural or ascitic fluid, bone marrow, or peripheral nodes obtained under local anesthesia may provide the diagnosis. Following the diagnosis of non-Hodgkin's lymphoma, studies should be obtained to determine the extent of disease. The rapid growth of these tumors and the life-threatening complications demand that studies be done expeditiously so that specific therapy is not delayed.

Table 26–6. Comparison of endemic and sporadic Burkitt's lymphoma.

	Endemic	**Sporadic**
Incidence	10 per 100,000	0.9 per 100,000
Cytogenetics	Chromosome 8 breakpoint upstream of c-*myc* locus	Chromosome 8 breakpoint within c-*myc* locus
EBV association	≥ 95%	≤ 20%
Disease sites at presentation	Jaw (58%), abdomen (58%), CNS (19%), orbit (11%), marrow (7%)	Jaw (7%), abdomen (91%), CNS (14%), orbit (1%), marrow (20%)

EBV = Epstein-Barr virus.

After a thorough physical examination, a CBC, liver and renal function tests, and a biochemical profile (electrolytes, calcium, phosphorus, uric acid) should be obtained. The LDH concentration reflects tumor burden and can serve as a marker of disease activity. Imaging studies should include a chest radiograph and chest CT scan if the plain films are abnormal, an abdominal ultrasound or CT scan, and possibly a gallium scan. Bone marrow and cerebrospinal fluid examinations are also essential.

Treatment

A. Supportive Care: The management of life-threatening problems at presentation is critical. The most common complications are the superior mediastinal syndrome and the acute tumor lysis syndrome. Patients with airway compromise require prompt initiation of specific therapy. Because of the risk of general anesthesia in these patients—and if a specific diagnosis cannot be made from peripheral studies—it is occasionally necessary to initiate steroids or low-dose radiation until the mass is small enough for a biopsy to be undertaken safely. Response to steroids and radiation is usually prompt (12–24 hours).

The tumor lysis syndrome should be anticipated in all non-Hodgkin's lymphoma patients with extensive disease. Maintaining a brisk urine output (> 3 mL/kg/h) with intravenous fluids and diuretics is the key to management. Allopurinol will reduce serum uric acid, and alkalinization of urine will increase its solubility. Because phosphate precipitates in an alkaline urine, alkali administration should be discontinued if hyperphosphatemia occurs. Renal dialysis may be necessary to control metabolic abnormalities. Every attempt should be made to correct or minimize metabolic abnormalities before initiating chemotherapy. However, this period of stabilization should not exceed 24–48 hours.

B. Specific Therapy: Chemotherapy is the bulwark of therapy for non-Hodgkin's lymphomas. Surgery has little to offer unless the entire tumor can be resected, which is rare. There is no role for partial resection or debulking surgery. Radiation therapy also has little to offer. Its use is confined to exceptional circumstances.

Therapy for lymphoblastic lymphoma is generally based on treatment protocols designed for ALL. Anthracyclines are usually an integral agent in effective treatment regimens for lymphoblastic lymphoma; cytarabine, etoposide, and teniposide are emerging as promising agents. Duration of therapy is determined by disease extent. Localized disease is treated for 6 months, whereas extensive disease is treated for 15 months.

Small non-cleaved cell lymphomas do not respond well to therapy based on ALL protocols even when bone marrow is involved. Protocols using alkylating agents and intermediate- to high-dose methotrexate administered on an intensive schedule produce the highest cure rates. Large cell lymphomas are treated similarly.

All non-Hodgkin's lymphoma patients require intensive intrathecal chemotherapy for prophylaxis.

Prognosis

A major predictor of outcome in non-Hodgkin's lymphoma is the extent of disease at diagnosis. Ninety percent of patients with localized disease can expect long-term disease-free survival, while patients with extensive disease on both sides of the diaphragm, CNS involvement, or bone marrow involvement in addition to a primary site have a 70–80% failure-free survival. Relapses occur early in non-Hodgkin's lymphoma; patients with lymphoblastic lymphoma rarely have recurrences after 30 months from diagnosis, whereas patients with small non-cleaved cell lymphomas essentially never have recurrences beyond 1 year.

Patients who experience relapse may have a chance for cure by autologous or allogeneic bone marrow transplantation.

Link MP et al: Treatment of children and young adults with early-stage non-Hodgkin's lymphoma. N Engl J Med 1997;337:1259.

Magrath I: Malignant non-Hodgkin's lymphomas in children. In: *Principles and Practice of Pediatric Oncology.* Pizzo PA, Poplack DG (editors). Lippincott, 1993.

Sandlund JT et al: Non-Hodgkin's lymphoma in childhood. N Engl J Med 1996;334:1238.

Toogood IRG et al: Effective multi-agent chemotherapy for advanced abdominal lymphoma and FAB L3 leukemia of childhood. Pediatr Oncol 1993;21:103.

NEUROBLASTOMA

Essentials of Diagnosis & Typical Features

- Bone pain, abdominal pain, anorexia, weight loss, fatigue, fever, irritability.
- Abdominal mass (65%), adenopathy, proptosis, periorbital ecchymosis, skull masses, subcutaneous nodules, hepatomegaly, spinal cord compression.

General Considerations

Neuroblastoma arises from neural crest tissue of the sympathetic ganglia or adrenal medulla. It is composed of small, fairly uniform cells with little cytoplasm and hyperchromatic nuclei that may form rosette patterns. Pathologic diagnosis is not always easy, and neuroblastoma must be differentiated from the other "small, round, blue cell" malignancies of childhood (Ewing's sarcoma, rhabdomyosarcoma, peripheral neuroepithelioma, lymphoma).

Neuroblastoma accounts for 7–10% of pediatric malignancies and is the most common solid neoplasm outside the CNS. Fifty percent of neuroblastomas are diagnosed in the first 2 years of life and 90% before age 5.

The biologic diversity of neuroblastoma makes this a fascinating tumor for study. Spontaneous regression in stage IV-S disease and spontaneous or induced differentiation to a benign neoplasm are examples of the unique behavior of this tumor. Unfortunately, neuroblastoma is also an extremely malignant neoplasm, and the overall survival in advanced disease has changed little in 20 years despite significant advances in our understanding of this tumor at a cellular and molecular level.

Clinical Findings

A. Symptoms and Signs: Clinical manifestations vary with the primary site of metastatic disease and the neuroendocrine function of the tumor. Many children present with constitutional symptoms such as fever, weight loss, and irritability. Bone pain suggests metastatic disease, which is present in 70% of children older than 1 year at diagnosis. Physical examination may reveal a firm, fixed, irregularly shaped mass that extends beyond the midline. The margins are often poorly defined. Although most children have an abdominal primary (40% adrenal gland, 25% paraspinal ganglion), neuroblastoma can arise wherever there is sympathetic tissue. In the posterior mediastinum, it is usually asymptomatic and discovered on a chest x-ray obtained for other reasons. Cervical neuroblastoma presents with a neck mass, often misdiagnosed as infection. Horner's syndrome or heterochromia iridis may accompany cervical neuroblastoma. Paraspinal tumors can extend through the spinal foramina, causing cord compression. Patients may present with paresis, paralysis, and bowel or bladder dysfunction.

The most common sites of metastases are bone, bone marrow, lymph nodes (regional as well as disseminated), liver, and subcutaneous tissue. Neuroblastoma has a predilection for metastasis to the skull, in particular the sphenoid bone and retrobulbar tissue. This causes orbital ecchymosis and proptosis. Liver metastasis, particularly in the newborn, can be massive. Subcutaneous nodules are bluish in color and associated with an erythematous flush followed by blanching when compressed, probably secondary to catecholamine release.

Neuroblastoma may also be associated with unusual paraneoplastic manifestations. Examples include chronic watery diarrhea associated with tumor secretion of vasoactive intestinal peptides and opsoclonus-myoclonus (dancing eyes, dancing feet). It is postulated that the neurologic manifestations are secondary to cross-reacting antibodies.

B. Laboratory Findings: Anemia is present in 60% of children with neuroblastoma and can be due to "chronic disease" or marrow infiltration. Thrombocytopenia may be present, but thrombocytosis is more common, even with metastatic disease in the marrow. Measures of tumor markers have prognostic significance and provide parameters for follow-up. LDH and ferritin can be elevated at diagnosis. Urinary catecholamines (vanillylmandelic acid, homovanillic acid) are elevated in at least 90% of patients at diagnosis and should be measured prior to surgery.

C. Imaging: Plain films or CT of the primary tumor may show stippled calcifications. CT scanning can evaluate the extent of the primary tumor, its effects on surrounding structures, and the presence of liver and lymph node metastases. Classically, in primary tumors originating from the adrenal, the kidney is displaced inferolaterally, which helps to differentiate neuroblastoma from Wilms' tumor. MRI is useful to evaluate for the presence of spinal cord involvement in tumors that appear to invade neural foramina.

Both skeletal survey and radionuclide bone scanning are obtained in the evaluation of bone metastases. On plain films, lesions are usually symmetric and appear irregular and lytic. Periosteal reaction and pathologic fractures may also be seen.

D. Staging: First a tissue diagnosis must be established and then the disease extent determined. In addition to the previously mentioned studies, bilateral bone marrow aspirates and biopsies are essential in evaluating for metastatic disease even if the CBC is normal. The appearance of neuroblastoma in the bone marrow may simulate the appearance of acute lymphoblastic leukemia; differentiation can be accomplished by monoclonal antibody phenotyping.

Molecular parameters are essential to supplement clinical staging and aid in treatment planning. Amplification of the N-*myc* proto-oncogene or its gene product can be detected in tumor tissue. Rapid disease progression is associated with N-*myc* amplification and necessitates aggressive therapy. Tumor DNA content is determined by flow cytometry. Hyperdiploidy is a favorable finding, whereas near-diploid DNA content is associated with advanced disease and a poor outcome. Double-minute chromosomes and homogeneous staining regions of DNA, manifestations of gene amplification, along with deletion of the short arm of chromosome 1, are cytogenetic characteristics of neuroblastoma.

Treatment & Prognosis

Since prognosis is independently influenced by age at diagnosis and stage of disease, both factors are taken into consideration when deciding on a treatment plan. Infants less than 1 year of age with stage 4S disease (small primary, with metastasis confined to liver, skin, or bone marrow) may need little if any therapy to effect a cure, though treatment may be initiated because of bulky disease causing mechanical complications.

Therapy is usually multimodal and involves surgery, radiation therapy, and chemotherapy. Bone marrow transplantation is being investigated as a means of improving the currently poor outcome for advanced neuroblastoma. Initial surgical efforts are aimed at resecting the primary tumor when feasible. The usually massive size of the tumor makes primary resection often impossible. Under these circumstances, only a biopsy may be performed. Following chemotherapy, a second surgical procedure may allow for resection of the primary tumor. Radiation may be given intraoperatively at the time of resection or postoperatively by external beam radiation therapy.

Effective chemotherapeutic agents in the treatment of neuroblastoma include cyclophosphamide, doxorubicin, etoposide, cisplatin, and vincristine. There is a clear dose-response relationship in neuroblastoma. About 80% of patients achieve complete or partial remission, though in advanced disease this is seldom durable. A current Children's Cancer Study Group (CCSG) treatment protocol compares aggressive conventional chemotherapy with chemotherapy plus autologous bone marrow transplantation. Clinical trials are also under way using radioactive monoclonal antibodies such as ^{131}I-meta-iodobenzylguanidine (MIBG) and [131]I-3F8 (a murine IgG antibody specific for ganglioside GD2, the predominant antigen on neuroblastoma cells). In another promising area of research, attempts are being made to manipulate the patient's immune system to eradicate residual disease.

For children with stage 1, 2, or 4S disease, the 5-year survival rate is 70–90%. Infants under 1 year of age who have stage 4 disease have a greater than 60% likelihood of long-term survival. Children over 1 year of age with stage 3 disease have an intermediate prognosis (approximately 40–70%), and those with stage 4 disease have a poor prognosis (5–20% survival 5 years from diagnosis).

Brodeur GM et al: Biology and genetics of human neuroblastomas. J Pediatr Hematol Oncol 1997;19:93.

Brodeur GM et al: Neuroblastoma. In: *Principles and Practice of Pediatric Oncology.* Pizzo PA, Poplack DG: (editors). Lippincott, 1997.

Kushner BH et al: Survival from locally invasive or widespread neuroblastoma without cytotoxic therapy. J Clin Oncol 1996;14:373.

Mattay KK et al: Allogenic versus autologous purge and bone marrow transplantation for neuroblastoma: A report from the Children's Cancer Study Group. J Clin Oncol 1994;12:2382.

Rubie H et al: N-*myc* gene amplification is a major prognostic factor in localized neuroblastoma: Results of the French NBL 90 study. J Clin Oncol 1997;15:1171.

WILMS' TUMOR (Nephroblastoma)

Essentials of Diagnosis & Typical Features

- Asymptomatic abdominal mass or swelling (83%).

- Fever (23%), hematuria (21%).
- Hypertension (25%), genitourinary malformations (6%), aniridia, hemihypertrophy.

General Considerations

Approximately 460 new cases of Wilms' tumor occur annually in the United States, representing 5–6% of cancers in children under 15 years of age. This is the second most common abdominal tumor in children following neuroblastoma. The tumor arises from kidney and is usually composed of three elements: blastema, epithelium, and stroma. The majority of Wilms' tumors are of sporadic occurrence. There are, however, several important associated malformations, syndromes, and cytogenetic disorders, including aniridia, hemihypertrophy, genitourinary malformations (eg, cryptorchism, hypospadias, gonadal dysgenesis, pseudohermaphroditism, horseshoe kidney), Beckwith-Wiedemann syndrome, Drash syndrome, and WAGR syndrome (Wilms', aniridia, ambiguous genitalia, mental retardation). Although most patients with Wilms' tumor are karyotypically normal, those with sporadic aniridia frequently have a constitutional deletion at the 11p13 locus. This deletion has also been found in the tumor cells of Wilms' patients without aniridia and who are karyotypically normal.

The median age at diagnosis is related both to gender and laterality, with bilateral tumors presenting at a younger age than unilateral tumors and males being diagnosed earlier than females. Wilms' tumor occurs most commonly between 2 and 5 years of age; it is unusual after 6 years of age. The mean age at diagnosis is 3 years.

Clinical Findings

A. Symptoms and Signs: Most children with Wilms' tumor present with increasing size of the abdomen or an abdominal mass incidentally discovered by a parent. The mass is usually smooth and firm, well demarcated, and rarely crosses the midline, though it can extend inferiorly into the pelvis. Gross hematuria is an uncommon presentation, though microscopic hematuria is found in approximately 25% of cases.

B. Laboratory Findings: The CBC is usually normal, but some patients have anemia secondary to hemorrhage into the tumor. BUN and serum creatinine are usually normal. Urinalysis may show some blood or leukocytes.

C. Staging: Ultrasonography or CT of the abdomen should establish the presence of an intrarenal mass. It is also essential to evaluate the contralateral kidney for presence and function as well as synchronous Wilms' tumor. The inferior vena cava needs to be evaluated for the presence and extent of tumor propagation. The liver should be imaged for the presence of metastatic disease. A plain chest radiograph (four views) should be obtained to determine whether pulmonary metastases are present. Approximately 10% of patients will have metastatic disease at diagnosis. Of these, 80% will have pulmonary disease and 15% liver metastases. Bone and brain metastases are very unusual and associated with certain unfavorable histologic types; hence, bone and brain scans are not routinely performed. The clinical stage is ultimately decided at surgery and confirmed by the pathologist.

Treatment & Prognosis

In the United States, treatment of Wilms' tumor begins with surgical exploration of the abdomen. The contralateral kidney is inspected and palpated for tumor involvement (one-third of patients with bilateral disease have no evidence of it on preoperative studies). The liver and lymph nodes are inspected and suspicious areas biopsied or excised. En bloc resection of tumor is performed. Every attempt is made to avoid tumor spillage at surgery. Because therapy is tailored to tumor stage, it is imperative that operation be done by a surgeon familiar with the staging requirements.

In addition to the staging, the histologic type has implications for therapy and prognosis. Favorable histology (FH; see below) refers to the class triphasic Wilms' tumor and its variants. Unfavorable histology (UH) refers to anaplasia, clear cell sarcoma of the kidney, and rhabdoid tumor of the kidney and is present in 10–12% of cases. Although clear cell sarcoma and rhabdoid tumor are no longer felt to be Wilms' tumor variants, these histologic types were identified in early Wilms' tumor studies as being associated with a worse outcome when compared with favorable histology tumors. Anaplasia is defined by extreme nuclear atypia. Only a few small foci of anaplasia in a Wilms' tumor is sufficient to impart a worse prognosis to stage II, III, or IV patients. Following excision and pathologic examination, the patient is assigned a stage that defines further therapy.

The progress and success in the treatment of Wilms' tumor is a result of the cooperative clinical trials of the National Wilms' Tumor Study (NWTS). Clinical trials that began in 1969 have resulted in an overall cure rate of approximately 90%. The NWTS-IV sought to further improve survival rate by intensifying therapy during the initial treatment phase while shortening overall treatment duration (6 versus 15 months of treatment). It is the first study of a pediatric population to evaluate the economic impact of two different treatment approaches.

Vincristine and dactinomycin are used in the treatment of all Wilms' tumor patients; doxorubicin is also administered to stage III and stage IV patients. NWTS-III showed that stage II Wilms' tumor patients did not benefit from flank irradiation, whereas stage III children had similar outcomes whether they received 10 Gy or 20 Gy. Chemotherapy is optimally begun within 5 days after surgery, whereas radiation therapy should be started within 10 days.

Using these approaches, survival at 4 years from diagnosis for patients treated on NWTS-III are as follows: stage I FH, 96.5%; stage II FH, 92.2%; stage III FH, 86.9%; and stage IV FH, 82.5%. Patients with unfavorable histology (UH) have only a 55–68% 4-year survival rate depending on stage. Patients with recurrent Wilms' tumor have approximately a 50% salvage rate with surgery, radiation therapy, and chemotherapy (singly or in combination). Bone marrow transplantation is also being explored as an way to improve the chances of survival post relapse.

Future Considerations

Although progress in the treatment of Wilms' tumor has been extraordinary, important questions remain to be answered. Questions are being raised about the role of prenephrectomy chemotherapy in the treatment of Wilms' tumor. Presurgical chemotherapy seems to decrease tumor rupture at resection but may unfavorably affect outcome by changing staging. Whether pulmonary radiation can be eliminated in metastatic pulmonary disease is also being investigated.

Beckwith JB: New developments in the pathology of Wilms tumor. Cancer Invest 1997;15:153.

Green DM et al: Wilms' tumor (nephroblastoma, renal embryoma). In: *Principles and Practice of Pediatric Oncology*. Pizzo PA, Poplack DG (editors). Lippincott, 1997.

Grundy P, Coppes M: An overview of the clinical and molecular genetics of Wilms' tumor. Med Pediatr Oncol 1996;27:394.

Paulino AC: Current issues in the diagnosis and management of Wilms' tumor. Oncology 1996;10:1553.

BONE TUMORS

Primary malignant bone tumors are uncommon in childhood. Osteosarcoma accounts for 60% of cases and is seen mostly in adolescents and young adults. Ewing's sarcoma is the second most common malignant tumor of bony origin. Both tumors have a male predominance.

The cardinal signs of bone tumor are pain at the site of involvement, often following slight trauma; mass formation; and fracture through an area of cortical bone destruction.

1. OSTEOSARCOMA

Although osteosarcoma is the sixth most common malignancy in childhood, it ranks third among adolescents and young adults. This peak occurrence during the adolescent growth spurt suggests a causal relationship between rapid bone growth and malignant transformation. Further evidence for this relationship is found in epidemiologic data showing patients with

osteosarcoma to be taller than their peers, osteosarcoma occurring most frequently at sites where the greatest increase in length and size of bone occurs, and osteosarcoma occurring at an earlier age in girls than boys, corresponding to their earlier growth spurt. Long tubular bones are primarily affected. The distal femur accounts for more than 40% of cases, with the proximal tibia, proximal humerus, and mid and proximal femur following in frequency. Typically, osteosarcoma arises in a metaphysis.

Radiographic findings show permeative destruction of the normal bony trabecular pattern with indistinct margins. In addition, periosteal new bone formation and lifting of the bony cortex may create a Codman triangle. A soft tissue mass plus calcifications in a radial or "sunburst" pattern are frequently noted. Despite this rather characteristic radiographic appearance, a tissue sample is needed to confirm the diagnosis. Radiographic studies to define the extent of the primary tumor include CT scan or MRI. A bone scan is useful for detecting "skip" lesions as well as distant bony metastasis (present in 10% of newly diagnosed patients). A chest CT scan is essential to look for lung metastases that are present in as many as 20% of patients at diagnosis and make the prognosis worse.

Placement of the incision for biopsy of a bone tumor is of critical importance. A misplaced incision could preclude a limb salvage procedure and necessitate amputation. Biopsy is best performed by the surgeon who would carry out the definitive surgical procedure. Histologically, osteosarcoma is characterized by the presence of malignant sarcomatous stroma associated with the production of tumor osteoid.

Once the diagnosis of osteosarcoma is established, treatment can be started. Over 70% of patients treated with surgery alone develop pulmonary metastases within 6 months after surgery. This suggests that micrometastatic disease is present at diagnosis though not detectable radiographically. Adjuvant chemotherapy trials have shown disease-free survival of 55–85% after 3–10 years of follow-up.

Chemotherapy is often administered prior to definitive surgery (neoadjuvant chemotherapy). This permits an early attack on micrometastatic disease. Presurgical chemotherapy may also shrink the tumor, facilitating a limb salvage procedure. Preoperative chemotherapy also makes possible detailed histologic evaluation of tumor response to the preoperative chemotherapeutic agents. If there is a poor histologic response, postoperative chemotherapy can be changed accordingly. Chemotherapy may be administered intra-arterially or intravenously. Agents having efficacy in the treatment of osteosarcoma include doxorubicin, cisplatin, high-dose methotrexate, and ifosfamide. A multi-agent regimen is most frequently employed.

Amputation and limb salvage are equally effective in achieving local control of osteosarcoma. Contraindications to limb-sparing surgery include major involvement of the neurovascular bundle by tumor; immature skeletal age, particularly for lower extremity tumors; infection in the region of the tumor; inappropriate biopsy site; and extensive muscle involvement that would result in a poor functional outcome.

Postsurgical chemotherapy is generally continued until the patient has received 1 year of treatment. Relapses are unusual beyond 3 years, but late relapses do occur. Histologic response to neoadjuvant chemotherapy is an excellent predictor of outcome. Patients having 90% tumor necrosis have a 70–90% long-term disease-free survival rate.

2. EWING'S SARCOMA

Ewing's sarcoma accounts for only 10% of primary malignant bone tumors; there are fewer than 200 new cases a year in the United States. It is a disease primarily of white males and almost never affects blacks.

The radiographic appearance of Ewing's sarcoma overlaps with osteosarcoma, though Ewing's sarcoma usually involves the diaphyses of long bones. The central axial skeleton gives rise to 40% of Ewing tumors.

Ewing's sarcoma is a "small, round, blue cell" malignancy. Although most commonly a tumor of bone, it may also occur in soft tissue (extraosseous Ewing's sarcoma or peripheral neuroepithelioma). Histologically, it consists of sheets of undifferentiated cells with hyperchromatic nuclei, well-defined cell borders, and scanty cytoplasm. Necrosis is common. The differential diagnosis includes rhabdomyosarcoma, lymphoma, and neuroblastoma. Electron microscopy, immunocytochemistry, and cytogenetics may be necessary to confirm the diagnosis. A generous tissue biopsy is often necessary for diagnosis but should not delay starting chemotherapy.

A consistent cytogenetic abnormality, t(11;22), has been identified in Ewing's sarcoma and in peripheral neuroepitheliomas. These tumors also express the proto-oncogene C-*myc*. Research suggests that these tumors arise from postganglionic parasympathetic cholinergic neurons.

Evaluation of a patient diagnosed with Ewing's sarcoma should include CT or MRI (or both) of the primary lesion to define the extent of local disease as precisely as possible. This is imperative for planning future surgical procedures or radiation therapy. Metastatic disease is present in 25% of patients at diagnosis. The lung (38%), bone (particularly the spine) (31%), and the bone marrow (11%) are the most common sites for metastasis. CT of the chest, bone scanning, and bilateral bone marrow aspirates and biopsies are all essential to the staging work-up.

Therapy usually commences with the administra-

tion of chemotherapy and is followed by local control measures. Depending on many factors, including the primary site of the tumor and the response to chemotherapy, local control could be achieved by surgery, radiation therapy, or a combination of these methods. Following local control, chemotherapy continues for 1 year. Agents that have been shown to have efficacy in the treatment of Ewing's sarcoma include dactinomycin, vincristine, doxorubicin, cyclophosphamide, etoposide, and ifosfamide. Modern therapy uses combinations of these drugs.

Patients with small localized primaries have a 50–70% long-term disease-free survival rate. For patients with metastatic disease and large pelvic primaries, survival is poor. Autologous bone marrow transplantation is being investigated for the management of these high-risk patients.

Damron TA, Pritchard DJ: Current combined treatment of high-grade osteosarcomas. Oncology 1995;9:327.

Horowitz ME et al: Ewing's sarcoma family of tumors: Ewing's sarcoma of bone and soft tissue and the peripheral primitive neuroectodermal tumors. In: *Principles and Practice of Pediatric Oncology.* Pizzo PA, Poplack DG (editors). Lippincott, 1997.

Link MP et al: Osteosarcoma. In: *Principles and Practice of Pediatric Oncology.* Pizzo PA, Poplack DG (editors). Lippincott, 1997.

RHABDOMYOSARCOMA

Essentials of Diagnosis & Typical Features

- Painless, progressively enlarging mass; proptosis; chronic drainage (nasal, aural, sinus, vaginal); cranial nerve palsies.
- Urinary obstruction, constipation, hematuria.

General Considerations

Rhabdomyosarcoma is the most common soft tissue sarcoma occurring in pediatrics and accounts for 10% of solid tumors in childhood. The peak incidence is between 2 and 5 years of age, with 70% of children diagnosed before 10 years of age. A second smaller peak is seen in adolescents with extremity tumors. Males are affected more commonly than females (1.4:1).

Arising from embryonic mesenchymal cells, rhabdomyosarcoma can occur anywhere in the body. When rhabdomyosarcoma imitates striated muscle and cross-striations are seen by light microscopy, the diagnosis is straightforward. Immunocytochemistry, electron microscopy, or chromosomal analysis is sometimes necessary to make the diagnosis. Rhabdomyosarcoma is further classified into subtypes based on pathologic features: embryonal (63%), of which botryoid is a variant; alveolar (19%); pleomorphic, which is seen in adults (1%); undifferentiated sarcoma (10%); and other (7%). These subtypes occur in characteristic locations and have different metastatic potentials and outcomes (Table 26–7).

Although the pathogenesis of rhabdomyosarcoma is unknown, in rare cases a genetic predisposition has been determined. Li-Fraumeni syndrome is an inherited mutation of the p53 tumor suppressor gene that results in a high risk of bone and soft tissue sarcomas in childhood plus breast cancer and other malignant neoplasms before age 45. A characteristic chromosomal translocation (t2;13) has been described in alveolar rhabdomyosarcoma, which may also shed light on the biology of this tumor.

Clinical Findings

A. Symptoms and Signs: The presenting signs and symptoms of rhabdomyosarcoma result from disturbances of normal body function due to tumor growth (Table 26–7). For example, orbital rhabdomyosarcoma presents as proptosis, while rhabdomyosarcoma of the bladder can present with hematuria, urinary obstruction, or a pelvic mass.

B. Imaging: A plain film as well as a CT scan or MRI should be obtained to determine the exact extent of the primary tumor and to assess regional lymph nodes. A lung CT is obtained to rule out pulmonary metastasis, the most common site of metastatic disease at diagnosis. A skeletal survey and a bone scan are obtained to determine whether bony metastasis is present. Bilateral bone marrow biopsies and aspirates are obtained to rule out bone marrow infiltration. Additional studies may be warranted in certain sites. For example, in parameningeal primaries, a lumbar puncture is performed to evaluate cerebrospinal fluid for tumor cells.

Treatment

Optimal management and treatment of children with rhabdomyosarcoma is complex and requires combined modality therapy. When feasible, the tumor should be excised, but this is not always possible because of site of origin and size of tumor. When only partial tumor resection is feasible, the operative procedure is usually limited to biopsy and sampling of lymph nodes. The role of debulking of unresectable tumor is unclear. Chemotherapy can often convert an inoperable tumor to a resectable one. A second-look procedure to remove residual disease and confirm the clinical response to chemotherapy and radiation therapy is generally performed at about week 20 of therapy.

Radiation therapy is an effective method of local tumor control for both microscopic and gross residual disease. It is generally administered to all patients, the only exception being group I nonalveolar rhabdomyosarcoma.

Chemotherapy is administered to all patients with rhabdomyosarcoma even when the tumor is fully resected at diagnosis. The exact regimen and duration of chemotherapy are determined by primary site, group, and TNM classification. Vincristine, dactinomycin, and cyclophosphamide have shown the greatest efficacy in the treatment of rhabdomyosarcoma.

Table 26–7. Characteristics of rhabdomyosarcoma.

Primary Site	Frequency	Symptoms and Signs	Three-Year Disease-Free Survival (Based on IRS-II)	Predominant Pathologic Subtype
Head and neck	**40%**			Embryonal
Orbit	10%	Proptosis	93%	
Parameningeal	20%	Cranial nerve palsies; aural or sinus obstruction with or without drainage	71%	
Other	10%	Painless, progressively enlarging mass	69%	
Genitourinary	**20%**			Embryonal (botryoid variant in bladder and vagina)
Bladder and prostate	12%	Hematuria, urinary obstruction	64–80%	
Vagina and uterus	2%	Pelvic mass, vaginal discharge	60–80%	
Paratesticular	6%	Painless mass	64–80%	
Extremities	**20%**	Adolescents, swelling of affected body part	56%	Alveolar (50%), undifferentiated
Trunk	**10%**	Mass	57%	Alveolar, undifferentiated

IRS = Intergroup Rhabdomyosarcoma Study.

Prognosis

The extent of tumor at diagnosis, the primary site, pathologic subtype, and response to treatment all influence long-term disease-free survival from the time of diagnosis. Children with localized disease in a favorable site have a 93% 3-year disease-free survival rate, whereas children with metastatic disease at presentation (group IV) have a poor outcome (Table 26–7).

Newer treatment strategies for high-risk patients include different drug combinations and dosing schedules, hematopoietic growth factor support, hyperfractionated radiation therapy, and autologous bone marrow transplantation.

Arndt C et al: A feasibility, toxicity, and early response study of etoposide, ifosfamide, and vincristine for the treatment of children with rhabdomyosarcoma: A report from the Intergroup Rhabdomyosarcoma Study IV pilot study. J Pediatr Hematol Oncol 1997;19:124.

Raney RB et al: Rhabdomyosarcoma and the undifferentiated sarcomas. In: *Principles and Practice of Pediatric Oncology.* Pizzo PA, Poplack DG (editors). Lippincott, 1997.

RETINOBLASTOMA

Retinoblastoma is a neuroectodermal malignancy arising from embryonic retinal cells and accounts for 3% of malignant disease in children under 15 years of age. It is the most common intraocular tumor in pediatric patients and causes 5% of cases of childhood blindness. There are 200–300 new cases per year in the United States. This is a malignancy of early childhood, with 90% of tumors diagnosed before 5 years of age. Bilateral disease typically presents at a younger age (median age 14 months) than unilateral disease (median age 23 months).

Retinoblastoma is the prototype of hereditary cancers due to mutation in the retinoblastoma gene *(RB1),* which is located on the long arm of chromosome 13 (13q14). This gene is a tumor suppressor gene or anti-oncogene that normally controls cellular growth. When the gene is inactivated, cellular growth is uncontrolled. Uncontrolled cell growth leads to tumor formation. Inactivation of both *RB1* alleles within the same cell is required for tumor formation.

Retinoblastoma is known to arise in heritable and nonheritable forms. Based on the different clinical characteristics of the two forms, Knudson proposed a two-mutation hypothesis for retinoblastoma tumor development. He postulated that two independent events were necessary for a cell to acquire tumor potential. Mutations at the *RB1* locus can be inherited or arise spontaneously. In heritable cases, the first mutation arises during gametogenesis, either spontaneously (90%) or through transmission from a parent (10%). This mutation is present in every retinal cell as well as all other somatic and germ cells. Ninety

percent of persons who carry this germline mutation will develop retinoblastoma. For tumor formation, the loss of the second *RB1* allele within a cell must occur; loss of only one allele is insufficient for tumor formation. The second mutation occurs in a somatic (retinal) cell. In nonheritable cases (60%), both mutations arise in a somatic cell after gametogenesis has taken place.

Clinical Findings

A. Symptoms and Signs: Children with retinoblastoma generally come to medical attention while the tumor is still confined to the globe. Although congenital, retinoblastoma is not usually detected until it has grown to a considerable size. Leukocoria (white pupillary reflex) is the most common manifestation (60% of cases). Parents may note an unusual appearance of the eye or asymmetry of the eyes in a photograph. The differential diagnosis of leukocoria includes *Toxocara canis* granuloma, astrocytic hamartoma, retinopathy of prematurity, Coats' disease, and persistent hyperplastic primary vitreous. Strabismus (20% of cases) is seen when tumor involves the macula and central vision is lost. Rarely (7% of cases), a painful red eye with glaucoma, a hyphema, or proptosis is the initial manifestation. A single focus or multiple foci of tumor may be seen in one or both eyes at diagnosis. Bilateral involvement occurs in 20–30% of children.

B. Evaluation: A child suspected of retinoblastoma must have a detailed ophthalmologic examination under anesthesia. An ophthalmologist makes the diagnosis of retinoblastoma by the appearance of the tumor within the eye without pathologic confirmation. A white to creamy pink mass protruding into the vitreous suggests the diagnosis; intraocular calcifications and vitreous seeding are virtually pathognomonic of retinoblastoma. A CT of the orbits detects intraocular calcification, evaluates the optic nerve for tumor infiltration, and detects extraocular extension of tumor. Metastatic disease of the marrow and meninges can be ruled out with a bone marrow aspirate and biopsy plus cerebrospinal fluid cytology. Under some circumstances, a bone scan or CT of the liver is indicated.

Treatment

Each eye is treated according to the potential for useful vision, and every attempt is made to preserve vision. The choice of therapy depends on the size, location, and number of intraocular lesions. Absolute indications for enucleation include no vision, neovascular glaucoma, inability to examine the treated eye, and inability to control tumor growth with conservative treatment. External beam irradiation is the mainstay of therapy. A total dose of 35–45 Gy is administered. Cryotherapy, photocoagulation, and radioactive plaques can be used for local tumor control.

Patients with metastatic disease also receive chemotherapy.

Children with retinoblastoma confined to the retina (whether unilateral or bilateral) have an excellent prognosis, with 5-year survival rates greater than 90%. Mortality is directly correlated with extent of optic nerve involvement, orbital extension of tumor, and massive choroid invasion. Patients who have disease in the optic nerve beyond the lamina cribrosa have only a 40% 5-year survival rate. Patients with meningeal or metastatic spread rarely survive, though intensive chemotherapy and autologous bone marrow transplants have produced long-term survivors.

Patients with the germinal mutation (heritable form) have a significant risk of developing second malignant neoplasms. Second tumors develop within as well as outside the field of radiation. Tumors also develop in patients who have received no radiation therapy. Sarcomas are the most commonly occurring second malignant neoplasm, with osteosarcoma accounting for 40% of such tumors. The risk for a second neoplasm is 10% at 10 years from diagnosis in patients who did not receive radiation therapy and 20% in patients who received external beam radiation therapy. The risk continues to increase over time. Although radiation contributes to the risk, it is the presence of the retinoblastoma gene itself that is primarily responsible for the development of nonocular tumors in these patients.

Donaldson SS et al: Retinoblastoma. In: *Principles and Practice of Pediatric Oncology.* Pizzo PA, Poplack DG (editors). Lippincott, 1997.
Kaelin WG: Recent insights into the functions of the retinoblastoma susceptibility gene product. Cancer Invest 1997;15:243.

Schwartzman E et al: Results of a stage-based protocol for the treatment of retinoblastoma. J Clin Oncol 1996; 14:1532.

HEPATIC TUMORS

The majority (57%) of liver tumors found in childhood are malignant. Ninety percent of hepatic malignancies are either hepatoblastoma or hepatocellular carcinoma. Hepatoblastomas are somewhat more frequent than hepatocellular carcinomas (51% versus 39%). A comparison of the features of these hepatic malignancies is presented in Table 26–8. Of the benign tumors, 60% are hamartomas or vascular tumors such as hemangiomas.

Children with hepatic tumors usually come to medical attention because of an enlarging abdomen. Approximately 10% of hepatoblastomas are first discovered on routine examination. Anorexia, weight loss, vomiting, and abdominal pain are seen more commonly in hepatocellular carcinoma. Serum alpha-fetoprotein is often elevated and is an excellent indicator for following response to treatment.

Imaging studies should include abdominal ultrasound as well as abdominal CT scan or MRI. Malignant tumors have a diffuse hyperechoic pattern on ultrasonography, whereas benign tumors are usually poorly echoic. Vascular lesions contain areas with varying degrees of echogenicity. Ultrasound is also useful for imaging the hepatic veins, portal veins, and inferior vena cava. CT scanning and in particular MRI are important for defining the extent of tumor within the liver. CT scanning of the chest and bone scan should be obtained to evaluate for metastatic spread.

Table 26–8. Comparison of hepatoblastoma and hepatocellular carcinoma in childhood.

	Hepatoblastoma	Hepatocellular Carcinoma
Median age at presentation	1 year (0–3 years)	12 years (5–18 years)
Male:female ratio	1.7:1	1.4:1
Associated conditions	Hemihypertrophy, Beckwith-Wiedemann syndrome	Hepatitis B virus infection, hereditary tyrosinemia, biliary cirrhosis, α_1-antitrypsin deficiency
Pathologic features	Fetal or embryonal cells; mesenchymal component (30%)	Large pleomorphic tumor cells and tumor giant cells
Solitary hepatic lesion	80%	20–50%
Unique features at diagnosis	Osteopenia (20–30%), isosexual precocity (3%)	Hemoperitoneum, polycythemia
Laboratory features Hyperbilirubinemia Elevated AFP Abnormal liver function tests	5% 60–70% 15–30%	25% 50% 30–50%

AFP = alpha-fetoprotein.

The prognosis for children with hepatic malignancies depends on the tumor type and the resectability of the tumor. Complete resectability is essential for survival. Chemotherapy can decrease the size of most hepatoblastomas. Following biopsy of the lesion, neoadjuvant chemotherapy is administered prior to attempting complete surgical resection. Chemotherapy can often convert an inoperable tumor to a completely resectable one and can also eradicate metastatic disease. Approximately 50–60% of hepatoblastomas are fully resectable, while only one-third of hepatocellular carcinomas can be completely removed. Even with complete resection, only one-third of patients with hepatocellular carcinoma are long-term survivors. A recent CCG/POG trial has shown cisplatin, fluorouracil, and vincristine to be as effective as but less toxic than cisplatin and doxorubicin. Other drugs that have demonstrated benefit include fluorouracil and cyclophosphamide. Etoposide, carboplatin, and ifosfamide are under investigation. Radiation as well as liver transplantation is being investigated for patients whose tumors cannot be completely resected following chemotherapy.

Greenberg M et al: Hepatic tumors. In: *Principles and Practice of Pediatric Oncology.* Pizzo PA, Poplack DG: (editors). Lippincott, 1997.

Raney B: Hepatoblastoma in children: A review. J Pediatr Hematol Oncol 1996;19:418.

LANGERHANS CELL HISTIOCYTOSIS

Langerhans cell histiocytosis (formerly called histiocytosis X) is a rare and poorly understood spectrum of disorders. It can occur as an isolated lesion or as widespread systemic disease involving virtually any body site. Eosinophilic granuloma, Hand-Schüller-Christian disease, and Letterer-Siwe disease are all syndromes encompassed by this disorder. Langerhans cell histiocytosis is not a true malignancy but a reactive proliferation of normal histiocytic cells, perhaps resulting from an immunoregulatory defect.

The distinctive pathologic feature is proliferation of histiocytic cells beyond what would be seen in a normal inflammatory process. Langerhans histiocytes have typical features: On light microscopy, the nuclei are deeply indented ("coffee bean"-shaped) and elongate, and the cytoplasm is pale, distinct, and abundant. Additional diagnostic characteristics include Birbeck granules on electron microscopy, expression of CD1 on the cell surface, and positive immunostaining for S-100 protein.

Clinical Findings

Because Langerhans cell histiocytosis encompasses a broad spectrum of diseases, its presentation can be variable, from a single asymptomatic lesion to widely disseminated disease. Although it is clearly a continuum of diseases, patients tend to present in distinct ways. Some present primarily with lesions limited to bone. Occasionally found incidentally on radiographs obtained for other reasons, these lesions are well-demarcated and frequently found in the skull, clavicles, ribs, and vertebrae. Lesions can be painful. Lesions are often solitary, but patients may develop other bone lesions and even visceral involvement.

Bony lesions, fever, weight loss, otitis media, exophthalmos, and diabetes insipidus are seen in a small number of children with the disease. Formerly called Hand-Schüller-Christian disease, this multifocal disease commonly presents with generalized symptoms and organ dysfunction.

Disseminated Langerhans cell histiocytosis (formerly called Letterer-Siwe disease) typically presents in children under 2 years of age with a seborrheic skin rash, fever, weight loss, lymphadenopathy, hepatosplenomegaly, and hematologic abnormalities.

Treatment & Prognosis

The outcome of Langerhans cell histiocytosis is extremely variable, but the process usually resolves spontaneously. Isolated lesions may need no therapy at all. Intralesional corticosteroids, curettage, or low-dose radiation therapy are useful local treatment measures for symptomatic lesions.

Multifocal disease is often treated with systemic chemotherapy. Prednisone, vinblastine, or etoposide, singly or in combination, can be given repeatedly or continuously until lesions heal and then reduced and finally stopped. Single-agent therapy is as effective as multi-agent therapy.

Patients with localized disease have an excellent prognosis. Multifocal disease is less predictable, but most cases resolve without sequelae. Age and degree of organ involvement are the most important prognostic factors. Infants with disseminated disease tend to do poorly, with mortality rates approaching 50%. New treatment approaches should be considered in this patient group. Cyclosporine is promising for this purpose.

Report of the Histiocyte Society workshop on central nervous system disease in Langerhans cell histiocytosis. Med Pediatr Oncol 1997;29:73.

Willman CL et al: Langerhans'-cell histiocytosis (histiocytosis X): A clonal proliferative disease. N Engl J Med 1994;331:154.

LATE EFFECTS OF PEDIATRIC CANCER THERAPY

Late effects of treatment by surgery, radiation, and chemotherapy have been identified in survivors of pediatric cancer. In some studies, up to 40% of survivors of pediatric cancer will have some disability secondary to treatment. Virtually any organ system can demonstrate sequelae related to previous cancer therapy. This has necessitated the creation of specialized oncology clinics whose function it is to identify and treat these patients.

GROWTH COMPLICATIONS

Growth complications of cancer therapy in the pediatric survivor are secondary to direct damage of endocrine tissue. Children with ALL, brain tumors, orbital tumors, and nasopharyngeal cancers who have received radiation are at highest risk.

Up to 90% of patients who receive greater than 30 Gy of radiation to the CNS will show evidence of growth hormone deficiency within 2 years. Approximately 50% of children receiving 24 Gy will have growth hormone problems. The effects of cranial radiation appear to be age-related, with children under 5 years at the time of therapy being particularly vulnerable. These patients may benefit from growth hormone therapy. There is currently no evidence that such therapy causes a recurrence of cancer.

Spinal radiation inhibits vertebral body growth. In 30% of such individuals, standing heights may be less than the fifth percentile. Asymmetric exposure of the spine to radiation may result in scoliosis. Chemotherapy alone may result in an attenuation of linear growth. This, however, is usually temporary, as a period of catch-up occurs when the drugs are discontinued.

Growth should be monitored closely. Follow-up studies should include height, weight, growth velocity, scoliosis examination, and, when indicated, growth hormone testing.

ENDOCRINE COMPLICATIONS

In addition to growth hormone deficiency, prepubertal children given cranial radiation may experience early puberty secondary to premature activation of the hypothalamic-pituitary-gonadal axis. This results in premature closure of the epiphyses, with decreased growth and height. This sequela appears to be more common in girls. Luteinizing hormone analog along with growth hormone is used to halt early puberty and facilitate continued growth.

Thyroid dysfunction is common in children receiving radiation therapy to the neck and those with brain tumors who receive more than 30 Gy. Up to 65–90% of patients receiving more than 25–30 Gy to the neck region will develop hypothyroidism. The average time to develop thyroid dysfunction is 12 months after exposure, but dysfunction can occur as early as 6 months or as late as 7 years following radi-

ation. Although signs and symptoms of hypothyroidism may be present, many patients will have a normal T_4 level with elevated TSH. These individuals should be considered for thyroid hormone replacement since persistent stimulation of the thyroid from an elevated TSH may predispose to thyroid nodules and carcinomas.

Gonadal dysfunction in males is usually the result of radiation to the testes, which can damage the germinal epithelium, producing azoospermia. Radiation to the testes can also produce Leydig cell damage with subsequent low testosterone levels and delayed sexual development. Patients who receive testicular radiation as part of their therapy for ALL, abdominal radiation for Hodgkin's disease, or total body irradiation in bone marrow transplantation are at highest risk. In boys, alkylating agents such as mechlorethamine and cyclophosphamide can also interfere with male gonadal function, resulting in oligospermia or azoospermia, low testosterone levels and abnormal FSH and LH levels. Determination of testicular size, semen analysis, and measurement of testosterone, FSH, and LH levels will help identify abnormalities in patients at risk.

Exposure of the ovaries during abdominal radiation may result in failure to undergo menarche, increased FSH and LH levels, and low estrogen levels. Girls given total body irradiation as preparation for bone marrow transplantation are at particularly high risk. Girls receiving craniospinal radiation for ALL (18–24 Gy) may also develop delayed menses and are at risk for early menopause. In patients at highest risk for development of gonadal complications, a detailed menstrual history should be obtained, and FSH and estrogen levels should be monitored if indicated.

There is no study to date that confirms an increased risk of miscarriage or spontaneous abortion, stillbirths or premature births, or congenital malformations in the offspring of childhood cancer survivors. Women who have received abdominal radiation and who develop uterine vascular insufficiency or fibrosis of the abdominal and pelvic musculature or uterus may have an increased risk of perinatal death or low-birth-weight premature infants, and their pregnancies should be high-risk.

CARDIOPULMONARY COMPLICATIONS

Several chemotherapeutic agents are known to cause pulmonary dysfunction as a late effect: bleomycin, the nitrosoureas, cyclophosphamide, methotrexate, and busulfan. Bleomycin has been implicated most frequently in chemotherapy-related lung injury. Ten percent of patients who receive a cumulative dose of this drug greater than 400 units will have pulmonary toxicity, which takes the form of pulmonary fibrosis. Pulmonary function tests in patients with chemotherapy-induced toxicity show restrictive lung disease, with decreased carbon monoxide diffusion and small lung volumes. Individuals exposed to this drug should be counseled to refrain from smoking and to give proper notification of the drug history if they should require general anesthesia.

Cardiac complications are usually due to anthracycline exposure (daunorubicin, doxorubicin), which destroys myocytes and leads to inadequate myocardial growth as the child ages. Inadequate left ventricular mass and decreased function can occur. Long-term survivors can present with arrhythmias or congestive heart failure. The latter is seen in at least 5% of patients who have received more than 550 mg/m^2 of anthracyclines (cumulative dose). In a recent study, complications from these agents appeared 6–19 years following administration of the drugs. Pregnant women who have received anthracyclines should be followed closely for signs and symptoms of congestive heart failure, since pregnancy is associated with an increase in intravascular volume.

Radiation therapy to the mediastinal region, which is common as part of therapy for Hodgkin's disease, has been linked to an increased risk of coronary artery disease, and chronic restrictive pericarditis may also occur in these patients.

Current recommendations include an echocardiogram and electrocardiogram every 2–3 years in patients who have received anthracyclines. Closer follow-up may be indicated for those who have received more than 500 mg/m^2 of these drugs. Holter monitoring, exercise testing, or gated radionuclide angiography is indicated in patients who have received large cumulative doses, have a history of cardiac dysfunction, have had mediastinal radiation, or who were treated with anthracyclines under 4 years of age.

RENAL COMPLICATIONS

Most of the renal long-term side effects stem from chemotherapy. Patients who have received cisplatin may develop an abnormal glomerular filtration rate and persistent tubular dysfunction with hypomagnesemia. Alkylating agents such as cyclophosphamide and ifosfamide can cause hemorrhagic cystitis, which may continue after chemotherapy has been terminated. Patients with a history of hemorrhagic cystitis may also be at risk for bladder carcinoma. Ifosfamide can also cause Fanconi's syndrome (proteinuria, glycosuria, phosphaturia with hypophosphatemia, aminoaciduria, and hyposthenuria), which may result in clinical rickets if adequate phosphate replacement is not provided.

Patients seen in long-term follow-up who have received nephrotoxic agents should be monitored with urinalysis, appropriate electrolyte profiles, and blood pressure. Urine collection for creatinine clearance or renal ultrasound may be indicated in individuals with suspected renal toxicity. Cystoscopy and cytologic study of urine sediment are recommended in patients with suspected malignancy.

NEUROPSYCHOLOGIC & PSYCHOSOCIAL COMPLICATIONS

Pediatric cancer survivors who have received cranial radiation for ALL or brain tumors appear to be at greatest risk for neuropsychologic problems. The severity of cranial radiation effects varies among individual patients and depends on the dose and dose schedule, the size and location of the radiation field, the amount of time elapsed after treatment, the age of the child when the radiation was administered, and the gender of the child. Girls may be more susceptible than boys to CNS toxicity since they have more rapid brain growth and development during childhood.

The main effects of CNS radiation appear to be related to nonverbal tasks such as visual processing speed, visual motor integration, sequencing ability, and short-term memory.

Psychosocial dysfunction can be traced to absenteeism from school, which is seen frequently in pediatric cancer patients. One study found that leukemia survivors were perceived as having more behavior problems and as being less socially competent than the sibling control group. Adolescent survivors of cancer demonstrate an increased sense of physical fragility and vulnerability that is manifested as hypochondriasis or phobic behaviors.

Pediatric cancer survivors may require ongoing counseling or other psychologic interventions once they have completed therapy. Children who have received CNS radiation may also require learning assistance in school, particularly in mathematics.

SECOND MALIGNANCIES

Approximately 3–12% of children treated for cancer will develop a new cancer within 20 years of their first diagnosis. This is a tenfold increased incidence when compared with age-matched controls. Exposure to alkylating agents and radiation therapy are risk factors in most second malignancies. Genetic and familial conditions associated with an increased risk of second malignancies include Li-Fraumeni syndrome, retinoblastoma, neurofibromatosis, nevoid basal cell carcinoma, and having a sibling with cancer.

Recently, acute nonlymphocytic leukemia has been reported as a second malignancy in patients treated with mitotic inhibitors such as etoposide and teniposide for ALL. The frequency of administration of the drug and the total dose may be important in the development of this secondary leukemia.

Children receiving radiation therapy as part of

treatment for ALL appear to be at an increased risk for developing brain tumors as a second malignancy. The population at highest risk appears to be patients who were 5 years old or less at the time of diagnosis.

A recent report examining the incidence of second neoplasms in a cohort of pediatric Hodgkin's disease patients showed the estimated actuarial incidence of a second neoplasm 15 years post diagnosis to be 7%. The most common solid tumor was breast cancer. Girls between the ages of 10 and 16 when they received radiation were at highest risk and had an actuarial incidence that approached 35% by 40 years of age. The majority of breast tumors were in the field of radiation.

Bhatia S et al: Breast cancer and other second malignant neoplasms after childhood Hodgkin's disease. N Engl J Med 1996;334:745.

Blatt J, Copeland DR, Bleyer WA: Late effects of childhood cancer and its treatment. In: *Principles and Practice of Pediatric Oncology.* Pizzo PA, Poplack DG (editors). Lippincott, 1997.

Green DM et al: Late effects of treatment for Wilms tumor. Hematol Oncol Clinics North Am 1995;9:1317.

Nvakovic B et al: Late effects of therapy in survivors of Ewing's sarcoma family tumors. J Pediatr Hematol Oncol 1997;19:220.

27

Immunodeficiency

Anthony R. Hayward, MD, PhD, & Erwin W. Gelfand, MD

Recurrent or severe infection is the most common symptom of immunodeficiency, but most children with recurrent minor infections do not have an immunodeficiency that is definable by currently available tests. Host defenses against infection depend mainly on excluding pathogens at surfaces, together with mechanical means to decontaminate them. Specific and nonspecific immune mechanisms are needed only after an organism gains access to the body. Specific immunity in this context consists of antibody and cell-mediated immunity. Nonspecific immune mechanisms include mechanical barriers, complement, phagocytes, and natural killer cells. Nonspecific mechanisms may be guided by specific responses, such as the ability of antibody to direct killing by natural killer cells or to promote phagocytosis by opsonizing bacteria.

Before investigating a patient for a defined primary immunodeficiency (most of which are rare), one should exclude the more common conditions that increase local susceptibility to infection, such as allergic rhinitis (causing sinusitis), cystic fibrosis, and asthma as causing pneumonia and conditions that interfere with the integrity of the skin or the normal flora of mucous membranes (Table 27–1). Common causes of secondary immunodeficiency (HIV infection, malnutrition, drugs, protein loss) must also be excluded.

Shearer WT et al: Practice parameters for the diagnosis and management of immunodeficiency. Ann Allergy Asthma Immunol 1996;76:282.

NONSPECIFIC FACTORS IN RESISTANCE TO INFECTION

DEFECTS OF COMPLEMENT

The complement series of proteins are activated by IgG or IgM antibody bound to surfaces. The split products of C3 and C5 activation attract neutrophils, and C3b bound to the surface of bacteria opsonizes them for phagocytosis by neutrophils. Deficiencies of individual classic pathway factors (C1–C9) occur as autosomal recessive traits and are rare. Deficiencies of factors 1, 4, and 2 are associated with immune complex disorders, particularly systemic lupus erythematosus, chronic glomerulonephritis, dermatomyositis, and cutaneous vasculitis. Primary deficiency of C3 interferes with the opsonization of bacteria by the classic and alternative pathways of complement activation and results in recurrent bacterial infections similar to those seen in antibody deficiency. Treatment is mostly with antibiotics. Serum levels of C3 are occasionally low enough in membranoproliferative glomerulonephritis with nephritic factor to increase susceptibility to infection. Deficiency of properdin (an alternative pathway factor) may also occasionally predispose to meningococcal infection.

C5, C6, C7, C8, and C9 deficiencies are associated with dissemination of neisserial infections, increasing the risks for arthritis in patients with gonorrhea and recurrences of meningitis. Survivors of meningococcal meningitis should probably have their complement function screened with a hemolytic assay

The serum "opsonizing defect" associated with Leiner's disease and originally attributed to C5a deficiency is now known to result from low plasma levels of mannan-binding protein. About 7% of the population has an allele associated with reduced function. Some affected infants have recurrent bacterial infections in infancy, which tend to get better with age.

Hereditary angioedema is a rare disorder, which causes recurrent angioedema without itching or wheals, usually beginning in late childhood or adolescence. It results from C1 esterase inhibitor deficiency in which susceptibility to infection is not increased. Transmission is autosomal dominant and there is an uncommon acquired form too. Affected persons typically have recurrent episodes of edema lasting 48–72 hours affecting the face or a limb. Edema affecting the bowel can be very painful. Laryngeal edema is life-threatening. Diagnosis is by

Table 27–1. Host defense mechanisms and examples of nonspecific defects.

Protection by	Defect
Intact skin	Burns, eczema, sinus tracks, indwelling catheters
Drainage	Auditory tube obstruction, cystic fibrosis, foreign body, urinary obstruction
Normal flora	Antibiotic-induced diarrhea, postantibiotic candidiasis

measurement of esterase inhibitor levels in serum; those who are symptomatic have levels below 30%. C4 levels are often low. Danazol, a synthetic androgen, prevents attacks by increasing C1 inhibitor levels. The diagnosis is suggested by decreased activity of whole complement, C4, and C2 and confirmed by direct assay of the C1 inhibitor.

Garred P et al: Increased frequency of homozygosity of abnormal mannan-binding-protein alleles in patients with suspected immunodeficiency. Lancet 1995;346:941.

He S et al: Epitope mapping of C1 inhibitor autoantibodies from patients with acquired C1 inhibitor deficiency. J Immunol 1996;156:2009.

Nishizaka H et al: Molecular bases for inherited human complement component C6 deficiency in two unrelated individuals. J Immunol 1996;156:2309.

Ruddy S: Rheumatic diseases and inherited complement deficiencies. Bull Rheum Diseases 1996;45:6.

CELLULAR DEFECTS

Defects of neutrophil function comprise adhesion defects, chemotaxis defects, and defects of bacterial killing. They are typically associated with bacterial infections in the first 6 months of life. These are fully discussed in Chapter 25, and their symptoms are summarized here in the context of the investigation of a child with recurrent infections. Patients with leukocyte adhesion defects present with infections ranging from progressive periumbilical necrosis with onset in infancy to recurrent surface infections starting in adult life. The severity of the clinical picture depends on the underlying defect. The infections are caused by a range of organisms, and although neutrophil count is normal or high, there is relatively little pus formation. In childhood, the infections are often around body orifices, but they also involve the skin, esophagus, and respiratory tract. Death in childhood is common. Other patients with a milder phenotype have survived for 20 or more years. Diagnosis is by phenotyping blood mononuclear cells for LFA-1 or Mac-1; this approach can also be used for antenatal diagnosis. Treatment is by bone marrow transplantation.

Chédiak-Higashi syndrome exemplifies a chemotaxis defect, resulting in progressive local infections without much pus formation. Most chemotaxis defects are probably secondary. A wide variety of other conditions also can be associated with depressed motility of phagocytic cells: burns; infections such as HIV, rubella, and influenza; metabolic and nutritional disorders, including diabetes mellitus; the hypophosphatemia associated with hyperalimentation; and uremia. The association of **impaired neutrophil chemotaxis with hyperimmunoglobulinemia E** (IgE levels are usually > 2000 units/mL), recurrent staphylococcal abscesses of the skin, eczema, and otitis media is clinically recognizable and sometimes called Job's syndrome. These patients can have impaired CMI, and the disorder also occurs in some patients with AIDS. Treatment is symptomatic.

Patients with bacterial killing defects (such as chronic granulomatous disease) usually have staphylococcal infections in the first months of life and develop groin, cervical, or axillary abscesses requiring incision and drainage. Sometimes they are infected by *Serratia* or *Nocardia* species. The infections cause high neutrophil counts and fever and sometimes spread to cause osteomyelitis or lung or liver abscesses. Colitis, leading to diarrhea and slow growth, is common. The abscesses require drainage and appropriate antibiotics for lengthy courses (3 weeks or more). As underlying tissues become damaged, fungal and *Pseudomonas cepacia* infections become increasingly common.

Defects of monocyte macrophage function occur in lysosomal storage diseases but infections are only a minor component of their symptomatology. **Natural killer cell** defects are now being reported, resulting either from autoantibodies (causing a low number in blood) or from lack of cell surface receptors for IgG. Symptoms result from infection, most notably severe herpesvirus infections.

Jawahar S et al: Natural killer (NK) cell deficiency associated with an epitope-deficient Fc receptor type IIIa (CD16-ii). Clin Exp Immunol 1996;103:408.

Witte T et al: Autoantibody against a 58 kD molecule in a patient with neutropenia and NK cell deficiency. Br J Haematol 1996;92:565.

DEFICIENCIES OF SPECIFIC IMMUNITY

Defects of specific immunity are broadly subdivided into those affecting predominantly antibody formation, those affecting cellular immunity, and those in which both mechanisms are impaired. The

Table 27–2. Classification of defects of specific immunity.

Deficiency of immunoglobulin	Deficiency of all Ig's = hypogamma-globulinemia Congenital (sometimes with high IgM) Acquired Unclassified (common variable hypogammaglobulinemia) Selective immunoglobulin deficiency IgA deficiency IgG subclass deficiencies IgM deficiency Antibody deficiency with immunoglobulins
Deficiency of cell-mediated immunity	Purine nucleoside phosphorylase DiGeorge syndrome Cartilage-hair hypoplasia Unclassified (common variable immunodeficiency affecting cell-mediated immunity)
Deficiency of both antibody and cell-mediated immunity	Severe combined immunodeficiency (various types) Ataxia-telangiectasia Wiskott-Aldrich syndrome

classification in Table 27–2 is based on combinations of clinical and laboratory results and includes only the more common conditions. Enormous advances are being made in identifying gene defects, and mechanisms of immunodeficiencies with simple mendelian inheritance and linkages are being mapped for some multifactorial conditions (common variable immunodeficiency, selective IgA deficiency).

Rosen FS et al: The primary immunodeficiencies. N Engl J Med 1995;333:431.

IMMUNOGLOBULIN & ANTIBODY DEFICIENCY SYNDROMES

1. HYPOGAMMAGLOBULINEMIA SYNDROMES

Patients who do not make antibodies have low immunoglobulin levels (hypogammaglobulinemia) and usually present with recurrent or severe bacterial infection of the respiratory tract (sinusitis, otitis, pneumonia) or skin (cellulitis, abscesses). Without antibiotic treatment, these infections tend to spread to cause septicemia and meningitis. There are several types of hypogammaglobulinemia (see Table 27–2) and in the **congenital X-linked agammaglobulinemia** infections usually start after 4 months of age, when passively acquired maternal IgG levels have declined. *Haemophilus influenzae* and *Streptococcus pneumoniae* cause most of the infections, but following courses of antibiotics, *Mycoplasma* family members such as *Ureaplasma* become important. Some boys have asymmetric arthritis, mostly of the knee or ankle, at the time of diagnosis, which may resolve after adequate IgG replacement. These patients typically have little or no tonsillar and adenoidal tissue. The severity of infections varies, so the diagnosis may not be made for many years. Congenital X-linked agammaglobulinemia results from mutations in the B cell tyrosine kinase gene (btk), and patients have few if any B cells in their blood, though they have normal blood lymphocyte counts. Carrier detection is available. Some of these patients have impaired growth resulting from primary or secondary deficiency of growth hormone.

Other types of hypogammaglobulinemia are more common and may develop at any age. The diagnosis of hypogammaglobulinemia is based on low serum immunoglobulin levels for age with absence of serum isohemagglutinins and of antibody response to immunization. Causes of secondary hypogammaglobulinemia (nephrotic syndrome, HIV infection, and protein-losing enteropathy) should be excluded by measuring serum albumin.

Borrelli S et al: Characterization of *Haemophilus influenzae* isolates from the respiratory tract of patients with primary antibody deficiencies: Evidence for persistent colonizations. Scand J Infect Dis 1995;27:303.

Shyur SD, Hill HR: Recent advances in the genetics of primary immunodeficiency syndromes. J Pediatr 1996;129:8.

Stewart DM et al: Molecular genetic analysis of X-linked hypogammaglobulinemia and isolated growth hormone deficiency. J Immunol 1995;155:2770.

Immunodeficiency With High IgM Levels

Affected boys have low IgG and IgA levels. Their IgM levels may start in the normal range but can rise to 1000 mg/dL or more. In addition to infections, these children often have lymphadenopathy and episodes of autoimmune neutropenia. The disease results from mutation in the CD40 ligand gene so that the patient's T cells are unable to switch their B cells from making IgM to making IgG and IgA. Cell-mediated immunity is also impaired, so these patients have *Pneumocystis* infections, cryptosporidiosis of the biliary tree and intestine, sclerosing cholangitis, and a high incidence of biliary tract carcinomas. Children with autosomal recessive forms of hyper-IgM immunodeficiency have normal expression of CD40L.

Kroczek RA et al: Defective expression of CD40 ligand on T cells causes "X linked Immunodeficiency with Hyper IgM (XHIM)." Immunol Rev 1994;138:39.

Common Variable Immunodeficiency Syndromes

Patients with congenital or acquired antibody deficiency syndromes not classified elsewhere are often included in this group, and they outnumber patients with all other types of antibody deficiency except selective IgA deficiency. Onset of the immunodeficiency may be at any age. Susceptibility to common variable immunodeficiency is inherited, linked with the same class III histocompatibility gene deletions (for C4 and 21-hydroxylase, on chromosome 6) as selective IgA deficiency, but the factors that precipitate expression of common variable immunodeficiency in susceptible individuals are not known. These patients usually have B cells that do not differentiate normally in tissue culture.

Infections follow the patterns described for other types of antibody deficiency. Some patients have remarkably few infections despite long-standing very low immunoglobulin levels. The laboratory findings are variable. Low levels of one or more immunoglobulin classes are associated with varying degrees of impairment of T cell proliferative responses. Autoantibody formation, raised IgE levels, and positive immediate hypersensitivity skin reactions occur, as do neutropenia and thrombocytopenia. Patients with hypogammaglobulinemia and facial anomalies may have the immunodeficiency-chromosome instability-facial anomaly (ICF) syndrome, in which a satellite DNA methylation anomaly is associated with instability of the pericentromeric heterochromatin of—in particular—chromosomes 1, 9, and 16. Inheritance of this variant is probably autosomal recessive.

Brown DC et al: ICF syndrome (immunodeficiency, centromeric instability and facial anomalies): Investigation of heterochromatin abnormalities and review of clinical outcome. Hum Genet 1995;96:411.
Jaffe JS et al: T-cell abnormalities in common variable immunodeficiency. Pediatr Res 1993;33(1 Suppl):S24.
Puck JM: Molecular basis for three X-linked immune disorders. Hum Mol Genet 1994;3:1457.
Sneller MC et al: NIH conference: New insights into common variable immunodeficiency. Ann Intern Med 1993;118:720.

Complications of Hypogammaglobulinemia

Many patients have B cell hyperplasia in the gut. About 10% of patients develop diarrhea and malabsorption that may be severe enough to resemble Crohn's disease. Infection is the likeliest cause of the diarrhea, and efforts should be made to exclude treatable agents such as *Giardia lamblia* or *Cryptosporidium*. In adult life, the patients often develop gastric atrophy with achlorhydria, sometimes followed by pernicious anemia. Affected boys occasionally develop optic atrophy or ataxia, evolving slowly or rapidly into fatal encephalitis. Echoviruses have sometimes been isolated from their cerebrospinal fluid or brains at biopsy or necropsy. A smaller proportion develop a dermatomyositis-like syndrome, with prominent peripheral cyanosis and myopathy

but little heliotrope coloration. There is an impression that both of these complications are less commonly seen now that much higher immunoglobulin replacements are given. There are reports of an increased rate of cancer in patients with antibody deficiency. The association is predominantly with lymphoreticular proliferation and may sometimes result from EBV infection. Lymphoreticular proliferations in hypogammaglobulinemic patients are not always malignant.

Some batches of intravenous IgG in use through 1995 were contaminated with hepatitis C virus, so patients with raised aminotransferases should be tested for C virus antigenemia. Many infected children fail to clear the virus and are at risk for chronic hepatitis and liver failure. The risk of hepatitis has been virtually eliminated since more stringent viral inactivation steps have been introduced, eg, solvent detergent.

Bresee JS et al: Hepatitis C virus infection associated with administration of intravenous immune globulin: A cohort study. JAMA 1996;276:1563.
Elenitoba-Johnson KS, Jaffe ES: Lymphoproliferative disorders associated with congenital immunodeficiencies. Semin Diagn Pathol 1997;14:35.
Jonas MM et al: Clinical and virologic features of hepatitis C virus infection associated with intravenous immunoglobulin. Pediatrics 1996;98:211.
Rudge P: Encephalomyelitis in primary hypogammaglobulinemia. Brain 1996;119:1.

Treatment of Hypogammaglobulinemia

Patients with hypogammaglobulinemia should have serum IgG replaced to protect against infection. IgG is usually given by intravenous infusions of specially prepared deaggregated IgG (200–600 mg/kg every 4 weeks). If intravenous treatment is very difficult in young children, they may be temporarily managed with intramuscular injections of IgG concentrate (0.6 mL/kg every 2–3 weeks). Some adults are managed more cheaply with subcutaneous infusions of the intramuscular IgG preparation, given overnight on several nights per week. The aim of treatment must be to avoid—or minimize progression of—chronic lung disease (bronchitis, bronchiectasis). Productive cough and purulent sputum or conjunctivitis must be taken seriously and antibiotics given until there has been radiologic and clinical resolution. *Mycoplasma* infections of the respiratory or urinary tract should be sought for and treated with doxycycline or other appropriate antibiotics.

Minor reactions to immunoglobulin infusions or injections are common, especially with the initial infusion. They include headache, back and limb pain, anxiety, and tightness of the chest. Signs are tachycardia, shivering, fever, and, in severe cases, shock. Reactions are frequent in some patients and rare in others; their occurrence is sporadic and not generally due to hypersensitivity (anti-IgA reactions may be an exception but are rare). Skin tests are not helpful. When indicated, immunoglobulin replacement should be maintained for life and the severity of the reactions limited by premedication with acetaminophen, an antihistamine, or intravenous hydrocortisone immediately before the infusion. Alternative brands of IgG should be tried if reactions persist despite premedication.

Abrahamsen TG et al: Home therapy with subcutaneous immunoglobulin infusions in children with congenital immunodeficiencies. Pediatrics 1996;98:1127.

2. OTHER TYPES OF HYPOGAMMAGLOBULINEMIA

Transient Hypogammaglobulinemia

Infants' IgG levels fall during the first 4–5 months of life, as maternal IgG is diluted and catabolized. The physiologic trough that occurs before the infant's IgG production maintains adult levels is accentuated in premature and dysmature infants. IgG levels of 250–300 mg/dL lie within 2 SD of the mean at 3–4 months of age, and the diagnosis of transient hypogammaglobulinemia is often made in infants with infections and IgG levels in this range. Immunoglobulin levels should return to normal by 30 months of age, and the diagnosis can only be made retrospectively. The only diagnostic laboratory findings are of low IgG—with or without low IgA and IgM—and subsequent return to normal levels. Salivary IgA is generally detectable, and, despite the low immunoglobulin levels, antibody activity (isohemagglutinin or antidiphtheria or tetanus antibody) is present in serum. IgG antibody is generally made following immunization, and tests for cellular immunity are normal. No treatment is usually required for infants who make antibody following immunization other than appropriate antibiotics for bacterial infections. Infants with severe infection and hypogammaglobulinemia could rationally be given IgG injections, since maternal antibody to the infecting organism will be rapidly depleted, but this is rarely necessary. The prognosis for affected infants is excellent provided they do not succumb to infection before normal immunity is achieved.

IgA Deficiency

This disorder is usually defined by a serum IgA < 5 mg/dL and occurs in about 1:800 whites, so it is by far the most common defect of specific immunity. Serum IgM and IgG are normal, as is cell-mediated immunity. Susceptibility is linked to HLA histocompatibility genes, perhaps because an autoimmune mechanism interferes with the differentiation of IgA B lymphocytes. Fifty percent or more of IgA-defi-

cient subjects have no symptoms arising from the deficiency, perhaps because they can protect their mucosa adequately with IgG and IgM antibodies. Failure of antibody responses in the IgG4 and IgG2 subclasses is reported in many symptomatic patients, but there is no simple relationship with IgA levels. When symptoms are present, they are predominantly upper respiratory tract infections or diarrhea. There are also strong associations with inflammatory bowel disease, allergy (mainly respiratory and gut), and autoimmune disorders (thyroiditis, arthritis, vitiligo, thrombocytopenia, and diabetes).

The selective lack of IgA antibody responses and the presence of normal antibody responses in other immunoglobulin classes distinguish IgA deficiency from unclassified variable immunodeficiency. IgA has a short half-life in serum, and replacement is impractical. It is conceivable but unproved that colostrum feeding could modify severe gut symptoms. Symptomatic IgA-deficient subjects who are also IgG2-deficient have sometimes been treated with IgG replacement. This approach has been both advocated and condemned on theoretical grounds but without controlled data. A subset of IgA-deficient patients make antibodies to IgA, which are an important cause of transfusion reactions. Most IgA-deficient patients manage reasonably well with antibiotics only; atopic or autoimmune symptoms should be treated conventionally.

French MA et al: Severity of infections in IgA deficiency: Correlation with decreased serum antibodies to pneumococcal polysaccharides and deceased serum IgG2 and/or IgG4. Clin Exp Immunol 1995;100:47.
Koskinen S et al: Long-term follow-up of anti-IgA antibodies in healthy IgA-deficient adults. J Clin Immunol 1995;15:194.

Other Selective Subclass Deficiencies

The possibility that deficiency of an IgG subclass might predispose to recurrent upper respiratory tract infections in patients who have normal serum immunoglobulin levels is still debated, and the issue is confused by the absence of any prospective studies. The IgG heavy chain genes on chromosome 11 (grouped with IgG1 close to IgG3 and IgG2 close to IgG4) are usually normal in subclass deficiencies. Normally, IgG1 comprises over 60% of total IgG and IgG2 over 10%. IgG3 accounts for about 5%, and IgG4 may be undetectable in up to 20% of healthy persons. Serum levels are age-related. When IgG1 is deficient, IgG2 and IgG3 are generally low also, giving the clinical picture of hypogammaglobulinemia. IgG1 and IgG2 contain much of the antibody to capsular polysaccharides. IgG2 (and IgG4) deficiency is also associated with IgA deficiency. IgG3 deficiency is less common but has been incriminated in subjects with antibody deficiency syndromes who have normal total IgG or IgG1 subclass levels. Even in adults it has been difficult to establish a link between IgG subclass deficiencies and any consistent pattern of infections. IgG replacement should be reserved for patients with defects of antibody production; many patients are managed with antibiotics alone.

Selective deficiencies of IgM, IgE, and kappa or lambda light chains due to gene deletions may be symptomless and are very rare. Selective IgM deficiency is reported in Bloom's syndrome and, in adults, predisposes to septicemia. Since IgM replacement is impractical on a long-term basis, reliance is placed mainly on antibiotics.

Avanzini MA et al: Qualitative and quantitative analyses of the antibody response elicited by *Haemophilus influenzae* type b capsular polysaccharide-tetanus toxoid conjugates in adults with IgG subclass deficiencies and frequent infections. Clin Exp Immunol 1994;96:54.

Herrod HG: Management of the patient with IgG subclass deficiency and/or selective antibody deficiency. Ann Allergy 1993;70:3.

Hoeger PH, Niggemann B, Haeuser G: Age related IgG subclass concentrations in asthma. Arch Dis Child 1994;70:179.

Mochizuki S et al: Systemic immunization against IgA in immunoglobulin deficiency. Clin Exp Immunol 1994; 94:334.

Plebani A et al: Extensive deletion of immunoglobulin heavy chain constant region genes in the absence of recurrent infections: When is IgG subclass deficiency clinically relevant? Clin Immunol Immunopathol 1993; 68:46.

Smith LJ et al: Familial enteropathy with villous edema and immunoglobulin G2 subclass deficiency. J Pediatr 1996;128:722.

SELECTIVE DEFECTS OF CELL-MEDIATED IMMUNITY

1. PURINE NUCLEOSIDE PHOSPHORYLASE DEFICIENCY

Purine nucleoside phosphorylase deficiency causes a relatively selective cell-mediated immunity defect. It results in increased intracellular deoxyguanosine triphosphate, which inhibits ribonucleotide reductase and interferes with DNA synthesis, especially in T cells. T cell help to B cells is not prevented, probably because it is not dependent on cell division. The gene for purine nucleoside phosphorylase is on chromosome 14, and transmission is recessive. Presenting features may be neurologic (developmental retardation, behavior disorders, and spasticity), with immunodeficiency (severe varicella, anemia, and growth deficiency) developing later. The age at presentation has ranged from 6 months to 7 years. Investigations show low serum uric acid, lymphopenia, absent delayed hypersensitivity skin responses, and low or absent lymphocyte responses to

mitogens. Serum immunoglobulins and antibody responses to injected antigens may be normal. Several patients developed an autoimmune hemolytic anemia. Diagnosis depends on enzyme measurement, and all patients with severely impaired cellular immunity who make immunoglobulin should probably be tested. Antenatal diagnosis is possible. It has been difficult to achieve stable engraftment following bone marrow transplantation.

Broome CB et al: Correction of purine nucleoside phosphorylase deficiency by transplantation of allogeneic bone marrow from a sibling. J Pediatr 1996;128:373.

Nelson DM et al: Correction of proliferative responses in purine nucleoside phosphorylase (PNP)-deficient T lymphocytes by retroviral-mediated PNP gene transfer and expression. J Immunol 1995;154:3006.

Tam DA Jr, Leshner RT: Stroke in purine nucleoside phosphorylase deficiency. Pediatr Neurol 1995;12:146.

2. THYMIC HYPOPLASIA (DiGeorge Syndrome)

DiGeorge syndrome is one of the "CATCH 22" disorders (cardiac defects, abnormal facies, thymic hypoplasia, cleft palate, and hypocalcemia) caused by microdeletions in the chromosome regions 22q11.2 and 10p12–13. Related syndromes are the velocardiofacial syndrome and isolated conotruncal cardiac disease. The defective chromosome is usually inherited from the mother. The hypocalcemia results from lack of parathyroid glands, and the common major vessel abnormalities are truncus arteriosus, anomalous pulmonary venous drainage, or right-sided aortic arch. Other features include a small jaw, low-set ears, and a short philtrum. The term "partial DiGeorge syndrome" is commonly applied to infants who have impaired rather than absent parathyroid or thymus function. Clinical presentation usually results from cardiac failure or, after 24–48 hours, from hypocalcemia, and the diagnosis is sometimes made during the course of cardiac surgery, when no thymus is found in the mediastinum. Postoperative hypocalcemia can be severe and persistent, requiring both calcium and vitamin D supplements. Despite receiving fresh blood transfusions during cardiopulmonary bypass, patients do not usually develop graft-versus-host disease. Their susceptibility to infection is variable—a few have died with septicemia, and some have had chronic candidiasis, but many appear to respond normally. This may reflect the tendency for the number of T cells in the patient's blood to rise spontaneously over the course of several years. The differential diagnosis includes hypocalcemia and a small or absent thymus on chest x-ray secondary to infection.

A subset of DiGeorge patients has severe problems with production of autoantibodies to red cells, white cells, and platelets. These may respond to intravenous IgG or to corticosteroids. Treatment of other DiGeorge features may require surgery for the cardiac defects and vitamin D and calcium to correct hypocalcemia. Blood for these patients should be irradiated. Grafting thymic hypoplasia patients with fetal thymus or thymic epithelial cells is often followed by rapid improvement in the lymphocyte response to mitogens. The improvement is so rapid that thymic humoral factors are thought to be responsible, but factors currently available for treatment have not been useful. Infusion of HLA-matched sibling blood or marrow has been tried in a few patients who did not improve spontaneously and carries a risk for graft-versus-host disease.

Guidelines on gamma irradiation of blood components for the prevention of transfusion-associated graft-versus-host disease. BCSH Blood Transfusion Task Force. Transfus Med 1996;6:261.

Leatherbury L, Kirby ML: Cardiac development and perinatal care of infants with neural crest-associated conotruncal defects. Semin Perinatol 1996;20:473.

Pignata C et al: Progressive deficiencies in blood T cells associated with a 10p12–13 interstitial deletion. Clin Immunol Immunopathol 1996;80:9.

3. OTHER DEFECTS OF CELL-MEDIATED IMMUNITY

Idiopathic CD4 lymphopenia is characterized by low CD4 counts with opportunistic infection but without HIV infection—increased sensitivity to apoptosis has been identified as one cause. Many patients with the American (but not Finnish) type of **cartilage-hair hypoplasia** have a moderate degree of lymphopenia, low lymphocyte responses to mitogens, and higher than normal morbidity and mortality rates from herpesvirus and poxvirus infections. Bone marrow transplantation can restore cell-mediated immunity but does not correct the cartilage abnormality. Short-limbed dwarfs who are immunodeficient should probably be tested for adenosine deaminase deficiency, which also is treatable. Other types of immunodeficiency affecting predominantly cellular immunity exist but are poorly classified. These are currently included in the "varied immunodeficiency" group. Infections in affected individuals resemble those described above, with the frequent addition of chronic diarrhea and malabsorption and lung infections due to atypical mycobacteria, fungi, and *Pneumocystis carinii*. Treatment is experimental.

Berthet F et al: Bone marrow transplantation in cartilage-hair hypoplasia: correction of the immunodeficiency but not of the chondrodysplasia. Eur J Pediatr 1996;155:286.

Brooks EG et al: Thymic hypoplasia and T-cell deficiency in ectodermal dysplasia: Case report and review of the literature. Clin Immunol Immunopathol 1994;71:44.

Dungan JS et al: Cartilage-hair hypoplasia syndrome: Implications for prenatal diagnosis. Fetal Diagn Ther 1996;11:398.

Fischer A et al: Bone marrow transplantation (BMT) in Europe for primary immunodeficiencies other than severe combined immunodeficiency: A report from the European Group for BMT and the European Group for Immunodeficiency. Blood 1994;83:1149.

Laurence J et al: Apoptotic depletion of CD4+ T cells in idiopathic CD4+ T lymphocytopenia. J Clin Invest 1996;97:672.

Le Deist F et al: A primary T-cell immunodeficiency associated with defective transmembrane calcium influx. Blood 1995;85:1053.

Sulisalo T et al: Uniparental disomy in cartilage-hair hypoplasia. Eur J Hum Genet 1997;5:35.

COMBINED IMMUNODEFICIENCY DISORDERS

Severe combined immunodeficiency disease (SCID) comprises a heterogeneous group of conditions that have in common a primary severe impairment of both antibody- and cell-mediated immunity. The term SCID is usually restricted to infants with congenital immunodeficiency, but equally severe defects can be caused by AIDS or lymphocyte loss. The heterogeneity of the congenital forms reflects the range of underlying defects that may interfere with lymphocyte development at different stages and the varying degrees of engraftment with maternal lymphocytes that can occur during gestation or at birth. X-linked SCID results from mutations in the gamma chain shared by the cell surface receptors for the cytokines IL-2, IL-4, IL-7, IL-9 and IL-15. These mutations vary in their interference with gamma chain function, and this allows for a range of clinical severity in X-linked SCID syndromes.

Diarrhea, vomiting, and cough are common symptoms. The diarrhea causes growth deficiency, and, although it may briefly remit after dietary changes, it recurs after a few days. The cough is usually persistent; it is often due to *P carinii* infection and can cause cyanosis. Skin rashes are common and frequently evanescent, except for rash following blood transfusion, which is due to graft-versus-host disease (see below). A *Candida* diaper rash is usual. Findings initially include absence of tonsils or palpable lymph nodes; later, there is emaciation.

All patients with SCID have some degree of hypogammaglobulinemia and failure of antibody production (though maternal IgG is present in infants). SCID infants with some immunoglobulin have been distinguished as having "Nezelof's syndrome," but this separation is not helpful in terms of pathogenesis or treatment. Lymphopenia is inconstant, but, with rare exceptions, all have very low or absent T (CD3) cells from blood, with normal numbers of NK (CD16) cells. B lymphocytes (with surface IgM) are usually present in blood. In vitro lymphocyte responses to mitogens are generally absent. Antigen-specific responses (T cell or antibody) are difficult to test for in infancy because of uncertainty about prior experience and because they are generally too time-consuming for clinical purposes. Antenatal diagnosis of X-linked SCID is possible by molecular methods. All other SCID syndromes may be detected by fetal blood sampling at 15 weeks of gestation and phenotyping the lymphocytes obtained.

Arpaia E et al: Defective T cell receptor signaling and CD8+ thymic selection in humans lacking zap-70 kinase. Cell 1994;76:947.

Leonard WJ: The defective gene in X-linked severe combined immunodeficiency encodes a shared interleukin receptor subunit: Implications for cytokine pleiotropy and redundancy. Curr Opin Immunol 1994;6:631.

Stephan JL et al: Severe combined immunodeficiency: A retrospective single-center study of clinical presentation and outcome in 117 patients. J Pediatr 1993;123:564.

Differential Diagnosis & Treatment

The combination of diarrhea and hypogammaglobulinemia in infancy is suggestive of SCID. The main differential is between severe varied immunodeficiency and secondary immunodeficiency due to HIV infection or severe gastrointestinal disease with loss of protein and cells. Some T cells are usually present in these secondary immunodeficiencies, with a weak lymphocyte response to phytohemagglutinin, and the serum albumin concentration may be low. Infants in whom the diagnosis is suspected should receive antibiotics for infection and IgG replacement. They should not be transfused with blood unless it has first been irradiated. With confirmation of the diagnosis, they may be started on trimethoprim-sulfamethoxazole for *Pneumocystis* prophylaxis. Bone marrow grafting offers the best hope for cure. If an HLA-matched sibling is available, there is a high chance of success; the treatment can be given without depleting the marrow of T cells or immunosuppressing the recipient. Most SCID patients do not have HLA-matched donors and are treated with grafts of parental bone marrow from which the T cells are removed by lectins or monoclonal antibodies. Pregraft suppression, with the attendant hazards of thrombocytopenia and neutropenia, may be required; reconstitution can take 4 months; and the overall rate of T cell engraftment is between 50% and 70%. Reconstitution for antibody responses may not occur even if B cells are produced.

Filipovich AH: Bone marrow transplantation from unrelated donors for congenital immunodeficiencies. Bone Marrow Transplant 1993;11(Suppl)1:78.

van Leeuwen JE et al: Relationship between patterns of engraftment in peripheral blood and immune reconstitution after allogeneic bone marrow transplantation for (severe) combined immunodeficiency. Blood 1994;84:3936.

VARIANTS OF SEVERE COMBINED IMMUNODEFICIENCY

1. ADENOSINE DEAMINASE DEFICIENCY

Adenosine deaminase converts adenosine and deoxyadenosine to inosine and deoxyinosine, respectively. Individuals homozygous for a null gene account for about 20% of cases of SCID. ADA deficiency impairs immunity through inhibition of ribonucleotide reductase by raised deoxy-ATP, so that T lymphocytes are prevented from dividing. There is also increased DNA fragmentation, interference with methylation reactions, and aberrant receptor signaling. Affected infants may be near-normal at birth (presumably because their mothers keep deoxyadenosine levels down in utero). Their cellular immunity fails first; they become lymphopenic and then become antibody-deficient, though they may continue to make immunoglobulin for months or years. Diagnosis is by assay of adenosine deaminase in red cell lysates. A bone marrow graft from a matched normal sibling is the ideal treatment (see below). Immune competence is also restored by weekly infusions of polyethylene glycol-stabilized ADA enzyme conjugate. Transfection of blood lymphocytes and stem cells is being evaluated for subjects who lack matched donors.

Hershfield MS: PEG-ADA replacement therapy for adenosine deaminase deficiency: An update after 8.5 years. Clin Immunol Immunopathol 1995;76:S228.

Resta R, Thompson LF: SCID: The role of adenosine deaminase deficiency. Immunol Today 1997;18:371.

2. SCID WITH LEUKOPENIA (Reticular Dysgenesis)

SCID with leukopenia occurs in infants with SCID who also have severe neutropenia, often with reduced numbers of granulocyte precursors in the marrow. Only about 20 cases have been reported. There is a familial trend, but the severity of the neutropenia varies between affected siblings, so this may be a secondary feature.

Gasparetto C et al: Dyshematopoiesis in combined immune deficiency with congenital neutropenia. Am J Hematol 1994;45:63.

3. SCID WITH DEFECTIVE EXPRESSION OF HLA ANTIGENS

Deficiency of class II (HLA-DR, -DP, and -DQ) histocompatibility antigen expression is difficult to diagnose because affected patients generally make immunoglobulins and have low to normal numbers of B and T cells in their blood, together with positive responses to phytohemagglutinin stimulation. Their clinical symptoms are nevertheless those of SCID, and the T cells do not make antigen-specific responses, so the patients remain antibody-deficient. There are at least four complementation groups, and diagnosis is by testing blood lymphocytes for HLA-DR antigen expression. A number of affected families has been of North African descent.

Defects of class I histocompatibility antigen range from abnormalities of antigen transport inside the cell to abnormal or unstable expression of HLA-A or HLA-B at the cell surface. In general, these conditions are associated with milder degrees of immunodeficiency.

de la Salle H et al: Human peptide transporter deficiency: Importance of HLA-B in the presentation of TAP-independent EBV antigens. J Immunol 1997;158:4555.
Elhasid R, Etzioni A: Major histocompatibility complex class II deficiency: A clinical review. Blood Reviews 1997;10:242.

4. T CELL KINASE DEFICIENCIES

Defects in several T cell receptor signaling enzymes (Zap-70, JAK 3) cause abnormal function of T cells. Infants lacking Zap-70 have CD4 but no CD8 cells in blood. Their lymphocytes do not proliferate in response to antigen or mitogens because they lack an essential kinase in the T cell activation pathway. Immunoglobulin production is variable.

Notarangelo LD: Immunodeficiencies caused by genetic defects in protein kinases. Curr Opin Immunol 1996;8:448.
Roifman CM: Selection transduction defect (STD) due to Zap-70 kinase deficiency. Immunodeficiency 1995; 5:193.

5. OTHER COMBINED IMMUNODEFICIENCY DISORDERS

There is a poorly defined group of infants with more severe impairment of antibody and cell-mediated immunity than occurs in common variable immunodeficiency disease but who have more T cells than are usually seen in SCID. These patients have severe and protracted infections, mainly of the respiratory tract and gut. A subgroup with multiple intestinal atresias, hypogammaglobulinemia, and impaired cell-mediated immunity has recently been recognized; the mechanism for this association is unknown. Many have severe herpesviruses infections. Autoimmune neutropenia, anemia, and thrombocytopenia are common, as are allergies as well. Immune deficiency in some of these patients has been corrected by bone marrow transplantation.

Moore SW et al: Immune deficiency in familial duodenal atresia. J Pediatr Surg 1996;31:1733.
Rothenberg ME et al: A syndrome involving immunodeficiency and multiple intestinal atresias. Immunodeficiency 1995;5:171.

6. SCID WITH RETICULOENDOTHELIOSIS (Omenn's Syndrome)

Omenn described a familial immunodeficiency with a severe eczematoid skin rash, lymphadenopathy, hepatosplenomegaly with diarrhea, and failure to thrive. Most of these patients have eosinophilia with high IgE and low IgG and IgM; blood B cells are low or absent. The blood T cell numbers may be normal or low, and a very restricted T cell repertoire is reported. At autopsy, the thymus has lacked Hassall's corpuscles. The absence of consistent laboratory abnormalities makes diagnosis difficult. Some cases have been successfully treated by marrow ablation followed by transplantation. The condition is probably different from maternal engraftment of an infant with SCID resulting in graft-versus-host disease.

Appleton AL et al: Differentiation of materno-fetal GVHD from Omenn's syndrome in pre-BMT patients with severe combined immunodeficiency. Bone Marrow Transplant 1994;14:157.
Loechelt BJ et al: Mismatched bone marrow transplantation for Omenn syndrome: A variant of severe combined immunodeficiency. Bone Marrow Transplant 1995;16:381.

OTHER DISORDERS ASSOCIATED WITH IMMUNODEFICIENCY

WISKOTT-ALDRICH SYNDROME

Wiskott-Aldrich syndrome patients have thrombocytopenia, eczema, and recurrent infection (originally draining ears) and results from deletion of the WASP gene at X11p. Inheritance is X-linked recessive; the incidence is about 4 per million male births. The disorder is associated with deficient expression of a 115 kDa cell surface sialophorin identified as CD43. Common presenting symptoms are bloody diarrhea, cerebral hemorrhage, or septicemia followed by severe infections with polysaccharide-encapsulated bacteria. However, some patients have little if any eczema, while others have few infections. The main causes of death in infancy are bleeding and infections, but with time lymphomas become increasingly common. Survival through the teens is rare in untreated patients, though partial syndromes are sometimes diagnosed in adults. A specific diagnosis should be easier now that the gene has been identified. Routine laboratory findings that suggest the diagnosis are a low platelet count, low or absent isohemagglutinins, and reduced antibody response to polysaccharides. IgM may be low; IgA and IgE are often high. Bone marrow transplantation with matched sibling marrow offers the best hope for long-term correction of the defect. The platelet count generally rises following splenectomy, but this operation must be followed by antibiotic prophylaxis because of the increased risk of septicemia and sudden death.

Featherstone C: The many faces of WAS protein. Science 1997;275:27.
Parolini O et al: Expression of Wiskott-Aldrich syndrome protein *(WASP)* gene during hematopoietic differentiation. Blood 1997;90:70.

ATAXIA-TELANGIECTASIA

Ataxia-telangiectasia is characterized by cerebellar ataxia (due to degeneration of Purkinje cells), usually developing between 2 and 5 years of age and followed by the appearance of telangiectases, particularly on the conjunctiva and over exposed areas, ie, the nose, ears, and shoulders. Defects in the gene for the ATM protein on chromosome 11 disrupt regulation of cell cycle regulation and result in failure of DNA repair. The Nijmegen breakage syndrome is probably a variant of ataxia-telangiectasia with more severe clinical features, including microcephaly and "bird-like" facies. Abnormal findings in ataxia-telangiectasia include raised serum α-fetoprotein levels (useful diagnostically), thymic hypoplasia, low or absent serum IgE, low IgA in 50%, abnormal carbohydrate tolerance, and defective ability to repair radiation-induced DNA fragmentation. Clinically, the most important symptom is progressive loss of motor coordination, followed by weakness. Respiratory tract infections and many types of malignancy (including carcinomas) are the major causes of death. About 10% of patients develop lymphomas, the majority of which are T cell-derived. Many of the lymphomas have translocations or inversions at sites where T cell receptor genes are normally rearranged. Radiotherapy has been followed by skin breakdown, presumably the result of the DNA repair defect. The heterozygote frequency is 0.5–5%, depending on geographic and ethnic factors, and these individuals have an increased incidence of breast cancer.

Lavin MF, Shiloh Y: The genetic defect in ataxia-telangiectasia. Annu Rev Immunol 1997;15:177.
Sullivan KE et al: Cell cycle checkpoints and DNA repair in Nijmegen breakage syndrome. Clin Immunol Immunopathol 1997;82:43.
Telatar M et al: Ataxia telangiectasia. Am J Hum Genet 1996;59:40.

CHRONIC MUCOCUTANEOUS CANDIDIASIS

This entity consists of chronic candidiasis affecting the skin or nails and mucous membranes not attributable to antibiotic treatment or another defined immunodeficiency disease. Involvement of the scalp and flexural creases is common, usually as erythema and scaling but occasionally as granulomas with skin hypertrophy. The recurrent candidiasis points to an underlying immunodeficiency, but the faulty mechanism has not been identified. Affected patients make anti-*Candida* antibodies, and their in vitro lymphocyte responses may be positive even when *Candida* skin tests are negative. Evidence for the complexity of this form of immunodeficiency includes the frequent association with endocrinopathy, sometimes autoimmune (affecting the parathyroids, thyroid, pituitary, or gonads), and, less commonly, increased susceptibility to staphylococcal infections with defective neutrophil mobility. Some control of the candidiasis can usually be achieved with continuous fluconazole treatment.

Tosti A et al: Itraconazole in the treatment of two young brothers with chronic mucocutaneous candidiasis. Pediatr Dermatol 1997;14:146.

X-LINKED LYMPHOPROLIFERATIVE SYNDROME

This term is applied to boys who develop bone marrow aplasia, hypogammaglobulinemia, or a lymphoproliferative syndrome following Epstein-Barr virus (EBV) infection. The gene responsible has been mapped to Xq2s, and antenatal diagnosis is possible. Affected boys are immunologically normal prior to EBV infection, and during acute mononucleosis they make some antibody to the EBV. In most instances, the EBV infection results in a lethal lymphoproliferative syndrome characterized by liver failure, disseminated intravascular coagulation, and multiple monoclonal serum IgM bands. Acyclovir is sometimes beneficial, and treatment with alpha interferon and monoclonal anti-B cell antibodies is being investigated. Only 10–20% of affected boys who are infected with EBV survive to develop hypogammaglobulinemia.

Pracher E et al: Successful bone marrow transplantation in a boy with X-linked lymphoproliferative syndrome and acute severe infectious mononucleosis. Bone Marrow Transplant 1994;13:655.
Purtilo DT et al: The X-linked lymphoproliferative disease: From autopsy toward cloning the gene, 1975–1990. Pediatr Pathol 1991;11:685.

GRAFT-VERSUS-HOST DISEASE

Graft-versus-host disease follows transfusion of immunocompetent but incompatible lymphocytes into a person incapable of rejecting them. It causes significant morbidity in about 30% of bone marrow transplant recipients and causes death in infants with SCID. It has been reported in infants receiving transfusions from HLA homozygous donors, so blood products for infants should be irradiated. An erythematous macular and then bullous skin rash is variably followed by diarrhea, hepatitis, nephritis, pulmonary infiltrates, and fever, whereas marrow damage results in neutropenia and then thrombocytopenia. Many patients develop high IgE levels. The diagnosis is suspected on the basis of transplantation and a history of an unirradiated blood or blood product transfusion, usually into an immunodeficient patient, and is confirmed by skin or lip biopsy. Prophylaxis in transplant recipients is with corticosteroids and cyclosporine, and when the disease becomes severe it may be slowed by high-dose corticosteroids or at least temporarily halted by anti-T cell antibodies (OKT3 or antilymphocyte serum). Chronic graft-versus-host disease after allogeneic bone marrow transplantation causes scleroderma and bile duct destruction. The liver damage can be severe enough to require transplantation.

Henslee-Downey PJ: Mismatched bone marrow transplantation. Curr Opin Oncol 1995;7:115.
Takanashi M et al: Graft-versus-host disease associated with transfusions of HLA-matched, HLA-homozygous platelets. Transfusion 1995;35:535.

BIOCHEMICAL DEFECTS SOMETIMES ASSOCIATED WITH IMMUNODEFICIENCY

Several primary errors of metabolism affect immunity adversely. **Transcobalamin 2 deficiency** causes a megaloblastic anemia with impaired bacterial killing by neutrophils and reduced serum immunoglobulins of all classes. **Biotin-dependent decarboxylase deficiencies** may be associated with convulsions, alopecia, candidiasis, low serum IgA, and a reduced number of T cells. Lymphopenia and impaired CMI are reported in **hereditary orotic aciduria.** Chromosomal instability syndromes impair cell-mediated immunity, as in Bloom's syndrome, which may be severe enough to cause antibody deficiency (mostly of IgM) and malabsorption. A systematic listing of genetic disorders with immunodeficiency is given in the review by Ming and others.

Ming JE, Stiehm ER, Graham JM Jr: Immunodeficiency as a component of recognizable syndromes. Am J Med Genet 1996;66:378.
Prigent C et al: Aberrant DNA repair and DNA replication due to an inherited enzymatic defect in human DNA ligase I. Mol Cell Biol 1994;14:310.

SECONDARY IMMUNODEFICIENCY

Secondary immunodeficiency is a common cause of pediatric illness. The mechanisms that may be impaired are summarized in Table 27–3, and the symptoms are generally those that would be anticipated from the combination of the primary disorder and the complicating immunodeficiency. Whenever possible, treatment should be directed at the primary disorder. Occasionally, immunologic methods may help—eg, varicella-zoster immune globulin may prevent varicella in patients with leukemia and intravenous immune globulin replacement might provide added protection where antibody production is diminished. IgG replacement is unlikely to help when loss (as in

Table 27–3. Mechanisms of secondary immunodeficiency.

Mechanism	Example
Loss	
Immunoglobulin	Renal, in nephrotic syndrome
Immunoglobulin	Skin, from burns
Immunoglobulin and cells	Gut, in intestinal lymphangiectasia
Phagocytes	Following splenectomy
Malnutrition	Kwashiorkor
Zinc deficiency	Impaired cell-mediated immunity
Copper and iron deficiency	Impaired neutrophil function
Drugs	Steroids, cancer chemotherapy
	Specific immunosuppressants
	Phenytoin → IgA deficiency
Infections	HIV, EBV, CMV, measles, rubella, hepatitis, malaria

nephrotic syndrome) is responsible for hypogamma-globulinemia.

Lee ML, Gale RP, Yap PL: Use of intravenous immunoglobulin to prevent or treat infections in persons with immune deficiency. Annu Rev Med 1997;48:93.

POST BONE MARROW TRANSPLANT IMMUNODEFICIENCY

In the months following a bone marrow transplant, patients remain highly susceptible to herpesvirus, *P carinii,* and other fungal infections even when their blood leukocyte counts recover. They require prophylaxis with trimethoprim-sulfonamide, acyclovir, and intravenous immune globulin, and pulmonary symptoms (cough, impaired oxygenation) must be investigated promptly. Their problems arise in part from immunosuppressive treatments used to reduce graft-versus-host disease (see below) and partly from delay in recovery of the B lymphocytes required for antibody responses.

Parra C, Roldan E, Brieva JA: Deficient expression of adhesion molecules by human CD5-B lymphocytes both after bone marrow transplantation and during normal ontogeny. Blood 1996;88:1733.

THERAPEUTIC IMMUNOSUPPRESSION

Therapeutic immunosuppression is increasingly used in pediatrics for transplant recipients and for autoimmune disease. Corticosteroids at doses equivalent to 2 mg/kg of prednisolone per day interfere with cytokine production and cause lymphopenia by directing lymphocytes to the marrow; the duration of action is about 24 hours. Much higher doses, equivalent to 20–30 mg/kg of prednisolone per day are used in 3- to 5-day courses for treatment of life-threatening conditions or to evaluate the potential for more powerful immunosuppressive agents. Corticosteroids are satisfactory anti-inflammatory and immunosuppressive agents when they can be given on alternate days as a single morning dose (as is sometimes the case for systemic lupus erythematosus or autoimmune anemias). Immunosuppression by corticosteroids is limited by the growth arrest and severe cushingoid changes, which occur even in dosages of 2 mg/kg of prednisolone per day. Transplant recipients require additional powerful immunosuppressives such as cyclosporine or tacrolimus (FK506). Both bind to immunophilins to form a complex that reversibly inhibits calcineurin-dependent signaling in lymphocytes, blocking cytokine production and release. Immunosuppression achievable by both agents is limited by their nephrotoxicity, and trough blood levels need to be monitored carefully and drugs that affect their metabolism (erythromycin, theophylline) tracked. Preventing organ rejection usually requires two drugs, such as cyclosporine and mycophenolate mofetil or azathioprine. Mycophenolate mofetil is a newer drug that inhibits purine synthesis and is relatively specific for lymphocytes. It is taken by mouth, and blood levels must be checked. Cost is one reason it has not replaced azathioprine, which causes much more general marrow suppression.

Severe organ rejection episodes, or graft-versus-host disease, can be controlled acutely with antibodies to T lymphocytes such as antithymocyte globulin and monoclonal CD3 antibody. Both deplete T cells and clear antigen receptors off the T cell surface. Some T cells are activated as well, causing a cytokine syndrome of fever, malaise, skin rash, and pulmonary edema. This syndrome is minimized by premedicating patients with an antihistamine, acetaminophen, corticosteroids, and even cyclosporine. Patients generally need to be tested for anti-horse, anti-rabbit, or anti-mouse antibodies after treatment.

Antimitotic agents (cyclophosphamide, chlorambucil) that block T cell proliferation are effective but toxic immunosuppressants. The risks of immunosuppression include reactivation of latent herpesviruses (CMV, HSV, VZV), though antiviral treatments have made these less life-threatening. EBV reactivation is hazardous if it results in a lymphoproliferative disease, which, when severe, is associated with marrow phagocytosis of red and white cells. The appearance of free EBV genome in the plasma probably provides the best advance warning of this dangerous complication. The usual treatment strategy is to reduce the dosage of agents such as cyclosporine and tacrolimus while continuing immunosuppression with steroids. Testing serum for oligoclonal immunoglobulin bands may give some indication of the progression or regression of lymphoproliferative disease. Combined immunosuppression with agents having different modes of action tends to be much more potent, with a greater potential for opportunistic infections, than immunosuppression by single agents. The risk of infection is greatest when the neutrophil count is depressed by antimitotic agents at the same time as specific immunity is suppressed by corticosteroids and cyclosporine.

Lake KD, Canafax DM: Important interactions of drugs with immunosuppressive agents used in transplant recipients. J Antimicrob Chemother 1995 36(Suppl B):11.

INVESTIGATION OF IMMUNODEFICIENCY

Physical and anatomic defects are the most common causes of recurrent infections, and if a single site is affected it should be searched for a local abnormality. The age at onset of infections is important because defects of phagocytes, C3, or cellular immunity become symptomatic in the first months of life, whereas maternal antibody protects infants with hypogammaglobulinemia for 3–6 months. Antibody, complement, and phagocyte defects predispose mainly to bacterial infections; diarrhea, superficial candidiasis, and severe herpesvirus infections are typical of cellular immunodeficiency. A simple protocol for testing these mechanisms is presented in Table 27–4, and the level of investigation should reflect the frequency and severity of infections. A complete blood count and quantitative immunoglobulin measurement will identify more than 90% of *primary* immunodeficiency syndromes.

Fleisher TA: Evaluation of the potentially immunodeficient patient. Adv Intern Med 1996;41:1.

PHAGOCYTE FUNCTION

Tests of phagocytic cell function should first rule out neutropenia with white blood cell count and differential. A blood film is useful to exclude the Howell-Jolly bodies of asplenia and to look for normal lysosomal granules in neutrophils. Myeloperoxidase deficiency is excluded by histochemical stains available in most oncology laboratories. The respiratory burst and generation of bactericidal factors can be tested by nitroblue tetrazolium reduction, so this test screens for most types of chronic granulomatous disease (the most common bacterial killing defect) and for leukocyte glucose-6-phosphate dehydrogenase deficiency. Leukocyte adhesion molecules are screened by flow cytometry—though the difference in symptoms of these various phagocyte defects should dictate which tests are used. Chemotaxis can be measured in migration chambers in the laboratory and can also be assessed by migration of cells from abraded skin onto a sterile coverslip. Results of chemotaxis tests must be interpreted cautiously, since secondary and transient defects in chemotaxis are

common. Quantitation of bacterial ingestion and microbicidal activity are mostly research procedures.

COMPLEMENT

Deficiency of a classic pathway component can be excluded by a normal hemolytic complement titer, for which the patient's serum must be separated and frozen to –70 °C within 30 minutes of collection. Alternative pathway function is tested by lysis of rabbit red blood cells. There is little point in measuring individual complement component levels if the hemolytic titer is normal—unless it is done to follow the activity of an immune complex-associated disease in which C4 and C3 may be low. The common form of opsonizing defect of yeast is now known to be due to allelic variants of mannan-binding protein.

Sumiya M, Summerfield JA: Mannose-binding protein, genetic variants and the risk of infection. Q J Med 1996;89:723.

ANTIBODIES & IMMUNOGLOBULINS

In patients who are not blood group AB, isohemagglutinins are the most easily tested naturally occurring antibodies. They are of the IgM class, become detectable by 6 months of age, and reach adult levels about 1 year later. The importance of antibody tests is illustrated by the inverse correlation between isohemagglutinin titer and susceptibility to meningitis in patients with hypogammaglobulinemia, regardless of their serum IgM levels. Tetanus and diphtheria antibody tests are widely available, as are antibodies to pneumococcal polysaccharide, rubella, and mumps. In practice, it is often easier to measure serum immunoglobulins as a screening procedure than to test for antibodies, but it should be appreciated that some patients with varied immunodeficiency syndromes and some infants with severely impaired cell-mediated immunity make immunoglobulin that does not have useful antibody activity.

Table 27–4. Hierarchy of tests for investigation of primary immunodeficiency.

Test Level	Complement	Phagocytes	Antibody	CMI
Screening	CH_{50}	Count, morphology	Ig measurement	Delayed hypersensitivity skin tests.
First level		NBT, LFA-1[1]	IHA,[2] TT	T-cell counts[3]
Second level	Factor assays	Killing and chemotaxis	Immunize	In vitro tests

[1]Only when chronic granulomatous disease or LFA-1 deficiency is suspected.
[2]IHA = isohemagglutinins, after age 1; TT = tetanus toxoid.
[3]Identify all T cells with CD3, subsets with CD4, CD8. CD45RO for memory cells.

Table 27–5. Blood lymphocyte phenotyping.[1]

Antigen	Commercial Antibodies	Cells Stained	Normal Range and Changes Seen Clinically
CD2	OKT11	T, NK	70–90%. Falls to 10–20% when T cells absent.
CD3	OKT3, Leu4	All T	55–85%. Falls when T-cell number reduced. Increases to 90% when B cells absent.
CD4	OKT4, Leu3	HLA-D restricted T cells	35–60%. Selectively reduced in HIV infections. Reduced with other T cells by steroids, defect of cell-mediated immunity.
CD5		T cells, immature B cells	55–85%. Falls when T-cell number reduced. Increased with immature B cells.
CD8	OKT8, Leu2	HLA-A/B restricted T cells	25–50%. Selectively increased in response to some viral infections. Reduced with other T-cell defects.
CD11	OKM1, Mac-1	Monocytes	Lacking in LFA-1 deficiency.
CD16	Leu11	NK cells	Increased by viral infections.
CD19		B cells	Absent or low in congenital X-linked agammaglobulinemia and common variable immunodeficiency disease. Increased when T cells are lacking.
CD20		B cells	Increased when T cells lacking.
CD25		IL-2 receptor	Activated T cells. Increased in graft-versus-host disease.
CD45RO	UCHL1	T cells	Memory T cells, low in newborns.
CD56	NKH-1	NK cells	Raised in active viral infections.

[1]From Thompson RA (editor): Laboratory investigation of immunological disorders. Clin Immunol Allergy 1985;5:No. 3. See also Spickett GP, Matamoros N, Farrant J: Lymphocyte surface phenotype in common variable immunodeficiency. Dis Markers 1992;10:67.

Properly performed immunoglobulin estimations are reproducible to ±10% for IgG and IgA and ±20% for IgM, so small changes are of no significance. Measurement of serum IgD is not generally of diagnostic value in pediatrics. Immunoglobulin concentrations are lower in infants than in adults, and laboratories may erroneously report normal children's values as low. Comparisons of results from different laboratories may be difficult, because few commercial kit suppliers calibrate their control sera against the international standard. Simple protein electrophoresis is not sufficiently sensitive to make a confident diagnosis of hypogammaglobulinemia, though it is valuable for identifying the monoclonal excesses seen in macroglobulinemia, in the oligoclonal gammopathy of EBV infections in X-linked lymphoproliferative syndrome, and in heavy chain diseases. Serum albumin should be measured at least once in patients with hypogammaglobulinemia to exclude secondary deficiencies due to loss. IgG or IgA subclass measurements may be abnormal in patients with varied immunodeficiency syndromes, but they are rarely helpful.

CELL-MEDIATED IMMUNITY

Positive delayed hypersensitivity skin tests give good evidence for antigen-specific T cell immunity. Only a positive response is interpretable—particularly in infancy, when prior immunization may not have been adequate to elicit good skin responses.

Blood T and B lymphocyte counts give a good assessment of specific immune function. Only small volumes of blood are required, and results are rapidly available. Some of the more useful antibodies—and common deviations from normal—are summarized in Table 27–5. When abnormalities are suspected, it is important to check absolute numbers of lymphocytes and their subsets. Tests of T cell proliferation and cytokine production are useful to characterize immunodeficiency detected by simpler tests, but they are not useful screening tests for children with recurrent infections.

Herrod HG et al: Cell-mediated immune status of children with recurrent infection. J Pediatr 1995;126:530.

28

Endocrine Disorders

Ronald W. Gotlin, MD, Michael S. Kappy, MD, PhD, Robert H. Slover, MD,
& Philip S. Zeitler, MD, PhD

GENERAL CONCEPTS

One of the major functions of the endocrine system is to regulate the enzymatic and other metabolic processes (eg, molecular transport) responsible for maintaining the equilibrium (homeostasis) of the internal environment to ensure survival of the individual. Other critical roles for the endocrine system are regulation of growth (in utero and postnatal), pubertal development and reproduction, energy production, regulation of blood pressure, and, to a lesser extent, behavior.

The classic concept of endocrine effects representing the result of hormones secreted into the blood to reach a target cell has been updated to account for other ways in which hormonal effects are realized. Specifically, some hormone systems involve the stimulation or inhibition (or both) of metabolic processes in neighboring (as opposed to distant) cells (eg, within the pancreatic islets or cartilage). This phenomenon is termed "paracrine."

Other hormone effects reflect the action of particular hormones on the same cells that produced them. This action is termed "autocrine." The discoveries of local production of insulin, glucagon, atrial natriuretic hormone, and many other hormones in the brain and gut support the concept of paracrine and autocrine processes in these tissues.

Another significant discovery in endocrine physiology was an appreciation of the role of specific hormone receptors in target tissues, without which the hormonal effects could not be manifested. In the complete androgen insensitivity (resistance) syndrome, androgen receptors are absent, and the individual develops normal female external genitalia despite the presence of testes (usually intra-abdominal) and adequate testosterone production. Similarly, in Albright's hereditary osteodystrophy (pseudohypoparathyroidism), affected persons have abnormal parathyroid hormone (PTH) receptor function and show the metabolic effects of hypoparathyroidism (low serum calcium and high serum phosphate), despite the secretion of more than adequate PTH. Alternatively, autonomous (abnormal) activation of a hormone receptor leads to the effects of the hormone without its abnormal secretion. Examples of this phenomenon include McCune-Albright syndrome (precocious puberty and hyperthyroidism) and familial male testotoxicosis (precocious pseudopuberty).

HORMONE TYPES

There are three main structural types of hormones: peptides and proteins, steroids, and amines. The peptide hormones include the releasing factors secreted by the hypothalamus, the hormones of the anterior and posterior pituitary gland, the pancreatic islet cells, the parathyroid glands, insulin-like growth factor I (IGF-I) from the liver and other tissues, angiotensin II, atrial natriuretic hormone, and many local growth factors. The steroid hormones are secreted primarily by the adrenal cortex, the gonads, and the liver (active vitamin D), whereas the amine hormones are secreted by the adrenal medulla (epinephrine) and the thyroid gland (T_4 and T_3).

As a general rule, the peptide hormones and epinephrine are more rapid-acting than the others and bind to specific receptors on the target cell surface. The metabolic effects of these hormones are usually manifested by their stimulation or inhibition of the activity of preexisting enzymes or transport proteins (posttranslational effects). The steroid hormones and active vitamin D, on the other hand, are more slow-acting and bind to their specific receptors within the target cell in the cytoplasm or directly to DNA in the nucleus. Their metabolic effects are generally caused by stimulating or inhibiting the synthesis of new enzymes or transport proteins (transcriptional effects), thereby increasing or decreasing the amount rather than the activity of these proteins in the target cell.

Metabolic processes that must be regulated rapidly (eg, blood glucose or calcium homeostasis) are usually under the control of the peptide hormones and epinephrine (Table 28–1), whereas those processes that may be regulated more slowly (eg, pubertal development, metabolic rate) are under the control of the steroid hormones (Table 28–1). The control of

Table 28–1. Hormonal regulation of metabolic processes.

First Level (Most Direct)

Metabolite or Other Parameter	Abnormality	Endocrine Gland	Hormone
Glucose	Hyperglycemia	Pancreatic beta cell	Insulin
Glucose	Hypoglycemia	Pancreatic alpha cell	Glucagon
Glucose	Hypoglycemia	Adrenal medulla	Epinephrine
Calcium	Hypercalcemia	Thyroid C cell	Calcitonin (?)
Calcium	Hypocalcemia	Parathyroid	PTH
Sodium/plasma osmolality	Hypernatremia/hyperosmolality	Hypothalamus (posterior pituitary gland)	ADH
Plasma volume	Hypervolemia	Heart	ANH

Second Level: Sodium and Potassium Balance

Metabolite or Other Parameter	Abnormality	Endocrine Gland	Hormone
Sodium/potassium	Hyponatremia	Kidney	Renin (an enzyme)
	Hyperkalemia	Liver and others	Angiotensin I
	Hypovolemia	Lung	Angiotensin II
		Adrenal cortex	Aldosterone

Third Level (Most Complex)

Releasing Hormone	Tropic Hormone	Endocrine Gland	Endocrine Gland Hormone
CRH	ACTH	Adrenal cortex	Cortisol
GHRH	GH	Liver	IGF-I
GnRH	LH	Testis	Testosterone
GnRH	FSH/LH	Ovary	Estradiol/progesterone
TRH	TSH	Thyroid gland	T_4 (some T_3)

ADH = antidiuretic hormone; ACTH = corticotropin; CRH = corticotropin-releasing hormone; FSH = follicle-stimulating hormone; GH = growth hormone; GHRH = growth hormone-releasing hormone; GnRH = gonadotropin-releasing hormone; IGF = insulin-like growth factor; LH = luteinizing hormone; PTH = parathyroid hormone; TRH = thyrotropin-releasing hormone; TSH = thyroid-stimulating hormone.

electrolyte homeostasis is intermediate and is regulated by a combination of peptide and steroid hormones (Table 28–1).

FEEDBACK CONTROL OF HORMONE SECRETION

Hormonal secretion is regulated, for the most part, by feedback in response to changes in the internal environment (Table 28–1). When the metabolic imbalance is corrected, stimulation of the initial hormone's secretion ceases and may even be inhibited. Overcorrection of the imbalance stimulates a counterregulatory hormone secretion, so the circulating concentrations of metabolites are kept within relatively narrow limits.

Hypothalamopituitary control of hormonal secretion is also regulated by feedback, so that end-organ failure (endocrine gland insufficiency) leading to decreased circulating concentrations of endocrine gland hormones results in increased secretion of hypothalamic releasing and pituitary hormones (Table 28–1; Figure 28–1). If restoration of normal circulating concentrations of endocrine gland hormones occurs, feed-back inhibition at the pituitary and hypothalamus results in cessation of the previously stimulated secretion of releasing and pituitary hormones and restoration of their circulating concentrations to normal.

Similarly, if there is autonomous endocrine gland hyperfunction (eg, in McCune-Albright syndrome, Graves' disease, and adrenal tumor), the specific hypothalamic releasing and pituitary hormones are suppressed (Figure 28–1). An understanding of the basic phenomenon of feedback control of hormonal secretion is fundamental to the understanding of endocrinologic disorders and their evaluation in children.

Sperling MA (ed): *Pediatric Endocrinology.* Saunders, 1996.

DISTURBANCES OF GROWTH

Disturbances of growth and development are the most common presenting complaints in the pediatric

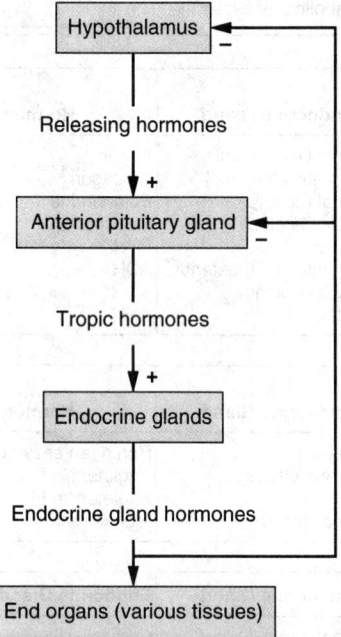

Figure 28–1. General scheme of the hypothalamus-pituitary-endocrine gland axis. Releasing hormones synthesized in the hypothalamus are secreted into the hypothalamohypophysial portal circulation. Tropic hormones are then secreted by the pituitary gland (hypophysis) in response, and they in turn act on specific endocrine glands to stimulate the secretion of their respective hormones. The endocrine gland hormones exert their respective effects on various target tissues (end organs) and exert an indirect negative feedback (feedback inhibition) on their own secretion by acting at the level of the pituitary gland and the hypothalamus. This system is characteristic of those hormones listed in Table 28–1.

endocrine clinic. Knowledge of the endocrine system is essential to differentiate disturbances in hormonal secretion and action from normal variations in the timing and pattern of development (ie, "constitutional" deviations from the average). It has been estimated that over 1 million children in the United States have abnormal short stature.

Tall stature has become an increasingly unusual presenting complaint in our society. Because of the preference for tallness in both males and females, the number of young people evaluated and treated for tall stature has decreased.

SHORT STATURE

Most short stature is familial, racial, or genetic. Pathologic short stature follows malnutrition, intrauterine growth retardation, dysmorphism, psy-

chosocial problems, and a wide range of systemic and chronic diseases (Table 28–2). The history, physical examination, growth curve, and radiographic bone age are most helpful in the differential diagnosis.

Differential Diagnosis of Short Stature

The following tests are useful when the history, physical examination, and growth chart do not point clearly to any of the conditions listed in Table 28–2.

(1) Complete blood count (to detect chronic anemia, infection, leukemia).

(2) Erythrocyte sedimentation rate (often elevated in collagen-vascular disease, cancer, chronic infection, inflammatory bowel disease).

(3) Urinalysis and microscopic examination (eg, occult pyelonephritis, glomerulonephritis, renal tubular disease).

(4) Stool examination for fat, occult blood, parasites, and parasite ova (inflammatory bowel disease, overwhelming parasitism).

(5) Serum electrolytes and phosphate (eg, mild adrenal insufficiency, renal tubular diseases, parathyroid disease, rickets); endomysial antibody (for celiac disease).

(6) Blood urea nitrogen and serum creatinine (occult renal insufficiency).

(7) Karyotyping (should be performed in all short girls with delayed sexual maturation with or without phenotypic features of Turner's syndrome).

(8) Thyroid function assessment: total thyroxine (T_4), free thyroxine (FT_4), and thyroid-stimulating hormone (TSH) concentrations (short stature may be the only sign of hypothyroidism).

(9) Controversy persists concerning the diagnosis of hGH deficiency. The authors prefer a combination of physiologic assessments: hGH levels obtained during natural sleep and following administration of the provocative agents clonidine, arginine, or glucagon. Measurement of IGF-I and IGF-binding protein-3 has proved to be a useful adjunct to diagnosis. Both are typically low in hGH deficiency, but they may also be reduced in malnutrition.

1. CONSTITUTIONAL SHORT STATURE

The term "familial" or "genetic" short stature implies that a child is small because he or she is "programmed" that way. In children with constitutional short stature, the growth pattern is normal and bone age correlates with chronologic age. Constitutional delay of growth, on the other hand, implies a delayed growth pattern with delayed maturity and normal final height. Bone age in these children is delayed relative to chronologic age, but it is more in keeping with height age and generally in agreement with the stage of puberty. Children with constitutional delay of

Table 28–2. Causes of short stature.

Familial, racial, or genetic
Constitutional short stature and delayed adolescence
Endocrine disturbances
  Growth hormone deficiency
    Hereditary—gene deletion
    Idiopathic—deficiency of growth hormone or growth hor-
      mone releasing hormone (or both) with and without
      associated abnormalities of midline structures of the
      central nervous system
    Acquired
      Transient—eg, psychosocial short stature
      Organic—tumor, irradiation of the central nervous
        system, infection, or trauma
  Hypothyroidism
  Adrenal insufficiency
  Cushing's disease and Cushing's syndrome (including
    iatrogenic causes)
  Sexual precocity (androgen or estrogen excess)
  Diabetes mellitus (poorly controlled)
  Diabetes insipidus
  Hyperaldosteronism
Primordial short stature
  Intrauterine growth retardation
    Placental insufficiency
    Intrauterine infection
  Primordial dwarfism with premature aging
    Progeria (Hutchinson-Gilford syndrome)
    Progeroid syndrome
      Werner's syndrome
      Cachectic (Cockayne's syndrome)
  Short stature without dysmorphism
  Short stature with dysmorphism (eg, Seckel's bird-headed
    dwarfism, leprechaunism, Silver's syndrome, Bloom's
    syndrome, Cornelia de Lange syndrome, Hallerman-
    Streiff syndrome)
Inborn errors of metabolism
  Altered metabolism of calcium or phosphorus (eg, hypo-
    phosphatemic rickets, hypophosphatasia, infantile hyper-
    calcemia, pseudohypoparathyroidism)
  Storage diseases
    Mucopolysaccharidoses (eg, Hurler's syndrome,
      Hunter's syndrome)
    Mucolipidoses (eg, generalized gangliosidosis,
      fucosidosis, mannosidosis)

Inborn errors of metabolism (cont'd)
    Sphingolipidoses (eg, Tay-Sachs disease, Niemann-Pick
      disease, Gaucher's disease)
    Miscellaneous (eg, cystinosis)
  Aminoacidemias and aminoacidurias
  Epithelial transport disorders (eg, renal tubular acidosis,
    cystic fibrosis, Bartter's syndrome, vasopressin-resistant
    diabetes insipidus, pseudohypoparathyroidism)
  Organic acidemias and acidurias (eg, methylmalonic acid-
    uria, orotic aciduria, maple syrup urine disease, isovaleric
    acidemia)
  Metabolic anemias (eg, sickle cell disease, thalassemia,
    pyruvate kinase deficiency)
  Disorders of mineral metabolism (eg, Wilson's disease,
    magnesium malabsorption syndrome)
  Body defense disorders (eg, Bruton's agammaglobulinemia,
    thymic aplasia, chronic granulomatous disease)
Constitutional (intrinsic) diseases of bone
  Defects of growth of tubular bones or spine (eg, achondro-
    plasia, metatropic dwarfism, diastrophic dwarfism, meta-
    physeal chondrodysplasia)
  Disorganized development of cartilage and fibrous compo-
    nents of the skeleton (eg, multiple cartilaginous exosto-
    ses, fibrous dysplasia with skin pigmentation, precocious
    puberty of McCune-Albright)
  Abnormalities of density of cortical diaphyseal structure or
    metaphyseal modeling (eg, osteogenesis imperfecta
    congenita, osteopetrosis, tubular stenosis)
Short stature associated with chromosomal defects
  Autosomal (eg, Down's syndrome, cri du chat syndrome,
    trisomy 18)
  Sex chromosomal (eg, Turner's syndrome-XO, penta X,
    XXXY)
Chronic systemic diseases, congenital defects, and can-
cers (eg, chronic infection and infestation, inflammatory
  bowel disease, hepatic disease, cardiovascular disease,
  hematologic disease, central nervous system disease, pul-
  monary disease, renal disease, malnutrition, cancers, colla-
  gen vascular disease)
Psychosocial short stature (deprivation dwarfism)
Miscellaneous syndromes (eg, arthrogryposis multiplex congenita, cerebrohepatorenal syndrome, Noonan's syndrome,
  Prader-Willi syndrome, Riley-Day syndrome)

growth (constitutional short stature) and skeletal maturation appear entirely normal in other respects. In children with constitutional short stature, birth weight and length are not abnormal but the rate of growth is typically decreased during infancy after the first year. There is often a history of a similar pattern of growth in one of the parents or in other members of the family. Puberty is delayed, and these children characteristically reach normal height at a later than average age.

Treatment with low doses of testosterone over a 3- to 6-month period in boys may be useful in hastening the timing of puberty and accelerating growth, but final adult height is not enhanced. Growth hormone does not have a place in treating these normal children, since its use does not increase ultimate height and it may actually decrease adult height by shortening the growth span.

2. GROWTH HORMONE & GROWTH HORMONE DEFICIENCY

The human growth hormone (hGH) gene on chromosome 17 codes for a 191-amino-acid peptide which is available as a pharmaceutical recombinant product.

hGH is released from the anterior pituitary in response to a delicate interplay of hypothalamic releasing and inhibitory factors. Moreover, a variety of stimuli, including adrenergic and dopaminergic agents, arginine, glucagon, and insulin-induced hypoglycemia, have been used clinically as provocative tests of hGH secretion. Serum concentrations of hGH vary considerably; episodic surges occur in relation to nutrients, to activity, and particularly to natural sleep. The latter typically is associated with significant sustained elevation of hGH during the first 2 hours after the onset of sleep. Electroencephalographic monitoring during this interval reflects slow wave or deep sleep, suggesting a role for specific neurotransmitter influence.

Following secretion, hGH binds to specific receptors in a large variety of tissues and triggers direct and indirect actions. The latter category is used to designate the activity of the IGFs generated in response to hGH (Figure 28–2).

Growth hormone deficiency occurs in approximately 1:4000 children. About two-thirds of cases are idiopathic (rarely familial); a deficiency or impairment in the hypothalamic secretion of hGH-releasing hormone is suspected. The remainder are secondary to pituitary or hypothalamic disease, infection, trauma, reticuloendotheliosis, and craniopharyngioma or other tumors (eg, gliomas). The deficiency of hGH may be an isolated defect, or it may occur in combination with other pituitary hormone deficiencies. Idiopathic hGH deficiency affects both sexes equally. There are also children who appear to be growth hormone-deficient but show normal responses to traditional provocative GH testing. This group includes children with hGH receptor defects. The most severely affected of these children have been called "Laron syndrome children," a group in whom the defective receptor for hGH leads to resistance to growth hormone. These children have benefited from treatment with IGF-I in experimental studies; however, the side effects and final height outcomes in these individuals are not known.

Other children who have defied traditional diagnostic criteria have been characterized as "idiopathic short children." These children seem to have normal growth hormone responses to testing but very poor growth rates. Recently, some of these children have been found to have lower serum IGF-I concentrations, suggesting again a partial insensitivity to hGH based on receptor gene defects. IGF-I may also help this group.

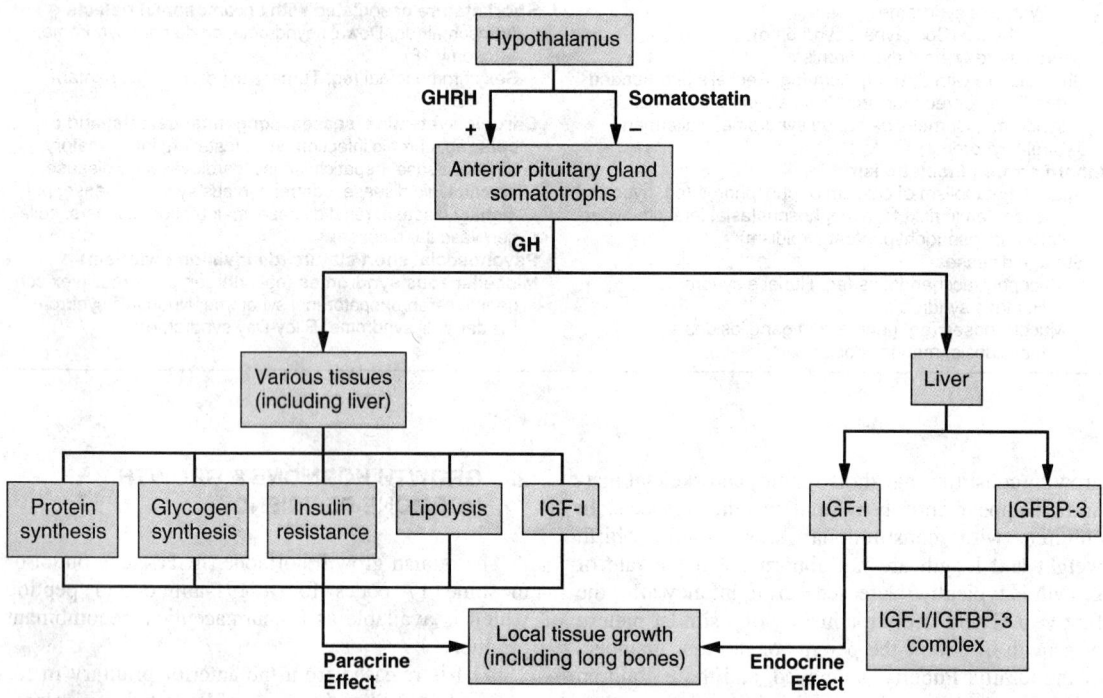

Figure 28–2. The GHRH/GH/IGF-I system. The effects of growth hormone (GH) on growth are partly due to its direct anabolic effects in muscle, liver, and bone. In addition, GH stimulates many tissues to produce IGF-I locally, which stimulates the growth of the tissue itself (paracrine effect of IGF-I). The action of GH on the liver results in the secretion of IGF-I (circulating IGF-I), which in turn stimulates growth in other tissues (endocrine effect of IGF-I). The action of growth hormone on the liver also enhances the secretion of IGF-binding protein-3 (IGFBP-3), which forms a high-molecular-weight complex with IGF-I. The function of this complex is to transport IGF-I to its target tissues, but the complex also serves as a reservoir and possible inhibitor of IGF-I action. In various chronic illnesses, the direct metabolic effects of growth hormone are inhibited; the secretion of IGF-I in response to GH is blunted, and in some cases IGFBP-3 synthesis is enhanced, resulting in marked inhibition in the growth of the child. (GHRH, growth hormone-releasing hormone; IGF, insulin-like growth factor.)

At birth, classic hGH-deficient children are of normal weight but length may be reduced slightly, suggesting that GH is not a major contributor to intrauterine growth. The most characteristic clinical feature of the child with hGH deficiency is a linear growth rate as low as 50% of that of the normal child of the same age. Growth retardation may begin during infancy or may be delayed until later childhood. Other findings include infantile fat distribution, inappropriately youthful facial features, midfacial hypoplasia, and delayed sexual maturation. Skeletal maturation (bone age) is delayed. Headaches, visual field defects, polyuria, and polydipsia may precede or accompany the onset of growth failure in cases resulting from central nervous system disease. Abnormalities on skull radiography, CT scans, and MRI are common in organic hypopituitarism.

The diagnosis of growth hormone deficiency continues to offer difficulties. Traditionally, provocative studies have been performed using a variety of agents including insulin-induced hypoglycemia, arginine, levodopa, clonidine, or glucagon. Alternatively, serum concentrations of IGF-I or IGF-binding protein 3 may give reasonable estimations of GH secretion in the adequately nourished child (Figure 28–2). When results of growth hormone testing are equivocal, a trial of hGH treatment may be useful in determining whether an abnormally short child will benefit from growth hormone. Currently, the treatment of choice for isolated GH deficiency is recombinant hGH in a dose of 0.15–0.3 mg/kg/wk administered subcutaneously divided into six or seven equal once-daily doses.

Results of clinical trials with hypothalamic hGH-releasing hormone have been encouraging, as have trials of peptide and nonpeptide GH secretagogues, some of which may be administered orally. IGF-I (somatomedin-C), as previously described, has proved useful in growth hormone-resistant conditions. Physiologic doses of protein anabolic agents (eg, oxandrolone) may be effective in promoting linear growth but may accelerate epiphysial closure, thus lessening adult height. Anabolic agents should be used, if at all, at the time of puberty and in combination with hGH.

The efficacy of hGH treatment for conditions associated with severe short stature and normal hGH secretion (eg, intrauterine growth retardation, chronic renal disease, steroid-dependent asthma) is currently under clinical investigation. In Turner's syndrome, results over the past 10 years have demonstrated significant improvement in final adult height. The role of hGH as an anabolic agent in GH-deficient adults is under investigation. Early studies demonstrate significant benefit in bone metabolism and sense of well-being.

Growth hormone therapy is expensive, and indications other than classic growth hormone deficiency remain controversial. Reported side effects of recombinant growth hormone therapy include benign intracranial hypertension, slipped capital femoral epiphysis, and leukemia, all subject to ongoing safety studies. Creutzfeld-Jakob disease has occurred in children previously treated with hGH before the recombinant form was available.

3. HYPOTHYROIDISM

Hypothyroidism in childhood (discussed in a subsequent section) is invariably associated with poor growth and delayed skeletal maturation. In occasional cases, short stature may be the principal finding.

4. INTRAUTERINE GROWTH RETARDATION

Intrauterine growth retardation may occur in craniofacial disproportion (eg, Seckel syndrome, Russell-Silver syndrome, Noonan's syndrome), in some cases of progeria (eg, Hutchinson-Gilford syndrome) and cachectic dwarfism, or in individuals with no accompanying significant dysmorphism. The birth weight and length of affected children are below normal for gestational age. They grow parallel with (but below) the fifth percentile. Most (85%) healthy full-term infants achieve catch-up in height during the first year of life, with half of those remaining short as adults. In most instances, skeletal maturation (bone age) corresponds to chronologic age or is only mildly delayed—in contrast to the striking delay often present in children with hGH and (especially) thyroid hormone deficiency.

There is no satisfactory long-term treatment for primordial short stature, though growth hormone in large doses may be efficacious and is being evaluated in clinical trials.

5. SHORT STATURE DUE TO EMOTIONAL FACTORS (Psychosocial Short Stature; Deprivation Dwarfism)

Psychologic deprivation with disturbances in motor and personality development may be associated with short stature. Undernutrition contributes to the growth retardation of some but not all affected persons. Sometimes the child has an increased or even voracious appetite; polydipsia and polyuria are sometimes present. These children are of normal size at birth and grow normally for a variable period of time before growth slows. A history of feeding problems in early infancy is common. Sleep is often restless. Emotional disturbances in the family are the rule. Skeletal maturation is delayed, and serum hGH concentrations during sleep or in response to pharmacologic stimulation may be diminished.

Foster home placement or a change in the psychologic and emotional environment at home usually results is significantly improved growth, normalization of personality, appetite, and dietary intake, and return of normal hGH secretion.

Goddard A, Covello R: Mutations of the growth hormone receptor in children with idiopathic short stature. J Pediatr 1995;127:244.

Kallberg J, Albertsson-Wikland K: Growth in full-term small-for-gestational age infants: From birth to final height. Pediatr Res 1995;38:733.

Kawaik M et al: Unfavorable effects of growth hormone therapy on the final height of boys with short stature not caused by growth hormone deficiency. J Pediatr 1997;130:205.

Pomerance H: Growth and its assessment. Adv Pediatr 1995;42:545.

Rosenfeld R: Recommendations for diagnosis, treatment, and management of individuals with Turner syndrome. The Endocrinologist 1994;4:351.

Rosenfeld R, Albertsson-Wikland K: Diagnostic controversy: The diagnosis of childhood growth hormone deficiency revisited. J Clin Endocrinol Metab 1995;80:1532.

Strauss RS, Dietz WH: Effects of intrauterine growth retardation in premature infants on early childhood growth. J Pediatr 1997;130:95.

Tillman V et al: Biochemical tests in the diagnosis of childhood growth hormone deficiency. J Clin Endocrinol Metab 1997;82:531.

Zadik Z, Chalen S: Effect of long-term growth hormone therapy on bone age and pubertal maturation in boys with and without classic growth hormone deficiency. J Pediatr 1995;126:478.

TALL STATURE

Tall stature has been of concern primarily to adolescent and preadolescent girls. However, the upper limit of acceptable height in both sexes appears to be increasing, and concerns about excessive growth for girls are infrequent. When such concerns arise, the family history, growth curve, pubertal stage, and assessment of epiphysial maturation (bone age) allow assessment of predicted final adult height. Although several conditions may produce tall stature, by far the most common cause is a constitutional or familial variation from the average (Table 28–3). Reassurance, counseling, and education may alleviate the subject's or family's concerns. In extremely rare instances in which the predicted height appears to be excessive and unacceptable, hormonal therapy may be attempted to accelerate bone maturation and shorten the growth period. Estrogens are ineffective when the physiologic age (as determined by stage of sexual maturity and epiphysial development) has reached the 12-year-old level and may be of little value even when administered at earlier ages. Of

Table 28–3. Causes of tall stature.

Constitutional (familial)
Endocrine causes
  Somatotropin excess (pituitary gigantism)
  Androgen excess (tall as children, short as adults)
    True sexual precocity
    Pseudosexual precocity
  Androgen deficiency (normal height as children, tall as adults)
    Klinefelter's syndrome
    Anorchia (infection, trauma, idiopathic)
  Hyperthyroidism
Genetic causes
  Klinefelter's syndrome
  Syndromes of XYY, XXYY (tall as adults)
Miscellaneous syndromes and entities
  Marfan's syndrome
  Cerebral gigantism (Soto's syndrome)
  Total lipodystrophy
  Diencephalic syndrome
  Homocystinuria

greater concern, however, are pathologic conditions that cause acceleration of growth (Table 28–3). Excessive growth in childhood warrants investigation to exclude early growth hormone excess, androgen excess, precocious puberty, and other genetic and syndromic causes.

GIGANTISM & ACROMEGALY

Although growth hormone treatment is being introduced for an increasing number of indications, endogenous hGH excess is rare in childhood. As with adults, hGH excess is the result of a pituitary adenoma, which may appear in response to excessive growth hormone-releasing hormone levels. The clinical presentation includes headaches and visual disturbance in most cases. Biochemical confirmation consists of elevations of serum concentrations of IGF-I and IGF-binding protein-3 and failure of hGH to be suppressed below 2 ng/mL during an oral glucose tolerance test.

Treatment consists of transsphenoidal surgery after localization by CT scanning or MRI. Somatostatin analogs or bromocriptine may be useful when resection is incomplete or there is a recurrence. Monitoring the serum concentration of IGF-I or IGF-binding protein-3 is useful in assessing efficacy of treatment.

Grinspoon S, Clemmons D: Serum insulin-like growth factor-binding protein-3 levels in the diagnosis of acromegaly. J Clin Endocrinol Metab 1995;80:927.

Zimmerman D, Young W: Congenital gigantism due to growth hormone-releasing hormone excess and pituitary hyperplasia with adenomatous transformation. J Clin Endocrinol Metab 1993;76:216.

THE POSTERIOR PITUITARY GLAND

The posterior pituitary (neurohypophysis) is an extension of the ventral hypothalamus. The two principal neurohormones of the posterior pituitary, oxytocin and vasopressin, are synthesized in the supraoptic and paraventricular nuclei. After synthesis, these neurohormones are packaged in granules with specific neurophysins and transported via the axons to their storage site in the neurohypophysis. Oxytocin is primarily important during parturition and breast feeding and is not discussed further here.

Antidiuretic Hormone (Vasopressin)

Osmoreceptors in the anterolateral hypothalamus and baroreceptors in the cardiac atria regulate antidiuretic hormone (ADH) release. The release of vasopressin is influenced by chemical mediators within the central nervous system, nausea and vomiting, and a variety of drugs and hormones. Disorders of vasopressin release and action include (1) central (neurogenic) diabetes insipidus (discussed in the following section), (2) nephrogenic diabetes insipidus (Chapter 21), and (3) the syndrome of inappropriate antidiuretic hormone (SIADH) (Chapter 39).

CENTRAL DIABETES INSIPIDUS

Essentials of Diagnosis & Typical Features

- Polydipsia and polyuria (> 4 L/d).
- Urine specific gravity (< 1.010; osmolality < 280 mOsm/kg).
- Inability to concentrate urine after fluid restriction.
- Hyperosmolality of plasma (> 300 mOsm/kg).
- Subnormal plasma ADH concentration.
- Responsiveness to ADH administration.

General Considerations

Hypofunction of the hypothalamus or posterior pituitary with deficiency of ADH (neurogenic or central diabetes insipidus) is usually due to loss of neurosecretory neurons in the neurohypophysis. The condition may be idiopathic, congenital, or acquired, or it may be associated with lesions of the posterior pituitary or hypothalamus (trauma, infections, suprasellar cysts, tumors, reticuloendotheliosis, or some developmental abnormality). Among the group previously considered to be idiopathic, improved imaging techniques and biopsies have demonstrated frequent lymphocytic infiltrates and infundibular neurohypophysitis. Familial ADH deficiency may be transmitted as an autosomal dominant or X-linked recessive trait.

In nephrogenic diabetes insipidus, the renal tubules fail to respond to physiologic or pharmacologic doses of vasopressin, and no lesion of the pituitary or hypothalamus can be demonstrated. This disease is believed to be X-linked with variable degrees of penetrance, with a milder variant present in carrier females.

Clinical Findings

The onset of diabetes insipidus is often sudden, with polyuria, intense thirst, constipation, fever, and dehydration, particularly in infants. A desire for very cold beverages is common. The child awakens at night to urinate, is very thirsty, and drinks copiously. It may be difficult to recognize polyuria and polydipsia in a young infant on an ordinary feeding regimen, and the infant may present with severe dehydration manifested by high fever, circulatory collapse, and convulsions. In long-standing cases, growth retardation, lack of sexual maturation, and central nervous system damage may occur. The serum osmolality exceeds 300 mOsm/kg. Familial diabetes insipidus may have a more insidious onset and a slowly progressive course.

Symptoms and signs of ADH deficiency may be absent in patients with panhypopituitarism. Treating these patients with glucocorticoids may unmask their polyuria and polydipsia.

Differential Diagnosis

Diabetes insipidus may be differentiated from psychogenic polydipsia (compulsive water drinking, potomania) and polyuria by limiting the usual excessive intake of fluid for 2–3 days and then withholding water for 7 hours. The test should be terminated if distress is clinically notable or if there is a weight loss exceeding 3% of body weight. The preliminary fluid limitation is necessary because patients with long-standing psychogenic polydipsia lose the ability to concentrate urine. Such a loss seems to correlate with the loss of the posterior pituitary signal (bright spot) on the MRI over time. Normal children and those with psychogenic polydipsia respond to dehydration with urinary osmolality above 450 mOsm/kg (specific gravity > 1.020). With neurogenic and nephrogenic diabetes insipidus, the urine osmolality usually does not increase above 280 mOsm/kg (specific gravity > 1.010) even after the period of dehydration. Measurement of serum ADH concentration at the time of dehydration and the administration of parenteral ADH help to distinguish between central neurogenic and nephrogenic forms of diabetes insipidus.

Decreased ability to concentrate urine may also occur with hypokalemia (eg, hyperaldosteronism) and with various forms of hypercalcemia (including hypervitaminosis D) and renal tubular abnormalities (eg, Fanconi's syndrome).

MRI may demonstrate anatomic abnormalities in central diabetes insipidus and may differentiate congenital from acquired (eg, posttraumatic) causes. The MRI in neurogenic diabetes insipidus demonstrates loss of the posterior pituitary bright spot. Gadolinium contrast is necessary to delineate small posterior pituitary tumors. Serial MRI is useful in following up posttraumatic diabetes insipidus.

Treatment

A. Medical Treatment: The treatment of choice for partial and total diabetes insipidus is desmopressin acetate (DDAVP) administered intranasally. More recently, an oral form has been shown to be effective in some children. Typically, the dose rather than the dose interval must be adjusted, because the duration of action of the intranasal form is generally at least 12 hours.

B. Other Therapy: Specific therapy is directed toward treatment of specific causative diseases when they are identified. Radiation therapy, surgery, and chemotherapy are used for such diseases as reticuloendotheliosis, histiocytosis, and craniopharyngioma.

Prognosis

In the absence of central nervous system damage in infancy resulting from severe dehydration and if there are no significant associated defects, life expectancy should be normal. Patients with infundibular neurohypophysitis may, in fact, have transient self-limited disease. Hydronephrosis and hydroureter are not uncommon sequelae of prolonged polyuria; patients should also be observed carefully for urinary tract infection.

Kappy M, Ganong C: Cerebral salt wasting in children. Adv Pediatr 1996;43: 271.
Perheentupa J, Czernichow P: Water regulation and its disorders. In: *Wilkins: The Diagnosis and Treatment of Endocrine Disorders in Childhood and Adolescence,* 4th ed. Kappy MS, Blizzard RM, Migeon CJ (editors). Thomas, 1994.

THE PINEAL GLAND

The pineal gland in animals other than humans may have parenchymal cells (pinealocytes) and is often assigned an endocrine function (eg, regulation of somatic growth, sexual maturation, body pigmentation, blood glucose regulation, and day/night-sensitive neuroendocrine regulatory function). In humans, the pineal gland does not grow after the first year of life, resulting in a drop in serum melatonin concen-

tration during the childhood years. About 25% of pineal glands are cystic. Pineal tumors are associated rarely with sexual precocity in the male. Cases of gonadotropin-secreting choriocarcinomas of the pineal gland with secondary Leydig cell activation and resultant sexual precocity have been reported.

Schmidt F, Penka B: Lack of pineal growth during childhood. J Clin Endocrinol Metab 1995;80:1221.

AUTOIMMUNE POLYGLANDULAR SYNDROMES

Two autoimmune syndromes (APS types I and II) causing multiple endocrine deficiencies are distinguished by their clinical, laboratory, and epidemiologic characteristics as well as by their associated nonendocrine pathologic features. Type I is thought to occur by autosomal recessive inheritance and usually presents in infancy. Males and females are equally affected, and there is no relation to HLA type. The children (often sibling pairs) have hypoparathyroidism, Addison's disease, or mucocutaneous candidiasis, singly or in combination. Other features include hypogonadism, alopecia, vitiligo, hepatitis, pernicious anemia, and insulin-dependent diabetes mellitus. Autoimmune thyroid disease is rare in type I.

Persons with type II are generally adults with the HLA-DR3 and DR4 haplotypes; there is a 2–3:1 female preponderance. In contrast with type I also, Addison's disease is common, but in contrast to type I autoimmune thyroid disease is often present, whereas diabetes mellitus is rare. Vitiligo, alopecia, hypogonadism, and pernicious anemia may be present (as in type I), and rheumatoid arthritis and celiac disease may occur.

Treatment is specific for each complication that occurs, and recognition of the associations of disorders in these syndromes may help to detect them early in their course.

Smith BR, Furmaniak J: Adrenal and gonadal autoimmune diseases. J Clin Endocrinol Metab 1995;80:1502.
Dyan CM, Daniel GH: Chronic autoimmune thyroiditis. N Engl J Med 1996;335:99.

THE THYROID GLAND

FETAL DEVELOPMENT OF THE THYROID

The thyroid is capable of hormone synthesis in the 14th week of gestation, when thyroid-stimulating hormone (TSH) is detected in the fetal serum and pituitary gland. TSH does not normally cross the placenta, T_4 and T_3 cross in limited amounts, and the fetal pituitary-thyroid axis functions largely independent of the maternal pituitary-thyroid axis. Antithyroid drugs, including propylthiouracil and methimazole, freely cross the placenta, and goitrous hypothyroid newborns may be born to hyperthyroid mothers who undergo treatment during pregnancy.

Mothers who have thyroid-stimulating immunoglobulins (TSI) can transmit these antibodies transplacentally, resulting in thyrotoxic newborns who may develop goiter and exophthalmos. Because TSI may be present in the serum of controlled, previously hyperthyroid mothers—or even in women who have had surgical or radioiodine-induced removal of their thyroid glands—the possible transmission of TSI should be considered in all mothers who are or have been hyperthyroid. In addition, thyroid-binding inhibitory immunoglobulins (TBIIs) can cross the placenta, so that the newborn is also at risk for hypothyroidism. Both maternal TSI and TBII usually disappear from the infant's circulation by 6–8 weeks.

Physiology

Pituitary TSH stimulates the thyroid gland to take up iodine and synthesize active thyroid hormones, ie, triiodothyronine (T_3) and tetraiodothyronine (T_4). Active hormone produced in excess of physiologic needs is stored within the thyroid follicles as colloid. The release of active thyroid hormones into the circulation is regulated by a negative feedback mechanism involving pituitary TSH and free thyroid hormone (Figure 28–1).

Most T_4 and T_3 circulate bound to thyroid hormone-binding globulin (TBG), albumin, and prealbumin, and less than 1% of T_3 and T_4 is free. T_4 is deiodinated in the tissues to either T_3 (active) or reverse T_3 (inactive), and the physiologic activity of thyroid hormone depends primarily on the amount of FT_4 presented to the cells. Receptors for T_3 are present on the cell surface, in the nucleus, in the cytosol, and on mitochondria.

At birth, the T_4 approximates that of the mother, but levels increase rapidly during the first to fifth days of life in response to a TSH surge following birth. TSH levels subsequently decrease to childhood levels by 2–4 weeks of age. This physiologic neonatal TSH surge can cause falsely positive neonatal screens for hypothyroidism (ie, "high" TSH), since most of the blood specimens for screening are collected on the first day of life.

The total T_4 is low in hypothyroidism and may be reduced in premature infants (particularly those with sepsis or respiratory distress), subacute and chronic thyroiditis, hypopituitarism, nephrosis, cirrhosis, hypoproteinemia, malnutrition, and following therapy with T_3. Prolonged administration of high doses of adrenocorticosteroids—as well as of sulfonamides,

testosterone, phenytoin, and salicylates—may also produce a decrease in total T_4. TSH and free T_4 levels remain in the normal range. Total T_3 and T_4 levels are high in hyperthyroidism and may be elevated in acute forms of thyroiditis and hepatitis; in some types of inborn errors of thyroid hormone synthesis, release, or binding of thyroid hormone; following the administration of estrogens or clofibrate or during pregnancy; and following the administration of various iodine-containing globulins.

TBG is increased in pregnancy, after estrogen therapy (including oral contraceptives), occasionally as a genetic variation, in certain hepatic disorders, following administration of phenytoin or phenothiazines, and occasionally from an unknown cause. TBG is decreased in familial TBG deficiency; following the administration of glucocorticoids, androgens, or anabolic steroids; in nephrotic syndrome with marked hypoproteinemia; in some forms of hepatic disease; or as an idiopathic finding.

HYPOTHYROIDISM (Congenital & Acquired Hypothyroidism)

Essentials of Diagnosis & Typical Features

- Growth retardation, diminished physical activity, impaired tissue perfusion, constipation, thick tongue, poor muscle tone, hoarseness, anemia, and intellectual retardation. (These findings can arise in the first 2 months of life.)
- Thyroid hormone concentrations low (total T_4, free T_4, and T_3 resin uptake [T_3RU]); TSH levels elevated in primary hypothyroidism.
- *Note:* Most newborns with congenital hypothyroidism appear normal at birth and gain weight normally, even if untreated, for the first 3–4 months of life. Since congenital hypothyroidism must be treated as early as possible to avoid intellectual impairment, the diagnosis should be based on the newborn screening test and not on abnormal physical findings.

General Considerations

Thyroid hormone deficiency may be either congenital or acquired (juvenile hypothyroidism). Although there are many causes of hypothyroidism in the newborn (Table 28–4), most cases result from hypoplasia or aplasia of the thyroid gland or failure of the gland to migrate into its normal anatomic location (ie, lingual or sublingual thyroid glands). Juvenile hypothyroidism, particularly if there is a history of goiter, usually results from chronic lymphocytic (Hashimoto's) thyroiditis (see below).

Of the genetically determined enzymatic defects that cause hypothyroidism (Table 28–4), only Pendred's syndrome (a defect in iodide organification

Table 28–4. Causes of hypothyroidism.

A. Congenital (cretinism):
1. Aplasia, hypoplasia, or associated with maldescent of thyroid
   a. Embryonic defect of development
   b. Autoimmune disease (?)
2. Familial iodine-induced goiter secondary to metabolic inborn errors—
   a. Iodide transport defect (defect 1)
   b. Organification defect (defect 2)—
      (1) Lack of iodine peroxidase
      (2) Lack of iodine transferase: Pendred's syndrome, associated with congenital nerve deafness
   c. Coupling defect (defect 3)
   d. Iodotyrosine deiodinase defect (defect 4)
   e. Abnormal iodinated polypeptide (defects 5a and 5b)
      (1) Resulting from defect in intrathyroidal proteolysis of thyroglobulin
      (2) Abnormal plasma binding preventing use of T_4 by peripheral cells
   f. Inability of tissues to convert T_4 to T_3
3. Maternal ingestion of medications during pregnancy
   a. Maternal radioiodine
   b. Goitrogens (propylthiouracil, methimazole)
   c. Iodides
4. Iodide deficiency (endemic cretinism)
5. Idiopathic

B. Acquired (juvenile hypothyroidism):
1. Thyroidectomy or radioiodine therapy for
   a. Thyrotoxicosis
   b. Cancer
   c. Lingual thyroid
   d. Isolated midline thyroid
2. Destruction by x-ray
3. Thyrotropin deficiency—
   a. Isolated
   b. Associated with other pituitary tropic hormone deficiencies
4. TRH deficiency due to hypothalamic injury or disease
5. Autoimmune disease (lymphocytic thyroiditis)
6. Chronic infections
7. Medications
   a. Iodides
      (1) Prolonged, excessive ingestion
      (2) Deficiency
   b. Cobalt
8. Idiopathic

with congenital nerve deafness) has distinguishing clinical features. In children who have enzymatic defects, thyroid enlargement is usually not present in the newborn period but occurs within the first 2 decades of life. Although thyroid function test (including radioactive iodide uptake studies) may be helpful in diagnosis, final clarification of the defect generally requires chromatographic fractionation of iodinated compounds in the serum, urine, and thyroid tissue.

Cabbage, soybeans, aminosalicylic acid, thiourea derivatives, resorcinol, phenylbutazone, cobalt, and iodides have been reported to cause goiter and hypothyroidism during pregnancy. Because many of these agents cross the placenta freely, they should be used with great caution during pregnancy.

Several hundred patients with clinical and laboratory features of resistance to thyroid hormone have been described. These syndromes are generally familial and are classified on the basis of the site of the resistance (eg, generalized; pituitary or peripheral tissue).

Clinical Findings

The severity of the findings in cases of thyroid deficiency depends on the age at onset and the degree of deficiency.

A. Symptoms and Signs: Even with congenital absence of the thyroid gland, the first finding may not appear for several days or weeks. Consequently, any suspected abnormality in the results of the newborn screen should be promptly investigated. Findings include physical and mental sluggishness; pale, gray, cool, or mottled skin; nonpitting myxedema; constipation; large tongue; poor muscle tone giving rise to a protuberant abdomen, umbilical hernia, and lumbar lordosis; hypothermia; bradycardia; diminished sweating (variable); decreased pulse pressure; hoarse voice or cry; delayed transient deafness; and a slow relaxation component of deep tendon reflexes (best appreciated in the ankles). Nasal obstruction and discharge and persistent jaundice may be present in the neonatal period.

The skin may be dry, thick, scaly, and coarse, with a yellowish tinge due to excessive deposition of carotene. The hair is dry, coarse, and brittle (variable) and may be excessive. Lateral thinning of the eyebrows may occur. The axillary and supraclavicular fat pads may be prominent in infants. Muscular hypertrophy (Kocher-Debré-Sémélaigne syndrome) is an unusual association with congenital hypothyroidism.

Growth changes include short stature; infantile skeletal proportions with relatively short extremities; infantile naso-orbital configuration (bridge of nose flat, broad, and underdeveloped; eyes seem to be widely spaced); delayed epiphysial development; delayed closure of fontanelles; and retarded dental eruption. Treatment of acquired hypothyroidism may not result in the predicted final adult target height. Menometrorrhagia may be seen in older girls; galactorrhea has been reported due to the action of thyrotropin-releasing hormone (TRH) on increasing pituitary prolactin secretion as well as TSH.

In hypothyroidism resulting from enzymatic defects, ingestion of goitrogens, or chronic lymphocytic thyroiditis, the thyroid gland may be enlarged. Thyroid enlargement in children is usually symmetric, and the gland is moderately firm and without nodularity. In chronic lymphocytic thyroiditis, however, a cobblestone surface frequently is present; size and shape are readily apparent on inspection in children. Slowing of mental responsiveness and retardation of development of the brain may occur in neonates and infants, and in some cases a coincidental congenital malformation of the brain is present.

B. Laboratory Findings: Total T_4 and free T_4 are decreased. Radioiodine uptake is below 10% (normal: 10–30%). The binding of T_3 by erythrocytes or resin in vitro (T_3RU test) is lowered. With primary hypothyroidism, the serum TSH concentration is elevated. Normocytic anemia is common, but microcytic or macrocytic anemia may occur as a result of decreased iron, folate, and cobalamin absorption. Serum cholesterol and carotene are usually elevated in childhood but may be low or normal in infants. Cessation of therapy in previously treated hypothyroid patients produces a marked rise in serum cholesterol levels in 6–8 weeks. Urinary creatinine excretion is decreased, and urinary hydroxyproline is low. Circulating autoantibodies to thyroid constituents may be present. Serum growth hormone may be decreased, with subnormal hGH response to insulin-induced hypoglycemia and arginine stimulation in children with severe primary hypothroidism.

C. Imaging: Skeletal maturation (bone age) is delayed. Centers of ossification, especially of the hip, may show multiple small centers or a single stippled, porous, or fragmented center (epiphysial dysgenesis). Vertebrae may show anterior beaking. Coxa vara and coxa plana may occur. Cardiomegaly is common.

Screening Programs for Neonatal Hypothyroidism

Congenital hypothyroidism should by diagnosed by neonatal screening within 10 days of birth. It may be clinically recognized during the first month of life or may be so mild that it remains unrecognized clinically for months. Adequate treatment started as soon as possible—but certainly before the second month of life—gives a better prognosis with respect to intellectual performance later in life.

Differential Diagnosis

The various causes of primary hypothyroidism due to intrinsic defects of the thyroid gland must be differentiated from pituitary and hypothalamic failure with secondary thyroid insufficiency. TSH and FT_4 levels are the most useful tests and are usually sufficient in directing treatment or the need for further investigations.

Down's syndrome, chondrodystrophy, generalized gangliosidosis, I-cell disease, Hurler's and Hunter's syndromes, and certain other causes of short stature and coarse features can all be readily distinguished by their clinical manifestations and by laboratory studies.

Treatment

Levothyroxine is the drug of choice in a dosage of 75–100 µg/m²/d as a single dose. In newborns and infants, the dose is 10–12 µg/kg. The hypothyroid patient may be very responsive to thyroid and may be sensitive to slight excesses of thyroid hormone. A dose of 0.025 mg (25 µg) of levothyroxine is often recommended initially, with subsequent increases to full replacement in 1–2 weeks. Serum T_4 or FT_4 concentrations should be used to monitor the adequacy of therapy initially, since the elevated TSH may not fall into the normal range for several days to weeks. Subsequently, elevations of serum TSH are sensitive early indicators of the need for increased medication (or increased compliance).

In the treatment of neonatal goiter with or without hypothyroidism resulting from drugs and goitrogens taken by the pregnant woman, temporary use of levothyroxine may be helpful in decreasing the size of the goiter.

Mortimer RH et al: Methimazole and propylthiouracil equally cross the perfused human term placental lobule. J Clin Endocrinol Metab 1997;82:3099.

Refetoff S, Weiss RE, Usala SJ: The syndrome of resistance to thyroid hormones. Endocr Rev 1993;14:348.

THYROIDITIS

Chronic lymphocytic (Hashimoto's) thyroiditis is perhaps the most common pediatric endocrinopathy, particularly in adolescent girls. Acute and subacute thyroiditis are rare in all age groups.

1. ACUTE SUPPURATIVE THYROIDITIS

Acute thyroiditis is rare. Oropharyngeal organisms are thought to reach the thyroid via a patent foramen cecum and thyroglossal duct tract. The most common pathogens are group A streptococci, pneumococci, *Staphylococcus aureus,* and anaerobes. The patient is invariably toxic, and the thyroid gland is exquisitely tender. There may be radiation of pain to adjacent areas of the neck or to the ear or chest. There is usually no consistently associated endocrine disturbance. Specific antibiotic therapy should be administered.

2. SUBACUTE NONSUPPURATIVE THYROIDITIS

Subacute thyroiditis (de Quervain's thyroiditis) is rare in the United States. In most cases, the cause is a virus (mumps, influenza, echovirus, coxsackievirus, Epstein-Barr virus, or adenovirus). Presenting features are similar to those of acute thyroiditis: fever, malaise, sore throat, dysphagia, pain in the thyroid gland that may radiate to the ears, and mild and transient manifestations of hyperthyroidism. In contrast to acute thyroiditis, the onset is generally insidious. The thyroid gland is firm, and the enlargement may be confined to one lobe. Radioiodine uptake is usually reduced, but thyroid hormone levels in the blood are normal or elevated. The differentiation from bacterial thyroiditis is difficult, and antibiotic therapy is therefore recommended.

3. CHRONIC LYMPHOCYTIC THYROIDITIS (Chronic Autoimmune Thyroiditis, Hashimoto's Thyroiditis)

Essentials of Diagnosis & Typical Features

- Firm, freely movable, nontender, and diffusely enlarged goiter.
- Serum T_4 concentrations are generally normal but may be elevated or decreased depending on the stage of the disease.

General Considerations

Chronic lymphocytic thyroiditis is being seen with increasing frequency in all age groups and currently is the most common cause of goiter and hypothyroidism in childhood. In children and adolescents, the incidence peaks between the ages of 8 and 15 years and occurs most commonly in females (4:1). The disease is the result of an autoimmune attack on the thyroid. Susceptibility to thyroid autoimmunity (and other endocrine autoimmune disorders) is associated with inheritance of certain histocompatibility alleles in autoimmune polyglandular syndrome type II (see above).

Clinical Findings

A. Symptoms and Signs: The goiter is characteristically firm, freely movable, nontender, and symmetric, with a pebbly consistency. Onset is usually insidious, and except for painless goiter clinical manifestations are unusual. Occasionally, a sensation of tracheal compression or fullness, hoarseness, and dysphagia are described by the patient. There are no local signs of inflammation and no evidence of systemic infection.

B. Laboratory Findings: Laboratory findings are variable. Serum concentrations of T_4, FT_4, and T_3RU are usually normal but may be elevated (hashitoxicosis) or depressed. Thyroid antibodies (antithyroglobulin, antithyroid peroxidase) are usually present, though titers are frequently low. A variety of abnormalities in radioactive iodide uptake studies have been described; thyroid scans usually

show a diffuse or patchy pattern, and cold (nonfunctioning) nodules have been reported. Thyroid scans and uptake studies add little to the diagnosis. Surgical or needle biopsy is diagnostic but seldom indicated.

Treatment

The treatment of chronic lymphocytic thyroiditis is controversial. Full therapeutic doses of thyroid hormone (levothyroxine, 100 $\mu g/m^2/d$) may decrease the size of the goiter within 3 months, but in controlled trials the efficacy of thyroid hormone therapy is unsupported in the euthyroid child. Hypothyroidism is believed to be a common end result of autoimmune thyroiditis in the second to third decades of life; consequently, patients with adolescent goiter require lifelong surveillance, and children with documented hypothyroidism should be treated with levothyroxine in full replacement doses.

Dayan CM, Daniels GH: Chronic autoimmune thyroiditis. N Engl J Med 1996;335:99.

HYPERTHYROIDISM

Essentials of Diagnosis & Typical Features

- Nervousness, irritability, emotional lability, tremor, excessive appetite, weight loss; smooth, moist, warm skin; increased perspiration, and heat intolerance.
- Goiter, exophthalmos, tachycardia, widened pulse pressure (systolic hypertension).
- Thyroid function studies elevated (eg, TT_4, FT_4, T_3RU). TSH concentration suppressed.

General Considerations

Most cases of hyperthyroidism in children are likely to have an autoimmune cause. Hyperthyroidism occurs with certain diseases that have an autoimmune basis, and a familial pattern with a predilection for females supports a role for a heritable and autoimmune basis. IgG antibody to thyroid receptors (TSI) stimulates thyroid hormone production in one form of hyperthyroidism accompanied by exophthalmos (Graves' disease). *Transient congenital hyperthyroidism may occur in infants of thyrotoxic mothers and is potentially life-threatening.* Hyperthyroidism may be associated with acute, subacute, or chronic thyroiditis, tumors of the thyroid, other tumors producing thyrotropin-like substances, and exogenous thyroid hormone excess.

Clinical Findings

A. Symptoms and Signs: Hyperthyroidism is four times more common in females than in males. The disease most frequently occurs in childhood between ages 12 and 14 years; only 2% of patients present before 10 years of age. The course of hyperthyroidism tends to be cyclic, with spontaneous remissions and exacerbations. A deterioration in school performance is a common feature in the history. Findings include weakness, dyspnea, dysphagia, amenorrhea, emotional instability, nervousness, marked variability in mood, personality disturbances, and (rarely) tremors and movements that may simulate chorea. The skin is warm and moist; the face is flushed. Palpitations, tachycardia, and systolic hypertension with increased pulse pressure are common. Proptosis and exophthalmos are common in hyperthyroid children. Goiter is present in more than 90% of cases and is characteristically diffuse and usually firm. A bruit and thrill may be present. Variable degrees of accelerated growth and development occur, and loss of weight is common despite polyphagia. In neonatal hyperthyroidism, hepatosplenomegaly and thrombocytopenia with antiplatelet antibodies are occasionally seen.

B. Laboratory Findings: TT_4, FT_4 and T_3RU are elevated except in rare cases in which only the serum T_3 radioimmunoassay concentration is elevated (T_3 thyrotoxicosis). Radioiodine uptake is elevated and does not suppress with T_3 (liothyronine). The basal metabolic rate is elevated, and serum cholesterol is low. Antibodies to thyroglobulin are found in most patients. Circulating TSH concentrations measured by very sensitive assays are depressed, and TSI is often present in plasma.

C. Imaging: Skeletal maturation assessed radiographically is advanced in younger children. In newborns, accelerated bone maturation may be associated with subsequent premature closure of the cranial sutures. Long-standing hyperthyroidism is associated with osteoporosis.

Differential Diagnosis

Although the well-established case of hyperthyroidism seldom presents a problem in diagnosis, the findings in the early stages of the disease may be confused with chorea or, more commonly, with euthyroid goiter. Typically, the patient is an adolescent with a recent decline in school performance, nervousness, emotional lability, and increased perspiration. Repeated clinical and laboratory evaluations may be required to make the diagnosis. Disease states associated with hypermetabolism (severe anemia, leukemia, chronic infections, pheochromocytoma, as well as muscle-wasting disease) may resemble hyperthyroidism clinically but differ in the thyroid function studies.

Treatment

The symptoms of hyperthyroidism can fluctuate and in some mild cases may not require treatment.

A. General Measures: Bed rest is advisable only in severe cases, in preparation for surgery, or at the beginning of a medical regimen. The diet should be high in calories, carbohydrates, and vitamins (particularly vitamin B_1).

B. Medical Treatment: It takes 2–3 weeks to see a clinical response, and adequate control may take 2–3 months. The thyroid frequently increases in size as treatment is started but then usually decreases within several months.

1. β-Adrenergic blocking agents (propranolol, atenolol)–These agents may be helpful in controlling symptoms of nervous instability and tachycardia and are indicated in severe disease with cardiovascular abnormalities (tachycardia, hypertension). In mild cases, beta-blockade without other antithyroid treatment may be adequate. In large doses, propranolol decreases the peripheral conversion of T_4 to T_3.

2. Propylthiouracil–This drug interferes with thyroid hormone synthesis and, in large doses, with the peripheral conversion of T_4 to T_3. The correct dose must always be individually determined. Propylthiouracil is frequently used in the initial treatment of children with hyperthyroidism. Short-term therapy is occasionally successful, but treatment usually must be continued for at least 2–3 years with the smallest drug dosage that will produce a euthyroid state. If T_4 levels rise rapidly with reduction in drug dosage after 18–24 months of therapy, continued or alternative therapy, such as radioablation of the thyroid gland, will be necessary. Relapse occurs in 10–30% of cases, and severe cases may not respond to initial treatment.

a. Initial dosage–Give 75–300 mg/d in three or four divided doses 6–8 hours apart until tests of thyroid function are normal and all signs and symptoms have subsided. Larger doses are frequently necessary.

b. Maintenance–Give 50–100 mg/d in two or three divided doses. Some authors recommend continuing the drug at higher levels until the euthyroid state is approached or reached and then, as the TSH level rises, adding thyroid hormone. The role of adjunctive thyroxine therapy in preventing recurrence of hyperthyroidism in Graves' disease is not proved. T_4 and TSH levels should be monitored during antithyroid treatment to determine whether the patient is becoming hypothyroid; thyroid hormone is added when indicated.

c. Toxicity–Granulocytopenia, fever, rash, and arthralgia may occur. The drug must be discontinued, and antibiotics and a short course of one of the adrenocorticosteroids should be prescribed if indicated.

3. Methimazole–This drug may be used in one-tenth the dosage of propylthiouracil and may be effective with a twice-daily dosage schedule. Toxic reactions are similar to those seen with propylthiouracil.

4. Iodide–Medical treatment with continuous iodide administration alone usually produces a rapid but brief response. Because the efficacy of iodide is short-lived, it is generally recommended only for acute management. A progressive increase in dosage is often required for satisfactory control, and toxic reactions to iodide are not uncommon.

C. Radiation Therapy: Radioactive iodide (^{131}I) ablation of the thyroid gland is currently being used as definitive therapy for children and adolescents whose hyperthyroidism does not remit after 2 years or so of medical therapy or where compliance with medication is poor. Reports do not support the fear of an increased incidence of thyroid cancer, particularly when an ablative dose of ^{131}I is used. Therapy with thyroid hormone is necessary after thyroid ablation.

D. Surgical Measures: Thyroidectomy is no longer considered a major form of treatment. An exception would be in the case of a noncompliant pregnant female in whom radioiodine would be contraindicated because it crosses the placenta. The patient should be prepared first with bed rest, diet, and propranolol (as above) and with iodide and propylthiouracil as follows: Propylthiouracil should be given for 2–4 weeks. Iodide (as saturated solution of potassium iodide) is added 10–21 days before surgery is scheduled. Iodides act by blocking the effect of TSH on the thyroid, with a resulting decrease in iodine trapping and reduction of vascularity, and by inhibiting the release of hormone, thus reducing the possibility of thyroid storm. Give 1–10 drops daily for 10–21 days. Continue the drug for 1 week after surgery.

Management of Congenital (Transient) Hyperthyroidism

Congenital hyperthyroidism has a significant death rate in the neonatal period, but the eventual prognosis in surviving infants is excellent. Temporary treatment of congenital hyperthyroidism may be necessary, in which case iodides appear to be the initial drug of choice, to be followed by propylthiouracil or methimazole. Reserpine or propranolol may be necessary to control cardiac arrhythmias. Transection of an enlarged thyroid isthmus may be of value if respiratory distress due to tracheal compression is present.

Course & Prognosis

Improvement may rarely occur without therapy, but partial remissions and exacerbations may continue for several years. With medical treatment alone, prolonged remissions may be expected in one-half to two-thirds of cases in the first 2 years or so.

Glaser NS, Styne DM: Predictors of early remission of hyperthyroidism in children. J Clin Endocrinol 1997;82: 1719.

CARCINOMA OF THE THYROID

Carcinoma of the thyroid is uncommon in child-hood. The presentation is usually with asymptomatic asymmetric thyroid enlargement. Neck discomfort, dysphagia, voice changes, and respiratory difficulty are unusual but may occur. Fifty percent of children have metastatic disease, usually to regional lymph nodes, at the time of presentation. Pulmonary metastasis occurs in 5% of cases.

Thyroid function tests are usually normal. A technetium or iodine scan of the thyroid shows a "cold" nodule and is the most definitive diagnostic test. Pulmonary metastases should be excluded by CT scan of the chest.

Papillary carcinoma is the most common form in childhood, and the prognosis with treatment is relatively good (survival rate greater than 80% after 10–20 years). The treatment of choice is surgical excision of the entire gland and removal of all involved lymph nodes. If metastatic disease is not identified at surgery or by radioactive iodide scan postoperatively, replacement thyroid hormone is generally the only additional therapy required. Follow-up thyroid scans every 2–5 years are recommended.

Less common malignant tumors of the thyroid are follicular, medullary, and undifferentiated carcinomas, lymphomas, and sarcomas. Medullary carcinoma of the thyroid may be familial (autosomal dominant), usually occurring as a component of type 2 multiple endocrine neoplasia (MEN). This condition may be associated with excessive elaboration of gastrin and calcitonin, with pheochromocytoma, parathyroid hyperplasia, "marfanoid habitus," and mucosal neuromas (MEN type 2b). The treatment and prognosis depend on the cell type present, but the outcome is generally less favorable.

Gagel RF et al: Medullary thyroid carcinoma: Recent progress. J Clin Endocrinol Metab 1993;76:809.

DISORDERS OF CALCIUM HOMEOSTASIS

The integrated action of parathyroid hormone (PTH) and vitamin D on bone, small intestine, and kidney maintains the serum calcium level within a narrow normal range and contributes to normal bone mineralization. Deficiencies and excesses of these agents, as well as abnormalities in their receptors or of vitamin D metabolism, lead to the clinical disturbances described below and shown in Tables 28–5, 28–6, and 28–7. Less important factors contributing to calcium homeostasis include calcitonin, magnesium, pyrophosphate, prostaglandins, and phosphate.

Table 28–5. Parathyroid deficiency states.

Disease or Condition	Synonym	Inheritance Pattern	Major Clinical Features	Metabolic Features							
				Serum Concentration				Urinary Excretion			
								Basal Conditions		Response to Parathyroid Hormone[1]	
				Ca^{2+}	P	Alk Ptase	PTH	Ca^{2+}	P	P	Cyclic AMP
"Idiopathic" (spontaneous), surgical, or "autoimmune" hypoparathyroidism	Autoimmune polyendocrinopathy. Thyroiditis and hypoparathyroidism (Schmidt's syndrome). Absence of parathyroid glands and thymic aplasia (DiGeorge's syndrome)	Familial in autoimmune type and associated with certain HLA types	Tetany, seizures, photophobia, diarrhea, positive Chvostek's and Trousseau's signs, candidiasis. In autoimmune type, other autoimmune diseases (eg, adrenal insufficiency, thyroiditis, pernicious anemia, diabetes mellitus).	↓(N)	↑	↓(N)	↓	N(↑,↓)	↓	N	N
Pseudohypoparathyroidism and pseudopseudohypoparathyroidism	Albright's syndrome	X-linked dominant	Brachymetacarpal and metatarsal short stature; mental subnormality; ectopic calcification of lenses, basal ganglia, and subcutaneous tissue.	↓(N)	↑(N)	↓↑(N)	↑	↓(N)	↓	↓	↓
Pseudohypoparathyroidism type II	PTH unresponsiveness	Unknown	Seizures. Phenotype normal.	↓	↑	N	↑	↓	↓	N	N
Pseudohypohyperparathyroidism with osteitis fibrosa[2]	Renal resistance to parathyroid hormone with osteitis fibrosa	Probably familial	Clinical features of hypocalcemia. Phenotype normal.	↓	N	N	N(↓)	N(↑)	↓(N)	↓(N)	↓
Pseudoidiopathic hypoparathyroidism[3]			Clinical features of hypoparathyroidism. Phenotype normal.	↓	↑	↑	↑	↓	↑	N	N

[1] PTH is not commercially available for testing.
[2] The opposite (ie, skeletal unresponsiveness to parathyroid hormone [PTH] with normal renal responsiveness) has been described.
[3] Structural anomaly of PTH molecule has been proposed.

Table 28–6. Rickets and disorders of calcium metabolism.[1]

Disease or Condition	Synonym	Inheritance Pattern	Clinical Features	Metabolic Features						Treatment
				Serum Concentrations				Urinary Excretion		
				Ca²⁺	P	Alk Ptase	PTH	Ca²⁺	P	
Hypoparathyroid states	See Table 29–5.			↓						Vitamin D and calcium
Transient tetany of the newborn			Tetany, focal seizures; more common in prematures and infants of diabetic mothers; rarely described in association with maternal hyperparathyroidism	↓ (N)	↓ (N)	↓ (N)	↓ (N)	↓ (N)	↑ (N)	Diet high in calcium, low in phosphate; vitamin D may be necessary
Malabsorption syndrome	Disease entities associated with malabsorption include cystic fibrosis, celiac disease, sprue, Shwachman syndrome; hypoplasia of cartilage and hair.	Generally familial with mode of inheritance related to specific disease	Steatorrhea, failure to thrive. Some forms associated with neutropenia, skeletal anomalies, immunologic deficiencies, and abnormalities of cartilage and hair	↓ (N)	(N) ↓	↑ (N)	↑ (N)	↓	N (↑ ↓)	Vitamin D, calcium, and magnesium (hypomagnesemic states)
Chronic renal insufficiency			Growth failure, undernutrition, skeletal changes	↓ (N)	↑	↑ (N)	↑	↓ (N)	↓	Diet high in calcium, low in phosphorus; vitamin D
Vitamin D-deficient rickets	Infantile rickets		Rickets	↓ (N)	↓	↑	↑	↑	↑	Vitamin D and calcium
Familial hypophosphatemic vitamin D-resistant rickets[2]	(1) Hereditary vitamin D-resistant rickets (2) Phosphate diabetes (3) X-linked hypophosphatemia	X-linked dominant (occasionally autosomal dominant or sporadic)	Skeletal deformities, growth retardation	N (↓)	↓	N	N (↑)	N	↑	Oral phosphate and vitamin D
Hereditary vitamin D-refractory rickets[3] Type I Type II	(1) Hypophosphatemic vitamin D-refractory rickets (2) Pseudo-vitamin D-deficiency rickets	Autosomal recessive	Severe rachitic bone changes; generalized aminoaciduria	↓	↓ (N)	↑	↑		↑	Vitamin D (calciferol) in large doses or approximately physiologic doses of 1,25-dihydroxycholecalciferol

[1]Normal tubular reabsorption of phosphate (TRP) is 83–98%; the lower values are associated with higher serum levels of phosphorus. In hypoparathyroidism, TRP varies from 40 to 70%. Low values for TRP are also found in some forms of inherited renal tubular disease, eg, vitamin D-resistant rickets.

[2]A variety of diseases (cystinosis, galactosemia, tyrosinosis, Wilson's disease, hereditary fructose intolerance) are associated with renal tubular defects and should be considered in the differential diagnosis.

[3]Type I has been shown to be the result of defective renal 1α-hydroxylation of 25-hydroxycholecalciferol; type II is due to tissue unresponsiveness to normal levels of 1,25-dihydroxycholecalciferol; in this type, the vitamin D receptor complex fails to bind to DNA.

Table 28–7. Hypercalcemic states.

I. **Primary hyperparathyroidism**
  A. Hyperplasia
  B. Adenoma
  C. Familial, including MEN I and II
  D. Ectopic PTH secretion
II. **Hypercalcemic states other than primary hyperpara-**
    thyroidism associated with increased intestinal or re-
    nal absorption of calcium
  A. Hypervitaminosis D (including idiopathic
     hypercalcemia of infancy)
  B. Familial hypocalciuric hypercalcemia
  C. Lithium therapy
  D. Sarcoidosis
  E. Phosphate depletion
  F. Aluminum intoxication
III. **Hypercalcemic states other than hyperparathyroid-**
     ism associated with increased mobilization of bone
     minerals
  A. Hyperthyroidism
  B. Immobilization
  C. Thiazides
  D. Vitamin A intoxication
  E. Malignant neoplasms
     1. Ectopic PTH secretion
     2. Prostaglandin-secreting tumor and perhaps
        prostaglandin release from subcutaneous fat necro-
        sis
     3. Tumors metastatic to bone
     4. Myeloma

MEN = multiple endocrine neoplasia; PTH = parathyroid hormone.

HYPOPARATHYROIDISM

Essentials of Diagnosis & Typical Features

- Tetany with facial and extremity numbness, tingling, cramps, spontaneous muscle contractures,
  carpopedal spasm, positive Trousseau and
  Chvostek signs, loss of consciousness, convulsions.
- Diarrhea, photophobia, prolongation of electrical
  systole (QT interval), and laryngospasm.
- Defective nails and teeth, cataracts, and ectopic
  calcification in the subcutaneous tissues and basal
  ganglia.
- Serum and urine calcium normal or low; serum
  phosphate high; urine phosphate low; alkaline
  phosphatase normal or low; azotemia absent. Inappropriately low ratio of PTH to ionized calcium.

General Considerations

PTH deficiency states result either from an absolute deficiency of PTH, an abnormality in the PTH
molecule, or from "hormone-resistant states." The
latter are related to abnormalities of the PTH-recep-
tor complex or its postreceptor action in the face of
normal hormonal secretion (ie, pseudohypoparathy-
roid states; see Table 28–5). Hypoparathyroidism
may be idiopathic or may result from autoimmune

damage or from parathyroidectomy. Hypoparathyroidism may develop following thyroidectomy with
either acute or insidious onset and may be transient
or permanent. Parathyroid deficiency has been reported following irradiation of the neck or the administration of therapeutic doses of radioactive iodine for
carcinoma of the thyroid.

Two types of transient hypoparathyroidism
("early" and "late") may be present in the newborn
due to a relative deficiency of PTH or hormone action. The early form occurs within the first 2 weeks
of life in newborns with a history of birth asphyxia or
those born to mothers with diabetes mellitus or hyperparathyroidism.

Hypomagnesemia may also be seen in the early
form and augments the severity of hypocalcemia.
The most common late form occurs almost exclusively in infants fed a milk formula with a high phos-
phate:calcium ratio.

Autoimmune hypoparathyroidism may be associated with candidal infection, Addison's disease, insulin-dependent diabetes mellitus, pernicious anemia,
alopecia, vitiligo, thyroiditis, hypogonadism, steatorrhea, and hepatitis (see autoimmune polyglandular
syndrome type I, above). This form of hypoparathyroidism is often familial (autosomal recessive). Infections resulting from lack of immune reaction to *Candida* may lead to severe intractable cutaneous and
gastrointestinal candidiasis. Because of the frequent
association of adrenocortical insufficiency with
parathyroid insufficiency, adrenocortical function
should be tested repeatedly.

Congenital absence of the parathyroids may occur
in association with congenital absence of the thymus
(with resultant thymus-dependent immunologic deficiency) and cardiovascular abnormalities (DiGeorge
syndrome), or, rarely, cerebral and ocular defects.

Clinical Findings

A. Symptoms and Signs: Prolonged hypocalcemia causes tetany, photophobia, blepharospasm,
and diarrhea.

Tetany is manifested by numbness, cramps, and
twitchings of the extremities; carpopedal spasm and
laryngospasm; a positive Chvostek sign (tapping of
the face in front of the ear produces spasm of the facial muscles); positive Trousseau sign (compression
of the upper arm with a blood pressure cuff inflated
to a pressure above systole for 2–4 minutes produces
carpopedal spasm); unexplained bizarre behavior; irritability; loss of consciousness; convulsions; and retarded physical and mental development. Headache,
vomiting, diarrhea, photophobia, increased intracranial pressure, papilledema, and pseudopapilledema
may occur. In early infancy, respiratory distress may
be the presenting finding.

B. Laboratory Findings: (Table 28–5.) Serum
calcium is decreased, serum phosphate is increased,
and serum alkaline phosphatase is usually low nor-

mal. Urinary excretion of calcium and phosphate is usually decreased but is influenced by the dietary intake. Renal clearance of phosphate is decreased, and the maximum tubular reabsorption of phosphate falls by 12–30% from a normal value of 85%. PTH levels are inappropriately reduced in relation to the ionized calcium concentration.

C. Imaging: Soft tissue and basal ganglia calcification may occur in idiopathic hypoparathyroidism or in pseudohypoparathyroidism.

Differential Diagnosis

The differential diagnosis of hypoparathyroid states is outlined in Table 28–5. Convulsions may suggest epilepsy and other chronic disorders of the central nervous system. Central nervous system features (headache, vomiting, increased intracranial pressure, and convulsions) may require differentiation from other causes of increased intracranial pressure, such as brain tumor.

Treatment

A. Acute or Severe Tetany: The objective of treatment is to correct hypocalcemia immediately with calcium intravenously and orally.

B. Maintenance Management of Hypoparathyroidism and Chronic Hypocalcemia: The objective of treatment is to maintain the serum calcium and phosphate at an approximately normal level.

1. Drugs–Give ergocalciferol (vitamin D_2), cholecalciferol (vitamin D_3), dihydrotachysterol, or calcitriol (1,25-dihydroxyvitamin D_3). These preparations may not reach their peak effects for 3–7 days; since they are fat-soluble and are stored in the adipose tissue and the liver, their activity persists for weeks or months. Careful control of dosage and frequent determinations of serum and urine calcium and the ability to concentrate urine are essential to avoid hypercalcemia with resultant nephrocalcinosis and renal damage.

2. Diet–A low-phosphate, high-calcium diet, supplemented with added calcium lactate or carbonate (300–1200 mg three or four times daily with meals) is the treatment of choice for prolonged oral therapy both for raising serum calcium and lowering serum phosphate. Because calcium is efficiently absorbed, large doses of vitamin D are rarely necessary.

Course & Prognosis

Abnormal mineral concentrations in extracellular fluid are easily corrected. Central nervous system manifestations are usually reversible, and the prognosis for intellectual development is excellent. Hypercalcemia and consequent renal damage must be avoided: patients receiving high doses of long-acting vitamin D preparations must be carefully monitored.

Cary AH et al: Molecular genetic study of the frequency of monosomy 22q11 in DiGeorge syndrome. Am J Hum Genet 1992;51:964.

PSEUDOHYPOPARATHYROIDISM (Albright's Syndrome, Albright's Hereditary Osteodystrophy, & Pseudopseudohypoparathyroidism)

Pseudohypoparathyroidism is an X-linked disease with a female:male ratio of approximately 2:1. PTH production is adequate, but there is failure of response of the target organ (renal tubule, bone, or both) to the hormone. The failure of responses results from deficiency of the G unit of the trimolecular cyclase complex. This messenger pathway is used in other hormone target tissues. Therefore, resistance to other adenylyl cyclase-dependent hormones (eg, ADH, TSH) has been described in pseudohypoparathyroidism.

Patients with pseudohypoparathyroidism may have the same clinical features and chemical findings seen in idiopathic hypoparathyroidism (Table 28–5). In addition, these patients have distinct phenotypes consisting of short stature; round, full faces; irregularly shortened hands and feet (with the index and third metacarpal bones often longer than the first, fourth, and fifth ones); a short, thick-set body; delayed and defective dentition; and mild mental retardation. The hair is dry and coarse, and nails and skin are thickened; candidiasis is not a feature. X-ray films may show thickening of the cortices of the long bones with limitation of growth at the metaphysial ends. There may be chondrodysplastic changes in the bones of the hands, demineralization of the bones, thickening of the cortices, and exostoses. Corneal and lenticular opacities and ectopic calcification of the basal ganglia and subcutaneous tissues may occur with or without abnormal serum calcium levels. Treatment is the same as that for hypoparathyroidism.

Similar phenotypic findings may be found in pseudopseudohypoparathyroidism, a variant of pseudohypoparathyroidism in which the blood chemistry findings are normal. No treatment is necessary.

In both pseudo- and pseudopseudohypoparathyroidism, the parathyroid glands are hyperplastic, serum levels of PTH are elevated, and the kidneys are relatively unresponsive to PTH.

Patten JL et al: Mutation in the gene encoding the stimulatory G protein of adenylate cyclase in Albright's hereditary osteodystrophy. N Engl J Med 1990;322:1412.

Spiegel AM, Shenker A, Weinstein LS: Receptor-effector coupling by G-proteins: Implications for abnormal signal transduction. Endocr Rev 1992;13:536.

HYPERPARATHYROIDISM & HYPERCALCEMIC STATES

Essentials of Diagnosis & Typical Features

• Abdominal pain, polyuria, polydipsia, hypertension, nephrocalcinosis, renal stones, intractable peptic ulcer, constipation, uremia, and pancreatitis.

- Bone pain and, rarely, pathologic fractures. X-ray film shows subperiosteal resorption, loss of the lamina dura of the teeth, renal parenchymal calcification or stones, and osteitis fibrosa cystica ("brown tumors").
- Unusual (often bizarre) behavior and mood swings.
- Elevated serum concentrations of PTH.
- Serum (and urine) ionized calcium elevated; urine phosphate high, with low or normal serum phosphate; alkaline phosphatase normal or elevated.
- Transient or mild hypercalcemia possibly entirely asymptomatic; hypercalcemia and mild hyperparathyroidism noted frequently as incidental findings in routine laboratory screening.

General Considerations

Over 80% of hypercalcemic children or adolescents have either hyperparathyroidism or a malignant tumor (Table 28–7). The latter condition is invariably associated with additional significant clinical features, and the diagnosis is readily established. Hyperparathyroidism is rare in childhood and may be primary or secondary. The most common cause of primary hyperparathyroidism is a parathyroid adenoma. The most common causes of the secondary form are chronic renal disease (glomerulonephritis, pyelonephritis), congenital anomalies of the genitourinary tract, or rickets (Table 28–6). Diffuse parathyroid hyperplasia or multiple adenomas has also been described in families. Familial hyperparathyroidism may be an isolated disease, or it may be associated with other endocrine neoplasias of the type I and, rarely, type II MEN syndromes.

Clinical Findings

A. Symptoms and Signs:

1. Due to hypercalcemia–Findings include hypotonicity and weakness of muscles; apathy, mood swings, and bizarre behavior; nausea, vomiting, abdominal pain, constipation, and loss of weight; hyperextensibility of joints; and hypertension, cardiac irregularities, bradycardia, and shortening of the QT interval. Coma occurs rarely. Calcium deposits may occur in the cornea or conjunctiva (band keratopathy) and may require slitlamp examination of the eye. Intractable peptic ulcer and pancreatitis occur in adults but rarely in children.

2. Due to increased calcium and phosphate excretion–Findings include loss of renal concentrating ability with polyuria, polydipsia, precipitation of calcium phosphate in the renal parenchyma or as urinary calculi, and progressive renal damage.

3. Due to changes in the skeleton–Findings may include bone pain, osteitis fibrosa cystica, subperiosteal absorption of the distal clavicles and phalanges, absence of lamina dura around the teeth,

spontaneous fractures, and a "moth-eaten" appearance of the skull. Later, there is generalized demineralization with a predilection for subperiosteal cortical bone.

B. Imaging: Bone changes may be subtle in children even when radiography shows nephrocalcinosis. Of the tumor-localizing options, technetium sestamibi scintigraphy is now shown to be more promising than conventional procedures such as ultrasonography, CT, and MRI).

Treatment

Treatment consists of complete removal of the tumor or subtotal removal of hyperplastic parathyroid glands. Preoperatively, intake of dietary calcium should be restricted and hypercalcemia controlled with normal saline infusion and nonthiazide diuretics. Postoperatively, hypocalcemia due to the remineralization of "hungry" bones may occur. A diet high in calcium and vitamin D is recommended immediately postoperatively and is continued until serum calcium concentrations are normal and stable.

Treatment of secondary hyperparathyroidism is directed at the underlying disease. Diminution in the absorption of phosphate with aluminum hydroxide orally is helpful. The hypocalcemia of severe renal disease (creatinine clearance less than 15 mL/min) results from increased complexing with the elevated phosphate, metabolic acidosis, and impaired renal activation of vitamin D. Calcitriol is the vitamin D preparation of choice in this disorder.

Course & Prognosis

The prognosis following removal of a single adenoma is excellent. The prognosis following subtotal parathyroidectomy for diffuse hyperplasia or removal of multiple adenomas is usually good and depends on correction of the underlying defect. In patients with multiple sites of parathyroid adenoma or hyperplasia, MEN is likely, and other family members may be at risk. Genetic counseling and DNA analysis to determine the specific gene defect are indicated.

A variety of drugs (excessive vitamin A or D, lithium, aluminum, thiazide diuretics) may result in hypercalcemia. Sarcoidosis, solid tumors, lymphomas, immobilization, hyperthyroidism, and hypothyroidism are additional disease conditions associated with hypercalcemia.

Pearce SHS et al: Calcium-sensing receptor mutations in familial benign hypercalcemia and neonatal hyperparathyroidism. J Clin Invest 1995;96:2683.

IDIOPATHIC FAMILIAL HYPOCALCIURIC HYPERCALCEMIA

As the name implies, this interesting condition is distinguished by extremely high renal calcium reabsorption with consequent low to normal urinary calcium excretion. PTH is normal or slightly elevated.

Familial hypocalciuric hypercalcemia is usually familial (autosomal dominant). In most cases, the gene defect has been identified as a mutation in the membrane-bound calcium-sensing receptor expressed on parathyroid and renal tubule cells. Patients are invariably asymptomatic, and treatment is unnecessary. The prognosis is excellent.

Pearce SH et al: Functional characterization of calcium-sensing receptor mutations expressed in human embryonic kidney cells. J Clin Invest 1996;98:1860.

HYPERVITAMINOSIS D

Exposure to sunlight and ingestion of vitamin D in a normal diet do not result in hypervitaminosis D and hypercalcemia except possibly in Williams syndrome or sarcoidosis. Vitamin D intoxication is the result of ingestion of excessive amounts of vitamin D, some forms of which may be stored for months in adipose tissue.

Signs, symptoms, and treatment of vitamin D-induced hypercalcemia are the same as those in other hypercalcemic states and include abdominal, renal, central nervous system, and bone findings. Renal insufficiency may be irreversible and is the result of renovascular effects of hypercalcemia and precipitation of calcium phosphate in renal interstitial tissue. Ectopic calcification can occur in many other tissues, including the cornea and the gastric mucosa.

Treatment depends on the stage of hypercalcemic toxicity. Because of adipose tissue storage of vitamin D, several months of treatment may be necessary. Dietary intake of foods fortified with vitamin D (eg, milk) and calcium should be reduced or, if possible, eliminated. Hypercalcemia can be treated with intravenous fluids and nonthiazide diuretics. Adrenocorticosteroids, salmon calcitonin, and the antineoplastic agent plicamycin have also been used with success.

The central nervous system manifestations may be dramatic, and deaths have occurred during acute crises. Chronic brain damage in young infants has been reported. Asymptomatic renal damage may cause failure before the diagnosis is made.

Adams J, Lee G: Gains in bone mineral density with resolution of vitamin D intoxication. Ann Intern Med 1997;127:203.

IDIOPATHIC HYPERCALCEMIA OF INFANCY

Idiopathic hypercalcemia (Williams syndrome) is an uncommon disorder of infancy characterized in its severe form by peculiar ("elfin") facies (receding mandible, depressed bridge of nose, relatively large mouth, prominent eyes, occasional esotropia, and hypertelorism). Failure to thrive, mental and motor retardation, cardiovascular abnormalities, irritability, purposeless movements, constipation, hypotonia, polyuria, polydipsia, and hypertension are common. Cardiac defects include supravalvular aortic stenosis, peripheral pulmonary stenosis, and aortic valve calcifications. An inability to follow directions and a tendency to get lost are common problems, and three-dimensional vision is impaired. A gregarious and affectionate personality is the rule in older children with the syndrome. Generalized osteosclerosis is common, and there may be premature craniosynostosis and nephrocalcinosis with evidence of urinary tract disease.

Clinical manifestations may not appear for several months after birth. Serum concentrations of 1,25-dihydroxycholecalciferol (1,25-dihydroxyvitamin D_3) were frequently elevated in cases reported after World War II in England when excessive vitamin D was introduced into the diet. Currently, a defect in the metabolism of—or responsiveness to—vitamin D is postulated rather than excessive dietary vitamin D intake and elevated serum 1,25-dihydroxycholecalciferol levels. Elastin deletions localized to chromosome 7 have been identified in over 90% of patients; thus, fluorescent in situ hybridization (FISH) analysis may be the best initial diagnostic tool.

Treatment consists of rigid restriction of dietary calcium and vitamin D and, in severe, unresponsive cases, moderate doses of glucocorticoids.

Russo AF et al: Characterization of the calcitonin/CGAP gene in Williams syndrome. Am J Med Genet 1991; 39:28.

IMMOBILIZATION HYPERCALCEMIA

Abrupt immobilization of a rapidly growing adolescent following injury may lead to a rapid decrease in bone deposition with continued bone resorption, calcium mobilization, and hypercalcemia. The condition is reversible when the patient becomes ambulatory.

HYPOPHOSPHATASIA

Hypophosphatasia is an uncommon inherited (autosomal recessive) condition characterized by a specific deficiency of alkaline phosphatase activity in serum, bone, and tissues. Radiographically, there is inadequate mineralization of epiphysial cartilage and osteoid, with localized areas of radiolucency. The disease is radiographically and histologically similar to rickets. The earlier the age at onset, the more severe the condition. Failure to thrive, feeding problems, dwarfing, hyperpyrexia, delayed dentition or premature loss of teeth, widening of the cranial sutures, bulging fontanelles, convulsions, bony deformities indistinguishable from rickets, hyperpigmentation, conjunctival calcification, band keratopathy, and renal lesions have been reported. Premature closure of cranial sutures may occur. Calcium and phosphate concentrations in the extracellular fluid are usually normal; calcium levels, however, may be elevated. In the latter case, signs and symptoms may be similar to those of idiopathic hypercalcemia; late features include osteoporosis, osteopenia, and pseudofractures. The plasma and urine of patients and heterozygote carriers contain phosphoethanolamine in excessive amounts. In some cases, marked metaphysial irregularities may occur. A condition known as pseudohypophosphatasia has been described in which the clinical features of hypophosphatasia are seen in association with normal levels of alkaline phosphatase.

No specific treatment is available, but glucocorticoids may be of value temporarily. The mortality rate is high in infancy. Adults are usually asymptomatic.

Whyte MP: Hypophosphatasia and the role of alkaline phosphatase in skeletal mineralization. Endocr Rev 1994;15:439.

THE GONADS (Ovaries & Testes)

DEVELOPMENT & PHYSIOLOGY

The gonads develop from a bipotential anlage in the genital ridge of the celomic cavity. The primordial germ cells, which will become oocytes and spermatocytes, arise in the yolk sac and migrate to the genital ridge by the fourth week after conception, when the gonad is identifiable. Between the fourth and eighth weeks of gestation, differentiation into an ovary or testis occurs; by 7–9 weeks, the fetal testis begins to produce androgens, and granulosa cells can be identified in the ovary. Testicular androgen production at this time occurs in response to placental human chorionic gonadotropin (hCG) and is necessary for male sexual differentiation. Between 9 and 12 weeks of gestational age, the fetal pituitary starts to produce luteinizing hormone (LH) and follicle-stimulating hormone (FSH); these fetal pituitary hormones are important for continued gonadal development. In response to fetal gonadotropins, ovarian development proceeds, and at the time of birth ovarian maturation has reached the follicular stage. In the testis, Leydig cell production of testosterone continues until several months after birth.

Throughout childhood, pulsatile secretion of FSH and LH occurs at 60- to 90-minute intervals and stimulates the output of gonadal hormones (Figure 28–1; Table 28–1). As puberty approaches, the amplitude and frequency of the peaks increase, initially at night during sleep. As puberty progresses, the basal serum LH concentrations rise, and estrogen production from the ovaries or testosterone production from the testes increases to adult levels.

SEXUAL DIFFERENTIATION

Normal Sexual Differentiation

Normal sexual differentiation requires a specific sequence of events. The bipotential gonad requires at least two X chromosomes to develop into an ovary; in the absence of a second X chromosome, a fibrous streak develops along the genital ridge (eg, in Turner's syndrome). Alternatively, in the presence of the testicular determining factor *(TDF)* gene located on the Y chromosome, a testis develops. Between the seventh and fourteenth weeks of gestation, testosterone produced locally by fetal Leydig cells transforms wolffian ducts into the male genital tract. In target tissues, the enzyme 5α-reductase converts circulating testosterone to dihydrotestosterone (DHT), which virilizes the urogenital sinus and external genitalia. The tissue response to testosterone and DHT is dependent on functional androgen receptors. The gene coding for androgen receptors is located on the X chromosome, and various point mutations and deletions have been described that result in complete or partial androgen insensitivity (see below). Growth of the penis occurs mainly in the late second and third trimesters, requiring stimulation of the testis by fetal pituitary gonadotropins. Müllerian duct inhibiting factor (MIF), a glycoprotein produced by Sertoli cells in the testes, causes regression of the internal female duct structures during the first 8 weeks of gestation. In the absence of this factor, the uterus and uterine (fallopian) tubes develop and mature. The homologous internal and external female and male genital structures are listed in Table 28–8.

Abnormal Sexual Differentiation

There are four major categories of abnormal sexual differentiation resulting in ambiguous external genitalia.

A. Abnormalities in Normal Gonadal Differentiation: These usually result from an abnormality in the number of sex chromosomes. Klinefelter's syndrome (Chapter 31), with a 47,XXY karyotype, is associated with a male phenotype but with poorly functioning testes. Turner's syndrome with a 45,XO karyotype (Chapter 31) is associated with a female phenotype but with streak ovaries (gonadal dysgenesis). Mosaic forms of gonadal dysgenesis that contain a Y-bearing cell line have variable ambiguous inter-

Table 28–8. Sexual differentiation in the female and male.

Internal Duct Derivatives

Müllerian Duct Derivatives	Wollfian Duct Derivatives[1]
Fallopian tubes (oviducts) and fimbria	Epididymis
Uterus	Vas deferens
Cervix	Seminal vesicles
Vagina (posterior two thirds)	Ejaculatory duct
	Prostatic urethra

External Genitalia Homologues

Primitive Structure	Female Genitalia	Male Genitalia[2]
Undifferentiated gonad	Ovary	Testis
Genital tubercle	Clitoris	Glans penis
Genital swelling	Labia majora	Scrotum
Genital/urethral fold	Labia minora	Penile urethra/corpora

[1]Normal wollfian duct development is dependent on the *local* production of testosterone by Leydig's cells of the adjacent testis and on *testosterone's diffusion into the surrounding embryonic tissues.* Thus, females with congenital adrenal hyperplasia who are virilized as the result of *circulating* androgens do not have wolffian duct development. Normal male development is also dependent on regression of müllerian duct derivatives through the *local action of müllerian inhibiting factor* elaborated by the Sertoli cells of the adjacent testis.

[2]The normal development of male external genitalia is dependent on an adequate circulating concentration of testosterone, which is then further converted to dihydrotestosterone in the target tissues through the action of the enzyme, 5α-reductase. Significantly elevated circulating concentrations of other (adrenal) androgens, as in females with congenital adrenal hyperplasia, can virilize the genital tubercle, genital swelling, and genital/urethral folds along the lines of their male homologues, resulting in varying degrees of female pseudohermaphroditism (ambiguity) (see text).

nal and external phenotypes. Idiopathic testicular failure prior to completion of sexual differentiation results in ambiguous genitalia (incomplete virilization). True hermaphroditism, with the presence of both testicular and ovarian tissue, is rare and associated with external genitalia that range from fully masculine to almost completely feminine.

B. Abnormalities in Testosterone Synthesis or Action: These disorders cause male pseudohermaphroditism in that only testicular tissue is present, but its decreased function results in incomplete virilization with ambiguous genitalia. The enzyme defects in testosterone synthesis may affect only testosterone synthesis or they may also affect the synthesis of cortisol, as in variants of congenital adrenal hyperplasia (Figure 28–3). Defects in testosterone action result from either absent or defective androgen receptors or a defect in the peripheral conversion of testosterone metabolism to DHT due to 5α-reductase deficiency. The androgen receptor defect may be complete or incomplete, resulting in varying degrees of ambiguity.

C. Presence of Excessive Androgens in a Female Fetus: These disorders cause female

pseudohermaphroditism (excessive virilization) and usually result in ambiguous genitalia. Excessive adrenal androgen production secondary to an enzyme defect in cortisol synthesis (ie, congenital adrenal hyperplasia; see below) is the cause of 95% of 46,XX patients with female pseudohermaphroditism and approximately 50% of all cases of patients with ambiguous genitalia. Occasionally, maternally derived androgens (eg, maternal congenital adrenal hyperplasia, adrenal tumor during pregnancy, luteoma of pregnancy) may cause virilization of the female fetus.

D. Miscellaneous Syndromes: These may be associated with multiple congenital anomalies, especially of the urinary tract and kidney. Occasionally, teratogenic agents (eg, drugs, radiation) may result in anomalous sexual development.

Migeon CJ, Berkovitz G, Brown T: Sexual differentiation and ambiguity. In: *Wilkins: The Diagnosis and Treatment of Endocrine Disorders in Childhood and Adolescence,* 4th ed. Kappy MS, Blizzard RM, Migeon CJ (editors). Thomas, 1994.

Quigley CA et al: Androgen receptor defects: Historical, clinical and molecular perspectives. Endocrine Rev 1995;16:271.

ABNORMALITIES IN OVARIAN FUNCTION

The ovary is composed of follicles (germ cells surrounded by granulosa cells), theca cells immediately surrounding the follicle, and stromal or supporting tissue. It produces several hormones, primarily estrogens and progesterone, but androgens are also produced. At least three natural estrogens have been identified: estrone, 17β-estradiol (the most potent), and estriol. Production of the major ovarian estrogen, estradiol, is stimulated by pituitary LH secretion (Figure 28–1; Table 28–1), but significant quantities of estrogen are not produced until the onset of puberty. Estrogens stimulate the growth of the uterus, vagina, and breasts. They also contribute to the normal adolescent growth spurt occurring in girls.

Patients with significant ovarian abnormalities (eg, McCune-Albright syndrome) in childhood may exhibit precocious puberty, delayed puberty (primary amenorrhea), or secondary amenorrhea.

1. PRECOCIOUS PUBERTY IN GIRLS

Puberty is considered precocious if the onset of secondary sexual characteristics occurs prior to 6–8 years of age, as shown in a recent study in girls. Precocious puberty is thought to be more common in girls than in boys, but this may be due to the inclusion of a large group of 6- to 8-year-old girls in published studies who have a benign, slowly progressing form that is probably a normal variant.

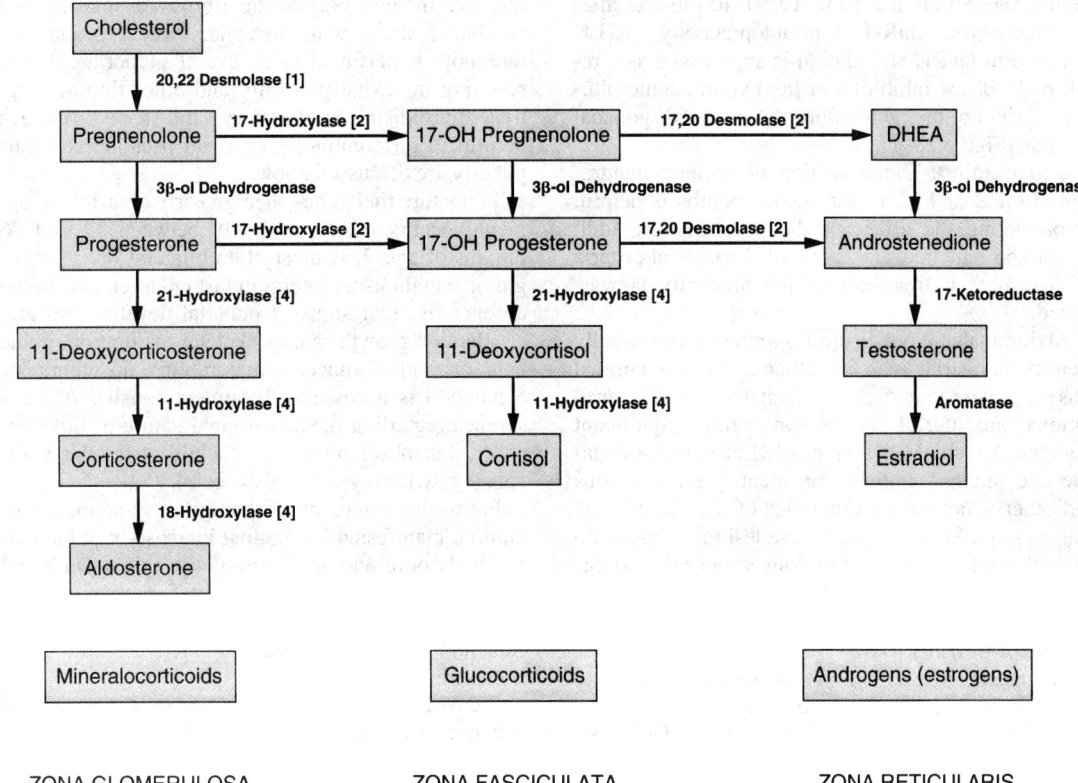

Figure 28–3. The corticosteroid hormone synthetic pathway. The pathways illustrated are present in differing amounts in the "steroid-producing" tissues: adrenal glands, ovaries, and testes. In the adrenal glands, mineralocorticoids from the zona glomerulosa, glucocorticoids from the zona fasciculata, and androgens (and estrogens) from the zona reticularis are produced. The major adrenal androgen is androstenedione, since the activity of 17-ketoreductase is relatively low. The adrenal gland does secrete some testosterone and estrogen, however. The pathways leading to the synthesis of mineralocorticoids and glucocorticoids are not present to any significant degree in the gonads; however, the testes and ovaries each produce both androgens and estrogens. Further metabolism of testosterone to dihydrotestosterone occurs in target tissues as a result of the action of the enzyme 5α-reductase. The current nomenclature for the adrenal steroidogenic enzymes is given as follows: [1], P450scc (side chain cleavage); [2], P450c17; [3], P450c21; [4], P450c11.

True (gonadotropin-releasing hormone [GnRH]-dependent) precocious puberty refers to early sexual maturation in response to hypothalamic-pituitary stimulation (GnRH, FSH, LH). In pseudoprecocity (ie, GnRH-independent precocity), the cause is elsewhere (eg, adrenal gland or ovary, or the result of exogenous estrogen). GnRH-dependent precocious puberty is always isosexual and may progress to the production of mature ova. In pseudoprecocity, sexual characteristics may be isosexual or heterosexual; secondary sexual characteristics develop, but the hypothalamic-pituitary gonadal axis (Figure 28–1) does not mature, and oocyte maturation does not occur.

Clinical Findings

A. Symptoms and Signs: Sexual development in girls usually starts with breast development, followed by pubic hair growth and menarche, but there are exceptions. The interval between breast development and menarche can range from 1 to 6 years but is usually about 2 years. Girls with ovarian or adrenal tumors may have a palpable abdominal mass, also visualized by ultrasonography. A history of excessive mood changes and emotional lability is common. Children with precocious puberty usually have accelerated growth and may be tall during childhood, but because skeletal maturation (bone age) advances at a more rapid rate than linear growth (particularly in the female), adult short stature may occur.

B. Laboratory Findings: In true precocious puberty, the basal serum concentrations of FSH and LH are usually in the prepubertal range. Thus, documentation of the maturity of the hypothalamic-pituitary axis depends on finding a pubertal LH response (serum concentration > 10 IU/L) 30–40 minutes after stimulation with GnRH. In pseudoprecocity, the LH response to GnRH stimulation is suppressed as a result of feedback inhibition of the hypothalamic-pituitary axis by the autonomously secreted gonadal steroids (Figure 28–1).

C. Imaging: Determination of skeletal maturation at onset and then every 6–12 months is helpful in predicting the effect of the precocity on adult height and may be used as one of the several criteria to determine if treatment of the precocity is warranted.

Abdominal and pelvic ultrasonography can usually identify an ovarian mass or follicular cysts or adrenal masses greater than 5 cm in diameter. Serial examinations are useful in demonstrating significant changes. A cranial CT scan or MRI of the hypothalamic and pituitary regions can identify mass lesions and other structural abnormalities of the central nervous system. Since some of these lesions produce no clinical manifestations for prolonged periods, examinations should be performed periodically.

Differential Diagnosis

The causes of true and pseudoprecocious puberty are listed in Table 28–9. Of girls with precocious puberty, 90% have true precocious puberty. Definable abnormalities on cranial CT or MRI are more commonly seen in the younger child. With newer scanning techniques, static (presumably congenital) mass lesions in the hypothalamus, including benign hypothalamic hamartomas, can be seen. The most common cause of pseudoprecocious puberty is McCune-Albright syndrome. Clinical manifestations of this

Table 28–9. Causes of isosexual precocious pubertal development.

True (GnRH-dependent) precocious puberty
 Constitutional (idiopathic)
 Hypothalamic lesions (hamartomas, tumors, congenital
  malformations)
 Dysgerminomas
 Hydrocephalus
 CNS infections
 CNS trauma, irradiation
 Pineal tumors (rare)
 Neurofibromatosis with CNS involvement
 Tuberous sclerosis
 hCG-secreting tumors (eg, hepatoblastomas,
  choriocarcinomas)
Pseudo (GnRH-independent)-precocious puberty
 CAH in males
 Adrenal tumors
 McCune-Albright syndrome (polyostotic fibrous dysplasia)
 Familial Leydig cell hyperplasia (testotoxicosis)—males
 Gonadal tumors
 Exogenous estrogen—oral (contraceptive pills) or topical
Premature adrenarche—males
Premature thelarche—females

CAH = congenital adrenal hyperplasia.

disorder include polyostotic fibrous dysplasia, café au lait lesions with irregular borders, and autonomous hyperfunction of several endocrine glands, resulting in sexual precocity and other findings (eg, hyperthyroidism). Laboratory and x-ray findings helpful in differentiating true and pseudoprecocious puberty are discussed above.

Premature thelarche—benign early breast development—occurs most commonly between 12 and 36 months of age. It is most often bilateral but may begin or remain as unilateral breast enlargement. In the absence of other signs of pubertal development (eg, accelerated growth rate or skeletal maturation, pubic hair, or vaginal mucosal maturation), no laboratory evaluation is necessary. Treatment consists of reassurance regarding the self-limited nature of this condition, but observation of the child at regular intervals (eg, twice a year) is also useful.

Premature adrenarche is benign early adrenal maturation, manifested by gradual increase in pubic hair and body odor and, less commonly, axillary hair and acne. The average age at onset is 5–6 years. Again, no increase in growth rate or skeletal maturation occurs, and no abnormal virilization (eg, clitoromegaly) is present.

Premature adrenarche requires only reassurance and regular observation.

Treatment

In pseudoprecocious puberty, removal of the adrenal or ovarian tumor or correction of the adrenal enzyme disorder usually halts abnormal pubertal development. True precocious puberty can be treated with analogs of GnRH but some long-term outcomes (eg, fertility rate) have not been established. The analogs—given either by daily injection or as a depot sustained-release preparations—interrupt the physiologic pulsatile effect of native GnRH on the pituitary. "Down-regulation" of the pituitary GnRH receptor also occurs, resulting in a block in pituitary LH secretion and release and the return of plasma estrogen concentrations to prepubertal values. If present initially, menses cease, secondary sexual development stabilizes or regresses, and linear growth and skeletal maturation slow to normal prepubertal rates.

In patients with McCune-Albright syndrome, analogs of GnRH are not initially helpful. Therapy with antiestrogens (eg, tamoxifen) or agents that block estrogen synthesis (eg, ketoconazole or testolactone), or both, may be effective. Regardless of the cause of precocious puberty or the medical therapy selected, attention to the psychologic needs of the patient and family is essential.

Ganong CA, Kappy MS: Advances in the treatment of precocious puberty. Adv Pediatr 1994;41:223.

Herman-Giddens ME et al: Secondary sexual characteristics and menses in young girls seen in office practice. Pediatrics 1997;99:505.

Reiter EO, Saenger P: Premature adrenarche. The Endocrinologist 1997;7:85.

2. AMENORRHEA

Primary amenorrhea is the absence of menarche in a female 14 years of age or older or in a female of any age who is over 3 years postpubertal maturation. Secondary amenorrhea is cessation of established menses after an interval of time equal to at least 6 months postmenarche or three menstrual cycles. A history and physical examination (including pelvic examination) often identify possible causes of amenorrhea (Table 28–10).

Primary Amenorrhea

The most common cause of primary amenorrhea is physiologic or constitutional delay. Turner's syndrome, chronic illness, and severe undernutrition or strenuous exercise are also common causes.

The term "pseudoamenorrhea" is used when the patient is menstruating but has a genital tract obstruction that prevents release of menstrual blood. Sexual development is usually at Tanner stage III or IV

Table 28–10. Causes of amenorrhea.

I. With obstruction of outflow tract
  A. Fusion or stenosis of labia, hymen (imperforate), vagina, or cervix
  B. Müllerian agenesis (Mayer-Rokitansky-Küster-Hauser)
  C. Postabortion infection, cesarean section, hysterectomy
  D. Complete androgen resistance syndrome (46,XY female)
II. Estrogen deficiency
  A. Primary ovarian insufficiency
    1. Gonadal agenesis
    2. Gonadal dysgenesis (Turner's syndrome variants, true gonadal dysgenesis)
    3. Ovarian steroid biosynthesis deficiency (enzyme defects)
    4. Premature ovarian failure
      a. Autoimmune disease
      b. Infection, surgery, radiation, chemotherapy
  B. Secondary/tertiary ovarian insufficiency
    1. Hypothalamic or pituitary tumor, infection, irradiation
    2. Kallman's syndrome (GnRH/FSH/LH deficiency associated with anosmia)
    3. Eating disorders (eg, anorexia nervosa, bulimia)
    4. Excessive exercise (swimmers, runners, gymnasts)
    5. Chronic illness, malnutrition
III. Androgen excess
  A. Polycystic ovary syndrome
  B. Adrenal androgen excess (CAH, Cushing's disease or syndrome)
IV. Ovarian tumors—granulosa-theca cell, and others

CAH = congenital adrenal hyperplasia, FSH = follicle-stimulating hormone; GnRH = gonadotropin-releasing hormone; LH = luteinizing hormone.

(where stage I is prepubertal and stage V is fully mature), and cyclic abdominal pain without menstruation is noted. Pelvic examination may reveal an imperforate hymen, transverse vaginal ridge, or other obstruction. Treatment is surgical.

Turner's syndrome (45,XO syndrome and its variants) should be considered in patients with short stature and sexual infantilism or adrenarche without normal pubertal progression. This is a form of hypergonadotropic hypogonadism in which serum concentrations of FSH and LH are elevated but plasma estrogen concentration is low owing to a total or relative lack of ovarian tissue. Skeletal maturation is usually delayed. The phenotypic features of Turner's syndrome (described in Chapter 31) may be absent in 40–50% of girls with the syndrome. Current treatment for short stature includes hGH with or without anabolic steroids. Low doses of estrogens are added to the treatment regimen when breast development is desired, but usually at a later age than the average girl, to ensure that maximal height will be achieved. After 2–3 years of estrogen therapy, a combination of estrogen and progesterone in physiologic doses is indicated, so that the patient does not have the increased risks associated with long-term unopposed estrogen treatment.

Mayer-Rokitansky-Küster-Hauser syndrome is characterized by congenital müllerian agenesis with normal ovaries, normal ovarian function, and normal breast development. Pelvic examination reveals an absent vagina and various uterine abnormalities with or without additional renal and skeletal anomalies. Full evaluation is necessary, including karyotyping, intravenous pyelography, and laparoscopy. Therapy for this syndrome is surgical vaginoplasty.

Androgen insensitivity syndrome (androgen receptor defect) may present as primary amenorrhea, since the affected individual (46,XY) has functioning testes that produce MIF during fetal life. Thus, no müllerian duct (oviduct, uterus) development occurs.

Secondary Amenorrhea

Common causes of secondary amenorrhea include stress, pregnancy, major weight loss, polycystic ovary syndrome, and hyperprolactinemia. Stress-induced amenorrhea is often noted in teenagers, but it should be diagnosed only after careful evaluation. Pregnancy is the most common cause of secondary amenorrhea in sexually active teenagers.

Irregular menses (oligomenorrhea) or amenorrhea may result from severe weight loss secondary to dieting, vigorous exercise (eg, in marathon runners, swimmers, ballet dancers, and gymnasts), depression, anorexia nervosa, or chronic illness. In the normally ovulating female, it is believed that a major source of estrogen is aromatization of androgens in peripheral adipose tissue. When the proportion of body weight represented by fat falls below a critical level

(15–25%), estrogen production is decreased. This hypothesis has been advanced to explain amenorrhea in athletes and in patients with anorexia nervosa.

In polycystic ovary syndrome, secondary amenorrhea is the result of chronic anovulation. Occasionally, dysfunctional uterine bleeding is the only finding; the full syndrome consists of obesity, hirsutism, secondary amenorrhea, bilaterally enlarged ovaries, and, in some cases, clitoromegaly, and it may be related to the excessive insulin secretion seen in these patients. Tests show normal circulating FSH concentrations, elevated LH, borderline to elevated adrenal or ovarian androgens, and increased plasma free testosterone concentrations. Laparoscopy, ovarian biopsy, endometrial biopsy, or a combination of these procedures may be necessary for diagnosis. Treatment consists of correction of the estrogen-androgen ratio by estrogen-progesterone combinations, with later induction of ovulation in adult patients who wish to become pregnant. Agents with antiandrogen activity (eg, spironolactone) may be helpful in controlling hirsutism, and newer regimens have included oral hypoglycemic agents that increase insulin sensitivity and reduce its secretion.

Other causes of amenorrhea are shown in Table 28–10. Chronic illness and central nervous system disorders should always be considered. When galactorrhea and amenorrhea occur together, hyperprolactinemia due to adenoma or ingestion of antidepressants or marijuana, hypothyroidism, stress, and hypothalamic injury should be considered.

Apter D et al: Metabolic features of polycystic ovary syndrome are found in adolescent girls with hyperandrogenism. J Clin Endocrinol Metab 1995;80:2966.

Constantini NW, Warner MP: Menstrual dysfunction in swimmers: A distinct entity. J Clin Endocrinol Metab 1995;80:2740.

Franks S: Polycystic ovary syndrome. Arch Dis Child 1997;77:89.

OVARIAN TUMORS

Ovarian tumors are not rare in children. They may occur at any age and are usually large, benign, and unilateral. They may be estrogen-producing; ovarian tumors account for about 1% of cases of female sexual precocity. The most common estrogen-producing tumor is the granulosa cell tumor. Others that may cause sexual precocity include thecomas, luteomas, mixed types, theca-lutein and follicular cysts, and ovarian tumors (teratomas, choriocarcinomas, and dysgerminomas). Ovarian tumors are usually palpated on rectal examination and readily seen by ovarian ultrasonography. Treatment is surgical removal. Recurrences are uncommon.

ABNORMALITIES IN TESTICULAR FUNCTION

The major testicular hormone, testosterone, is produced by Leydig (interstitial) cells. Production of testicular androgens is stimulated by LH secretion (Figure 28–1; Table 28–1). Testicular androgen (testosterone) is responsible wholly or in part for growth of the internal (wolffian) duct derivatives (Table 28–8), and dihydrotestosterone for the development of the external genitalia in utero. Testosterone and dihydrotestosterone (from the testes and peripheral tissues, respectively) and adrenal androgens are necessary for development of secondary sexual characteristics, including pubic, axillary, and facial hair during puberty. Androgens induce nitrogen retention, accelerated growth rate (pubertal growth spurt), and skeletal maturation.

The seminiferous tubules are composed of germinal epithelium and Sertoli cells. Testicular androgens in combination with pituitary FSH stimulate the development and maturation of the germinal epithelium and thus promote spermatogenesis. Sertoli cells provide structural support for the germinal epithelium.

Patients with abnormalities in testicular function may present with delayed or precocious sexual development or cryptorchism.

1. PRECOCIOUS PUBERTY IN BOYS

Puberty is considered precocious in boys if secondary sexual characteristics appear prior to 9 years of age. Precocious puberty appears to be much less common in boys than in girls, but this may be more apparent than real. In boys presenting with sexual precocity, pseudoprecocious puberty is as common as true, GnRH-dependent, precocious puberty. In addition, boys with true precocious puberty are more likely to have an identifiable pathologic process (eg, central nervous system abnormality) rather than idiopathic precocious puberty.

Two main GnRH-independent forms of precocious puberty have been described in boys: McCune-Albright syndrome (described previously) and familial Leydig cell hyperplasia, or testotoxicosis, a condition in which the LH receptor on the Leydig cell is hypersensitive to LH, resulting in testicular overproduction of testosterone in the face of prepubertal LH concentrations. As in McCune-Albright syndrome or other causes of autonomous gonadal or adrenal androgen secretion, the LH response to GnRH stimulation testing is suppressed.

Clinical Findings

A. Symptoms and Signs: In precocious development, increases in growth rate and growth of pubic hair are the common presenting signs. Testicular size may differentiate true precocity, in which the testes enlarge, from pseudoprecocity (most commonly due to congenital adrenal hyperplasia), in which the testes usually remain small. There are some exceptions: In advanced cases of pseudoprecocity, for example, some testicular enlargement may occur because seminiferous tubule elements may be stimulated by prolonged elevated androgen levels. In the very young child with early true precocity, minimal increases of testosterone may result in dramatic increases in penis size and pubic hair growth with very little testicular enlargement. Tumors of the testis present with asymmetric testicular enlargement.

B. Laboratory Findings: Basal serum LH and FSH concentrations are usually not in the pubertal range in boys with true sexual precocity, but the LH response to GnRH stimulation testing is pubertal (> 10 IU/L). Sexual precocity caused by congenital adrenal hyperplasia is usually associated with abnormal plasma concentrations of dehydroepiandrosterone (DHEA), androstenedione, 17-hydroxyprogesterone (in congenital adrenal hyperplasia due to 21-hydroxylase deficiency), 11-deoxycortisol (in congenital adrenal hyperplasia due to 11-hydroxylase deficiency), or a combination of these steroids (see Adrenal Cortex section, below). Determining serum hCG concentrations to confirm the presence of an hCG-producing tumor (eg, central nervous system dysgerminoma, hepatoma) may be necessary in boys who present with apparent true sexual precocity (accompanied by testicular enlargement).

C. Imaging: Diagnostic studies are similar to those used to evaluate sexual precocity in girls (see previous text). Ultrasonography may be useful in detection of hepatic, presacral, and testicular tumors.

Differential Diagnosis

The causes of isosexual precocity are outlined in Table 28–9. In boys, it is particularly important to differentiate pseudoprecocity from true sexual precocity. Seventy percent of boys with pseudoprecocious puberty have an adrenal enzyme abnormality (congenital adrenal hyperplasia). Of boys with true precocious puberty, 70% have benign central nervous system mass lesions. Premature adrenarche (described above) may occur in males as well as females.

Treatment

Specific therapy should be provided whenever possible. Treatment of idiopathic true precocious puberty in boys is similar to that in girls (see above). Treatment of McCune-Albright syndrome or familial Leydig cell hyperplasia with agents that block steroid synthesis (eg, ketoconazole), with an antiandrogen (eg, spironolactone), or with a combination of both has been successful.

Blizzard RM, Rogol AD: Variations and disorders of pubertal development. In: *Wilkins: The Diagnosis and Treatment of Endocrine Disorders in Childhood and Adolescence,* 4th ed. Kappy MS, Blizzard RM, Migeon CJ (editors). Thomas, 1994.

Ganong CA, Kappy MS: Advances in the treatment of precocious puberty. Adv Pediatr 1994;41:223.

Latronico AC et al: A novel mutation of the LH receptor gene causing male gonadotropin-independent precocious puberty. J Clin Endocrinol Metab 1995;80:2490.

2. SEXUAL INFANTILISM (Primary & Secondary Testicular Failure)

Lack of development of secondary sexual characteristics after the age of 15 years suggests abnormal testicular maturation. Although delay of puberty until 15 years of age may be physiologically normal, boys generally become concerned if pubertal changes do not occur by then, and evaluation should be initiated at that time. Sexual infantilism may be difficult to differentiate from constitutionally delayed adolescence. Although the latter may be associated with a delay in testicular function, normal puberty occurs at a later date.

Testicular failure or insufficiency may be primary, resulting from the absence, malfunction, or destruction of testicular tissue, or secondary, due to pituitary (or hypothalamic) insufficiency. Primary testicular failure may be due to anorchia, surgical castration, Klinefelter's syndrome or other sex chromosome abnormalities, enzymatic defects in testosterone synthesis or action, or inflammation and destruction of the testes following infection (eg, mumps), autoimmune disorders, radiation, trauma, or tumor.

Secondary testicular failure may accompany panhypopituitarism, empty sella syndrome, Kallmann's syndrome (gonadotropin deficiency accompanied by anosmia), or isolated deficiencies of LH or FSH. Destructive lesions in or near the anterior pituitary, especially craniopharyngiomas, gliomas, or infection, may also result in hypothalamic or pituitary dysfunction. Prader-Willi syndrome and Laurence-Moon syndrome (Bardet-Biedl syndrome) are frequently associated with LH and FSH deficiency secondary to deficiency of GnRH. Miscellaneous causes of secondary testicular failure include chronic debilitating disease and hypothyroidism.

Clinical Findings

A. Symptoms and Signs: Physical examination may not be helpful in differentiating primary from secondary testicular insufficiency. Whereas cryptorchism suggests primary testicular failure, hypothalamic or pituitary insufficiency as well as anatomic abnormalities may also lead to failure of testicular descent.

B. Laboratory Findings: In primary testicular failure, the plasma testosterone concentration is low, whereas LH and FSH values are elevated into the castrate range. In secondary testicular failure, circulating concentrations of all three hormones are below the normal adult range. To establish the presence of the testes and their ability to respond to stimulation, four daily doses of chorionic gonadotropin, 3000 units/m^2 each, are given intramuscularly. The plasma testosterone should rise to above 200 mg/dL 24 hours after the final dose. A karyotype should be determined in primary testicular failure of unknown cause.

C. Imaging: Skeletal (epiphysial) maturation is usually delayed. A cranial CT scan or MRI should be performed in cases of secondary testicular failure.

Treatment

Specific therapy is indicated when the cause of testicular failure is known. Treatment with depot testosterone (eg, testosterone enanthate), beginning with 75–100 mg intramuscularly and increasing to 200 mg every 3–4 weeks, may be continued indefinitely. Specific therapy (pulsatile subcutaneous delivery of GnRH) may result in fertility in patients with hypothalamic-pituitary insufficiency.

Ghaik K, Cara JF, Rosenfield RL: GnRHa (nafarelin) test to differentiate gonadotropin deficiency from constitutionally delayed puberty in teenage boys: A clinical research study. J Clin Endocrinol Metab 1995;80:2980.
Lanes R et al: Effectiveness and limitations of the use of the GnRH agonist leuprolide acetate in the diagnosis of delayed puberty in males. Horm Res 1997;48:1.

3. CRYPTORCHISM

Cryptorchism (undescended testis) is a common disorder in children. It may be unilateral or bilateral and may be classified as ectopic or true cryptorchism.

Approximately 3% of term male newborns and 10% of premature males have undescended testes at birth. In over 50% of these cases, the testes descend by the second month; by the age of 1 year, 80% of all undescended testes are in the scrotum. Further descent may occur through puberty, the latter perhaps stimulated by endogenous gonadotropins. If cryptorchism persists into adult life, failure of spermatogenesis occurs, but testicular androgen production usually remains intact. The incidence of malignant neoplasm (usually seminoma) is appreciably greater in testes that remain in the abdomen after puberty.

Ectopic testes are presumed to develop normally but are diverted as they descend through the inguinal canal. They are subclassified on the basis of their location; surgery is indicated once the diagnosis is established.

True cryptorchism is thought in most cases to be the result of an abnormality in testicular development (dysgenesis). Cryptorchid testes frequently have a short spermatic artery, poor blood supply, or both. Although early scrotal positioning of these testes will obviate further damage related to intra-abdominal location, the testes generally remain abnormal, spermatogenesis is rare, and the risk of malignant neoplasm is increased. These testes should probably be removed if spermatogenesis does not occur after a reasonable period of observation.

Bilateral cryptorchism is a common feature in prepubertal castrate syndrome (the vanishing testes syndrome), Noonan's syndrome, and disorders of androgen synthesis or action; it is seen less commonly with Klinefelter's syndrome, Sertoli cell only syndrome, and hypogonadotropic states.

Note: The diagnosis of bilateral cryptorchism in an apparently male newborn should never be made until the possibility that the child is actually a fully virilized female with potentially fatal salt-losing congenital adrenal hyperplasia has been ruled out (see Adrenal Cortex, below).

Clinical Findings

Plasma testosterone concentrations may be obtained after hCG stimulation to confirm the presence or absence of abdominal testes (see previous text). The child with bilaterally undescended testes should be evaluated for sex chromosome abnormalities; evaluation should include consideration of the possibility that the child is actually a virilized female.

Differential Diagnosis

In palpating for the testes, the cremasteric reflex may be elicited, with a resultant ascent of the testes into the inguinal canal or abdomen (pseudocryptorchism). To prevent this, the fingers first should be placed across the abdominal ring and the upper portion of the inguinal canal, obstructing ascent. Examination while the child is in the squatting position or in a warm bath is also helpful. No treatment for retractile testes is necessary, and the prognosis for testicular descent and competence is excellent.

Treatment

The best age for medical or surgical treatment has not been determined, but there is a trend toward operation in infancy or early childhood. Surgical repair is indicated for cryptorchism persisting beyond puberty.

Gonadotropin therapy (chorionic gonadotropin, 4000–5000 units intramuscularly three to five times per week for 2 or 3 weeks) is generally ineffective unless the child has retractile testes (pseudocryptorchism) rather than true cryptorchism.

Androgen treatment (eg, depot testosterone) is indicated as replacement therapy in the male beyond the normal age of puberty who has been shown to lack functional testes.

4. GYNECOMASTIA

Adolescent gynecomastia is a common, self-limited finding in boys. It may sometimes be seen as part of Klinefelter's syndrome, or it may be seen in boys who are taking certain drugs such as antidepressants or marijuana. This topic is discussed in more detail in Chapter 5.

TESTICULAR TUMORS

The major primary malignant tumors of the testis are seminomas and teratomas. Seminomas are rare in childhood; they may be hormone-producing. The major hormone-producing tumor of the testis is Leydig cell tumor. It is frequently associated with sexual precocity. Other testicular tumors (choriocarcinomas and dysgerminomas) have been reported in association with sexual precocity.

Treatment of testicular tumors is surgical removal; chemotherapy and radiation therapy are not used in childhood unless there is a high-grade malignancy or metastasis. The prognosis in patients with Leydig cell tumors is generally good.

ADRENAL CORTEX

The adult adrenal cortex displays relative regional specificity of terminal steroid production. The outermost zona glomerulosa is the predominant source of aldosterone, while the zona fasciculata makes cortisol, the major glucocorticoid, as well as small amounts of mineralocorticoids. The innermost zona reticularis produces mainly adrenal androgens and estrogens. During fetal life, a fetal zone, or provisional cortex, predominates. This fetal zone produces glucocorticoids, mineralocorticoids, androgens, and estrogens but is relatively deficient in 3β-ol dehydrogenase (Figure 28–3). Therefore, placentally produced progesterone serves as the major precursor for the fetal adrenal production of cortisol and aldosterone.

The adrenal cortex produces cortisol under the control of pituitary ACTH (Figure 28–1; Table 28–1), which is, in turn, regulated by corticotropin-releasing hormone (CRH), a hypothalamic peptide. The complex interaction of central nervous system influences on CRH secretion coupled with negative feedback of serum cortisol leads to a marked diurnal pattern of ACTH and cortisol release. ACTH concentrations are greatest during the early morning hours, display a smaller peak in the late afternoon, and are lowest during the night. The pattern of serum cortisol concentration closely follows this diurnal pattern

with a lag of a few hours. In the absence of cortisol feedback, both CRH and ACTH display dramatic hypersecretion.

At the cellular level, glucocorticoids are critical for normal gene expression in a wide variety of cells. In excess, glucocorticoids are both catabolic and antianabolic; ie, they promote the release of amino acids from muscle and increase gluconeogenesis while decreasing incorporation of amino acids into muscle protein. They also antagonize insulin action and facilitate lipolysis. Glucocorticoids help maintain blood pressure through their "permissive" effect on peripheral vascular tone and by promoting sodium and water retention.

Mineralocorticoids (primarily aldosterone in humans) promote sodium retention and stimulate potassium excretion in the distal tubule. Although ACTH can stimulate aldosterone production, the predominant regulator of aldosterone secretion is the volume- and sodium-sensitive renin-angiotensin-aldosterone system. Elevations of serum potassium concentrations also directly influence aldosterone release from the cortex.

Androgen (DHEA and androstenedione) production by the zona reticularis is insignificant in prepubertal children. At the onset of puberty, androgen production increases and may be an important factor in the dynamics of puberty in both sexes. The adrenal gland is a major source of androgen in the pubertal and adult female.

ADRENOCORTICAL INSUFFICIENCY (Adrenal Crisis, Addison's Disease)

The leading causes of adrenal insufficiency today are hereditary enzymatic defects (congenital adrenal hyperplasia), loss of adrenal function due to autoimmune destruction of the glands (Addison's disease), and central adrenal insufficiency following an intracranial neoplasm or its treatment. A rare form of familial adrenal insufficiency can be seen in association with cerebral sclerosis and spastic paraplegia (adrenoleukodystrophy). Autoimmune Addison's disease may be familial and has been described in association with hypoparathyroidism, candidiasis, hypothyroidism, pernicious anemia, hypogonadism, and diabetes mellitus as one of the polyglandular autoimmune syndromes. The finding of circulating antibodies to adrenal tissue and other tissues involved in these conditions suggests that an autoimmune mechanism is the cause. Less commonly, the gland is destroyed by tumor, calcification, or hemorrhage (Waterhouse-Friderichsen syndrome). Adrenal disease secondary to opportunistic infections (fungal, tuberculous) is again being reported in adults with AIDS. A similar relationship is likely in children. In children, central adrenal insufficiency due to a primary anterior pituitary tumor is rare.

A temporary salt-losing disorder due to partial mineralocorticoid deficiency or renal underresponsiveness (pseudohypoaldosteronism) may occur during infancy.

Any acute illness, surgery, trauma, or exposure to excessive heat may precipitate an adrenal crisis in susceptible individuals. Patients with primary adrenal insufficiency are generally at greater risk of life-threatening crisis than patients with central ACTH deficiency. This is a consequence of intact mineralocorticoid secretion and low-level autonomous cortisol secretion in central ACTH deficiency.

Clinical Findings

A. Symptoms and Signs:

1. Acute form (adrenal crisis)–Manifestations include nausea and vomiting, diarrhea, abdominal pain, dehydration, fever (which may be followed by hypothermia), weakness, hypotension, circulatory collapse, and confusion or coma. Increased pigmentation may be seen in primary adrenal insufficiency as a result of the melanocyte-stimulating activity of the hypersecreted parent molecule of ACTH.

2. Chronic form–Manifestations include fatigue, hypotension, weakness, failure to gain or loss of weight, increased appetite for salt (primary insufficiency), vomiting (which may become forceful and sometimes projectile), and dehydration. Diffuse tanning with increased pigmentation over pressure points, scars, and mucous membranes may be present in primary adrenal insufficiency. A small heart may be seen on chest x-ray.

B. Laboratory Findings:

1. Suggestive of adrenocortical insufficiency–In primary adrenal insufficiency, serum sodium and bicarbonate, $PaCO_2$, blood pH, and blood volume are decreased. Serum potassium and urea nitrogen are increased. Urinary sodium and sodium:potassium ratio are elevated for the degree of hyponatremia. In central adrenal insufficiency, serum sodium may be mildly decreased as a result of impaired water excretion. Eosinophilia and moderate lymphopenia may be present in either form of insufficiency.

2. Confirmatory tests–The following tests measure the functional capacity of the adrenal cortex:

a. The ACTH (cosyntropin) stimulation test is the most direct test of adrenal gland function. In primary adrenal insufficiency (ie, originating in the gland itself), plasma cortisol and aldosterone concentrations fail to increase significantly over baseline 60 minutes after an intravenous dose of ACTH.

b. Baseline serum ACTH concentrations are elevated in primary adrenal failure.

c. Urinary free cortisol and 17-hydroxycorticosteroid excretion are decreased.

d. The metyrapone (an inhibitor of 11-hydroxylase) test may helpful in diagnosing adrenal insufficiency due to pituitary or hypothalamic disease. Af-

ter a dose of metyrapone at midnight, the transient inhibition of cortisol biosynthesis will lead to elevation of ACTH and subsequent increase in the morning 11-deoxycortisol concentration in patients with an intact CRH-ACTH-adrenal axis. In children with pituitary or hypothalamic disease, ACTH secretion is compromised, and the 11-deoxycortisol does not rise. *Caution:* This test may provoke acute adrenal insufficiency in an individual with compromised hypothalamic, pituitary, or adrenal function, and the test is best done in the hospital with monitoring of the patient's vital signs.

e. CRH test–The recently introduced CRH test can be used to assess responsiveness of the entire hypothalamic-pituitary-adrenal axis. After administration of ovine CRH, serum concentrations of ACTH and cortisol can be measured over a period of 2 hours. Verification of the presence of an intact axis or localization of the site of impairment is possible with careful interpretation of these results.

Differential Diagnosis

Acute adrenal insufficiency must be differentiated from severe acute infections, diabetic coma, various disturbances of the central nervous system, and acute poisoning. In the neonatal period, adrenal insufficiency may be clinically indistinguishable from respiratory distress, intracranial hemorrhage, or sepsis.

Chronic adrenocortical insufficiency must be differentiated from anorexia nervosa, certain muscular disorders (eg, myasthenia gravis), salt-losing nephritis, and chronic debilitating infections (eg, tuberculosis) and must be considered in cases of recurrent spontaneous hypoglycemia.

Treatment

A. Acute (Adrenal Crisis):

1. Hydrocortisone sodium succinate, 2 mg/kg intravenously over 2–5 minutes initially; thereafter, it is given intravenously, 1.5 mg/kg in infants or 12.5 mg/m^2 in older children, every 4–6 hours until stabilization is achieved and oral therapy can be tolerated.

2. Fluids and electrolytes–In primary adrenal insufficiency, 5–10% glucose in normal saline, 10–20 mL/kg intravenously, is given over the first hour and repeated if necessary to reestablish vascular volume. Normal saline is continued thereafter at one and one-half to two times the maintenance fluid requirements. In addition, intravenous boluses of glucose (10% glucose, 2 mL/kg) may be needed every 4–6 hours for hypoglycemia. In central adrenal insufficiency, routine fluid management is generally adequate following reinstatement of vascular volume and institution of cortisol replacement.

3. Fludrocortisone–When oral intake is tolerated, fludrocortisone, 0.1 mg daily, is started and continued as necessary every 12–24 hours for primary adrenal insufficiency.

4. Rarely, inotropic agents such as dopamine or

dobutamine are needed. However, adequate cortisol replacement is critical since pressor agents may be ineffective in adrenal insufficiency.

5. Waterhouse-Friderichsen syndrome with fulminant infections–The use of adrenocorticosteroids and norepinephrine in the treatment or prophylaxis of fulminant infections remains controversial; corticosteroids may augment the generalized Shwartzman reaction in fatal cases of meningococcemia. However, corticosteroids should be considered in the presence of possible adrenal insufficiency, particularly with hypotension and circulatory collapse.

B. Maintenance Therapy: Following initial stabilization, the most effective substitution therapy is hydrocortisone, combined with fludrocortisone in primary adrenal insufficiency. Overtreatment should be avoided because it may result in obesity, growth retardation, and other cushingoid features. Additional hydrocortisone, fludrocortisone, or sodium chloride, singly or in combination, may be necessary with acute illness, surgery, trauma, or other stress reactions.

Supportive adrenocortical therapy should be given whenever surgical operations are performed in patients who have at some time received prolonged therapy with adrenocorticosteroids (see below).

1. Glucocorticoids–A maintenance dosage of 8–10 mg/m^2/d of hydrocortisone (or equivalent) is given orally in two or three divided doses. For adrenal enzyme defects (see below), this dosage may need to be increased to 18–22 mg/m^2/d to obtain adequate suppression of the adrenal axis, with two-thirds given at night (the time of greatest axis suppressibility). The dosage of all glucocorticoids is increased to 30–50 mg/m^2/d during intercurrent illnesses or other times of stress.

2. Mineralocorticoids–In primary adrenal insufficiency, give fludrocortisone, 0.05–0.15 mg orally daily as a single dose or in two divided doses. Periodic monitoring of blood pressure is recommended to avoid overdosing.

3. Salt–The child should be given ready access to table salt. Frequent blood pressure determinations in the recumbent position should be made to ensure that hypertension is avoided. In the infant, supplementation of formula with 3 mEq Na$^+$/kg is generally required until table foods are introduced.

C. Corticosteroids in Patients With Adrenocortical Insufficiency Who Undergo Surgery:

1. Before operation–Hydrocortisone sodium succinate, 30–50 mg/m^2/d intravenously, is given 1 hour before surgery.

2. During operation–Hydrocortisone sodium succinate, 25–100 mg intravenously, is administered with 5–10% glucose in saline throughout surgery.

3. During recovery–Hydrocortisone sodium succinate, 12.5 mg/m^2 intravenously, is given every 4–6 hours until oral doses are tolerated. The oral

dose of three to five times the maintenance dose is continued until the acute stress is over, at which time the patient can be returned to their maintenance dose.

Course & Prognosis

A. Acute Adrenal Insufficiency: The course of acute adrenal insufficiency is rapid, and death may occur within a few hours, particularly in infants, unless adequate treatment is given. Spontaneous recovery is unlikely. Patients who have received long-term treatment with adrenocorticosteroids may exhibit adrenal collapse if they undergo surgery or other acute stress. Pharmacologic doses of glucocorticoids during these episodes may be needed throughout life.

In all forms of acute adrenal insufficiency, the patient should be observed carefully once the crisis has passed and evaluated with laboratory tests to assess the degree of permanent adrenal insufficiency.

B. Chronic Adrenal Insufficiency: Adequately treated, chronic adrenocortical insufficiency is consistent with a relatively normal life. Patients receiving maintenance doses of glucocorticoids may require increases (two- to fourfold) during severe illnesses and operations.

August GP: Treatment of adrenocortical insufficiency. Pediatr Rev 1997;18:59.

Migeon CJ, Donohoue P: Adrenal disorders. In: *Wilkins: The Diagnosis and Treatment of Endocrine Disorders in Childhood and Adolescence,* 4th ed. Kappy MS, Blizzard RM, Migeon CJ (editors). Thomas, 1994.

Smith BB, Furmaniak J: Adrenal and gonadal autoimmune disease. J Clin Endocrinol Metab 1995;80:1502.

Winter WE: Autoimmune endocrinopathies. In: *Wilkins: The Diagnosis and Treatment of Endocrine Disorders in Childhood and Adolescence,* 4th ed. Kappy MS, Blizzard RM, Migeon CJ (editors). Thomas, 1994.

CONGENITAL ADRENAL HYPERPLASIAS

Essentials of Diagnosis & Typical Features

- Pseudohermaphroditism in females, with urogenital sinus, enlargement of the clitoris, or other evidence of virilization.
- Salt-losing crisis in infant males or isosexual precocity in older males with infantile testes.
- Increased linear growth in young children; advancement of skeletal maturation.
- Urinary and plasma androgen elevation; plasma 17-hydroxyprogesterone and urinary pregnanetriol concentrations increased in the common form; may be associated with electrolyte and water disturbances (hyponatremia, hyperkalemia, and metabolic acidosis), particularly in the newborn period.

General Considerations

Autosomal recessive enzyme defects involved in

adrenal steroidogenesis have in common a defect in cortisol biosynthesis with resultant increased ACTH secretion during fetal life. ACTH excess subsequently results in adrenal hyperplasia with increased production of various adrenal hormone precursors, including androgens, and increased urinary excretion of their metabolites. Increased pigmentation, especially of the scrotum, labia majora, and nipples, frequently results from excessive ACTH secretion. Congenital adrenal hyperplasia (CAH) is most commonly (> 80%) the result of homozygous 21-hydroxylase (P450c21) deficiency (Figure 28–3), an autosomal recessive disorder. In its severe form, excess adrenal androgen production beginning in the first trimester of fetal development results in virilization of the female infant and life-threatening hypovolemic, hyponatremic shock (adrenal crisis) in the newborn. Other enzyme defects that less commonly result in congenital adrenal hyperplasia include 20,22-desmolase, 3β-ol dehydrogenases, 18-hydroxylase-17,22-desmolase, and 11-hydroxylase deficiencies. The clinical syndromes associated with each of these defects can be predicted from Figure 28–3 and Table 28–11. Recently, all of these enzymes except 3β-ol dehydrogenase have been shown to be associated with the cytochrome P450 complex. A new enzyme nomenclature has been established, and it is given along with the older, more familiar nomenclature in Figure 28–3 to avoid confusion.

Studies in patients with 21-hydroxylase deficiency indicate that the clinical type (salt-wasting versus non-salt-wasting) is usually consistent within a family and that there is a close genetic linkage of the 21-hydroxylase gene to the HLA complex on chromosome 6. The latter finding has allowed more precise heterozygote detection and prenatal diagnosis. Population studies indicate that the defective gene is present in 1:250–1:100 people and that the incidence of the disorder is 1:15,000–1:5000. Hormonal evaluation of unaffected family members following ACTH stimulation allows detection of the heterozygote with a certainty of 80–90%, and a combination of hormonal and HLA studies can increase the number of cases detected. HLA typing in combination with the measurement of 17-hydroxyprogesterone and androstenedione in amniotic fluid has been used in the prenatal diagnosis of 21-hydroxylase deficiency. Mass screening for this enzyme defect, using a microfilter paper technique to measure 17-hydroxyprogesterone, has been established in some states.

Nonclassic presentations of 21-hydroxylase deficiency have been reported with increasing frequency. Affected persons have a normal phenotype at birth and develop evidence of virilization during later childhood, adolescence, or early adulthood. In these cases, previously referred to as late-onset or acquired enzyme deficiencies, results of hormonal studies are characteristic of 21-hydroxylase deficiency. An asymptomatic form has also been identified in which individuals have none of the phenotypic features of

Table 28–11. Clinical and laboratory findings in adrenal enzyme defects resulting in CAH.

Enzyme Deficiency[1]	Urinary 17-Ketosteroids	Elevated Plasma Metabolite	Plasma Androgens	Aldosterone	Hypertension/ Salt Loss	External Genitalia
20,22-Desmolase [1]	↓↓↓	—	↓↓↓	↓↓↓	–/+	Males: ambiguous Females: normal
3β-ol dehydrogenase	↑↑ (DHEA)	17-OH pregnenolone (DHEA)	↑ (DHEA)	↓↓↓	–/+	Males: ambiguous Females: virilized (?)
17-Hydroxylase [2]	↓↓↓	Progesterone	↓↓	Normal to ↑	+/–	Males: ambiguous Females: normal
21-Hydroxylase [3][2]	↑↑↑	17-OHP	↑↑	↓↓	–/+	Males: normal Females: virilized
11-Hydroxylase [4]	↑↑	11-Deoxycortisol	↑↑	↓↓ (↑ Deoxycorticosterone)	+/–	Males: normal Females: virilized
17,20-Desmolase [2]	↓↓↓	17-Hydroxysteroids (?)	↓↓	Normal	–/–	Males: ambiguous Females: normal

[1]Bracketed numbers correspond to those in Figure 29–3.
[2]Children with "simple virilizing (non–salt-wasting)" forms of 21-hydroxylase deficiency congenital adrenal hyperplasia (CAH) may have normal aldosterone production and serum electrolytes, but some children have normal aldosterone production and serum electrolytes at the expense of elevated plasma renin activity and are therefore *compensated salt-wasters* by definition. These children are usually treated with mineralocorticoid as well as glucocorticoid. Children with 21-hydroxylase deficiency CAH should therefore have documented normal plasma renin activity in addition to normal serum electrolytes before they are considered non–salt-wasters.

the disorder but have hormonal study results identical with those in patients with nonclassic 21-hydroxylase deficiency. The nonclassic form appears to be less severe than the classic form. Because members of the same family may have classic, nonclassic, and asymptomatic forms, the disorders may be due to allelic variations of the same enzyme.

Female pseudohermaphroditism can be caused by factors other than enzyme deficiencies. In females, these include virilizing maternal conditions or related hormones taken by the mother during the first trimester of pregnancy. In such cases, the condition does not progress after birth, and cortisol deficiency with abnormal steroidogenesis is not present. Male pseudohermaphroditism may be seen in children with 17,20-desmolase deficiency since that enzyme is necessary for normal androgen biosynthesis (Table 28–11). Male pseudohermaphroditism can also be a consequence of androgen receptor abnormalities.

Virilization of the female or male fetus may result from tumors of the adrenal gland, ovary, or testis or from nonclassic congenital adrenal hyperplasia later in life. Symptoms begin after birth and progress until treated.

Clinical Findings

A. Symptoms and Signs:

1. In females–In the female with potentially normal ovaries and uterus, virilization occurs, and sexual development is therefore along heterosexual lines. The abnormality of the external genitalia may vary from mild enlargement of the clitoris to complete fusion of the labioscrotal folds, forming a scrotum, a penile urethra, a penile shaft, and enlargement of the clitoris to form a normal-sized glans (Table 28–8). Signs of adrenal insufficiency (salt loss) may be present during the first days of life (typically in the first or second week). In rare cases, adrenal insufficiency does not occur for months or years. When the enzyme defect is milder, salt loss may not occur, and evidence of virilization predominates (simple virilizing form). In untreated, non-salt-losing 21-hydroxylase or 11-hydroxylase deficiency, growth rate and skeletal maturation are accelerated, and patients may become muscular. Pubic hair appears early (often before the second birthday); acne may be excessive; and the voice may deepen. Excessive pigmentation may develop.

2. In males–In males, sexual development proceeds normally. The male infant usually appears normal at birth but may present with a salt-losing crisis in the first 2–4 weeks of life. However, in milder forms, salt-losing crises may not occur. In this circumstance, enlargement of the penis and increased pigmentation may be noted during the first few months. Other symptoms and signs are similar to those seen in females. The testes are soft and not enlarged except in the rare male in whom aberrant adrenal cells (adrenal rests) are present in the testes

and produce unilateral or bilateral enlargement, often asymmetric. In the rare isolated defect of 17,20-desmolase activity, ambiguous genitalia may be present because of the compromise in androgen production (Figure 28–3).

B. Laboratory Findings:

1. Blood and urine–Hormonal studies are essential for accurate diagnosis. Findings characteristic of the enzyme deficiencies are shown in Table 28–11. With adrenal tumor, secretion of DHEA is greatly elevated, and determining plasma concentrations of DHEA sulfate may be useful in the differential diagnosis.

2. Genetic studies–When available, rapid chromosomal diagnosis should be obtained in any newborn with ambiguous genitalia.

C. Imaging: Adrenal ultrasonography, CT scanning, and MRI may be useful in defining pelvic anatomy or enlarged adrenals or in localizing an adrenal tumor. Vaginograms using contrast material and pelvic ultrasonography may be helpful in delineating the internal anatomy in a newborn with ambiguous genitalia.

Treatment

A. Medical Treatment: Treatment goals in congenital adrenal hyperplasia consist of normalizing growth velocity and skeletal maturation using the smallest dose of glucocorticoids that will suppress adrenal function. The use of excessive amounts of glucocorticoids results in the undesirable side effects of Cushing's syndrome. Mineralocorticoid replacement helps to sustain normal electrolyte homeostasis, though excessive mineralocorticoid dosing results in hypertension. (See Uses of Glucocorticoids & ACTH in Treatment of Nonendocrine Diseases, below, for a more complete discussion of the effects of pharmacologic glucocorticoid therapy.)

1. Glucocorticoids–Initially, hydrocortisone given in a dosage of 30–50 $mg/m^2/d$ parenterally or orally suppresses abnormal adrenal steroidogenesis within 2 weeks. When adrenal suppression has been accomplished, as evidenced by normalization of serum 17-hydroxyprogesterone, the patients are placed on maintenance doses of 15–20 $mg/m^2/d$ in two or three divided doses. Fifty to 60 percent of the daily dose should be given in the late evening to suppress the early morning ACTH rise. Dosage is adjusted to maintain a normal growth rate and a normal rate of skeletal maturation. A variety of serum and urine androgens have been used to monitor adequacy of therapy, including 17-hydroxyprogesterone, androstenedione, and urinary pregnanetriol. However, none of these have been universally accepted. In adolescent females, normal menses are a sensitive index of the adequacy of therapy. Therapy should be continued throughout life in both males and females because of the possibility of malignant degeneration of the hyperplastic adrenal gland. In the pregnant female with congenital adrenal hyperplasia, adequate suppression of adrenal androgen secretion is critical to avoid virilization of the fetus, particularly a female fetus.

2. Mineralocorticoids–Fludrocortisone in a dose of 0.05–0.15 mg is given orally once a day or in two divided doses. Periodic monitoring of blood pressure is recommended to avoid overdosing.

B. Surgical Treatment: Consultation with a urologist experienced with female genital reconstruction is indicated in affected females as soon as possible during infancy.

Course & Prognosis

When therapy is initiated in early infancy, abnormal metabolic effects and progression of masculinization can be avoided. Treatment with glucocorticoids permits normal growth, development, and sexual maturation. However, if not adequately controlled, congenital adrenal hyperplasia results in sexual precocity and masculinization throughout childhood. Affected individuals will be tall as children but short as adults because the rate of skeletal maturation is excessive and leads to premature closure of the epiphyses. If treatment is delayed or inadequate until somatic development is over 12–14 years as determined by skeletal maturation (bone age), true central sexual precocity may occur in males and females.

Patient education stressing lifelong therapy is important to ensure compliance in adolescence and later life.

Virilization and multiple surgical genital reconstructions are associated with a high risk of psychosexual disturbances in female patients. Ongoing psychologic evaluation and support is a critical component of care.

When virilization of the patient (male or female) is caused by a tumor, the progression of signs and symptoms ceases after surgical removal; however, evidence of masculinization, particularly deepening of the voice, may persist.

Jaakskelainen J, Voutilainen R: Growth of patients with 21-hydroxylase deficiency: An analysis of the factors influencing adult height. Pediatr Res 1997;41:30

Mercado AB et al: Prenatal treatment and diagnosis of congenital adrenal hyperplasia owing to steroid 21-hydroxylase deficiency. J Clin Endocrinol Metab 1995;80:2014.

Merke DP, Cutler GB: New approaches to the treatment of congenital adrenal hyperplasia. JAMA 1997;277:1073.

Migeon CJ, Donohoue P: Adrenal disorders. In: *Wilkins: The Diagnosis and Treatment of Endocrine Disorders in Childhood and Adolescence*, 4th ed. Kappy MS, Blizzard RM, Migeon CJ (editors). Thomas, 1994.

Zucker KJ et al: Psychosexual development of women with congenital adrenal hyperplasia. Horm Behav 1996; 30:300.

ADRENOCORTICAL HYPERFUNCTION (Cushing's Disease, Cushing's Syndrome)

Essentials of Diagnosis & Typical Features

- "Truncal type" adiposity with thin extremities, moon facies, muscle wasting, weakness, plethora, easy bruisability, purplish striae, decreased growth rate, delayed skeletal maturation.
- Hypertension, osteoporosis, glycosuria.
- Elevated serum and urine adrenocorticosteroids; low serum potassium; eosinopenia, lymphopenia.

General Considerations

Cushing's syndrome is nonspecific. It may result from excessive secretion of adrenal steroids autonomously (adenoma or carcinoma), from excessive ACTH secretion from the pituitary (Cushing's disease) or from ectopic sources, or from chronic exposure to pharmacologic doses of glucocorticoids.

In children under age 12 years, Cushing's syndrome is usually iatrogenic (secondary to pharmacologic doses of ACTH or one of the glucocorticoids). It may rarely be due to an adrenal tumor, adrenal hyperplasia, an adenoma of the pituitary gland, or, even more rarely, an extrapituitary (ectopic) ACTH-producing tumor.

Clinical Findings

A. Symptoms and Signs:

1. Excess glucocorticoid–"Buffalo type" adiposity, most marked on the face, neck, and trunk (a fat pad in the interscapular area is characteristic); easy fatigability and weakness, plethoric facies, purplish striae, easy bruisability, ecchymoses, hirsutism, osteoporosis, hypertension, diabetes mellitus (usually latent), pain in the back, muscle wasting and weakness, and marked retardation of growth and skeletal maturation.

2. Excess mineralocorticoid–Hypokalemia, mild hypernatremia with water retention, increased blood volume, edema, and hypertension.

3. Excess androgen–Hirsutism, acne, and varying degrees of virilization. Menstrual irregularities occur during puberty in older girls.

B. Laboratory Findings:

1. Blood–

a. Plasma cortisol concentrations are elevated, with loss of the normal diurnal variation in cortisol secretion. Determination of cortisol level between midnight and 2 AM may be a sensitive indicator of loss of variation.

b. Serum chloride and potassium may be lowered. Serum sodium and bicarbonate concentrations may be elevated (metabolic alkalosis).

c. Serum ACTH concentrations are slightly elevated with adrenal hyperplasia (Cushing's disease), decreased in cases of adrenal tumor, and greatly increased with ACTH-producing pituitary or extrapituitary tumors.

d. The leukocyte count shows polymorphonuclear leukocytosis with lymphopenia, and the eosinophil count is low. The erythrocyte count may be elevated.

2. Urine–

a. Urinary free cortisol excretion is elevated. This is currently considered the most useful diagnostic test.

b. Urinary 17-hydroxycorticosteroid excretion (excretion products of the glucocorticoids) is elevated.

c. Urinary 17-ketosteroid excretion is usually elevated in association with adrenal tumors.

d. Glycosuria may be present.

3. Response to dexamethasone suppression testing–There is diminished suppression of adrenal function after a small dose (0.5 mg) of dexamethasone; larger doses of dexamethasone cause suppression of adrenal activity when the disease is due to adrenal hyperplasia. Adenomas and adrenal carcinomas may rarely be suppressed by large doses of dexamethasone (4–16 mg/d in four divided doses).

4. CRH test–The recently introduced CRH stimulation test may replace the high-dose dexamethasone test for differentiating pituitary and ectopic sources of ACTH excess.

C. Imaging: Pituitary imaging may demonstrate a pituitary adenoma. This can be used in conjunction with pituitary venous sampling for localization of ACTH-secreting adenomas. Adrenal imaging (eg, CT scan) may demonstrate adenoma or bilateral hyperplasia. Radionuclide studies of the adrenals may be useful in complex cases. Osteoporosis (evident first in the spine and pelvis) with compression fractures may be seen in advanced cases, and skeletal maturation is usually delayed.

Differential Diagnosis

Children with exogenous obesity, particularly when accompanied by striae and hypertension, are frequently suspected of having Cushing's syndrome. The child's height, growth rate, and skeletal maturation are helpful in differentiating the two, since children with Cushing's syndrome have a poor growth rate, relatively short stature, and delayed skeletal maturation, whereas those with exogenous obesity usually have a normal or slightly increased growth rate, normal to tall stature, and advanced skeletal maturation. In addition, the color of the striae (purplish in Cushing's syndrome, pink in obesity) and the distribution of the obesity assist in the differentiation. The urinary free cortisol excretion (mg/g creatinine) is always normal in obesity.

Treatment

In all cases of primary adrenal hyperfunction due to tumor, surgical removal, if possible, is indicated.

Corticotropin (ACTH) should be given preoperatively and postoperatively to stimulate the nontumorous contralateral adrenal cortex, which is generally atrophied. Glucocorticoids should be administered parenterally in pharmacologic doses during and after surgery until the patient is stable. Supplemental oral glucocorticoids, potassium, salt, and mineralocorticoids may be necessary until the suppressed contralateral adrenal gland has recovered, sometimes over a period of several months. (See above section on corticosteroid administration in surgical patients.)

The use of mitotane, a DDT derivative toxic to the adrenal cortex, and aminoglutethimide, an inhibitor of steroid synthesis, has been suggested, but the efficacy of these agents in children with adrenal tumors has not been determined.

Adrenal hyperplasia resulting from a pituitary microadenoma may respond to pituitary surgery or irradiation.

Prognosis

If the tumor is malignant, the prognosis is poor if it cannot be completely removed. If it is benign, cure is to be expected following proper preparation and surgery.

Leinung MC et al: Long term follow-up of transsphenoidal surgery for the treatment of Cushing's disease in children. J Clin Endocrinol Metab 1995;80:2475.

Migeon CJ, Donohoue P: Adrenal disorders. In: *Wilkins: The Diagnosis and Treatments of Endocrine Disorders in Childhood and Adolescence,* 4th ed. Kappy MS, Blizzard RM, Migeon CJ (editors). Thomas, 1994.

Tsigos C, Chrousos GP: Differential diagnosis and management of Cushing's syndrome. Ann Rev Med 1996; 47:443.

PRIMARY HYPERALDOSTERONISM

Primary hyperaldosteronism may be caused by a benign adrenal tumor or by adrenal hyperplasia. It is characterized by paresthesias, tetany, weakness, polyuria (nocturnal enuresis is common in young children), periodic paralysis, low serum potassium, elevated serum sodium, hypertension, metabolic alkalosis, and production of a large volume of alkaline urine with a low fixed specific gravity; the latter does not respond to vasopressin. Edema is rare. The glucose tolerance test is frequently abnormal. Plasma and urinary aldosterone are elevated, but other steroid levels are variable. Plasma renin activity is suppressed, in contrast to the secondary hyperaldosteronism due to renal vascular disease and Bartter's syndrome). In patients with adrenal tumor, the administration of ACTH may further increase the excretion of aldosterone. Marked decrease of aldosterone-induced hypokalemia, alkalosis, hypochloremia, or hypernatremia after the administration of an aldosterone antagonist such as spironolactone, may be of diagnostic value.

Treatment is with glucocorticoids or spironolactone, subtotal or total adrenalectomy for hyperplasia, and surgical removal if a tumor is present.

White PC: Disorders of aldosterone biosynthesis and action. N Engl J Med 1994;331:250.

USES OF GLUCOCORTICOIDS & ACTH IN TREATMENT OF NONENDOCRINE DISEASES

Glucocorticoids are used for their anti-inflammatory and immunosuppressive properties in a variety of conditions in childhood. Pharmacologic doses are necessary to achieve these effects, and side effects are common. Numerous synthetic preparations possessing variable ratios of glucocorticoid to mineralocorticoid activity are available (Table 28–12).

Actions
Glucocorticoids exert a direct or permissive effect on virtually every tissue of the body; major known effects include the following:

(1) Gluconeogenesis in the liver.

(2) Stimulation of fat breakdown (lipolysis) and redistribution of body fat.

(3) Catabolism of protein with an increase in nitrogen and phosphorus excretion.

(4) Decrease in lymphoid and thymic tissue and a decreased cellular response to inflammation and hypersensitivity.

(5) Alteration of central nervous system excitation.

(6) Retardation of connective tissue mitosis and migration, decreased wound healing.

(7) Improved capillary tone and increased vascular compartment volume and pressure.

Uses
Glucocorticoids are used in physiologic doses to treat adrenal insufficiency (eg, Addison's disease and congenital adrenal hyperplasia) but in pharmacologic doses to treat a wide variety of inflammatory and autoimmune malignant conditions in childhood. Corticosteroid use is contraindicated in active, questionably healed, or suspected tuberculosis. Corticosteroids should be used with extreme caution in the presence of herpes simplex infection of the eye, osteoporosis, peptic ulcer, active systemic infections, emotional instability, and thrombophlebitis.

Side Effects of Therapy
When prolonged use of pharmacologic doses of glucocorticoids are necessary, clinical manifestations of Cushing's syndrome are common. Side effects may result either from the use of synthetic exogenous agents by any route, including inhalation and topical administration (inflamed skin), or from the use of ACTH, which stimulates excessive production of endogenous corticosteroids. Use of a larger dose of glucocorticoids given once every 48 hours (alternate-day therapy) lessens the incidence and severity of some of their side effects.

A. Endocrine and Metabolic Effects:

1. Hyperglycemia and glycosuria (chemical diabetes).

2. Cushing's syndrome.

3. Persistent suppression of pituitary-adrenal responsiveness to stress with resultant hypoadrenocorticism.

B. Effects on Electrolytes and Minerals:

Table 28–12. Potency equivalents for adrenocorticosteroids.

Adrenocorticosteroid	Trade Names	Potency/mg Compared With Cortisol (Glucocorticoid Effect)	Potency/mg Compared With Cortisol (Sodium-Retaining Effect)
Glucocorticoids Hydrocortisone (cortisol)	Cortef	1	1
Cortisone	Cortone Acetate	0.8	1
Prednisone	Meticorten, others	4–5	0.4
Methylprednisolone	Medrol, Meprolone	5–6	Minimal
Triamcinolone	Aristocort, Kenalog Kenacort, Atolone	5–6	Minimal
Dexamethasone	Decadron, others	25–40	Minimal
Betamethasone	Celestone	25	Minimal
Mineralocorticoid Fludrocortisone	Florinef	15–20	300–400

1. Marked retention of sodium and water, producing edema, increased blood volume, and hypertension (more common in endogenous hyperadrenal states).

2. Potassium loss with symptoms of hypokalemia.

3. Hypocalcemia, tetany.

C. Effects on Protein Metabolism and Skeletal Maturation:

1. Negative nitrogen balance, with loss of body protein and bone protein, resulting in osteoporosis, pathologic fractures, and aseptic bone necrosis.

2. Suppression of growth, retarded skeletal maturation.

3. Muscular weakness and wasting.

D. Effects on the Gastrointestinal Tract:

1. Excessive appetite and intake of food.

2. Activation or production of peptic ulcer.

3. Gastrointestinal bleeding from ulceration or from unknown cause (particularly in children with hepatic disease).

4. Fatty liver with embolism, pancreatitis, nodular panniculitis.

E. Lowering of Resistance to Infectious Agents; Silent Infection; Decreased Inflammatory Reaction:

1. Susceptibility to fungal infections; intestinal parasitic infections.

2. Activation of tuberculosis; false-negative tuberculin reaction.

3. Stimulation of activity of herpes simplex virus.

F. Neuropsychiatric Effects:

1. Euphoria, excitability, psychotic behavior, and status epilepticus with electroencephalographic changes.

2. Increased intracranial pressure with pseudotumor cerebri syndrome.

G. Hematologic and Vascular Effects:

1. Bleeding into the skin as a result of increased capillary fragility.

2. Thrombosis, thrombophlebitis, cerebral hemorrhage.

H. Miscellaneous Effects:

1. Myocarditis, pleuritis, and arteritis following abrupt cessation of therapy.

2. Cardiomegaly.

3. Nephrosclerosis, proteinuria.

4. Acne (in older children), hirsutism, amenorrhea, irregular menses.

5. Posterior subcapsular cataracts; glaucoma.

Tapering of Pharmacologic Doses of Steroids

Prolonged use of pharmacologic doses of glucocorticoids results in suppression of ACTH secretion and consequent adrenal atrophy. Thus, the abrupt discontinuation of glucocorticoids may result in adrenal insufficiency. Furthermore, ACTH secretion gener-

ally does not occur until the administered steroid has been given in subphysiologic doses (< 8 mg/m^2/d orally) for several weeks.

If pharmacologic glucocorticoid therapy has been given for less than 2–3 weeks, the drug can be discontinued abruptly (if the condition for which it was prescribed allows) because adrenal suppression will be short-lived. However, it is advisable to educate the patient and family about the signs and symptoms of adrenal insufficiency in case problems arise.

If tapering is necessary for treatment of the underlying disease for which the glucocorticoid is being prescribed, a reduction of 25–50% every 2–7 days is sufficiently rapid to permit observation of clinical symptomatology. Moreover, the use of an alternate-day schedule (ie, a single dose given every 48 hours) will allow for a 50% decrease in the total 2 days' dosage while providing the desired pharmacologic effect. If tapering is not necessary for the underlying disease, the dosage can be safely decreased to the physiologic range. However, while a rapid decrease in dose to the physiologic range will not lead to frank adrenal insufficiency (since adequate exogenous cortisol is being provided), some patients may experience "steroid withdrawal syndrome" characterized by malaise, fatigue, and loss of appetite. The occurrence of these symptoms may necessitate a two- or three-step decrease in dose to the physiologic range.

Once a physiologic equivalent dose (8–10 mg/m^2/d hydrocortisone or equivalent) is achieved and the patient's underlying disease is stable, the dosage can be decreased to 4–5 mg/m^2/d given only in the morning. This will allow the adrenal axis to recover. After this dosage has been given for 4–6 weeks, assessment of endogenous adrenal activity can be estimated by obtaining fasting plasma cortisol concentrations between 7 and 8 AM prior to the morning steroid dose. When an alternate-day schedule is followed, plasma cortisol is measured the morning prior to treatment. A plasma cortisol concentration within the physiologic range (> 10 mg/dL) demonstrates return of basal physiologic adrenal rhythm. Exogenous steroids may then be safely discontinued, though it is advisable to continue to treat the patient with stress doses of glucocorticoids when appropriate until recovery of the response to stress has been documented.

After basal physiologic adrenal function returns, the adrenal reserve or capacity to respond to stress and infection can be estimated by the ACTH stimulation test, in which 0.25 mg/m^2 of synthetic ACTH (cosyntropin) is administered intravenously. Plasma cortisol is measured prior to (zero time) and at 45–60 minutes after the infusion. A plasma cortisol concentration of greater than 18 mg/dL at 60 minutes indicates a satisfactory adrenal reserve.

Even if the results of testing are normal, patients who have received prolonged treatment with glucocorticoids may exhibit signs and symptoms of adrenal insufficiency during acute stress, infection, or surgery for months to years after they have been withdrawn. Careful monitoring and, when necessary, the use of stress doses of glucocorticoids should be considered during severe illnesses and surgery.

Allen DB: Growth suppression by glucocorticoid therapy. Pediatr Rounds 1995;4:1.

Loke KY et al: Efficacy and safety of one year of growth hormone therapy in steroid-dependent nephrotic syndrome. J Pediatr 1997;130:793.

Rivkees SA, Danon M, Herrin J: Prednisone dose limitation of growth hormone treatment of steroid-induced growth failure. J Pediatr 1994;125:322.

Sarna S et al: Methylprednisolone exposure, rather than dose, predicts adrenal suppression and growth inhibition in children with liver and renal transplants. J Clin Endocrinol Metab 1997;82:75.

ADRENAL MEDULLA

PHEOCHROMOCYTOMA

Pheochromocytoma is an uncommon tumor in childhood. Only 10% of the total number of reported cases occur in pediatric patients. The tumor may be located wherever there is any chromaffin tissue (eg, adrenal medulla, sympathetic ganglia, carotid body). It may be multiple, familial (autosomal dominant, in which case a high prevalence of MEN exists), recurrent, and sometimes malignant.

Although the clinical manifestations of pheochromocytoma may result from physical expansion of lesions into surrounding tissue (eg, spinal cord), they are generally due to excessive secretion of epinephrine or norepinephrine. Attacks of anxiety, unexplained perspiration, and headaches should arouse suspicion. Other findings are palpitation and tachycardia, dizziness, weakness, nausea and vomiting, diarrhea, dilated pupils with blurring of vision, abdominal and precordial pain, hypertension (usually persistent), heat intolerance, and vasomotor instability (flushing, postural hypotension). The symptoms may be sustained, producing all of the above findings plus papilledema, retinopathy, and enlargement of the heart. There is an increased incidence of pheochromocytomas in patients and families with neurofibromatosis, and MEN type 2 (see above). Neuroblastomas, neurogangliomas, and other neural tumors may cause increased secretion of pressor amines and may occasionally simulate the findings of pheochromocytoma. Carcinoid tumors may produce cardiovascular changes similar to those associated with pheochromocytoma.

Laboratory diagnosis is possible in over 90% of cases. Serum catecholamines are elevated, particularly while the patient is symptomatic, and urinary excretion of catecholamines parallels this elevation. Catecholamine levels are characteristically high enough to be diagnostic but may be limited to the period of a paroxysm. The 24-hour urine excretion of metanephrines and vanilmandelic acid is increased. Provocative tests employing histamine, tyramine, or glucagon and the phentolamine tests may be abnormal but are dangerous, and these agents are rarely necessary for diagnosis. Displacement of the kidney may be shown by intravenous urography, and the tumor may be identified by CT scans or MRI. Angiocatheterization with localized measurement of circulating concentrations of catecholamines may be helpful in localizing the tumor prior to surgery.

Surgical removal of the tumor is the treatment of choice; however, the procedure must be undertaken with great caution and with the patient properly stabilized because manipulation of the tumor may cause sudden and profound, potentially fatal changes in blood pressure. Oral phenoxybenzamine or intravenous phentolamine is used preoperatively. Profound hypotension may occur as the tumor is removed but may be controlled with an infusion of norepinephrine, which may have to be continued for 1–2 days.

Unless irreversible secondary vascular changes have occurred, complete relief of symptoms is to be expected after recovery from removal of a benign tumor. Without treatment, severe cardiac, renal, and cerebral damage may result.

Eng C: The *RET* protooncogene in multiple endocrine neoplasia type 2 and Hirschsprung's disease. N Engl J Med 1996;335:943.

Migeon CJ, Donohoue P: *Wilkins: The Diagnosis and Treatments of Endocrine Disorders in Childhood and Adolescence,* 4th ed. Kappy MS, Blizzard RM, Migeon CJ (editors). Thomas, 1994.

Werbel SS, Ober KP: Pheochromocytoma: Update on diagnosis, localization, and management. Med Clin North Am 1995;79:131.

Diabetes Mellitus

29

H. Peter Chase, MD, & George S. Eisenbarth, MD, PhD

Essentials of Diagnosis & Typical Features

- Polyuria, polydipsia, and weight loss.
- Hyperglycemia and glucosuria with or without ketonuria.

General Considerations

Type 1a diabetes mellitus (previously called juvenile diabetes or insulin-dependent diabetes) is the most common type of diabetes in people under age 40 years. It is associated with immunologic markers, diminished insulin production, and being ketosis-prone. About 85% of affected persons still make some insulin a year after diagnosis, and 42% still make small amounts 3 years after diagnosis. Type 2 (non-insulin-dependent) diabetes is the most common type in persons over age 40; it is associated with being overweight, not being prone to ketosis, and insensitivity to insulin. Type 2 and type 1b (non-immune-mediated insulin-deficient diabetes) are found in up to half of black and Hispanic children who develop diabetes. Cases occur most frequently in overweight teenagers. Maturity-onset diabetes of youth (MODY) comprises several forms of diabetes in children with identified genetic mutations (eg, mutations of glucokinase and hepatic nuclear factor 1 and 2 genes). Initially for children with non-type 1a diabetes, insulin therapy is often required, particularly if ketonuria or a very high glycohemoglobin level (HbA$_{1c}$; see below) is present. Later, diet, exercise, and oral hypoglycemic agents are the main therapeutic resources for patients with MODY—as for adults with type 2 diabetes. The remainder of this discussion deals with type 1a diabetes.

Etiology

Type 1a diabetes results from immunologic damage to the insulin-producing B cells of the pancreatic islets. This damage occurs gradually—over months or years in most people—and symptoms do not appear until about 90% of the pancreatic islets have been destroyed. The immunologic damage requires a genetic predisposition and is probably affected by environmental factors.

The importance of genetics is shown by the fact that 35–70% of second identical twins develop diabetes after the first twin develops the disease. About 6% of siblings or offspring of persons with type 1 diabetes also develop diabetes (compared with the incidence in the general population of 2–3:1000). The condition is more common in white children but occurs in all racial groups. There is an association with HLA-DR3 and -DR4, and about 95% of white diabetic children have at least one of these HLA types. Forty percent have both HLA-DR3 and -DR4 (one from each parent), compared with only 3% of the general population with this combination. The presence of aspartic acid on position 57 of the -DQ beta chain of the HLA complex is associated with protection from type 1 diabetes; conversely, its absence provides a marker for susceptibility, but there are important exceptions to this rule.

The importance of environmental factors is suggested because fewer than 50% of second identical twins develop diabetes—if the condition were purely genetic and had no random factors, the second twin would always develop the disease. Important environmental factors may be viral infections or chemicals in the diet. For example, 40% of infants with congenital rubella develop diabetes or an abnormal glucose tolerance test by age 20 years, and the incidence of diabetes was high after eating foods accidentally preserved with excessive nitrates. The early introduction of cow's milk has also been suggested as a possible environmental factor, but recent prospective studies have failed to confirm this association.

The immunologic basis of diabetes is demonstrated by the ability of cyclosporine, a potent immunosuppressive agent, to preserve islet tissue for 1–2 years when given to newly diagnosed patients. However, renal damage from cyclosporine precludes its long-term use. White blood cells are found in the islets of newly diagnosed patients and may release toxic products (free radicals, interleukin-1, tumor necrosis factor) that injure the islets. Antibodies to islet cells (ICA), insulin, "64 K" or glutamic acid decarboxylase, ICA512, and other antibodies may be present in the serum of over 90% of patients who will develop type 1a diabetes for months to years prior to diagnosis. These antibodies are probably the effect and not the cause of islet B cell destruction.

Many centers now screen for prediabetes using an ICA test or other antibody test, and—especially for children—the biochemical tests are replacing the ICA tests. An intravenous glucose tolerance test helps to define those at highest risk so that they may be enrolled in prevention trials.

Intervention trials on antibody-positive first-degree relatives based on data from pilot trials have been started. European investigators are conducting a double-blind study of nicotinamide, whereas United States centers are conducting a randomized study of intravenous and subcutaneous insulin compared with no therapy (see Keller, 1993) and of oral insulin versus placebo.

Diagnosis

The classic symptoms of polyuria, polydipsia, and weight loss are now so well recognized that friends or family members often suspect the diagnosis of type 1 diabetes. Other cases may be detected by finding glucosuria on routine office urinalysis. Up to 50% of new cases of diabetes used to present in coma, but most are now diagnosed before developing severe ketonuria, ketonemia, and secondary acidosis. An oral glucose tolerance test is rarely necessary in children. A random blood glucose level above 300 mg/dL (16.6 mmol/L) or a fasting blood glucose above 200 mg/dL (11 mmol/L) is all that is needed to make the diagnosis of type 1 diabetes. The 1997 revised guidelines for the diagnosis of diabetes are a fasting plasma glucose level over 126 mg/dL (7 mmol/L) or a plasma glucose level above 200 mg/dL (11.1 mmol/L) taken randomly or 2 hours after an oral glucose load (1.75 g glucose/kg up to a maximum of 50 g). "Impaired" 2-hour glucose values are from 140 mg/dL (7.8 mmol/L) to 200 mg/dL (11.1 mmol/L). If the presentation is mild, hospitalization is usually not necessary.

Education about diabetes for all family members is essential for proper handling of the problems of diabetes care in the home. All caregivers need to learn about diabetes and how to give insulin injections and perform home blood glucose monitoring. The stress imposed on the family around the time of initial diagnosis may lead to feelings of shock, denial, sadness, anger, fear, and guilt. Meeting with a counselor to express these feelings at the time of diagnosis helps with long-term adaptation.

Treatment

The five major variables in the treatment of type 1 diabetes are (1) insulin dosage, (2) diet, (3) exercise, (4) stress management, and (5) blood glucose and urine ketone monitoring. All must be taken into account to obtain safe and effective metabolic control.

Although teenagers can be taught to perform many of the tasks of diabetes management, they do better when supportive—not overbearing—parents continue to be involved in management of the disease. Children younger than 10 or 11 years of age cannot reliably administer insulin without adult supervision because they lack fine motor control and may not understand the importance of accurate dosage.

A. Insulin: Insulin functions (1) to allow glucose to pass into the cell; (2) to decrease the physiologic production of glucose, particularly in the liver and muscles; and (3) to turn off ketone production.

1. Treatment of new-onset diabetes–If ketonuria is large, the venous blood pH low (< 7.30), and the patient dehydrated, intravenous insulin and fluid therapy should be given as described below in the section on ketoacidosis. If moderate or large ketonuria is present at first diagnosis and the child is adequately hydrated and has a normal venous blood pH, one or two intramuscular or subcutaneous injections of 0.1–0.2 unit of regular insulin or insulin lispro (Humalog) (short-acting) insulin per kilogram of body weight about 1 hour apart will help shut down ketone production. If ketonuria is small or absent, this regimen is not necessary, and subcutaneous injections can be started.

When ketonuria is not present, the child is usually more sensitive to insulin, and a total daily dose of 0.25–0.5 unit/kg/24 h (by subcutaneous injection) can be used. If ketonuria is or was present, the child usually does not produce as much insulin and will require 0.5–1 unit/kg of total insulin per 24 hours.

These doses are adjusted with each injection during the first week. Most physicians begin newly diagnosed children with synthetic human insulin and insulin lispro (Humalog). About two-thirds of the total dose is usually given before breakfast and the remainder before dinner. If human regular insulin is used, the injections are given 30–60 minutes before meals; when Humalog is the short-acting insulin, they are given just before eating. In young children who eat irregular amounts of food, it is often helpful to wait until after the meal to decide on the dose of Humalog and to give the injection. Children under age 4 years usually need 1 or 2 units of regular insulin to cover meals, and the remainder of the dosage is neutral protamine Hagedorn (NPH) insulin. Children 4–10 years of age may require up to 4 units of regular insulin to cover breakfast and dinner (Table 29–1), whereas proportionately higher doses (usually 4–10 units) of regular or Humalog insulin are used for older children.

The new more rapid-acting form of regular insulin called insulin lispro (Humalog) is now available. Humalog's onset of activity is 10–15 minutes rather than 30–60 minutes, as with regular insulin (see Table 29–2). It is thus not necessary to wait 30–60 minutes to eat after injection of Humalog. Humalog also peaks sooner than regular insulin and is gone

Table 29–1. Example of a "thinking" scale to adjust regular insulin or Humalog (insulin lispro) dose for a child 4–10 years of age[1]

Active			Not Active		
Blood Sugar (mg/dL)	Blood Sugar (mmol/L)	Insulin Units	Blood Sugar (mg/dL)	Blood Sugar (mmol/L)	Insulin Units
< 100	< 5.5	0	< 70	< 3.9	0
100–200	5.5–11.1	1	70–150	3.9–8.3	1
201–300	11.2–16.6	2	151–200	8.4–11.1	2
> 300	> 16.6	3	201–250	11.2–13.9	3
			> 250	> 13.9	4

[1]The family must think about each dosage. If the child does not eat well, it may be wise to use Humalog and to give the shot after the meal—reducing the dose with lower food intake.

within 4 hours. The shorter duration reduces the risk of later hypoglycemia. It is likely that most patients will benefit from the use of Humalog at some time during the day. Many children continue to receive regular insulin in the morning (to last long enough to help cover lunch) and Humalog insulin prior to dinner (with activity mostly dissipated by bedtime). Low glucose levels during the night are less frequent when Humalog rather than regular insulin is used with the dinnertime injection.

2. Continuing insulin dosage–The total daily insulin dosage may need to be increased gradually to 1 unit/kg (especially if ketonuria is present at onset). When gluconeogenesis and glycolysis are suppressed by insulin, a "honeymoon" or "grace" period is a common phenomenon. This may occur 1–8 weeks after diagnosis in over 50% of children. Continuing

Table 29–2. Times of insulin action.

Type of Insulin	Begins Working	Main Effect	All Gone
Short-acting			
Regular	½ hour	2–4 hours	4–8 hours
Humalog	10–15 minutes	30–60 minutes	4 hours
Semilente	1–2 hours	2–5 hours	8–12 hours
Longer-acting			
NPH	2–4 hours	6–8 hours	12–15 hours
Ultralente	4–6 hours	8–15 hours	15–18 hours
Premixed			
Lente (3 parts semilente and 7 parts Ultralente)	1–2 hour	6–12 hour	15–18 hours
NPH/ Regular	½ hour	Variable[1]	12–15 hours

[1]Available in various combinations to fit individual needs.

small doses of insulin at levels that do not cause frequent episodes of hypoglycemia may be important at this time to help preserve later B cell function.

In helping families with day-to-day dosing of regular or Humalog insulin, some physicians use sliding scales, more recently referred to as "thinking scales," to emphasize that the family must always be thinking about food recently eaten or to be eaten and recent or forthcoming exercise—in addition to the blood glucose level. Table 29–1 is an example of a thinking scale for a child 4–10 years old.

After the initial correct dosage of NPH (long-acting) insulin is achieved, daily adjustments usually are not needed. However, small decreases may be made for heavy activity (eg, afternoon sports or overnight events). Many families gradually learn to make small (0.5–1 unit) weekly adjustments in insulin dosage based on home blood glucose testing. Understanding the onset, peak and duration of insulin activity is essential (Table 29–2).

Most children receive at least two injections of insulin daily. The most common combinations are mixtures of regular or Humalog and NPH insulins twice daily (Table 29–2) or regular and NPH insulin in the morning and Humalog or regular and ultralente insulin at dinner. Ultralente insulin is sometimes preferred at dinner because it does not peak as much as NPH insulin during the night and because it is also more apt to last through the night. Ultralente insulin delays the action of regular insulin slightly but not the action of Humalog.

When children and families are willing to deal with three insulin injections per day, the evening dose is often split, with Humalog or regular insulin given before dinner and NPH insulin at bedtime (to help maintain coverage through the night). Some physicians use injections of Humalog and ultralente insulin before breakfast and dinner and an injection of Humalog insulin before lunch. Continuous subcutaneous insulin injection therapy by insulin pump is sometimes used in emotionally mature, older teens who are willing to invest more time in blood glucose monitoring and dietary therapy. This is particularly true when glucose control (monitored by HbA_{1c} levels; see following text) remains suboptimal despite three or more injections per day.

The following constitutes **"intensive diabetes management":** (1) three or more insulin injections per day, or insulin pump therapy; (2) four or more blood sugar determinations per day; (3) careful attention to dietary intake; and (4) frequent contact with the health care provider. This was shown in the Diabetes Control and Complications Trial (DCCT; see below) to result in improved glucose control and to reduce the risk for retinal, renal, and neurologic complications of diabetes. All teenagers with suboptimal glucose control who are willing to comply should be considered for intensive diabetes management.

B. Diet: The mainstays of dietary treatment are listed in the accompanying box. They are discussed in detail in *Understanding Insulin Dependent Diabetes,* the entire text of which is also to be found at http://www.uchsc.edu./misc/diabetes/bdc.html. Of these recommendations, No. 2 (consistency) and No. 5 (careful management of carbohydrate intake) are essential to any regimen of dietary treatment.

Mainstays of Dietary Treatment

1. Eat a well-balanced diet.
2. Keep the day-to-day intake consistent.
3. Eat meals and snacks at the same time each day.
4. Use snacks to prevent insulin reactions (encourage solid protein at bedtime every night).
5. Manage carbohydrate intake carefully.
6. Avoid overtreating low blood sugar.
7. Reduce cholesterol, total fat, and saturated fat intake.
8. Maintain appropriate weight for height; avoid becoming overweight.
9. Increase fiber intake.
10. Avoid foods high in salt.
11. Avoid excessive protein intake.

The American Diabetes Association (ADA) no longer recommends any one "diabetic diet" or "ADA diet." Instead, nutrition therapy for diabetics should be individualized, with consideration given to the patient's customary cultural eating habits and other lifestyle matters. Some families and children (particularly those with weight problems) find exchange diets helpful initially while they are learning categories of foods. An exchange diet is a food plan in which foods are grouped into one of six food lists having similar nutritional compositions. Caloric intake and numbers of exchanges are established, but foods within a group can be exchanged with one another. Working with a dietitian familiar with the problems of diabetes care is important in diabetes management.

The DCCT found that four nutrition factors contributed to better sugar control (lower hemoglobin A_{1c} levels). These factors are (1) adherence to a meal plan, (2) avoidance of extra snacks, (3) avoidance of overtreatment of low blood sugars (hypoglycemia), and (4) prompt treatment of high blood sugars. Two other nutritional factors include adjusting insulin levels for meals and maintaining a consistent schedule of nighttime snacks. The DCCT did popularize a "carbohydrate-counting" dietary plan in which the dosage of regular insulin is altered with each injection to adjust for the amount of carbohydrate to be eaten and the amount of exercise contemplated.

C. Exercise: Regular aerobic exercise—at least 25 minutes a day—is important for children with diabetes. Exercise fosters a sense of well-being, helps increase insulin sensitivity, and helps maintain proper weight, blood pressure, and blood fat levels. Exercise may also help maintain normal peripheral circulation in later years.

Hypoglycemia during exercise or in the 2–8 hours after exercise (delayed hypoglycemia) should be prevented by careful monitoring of blood sugar before, during, and after exercise; sometimes by reducing the dosage of the insulin having activity at the time of the exercise; and by providing extra snacks. In general, the longer and more vigorous the activity, the more food should be eaten before exercising. One "carbohydrate count" is 15 g of glucose in the United States (10 g in Canada and the United Kingdom); 15 g of glucose usually covers about 30 minutes of exercise. The use of drinks containing 5–10% dextrose, such as Gatorade, during the period of exercise is often beneficial.

D. Stress Management: Management of stress is important on a short-term basis because stress hormones increase blood glucose levels. Chronic emotional upsets may lead to missed injections or other compliance problems. When this happens, counseling for the family and child becomes an important part of diabetes management.

E. Blood Glucose Measurements: All families must be able to monitor blood glucose levels three or four times daily—and more frequently in small infants or patients who have glucose control problems or intercurrent illnesses. Blood glucose levels can be monitored using visual strips or by meters with an accuracy of 10% or better. Levels to aim for when no food has been eaten for 2 or more hours vary according to age (Table 29–3).

Blood glucose results must be recorded even if the meter has a memory feature. This allows the family to look for patterns and make changes in insulin dosage. If more than 50% of the values are above the desired range for age or more than 12% below the desired range, the insulin dosage usually needs to be adjusted. Some families are able to make these changes independently (particularly after the first year), whereas others need help from the physician.

Table 29–3. Ideal glucose levels after 2 or more hours of fasting.

Age	Glucose Level
≤ 4 years	100–200 mg/dL (5.5–11 mmol/L)
5–12 years	80–180 mg/dL (4.6–10 mmol/L)
≥ years	70–150 mg/dL (3.9–8.3 mmol/L)

[1]At least half of the values must be "within range" to have a good HbA_{1c} value.

The recommendation of the ADA in the 1994 Standards of Care is that children with diabetes have clinic visits every 3 months. This provides an opportunity to adjust insulin dosages according to changes in growth and blood glucose levels as well as to check for changes noted on physical examination (eg, eyes, thyroid).

Laboratory Evaluations

In addition to home measurements of blood glucose and urine ketone levels, glycosylated hemoglobin should be measured every 3 months. This test reflects the frequency of elevated blood glucose levels over the previous 3 months. Normal values vary among laboratories but are usually below 6.2% (HbA_{1c}) or below 8% (total glycosylated hemoglobin). The desired ranges vary according to age. For the HbA_{1c} method, these ranges are as follows: 12 years or older, less than 7.8%; 5–11 years, less than 8.5%; and under 5 years, 7.5–9%. Higher levels are allowed in younger children to reduce the risk of hypoglycemia because their brains are still developing and they may not relate symptoms of hypoglycemia to a need for treatment. Low HbA_{1c} values are generally associated with a greater risk for low blood sugars (see Hypoglycemia, below). Using either method, longitudinal averages more than 33% above the upper limit of normal are associated with a higher risk for later renal and retinal complications. In the intensive treatment group of the DCCT, the lower HbA_{1c} values resulted in greater than 50% reductions in the retinal, renal, and neurologic complications of diabetes.

It is also important to measure serum cholesterol levels once yearly, though elevations may be secondary to poor glucose control. Thus, if both the cholesterol and the hemoglobin A_{1c} levels are elevated, it is important to determine if the cholesterol level declines as the HbA_{1c} value declines.

When puberty is reached and the individual has had diabetes for 5 years or longer, the 24-hour urinary excretion of albumin should be measured (as "microalbumin") in two separate urines once yearly (see Chronic Complications, below). This can be done using timed overnight urine collections, since teens hate collecting 24-hour specimens. Normal val-

ues vary with the methodology of the laboratory but are generally below 20 μg/min.

If the thyroid is enlarged (about 20% of patients with type 1 diabetes), the thyroid-stimulating hormone level should be measured once or twice yearly. This is the first test to become abnormal in the autoimmune thyroiditis that is commonly associated with type 1 diabetes.

In recent years the antiendomysial antibody, which has been shown to be a reliable predictor of celiac disease, has been shown to be more common in children with diabetes as well as in their siblings. It is carried on HLA-DR3 and is more frequent in children with diabetes (occurring in about 5%). The antibody should be checked in diabetic children with poor growth (especially when not related to poor glucose control) or those who present with gastrointestinal symptoms. 21-Hydroxylase autoantibody, a marker of increased risk of Addison's disease, is present in approximately 1:60 patients with type 1a diabetes.

A checklist of the physician's contributions to good diabetes care is presented in Table 29–4.

Acute Complications

A. Hypoglycemia: Hypoglycemia (or insulin reaction) is defined as a blood glucose level below 60 mg/dL (or 3.3 mmol/L). For preschool children, values below 70 mg/dL (3.9 mmol/L) should be cause for concern. The common symptoms of hypoglycemia are hunger, weakness, shakiness, sweating, drowsiness (at an unusual time), headache, and behavioral changes. Children learn to recognize hypoglycemia at different ages but can often report "feeling funny" as young as 4–5 years of age. If low blood sugar is not treated immediately with simple

Table 29–4. Physician's checklist of good diabetes management.

Variable	Frequency of Measurement	Tests and Values
Blood sugars	3–4 times daily	See age-appropriate values.
Hemoglobin A_{1c}	Every 3 months	See age-appropriate values.
Urine microalbumin	Annually after 5 years of diabetes (pubertal patients)	< 20 μg/min
Ophthalmology referral	Annually after 5 years of diabetes (pubertal patients)	Retinal photographs
Signs of other endocrinopathy	Evaluate annually (eg, thyroid enlargement)	(eg, TSH: 0.5–5.0 mU/L)

TSH = thyroid-stimulating hormone.

sugar, the hypoglycemia may result in loss of consciousness or convulsions. If hypoglycemia is left untreated for several hours, brain damage or death can occur.

Consistency in daily routine, correct insulin dosage, regular blood glucose monitoring, controlled snacking, compliance of patients and parents, and good education—all are important in preventing severe hypoglycemia.

The treatment of mild hypoglycemia involves giving 4 oz of juice, a sugar-containing soda drink, or milk and waiting 10 minutes. If the blood glucose level is still below 60 mg/dL (3.3 mmol/L), the liquids are repeated. If the glucose level is above 60 mg/mL, solid foods are given. Moderate hypoglycemia, in which the person is conscious but incoherent, is treated by squeezing one-half tube of concentrated glucose (eg, Insta-Glucose) or cake frosting between the gums and lips and stroking the throat to encourage swallowing.

In the DCCT study, 10% of patients with standard management and 25% of those with intensive insulin management—insulin pumps or three or more insulin shots per day—had one or more severe hypoglycemic reactions each year. Families are advised to have glucagon in the home and to treat hypoglycemia by giving subcutaneous or intramuscular injections of 0.3 mL (0.3 mg) for children under 5 years of age and 0.5 mL (0.5 mg) to those over 5 years. Some patients (usually those who have had diabetes for more than 10 years) fail to recognize the symptoms of low blood sugar ("hypoglycemic unawareness"). For these individuals, glucose control must be liberalized to prevent severe hypoglycemic reactions. School personnel, sports coaches, and baby-sitters must be trained to recognize and treat hypoglycemia.

B. Ketonuria and Ketoacidosis: Families must be educated to check urine ketones during any illness (including vomiting even once) or any time a blood glucose level is above 240 mg/dL (13.3 mmol/L). If moderate or large ketonuria is detected, the physician must be called and 10–20% of the total daily insulin dose given subcutaneously as Humalog or regular insulin every 2–3 hours until the urine ketones are small or negative. This prevents ketonuria from progressing to ketoacidosis and allows most patients to be treated at home by telephone management. Juices and other fluids are encouraged, and suppositories of promethazine to prevent vomiting may be indicated. If deep breathing (Kussmaul respirations) or excessive weakness occurs, the patient should be evaluated promptly by a physician.

Acidosis (venous blood pH < 7.30) is now present in fewer than 25% of newly diagnosed children. Acidosis may also occur in those with known diabetes who do not check for ketonuria and call the physician when moderate or large urine ketones are present. Repeated episodes of ketoacidosis usually result from missed insulin injections and signify that a re-

sponsible adult must take over the diabetes management. If for any reason this is not possible, a change in the child's living situation may be necessary.

Treatment of diabetic ketoacidosis (DKA) is based on four physiologic principles: (1) restoration of fluid volume, (2) inhibition of lipolysis and return to glucose utilization, (3) replacement of body salts, and (4) correction of acidosis. Laboratory tests at the start of treatment should include venous blood pH, blood glucose, and an electrolyte panel. Mild DKA is defined as a venous blood pH of 7.2–7.3; moderate DKA, a pH of 7.10–7.19; and severe DKA, a pH below 7.10. Patients with severe DKA should be hospitalized and not treated in a clinic or emergency room. More severe cases may benefit from determination of osmolality, calcium and phosphorus, and BUN levels. Severe and moderate episodes of DKA generally require hourly determinations of serum glucose, electrolyte, and venous pH levels, whereas these parameters can be measured every 2 hours if the pH level is between 7.20 and 7.30.

1. Restoration of fluid volume–Dehydration is judged by (1) acute loss of body weight (if a recent weight is known), (2) dryness of oral mucous membranes, (3) low blood pressure, and (4) tachycardia. Initial treatment is with physiologic saline (0.9%), 10–20 mL/kg during the first hour. If indicated by continued signs of dehydration, this is repeated during the second hour. The total volume of initial reexpansion fluid should not exceed 40 mL/kg because of the danger of cerebral edema (see Management of Cerebral Edema, below). Human albumin, 10 mL/kg of 5% solution, can be given over 30 minutes if the patient is in shock. After initial reexpansion, half-physiologic (0.45%) saline usually is given at 1.5 times maintenance. Maintenance fluids are calculated as follows:

Body Weight (kg)	Fluid Maintenance Requirements
Up to 10	100 mL/kg
10–20	1000 mL + 50 mL/kg over 10 kg
> 20	1500 mL + 20 mL/kg over 20 kg

2. Inhibition of lipolysis and return to glucose utilization–Insulin turns off fat breakdown and ketone formation. Regular insulin is usually given intravenously at a rate of 0.1 unit/kg/h. The insulin solution should be administered by pump and can be made by diluting 30 units of regular insulin in 150 mL of 0.9% saline (1 unit/5 mL). If the glucose level falls below 250 mg/dL (13.9 mmol/L), 5% dextrose is added to the intravenous fluids. If the glucose level continues to decrease below 120 mg/dL (6.6 mmol/L), 10% dextrose can be added. If necessary, the insulin dose can be reduced to 0.05 unit/kg/h, but it should not be discontinued before the venous blood pH reaches 7.30. The half-life of intravenous insulin when discontinued is 6 minutes, whereas subcutaneous insulin takes 30–60 minutes to act. Thus, it is often better to continue intravenous insulin until subcutaneous insulin can begin acting.

3. Replacement of body salts–In patients with DKA, both sodium and potassium pass into the urine with the ketones and are depleted. Serum sodium concentrations may be falsely lowered by hyperglycemia, causing water to be drawn into the intravenous space, and by hyperlipemia if fat replaces some of the water in the serum used for electrolyte analysis. Sodium is usually replaced adequately by the use of physiologic and half-physiologic saline in the rehydration fluids as previously discussed.

Serum potassium levels may be elevated initially because of inability of potassium to stay in the cell in the presence of acidosis (though total body potassium is low). Potassium should not be given until the serum potassium level is known to be low or normal and the pH is above 7.10. It is then usually given at a concentration of 40 mEq/L, with 50% of the potassium (20 mEq/L) either as potassium acetate or potassium chloride and the other half as potassium phosphate (20 mEq/L). Hypocalcemia can occur if all of the potassium is given as the phosphate salt; hypophosphatemia occurs if none of the potassium is of the phosphate salt.

4. Correction of acidosis–Acidosis is corrected as the fluid volume and aerobic glycolysis are restored and as insulin is administered to inhibit ketogenesis. As noted earlier, measuring the venous blood pH (identical with arterial blood pH) reveals the severity of acidosis. Bicarbonate is usually reserved for patients with a pH lower than 7.00 and is given as 1–2 mEq/kg over 1 or 2 hours. The pH is monitored every hour and the bicarbonate discontinued when the pH reaches 7.10.

5. Management of cerebral edema–Some degree of cerebral edema has been shown by CT scan to be common in DKA. Associated clinical symptoms are rare, unpredictable, and often associated with demise. Cerebral edema may be related to overhydration with hypotonic fluids, though the cause is not well understood. Early neurologic signs may include headache, excessive drowsiness, and dilated pupils. Prompt initiation of therapy should include elevation of the head of the bed, hyperventilation, mannitol (1 g/kg by intravenous bolus), and fluid restriction. If the cerebral edema is not recognized early, over 50% of patients will die or have permanent brain damage.

Chronic Complications

About 30–40% of persons with type 1 diabetes eventually develop renal failure or loss of vision. Factors that greatly reduce this likelihood are longitudinal hemoglobin A_{1c} levels in a good range, maintenance of blood pressure below the 90th percentile for age, and abstinence from smoking or chewing tobacco. Annual retinal examinations and urine microalbumin measurements are important for pubertal children who have had diabetes for 5 years or longer (see Laboratory Evaluations, above). Preliminary data now show that the use of angiotensin-converting enzyme (ACE) inhibitors may reverse or delay kidney damage when it is detected in the microalbuminuria stage (20–300 µg/min). Similarly, laser treatment to coagulate proliferating capillaries prevents bleeding and leakage of blood into the vitreous fluid or behind the retina. This treatment thus prevents retinal detachment and preserves useful vision for many diabetics with proliferative diabetic retinopathy.

American Diabetes Association: Standards of medical care for patients with diabetes mellitus. Diabetes Care 1994;17:616.

Chase HP, Garg SK, Jelley DH: Diabetic ketoacidosis in children and the role of outpatient management. Pediatr Rev 1990;11:297.

Chase HP: *Understanding Insulin Dependent Diabetes,* 8th ed. Hirschfeld Press, 1995. [Available also at http://www.uchsc.edu./misc/diabetes/bdc.html.]

Davies JL et al: A genome-wide search for human type I diabetes susceptibility genes. Nature 1994;371:130.

Delahanty LM, Halford BN: The role of diet behaviors in achieving improved glycemic control in intensively treated patients in the Diabetes Control and Complications Trial. Diabetes Care 1994;16:1453.

The Diabetes Control and Complications Trial Research Group: The effect of intensive treatment of diabetes on the development and progression of long-term complications in insulin-dependent diabetes mellitus. N Engl J Med 1993;329:977.

Keller RJ, Eisenbarth GS, Jackson RA: Insulin prophylaxis in individuals at high risk of type I diabetes. Lancet 1993;341:927.

Krane EJ et al: Subclinical brain swelling in children during treatment of diabetic ketoacidosis. N Engl J Med 1985;312:1147.

Leslie RDG, Elliott RB: Early environmental events as a cause of IDDM: Evidence and implications. Diabetes 1994;43:843.

Nutrition recommendations and principles for people with diabetes mellitus. Position Statement of the American Diabetes Association. Diabetes Care 1994;17:519.

Polonsky KS, Sturis J, Bell GI: Non-insulin-dependent diabetes mellitus: A genetically programmed failure of the beta cell to compensate for insulin resistance. N Engl J Med 1996;334:777.

Report of the Expert Committee on the Diagnosis and Classification of Diabetes Mellitus. Diabetes Care 1997;20:1183.

Rutledge SK et al: Effectiveness of postprandial Humalog in toddlers with diabetes. Pediatrics 1997;100:968.

30

Inborn Errors of Metabolism

Carol L. Greene, MD, & Stephen I. Goodman, MD

Disorders in which defects of single genes cause clinically significant blocks in metabolic pathways are called **inborn errors of metabolism.** For many years after Garrod first described them in 1908, these conditions were considered esoteric and rare. The number of known inborn errors has increased rapidly in recent years, however, and they are now recognized as important causes of disease in the pediatric age group. Many of them can now be treated effectively. Even when treatment is not available, correct diagnosis permits couples to make informed decisions about future offspring.

The pathology is almost always due to accumulation of enzyme substrate behind the metabolic block or to deficiency of the reaction product. In some cases, the accumulated enzyme substrate is diffusible and has an adverse effect on distant organs; in others, as in lysosomal storage diseases, the substrate accumulates only locally.

The clinical manifestations of inborn errors vary widely; there are mild and severe forms of virtually every disorder, and many patients do not match the classic phenotype. In many cases, this is because the mutations in different patients, even though they are in the same gene, are not identical.

Strategies used to treat inborn errors include avoiding enzyme substrate in the diet (eg, low-phenylalanine diet for phenylketonuria), removing accumulated substrate by pharmacologic means (eg, glycine therapy for isovaleric acidemia), supplementing an inadequately produced metabolite (eg, arginine administration for urea cycle disorders), providing additional coenzyme (eg, vitamin B_{12} therapy for methylmalonic acidemia), and providing normal enzyme (eg, enzyme infusion in Gaucher's disease or liver transplantation for Wilson's disease). Gene replacement is a long-term goal, and trials of treatment of adenine deaminase deficiency began in 1990. However, problems of delivery to target organs and control of gene action make this an unrealistic option at present for most of these disorders.

Inborn errors can present at any time, affect virtually any organ system, and cause all but the most common pediatric problems. This chapter focuses

first on when these conditions should be considered in the differential diagnosis of common pediatric problems. A few of the more important disorders are then discussed in greater detail.

DIAGNOSIS

SUSPECTING INBORN ERRORS

Some important clinical situations are considered later in this section. In general, inborn errors must be considered in the differential diagnosis of the critically ill newborn and of the child with seizures, mental retardation or developmental delay, recurrent vomiting, Reye-like syndromes, parenchymal liver disease, unusual odor, unexplained acidosis, hyperammonemia, and hypoglycemia.

Inborn errors should be strongly suspected when (1) symptoms accompany changes in diet, (2) there is developmental slowing or regression, (3) there is a history of food preferences or aversions, or (4) there is a history of parental consanguinity or of problems that could be due to an inborn error, such as retardation or unexplained deaths in sibs, cousins, or other relatives.

Physical findings that should always arouse suspicion of an inborn error include alopecia or abnormal hair, retinal cherry-red spot or retinitis pigmentosa, cataracts or corneal opacity, hepatomegaly or splenomegaly, coarse features, skeletal changes (including gibbus), and ataxia. Features that may be important, in combination with a suspicious history, include failure to thrive, microcephaly, rash, jaundice, hypotonia, and hypertonia.

Finding an immediate cause of symptoms does not rule out an underlying inborn error. Renal tubular acidosis and cirrhosis are often due to an underlying inborn error. Some inborn errors predispose to infection, eg, gram-negative septicemia in patients with galactosemia. In other inborn errors, acute crises may be brought on by intercurrent infections. Presentation of some inborn errors has been mistaken for nonaccidental trauma (eg, glutaric acidemia type I) or poisoning (eg, methylmalonic acidemia); in addition, children with inborn errors of metabolism may be at higher risk of child abuse or neglect because of the much greater irritability that some of these infants often demonstrate.

LABORATORY STUDIES

Table 30–1 lists common clinical and laboratory features of different groups of inborn errors. Table 30–2 lists laboratory tests used to diagnose these diseases and offers some comments about their use.

Laboratory studies are almost always needed for the diagnosis of inborn errors. Serum electrolytes and pH can be determined in any hospital laboratory and should be used to estimate anion gap as well as acid-base status. Analysis of serum lactate, pyruvate, and ammonia may be available in large hospitals. Amino acid and organic acid studies must be performed at specialized facilities to ensure adequate analysis and interpretation. It is becoming possible to diagnose an increasing number of inborn errors with DNA probes. For most disorders, this requires an extensive genealogic chart or a knowledge of the precise mutation carried in the family.

The physician should know what conditions a test will detect and when it will detect them. For example, urine organic acids may be normal in patients with medium-chain acyl-CoA dehydrogenase deficiency or biotinidase deficiency; glycine may be elevated only in cerebrospinal fluid in patients with glycine encephalopathy; and a result that is normal in one physiologic state may be abnormal in another. For instance, the urine of a hypoglycemic child should be positive for ketones; in such children, a ketone-negative urine test may suggest the presence of a defect in fatty acid oxidation.

Samples used to diagnose metabolic disease may be obtained at autopsy. They may be analyzed directly or stored frozen until a particular analysis is justified by the results of postmortem examination, new clinical information, or new developments in the field. Studies of other family members may also help to establish the diagnosis in a deceased patient; these include demonstrating that the parents are heterozygous carriers of a particular disorder or showing that another sibling has the condition.

COMMON CLINICAL SITUATIONS

Mental Retardation
Many inborn errors can cause mental retardation without other distinguishing characteristics. Labora-

tory studies of serum and urine amino acids should be obtained for every patient with nonspecific mental retardation. Because physical stigmas of certain mucopolysaccharidoses are subtle, urine screens for mucopolysacchariduria are also useful. Electrolytes should be examined because the presence of a high anion gap or renal tubular acidosis significantly increases the chance of finding an underlying inborn error. If developmental regression or specific neurologic findings are present, the evaluation should be expanded accordingly.

Acute Presentation in Neonate
Acute metabolic disease in the newborn may be clinically indistinguishable from sepsis and is most often caused by disorders of protein or carbohydrate metabolism. Initial symptoms may be poor feeding or vomiting, altered mental status or tone, jitteriness or seizures, and jaundice. Acidosis or altered mental status out of proportion to systemic symptoms should increase suspicion of metabolic disorder. Laboratory studies should include determination of electrolytes, ammonia, glucose, urine pH, and urine ketones. Glycine in cerebrospinal fluid should be measured if glycine encephalopathy is suspected. Serum and urine to be used for amino acid and organic acid analysis should be collected before oral intake is stopped and sent for analysis if indicated by the results of initial studies.

Vomiting & Encephalopathy in the Infant or Older Child
Even though vomiting and altered consciousness in the infant or child are more often due to infection and trauma than to an inborn error, the physician should order laboratory studies of electrolytes, ammonia, glucose, urine pH, urine-reducing substances, and urine ketones in all patients before the results are altered by treatment. Samples for amino and organic acid analysis should be obtained early and frozen pending the results of initial studies. An inborn error is even more likely when the presentation is judged "typical" of Reye's syndrome (vomiting, encephalopathy, and hepatomegaly), and amino acids and organic acids should be studied immediately. If there is hypoglycemia with inappropriately low urine or serum ketones, disorders of fatty acid oxidation should be considered.

Hypoglycemia
Studies of electrolytes, ammonia, uric acid, urine-reducing substances, and urine ketones should be performed, and urine should be obtained to measure levels of organic acids. Ketone body production is usually not efficient in the neonate, and ketonuria in a hypoglycemic neonate suggests an inborn error. In the older child, however, the absence of ketonuria suggests inborn error, particularly of fatty acid oxidation.

Hyperammonemia
Symptoms of hyperammonemia may appear and

Table 30–1. Presenting clinical and laboratory features of inborn errors.[1]

	Defects of Carbohydrate Metabolism	Defects of Amino Acid Metabolism[2]	Organic Acid Disorders[3]	Defects of Fatty Acid Oxidation	Defects of Purine Metabolism	Lysosomal Storage Diseases	Disorders of Peroxisomes
Neurodevelopmental							
Mental/developmental retardation	+++	+++	+++	+	++	+++	+++
Developmental regression	-	-	+	-	-	+++	+++
Acute encephalopathy	+++	+++	+++	+++	-	-	-
Seizures	++	+++	+++	+	-	+++	++
Ataxia/movement disorder	-	+	++	-	+++	-	-
Hypotonia	++	++	+++	+++	-	+	+++
Hypertonia	-	++	+++	-	++	+	-
Abnormal behavior	-	++	++	-	++	+++	-
Growth							
Failure to thrive	+++	+++	+++	+	-	+	-
Short stature	++	-	+	-	-	++	-
Macrocephaly	-	-	+	-	-	+++	++
Microcephaly	+	++	+++	-	-	+	-
General							
Vomiting/anorexia	++	+++	+++	+++	-	-	++
Food aversion or craving	++	+++	+++	+++	-	-	-
Odor	-	++	++	-	-	-	-
Dysmorphic features	-	+	+	-	-	++	++
Congenital malformations	-	++	++	-	-	-	++

Organ-specific

Hepatomegaly	+++	–	++	+++	–	+++	+++
Liver disease/cirrhosis	++	+	–	+	–	–	+
Splenomegaly	–	–	–	–	–	++	+
Skeletal dysplasia	–	–	–	–	–	++	++
Cardiomyopathy	++	–	+	+++	–	++	–
Tachypnea/hyperpnea	++	++	++	++	–	–	–
Rash	–	++	++	–	–	–	–
Alopecia or abnormal hair	–	+	++	–	–	–	+
Cataracts or corneal opacity	++	–	–	–	–	++	–
Retinal abnormality	–	+	+	+	–	++	++
Frequent infections	++	–	++	–	++	–	–
Deafness	–	–	+	–	–	++	–
Laboratory							
Hypoglycemia	+++	+	++	++	–	–	–
Hyperammonemia	–	++	++	++	–	–	–
Metabolic acidosis	++	++	+++	+++	–	–	–
Respiratory alkalosis	–	++	–	–	–	–	–
Elevated lactate/pyruvate	++	–	+++	++	–	–	–
Elevated liver enzymes	++	++	++	+++	–	+	+
Neutropenia or thrombocytopenia	+	–	+	–	++	+	–
Ketosis	+++	++	+++	–	–	–	–
Hypoketosis	–	–	+	+++	–	–	–

[1] +++, most conditions in group; ++, some; +, one or few; –, not found.
[2] Includes disorders of urea cycle but not maple syrup urine disease.
[3] Includes maple syrup urine disease and disorders of pyruvate oxidation.

Table 30–2. Obtaining and handling samples to diagnose inborn errors.

Test	Comments
Acid-base status	Accurate estimation of anion gap must be possible. Samples for blood gases should be kept on ice and analyzed immediately.
Blood ammonia	Sample should be collected without a tourniquet, kept on ice, and analyzed immediately.
Blood lactic acid and pyruvic acid	Sample should be collected without a tourniquet, kept on ice, and analyzed immediately. Reduction of pyruvic acid to lactic acid must be prevented. Normal literature values are for the fasting, rested state.
Amino acids	Blood and urine should be examined. CSF glycine should be measured if nonketotic hyperglycinemia is to be ruled out. Normal literature values are for the fasting state. Growth of bacteria in urine should be prevented. At autopsy: liver, kidney, or aqueous humor may be analyzed if urine is not available.
Organic acids	Urine preferred for analysis. At autopsy: liver, kidney, or aqueous may be analyzed if urine is not available.
Carnitine and acylcarnitine profile	Blood (plasma) may be analyzed for total, free, and esterified carnitine; normal values are for the healthy, nonfasted state. Acylcarnitine profile in blood may identify compounds esterified to carnitine, and urine and tissue studies may be needed for certain conditions.
Urine mucopolysaccharides	Variations in urine concentration may cause errors in screening tests. Diagnosis requires knowing which mucopolysaccharides are increased. Some patients with Morquio's disease do not have abnormal mucopolysacchariduria.
Enzyme assays	Specific assays must be requested. Exposure to heat may cause loss of enzyme activity. Enzyme activity in whole blood may become normal after transfusion or vitamin therapy. Leukocyte or fibroblast pellets should be kept frozen prior to assays. Fibroblasts may be grown from skin biopsies taken up to 72 hours after death. Tissues such as liver and kidney should be taken as soon as possible after death, frozen immediately, and kept at –70 °C until assayed.

progress rapidly or insidiously. Decreased appetite and irritability usually appear first, with vomiting, lethargy, seizures, and coma appearing as ammonia levels increase. Tachypnea is caused by a direct effect on respiratory drive. Physical examination cannot exclude the presence of hyperammonemia, and serum ammonia should be measured whenever hyperammonemia is possible.

Severe hyperammonemia may be due to urea cycle disorders, to organic acidemias, or, in the neonate, to transient hyperammonemia of the newborn. The cause can usually be ascertained by measuring citrulline and electrolytes in serum and measuring amino acids, organic acids, and orotic acid in urine. Respiratory alkalosis is usually present in transient hyperammonemia of the newborn and hyperammonemia due to a urea cycle defect, whereas metabolic acidosis is usually associated with hyperammonemia due to organic acidemia. Urine organic acid analysis will demonstrate the cause if the condition is due to organic acidemia. Serum citrulline is usually low or undetectable in early urea cycle defects; normal or slightly high in transient hyperammonemia of the newborn; and very high in citrullinemia and argininosuccinic acidemia. Argininosuccinic acid is found in urine only in the latter. Of infants with early urea cycle defects, only those with hyperammonemia due to ornithine transcarbamoylase deficiency have increased urine orotic acid levels and (often) a family history of male newborn deaths due to defects that appear to be transmitted as an X-linked trait.

Acidosis

Inborn errors may cause chronic or acute acidosis at any age, and with or without an increased anion gap. Inborn errors should be considered when acidosis occurs with recurrent emesis or hyperammonemia and when acidosis is out of proportion to the clinical status. Acidosis due to an inborn error is usually (not always) difficult to correct. The presence of renal tubular acidosis does not exclude an underlying inborn error.

Serum glucose and ammonia and urine pH and ketones should always be examined. Samples for amino acids and organic acids should be obtained at once and sent to the laboratory or saved in the freezer, depending on how strongly an inborn error is suspected. It is useful to test blood lactate and pyruvate levels in the chronically acidotic patient even if urine organic acid levels are normal. Lactate and pyruvate levels are difficult to interpret in the acutely ill patient, but in the absence of shock very high levels of lactic acid suggest primary lactic acidosis.

MANAGEMENT OF METABOLIC EMERGENCIES

Patients with severe acidosis, hypoglycemia, and hyperammonemia may be very ill; initially mild symptoms may worsen quickly, and coma and death may ensue within hours. With prompt and vigorous treatment, however, patients can recover completely, even from deep coma. All oral intake should be stopped. Glucose should be given intravenously in amounts sufficient to stop catabolic processes or to prevent development of catabolism in a patient with a known inborn error at risk for crisis. Most conditions respond favorably to glucose administration, and few (eg, primary lactic acidosis due to pyruvate dehydrogenase deficiency) do not. Severe or increasing hyperammonemia should be treated pharmacologically or with dialysis, and severe acidosis should be treated with bicarbonate administration. More specific measures can be instituted when a diagnosis is established.

NEWBORN SCREENING

Criteria used to decide whether or not to screen newborns for a disorder include its frequency, the significance of consequences if it is not treated, the availability and cost of screening and diagnostic tests, and the availability and cost of treatment. All states in the United States screen newborns for phenylketonuria and hypothyroidism, and most states also screen for galactosemia. Other metabolic disorders for which newborns are frequently screened include maple syrup urine disease, homocystinuria due to cystathionine synthase deficiency, and biotinidase deficiency.

Some screening tests measure a metabolite (eg, phenylalanine) that becomes abnormal only with time and exposure to diet, and in such instances the disease cannot be detected reliably until intake of the enzyme substrate has become established. Other tests (eg, for biotinidase deficiency) assay an enzyme and can be performed at any time; however, transfusions may cause false-negative results, and exposure of the sample to heat may cause false-positive results. Screening tests are not diagnostic, and diagnostic tests must be undertaken when an abnormal screening result is obtained. Furthermore, because false-negative results are not unknown, a normal newborn screening test does not rule out a condition if symptoms develop.

The timing of newborn screening recommended by the American Academy of Pediatrics is appropriate for the detection of phenylketonuria, but hypothyroidism, for instance, can be missed when screening is carried out at the same time. Early discharge of neonates causes significant problems with newborn screening, both with false-negative and false-positive results. Nevertheless, all babies should be screened before discharge from hospital. Physicians should combine current AAP recommendations and law and regulations in each state to arrive at appropriate strategies for each hospital and practice.

American Academy of Pediatrics, Committee on Genetics: Newborn screening fact sheets. Pediatrics 1996;98:473.

Buist NRM, Tuerck JM: The practitioner's role in newborn screening. Pediatr Clin North Am 1992;39:199.

Chaves-Carballo E: Detection of inherited neurometabolic disorders: A practical clinical approach. Pediatr Clin North Am 1992;39:801.

Childs B: Sir Archibald Garrod's conception of chemical individuality: A modern appreciation. N Engl J Med 1970;282:71.

Emery JL et al: Investigation of inborn errors of metabolism in unexpected infant deaths. Lancet 1988;2:29.

Fernandez J et al (editors): Inborn Metabolic Diseases: Diagnosis and Treatment, 2nd ed. Springer, 1995.

Goodman SI, Greene CL: Metabolic disorders of the newborn. Pediatr Rev 1994;15:359.

Greene CL, Blitzer MG, Shapira E: Inborn errors of metabolism and Reye syndrome: Differential diagnosis. J Pediatr 1988;113:156.

Ozand PT, Gascon GG: Organic acidurias: A review. Part 1. J Child Neurol 1991;6:196.

Roth KS: Inborn errors of metabolism: The essentials of clinical diagnosis. Clin Pediatr 1991;30:183.

Rowe PC, Valle D, Brusilow SW: Inborn errors of metabolism in children referred with Reye's syndrome: A changing pattern. JAMA 1988;260:3167.

Scriver CR et al (editor): *The Molecular and Metabolic Bases of Inherited Disease,* 7th ed. McGraw-Hill, 1995.

Shih VE: Detection of hereditary metabolic disorders involving amino acids and organic acids. Clin Biochem 1991;24:301.

Surtees R, Leonard JV: Acute metabolic encephalopathy: A review of causes, mechanism and treatment. J Inherit Metab Dis 1989;12:42.

Valle D: Treatment of genetic disease: Current status and prospects for the future. Semin Perinatol 1991;15:52.

Ward JC: Inborn errors of metabolism of acute onset in infancy. Pediatr Rev 1990;11:205.

DISORDERS OF CARBOHYDRATE METABOLISM

GLYCOGEN STORAGE DISEASES

Glycogen is a highly branched polymer of glucose that is stored in liver and muscle. Many different disorders of its biosynthesis and degradation have been described, and the enzyme defects responsible have been identified. The most common forms of glycogenosis are characterized by growth failure, hepatomegaly, and fasting hypoglycemia. Defects that cause these so-called hepatic forms of the disease include glucose-6-phosphatase (type I; von Gierke disease), debrancher enzyme (type III), hepatic phosphorylase (type VI), and phosphorylase kinase (type IX), which normally regulates hepatic phosphorylase activity. Further, there are two forms of glucose-6-phosphatase deficiency: In one, the enzyme defect can be demonstrated in fresh or frozen liver; in the other, the defect can be demonstrated only in fresh tissue.

Forms of the disease affecting primarily muscle include acid maltase deficiency (type II; Pompe's disease), which may be seen in infancy with cardiomegaly and macroglossia, and muscle phosphorylase (type V) and phosphofructokinase (type VII) deficiencies, in which the most striking features are easy fatigability and muscle weakness and stiffness.

Diagnosis

Precise diagnosis is by biochemical tests, such as responsiveness of blood glucose to fasting and glucagon, and enzyme assays on leukocytes, liver, or muscle. Disorders that can be diagnosed using red or white blood cells include deficiencies of debrancher enzyme (type III) and phosphorylase kinase (IX). Pompe's disease can usually be diagnosed by assaying acid maltase in fibroblasts.

Treatment

In general, treatment is designed to prevent hypoglycemia while avoiding storage of even more glycogen in the liver. In the most severe hepatic forms, this requires careful monitoring of specific diets, using restriction of free sugars and measured amounts of cornstarch, and some good results have been reported following continuous nighttime carbohydrate feeding.

Fernandes J, Chen Y-T: Glycogen storage diseases: In: *Inborn Metabolic Diseases: Diagnosis and Treatment,* 2nd ed. Fernandez J et al (editors). Springer, 1995.
Greene HL et al: Type I glycogen storage disease: A metabolic basis for advances in treatment. Adv Pediatr 1979;26:63.
Hers HG et al: Glycogen storage diseases. In: The Molecular and Metabolic Bases of Inherited Disease, 7th ed. Scriver CR et al (editors). McGraw-Hill, 1995.

GALACTOSEMIA

Classic galactosemia is caused by almost total deficiency of galactose-1-phosphate uridyltransferase. Accumulation of galactose-1-phosphate in liver, brain, and renal tubules causes hepatic parenchymal disease, mental retardation, and renal Fanconi's syndrome. Accumulation of galactitol (dulcitol) in the lens produces cataracts. With prompt institution of a galactose-free diet, the prognosis for life is excellent.

In the severe form of the disease, onset is marked by vomiting, jaundice, and hepatomegaly in the newborn period after milk feeding. Without treatment, death frequently occurs in the first month of life, often from *Escherichia coli* sepsis. Cataracts usually develop within 2 months in untreated cases, and hepatic cirrhosis is progressive. In less severe cases, survival is possible but mental retardation is irreversible. Even when dietary restrictions are instituted early, patients with galactosemia are at increased risk for speech and language deficits and ovarian failure, and some patients develop progressive delay, tremor, and ataxia. Clinical and laboratory evidence of the disease abates gradually with effective treatment.

The disorder is inherited as an autosomal recessive trait with an incidence of approximately one in 40,000 live births. Because disease in infancy may be severe and diagnosed late, newborn screening is becoming increasingly common. Screening is accomplished by demonstrating enzyme deficiency in red cells with the Beutler test or by demonstrating increased serum galactose. Prenatal diagnosis is possible if a specific DNA mutation in a family is known.

Diagnosis

In infants receiving foods containing galactose, laboratory findings include galactosuria and hypergalactosemia together with proteinuria and aminoaciduria. It is important not to exclude the diagnosis simply because the urine does not contain reducing substances. When the diagnosis is suspected, galactose-1-phosphate uridyltransferase should be assayed in erythrocytes; only blood transfusions will cause this test to be falsely negative, and only sample deterioration will cause it to be falsely positive.

Treatment

A galactose-free diet should be instituted as soon as the diagnosis is made. Compliance with the diet must be monitored because it is not a simple exclusion of milk and requires extensive knowledge about the galactose content of foods. Avoidance of galactose should be lifelong in severe cases, with appropriate calcium replacement. Additional therapies, such as supplementation with uridine, are under investigation. Heterozygous mothers may be advised to maintain a galactose-free diet during pregnancies.

Donnel G (editor): Galactosemia: New frontiers in research. NIH Publication No. 93-3438, 1993.
Gross KC, Acosta PB: Fruits and vegetables are a source of galactose: Implications in planning the diets of patients with galactosemia. J Inherit Metab Dis 1991:253.
Kaufman FR et al: Correlation of ovarian function with galactose-1-phosphate uridyl transferase levels in galactosemia. J Pediatr 1988;112:755.
Levy HL et al: Sepsis due to *Escherichia coli* in neonates with galactosemia. N Engl J Med 1977;297:823.

Lo W et al: Neurologic sequelae in galactosemia. Pediatrics 1984;73:309.

Sardharwalla IB, Wraith JE: Galactosemia. Nutr Health 1987;5:175.

HEREDITARY FRUCTOSE INTOLERANCE

Hereditary fructose intolerance is an autosomal recessive disorder in which deficient activity of fructose-1-phosphate aldolase causes hypoglycemia and tissue accumulation of fructose-1-phosphate on fructose ingestion. Other abnormalities include failure to thrive, vomiting, jaundice, hepatomegaly, proteinuria, and generalized aminoaciduria. The untreated condition can progress to death as a result of liver failure.

Diagnosis

The diagnosis is supported by the demonstration of fructosuria following an inpatient, closely monitored fructose load. The appearance of hypoglycemia and hypophosphatemia after fructose loading (200 mg/kg) is diagnostic, as is reduced activity of fructose-1-phosphate aldolase in the liver. Some patients may be diagnosed by identification of one of the common mutations on DNA analysis.

Treatment

Treatment consists of eliminating fructose from the diet and is complicated by the fact that many proprietary drugs and vitamins are in a sucrose base. If the diet is relaxed, there may be retardation of physical growth, but growth will resume when more stringent dietary restrictions are instituted. If the disorder is recognized early, the prospects for normal development are good. As affected individuals grow up, they may recognize the association of nausea and vomiting with fructose-containing foods and selectively avoid them.

Brooks CC, Tolan DR: Association of the widespread A149P hereditary fructose intolerance mutation with newly identified sequence polymorphisms in the aldolase B gene. Am J Hum Genet 1993;52:835.

Odierre M et al: Hereditary fructose intolerance in childhood: Diagnosis, management and course in 55 patients. Am J Dis Child 1978;132:605.

Steinmann B, Gitzelmann R: The diagnosis of hereditary fructose intolerance. Helv Paediatr Acta 1981;36:297.

PRIMARY LACTIC ACIDEMIAS & OTHER DISORDERS OF ENERGY METABOLISM

Primary lactic acidemia is a diagnosis being made with increasing frequency and may be one of the more common causes of static, progressive, or self-limited neurodevelopmental problems in children. The range of severity and prognosis in these disorders is illustrated by extremes. For example, defects in the mitochondrial respiratory chain, including complex IV deficiency, may cause Leigh's disease, a fatal neurodegenerative disorder, whereas another presentation of complex IV deficiency is benign resolving congenital hypotonia. Lactic acidemia is said to be primary when it is due to a defect in the metabolism of pyruvic acid and secondary when a change in cellular redox potential favors the reduction of pyruvate to lactate (as in shock). Some causes of primary lactic acidosis are shown in Table 30–3. In general, such disorders may present at any age with neurologic findings and, when the defect is in gluconeogenesis, with hypoglycemia. Patients with a defect in the E_1 component of the pyruvate dehydrogenase complex often show central nervous system malformations or mild facial dysmorphism. Recurrent altered mental status, recurrent ataxia, and recurrent acidosis are typical of many disturbances of pyruvate metabolism.

Defects in the mitochondrial respiratory chain also may present with nonspecific findings such as hypotonia or renal tubular acidosis or with more specific features such as ophthalmoplegia. Ragged red fibers and mitochondrial abnormalities may be noted on histologic examination of muscle. Thirteen of the more than 100 genes that control activity of the respiratory chain are part of the mitochondrial genome. Therefore, inheritance of defects in the respiratory chain may be mendelian or maternal.

Diagnosis

Diagnosis of primary lactic acidemia may be based on (1) demonstration of significant elevations of blood lactic acid concentration (more than 2

Table 30–3. Causes of primary lactic acidosis in childhood.

Defects of the pyruvate dehydrogenase complex
  E_1 (pyruvate decarboxylase) deficiency
  E_2 (dihydrolipoyl transacetylase) deficiency
  E_3 (lipoamide dehydrogenase) deficiency
  Pyruvate decarboxylase phosphate phosphatase
    deficiency
Abnormalities of gluconeogenesis
  Pyruvate carboxylase deficiency
    Isolated
    Biotinidase deficiency
    Holocarboxylase synthetase deficiency
  Fructose-1,6-diphosphatase deficiency
  Glucose-6-phosphatase deficiency (von Gierke's disease)
Defects in mitochondrial respiratory chain
  Complex I deficiency
  Complex IV deficiency (cytochrome C oxidase deficiency; frequent cause of Leigh's disease)
  ATPase deficiency (frequent cause of Leigh disease)
  Other respiratory chain disorders

mmol/L in a fasting, resting, free-flowing venous sample) or pyruvic acid in blood or spinal fluid and excluding secondary lactic acidemia; or (2) demonstration of classic features of mitochondrial disorder such as ragged red fibers. Primary lactic acidemia may be present even if the blood lactic acid concentration is normal, since lactate levels may vary according to the state of the patient (eg, resting versus active; fasting versus fed). Carefully controlled and monitored provocative testing such as fasting, challenge with carbohydrates, or exercise may identify clinical categories leading to suggestions for diagnosis and treatment. If a specific diagnosis is suggested by clinical symptoms, diagnostic tests of blood samples for enzyme assays (eg, biotinidase, pyruvate carboxylase) may lead to diagnosis, but enzyme analysis of fibroblasts or skeletal muscle is often required. For some clinical presentations, mitochondrial DNA analysis of blood or tissue may identify a diagnostic mutation. In many patients, the cause of the disorder cannot be defined. For some diagnoses, the genetics and prognosis may be clear, but in many cases neither recurrence risk nor prognosis can be predicted.

Treatment

In some patients, defects in gluconeogenesis can be treated with glucose administration, fructose avoidance, or administration of pharmacologic amounts of biotin. Modified ketogenic diet has been reported to be useful in some cases of proved or presumed pyruvate dehydrogenase deficiency. Other treatments are of theoretic or empiric value, with little data on efficacy. Thiamine or lipoic acid can be tried in patients with pyruvate dehydrogenase complex deficiencies, and coenzyme Q and riboflavin have been reported to be helpful in some patients with respiratory chain defects. Dichloroacetic acid has been tried in pyruvate dehydrogenase complex deficiencies and in respiratory chain disorders, with variation in both clinical response and adverse effects.

Brown GK et al: "Cerebral" lactic acidosis: Defects in pyruvate metabolism with profound brain damage and minimal systemic acidosis. Eur J Pediatr 1988;147:10.

Clarke LA: Mitochondrial disorders in pediatrics: Clinical, biochemical and genetic implications. Pediatr Clin North Am 1992;39:319.

Eymard B, Hauw J-J: Mitochondrial encephalomyopathies. Curr Opin Neurol Neurosurg 1992;5:909.

Hart Z, Chang C: A newborn infant with respiratory distress and persistent stridulous breathing. J Pediatr 1988;113:150.

Kerr DS: Lactic acidosis and mitochondrial disorders. Clin Biochem 1991;24:33.

Munnich A et al: Clinical aspects of mitochondrial disorders. J Inherit Metab Dis 1992;15:448.

Rahman S et al: Clinical features and biochemical and DNA abnormalities. Ann Neurol 1996;39:343.

Robinson BH et al: Variable clinical presentation in patients with defective E$_1$ component of pyruvate dehydrogenase complex. J Pediatr 1987;111:525.

Shoffner JM, Wallace DC: Mitochondrial genetics: Principles and practice. Am J Hum Genet 1992;51:1179.

Tulinius MH et al: Mitochondrial encephalomyopathies in childhood: I. Biochemical and morphologic investigations. J Pediatr 1991;119:242.

Tulinius MH et al: Mitochondrial encephalomyopathies in childhood: II. Clinical manifestations and syndromes. J Pediatr 1991;119:251.

DISORDERS OF AMINO ACID METABOLISM

DISORDERS OF THE UREA CYCLE

Ammonia is converted to an amino group in urea by enzymes of the urea cycle. Defects in early urea cycle enzymes, such as carbamoyl phosphate synthetase or ornithine transcarbamoylase, usually present in infancy with severe and rapidly fatal hyperammonemia, vomiting, and encephalopathy, but the course may also be milder, with vomiting and encephalopathy following protein ingestion or infections. Although defects in argininosuccinic acid synthetase (citrullinemia) and argininosuccinic acid lyase (argininosuccinic acidemia) may also present with severe hyperammonemia in infancy, a chronic course with mental retardation is more usual in these conditions.

Except for ornithine transcarbamoylase deficiency, which is X-linked, urea cycle disorders are inherited as autosomal recessive traits. Citrullinemia and argininosuccinic acidemia can be diagnosed in utero by appropriate enzyme assays, but carbamoyl phosphate synthetase and ornithine transcarbamoylase deficiency states can be diagnosed in utero only by using specific gene probes, and then only in certain families.

Diagnosis

Blood ammonia levels should be measured in any newborn who is acutely ill without obvious cause. A urea cycle defect should be suspected when severe hyperammonemia is associated with respiratory alkalosis. Serum citrulline is low or undetectable in carbamoyl phosphate synthetase and ornithine transcarbamoylase deficiency, high in argininosuccinic acidemia, and very high in citrullinemia. Large amounts of argininosuccinic acid are found in the urine of patients with argininosuccinic acidemia. Urine orotic acid is increased in infants with ornithine transcarbamoylase deficiency, and there may also be a family history of male newborn deaths that appear to be transmitted as an X-linked trait.

Age of onset of symptoms varies with protein intake, growth, and stress such as infection. Even within a family, affected males may differ by decades in their age at onset of symptoms. Many female carriers of ornithine transcarbamoylase deficiency show protein intolerance; some develop migraine-like symptoms after protein loads, and others develop potentially fatal episodes of vomiting and encephalopathy after protein ingestion, certain infections, or labor and delivery. Trichorrhexis nodosa is common in patients with the chronic form of argininosuccinic acidemia.

Treatment

In the newborn, measures to reduce serum ammonia by hemodialysis, peritoneal dialysis, or double-volume exchange transfusion should be instituted as soon as hyperammonemia is documented. Protein intake should be stopped, and glucose should be given to reduce endogenous protein breakdown. Arginine should be given intravenously, both because it is an essential amino acid for patients with urea cycle defects and because it increases the excretion of waste nitrogen in patients with citrullinemia and argininosuccinic acidemia. Sodium benzoate, sodium phenylacetate, and sodium phenylbutyrate can also be given intravenously, and one or more of these drugs is needed intravenously for treatment of hyperammonemic coma.

Long-term treatment includes oral administration of arginine (or citrulline), adherence to a low-protein diet, and administration of sodium benzoate and sodium phenylacetate or sodium phenylbutyrate to increase excretion of nitrogen as hippuric acid and phenylacetylglutamine. Female ornithine transcarbamoylase-deficient heterozygotes who develop hyperammonemia should also receive such treatment.

The outcome of argininosuccinic acidemia and citrullinemia is better than that of ornithine transcarbamoylase and carbamoyl phosphate synthetase deficiency. Most patients with urea cycle defects, no matter what the enzyme defect, develop permanent neurologic and intellectual impairments, with cortical atrophy and ventricular dilation seen on CT scan. The prognosis may be improved if the initial hyperammonemic episode is rapidly identified and treated.

Batshaw ML et al: Risk of serious illness in heterozygotes for ornithine transcarbamylase deficiency. J Pediatr 1986;108:236.

Brusilow SW et al: Treatment of episodic hyperammonemia in children with inborn errors of urea synthesis. N Engl J Med 1984;310:1630.

Cederbaum SD: The treatment of urea cycle disorders. Int Pediatr 1992;7:61.

Leonard JV: Urea cycle disorders. In: *Inborn Metabolic Disorders: Diagnosis and Treatment,* 2nd ed. Fernandez et al (editors). Springer, 1995.

Nagata N et al: Retrospective survey of urea cycle disorders: Part 2. Neurological outcome in forty-nine Japanese patients with urea cycle enzymopathies. Am J Med Genet 1991;40:477.

PHENYLKETONURIA & THE HYPERPHENYLALANINEMIAS

Probably the best-known disorder of amino acid metabolism is the classic form of phenylketonuria. It was first recognized in 1934 by Fölling in several retarded children who excreted phenylpyruvic acid in the urine. The disorder is due to decreased activity of phenylalanine hydroxylase, the enzyme that converts phenylalanine to tyrosine. Phenylketonuria is inherited as an autosomal recessive trait, with an incidence in whites of approximately 1:10,000 live births. On normal phenylalanine intake, affected patients develop hyperphenylalaninemia and produce and excrete phenylpyruvic, phenyllactic, phenylacetic, and 2-hydroxyphenylacetic acid. The untreated patient shows severe mental retardation, hyperactivity, seizures, a light complexion, and eczema. The patient's urine has a "mouse-like" odor.

Clinicians had early success preventing severe mental retardation in phenylketonuric children by restricting phenylalanine from the diet starting in early infancy. This success led to the development of screening programs to detect the disease early. Since the outcome is best when treatment is begun in the first month of life, infants should be screened during the first few days. A second test is necessary when newborn screening is done before 24 hours of age, and in such cases the second test should be completed by the third week of life. Infants receiving hyperalimentation and premature infants should be screened at or near 7 days, and rescreened if they were transfused or not fed at the time of the initial test.

Enzymes involved with the interconversion of phenylalanine and tyrosine and whose deficiencies can produce hyperphenylalaninemia are shown in Figure 30–1. In classic phenylketonuria, there is little or no phenylalanine hydroxylase activity, but in the less severe hyperphenylalaninemias there is significant residual activity. Rare variants can be due to deficiency of dihydrobiopterin reductase or to defects in biopterin synthesis. All are inherited as autosomal recessive traits.

Prenatal diagnosis of phenylketonuria is often possible using DNA probes. Molecular approaches are replacing serum measurements of phenylalanine and tyrosine to determine carrier status. Prenatal diagnosis of defects in pterin metabolism can often be made.

Diagnosis & Treatment

The diagnosis of phenylketonuria in a severely re-

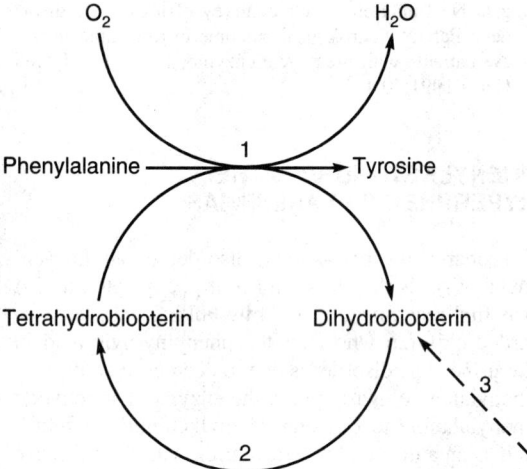

O$_2$ H$_2$O

Phenylalanine ⟶ **1** ⟶ Tyrosine

Tetrahydrobiopterin   Dihydrobiopterin

3

2

Figure 30–1. Oxidation of phenylalanine to tyrosine. **1.** Phenylalanine hydroxylase. **2.** Dihydropteridine reductase. **3.** Enzymes of biopterin biosynthesis.

tarded older child with typical biochemical and physical characteristics is straightforward, but in the newborn period, especially when there is no family history, the condition must be differentiated from other forms of hyperphenylalaninemia. This is usually done by determining serum phenylalanine and tyrosine levels on a normal diet and by examining pterins and metabolites of phenylalanine in urine.

A. Classic Phenylketonuria: Findings include persistently elevated serum levels of phenylalanine (> 20 mg/dL on a regular diet), normal or low serum levels of tyrosine, urinary excretion of phenylpyruvic and 2-hydroxyphenylacetic acids, and normal pterins. Poor phenylalanine tolerance persists throughout life. Restriction of dietary phenylalanine intake (see below) is indicated, and a favorable outcome is the rule.

B. Persistent Hyperphenylalaninemia: In infants receiving a normal protein intake, serum phenylalanine levels are usually 4–20 mg/dL, and pterins are normal. Phenylalanine restriction may or may not be indicated, depending on the phenylalanine tolerance.

C. Transient Hyperphenylalaninemia: Serum phenylalanine levels are elevated early but progressively decline toward normal. If required at all, dietary restriction is only temporary.

D. Dihydropteridine Reductase Deficiency: Serum phenylalanine levels vary. The pattern of pterin metabolites is abnormal. Seizures and psychomotor regression occur even with diet therapy, probably because the enzyme defect also causes neuronal deficiency of serotonin and dopamine. These deficiencies require treatment with levodopa, carbidopa, and 5-hydroxytryptophan, and possibly also with tetrahydrobiopterin.

E. Defects in Biopterin Biosynthesis: Serum phenylalanine levels vary. Total pterins are low, and their pattern may suggest the specific defect, which can be at one of several steps in the biosynthetic pathway. Clinical findings include myoclonus, tetraplegia, and other movement disorders. Treatment is the same as for dihydropteridine reductase deficiency but in general is not as effective.

F. Tyrosinemia of the Newborn: Serum phenylalanine levels are lower than those seen in phenylketonuria and are accompanied by marked hypertyrosinemia. This usually occurs in premature infants and is due to immaturity of 4-hydroxyphenylpyruvic acid oxidase. The condition resolves spontaneously within 3 months, almost always without sequelae. If necessary, intramuscular injection of 100 mg ascorbic acid will normalize serum tyrosine (and phenylalanine) within 48 hours.

G. Maternal Phenylketonuria: Offspring of phenylketonuric mothers may have transient hyperphenylalaninemia at birth. Elevated maternal phenylalanine causes mental retardation, microcephaly, growth retardation, and often congenital heart disease or other malformations. The risk to the fetus is considerably lessened if phenylalanine restriction is begun before conception and maintained throughout pregnancy.

Treatment of Classic Phenylketonuria

Treatment of classic phenylketonuria is to limit dietary phenylalanine intake to amounts that permit normal growth and development. Products deficient in phenylalanine but otherwise similar to milk are commercially available but must be supplemented with normal milk and other foods to supply enough phenylalanine to permit normal growth and development. Serum phenylalanine concentrations must be monitored frequently while ensuring that growth, development, and nutrition are adequate. This monitoring is best done in clinics experienced in dealing with such problems. Although dietary treatment is most effective when initiated during the first months of life, it may also be of benefit in reversing behaviors such as hyperactivity, irritability, and distractibility when started later in life.

Phenylalanine restriction should continue throughout life, both because of subtle changes in IQ and behavior in persons treated early who go off diet and because of the risk of late development of potentially irreversible neurologic damage after stopping the diet. Females with phenylketonuria merit special attention during the childbearing years. Counseling should be given during adolescence, and the woman's diet should be closely monitored prior to conception and throughout pregnancy.

Children with classic phenylketonuria who are treated promptly after birth and achieve phenylalanine and tyrosine homeostasis will develop well physically and can be expected to have normal or nearly normal intellectual development.

Blau N et al: Tetrahydrobiopterin deficiency: From phenotype to genotype. Pteridines 1993;4:1.

Cleary MA et al: Magnetic resonance imaging in phenylketonuria: Reversal of cerebral white matter change. J Pediatr 1995;127:251.

Hanley WB et al: Malnutrition with early treatment of phenylketonuria. Pediatr Res 1970;4:318.

Koch R et al: The effects of diet discontinuation in children with phenylketonuria. Eur J Pediatr 1987;146(Suppl): A12.

Matalon R, Michals K: Phenylketonuria: Screening, treatment and maternal PKU. Clin Biochem 1991;24:337.

O'Flynn ME: Newborn screening for phenylketonuria: Thirty years of progress. Curr Probl Pediatr 1992:159.

Potocnik U, Widhalm K: Long-term follow-up of children with classical PKU after diet discontinuation: A review. J Am Coll Nutr 1994;13:232.

Thompson AJ et al: Neurologic deterioration in young adults with phenylketonuria. Lancet 1990;336:602.

Villasana D et al: Neurological deterioration in adult phenylketonuria. J Inherited Metab Dis 1989;12:451.

HEREDITARY TYROSINEMIA

Hereditary tyrosinemia is caused by deficiency of fumarylacetoacetase and is characterized by progressive hepatic parenchymal damage, renal tubular dystrophy with generalized aminoaciduria and hypophosphatemic rickets, hypermethioninemia, and tyrosine metabolites, succinylacetone, and δ-aminolevulinic acid in the urine. The course may be rapidly fatal in infancy or somewhat more chronic, with liver cell carcinoma almost invariable.

The condition is inherited as an autosomal recessive trait and is especially common in Scandinavia and in the Chicoutimi-Lac St. Jean region of Quebec. Prenatal diagnosis can be established.

Diagnosis

Similar clinical and biochemical findings may occur in galactosemia and hereditary fructose intolerance, but increased succinylacetone occurs only in fumarylacetoacetase deficiency, and diagnosis is based on demonstrating this compound in urine.

Treatment

A diet low in phenylalanine and tyrosine is indicated but not usually successful in preventing or reversing liver disease, and liver transplantation appears to be the only effective therapy for these children. Pharmacologic therapy to inhibit 4-hydroxyphenylpyruvate dehydrogenase improves the biochemical profile and acute clinical status, and studies are in progress to determine to what extent the risk of hepatocellular carcinoma is altered.

Kvittingen EA et al: Tyrosine. In: *Metabolic Diseases: Diagnosis and Treatment.* Fernandez J et al (editors). Springer, 1995.

Lindstedt S et al: Treatment of hereditary tyrosinaemia type I by inhibition of 4-hydroxyphenylpyruvate dioxygenase. Lancet 1992;340:813.

MAPLE SYRUP URINE DISEASE (Branched-Chain Ketoaciduria)

Maple syrup urine disease is due to deficiency of the enzyme that catalyzes oxidative decarboxylation of the branched-chain keto acid derivatives of leucine, isoleucine, and valine. The accumulated keto acids of leucine and isoleucine cause the characteristic odor, while only the keto acid of leucine has been implicated in causing central nervous system dysfunction. Many variants of this disorder have been described, including mild, intermittent, and thiamin-dependent forms, and all are inherited as autosomal recessive traits.

Patients with classic maple syrup urine disease are normal at birth but soon develop the characteristic odor, lethargy, feeding difficulties, coma, and seizures. Unless diagnosis is made and dietary restriction of branched-chain amino acids is begun, most will die in the first month of life, but nearly normal growth and development may be achieved if treatment is begun before about 10 days of age.

Diagnosis

Marked elevations of branched-chain amino acids (including alloisoleucine) in serum and urine are characteristic. Alloisoleucine, a transamination product of the keto acid of isoleucine, is almost pathognomonic. The magnitude and consistency of amino acid and organic acid changes are altered in mild and intermittent forms of the disease. Prenatal diagnosis is possible.

Treatment

Products deficient in branched-chain amino acids but in other respects similar to milk are commercially available S but must be supplemented with normal milk and other foods to supply enough branched-chain amino acids to permit normal growth and development. Serum levels of branched-chain amino acids must be monitored frequently—even at intervals of 1 or 2 days—in the first months of life to deal with changing protein requirements. Acute episodes must be aggressively treated to *prevent* catabolism and negative nitrogen balance.

Biggeman B, Zass R, Wendel U: Postoperative metabolic decompensation in maple syrup urine disease is completely prevented by insulin. J Inherited Metab Dis 1993;16:912.

Giacoia GP, Berry GT: Acrodermatitis enteropathic-like syndrome secondary to isoleucine deficiency during treatment of maple syrup urine disease. Am J Dis Child 1993;147:954.

Nord A et al: Developmental profile of patients with maple syrup urine disease. J Inherit Metab Dis 1991;14:881.

Ogier deBaulny H et al: Branched chain organic acidurias. In: *Inborn Metabolic Disease: Diagnosis and Treatment,* 2nd ed. Fernandez J et al (editors). Springer, 1995.

Treacy E et al: Maple syrup urine disease: Interrelation between branched-chain amino, oxo, and hydroxy acids; implications for treatment; associations with CNS dysmyelination. J Inherit Metab Dis 1992;15:121.

HOMOCYSTINURIA

Homocystinuria is most often due to deficiency of cystathionine synthase, but it may also be due to deficiency of methylenetetrahydrofolate reductase (MTHR) or to defects in the biosynthesis of methyl-B_{12}, which is the coenzyme for N^5-methyltetrahydrofolate methyltransferase. All known inherited forms of homocystinuria are transmitted as autosomal recessive traits and can be diagnosed in the fetus.

About half of untreated patients with cystathionine synthase deficiency are retarded, and most have arachnodactyly, osteoporosis, and a tendency to develop dislocated lenses and thromboembolic phenomena. Milder elevations of homocystine, detectable only by special studies measuring total plasma homocysteine, are increasingly recognized to be a factor in the etiology of vascular disease leading to myocardial infarction and stroke. These mild elevations are often caused by mutations leading to heat-sensitive defects in MTHR. Patients with remethylation defects usually show failure to thrive and a variety of neurologic symptoms, including microcephaly and seizures in infancy and early childhood.

Diagnosis

Diagnosis is made by demonstrating homocystinuria in a patient who is not severely deficient in vitamin B_{12}. Serum methionine levels are usually high in patients with cystathionine synthase deficiency and often low in patients with remethylation defects. When the remethylation defect is due to deficiency of methyl-B_{12}, megaloblastic anemia may be present, and an associated deficiency of adenosyl-B_{12} may cause methylmalonic aciduria. Studies of cultured fibroblasts may be necessary to make a specific diagnosis.

Treatment

About 50% of patients with cystathionine synthase deficiency respond to large oral doses of pyridoxine. Early treatment of pyridoxine nonresponders by dietary methionine restriction may prevent mental retardation and delay lens dislocations, perhaps justifying screening of newborn infants for the condition. Oral administration of betaine (250 mg/kg/d) will increase methylation of homocystine to methionine in patients with remethylation defects and may also improve neurologic function. Large doses of vitamin B_{12} (eg, 1 mg hydroxocobalamin) administered intramuscularly every other day) are indicated in some patients.

Andrea G, Sebastio G: Homocystinuria due to cystathionine β-synthase deficiency and related disorders. In: *Inborn Metabolic Diseases: Diagnosis and Treatment,* 2nd ed. Fernandez J et al (editors). Springer, 1995.

Guttormsen AB et al: Determinants and vitamin responsiveness of intermediate hyperhomocysteinemia (≥ 40 micromol/liter). J Clin Invest 1996;98:2174.

Mudd SH et al: The natural history of homocystinuria due to cystathionine β-synthase deficiency. Am J Hum Genet 1985;37:1.

Rosenblatt DS, Shevell MI: Inherited disorders of cobalamin and folate absorption and metabolism. In: *Inborn Diseases: Diagnosis and Treatment,* 2nd ed. Fernandez J et al (editors). Springer, 1995.

NONKETOTIC HYPERGLYCINEMIA

Inherited deficiency of various subunits of the glycine cleavage enzyme causes nonketotic hyperglycinemia. In its most severe form, also termed **glycine encephalopathy,** the condition presents in the newborn period with unremitting seizures, hypotonia, hiccups, a burst suppression pattern on EEG, and (usually) death in infancy. Forms that present with seizures later in infancy or with developmental delay in childhood are observed. All forms of the condition are inherited as autosomal recessive traits.

Diagnosis

This deficiency should be suspected in any infant with intractable seizures, especially when hiccupping, and is confirmed by demonstrating a large increase in glycine in cerebrospinal fluid, with the CSF:serum glycine ratio being abnormally high. Demonstrating the specific enzyme defect by liver biopsy is necessary only if the couple is contemplating having more children, as prenatal diagnosis is possible only by assaying the enzyme in chorionic villus samples.

Treatment

Treatment is generally unsuccessful. Early efforts to use sodium benzoate therapy were thought to be without effect on long-term outcome, but recent studies suggest that this drug may be useful in seizure control.

Eyskens FJM et al: Neurologic sequelae in transient nonketotic hyperglycinemia of the neonate. J Pediatr 1992; 121:620.

Hamosh et al: Dextromethorphan and high dose benzoate therapy for nonketotic hyperglycinemia in an infant. J Pediatr 1992;121:131.

Hayasaka K et al: Nonketotic hyperglycinemia: Analyses of glycine cleavage system in typical and atypical cases. J Pediatr 1987;110:873.

Tada K, Hayasaka K: Non-ketotic hyperglycinaemia: Clinical and biochemical aspects. Eur J Pediatr 1987;146: 221.

Toone JR, Applegate DA, Levy HL: Prenatal diagnosis of non-ketotic hyperglycemia: Experiences in 50 at risk pregnancies. J Inherited Metab Dis 1994;17:342.

ORGANIC ACIDEMIAS

Organic acidemias are disorders of amino and fatty acid metabolism in which nonamino organic acids accumulate in serum and urine. These conditions are usually diagnosed by examining organic acids in urine, a complex procedure that requires considerable interpretive expertise and is usually performed only in specialized laboratories. The clinical features of organic acidemias are listed in Table 30–4, together with the urine organic acid patterns typical of each. Additional details about some of the more important organic acidemias are provided below.

KETOTIC HYPERGLYCINEMIAS (Propionic & Methylmalonic Acidemia)

Idiopathic hyperglycinemia was first reported in 1961 as a syndrome of mental retardation and episodic ketoacidosis, neutropenia, thrombocytopenia, osteoporosis, and hyperglycinemia induced by protein intake or infection. It was then renamed ketotic hyperglycinemia to distinguish it from nonketotic hyperglycinemia, described above. It is now known that the syndrome is almost always due to propionic or methylmalonic acidemia.

The oxidation of threonine, valine, isoleucine, and methionine through propionyl- and L-methylmalonyl-CoA is diagrammed in Figure 30–2. Propionic acidemia is due to a defect in the biotin-containing enzyme propionyl-CoA carboxylase, and methylmalonic acidemia is due to a defect in methylmalonyl-CoA mutase. In most cases the latter is due to a defect in the mutase apoenzyme, but in others it is due to a defect in the biosynthesis of its adenosyl-B_{12} coenzyme. In some of these defects, only the synthesis of adenosyl-B_{12} is blocked; in others, the synthesis of methyl-B_{12} is also blocked.

Clinical symptoms in propionic and methylmalonic acidemia vary according to the location and severity of the enzyme block. Those with severe blocks present with acute, life-threatening metabolic acidemia and hyperammonemia early in infancy or with metabolic acidemia, vomiting, and failure to thrive during the first few months of life. Children with less severe blocks may show only mild or moderate mental retardation.

All known forms of propionic and methylmalonic acidemia are transmitted as autosomal recessive traits and can be diagnosed in utero.

Diagnosis

Laboratory findings include hyperglycinemia and hyperglycinuria, a positive methylmalonic aciduria screening test, the presence of diagnostic changes on urine organic acid chromatography (Table 30–4), and, in certain blocks of vitamin B_{12} metabolism, hypomethioninemic homocystinuria.

Treatment

Patients with enzyme blocks in B_{12} metabolism usually respond to massive (up to 1 mg/d) doses of vitamin B_{12} as given intramuscularly, whereas nonresponders require amino acid restriction and correction of their rather constant metabolic acidemia. Secondary carnitine deficiency has been reported, and blood carnitine should be measured and supplemented if required.

Ogier deBaulny H et al: Branched chain organic acidurias. In: *Inborn Metabolic Disease: Diagnosis and Treatment,* 2nd ed. Fernandez J et al (editors). Springer, 1995.

Shevell MI et al: Varying neurological phenotypes among mut[E] and mut[−] patients with methylmalonyl-CoA mutase deficiency. Am J Med Genet 1993;45:619.

Shinnar S, Singer HS: Cobalamin C mutation (methylmalonic aciduria and homocystinuria) in adolescence: A treatable cause of dementia and myelopathy. N Engl J Med 1984;311:451.

Werlin SL: *E. coli* sepsis as a presenting sign in neonatal propionic acidemia. Am J Med Genet 1993;46:455.

ISOVALERIC ACIDEMIA

This condition, due to deficiency of isovaleryl-CoA dehydrogenase in the leucine oxidative pathway, was the first organic acidemia to be described in humans. It usually presents with poor feeding, metabolic acidosis, seizures, and an odor of "sweaty feet" during the first few days of life, with coma and death occurring if the condition is not recognized and appropriate therapy quickly started. Other patients show a more chronic course, with episodes of vomiting, lethargy, and urine (and body) odor precipitated by intercurrent infections or increased protein intake. The condition is inherited as an autosomal recessive trait and can be diagnosed in utero.

Diagnosis

Isovaleric acidemia and glutaric acidemia type II

Table 30–4. Clinical and laboratory features of organic acidemias.

Disorder	Enzyme Defect	Clinical and Laboratory Features
Isovaleric acidemia	Isovaleryl-CoA dehydrogenase	Acidosis and "odor of sweaty feet" in infancy, or growth retardation and episodes of vomiting, lethargy, acidosis, and odor. Isovalerylglycine always present in urine, with 3-hydroxyisovaleric acid during acute episodes.
3-Methylcrotonyl-CoA carboxylase deficiency	3-Methylcrotonyl-CoA carboxylase	Acidosis and feeding problems in infancy, or Reye-like episodes in older child. 3-Methylcrotonylglycine in urine, usually with 3-hydroxyisovaleric acid.
Combined carboxylase deficiency	Holocarboxylase synthetase	Hypotonia and lactic acidosis in infancy. 3-Hydroxyisovaleric acid in urine, often with small amounts of 3-hydroxypropionic and methylcitric acids. Often biotin-responsive.
	Biotinidase	Alopecia, seborrheic rash, and ataxia in infancy or childhood. Urine organic acids as above. Usually biotin-responsive.
3-Hydroxy-3-methylglutaric acidemia	Hydroxymethylglutaryl-CoA lyase	Hypoglycemia and acidosis in infancy; Reye-like episodes with non-ketotic hypoglycemia in older children. 3-Hydroxy-3-methylglutaric, 3-methylglutaconic, and 3-hydroxyisovaleric acids in urine.
3-Ketothiolase deficiency	3-Ketothiolase	Ketotic hyperglycinemia syndrome in infancy, or developmental and growth retardation with episodes of vomiting, acidosis, and encephalopathy. 2-Methyl-3-hydroxybutyric and 2-methylacetoacetic acids and tiglylglycine in urine, especially after isoleucine load.
Propionic acidemia	Propionyl-CoA carboxylase	Hyperammonemia and metabolic acidosis in infancy; ketotic hyperglycinemia syndrome later. 3-Hydroxypropionic and methylcitric acids in urine, with 3-hydroxy- and 3-ketovaleric acids during ketotic episodes.
Methylmalonic acidemia	Methylmalonyl-CoA mutase	Clinical features same as in propionic acidemia. Methylmalonic acid in urine, often with 3-hydroxypropionic and methylcitric acids.
	Defects in B_{12} biosynthesis	Clinical features same as above when only adenosyl-B_{12} synthesis is decreased: early neurologic features prominent when accompanied by decreased synthesis of methyl-B_{12}. In latter instance, hypomethioninemia and homocystinuria accompany methylmalonic aciduria.
Pyroglutamic acidemia	Glutathione synthetase	Acidosis and hemolytic anemia in infancy; chronic acidosis later. Pyroglutamic acid in urine.
Glutaric acidemia type I	Glutaryl-CoA dehydrogenase	Progressive extrapyramidal movement disorder in childhood, with episodes of acidosis, vomiting, and encephalopathy. Glutaric acid in urine, usually with 3-hydroxyglutaric acid.
Glutaric acidemia type II	Electron transfer flavoprotein (ETF) ETF:ubiquinone oxidoreductase (ETF dehydrogenase)	Hypoglycemia, acidosis, hyperammonemia, and "odor of sweaty feet" in infancy, often with polycystic and dysplastic kidneys. Later onset may be with episodes of hypoketotic hypoglycemia or slowly progressive skeletal myopathy. Glutaric, ethylmalonic, 3-hydroxyisovaleric, isovalerylglycine, and 2-hydroxyglutaric acids in urine, often with sarcosine in serum and urine.
4-Hydroxybutyric acidemia	Succinic semialdehyde dehydrogenase	Seizures and developmental retardation. 4-Hydroxybutyric acid in urine.

are the only conditions in which the characteristic odor of "sweaty feet" occurs. Isovalerylglycine is consistently detected in the urine by organic acid chromatography.

Treatment

Providing a low-protein diet or diets low in leucine or all three branched-chain amino acids is effective. Oral administration of glycine appears to prevent complications during acute infections but poses a risk of neurotoxicity due to severe hyper-glycinemia. Oral administration of L-carnitine may also be indicated.

Cohn RM et al: Isovaleric acidemia: Use of glycine therapy in neonates. N Engl J Med 1978;299:996.

de Sousa C et al: The response to L-carnitine and glycine therapy in isovaleric acidaemia. Eur J Pediatr 1986; 144:451.

Ogier deBaulny H et al: Branched chain organic acidurias. In: *Inborn Metabolic Disease: Diagnosis and Treatment*, 2nd ed. Fernandez J et al (editors). Springer, 1995.

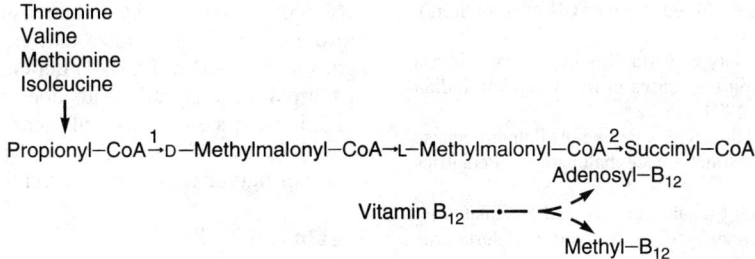

Figure 30–2. Oxidation of propionyl-CoA to succinyl-CoA. **1.** Propionyl-CoA carboxylase. **2.** Methylmalonyl-CoA mutase.

COMBINED CARBOXYLASE DEFICIENCY

Holocarboxylase synthetase and biotinidase are two enzymes of biotin metabolism in mammals. Holocarboxylase synthetase covalently binds biotin to the apocarboxylases for pyruvate, 3-methylcrotonyl-CoA, and propionyl-CoA; and biotinidase releases biotin from these proteins and from proteins in the diet. Recessively inherited deficiency of either enzyme causes deficiency of all three carboxylases, ie, multiple carboxylase deficiency. Holocarboxylase synthetase deficiency usually presents in the neonatal period with hypotonia, and biotinidase deficiency more often presents somewhat later with a syndrome of ataxia, seborrhea, and alopecia. Because many patients with biotinidase deficiency do not show typical symptoms but do develop neurologic sequelae, newborn screening for the condition may be justified.

Diagnosis

This diagnosis should be considered in patients with typical symptoms or in those with primary lactic acidosis. Urine organic acids are usually but not always abnormal (Table 30–4). Diagnosis is usually by enzyme assay. Biotinidase can be assayed in serum; holocarboxylase synthetase, in leukocytes or fibroblasts.

Treatment

Oral administration of biotin in large doses, 10–20 mg/d, often reverses the organic aciduria within days and the clinical symptoms within days to weeks. The incidence of hearing loss is high even in treated patients.

Burri BJ, Sweetman L, Nyhan WL: Heterogeneity of holocarboxylase synthetase in patients with biotin-responsive multiple carboxylase deficiency. Am J Hum Genet 1985;37:326.

Kalayci O et al: Infantile spasms as the initial symptom of biotinidase deficiency. J Pediatr 1994;124:103.

McVoy JRS et al: Partial biotinidase deficiency: Clinical and biochemical features. J Pediatr 1990;116:78.

Wolf B, Heard GS: Screening for biotinidase deficiency in newborns: Worldwide experience. Pediatrics 1990;-85:512.

GLUTARIC ACIDEMIA TYPE I

Glutaric acidemia type I is due to deficiency of glutaryl-CoA dehydrogenase and causes a progressive extrapyramidal movement disorder in childhood, with dystonia and athetosis and neuronal degeneration in the caudate and putamen. Macrocephaly at birth is common. Death often occurs during the first decade, but the clinical course is highly variable, and several patients have had only mild neurologic abnormalities. Children with glutaric acidemia type I may present with retinal hemorrhages and intracranial bleeding, strongly resembling shaken baby syndrome. The condition is inherited as an autosomal recessive trait.

Diagnosis

Glutaric acidemia type I should be suspected in any patient with progressive dystonia or athetosis. The diagnosis is confirmed by demonstration of glutaric and 3-hydroxyglutaric acids in urine by organic acid analysis. Deficiency of glutaryl-CoA dehydrogenase can be demonstrated in fibroblasts, leukocytes, and, for prenatal diagnosis, amniotic cells.

Treatment

Restriction of dietary lysine and tryptophan is indicated, but neurologic symptoms, once present, may not resolve. A variety of drugs that alter neurotransmitter levels, especially GABA, may be used to control dystonia. Studies suggest that early dietary treatment and aggressive management of intercurrent illness may prevent neurologic deterioration in some patients.

Goodman SI, Frerman FE: Organic acidemias due to defects in lysine oxidation: 2-ketoadipic acidemia and glutaric acidemia. In: The Molecular and Metabolic Bases of Inherited Disease, 7th ed. Scriver CR et al (editors). McGraw-Hill, 1995.

Haworth JC et al: Phenotypic variability in glutaric aciduria type I: Report of fourteen cases in five Canadian Indian kindreds. J Pediatr 1991;118:52.

Hoffman GF et al: Glutaryl-coenzyme A dehydrogenase deficiency: A distinct encephalopathy. Pediatrics 1991;88:1194.

Iafolla AK, Kahler SG: Megalencephaly in the neonatal period as the initial manifestation of glutaric aciduria type I. J Pediatr 1989;115:1004.

DISORDERS OF FATTY ACID OXIDATION & CARNITINE

LONG-CHAIN & MEDIUM-CHAIN ACYL-CoA DEHYDROGENASE DEFICIENCIES

Deficiencies of long-chain and medium-chain acyl-CoA dehydrogenase (LCAD, MCAD) and long-chain hydroxyacyl-CoA dehydrogenase (LCHAD), three enzymes of fatty acid β-oxidation, usually cause Reye-like episodes of hypoketotic hypoglycemia, mild hyperammonemia, hepatomegaly and encephalopathy, or, less often, sudden death in infancy. The long- and medium-chain defects can usually be distinguished clinically, with the long-chain defects more often causing early severe hypotonia and cardiomyopathy. MCAD deficiency is common, occurring in perhaps 1:5000 live births, and recent studies suggest that LCHAD deficiency may also be common. Although Reye-like episodes may be fatal, they tend to become less frequent and severe with time, and prolonged survival is typical of MCAD deficiency, with few deaths after diagnosis is made and treatment instituted. In LCAD and LCHAD deficiency, cardiomyopathy is the direct result of the defect in the oxidation of long-chain fatty acids, and progressive liver disease and renal tubular acidosis may also be present. These conditions are inherited as autosomal recessive traits.

Diagnosis

Suspicion should be aroused by the lack of an appropriate ketone response to fasting. Patients with MCAD deficiency excrete phenylpropionylglycine and hexanoylglycine in the urine, and the acylcarnitine profile is abnormal in blood; urine and blood findings may be highly variable in LCAD and LCHAD deficiency. A common mutation has been found in MCAD deficiency, which may be useful to prove the diagnosis. Reports suggest a common mutation in LCHAD deficiency may be similarly used. Assays of MCAD activity in fibroblasts are neces-

sary only when typical biochemistry is not found. However, fibroblast studies may be required for diagnosis of LCAD or LCHAD deficiency. The finding of normal urine organic acids does not exclude these conditions, since excretion of dicarboxylic acids and other products of microsomal and peroxisomal oxidation of fatty acids can be intermittent.

Treatment

Acute management is directed toward preventing or reversing catabolism and hypoglycemia. Long-term measures include providing carbohydrate snacks before bedtime and vigorous treatment of intercurrent infections. Because cardiomyopathy and muscle weakness in MCAD deficiency may be due to secondary carnitine deficiency, oral administration of carnitine is typically prescribed. Medium-chain triglycerides are contraindicated in MCAD deficiency because they may cause serum octanoic acid to rise to neurotoxic concentrations, but they appear to be a useful energy source for patients with LCAD and LCHAD deficiency.

Duran M et al: Sudden child death and "healthy" affected family members with medium-chain acyl-coenzyme A dehydrogenase deficiency. Pediatrics 1986;78:1052.

Hale DE, Bennett MJ: Fatty acid oxidation disorders: A new class of metabolic diseases. J Pediatr 1992;121:1.

Pollitt RJ: Disorders of mitochondrial β-oxidation: Prenatal and early postnatal diagnosis and their relevance to Reye's syndrome and sudden infant death. J Inherited Metab Dis 1989;12:215.

Rhead WJ: Inborn errors of fatty acid oxidation in man. Clin Biochem 1991;24:319.

Stanley CA: Disorders of fatty oxidation. In: *Inborn Metabolic Disease: Diagnosis and Treatment*, 2nd ed. Fernandez J et al (editors). Springer, 1995.

Taubman B, Hale DE, Kelley RI: Familial Reye-like syndrome: A presentation of medium-chain acyl-coenzyme A dehydrogenase deficiency. Pediatrics 1987;79:382.

Vockley J: The changing face of disorders of fatty acid oxidation. Mayo Clin Proc 1994;69:249.

Wanders RJ et al: Long chain 3-hydroxyacyl-CoA dehydrogenase deficiency: Different clinical expression in three unrelated patients. J Inherited Metab Dis 1991; 14:325.

GLUTARIC ACIDEMIA TYPE II

Glutaric acidemia type II (multiple acyl-CoA dehydrogenation deficiency) was first described in 1976 in a baby who died at 3 days of age with profound hypoglycemia, metabolic acidosis, and the "smell of sweaty feet." Since that time, many others have been diagnosed. Some have renal cysts and die in early infancy, and others have Reye-like episodes or skeletal muscle weakness (or both) beginning in childhood or adolescence. Some patients are deficient in electron transfer flavoprotein and others in ETF:ubiquinone oxidoreductase, proteins that transfer electrons from many flavin-containing enzymes of fatty acid and amino acid oxidation into the respiratory chain. Both enzyme deficiencies are inherited as autosomal recessive traits, and the infantile form of the disease can be diagnosed in utero.

Diagnosis

Diagnosis can be made by demonstrating derivatives of the substrates of mitochondrial flavin-containing dehydrogenases on organic acid analysis of urine (Table 30–4). Tissue assays of electron transfer flavoprotein and ETF:ubiquinone oxidoreductase are not usually necessary.

Treatment

Dietary measures (carbohydrate feedings before bedtime, provision of bicarbonate, and restriction of fat) are variably effective, and administration of riboflavin and carnitine has shown promise, usually in older patients.

Frerman FE, Goodman SI: Glutaric acidemia type II and defects of the mitochondrial respiratory chain. In: *The Molecular and Metabolic Bases of Inherited Disease,* 7th ed. Scriver CR et al (editors). McGraw-Hill, 1995.

Goodman SI, Loehr JP, Frerman FE: Clinical and biochemical aspects of glutaric acidemia Type II. In: *Fatty Acid Oxidation: Clinical, Biochemical, and Molecular Aspects.* Liss, 1990.

CARNITINE

Carnitine is an essential nutrient that is found in highest concentrations in red meats. Its primary function is to transport long-chain fatty acids into mitochondria for oxidation. Primary defects of carnitine biosynthesis and transport exist and may present with Reye's syndrome, myoglobinuria, hypotonia, or cardiomyopathy. These disorders are exceedingly rare compared with secondary carnitine deficiency or insufficiency, which may be due to diet (especially hyperalimentation), renal losses, drug therapy (especially valproic acid), and other metabolic disorders (especially disorders of fatty acid oxidation and organic acidemias). The prognosis depends on the cause of the carnitine abnormality.

Carnitine can be measured in blood. Unless the purpose is solely to monitor dietary deficiency, amounts of free and esterified carnitine should be determined. In some situations, muscle carnitine may be low despite normal blood levels. Free and esterified carnitine also can be measured in urine, and specialized laboratories can identify the specific ester present. If carnitine insufficiency is suspected, the patient should be evaluated to rule out disorders that might cause secondary carnitine deficiency.

Oral levocarnitine is used in carnitine deficiency or insufficiency in doses of 25–100 mg/kg/d or higher. Intravenous levocarnitine may be added to hyperalimentation, and high-dose intravenous levocarnitine is available. Treatment is aimed at maintaining normal free carnitine levels. Carnitine supplementation in patients with disorders of fatty acid oxidation and organic acidosis may also augment excretion of accumulated metabolites in addition to ameliorating carnitine insufficiency. Supplementation may not prevent metabolic crises in such patients, however, even when serum carnitine has been normalized.

DeVivo DC, Tein I: Primary and secondary disorders of carnitine metabolism. Int Pediatr 1990;5:134.

Kelly KJ et al: Fatal rhabdomyolysis following influenza infection in a girl with familial carnitine palmityl transferase deficiency. Pediatrics 1988;84:312.

Matsuda I et al: Carnitine deficiency and hyperammonemia with valproate therapy. J Pediatr 1986;109:131.

Moukarzel AA et al: Carnitine status of children receiving long-term total parenteral nutrition: A longitudinal prospective study. J Pediatr 1992;120:759.

Schmidt-Sommerfeld E, Werner D, Penn D: Carnitine plasma concentrations in 353 metabolically healthy children. Eur J Pediatr 1988;147:356.

Shapira Y, Glick B, Gutman A: Carnitine deficiency. Int Pediatr 1993;8:219.

Stanley CA: Disorders of fatty acid oxidation. In: *Inborn Metabolic Disorders: Diagnosis and Treatment,* 2nd ed. Fernandez J et al (editors). Springer, 1995.

DISORDERS OF PURINE METABOLISM

HYPOXANTHINE-GUANINE PHOSPHORIBOSYLTRANSFERASE DEFICIENCY (Lesch-Nyhan Syndrome)

Hypoxanthine-guanine phosphoribosyltransferase (HPRT) is the enzyme that converts the purine bases hypoxanthine and guanine to inosine monophosphate (IMP) and guanosine monophosphate (GMP), respectively. The X-linked recessive disorder with complete deficiency is characterized by central nervous system dysfunction and purine overproduction with hyperuricemia and hyperuricuria. Depending on the residual activity of the mutant enzyme, male hemizygotes may be severely retarded and show choreoathetosis, spasticity, and compulsive, mutilating lip and finger biting, or they may present with only gouty arthritis and urate ureterolithiasis. The enzyme deficiency can be demonstrated in erythrocytes, fibroblasts, and cultured amniotic cells; this disorder can thus be diagnosed in utero.

Although the cause of the central nervous system dysfunction in Lesch-Nyhan syndrome remains obscure, the absent or less severe central nervous system manifestations of purine nucleoside phosphorylase deficiency suggest that the problem relates to accumulation of substrate behind the block.

Diagnosis

Diagnosis is made by demonstrating an elevated uric acid:creatinine ratio in urine, followed by demonstration of enzyme deficiency in red blood cells.

Treatment

Allopurinol and probenecid may be given to reduce hyperuricemia but do not affect the neurologic status. Insertion of the HPRT gene into cultured cells from affected patients and into experimental animals has been effective, and such experiments offer promise as models for human gene therapy in the future.

Van den Berghe G, Vincent MF: Disorders of purine and pyrimidine metabolism. In: *Inborn Metabolic Disorders: Diagnosis and Treatment,* 2nd ed. Fernandez J et al (editors). Springer-Verlag, 1995.

LYSOSOMAL DISEASES

Lysosomes are cellular organelles in which complex macromolecules are degraded by specific acid hydrolases. Deficiency of a lysosomal enzyme causes its substrate to accumulate in lysosomes of tissues that degrade it, creating a characteristic clinical picture. These so-called storage disorders are classified as mucopolysaccharidoses, lipidoses, or mucolipidoses depending on the nature of the stored material. Two additional disorders, cystinosis and Salla disease, are caused by defects in lysosomal proteins that normally transport material from the lysosome to the cytoplasm.

Clinical and laboratory features of these conditions are set forth in Table 30–5. Most are autosomal recessive traits, and all can be diagnosed in utero.

The diagnosis of mucopolysaccharidosis is suggested by certain clinical and radiologic findings and urine screening tests. Further tests are needed to determine which particular mucopolysaccharides are present. Diagnosis should be confirmed by enzyme assays of cultured fibroblasts or leukocytes; this is especially important when the parents are contemplating having more children.

When a lipidosis or mucolipidosis is suspected, diagnosis is made by appropriate enzyme assays of biopsy specimens, cultured skin fibroblasts, and peripheral leukocytes.

Most of these conditions cannot be treated effectively, though there is increasing evidence that bone marrow transplantation may affect the course of some lysosomal diseases. Gaucher's disease is treated effectively with infusions of natural enzyme modified to allow uptake of the enzyme by lysosomes.

Barth PG: Sphingolipids. In: *Inborn Metabolic Disorders: Diagnosis and Treatment,* 2nd ed. Fernandez J et al (editors). Springer, 1995.

Beck M, Spranger J: Mucopolysaccharides and oligosaccharides. In: *Inborn Metabolic Disorders: Diagnosis and Treatment,* 2nd ed. Fernandez J et al (editors). Springer, 1995.

Grabowski G: Clinical and therapeutic perspectives on Gaucher disease. Int Pediatr 1993;8:22.

Muenzer J: Mucopolysaccharidoses. Acta Pediatr 1986;33:269.

Sidransky E, Ginns EI: Clinical heterogeneity among patients with Gaucher's disease. JAMA 1993;269:1154.

Whitley CB et al: Long-term outcome of Hurler syndrome following bone marrow transplantation. Am J Med Genet 1993;46:209.

PEROXISOMAL DISEASES

Peroxisomes are intracellular organelles that contain a large number of enzymes, many of which are oxidases linked to catalase or peroxidase. Among the enzyme systems in peroxisomes is one for β-oxidation of very long chain fatty acids (which is analogous in many ways to the system for fatty acid oxidation in mitochondria) and another for plasmalogen biosynthesis. In addition, peroxisomes contain oxidases for D- and L-amino acids, pipecolic acid and phytanic acid, and an enzyme (alanine-glyoxylate aminotransferase) that effects transamination of glyoxylate to glycine.

In some peroxisomal diseases, many enzymes are deficient. Zellweger (cerebrohepatorenal) syndrome, the best known among these, is probably due to a defect in organelle assembly. Patients present in infancy with seizures, hypotonia, characteristic facies with a large forehead, and hepatomegaly and at autopsy show renal cysts and absent peroxisomes. Neonatal adrenoleukodystrophy and hyperpipecolic acidemia have similar clinical and laboratory findings and multiple enzyme deficiencies in cultured fibroblasts, but peroxisomes are usually detected in tissues.

In other peroxisomal diseases, only a single enzyme is deficient. Primary hyperoxaluria (alanine-

Table 30–5. Clinical and laboratory features of lysosomal storage diseases.

Disorder	Enzyme Defect	Clinical and Laboratory Features
I. Mucopolysaccharidoses		
Hurler syndrome	α-Iduronidase	Autosomal recessive. Mental retardation, hepatosplenomegaly, umbilical hernia, coarse facies, corneal clouding, dorsolumbar gibbus, severe heart disease. Heparan sulfate and dermatan sulfate in urine.
Scheie syndrome	α-Iduronidase (incomplete)	Autosomal recessive. Corneal clouding, stiff joints, normal intellect. Clinical types intermediate between Hurler and Scheie common. Heparan sulfate and dermatan sulfate in urine.
Hunter syndrome	Sulfoiduronate sulfatase	X-linked recessive. Coarse facies, hepatosplenomegaly, mental retardation variable. Corneal clouding and gibbus not present. Heparan sulfate and dermatan sulfate in urine.
Sanfilippo syndrome: Type A Type B Type C Type D	 Sulfamidase α-N-Acetylglucos-aminidase Acetyl-CoA: α-glucosaminide-N-acetyltransferase α-N-acetylglucosamine-6-sulfatase	Autosomal recessive. Severe mental retardation with comparatively mild skeletal changes, visceromegaly, and facial coarseness. Types cannot be differentiated clinically. Heparan sulfate in urine.
Morquio syndrome	N-Acetylgalactosamine-6-sulfatase	Autosomal recessive. Severe skeletal changes, platyspondylisis, corneal clouding. Keratan sulfate in urine.
Maroteaux-Lamy syndrome	N-Acetylgalactosamine-4-sulfatase	Autosomal recessive. Coarse facies, growth retardation, dorsolumbar gibbus, corneal clouding, hepatosplenomegaly, normal intellect. Dermatan sulfate in urine.
β-Glucuronidase deficiency	β-Glucuronidase	Autosomal recessive. Varies from mental retardation, dorsolumbar gibbus, corneal clouding, and hepatosplenomegaly to mild facial coarseness, retardation, and loose joints. Hearing loss common. Dermatan sulfate or heparan sulfate in urine.
II. Mucolipidoses		
Mannosidosis	α-Mannosidase	Autosomal recessive. Varies from severe mental retardation, coarse facies, short stature, skeletal changes, and hepatosplenomegaly to mild facial coarseness and loose joints. Hearing loss common. Abnormal oligosaccharides in urine.
Fucosidosis	α-Fucosidase	Autosomal recessive. Variable: coarse facies, skeletal changes, hepatosplenomegaly, occasional angiokeratoma corporis diffusum. Abnormal oligosaccharides in urine.
I-cell disease (mucolipidosis II)	N-Acetylglucosaminyl-phosphotransferase	Autosomal recessive; severe and mild forms known. Very short stature, mental retardation, early facial coarsening, clear cornea, stiffness of joints. Increased lysosomal enzymes in serum. Abnormal sialyl oligosaccharides in urine.
Sialidosis	N-Acetylineuraminidase (sialidase)	Autosomal recessive. Mental retardation, coarse facies, skeletal dysplasia, myoclonic seizures, cherry-red macular spot. Abnormal sialyl oligosaccharides in urine.
III. Lipidoses		
Niemann-Pick disease	Sphingomyelinase	Autosomal recessive. Acute and chronic forms known. Acute neuronopathic form common in eastern European Jews. Accumulation of sphingomyelin in lysosomes of RE system and CNS. Hepatosplenomegaly, developmental retardation, macular cherry-red spot. Death by 1–4 years.
Metachromatic leukodystrophy	Arylsulfatase A	Autosomal recessive. Late infantile form, with onset at 1–4 years, most common. Accumulation of sulfatide in white matter. Gait disturbances (ataxia), motor incoordination, and dementia. Death usually in first decade.
Krabbe disease (globoid cell leukodystrophy)	Galactocerebroside β-galactosidase	Autosomal recessive. Globoid cells in white matter. Onset at 3–6 months with seizures, irritability, and retardation. Death by 1–2 years. Juvenile and adult forms are rare.

(*continued*)

Table 30–5. Clinical and laboratory features of lysosomal storage diseases. (continued)

Disorder	Enzyme Defect	Clinical and Laboratory Features
Fabry disease	α-Galactosidase A	X-linked recessive. Storage of trihexosylceramide in endothelial cells. Pain in extremities, angiokeratoma corporis diffusum and (later) poor vision, hypertension, and renal failure.
Farber disease	Ceramidase	Autosomal recessive. Storage of ceramide in tissues. Subcutaneous nodules, arthropathy with deformed and painful joints, and poor growth and development. Death within first year.
Gaucher disease	Glucocerebroside β-glucosidase	Autosomal recessive. Acute neuronopathic form: Accumulation of glucocerebroside in lysosomes of RE system and CNS. Retardation, hepatosplenomegaly, macular cherry-red spot, and Gaucher cells in bone marrow. Death by 1–2 years. Chronic form common in eastern European Jews. Accumulation of spingomyelin in lysosomes of RE system. Hepatosplenomegaly and flask-shaped osteolytic bone lesions. Consistent with normal life expectancy.
G_{M1} gangliosidosis	GM_1 ganglioside β-galactosidase	Autosomal recessive. Accumulation of G_{M1} ganglioside in lysosomes of RE system and CNS. Infantile form: Abnormalities at birth with dysostosis multiplex, hepatosplenomegaly, macular cherry-red spot, and death by 2 years. Juvenile form: Normal development to 1 year of age, then ataxia, weakness, dementia, and death by 4–5 years. Occasional inferior beaking of vertebral bodies of L1 and L2.
G_{M2} gangliosidoses Tay-Sachs disease Sandhoff disease	β-N-Acetylhexos-aminidase A β-N-Acetylhexos-aminidase A & B	Autosomal recessive. Tay-Sachs disease common in eastern European Jews; Sandhoff disease is panethnic. Clinical phenotypes are identical, with accumulation of G_{M2} ganglioside in lysosomes of CNS. Onset at age 3–6 months, with hypotonia, hyperacusis, retardation, and macular cherry-red spot. Death by 2–3 years. Juvenile and adult onset forms of Tay-Sachs disease are rare.
Wolman disease	Acid lipase	Autosomal recessive. Accumulation of cholesterol esters and triglycerides in lysosomes of reticuloendothelial system. Onset in infancy with gastrointestinal symptoms and hepatosplenomegaly, and death by 3–6 months. Adrenals commonly enlarged and calcified.

glyoxalate aminotransferase deficiency), X-linked adrenoleukodystrophy and adrenomyeloneuropathy (very long chain acyl-CoA ligase deficiency), and adult Refsum's disease (phytanic acid oxidase deficiency) are disorders due to deficiency of single peroxisomal enzymes.

Except for childhood adrenoleukodystrophy, which is X-linked, all peroxisomal diseases are transmitted as autosomal recessive traits and can be diagnosed in utero. Bone marrow transplantation may be effective treatment for males with adrenoleukodystrophy. Dietary treatment may have some promise for female carriers of X-linked adrenomyeloneuropathy, and diet therapy is being attempted in other peroxisomal disorders.

Diagnosis

The best screening test for Zellweger syndrome, hyperpipecolic acidemia, X-linked adrenoleukodystrophy, neonatal adrenoleukodystrophy, and infantile Refsum's disease is determination of very long chain fatty acids in serum or plasma; these acids are increased in all of these conditions. Urine bile acids are abnormal in other peroxisomal disorders; together, these studies identify most peroxisomal diseases. Tis-

sue biopsy and appropriate enzyme assays are needed for confirmation, especially when a family plans further pregnancies.

Aubourg P et al: A two-year trial of oleic and erucic acids ("Lorenzo's oil") as treatment for adrenomyeloneuropathy. N Engl J Med 1993;329:745.

Moser HW et al: Adrenoleukodystrophy: Phenotypic variability and implications for therapy. J Inherit Metab Dis 1992;15:645.

Moser HW: Peroxisomal disorders. Clin Biochem 1991; 24:343.

Sadeghi-Nejad A, Senior B: Adreno-myeloneuropathy presenting as Addison's disease in childhood. N Engl J Med 1990;322:13.

CARBOHYDRATE-DEFICIENT GLYCOPROTEIN SYNDROMES

A variety of proteins, including many enzymes, require glycosylation with various carbohydrate moieties for normal function. The carbohydrate-deficient glycoprotein syndromes are a family of disorders that result from failures of glycosylation. Type I usually presents with prenatal growth disturbance, often with abnormal fat, cerebellar hypoplasia, typical facial dysmorphic features, and mental retardation. The typical course is remarkable for chronic liver disease, peripheral neuropathy, endocrinopathies, retinopathy, and, in some patients, acute life-threatening events. Biochemical differences and variations in clinical course, eg, the absence of peripheral neuropathy, characterize the other types. Pathophysiology probably relates to defects of those biochemical pathways that require glycosylated proteins. The syndromes appear so far to be inherited in an autosomal recessive manner, and frequency was initially estimated to be as high as 1:20,000 in northern Europe.

Diagnosis

Diagnosis is supported by finding altered levels of glycosylated enzymes or other proteins such as transferrin, thyroxine-binding globulin, lysosomal enzymes, clotting factors, etc, but these may be normal in carbohydrate-deficient glycoprotein syndromes or altered in other conditions. Diagnosis is confirmed by demonstration of typical patterns of altered isoelectric focusing of selected proteins, with most diagnostic laboratories examining serum transferrin. Some patients with type I carbohydrate-deficient glycoprotein syndrome may be demonstrated to have deficient activity of phosphomannomutase in fibroblasts.

Treatment

Treatment is supportive, with opportunity to monitor and provide early treatment for expected clinical features. Trials of therapy with mannose supplementation for patients with demonstrated defects of mannose incorporation into glycoproteins are under way.

Jaeken J, Carchon H: The carbohydrate-deficient glycoprotein syndromes: An overview. J Inherit Metab Dis 1993;16:813.

Petersen MB et al: Early manifestations of the carbohydrate-deficient glycoprotein syndrome. J Pediatr 1993;122:66.

growth, mental retardation, typical dysmorphic features of face and extremities, and frequent malformations of the heart and genitourinary system. Severity ranges from survival with moderate to severe mental retardation to early death. In 1994, thirty years after the initial report of this syndrome, decreased levels of cholesterol with increased levels of precursor 7-dehydrocholesterol was found in affected individuals. Deficient synthesis of cholesterol leads directly to deficiency of some hormones and all bile acids. Animal models show abnormal organogenesis, but pathophysiology remains unclear with respect to the question whether birth defects are due to decrease in cholesterol or to increase in levels of the 7-hydroxy precursor and its isomers. Frequency is estimated to be between 1:40,000 and 1:20,000.

Diagnosis

Elevated 7- and 8-dehydrocholesterol in serum or other tissues, including amniotic fluid, is diagnostic. Serum cholesterol is typically low but may be in the normal range, especially in older individuals. 7-Dehydrocholesterol Δ^7-reductase may be measured in cultured fibroblasts or amniocytes.

Treatment

Supplementation with cholesterol has been reported to lead to improvements in growth and behavior, and the role (if any) of supplementation with bile acids is controversial. Studies are in progress to consider the extent to which postnatal treatment alters the course of a condition in which prenatal biochemical abnormality has altered development of multiple organs, including the brain.

Irons M et al: Clinical features of the Smith-Lemli-Opitz syndrome and treatment of the cholesterol metabolic defect. Int Pediatr 1995;10:28.

Tint GS et al: Defective cholesterol biosynthesis associated with the Smith-Lemli-Opitz syndrome. N Engl J Med 1994;330:107.

Xu G et al: Reproducing abnormal cholesterol biosynthesis as seen in the Smith-Lemli-Opitz syndrome by inhibiting the conversion of 7-dehydrocholesterol to cholesterol in rats. J Clin Invest 1995;95:76.

SMITH-LEMLI-OPITZ SYNDROME

Smith-Lemli-Opitz syndrome is an autosomal recessive disorder characterized by microcephaly, poor

REFERENCES

Clark JTR: *A Clinical Guide to Inherited Metabolic Diseases.* Cambridge Univ Press, 196.

Cohn RM, Roth KS: *Metabolic Disease: A Guide to Early Recognition. Saunders,* 1983.

Fernandez J, Saudubray J-M, Tada K (editors): *Inborn Metabolic Diseases: Diagnosis and Treatment,* 2nd ed. Springer, 1995.

Goodman SI, Markey SP: *Diagnosis of Organic Acidemias by Gas Chromatography-Mass Spectrometry.* Liss, 1981.

Scriver CR et al (editor): *The Molecular and Metabolic Bases of Inherited Disease,* 7th ed. McGraw-Hill, 1995.

Genetics & Dysmorphology

31

Eva Sujansky, MD, Janet M. Stewart, MD, & David K. Manchester, MD

New techniques in molecular biology and biochemistry have changed the way clinicians think about and approach birth defects. Molecular approaches to clinical problems now support "reverse genetics," the characterization of human disorders at the level of the gene before their clinical biochemistry and pathophysiology are described. The clinical implications of these advances are too numerous and extensive to be discussed completely in this text. The present chapter reviews human chromosomes and chromosome abnormalities, briefly describes diagnostic and therapeutic applications of recombinant DNA technology, and then outlines clinically important aspects of mendelian genetics, dysmorphology, and teratology. The chapter concludes with a review of the scope and approach of genetic counseling. The reader is directed to the referenced publications for more comprehensive discussion of the rapidly expanding field of clinical genetics.

I. CHROMOSOMES & CELL DIVISIONS

Human chromosomes consist of DNA and specific proteins. In a nondividing cell, chromosomes are tightly packaged in the nucleus. Chromosomes contain most of the genetic information necessary for growth and differentiation. Chromosome aberrations lead to physical and mental abnormalities. Documentation of chromosome abnormalities is important for appropriate management of the affected child and for assessment of the risk of recurrence; sometimes this risk affects many family members.

The nuclei of all normal human cells, with the exception of gametes, contain 46 chromosomes, consisting of 23 pairs (Figure 31–1). Of these, 22 pairs are called **autosomes.** They are numbered according to their size; chromosome 1 is the largest and chro-

mosome 22 the smallest. In addition, there are two **sex chromosomes:** two X chromosomes in females and one X and one Y chromosome in males. The two members of a chromosome pair are called **homologous chromosomes.** One homolog of each chromosome pair is maternal in origin (from the egg); the second is paternal (from the sperm). The egg and sperm each contain 23 chromosomes (**haploid cells).** During formation of the zygote, they fuse into a cell with 46 chromosomes (**diploid cell).** Subsequent prenatal and postnatal growth of the human organism is through somatic cell divisions called "mitoses."

Mitosis (Figure 31–2) is division of somatic cells. The process occurs in stages during which DNA replication takes place and two daughter cells, genetically identical to the original parent cells, are formed. During **metaphase**—the phase following DNA replication but preceding cell division—individual chromosomes can be visualized. They consist of two arms, a short arm and a long arm, separated by a centromere. Each arm consists of two identical parts, called **chromatids.** Chromatids of the same chromosome are called **sister chromatids.**

Meiosis (Figure 31–3), during which eggs and sperm are formed, is cell division limited to gametes. During meiosis, three unique processes take place:

(1) Crossing over of genetic material between two homologous chromosomes. This is preceded by pairing of both members of each chromosome pair, thus facilitating the physical exchange of homologous genetic material.

(2) Random assortment of maternally and paternally derived homologous chromosomes into the daughter cells. The distribution of maternal or paternal chromosomes to a particular daughter cell is independent for each such cell.

(3) Two cell divisions, the first of which is a **reduction division,** ie, a diploid parental cell with 46 chromosomes divides into two haploid daughter cells with 23 chromosomes each. The second meiotic division is like mitosis, ie, it consists of DNA replication in haploid cells and the formation of two genetically identical daughter cells.

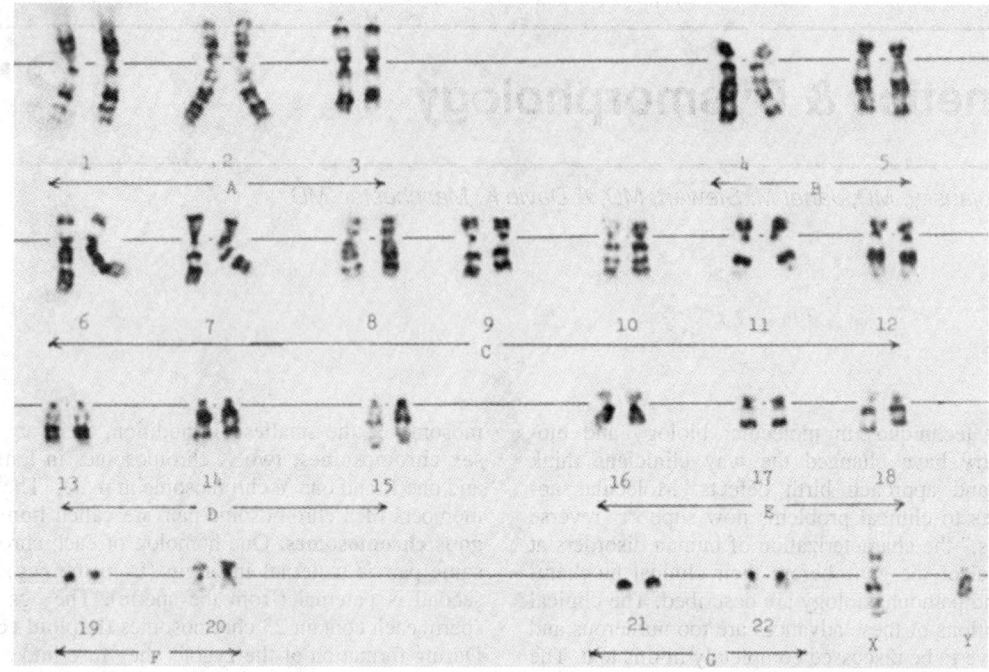

Figure 31–1. Normal male human karyotype.

CHROMOSOME PREPARATION & ANALYSIS

Chromosome structure is seen only during mitosis, most frequently achieved by stimulating for 3 days a blood lymphocyte culture with a mitogen. Other tissues used for this purpose include skin or internal organs, such as thymus or gonads. Chorionic villi or amniocytes are used for prenatal diagnosis. Spontaneously dividing cells without a mitogen are present in numbers sufficient for chromosome analysis only in the bone marrow. Because bone marrow is not readily accessible, it is used for chromosome analysis only when immediate identification of a patient's chromosome constitution is necessary for appropriate management (eg, to rule out trisomy 13 in a newborn with a complex congenital heart disease requiring immediate intervention).

Cells processed for routine chromosome analysis are stained on glass slides to yield a light-and-dark band pattern across the arms of the chromosomes (Figure 31–1). This band pattern is characteristic and reproducible for each chromosome, allowing the chromosomes to be arranged in homologous pairs and numeric and structural abnormalities to be identified. The layout of chromosomes on a sheet of paper in a predetermined order is called a **karyotype.** Other special chromosome studies include the following:

(1) **High-resolution chromosome analysis** of more elongated chromosomes, allowing visualization of more detailed chromosome bands and detection of abnormalities in a smaller segment of chromosome.

(2) **Fluorescent in situ hybridization (FISH).** Specific fluorescent-labeled DNA probes that hy-

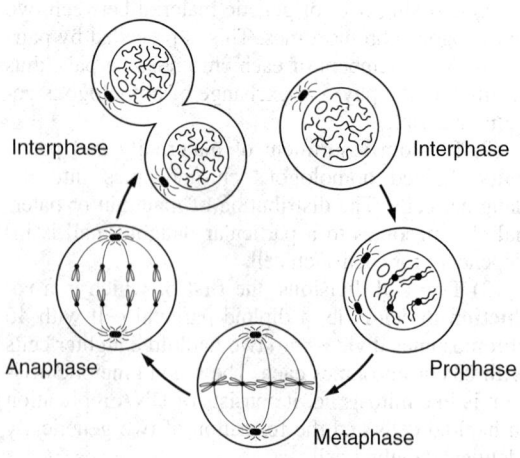

Figure 31–2. Stages of the mitotic cycle.

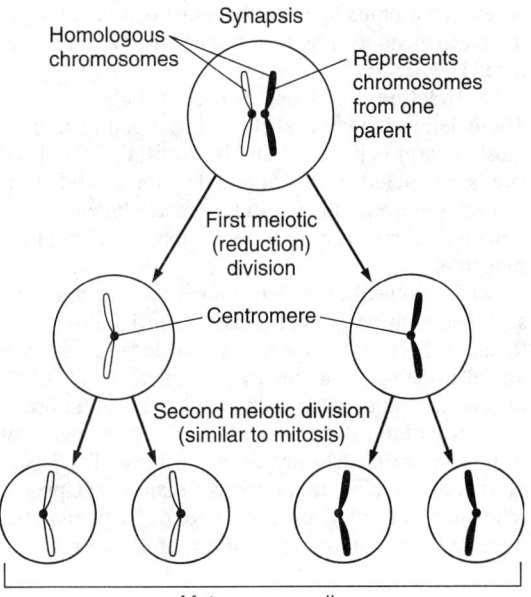

Figure 31–3. Meiosis—demonstrating conversion from the diploid somatic cell to the haploid gamete.

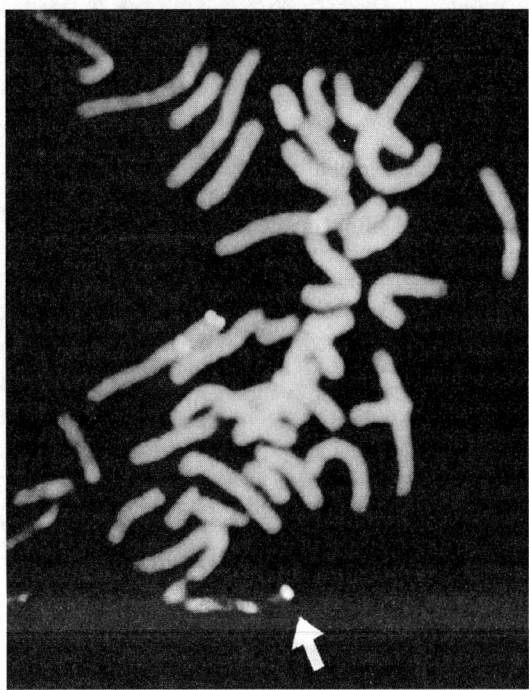

Figure 31–4. Fluorescent in situ hybridization (FISH), showing the brightly fluorescent probes of Wolf-Hirschhorn syndrome (4p deletion syndrome). One probe is hybridized to the normal location on chromosome 4; the other (arrow) documents 4/11 translocation, which was not detectable by a classic cytogenetic analysis.

bridize to the corresponding regions of chromosomes allow their visualization under a fluorescent microscope. If a cocktail of probes from the same chromosome is used, the whole chromosome may be stained (**chromosome painting**). FISH can detect submicroscopic structural rearrangements undetectable by classic cytogenetic techniques and can identify marker chromosomes in metaphase cells (Figure 31–4). It also allows interphase cells (lymphocytes, amniocytes) to be screened for numerical abnormalities such as trisomy 21. However, the study of interphase nuclei is not completely accurate, and any abnormality must be confirmed by conventional chromosome analysis.

(3) **Fragile X study** (see the section on fragile X syndrome, below).

(4) **Assessment of chromosome breaks and sister chromatid exchanges** requires special techniques that may lead to enhancement of the breaks or special staining that allows visualization of the exchanged chromatids.

CHROMOSOME NOMENCLATURE

Internationally accepted symbols for normal male and female constitution are 46,XY and 46,XX, re-

spectively. The sign (+) or (–) preceding the chromosome number indicates increased or decreased number, respectively, of that particular whole chromosome in a cell. For example, 47,XY+21 designates a male with three copies of chromosome 21. The sign (+) or (–) after the chromosome number signifies extra material or missing material, respectively, on one of the arms of the chromosome. The symbol for the short arm is p; for the long arm, q. Thus, 46,XX,8q– denotes a deletion on the long arm of chromosome 8. More detailed descriptions of structural abnormalities include break points in the rearrangement. For example, 46,XY,t(4:8)(q22;p21) means a reciprocal translocation (letter *t*) between the long arm of chromosome 4, at band 22, and the short arm of chromosome 8, at band 21. Examples of other common symbols include *del* (deletion), *dup* (duplication), *inv* (inversion), *ish* (in situ hybridization), *i* (isochromosome), *pat* (paternal origin), *mat* (maternal origin), and *r* (ring chromosome).

CHROMOSOME ABNORMALITIES

Errors during cell division may result in numerical or structural abnormalities of chromosomes.

Numerical abnormalities are the result of unequal division, called **nondisjunction,** of chromosomes into the daughter cells. Any deviation from the normal diploid number of chromosomes is called **aneuploidy.** This most frequently involves the presence of an additional chromosome, called **trisomy** (eg, trisomy 21, Down syndrome), or the presence of only a single copy of a chromosome, called **monosomy** (eg, monosomy X, Turner syndrome). Rarely, three copies **(triploidy)** of the whole set of 23 chromosomes are found. Four sets of chromosomes **(tetraploidy)** are not found in liveborn neonates.

Structural abnormalities are the result of breaks in chromosomes, which join randomly to form new combinations. In contrast to the numerical abnormalities, which result in trisomy or monosomy of a whole chromosome, structural chromosome abnormalities result in trisomy or monosomy (or both) of only part of a chromosome. The number of possible chromosome abnormalities is infinite. The following types of chromosome rearrangements, according to the mechanism leading to the abnormality, are recognized (Figure 31–5):

(1) **Deletion** is absence of part of a chromosome. The deletion is **terminal** if the distal end of a chromosome arm is included and **interstitial** if the distal end is not included. A terminal deletion of both arms of a chromosome may result in reattachment of the remaining arms, leading to formation of a **ring chromosome.**

(2) **Translocation** is detachment of a chromosome segment from its normal location and its attachment to another chromosome. The translocation is **balanced** if the cell contains two complete copies of all the chromosome material, though in a different order. In an **unbalanced translocation,** the rearrangement results in partial trisomy or monosomy. Translocations can be reciprocal or robertsonian. A **reciprocal translocation** involves exchange of segments between two chromosomes; for example, part of the short arm of chromosome 4 trades places with part of the long arm of chromosome 10. In **robertsonian translocations,** two acrocentric chromosomes fuse at their centromeres. The most frequent robertsonian translocation is formed between chromosomes 14 and 21.

(3) **Inversion** is the result of a double break in the

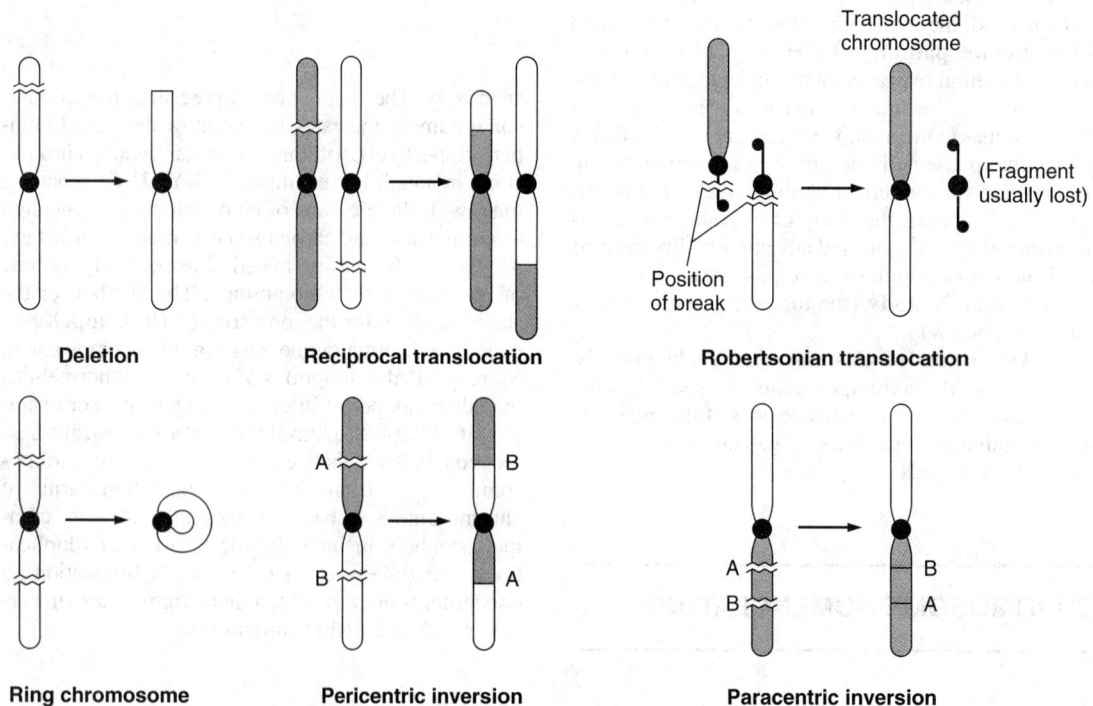

Deletion   **Reciprocal translocation**   **Translocated chromosome**   **Position of break**   **(Fragment usually lost)**   **Robertsonian translocation**

Ring chromosome   **Pericentric inversion**   A B   B A   **Paracentric inversion**   A B   B A

Figure 31–5. Examples of structural chromosome abnormalities.

same chromosome. The detached middle section turns upside down before reattaching. If both breaks are on the same side of the centromere, the inversion is **paracentric;** if the breaks are on the opposite arms of a chromosome, the inversion is **pericentric.**

MOSAICISM

Mosaicism is the presence of two or more different chromosome constitutions in different cells of the same individual. For example, a patient may have some cells with 47 chromosomes and others with 46 chromosomes; 46,XX/47,XX,+21 indicates mosaicism for trisomy 21; 45,X/46,XX/47,XXX indicates mosaicism for a monosomy and a trisomy X. Mosaicism should be suspected if clinical symptoms are milder than expected in a nonmosaic patient with the same chromosome abnormality or if the patient's skin shows patchy or streaky hyper- or hypopigmentation. The prognosis is frequently better for a patient with mosaicism than for one with a corresponding chromosome abnormality without mosaicism. In general, the smaller the proportion of the abnormal cell line, the better the prognosis. In the same patient, however, the proportion of normal and abnormal cells in various tissues, such as in skin and peripheral blood, may be significantly different. A prognosis frequently cannot be reliably assessed and should be made with caution or deferred. Mosaicism for structural abnormalities is very rare.

UNIPARENTAL DISOMY

Under normal circumstances, one member of each homologous pair of chromosomes is of maternal origin from the egg and the other is of paternal origin from the sperm (Figure 31–6A). In uniparental **disomy,** both copies of a particular chromosome pair originate from the same parent. If uniparental disomy is caused by chromosome error in the first meiotic division, both homologous chromosomes of that parent will be present in the gamete. This is called **heterodisomy** (Figure 31–6B). If the disomy is caused by an error in the second meiotic division, two copies of the same chromosome will be present. This is called **isodisomy** (Figure 31–6C). The union of a disomic gamete with a nullisomic gamete from the other parent will result in a zygote with a normal karyotype. Therefore, uniparental disomy would not be detected by chromosome analysis. However, DNA analysis would reveal that the child inherited two copies of DNA of a particular chromosome from one parent without the contribution from the other parent. Uniparental disomy has been documented for human chromosomes 7, 11, 15, and X. It has been found in patients with Prader-Willi, Angelman, and Beckwith-Wiedemann syndromes. In addition, cystic fibrosis with only one carrier parent (caused by maternal isodisomy) has been reported. Hemophilia A has been passed from father to son as a result of paternal heterodisomy of X and Y.

Uniparental disomy causes severe prenatal and postnatal growth retardation. Furthermore, it is sus-

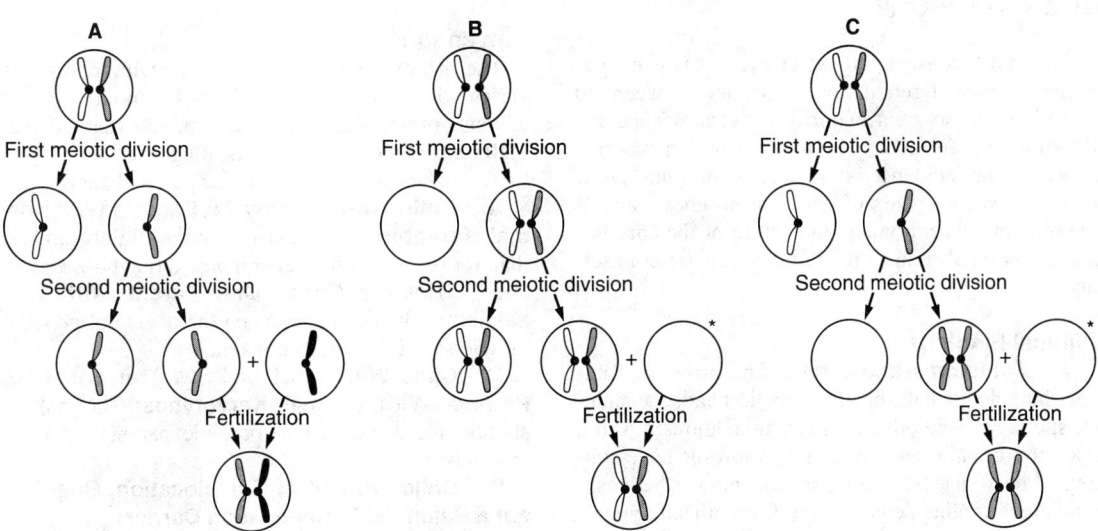

Figure 31–6. The assortment of homologous chromosomes during normal gametogenesis and uniparental disomy. **A:** Fertilization of normal gametes. **B:** Heterodisomy. **C:** Isodisomy. The asterisks in **B** and **C** indicate nullisomic gametes from the other parent.

pected that uniparental disomy of some chromosomes is lethal. The possible mechanisms for the adverse effects of uniparental disomy include possible homozygosity for deleterious recessive genes and the consequences of imprinting. (See principles of imprinting in the section on dysmorphology, below.)

CLINICAL SIGNIFICANCE OF CHROMOSOME ABNORMALITIES

Chromosome abnormalities result in dysmorphic features, major malformations, developmental delays, or mental retardation. As a rule, abnormalities of autosomes have more severe consequences than abnormalities of sex chromosomes, some of which result only in behavioral problems. Numerical abnormalities resulting in complete trisomy or monosomy are more deleterious than structural chromosome abnormalities resulting in duplication or deletion of a chromosome segment. It often happens that the smaller the duplicated or deleted segment, the milder the clinical symptoms. However, comparison of patients with duplications or deletions of different sizes in a particular chromosome indicates that involvement of a small specific segment sometimes has a disproportionately greater effect on mortality and morbidity.

ABNORMALITIES OF AUTOSOMES

DOWN SYNDROME

The most constant characteristic of Down syndrome is mental retardation. IQs vary between 20 and 80, with the great majority between 45 and 55. Down syndrome occurs in about 1:600 newborns; however, the incidence is greater among children of mothers over 35 years of age. The mother's age at the time of conception and the nature of the chromosome abnormality are important in genetic counseling.

Clinical Findings

A. Symptoms and Signs: The principal findings include a small, brachycephalic head, a characteristic facies, and other dysmorphic features.* About one-third of children with Down syndrome have congenital heart disease, most often an endocardial cushion defect or other septal defect. Generalized hypoto-

---

*For details, see Jones KL: *Smith's Recognizable Patterns of Human Malformation,* 5th ed. Saunders, 1996.

nia is common. Sexual development is retarded, especially in males, who are usually sterile. The affected newborn is likely to have prolonged physiologic jaundice, polycythemia, and a transient leukemoid reaction. Later, there is an increased tendency for thyroid dysfunction, hearing loss, and atlantooccipital instability. Leukemia is 20 times more common in Down syndrome than in unaffected children. Under 2 years of age, this is often a megakaryocytic acute myelogenous leukemia; over 2 years, it is usually acute lymphoblastic leukemia; and by age 15, the risk of leukemia diminishes. Susceptibility to intercurrent infections is increased. Patients with Down syndrome have heightened sensitivity to the mydriatic effects of atropine instilled into the conjunctiva.

B. Laboratory Findings: The chromosome abnormalities are pathognomonic. In the great majority of cases (95%) there are 47 chromosomes with trisomy of chromosome 21. However, about 4% of sporadic cases and about one-third of familial cases have 46 chromosomes, including an abnormal translocated chromosome formed as the result of a centric fusion between two acrocentric chromosomes (robertsonian translocation), one of which is chromosome 21. The translocation is found in 10% of patients whose mothers are younger but in only 3% of those with older mothers. In structural chromosome rearrangements, only band q22 on the long arm of chromosome 21 need be trisomic for Down syndrome to occur.

Mosaicism of the 46/47 type can also occur in persons with Down syndrome. These patients may have milder symptoms, especially higher than expected IQs. Occasionally, normal parents of affected children have inapparent mosaicism.

Prevention

The risk of having a child affected with trisomy 21 varies with maternal age (1:2000 for mothers under 25 years of age; 1:50 for mothers 35–39 years of age; 1:20 for mothers over 40 years of age).

The risk is also affected by the parental karyotype:

A. Child With Trisomy 21, Parents With Normal Karyotypes: The risk is only slightly greater than for parents in the general population (1–2%).

B. Trisomic Child, One Parent With Mosaicism: The risk depends on the degree of gonadal mosaicism of the affected parent.

C. Child With 14/21 or 21/21 Translocation, Parents With Normal Karyotypes: The risk is slightly increased due to possible parental gonadal mosaicism.

D. Child With 14/21 Translocation, One Parent a Balanced Translocation Carrier:

1. When the mother is the carrier, there is a 10–15% chance that the child will be affected and a 33% chance that the child will be a balanced translocation carrier.

2. When the father is the carrier, there is a 3–5% chance of having another affected child, and 50% of the apparently unaffected children have a 50% chance of being carriers.

E. Child With 21/21 Translocation and One Parent With the Translocation: The recurrence risk is 100%.

Treatment

There is no convincing documentation of the merit of any of the forms of specific therapy that have been attempted, ranging from megadoses of vitamins to exercise programs proposed to overcome the physical and developmental abnormalities of the syndrome. Therapy is thus directed toward specific problems, eg, cardiac surgery or digitalis administration for heart problems, antibiotic administration for infections, tests of thyroid function, infant stimulation programs, special education, and occupational training. The goal of treatment is to help affected children develop to their full potential. Parents' participation in support groups should be encouraged.

Takashima S: Down syndrome. Curr Opin Neurol 1997;10:148.

TRISOMY 18 SYNDROME

The incidence of trisomy 18 syndrome is about 1:4000 live births, and the ratio of affected males to females is approximately 1:3. The mean maternal age is advanced. Affected babies frequently die in early infancy, though patients occasionally survive into childhood.

Clinical Findings

A. Symptoms and Signs: Trisomy 18 is characterized by prenatal and postnatal growth retardation; hypertonicity; dysmorphic features, including a characteristic face (Figure 31–7) and extremities;* and congenital heart disease (often ventricular septal defect or patent ductus arteriosus). Surviving children show significant developmental delay and mental retardation.

B. Laboratory Findings: In place of uniform trisomy 18, chromosome analysis occasionally reveals mosaicism for trisomy 18 or an unbalanced translocation involving a third number 18 and another chromosome. Rarely, double trisomies have been found in which trisomy X or trisomy 21 is present in addition to trisomy 18.

Complications

Complications are related to associated birth de-

fects. Death is often caused by heart failure or pneumonia.

Treatment & Prognosis

There is no treatment other than general supportive care. Death usually occurs in infancy or early childhood, though some patients have reached adulthood.

TRISOMY 13 SYNDROME

The incidence of trisomy 13 is about 1:12,000 live births, and 60% of affected individuals are female. The mean maternal age is increased. Death usually occurs in early infancy or by the second year of life, commonly as a result of heart failure or infection.

The symptoms and signs include prenatal and postnatal growth deficiency, arrhinencephaly, eye malformations (anophthalmia, colobomas), cleft lip and palate, polydactyly or syndactyly, and congenital heart disease (usually ventricular septal defect). The facies of an infant with trisomy 13 is shown in Figure 31–8.* Surviving children demonstrate failure to thrive, developmental retardation, apneic spells, seizures, and deafness.

Treatment is supportive. Because it is sometimes necessary to decide immediately after birth how extensive therapy should be for a severely malformed infant, this diagnosis (as well as one of trisomy 18) can be immediately confirmed by direct chromosome analysis of mitotic figures obtained from bone marrow. Prevention by genetic counseling is indicated. Prenatal diagnosis is available. The recurrence risks are analogous to those of similar chromosome situations in Down syndrome.

ABNORMALITIES OF SEX CHROMOSOMES

TURNER SYNDROME

The incidence of Turner syndrome is 1:10,000 females. However, it is estimated that 95% of conceptuses with monosomy X are miscarried and only 5% are liveborn. Turner syndrome should be ruled out in all females with short stature, webbing of the neck, coarctation of the aorta, or amenorrhea. Patients with pseudohypoparathyroidism and Noonan syndrome have a similar phenotype with normal chromosomes.

---

*For details, see Jones KL: *Smith's Recognizable Patterns of Human Malformation,* 5th ed. Saunders, 1996.

*For other abnormal findings, see Jones KL: *Smith's Recognizable Patterns of Human Malformation,* 5th ed. Saunders, 1996.

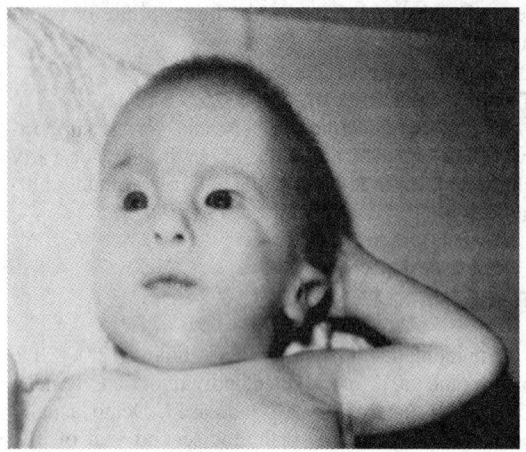 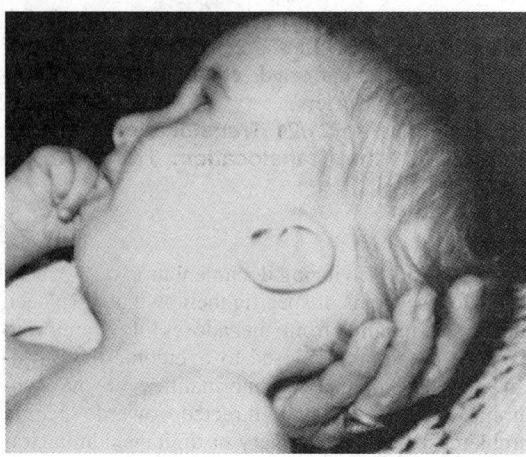

Figure 31–7. Child with trisomy 18.

Clinical Findings

A. Symptoms and Signs: Newborns with Turner syndrome may have webbed neck, edema of the hands and feet, coarctation of the aorta, and a characteristic triangular facies. Later symptoms include short stature, a shield chest with wide-set nipples, streak ovaries, amenorrhea, absence of secondary sex characteristics, and infertility. Some affected girls have only short stature and amenorrhea.

Complications relate primarily to coarctation of the aorta, when present. Rarely, the dysgenetic gonads may become neoplastic (gonadoblastoma). The incidence of malformations of the urinary tract is increased. Psychologic problems can arise from sexual infantilism and perceptual motor difficulties.

B. Laboratory Findings: Monosomy X (45,X) is found in a majority of patients. Mosaicism 45,X/46,XX or 45,X/46, XX/47,XXX may be present. Occasionally, the patient has two X chromosomes one of which has a structural abnormality, eg, deletion or translocation of part of one X to one of the autosomal chromosomes. Rarely, mosaicism 45,X/46,XY is found. The presence of a Y chromosome significantly increases the risk for gonadoblastoma.

Treatment & Prognosis

Treatment consists of identifying and treating perceptual problems before they become established. Estrogen replacement therapy will permit development of secondary sex characteristics and normal menstruation and prevent osteoporosis. Teenage patients need counseling to cope with the stigma of their condition and to understand the need for hormone therapy. Growth hormone therapy has been used to increase the height of affected girls. Females with 45,X or 45,X mosaicism have a low fertility rate, and those who become pregnant have a high risk of fetal wastage (spontaneous miscarriage, approximately 30%; stillbirth, 6–10%). Furthermore, their liveborn offspring have an increased frequency of chromosome abnormalities involving either sex chromosomes or autosomes and congenital malformations. Thus, prenatal ultrasonography and chromosome analysis are indicated for the offspring of females with sex chromosome abnormalities.

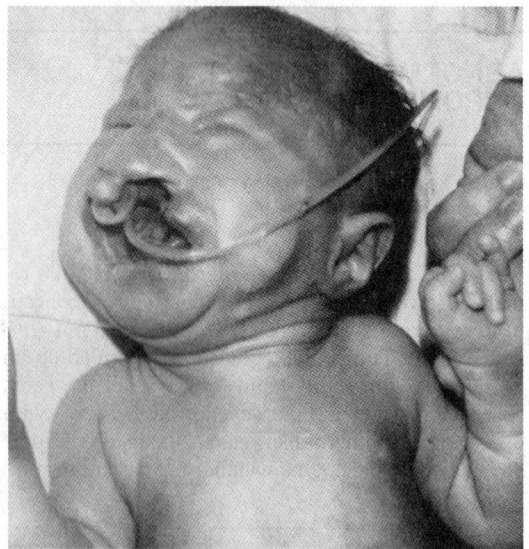

Figure 31–8. Child with trisomy 13.

KLINEFELTER SYNDROME

The incidence of Klinefelter syndrome in the newborn population is roughly 1:500, but it is about 1% among mentally retarded males and about 3% among males seen at infertility clinics. The maternal age at birth is often advanced. The diagnosis is rarely made before puberty except as a result of prenatal diagnosis. Unlike gonadal dysgenesis, Klinefelter syndrome is rarely the cause of spontaneous abortions.

Clinical Findings

A. Symptoms and Signs: Prepubertal boys have a normal phenotype. The characteristic findings after puberty include micro-orchidism associated with otherwise normal external genitalia, azoospermia, sterility, gynecomastia, normal to borderline IQ, diminished facial hair, lack of libido and potency, and a tall, eunuchoid build. In chromosome variants with three or four X chromosomes (XXXY and XXXXY), mental retardation may be severe, and radioulnar synostosis may be present as well as anomalies of the external genitalia and cryptorchidism. In the XXXXY cases, these findings are especially prominent, and there are also microcephaly, short stature, and dysmorphic features.

The adult XXYY patient tends to be taller and more retarded than the average XXY patient.

In general, the physical and mental abnormalities associated with Klinefelter syndrome increase as the number of sex chromosomes increases.

B. Laboratory Findings: The majority of cases have a 47,XXY constitution. Rare variants are 48,XXXY, 49,XXXXY, and 48,XXYY. A variety of mosaicisms containing combinations of the above, as well as 46,XY/47,XXY mosaicism, have been reported. Some patients with 46,XY/47,XXY mosaicism are fertile.

Urinary excretion of gonadotropins is high in adults. Levels are comparable to those found in postmenopausal women.

Linden MG, Bender BG, Robinson A: Sex chromosome tetrasomy and pentasomy. Pediatrics 1995;96:672.
Sotos JF: Genetic disorders associated with overgrowth. Clin Pediatr 1997;36:39.

XYY SYNDROME

The incidence of the 47,XYY karyotype in the newborn population is estimated at 1:1000 male births. Affected newborns in general are normal. Affected individuals may on occasion exhibit an abnormal behavior pattern from early childhood and may be slightly retarded. Fertility may be normal.

There is no treatment. Many males with an XYY karyotype are normal. Long-term problems may relate to low IQ and environmental stress.

RECURRENCE RISKS

Most numerical chromosome abnormalities occur sporadically. However, occurrences in siblings or other relatives have been reported, suggesting a hereditary predisposition to nondisjunction in some kindreds. Attempts to identify a single cause have been unsuccessful. It is reasonable to assign parents of a child with aneuploidy an empirical recurrence risk of 1–2% and offer prenatal diagnosis for subsequent pregnancies. Determination of the recurrence risk in structural chromosome abnormalities requires chromosome analysis of the parents to assess whether the abnormality was a sporadic occurrence or if a balanced rearrangement of chromosomes exists in one of the parents. If a balanced rearrangement is found, chromosome analysis of other family members must be attempted until all family members with the rearrangement have been identified. This analysis is important because—although members of kindreds with normal chromosomes are not at increased risk of recurrence (except in a rare case of gonadal mosaicism)—those with balanced structural rearrangements are at risk. The specific degree of risk varies according to the type of rearrangement and the chromosomes involved.

OTHER CHROMOSOME ABNORMALITIES

FRAGILE X SYNDROME

Fragile X syndrome, present in approximately 1:1000 males, accounts for 30–50% of cases of X-linked mental retardation. The responsible gene is named *FMR-1* and has unstable CGG repeats at the 5' end. Normal individuals have up to a 200 bp (base pair) fragment of cytidine phosphate guanosine dinucleotides. In asymptomatic carriers, this fragment is increased up to 500 bp (**premutation**) and in persons expressing the fragile X phenotype to over 600 bp (**full mutation**). Abnormal methylation of this region, found in persons with the full mutation, shuts off expression of the adjacent genes. DNA analysis is more reliable in detecting fragile X than the cytogenetic study and should be used when suspicion of fragile X is high, especially in known fragile X families. However, in the case of isolated developmental delay or behavioral problems, cytogenetic analysis is preferable since it may detect another chromosome abnormality.

The fragile site is visible only when the tissue culture medium used for chromosome analysis is deficient in folate or thymidine, so the cytogenetic laboratory must be informed in advance that a fragile X study is desired. Even under optimal circumstances, the fragile site is not expressed in all cells. In affected males, up to 50% of cells are positive. In female carriers of the gene, the fragile site is usually expressed in a low percentage of cells. Furthermore, approximately 40% of carrier females and 20% of males who carry the gene do not express the fragile site at all.

Most males with fragile X syndrome present with mental retardation, oblong face with large ears, and large testicles, especially after puberty. Other physical signs include evidence of connective tissue disorder, eg, hyperextensible joints and mitral valve prolapse. Most affected individuals are hyperactive and exhibit infantile autism or autistic-like behavior. However, some males with the abnormal gene are of normal phenotype.

In contrast, only about one-third of females with the fragile X chromosome show any degree of mental retardation. Abnormal physical features and behavioral problems are also less common. There is a difference in the clinical expression of fragile X in male and female offspring depending on which parent is transmitting the gene. The premutation can change into the full mutation only when passed through a female. Persons with the premutation have minimal or no risk of retardation.

Genetic counseling in families with this disorder used to be difficult because the incomplete penetrance of cytogenetic and clinical symptoms in both sexes precluded identification of all carriers. Identification of the abnormal DNA amplification by direct DNA analysis can detect nearly all asymptomatic gene carriers of both sexes. Therefore, DNA analysis is a reliable test for prenatal and postnatal diagnosis of fragile X and facilitates genetic counseling.

SYNDROMES ASSOCIATED WITH CHROMOSOME FRAGILITY

It is well known that such environmental factors as exposure to radiation, certain chemicals, and viruses contribute to chromosome breaks and rearrangements. However, some well-defined autosomal recessive syndromes are associated with a greatly increased risk of chromosome aberrations. These include **Bloom syndrome,** characterized by small stature and development of telangiectasia upon exposure to sunlight; **Fanconi anemia,** frequently associated with a radial ray defect, pigmentary changes, hypogonadism, mild mental retardation, and development of pancytopenia; **ataxia-telangiectasia** (Louis-Bar syndrome), characterized by telangiectasia of the skin and eyes, immunodeficiency, and progressive ataxia; **xeroderma pigmentosum,** resulting in for-

mation of skin lesions secondary to sun exposure; and **Werner syndrome,** which is associated with premature senility.

The knowledge that specific chromosome aberrations are associated with these syndromes is frequently the basis for cytogenetic confirmation of their diagnosis. For example, Bloom syndrome is associated with an increased tendency to exchange segments between homologous chromosomes during mitosis; this tendency is called "sister chromatid exchange." In Fanconi anemia, translocations between nonhomologous chromosomes take place, resulting in the formation of so-called quadriradii.

CONTIGUOUS GENE SYNDROMES

Syndromes are disorders with recognizable patterns of malformations. Some are caused by chromosome abnormalities, others by single-gene defects. In many syndromes, the cause is unknown. In some of these syndromes, which usually occur sporadically but in rare instances are familial, high-resolution chromosome analysis can lead to identification of small interstitial deletions. The deletion is visible under the microscope in the chromosomes of some but not all affected individuals. It is postulated that the syndrome is caused by absence of a cluster of genes located in the deleted segment. In some cases with normal karyotypes, the deletion is submicroscopic, subject to detection by FISH (Figure 31–4) or DNA analysis. In other cases, other mechanisms interfere with the normal activity of the genes believed to be responsible for the syndrome. Uniparental disomy has been documented in some patients with Prader-Willi syndrome (short stature, obesity, hypogonadism, mental retardation), Angelman syndrome ("happy puppet syndrome," with mental retardation, inappropriate laughter, and hand flapping), and Beckwith-Wiedemann syndrome (overgrowth, macroglossia, omphalocele, mental retardation) with normal high-resolution chromosomes. Abnormal imprinting, caused by the uniparental origin of the responsible chromosome segment, is implicated in the etiology. (See the discussion on imprinting in the section on dysmorphology, below.) The genes causing the syndrome are related only through their linear placement on the same chromosome segments and do not influence each other's functions directly (thus the term "contiguous gene syndrome"). Table 31–1 lists examples of the currently known contiguous gene syndromes and their associated chromosome abnormalities.

CHROMOSOME ABNORMALITIES IN CANCER

Numerical and structural chromosome abnormalities have been identified in numerous hematopoietic

Table 31–1. Examples of contiguous gene syndromes.

Syndrome	Abnormal Chromosome Segment
Prader-Willi syndrome	del 15q11
Shprintzen/DiGeorge spectrum	del 22q11
Langer-Gideon syndrome	del 8q24
Miller-Dieker syndrome	del 17p13
Retinoblastoma/mental retardation	del 13q14
Beckwith-Wiedemann syndrome	11p15
Wilms tumor with aniridia, genitourinary malformations, and mental retardation	del 11p13

and solid tumor malignancies of individuals with otherwise normal chromosomes. The cytogenetic abnormalities have been categorized as follows: In **primary abnormalities,** their presence is necessary for initiation of the malignancy. (*Example:* 13q– in retinoblastoma.) **Secondary abnormalities** appear only after the malignancy has developed. (*Example:* Philadelphia chromosome, t[9;22][q34;q11], in acute and chronic myeloid leukemia.) **Cytogenetic noise** is the term used to denote a variety of random chromosome abnormalities.

The primary and secondary chromosome abnormalities are specific for particular malignancies and can be utilized for diagnosis or prognosis. For example, the presence of Philadelphia chromosome is a good prognostic sign in chronic myelogenous leukemia and indicates a poor prognosis in acute lymphoblastic leukemia. The sites of chromosome breaks coincide with the known loci of oncogenes and antioncogenes.

Clarke A: Genetic imprinting in clinical genetics. Dev Suppl 131.

Emanuel BS: Molecular cytogenetics: Toward dissection of the contiguous gene syndrome. Am J Hum Genet 1988;43:575.

Hagerman RJ, Cronister-Silverman A (editors): *Fragile X Syndrome.* Johns Hopkins Univ Press, 1991.

Hall JG: How imprinting is relevant to human disease. Development 1990(Suppl 141).

Jones KL: *Smith's Recognizable Patterns of Human Malformation,* 5th ed. Saunders, 1996.

Kaneko N, Kawagoe S, Hiroi M: Turner's syndrome: Review of the literature with reference to a successful pregnancy outcome. Gynecol Obstet Invest 1990;29:81.

Mittleman F, Heim S: Chromosome abnormalities in cancer. Cancer Detect Prev 1990;14:527.

Rooney DE, Czepulkowski BH (editors): *Human Cytogenetics: A Practical Approach.* Oxford Univ Press, 1986.

Rousseau F et al: Direct diagnosis by DNA analysis of the fragile X syndrome of mental retardation. N Engl J Med 1991;325:1673.

Smith AN, Scott JA (editors): *Genetic Applications: A Health Perspective.* Learner Managed Designs, 1988.

Spence JE et al: Uniparental disomy as a mechanism for human genetic disease. Am J Hum Genet 1988;42:217.

Tkachuk DC et al: Clinical applications of fluorescence in situ hybridization. Genet Anal Tech Appl 1991;8:67.

Trask BJ: Fluorescence in situ hybridization: Applications in cytogenetics and gene mapping. Trends Genet 1991;7:149.

II. PRINCIPLES OF RECOMBINANT DNA

Recombinant DNA technology has major implications for all medical disciplines and especially for human genetics, since it makes possible determination of the location of genes on chromosomes, isolation and characterization of genes, and determination of DNA sequences and encoded protein sequences. Recombinant DNA technology was developed using bacterial enzymes (restriction enzymes that cleave DNA at sites specific for each enzyme). Each restriction endonuclease recognizes a specific nucleotide sequence consisting of four, six, eight, or ten nucleotides and cleaves DNA within that sequence, thus producing DNA fragments. A difference in DNA sequence caused by a normal variation of DNA or by a gene mutation either produces or eliminates an endonuclease recognition site, resulting in a DNA fragment of different size. Thus, the number and arrangement of restriction sites (called a "restriction map") are characteristic of a given DNA sequence.

Before a DNA fragment of interest can be analyzed, multiple copies of it must be produced. This can be achieved by incorporating the human DNA fragment into a **vector,** ie, a DNA segment containing the means of replication and selection in bacteria. The vector-containing human DNA insert is replicated, thus producing multiple copies of the segment of interest. The source of inserts can be **genomic DNA,** obtained directly from cleaving of the target organism, or **complementary DNA** (cDNA), obtained by copying messenger RNA (mRNA) into DNA by reverse transcription.

A **genomic library** can be assembled by randomly fragmenting human genomic DNA with restriction enzymes and then inserting the fragments into a vector. Such a library contains large numbers of different DNA sequences. Some of these specific DNA fragments are used to manufacture human proteins (eg, insulin, growth hormone, interferon, and blood clotting factors) for pharmacologic applications; others are used as **probes,** which may be thought of as

DNA segment-specific, radioactively labeled reagents for mapping and diagnosis.

Molecular genetics is most commonly used to look for changes in genomic DNA detected by Southern blot analysis, but a similar technique of Northern blot analysis is being used increasingly to look for mRNA abnormalities. **Southern blot analysis** relies on the use of restriction endonucleases to cleave human genomic DNA at specific nucleotide sequences and to produce DNA fragments of different lengths. These DNA fragments are then separated by agarose gel electrophoresis, transferred to a membrane, and overlaid with a radioactive probe, which hybridizes only with a fragment having cDNA. This fragment is identified by autoradiography, and its size is determined.

Gene amplification by **polymerase chain reaction (PCR)** has an increasing effect on DNA diagnosis because it is simpler and less time-consuming than older methods. PCR substantially increases the amount of DNA sequence to be analyzed by easy enzymatic synthesis of 0.1–1 million copies of the original DNA segment in a short time. Oligonucleotides, which usually consist of 120 bases and are complementary to the DNA flanking the target segment, are synthesized and used to prime DNA synthesis by DNA polymerase. Each cycle, consisting of denaturation of genomic DNA, primer annealing, and polymerase extension, produces new DNA strands complementary to the target DNA. During each cycle, the amount of amplified DNA doubles, accumulating rapidly in an exponential fashion. After 20 cycles, the DNA is amplified 1 million-fold.

The amplified DNA can be labeled with synthetic oligonucleotide probes. DNA sequence variation can be analyzed in a crude cell lysate of fewer than 100 cells in a dot blot format. This method, therefore, eliminates the need for DNA purification, gel electrophoresis, and the use of radioactive probes. It can be performed on a small DNA sample in a short time. The disadvantage is that a small contamination with a foreign DNA can result in an incorrect diagnosis.

APPLICATION OF RECOMBINANT DNA TECHNOLOGIES IN CLINICAL GENETICS

GENETIC DIAGNOSIS

Genetic diagnosis can be performed by direct detection of a mutant gene or by indirect methods.

Direct detection of an abnormal gene is possible only when the nature of the mutation is known. If the abnormal gene has a partial deletion, insertion, or re-

arrangement, restriction endonuclease analysis with the Southern blot technique is used. Cloned DNA fragments of the gene are used as molecular probes to label the gene, demonstrating the altered size of the gene in comparison with a normal control. Gene mutations have been found in α- and β-thalassemia, antithrombin III deficiency, congenital adrenal hyperplasia secondary to 21-hydroxylase deficiency, Duchenne muscular dystrophy, hemophilias A and B, Lesch-Nyhan syndrome, ornithine transcarbamoylase deficiency, neurofibromatosis, and other disorders.

An abnormal gene with a point mutation can be diagnosed by restriction analysis if the mutation either created or abolished a restriction recognition site, but a restriction recognition site is created or abolished in only 5–10% of point mutations. In the remainder, PCR can be used for DNA amplification, and the mutation can be documented by a mutant-specific oligonucleotide probe, which recognizes the mutant but not the normal alleles. In addition to point mutations, deletions, and insertions, a phenomenon called **unstable expansion of trinucleotide repeats** has been found to be responsible for human gene mutations. These repeats were found to be CGG in fragile X syndrome, CTG in myotonic dystrophy (autosomal dominant), and CAG in both Huntington disease (autosomal dominant) and spinobulbar muscular atrophy (Kennedy disease, X-linked). The repeats are found in the 3′ or 5′ region of the genes, and their size varies within the normal population. Mutations result in increase in the number of repeats; the number of repeats frequently corresponds with the severity of the disorder. The tendency of the repeats to increase in number in each successive generation is the molecular basis for so-called anticipation, ie, increased severity of the disorder in successive generations.

The advantage of a diagnostic study using the direct detection of the mutant gene is that it requires the affected individual only and need not involve other family members.

Indirect detection of abnormal genes is used (1) when the gene is known but there is extensive heterogeneity of the molecular defect between families, and (2) when the gene responsible for a disease is unknown but its chromosome location is known. In the former situation—when the gene is known—it is not always necessary to know the exact molecular defect to determine the presence of the gene. It is, however, necessary to mark and trace the inheritance of the abnormal gene. This can be done on the basis of intragenic DNA polymorphism, which is characterized by the addition or removal of a restriction site and is thus identifiable by restriction fragment length polymorphism (RFLP) analysis. This DNA polymorphism, though it is intragenic, is not the mutation that causes the disorder—it simply marks and helps to differentiate the abnormal gene from the normal one. RFLP cannot be used, however, unless both parents of the tested individual are heterozygous. Thus, a family study is necessary to determine the haplotypes of the chromosomes with and without the mutant gene. However, crossover and recombination are not a problem, because the polymorphism is intragenic or in very close proximity to the gene. Examples of disorders that can be screened by this method are phenylketonuria, hemophilia, β-thalassemia, and Fabry disease.

The latter situation—when the abnormal gene is unknown—prevails in the majority of single-gene disorders. In this case, linkage analysis using a large number of DNA polymorphic markers may reveal a close link between one or more such markers and the presence of the clinical disorder. Such a linkage study localizes the gene of interest to a specific chromosome or to a specific region of a chromosome. Once the location of the gene is known, the same technique (using probes known to be linked to the gene locus of interest) can be used to trace the presence or absence of the gene through the family. This method assumes that the two loci—the locus of the gene and the locus of the DNA polymorphism used to mark the gene—are so close that they will not segregate independently but will be transmitted together. The presence of the marker, therefore, is a reliable indication of the presence of the gene of interest. Thus, the distance between the two loci is of utmost importance in determining the reliability of any linkage analysis, because crossing over and recombination between the gene and the marker during meiosis will result in an error in the diagnosis. To minimize the errors, multiple linked markers should be used in linkage analysis of any gene.

DETECTION OF GENETIC HETEROGENEITY

Genetic heterogeneity is occasionally suspected on the basis of clinical variability. In other instances, there is no clinical clue. For example, enzyme deficiencies may be caused by a number of different mutations, such as an abnormal active site in one case and an abnormal coenzyme in another. Alternatively, the phenotype may be caused in different families by different enzyme defects. Such heterogeneity cannot be suspected on a clinical basis; however, it can be detected using DNA technology.

PREVENTION

Recombinant DNA technology has the potential for preventing genetic disease by facilitating the detection of carriers of defective genes and permitting prenatal diagnosis. Family studies can also clarify the mode of inheritance, thus allowing more accurate determination of recurrence risks and appropriate options. For example, differentiation of gonadal mo-saicism from decreased penetrance of a dominant gene has important implications for genetic counseling.

In the past, the diagnosis of a genetic disease characterized by a late onset of symptoms (eg, Huntington disease) could not be made prior to the appearance of clinical symptoms. In some inborn errors of metabolism, diagnostic tests (eg, measurement of enzyme activities) could be conducted only on inaccessible tissues. Gene identification techniques can enormously enhance our ability to diagnose symptomatic and presymptomatic individuals, conduct prenatal diagnosis, and detect heterozygous carriers. However, presymptomatic DNA testing is associated with psychologic, ethical, and legal implications and therefore should be used only with informed consent.

TREATMENT

Recombinant DNA technology could facilitate treatment in the following ways:

(1) By production of large amounts of therapeutic agents, eg, growth hormone and interferon, which are present naturally in small quantities and are therefore very expensive. This is already being done.

(2) By gene therapy, ie, the introduction of a normal gene into an individual affected with a serious inherited disorder. In principle, genes could be introduced either during embryonic life (germ line therapy), in which case it could be transmitted to future generations; or it could be introduced only into somatic cells (somatic therapy), in which case it would be present only during the life of the recipient. Gene therapy through bone marrow transplantation has been done experimentally in patients with severe combined immunodeficiency disease and with the nonneurologic form of Gaucher disease.

Korf B: Molecular medicine: Molecular diagnosis. (Two parts.) N Engl J Med 1995;332:1218, 1499.
Mandel JL: Questions of expansion. Nat Genet 1993;4:8.
Nelson DL: Fragile X syndrome: Review and current status. Growth Genet Horm 1993;9:1.

III. MENDELIAN GENETICS

SINGLE-GENE DEFECTS

A **gene** is the unit of inheritance that determines the genetic makeup of an individual. Genes occur in pairs at a single locus or site on specific chromosomes. These paired genes, called **alleles,** determine the genotype of an individual at that locus. If the genes at a specific locus are identical, the individual is **homozygous;** if they are different, **heterozygous.** During normal meiosis, these alleles separate, one going to each of the two gametes. An understanding of this process is necessary for an understanding of single-gene inheritance.

Disorders caused by an abnormality in a single gene are either autosomal or X-linked, depending on the location of the gene on an autosome in the former and on the X chromosome in the latter. If the abnormality is present when the defective gene is in either the heterozygous or the homozygous state, it is dominantly inherited. If, however, it is present only when the gene involved is in the homozygous state, the disorder is recessively inherited.

AUTOSOMAL DOMINANT INHERITANCE

Autosomal dominant inheritance has the following characteristics:

(1) Affected individuals in the same family may show very different manifestations. This phenomenon is called **variable expressivity.** Typically, at least some persons who carry the gene are mildly affected, because an individual must be healthy enough and fertile enough to reproduce and pass on the trait. In some disorders, such as Huntington disease, manifestations do not appear until after the childbearing years. In others, which tend to be more severe (eg, achondroplasia), there is a high mutation rate.

(2) Some persons who are obligatory carriers of the gene (ie, both their parent and their child are affected) may have no apparent manifestations. This phenomenon is called **nonpenetrance,** and the penetrance rate varies for each dominantly inherited condition.

(3) Males and females are equally affected, though the manifestations may vary according to sex. For example, baldness is a dominant trait but affects only males. In this case, the trait is said to be **sex-limited.** Both males and females can pass on the abnormality to children of either sex.

(4) Dominant inheritance is typically said to be "vertical," ie, the condition passes from one generation to the next in a vertical fashion (Figure 31–9).

(5) In some cases, the family history seems to be completely negative, and the affected individual appears to be the first abnormal case. This spontaneous appearance may be caused by a point mutation or a change in the structure of a specific gene. Such a change may be a deletion, a duplication, or an amino acid substitution. The mutation rate varies with each dominant condition, and in some cases the mutation

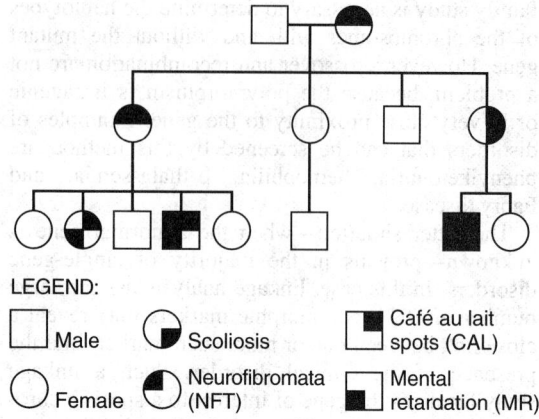

LEGEND:

☐ Male
◔ Scoliosis
◳ Café au lait spots (CAL)
○ Female
◔ Neurofibromata (NFT)
▣ Mental retardation (MR)

Figure 31–9. Autosomal dominant inheritance: Neurofibromatosis, showing variable expressivity.

rate increases with advancing paternal age. There are, however, several other possible explanations for a negative family history:

(a) Nonpaternity.

(b) Decreased penetrance or mild manifestations in one of the parents. For this reason, both parents must be carefully examined and a thorough family history taken.

(c) Germ cell mosaicism. In rare cases, there may be mosaicism in the germ cell line of either parent, in which case the risk of recurrence increases. This is a proposed explanation for cases in which two children of completely normal parents are affected with a dominant condition. The best example of this is osteogenesis imperfecta. Earlier it was thought that there were two forms of the disorder—one autosomal dominant, milder and later in onset; and one autosomal recessive, perinatal in onset and severe (often lethal). The latter was felt to be recessive because of affected siblings born to clinically normal parents. However, newer studies have shown that only one of the paired collagen genes is abnormal in the severe form instead of two, as would be expected in a recessive disease. Recurrent cases, therefore, must be the result of germ cell mosaicism, and indeed, prenatal diagnosis has shown that the actual recurrence risk in this form of osteogenesis imperfecta is 7%.

It is not known how common germ cell mosaicism is, but it has been described in two X-linked disorders as well (Duchenne muscular dystrophy and hemophilia A). The incidence of germ cell mosaicism may depend on many factors that are just beginning to be understood.

(d) The possibility that the abnormality is not truly an autosomal dominant condition. It may be a phenocopy—ie, a nongenetic condition that mimics a certain genotype—or it may be a similar but genetically different abnormality with a different mode of inheritance.

(6) As a general rule, dominant conditions are not caused by enzyme defects, since most biochemical defects are substrate-limited rather than enzyme-limited. Therefore, enzyme levels at 50% of the normal value are sufficient for normal function. There are exceptions, such as acute intermittent porphyria. Dominant traits are more often related to structural abnormalities of protein, as for example in the Marfan syndrome.

(7) For a parent who is affected, the risk of any offspring's carrying an abnormal dominant gene is 50%, or 1:2 for each pregnancy. This is true whether the gene is penetrant or not, and the severity in the offspring is not related to the severity in the affected parent but may be related to the sex of the parent transmitting the gene. For example, if the gene for myotonic dystrophy is passed through the mother, there is a 10–20% chance that the child (regardless of sex) may have a severe congenital form of the disease. Conversely, if the gene for Huntington disease is passed through the father, there is a 5–10% possibility that the offspring may have the severe, rigid juvenile form. This is independent of the severity of the condition in the transmitting parent. It has been attributed to imprinting, though we know in these two conditions that it is associated with expansion of the repeat segment that causes the disease in question. There are certainly other mechanisms of imprinting in other conditions. If an abnormality represents a new mutation of a dominant trait, the parents of the affected individual run a low risk during subsequent pregnancies (see Germ Cell Mosaicism, above), but the risk for the offspring of the affected individual is 50%.

(8) Options available for future pregnancies include prenatal diagnosis in an increasing number of cases and artificial insemination or egg donation, depending on which parent carries the abnormal gene.

NEUROFIBROMATOSIS TYPE 1

Essentials of Diagnosis
& Typical Features

Two or more of the following:
- Six or more café au lait macules, at least 15 mm in diameter in postpubertal and 5 mm in prepubertal individuals.
- Two or more neurofibromas of any type or one plexiform neurofibroma.
- Axillary or inguinal freckling.
- Two or more Lisch nodules (iris hamartomas).
- Distinctive bony lesions such as sphenoid dysplasia or pseudarthrosis.
- An affected first-degree relative.

General Considerations

Neurofibromatosis is one of the most common

autosomal dominant disorders, occurring in 1:4000–1:3000 births and seen in all races and ethnic groups. It has a wide range of variability and can present in many ways. In general, however, the disorder is progressive, and new manifestations appear over time. There are at least two types of neurofibromatosis: Neurofibromatosis 1 is characterized by multiple skin findings and neurofibromatosis 2 by bilateral acoustic neuromas, with minimal or no skin manifestations. A third category includes all of the atypical forms. Because neurofibromatosis 2 is less common and rarely presents before late adolescence, the discussion here is limited to neurofibromatosis type 1.

Clinical Findings

Café au lait macules may be present at birth, and in about 80% of individuals with neurofibromatosis 1 they are apparent by 1 year of age. The typical skin lesion is 10–30 mm, ovoid, and smooth-bordered, but there is great variation. Neurofibromas are benign tumors consisting of Schwann cells, nerve fibers, and fibroblasts; they may be discrete or plexiform. Discrete tumors are more common and can occur at any age. They are well demarcated and can present in cutaneous, subcutaneous, or internal tissues. Plexiform neurofibromas are more diffuse and can invade normal tissue. They are congenital and are frequently detected during periods of rapid growth. If the face or a limb is involved, there may be associated hypertrophy or overgrowth. The incidence of Lisch nodules, which can be seen with a slitlamp, also increases with age. Common features of affected individuals include a large head (though only a small percentage have true hydrocephalus), bony abnormalities on x-ray studies, scoliosis, and a wide spectrum of developmental problems ranging from learning disabilities to true mental retardation. The most common problems in childhood are secondary to plexiform neurofibromas and learning disabilities. Although the average IQ is within the normal range, it is lower than in unaffected family members. The learning problem seems to be specific and involves a visual-perceptual disability that could lead to difficulties in reading and writing or to behavioral impulsivity.

Differential Diagnosis

Areas of hyperpigmentation can be seen in other conditions (eg, the Albright, Noonan, and LEOPARD syndromes), but the lesions are either single or different in character. Isolated neurofibromas and familial café au lait spots (fewer than six and with no other manifestations of neurofibromatosis) have been described. The relationship of such cases to classic neurofibromatosis type 1 is uncertain.

Complications

It is difficult to differentiate a complication from a rare manifestation of the underlying disorder. Seen in less than 25% of persons with neurofibromatosis are seizures, optic glioma, deafness, constipation, short stature, early puberty, and hypertension. Optic glioma seems to occur in about 15% of individuals with neurofibromatosis 1. Although the tumor may be apparent at an early age, it rarely causes functional problems and is usually nonprogressive. There is an increased risk for a variety of malignancies. Other tumors may be benign but may cause significant morbidity and mortality because of their location in a vital and closed space.

Treatment

Appropriate therapy should be initiated as each new manifestation arises. Neurofibromas can be removed, but removal is of limited help if they are multiple or in a vital area. The most important part of therapy is close, ongoing follow-up. Because this disorder is progressive, affected individuals should be seen at regular intervals and have regular eye examinations, hearing tests, and developmental screening as well as other evaluations (eg, CT scans) as indicated. This is best done in a multidisciplinary neurocutaneous clinic.

Prognosis

Because there is such variability in neurofibromatosis, it is difficult to assess the prognosis. However, most affected persons have only skin lesions and few other problems. Severely affected individuals are rare in the pediatric age range, and close follow-up and early intervention may ameliorate some complications.

Genetic Counseling

The gene for neurofibromatosis 1 is on the long arm of chromosome 17 and seems to code for a protein similar to a tumor suppressor factor. Neurofibromatosis results from a variety of mutations, including substitutions, deletions, and additions. Only a small percentage of the mutations can be identified, but the majority seem to code for a truncated protein. There are numerous informative, flanking DNA probes that can be used in a high percentage of families for linkage analysis to identify those carrying the gene, including affected fetuses through prenatal diagnosis.

Approximately 50% of all cases of neurofibromatosis are felt to be caused by new mutations. Before attributing an individual case to a new mutation, however, both parents must be carefully evaluated, including a thorough examination of the skin and a slitlamp examination to look for Lisch nodules. Recent evidence suggests that penetrance is close to 100% in those who carry the gene if individuals are carefully examined.

AUTOSOMAL RECESSIVE INHERITANCE

Autosomal recessive inheritance also has some distinctive characteristics:

(1) There is less variability among affected persons. Parents are carriers and are clinically normal. (There are exceptions to this rule, however. For example, sickle cell disease is considered recessive. Under normal circumstances, carriers—those with the sickle cell trait—are normal but may become symptomatic if they become hypoxic.)

(2) Males and females are affected equally.

(3) Inheritance is horizontal; siblings may be affected (Figure 31–10).

(4) Recessive conditions are frequently rare; the rarer the condition, the more likely it is that consanguinity is present. Conversely, if a child whose parents are related presents with an unrecognized abnormality, a recessive condition is likely.

(5) The family history is usually negative. In common conditions such as cystic fibrosis, there may be an affected second- or third-degree relative, but usually not.

(6) Recessive conditions are frequently associated with enzyme defects. (See Chapter 25.)

(7) The recurrence risk for parents of an affected

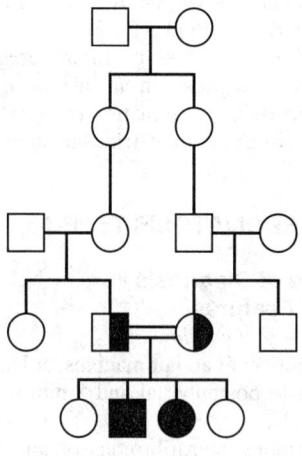

LEGEND:

■ Affected (Dwarfism)

◑ Carrier

□═○ Consanguineous marriage

Figure 31–10. Autosomal recessive inheritance: Rare form of dwarfism.

child is 25%, or 1:4 for each pregnancy, The gene carrier frequency in the general population can be used to assess the risk of having an affected child with a new partner, for unaffected siblings, and for the affected individuals themselves.

(8) In rare instances, a child with a recessive disorder and a normal karyotype may have inherited both copies of the abnormal gene from one parent and none from the other. This **uniparental disomy** was first described in a girl with cystic fibrosis and growth retardation. This phenomenon is of unknown frequency, but it is more likely to be present in a child with several autosomal recessive conditions or one who has some unexpected and seemingly unrelated abnormalities or severe growth retardation. Molecular testing can confirm the presence of uniparental disomy. The recurrence risk is obviously lower in such a situation, though it is not known what factors predispose to uniparental disomy. In at least some cases, the fetus starts as a trisomy for the involved chromosome and then loses one of the chromosomes, resulting in what appears to be a normal karyotype. However, there is 33% chance that the fetus now has uniparental disomy for the parent who contributed the extra chromosome. Maternal age may play a role in these situations.

(9) Options available for future pregnancies include prenatal diagnosis in many cases and artificial insemination.

CYSTIC FIBROSIS

The gene for cystic fibrosis is one of the most common abnormal genes in the white population. Approximately 1:22 persons is a carrier. Over 600 mutations have been identified: the commonest in the Caucasian population, known as *delta F508,* is a three-base deletion coding for phenylalanine. The identification of this gene has raised the possibility of therapy by attaching the gene to a vector and delivering it to the respiratory or nasal epithelium via an aerosol. Early trials, however, have been disappointing. This therapy is directed at somatic cells and will not affect the cystic fibrosis gene in germ cells.

Cloning of the gene for cystic fibrosis and identification of the mutation in the majority of cases have completely changed genetic counseling and prenatal diagnosis for this disorder. Today, the affected child is studied using PCR techniques to search for an identifiable mutation. If this is found, carriers can be identified and specific prenatal diagnosis can be performed, identifying both carriers and affected fetuses. If a mutation cannot be identified, linkage analysis, DNA haplotyping, and amniotic fluid enzyme studies can be done. With continuing research, more mutations are being identified, but linkage analysis available today can achieve 90–99% accuracy.

The identification of the mutation in the cystic fibrosis gene has also raised the issue of mass screening because of the high frequency of this gene in the white population. A 1997 task force did not recommend mass population screening but did recommend screening for those with affected family members, for partners of individuals with cystic fibrosis, and perhaps for couples seeking prenatal diagnosis. Because all of the mutations have not yet been identified, a significant number of "negative" individuals will still carry a gene for cystic fibrosis. Although a specific risk could be calculated for each couple, the high false-negative rate and the counseling required for each couple tested make the value and cost-effectiveness of mass screening questionable at this time.

X-LINKED INHERITANCE

When a gene for a specific disorder is on the X chromosome, the condition is said to be X-linked, or sex-linked. Females may be either homozygous or heterozygous, because they have two X chromosomes. Males, by contrast, have only one, and an affected male is said to be hemizygous. The severity of any disorder is more consistent in males than in females (within a specific family). According to the Lyon hypothesis, because one of the two X chromosomes is inactivated and because this inactivation is random, the clinical picture in females depends on the percentage of mutant versus normal alleles inactivated. The X chromosome is not inactivated until about 14 days of gestation, and parts of the short arm remain active throughout life.

X-LINKED RECESSIVE INHERITANCE

The following features are characteristic of X-linked recessive inheritance:

(1) Males are affected, and heterozygous females are either normal or have mild manifestations.

(2) Inheritance is "diagonal" through the maternal side of the family (Figure 31–11).

(3) A female carrier has a 50% chance of having carrier daughters and a 50% chance of having affected sons.

(4) All of the daughters of an affected male are carriers, and none of his sons are affected. Because a father can give only his Y chromosome to his sons, male-to-male transmission excludes X-linked inheritance except in the rare case of uniparental disomy, where a son receives both the X and the Y from his father.

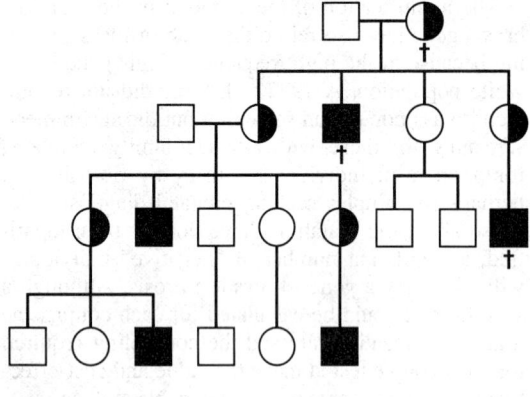

LEGEND:

■ Duchenne muscular dystrophy (DMD)

◐ Carrier

† Deceased

Figure 31–11. X-linked recessive inheritance: Duchenne-type muscular dystrophy.

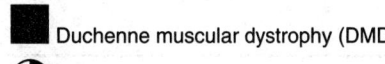

(5) The mutation rate is high in some X-linked disorders, particularly when the affected male is infertile. In such instances, the mutation is felt to occur in the propositus in one-third of cases, in the mother in one-third of cases, and in earlier generations in one-third of cases. For this reason, genetic counseling may be difficult in families with an isolated case.

(6) On rare occasions, a female may be fully affected. Several possible mechanisms may account for a fully affected female: (a) unfavorable lyonization, (b) 45,X karyotype, (c) homozygosity in the female, (d) an X-autosome translocation in which the X chromosome of normal structure is preferentially inactivated, (e) uniparental disomy, and (f) nonrandom inactivation, which may be controlled by an autosomal gene.

DUCHENNE-TYPE MUSCULAR DYSTROPHY

Duchenne-type muscular dystrophy has been recognized as an X-linked recessive condition for many years. There is also a milder type, Becker muscular dystrophy, which is allelic. The gene, now known to be in band Xp21, is one of the largest genes in the human genome, which may explain its high mutation rate. About 60–65% of families have a deletion in the gene. In rare cases, this may be visible on cytogenetic analysis, but molecular studies are usually re-

quired. Because of the length of the gene, many informative RFLPs exist, both flanking and within the gene itself. This gene has been shown to encode mRNA for a protein called dystrophin, which is localized to the muscle surface membrane, the sarcolemma. Males with low or undetectable levels of dystrophin have Duchenne-type muscular dystrophy, whereas those with nearly normal levels but an abnormal size of dystrophin have Becker muscular dystrophy. New treatments, such as corticosteroids and even gene therapy, are being tried, but this should be done only in the context of a research protocol in a center for muscle disease.

If a deletion is present, it is usually apparent in the female carrier as well, using gene dosage studies. If there is no deletion, linkage studies, combined with creatine kinase levels, help to predict female carriers in informative families with a high degree of probability. Negative studies in the mother, however, do not guarantee a negligible risk because of germ cell mosaicism. This may be present in 20–25% of the women, giving an actual recurrence risk of about 5–7% even with negative studies. Both deletion testing and linkage studies can be used to identify an affected fetus. In noninformative families, a fetal muscle biopsy can be done to look for dystrophin.

X-LINKED DOMINANT INHERITANCE

The X-linked dominant inheritance pattern is much less common than the X-linked recessive type. Examples include incontinentia pigmenti and hypophosphatemic or vitamin D-resistant rickets.

(1) The heterozygous female is symptomatic, and the disease is twice as common in females because they have two X chromosomes that can be affected.

(2) Clinical manifestations are more variable in females than in males.

(3) The risk for the offspring of heterozygous females is 50% regardless of sex.

(4) All of the daughters but none of the sons of affected males will have the disorder.

(5) Although a homozygous female is possible (particularly in an inbred population), she would be severely involved. All of her children would also be affected, but more mildly.

(6) Some disorders (eg, incontinentia pigmenti) are lethal in males (and in homozygous females). Affected women have twice as many daughters as sons and an increased incidence of miscarriages, because affected males will be spontaneously aborted. A 47,XXY karyotype has allowed affected males to survive.

For more complete information about specific single-gene defects, see the McKusick reference cited at the end of this chapter.

MITOCHONDRIAL INHERITANCE

Some unusual disorders seem to be transmitted only by female members of a family and affect a high proportion of offspring, both male and female. Examples include Leber hereditary optic neuropathy, Leigh disease, MELAS (mitochondrial encephalomyopathy, lactic acidosis, and stroke-like episodes), and MERRF (myoclonic epilepsy and ragged red fibers). It is now known that these diseases are caused by mutations in mitochondrial DNA (mtDNA). Mitochondrial DNA is double-stranded, circular, and smaller than nuclear DNA and is found in the cytoplasm. It codes for enzymes involved in oxidative phosphorylation, which generates ATP.

There are several characteristics of mitochondrial disorders:

(1) Mitochondrial disorders show remarkable phenotypic variability.

(2) They are maternally inherited, because only the egg has any cytoplasmic material.

(3) In most mitochondrial disorders, cells are heteroplasmic—ie, all cells contain both normal and mutated or abnormal mtDNA. The proportion of normal to abnormal mtDNA seems to determine the severity of the disease and the age at onset in most cases.

(4) Those tissues with the highest ATP requirements—specifically, central nervous system and skeletal muscle—seem to be most susceptible to mutations in mtDNA.

(5) There is an increase in somatic cell mtDNA mutations and a decline in oxidative phosphorylation function with age. This explains the later onset of some of these disorders and may indeed be a clue to the whole aging process.

Mitochondrial dysfunction due to mutations in nuclear genes encoding mitochondrial proteins can be inherited as dominant, recessive, or X-linked. Some mitochondrial disorders are associated with deletions or duplications in mitochondrial DNA. Large deletions are usually sporadic, but smaller deletions may be secondary events due to defects in dominantly inherited nuclear genes. Because of the difficulty in diagnosing a mitochondrial disorder and the variability of the clinical course, it is often difficult to calculate specific recurrence risks.

POLYGENIC DISEASE
(Multifactorial Inheritance)

The inheritance of many common traits and abnormalities does not seem to be caused by a single gene. In the past, multiple genes, each with a small effect, as well as a variety of environmental factors were felt to be important, and the terms "polygenic inheritance" and "multifactorial inheritance" have been used. It is now felt that there may be a smaller number of genes involved, with one or more major genes important in each condition. The terms "oligogenic" and "multilocus" have been used to characterize this more limited concept. Inherited in this way are a variety of normal traits—eg, height and intelligence—as well as a variety of common abnormalities such as hypertension and allergies. It is important to realize that many of these conditions do not have a single cause and represent genetic heterogeneity or a group of diseases with common manifestations and different causes. In some conditions, there is an association with certain HLA types. For example, there is a high correlation between ankylosing spondylitis and HLA-B27. It is important to understand the difference between an association such as this and linkage of a certain disease with the HLA locus. In the latter instance, the gene for the disease is on chromosome 6, close to the HLA locus, but there is no association with a specific HLA type. Although the concept of polygenic inheritance has been questioned, many of the principles still hold true. The actual recurrence risks remain the same unless a broad category (eg, coronary artery disease, diabetes) can be subdivided and the consultand can be identified as being in a higher or lower risk group. For these reasons, the earlier terminology will be used in this section.

Many common congenital abnormalities, such as cleft lip and palate, neural tube defects, and some kinds of congenital heart disease, are inherited in a polygenic manner. If the combination of predisposing genes from both parents and certain environmental factors (mostly unknown) exceeds the "threshold," the abnormality then becomes manifest. Twin studies have been helpful in determining the relative importance of genetic versus environmental factors. If genetic factors are of little or no importance, then the concordance between monozygotic and dizygotic twins should be the same. (Dizygotic twins are no more genetically similar to each other than to other siblings.) If an abnormality is completely genetic, the concordance between identical twins should be 100%. In polygenic conditions, the concordance rate for identical twins is higher than that seen in dizygotic twins but still not 100%, indicating both genetic and environmental factors.

Polygenic or multifactorial inheritance has some distinctive characteristics:

(1) The risk for relatives of affected persons is increased, and the risk is higher for first-degree relatives (those who have 50% of their genes in common) and lower for more distant relations, though the risk for the latter is higher than for the general population (Table 31–2).

(2) The recurrence risk varies with the number of affected family members. For example, after one child is born with a neural tube defect, the recurrence risk is 2–3%. If a second affected child is born, the risk increases to 10–12%. This is in contrast to single-gene disorders, in which the risk is the same no matter how many family members are affected.

(3) The risk is higher if the defect is more severe. In Hirschsprung disease, another polygenic condition, the longer the aganglionic segment, the higher the recurrence risk.

(4) Sex ratios may not be equal. If there is a marked discrepancy, the recurrence risk is higher if a child of the less commonly affected sex has the disorder. This assumes that more genetic factors are required to raise the more resistant sex above the threshold. For example, pyloric stenosis is more common in males. If the first affected child is a female, the recurrence risk is higher than if the child is a male.

(5) The risk for the offspring of an affected person is approximately the same as the risk for siblings, assuming that the spouse of the affected person has a negative family history.

CLEFT LIP & CLEFT PALATE

From a genetic standpoint, cleft lip with or without cleft palate is distinct from isolated cleft palate. The former is more common in males, the latter in females. Although both can occur in a single family, particularly in association with certain syndromes, this pattern is unusual. There is racial variation in the incidence of facial clefting. Among Asians, whites, and blacks, the incidence is 1.61, 0.9, and 0.31, respectively, per 1000 live births.

Clinical Findings

A cleft lip may be unilateral or bilateral and complete or incomplete. It may occur with a cleft of the entire palate or just the primary (anterior and gingival ridge) or secondary (posterior) palate. An isolated cleft palate can involve only the soft palate or both the soft and hard palates. It can be a V-shaped or wide horseshoe cleft. A cleft associated with micrognathia and glossoptosis (a tongue that falls back and causes respiratory or feeding problems) is called **Pierre Robin syndrome.** Among individuals with facial clefts—more commonly those with isolated cleft palate—there is an increased incidence of other congenital abnormalities. The incidence of congenital heart disease, for example, is between 1% and 2% in liveborn infants, but among those with Pierre Robin syndrome it can be as high as 15%. Associated abnormalities should be identified in the period immediately after birth and before surgery.

Differential Diagnosis

A facial cleft may occur in many different circumstances. It may be an isolated abnormality or part of a more generalized syndrome. Prognosis, management, and accurate determination of recurrence risks all depend on accurate diagnosis. In evaluating a child with a facial cleft, one must determine if the cleft is nonsyndromic or syndromic.

(1) Nonsyndromic. In the past, nonsyndromic cleft lip or cleft palate has been considered a classic example of polygenic or multifactorial inheritance. More recently, however, this mode of inheritance has been questioned, and several studies have suggested one or

Table 31–2. Empiric risks for some congenital disorders.

Anencephaly and spina bifida: Incidence (average) 1:1000
    One affected child: 2–3%
    Two affected children: 10–12%
    One affected parent: 2–3%
Hydrocephalus: Incidence 1:2000 newborns
    Occasional X-linked recessive
    Often associated with neural tube defect
    Some environmental etiologies (eg, toxoplasmosis)
    Recurrence risk, one affected child
        Hydrocephalus: 1%
        Some central nervous system abnormality: 3%
Non-syndrome cleft lip and/or palate: Incidence (average) 1:1000
    One affected child: 2–4%
    One affected parent: 2–4%
    Two affected children: 10%
    One affected parent, one affected child: 10–20%
Non-syndrome cleft palate: Incidence 1:2000
    One affected child: 2%
    Two affected children: 6–8%
    One affected parent: 4–6%
    One affected parent, one affected child: 15–20%
Congenital heart disease: Incidence 8:1000
    One affected child: 2–3%
    One affected parent, one affected child: 10%
Clubfoot: Incidence 1:1000 (male:female = 2:1)
    One affected child: 2–3%
Congenital dislocated hip: Incidence 1:1000
    (female > male) with marked regional variation
    One affected: 2–14%
Pyloric stenosis: Incidence, males: 1:200; females: 1:1000
    Male index parent

Brothers	3.2%
Sons	6.8%
Sisters	3.0%
Daughters	1.2%

    Female index patient

Brothers	13.2%
Sons	20.5%
Sisters	2.5%
Daughters	11.1%

more major autosomal loci, both recessive and dominant or codominant. Empirically, however, the recurrence risk is still in the range of 2–3% because of nonpenetrance or the presence of other contributing genes.

(2) Syndromic. (See Table 31–3.) Cleft lip with or without cleft palate and isolated cleft palate may be seen in a variety of syndromes that may be environmental, chromosomal, single-gene, or of unknown origin. Prognosis and accurate recurrence risks depend upon the correct diagnosis.

Complications & Treatment

Problems associated with facial clefts include early feeding difficulties, which may be severe; recurrent serous otitis media associated with fluctuating hearing and language delays; speech problems, including hypernasality and articulation errors; and dental and orthodontic complications. Long-term management should ideally be through a multidisciplinary cleft palate clinic.

Genetic Counseling

Accurate counseling depends on accurate diagnosis and the differentiation of syndromic from nonsyndromic clefts. A complete family history must be taken, and both parents must be examined. The choice of laboratory studies is guided by the presence of other abnormalities and clinical suspicions. They may include chromosome analysis, eye examination, and x-ray studies. Clefts of both the lip and the palate have been detected on ultrasound prenatally, but intrauterine diagnosis is most likely in syndromes in which other more serious abnormalities can be identified.

NEURAL TUBE DEFECTS

The neural tube defects comprise a variety of malformations, including anencephaly, spina bifida or

Table 31–3. Syndromic isolated cleft palate (CP) and cleft lip with or without cleft palate (CL/CP)

Environmental
  Maternal seizures, anticonvulsant usage (CL/CP or CP)
  Fetal alcohol syndrome (CP)
  Amniotic band syndrome (CL/CP)
Chromosomal
  Trisomies 13 and 18 (CL/CP)
  Wolf-Hirschorn or 4p- syndrome (CL/CP)
  Shprintzen or 22q11.2 deletion syndrome (CP)
Single gene disorders
  Van der Woude syndrome, AD (CL/CP or CP)
  Treacher Collins syndrome, AD (CP)
  Stickler syndrome, AD (CP)
Unknown etiology
  Möbius syndrome (CP)
  Cornelia de Lange syndrome (CP)

myelomeningocele, sacral agenesis, sacral lipomas, and other spinal dysraphisms. Hydrocephalus associated with the Arnold-Chiari malformation is commonly seen with spina bifida at all levels. Sacral agenesis, also called the caudal regression syndrome, is seen more frequently in infants of diabetic mothers.

Clinical Findings

At birth, neural tube defects can present as rachischisis at any level, as a fluid-filled sac that may or may not be leaking, or as a variety of skin-covered lesions associated with a fatty mass, a hemangioma, a tuft of hair, or asymmetric buttock creases. In the latter cases, CT or MRI studies should be conducted to look for bony and neural involvement. The extent of associated abnormalities depends on the level of the lesion and may include a variety of foot deformities, flexion contractures, dislocated hips, or total flaccid paralysis below the level of the lesion. Hydrocephalus may be apparent at birth, but more often there is an increase in head circumference, irritability, and poor feeding, with vomiting beginning shortly after the back has been closed. Neurogenic bladder and bowel may present as constant urinary dribbling, frequent stooling, and occasionally rectal or even vaginal prolapse. Urinary retention may also occur, particularly in the immediate postoperative period. There is also a higher incidence of unassociated abnormalities, particularly with higher lesions and anencephaly.

Differential Diagnosis

It is important to look for syndromes that may present as neural tube defects. Some chromosome abnormalities, congenital rubella, and the fetal valproic acid syndrome have been associated with neural tube defects.

Complications & Management

If the spinal defect is leaking or open at birth, the major concerns are infection and drying of the nerve roots, leading to further loss of function. For this reason, surgical closure is recommended as soon as possible. The infant should be closely monitored, and a shunt, usually ventriculoperitoneal, should be inserted as soon as signs of hydrocephalus become apparent. The shunt may need to be replaced if it becomes obstructed, infected, or separated, or it may need to be lengthened as the child grows. There has been much discussion about whether true shunt independence ever develops. The signs and symptoms of chronic shunt malfunction may be very insidious and consist only of slow deterioration of school performance or staring spells. Hydromyelia may develop and lead to progressive scoliosis; sudden death has also been ascribed to shunt malfunction in adults with spina bifida.

The child's ability to walk varies according to the level of the lesion. Children with low lumbar and sacral lesions walk with minimal support; those with high lumbar and thoracic lesions are rarely functional walkers; and in those with midlumbar lesions the effects are variable. In any case, the child should receive physical therapy and assume the upright position at the appropriate developmental age. Orthopedic surgery may be necessary to get the child upright and ambulatory.

Concerns about the bladder begin at birth. The bladder may be small and spastic or large and hypotonic; the sphincter may be flaccid or tight. The child may therefore be constantly wet because the bladder holds little urine, or there may be incomplete emptying of the bladder and ureteral reflux. In the latter case, there is a high risk for urinary tract infections. In addition, there may be a problem called "bladder dyssynergy." Normally, when the bladder contracts, the sphincter relaxes, allowing for an unimpeded flow of urine. In a dyssynergic state, the sphincter also contracts, predisposing the patient to urethral reflux. Management is guided by the results of early studies to determine the type of bladder present. Continence can be achieved in a variety of ways. In most cases, medications are necessary, such as anticholinergic agents to relax the smooth muscle of the bladder or alpha-sympathomimetic drugs to increase bladder outlet resistance. The mother and ultimately the child are taught the technique for clean intermittent catheterization. If the bladder is small, with increased tone, augmentation using a portion of bowel may be necessary to prevent reflux and upper tract deterioration. If the child still cannot achieve continence, there are a variety of surgical procedures to improve urinary retention and decrease leakage, but they usually require intermittent catheterization as well to ensure complete emptying. Renal function should be monitored regularly, and an ultrasound examination should be performed annually. Symptomatic infections should be treated.

Bowel control can be more of a problem, because a lax sphincter and poor peristalsis predispose to constipation and poor emptying. The principles of management include increasing the bulk of the stool to facilitate spontaneous and more complete evacuation while keeping the child as free from accidents as possible. This is done with a combination of a high-fiber diet, fluids, and suppositories. Enemas, digital stimulation or evacuation, and surgical procedures have been used as well. A recently developed surgical procedure called ACE (antegrade continent enema) uses the appendix to create a conduit from the upper colon to the surface at the umbilicus. An enema is then given through the conduit, cleaning out the colon from above rather than from below. Early results with respect to continence and patient satisfaction have been encouraging.

Areas of skin anesthesia or hypesthesia correlate roughly with motor level. Skin breakdown is always a threat, and skin care must be meticulous. If skin breakdown does occur, all pressure must be relieved, the wound kept clean, and an artificial skin dressing used to promote healing. Surgical closure is sometimes required. The advantages of prevention over treatment cannot be overemphasized.

Children with spina bifida and urinary tract anomalies have a significant risk for type I (IgE-mediated) allergic reactions to latex. Symptoms may vary from urticaria to anaphylaxis during surgery. Some but not all children will have a history of allergic reactions to rubber. It is difficult to predict who has this sensitivity. Skin tests are poorly standardized and carry some risk. The IgE radioallergosorbent test (RAST) is helpful if positive, but it is not 100% sensitive. It has been predicted that up to 40% of children with spina bifida are latex-sensitive, with the incidence increasing with age. Recognition of this problem and avoidance of latex products are essential.

There is a wide range of intellectual capacity in children with neural tube defects, but most function at the low normal to borderline levels. Most children are now mainstreamed, but they have a higher incidence of fine motor and visual-perceptual problems. Because of early aggressive care, most children with neural tube defects now survive into adolescence, when different problems become apparent. MRI has demonstrated that most individuals with spina bifida have tethered cords. Many are asymptomatic, but others develop back or leg pain, change in bladder function, change in motor or sensory level, spasticity, or scoliosis. These symptoms may develop at any age, and prompt surgical intervention is necessary because lost function may not be regained. Scoliosis may also become apparent in adolescence and may be associated with syringomyelia or a tethered cord. Neurologic evaluation is indicated before scoliosis surgery. Respiratory compromise and even sleep apnea may occur. A small percentage of patients have progressive loss of renal function secondary to chronic infection and stones despite aggressive treatment, and some develop renal failure. Problems with bowel management and skin breakdown increase as individuals become obese and less ambulatory. The major problems, however, are psychosocial. The transition into independent adulthood is very difficult because of poor social skills, limited social contacts, inferior education, and poor preparation for the competitive work world.

Individuals with closed spinal cord abnormalities (eg, sacral lipomas) have similar problems, though hydrocephalus is seen less often and intelligence is usually normal. Early surgical treatment is important to preserve function and prevent further disability secondary to cord tethering. Because needs are ongoing and management approaches change with time, all children with spinal defects of any type should be followed in a multidisciplinary clinic. However, the increase in managed health care, both in the private and in the public sectors, has made referral to such clinics more difficult. It is the responsibility of the primary health care provider to see that all children with a chronic disability such as a neural tube defect receive coordinated and timely care from experienced specialists.

Genetic Counseling

Recurrence risks vary according to etiology, but most neural tube defects are polygenic, with a recurrence risk of 2–3%. The risk for the offspring of an affected person is essentially the same. There would be a considerably higher risk if the anencephaly or encephalocele were associated with renal abnormalities or polydactyly, as seen in Meckel-Gruber syndrome, which is autosomal recessive. Prenatal diagnosis is available, and pregnancies can be monitored in a variety of ways. In fetuses with open neural tube defects, serum alpha-fetoprotein levels, measured at 16–18 weeks of gestation, are elevated. Routine screening has been recommended by the American Academy of Obstetrics and Gynecology. Alpha-fetoprotein levels in amniotic fluid are also elevated, and amniocentesis combined with ultrasound studies will detect more than 90% of neural tube defects. Recent studies have shown that folic acid can significantly lower the incidence and recurrence rate of neural tube defects, but the folic acid must be taken prior to conception. It is now recommended that all women of childbearing age take 0.4 mg of folic acid daily. This can be achieved by dietary modification (see Table 10–8) or by taking a multivitamin capsule once daily that contains 0.4 mg of folic acid. As of January 1998, folic acid will be added to wheat products, but the amount added will not be sufficient to provide the recommended daily dose of 0.4 mg; other folate-rich foods or a supplemental vitamin will be needed. For the woman at increased risk because of a previous child with a neural tube defect, the current recommendation is to increase folic acid intake to 4 mg daily when pregnancy is planned. While the data are inconsistent, there is some evidence that preconceptual folic acid supplementation may lower the incidence of other congenital malformations such as conotruncal heart defects.

American Academy of Pediatrics Committee on Genetics: Health supervision for children with neurofibromatosis. Pediatrics 1995;96:368.

Austin KD, Hall JG: Nontraditional inheritance. Pediatr Clin North Am 1992;39:335.

Carey JC: Health supervision and anticipatory guidance for children with genetic disorders (including specific recommendations for trisomy 21, trisomy 18, and neurofibromatosis 1). Pediatr Clin North Am 1992;39:25.

Gutmann DH et al: The diagnostic evaluation and multidisciplinary management of neurofibromatosis 1 and neurofibromatosis 2. JAMA 1997;278:51.

Ireys HT, Grason HA, Guyer: Assuring quality of care for children with special needs in managed care organizations: Roles for pediatricians. Pediatrics 1996;98:178.

Korf B: Molecular medicine: Molecular diagnosis. (Two parts.) N Engl J Med 1995;332:1218, 1499.

Miller RG, Hoffman EP: Molecular diagnosis and modern management of Duchenne muscular dystrophy. Neurol Clin 1994;12:699.

Recommendations for use of folic acid to reduce number of spina bifida cases and other neural tube defects. JAMA 1993;269:1233.

Shoffner JM, Wallace DC: Mitochondrial genetics: Principles and practice. Am J Hum Genet 1992;51:1179.

Turvey TA, Vig KWL, Fonesca RJ: *Facial Clefts and Craniosynostosis: Principles and Management.* Saunders, 1996.

Winn HR, Mayberg MR, Pang D (editors): Spinal dysraphism. Neurosurg Clin North Am 1995;6(2).

IV. DYSMORPHOLOGY

With advances in perinatal medicine and treatment of infectious diseases, **birth defects** have now become the leading cause of death in the first year. Birth defects are evident in 2–3% of newborns and by adulthood will be detected in 7% of the population. The science of maldevelopment is called teratology. Dysmorphology is its clinical arm.

MECHANISMS

Most birth defects are multifactorial—ie, they result from miscommunication between genetically regulated morphogenic processes and the environments in which they unfold. Specific causes of maldevelopment can be identified in about 30% of cases, but advances in developmental biology and human genetics promise better understanding.

GENETIC REGULATION

Single gene mutations and chromosomal abnormalities explain approximately 25% of birth defects. These result in recurring phenotypes—syndromes—many of which have been mapped to specific chromosomal locations.

Because the major themes of morphogenesis and the genes that regulate them have been conserved through evolution, experiments in zebra fish and *Drosophila* (fruit flies) are highly relevant to human development. Genes discovered in these organisms become candidate genes for human birth defects.

Among the better examples of this connection are *pax* genes that are involved in eye development in *Drosophila* and have been conserved in mice and humans. Mutations in one of these, *Pax 6,* produce "small eye" in mice and aniridia and other anterior chamber eye abnormalities in humans.

Other advances in molecular genetics that contribute to rapidly accumulating knowledge about morphogenesis include in situ hybridization for visualizing the expression of genes in embryos and transgenic animals in which genes of interest can be "knocked out" in order to determine their contributions to development. Combinations of these techniques have uncovered, for example, very important roles for "sonic hedgehog," a humorously named gene that determines morphologic patterns in organs as diverse as limbs and the central nervous system. Mutations in this evolutionarily conserved gene are among the genetic factors that can contribute to **holoprosencephaly,** a birth defect in which the central nervous system fails to complete hemispheric division.

Among the most fundamental genetic programs in cells are those that regulate cell division, **proliferation,** and those that program cell death, **apoptosis.** The development of structure is as dependent upon the loss of cells and the regression of tissues as it is upon their proliferation. Both proliferation and apoptosis are very active in embryogenesis. The balance between these processes can be disrupted by a variety of factors and is emerging as an important determinant of birth defects. The picture emerging from recent studies of morphogenesis is one of a hierarchy of gene expression during development. The genetic organization of morphogenesis begins with expression of genes encoding **transcription factors.** These proteins bind to critical regions within the genomes of undifferentiated embryonic cells, thereby recruiting them into **developmental fields,** groups of cells primed to respond to specific signals later in development. This recruitment also establishes spatial relationships and orients cells with respect to their neighbors. As fields differentiate into identifiable tissues (eg, ectoderm, mesoderm, and endoderm), cellular proliferation, migration, and further differentiation are mediated through genes encoding proteins that send signals through interactions with other proteins (receptors). Products of these genes include **growth factors** and their receptors, **cellular adhesion molecules,** and **extracellular matrix** proteins that both provide structure and localize signals for further differentiation. Motifs in which fields of primed cells proliferate, migrate, and then interact through locally expressed proteins and receptors can be recognized repeatedly in the progression of mammalian development. Within them lie clues to understanding not only of many birth defects but also of the disorganization of developmental processes that underlies cancer.

EPIGENETIC INTERACTIONS

Development is regulated by genes but is initiated and sustained by nongenetic processes. **Epigenetic events** are points of interaction between evolutionarily conserved programs and the physicochemical environments in which genes and cells exist. Human development is set in motion through the physical events of fertilization. Temperature, concentration, charge, and energy state are as important to differentiation as the genetic programs that are being read.

Genetic imprinting and **DNA methylation** are examples of epigenetic processes that impact development. Certain genes important in regulation of growth and differentiation are themselves regulated by chemical modification—methylation—that occurs in specific patterns in gametes: eggs and sperm cells. The pattern of genes methylated is determined by the sex of the parent of origin. This process—imprinting—leads to the expression of one gene in preference to its homolog. Recent experiments indicate that expression of imprinted genes may be limited to specific organs (eg, the brain) and that imprinting can be relaxed and methyl groups lost as development progresses. Disruption of imprinting is now recognized as contributing to a number of maldevelopment syndromes (see below).

DNA methylation also occurs after fertilization. Embryonic methylation is less specific with respect to the genes modified and is independent of parent of origin. It is very active early in development and appears to serve as a mechanism for silencing genes in order to maintain differentiated programs. Both imprinted and embryonic patterns of methylation can be preserved through cell division, but with age, DNA methylation and hence maintenance of cell differentiation can be lost.

ENVIRONMENTAL FACTORS

The effects of exogenous agents during development are mediated through genetic and developmentally regulated pathways. At the cellular level, environmental effects occur because **xenobiotics,** compounds foreign to nature, either interact with signaling pathways or receptors and misdirect morphologically important cellular functions or are cytotoxic and lead to cell death in excess of the usual developmental cell formation processes.

In general, pharmacologically active receptors expressed in embryos and fetuses are the same molecules that mediate effects in adults. However, because differentiation pathways are active and embryonic and fetal physiology differs from that of mature organisms, pharmacologic effector systems may be different. These properties predict dose-response relationships for drug and chemical exposures during development but, for now, also mean that unanticipated effects are possible.

In order to affect human embryonic and fetal tissues, xenobiotics must traverse the placenta. While the human placenta is a relatively effective barrier to microorganisms, it is ineffective at excluding drugs and chemicals. The physicochemical properties (molecular size, solubility, charge, etc) that allow foreign chemicals to be absorbed into the maternal circulation also allow them to cross the placenta. Xenobiotic metabolism occurs in the human placenta but is more active toward steroid hormones and low level environmental contaminants than toward drugs.

The timing of xenobiotic exposures is also an important determinant of effect. Individual organs express so-called **critical periods** of development during which they may be particularly susceptible to maldevelopment if programs for differentiation are disrupted or unbalanced. Figure 31–12 shows critical periods of development for several organs. It is not the case that these periods are confined to early gestation. Note, for instance, that the developing brain is susceptible to toxicity throughout pregnancy.

Prescribed and over-the-counter drugs can be expected to reach pharmacologically active levels in maternal blood and will, in general, equilibrate to the same levels across the placenta. Agents known to produce cytotoxicity in adults are therefore likely to be teratogenic. Drugs generally safe in adults will be generally safe for fetuses, but the capacity for embryologic maldevelopment will depend upon specific drug-effector actions and may be less predictable. Risk assessment requires continuous monitoring of populations exposed to drugs during pregnancy. Abused substances achieve pharmacologically and toxicologically active levels on both sides of the placenta. As they are frequently toxic to adults, they will be predictably toxic to embryos and fetuses.

As cytotoxic agents accumulate in the environment, concerns about adverse developmental effects increase. However, like drugs, effects of environmental agents on the embryo and fetus are also dose-dependent, and the level of exposure frequently becomes the primary determinant of risk. In general, exposures producing symptoms in mothers can be assumed to be potentially toxic to the fetus.

Mutagens in the environment may be a special problem. Experiments at high levels of exposure indicate that mutagenic agents are also teratogenic. Specific phenotypes, however, are difficult to predict. Mutations induced in embryonic tissues produce mosaicism that may not be visible, but they may also contribute to diseases such as cancer later in life. On the other hand, DNA damage alone can induce cells to switch to apoptotic pathways and may therefore have more immediate effects. The extent of this problem for humans is incompletely understood. Maternal exposure to mutagenic chemotherapy is predictably associated with abnormalities of fetal growth or birth defects. However, transplacental effects specific to lower levels of chemical mutagens such as those absorbed from tobacco smoke have yet to be demonstrated.

Not all transplacental pharmacologic effects are toxic. There is increasing potential for therapeutic transplacental uses of drugs in pregnancy. Folic acid supplementation may lower risks for birth defects such as spina bifida (see above) through pharmacologic as well as nutritional mechanisms. Maternal administration of corticosteroids to induce synthesis and secretion of surfactants provides another example of a transplacental therapy.

MECHANICAL FACTORS

Much of embryonic development and all of fetal growth occurs normally with the conceptus surrounded by amniotic fluid held in place by placental membranes. The low pressure and the space provided by this fluid is critical to the development of most organs. Disruption of formation or integrity of placental membranes for whatever reason leads to major, usually lethal distortion of the embryo (**early amnion disruption sequence**) and to deformation or even amputation of fetal extremities (**amniotic band sequence**). Dislocation of structures and abnormal histogenesis may also occur, reflecting malalignment of important cell surface and extracellular matrix interactions.

Fetal movement also contributes to morphogenesis. Normal movement is necessary for normal development of joints and is a principal determinant of folds and creases present at birth in the face, hands, feet, and other areas of the body.

Mechanical forces play prominent roles in the development of many important birth defects. **Clubfoot** is an etiologically heterogeneous condition in which the foot at birth is malpositioned, limited in motion, and may be undergrown. This condition more often results from mechanical constraint secondary to intrauterine position and crowding, decreased muscle strength or tone, or abnormal neurologic function than from primary skeletal maldevelopment.

Lung and kidney development are particularly sensitive to mechanical forces. Constriction of the chest through maldevelopment of the ribs, lack of surrounding amniotic fluid, or lack of movement (fetal breathing) leads to varying degrees of **pulmonary hypoplasia** in which lungs are smaller than normal and develop fewer alveoli. Mechanically induced pulmonary hypoplasia is a common cause of respiratory distress at birth and may be lethal. **Cystic renal dysplasia** commonly accompanies birth defects that obstruct ureters or outflow from the bladder. In such cases, as the kidneys become functional, urinary pressure within obstructed collecting systems increases and is propagated back into developing tissues. Here again, distortion of cell surface interac-

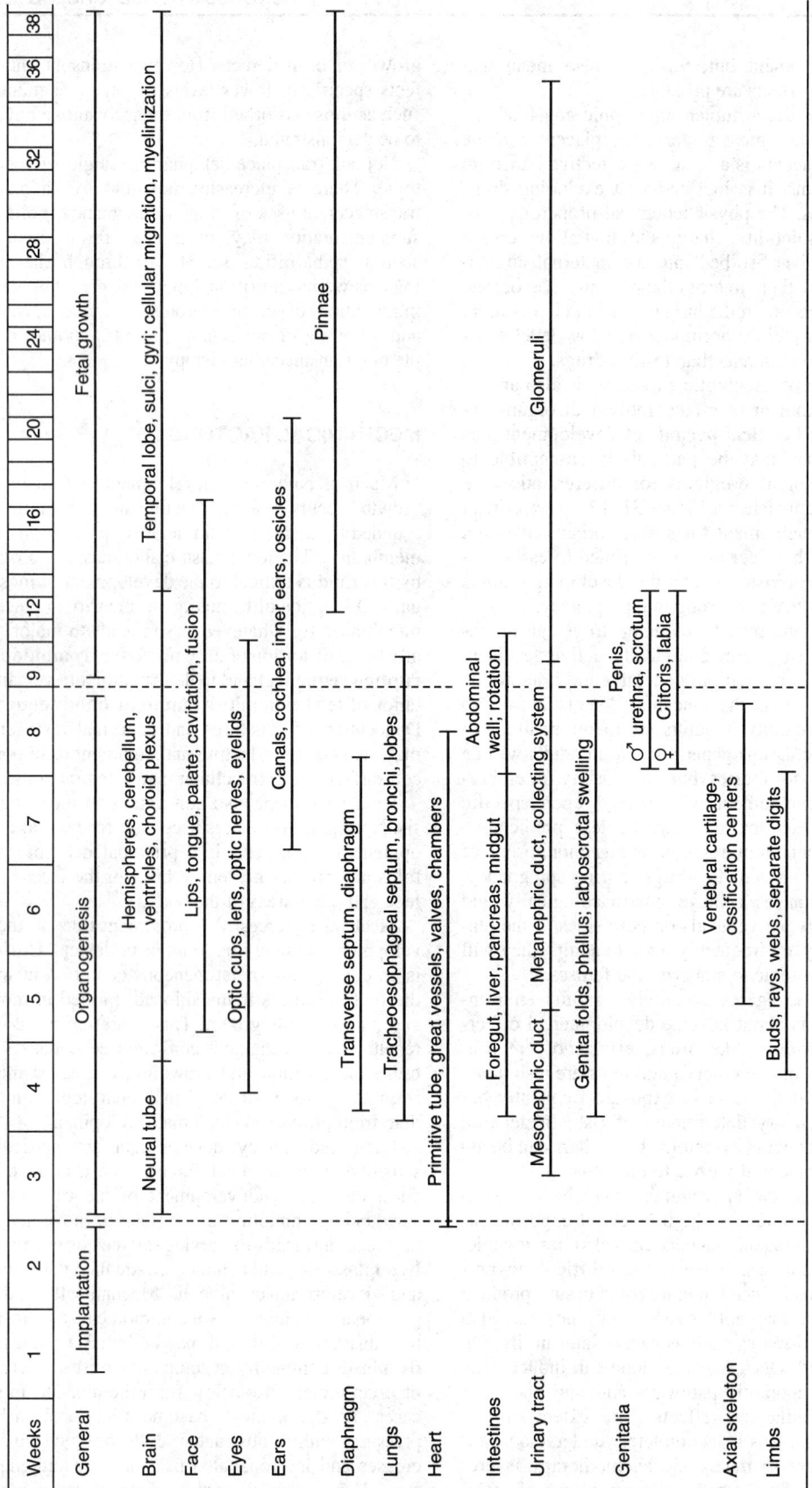

Figure 31–12. Critical periods in human gestation.

tions and malalignment of extracellular matrix leads to abnormal histogenesis. Developing kidneys exposed for long periods to increased internal pressures eventually become nonfunctional.

CLINICAL APPLICATIONS

Classification of dysmorphic features is beginning to reflect better understanding of mechanisms of maldevelopment. However, the recognition of many patterns prior to the advances of molecular genetics and cell biology that now explain them may be reflected in preserved acronyms or nomenclature that acknowledge historical observations.

Structural alterations during development are referred to as **malformations** when they result from altered genetic or developmental processes. When physical forces interrupt or distort morphogenesis, their effects are termed **disruptions** and **deformations,** respectively. The term **dysplasia** is used to denote abnormal histogenesis.

Congenital abnormalities are often multiple and recur in patterns recognized through classification as **syndromes.** Current understanding of maldevelopment recognizes that recurrent patterns most often reflect either the neighboring chromosomal location of duplicated or deleted genes, **contiguous gene syndromes;** or the alteration of genetically regulated developmental programs, **developmental field defects.** The term **sequences** is preferred to "syndromes" when secondary factors (eg, mechanical distortion) are major determinants of abnormal patterns. Malformations occurring together more frequently than would be expected by chance alone, whether within a currently recognized developmental field or not, may be classified as belonging to **associations.**

COMMON SYNDROMES & SEQUENCES

In the text that follows the important and commonly occurring human malformation syndromes are described, with emphasis on clinical findings that should suggest their inclusion in differential diagnoses and on brief explanations of causes. The reader is again referred to *Smith's Recognizable Patterns of Human Malformation* to examine what have become standard photographs of these conditions.

1. IN NEWBORNS

Chromosomal abnormalities most often present in newborns as multiple congenital anomalies in association with intrauterine growth retardation. Common aneuploid syndromes (trisomy 13, 18, and 21) have been described elsewhere in this chapter. Chromosomal deletions producing contiguous gene syndromes recognizable in newborns include **cri du chat syndrome (del 5p),** in which growth retardation and microcephaly coexist with an unusual cat-like cry; **Wolf-Hirschhorn syndrome (del 4p16),** characterized by prominent ears and unusual development of the nose and orbits that produces an appearance suggesting an ancient Greek warrior's helmet, often in association with cleft lip and palate; and **Miller-Dieker syndrome (del 17p13),** in which microcephaly and an unusually developed face and forehead reflect abnormal migration of neuronal germinal matrix cells (lissencephaly). In the presence of apparently normal chromosomes, each of these conditions can be detected by FISH.

Cornelia de Lange Syndrome

Cornelia de Lange syndrome is a sporadically occurring malformation syndrome whose etiology remains obscure. It is characterized by severe growth retardation; limb, especially hand, reduction defects (50%); congenital heart disease (25%); and stereotypical facies with hirsutism, medial fusion of eyebrows (synophrys), and thin, downturned lips.

The course and severity are variable, but the prognosis for survival and normal development is poor. Chromosomal analysis is usually normal.

DiGeorge Syndrome

DiGeorge syndrome (del 22q11) was originally described in newborns presenting with cyanotic congenital heart disease, usually involving great vessel abnormalities; thymic hypoplasia leading to immunodeficiency; and hypocalcemia due to absent parathyroid glands. The disorder is now known to result most often from deletions of chromosome 22q11 and to be phenotypically highly variable. Chromosome 22q11 deletions also produce less severe phenotypes (velocardiofacial syndrome, Shprintzen syndrome) that may be more easily recognized in older children (see below). However, a high level of suspicion and use of FISH to detect cryptic deletions is warranted since this deletion may account for as much as 5% of cases of congenital heart disease and is present in approximately 40% of cases when tetralogy of Fallot occurs in association with another congenital abnormality.

Smith-Lemli-Opitz Syndrome

This syndrome also combines intrauterine growth retardation; syndactyly or polydactyly (or both) of the toes; hypogenitalism (with hypospadias in males); microcephaly, ptosis, and characteristic facies; and neurologic dysfunction, especially feeding difficulties.

The disorder is recessive and results from inability

to complete cholesterol synthesis. Diagnosis is based on elevation of the cholesterol precursor 7-dehydrocholesterol. Treatment with cholesterol dietary supplementation is under investigation. This is an important syndrome to recognize in newborns in whom chromosomal studies are normal.

VACTERL Association

VACTERL association is described by an acronym denoting the association of *v*ertebral defects (segmentation anomalies), imperforate *a*nus, *c*ardiac malformation (most often ventricular septal defect), *t*racheo*e*sophageal fistula, *r*enal anomalies, and *l*imb (most often radial ray) anomalies.

The disorder is sporadic and the defects life-threatening, thus calling for immediate attention. The prognosis for normal later development is good. The cause is unknown, but association of the syndrome with monozygotic twinning—in which case it is frequently discordantly expressed—suggests a mechanism dating back to events perhaps as early as blastogenesis. Careful examination and follow-up are important, since numerous other syndromes with more complicated prognoses also include features present in VACTERL association. Intrauterine growth is usually normal, and no abnormalities should occur above the neck. Chromosomal studies and genetic consultation are warranted, because the condition is overdiagnosed.

CHARGE Association

CHARGE association involves numerous structures derived from developmental fields involving rostral neural crest cells but also includes abnormal development of the eyes and midbrain. It is a sporadic condition whose etiology is not understood. The acronym serves as a mnemonic for associated abnormalities that include *c*olobomas, congenital *h*eart disease, choanal *a*tresia, growth *r*etardation, *g*enital abnormalities (hypogenitalism), and *e*ar abnormalities.

Abnormally shaped or placed ears are almost invariable in this condition, and that deformity should always lead to careful physical assessment, including ophthalmologic consultation. Neurologic dysfunction is frequently present at birth and may raise ethical issues about limiting interventions. Studies of surviving patients indicate that neuronal damage due to airway and feeding complications contribute substantially to developmental delays. Again, numerous other syndromes present with features of this condition, many with better prognoses. Chromosomal studies are normal but are usually necessary to distinguish this condition from other disorders.

Oligohydramnios Sequence (Potter Sequence)

This condition presents in newborns as severe respiratory distress due to pulmonary hypoplasia in association with positional deformities of the extremities, usually bilateral clubfeet, and typical facies consisting of suborbital creases, depressed nasal tip and low-set ears, and retrognathia. The sequence may be due to prolonged lack of amniotic fluid. Most often it is due to leakage, renal agenesis, or severe obstructive uropathy.

Arthrogryposis Multiplex

Arthrogryposis multiplex is due to lack of fetal movement. Causes most often involve constraint, central nervous system maldevelopment or injury, or neuromuscular disorders. In the neuromuscular disorders, polyhydramnios is often present as a result of lack of fetal swallowing. Pulmonary hypoplasia may also be present, reflecting lack of fetal breathing. The workup will usually include brain imaging, careful consideration of metabolic disease—especially peroxisomal disorders presenting with elevated very long chain fatty acids—neurologic consultation, and, in some cases, electrophysiologic studies and muscle biopsy. The family history should be carefully reviewed for findings such as muscle weakness or cramping, cataracts, and early-onset heart disease, suggesting myotonic dystrophy. Parents should have careful neurologic examinations that include testing for myotonia.

Skeletal Dysplasias

Skeletal dysplasias in newborns present with disproportionate growth (Figure 31–13) with or without respiratory compromise. Impaired growth of the chest wall is an ominous sign and when responsible for pulmonary hypoplasia invariably presages early demise. However, it is important to recognize that treatable airway compromise may also cause respiratory distress. The diagnosis of skeletal dysplasia is made through careful physical examination and evaluation of skeletal films. Consultation with clinical geneticists and radiologists experienced with skeletal dysplasias is usually necessary. **Achondroplasia,** the most common type of skeletal dysplasia in infants surviving the newborn period, can be confirmed through molecular genetic studies for specific mutations in the gene for fibroblast growth factor receptor 3 *(FGFR3)*.

2. MATERNAL DRUG EXPOSURES

Anticonvulsant exposure during pregnancy is now recognized as being associated with adverse outcomes in approximately 10% of cases. A syndrome characterized by small head circumference, anteverted nares, cleft lip and palate (occasional), and distal digital hypoplasia was first described in association with maternal use of phenytoin but can also been seen with other anticonvulsants. Risks for spina bifida are increased, especially in pregnancies exposed to valproic acid.

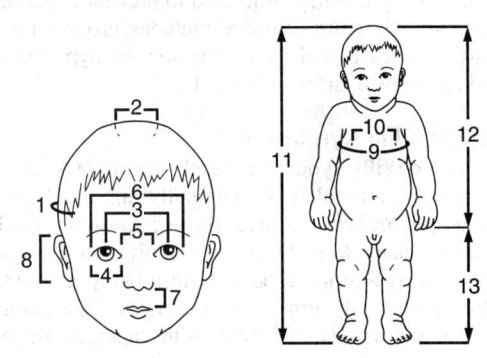

Measurement	Range (cm)	
	Term (38–40 weeks)	Preterm (32–33 weeks)
1 Head circumference	32–37	27–32
2 Anterior fontanelle $\left(\frac{L-W}{2}\right)$	0.7–3.7	. . .
3 Interpupillary distance	3.3–4.5	3.1–3.9
4 Palpebral fissure	1.5–2.1	1.3–1.6
5 Inner canthal distance	1.5–2.5	1.4–2.1
6 Outer canthal distance	5.3–7.3	3.9–5.1
7 Philtrum	0.6–1.2	0.5–0.9
8 Ear length	3–4.3	2.4–3.5
9 Chest circumference	28–38	23–29
10 Internipple distance*	6.5–10	5–6.5
11 Height	47–55	39–47
12, 13 Ratio Upper body segment / Lower body segment	1.7	. . .
14 Hand (palm to middle finger)	5.3–7.8	4.1–5.5
15 Ratio of middle finger to hand	0.38–0.48	0.38–0.5
16 Penis (pubic bone to tip of glans)	2.7–4.3	1.8–3.2

*Internipple distance should not exceed 25% of chest circumference.

Figure 31–13. Neonatal measurements.

Fetal alcohol syndrome results from excessive exposure to alcohol during gestation and affects 30–40% of offspring of mothers whose daily intake of alcohol exceeds 3 oz. Features of the syndrome include short stature, poor head growth (may be postnatal in onset), developmental delay, and mid face hypoplasia characterized by a poorly developed long philtrum, narrow palpebral fissures, and short nose with anteverted nares. Facial findings may be subtle, but careful measurements and comparisons with standards (Figure 31–13) can be useful. Structural abnormalities occur in half of affected children. Genitourinary tract anomalies are frequent. The consensus now among scientists and clinicians is that the term "fetal alcohol effect" is misleading and should not be applied to apparently incomplete phenotypes. Careful evaluation for other syndromes and chromosomal disorders should be included in the workup. Behavioral abnormalities may or may not be directly attributable to alcohol, since psychiatric disorders, many with recognized inherited predisposition, affect a large number of women and their partners who abuse.

Vitamin A and its analogs are potent embryologic morphogens that interact with specific receptors and therefore have considerable teratogenic potential. Developmental toxicity occurs in approximately one-third of pregnancies exposed in the first trimester to the synthetic retinoid isotretinoin. Exposure disrupts developmental fields to which rostral neural crest cells contribute and produces central nervous system maldevelopment, especially of the posterior fossa; ear anomalies (often absence of pinnae); congenital heart disease (great vessel anomalies); and tracheoesophageal fistula. These findings constitute a partial phenocopy of DiGeorge syndrome and demonstrate the continuum of contributing genetic and epigenetic factors in morphogenesis. It is now recognized that vitamin A itself, when taken during pregnancy in the active form of retinoic acid in doses exceeding 10,000 IU/d, can produce partially affected phenotypes. Maternal ingestion of even large amounts of "vitamin A" taken as *retinol* during pregnancy does not increase risks, since conversion of this precursor to active retinoic acid is regulated by the body.

Maternally abused substances in general are associated with increased risks for adverse perinatal outcomes, including miscarriage, preterm delivery, growth retardation, and increased risk for injury to the developing central nervous system. For most abused substances, the link between exposures and adverse outcomes is less well demonstrated than with alcohol. Multiple factors are probably involved, and it should be recognized that substance abuse often involves more than one drug. Maternal inhalant abuse appears to be associated with findings similar to those of fetal alcohol syndrome. Reports of outcomes of cocaine abuse (and the "crack baby" syndrome) have been contradicted by studies finding no effects. The form of the drug used and its route of administration may be important determinants of risk.

3. IN CHILDREN

Chromosomal Abnormalities

Chromosomal abnormalities are, again, an important consideration in children who present with the triad of growth failure, developmental delay, and dysmorphic features. High-resolution cytogenetic studies are very useful in evaluation of these children and may detect abnormalities not evident in karyotypes from amniotic fluid or newborn blood samples. FISH studies can also be very useful when directed by experienced clinical geneticists.

Short Stature

Short stature is an important component of numerous syndromes or may be an isolated finding. In the absence of nutritional deficiencies, endocrine abnormalities, evidence for skeletal dysplasia (disproportionate growth with abnormal skeletal films), or a positive family history, intrinsic short stature can be due to uniparental disomy (see above) such that only imprinted (silenced) copies of specific sequences are present. The phenotype of **Russell-Silver syndrome**—short stature with normal head growth (pseudohydrocephalus), normal development, and minor dysmorphic features (especially fifth finger clinodactyly)—has been associated in some cases with maternal uniparental disomy for chromosome 7.

Overgrowth Syndromes

Overgrowth syndromes are becoming increasingly recognized as important childhood conditions. They present at birth and are characterized by macrocephaly, motor delays (cerebral hypotonia), and, in many cases, asymmetry of extremities. Bone age may be advanced. Hemihypertrophy may be an important feature because its presence is associated with increased risks for Wilms tumors. Overgrowth syndromes include recognizable phenotypes of unknown cause *(Soto syndrome),* single gene disorders **(Simpson-Golabi-Behmel syndrome, Bannayon-Zanoni-Ruvalcaba syndrome),** and disorders that overexpress *IGF2* through duplication or relaxation of maternal imprinting **(Beckwith-Wiedemann syndrome, hemihypertrophy).**

Noonan Syndrome

Noonan syndrome is an autosomal dominant disorder characterized by short stature, congenital heart disease, abnormalities of cardiac conduction and rhythm, webbed neck, downslanting palpebral fissures, and low-set ears. Affected children may be large at birth and have mild subcutaneous edema. The phenotype evolves with age and may be difficult to recognize in older relatives. Mild developmental delays are often present. No candidate genes have yet been identified.

Williams Syndrome

Williams syndrome (del 7q) is a contiguous gene disorder characterized by short stature, congenital heart disease (supravalvular aortic stenosis), coarse, elfin-like facies with prominent lips, hypercalcemia or hypercalciuria in infancy, developmental delay, and neonatal irritability evolving into an overly friendly personality.

FISH studies are nearly always necessary to confirm the clinical diagnosis. Calcium restriction may

be necessary in early childhood to prevent nephrocalcinosis. The natural history includes progression of cardiac disease and predisposition to hypertension and spinal osteoarthritis in adults.

Prader-Willi Syndrome

Prader-Willi syndrome results from lack of expression of a number of maternally imprinted genes, including *SNRPn,* located on chromosome 15q11. Clinical characteristics include short stature; weakness and hypotonia, especially in infancy; characteristic facies with almond-shaped eyes; hypogenitalism; small hands and feet with tapering fingers; hypopigmentation (occasionally); developmental delay (variable); obsessive hyperphagia (onset as late as age 6); and type 2 (adult-onset) diabetes mellitus

Multiple chromosomal rearrangements and mutations have been reported to disrupt expression of the genes that contribute to this syndrome. Of these, deletion of paternal chromosome 15q11 is most common, followed by maternal uniparental disomy. Molecular techniques that analyze patterns of methylation of involved DNA sequences provide a practical approach to diagnosis when clinical suspicion is aroused, but additional studies (eg, FISH) to determine the genetic mechanisms responsible are necessary in confirmed cases for reproductive risk counseling.

Angelman Syndrome

Angelman syndrome also involves imprinting. It is most commonly caused when sequences detectable by FISH on 15q11 are deleted from the maternal homolog. Uniparental paternal disomy 15 is the least common cause. Mutations in a single gene that is paternally imprinted (methylated) and expressed only in the central nervous system during development cause the disorder in perhaps one-fourth of cases.

The classic phenotype includes severe mental retardation with marked delay in motor milestones, prognathism, seizures; abnormal puppet-like gait and posturing; poor language development; and paroxysmal laughter and tongue thrusting.

With additional studies of mutations in the gene responsible for this syndrome, it is possible that its clinical description will be expanded to include less severely delayed individuals. Recurrence is possible when mothers inherit mutations that are paternally imprinted and therefore silent.

Shprintzen Syndrome

Shprintzen syndrome (del 22q11), also known as **velocardiofacial syndrome,** is commonly associated with deletion in the same region as that causing DiGeorge syndrome. Characteristics include mild microcephaly, palatal clefting or incompetence, speech and language delays, congenital heart disease (ventricular or atrial septal defect), buildup of tissue lateral to the nose, long, tapering fingers, and emotional lability.

The reasons for the phenotypic variability encountered in patients with contiguous genes deleted at 22q11 are not clear. Phenotypic variability occurs within affected families. Use of FISH to detect deletions is helping to define the range of phenotypes. Emotional lability and mood swings are prominent features, and there is an apparent predisposition to psychosis.

Disorders of Connective Tissue

Connective tissue disorders affect children in a variety of ways that bring them to medical attention. These include excessive or disproportionate growth, unusual scarring and poor wound healing, bruising and bleeding, scoliosis, venous varicosities, and joint hyperextension and injury.

A common clinical dilemma involves distinguishing between several of the forms of *Ehlers-Danlos syndrome,* each with its own characteristic predispositions to medical complications, and *Marfan syndrome,* which carries with it a significant risk for aortic root widening and dissection. Although genes and mutations for several of these conditions have been described, molecular diagnostic testing is limited. Collagen analyses in cultured fibroblasts are available if Ehlers-Danlos syndrome type IV or osteogenesis imperfecta is suspected, but diagnoses are made largely on clinical grounds, and referral to clinical geneticists with experience in examining patients with connective tissue disorders is indicated.

Marfan Syndrome

Marfan syndrome is caused by mutations in genes for the connective tissue protein fibrillin, but laboratory detection of mutations in clinical practice remains, for the time being, difficult. Clinical diagnostic criteria have therefore been developed that include disproportionate growth (arachnodactyly and other manifestations), joint hyperextensibility, lens dislocation, and dilation of the aortic root. The latter two characteristics are considered major criteria and are diagnostic when accompanied by evidence of connective tissue involvement, usually joint hyperextensibility. When the family history is positive for major criteria, the diagnosis can be made in relatives on the basis of minor criteria. Minor criteria alone are not sufficient for diagnosis. In sporadic cases with major criteria, it is important to exclude homocystinuria through careful metabolic testing.

CLINICAL APPROACH TO THE DYSMORPHIC INFANT

Physicians caring for neonates with birth defects must frequently provide care and make accurate diagnoses under conditions of great stress. The extent of an infant's abnormalities may not be immediately apparent, and parents who feel grief and guilt are often desperate for information. As with any medical problem, however, the history and physical examination provide most of the clues to diagnosis. Special aspects of these procedures are outlined below.

HISTORY

Environmental, family, and pregnancy histories may contain important clues to the diagnosis. Parental recall after delivery of an infant with an anomaly is better than recall after a normal birth. An obstetric wheel can help document gestational age and events of the first trimester: the last menstrual period, the onset of symptoms of pregnancy, the date of diagnosis of the pregnancy, the date of the first prenatal visit, and the physician's impressions of fetal growth at that time.

To investigate fetal growth and development, prenatal visits should be noted and, with the aid of the obstetric wheel, a record should be made of the patterns of fetal growth, the onset of fetal movement (usually at 16 weeks), and the mother's perceptions of fetal movements. Normal fetal movement is usually strong enough to hurt the mother and be visible to the father. Abnormal fetal movement may indicate neuromuscular dysfunction or fetal constraint. A history of decreased fetal movement will often distinguish neuromuscular abnormalities (which result in a low Apgar score) from intrapartum events (which depress the infant).

Abnormal patterns of uterine growth may also provide clues to fetal function. Increased uterine size may indicate accumulation of amniotic fluid (hydramnios). Fluid may accumulate if the fetus fails to swallow as a result of a neuromuscular disorder, obstruction of the fetal esophagus or proximal small bowel, or fetal heart failure. Hydramnios is also associated with diabetes and high-output renal failure in the fetus. Lack or delay of uterine growth may reflect fetal growth directly or may be a sign of too little amniotic fluid (oligohydramnios). Amniotic fluid may be lost through premature rupture of membranes with or without formation of amniotic bands, or it may be the result of compromised function of fetal kidneys. The mother should be questioned about loss or leakage of amniotic fluid, which may have been mistaken for a vaginal discharge.

The history should also include details about the onset and progression of labor. Breech presentation at term may indicate a uterine anomaly or abnormality of the fetal central nervous system.

Family histories should always be included but may seem threatening to parents or relatives attempting to cope with strong feelings about birth defects. The interviewer should be prepared to respond to specific questions from family members.

Finally, an environmental history that includes descriptions of parental habits, their work, and the home should be obtained.

PHYSICAL EXAMINATION

Meticulous physical examination is crucial to accurate diagnosis in dysmorphic infants. Delivery of an affected infant may necessitate immediate attention to potentially life-threatening problems, but it is precisely because intensive support may be required that a complete examination becomes urgent. The examination should be performed as soon as possible.

In addition to the routine procedures described in Chapter 3, special attention should be paid to the neonate's physical measurements (Figure 31–13). Photographs are helpful and should include a scale of measurements for reference. The placenta should also be examined.

IMAGING & LABORATORY STUDIES

Radiologic and ultrasonographic examinations can be extremely helpful in the evaluation of dysmorphic infants. In general, films of infants with apparent limb or skeletal anomalies should include views of the skull and all of the long bones in addition to frontal and lateral views of the axial skeleton. Chest and abdominal films should be obtained when indicated. The pediatrician should consult a radiologist for further workup. Nuclear scans and imaging by CT, MRI, and ultrasonography are all useful diagnostic tools, but their interpretation in the presence of birth defects may require considerable experience.

Cytogenetic analysis provides specific diagnoses in approximately 5% of dysmorphic infants who survive the newborn period. Chromosome abnormalities are recognized in 10–15% of infants who die. Karyotypes can be determined rapidly through analysis of cells in bone marrow. These allow limited interpretation and should always be accompanied by complete analysis of cultured cells. Any case requiring rapid diagnosis should be discussed with an experienced dysmorphologist. A normal karyotype does not rule out the presence of significant genetic disease.

PERINATAL AUTOPSY

When a dysmorphic infant dies, postmortem examination can provide important diagnostic information and should include sampling of tissue for cytogenetic analysis. The pediatrician and the pathologist should consider whether samples of blood, urine, or tissue should be obtained for metabolic analyses.

X-ray studies should be done whenever limb anomalies or disproportionate growth is present. Pla-

cental as well as fetal tissue can be used for viral culture. The pediatrician should discuss the case thoroughly with the pathologist, and photographs should always be taken.

DYSMORPHOLOGIC EVALUATION OF THE DEVELOPMENTALLY DELAYED CHILD

Mental retardation or developmental delays affect 8% of the population. Disorders presenting with symptoms of delayed development are heterogeneous but frequently include heritable components. Evaluation should be multidisciplinary; Table 31–4 lists its main features, emphasizing the major clinical and genetic considerations.

Table 31–4. Evaluation of the developmentally delayed child.

History
 Pregnancy history
 Growth parameters at birth
 Neonatal complications
 Feeding history
 History of somatic growth
 Motor, language and psychosocial milestones
 Seizures
 Loss of skills
 Abnormal movements
 Results of previous tests and examinations
Family history
 Developmental and educational histories
 Psychiatric disorders
 Pregnancy outcomes
 Medical history
 Consanguinity
Physical examination
 General pediatric examination
 Focused dysmorphologic evaluation including
  measurement of facial features and assessment of
  dermatoglyphics
 Complete neurologic examination
 Parental growth parameters (especially head
  circumferences) and dysmorphic features should also be
  assessed.
Imaging studies
 See text.
Laboratory assessment[1]
 Chromosomes (high resolution analyses)
 Fragile X testing (analysis of FMR1 gene for triplet repeats)
 FISH analyses guided by dysmorphic features
 Other blood analyses: CBC, electrolytes, liver function
  tests
 Serum amino acid analyses
 Urine amino and organic acid analyses
 Urine analyses for mucopolysaccharides

[1]In many cases, negative results may be important.

Patterns and timing of growth and development are particularly important to discern. For example, prenatal-onset growth retardation is less likely to have a metabolic origin than postnatal growth delay. Loss of skills raises suspicion about possible metabolic or neurodegenerative disorders.

Behavioral abnormalities are commonly associated with developmental delays, but behavioral diagnoses such as attention deficit disorder, obsessive-compulsive disorder, autism, or autistic-like behaviors are better viewed as descriptive rather than etiologically informative diagnoses.

Standard pedigrees in clinical genetic practice include specific information at least three generations antecedent to the individual being evaluated.

Examination for diagnosis of dysmorphologic disorders is a clinical skill that requires practice. Referral to a clinical geneticist is indicated whenever unusual features are encountered. Neurologic, ophthalmologic, and audiologic consultation should be sought when indicated. Brain imaging should be requested in most cases involving otherwise unexplained deviations from normal head growth. Neuroimaging and skeletal studies may also be suggested by dysmorphic features. Neurologic consultation can often help sort through indications for imaging.

As molecular explanations for genetic disorders accumulate, opportunities for molecular genetic testing increase. Unlike the majority of the studies listed in Table 31–4, these are not screening tests—they may confirm but often do not entirely rule out specific diagnoses. In general, it will not be cost-effective to proceed with molecular genetic testing without clinical genetic consultation.

Metabolic and genetic testing procedures other than what are listed in the table may also be indicated. Appropriate consultations should be sought to coordinate these investigations.

Interpretation & Follow-Up

Clinical experience indicates that specific diagnoses can be made in approximately half the patients evaluated according to the protocol presented here. With specific diagnosis comes prognosis, ideas for management, and insight into recurrence risks. Prenatal diagnosis may also become possible.

Follow-up is important both for patients in whom diagnoses have been made and for those initially undiagnosed. Genetic information is rapidly accumulating and can be translated into new diagnoses and better understanding with periodic review of clinical cases.

Astley SJ, McLarren SK: A case definition and photographic screening tool for the facial phenotype of fetal alcohol syndrome. J Pediatr 1996;129:33.

Cohen MM: *The Child With Multiple Birth Defects.* Oxford Univ Press, 1997.

Hall JG, Fnoster-Iskenium UG, Allanson JE: *Handbook of Normal Physical Measurements.* Oxford Univ Press, 1989.

Thomas JA, Graham JM: Chromosome 22q11 deletion syndrome: An update and review for the primary pediatrician. Clin Pediatr 1997;36:253.

Stevenson RE, Hall JG, Goodman RM (editors): *Human Malformations and Related Anomalies.* 2 vols. Oxford Univ Press, 1993.

Wynne-Davies R, Hall C, Apley A: *Atlas of Skeletal Dysplasias.* Churchill Livingstone, 1987.

V. GENETIC COUNSELING

THE PROCESS OF COUNSELING

Genetic counseling is more than just a communication process about the risk for recurrence of genetic disorders in a family. It is the culmination of a genetic evaluation when a specific diagnosis has been made (if possible) and the etiology, prognosis, and management of the disorder in question have been discussed. At the time of formal genetic counseling, this information should be reviewed and recurrence risk assessments presented. If a specific diagnosis has been made, specific risks for future pregnancies can be quantitated. It is often useful at this time to review with the family some basic genetic information, showing pictures of chromosomes, explaining the difference between chromosomes and genes, and diagramming the common mechanisms of inheritance. If a specific diagnosis has not been made, empiric risk figures can be presented. The final step in the genetic counseling process is the discussion of possible prevention or prenatal diagnosis in future pregnancies.

Much has been written about directive versus nondirective genetic counseling, but in the United States at least, the latter is recommended and more widely practiced. Although it is difficult to be completely objective—particularly if the geneticist is familiar with the long-term burden of a disorder—it is important to remember that the ultimate choice about reproduction will be made by the parents. A geneticist may have concerns about society at large, but a counselor should be the advocate for the family, not for society.

The timing of genetic counseling is also important. There is a fine line between counseling that is too early (because the family, still concerned about the welfare of the affected individual, is emotionally unprepared) and counseling that is too late (because another at-risk fetus has already been conceived). The possibility of a genetic basis for the mishap should be mentioned early, but continuing contact is needed to refine the diagnosis and help the family understand the implications.

There are many ways to communicate information to the parents, but all explanations should be given in plain language and in a relaxed and unhurried atmosphere. The baseline risk for congenital abnormalities should be discussed and put into the perspective of the risk being quoted. The actual risk should be compared with the burden (or the parents' perception of the burden) of the abnormality. Examples can be helpful. Issues of guilt and blame must be addressed. This part of counseling can be difficult if one of the parents carries an abnormal gene or used a teratogenic substance, such as alcohol. Ongoing psychologic counseling may be needed. It may be difficult for parents to understand how an isolated abnormality in a family can still be genetic and be associated with a significant recurrence risk; it may be necessary to review with them such concepts as phenocopy, new mutations, decreased penetrance, and variable expressivity.

All too often, no specific diagnosis can be made and no cause for a specific genetic disorder or malformation can be determined. In such cases, recurrence risks can only be estimated. It may be helpful for families to explore possible mechanisms and for the geneticist to discuss the implications for subsequent pregnancies. Parents should think about and give weight to their own emotional response to the birth of a second affected child.

Genetic counseling is not a static process. Families often continue to have questions. A letter sent to them explaining clearly and concisely the information covered in the counseling session is helpful. Although a geneticist cannot assume responsibility for all problems a family may have, appropriate referrals can be made. Periodic contact by a member of the counseling team—social worker, genetic nurse, or genetic counselor—is advisable to ensure adequate understanding and to reopen counseling as new information and testing become available.

A word should be said about responsibility to the extended family. As more genetic disorders become diagnosable by new molecular techniques, counseling needs to be expanded to the family at large. This requires both the cooperation of the consultant and collaboration between genetic units throughout the country. During counseling, it is necessary to educate families concerning this need and at the same time respect confidentiality.

COUNSELING OPTIONS

In situations of increased risk for inherited disorders, families have a variety of options. They can have no further children or they can take the risk, but in many cases there are other choices. Some families for whom prenatal diagnosis is unacceptable or un-

available may prefer adoption. Artificial insemination is genetically appropriate if a disease is recessive or if the father is the carrier, and in vitro fertilization with donor ova if the mother is the carrier. Preimplantation diagnosis of an embryo obtained after in vitro fertilization with maternal eggs and paternal sperm is possible for some single-gene disorders and for sex determination using molecular and FISH technology. However, this option is still experimental and thus of limited availability. Even if it were more widely available, cost might be a determining factor in its application. Some families may consider sterilization, but they should realize that the risk for each of the parents may drop markedly if the couple should separate and remarry. For most families, however, some type of prenatal diagnosis is requested and often available.

All of these options are expensive. Prevention of an abnormality is, of course, the ideal result. To date, the use of periconceptional folic acid and rubella vaccine are the only known effective preventive measures other than the avoidance of teratogenic substances such as alcohol.

VI. PRENATAL DIAGNOSIS

It has been estimated that prenatal diagnosis is indicated in 7–8% of all pregnancies. As technology improves, the indications for and the accuracy of prenatal diagnosis can only increase. Today, a large proportion of pregnant women undergo at least one ultrasound study during pregnancy, and congenital abnormalities are being detected more frequently prior to birth even in low-risk women. Prenatal diagnosis introduces options for management that range from interruption of abnormal pregnancies to preparation for specialized perinatal care.

METHODS

Prenatal diagnosis techniques analyze maternal blood, image the conceptus, and sample fetal and placental tissues. See Table 31–5.

Maternal Blood

The use of maternal serum α-fetoprotein as a screening test was originally introduced because higher than normal values were found in association with neural tube defects. It was also noted that women who carried a fetus with Down syndrome had a 25% lower α-fetoprotein value than those in whom the fetus was normal. Subsequent studies have shown that adding measurements of human chorionic go-

Table 31–5. Prenatal diagnostic techniques.

Maternal blood screening such as alpha-fetoprotein, estriol,
  hCG ("triple screen")
  Trisomy 21 and 18
  Neural tube defects
Fetal cells in maternal blood (research only)
Fetal ultrasound
  Structural defects
  Fetal hydrops
  Poly- or oligohydramnios
Fetal x-ray
  Skeletal defects
Fetal MRI
Amniocentesis
  Karyotyping
  Fetal cells for molecular or metabolic studies
  Amniotic fluid alpha-fetoprotein level for neural tube
    defects
  Biochemical studies on fluid
Chorionic villus sampling
  Karyotyping
  Fetal cells for molecular or metabolic studies
Fetal tissues
  Blood per percutaneous umbilical blood sampling
  Biopsy of other fetal tissues
Direct fetal visualization via fetoscopy (rarely used today) be-
  cause of the advances in fetal visualization by ultrasound
  and MRI)

nadotropin and unconjugated estradiol can increase rates of detection for trisomy 21 and predict some cases of trisomy 18 as well.

Fetal cells, including lymphocytes, trophoblasts, and nucleated red blood cells, are present in the maternal circulation. Research is being directed toward isolating these cells for prenatal diagnosis using culture, hybridization, and PCR-based techniques.

Testing of Fetal Tissue

Amniocentesis has been available for many years. Its accuracy and safety are well established. Fluid surrounding the fetus is sampled, and cells are cultured for cytogenetic, molecular, or metabolic analysis. Alpha-fetoprotein and other molecules can also be measured. This is a safe procedure with a complication rate (primarily for miscarriage) of less than 1% in experienced hands.

Chorionic villus sampling (placental) is now available in most centers and can be performed late in the first trimester. Tissue obtained by chorionic villus sampling provides more DNA for molecular analysis and contains dividing cells (cytotrophoblast) that can be rapidly karyotyped. However, direct cytogenetic preparations may be of poor quality. In addition, chromosomal abnormalities detected by this technique may be confined to the placenta (confined placental mosaicism). Cultured preparations may be more accurate. Certainly, if an unusual cytogenetic picture is found on chorionic villus sampling, further studies should be considered before management de-

cisions are made. Numerous studies have been done comparing the safety of first-trimester chorionic villus sampling with amniocentesis. Of some concern is the possible association of chorionic villus sampling prior to 11 weeks with terminal transverse limb defects, perhaps secondary to vascular disruption.

Fetal blood can be directly sampled in late gestation through ultrasound-guided percutaneous umbilical blood sampling (PUBS).

It is occasionally necessary to biopsy fetal tissues such as liver or muscle for accurate prenatal diagnosis. These procedures are available in only a few perinatal centers.

Fetal Visualization

Transabdominal real-time ultrasonography can visualize all major fetal organs, including the kidneys, heart, brain, spinal cord, bladder, and limbs, beginning as early as 16–18 weeks of gestation. Transvaginal ultrasonography is now providing even earlier imaging. It is therefore possible to look for almost any genetic syndrome that includes a specific defect. Routine ultrasound screening has demonstrated many unexpected abnormalities. Most of these are major defects, however, and minor anomalies are easily missed, especially if unexpected.

Fetal motion has been a major deterrent to the use of MRI as a tool for prenatal diagnosis. However, new techniques are being developed to overcome this problem, making MRI a potentially valuable noninvasive means of fetal assessment.

X-ray studies of the fetus are rarely necessary because ultrasonography has improved so greatly. If a skeletal abnormality or bone dysplasia is suspected, however, x-ray films may be helpful.

INDICATIONS

Amniocentesis or chorionic villus sampling is indicated in the following circumstances:

(1) Maternal age over 35 years.

(2) Previous child with a chromosome abnormality.

(3) Either parent a translocation carrier. In this case, the risk for a fetus with an unbalanced chromosome abnormality depends on the type of translocation.

(4) A history of any genetic disorder diagnosable by biochemical techniques or by DNA analysis. The list of such conditions changes daily, and a genetic center should be contacted for the most recent information.

(5) A request by the parents for fetal sex determination because of a history of an X-linked disorder that is not otherwise diagnosable.

(6) Maternal blood testing (eg, triple screen) indicating increased risks for chromosomal abnormalities.

(7) As part of the workup of fetal anomalies found by ultrasonography.

Fetal ultrasonography is indicated whenever an abnormality characterized by a structural defect is suspected. The defect may be suspected because of the family history, potential exposure to teratogens during pregnancy, or questionable abnormalities noted on a routine ultrasound examination done in the obstetrician's office. In any case, the patient should be referred for further evaluation to a medical center staffed by personnel experienced in fetal ultrasonography.

ETHICAL CONSIDERATIONS

Much has been written about the conflict surrounding elective termination of pregnancy and concerns about "genetic engineering," but there are other important issues of immediate concern. The question of privacy and confidentiality is raised by many families. They are worried about genetic discrimination both in employment and health insurance. While efforts are made to keep records confidential and laws are being passed to prevent such discrimination, there are still potential problems. Many commentators question the ethics of presymptomatic testing where there is no effective intervention at this time.

Such testing may lead to significant psychologic problems as well as genetic discrimination and should only be done in a carefully controlled setting. However, as molecular tests become more widely and economically available and there is increasing emphasis on cost containment, there may be a greater temptation to perform these tests in an office setting, with potentially harmful consequences.

Another issue that has raised concern is the presymptomatic or carrier testing of minors. Most genetic centers do not perform these tests except under very unusual circumstances.

These are only a few of the current pressing concerns. Others will no doubt arise as technology advances.

Eisenberg VH, Schenker JJ: The moral aspects of prenatal diagnosis. Obstet Gynecol 1997;72:35.

Ferguson-Smith MA: Editorial: DNA for diagnosis. Prenat Diagn 1996;16:1175.

Hogge JS, Hogge WA: Preconceptual genetic counseling. Clin Obstet Gynecol 1996;39:751.

Poulton J, Marchington DR: Prospects for DNA-based prenatal diagnosis of mitochondrial disorders. Prenat Diagn 1996;16:1247.

Stranc LC, Evans JA, Hamerton JL: Chorionic villus sampling and amniocentesis for prenatal diagnosis. Lancet 1997;349:711.

REFERENCES

Emery AEH, Rimoin DL: *Principles and Practice of Medical Genetics,* 2nd ed. Churchill Livingstone, 1990.

Jones KL: *Smith's Recognizable Patterns of Human Malformation,* 5th ed. Saunders, 1996.

King RA, Rotter JI, Motulsky AG: *The Genetic Basis of Common Diseases.* Oxford Univ Press, 1993.

McKusick VA: *Mendelian Inheritance in Man,* 11th ed. Johns Hopkins Univ Press, 1994.

Stevenson RE, Hall JG, Goodman RM (editors): *Human Malformations and Related Anomalies,* vols 1 and 2. Oxford Univ Press, 1993.

Allergic Disorders

32

Mark Boguniewicz, MD, & Donald Y.M. Leung, MD, PhD

Allergic disorders are among the most common problems seen by pediatricians and primary care physicians, affecting over 25% of the population in developed countries. The economic impact of these illnesses can be measured in billions of dollars.

The prevalence of asthma, allergic rhinitis, and atopic dermatitis has increased in recent years. Among school-age children and adolescents, these illnesses result in significant morbidity and school absenteeism, with adverse consequence for school performance and quality of life, and may cause emotional stress. Understanding the language of allergy and the basic mechanisms involved may help physicians when treating these patients.

Anaphylaxis was first described as a fatal reaction following repeated injection of dogs with jellyfish venom—which was the opposite of the expected **prophylaxis.** Subsequently, allergic rhinitis and asthma were described as **human anaphylaxis. Allergy** is altered reactivity to a foreign substance after prior exposure to that substance. **Atopy** is a term first introduced to denote end organ hypersensitivity to environmental proteins in familial allergic rhinitis and asthma—later extended to include the propensity to produce heat-labile reaginic antibody, subsequently identified as IgE, to common allergens and to include allergic eczema as well. **Atopic dermatitis** denotes both the weeping eczema of infancy and childhood and the chronic xerosis and lichenified lesions more typically seen in older patients. This term also recognizes the close relationship between atopic dermatitis, allergic rhinitis, and asthma. Much progress has been made in the understanding of atopic diseases since the introduction of these terms, and much remains to be learned about the complex interrelationship of genetic, environmental, and immunologic factors in their pathogenesis.

THE ALLERGIC CASCADE

Allergic responses begin with sensitization to an allergen in a genetically susceptible host. The CD4 cells of allergic patients respond to allergens by producing predominantly interleukin-3, IL-4, IL-5, and IL-13 (a so-called Th-2-like profile). These cytokines are involved in IgE synthesis and in the differentiation and activation of eosinophils (Figure 32–1).

Allergen-specific IgE binds to receptors on mast cells, basophils, and Langerhans cells distributed throughout the skin and respiratory tract and in the circulation. Cross-linking of receptor-bound IgE by allergen activates effector cells to release allergic mediators, including histamine and newly synthesized mediators such as prostaglandins and leukotrienes. Effector cells may also release other enzymes and cytokines. This immediate allergic reaction may be manifested clinically as sneezing, hives, wheezing, vomiting, or anaphylaxis. As part of the allergic cascade, mononuclear cells and eosinophils are recruited to the site of the acute reaction and can cause late phase responses. Activated eosinophils in particular release toxic mediators that cause many of the clinical symptoms in allergic diseases. It is likely that a number of infiltrating cells such as monocytes, neutrophils, and basophils and resident cells such as epithelial cells and fibroblasts participate in perpetuating this inflammatory process even in the absence of allergens.

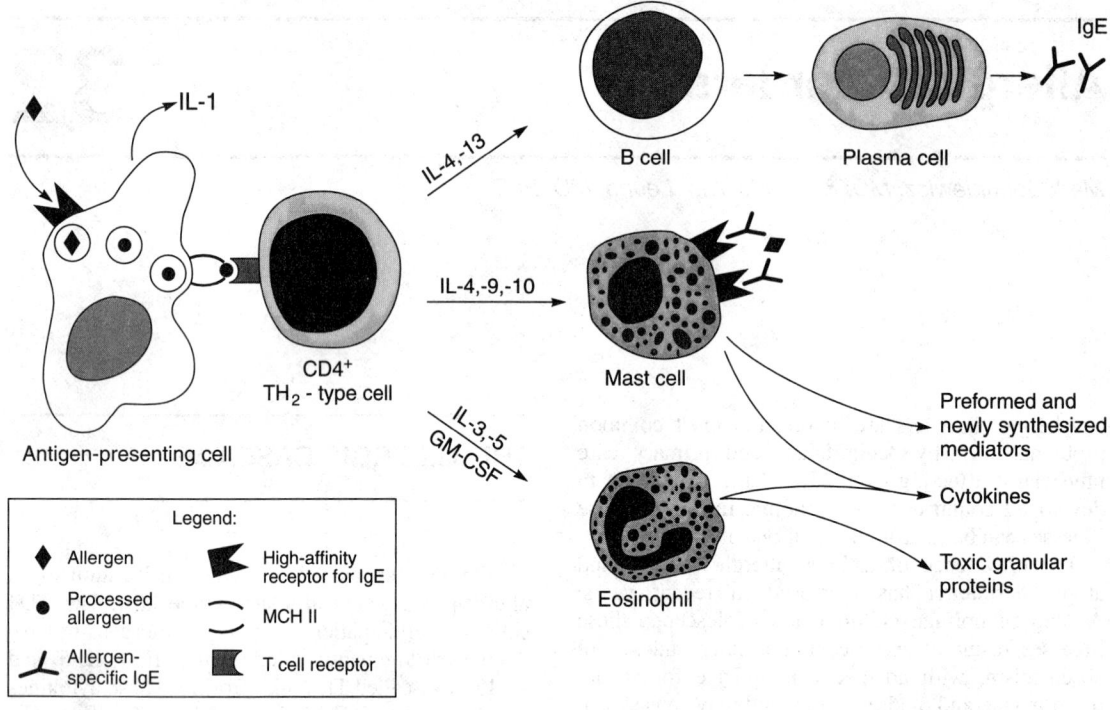

Figure 32–1. Cellular interactions in allergic responses.

MAJOR ALLERGIC DISORDERS SEEN IN PEDIATRIC PRACTICE

ASTHMA

Essentials of Diagnosis & Typical Features

• Episodic symptoms of airflow obstruction including wheezing, cough, or chest tightness.
• Airflow obstruction at least partially reversible.
• Exclusion of alternative diagnoses.

General Considerations

Asthma is the most common chronic disease of childhood, affecting an estimated 4.8 million children in the United States. Despite advances in the understanding of asthma, associated morbidity has increased over the past decade and mortality rates have remained relatively stable. Asthma hospitalization rates have been highest in the black population, with death rates consistently highest among African-Americans ages 15–24 years. The reasons for this are not clear but may be related to a combination of poor access to health care together and such environmental factors as smoke and perennial allergen exposure.

Up to 80% of children with asthma develop symptoms before their fifth birthday. Atopy, the genetic predisposition for the development of an IgE-mediated response to common allergens, is the strongest identifiable predisposing factor. Exposure to tobacco smoke, especially by the mother, is also a risk factor for asthma. About 40% of infants and young children who have wheezing with viral infections in the first few years of life will have continuing asthma through childhood. Sensitization to inhalant allergens increases over time and is found in the majority of children with asthma. The most important allergens associated with increased risk for asthma include perennial aeroallergens such as dust mites, animal danders, cockroaches, and *Alternaria*. Rarely, foods may provoke isolated asthma symptoms. Other triggers include exercise, cold air, cigarette smoke, pollutants, strong chemical odors, and rapid changes in barometric pressure. Aspirin sensitivity is uncommon in children. Psychologic factors may precipitate asthma exacerbations and in addition place the patient at high risk from the disease.

Pathologic features of asthma include shedding of airway epithelium, edema, mucus plug formation, mast cell activation, and collagen deposition beneath the basement membrane. The inflammatory cell infiltrate includes eosinophils, lymphocytes, and neutrophils, especially in fatal asthma exacerbations.

Airway inflammation contributes to airway hyperresponsiveness, airflow limitation, and disease chronicity. Persistent airway inflammation can lead to airway wall remodeling and irreversible changes.

Clinical Findings

A. Symptoms and Signs: Wheezing is the most characteristic sign of asthma though it may be absent in some children, especially with cough variant asthma. Patients may also have cough and shortness of breath. Complaints may include "chest congestion," prolonged cough, exercise intolerance, dyspnea, and recurrent bronchitis or pneumonia. If symptoms are absent or mild, chest auscultation during forced expiration may reveal prolongation of the expiratory phase and wheezing. As the obstruction becomes more severe, wheezes become more high-pitched and breath sounds diminished. With severe obstruction, wheezes may not be heard because of poor air movement. Flaring of nostrils, intercostal and suprasternal retractions, and use of accessory muscles of respiration are signs of severe obstruction. Flushed, moist skin may be noted, with dry mucous membranes. Cyanosis of the lips and nail beds may be seen with underlying hypoxia. Tachycardia and pulsus paradoxus are also observed. Agitation or lethargy may be signs of impending respiratory failure.

B. Laboratory Findings: Airway hyperresponsiveness to nonspecific stimuli is considered a hallmark of asthma. These include inhaled pharmacologic agents such as histamine and methacholine as well as physical stimuli such as exercise and cold air. Airways may exhibit hyperresponsiveness or twitchiness even when pulmonary function tests are normal. Giving increasing amounts of a bronchoconstrictive agent to induce a decrease in lung function (usually a 20% drop in forced expiratory volume in 1 second [FEV_1]) is the most common method of testing airway responsiveness. Hyperresponsiveness in normal children less than 5 years of age is greater than in older children. The level of airway hyperresponsiveness usually correlates with the severity of asthma.

During acute asthma exacerbations, FEV_1 is diminished and the flow-volume curve shows a "scooping out" of the distal portion of the expiratory portion of the loop. The residual volume, functional residual capacity, and total lung capacity are usually increased, while the vital capacity is decreased. Reversal or significant improvement of these abnormalities in response to inhaled bronchodilator therapy alone or with anti-inflammatory therapy is observed. Increased airway resistance also results in a decreased peak expiratory flow rate (PEFR). Diurnal variation in PEFR (ie, the difference between morning and evening measurements) of greater than 15–20% has been used as a defining feature of asthma. Significant changes in PEFR may occur before symptoms become evident. In more severe cases, PEFR monitoring enables earlier recognition of suboptimal asthma control. Exercise, cold air, and methacholine or histamine challenges may be helpful in establishing the diagnosis of suspected asthma when the history, examination, and pulmonary function tests are not definitive. Alternatively, a diagnostic trial of inhaled bronchodilators and anti-inflammatory medications may be helpful, especially in infants and young children in whom underdiagnosis and undertreatment are difficult problems.

Hypoxemia is present early with a normal or low P_{CO_2} level and respiratory alkalosis. Hypoxemia may be aggravated during treatment with a β_2-agonist due to ventilation-perfusion mismatch. Oxygen saturation less than 91% is indicative of significant obstruction. Respiratory acidosis and increasing CO_2 tension may ensue with further airflow obstruction and signal impending respiratory failure. Hypercapnia is usually not seen until the FEV_1 falls below 20% of predicted value. Metabolic acidosis has also been noted in combination with respiratory acidosis in children with severe asthma and indicates imminent respiratory failure. A PaO_2 less than 60 mm Hg despite oxygen therapy and a $PaCO_2$ over 60 mm Hg and rising to more than 5 mm Hg per hour are relative indications for mechanical ventilation in a child in status asthmaticus.

Pulsus paradoxus may be present with moderate or severe asthma. In moderate asthma in a child, this may be between 10 and 25 mm Hg, and in severe asthma between 20 and 40 mm Hg. Absence of pulsus paradoxus in a child with severe asthma exacerbation may be an indication of respiratory muscle fatigue.

Clumps of eosinophils on sputum smear and blood eosinophilia are frequent findings. Their presence tends to reflect disease activity and does not necessarily mean that allergic factors are involved. Leukocytosis is common in acute severe asthma without evidence of bacterial infection and may be more pronounced after epinephrine administration. Hematocrit can be elevated with dehydration during prolonged exacerbations or in severe chronic disease.

C. Imaging: On chest x-rays, bilateral hyperinflation with flattening of the diaphragms, peribronchial thickening, prominence of the pulmonary arteries and areas of patchy atelectasis may be present. Atelectasis is often misinterpreted as pneumonia.

Allergy testing is discussed below.

Differential Diagnosis

Diseases that may be mistaken for asthma are often related to the age of the patient (Table 32–1). Congenital abnormalities are most often seen in infants and young children. Asthma can be confused with croup, acute bronchiolitis, pneumonia, and pertussis. Immunodeficiency may be associated with cough and wheezing. Foreign bodies in the airway

Table 32–1. Differential diagnosis of asthma in infants and children.

Viral bronchiolitis
Aspiration
Laryngotracheomalacia
Vascular rings
Airway stenosis or web
Enlarged lymph nodes
Mediastinal mass
Foreign body
Bronchopulmonary dysplasia
Obliterative bronchiolitis
Cystic fibrosis
Vocal cord dysfunction
Cardiovascular disease

may cause dyspnea or wheezing of sudden onset, and on auscultation wheezing may be unilateral. Asymmetry of the lungs secondary to air trapping may be seen on a chest x-ray, especially with forced expiration. Cystic fibrosis can be associated with or mistaken for asthma.

Vocal cord dysfunction is an important masquerader of asthma, though the two can occasionally coexist. It is characterized by the paradoxic closure of the vocal cords that can result in dyspnea and wheezing. Diagnosis is made by direct visualization of the vocal cords. In normal individuals, the vocal cords abduct during inspiration and may adduct slightly during expiration. Asthmatic patients may have narrowing of the glottis during expiration as a physiologic adaptation to airway obstruction. In contrast, patients with isolated vocal cord dysfunction typically show adduction of the anterior two-thirds of their vocal cords during inspiration, with a small diamond-shaped aperture posteriorly. Since this abnormal vocal cord pattern may not be seen in the absence of symptoms, a normal examination does not exclude the diagnosis. Exercise or methacholine challenges can often precipitate symptoms of vocal cord dysfunction. The flow-volume loop may provide additional clues to the diagnosis of vocal cord dysfunction. Truncation of the inspiratory portion can be demonstrated in most patients during an acute episode, and some patients continue to show this pattern even when they are asymptomatic. In contrast to adults with vocal cord dysfunction where a high incidence of abuse has been reported, children and especially adolescents tend to be overly competitive, especially in athletics and scholastics. A psychiatric consultation may help define underlying psychologic issues and provide appropriate therapy.

Treatment of patients with isolated vocal cord dysfunction includes education regarding the syndrome and appropriate breathing exercises. Hypnosis, biofeedback, and psychotherapy have been effective for some patients. During an acute episode, a helium-oxygen mixture can be administered because the low density of the gas mixture facilitates movement of air through the adducted vocal cords.

Conditions That May Increase Asthma Severity

Chronic hyperplastic sinusitis is frequently found in association with asthma. Upper airway inflammation has been shown to contribute to the pathogenesis of asthma, and asthma may improve after treatment of sinusitis. However, sinus surgery is usually not indicated for initial treatment of chronic mucosal disease associated with allergy.

A significant correlation has been observed between nocturnal asthma and gastroesophageal reflux. Patients may not complain of epigastric burning or have reflux symptoms—cough may be the only sign. For patients with poorly controlled asthma, particularly with a nocturnal component, investigation for gastroesophageal reflux may be warranted even in the absence of suggestive symptoms.

The risk factors for death from asthma include psychologic and sociologic factors. They are probably related to the consequences of illness minimalization or denial as well as to noncompliance with the medical regimen. Recent studies have shown that less than 50% of inhaled asthma medications are taken as prescribed and that compliance does not improve with increasing severity of illness. Moreover, children requiring hospitalization for asthma have often failed to institute appropriate early home treatment.

Complications

With acute asthma, complications are primarily related to hypoxemia and acidosis and can include generalized seizures. Pneumomediastinum or pneumothorax can be a complication in status asthmaticus. Recent studies point to airway wall remodeling and loss of pulmonary function with persistent airway inflammation. Childhood asthma independent of any corticosteroid therapy has been shown to be associated with delayed maturation and an extended slowing of prepubertal growth velocity. However, attainment of final predicted adult height does not appear to be compromised.

Treatment

A. Chronic Asthma:

1. General measures—Patients should avoid exposure to tobacco smoke and allergens to which they are sensitized, exertion outdoors when levels of air pollution are high, beta-blockers, and sulfite-containing foods. Patients with persistent asthma should be given influenza vaccine yearly.

For patients with persistent asthma, the clinician should use the patient's history to assess sensitivity to seasonal allergens; use skin testing or in vitro testing to assess sensitivity to perennial indoor allergens; assess the significance of positive tests in the context of the patient's history; and identify relevant allergen exposures. For dust mite-allergic children, important environmental control measures include encasing the pillow and mattress in an allergen-impermeable cover and washing the sheets and blankets on the patient's bed weekly in hot water. Other measures include keeping indoor humidity below 50%, minimizing the number of stuffed toys, and washing such toys weekly in hot water. Children allergic to furred animals or feathers should avoid indoor exposure, especially for prolonged periods of time. If removal of the pet is not possible, the animal should be kept out of the bedroom with the door closed. Carpeting and upholstered furniture should be removed. The use of a high-efficiency particle-arresting (HEPA) filter unit in the bedroom may be of benefit. For cockroach-allergic children, control measures need to be instituted when infestation is present in the home. Poison baits, boric acid, and traps are preferred to chemical agents, which can be irritating if inhaled by asthmatics. Indoor molds are especially prominent in humid environments or in homes with dampness. Measures to control dampness or fungal growth in the home may be of benefit. Patients can reduce exposure to outdoor allergens by staying in an air-conditioned environment. Allergen immunotherapy may be useful for implicated aeroallergens that cannot be avoided. However, it should be administered only in a facility where a physician and trained personnel are available to treat life-threatening reactions if they occur.

The patient and family must understand the role of asthma triggers, the importance of disease activity even without obvious symptoms, how to use objective measures to gauge disease activity, and the importance of airway inflammation—and must learn to recognize the warning signs of worsening asthma, allowing for early intervention. A stepwise care plan should be developed for all patients with asthma. This educational process extends to school personnel and all those who care for the child with asthma.

Since the degree of airflow limitation is poorly perceived by many patients, peak flow meters can aid in the assessment of airflow obstruction and day-to-day disease activity. Peak flow rates may provide early warning of worsening asthma. They are also helpful in monitoring the effects of medication changes. Spacer devices optimize delivery of medication from metered-dose inhalers to the lungs and, with inhaled steroids, minimize side effects. Large-volume spacers are preferred.

Patients should be treated for confounding rhinitis, sinusitis, or gastroesophageal reflux, if present. Treatment of upper respiratory tract symptoms is an integral part of asthma management. Intranasal corticosteroids are recommended for the treatment of chronic rhinitis in patients with persistent asthma. Intranasal corticosteroids have been shown to reduce lower-airway hyperresponsiveness and asthma symptoms. Intranasal cromolyn has been shown to reduce

symptoms of asthma during the ragweed season but to a lesser extent than intranasal corticosteroids. Treatment of sinusitis includes medical measures to promote drainage and the use of antibiotics for acute bacterial infections. Medical management of gastroesophageal reflux includes avoiding eating or drinking 2 hours before bedtime, elevating the head of the bed with 6- to 8-inch blocks, and using appropriate pharmacologic therapy.

2. Pharmacologic therapy–A stepwise approach to pharmacologic therapy is recommended in the most recent Expert Panel Report 2: Guidelines for the Diagnosis and Management of Asthma. In this approach, the choice of therapy is based on assessment of clinical features prior to treatment (Table 32–2). The preferred strategy is to initiate therapy at a higher level at the onset to gain prompt control and then step down, rather than gradually stepping up treatment if control is not achieved. A rescue course of systemic corticosteroids may be necessary at any step. A short course of systemic corticosteroids is recommended for patients with intermittent asthma who experience infrequent but severe exacerbations—typically triggered by respiratory infections—with normal lung function between episodes.

Medications are now classified as long-term control medications and quick-relief medications (Table 32–3). The former include anti-inflammatory agents, long-acting bronchodilators, and leukotriene modifiers. Inhaled corticosteroids are the most potent inhaled anti-inflammatory agents currently available (Table 32–4). Recent data suggest that different inhaled corticosteroids are not equivalent on a per puff or microgram basis. Early intervention with inhaled corticosteroids can improve asthma control and normalize lung function and may prevent irreversible airway injury. High doses of inhaled corticosteroids may be associated with growth retardation in children, though the clinical significance of this potential systemic effect has yet to be determined. Possible risks from inhaled corticosteroids need to be weighed against the risks from undertreated asthma. Only inhaled corticosteroids have been shown to be effective in long-term clinical studies with infants, though symptom control and reduced airway hyperresponsiveness have been demonstrated with cromolyn in a number of pediatric studies. Fewer data are available with nedocromil, but benefit has been demonstrated. Sustained-release theophylline, an alternative long-term control medication for older children, may have particular risks of adverse side effects in infants, who frequently have febrile illnesses that increase theophylline concentrations. Salmeterol, a long-acting β_2-agonist, is approved for patients 12 years and older and can be used as adjunctive therapy with anti-inflammatory medications for long-term symptom control, especially at night. Salmeterol should not be used for treatment of acute symptoms and anti-inflammatory medication should not be discontinued

Table 32–2. Assessment of asthma severity prior to starting treatment.[1]

	Symptoms	Nighttime Symptoms	Lung Function
Step 1: Mild Intermittent	Symptoms 2 times a week Asymptomatic and normal PEF between exacerbations Exacerbations brief (from a few hours to a few days); intensity may vary	≤ 2 times a month	FEV$_1$ or PEF ≥ 80% of predicted PEF variability < 20%
Step 2: Mild Persistent	Symptoms > 2 times a week but < 1 time a day Exacerbations may affect activity	> 2 times a month	FEV$_1$ or PEF ≥ 80% of predicted PEF variability 20–30%
Step 3: Moderate Persistent	Daily symptoms Daily use of inhaled short-acting beta2-agonist Exacerbations affect activity Exacerbations ≥ 2 times a week; may last days	> 1 time a week	FEV$_1$ or PEF > 60% to < 80% of predicted PEF variability > 30%
Step 4: Severe Persistent	Continual symptoms Limited physical activity Frequent exacerbations	Frequent	FEV$_1$ or PEF ≤ 60% of predicted PEF variability > 30%

[1]Adapted from Expert Panel Report 2: *Guidelines for the Diagnosis and Management of Asthma.* NIH Publication No. 97–4051, 1997.

when salmeterol is initiated, even if the patient feels better.

Zafirlukast, a leukotriene receptor antagonist, and zileuton, a 5-lipoxygenase inhibitor, are leukotriene modifiers available in oral tablet formulations for patients age 12 and older. Zafirlukast is given in a dosage of 20 mg twice daily and should be taken 1 hour before or 2 hours after meals. The dosage of zileuton is 200 mg four times daily. Zafirlukast has recently been associated with several cases of Churg-Strauss syndrome in patients with severe asthma whose steroids were being tapered. Zileuton can cause hepatic toxicity, and ALT levels should be monitored. Zileuton may also increase serum theophylline levels.

Montelukast, a recently introduced leukotriene receptor antagonist is given in once-daily dosage and has been approved for children age 6 and older. To date, no drug interactions have been noted. The dosage is 5 mg for children aged 6–14 years and 10 mg for those aged 15 and older. The drug is given without regard to mealtimes, preferably in the evening.

Quick-relief medications include short-acting inhaled β_2-agonists such as albuterol, pirbuterol, or terbutaline, 1–2 puffs by inhaler. Albuterol can be given by nebulizer, 0.05 mg/kg (with a minimal dose of 1.25 mg and a maximum 2.5 mg) in 2–3 mL saline. It is better to use β_2-agonists as needed rather than on a regular basis. Increasing use, including more than one canister per month, may signify inadequate asthma control and the need to intensify anti-inflammatory therapy. Anticholinergic agents such as ipratropium, 1–3 puffs or 0.25–0.5 mg by nebulizer every 6 hours, may provide additive benefit when used together with inhaled β_2-agonists. Systemic cor-

ticosteroids such as prednisone, prednisolone, or methylprednisolone can be given in a dosage of 1–2 mg/kg, usually up to 60 mg/d in single or divided doses for 3–10 days. There is no evidence that tapering the dose following a "burst" prevents relapse.

Continual monitoring is necessary to ensure that control of asthma is achieved and sustained. Once control is established, gradual reduction in therapy is appropriate and may help determine the minimum amount of medication necessary to maintain control. Regular follow-up visits with the clinician are important to assess the degree of control and consider appropriate adjustments in therapy. At each step, patients should be instructed to avoid or control allergens, irritants, or other factors that contribute to asthma severity. Referral to an asthma specialist for consultation or comanagement is recommended if there are difficulties in achieving or maintaining control or if the patient has severe persistent asthma. Referral is also recommended if allergen immunotherapy is being considered.

Referral may be considered for patients with moderate persistent asthma. For children under 3 years of age, referral is recommended if the patient requires step 3 or 4 care and should be considered if the patient requires step 2 care (Table 32–3).

2. Exercise induced bronchospasm–Exercise-induced bronchospasm should be anticipated in all asthma patients. It typically occurs during or minutes after vigorous activity, reaches its peak 5–10 minutes after stopping the activity, and usually resolves over the next 20–30 minutes. Participation in physical activity should be encouraged in children with asthma, though the choice of activity may need to be modified based on the severity of illness, triggers such as cold air, and, rarely, confounding factors

Table 32–3. Stepwise approach for managing asthma in children.[1]

	Long-Term Control[2]	Quick Relief[2]	Education
Step 1: Mild Intermittent	No daily medication needed.	Short-acting bronchodilator: **inhaled β_2-agonist** or oral β_2-agonist as needed for symptoms. Use of short-acting inhaled β_2-agonist more than 2 times a week may indicate the need to initiate long-term control therapy. With viral respiratory infection: bronchodilator every 4–6 hours up to 24 hours (longer with physician consult) but, in general, repeat no more than once every 6 weeks. Consider systemic corticosteroid if current exacerbation is severe or patient has a history of previous severe exacerbations.	Teach basic facts about asthma. Teach inhaler and spacer technique. Discuss roles of medications. Develop self-management plan. Develop an action plan for when and how to take rescue actions. Discuss appropriate environmental control measures to avoid exposure to known allergens and irritants.
Step 2: Mild Persistent	*Daily medication:* **Anti-inflammatory:** either **inhaled corticosteroid** (low-dose) or **cromolyn** or **nedocromil** (infants and young children usually begin with a trial of cromolyn or nedocromil). Sustained-release theophylline (serum concentration of 5–15 µg/mL) is an alternative, but not preferred therapy. Zafirlukast or zileuton may also be considered for patients age 12 or older, though their position in therapy is not fully established.	Short-acting bronchodilator: **inhaled β_2-agonist** as needed for symptoms. Use of short-acting inhaled β_2-agonist on a daily basis or increasing use indicates the need for additional long-term control therapy.	Step 1 actions as above. Teach self-monitoring. Refer for group education if available. Review and update self-management plan.
Step 3: Moderate Persistent	*Daily medication:* **Anti-inflammatory:** either **inhaled corticosteroid** (medium dose) or inhaled corticosteroid (low-medium dose) and add nedocromil or a long-acting bronchodilator, especially for nighttime symptoms: either **long-acting inhaled β_2-agonist** (age 12 or older), sustained-release theophylline, or long-acting β_2-agonist tablets. *If needed:* **Anti-inflammatory: inhaled corticosteroid** (medium-high dose) and long-acting **bronchodilator,** especially for nighttime symptoms; either **long-acting inhaled β_2-agonist,** sustained-release theophylline or long-acting β_2-agonist tablets.	Short-acting bronchodilator: **inhaled β_2-agonist** as needed for symptoms. Use of short-acting inhaled β_2-agonist on a daily basis or increasing use indicates the need for additional long-term-control therapy.	Step 1 and 2 actions as above.

(*continued*)

Table 32–3. Stepwise approach for managing asthma in children.[1] (continued)

	Long-Term Control[2]	Quick Relief[2]	Education
Step 4: Severe Persistent	*Daily medication:* **Anti-inflammatory: inhaled corticosteroid** (high-dose) and long-acting bronchodilator: either **long-acting inhaled β$_2$-agonist,** sustained-release theophylline, or long acting β$_2$-agonist tablets. *and* Corticosteroid tablets or syrup (2 mg/kg/d, generally not to exceed 60 mg/d) and reduce to lowest daily or alternate-day dose that stabilizes symptoms.	Short-acting bronchodilator: **inhaled β$_2$-agonist** as needed for symptoms. Use of short-acting inhaled β$_2$-agonist on a daily basis or increasing use indicates the need for additional long-term control therapy.	Step 1 and 2 actions as above Refer for individual education/ counseling

Step down
Review therapy every 1–6 months; a gradual stepwise reduction in treatment may be possible.

Step up
If control is not maintained, consider stepping up. First, review patient's medication technique, compliance and environmental control (avoidance of allergens or other factors that contribute to asthma severity).

[1]Adapted from Expert Panel Report 2: *Guidelines for the Diagnosis and Management of Asthma.* NIH Publication No. 97-4051, 1997.
[2]Preferred treatment is indicated by bold type.

such as osteoporosis. Treatment immediately prior to vigorous activity or exercise is usually effective. Short-acting inhaled β$_2$-agonists such as cromolyn or nedocromil can be used shortly before exercise. The combination of a short-acting inhaled β$_2$-agonist with either cromolyn or nedocromil is more effective than either drug alone. Salmeterol may block exercise-induced bronchospasm for up to 12 hours. Occasion-ally, an extended warm-up period may induce a refractory state, allowing patients to exercise without a need for repeat medications. If symptoms occur during usual play activities, a step-up in long-term therapy is warranted. Poor endurance or exercise-induced bronchospasm can be an indication of poorly controlled persistent asthma.

B. Acute Asthma:

1. General measures–The most effective strategy in managing asthma exacerbations involves early recognition of warning signs and early treatment. For patients with moderate or severe persistent asthma or a history of severe exacerbations, this should include a written action plan. The latter usually defines the patient's peak flow zones and what steps to take if peak flows are between 50% and 80% or below 50% of personal best. The child, parents, and other caregivers must be able to assess asthma severity accurately. Prompt communication with the clinician is indicated with severe symptoms or a drop in peak flow or with decreased response to inhaled β$_2$-agonists. At such times, intensification of therapy may include a short course of oral corticosteroids. The child should be removed from exposure to any irritants or allergens that could be contributing to their exacerbation.

2. Management at home–Early treatment of asthma exacerbations may prevent progression to severe disease. Initial treatment should be with a short-acting inhaled β$_2$-agonist such as albuterol; 2–4 puffs from a metered-dose inhaler can be given every 20

Table 32–4. Comparative daily doses of inhaled steroids for children.[1]

Drug	Low dose (μg)	Medium dose (μg)	High dose (μg)
Beclomethasone 42,84 μg/puff	84–336	336–672	> 672
Budesonide 200 μg/dose	100–200	200–400	> 400
Flunisolide 250 μg/puff	500–750	1000–1250	> 1250
Fluticasone 44, 110, 220 μg/puff	88–176	176–440	> 440
Triamcinolone 100 μg/puff	400–800	800–1200	> 1200

[1]Adapted from Expert Panel Report 2: *Guidelines for the Diagnosis and Management of Asthma.* NIH Publication No. 97–4051, 1997.

minutes up to three times, or a single treatment can be given by nebulizer (0.05 mg/kg; minimum 1.25 mg, maximum 2.5 mg of 0.5% solution of albuterol in 2–3 mL saline). If the response is good as assessed by sustained symptom relief or improvement in PEFR to over 80% of the patient's best, the β_2-agonist can be continued every 3–4 hours for 24–48 hours. For patients taking inhaled corticosteroids, the dose may be doubled for 7–10 days. If there is incomplete improvement from the initial therapy, with PEFR between 50% and 80%, the β_2-agonist should be continued, an oral corticosteroid should be added, and the patient should contact the physician. If there is marked distress or if PEFR persists at under 50%, the patient should repeat the β_2-agonist immediately and go to the emergency department or call 911 or other emergency number for assistance.

3. Management in the office or emergency department–Functional assessment of the patient includes obtaining objective measures of airflow limitation with PEFR or FEV_1 and monitoring the patient's response to treatment. Other tests may include oxygen saturation and blood gases. If the initial FEV_1 or PEFR is over 50%, initial treatment can be with an inhaled β_2-agonist by inhaler (albuterol, 4–8 puffs) or nebulizer (0.15 mg/kg of albuterol 0.5% solution, minimum dose 2.5 mg), up to three doses in the first hour. Oxygen should be given to maintain oxygen saturation at greater than 90%. Oral corticosteroids (1 mg/kg every 6 hours for 48 hours, then 1–2 mg/kg/d in divided doses, maximum 60 mg/d) should be instituted if the patient has responds poorly to therapy or if the patient has been on oral corticosteroids recently. Sensitivity to adrenergic drugs may improve after initiation of corticosteroids. If the initial FEV_1 or PEFR is under 50%, initial treatment should be with a high-dose inhaled β_2-agonist by nebulizer every 20 minutes or continuously for the first hour (0.5 mg/kg/h). Ipratropium can be added to albuterol, 0.25 mg every 20 minutes for three doses, then every 2–4 hours. Oxygen should be given to maintain oxygen saturation at greater than 90%, and systemic corticosteroids should be instituted. In severe asthma unresponsive to initial aerosolized therapy or in patients who cannot cooperate with or those who resist inhalation therapy, epinephrine 1:1000 or terbutaline 1 mg/mL (both 0.01 mg/kg up to 0.3–0.5 mg) may be administered subcutaneously every 20 minutes for three doses. Theophylline or aminophylline does not appear to provide additional benefit to optimal inhaled β_2-agonist therapy and may be associated with adverse events. For impending or ongoing respiratory arrest, patients should be intubated and ventilated with 100% oxygen and admitted to an intensive care unit (see Chapter 12). Further treatment is based on clinical response and objective laboratory findings. Hospitalization should be strongly considered for any patient with a history of respiratory failure.

4. Hospital management–For patients who do not respond to outpatient therapy, admission to the hospital becomes necessary for more aggressive care and support. Fluids should be given at maintenance requirements unless the patient has poor oral intake secondary to respiratory distress or vomiting, since overhydration may contribute to pulmonary edema associated with high intrapleural pressures generated in severe asthma. Potassium requirements should be kept in mind as both corticosteroids and β_2-agonists can cause potassium loss. Moisturized oxygen should be titrated by oximetry to maintain SaO_2 above 90%. Inhaled β_2-agonist should be continued by nebulization in single doses as needed or by continuous therapy, along with ipratropium and systemic corticosteroids. As discussed above, therapy with methylxanthines does not appear to provide additional benefit for hospitalized children. Antibiotics may be necessary for coexisting bacterial infection. Sedatives and anxiolytic agents are contraindicated in severely ill patients owing to their depressant effects on respiration. Chest physiotherapy is usually not recommended for acute exacerbations.

5. Patient discharge–Criteria for discharging patients home from the office or emergency department should include a sustained response of at least 1 hour to bronchodilator therapy with FEV_1 or PEFR greater than 70% and oxygen saturation greater than 90% in room air. Prior to discharge, the ability of the patient or caregiver to continue therapy and assess symptoms appropriately needs to be considered. Patients should be given an action plan for management of recurrent symptoms or exacerbations, and instructions about medications should be reviewed. The inhaled β_2-agonist and oral corticosteroids should be continued, the latter for 3–10 days. Finally, the patient or caregiver should be instructed about the follow-up visit, typically within 1 week. Hospitalized patients should receive more intensive education prior to discharge. Referral to an asthma specialist should be considered for all children with severe exacerbations or multiple emergency department visits or hospitalizations.

Prognosis

In the past 25–30 years, morbidity and mortality rates for asthma have increased. Mortality statistics indicate that a high percentage of deaths have resulted from underrecognition of asthma severity and undertreatment, particularly in labile asthmatics and asthmatics whose perception of pulmonary obstruction is poor. Long-term outcome studies suggest that children with mild symptoms generally outgrow their asthma, while patients with more severe symptoms, marked airway hyperresponsiveness, and a greater degree of atopy tend to have persistent disease. It is possible that early intervention with anti-inflammatory therapy and environmental control measures may alter the natural history of childhood asthma. In this respect, the pediatrician or primary care provider together with the asthma specialist have a critical opportunity to affect the course of this increasingly common disease.

Resources for patients and families:

Asthma and Allergy Foundation of America
1125 15th St NW, Suite 502
Washington, DC 20005; (800) 7-ASTHMA

Asthma and Allergy Network/Mothers of Asthmatics
3554 Chain Bridge Rd, Suite 200
Fairfax, VA 22030-2709; (800) 878-4403

Agertoft L, Pedersen S: Effects of long-term treatment with an inhaled corticosteroid on growth and pulmonary function in asthmatic children. Respir Med 1994;88:373.

Busse WW, Gern JE: Viruses in asthma. J Allergy Clin Immunol 1997;100:147.

Expert Panel Report 2: Guidelines for the diagnosis and management of asthma. NIH Publication No. 97-4051, 1997.

Landwehr LP et al: Vocal cord dysfunction presenting as exercise-induced bronchospasm in adolescents. Pediatrics 1996;98:971.

Martinez FD et al: Asthma and wheezing in the first six years of life. N Engl J Med 1995;332:133.

Milgrom H et al: Non-compliance and treatment failure in children with asthma. J Allergy Clin Immunol 1996;98:1051.

Rosenstreich DL et al: The role of cockroach allergy and exposure to cockroach allergen in causing morbidity among inner-city children with asthma. N Engl J Med 1997;336:1356.

Sears MR: Epidemiology of childhood asthma. Lancet 1997;350:1015.

ALLERGIC RHINITIS

Essentials of Diagnosis & Typical Features

After exposure to allergen:
- Sneezing.
- Itching of nose and eyes.
- Clear rhinorrhea or nasal congestion.

General Considerations

Allergic rhinitis is the most common allergic disease and has significant impact on quality of life as well as school performance and attendance. It frequently coexists with asthma and is a risk factor for subsequent development of asthma. Prevalence of this disease increases during childhood, peaking at 15% in the postadolescent years. Although allergic rhinitis is more common in boys during early childhood, there is little difference in incidence between the sexes after adolescence. Race and socioeconomic status are not considered to be important factors in this common disease.

The pathologic changes in allergic rhinitis are chiefly hyperemia, edema, and increased serous and mucoid secretions caused by mediator release, all of which lead to variable degrees of nasal obstruction, pruritus, and rhinorrhea. This process may involve the eyes and other structures, including the sinuses and possibly the middle ear. Inhalant allergens are primarily responsible for symptoms, but food allergens can cause symptoms as well. Children with allergic rhinitis seem to be more susceptible to—or at least may experience more symptoms from—upper respiratory infections, which, in turn, may aggravate the allergic rhinitis.

Allergic rhinitis may be perennial, seasonal ("hay fever"), or episodic. Perennial allergic rhinitis occurs to some degree all year long but may be more severe in winter. Greater exposure to indoor allergens results from well-insulated homes, an increase in the amount of time spent indoors, and heating systems that disperse the allergens. Seasonal allergic rhinitis occurs as a result of exposure to specific aeroallergens, including pollens and molds. The major pollen groups in the temperate zones include trees (late winter to early spring), grasses (late spring to early summer), and weeds (late summer to early fall), but seasons can vary significantly in different parts of the country. Mold spores also cause seasonal allergic rhinitis, principally in the summer and fall. Seasonal allergy symptoms may be aggravated by coincident exposure to perennial allergens.

Clinical Findings

A. Symptoms and Signs: Patients may complain of itching of the nose, eyes, palate, or pharynx. Nasal itching can cause paroxysmal sneezing and epistaxis. Repeated rubbing of the nose ("allergic salute") may lead to a horizontal crease across the lower third of the nose. Nasal obstruction is manifested by mouth breathing, nasal speech, "allergic salute," and snoring. Nasal turbinates may appear pale blue and swollen, with dimpling, or injected, with minimal edema. Typically, clear and thin nasal secretions are increased, with anterior rhinorrhea, sniffling, postnasal drip, and congested cough. Nasal secretions often cause poor appetite, fatigue, and pharyngeal irritation. Conjunctival injection, tearing, periorbital edema, and infraorbital cyanosis ("allergic shiners") are frequently observed. Increased pharyngeal lymphoid tissue ("cobblestoning") from chronic drainage and enlarged tonsillar and adenoidal tissue may be present.

B. Laboratory Findings: Eosinophilia often can be demonstrated on smears of nasal secretions or blood. This is a frequent but nonspecific finding and may occur in nonallergic conditions. Although serum IgE may be elevated, measurement of total IgE is a poor screening tool owing to wide overlap between atopic and nonatopic subjects. Skin testing to identify allergen-specific IgE is the most sensitive and specific test for inhalant allergies; alternatively, RAST,

CAP, or other in vitro tests can be done for suspected allergens.

Differential Diagnosis

Disorders that need to be differentiated from allergic rhinitis include infectious rhinitis and sinusitis. Foreign bodies and structural abnormalities such as choanal atresia, marked septal deviation, nasal polyps, and adenoidal hypertrophy may cause chronic symptoms. Overuse of topical nasal decongestants may result in rhinitis medicamentosa. Use of medications such as propranolol, clonidine, and some psychoactive drugs may cause nasal congestion. Illicit drugs like cocaine can cause rhinorrhea. Spicy or hot foods may cause gustatory rhinitis. Nonallergic rhinitis with eosinophilia syndrome is usually not seen in young children. Vasomotor rhinitis is associated with persistent symptoms but without allergen exposure. Less common causes of symptoms that may be confused with allergic rhinitis include pregnancy, congenital syphilis, hypothyroidism, tumors, and cerebrospinal fluid rhinorrhea.

Complications

Sinusitis may accompany allergic rhinitis. Allergic mucosal swelling of the sinus ostia can obstruct sinus drainage, interfering with normal sinus function and predisposing to chronic mucosal disease. Nasal polyps due to allergy are unusual in children, and cystic fibrosis should be considered if they are present.

Treatment

A. General Measures: The value of identification and avoidance of causative allergens cannot be overstated. Reducing indoor allergens through environmental control measures as discussed above in the section on asthma can be very effective. Nasal saline irrigation may be useful.

B. Pharmacologic Therapy:

1. Antihistamines–Antihistamines help control itching, sneezing, and rhinorrhea. Sedating antihistamines include diphenhydramine, chlorpheniramine, hydroxyzine, and clemastine. Sedating antihistamines may cause daytime somnolence and negatively impact on school performance and activities, especially driving. Nonsedating antihistamines include terfenadine, astemizole, loratadine, cetirizine, and fexofenadine. Because terfenadine and astemizole have been associated with prolongation of the QT interval and cardiac arrhythmias and patients must be cautioned about their use with other drugs, these agents are generally less used nowadays. Loratadine and cetirizine are approved for use in children age 6 years or older and are available in tablet and liquid formulations, both 10 mg once daily. Loratadine is also available as a 10 mg rapidly disintegrating tablet. Loratadine is available in combination with pseudoephedrine for patients age 12 years or older in extended-release tablets for twice-daily or once-daily use, though the 24-hour preparation has been associated with a few cases of gastric outlet obstruction. Azelastine is available in a nasal spray and levocabastine as an ophthalmic preparation.

2. Decongestants–Alpha-adrenergic agents help to relieve nasal congestion. Topical decongestants such as phenylephrine or oxymetazoline should not be used for more than 4 days for severe episodes since prolonged use may be associated with a rebound congestion (rhinitis medicamentosa). Oral decongestants, including pseudoephedrine and phenylpropanolamine, are often combined with antihistamines or expectorants and cough suppressants in "cold medications." They may cause insomnia, agitation, tachycardia, and, rarely, cardiac arrhythmias.

3. Corticosteroids–Intranasal corticosteroid sprays are extremely effective in controlling allergic rhinitis. They are minimally absorbed in usual doses and are available in pressurized nasal inhalers and aqueous sprays (Table 32–5). Side effects include nasal irritation, soreness, and bleeding, though epistaxis occurs commonly in patients with allergic rhinitis. Rarely, they can cause septal perforation, and excessive doses may produce systemic effects. Onset of action is within hours, though clinical benefit is usually not observed for a week or more. They may be effective alone or together with antihistamines.

4. Other pharmacologic agents–Intranasal cromolyn may be used alone or in conjunction with oral antihistamines and decongestants. It is most effective when used prophylactically, 1-2 sprays per nostril, four times a day. This dose may be tapered if symptom control is achieved. Rarely, patients complain of nasal irritation or burning. The four times daily dosing is difficult for most patients to comply with. Cromolyn is also available in an ophthalmic solution. Another ophthalmic mast cell stabilizer is lo-

Table 32–5. Intranasal corticosteroid preparations.

Medication	Dose per Inhalation	Daily Dose per Nostril
Beclomethasone Inhaler Aqueous spray	42 μg 84 μg	1 spray bid–qid 1 or 2 sprays qd
Budesonide inhaler	32 μg	2 sprays bid or 4 sprays qd
Dexamethasone	84 μg	1 or 2 sprays bid
Flunisolide	25 μg	2 sprays bid
Fluticasone	50 μg	1 or 2 sprays qd
Triamcinolone Inhaler Aqueous spray	55 μg 55 μg	1 or 2 sprays qd 1 or 2 sprays qd

doxamide 0.1% solution and dosed 1-2 drops 4 times daily. Intranasal ipratropium can be used as adjunctive therapy for rhinorrhea.

C. Surgical Therapy: Surgical procedures, including turbinectomy, polypectomy and functional endoscopic sinus surgery, are rarely indicated in allergic rhinitis or chronic hyperplastic sinusitis.

D. Immunotherapy: Allergen immunotherapy should be considered when symptoms are severe and due to unavoidable exposure to inhalant allergens, especially if symptomatic measures have failed. Immunotherapy is the only form of therapy that may alter the course of the disease. It should not be prescribed by sending serum to a laboratory where extracts based on in vitro tests are prepared for the patient, ie, "the remote practice of allergy." Immunotherapy should be done in a facility where a physician prepared to treat anaphylaxis is present. Patients with concomitant asthma should not receive an injection if their asthma is not under good control, ie, peak flows preinjection below the "green zone" and the patient should wait for 25–30 minutes before leaving the facility.

Outcomes with single allergen immunotherapy show success rates of approximately 80%. The optimal duration of therapy is unknown, but data suggest that immunotherapy may have lasting benefit when it is discontinued in most patients after 3–5 years of maintenance therapy.

Prognosis

Perennial allergic rhinitis tends to be protracted unless specific allergens can be identified and eliminated from the environment. In seasonal allergic rhinitis, symptoms are usually most severe from adolescence through mid adult life. After moving to a region devoid of problem allergens, patients may be symptom-free for several years, but they can develop new sensitivities to local aeroallergens.

ATOPIC DERMATITIS

Essentials of Diagnosis & Typical Features

- Pruritus.
- Facial and extensor involvement in infants and young children.
- Flexural lichenification in older children and adolescents.
- Chronic or relapsing dermatitis.
- Personal or family history of atopic disease.

General Considerations

Atopic dermatitis is a chronically relapsing inflammatory skin disease typically associated with respiratory allergy. Like asthma and allergic rhinitis, atopic dermatitis is associated with the local infiltration of T cells secreting IL-4 and IL-5. Over half of

patients with atopic dermatitis will develop asthma and allergic rhinitis—often as they outgrow their atopic dermatitis. Atopic dermatitis may result in significant morbidity, leading to school absenteeism, occupational disability, and emotional stress. Atopic dermatitis typically presents in early childhood, with onset rarely before 2 months of age but prior to 5 years of age in approximately 90% of patients.

Recent studies have shown that exotoxins such as enterotoxins A, B, and toxic shock syndrome toxin-1, secreted by *Staphylococcus aureus,* can act as superantigens, contributing to persistent inflammation or exacerbations of atopic dermatitis. Over half of atopic dermatitis patients studied have toxin-secreting *S aureus* cultured from their skin. These patients make specific IgE antibodies directed against the toxins found on their skin.

Clinical Findings

A. Symptoms and Signs: Atopic dermatitis has no pathognomonic skin lesions or unique laboratory parameters. Diagnosis is based on the presence of major and associated clinical features, including severe pruritus, a chronically relapsing course, and typical morphology and distribution of the skin lesions. Acute atopic dermatitis is characterized by intensely pruritic, erythematous papules associated with excoriations, vesiculations, and serous exudate. Subacute atopic dermatitis is characterized by erythematous, excoriated, scaling papules, chronic atopic dermatitis by thickened skin with accentuated markings (lichenification) and fibrotic papules. Patients with chronic atopic dermatitis may have all three types of lesions present concurrently. Patients usually have dry, "lackluster" skin. During infancy, atopic dermatitis involves primarily the face, scalp, and extensor surfaces of the extremities. The diaper area is usually spared. When involved, it may be secondarily infected with *Candida,* in which case the dermatitis does not spare the inguinal folds. In older patients with long-standing disease, the flexural folds of the extremities are the predominant location of lesions.

B. Laboratory Findings: Identification of allergens involves taking a careful history and performing selective immediate hypersensitivity skin tests or in vitro tests when appropriate. Negative skin tests with proper controls have a high predictive value for ruling out a suspected allergen. Positive skin tests have a lower correlation with clinical symptoms in suspected food allergen-induced atopic dermatitis and should be confirmed with double-blind, placebo-controlled food challenges unless there is a coincidental history of anaphylaxis to the suspected food.

Elevated serum IgE levels can be demonstrated in 80–85% of patients with atopic dermatitis, and a similar number have positive immediate skin tests or in vitro tests with food and inhalant allergens. A number of well-controlled studies suggest that specific allergens can influence the course of this disease. However, triggers for clinical disease cannot be predicted simply by performing allergy testing. Double-blind, placebo-controlled food challenges have demonstrated that food allergens can cause exacerbations in a subset of patients with atopic dermatitis. Although lesions induced by single positive challenges are usually transient, repeated challenges, more typical of real life exposure, can result in eczematous lesions. Furthermore, elimination of food allergens results in amelioration of skin disease and a decrease in spontaneous basophil histamine release. Exacerbation of atopic dermatitis can occur with exposure to aeroallergens such as house dust mites, animal danders, and pollens. Environmental control measures have been shown to result in clinical improvement. Eosinophilia may occur. Routine skin biopsy does not differentiate atopic dermatitis from other eczematous processes and is not usually indicated.

A subset of patients with atopic dermatitis have elevated specific IgE to the yeast *Pityrosporum ovale* and the superficial dermatophyte *Trichophyton rubrum*. Patients with atopic dermatitis predominantly of the head and neck more often demonstrate positive skin tests, positive RAST, and specific histamine release to *P ovale*. The clinical significance of these findings is suggested by clinical improvement of such patients following treatment with antifungal therapy.

Differential Diagnosis

Scabies can present as a pruritic skin disease. However, distribution in the genital and axillary areas and the presence of linear lesions as well as skin scrapings may help to distinguish it from atopic dermatitis. Seborrheic dermatitis may be distinguished by a lack of significant pruritus, its predilection for the scalp ("cradle cap"), and its coarse, yellowish scales. Allergic contact dermatitis may be suggested by the distribution of lesions with a greater demarcation of dermatitis than in atopic dermatitis. Occasionally, allergic contact dermatitis superimposed on atopic dermatitis may appear as an acute flare of the underlying disease. Nummular eczema is characterized by coin-shaped plaques. In an older patient with an eczematous dermatitis and no history of childhood eczema or other atopic features, cutaneous T cell lymphoma needs to be considered. Eczematous rash has been reported with HIV. Other disorders that may resemble atopic dermatitis include Wiskott-Aldrich syndrome, severe combined immunodeficiency disease, hyper-IgE syndrome, zinc deficiency, phenylketonuria, and Letterer-Siwe disease.

Complications

Ocular complications associated with atopic dermatitis can lead to significant morbidity. Atopic keratoconjunctivitis is always bilateral, and symptoms include itching, burning, tearing, and copious mucoid discharge. It is frequently associated with eyelid dermatitis and chronic blepharitis and may result in visual impairment from corneal scarring. Vernal conjunctivitis is a severe bilateral recurrent chronic inflammatory process of the upper eyelid conjunctiva, occurring primarily in younger patients. It has a marked seasonal incidence, often in the spring. The associated intense pruritus is exacerbated by exposure to irritants, light, or perspiration. Examination of the eye reveals a papillary hypertrophy or "cobble-stoning" of the upper inner eyelid surface. Keratoconus is a conical deformity of the cornea believed to result from persistent rubbing of the eyes in patients with atopic dermatitis and allergic rhinitis. Anterior subcapsular cataracts may develop during adolescence or early adult life.

Patients with atopic dermatitis have increased susceptibility to infection or colonization with a variety of organisms. These include viral infections with herpes simplex, molluscum contagiosum, and human papillomavirus. Superimposed dermatophytosis may cause atopic dermatitis to flare. A number of studies have elucidated the importance of S aureus in atopic dermatitis. S aureus can be cultured from the skin of more than 90% of patients with atopic dermatitis, compared with only 5% of normal subjects. Patients without obvious superinfection may show a better response to combined antistaphylococcal and topical corticosteroid therapy than to corticosteroids alone. Although recurrent staphylococcal pustulosis can be a significant problem in atopic dermatitis, invasive S aureus infections occur rarely and should raise the possibility of an immunodeficiency such as hyper-IgE syndrome.

Patients with atopic dermatitis often have a nonspecific hand dermatitis. This is frequently irritant in nature and aggravated by repeated wetting, especially in the occupational setting.

Nutritional disturbances may result from unwarranted and unnecessarily vigorous dietary restrictions imposed by physicians and parents.

Poor academic performance and behavioral disturbances may be a result of uncontrolled intense or frequent itching, sleep loss, and poor self-image. Severe disease may lead to problems with social interactions and self-esteem.

Treatment

A. General Measures: Patients with atopic dermatitis have a lowered threshold of irritant responsiveness. Avoidance of irritants such as detergents, chemicals, and abrasive materials as well as extremes of temperature and humidity is important in managing this disease. Soaps should have minimal defatting activity and a neutral pH. New clothing should be washed to reduce the content of formaldehyde and other chemicals. Since residual laundry detergent in clothing may be irritating, using a liquid rather than powder detergent and adding an extra rinse cycle is beneficial. Occlusive clothing should be avoided in favor of cotton or cotton blends. Temperature in the home and work environments should be controlled to minimize sweating. Swimming is usually well tolerated; however, since swimming pools are treated with chlorine or bromine, patients should shower and use a mild soap to remove these irritating chemicals, then apply a moisturizer or occlusive agent. While sunlight may be beneficial to some patients with atopic dermatitis, nonsensitizing sunscreens should be used to avoid sunburn. Prolonged sun exposure can cause evaporative losses, overheating, and sweating, all of which can be irritating.

In children who have undergone controlled food challenges, eggs, milk, peanuts, soy, wheat, and fish account for approximately 90% of the food allergens that exacerbate atopic dermatitis. Avoidance of foods implicated in controlled challenges can lead to clinical improvement. Extensive elimination diets, which can be nutritionally unsound and burdensome, are almost never warranted since even patients with multiple positive skin tests rarely react to more than three foods on blinded challenges.

In patients who demonstrate specific IgE to dust mite allergen, environmental control measures aimed at reducing the dust mite load have been shown to improve atopic dermatitis. These include use of dust mite-proof covers on pillows and mattresses, washing linens weekly in hot water, decreasing indoor humidity levels, and in some cases removing bedroom carpeting.

Counseling may be of benefit when dealing with the frustrations associated with atopic dermatitis. Relaxation, behavioral modification, or biofeedback training may help patients with habitual scratching. Patients with severe or disfiguring disease may require psychotherapy.

Clinicians should provide the patient and family with both general information and specific written skin care recommendations. The patient or parent should demonstrate an appropriate level of understanding to help ensure a good outcome. Counseling should include the natural history and prognosis of the disease along with vocational counseling. Educational pamphlets and a video about atopic dermatitis can be obtained from the Eczema Association for Science and Education, 1221 SW Yamhill, Suite 303, Portland, OR 97205; (503) 228-4430—a national nonprofit, patient-oriented organization.

B. Hydration: Patients with atopic dermatitis have evaporative losses due to a defective skin barrier, so soaking the affected area or bathing for 15–20 minutes in lukewarm water, then applying an occlusive agent to retain the absorbed water, is an essential component of therapy. Oatmeal or baking soda added to the bath may feel soothing to certain patients but do not improve water absorption. The face or neck can be treated by applying a wet facecloth or towel to the involved area for 15–20 minutes. The washcloth may be more readily accepted by a child if it is turned into a mask. This also allows the older patient to remain functional. Lesions limited to the hands or feet can be treated by soaking in a basin. Daily baths may need to be taken on a chronic basis and increased to several times daily during flares of atopic dermatitis, while showers may be adequate for patients with mild disease. It is important to use an occlusive preparation within a few minutes after soaking the skin to prevent evaporation, which is both drying and irritating.

C. Moisturizers and Occlusives: An effective emollient combined with hydration therapy will help skin healing and can reduce the need for topical corticosteroids. Moisturizers are available as lotions, creams, and ointments. Since lotions contain more water than creams, they are more drying because of their evaporative effect. Preservatives and fragrances in lotions and creams may cause skin irritation. Since moisturizers often need to be applied several times daily on a long-term basis, they should be obtained in the largest size available. Crisco shortening can be substituted as an inexpensive alternative. Petroleum jelly (Vaseline) is an effective occlusive agent when used to seal in water after bathing.

D. Corticosteroids: Corticosteroids reduce the inflammation and pruritus in atopic dermatitis. Topical corticosteroids can decrease *S aureus* colonization. Systemic corticosteroids, including oral prednisone, should be avoided in the management of this chronic relapsing disease. The dramatic improvement observed with systemic corticosteroids may be associated with an equally dramatic flaring of atopic dermatitis following their discontinuation. If a short course of oral corticosteroids is given, it is usually best to prescribe a tapering dose.

Topical corticosteroids are available in a wide variety of formulations, ranging from extremely high-potency to low potency preparations (see Table 13–3). Choice of a particular product depends on the severity and distribution of skin lesions. Patients need to be counseled regarding the potency of their corticosteroid preparation and its potential side effects. In general, the least potent agent that is effective should be used. However, choosing a preparation that is too weak may result in persistence or worsening of the atopic dermatitis. Side effects include thinning of the skin, telangiectasias, bruising, hypopigmentation, acne, and striae, though these occur infrequently when low- to medium-potency topical corticosteroids are used appropriately. In contrast, use of potent topical corticosteroids for prolonged periods—especially under occlusion—may result in significant atrophic changes as well as systemic side effects. The face (especially the eyelids) and intertriginous areas are especially sensitive to corticosteroid side effects, and only low-potency preparations should be used routinely on these areas. Since topical corticosteroids are commercially available in a variety of bases, including ointments, creams, lotions, solutions, gels, and sprays, there is no need to compound them. Ointments are most occlusive and in general provide better delivery of the medication while preventing evaporative losses. However, in a humid environment, creams may be better tolerated than ointments since the increased occlusion may cause itching or even folliculitis. Creams and lotions, while easier to spread, can contribute to skin dryness and irritation. Solutions can be used on the scalp and hirsute areas, though they can be irritating, especially to open lesions. With clinical improvement, a less potent corticosteroid should be prescribed and the frequency of use decreased. Topical corticosteroids can be discontinued when inflammation resolves, but hydration and moisturizers need to be continued.

E. Tar Preparations: Crude coal tar extracts have less anti-inflammatory effects than topical corticosteroids. Tar preparations used in conjunction with topical corticosteroids in chronic atopic dermatitis may reduce the need for more potent corticosteroid preparations. However, their use has declined significantly other than in shampoos. Side effects associated with tar products include skin dryness or irritation, especially if applied to inflamed skin, and, less commonly, photosensitivity reactions and folliculitis.

F. Wet Dressings: Wet dressings are used together with hydration and topical corticosteroids primarily for the treatment of severe atopic dermatitis. They can also serve as an effective barrier against the persistent scratching that often undermines therapy. Total body dressings can be applied by using wet pajamas or long underwear with dry pajamas or a sweat suit on top. Hands and feet can be covered by wet tube socks with dry tube socks on top. Alternatively, wet gauze with a layer of dry gauze over it can be used and secured in place with an elastic bandage. Dressings can be removed when they dry out, usually after several hours, and are often best tolerated at bedtime. Incorrect use of wet dressings can result in chilling, maceration of the skin, or secondary infection.

G. Anti-infective Therapy: Systemic antibiotic therapy may be important when treating atopic dermatitis secondarily infected with *S aureus*. For limited areas of involvement, a topical antibiotic such as mupirocin may be effective. Erythromycin or a semisynthetic penicillin is usually the first choice for oral therapy. However, erythromycin-resistant organisms are fairly common. First- or second-generation cephalosporins are an alternative. Maintenance antibiotic therapy is rarely indicated and may result in colonization by methicillin-resistant bacteria.

Patients with disseminated eczema herpeticum (also referred to as Kaposi's varicelliform eruption) usually require treatment with systemic acyclovir. Patients with recurrent cutaneous herpetic lesions can be treated with prophylactic oral acyclovir. Superficial dermatophytosis and *P ovale* can be treated with topical or (rarely) systemic antifungal agents.

H. Antihistamines: Pruritus is usually the least well tolerated symptom of atopic dermatitis. Oral antihistamines and anxiolytics may be effective owing to their tranquilizing and sedating effects and can be taken mostly in the evening to avoid daytime somnolence. Nonsedating antihistamines may be less effective in treating pruritus, though beneficial effects have been reported in blinded studies. Use of topical antihistamines and local anesthetics should be avoided because of potential sensitization.

I. Recalcitrant Disease: Patients who are erythrodermic or who appear toxic may need to be hospitalized. Hospitalization may be appropriate for patients with more severe disease who fail outpatient management. Marked clinical improvement often occurs when the patient is removed from environmental allergens or stressors. In this setting, then, compliance with therapy can be monitored, the patient and family can receive intense education, and controlled provocative challenges can be conducted to help identify potential triggering factors. Ultraviolet light therapy can be useful for chronic recalcitrant atopic dermatitis. Patients who do not experience photoexacerbations of their atopic dermatitis and who are not fair-complexioned may benefit from moderate amounts of natural sunlight. However, they should be cautioned to avoid sunburn and to avoid sweating, which can induce pruritus. Under medical supervision, UVB has been shown to be effective in the treatment of atopic dermatitis. Photochemotherapy with oral methoxypsoralen therapy followed by UVA (PUVA) has been used in a limited number of children with severe atopic dermatitis unresponsive to other therapy, and significant improvement has been noted. However, the increased long-term risk of cutaneous malignancies from this therapy has prevented its widespread use.

Therapy directed toward correction of the immune dysfunction represents an alternative approach for patients unresponsive to conventional therapies. In an open study, children treated with cyclosporine, 5 mg/kg daily for 6 weeks, improved significantly and tolerated the treatment well. Unfortunately, discontinuation of treatment resulted in relapse, though the rate of relapse was variable. Tacrolimus (FK506) is an immunosuppressive agent with a spectrum of activity similar to that of cyclosporine. The therapeutic effects of this agent may be due to inhibition of IL-4 and IL-5 gene transcription. Use in children in a blinded, vehicle-controlled phase II trial showed significant clinical improvement. Other than local burning at the site of application, no significant side effects were noted over the 21 days of treatment. Phosphodiesterase inhibitors such as Ro 20–1724 have been shown to decrease IgE synthesis and basophil histamine release in vitro and to significantly reduce abnormal levels of IL-4, IL-10, and PGE_2 found in atopic dermatitis. Recently, patients treated with a potent inhibitor of phosphodiesterase type IV applied topically in a blinded, placebo-controlled paired-lesion study showed significant clinical improvement with the active drug.

J. Experimental and Unproved Therapies: A number of uncontrolled trials have suggested that desensitization to specific allergens may improve atopic dermatitis; however, controlled trials with standardized extracts of relevant allergens in atopic dermatitis are needed before this form of therapy can be recommended.

Traditional Chinese herbal therapy in the form of decoctions has also been proposed for atopic dermatitis. The herbs used may have antimicrobial, sedative, anti-inflammatory, and corticosteroid-like activities. Despite studies showing clinical efficacy, toxicity or idiosyncratic reactions remain a concern, and traditional Chinese herbal therapy should be considered investigational at best. Finally, although disturbances in the metabolism of essential fatty acids have been reported in patients with atopic dermatitis, well-controlled trials with fish oil and evening primrose have shown no clinical benefit.

Prognosis

Although it has been held that most children outgrow atopic dermatitis by adolescence, recent studies present less optimistic outcomes. In one, atopic dermatitis had disappeared in only 18% of children who had been followed from infancy until 13 years of age, though the symptoms had become less severe in 65%. In a prospective study from Finland, between 77% and 91% of adolescent patients treated for moderate or severe atopic dermatitis had persistent or frequently relapsing dermatitis as adults, though only 6% had severe disease. More than half of adolescents treated for mild dermatitis experienced a relapse of disease as adults. Adults whose childhood atopic dermatitis has been in remission for a number of years may present with hand dermatitis, especially if daily activities require repeated hand wetting.

Boguniewicz M, Leung DYM: Atopic dermatitis. In: *Allergy: Principles and Practice.* Middleton E Jr et al (editors). Mosby, 1998.

Boguniewicz M, Leung DYM: Management of atopic dermatitis. In: *Atopic Dermatitis: From Pathogenesis to Treatment.* Leung DYM (editor). RG Landes, 1996.

Boguniewicz M: Advances in the understanding and treatment of atopic dermatitis. Curr Opin Pediatr 1997;9:577.

Tan BB et al: Double-blind controlled trial of effect of house dust-mite allergen avoidance on atopic dermatitis. Lancet 1996;347:15.

URTICARIA & ANGIOEDEMA

Essentials of Diagnosis & Typical Features

- Urticaria: Erythematous, blanchable, circumscribed, pruritic, edematous papules ranging from 1–2 mm to several centimeters in diameter and involving the superficial dermis. Individual lesions can coalesce.
- Angioedema: Edema extending into the deep dermis or subcutaneous tissues.
- Both resolve without sequelae—urticaria usually within hours (individual lesions rarely lasting up to 24 hours), angioedema within 72 hours.

General Considerations

Urticaria and angioedema are common dermatologic conditions, occurring at some time in up to 25% of the population. About half of patients will have concomitant urticaria and angioedema, whereas 40% will have only urticaria and 10% only angioedema. Urticarial lesions are arbitrarily designated as acute, lasting less than 6 weeks, or chronic, lasting more than 6 weeks. Acute versus chronic urticaria can also be distinguished by differences in histologic features. A history of atopy is common with acute urticaria or angioedema. In contrast, atopy does not appear to be a factor in chronic urticaria.

Mast cell degranulation, dilated venules, and dermal edema are present in most forms of urticaria or angioedema. The dermal inflammatory cells may be sparse or dense depending on the chronicity of the lesions. Mast cells are thought to play a critical role in the pathogenesis through release of a variety of vasoactive mediators. Mast cell activation and degranulation can be triggered by different stimuli, including cross-linking of Fc receptor bound IgE by allergens or anti-FcεRI antibodies. Non-IgE-mediated mechanisms have also been identified, including complement anaphylatoxins (C3a, C5a), radiocontrast dyes, or physical stimuli. Chronic urticarial lesions have greater numbers of perivascular mononuclear cells, consisting primarily of T cells. There is also a marked increase in cutaneous mast cells.

The cause of acute disease can be identified in about half of cases and include allergens such as foods, aeroallergens, latex, drugs, and insect venoms. Infectious agents, including streptococci, mycoplasmas, hepatitis B virus, or Epstein-Barr virus, can cause acute urticaria. Urticaria or angioedema can occur after the administration of blood products or immunoglobulin. This results from immune complex formation with complement activation, vascular alterations, and triggering of mast cells by anaphylatoxins. A number of drugs and diagnostic agents, including opiate analgesics, polymyxin B, tubocurarine, and radiocontrast media, can induce acute urticaria by direct mast cell activation. These disorders can also occur following ingestion of aspirin or nonsteroidal anti-inflammatory agents (see section on Adverse Drug reactions below).

Physical urticarias represent a heterogeneous group of disorders in which urticaria or angioedema is triggered by physical stimuli, including pressure, cold, heat, water, or vibrations. Dermographism is the most common form of physical urticaria, affecting up to about 4% of the population and occurring at skin sites subjected to mechanical stimuli. Many physical urticarias are considered to be acute in nature because the lesions are usually rapid in onset, with resolution within hours. However, symptoms can recur for months to years.

The underlying cause of chronic urticaria cannot determined in the great majority of cases. Typically, this occurs in older patients, and recent studies have detected the presence of autoantibodies directed at IgE or the high-affinity receptor for IgE, suggesting that chronic urticaria may be an autoimmune disease. Urticaria can also occur in association with other disorders, such as hepatitis, thyroid disease, and neoplasms.

Clinical Findings

A. Symptoms and Signs: The main features of these disorders are listed above. Cold-induced urticaria or angioedema can occur within minutes of exposure to a decreased ambient temperature or as the skin is warmed following direct cold contact. Systemic features include headache, wheezing, and syncope. If the entire body is cooled, as may occur during swimming, hypotension and collapse can occur. Two forms of dominantly inherited cold urticaria have been described. The immediate form is known as familial cold urticaria, in which erythematous macules appear rather than wheals, along with fever, arthralgias, and leukocytosis. The delayed form consists of erythematous, deep swellings which develop 9–18 hours after local cold challenge without immediate lesions.

In solar urticaria, which occurs within minutes after exposure to light of appropriate wavelength, pruritus is followed by morbilliform erythema and urticaria.

Cholinergic urticaria occurs after increases in core body and skin temperatures and typically develops after a warm bath or shower, exercise, or episodes of fever. Occasional episodes are triggered by stress or the ingestion of certain foods. The eruption appears as small punctate wheals surrounded by extensive areas of erythema. Rarely, the urticarial lesions become confluent and angioedema develops. Associated features can include one or more of the following: headache, syncope, bronchospasm, abdominal pain, vomiting, and diarrhea. In severe cases, systemic anaphylaxis may develop. Pressure urticaria or angioedema is manifested by red, deep, painful swelling occurring immediately or 4–6 hours after the skin has been exposed to pressure. The immediate form is often associated with dermographism. The delayed form, which may be associated with fever, chills, and arthralgias, may be accompanied by elevated erythrocyte sedimentation rate and leukocytosis. Lesions are frequently diffuse, tender, and painful rather than pruritic. They typically resolve within 48 hours.

B. Laboratory Findings: Laboratory tests are selected on the basis of the history and physical findings. Testing for specific IgE antibody to food or inhalant allergens may be helpful in implicating a potential cause. Specific tests for physical urticarias, such as an ice cube test or a pressure test, may be indicated. Intradermal injection of methacholine reproduces clinical symptoms locally in about one-third of patients with cholinergic urticaria. A throat culture for streptococcal infection may be warranted with acute urticaria. In chronic urticaria, selected "screening" studies to look for an underlying disease may be indicated, including a complete blood count, erythrocyte sedimentation rate, biochemistry panel, and urinalysis. Antithyroid antibodies may be considered, as well as anti-IgE and anti-FcεRIα, though the latter two are not commercially available. Other tests should be done based on suspicion of a specific underlying disease. If the history or appearance of the urticarial lesions suggests vasculitis, a skin biopsy for immunofluorescence is indicated. Patient diaries occasionally may be helpful to determine the cause of recurrent hives. A trial of food or drug elimination may be considered.

Differential Diagnosis

Urticarial lesions are usually easily recognized—the major dilemma is the etiologic diagnosis. Lesions of urticarial vasculitis typically last for more than 24 hours. "Papular urticaria" is a term used to characterize multiple papules from insect bites, found especially on the extremities, and is not true urticaria. Angioedema can be distinguished from other forms of edema because it is transient, asymmetric, and nonpitting and does not occur predominantly in dependent areas. Hereditary angioedema is a rare autosomal dominant disorder caused by a quantitative or functional deficiency of C1-esterase inhibitor and characterized by episodic, frequently severe, nonpruritic angioedema of the skin, gastrointestinal tract, or upper respiratory tract. Life-threatening laryngeal angioedema may occur.

Complications

In severe cases of cholinergic urticaria, systemic anaphylaxis may develop. In cold-induced disease, sudden cooling of the entire body as can occur with swimming can result in hypotension and collapse.

Treatment

A. General Measures: The most effective treatment is identification and avoidance of the triggering agent. Underlying infection should be treated appropriately. Patients with physical urticarias should avoid the relevant physical stimulus. Epinephrine can be used for treatment of acute episodes, especially when laryngeal edema complicates an attack (see below under Anaphylaxis). Intubation may be indicated for life-threatening laryngeal edema.

B. Antihistamines: For the majority of patients, H_1 antihistamines given orally or systemically are the mainstay of therapy. Antihistamines are more effective when given on an ongoing basis rather than after lesions appear. For breakthrough symptoms, the dose may need to be increased. In the case of cold urticaria, the best treatment appears to be cyproheptadine. Cholinergic urticaria can be treated with hydroxyzine and dermographism with hydroxyzine or diphenhydramine. The addition of H_2 antihistamines may benefit some patients who fail to respond to H_1 receptor antagonists alone. Second-generation antihistamines are minimally sedating at usual dosing and lack anticholinergic effects. Nonsedating antihistamines approved for use in children 6 years of age and older include cetirizine and loratadine, both given in a dosage of 10 mg once daily. Both are available in liquid and tablet form, and loratadine comes in a rapidly dissolving tablet. Both appear to be devoid of the serious adverse effects, including QT interval prolongation and cardiac arrhythmias, seen with terfenadine and astemizole. Fexofenadine, the active metabolite of terfenadine is approved for patients age 12 or older in a dosage of 60 mg twice daily.

C. Corticosteroids: Although corticosteroids are usually not indicated in the treatment of acute or chronic urticaria, severe recalcitrant cases may require alternate-day therapy in an attempt to diminish disease activity and facilitate control with antihistamines. Systemic corticosteroids may also be needed in the treatment of patients with urticaria or angioedema secondary to necrotizing vasculitis, an uncommon occurrence in patients with serum sickness or collagen-vascular disease.

D. Other Pharmacologic Agents: The tricyclic anti-depressant doxepin blocks both H_1 and H_2 histamine receptors and may be particularly useful in chronic urticaria, though use may be limited by the sedating side-effect. A limited number of patients—including euthyroid patients—with chronic urticaria and antithyroid antibodies have improved when given thyroid hormone. Treatment of chronic urticaria with nifedipine, colchicine, dapsone, sulfasalazine, cyclosporine, or intravenous immune globulin should be considered investigational.

Prognosis

Spontaneous remission of urticaria and angioedema is frequent, but some patients have a prolonged course. Reassurance is important, since this disorder can cause significant frustration. Periodic follow-up is indicated, particularly for patients with laryngeal edema, to monitor for possible underlying cause.

Charlesworth EN: Urticaria and angioedema: A clinical spectrum. Ann Allergy Asthma Immunol 1996;76:484.

Dreyfus DH, Schocket AL, Milgrom H: Steroid-resistant chronic urticaria associated with anti-thyroid microsomal antibodies in a nine year old boy. J Pediatr 1996;128:576.

Greaves MW: Chronic urticaria. N Engl J Med 1995; 332:1767.

Tong LJ et al: Assessment of autoimmunity in patients with chronic urticaria. J Allergy Clin Immunol 1997;99:461.

ANAPHYLAXIS

Essentials of Diagnosis & Typical Features

- Rapid onset of allergic symptoms after exposure to allergen in a previously sensitized person.
- Generalized pruritus, anxiety, urticaria, angioedema, throat fullness, dyspnea, hypotension, and collapse.

General Considerations

Anaphylaxis is an acute life-threatening clinical syndrome that occurs when large quantities of inflammatory mediators are rapidly released from mast cells and basophils after exposure to an allergen in a previously sensitized patient. **Anaphylactoid reactions** mimic anaphylaxis but are not mediated by IgE. They may be mediated by anaphylatoxins such as C3a or C5a or through nonimmune mast cell degranulating agents. Some of the common causes of anaphylaxis or anaphylactoid reactions are listed in Table 32–6. "Idiopathic anaphylaxis" by definition has no recognized external cause.

Clinical Findings

A. Symptoms and Signs: The signs and symptoms of anaphylaxis or anaphylactoid reactions depend on the organs affected. Onset typically occurs within minutes after exposure to the offending agent

Table 32–6. Common causes of systemic allergic and pseudoallergic reactions.

Causes of anaphylaxis
Drugs
Antibiotics
Anesthetic agents
Foods
Peanuts, tree nuts, shellfish, and others
Biologicals
Latex
Insulin
Allergen extracts
Antisera
Blood products
Enzymes
Insect venoms
Causes of anaphylactoid reactions
Radiocontrast media
Aspirin and other nonsteroidal anti-inflammatory drugs
Anesthetic agents

and can be short-lived, protracted, or biphasic, with recurrence after several hours despite treatment. Patients may report a feeling of "impending doom" or generalized pruritus. Cutaneous signs include erythema, urticaria, and angioedema. Tearing, rhinorrhea, sneezing, and nasal congestion may occur. Respiratory symptoms include "a lump in the throat" or shortness of breath, with signs including uvular edema, hoarseness, dysphonia, stridor, tachypnea, and wheezing. Cardiovascular findings include tachycardia, arrhythmias, hypotension and collapse. The patient may complain of nausea and cramping pain with associated vomiting, and diarrhea. There may be anxiety or generalized seizures. Shock, upper airway edema, and bronchial obstruction are the principal life-threatening manifestations.

B. Laboratory Findings: Tryptase released by mast cells can be measured in the serum and may remain elevated for up to 24 hours after an acute reaction. This may be helpful when the diagnosis of anaphylaxis is in question. The CBC may show an elevated hematocrit due to hemoconcentration. Elevation of serum creatine kinase, aspartate aminotransferase, and lactic dehydrogenase may be seen with myocardial involvement. Electrocardiographic abnormalities may include S–T wave depression, bundle branch block, and various arrhythmias. Arterial blood gases may show hypoxemia, hypercapnia, and acidosis. The chest x-ray may show hyperinflation.

Differential Diagnosis

Although shock may be the only sign of anaphylaxis, other diagnoses should be considered, especially in the setting of sudden collapse without typical allergic findings. Other causes of shock along with cardiac arrhythmias must be ruled out (see Chapters 11 and 12). Respiratory failure associated with asthma may be confused with anaphylaxis. Mastocytosis, hereditary angioedema, scombroid poisoning, vasovagal reactions, vocal cord dysfunction, and anxiety attacks may cause symptoms mistaken for anaphylaxis.

Complications

Depending on the organs involved and the severity of the reaction, complications may vary from none to aspiration pneumonitis, acute tubular necrosis, bleeding diathesis, or sloughing of the intestinal mucosa. With irreversible shock, heart and brain damage can be terminal.

Treatment

A. General Measures: Anaphylaxis is a medical emergency that requires rapid assessment and treatment. Exposure to the triggering agent should be discontinued. Airway patency should be maintained and blood pressure and pulse monitored. The patient should be placed in a supine position with the legs elevated. Oxygen should be delivered by mask or nasal cannula with pulse oximetry monitoring. If the reaction is secondary to a sting or injection into an extremity, a tourniquet may be applied proximal to the site, briefly releasing it every 10–15 minutes.

B. Epinephrine: Epinephrine 1:1000, 0.01 mL/kg to a maximum of 0.3 mL, should be injected subcutaneously without delay. This dose may be repeated at intervals of 15–20 minutes two or three times as necessary. If the precipitating allergen has been injected intradermally or subcutaneously, absorption may be delayed by giving 0.1 mL of epinephrine subcutaneously at the injection site unless the site is a digit.

C. Antihistamines: Diphenhydramine, an H_1-blocker, 1–2 mg/kg up to 50 mg, can be given intramuscularly or intravenously. Intravenous antihistamines should be infused over a period of 5–10 minutes to avoid inducing hypotension. Addition of ranitidine, an H_2-blocker, 1 mg/kg up to 50 mg intravenously, may be more effective than an H_1-blocker alone, especially for hypotension.

D. Fluids: Treatment of persistent hypotension requires restoration of intravascular volume by fluid replacement, initially with a crystalloid solution, 20–30 mL/kg in the first hour.

E. Bronchodilators: Nebulized β_2-agonists such as albuterol 0.5% solution, 2.5 mg (0.5 mL) diluted in 2–3 mL saline, may be useful for reversing bronchospasm. Intravenous methylxanthines are generally not recommended since they provide little benefit over inhaled β_2-agonists and may contribute to toxicity.

F. Corticosteroids: Although corticosteroids do not provide immediate benefit, when given early they may prevent protracted or biphasic anaphylaxis. Intravenous methylprednisolone, 1–2 mg/kg, or hydrocortisone, 5 mg/kg, can be given every 4–6 hours.

G. Vasopressors: Refractory hypotension should be treated with intravenous vasopressors such as dopamine or epinephrine (see Chapter 12).

H. Observation: The patient should be monitored after the initial symptoms have subsided, since biphasic or protracted anaphylaxis can occur despite ongoing therapy.

Prevention

Strict avoidance of the causative agent is extremely important. If the cause of anaphylaxis is not known, an effort to determine its cause should be made, beginning with a thorough history. Typically, there is a strong temporal relationship between exposure and onset of symptoms. Testing for specific IgE to allergen either with in vitro or skin testing may be indicated. With exercise-induced anaphylaxis, patients should be instructed to exercise with another person and to stop exercising at the first sign of symptoms. If prior ingestion of food has been implicated, eating within 4 hours—perhaps up to 12 hours—before exercise should be avoided. Patients with a history of anaphylaxis should carry epinephrine for self-administration (eg, EpiPen, EpiPen Jr, Ana-Kit), and they and all caretakers should be instructed on its use. They should also carry an oral antihistamine such as diphenhydramine and wear a medical alert bracelet. Patients with idiopathic anaphylaxis may require prolonged treatment with oral corticosteroids. Specific measures for dealing with food, drug, latex, and insect venom allergies as well as radiocontrast media reactions are discussed below.

Prognosis

Anaphylaxis can be fatal. In one study of children and adolescents who died from food-induced anaphylaxis (peanuts, tree nuts, egg), treatment with epinephrine was delayed for more than 1 hour after onset. The prognosis is good when signs and symptoms are promptly recognized and aggressively treated and the offending agent is subsequently avoided. Exercise-induced and idiopathic anaphylaxis may be recurrent. Accidental exposure to the causative agent may occur, so patients, parents, and care providers must be prepared to recognize and treat anaphylaxis.

Ditto AM et al: Pediatric idiopathic anaphylaxis: Experience with 22 patients. J Allergy Clin Immunol 1997;100:320.

Kemp SF et al: Anaphylaxis: A review of 266 cases. Arch Intern Med 1995;155:1749.

Sampson HA, Mendelson L, Rosen JP: Fatal and near-fatal anaphylactic reactions to food in children and adolescents. N Engl J Med 1992;327:380.

Tilles S, Schocket AL, Milgrom H: Exercise-induced anaphylaxis related to specific foods. J Pediatr 1995; 127:587.

ADVERSE REACTIONS TO DRUGS & BIOLOGICALS

The majority of adverse drug reactions are not immunologically mediated and may instead involve or be due to idiosyncratic reactions, overdosage, pharmacologic side effects, nonspecific release of pharmacologic effector molecules, or drug interactions.

Patients often describe themselves as being "allergic" to medications or biologicals, and clinicians may document a drug allergy in the patient's medical record based solely on this history. The term "allergic" is used also to describe a number of different adverse reactions to these agents. Adverse drug reactions are any undesirable and unintended response elicited by a drug. Allergic or hypersensitivity drug reactions are adverse reactions involving immune mechanisms. Although hypersensitivity reactions account for only 5–10% of all adverse drug reactions, they are the most serious, with 1:10,000 resulting in death.

1. ANTIBIOTICS

Antibiotics constitute the most frequent cause of allergic drug reactions. Amoxicillin, trimethoprim-sulfamethoxazole, and ampicillin are the most common causes of cutaneous drug reactions.

Most antibiotics and their metabolites are low-molecular-weight compounds that are not immunologically detectable until they have become covalently bound to a carrier protein. The penicillins and other β-lactam antibiotics, including cephalosporins, carbacephems, carbapenems, and monobactams, share a common β-lactam ring structure and a marked propensity to couple to carrier proteins. Penicilloyl is the predominant metabolite of penicillin and is called the major determinant. The other penicillin metabolites are present in low concentrations and are referred to as minor determinants. Sulfonamide reactions are mediated presumably by a reactive metabolite (hydroxylamine) produced by cytochrome P450 oxidative metabolism. Slow acetylators appear to be at increased risk. Other risk factors for drug reactions include previous exposure, previous reaction, age (20–49 years), route (parenteral), and dose (high, intermittent) of administration. Atopy does not predispose to development of a reaction, but atopic individuals have more severe reactions.

Immunopathologic reactions to antibiotics include type I (IgE-mediated) reactions resulting from a drug or metabolite interaction with preformed specific IgE bound to the surfaces of tissue mast cells or circulating basophils. Release of mediators such as histamine and leukotrienes contributes to the clinical development of angioedema, urticaria, bronchospasm, or anaphylaxis. Type II (cytotoxic) reactions involve IgG or IgM antibodies that recognize drug bound to cell membranes. In the presence of serum complement, the antibody-coated cell is either cleared or destroyed, causing drug-induced hemolytic anemia or thrombocytopenia. Type III (immune complex) reactions are caused by soluble complexes of drug or metabolite with IgG or IgM antibody. If the immune complex is deposited on blood vessel walls and activates the complement cascade, serum sickness may result. Type IV (T cell-mediated) reactions require activated T lymphocytes that recognize a drug or its metabolite as seen in allergic contact dermatitis.

Sensitization usually occurs via the topical route of administration. Immunopathologic reactions not fitting into the type I–IV classification include Stevens-Johnson syndrome, exfoliative dermatitis, and the maculopapular rash associated with penicillin or ampicillin. The prevalence of morbilliform rashes in patients treated with ampicillin is between 5.2% and 9.5% of treatment courses. However, patients given ampicillin during EBV and CMV infections or with acute lymphoblastic anemia have a 69–100% incidence of non-IgE-mediated rash. Serum sickness-like reactions resemble type III reactions, though immune complexes are not documented; β-lactams, especially cefaclor and sulfonamides have been implicated most often. They may result from an inherited propensity for hepatic biotransformation of drug into toxic or immunogenic metabolites. The incidence of "allergic" cutaneous reactions to trimethoprim-sulfamethoxazole in patients with AIDS has been reported to be as high as 70%. The mechanism is thought to relate to the severe immune dysregulation, though it may be due to glutathione deficiency resulting in toxic metabolites.

Clinical Findings

A. Symptoms and Signs: Hypersensitivity reactions can result in pruritus, urticaria, angioedema, or anaphylaxis. Serum sickness is characterized by fever, rash, lymphadenopathy, myalgias, and arthralgias. Cytotoxic drug reactions can result in signs and symptoms associated with the underlying anemia or thrombocytopenia. Delayed-type hypersensitivity may cause contact dermatitis.

B. Laboratory Findings: Skin testing is the most rapid, useful, and sensitive method of demonstrating the presence of IgE antibody to a specific allergen. Skin testing to nonpenicillin antibiotics may be difficult, however, because many immunologic reactions are due to metabolites rather than to the parent drug and because the relevant metabolites for most drugs other than penicillin have not been identified. Since metabolites are usually low-molecular-weight haptens, they must combine with carrier proteins to be useful for diagnosis. In the case of contact sensitivity reactions to topical antibiotics, a 48-hour patch test can be useful.

Solid-phase in vitro RAST immunoassays for IgE to penicillins are available for identification of IgE to the major (penicilloyl) determinant of penicillin but are considerably less sensitive and give less information than skin testing. Assays for specific IgG and IgM have been shown to correlate with a drug reaction in immune cytopenias, but in most other instances such assays are not clinically useful. It should be noted that skin testing for immediate hypersensitivity is helpful only in predicting reactions caused by IgE antibodies. Most nonpruritic maculopapular rashes will not be predicted by skin testing.

Approximately 80% of patients with a history of penicillin allergy will be skin test-negative. Penicillin therapy of patients with a history of an immediate hypersensitivity reaction to penicillin but with negative skin tests to both penicilloyl and the minor determinant mixture is accompanied by a 1–3% chance of urticaria or other mild allergic reactions at some time during therapy, with anaphylaxis occurring in less than 0.1%. On the other hand, the predictive value of a positive skin test is approximately 60%. Testing with penicilloyl linked to polylysine (PPL) alone carries about a 76% sensitivity, while use of both PPL and penicillin G (used as a minor determinant) in-

creases sensitivity to about 95%. Not using minor determinant mixture in skin testing can result in failure to predict potential anaphylactic reactions. Unfortunately, the minor determinant mixture is still not commercially available, though most academic allergy centers make their own. Approximately 4% of subjects tested with no history of penicillin allergy have positive skin tests, and most fatalities occur in patients with no prior history of reaction. Rarely, patients may have skin test reactivity only to a specific semisynthetic penicillin. Resensitization in skin test-negative children occurs infrequently (< 1%) after a course of oral antibiotic.

The degree of cross-reactivity of determinants formed from cephalosporins with IgE to other β-lactam drugs remains unresolved, especially since haptens that may be unique to cephalosporin metabolism remain unknown. The degree of clinical cross-reactivity is much lower than the in vitro cross-reactivity. A clinical adverse reaction rate of 3–7% for cephalosporins may be expected in patients with positive histories of penicillin allergy. Antibodies to the second- and third-generation cephalosporins appear to be directed at the unique side chains rather than at the common ring structure. The present literature suggests that a positive skin test to a cephalosporin used at a concentration of 1 mg/mL would place the patient at increased risk for an allergic reaction to that antibiotic. However, a negative skin test would not exclude sensitivity to a potentially relevant metabolite. A recent review concluded that there is no increased incidence of allergy to second- and third-generation cephalosporins in patients with penicillin allergy and that penicillin skin testing does not identify patients who develop cephalosporin allergy.

Carbacephems (loracarbef) are similar to cephalosporins, though the degree of cross-reactivity is undetermined. Carbapenems (imipenem) represent another class of β-lactam antibiotics with a bicyclic nucleus and a high degree of cross-reactivity with penicillin. On the other hand, monobactams (aztreonam) contain a monocyclic rather than bicyclic ring structure and limited data suggests that aztreonam can be safely administered to most penicillin-allergic subjects.

Skin testing for non-β-lactam antibiotics is less reliable, since the relevant degradation products are for the most part unknown or multivalent reagents are unavailable. Evidence that the N4 sulfonamidoyl determinant is the major determinant formed from sulfamethoxazole has led to the assessment of a multivalent form for use in skin tests for IgE to sulfamethoxazole.

Treatment

A. General Measures: Withdrawal of the implicated drug is usually a central component of management. Acute IgE-mediated reactions such as anaphylaxis, urticaria, and angioedema are treated according to established therapeutic guidelines that include the use of epinephrine, H_1 and H_2 receptor blocking agents, volume replacement, and systemic corticosteroids (see sections above). Antibiotic-induced immune cytopenias can be managed by withdrawal of the offending agent or reduction in dose. Drug-induced serum sickness can be suppressed by drug withdrawal, antihistamines, and corticosteroids. Contact allergy can be managed by avoidance and treatment with antihistamines and topical corticosteroids. Reactions such as toxic epidermal necrolysis and Stevens-Johnson syndrome require immediate drug withdrawal and supportive care.

B. Alternative Therapy: If possible, subsequent therapy should be with an alternative drug that has therapeutic actions similar to the drug in question but with no immunologic cross-reactivity.

C. Desensitization: Administering gradually increasing doses of an antibiotic either orally or parentally over a period of hours to days may be considered if alternative therapy is not acceptable. This should only be done by a physician familiar with desensitization, typically in an intensive care setting. Desensitization does not reduce or prevent non-IgE-mediated reactions. Patients with Stevens-Johnson syndrome should not be desensitized because of the high mortality rate.

Prognosis

The prognosis is good when drug allergens are identified early and avoided. Stephens-Johnson syndrome and toxic epidermal necrolysis may be associated with a high mortality rate.

2. LATEX ALLERGY

Essentials of Diagnosis & Typical Features

- Immediate hypersensitivity reaction after exposure to latex, including on airborne particles.
- Allergic contact dermatitis 24–48 hours after exposure to rubber accelerators or antioxidants.

General Considerations

Allergic reactions to latex and rubber products have become increasingly common since the institution of universal precautions for exposure to bodily fluids. Children with spina bifida appear to have a unique sensitivity to latex, perhaps because of early and frequent latex exposure as well as altered neuroimmune interactions. Atopy—especially symptomatic latex allergy—appears to be significantly increased in patients with spina bifida experiencing anaphylaxis during general anesthesia. Other conditions requiring chronic or recurrent exposure to latex such as urogenital anomalies and ventriculoperitoneal shunt have also been associated with latex hypersensitivity. The combination of atopy and frequent exposure seems to synergistically increase the risk of latex hypersensitivity.

Latex is the milky fluid obtained by tapping the cultivated rubber tree, *Hevea brasiliensis*. During manufacture of latex products, various antioxidants and accelerators such as thiurams, carbamates, and mercaptobenzothiazoles are added. Latex products are typically produced by dipping a porcelain mold into a tank of latex and then vulcanizing it to enhance mechanical stability. The product is washed or "leached" of excess proteins, then dry-lubricated with a powder such as corn starch.

Latex is a complex biologic mixture composed of rubber particles in a phospholipoprotein envelope and a serum containing sugars, lipids, nucleic acids, minerals, and various proteins. The protein component is thought to contain the allergenic properties. Extra leaching steps may reduce the protein content and hence the allergenicity of the final product. IgE from latex-sensitized individuals reacts with different protein components, supporting the notion that there is more than one clinically important latex antigen. New allergenic epitopes are generated during the manufacturing process. Thus, polypeptides from latex glove extracts vary both quantitatively and qualitatively with different brands and lots of gloves. Identification of the causative antigens is important because it may be possible to alter the manufacturing process to reduce the final allergen content.

Latex is ubiquitous in medical settings, and many sources may be inconspicuous. Synthetic alternatives to some latex products are available, including gloves, dressings, and tape. Avoidance of contact with latex-containing items, however, may be insufficient to prevent allergic reactions, since lubricating powders may serve as vehicles for aerosolized latex antigens. The use of powder-free latex gloves is an important control measure for airborne latex allergen.

Nonmedical sources of latex are also common and include balloons, toys, rubber bands, erasers, condoms, and shoe soles. Pacifiers and bottle nipples have also been implicated as sources of latex allergen, though these products are molded rather than dipped, and allergic reactions to molded products are less common. Latex-allergic patients and their caretakers must be continuously vigilant for hidden sources of exposure.

Clinical Findings

A. Symptoms and Signs: The clinical manifestations of IgE-mediated reactions to latex can involve the full spectrum of symptoms associated with mast cell degranulation. Localized pruritus and urticaria occur after cutaneous contact, while conjunctivitis and rhinitis can result from aerosol exposure or direct facial contact. Systemic reactions, including bronchospasm, laryngospasm, and hypotension, may occur with more substantial exposure or in the case of an exquisitely sensitive individual. Finally, vascular collapse and shock leading to fatal cardiovascular events may occur. Intraoperative anaphylaxis represents a common and very serious manifestation of latex allergy.

Allergic contact dermatitis to rubber products typically appears 24–48 hours after contact with the allergen. The primary allergens include accelerators and antioxidants used in the manufacturing process. The diagnosis is established by patch testing. Shoe soles are an important source of exposure. The skin lesions appear primarily as a patchy eczema on exposed surfaces, though reactions can become generalized.

B. Laboratory Findings: Epicutaneous prick testing is a rapid, inexpensive, and sensitive test that detects the presence of latex-specific IgE on skin mast cells. Obstacles to its use include lack of a standardized antigen. Reports of life-threatening anaphylactic events have been associated with skin testing to latex, and intradermal testing may be especially dangerous. A commercially available extract is pending FDA approval.

Immunoassay testing involves the in vitro measurement of specific IgE, which binds latex antigens. Antigen sources used for testing have included native plant extracts, raw latex, and finished products. Although radioimmunoassay and enzyme-linked assays are most often used, a number of other in vitro assays have been developed, including an assay using a soluble allergen matrix. When compared with a history of latex-induced symptoms or positive skin tests, the sensitivity of immunoassays testing for latex antigens ranges from 50% to 100% with specificity between 63% and 100%. These broad ranges may reflect the patient population studied and the source of latex antigen as well as the assay employed. A positive immunoassay test to latex in the presence of a highly suggestive latex allergy history is very useful and may circumvent the potential concerns associated with prick skin testing in certain patients.

Cross-reactivity has been demonstrated between latex and a number of other antigens such as foods. Banana, avocado, and chestnut have been found to be antigenically similar to latex both immunologically and clinically.

Complications

Complications may be similar to those caused by other allergens. Prolonged exposure to aerosolized latex may lead to persistent asthma. Chronic allergic contact dermatitis, especially on the hands, can lead to functional disability.

Treatment

Avoidance remains the cornerstone of treatment for latex allergy. Prevention and supportive therapy are the most common methods for managing this problem. Patients identified as being allergic to latex may need to have a personal supply of vinyl or latex-free gloves for use when visiting a physician or dentist. "Hypoallergenic" gloves are poorly classified with respect to their ability to induce IgE-mediated reactions; the FDA currently uses this term to designate products that have a reduced capacity to induce contact dermatitis. Gloves made from synthetic materials include Neolon (Becton-Dickinson), Tactyl 1 (Smart Practice), and Elastyren (Hermal). Autoinjectable epinephrine and medical identification bracelets may be prescribed for latex-allergic patients along with avoidance counseling.

Prophylactic premedication of latex-allergic individuals has been used in some surgical patients at high risk for latex allergy. The rationale for this therapy is derived from the pretreatment protocols developed for iodinated radiocontrast media and anesthetic reactions. Although there has been some success using this regimen, anaphylaxis has occurred despite pretreatment. This approach should not substitute for careful avoidance measures.

Prognosis

Owing to the ubiquitous nature of natural rubber, the prognosis is guarded for patients with severe latex allergy. Chronic exposure to airborne latex particles may lead to chronic asthma. Chronic dermatitis can lead to functional disability.

3. VACCINES

MMR vaccine has been shown to be safe in egg-allergic patients. The ovalbumin content in influenza vaccine is variable, and skin testing with the specific vaccine lot is warranted in patients with egg allergy.

4. RADIOCONTRAST MEDIA

Non-IgE-mediated anaphylactoid reactions may occur with radiocontrast media with up to 30% reaction rate on reexposure. Management involves using a low-molarity agent and premedication with prednisone, diphenhydramine, and possibly an H_2-blocker.

5. INSULIN

Approximately 50% of patients receiving insulin have positive skin tests, but IgE-mediated reactions occur rarely. Insulin resistance is mediated by IgG. If less than 24 hours have elapsed after an allergic reaction to insulin, do not discontinue insulin but rather reduce the dose by one-third, then increase by 2–5 units per injection. Skin testing and desensitization are necessary if the interval between the allergic reaction and subsequent dose is greater than 24 hours.

6. LOCAL ANESTHETICS

Less than 1% of reactions to local anesthetics are IgE-mediated. Management involves selecting a local anesthetic from another class. Esters of benzoic acid include benzocaine and procaine; amides include lidocaine and mepivacaine. Alternatively, the patient can be skin tested with the suspected agent, followed by a provocative challenge. To rule out paraben sensitivity, skin testing can be done with 1% lidocaine from a multidose vial.

7. ASPIRIN & OTHER NONSTEROIDAL ANTI-INFLAMMATORY DRUGS

Reactions to aspirin and other nonsteroidal anti-inflammatory drugs are non-IgE-mediated and include urticaria and angioedema; rhinosinusitis, nasal polyps, and asthma; anaphylactoid reactions; and NSAID-related hypersensitivity pneumonitis. After a systemic reaction, a refractory period of 2–7 days occurs. Most aspirin-sensitive patients tolerate sodium salicylate. All NSAIDs inhibiting cyclooxygenase cross-react with aspirin. Cross-reactivity between aspirin and tartrazine (yellow dye No. 5) has not been substantiated in controlled trials. No skin test or in vitro test is available to diagnose aspirin sensitivity. Oral challenge can induce severe bronchospasm. "Desensitization" and "cross-desensitization" to NSAIDs can be achieved in most patients and maintained long-term. Leukotriene receptor antagonists or 5-lipoxygenase inhibitors attenuate or ablate the reaction to aspirin challenge and may be the drugs of choice for aspirin-sensitive asthmatics.

Boguniewicz M, Leung DYM: Hypersensitivity reactions to antibiotics commonly used in children. Pediatr Inf Dis J 1995; 14:221.

James JM et al: Safe administration of the measles vaccine to children allergic to eggs. N Engl J Med 1995; 332:1262.

Landwehr LP, Boguniewicz M: Current perspective on latex allergy. J Pediatr 1996;128:305.

FOOD ALLERGY

Essentials of Diagnosis & Typical Features

- Temporal relationship between ingestion of a suspected food and onset of allergic symptoms.
- Positive prick skin test or in vitro test to a suspected food allergen confirmed by a double-blind, placebo-controlled food challenge (except in cases of anaphylaxis).

General Considerations

Adverse reactions to foods are common in young children, especially in the first 3 years of life. The highest prevalence of food allergy is found in children with moderate to severe atopic dermatitis, with up to 33% affected. Up to 16% of children with asthma have been found to have food-induced wheezing in some studies. The most common food allergens in young children are eggs, milk, peanuts, soy, and wheat. In older children and adolescents, fish, shellfish, and nuts are most often involved in allergic reactions, and these may be lifelong.

Other reactions often diagnosed by patients or physicians as "allergic" involve pharmacologic or metabolic mechanisms and reactions to food toxins. Foods containing significant amounts of vasoactive amines such as chocolate, cheese, and some wines and beers may precipitate migraine headaches in some patients. Claims that dyes, sugar, and food additives may contribute to hyperactivity in children with attention deficit hyperactivity disorder are controversial. In the occasional case in which a child appears to benefit from a restricted diet, there is no evidence for an IgE-mediated reaction.

Clinical Findings

A. Symptoms and Signs: Most reactions to foods occur minutes to 2 hours after ingestion. A history of a temporal relationship between the ingestion of a suspected food and onset of a reaction—as well as the nature and duration of symptoms observed—are important in establishing the diagnosis of food allergy. With chronic atopic dermatitis or persistent urticaria, the association with food may be less obvious (see sections on Atopic Dermatitis and Urticaria, above). At times, acute symptoms may occur, but the cause may not be obvious because of hidden food allergens. A symptom diary kept for 7–14 days may be helpful in establishing an association between ingestion of foods and symptoms and also serves to provide a baseline observation for the pattern of symptom expression. It is important to record both the form in which the food was ingested and the foods ingested concurrently.

Hives, flushing, facial angioedema, and mouth or throat itching are common. In severe cases, angioedema of the tongue, uvula, pharynx, or upper airway can occur. Contact urticaria can occur without systemic symptoms in some children. Gastrointestinal symptoms include abdominal discomfort or pain, nausea, vomiting, and diarrhea. Food allergy may occasionally be manifested as isolated rhinoconjunctivitis or wheezing. Rarely, anaphylaxis to food may present only as cardiovascular collapse (see Anaphylaxis, above). Anaphylactoid reactions can occur after ingestion of foods such as certain fish containing high amounts of histamine.

B. Laboratory Findings: Typically, fewer than 50% of histories of food allergy will be confirmed by blinded challenge. Prick skin testing is useful to rule out a suspected food allergen, since the predictive value is very high for a properly performed negative test with an extract of good quality. On the other hand, the predictive value for a positive test is approximately 50%. RAST and other in vitro tests have low specificity and positive predictive value. Recently, the CAP System (Pharmacia) has been shown to be comparable to prick skin testing for egg, milk, peanut, and fish. Measurement of IgG to foods is not clinically useful. Eosinophilia of stool mucus may be present in cases of gastrointestinal allergy; elevated circulating eosinophils may be present as well.

Double-blind, placebo-controlled food challenge is considered the standard method for diagnosing food allergy except in cases of severe reactions. Even when multiple food allergies are suspected, most patients will be positive to three or fewer foods on blinded challenge. Therefore, extensive elimination diets are almost never indicated. Elimination without controlled challenge is a less desirable but at times more practical approach for suspected food allergy.

Differential Diagnosis

Repeated vomiting in infancy may be due to pyloric stenosis or gastroesophageal reflux. With chronic gastrointestinal symptoms, enzyme deficiency (eg, lactase), cystic fibrosis, celiac disease, chronic intestinal infections, gastrointestinal malformations, and irritable bowel syndrome should be considered.

Treatment

Treatment consists of eliminating and avoiding foods that have been documented to cause allergic reactions. This involves educating the patient, parent, and caregivers regarding hidden food allergens, the necessity for reading labels, and the signs and symptoms of food allergy and its appropriate management. Examples of labels that may indicate an implicated food protein include "emulsifier" (egg), "lecithin" (egg or soy), "natural flavoring" (milk), and "thickener" (soy). Consultation with a dietician familiar with food allergy may be helpful, especially when common foods such as milk, egg, peanut, soy, or wheat are involved. Patients with a history of food-induced anaphylaxis or respiratory distress should carry epinephrine (see Anaphylaxis, above).

Prognosis

The prognosis is good if the offending food can be identified and avoided. Unfortunately, accidental exposure to food allergens in severely allergic patients can result in death. Most children "outgrow" their food allergies to egg, milk, or soy but not to peanut or tree nuts. Approximately 2% will have food allergy as adults. Resources for food-allergic patients include the Food Allergy Network and the National Peanut and Tree Nut Registry (800-929-4040).

Sampson HA, Ho DG: Relationship between food-specific IgE concentrations and the risk of positive food chal-

lenges in children and adolescents. J Allergy Clin Immunol 1997;100:444.
Steinman HA: Hidden allergens in food. J Allergy Clin Immunol 1996;98:241.
Zeiger RS, Heller S: The development and prediction of atopy in high-risk children: Follow-up at age seven years in a prospective randomized study of combined maternal and infant food allergen avoidance. J Allergy Clin Immunol 1995;95:1179.

INSECT ALLERGY

Allergic reactions to insects include symptoms of respiratory allergy as a result of inhalation of particulate matter of insect origin, local cutaneous reactions to insect bites, and anaphylactic reactions to stings. The latter are almost exclusively caused by Hymenoptera and result in approximately 40 deaths each year in the United States. The order Hymenoptera includes honey bees, yellow jackets, yellow hornets, white-faced hornets, wasps, and fire ants. Africanized honey bees, also known as "killer bees," are a concern because of their aggressive behavior and excessive swarming and not because their venom is more toxic. Rarely, patients sensitized to reduviid ("kissing") bugs may have episodes of nocturnal anaphylaxis. Lepidopterism is adverse effects secondary to contact with larval or adult butterflies and moths. Salivary gland antigens are responsible for immediate and delayed skin reactions in mosquito-sensitive patients.

Clinical Findings

A. Symptoms and Signs: Insect bites or stings can cause local or systemic reactions ranging from mild to fatal responses in susceptible persons. The frequency increases in the summer months and with outdoor exposure. Local cutaneous reactions include urticaria as well as papulovesicular eruptions and lesions that resemble delayed hypersensitivity reactions. Papular urticaria is almost always the result of insect bites, especially of mosquitoes, fleas, and bedbugs. Toxic systemic reactions consisting of gastrointestinal symptoms, headache, vertigo, syncope, convulsions, or fever can occur following multiple stings. These reactions result from histamine-like substances in the venom. In children with hypersensitivity to fire ant venom, sterile pustules occur at sting sites on a nonimmunologic basis due to the inherent toxicity of piperidine alkaloids in the venom. Mild systemic reactions include itching, flushing, and urticaria. Severe systemic reactions may include dyspnea, wheezing, chest tightness, hoarseness, fullness in the throat, hypotension, loss of consciousness, incontinence, nausea, vomiting, and abdominal pain. Delayed systemic reactions occur from 2 hours to 3 weeks following the sting and include serum sickness, peripheral neuritis, allergic vasculitis, and coagulation defects.

B. Laboratory Findings: Skin testing is indicated for children with systemic reactions. Venoms of honeybee, yellow jacket, yellow hornet, white-faced hornet, and wasp are available for skin testing and treatment. Fire ant venom is not yet commercially available, but an extract made from fire ant bodies appears adequate to establish the presence of IgE antibodies to fire ant venom. Ideally, skin testing should be deferred for several weeks following a systemic reaction to outwait a possible refractory period. The presence of a positive skin test denotes prior sensitization but does not predict whether a reaction will occur with the patient's next sting, nor does it differentiate between local and systemic reactions. It is common for children who have had an allergic reaction to have positive skin tests to more than one venom. This might reflect sensitization from prior stings that did not result in an allergic reaction or cross-reactivity between closely related venoms. In vitro testing (compared with skin testing) has not substantially improved the ability to predict anaphylaxis. With venom RAST, there is a 15–20% incidence of both false-positive and false-negative results. Tests for mosquito saliva antigens or other insect allergy are not commercially available.

Complications

Secondary infection can complicate allergic reactions to insect bites or stings. Serum sickness, nephrotic syndrome, vasculitis, neuritis, or encephalopathy may be seen as late sequelae of reactions to stinging insects.

Treatment

For cutaneous reactions caused by biting insects, symptomatic therapy includes cold compresses, antipruritics (including antihistamines), and occasionally potent topical corticosteroids. Treatment of stings includes careful removal of the stinger, if present, by flicking it away from the wound and not by grasping to prevent further envenomation. Topical application of monosodium glutamate, baking soda, or vinegar compresses is of questionable efficacy. Local reactions can be treated with ice, elevation of the affected extremity, oral antihistamines, and nonsteroidal anti-inflammatory drugs as well as potent topical corticosteroids. Large local reactions in which swelling extends beyond two joints or an extremity, may require a short course of oral corticosteroids. Anaphylactic reactions following Hymenoptera stings should be managed essentially the same as anaphylaxis (see Anaphylaxis, above). Children who have had severe or anaphylactic reactions to Hymenoptera stings—or their parents and caregivers—should be instructed in the use of epinephrine. Patients at risk for anaphylaxis from an insect sting should also wear an identification bracelet indicating their allergy. Children at risk from insect stings should avoid wearing bright-colored clothing and perfumes when outdoors and should wear long pants and shoes when walking in the grass. Patients who experience severe systemic reactions and have a positive skin test should receive venom immunotherapy. Immunotherapy is not indicated for children with only urticarial or local reactions.

Prognosis

Children generally have milder reactions than adults after insect stings, and fatal reactions are extremely rare. Patients aged 3–16 years with reactions limited to the skin, such as urticaria and angioedema, appear to be at low risk for more severe reactions with subsequent stings.

Demain JG, Taylor TM: Reactions to stinging and biting arthropods. In: *Cutaneous Allergy.* Charlesworth EN (editor). Blackwell Science, 1996.
Valentine MD et al: The value of immunotherapy with venom in children with allergy to insect stings. N Engl J Med 1990;323:1601.

Antimicrobial Therapy

33

John W. Ogle, MD

PRINCIPLES OF ANTIMICROBIAL THERAPY

Antimicrobial therapy of bacterial infections is arguably the most important scientific development of 20th century medicine. It contributes significantly to the quality of life of many people and reduces the morbidity and mortality due to infectious diseases. The remarkable success of antimicrobial therapy has been achieved with comparatively little toxicity and expense. The relative ease of administration and the widespread availability of these drugs have led many to adopt a philosophy of broad-spectrum empiric antimicrobial therapy for many common infections.

Unfortunately, this era of cheap, safe, and reliable therapy may be coming to a close owing to the increasing frequency of antimicrobial resistance being encountered in previously susceptible microorganisms. The problem of antimicrobial resistance is certainly not new—resistance was recognized in sulfonamides and penicillins shortly after their introduction. What is new is the worldwide dissemination of resistant clones of microorganisms, such as *Streptococcus pneumoniae* and *Staphylococcus aureus,* which are inherently virulent and common causes of serious infections not only among hospitalized patients but also among outpatients.

Until recently, the recognition of new resistance clones was balanced by the promise of newer and more potent antimicrobial agents. Today, since fewer new agents are under development, clinicians are beginning to encounter limitations in their ability to treat some serious bacterial infections. Many factors contribute to the selection of resistant clones. Our success in treating patients with chronic diseases and immune-compromising conditions has resulted in additional years of life for such patients but has favored selection of resistant strains in inpatient units and chronic care facilities.

Overuse of antimicrobial agents by well-intentioned clinicians contributes also to the selection of resistant strains. Examples include medications for mildly ill patients with self-limited conditions such as viral infections and administration of broad-spec-

trum antimicrobials for patients whose condition can be treated with narrow-spectrum agents. Similarly, failure to document infection with cultures of samples obtained prior to starting therapy limits our willingness to stop or narrow the spectrum of antimicrobials. Little research has been conducted to determine the necessary duration of therapy, with the result that we probably often treat longer than is necessary. Prophylactic strategies, as used for prevention of recurrent otitis media, create a selection pressure for antibiotic resistance.

The decision-making process for choosing an appropriate antimicrobial agent is summarized in Table 33–1. Accurate clinical diagnosis is based on the history, physical examination, and initial laboratory tests. The clinical diagnosis then leads to a consideration of the organisms that are most commonly associated with the clinical condition, the usual pattern of antimicrobial susceptibility of the most likely organism or organisms, and past experience with successful treatment regimens.

Cultures should be obtained in potentially serious infections. Empiric antimicrobial therapy may be initiated, then modified according to the patient's response and the culture results. Often there are several equally safe and efficacious antimicrobials. In this circumstance, the relative cost and ease of administration of the different choices should be considered.

Other important considerations include the patient's age, immune status, and exposure history. Neonates and young infants may present with nonspecific signs of infection, making the differentiation of serious disease from mild illness difficult. In older children, clinical diagnosis is more precise, which may allow no therapy or use of a narrower-spectrum antibiotic. Immune deficiency may increase the number and types of potential infecting organisms that need to be considered, including organisms that are usually avirulent but that may be serious and difficult to treat once infection is established. An abnormal immune response may also diminish the severity of the clinical signs and symptoms of infection and thus lead to underestimation of the severity of illness. The exposure history may suggest the greater likelihood

Table 33–1. Steps in decision making for use of antimicrobial agents.

Step	Action	Example
1	Determine diagnosis.	Septic arthritis
2	Consider age and preexisting condition.	Normal 2-year-old child
3	Consider common organisms.	*Staphylococus aureus, Kingella kingae*
4	Consider organism susceptibility.	Penicillin- or ampicillin-resistant
5	Obtain proper cultures.[1]	Blood, joint fluid
6	Initiate empiric therapy based on above considerations and past experience (eg, personal, literature).	Nafcillin and cefotaxime
7	Modify therapy based on culture results and patient response.	*S aureus* isolated. Discontinue cefotaxime.
8	Follow clinical response.	Interval physical examination
9	Stop therapy.	Clinically improved or well, minimum 3–4 weeks

[1]Indicated for serious or unusual infections or those with unpredictable clinical response to empiric therapy.

of certain types of infecting organisms. This history includes exposures from family members, classmates, or day care environments or exposure to unusual organisms by virtue of travel, diet, or contact with animals.

Final important considerations are the pace and seriousness of the illness. A rapidly progressive and severe illness should be treated initially with broad-spectrum antimicrobials until a specific etiologic diagnosis is made. A mildly ill outpatient should be treated preferentially with narrow-spectrum antimicrobials.

Antimicrobial susceptibility, antimicrobial families, and dosing recommendations are listed in Tables 33–2 to 33–6.

ANTIMICROBIAL SUSCEPTIBILITY TESTING

Cultures and other diagnostic material must be obtained prior to initiating antimicrobial therapy—especially when the patient has a serious infection, initial attempts at therapy have failed, or multi-agent therapy is anticipated. Whenever cultures identify the causative agent, therapy can be narrowed or optimized according to susceptibility results. Antimicrobial susceptibility testing should be done in a laboratory using carefully defined procedures (National Committee for Clinical Laboratory Standards). The use of nonstandard media, inoculum size, or growth conditions may give markedly different and undependable results.

There are several ways to test antimicrobial sus-

ceptibility. Identification of an antibiotic-destroying enzyme (eg, β-lactamase) implies resistance to that group of antimicrobial agents. Tube or microtiter broth dilution techniques can be used to determine the minimum inhibitory concentration (MIC) of antibiotic, which is the amount of antibiotic (in μg/mL) necessary to inhibit the organism under specific laboratory conditions. With knowledge of the clinical pharmacology of the antimicrobial agent, the clinician can infer antibiotic susceptibility if the MIC is less than the antibiotic concentration achievable in the patient using appropriate antibiotic dosages. Disk susceptibility testing (again, only under carefully controlled conditions) yields similar results. The E-test is a newly standardized test for some organisms and correlates well with MICs. Clinical laboratories usually define antimicrobial susceptibility (susceptible, intermediate, resistant) in relation to levels of the test antibiotic achievable in the blood (or serum).

In general, organisms are considered susceptible to an antibiotic if the MIC of the antibiotic for the organism is lower than levels of that agent achievable in the blood using appropriate parenteral dosages. This assumption of susceptibility should be reconsidered whenever the patient has a focus of infection (eg, meningitis, osteomyelitis, abscess) in which poor antibiotic penetration might occur, since the levels of antibiotic might be lower than the MIC in such areas. Conversely, although certain organisms may be reported resistant to an antibiotic because sufficiently high blood concentrations cannot be achieved, urine concentrations may be much higher. If so, a urinary tract infection would respond to that antibiotic whereas septicemia would not.

Table 33–2. Susceptibility of some common pathogenic microorganisms to various antimicrobial drugs.

Organism	Potentially Useful Antibiotics[1]
BACTERIA	
Anaerobic bacteria[2]	Cefoxitin,[3] cefotetan,[3] clindamycin, imipenem[3] meropenem, metronidazole, penicillins with or without β-lactamase inhibitor
Bartonella henselae	Azithromycin, clarithromycin, doxycycline, erythromycin
Bordetella pertussis	Amoxicillin, azithromycin, erythromycin, clarithromycin, trimethoprim-sulfamethoxazole
Borrelia burgdorferi	Amoxicillin, cephalosporins (III), doxycycline
Campylobacter spp	Erythromycin, tetracyclines
Clostridium spp	Clindamycin, metronidazole, penicillins, tetracyclines
Clostridium difficile	Bacitracin (PO), metronidazole, vancomycin (PO)
Corynebacterium diphtheriae	Erythromycin, penicillins
Enterobacteriaceae[4]	Aminoglycosides,[5] ampicillins, aztreonam, cephalosporins, imipenem, meropenem, quinolones,[3,6] trimethoprim-sulfamethoxazole
Enterococcus	Ampicillin (with aminoglycoside), carbapenems (not *E faecium*), vancomycin
Haemophilus influenzae	Amoxicillin/clavulanate, ampicillins (if β-lactamase negative),[7] cephalosporins (II and III),[8] chloramphenicol, rifampin, trimethoprim-sulfamethoxazole
Listeria monocytogenes	Ampicillin with aminoglycoside, trimethoprim-sulfamethoxazole
Moraxella catarrhalis	Amoxicillin/clavulanate, ampicillins (if β-lactamase-negative),[7] cephalosporins (III),[8] erythromycin, trimethoprim-sulfamethoxazole
Neisseria gonorrhoeae	Ampicillins (if β-lactamase-negative),[7] cephalosporins (II and III),[8] penicillins, quinolones,[3,6] spectinomycin, tetracyclines, trimethoprim-sulfamethoxazole
Neisseria meningitidis	Ampicillins, cephalosporins (II and III),[8] chloramphenicol, penicillins, rifampin
Pasteurella multocida	Amoxicillin/clavulanate, ampicillins, penicillins, tetracyclines
Pseudomonas aeruginosa	Aminoglycosides,[5] anti-*pseudomonas* penicillins,[9] aztreonam, cefepime, ceftazidime, imipenem, meropenem, quinolones[3,6]
Salmonella spp	Ampicillin, cephalosporins (III),[8] trimethoprim-sulfamethoxazole
Shigella spp	Ampicillin, cephalosporins (III),[8] tetracyclines, trimethoprim-sulfamethoxazole
Staphylococcus aureus	Antistaphylococcal penicillins,[10] cephalosporins (I and II), clindamycin, erythromycin, rifampin, trimethoprim-sulfamethoxazole, vancomycin
S aureus (methicillin resistant)	Vancomycin
Staphylococci (coagulase-negative)	Cephalosporins (I and II),[11] clindamycin, rifampin, vancomycin
Streptococci (most species)	Ampicillins, cephalosporins, clindamycin, erythromycin, penicillins, vancomycin
Streptococcus pneumoniae[12]	Ampicillins, cephalosporins, erythromycin, penicillin, meropenem, vancomycin[12]
INTERMEDIATE ORGANISMS	
Chlamydia spp	Clarithromycin, erythromycin, quinolones,[3,6] tetracyclines
Mycoplasma spp	Erythromycin, tetracyclines
Rickettsia spp	Chloramphenicol, tetracyclines
FUNGI	
Candida spp	Amphotericin B, fluconazole, flucytosine, ketoconazole
Fungi, systemic[2]	Amphotericin B, fluconazole, itraconazole,[3] ketoconazole, miconazole
Dermatophytes	Ciclopirox olamine, clotrimazole, econozole, griseofulvin, itraconazole[3] miconazole, naftifine, oxiconazole, sulconazole, terbinafine
Pneumocystis carinii	Dapsone, pentamidine, trimethoprim-sulfamethoxazole

(*continued*)

Table 33–2. Susceptibility of some common pathogenic microorganisms to various antimicrobial drugs. (continued)

Organism	Potentially Useful Antibiotics[1]
VIRUSES	
Herpes simplex	Acyclovir, famciclovir[3], valacyclovir[3]
Human immunodeficiency virus	Dideoxyinosine (ddl), dideoxycytodine (ddC), lamivudine (3TC), stavudine (d4T), zidovudine (AZT), indinavir, nelfinavir, nevirapine, ritonavir, saquinavir
Influenza A virus	Amantadine, rimantidine
Respiratory syncytial virus	Ribavirin[13]
Varicella-zolster virus	Acyclovir, famciclovir,[3] valacyclovir[3]
Cytomegalovirus	Foscarnet, ganciclovir

[1]In alphabetical order. Selection depends on patient's age, diagnosis, site of infection, severity of illness, antimicrobial susceptibility of suspected organism, and drug risk.
[2]Species-dependent.
[3]Not FDA-approved for use in children.
[4]Includes *E coli, Klebsiella* spp, *Enterobacter* spp, and others; antimicrobial susceptibilities should always be measured.
[5]Amikacin, gentamicin, kanamycin, tobramycin.
[6]Includes ciprofloxacin, enoxacin, levofloxacin, lomefloxacin, norfloxacin, ofloxacin, sparfloxacin.
[7]Also applies to amoxicillin and related compounds.
[8]Refer to second- (II) or third- (III) generation cephalosporins.
[9]Carbenicillin, mezlocillin, piperacillin, ticarcillin.
[10]Cloxacillin, dicloxacillin, methicillin, nafcillin, oxacillin.
[11]Only if the coagulase-negative *Staphylococcus* is also methicillin- or oxacillin-sensitive.
[12]Because of increasing frequency of *S pneumoniae* strains resistant to penicillin and cephalosporins, therapy for presumed severe infections (eg, meningitis) should include vancomycin until susceptibility studies are available.
[13]FDA-approved for therapy of RSV by aerosol, but clinical studies show variable efficacy.

Thus, antimicrobial susceptibility testing, although a very important part of therapeutic decision making, reflects assumptions that the clinician must understand, especially for management of patients with serious infections. Ultimately, the true test of the efficacy of therapy is patient response. Patients who do not respond to seemingly appropriate therapy may require reassessment, including reculturing and repeat susceptibility testing, to determine whether resistant strains have evolved or superinfection with a resistant organism is present. Antimicrobial therapy cannot be expected to cure some infections unless additional supportive treatment (usually surgical) is undertaken.

ALTERATION OF DOSE & MEASUREMENT OF BLOOD LEVELS

Certain antimicrobial agents have not been approved (and often not tested) for use in newborns. For those that have been approved, it is important to recognize that both dose and frequency of administration may need to be altered (Tables 33–4 and 33–5), especially in young (7 days or less) or low-birth-weight neonates (≤ 2000 g).

Antimicrobial agents are excreted or metabolized through various physiologic mechanisms (eg, renal, hepatic). It is important to consider these routes of excretion and alter the antimicrobial dosage appropriately in any patient with some degree of organ dysfunction (see Chapter 40). As indicated in Table

33–4, an assessment of renal or hepatic function may be routinely necessary for patients receiving certain drugs (eg, renal function for aminoglycosides, hepatic function for erythromycin or clindamycin); otherwise, harmful drug levels may accumulate. If significant organ dysfunction is present, dosage modification may be necessary (see detailed descriptions in individual drug information packets), and measurement of drug levels may be indicated.

Serum levels of drugs posing a high risk of toxicity (eg, aminoglycosides) are ordinarily measured, and measurement of other drugs (eg, vancomycin) may be useful in selected circumstances. For certain other serious bacterial infections (eg, bacterial endocarditis), measurement of the serum concentration of an antimicrobial may be important to deliver optimal therapy.

Certain drug interactions may require modification of drug dosage or other therapeutic alterations. For example, rifampin stimulates the metabolism of warfarin, birth control pills, and anticonvulsants by stimulating the P450 metabolic pathway. Dosage adjustments or alternative medications may be necessary to avoid significant adverse events. Another common example is erythromycin, which may inhibit the metabolism of theophylline, resulting in toxic theophylline levels. Although many drug interactions are known and well documented, it may be difficult to predict interactions that result from a combination of four, five, or more than five different medications. A high level of suspicion regarding adverse clinical events should be maintained.

Table 33–3. Groups of common antibacterial agents.

Group	Examples	Some Common Susceptible Organisms[1]	Common Resistant Organisms	Common or Unique Adverse Reactions
PENICILLIN GROUP				
Penicillins	Penicillin G, V	*Streptococcus, Neisseria*	*Staphylococcus, Haemophilus,* Enterobacteriaceae	Rash, anaphylaxis, drug fever, bone marrow suppression
Ampicillins	Ampicillin, amoxicillin	(Same as penicillins), plus *Haemophilus* (β-lactamase negative), *Escherichia coli, Enterococcus*	*Staphylococcus,* many Enterobacteriaceae	Diarrhea
Antistaphylococcal penicillins	Cloxacillin, dicloxacillin, methicillin, nafcillin, oxacillin	*Streptococcus, Staphylococcus aureus*	Gram-negative, *Staphylococcus* (coagulase-negative), enterococci	Renal (interstitial nephritis)
Anti-*Pseudomonas* penicillins	Azlocillin, piperacillin, ticarcillin	(Same as ampicillins), plus *Pseudomonas*	(Same as ampicillins)	Decreased platelet adhesiveness, hypokalemia, hypernatremia
Penicillin and β-lactamase inhibitor combination	Amoxicillin-clavulanate, ampicillin-sulbactam, ticarcillin-clavulanate	Broad-spectrum	Some enterobacteriaceae, *Pseudomonas*	Diarrhea
Carbapenems	Imipenem/cilastatin meropenems	Broad-spectrum, gram-negative rods, anaerobes, *Pseudomonas*	MRSA,[2] many enterococci	CNS, seizures
CEPHALOSPORIN GROUP				
First generation (I)	Cefazolin, cephalexin, cephalothin, cephapirin, cephradine	Gram-positive	Gram-negative, enterococci, some staphylococci (coagulase-negative)	Rash; anaphylaxis, drug fever
Second generation (II)	Cefaclor, cefamandole, cefonicid, cefuroxime loracarbef	Gram-positive, some *Haemophilus,* some Enterobacteriaceae	*Enterococcus, Pseudomonas,* some staphylococci (coagulase-negative)	Serum sickness (cefaclor)
	Cefoxitin, cefotetan	Same as second-generation plus anaerobes		
Third generation (III)	Cefotaxime, ceftizoxime, ceftriaxone, cefixime, cefpodoxime, ceftibuten	*Streptococcus, Haemophilus,* Enterobacteriaceae, *Neisseria*	*Pseudomonas,* staphylococci	Biliary sludging (ceftriaxone)
	Ceftazidime, cefepime	(Same as other third-generation cephalosporisn), plus *Pseudomonas*	Staphylococci	
OTHER DRUGS				
Clindamycin	Clindamycin	Gram-positive, anaerobes	Gram-negative, *Enterococcus*	Nausea, vomiting, hepatotoxicity
Vancomycin	Vancomycin	Gram-positive	Gram-negative	"Red man" syndrome, shock, ototoxicity, renal
Macrolide agents	Erythromycin, clarithromycin, azithromycin	Gram-positive *Bordetella, Haemophilus, Mycoplasma, Chlamydia*	Gram-negative	Nausea and vomiting
Quinolones[3]	Ciprofloxacin, norfloxacin, ofloxacin	Gram-negative, *Staphylococcus*	*Enterococcus, Streptococcus S pneumoniae,* anaerobes	GI, rash, CNS

(continued)

Table 33–3. Groups of common antibacterial agents. (continued)

Group	Examples	Some Common Susceptible Organisms[1]	Common Resistant Organisms (Genus)	Common or Unique Adverse Reactions
Tetracyclines	Chlortetracycline, tetracycline, doxycycline, minocycline	Anaerobes, *Mycoplasma, Chlamydia, Rickettsia*	Many Enterobacteriaceae, *Staphylococcus*	Teeth staining,[4] rash, flora overgrowth, hepatotoxicity, pseudotumor cerebri
Chloramphenicol	Chloramphenicol	*S pneumoniae, H influenzae, Salmonella*	*Staphylococcus*, many Enterobacteriaceae	Bone marrow suppression, gray syndrome, neuritis
Sulfonamides	Many	Gram-negative (urine)	Gram-positive	Rash, renal, bone marrow suppression, Stevens-Johnson syndrome
Trimethoprim-sulfamethoxazole	Trimethoprim-sulfamethoxazole	*S aureus*, gram-negative *S pneumoniae H influenzae*	*Streptococcus, Pseudomonas* anaerobes	Rash, renal, bone marrow suppression, Stevens-Johnson syndrome
Rifampin	Rifampin	*Neisseria, Haemophilus, Staphylococcus Streptococcus*	Resistance develops rapidly if used as sole agent	Rash, GI, hepatotoxicity, CNS, bone marrow suppression, alters metabolism of other drugs
Aminoglycosides	Amikacin, gentamicin, kanamycin, streptomycin, tobramycin	Gram-negative, including *P aeruginosa*	Gram-positive, anaerobes, some pseudomonads	Renal, ototoxicity, potentiates neuromuscular blocking agents

[1]Not all strains susceptible; always obtain antimicrobial susceptibility tests on significant isolates.
[2]Methicillin-resistant S aureus
[3]Not approved for children.
[4]Tooth staining is dose-dependent in children < 9 years of age.

THE USE OF NEW ANTIMICROBIAL AGENTS

New antibiotics are introduced frequently, often with claims about unique features that distinguish these usually more expensive products from existing compounds. The role that any new antimicrobial will play can only be determined over time, during which new or previously unrecognized side effects might be described and the clinical efficacy established in large numbers of patients. Because this may take many years, a conservative approach to using new antibiotics seems fitting, especially since the costs are often higher and appropriate antimicrobial choices for most common infections already exist. It is appropriate to ask if a new antimicrobial has been proved to be as effective as (or more effective than) the current drug of choice and, if so, whether its side effects are comparable or less common and its cost reasonable.

The development of new antibiotics is important as a response to the emergence of resistant organisms and for treatment of infections that are clinically difficult to treat (eg, viruses, fungi, and some resistant bacteria). Fortunately, these infections are either rare or (usually) self-limited in normal hosts.

PROPHYLACTIC ANTIMICROBIAL AGENTS

Antimicrobials can be used to decrease the incidence of postoperative infections (Table 33–7). A dose of an antimicrobial is given 30 minutes to 2 hours prior to surgery. The goal is to achieve high levels in the serum at the time of incision and by this means—along with good surgical technique—to minimize bacterial contamination of the wound. During a lengthy procedure, a second dose may be given. No evidence exists that multiple subsequent doses of antimicrobials confer additional benefit. The antimicrobial used for prophylaxis is directed toward the flora that most commonly cause postoperative infection. Gram-positive cocci such as *S aureus* are usually targeted, and a first-generation cephalosporin (such as cefazolin) is a cost-effective choice. Third-generation cephalosporins and other broad-spectrum agents are more expensive and offer less benefit because they are less active than cefazolin against *S aureus*. Cefoxitin or cefotetan is useful for procedures such as colorectal surgery, though cefazolin is appropriate for most gynecologic patients. In colorectal surgery, oral antimicrobials such as neomycin and erythromycin may be more effective than parenteral therapy.

Table 33–4. Guidelines for use of common parenteral antibacterial agents[1] in children ≥ 1 month of age.

	Route	Dose[2] (mg/kg/d)	Maximum Daily Dose	Interval (hours)	Adjustment[3]	Blood Levels[4] (μg/mL) Peak	Trough
Amikacin	IM, IV	15–22.5	1.5 g	8	R	15–25	5–10
Ampicillin	IM, IV	100–400	12 g	4–6	R		
Aztreonam	IM, IV	90–120	6 g	6–8	R		
Cefazolin	IM, IV	50–100	6 g	8	R		
Cefotaxime	IM, IV	100–200	12 g	6–8	R		
Cefoxitin	IM, IV	80–160	12 g	4–6	R		
Ceftazidime	IM, IV	100–150	6 g	8	R		
Ceftizoxime	IM, IV	150–200	12 g	6–8	R		
Ceftriaxone	IM, IV	50–100	4 g	12–24	R		
Cefuroxime	IM, IV	100–150	6 g	6–8	R		
Cephalothin	IM, IV	75–125	12 g	4–6	R		
Cephradine	IM, IV	50–100	8 g	6	R		
Chloramphenicol	IV	50–100	4 g	6	R, H	15–25	5–10
Clindamycin	IM, IV	25–40	4 g	6–8	R, H		
Gentamicin	IM, IV	3–7.5	300 mg	8	R	5–10	< 2
Meropenem	IV	60–120	2g	8	R		
Methicillin	IM, IV	150–200	12 g	6	R		
Metronidazole	IV	30	4 g	6	H		
Nafcillin	IM, IV	150	12 g	6	None		
Penicillin G	IV	100,000–250,000 units/kg	20 million units	4–6	H, R		
Pencillin G (benzathine)	IM	50,000 units/kg	2.4 million units	Single dose	None		
Penicillin G (procaine)	IM	25,000–50,000 units/kg	4.8 million units	12–24	R		
Tetracycline[5]	(IV)[5]	20–30	2 g	12	R		
Ticarcillin	IV	200–300	24 g	4–6	R		
Tobramycin	IM, IV	3–6	300 mg	8	R	5–10	< 2
Vancomycin	IV	40–60	2 g	6	R	20–40[6]	

[1]Not including some newly released drugs, ones not recommended for use in children, or ones not widely used.
[2]Always consult package insert for complete prescribing information. Dosage may differ for alternative routes, newborns (see Table 33–6), or patients with liver or renal failure (see Adjustment column) and may not be recommended for use in pregnant women or newborns. Maximum dosage may be indicated only in severe infections or by parenteral routes.
[3]Mode of excretion (R = renal, H = hepatic) of antimicrobial agent should be assessed at the onset of therapy and dosage modified or levels determined as indicated in package insert.
[4]Suggested levels to reduce toxicity.
[5]Use with caution in children < 9 years of age because of tooth staining with repeated doses.
[6]Target peak and trough vancomycin levels are not well correlated with either toxicity or outcome. Measure selectively in meningitis, impaired or changing renal function, or altered volume of distribution.

In hospitals where the predominant *S aureus* strains are methicillin-resistant or in cases where the patient is allergic to penicillin and cephalosporins, vancomycin can be considered. However, prophylactic vancomycin has caused hypotension at the time of induction of general anesthesia. Frequent use of vancomycin as a prophylactic antimicrobial will undoubtedly contribute also to the development of vancomycin-resistant strains such as *Enterococcus faecalis*. For these reasons, vancomycin should generally not be used for prophylaxis, though it might prove useful for individual patients at extremely high risk.

Table 33–5. Guidelines for use of common oral antibacterial agents in children ≥ 1 month of age.

Agent[1]	Dose[2] (mg/kg/d)	Interval (hours)	Other Considerations
Amoxicillin	40	8	GI side effects
Amoxicillin-clavulanate	45	12	GI side effects
Ampicillin	50	6	GI side effects
Azithromycin	10 (first dose) then 5; 12 for pharyngitis	24	GI side effects
Cefaclor	40	8	Serum sickness-like illness
Cefadroxil	30	12	
Cefixime	8	12–24	
Cefpodoxime	10	12	Taste (suspension)
Cefprozil	30	12	GI side effects
Ceftibuten	9	24	GI side effects
Cefuroxime	30–40	12	GI side effects
Cephalexin	25–50	6	
Cephradine	25–50	6	
Chloramphenicol	50–75	6	Aplastic anemia
Clarithromycin	15	12	GI side effects
Clindamycin	20–30	6	GI side effects
Cloxacillin	50–100	6	GI side effects
Dicloxacillin	12–25	6	GI side effects
Doxycycline[3]	2–4	12–24	Teeth staining < 9 years
Erythromycin[4]	20–50	6–12	GI side effects
Erythromycin-sulfisoxazole	40 (erythromycin)	6–8	
Furazolidone	5–8	6	
Loracarbef	15; 30 for otitis	12	
Metronidazole	15–35	8	
Nitrofurantoin	5–7	6	
Oxacillin	50–100	6	
Penicillin V	25–50	6	Taste (suspension)
Rifampin	10–20	12–24	
Sulfisoxazole	120–150	6	
Tetracycline[3]	25–50[3]	6	Teeth staining < 9 years
Trimethoprim-sulfamethoxazole	8–12 (TMP)	12	Stevens-Johnson syndrome

[1]Not including some newly released drugs, ones not recommended for use in children, or ones not widely used.
[2]Always consult package insert for complete prescribing information. Dosage may differ for alternative routes, newborns (see Table 33–6), or patients with liver or renal failure (see Table 33–4, Adjustment column) and may not be recommended for use in pregnant women or newborns. Maximum dosage may be indicated only in severe infections or by parenteral routes.
[3]Use with caution in children < 9 years of age because of tooth staining with repeated doses.
[4]Preparation-dependent.

Table 33–6. Guidelines for use of selected antimicrobial agents in newborns.[1]

	Route	Body Wt (g)	Maximum Dosage (mg/kg/d) [Frequency] < 7 Days	8–30 Days	Blood Levels (μg/mL) Peak	Trough
Amikacin[2]	IV, IM	< 2000	15 [q12h]	22.5 [q8h]	15–25	5–10
		> 2000	20 [q12h]	30 [q8h]		
Ampicillin	IV, IM	< 2000	100 [q12h]	150 [q8h]		
		> 2000	150 [q8h]	200 [q6h]		
Cefotaxime	IV, IM		100 [q12h]	150 [q8h]		
Ceftazidime	IV, IM	< 2000	100 [q12h]	150 [q8h]		
		> 2000	150 [q8h]	150 [q8h]		
Clindamycin	IV, IM, PO	< 2000	10 [q12h]	15 [q8h]		
		> 2000	15 [q8h]	20 [q6h]		
Erythromycin	PO		20 [q12h]	30 [q8h]		
Gentamicin[2]	IV, IM		5 [q12–18h]	7.5 [q8h]	5–10	< 2
Methicillin	IV, IM	< 2000	100 [q12h]	150 [q8h]		
		> 2000	150 [q8h]	200 [q6h]		
Nafcillin	IV	< 2000	50 [q12h]	75 [q8h]		
		> 2000	60 [q8h]	150 [q6h]		
Oxacillin	IV, IM	< 2000	50 [q12h]	75 [q8h]		
		> 2000	75 [q8h]	150 [q6h]		
Penicillin G[3]	IV	< 2000	100,000 [q12h]	150,000 [q8h]		
		> 2000	150,000 [q8h]	200,000 [q6h]		
Ticarcillin	IV, IM	< 2000	150 [q12h]	225 [q8h]		
		> 2000	225 [q8h]	300 [q6h]		
Tobramycin[2]	IV, IM		4 [q12–18h]	6 [q8h]	5–10	< 2
Vancomycin[4]	IV		20 [q12h]	30 [q8h]	20–40	

[1]Adapted from Nelson JD: *Pocketbook of Pediatric Antimicrobial Therapy,* 11th ed. Williams & Wilkins, 1995.
[2]Neonates weighting < 1200 g may require even smaller doses. Antibiotic levels should be closely monitored.
[3]Penicillin dosages are in units/kg/d. Other preparations (eg, benzathine penicillin) may be given IM. See specific diseases for dosage.
[4]Target peak and trough vancomycin levels are not well correlated with either toxicity or outcome.

Prophylactic antimicrobials are given in several other circumstances. Endocarditis prophylaxis is indicated during dental and colorectal or genitourinary procedures on patients with high-risk heart lesions. Patients with indwelling vascular catheters such as Broviac catheters should receive prophylaxis. Prophylaxis against infection with group A streptococcal infection reduces the recurrence rate for acute rheumatic fever. Postexposure prophylaxis is given after exposure to pertussis, *Haemophilus influenzae* type b infection (depending on age), meningococcus, household exposure to tuberculosis, plague, aerosolized tularemia, and other high-risk infections. Family or close contacts of patients with severe invasive streptococcal disease should also receive prophylaxis. Silver nitrate, erythromycin, or tetracycline can be used in ophthalmic preparations for prevention of gonococcal ophthalmia neonatorum. Children with asplenia and sickle cell disease receive prophylactic penicillin to protect against overwhelming *S pneumoniae* sepsis.

Prophylactic antimicrobials are also useful during the viral respiratory season in children at high risk for recurrent otitis media and for some children with recurrent urinary tract infection. However, because of the emergence of resistant *S pneumoniae* as well as its frequency, decisions for antimicrobial prophylaxis should be carefully considered for each child.

INITIAL EMPIRIC ANTIMICROBIAL CHOICES FOR SELECTED CONDITIONS

General recommendations for specific conditions are included in the paragraphs that. A specific selection de-

Table 33–7. Antimicrobial prophylaxis and preferred prophylactic agents: Selected conditions and pathogens.[1,2]

Pathogen (Indication)	Prophylactic Agent
Bacterial endocarditis[3]	Ampicillin, ampicillin and gentamicin, amoxicillin, or other approved regimens
Bordetella pertussis (exposure to respiratory secretions)	Azithromycin, clarithromycin, erythromycin
Chlamydia trachomatis (genital contact or neonate)	Erythromycin
Haemophilus influenzae type b[4] (household exposure)	Rifampin
Mycobacterium tuberculosis (household exposure)	Isoniazid
Neisseria meningitidis (household exposure)	Rifampin, sulfadiazine[5]
N gonorrhoeae (ophthalmia neonatorum)	Erythromycin, silver nitrate ophthalmic
N gonorrhoeae (sexual contact)	Ceftriaxone, cefixime, cefpodoxime, quinolone
Treponema pallidum (sexual contact)	Penicillin
Streptococcus pneumoniae (sickle cell disease, asplenia)	Penicillin
Postoperative wound infection[6]	Cefazolin, other regimens
Group A streptococci (rheumatic fever)[7]	Benzathine penicillin G, penicillin, sulfadiazine
Group B streptococcal sepsis	Ampicillin to mother prior to delivery
Pneumonic *Yersinia pestis*[8] (exposure)	Tetracycline,[9] chloramphenicol
Francisella tularensis[8] (aerosolized exposure)	Tetracycline,[9] chloramphenicol
Vibrio cholera	Tetracycline,[9] trimethoprim-sulfamethoxazole
Recurrent otitis media	Amoxicillin, sulfadiazine
Recurrent urinary tract infection	Nitrofurantoin, trimethoprim-sulfamethoxazole
Pneumocystis carinii—(HIV, some immunocompromised patients)	Trimethoprim-sulfamethoxazole, pentamidine

[1]Modified, with permission, from Peter G, Hall CB, Orenstein WA (editors): *1997 Red Book: Report of the committee on Infectious Diseases,* 24th ed. American Academy of Pediatrics, 1997.
[2]Decisions for prophylaxis must take a number of factors into account, including the evidence for efficacy of therapy, the degree of the exposure to an infecting agent, the risk and consequences of infection, the susceptibility of the infecting agent to antimicrobials, and the patient's ability to tolerate and comply with the antimicrobial agent. See individual chapters of the text for discussion.
[3]See discussion in chapter 18.
[4]Prophylaxis provided to family if contacts include children < 4 years old. Some experts provide prophylaxis in day care settings after one case and some after two cases of HiB.
[5]Only for known sulfadiazine-susceptible strains.
[6]Alternative regimens may be used, depending on the site of surgery and the degree of contamination.
[7]Oral prophylaxis may be indicated in some patients. Alternative regimens indicated for penicillin-allergic patients. See discussion in chapter.
[8]Prophylaxis not well established. Carefully assess risk on a case-by-case basis.
[9]Usually not indicated for children < 9 years old because of tooth staining with repeated doses.

pends on the patient's age, diagnosis, site of infection, severity of illness, antimicrobial susceptibility of bacterial isolates, and history of drug allergy. Always consult the package insert for detailed prescribing information. Tables 33–2 to 33–6 include further information.

Neonatal Sepsis & Meningitis

The newborn with sepsis may have signs of focal infection such as pneumonia or respiratory distress syndrome or may have subtle nonfocal signs. Group B streptococci, *E coli,* other gram-negative rods, and *Listeria monocytogenes* are commonly encountered. Ampicillin and gentamicin (or another aminoglycoside) are preferred. If meningitis is present, many clinicians substitute a third-generation cephalosporin for the aminoglycoside. In the newborn with cellulitis, *S aureus* and group A streptococci are additional considerations. Nafcillin, oxacillin, or a first-generation cephalosporin is usually added.

Omphalitis is often polymicrobial, and *Enterococcus* species, gram-negative aerobes, and anaerobes may be causative. Clindamycin, ampicillin, and an aminoglycoside or third-generation cephalosporin cover the most likely organisms; early surgical intervention is indicated.

Sepsis in an Infant

S pneumoniae and *Neisseria meningitidis* are most commonly encountered in infants. *H influenzae* type b infection may occur in unimmunized children. A third-generation cephalosporin is appropriate. Intermediate-level penicillin and cephalosporin resistance in *S pneumoniae* usually do not cause therapy to fail unless meningitis or another difficult-to-treat infection such as endocarditis or osteomyelitis is present.

Nosocomial Sepsis

Many bacterial pathogens are possible causes of infection in hospitalized patients. Recent local experience is usually the best guide to etiologic diagnosis. For example, some neonatal units experience frequent infections due to *Enterobacter cloacae,* whereas in other units *Klebsiella pneumoniae* is the most common nosocomial isolate. Initial therapy should be effective for methicillin-resistant *S aureus* (MRSA) and resistant *Pseudomonas aeruginosa* if these are frequent isolates. *E faecalis* is a common cause of nosocomial bacteremia in patients with central catheters, particularly in units where cephalosporins are heavily used. Coagulase-negative staphylococci are commonly isolated from patients with indwelling central catheters. In seriously ill patients when the local experience suggests that *Enterococcus* species or coagulase-negative staphylococci are common, the initial regimen should include vancomycin. Because *Enterococcus* species and coagulase-negative staphylococci commonly cause fever without significant morbidity or mortality, initial regimens without vancomycin are appropriate, with adjustment of treatment after susceptibility is known. Regimens containing ampicillin are effective for *Enterococcus* species unless the local isolates have a high rate of resistance.

Meningitis

Bacterial meningitis in neonates is usually caused by infection with group B streptococci, *E coli,* or *L monocytogenes*. A combination of ampicillin and gentamicin or another aminoglycoside—or ampicillin and a third-generation cephalosporin—is started initially. In an infant or older child, *S pneumoniae* or *N meningitidis* is the most commonly isolate. *H influenzae* type b is uncommon now because of widespread immunization. Increasingly, *S pneumoniae* with multiple resistances to penicillin,

cephalosporins, and other drugs is isolated. In some communities, 30–40% of *S pneumoniae* isolates have intermediate susceptibility to penicillin (MIC between 0.1 and 2 μg/mL) and 5–10% of isolates may be highly resistant to penicillin (MIC > 2 μg/mL). Resistance to a third-generation cephalosporin (MIC > 2 μg/mL) may be seen in 3–5% of isolates.

In bacterial meningitis, peak cerebrospinal fluid antimicrobial concentrations ten or more times greater than the MIC of the organism are desirable, but this may be difficult to achieve if organisms are resistant. The therapeutic problem is complicated if dexamethasone, which reduces the entry of some antimicrobials into the cerebrospinal fluid, is also given.

Initial therapy of bacterial meningitis in an older child thus should include vancomycin and a third-generation cephalosporin. Alternatively, limited clinical experience with meropenem has also been successful. A lumbar puncture should be repeated 24–48 hours after start of therapy to assess the sterility of the cerebrospinal fluid. Rifampin should be added if the Gram stain or cultures of cerebrospinal fluid are positive upon repeated lumbar puncture; if the child has failed to improve; or if an organism with a very high MIC to ceftriaxone is isolated. The optimal therapy of highly resistant *S pneumoniae* meningitis is not well established by clinical data..

Meningitis in a child with a ventriculoperitoneal shunt is most commonly caused by coagulase-negative staphylococci, many of which are methicillin-resistant. Many of these patients are not seriously ill, and therapy should be postponed while awaiting the appropriate shunt fluid for Gram's stain and culture. Seriously ill patients should be treated initially with vancomycin and a third-generation cephalosporin, because *S aureus* and gram-negative rods are also possible and more serious causes of infection.

Urinary Tract Infection

E coli is the most common isolate in the urinary tract. Outpatients with symptoms of lower urinary tract disease or with mild illness can be treated with ampicillin, cephalexin, or a sulfonamide. For hospitalized patients with suspected bacteremia, ampicillin and gentamicin or a cephalosporin is appropriate. Gram's stain may be used to guide the initial choice. For patients with known or suspected resistant organisms, such as *P aeruginosa,* or for patients with urosepsis, an aminoglycoside or ceftazidime and ticarcillin may be started. Unit-specific data on typical bacterial species and their patterns of susceptibility should guide the antimicrobial choice for nosocomial urinary tract infections.

Bacterial Pneumonia

Bacterial pneumonia in newborn generally should be treated in the same way as for sepsis. Infants and older children are frequently infected with *S pneumo-*

niae. Ampicillin, a second- or third-generation cephalosporin, erythromycin-sulfisoxazole, or trimethoprim-sulfamethoxazole may be used depending on the local rates of resistant organisms and the seriousness of the illness. A rapidly progressive pneumonia, with pneumatoceles or large pleural effusions, may be due to *S aureus* or group A streptococci, *H influenzae* type b, or another gram-negative rod. Oxacillin, nafcillin, or another effective antistaphylococcal agent should be used in addition to a third-generation cephalosporin.

Children aged 6 years and older frequently have infection with *Mycoplasma pneumoniae, Chlamydia pneumoniae,* or *S pneumoniae.* Erythromycin or some other macrolide antibiotic is usually indicated for initial empiric therapy.

SPECIFIC ANTIMICROBIAL AGENTS

PENICILLINS

1. AMINOPENICILLINS

Penicillin remains the drug of choice for streptococcal infections, acute rheumatic fever prophylaxis, syphilis, oral anaerobic infections, dental infections, *N meningitidis* infection, leptospirosis, rat-bite fever, actinomycosis, and infections due to *Clostridium* and *Bacillus* species. For oral therapy of minor infections, amoxicillin or ampicillin is usually equivalent. For systemic therapy, aqueous penicillin G is preferable. Amoxicillin is preferred for oral therapy of Lyme disease in children. For dog or cat bites, where *Pasteurella multocida* is commonly encountered, amoxicillin-clavulanate provides good coverage of *Pasteurella* as well as *Staphylococcus.* An alternative is separate prescriptions for penicillin and an antistaphylococcal drug such as cephalexin. As for human bites, amoxicillin-clavulanate provides adequate therapy for *Eikenella corrodens* and other mixed oral aerobes and anaerobes.

2. PENICILLINASE-RESISTANT PENICILLINS (PRPs)

S aureus is usually resistant to penicillin and amoxicillin owing to penicillinase production by these organisms. Nafcillin, oxacillin, methicillin, and first- and second-generation cephalosporins are stable to penicillinase and are usually equivalent for intravenous therapy. Methicillin is associated with more frequent interstitial nephritis. Oxacillin and methicillin are renally excreted, whereas nafcillin is

excreted through the biliary tract. These properties are occasionally advantageous in children with renal or liver failure. Cost should usually be the deciding factor for choosing one agent over another. Often both *S aureus* and *S pyogenes* are suspected initially, eg, in cellulitis or postoperative wound infections. The PRPs and first- and second-generation cephalosporins are efficacious for most streptococcal infections.

Methicillin-resistant *S aureus* (MRSA) is an uncommon community-acquired infection in children but may cause nosocomial infection. MRSA infections are also resistant to other PRPs and to first- and second-generation cephalosporins. Vancomycin is effective against MRSA and coagulase-negative staphylococci.

For outpatient therapy, cloxacillin, dicloxacillin, and first- or second-generation cephalosporins are usually equally effective for infections due to *S aureus.* Cost may determine the choice between drugs.

3. ANTI-*PSEUDOMONAS* PENICILLINS

Ticarcillin, mezlocillin, and piperacillin are active intravenously against streptococci, ampicillin-susceptible enterococci, *H influenzae,* gram-negative rods—including more resistant gram-negative rods such as *Enterobacter, Proteus,* and *P aeruginosa*—and gram-negative anaerobes such as *Bacteroides fragilis. P aeruginosa* is inherently resistant to most antimicrobials, and high levels of these drugs are usually required. Carbenicillin is rarely used except for oral therapy of *P aeruginosa* urinary tract infections. The combination of ticarcillin and an aminoglycoside is synergistic against *P aeruginosa* and many other enteric gram-negative rods. Ticarcillin in a fixed combination with clavulanic acid has activity against β-lactamase-producing strains of *Klebsiella, S aureus,* and *Bacteroides.* Piperacillin is more active in vitro against many gram-negative enteric infections and may be advantageous in some circumstances, but it is not approved in children. Piperacillin-tazobactam is another combination antimicrobial and β-lactamase inhibitor that has enhanced activity against many β-lactamase producers.

Antipseudomonal penicillins cause the same toxicities as penicillin and therefore are usually very safe. Carbenicillin, ticarcillin, and piperacillin contain large amounts of sodium, which may cause problems for some patients with cardiac or renal disease.

GLYCOPEPTIDE AGENTS

Vancomycin and teicoplanin are glycopeptide antimicrobial agents active against the cell wall of gram-positive organisms. Only vancomycin is licensed in the United States. Vancomycin is useful for parenteral therapy of resistant gram-positive cocci such as MRSA, methicillin-resistant coagulase-negative staphylococci, and ampicillin-resistant enterococci. Vancomycin is also used orally for therapy of colitis due to *Clostridium difficile,* though it should not be used as the drug of first choice. The empiric use of vancomycin has increased tremendously over the last several years. As a result, vancomycin-resistant enterococci and coagulase-negative staphylococci have become problems, particularly in inpatient units, intensive care units, and oncology wards. *S aureus* with increased MICs to vancomycin has been reported in the United States and Japan. This resistance is of concern because of the inherent virulence of many *S aureus* strains. Vancomycin use should be carefully monitored in hospitals and in their intensive care units. It should not be used empirically when an infection is mild or when other antimicrobial agents are likely to be effective. Vancomycin should be stopped promptly if infection is found to be due to organisms susceptible to other antimicrobials.

Infection control guidelines for prevention of spread of vancomycin-resistant enterococci were recently published by the Centers for Disease Control and Prevention. Laboratory-based monitoring for vancomycin-resistant enterococci and vancomycin-resistant *S aureus* is appropriate in most communities.

Rapid infusion of vancomycin is associated with the "red man syndrome," characterized by diffuse red flushing, at times pruritus, and occasionally tachycardia and hypotension. As a result, vancomycin is infused slowly over 1 hour or longer in some cases. Diphenhydramine or hydrocortisone (or both) may also be used as premedication.

Vancomycin peak-and-trough serum concentrations are commonly measured despite the absence of data associating these levels either with toxicity or with a favorable therapeutic outcome. Vancomycin accumulation may occur in patients with abnormal or unpredictable renal function. Similarly, vancomycin dosing may be unpredictable in patients with an altered volume of distribution such as nephrotic syndrome or in patients in shock. Measuring vancomycin peak serum concentrations is helpful in these patients.

CEPHALOSPORINS

Cephalosporin agents make up a large and often confusing group of antimicrobials. Many of these drugs are similar in antibacterial spectrum and side effects and may have similar names. Clinicians should learn well the properties of one or two drugs in each class. Cephalosporins are often grouped as "generations" to signify their similar antimicrobial activity. First-generation cephalosporins such as cephapirin intravenously and cephalexin orally are

useful mainly for *S aureus* infection and urinary tract infection due to susceptible *E coli.* Second-generation cephalosporins, such as cefuroxime intravenously and cefaclor orally, have somewhat reduced but acceptable activity against gram-positive cocci but greater activity against gram-negative rods. They are active against *H influenzae, Moraxella catarrhalis,* and *N gonorrhoeae,* including strains that produce β-lactamase capable of inactivating ampicillin. Third-generation cephalosporins have substantially less activity against gram-positive cocci such as *S aureus* but greatly augmented activity against aerobic gram-negative rods. Cefotaxime and ceftriaxone are examples of intravenous drugs, whereas cefixime, cefpodoxime, cefprozil, and ceftibuten are representative oral drugs.

No cephalosporin agent has substantial activity against *L monocytogenes,* enterococci, or MRSA. The cephalosporins have little value for treating anaerobic infections except for cefoxitin and cefotetan, two second-generation cephalosporins with excellent activity against *B fragilis.* Ceftazidime is a third-generation cephalosporin with appreciable activity against *P aeruginosa.*

Cefepime is a new antimicrobial often described as "fourth-generation" because of its broad activity against gram-positive and gram-negative organisms, including *P aeruginosa.* Cefepime is stable to β-lactamase degradation and is a poor inducer of β-lactamase. Cefepime will be most useful for organisms resistant to other drugs. Cefepime is not approved for use in children under 12 years of age.

Cephalosporins are seldom the drug of choice for therapy of ambulatory infections, and despite their popularity they are often more expensive than other antimicrobials with similar side effects. Resistance to cephalosporins is common among aerobic gram-negative rods. The presence of inducible cephalosporinases in the chromosome of some gram-negative rod organisms such as *P aeruginosa, Serratia marcescens, Citrobacter,* and *Enterobacter* has led to clinical failures because of the emergence of resistance during therapy. Many clinicians treat infections due to these organisms with a second effective drug to attempt to limit the emergence of resistant strains. Similarly, extended-spectrum cephalosporinases that hydrolyze third-generation cephalosporins have become widespread in some hospitals. Active laboratory-based surveillance is necessary to predict the usual susceptibility encountered in gram-negative infections.

AZTREONAM

Aztreonam is the only monobactam antimicrobial agent that is approved in the United States. Although it is not approved for use in children, there is considerable pediatric experience with its use, including in neonates and premature infants. Aztreonam is active against streptococcal species and aerobic gram-negative rods, including *P aeruginosa*. Aztreonam has activity against *H influenzae* and *M catarrhalis,* including those that are β-lactamase producers. Most patients with allergy to penicillin or cephalosporins are not sensitized to aztreonam, except that children with prior reactions to ceftazidime may have reactions to aztreonam because aztreonam and ceftazidime have a common side chain.

CARBAPENEMS

Meropenem and imipenem are broad-spectrum β-lactam antimicrobials. Imipenem-cilastatin is a combination of an active antibiotic and cilastatin, which inhibits the metabolism of imipenem in the kidney and thereby results in high serum and urine levels of imipenem. Although imipenem-cilastatin is not approved for children younger than 12 years, there is considerable experience with its use. Meropenem is approved for use in children. These agents are broadly active against streptococci, methicillin-susceptible staphylococci, some enterococci, and gram-negative rods such as *P aeruginosa,* β-lactamase-producing *H influenzae,* and gram-negative anaerobes. Because carbapenems are active against so many species of bacteria, there is a strong temptation to use them as single-drug empiric therapy. Units that have used carbapenems heavily have encountered resistance in many different species of gram-negative rods. A more appropriate practice is to reserve carbapenems for patients who have infections that are unresponsive or have proved resistant to other antimicrobial agents.

MACROLIDES

Erythromycin is the most commonly used macrolide antimicrobial agent. It is active against many bacteria that are resistant to cell wall-active antimicrobials and is the drug of choice for *Bordetella pertussis, Legionella pneumophila, C pneumoniae, M pneumoniae,* and *C trachomatis* infections (in children for whom tetracycline is not an option). Erythromycin is used for outpatient therapy of mild infections and streptococcal and staphylococcal infections and in patients with penicillin allergy. More serious infections due to streptococci and staphylococci are usually treated with penicillins, clindamycin, PRPs, or cephalosporins because of a significant incidence of erythromycin resistance in both species. The combination erythromycin-sulfisoxazole is very useful for otitis media, but erythromycin alone does not have sufficient activity against *H influenzae* to be recommended. Gastrointestinal side effects are common.

Erythromycin is available in many formulations, including the base, estolate, ethyl succinate, and stearate. Transient hepatic toxicity is seen in adults but is much less common in children. Erythromycin base and stearate should be taken with meals for best absorption.

Clarithromycin and azithromycin are macrolide antimicrobials that are much less likely than erythromycin to cause nausea, vomiting, and diarrhea. Therefore, these agents are useful in children who cannot tolerate erythromycin. Clarithromycin is more active than erythromycin against *H influenzae, M catarrhalis,* and *N gonorrhoeae* and is the drug of choice, sometimes in combination, for atypical mycobacterial infections. Clarithromycin is effective against Lyme disease, but 7 days of azithromycin for that indication was inferior to amoxicillin. Clarithromycin and azithromycin are alternative drugs for toxoplasmosis in sulfonamide-allergic patients and as alternatives to erythromycin in legionellosis. In vitro and limited clinical experience in treatment of contacts of pertussis cases suggest efficacy equal to that of erythromycin. Azithromycin can be used for single-dose therapy of *C trachomatis* infections. It is beneficial in adolescents when compliance with erythromycin is a concern. Clarithromycin and azithromycin are considerably more expensive than most erythromycin formulations, which for that reason are usually preferred, but they are advantageous by virtue of their twice-daily and once-daily dosing, respectively. Some failures of the newer macrolides have occurred in *S pneumoniae* sepsis and meningitis, perhaps because of low serum levels despite the high tissue levels achieved.

CLINDAMYCIN

Clindamycin is active against *S aureus, S pyogenes,* other streptococcal species except enterococci, and both gram-positive and gram-negative anaerobes. Clindamycin and metronidazole are frequently combined with other antimicrobials for empiric therapy of suspected anaerobic or mixed anaerobic and aerobic infections. Examples are pelvic inflammatory disease, necrotizing enterocolitis, other infections in which the integrity of the gastrointestinal or genitourinary tracts is compromised, and sinusitis. Clindamycin may be superior for treatment of serious streptococcal infections that appear to be toxin-mediated. For the usual oral anaerobes, penicillin is more active than clindamycin. Empiric use of clindamycin is justified in suspected anaerobic infections because cultures frequently cannot be obtained and, if obtained, may be slow in confirming anaerobic infection. Clindamycin has been associated with the occurrence of pseudomembranous colitis. Although diarrhea is a frequent side effect, pseudomembranous colitis is uncommonly due to clindamycin in children.

SULFONAMIDES

Sulfonamides—the oldest class of antimicrobials—remain useful for many infections. They are often used to treat urinary tract infections and otitis media in combination with erythromycin or trimethoprim. They are used also for other infections due to *E coli* and for *Nocardia*. Although useful for rheumatic fever prophylaxis in penicillin-allergic patients, sulfonamides fail to eradicate group A streptococci and cannot be used for treatment of acute infections.

Trimethoprim-sulfamethoxazole (TMP-SMZ) is a fixed combination which is more active than either drug alone. Gram-positive cocci, including *S pneumoniae,* some staphylococci, *Haemophilus,* and many gram-negative rods, are susceptible. Unfortunately, resistance to TMP-SMZ has developed in recent years. *S pneumoniae* resistant to penicillin and cephalosporins is often also resistant to TMP-SMZ and erythromycin. Most *Shigella* and *Salmonella enteritidis* strains remain susceptible, as do most *E coli*. TMP-SMZ is therefore very useful for treatment of urinary tract infections, respiratory infections such as otitis media, sinusitis, and pneumonia, and bacterial dysentery. TMP-SMZ is also the drug of choice for treatment of and prophylaxis against *Pneumocystis carinii* infection. Dermatologic and myelosuppressive side effects limit the use of TMP-SMZ in some children infected with HIV.

Sulfonamide is associated with several cutaneous reactions, including urticaria, photosensitivity, Stevens-Johnson syndrome, purpura, and maculopapular rashes. Hematologic side effects such as leukopenia, thrombocytopenia, and hemolytic anemia are uncommon. Common gastrointestinal side effects are nausea and vomiting. The dermatologic and hematologic side effects are thought to be more common with TMP-SMZ than with sulfonamide alone.

TETRACYCLINES

Tetracyclines are effective against a broad range of bacteria but are not commonly used in children because alternative effective drugs are available. Many different tetracycline formulations are available. Tetracycline agents are effective against *B pertussis* and *E coli* and many species of *Rickettsia, Chlamydia,* and *Mycoplasma.* Doxycycline or minocycline is the drug of choice for eradication of *C trachomatis* in pelvic inflammatory disease and nongonococcal urethritis.

Staining of the permanent teeth was noted in young children treated with repeated courses of tetracyclines. As a result, tetracyclines are generally not given to children younger than 9 years of age unless alternative drugs are unavailable. A single course of tetracycline does not pose a significant risk of tooth staining. Mucous membrane candidiasis, photosensitivity, nausea, and vomiting are other common side effects. Tetracycline should be taken on an empty stomach, either 1 hour before or 2 hours after a meal. Doxycycline is well absorbed even in the presence of food; administration with food may minimize gastrointestinal side effects.

Tetracycline is used for therapy of rickettsial infections such as Rocky Mountain spotted fever, rickettsialpox, typhus, and Q fever; as an alternative to erythromycin for *M pneumoniae* and *C pneumoniae;* and for treatment of psittacosis, chancroid, melioidosis, brucellosis, *P multocida* infection, and relapsing fever.

AMINOGLYCOSIDES

The aminoglycosides are protein synthesis inhibitors and are active against aerobic gram-negative rods, including *P aeruginosa.* Streptomycin was the first drug in this class, but today it is used only for tuberculosis and the occasional cases of plague and tularemia. Kanamycin was subsequently introduced and used extensively in newborn nurseries, but when resistance developed, gentamicin, tobramycin, and then amikacin supplanted kanamycin.

Aminoglycosides are used for serious gram-negative infections and are given intravenously or intramuscularly. Aminoglycosides are used for pyelonephritis, suspected gram-negative sepsis, *P aeruginosa* infections in patients with cystic fibrosis or burns, and other gram-negative pneumonias. Aminoglycosides also have activity against gram-positive organisms and, combined with penicillin or ampicillin, may achieve synergistic killing of *L monocytogenes* and group B streptococci. Penicillin or ampicillin combined with an aminoglycoside is indicated for therapy of serious enterococcal infections, such as sepsis or endocarditis. Aminoglycosides have activity against *S aureus* but are not used for therapy except in combination with other antistaphylococcal antibiotics.

Aminoglycosides are not active in an acidic environment and may not be effective against loculated abscesses. Aminoglycosides diffuse poorly into the cerebrospinal fluid and achieve there only about 10% of serum concentrations. As a result, a third-generation cephalosporin is preferred for bacillary meningitis.

Aminoglycosides kill bacteria in a concentration-dependent manner. Aminoglycosides also have a prolonged suppressive effect on the regrowth of susceptible organisms ("postantibiotic effect"). These principles have led some investigators to establish guidelines for once-daily dosing of aminoglycosides, using larger initial doses given every 24 hours. Although aminoglycosides are associated with both renal and eighth nerve toxicity, the entry of the drug into renal and cochlear cells is saturable. It therefore was predicted that once-daily dosing would result in less toxicity than traditional twice-daily or three times daily dosing.

Studies in adult patients suggest that once-daily dosing is as efficacious as traditional dosing and is associated with less toxicity. Although there is extensive experience with dosing intervals of 18–36 hours in premature babies, small total daily doses are customarily used (2–2.5 mg/kg/dose). A convenient and cost-effective approach in children is based on the experience with adult patients and uses larger daily doses (4–7 mg/kg/dose every 24 hours). Unfortunately, there is little published information on the efficacy and safety of this approach in children.

Accordingly, traditional twice-daily or three times daily dosing regimens of aminoglycosides, with monitoring of serum levels, are still widely used. Careful monitoring is necessary, particularly in children with abnormal or changing renal function, premature infants, and infants with rapidly changing volumes of distribution. Aminoglycosides are usually infused over 30–45 minutes, and the peak serum concentration is measured 30–45 minutes after the end of the infusion. A trough serum concentration is measured prior to the next dose. The efficacious and nontoxic serum concentrations for gentamicin and tobramycin are trough less than 2 μg/mL and peak 5–10 μg/mL; for amikacin, trough less than 10 μg/mL and peak 15–25 μg/mL.

QUINOLONES

Nalidixic acid was the prototype quinolone antimicrobial, but it is not frequently used today. Modification of the quinolone structure has led to the introduction of many new compounds called fluoroquinolones, which are well absorbed after oral administration and possess excellent antibacterial activity against resistant gram-negative pathogens. The many different fluoroquinolones vary in their activity against specific organisms. Fluoroquinolones are active against most of the Enterobacteriaceae, including *E coli, Enterobacter, Klebsiella,* in some cases *P aeruginosa,* and many other gram-negative bacteria such as *H influenzae, M catarrhalis, N gonorrhoeae,* and *N meningitidis.* The fluoroquinolones are active against some enterococci, *S aureus* and coagulase-negative staphylococci but not against methicillin-resistant *S aureus.* The activity of fluoroquinolones against streptococci and anaerobic organisms is too limited for clinical usefulness.

Quinolones are contraindicated in children, though they are potentially attractive alternatives to currently approved agents. The objection is based on the recognition that nalidixic acid and other quinolones cause arthropathy when used experimentally in newborn animals of many species. The fear that children would also be susceptible to cartilage injury has not been realized in clinical experience. Both retrospective long-term follow-up studies of children treated with nalidixic acid and prospective studies of children treated under protocols with fluoroquinolones have shown no toxicity. For these reasons, quinolones should be considered for use in children when the benefit clearly outweighs the risk; when no alternative drug is available; and after discussion with the parents followed by informed consent.

Quinolones are useful for oral therapy of resistant gram-negative urinary tract infections such as *P aeruginosa,* single-dose therapy of gonorrhea, therapy of resistant cases of shigellosis, of patients with cystic fibrosis infected with *P aeruginosa,* for patients with chronic suppurative otitis media, and in some cases atypical mycobacterial infection. They are used as alternatives to other drugs in treatment of *C trachomatis* infections.

METRONIDAZOLE

Metronidazole has excellent activity against most anaerobes, particularly gram-negative anaerobes such as *Bacteroides* and *Fusobacterium,* and gram-positive anaerobes such as *Clostridium, Prevotella,* and *Porphyromonas.* Gram-positive anaerobic cocci such as *Peptococcus* and *Peptostreptococcus* are often more susceptible to penicillin or to clindamycin. Because metronidazole lacks activity against aerobic organisms, it is usually given with one or more other antibiotics.

Metronidazole is well absorbed after oral administration and has excellent penetration into the central nervous system.

CHLORAMPHENICOL

Chloramphenicol has been used for many years to treat infections with a broad range of bacteria. Streptococci, many enterococci, gram-negative rods such as *E coli, H influenzae,* gram-negative cocci such as *Neisseria,* and anaerobic organisms are usually susceptible. Cerebrospinal fluid levels are about 70% of serum levels. Although oral chloramphenicol results in predictable serum levels, the oral preparation is not available.

Chloramphenicol causes a reversible suppression of bone marrow with prolonged use. Aplastic anemic is a rare idiosyncratic (non-dose-related) complication that occurs in about 1:100,000–1:20,000 patients. Chloramphenicol given by any route may cause aplastic anemia, but most cases of aplastic anemia follow oral therapy. Because of this toxicity and because other antimicrobials are usually equally efficacious, chloramphenicol is not often used in general practice. However, Rocky Mountain spotted fever and resistant *S typhi* infections are treated with chloramphenicol. Chloramphenicol is an alternative drug for penicillin-allergic and cephalosporin-allergic patients with serious bacterial infections.

The "gray baby syndrome" consists of cardiovascular collapse associated with high serum levels of chloramphenicol. Accordingly, serum concentrations of chloramphenicol should be monitored whenever the drug is used. Peak serum concentrations between 15 and 30 µg/mL are safe and efficacious.

REFERENCES

Ahmend A: A critical evaluation of vancomycin for treatment of bacterial meningitis. Pediatr Inf Dis J 1997;16: 895.

Antimicrobial prophylaxis in surgery. Med Lett Drugs Ther 1992;34:5.

Bradley JS: Meropenem: A new extremely broad spectrum beta-lactam antibiotic for serious infections in pediatrics. Pediatr Inf Dis J 1997;16:263.

Classen DC et al: The timing of prophylactic administration of antibiotics and the risk of surgical-wound infection. N Engl J Med 1992;326:281.

Edmond MB, Wenzel RP, Pasculle AW: Vancomycin-resistant *Staphylococcus aureus*: Perspectives on measures needed for control. Ann Intern Med 1996;124:329.

Jacobson KL et al: The relationship between antecedent antibiotic use and resistance to extended-spectrum cephalosporins in group I β-lactamase-producing organisms. Clin Infect Dis 1995;21:1107.

Moellering RCJ: Monitoring serum vancomycin levels: Climbing the mountain because it is there? (Editorial.) Clin Infect Dis 1994;18:544.

Nelson JD: *Pocketbook of Pediatric Antimicrobial Therapy,* 12th ed. Williams & Wilkins, 1996.

Peter G, Hall CB, Orenstein WA (editors): *1997 Red Book: Report of the Committee on Infectious Diseases,* 24th ed. American Academy of Pediatrics, 1997.

Recommendations for preventing the spread of vancomycin resistance: Recommendations of the Hospital Infection Control Practices Advisory Committee. Am J Infect Control 1995;23:87.

Rice LB, Chales DM: Vancomycin resistance in the *Enterococcus.* Pediatr Clin North Am 1995;42:601.

Saez-Llorens X et al: Prospective randomized comparison of cefepime and cefotaxime for treatment of bacterial meningitis in infants and children. Antimicrob Agents Chemother 1995;39:937.

Sanford JP et al: *Sanford Guide to Antimicrobial Therapy.* 27th ed. Antimicrobial Therapy, 1997.

Schaad JB et al: Use of fluoroquinolones in pediatrics: Consensus report of an International Society of Chemotherapy Commission. Pediatr Infect Dis J 1995; 14:1.

Skopnik H, Heimann G: Once daily aminoglycoside dosing in full term neonates. Pediatr Infect Dis J 1995;14:71.

Staphylococcus aureus with reduced susceptibility to Vancomycin—United States, 1997. MMWR Morb Mortal Wkly Rep 1997;46:813.

Todd JK: Antimicrobial susceptibility testing in the office laboratory. Pediatr Infect Dis 1983;2:481.

Tomasz A: Multiple-antibiotic-resistant pathogenic bacteria: A report on the Rockefeller University Workshop. N Engl J Med 1994;330:1247.

34

Infections: Viral & Rickettsial

Myron J. Levin, MD

I. VIRAL INFECTIONS

Viruses cause most pediatric infections. Although immunizations have decreased the incidence of some viral infections, new viruses have been discovered, and some previously unexplained diseases have been associated with familiar viruses. Mixed viral or viral-bacterial infections of the respiratory and intestinal tracts are rather common, as is prolonged asymptomatic shedding of some viruses in childhood. Thus, the detection of a virus is not always proof that it is the cause of a given illness. Viruses are often a predisposing factor for bacterial respiratory infections (eg, otitis, sinusitis, and pneumonia).

Diagnosis of many viral illnesses is now possible through antigen or nucleic acid detection techniques. These are more rapid than isolation of viruses in tissue culture and in many cases are equally sensitive or more so. Polymerase chain reaction (PCR) amplification of viral genes has led to recognition of previously undetected infections. New diagnostic tests have changed some basic concepts about viral diseases and made diagnosis of viral infections increasingly complex. Only laboratories with excellent quality control procedures should be used, and the results of new tests must be interpreted cautiously. The availability of specific antiviral agents increases the value of early diagnosis for some serious viral infections. Table 34–1 lists viral agents associated with common clinical signs, and Table 34–2 lists diagnostic tests. The viral diagnostic laboratory should be contacted for details regarding specimen collection, handling, and shipping. Table 34–3 lists common causes of red rashes in children that should be considered in the differential diagnosis of certain viral illnesses.

Respiratory Infections

Many virus infections cause upper or lower respiratory tract signs and symptoms. Those that produce a predominance of these signs and symptoms are described in the text that follows. However, many "respiratory" viruses can also produce distinct nonrespiratory disease (eg, enteritis or cystitis caused by adenoviruses; parotitis caused by parainfluenza viruses). Respiratory viruses can cause disease in any area of the respiratory tree. Thus, they can cause coryza, pharyngitis, sinusitis, tracheitis, bronchitis, bronchiolitis, and pneumonia—though certain viruses tend to be closely associated with one anatomic area (eg, parainfluenza with croup; respiratory syncytial virus with bronchiolitis) or discrete epidemics (eg, influenza, RSV, parainfluenza). Nevertheless, it is not possible on clinical grounds to be certain of the viral cause of an infection in a given child. This information is provided by the virology laboratory and is often important for epidemiologic, therapeutic, and preventive reasons.

VIRUSES CAUSING THE COMMON COLD

The common cold syndrome ("upper respiratory infection") is characterized by various combinations of runny nose, nasal congestion, sore throat, tearing, cough, and sneezing. Low-grade fever may be present. The etiologic agent is usually not sought or determined. Epidemiologic studies indicate that rhinoviruses, which are the most common cause, are present throughout the year. Adenoviruses also cause colds in all seasons, but epidemics are common. Respiratory syncytial, parainfluenza, and influenza viruses cause the cold syndrome during epidemics from late fall through winter. Coronaviruses also cause colds in winter, while enteroviruses cause the "summer cold." One significance of these infections is morbidity continuing for 5–7 days. It is likely also that changes in respiratory epithelium, local obstruc-

Table 34–1. Common viral causes of clinical syndromes.

Rash	**Pneumonia**
Enterovirus	Respiratory syncytial virus[7]
Adenovirus	Adenovirus
Measles	Parainfluenza
Rubella	Dengue
Human herpes virus type 6[1] or 7	Measles
Varicella	Varicella[8]
Parvovirus B19[2]	Cytomegalovirus[7,9]
Epstein-Barr virus	**Enteritis**
Fever	Rotavirus
Enterovirus	Enteric adenovirus
Adenovirus	Hepatitis A[10]
Epstein-Barr virus	Enterovirus
Human herpes virus type 6[1] or 7	Norwalk agent
Cytomegalovirus	Calicivirus
Influenza	**Hepatitis**
Rhinovirus	Hepatitis A,[10] B, C, D, E
Most others	Epstein-Barr virus
Conjunctivitis	Adenovirus
Adenovirus	Cytomegalovirus
Enterovirus 70	Varicella[11]
Measles	**Arthritis**
Herpes simplex[3]	Parvovirus B19
Parotitis	Rubella
Mumps	Hepatitis B
Parainfluenza	**Congenital or perinatal infection**
Enterovirus	Cytomegalovirus
Cytomegalovirus	Hepatitis B
Epstein-Barr virus	Hepatitis C[12]
Human immunodeficiency virus	Rubella
Pharyngitis	Human immunodeficiency virus
Adenovirus	Parvovirus B19
Enterovirus	Enterovirus
Epstein-Barr virus	Varicella
Herpes simplex virus[4]	Herpes simplex virus
Influenza	**Meningoencephalitis**
Other respiratory viruses	Enterovirus
Adenopathy	Mumps
Epstein-Barr virus	Arthropod-borne viruses
Cytomegalovirus	Herpes simplex virus
Rubella[5]	Cytomegalovirus
Human immunodeficiency virus	Lymphocytic choriomeningitis virus
Croup	Measles
Parainfluenza	Varicella
Influenza	Adenovirus
Adenovirus	Human immunodeficiency virus
Measles	Epstein-Barr virus
Bronchiolitis	
Respiratory syncytial virus[6]	
Adenovirus	
Parainfluenza	
Influenza	

[1]Roseola agent.
[2]Erythema infectiosum agent.
[3]Conjunctivitis rare, only in primary infections; keratitis in older patients.
[4]May cause isolated pharyngeal vesicles at any age.
[5]May cause adenopathy without rash.
[6]Over 70% of cases.
[7]Usually only in young infants.
[8]Immunosuppressed, pregnant, rarely other adults.
[9]Severely immunosuppressed at risk.
[10]Anicteric cases more common in children; these may resemble viral gastroenteritis.
[11]Common, but only mild laboratory abnormalities.
[12]Especially when the mother is HIV-positive.

Table 34–2. Diagnostic tests for viral infections.

Agent	Rapid Antigen Detection (Specimen)	Tissue Culture Mean Days to Positive (Range)	Serology Acute	Serology Paired	Polymerase Chain Reaction[1]	Comments
Adenovirus	+ (respiratory secretions)	10 (1–21)	–	+	RL	"Enteric" strains detected by culture on special cell line, or antigen detection
Arboviruses	–	–	+	+		Acute serum may diagnose many forms
Astrovirus	–	–	–	–		Diagnosis by electron microscopy
Calicivirus	–	–	–	–		Diagnosis by electron microscopy
Colorado tick virus	On RBC	–	–	RL, CDC	+	
Cytomegalovirus	+ (tissue biopsy, blood, respiratory secretions)	2	+	+	+	Diagnosis by presence of IgM antibody
Enterovirus	–	4 (2–15)	–	+	+	Serology for coxsackie B viruses
Epstein-Barr virus	–	–	+	+	+	Single serologic panel defines infection status; heterophil titer less sensitive
Hantavirus	–	–	+	ND		Diagnosis by presence of IgM antibody
Hepatitis A virus	–	–	+	ND		Diagnosis by presence of IgM antibody
Hepatitis B virus	+ (blood)	–	+	ND	+	Diagnosis by presence of surface antigen or anti-core IgM antibody
Hepatitis C virus	–	–	+	ND	+	Postitive serology suggests that hepatitis C may be the causative agent. PCR is confirmatory
Herpes simplex virus	+ (skin)	1	+	+	+	Serology rarely used for herpes simplex. IgM antibody used in selected cases. Tzanck preparation 70% sensitive
Human herpesvirus-6	–	2	RL, CDC	RL, CDC	+	Roseola agent
Human immunodeficiency virus	+ (blood) (acid dissociation of immune complexes)	15 (5–28)	+		+	Antibody proves infection unless passively acquired (< age 15 months); culture not widely available; PCR definitive early for infant diagnosis
Influenza virus	+ (respiratory secretions)	2	–	+	RL	Antigen detection 70–90% sensitive
Lymphocytic choriomeningitis virus	–	Blood, CSF 7 (5–20)	–	+		Can be isolated in suckling mice
Measles virus	+ (respiratory secretions)	5 (3–14)	+	+	RL	Difficult to grow; IgM serology diagnostic
Mumps virus	–	>5	+	+		Complement fixation titers may allow single-specimen diagnosis
Parvovirus B19	–	–	+	+	+	Erythema infectiosum agent
Parainfluenza virus	+ (respiratory secretions)	2	–	+		
Rabies virus	+ (skin, conjunctiva, tissue biopsy)	–	+	+	CDC	Usually diagnosed by antigen detection
Respiratory syncytial virus	+ (respiratory secretions)	2	–	+		Rapid antigen detection; 85–90% sensitive
Rhinovirus	–	4 (2–7)	–	–		Too many viruses to diagnose serologically
Rotavirus	+ (feces)	–	–	–		Electron microscopy useful for many enteric viruses
Rubella virus	–	> 10	+	+		Recommended that paired sera be tested simultaneously
Varicella-zoster virus	+ (skin scraping)	8 (5–14)	RL	+	+	Tzanck preparation 70% sensitive

[1]Useful only when performed on selected specimens by qualified laboratories.

Key:

Plus signs signify commercially or widely available; **minus signs** signify not commercially available. **Note:** Results from some commercial laboratories are unreliable.

RL, CDC: Specific antibody titers or PCR available by arrangement with individual research laboratories or the Centers for Disease Control and Prevention.

ND: Not done.

Table 34–3. Red rashes in children.

Condition	Incubation Period (Days)	Prodrome	Rash	Laboratory Tests	Comments, Other Diagnostic Features
Measles	9–14	Cough, rhinitis, conjunctivitis	Maculopapular; face to extremities; lasts 7–10 days; Koplik's spots in mouth	Leukopenia	Toxic. Bright red rash becomes confluent, may desquamate.
Rubella	14–21	Usually none	Mild maculopapular; rapid spread face to extremities; gone by day 4	Normal or leukopenia	Postauricular, occipital adenopathy common. Polyarthralgia in some older girls. Mild clinical illness.
Roseola (exanthem subitum)	10–14	Fever (3–4 days)	Pink, macular rash occurs at end of illness; transient	Normal	Fever often high; disappears when rash develops; child appears well. Usually occurs in children 6 months to 2 years of age.
Erythema infectiosum	13–18	None	Erythematous "slapped" cheeks; then reticular rash on extremities, trunk	Normal (reticulocytopenia)	Rash may reappear over weeks, especially with exposure to heat, sunlight. May cause arthralgia/arthritis, usually in older children or adults. Red cell maturation arrest in children with chronic hemolysis can cause aplastic crisis.
Enterovirus	2–7	Variable fever, chills, myalgia, sore throat	Usually macular, maculopapular on trunk or palms, soles; vesicles; petechiae also seen	Variable	Varied rashes may resemble those of many other infections. Pharyngeal or hand-foot-mouth vesicles may occur.
Streptococcal scarlet fever	1–7	Fever, abdominal pain, headache, sore throat	Diffuse erythema, "sandpaper" texture; neck, axillae, inguinal areas; spreads to rest of body; desquamates 7–14 days	Leukocytosis; positive group A streptococcus culture of throat or wound	Strawberry tongue, red pharynx with or without exudate. Eyes, perioral and periorbital area, palms, and soles spared. Pastia's lines. Brief prodrome. Cervical adenopathy. Usually occurs in children 2–10 years of age.
Staphylococcal scarlet fever	1–7	Variable fever	Diffuse erythroderma; resembles streptococcal scarlet fever except eyes may be hyperemic, no "strawberry" tongue, pharynx spared	Variable leukocytosis if infected	Focal infection usually present.

(continued)

Table 34-3. Red rashes in children. (continued)

Condition	Incubation Period (Days)	Prodrome	Rash	Laboratory Tests	Comments, Other Diagnostic Features
Staphylococcal scalded skin	Variable	Irritability, absent to low fever	Painful erythroderma, followed in 1–2 days by cracking around eyes, mouth; bullae form with friction (Nikolsky's sign)	Normal if only colonized by staphylococci, leukocytosis and sometimes bacteremia if infected	Normal pharynx. Look for focal staphylococcal infection. Usually occurs in infants.
Toxic shock syndrome	Variable	Fever, myalgia, headache, diarrhea, vomiting	Nontender erythroderma; red eyes, palms, soles, pharynx, lips	Leukocytosis; abnormal liver enzymes, coagulation tests; proteinuria	*S aureus* infection, multiorgan involvement. Swollen hands, feet. Hypotension or shock.
Erythema multiforme	–	Usually none or related to underlying cause	Discrete, red maculopapular lesions; symmetric, distal, palms and soles; target lesions classic	Normal or eosinophilia	Reaction to drugs (especially sulfonamides), or infectious agents. Urticaria, arthralgia also seen.
Stevens-Johnson syndrome	–	Pharyngitis, conjunctivitis, fever, malaise	Bullous erythema multiforme; may slough in large areas; hemorrhagic lips; purulent conjunctivitis	Leukocytosis	Classic precipitants are drugs (especially sulfonamides), *Mycoplasma pneumoniae* and herpes simplex infections. Pneumonitis and urethritis also seen.
Drug allergy	–	None, fever alone, or with myalgia, pruritus	Macular, maculopapular, urticarial, or erythroderma	Leukopenia, eosinophilia	Rash variable. Severe reactions may resemble measles, scarlet fever; adenopathy, hepatosplenomegaly; marked toxicity possible.
Kawasaki disease	Unknown	Fever, cervical adenopathy, irritability	Polymorphous (may be erythroderma) on trunk and extremities; red palms and soles; lips, tongue, pharynx	Leukocytosis, thrombocytosis, elevated ESR; pyuria; negative cultures and streptococcal serology; resting tachycardia	Swollen hands, feet; prolonged illness; bulbar hyperemia; uveitis; aseptic meningitis; no response to antibiotics. Vasculitis and aneurysms of coronary and other arteries occur.
Leptospirosis	4–19	Fever (biphasic), myalgia, chills	Variable erythroderma	Leukocytosis; hematuria, proteinuria; hyperbilirubinemia	Conjunctivitis; Hepatitis, aseptic meningitis may be seen. Rodent, dog contact.

tion, and altered local immunity are sometimes the precursors of more severe illnesses such as otitis media, pneumonia, or sinusitis. Asthma attacks are also provoked by viruses that cause the common cold. Nevertheless, there is no evidence that antibiotics will prevent these complications, and the unjustified widespread use of antibiotics for cold symptoms has contributed to the emergence of antibiotic-resistant respiratory flora.

In 5–10% of children, symptoms from these virus infections persist for more than 10 days. This overlap with the symptoms of bacterial sinusitis presents a difficult problem for clinicians, especially since colds can produce an abnormal CT scan of the sinuses. Viruses that cause a minor illness in normal children, such as rhinoviruses, can cause severe lower respiratory disease in immunologically or anatomically compromised children.

There is no evidence that symptomatic relief can be achieved with oral antihistamines or cough suppressants. Topical decongestants provide temporary improvement in nasal symptoms.

Chidekel AS et al: Rhinovirus infection associated with serious lower respiratory illness in patients with bronchopulmonary dysplasia. Pediatr Infect Dis J 1997; 16:43.

Gadomski A: Rational use of over-the-counter medications in young children. JAMA 1994;272:1063.

Gaffey MJ, Kaiser DL, Hayden FG: Ineffectiveness of oral terfenadine in natural colds: Evidence against histamine as a mediator of common cold symptoms. Pediatr Infect Dis J 1988;7:215.

Gwaltney JM Jr et al: Computed tomographic study of the common cold. N Engl J Med 1994;330:25.

Taylor JA et al: Efficacy of cough depressants in children. J Pediatr 1993;122:79.

Wald ER et al: Upper respiratory tract infections in young children: Duration of and frequency of complications. Pediatrics 1991;87:129.

INFECTIONS DUE TO ADENOVIRUSES

There are over 45 types of adenoviruses, which account for 2–10% of all respiratory illnesses. Enteric adenoviruses are an important cause of childhood diarrhea. Adenoviral infections are common early in life. Epidemic disease occurs in winter and spring, especially in closed environments such as day care centers and institutions. Because of latent infection in lymphoid tissue, asymptomatic shedding from the respiratory or intestinal tract is common.

Diagnosis is by culture of conjunctival, respiratory, or stool specimens. Several days to weeks are required for growth in conventional cultures. Rapid culture using the shell vial technique and immunodiagnostic reagents detects virus in 48 hours. Adenovirus infection can also be diagnosed using these reagents directly on respiratory secretions. This is quicker, but less sensitive than the culture methods. Special cells are needed to isolate enteric adenoviruses. Respiratory adenovirus infections can be detected by serologic tests using acute and convalescent serum. Detection of enteric adenoviruses in diarrheal specimens can now be done rapidly with EIA.

Specific Adenoviral Syndromes

A. Pharyngitis: Pharyngitis is the most common adenoviral disease in children. Fever and adenopathy are common. Tonsillitis may be exudative. An influenza-like systemic illness may be present. Laryngotracheitis or bronchitis may accompany pharyngitis.

B. Follicular Conjunctivitis: This form of conjunctivitis may be prolonged and associated with preauricular adenopathy and corneal damage. Association with fever, pharyngitis, and cervical adenopathy is called "pharyngoconjunctival fever."

C. Epidemic Keratoconjunctivitis: Symptoms are severe conjunctivitis with punctate keratitis and occasionally visual impairment. A foreign body sensation, photophobia, and swelling of conjunctiva and eyelids are characteristic. Preauricular adenopathy and subconjunctival hemorrhage are common.

D. Pneumonia: Severe pneumonia may occur at all ages. It is especially common in young children (< age 3 years). Chest radiographs show bilateral peribronchial and interstitial infiltrates. Symptoms persist for 2–4 weeks. Adenoviral pneumonia can be necrotizing and cause permanent lung damage.

E. Rash: A diffuse morbilliform (rarely petechial) rash resembling measles, rubella, or roseola may be present. Koplik's spots are absent.

F. Diarrhea: Enteric adenoviruses (types 40 and 41) are the second most common cause of short-lived diarrhea in an afebrile child.

G. Mesenteric Lymphadenitis: Fever and abdominal pain may mimic appendicitis. Pharyngitis is often associated. Adenovirus-induced adenopathy may be a factor in appendicitis and intussusception.

H. Other Syndromes: Immunosuppressed patients, including neonates, may develop severe or fatal pulmonary or gastrointestinal infections or multisystem disease. Other rare complications include encephalitis, hepatitis, and myocarditis. Hemorrhagic cystitis can be a serious problem in immunocompromised children.

Treatment

There is no specific treatment for adenovirus infections. Intravenous immune globulin may be tried in immunocompromised patients with severe pneumonia. There are anecdotal reports of successful treatment of immunocompromised patients with ribavirin or cidofovir.

Abzug M, Levin MJ: Neonatal adenovirus infection: Four patients and a review of the literature. Pediatrics 1991;87:890.

Krajden M et al: Clinical features of adenoviral enteritis: A review of 127 proven cases. Pediatr Infect Dis J 1990;9:636.

Krilov LR et al: Disseminated adenovirus infection with hepatic necrosis in patients with human immunodeficiency virus infection and other immunodeficiency states. Rev Infect Dis 1990;12:303.

Murtagh P et al: Adenovirus type 7H respiratory infections: A report of 29 cases of acute lower respiratory disease. Acta Paediatr 1993;82:557.

INFLUENZA

Because young children have little prior experience with influenza viruses, clinical infections are common. Infection rates in children are greater than those of young adults during epidemics, and infections in children are instrumental in facilitating community outbreaks. Although only three main types of influenza viruses (A/H1N1, A/H3N2, B) have been prevalent recently, antigenic shift and drift ensure a supply of susceptible hosts of all ages. Outbreaks occur in fall and winter. Each year's strain tends to arise first in the Far East.

Clinical Findings

Spread of influenza occurs by way of airborne respiratory secretions. The incubation period is 2–7 days. Influenza infections are easily recognized during epidemics.

A. Symptoms and Signs: Influenza infection in older children and adults produces a characteristic syndrome of sudden onset of high fever, severe myalgia, headache, and chills. These overshadow the associated coryza, pharyngitis, and cough. Usually absent are rash, marked conjunctivitis, adenopathy, exudative pharyngitis, and dehydrating enteritis. Fever, diarrhea, vomiting, and abdominal pain are common in young children. Infants may develop a sepsis-like illness and apnea. Chest examination is usually unremarkable. Unusual clinical findings or variants include croup (most severe with type A influenza), exacerbation of asthma, myositis (especially calf muscles), myocarditis, parotitis, encephalopathy (distinct from Reye's syndrome), nephritis, and a transient maculopapular rash. Acute illness lasts 2–5 days. Cough and fatigue may last several weeks. Viral shedding may persist for several weeks in young children.

B. Laboratory Findings: The leukocyte count is normal to low, with variable shift. The virus may be found in respiratory secretions by fluorescent antibody staining or enzyme immunoassay (EIA; for influenza A only). It can also be cultured within 3–5 days from pharyngeal swabs or throat washings. Many laboratories obtain positive cultures within 48 hours by centrifuging specimens onto cell layers and using antigen detection. Other body fluids or tissues (except lung) rarely yield the virus. A late diagnosis may be made with paired serology, using hemagglutination inhibition assays.

C. Imaging: The chest radiograph is nonspecific; it may show hyperaeration, peribronchial thickening, diffuse interstitial infiltrates, or bronchopneumonia in severe cases. Pneumothorax may occur. Hilar nodes are not enlarged. Pleural effusion is rare in uncomplicated influenza.

Differential Diagnosis

The following may be considered: all other respiratory viruses, *Mycoplasma pneumoniae* or *Chlamydia pneumoniae* (longer incubation period, prolonged illness), streptococcal pharyngitis (pharyngeal exudate or petechiae, adenitis, no cough), bacterial sepsis (petechial or purpuric rash may occur), toxic shock syndrome (rash, hypotension), and rickettsial infections (rash, different season, insect exposure). High fever, the nature of preceding or concurrent illness in family members, and the presence of influenza in the community are distinguishing features from parainfluenza or respiratory syncytial virus infections.

Complications & Sequelae

Lower respiratory tract symptoms are most common in children younger than 5 years. Influenza can cause croup in these children. Secondary bacterial infections (classically staphylococcal) of the middle ear, sinuses, or lungs are most common. Of the viral infections that precede Reye's syndrome, varicella and influenza (usually type B) are most notable. During an influenza outbreak, ill children who develop protracted vomiting or irrational behavior should be evaluated for Reye's syndrome (see Chapter 20). Influenza can also cause a viral or postviral encephalitis, with cerebral symptoms much more prominent than those of the accompanying respiratory infection. Although the myositis is usually mild and resolves promptly, severe rhabdomyolysis and renal failure have been reported.

Children with underlying cardiopulmonary, metabolic, neuromuscular, or immunosuppressive disease may develop severe viral pneumonia.

Prevention

Influenza vaccine is moderately protective in older children (see Chapter 9). All high-risk children should be immunized, and medical staff and family members should also be immunized to protect high-risk patients. Type A infections may be prevented by amantadine or rimantadine (5 mg/kg; maximum 150 mg/d under age 10; 200 mg/d if older). Amantadine is divided into two daily doses; rimantadine can be given in a single dose. The physician should consider administering chemoprophylaxis during an epidemic to high-risk children who cannot be immunized or who have not yet developed immunity (about 6 weeks after primary vaccination or 2 weeks after a booster dose). These agents are inactive against influenza B.

Treatment & Prognosis

Treatment consists of general support and management of pulmonary complications, especially bacterial superinfections. Amantadine and rimantadine are of some benefit against influenza A if begun within 48 hours after onset. A new class of drugs—neuraminidase inhibitors—is licensed for treatment within 36 hours of onset. Their value in compromised hosts or others with severe disease is uncertain. Ribavirin is active in vitro against influenza A and B. The efficacy of aerosolized ribavirin in humans is controversial, but it may be tried in severe infections, especially in compromised hosts.

Recovery is usually complete unless severe cardiopulmonary or neurologic damage has occurred. Fatal cases occur in immunodeficient and anatomically compromised children.

Advisory Committee on Immunization Practices (Centers for Disease Control and Prevention). Prevention and control of influenza. MMWR Morb Mortal Wkly Rep 1998;47(RR-6):1.

Brady MT: Amantadine and rimantadine. Rep Pediatr Infect Dis 1994;4:29.

Christenson JC, San Joaquin VH: Influenza-associated rhabdomyolysis in a child. Pediatr Infect Dis J 1990;9:60.

Kondos AK: The effects of influenza virus infection on FEV_1 in asthmatic children. Chest 1991;100:1235.

Rodriguez WJ et al: Efficacy and safety of aerosolized ribavirin in young children hospitalized with influenza: A double-blind, multicenter, placebo-controlled trial. J Pediatr 1994;125:129.

Serwint JR, Hiller RM, Korsch BM: Influenza type A and B infections in hospitalized pediatric patients who should be immunized. Am J Dis Child 1991;145:623.

Sugaya N et al: Impact of influenza virus infection as a cause of pediatric hospitalization. J Infect Dis 1992; 165:373.

PARAINFLUENZA

Parainfluenza viruses (types 1–4) are the most important cause of croup. Most infants are infected with type 3 within the first 3 years of life; all types may cause outbreaks. Infection with types 1 and 2 are experienced gradually over the first 5 years of life. Types 1 and 2 occur in the fall; type 3 appears annually, with a peak in the spring or summer. Most primary infections are symptomatic and frequently involve the lower respiratory tract.

Clinical Findings

A. Symptoms and Signs: Clinical diseases include febrile upper respiratory infection (especially in older children with reexposure), laryngitis, tracheobronchitis, croup, and bronchiolitis (second most common cause after respiratory syncytial virus). The relative incidence of these manifestations is type-specific. Parainfluenza viruses (especially type 1) cause 65% of cases of croup in young children, 25% of tracheobronchitis, and 50% of laryngitis. Pneumonia occurs in infants and immunodeficient children. Onset is acute. Most children are febrile. Symptoms of upper respiratory tract infection often accompany croup.

B. Laboratory Findings: Diagnosis is often based on clinical findings. These viruses can be identified by rapid culture techniques (48 hours) and by direct immunofluorescence on nasopharyngeal epithelial cells in respiratory secretions (under 3 hours).

Differential Diagnosis

Parainfluenza-induced respiratory syndromes are difficult to distinguish from those caused by other respiratory viruses. Croup must be distinguished from epiglottitis caused by *Haemophilus influenzae* (abrupt onset, toxicity, drooling, dyspnea, little cough, left shift of blood smear, and a history of inadequate immunization).

Treatment

There is no specific therapy or vaccine. Croup management is discussed in Chapter 17. Ribavirin is active in vitro and has been used in immunocompromised children, but its efficacy is unproved.

Heidemann SM: Clinical characteristics of parainfluenza virus infection in hospitalized children. Pediatr Pulmonol 1992;13:86.

Husby et al: Treatment of croup with nebulized steroid (budesonide): A double blind, placebo controlled study. Arch Dis Child 1993;68:352.

Knott AM, Long CE, Hall CB: Parainfluenza viral infections in pediatric outpatients: Seasonal patterns and clinical characteristics. Pediatr Infect Dis J 1994;13:269.

Welliver RC et al: Parainfluenza virus bronchiolitis. Am J Dis Child 1986;140:34.

RESPIRATORY SYNCYTIAL VIRUS (RSV) DISEASE

Essentials of Diagnosis & Typical Features

- Diffuse wheezing and tachypnea following upper respiratory symptoms in an infant (bronchiolitis).
- Epidemics in late fall to early spring (January-February peak).
- Hyperinflation on chest radiograph.
- RSV antigen detected in nasal secretions.

General Considerations

Respiratory syncytial virus is the most important cause of lower respiratory tract illness in young children, accounting for more than 70% of cases of bronchiolitis and 40% of cases of pneumonia. Outbreaks occur annually, and attack rates are high; 60% of children are infected in the first year of life. During peak season, the clinical diagnosis of RSV infection in infants with bronchiolitis is as accurate as most laboratory tests. Despite the presence of serum antibody, reinfection is common. However, reinfection generally causes only upper respiratory symptoms. No vaccine is available. Immunosuppressed patients may develop progressive severe pneumonia. Children with congenital heart disease with increased pulmonary blood flow, children with chronic lung disease, and premature infants under 6 months of age are also at higher risk for severe illness.

Clinical Findings

A. Symptoms and Signs: Initial symptoms are those of upper respiratory infection. Fever may be present. The classic disease is bronchiolitis, characterized by diffuse wheezing, variable fever, cough, tachypnea, difficulty feeding, and cyanosis in severe cases. Hyperinflation, crackles, prolonged expiration, wheezing, and retractions are present. The liver and spleen may be palpable because of lung hyperinflation but are not enlarged. The disease usually lasts 3–7 days in previously healthy children.

Apnea may be the presenting manifestation, especially in premature infants, in the first few months of life; it usually resolves after a few days, often being replaced by obvious signs of bronchiolitis. No explanation for apnea has been found.

RSV infections in subsequent years are more likely to cause tracheobronchitis or upper respiratory tract infection. Exceptions are immunocompromised hosts and children with severe chronic lung or heart disease, who may have especially severe or prolonged primary infections and are subject to additional attacks of severe pneumonitis.

B. Laboratory Findings: Routine tests are nonspecific. Rapid detection of RSV antigen in nasal or pulmonary secretions by fluorescent antibody staining or EIA is more than 90% sensitive and specific. These tests provide an etiologic diagnosis within several hours after the specimens are processed. Rapid tissue culture methods take 48 hours and have comparable sensitivity.

C. Imaging: Diffuse hyperinflation and peribronchiolar thickening are most common; atelectasis and patchy infiltrates also occur in uncomplicated infection, but pleural effusions are rare. Consolidation occurs in 25% of children with lower tract disease.

Differential Diagnosis

Although almost all cases of bronchiolitis are due to RSV during an epidemic, other viruses cannot be excluded. Mixed infections with other viruses, chlamydiae, or bacteria are not uncommon. Wheezing may be due to asthma, a foreign body, or other airway obstruction. RSV infection may closely resemble chlamydial pneumonitis when fine crackles are present and fever and wheezing are not prominent. The two may also coexist. Cystic fibrosis may resemble RSV infection; a positive family history or failure to thrive associated with hyponatremia or hypoalbuminemia should prompt a sweat chloride test. Pertussis should also be considered in this age group, especially if cough is prominent and if the infant is under 6 months of age. A markedly elevated leukocyte count should suggest bacterial superinfection (neutrophilia) or pertussis (lymphocytosis).

Complications

Secondary bacterial infection of the middle ear (usually due to pneumococci or *H influenzae*) is the most common complication. However, bacterial pneumonia occurs in only 0.5–1% of hospitalized cases. Sudden exacerbations of fever and leukocytosis should suggest bacterial infection. Respiratory failure or apnea may require mechanical ventilation. Cardiac failure may occur as a complication of pulmonary disease or myocarditis. Respiratory syncytial virus—as well as parainfluenza and influenza viruses—commonly causes acute exacerbations of asthma. Nosocomial infection is so common during outbreaks that elective hospitalization or surgery, especially for those with underlying illness, should be postponed. Well-designed hospital programs to prevent nosocomial spread are imperative (see below).

Treatment

Children who are very hypoxic or cannot feed because of respiratory distress must be hospitalized and given humidified oxygen and tube or intravenous feedings. Antibiotics, decongestants, expectorants, and steroids are of no value in routine infections. The child should be kept in respiratory isolation. Cohorting ill infants in respiratory isolation during peak season (with or without rapid diagnostic attempts) and emphasizing good hand-washing may greatly decrease nosocomial transmission.

Often a trial of bronchodilator therapy is given to determine if bronchospasm coexists. Patients appear to respond differently to bronchodilator therapy. Discontinue bronchodilators if there is no improvement. If they do help, nebulized salbutamol, 0.1 mg/kg every 2–6 hours as needed, may be tried (see Chapter 17).

Ribavirin is the only licensed antiviral therapy used for RSV infection. It is given by continuous aerosolization (6 g in a 300 mL vial of water) by a special nebulizer for 12–18 hours of every day for 3–5 days. This agent has minimal effect on virus shedding. There is controversy about its efficacy. At best, there is a very modest effect on disease severity in normal infants. Even in high-risk infants, clinical response to ribavirin therapy was not demonstrated in several studies. Nevertheless, ribavirin is often used in severely ill children who are immunologically or anatomically compromised. It is expensive. It should be used in a negative-pressure room, preferably equipped with additional respiratory care equipment capable of preventing contamination of room air. Caregivers should wear masks, and pregnant women should not be in the room when ribavirin is being administered.

Bronchospasm may be exacerbated by this drug. It should be used with extreme caution in ventilated patients and only by therapists expert in pediatric ventilator management. In general, it should be considered for use only for very young infants ($\leq$ 8 weeks), former premature infants (< 35 weeks) who are under 6 months old, children with underlying cardiopulmonary or immunologic diseases, and normal infants with evidence of severe RSV infection (ventilated or with Po_2 < 65 mm Hg; Pco_2 rising).

Monthly administration of intravenous immune globulin containing high titers of anti-RSV antibody is now recommended to prevent severe disease in high-risk patients during epidemic periods. Monthly administration should be considered during the RSV season for children with bronchopulmonary dysplasia up to 24 months of age who received O_2 supplementation in the prior 6 months and for children under 6 months of age who were born before 32 weeks gestation. Use of passive immunization for immunocompromised children is logical but not established. Use in children with congenital heart disease is not recommended, based on recent studies.

Prognosis

Although mild bronchiolitis does not produce long-term problems, 30–40% of patients hospitalized with this infection will wheeze later in childhood. Chronic restrictive lung disease and bronchiolitis obliterans are rare sequelae.

Hall CB et al: Risk of secondary bacterial infection in infants hospitalized with respiratory syncytial viral infection. J Pediatr 1988;113:266.

Hammer J, Numa A, Newth CJL: Albuterol responsiveness in infants with respiratory failure caused by respiratory syncytial virus infection. J Pediatr Med 1995;127:485.

La Via WV, Marks MI, Stutman HR: Respiratory syncytial virus puzzle: Clinical features, pathophysiology, treatment, and prevention. J Pediatr 1992;121:503.

MacDonald NE et al: Respiratory syncytial viral infection in infants with congenital heart disease. N Engl J Med 1982;307:397.

Madge P et al: Prospective controlled study of four infection-control procedures to prevent nosocomial infection with respiratory syncytial virus. Lancet 1992;340:1079.

Meart KL et al: Aerosolized ribavirin in mechanically ventilated children with respiratory syncytial virus lower respiratory tract disease: A prospective, double-blind, randomized trial. Intensive Care Med 1994;22:566.

Meissner HC, Groothuis JR: Immunoprophylaxis and the control of respiratory syncytial virus disease. Pediatrics 1997;100:260.

Smith DW et al: A controlled trial of aerosolized ribavirin in infants receiving mechanical ventilation for severe respiratory syncytial virus infection. N Engl J Med 1991;325:24.

Wildin SR, Chonmaitree T, Swischuk LE: Roentgenographic features of common pediatric viral respiratory infections. Am J Dis Child 1988;142:43.

MEASLES
(Rubeola)

Essentials of Diagnosis
& Typical Features

- Exposure to measles 9–14 days previously.
- Prodrome of fever, cough, conjunctivitis, and coryza.
- Koplik's spots (few to countless small white papules on a diffusely red base on the buccal mucosa) 1–2 days prior to and after onset of rash.
- Maculopapular rash spreading down from the face and hairline over 3 days and later becoming confluent.
- Leukopenia.

General Considerations

This childhood exanthem has greatly decreased in incidence in the United States because of vaccination. Sporadic clusters of cases are the result of improper immunization more so than of vaccine failures. It is now recommended that all children be revaccinated upon entrance into primary or secondary school (Chapter 9). The attack rate in susceptibles is extremely high; spread is respiratory. Morbidity and mortality rates in the developing world are substantial because of underlying malnutrition and secondary infections.

Clinical Findings

A history of contact with a suspected case is often obtainable during an epidemic, but since airborne spread is efficient and patients are contagious during the prodrome, no contact history may be obtained. In temperate climates, measles is a winter-spring disease. Many suspected cases are misdiagnoses of other viral infections.

A. Symptoms and Signs: High fever and lethargy are prominent. Sneezing, eyelid edema, tearing, copious coryza, photophobia, and harsh cough ensue and worsen. Koplik's spots are white macular lesions on the buccal mucosa, typically opposite the lower molars. These are almost pathognomonic for rubeola, though they may be absent. A discrete maculopapular rash begins when the respiratory symptoms are maximal and spreads quickly over the face and trunk, coalescing to a bright red. As it involves the extremities, it fades from the face and is completely gone within 6 days; fine desquamation may occur. Fever peaks when the rash appears and usually falls 2–3 days thereafter.

B. Laboratory Findings: Lymphopenia is characteristic. Total leukocyte counts may fall to 1500/μL. An experienced cytologist may see multinucleated giant cells in oral mucosal scrapings and in nasal secretions, but the diagnosis is usually made by detection of measles IgM antibody in serum drawn at least 3 days after the onset of rash or by detection of a significant rise in antibody. Tissue culture may also be used, but it takes longer and is less sensitive. Direct detection of measles antigen by fluorescent antibody staining of nasopharyngeal cells is a useful rapid method.

C. Imaging: Chest radiographs often show hyperinflation, perihilar infiltrates, or parenchymal patchy, fluffy densities. Secondary bacterial infection produces consolidation or effusion.

Differential Diagnosis

Table 34–3 lists other illnesses that may resemble measles.

Complications & Sequelae

A. Respiratory Complications: These occur in up to 15% of cases. Bacterial superinfections of lung, middle ear, sinus, and cervical nodes are most common. Fever that persists after the third or fourth day of rash suggests such a complication, as does leukocytosis. Bronchospasm, severe croup, and progressive viral pneumonia or bronchiolitis (in infants) also occur. Immunosuppressed patients are at much greater risk for fatal pneumonia.

B. Cerebral Complications: Encephalitis occurs in 1:2000 cases. Onset is usually within a week after appearance of rash. Symptoms include combativeness, ataxia, vomiting, seizures, and coma. Lymphocytic pleocytosis and a mildly elevated protein are usual cerebrospinal fluid findings, but the fluid may be normal. Forty percent of patients so affected die or are severely damaged.

Subacute sclerosing panencephalitis is a slow measles virus infection of the brain that becomes symptomatic years later in about 1:100,000 previously infected children. This progressive cerebral deterioration is associated with myoclonic jerks and a typical electroencephalographic pattern. It is fatal in 6–12 months. It rarely occurs following administration of vaccine, with an estimated incidence of < 1:1,000,000. High titers of measles antibody are present in serum and spinal fluid.

C. Other Complications: These include hemorrhagic or "black" measles (severe disease with multiorgan bleeding, fever, cerebral symptoms), thrombocytopenia, appendicitis, keratitis, myocarditis, reactivation or progression of tuberculosis in untreated children (including transient cutaneous anergy), and premature delivery or stillbirth.

Mild liver function test elevation has been detected in up to 50% of cases in young adults; frank jaundice may also occur.

Treatment, Prognosis, & Prevention

Recovery generally occurs 7–10 days after onset of symptoms. Therapy is supportive: eye care, cough relief (avoid opioid suppressants in infants), and fever reduction (acetaminophen, lukewarm baths; avoid salicylates). Secondary bacterial infections should be treated promptly; antimicrobial prophylaxis is not indicated. Ribavirin is active in vitro and may be useful in infected immunocompromised children. In malnourished children, vitamin A supplementation should be given to attenuate the illness.

The current two-dose active vaccination strategy is successful. Vaccine should not be withheld for concurrent mild acute illness, tuberculosis or positive PPD, breast feeding, or exposure to an immunodeficient contact.

Vaccination prevents the disease in susceptible exposed individuals if given within 72 hours (see Chapter 9). Immune globulin (0.25 mL/kg intramuscularly; 0.5 mL/kg if immunocompromised) will prevent or modify measles if given within 6 days. Suspected cases should be diagnosed promptly and reported to the local health department.

Gellin BG, Katz SL: Measles: State of the art and future directions. J Infect Dis 1994;170(Suppl):53.

Helfand RF et al: Diagnosis of measles with an IgM capture EIA: The optimal timing of specimen collection after rash onset. J Infect Dis 1997;175:195.

Hussey GD, Klein M: Randomized, controlled trial of vitamin A in children with severe measles. N Engl J Med 1990;323:160.

Kaplan LJ et al: Severe measles in immunocompromised patients. JAMA 1992;267:1237.

Kipps A, Dick G, Moodie JW: Measles and the central nervous system. Lancet 1983;2:1406.

Mason WH et al: Epidemic measles in the postvaccine era: Evaluation of epidemiology, clinical presentation and complications during an urban outbreak. Pediatr Infect Dis J 1993;12:42.

INFECTIONS DUE TO ENTEROVIRUSES

Enteroviruses are a major cause of illness in young children. The multiple types are physically and biochemically similar and may produce identical syndromes. The multiplicity of types makes vaccine development impractical and has hindered development of antigen detection and serologic tests. However, common

RNA sequences and group antigens have led to diagnostic tests for viral nucleic acid and proteins. A polymerase chain reaction assay is available in some medical centers, but tissue culture is the most commonly used diagnostic method for echoviruses, polioviruses, and coxsackie B viruses. Since cultures may turn positive in 2–4 days, they should be inoculated promptly and may be clinically useful, particularly in cases of meningoencephalitis. Many coxsackie A viruses fail to grow.

Transmission is fecal-oral or from upper respiratory secretions. Multiple enteroviruses circulate in the community at any one time; summer-fall outbreaks are common in temperate climates, but illness is seen year-round. After poliovirus, coxsackie B virus is most virulent, followed by echovirus. Neurologic, cardiac, and overwhelming neonatal infections are the severest forms of illness.

ACUTE FEBRILE ILLNESS

Accompanied by nonspecific upper respiratory or enteric symptoms, sudden onset of fever and irritability in infants or young children is often enteroviral in origin, especially in late summer and fall. Occasionally, a petechial rash is seen; more often, a diffuse maculopapular eruption (often prominent on palms and soles) occurs on the second to fourth days of fever. Purpura is rare and should suggest bacterial sepsis. Rapid recovery is the rule. More than one febrile enteroviral illness can occur in the same patient in one season. The leukocyte count is usually normal. Infants, because of fever and irritability, may undergo an evaluation for bacteremia or meningitis and be hospitalized to rule out sepsis. Approximately one-half of these infants have aseptic meningitis.

Dugan R: Nonpolio enteroviruses and the febrile young infant: Epidemiologic, clinical, and diagnostic aspects. Pediatr Infect Dis J 1996;15:67.

RESPIRATORY TRACT ILLNESSES

1. FEBRILE UPPER RESPIRATORY INFECTION WITH PHARYNGITIS

This syndrome is most common in older children, who complain of headache, sore throat, myalgia, and abdominal discomfort. The usual duration is 3–4 days. Vesicles or papules may be seen in the pharynx. There is no exudate. Occasionally, enteroviruses are the cause of croup, bronchitis, or pneumonia. They may also exacerbate asthma.

2. HERPANGINA

Herpangina is characterized by an acute onset of fever and posterior pharyngeal ulcers, often linearly arranged on the anterior fauces. Bilateral faucial ulcers may also be seen. Dysphagia, vomiting, and anorexia also occur and, rarely, parotitis or vaginal ulcers. Symptoms disappear in 1 week. The epidemic form is due to a variety of coxsackie A viruses; coxsackie B viruses and echoviruses cause sporadic cases.

The differential diagnosis includes primary herpes simplex gingivostomatitis (ulcers are more prominent anteriorly, and gingivitis is present), aphthous stomatitis (fever absent, recurrent episodes, anterior lesions), trauma, hand-foot-and-mouth disease (see below), and Vincent's angina (painful gingivitis spreading from the gum line, underlying dental disease).

3. ACUTE LYMPHONODULAR PHARYNGITIS

Coxsackievirus A10 has been associated with a febrile pharyngitis characterized by nonulcerating yellow-white posterior pharyngeal papules. The duration is 1–2 weeks; therapy is supportive.

4. PLEURODYNIA (Bornholm Disease, Epidemic Myalgia)

Caused by coxsackie B virus (epidemic form) or many nonpolio enteroviruses (sporadic form), pleurodynia presents with an abrupt onset of unilateral pleuritic pain of variable intensity. Symptoms are episodic, and relapses occur. Associated symptoms include headache, fever, vomiting, myalgias, and abdominal and neck pain. Physical findings include fever, chest muscle tenderness, decreased thoracic excursion, and occasionally a friction rub. The chest radiograph is normal. Hematologic tests are nondiagnostic. The illness generally lasts less than 1 week.

The differential diagnosis includes bacterial pneumonia, empyema, tuberculosis, and coccidioidomycosis (all excluded radiographically), costochondritis (no fever or other symptoms), and a variety of abdominal problems, especially those causing diaphragmatic irritation.

There is no specific therapy. Potent analgesic agents and chest splinting alleviate the pain.

RASHES (Including Hand-Foot-and-Mouth Disease)

The rash may be macular, maculopapular, urticarial, scarlatiniform, petechial, or vesicular. One of the most characteristic is that of hand-foot-and-mouth disease (caused by coxsackieviruses, especially types A5, A10, and A16), in which vesicles or red papules are found on the tongue, oral mucosa, hands, and feet. Associated fever and malaise are mild. The rash may appear when fever abates, simulating roseola.

CARDIAC INVOLVEMENT

Myocarditis and pericarditis may be caused by a number of nonpolio enteroviruses, particularly type B coxsackieviruses. Most commonly, upper respiratory symptoms are followed by substernal pain, dyspnea, and exercise intolerance. A friction rub or gallop may be detected. Ultrasound will define ventricular dysfunction, and electrocardiography may show pericarditis or ventricular irritability. Creatine kinase may be elevated. The disease may be mild or fatal, but most children recover completely. In infants, other organs may be involved at the same time; in older patients, cardiac disease is usually isolated (see Chapter 18 for therapy). Enteroviral RNA is present in cardiac tissue in some cases of dilated cardiomyopathy or myocarditis; the significance of this finding is not known.

SEVERE NEONATAL INFECTION

Sporadic and nosocomial nursery cases of severe systemic enteroviral disease occur. Clinical manifestations include combinations of fever, rash, pneumonitis, encephalitis, hepatitis, gastroenteritis, myocarditis, pancreatitis, and myositis. The infants may appear septic, with cyanosis, dyspnea, and seizures. The differential diagnosis includes bacterial and herpes simplex infections, necrotizing enterocolitis, other causes of heart or liver failure, and metabolic diseases. Diagnosis is suggested by the finding of cerebrospinal fluid mononuclear pleocytosis and confirmed by the isolation of virus from urine, stool, cerebrospinal fluid, or pharynx. Therapy is supportive. Intravenous immune globulin is often administered, but its value is uncertain. Passively acquired maternal antibody may protect newborns from severe disease. For this reason, labor should not be induced in pregnant women near term who have suspected enteroviral disease.

Abzug M, Levin MJ, Rotbart HA: Profile of enterovirus disease in the first two weeks of life. Pediatr Infect Dis J 1993;12:820.

Dagan R: Nonpolio enteroviruses and the febrile young infant: Epidemiology, clinical, and diagnostic aspects. Pediatr Infect Dis J 1996;15:67.

Modlin JF: Perinatal echovirus and group B coxsackie infections. Clin Perinatol 1988;15:233.

CENTRAL NERVOUS SYSTEM ILLNESSES

1. POLIOMYELITIS

Essentials of Diagnosis & Typical Features

- Inadequate immunization or underlying immune deficiency.
- Headache, fever, muscle weakness.
- Aseptic meningitis.
- Asymmetric, flaccid paralysis; muscle tenderness and hyperesthesia; intact sensation; late atrophy.

General Considerations

Poliovirus infection is subclinical in 90–95% of cases; causes nonspecific febrile illness in about 5%; and causes aseptic meningitis or paralytic disease in 1–3%. In endemic areas, most older children and adults are immune because of prior inapparent infections. Occasional cases in the United States occur in patients who have traveled to foreign countries; most cases are in immunodeficient patients who receive the poliovirus vaccine or are exposed to recent vaccinees. Severe poliovirus infections rarely follow oral poliovirus vaccination as a result of reversion of the vaccine virus. The incidence varies from 1:10,000,000 to 1:1,000,000, depending on virus type and the age of the vaccinee. The risk of this complication is about 2600 times greater in immunodeficient children.

Clinical Findings

A. Symptoms and Signs: The initial symptoms are fever, myalgia, sore throat, and headache for 2–6 days. In less than 10% of infected children, several symptom-free days are followed by recurrent fever and signs of aseptic meningitis: headache, stiff neck, spinal rigidity, and nausea. Mild cases resolve completely. In only 1–2% of children does high fever, severe myalgia, and anxiety portend progression to loss of reflexes and subsequent flaccid paralysis. Sensation remains intact, though hyperesthesia of skin overlying paralyzed muscles is common and pathognomonic.

Paralysis is usually asymmetric. Proximal limb muscles are more often involved than distal, and lower limb involvement is more common. Bulbar involvement affects swallowing, speech, and cardiorespiratory function and accounts for most deaths. Bladder distention and marked constipation characteristically accompany lower limb paralysis. Paralysis is usually complete by the time the temperature normalizes. Weakness often resolves completely. Atrophy is usually apparent by 4–8 weeks. Most improvement of muscle paralysis will take place within 6 months.

B. Laboratory Findings: In patients with meningeal symptoms, the cerebrospinal fluid contains up to several hundred leukocytes (mostly lymphocytes) per microliter; the glucose level is normal, and protein concentration is mildly elevated. Poliovirus is easy to grow in cell culture and can be readily differentiated from other enteroviruses. It is rarely isolated from spinal fluid but is often present in the throat and stool for several weeks following infection. Paired serology is also diagnostic. Laboratory methods are available to differentiate wild from attenuated vaccine isolates.

Differential Diagnosis

Aseptic meningitis due to poliovirus is indistinguishable from that due to other viruses. Paralytic disease in the United States is usually due to nonpolio enteroviruses. Polio may resemble Guillain-Barré syndrome (variable sensory loss, symmetric loss of function; minimal pleocytosis, high protein concentration in spinal fluid), polyneuritis (sensory loss), pseudoparalysis due to bone or joint problems (eg, trauma, infection), botulism, or tick paralysis.

Complications & Sequelae

Complications are the result of the acute and permanent effects of paralysis. Respiratory, pharyngeal, bladder, and bowel malfunction are most critical. Deaths are usually due to complications arising from respiratory dysfunction. Limbs injured near the time of infection, such as intramuscular injections, excessive prior use, or trauma, tend to be most severely involved and have the worst prognosis for recovery (provocation paralysis). Postpolio muscular atrophy occurs in 30–40% of paralyzed limbs 20–30 years later, characterized by increasing paralysis and fasciculations in previously affected, partially recovered limbs.

Treatment & Prognosis

Therapy is supportive. Bed rest, fever and pain control (heat therapy is helpful), and careful attention to progression of weakness (particularly of respiratory muscles) are important. No intramuscular injections should be given during the acute phase. Intubation or tracheostomy for secretion control and catheter drainage of the bladder may be needed. Assisted ventilation and enteral feeding may also be needed. Paralysis is mild in about 30%, permanent in 15%, and results in death in 5–10%. Disease is worse in adults and pregnant women than in children.

Agre JC, Rodriguez AA: Neuromuscular function in polio survivors at one-year follow-up. Arch Phys Med Rehabil 1991;72:7.

Nikowane BM et al: Vaccine associated paralytic poliomyelitis. JAMA 1987;257:1335.

Strebel PM et al: Intramuscular injections within 30 days of immunization with oral poliovirus vaccine: A risk factor for vaccine-associated paralytic poliomyelitis. N Engl J Med 1995;332:500.

Wright PF et al: Strategies for the global eradication of poliomyelitis by the year 2000. N Engl J Med 1991; 325:1774.

2. ASEPTIC MENINGITIS

Nonpolio enteroviruses cause over 80% of cases of aseptic meningitis at all ages. In the summer and fall, multiple cases may be seen associated with circulation of neurotropic strains. Nosocomial outbreaks also occur.

Clinical Findings

The usual enteroviral incubation period is 4–6 days. Since enteroviral infections are often subclinical, a history of contact with a patient with meningitis is unusual. Neonates may acquire infection from maternal blood, vaginal secretions, or feces at birth; occasionally, the mother has had a febrile illness just prior to delivery.

A. Symptoms and Signs: Onset is usually acute with variable fever, marked irritability, and lethargy in infants. Incidence is much greater in children less than 1 year of age. Older children also describe frontal headache, photophobia, and myalgia. Abdominal pain, diarrhea, and vomiting may occur. The incidence of rash varies with the infecting strain. If rash occurs, it is usually seen after several days of illness and is diffuse, macular or maculopapular, occasionally petechial, but not purpuric. Oropharyngeal vesicles and rash on the palms and soles suggest an enteroviral cause. The anterior fontanelle may be full. In older children, it is easier to demonstrate meningeal signs. Seizures are unusual, and focal neurologic findings are so rare that they suggest another agent or diagnosis. Frank encephalitis is rare at all ages, though more common in neonates. Nevertheless, because of the overall frequency of enteroviral disease in children, 10–20% of all cases of encephalitis of proved viral etiology are caused by enteroviruses. Rarely, nonpolio enteroviruses can cause acute motor weakness similar to that seen with poliovirus infection.

B. Laboratory Findings: Blood leukocyte counts are nonspecific and often normal. The spinal fluid leukocyte count is 100–1000/μL. Early in the illness, polymorphonuclear cells predominate; a shift to mononuclear cells occurs within 8–36 hours. In about 95% of cases, spinal fluid parameters include a total leukocyte count less than 3000/μL, protein less than 80 mg/dL, and glucose more than 40% of serum values. Marked deviation from any of these findings should prompt consideration of another diagnosis (see below). The syndrome of inappropriate secretion of antidiuretic hormone may occur but is rarely clinically significant.

Culture of cerebrospinal fluid may yield an enterovirus within a few days; virus may be found in acellular spinal fluids. Polymerase chain reaction for enteroviruses is a useful diagnostic method in centers where it is available. This can give an answer within 48 hours. Isolation of an enterovirus from throat or stool suggests but does not prove enteroviral meningitis. Vaccine poliovirus present in feces in infants being evaluated for aseptic meningitis may confuse the diagnosis but can usually be distinguished by growth characteristics. Rarely, vaccine poliovirus causes ventriculoperitoneal shunt infections.

C. Imaging: Cerebral imaging is not often indicated; if done, it is usually normal; subdural effusions, infarcts, edema, or focal abnormalities seen in bacterial meningitis are absent except for the very rare case of focal encephalitis.

Differential Diagnosis

In the prevaccine era, mumps and polio were leading causes of aseptic meningitis. Other causative viruses are mosquito-borne viruses and herpes simplex. In adolescents, herpesvirus type 2 may cause aseptic meningitis with initial genital infection. In neonates, early herpes simplex meningoencephalitis may mimic enteroviral disease (see the section on herpesviruses, below). This is an important alternative diagnosis to exclude because of the need for urgent specific therapy.

Other causes of aseptic meningitis that may resemble enteroviral infection include partially treated bacterial meningitis (recent antibiotic treatment; spinal fluid parameters resembling those seen in bacterial disease and bacterial antigen sometimes present); parameningeal foci of bacterial infection such as brain abscess, subdural empyema, mastoiditis (predisposing factors, glucose level in cerebrospinal fluid may be lower, focal neurologic signs, and imaging); tumors or cysts (malignant cells detected by cytologic examination, a history of neurologic symptoms, higher protein concentration or lower glucose level in cerebrospinal fluid); trauma (presence, without exception, of red blood cells, which may be erroneously assumed to be due to traumatic lumbar puncture but are crenated and fail to clear); vasculitis (other systemic or neurologic signs; older children); tuberculous or fungal meningitis (see Chapters 36 and 37); cysticercosis; parainfectious encephalopathies (*Mycoplasma pneumoniae*, respiratory viruses); Lyme disease; leptospirosis; and rickettsial diseases.

Treatment & Prevention

There is no specific therapy. Infants are usually hospitalized, isolated, and treated with fluids and antipyretics. Moderately to severely ill infants are given appropriate antibiotics for bacterial pathogens until cultures are negative for 48–72 hours. This practice will change somewhat in areas where the polymerase chain reaction assay for enteroviruses becomes available. If patients—especially older children—are mildly ill, antibiotics may be withheld and the child observed. A repeat lumbar puncture in 8–12 hours may be helpful; with viral infection, the Gram stain is again negative, the cell count does not rise substantially, and there is a further shift to mononuclear cells. In these cases, children who are clinically sta-

ble may be closely observed in the hospital or at home. The illness usually lasts less than 1 week. Adequate analgesia, including codeine compounds or other strong pain relievers, may be needed. C-reactive protein and lactate levels are usually low in the cerebrospinal fluid of children with viral meningitis; both may be elevated with bacterial infection. With clinical deterioration, repeat lumbar puncture, cerebral imaging, neurologic consultation, and more aggressive diagnostic tests should be considered. Herpesvirus encephalitis is an important consideration in such cases, particularly in infants under 1 month of age. Newborns may receive empiric acyclovir therapy until an etiologic diagnosis is made.

Measures to prevent enteroviral infection include good hygiene, scrupulous hand washing, and proper isolation in the hospital.

Prognosis

In general, enteroviral meningitis has no significant short-term neurologic or developmental sequelae. Encephalitis due to other viruses may cause diffuse brain damage. Developmental delay may follow severe neonatal infections. Unlike mumps, enterovirus infections rarely cause hearing loss.

Dalton M, Newton RW: Aseptic meningitis. Dev Med Child Neurol 1991;33:446.

Modlin JF et al: Focal encephalitis with enterovirus infections. Pediatrics 1991;88:841.

Rotbart HA: Enteroviral infections of the central nervous system. Clin Infect Dis 1995;20:971.

Schlesinger Y, Sawyer MM, Storch GA: Enteroviral meningitis in infancy: Potential role for polymerase chain reaction in patient management. Pediatrics 1994;94:157.

Sumaya CV, Corman LI: Enteroviral meningitis in early infancy: Significance in community outbreaks. Pediatr Infect Dis J 1982;1:151.

INFECTIONS DUE TO HERPESVIRUSES

HERPES SIMPLEX

Essentials of Diagnosis & Typical Features

- Grouped vesicles on an erythematous base.
- Tender regional adenopathy, especially with primary infection.
- Fever and malaise with primary infection.
- Recurrent episodes in many patients.

General Considerations

There are two types of herpes simplex viruses.

Type 1 causes most cases of oral, skin, and cerebral disease. Type 2 causes most (80–85%) genital and congenital infections. Latent infection in sensory ganglia routinely follows primary infection. Recurrences may be spontaneous or induced by external events (eg, fever, menstruation, or sunlight) or immunosuppression. Transmission is by direct contact with infected secretions. Herpes simplex viruses are very susceptible to antiviral drugs.

Primary infection usually occurs early in childhood, though many adults (20–50%) have never been infected. Primary infection with HSV-1 is subclinical in 80% of cases and causes gingivostomatitis in the remainder. Type 2 HSV, which is transmitted sexually, is also usually (80%) subclinical or produces mild, nonspecific symptoms. Infection with one type usually precludes clinically apparent reinfection with other strains of the same type, but individuals can be infected with both type 1 and type 2 HSV. Recurrent episodes are due to reactivation of latent HSV.

Clinical Findings

The source of primary infection is often an asymptomatic excreter; at any one time, 1–3% of normal seropositive adults excrete HSV-1 in the saliva, and a higher percentage of recently infected children are shedding HSV. HSV-2 shedding in genital secretions occurs with a point prevalence of 8–28%, depending on the method of detection. A history of contact with an active HSV infection is rarely obtained.

A. Symptoms and Signs:

1. Gingivostomatitis–High fever, irritability, and drooling are seen in infants. Multiple oral ulcers are seen on the tongue and on the buccal and gingival mucosa, occasionally extending to the pharynx. Pharyngeal ulcers may predominate in older children and adolescents. Diffusely swollen red gums that are friable and bleed easily are typical. Cervical nodes are swollen and tender. Duration is 7–14 days. Herpangina, aphthous stomatitis, thrush, and Vincent's angina should be excluded.

2. Vulvovaginitis or urethritis–Genital herpes (especially type 2) in a prepubertal child should suggest sexual abuse. Vesicles or painful ulcers on the vulva, vagina, or penis and tender adenopathy are seen. Systemic symptoms (fever, flu-like illness, myalgia) are common with the initial episode. Painful urination may cause retention. Primary infections last 10–21 days. Lesions may resemble trauma, syphilis (ulcers are painless), or chancroid (ulcers are painful and nodes are very tender, erythematous, and fluctuant) in the adolescent, and bullous impetigo, trauma, and severe chemical irritation in younger children.

3. Cutaneous infections–Direct inoculation onto cuts (eg, herpetic whitlow on a thumb) or abrasions may produce localized or extensive vesicles or ulcers. A deeper HSV infection on the fingers may be mistaken for a bacterial felon or paronychia; surgical drainage is of no value and is contraindicated.

HSV infection of eczematous skin may result in extensive areas of vesicles and shallow ulcers (eczema herpeticum), which may be mistaken for impetigo or varicella.

4. Recurrent mucocutaneous infection–Recurrent oral shedding is usually asymptomatic. Perioral recurrences often begin with a prodrome of tingling or burning limited to the vermilion border, followed by vesiculation, scabbing, and crusting around the lips over the next few days. Intraoral lesions rarely recur. Fever, adenopathy, and other symptoms are absent. Recurrent cutaneous herpes most closely resembles impetigo; the latter is often outside the perinasal and perioral region, responds to antibiotics, and yields *Streptococcus pyogenes* or *Staphylococcus aureus* on culture. Recurrent genital disease is common after the initial infection with type 2 herpes simplex. The disease is shorter (5–7 days) and milder (mean, four lesions) and is not associated with systemic symptoms.

5. Keratoconjunctivitis–Keratoconjunctivitis may be part of a primary infection due to spread from infected saliva. Most cases are caused by reactivation of virus latent in the ciliary ganglion. Keratoconjunctivitis produces photophobia, pain, and conjunctival irritation. With recurrences, dendritic corneal ulcers may be demonstrable with fluorescein staining. Stromal invasion may occur. Steroids should never be used for unilateral keratitis without ophthalmologic consultation. Other causes of these symptoms include trauma, bacterial infections, and other viral infections (especially adenovirus if pharyngitis is present). (See Chap. 14.)

6. Encephalitis–Although unusual in infants outside the neonatal period, encephalitis may occur at any age, usually without cutaneous herpes lesions. In older children, HSV encephalitis often represents a reactivation of latent virus. HSV is probably the most common cause of sporadic severe encephalitis. It is the most important because it can be treated with specific antiviral therapy. Fever, headache, behavioral changes, and neurologic deficits or focal seizures occur. Mild mononuclear pleocytosis is typically present along with an elevated protein concentration, which continues to rise on repeat lumbar punctures. Hypodense areas with a temporal lobe predilection are seen on CT scan, especially after 3–5 days. MRI is more sensitive and is positive sooner. Periodic focal epileptiform discharges are seen on EEGs but are not diagnostic of HSV infection. Viral cultures of spinal fluid are rarely positive. The polymerase chain reaction to detect HSV DNA in spinal fluid is a sensitive and specific rapid test. Without early antiviral therapy, the prognosis is very poor. The differential diagnosis includes mumps and mosquito-borne encephalitis, rabies, parainfectious and postinfectious encephalopathy, brain abscess, acute demyelinating syndromes, and bacterial meningoencephalitis.

7. Neonatal infections–The infection is acquired by ascending spread prior to delivery (5–10% of cases) or at the time of vaginal delivery from a mother with genital infection. Occasionally, the infection is acquired in the postpartum period from oral secretions of family members or hospital personnel. A history of genital herpes in the mother is usually absent. Within a few days to weeks, skin vesicles (especially at sites of trauma, such as where scalp monitors were placed) appear in infected infants. Some infants are acutely ill, presenting with jaundice, shock, bleeding, or respiratory distress. Others appear well initially, but dissemination to brain or other organs becomes evident during the ensuing week if the infection is untreated. Some infants present with only neurologic symptoms at 2–3 weeks after delivery: apnea, lethargy, fever, poor feeding, or persistent overt seizures. The brain infection in these children is often diffuse and is best appreciated by MRI. The skin lesions may resemble impetigo, bacterial scalp abscesses, or miliaria, and some children may fail to develop skin lesions. Skin lesions may recur over weeks or months. The systemic signs are nonspecific.

B. Laboratory Findings: Routine test results are nonspecific. With multisystem disease, abnormalities in platelets, clotting factors, and liver function tests are often present. A finding of lymphocytic pleocytosis is the rule in aseptic meningitis or encephalitis. Virus may be cultured from infected epithelial sites (vesicles, ulcers, or corneal scrapings) and from infected tissue (skin, brain) obtained by biopsy. Cultures of spinal fluid are positive in about 50% of neonatal cases. Isolation from throat, eye, urine, or stool of a newborn is diagnostic. Vaginal culture of the mother may offer circumstantial evidence for the diagnosis.

Herpes simplex virus will be detected within 2 days by rapid tissue culture methods. Rapid diagnostic tests include cytology of scrapings from the bases of vesicles or ulcers, using chemical stains (Tzanck test) to look for characteristic multinucleated giant cells, immunofluorescent stains to detect viral antigen, or EIA. The polymerase chain reaction for HSV DNA is positive in the cerebrospinal fluid when there is brain involvement. Serum is often positive in the presence of multisystem disease.

Complications, Sequelae, & Prognosis

Gingivostomatitis may result in dehydration due to dysphagia; severe chronic oral disease and esophageal involvement may occur in immunosuppressed patients.

Primary vulvovaginitis may be associated with aseptic meningitis, paresthesias, autonomic dysfunction due to neuritis (urinary retention, constipation), and secondary candidal infection.

Extensive cutaneous disease (as in eczema) may be associated with dissemination, and bacterial superinfection.

Keratitis may result in corneal opacification or perforation.

Untreated encephalitis is fatal in 70% of patients and causes severe damage in most of the remainder. When acyclovir treatment is instituted early, 20% die and 40% are neurologically impaired.

Disseminated neonatal infection is often fatal in spite of therapy.

Treatment

A. Specific Measures: Herpes simplex virus is very sensitive to antiviral therapy. Topical antivirals are most effective for corneal disease and include 1% trifluridine, 5% acyclovir, and 3% vidarabine. Trifluridine appears superior; cure rates over 95% are reported. These should be used with the guidance of an ophthalmologist.

Mucocutaneous HSV infections respond to administration of oral nucleoside analogs (acyclovir, valacyclovir, or famciclovir). The main indication is severe genital HSV infection in adolescents (See Chapter 38). Antiviral therapy is beneficial for primary disease when begun early. Recurrent disease rarely requires therapy. Frequent genital recurrences may be suppressed by oral administration of nucleoside analogs, but this approach should be used sparingly. Other forms of severe cutaneous disease, such as eczema herpeticum and HSV infections in immunocompromised children, also respond to these antivirals. Intravenous acyclovir may be required when disease is extensive in immunocompromised children (250 mg/m^2 every 8 hours). Oral acyclovir, which is available in suspension, is also used for severe primary gingivostomatitis in young children (5–10 mg/kg per dose four times a day for 5–7 days).

Severe HSV infections are treated with acyclovir, 500 mg/m^2 every 8 hours intravenously for 14 days for encephalitis and 14–21 days for neonates. Neonates now receive 20 mg/kg every 8 hours.

Antiviral therapy does not alter the incidence or severity of subsequent recurrences of genital infection. Development of resistance to antivirals is rare after standard courses but is increasingly reported in immunocompromised patients after prolonged therapy.

B. General Measures:

1. Gingivostomatitis–Gingivostomatitis is treated with pain relief and temperature control. Maintaining hydration is important because of the long duration of illness (7–14 days). Nonacidic, cool fluids are best. Topical anesthetic agents (such as viscous lidocaine or an equal mixture of Kaopectate, diphenhydramine, and viscous lidocaine) may be used as a mouthwash for older children who will not swallow it; ingested lidocaine may be toxic to infants or may lead to aspiration. Antiviral therapy is indicated in normal hosts with severe disease. Antibiotics are not helpful.

2. Genital infections–Genital infections require pain relief, assistance with voiding (warm baths, topical anesthetics, rarely catheterization), and psychologic support. Lesions should be kept clean; drying decreases the potential for spread and may shorten the duration of infection. Sexual contact should be avoided during the interval from prodrome to crusting stages.

3. Cutaneous lesions–Skin lesions should be kept clean, dry, and covered if possible to prevent spread. Systemic analgesics may be helpful. Secondary bacterial infection is uncommon in patients with lesions on the mucosa or involving small areas. Secondary infection should be considered and treated if necessary (usually with an antistaphylococcal agent) in patients with more extensive lesions. Candidal superinfection occurs in 10% of women with primary genital infections.

4. Recurrent cutaneous disease–Recurrent disease is usually milder than primary infection. Sun block lip balm helps prevent labial recurrences after intense sun exposure. There is no evidence that the many popular topical or vitamin therapies are efficacious.

5. Keratoconjunctivitis–An ophthalmologist should be consulted regarding the use of cycloplegics, anti-inflammatory agents, local debridement, and other therapies.

6. Encephalitis–See Chapter 22.

7. Neonatal infection–The affected infant should be isolated and treated with acyclovir for 14–21 days. Cesarean section is indicated if there are obvious maternal cervical or vaginal lesions, especially if these represent primary infection. In women with a history of genital herpes infection, vaginal delivery with peripartum cultures of maternal cervix is the standard. Clinical follow-up is recommended when maternal cultures are positive. Repeated cervical cultures during pregnancy are not useful.

Corey L, Spear PG: Infections with herpes simplex viruses. (Two parts.) N Engl J Med 1986;314:686, 749.

Gasecki AP, Steg RE: Correlation of early MRI with CT scan, EEG, and CSF: Analyses in a case of biopsy-proven herpes simplex encephalitis. Eur Neurol 1991;31:372.

Grose C, Wiedeman J: Generic acyclovir vs famciclovir and valacyclovir. Pediatr Infect Dis J 1997;16:838.

Jeffery KJM et al: Diagnosis of viral infections of the central nervous system: Clinical interpretations of PCR results.Lancet 1997;349:313.

Kimura H et al: Relapse of herpes simplex encephalitis in children. Pediatrics 1992;89:891.

Koskiniemi M et al: Neonatal herpes simplex virus infection: A report of 43 patients. Pediatr Infect Dis 1989;8:30.

Kuzushima K et al: Clinical manifestations of primary herpes simplex type 1 infection in a closed community. Pediatrics 1991;87:152.

Monney MA, Janniger CK, Schwartz RA: Kaposi's varicelliform eruption. Cutis 1994;53:243.

Prober C: Herpes simplex virus infections in neonates. Rep Pediatr Infect Dis 1997;7:9.

VARICELLA & HERPES ZOSTER

Essentials of Diagnosis & Typical Features

Varicella (chickenpox):
- Exposure to varicella or herpes zoster 10–20 days previously; no prior history of varicella.
- Widely scattered red macules and papules concentrated on the face and trunk, rapidly progressing to clear vesicles, pustules, and then crusting, over 5–6 days. Variable fever and nonspecific systemic symptoms.

Herpes zoster (shingles):
- History of varicella.
- Local paresthesias and pain prior to eruption (more common in older children).
- Dermatomal distribution of grouped vesicles on an erythematous base.

General Considerations

Primary infection with varicella-zoster virus results in varicella, which almost always confers life-long immunity; the virus remains latent in sensory ganglia and reappears as herpes zoster in 10–15% of individuals. The incidence of herpes zoster is increased in immunosuppressed patients. Spread from a contact with varicella during primary infection is by respiratory secretions or fomites from vesicles or pustules, with a greater than 95% infection rate in susceptibles. Herpes zoster is about one-third as infectious. Over 95% of young adults with a history of varicella are immune, as are 90% of native-born Americans who are unaware of having had varicella. Many individuals from tropical or subtropical areas never have childhood exposure and thus are susceptible. Humans are the only reservoir.

Clinical Findings

Exposure to varicella or herpes zoster has usually occurred 14–16 days previously (range, 10–21 days). Contact may not have been recognized. Although varicella is the most distinctive childhood exanthem, inexperienced observers may mistake other diseases for varicella. A 1- to 3-day prodrome of fever, respiratory symptoms, and headache may occur, especially in older children. The preeruptive pain of herpes zoster may last several days and be mistaken for other illnesses.

A. Symptoms and Signs:

1. Varicella–The usual case consists of mild systemic symptoms followed by crops of red macules that rapidly become tiny vesicles with surrounding erythema ("dew drop on a rose petal"), form pustules, become crusted and then scab over, and leave no scar. The rash appears predominantly on the trunk and face. Lesions occur in the scalp, nose, mouth (where they are nonspecific ulcers), conjunctiva, and vagina. The magnitude of systemic symptoms usually parallels skin involvement. Up to five crops of lesions may be seen. New crops usually stop forming after 5–7 days. Pruritus is often intense. If varicella occurs in the first few months of life, it is often mild as a result of persisting maternal antibody. Once crusting begins, the patient is no longer contagious.

2. Herpes zoster–The eruption of shingles involves a single dermatome, usually truncal or cranial. The rash does not cross the midline. Ophthalmic zoster may be associated with corneal involvement. The closely grouped vesicles, which resemble a localized version of varicella or herpes simplex, often coalesce. The duration is 7–10 days before crusting. Postherpetic neuralgia is rare in children. A few vesicles are occasionally seen outside the involved dermatome. This disease is a common problem in HIV-infected or other immunocompromised children. Herpes zoster is also common in children who had varicella in early infancy or whose mothers had varicella during pregnancy.

B. Laboratory Findings: Leukocyte counts are normal or low. Leukocytosis suggests secondary bacterial infection. Multinucleated giant cells in a stained cytologic scraping from a vesicle base (Tzanck test) will indicate the presence of either a varicella-zoster virus or herpes simplex infection. Further distinction is usually made on clinical grounds. The virus may also be identified by fluorescent antibody staining of a lesion smear. Rapid culture methods take 48 hours. Diagnosis can be made with paired serology. Serum aminotransferase levels may be modestly elevated during normal varicella.

C. Imaging: Varicella pneumonia classically produces numerous bilateral nodular densities and hyperinflation. This is very rare in normal children. Abnormal chest radiographs are seen more frequently in adults.

Differential Diagnosis

Varicella is usually distinctive. Similar rashes include those of coxsackievirus infection (fewer lesions, lack of crusting), impetigo (fewer lesions, no classic vesicles, positive Gram stain, response to antimicrobial agents, perioral or peripheral lesions), papular urticaria (insect bite history, nonvesicular rash), scabies (burrows, no typical vesicles), parapsoriasis (rare in children under 10 years of age; chronic or recurrent; often a history of prior varicella), rickettsialpox (eschar where the mite bites, smaller lesions, no crusting), dermatitis herpetiformis (chronic, urticaria, residual pigmentation), and folliculitis. Herpes zoster is sometimes confused with a linear eruption of herpes simplex or a contact dermatitis (eg, *Rhus* dermatitis).

Complications & Sequelae

Secondary bacterial infection with staphylococci or group A streptococci is most common, presenting as impetigo, cellulitis or fasciitis, abscesses, scarlet fever, or sepsis.

Protracted vomiting or a change in sensorium suggests Reye's syndrome or encephalitis. Since Reye's syndrome usually occurs in patients who are also using salicylates, this drug should be avoided in patients with varicella. Encephalitis occurs in less than 0.1% of cases, usually in the first week of illness. It is usually limited to cerebellitis with ataxia, which resolves completely. Diffuse encephalitis can be severe.

Varicella pneumonia usually afflicts immunocompromised, pregnant, or older patients and may be fatal. Cough, dyspnea, tachypnea, rales, and cyanosis occur several days after onset of rash. Varicella may be life-threatening in immunosuppressed patients (especially those with leukemia or lymphoma or those receiving high doses of steroids). Their disease is complicated by severe pneumonitis, hepatitis, and encephalitis. Varicella exposure in such patients must be evaluated immediately (see Chapter 9).

Hemorrhagic varicella lesions may be seen without other complications. This is most often caused by autoimmune thrombocytopenia, but hemorrhagic lesions can occasionally represent idiopathic disseminated intravascular coagulation (purpura fulminans).

Neonates born to mothers who develop varicella from 5 days before to 2 days after delivery are at high risk for severe or fatal (5%) disease and must be given varicella-zoster immune globulin and followed closely (see Chapter 9).

Varicella occurring during the first 20 weeks of pregnancy may cause (2% incidence) congenital infection associated with cicatricial skin lesions, associated limb anomalies, and cortical atrophy.

Unusual complications of varicella include optic neuritis, myocarditis, transverse myelitis, orchitis, and arthritis.

Complications of herpes zoster include secondary bacterial infection, motor or cranial nerve paralysis, encephalitis, keratitis, and dissemination in immunosuppressed patients. These complications are rare in normal children, and they do not develop prolonged pain. Postherpetic neuralgia does occur in immunocompromised children.

Treatment

A. General Measures: Supportive measures include maintenance of hydration, administration of acetaminophen for discomfort, cool soaks or antipruritics for itching (diphenhydramine, 1.25 mg/kg every 6 hours; or hydroxyzine, 0.5 mg/kg every 6 hours), and observance of general hygiene measures (keep nails trimmed and skin clean). Care must be taken to avoid overdosage with antihistaminic agents. Topical or systemic antistaphylococcal antibiotics may be needed.

B. Specific Measures: Although acyclovir is more active against herpes simplex, it is the preferred drug for varicella and herpes zoster infections. Recommended parenteral acyclovir dosage for severe disease is 30 mg/kg/d intravenously in three divided doses, each infused over 1 hour. Parenteral therapy should be started early in immunosuppressed patients or high-risk infected neonates. Varicella-zoster immune globulin is of no value for established disease. The effect of oral acyclovir (80 mg/kg/d in four doses) on varicella in normal children was modestly beneficial and nontoxic, but only when administered within 24 hour after the onset of varicella. This should be used selectively in normal children (intercurrent illness; possibly second attacks in the household or adolescent age—both of which are associated with more severe disease) and in children with underlying chronic illnesses. Valacyclovir and famciclovir are new antiviral agents that are superior because of better absorption; acyclovir is available as a pediatric suspension. Herpes zoster in an immunocompromised child is treated with intravenous acyclovir if it is severe or with oral valacyclovir or famciclovir when the nature of the illness and the immune status support this decision.

Prevention

Varicella-zoster immune globulin (VZIG) is available for postexposure prevention of varicella in high-risk susceptible persons (see Chapter 9). The live attenuated vaccine is recommended for all susceptible children and adults.

Prognosis

Except for secondary bacterial infections, serious complications are rare and recovery complete in normal hosts.

Abzug MJ, Cotton MF: Severe chickenpox after intranasal use of corticosteroids. J Pediatr 1993;123:577.

Brady MB, Mayer D: Varicella-zoster virus infection. The complex prevention-treatment picture. Postgrad Med 1997;102:187.

Fleischer G et al: Life-threatening complications of varicella. Am J Dis Child 1981;135:896.

Peterson CL et al: Children hospitalized for varicella: A prevaccine review. J Pediatr 1996;129:529.

Srugo I et al: Clinical manifestations of varicella-zoster virus infections in human immunodeficiency virus-infected children. Am J Dis Child 1993;147:742.

Vugia DJ et al: Invasive group A streptococcal infections in children with varicella in Southern California. Pediatr Infect Dis J 1996;15:146.

Wurzel CL et al: Prognosis of herpes zoster in healthy children. Am J Dis Child 1986;140:477.

ROSEOLA INFANTUM (Exanthema Subitum)

Roseola infantum is a benign illness caused by human herpesvirus 6 (HHV-6). HHV-6 is a major cause of acute febrile illness in young children. Its significance is its ability to mimic more serious causes of high fever and its role in inciting febrile seizures. This disease may also result from infection with human herpesvirus 7 (HHV-7).

Clinical Findings

The most prominent historical feature is the abrupt onset of fever, often reaching 40.6 °C, which lasts up to 8 days (mean, 4 days) in an otherwise mildly ill child. The fever then ceases abruptly, and a characteristic rash may appear. Roseola occurs predominantly in children 6 months to 3 years old, with 90% of cases occurring before the second year. It is the most common recognized cause of exanthematous fever in this age group and is responsible for 20% of emergency room visits by children 6–12 months old.

A. Symptoms and Signs: Mild lethargy and irritability may be present, but generally there is a dissociation between systemic symptoms and the febrile course. The pharynx, tonsils, and tympanic membranes may be injected. Conjunctivitis and pharyngeal exudate are notably absent. Diarrhea and vomiting occur in one-third. Adenopathy of the head and neck often occurs. The anterior fontanelle is bulging in one-quarter of HHV-6 infected infants. If rash appears (10–20% incidence), it begins on the trunk and spreads to the face, neck, and extremities. Rose-pink macules or maculopapules, 2–3 mm in diameter, are nonpruritic, tend to coalesce, and disappear in 1–2 days without pigmentation or desquamation. Rash may occur without fever.

B. Laboratory Findings: Leukopenia and lymphocytopenia are present early. Laboratory evidence of hepatitis occurs in some patients, especially adults.

Differential Diagnosis

The initial high fever may require exclusion of serious bacterial infection. However, the relative wellbeing of most children and the typical course and rash soon clarify the diagnosis. The erythrocyte sedimentation rate is normal. If the child has a febrile seizure, it is important to exclude bacterial meningitis. The cerebrospinal fluid is normal in children with roseola. In children who receive antibiotics or other medication at the beginning of the fever, the rash may be incorrectly attributed to drug allergy.

Complications & Sequelae

Febrile seizures occur in 10% of cases. There is some evidence that HHV-6 can directly infect the central nervous system, causing meningoencephalitis or aseptic meningitis. Multiorgan disease (pneumonia, hepatitis, encephalitis) may occur in immunocompromised patients.

Treatment & Prognosis

Fever is readily managed with acetaminophen and sponge baths. Fever control should be a major consideration in children with a history of febrile seizures. Roseola infantum is otherwise entirely benign.

Barone SR, Kaplon MH, Krilov LR: Human herpesvirus 6 infection in children with first febrile seizures. J Pediatr 1995;127:95.

Hall CB et al: Human herpesvirus 6 infection in children: A prospective study of complications and reactivation. N Engl J Med 1994;331:432.

Levy JA: Three new human herpesviruses (HHV 6, 7, 8). Lancet 1997;349:558.

Okada K et al: Exanthema subitum and human herpesvirus 6 infection: Clinical observations in fifty-seven cases. Pediatr Infect Dis J 1993;12:204.

Suga S et al: Clinical and virological analyses of 21 infants with exanthem subitum (roseola infantum) and central nervous system complications. Ann Neurol 1993; 33:597.

CYTOMEGALOVIRUS (CMV) INFECTIONS

Cytomegalovirus is a ubiquitous herpesvirus transmitted by many routes. It can be acquired in utero following maternal viremia or postpartum from birth canal secretions or maternal milk. Young children are infected by the saliva of playmates; older individuals are infected by sexual partners (saliva, vaginal secretions, and semen). Transfused blood products and transplanted organs can be a source of CMV infection. Clinical illness is largely determined by the immune competence of the patient. Normal individuals usually develop a mild self-limited illness, whereas immunocompromised children can develop severe, progressive, often multiorgan disease. In utero infection can be teratogenic.

1. IN UTERO CYTOMEGALOVIRUS INFECTION

Approximately 0.5–1.5% of children are born with CMV infections acquired during maternal viremia. Over 90% of them are asymptomatic and are usually born to mothers who had experienced reactivation of latent CMV infection during the pregnancy. Symptomatic infants are born to mothers with primary CMV infection. Even when exposed to a primary maternal infection, less than 50% of fetuses are infected, and only 10% of those infected are symptomatic at birth. Primary infection in the first half of pregnancy poses the greatest risk for severe fetal damage. Congenital CMV is more common in HIV-infected infants born to HIV-infected mothers.

Clinical Findings

A. Symptoms and Signs: Severely affected infants are born ill; they are often small for gestational age, floppy, and lethargic. They feed poorly and have poor temperature control. Hepatosplenomegaly, jaundice, petechiae, seizures, and microcephaly are common. Characteristic signs are a distinctive chorioretinitis and periventricular calcification. A purpuric ("blueberry muffin") rash similar to that seen with congenital rubella may be present. The mortality rate is 10–20%. Survivors usually have significant sequelae, especially retardation, neurologic deficits, retinopathy, and hearing loss. Isolated hepatosplenomegaly or thrombocytopenia may occur. Even mildly affected children may subsequently manifest mental retardation and psychomotor delay. However, most infected infants (90%) are born to mothers with preexisting immunity who had a reactivation of latent CMV during pregnancy. These children have no clinical manifestations at birth. Of these, 10–15% develop sensorineural hearing loss, which is often bilateral, and may appear several years after birth.

B. Laboratory Findings: In severely ill infants, anemia, thrombocytopenia, hyperbilirubinemia, and elevated aminotransferase levels are common. Lymphocytosis is occasionally seen. Pleocytosis and elevated protein are seen in cerebrospinal fluid. The diagnosis is readily confirmed by isolation of CMV from urine or saliva within 48 hours, using rapid culture methods combined with immunoassay. The presence in the infant of IgM-specific CMV antibodies suggests the diagnosis. Some commercial EIA kits are 90% sensitive and specific for these antibodies.

C. Imaging: Skull radiographs show microcephaly and periventricular calcification. CT scan shows calcification and ventricular dilation. This correlates strongly with neurologic sequelae and retardation. Long bone films show the "celery stalk" pattern characteristic of congenital viral infections. Interstitial pneumonia may be present.

Differential Diagnosis

Cytomegalovirus infection should be considered in any newborn who is seriously ill shortly after birth, especially once bacterial sepsis, metabolic disease, intracranial bleeding, and cardiac disease have been excluded. Other congenital infections to be considered in the differential diagnosis include toxoplasmosis (serology, more diffuse calcification of the central nervous system, specific type of retinitis, macrocephaly), rubella (serology, specific type of retinitis, cardiac lesions, eye abnormalities), enteroviral infections (time of year, maternal illness, severe hepatitis), herpes simplex (skin lesions, cultures, severe hepatitis, macular rash), and syphilis (serology for both infant and mother, skin lesions, bone involvement).

Treatment & Prevention

Support is rarely required for anemia and thrombocytopenia. The antiviral drug ganciclovir is under study in severely ill children. Most children with symptoms at birth have significant neurologic, intellectual, visual, or auditory impairment. Children who are asymptomatic at birth have a 5–15% incidence of hearing loss but few other sequelae. It is possible that the late sequelae of CMV infection—including abnormalities occurring in initially asymptomatic infants—may be ameliorated by ganciclovir use. Delayed development and hearing loss should be discovered and treated as soon as possible.

2. PERINATAL CYTOMEGALOVIRUS INFECTION

Cytomegalovirus infection can be acquired from birth canal secretions or shortly after birth from maternal milk. In some socioeconomic groups, 10–20% of infants are infected at birth and excrete CMV for many months. Infection can also be acquired in the postnatal period from unscreened transfused blood products.

Clinical Findings

A. Symptoms and Signs: Ninety percent of normal infants infected by their mothers at birth develop subclinical illness (ie, virus excretion only) or a minor illness within 1–3 months. The remainder develop an illness lasting several weeks which is characterized by hepatosplenomegaly, lymphadenopathy, and interstitial pneumonitis in various combinations. The severity of the pneumonitis may be increased by the simultaneous presence of *Chlamydia trachomatis.* Infants who receive blood products are often premature and immunologically impaired. If they are born to CMV-negative mothers and subsequently receive CMV-containing blood, they frequently develop severe infection and pneumonia after a 2- to 6-week incubation period.

B. Laboratory Findings: Lymphocytosis, atypical lymphocytes, anemia, and thrombocytopenia may be present, especially in premature infants. Liver function is abnormal. CMV can be isolated from urine and saliva. Secretions obtained at bronchoscopy contain CMV and epithelial cells bearing CMV antigens. Serum levels of CMV antibody rise significantly.

C. Imaging: Chest films show a diffuse interstitial pneumonitis in severely affected infants.

Differential Diagnosis

Cytomegalovirus infection should be considered as a cause of any prolonged illness in early infancy, especially if hepatosplenomegaly, lymphadenopathy, or atypical lymphocytosis is present. This must be distinguished from granulomatous or malignant diseases and from congenital infections (syphilis, toxoplasmosis, hepatitis B) not previously appreciated. Other viruses (Epstein-Barr virus, HIV, adenovirus) can cause this syndrome. CMV is a recognized cause

of viral pneumonia in this age group. However, since asymptomatic CMV excretion is common in early infancy, care must be taken to establish the diagnosis and to rule out concomitant pathogens such as *Chlamydia* and RSV.

Treatment & Prevention

The self-limited disease of normal infants requires no therapy. Severe pneumonitis in premature infants requires oxygen administration and often intubation. Very ill infants should receive ganciclovir (6 mg/kg every 12 hours). CMV infection acquired by transfusion can be prevented by excluding CMV-seropositive blood donors. Milk donors should also be screened for prior CMV infection. It is likely that high-risk infants receiving large doses of intravenous immune globulin for other reasons will be protected against severe CMV disease.

3. CYTOMEGALOVIRUS INFECTION ACQUIRED IN CHILDHOOD & ADOLESCENCE

Young children are readily infected by playmates, especially since CMV continues to be excreted in saliva and urine for many months after infection. The annual incidence of CMV excretion by children in day care centers exceeds 75%. In fact, young children in a family are often the source of primary CMV infection of their mothers during subsequent pregnancies. An additional peak of CMV infection occurs in sexually active individuals.

Clinical Findings

A. Symptoms and Signs: Most young children who acquire CMV are asymptomatic or have a minor febrile illness, occasionally with adenopathy. They provide an important reservoir of virus shedders that facilitates spread of CMV. Occasionally, a child may have prolonged fever with hepatosplenomegaly and adenopathy. Older children and adults, many of whom are infected during sexual activity, are more likely to be symptomatic in this fashion and can present with a syndrome that mimics the infectious mononucleosis syndrome which follows infection by Epstein-Barr virus (1–2 weeks of fever, malaise, anorexia, splenomegaly, mild hepatitis, and some adenopathy). This syndrome can also occur 2–4 weeks after transfusion of CMV-infected blood.

B. Laboratory Findings: In the CMV mononucleosis syndrome, lymphocytosis and atypical lymphocytes are common, as is a mild rise in aminotransferase levels. CMV is present in saliva and urine, and diagnosis is made as above.

Differential Diagnosis

In older children, CMV infection should be included as a possible cause of fever of unknown origin, especially when lymphocytosis and atypical lymphocytes are present. CMV infection is distinguished from Epstein-Barr virus infection by the absence of pharyngitis, the relatively minor adenopathy, and the absence of serologic evidence of acute Epstein-Barr virus infection. Mononucleosis syndromes are also caused by *Toxoplasma gondii*, rubella virus, adenovirus, hepatitis A virus, and HIV.

Prevention

Screening of transfused blood or using filtered blood (thus removing CMV-containing lymphocytes) prevents cases related to this source.

4. CYTOMEGALOVIRUS INFECTION IN IMMUNOCOMPROMISED CHILDREN

Cytomegalovirus infection in this setting can be acquired from infused blood products or transplanted tissue as well as from playmates. In addition, reactivation of latent CMV can cause symptomatic disease. This is clearly seen in children with AIDS or congenital immunodeficiencies. However, in most immunocompromised patients, primary infection is more likely to cause severe symptoms than is reactivation disease. The severity of the resulting disease is generally proportionate to the degree of immunosuppression.

Clinical Findings

A. Symptoms and Signs: A mild febrile illness with myalgia, malaise, and arthralgia may occur, especially with reactivation disease. Severe disease often includes subacute onset of dyspnea and cyanosis as manifestations of interstitial pneumonitis. Auscultation reveals only coarse breath sounds and scattered rales. A rapid respiratory rate may precede clinical or x-ray evidence of pneumonia. Hepatitis without jaundice or hepatomegaly is common. Diarrhea, which can be severe, occurs with CMV colitis, and CMV can cause esophagitis with symptoms of odynophagia or dysphagia. These enteropathies are most common in AIDS, as is the presence of a retinitis that often progresses to blindness. Encephalitis and polyradiculitis also occur in AIDS.

B. Laboratory Findings: Neutropenia and thrombocytopenia are common. Atypical lymphocytosis is not frequent. Serum aminotransferase levels are often elevated. The stools may contain occult blood if enteropathy is present. CMV is readily isolated from saliva, urine, buffy coat, and bronchial secretions. Results are available in 48 hours. Interpretation of positive cultures is made difficult by asymptomatic shedding of CMV in saliva and urine in many immunocompromised patients. CMV disease correlates more closely with the presence of CMV in the blood or lung lavage fluid. Detection of

CMV DNA in plasma or CMV antigen in blood mononuclear cells can be used as a guide to early antiviral therapy.

C. Imaging: Bilateral interstitial pneumonitis is present on chest radiographs.

Differential Diagnosis

The initial febrile illness must be distinguished from treatable bacterial or fungal infection. Similarly, the pulmonary disease must be distinguished from intrapulmonary hemorrhage, drug-induced or radiation pneumonitis, pulmonary edema, and bacterial, fungal, parasitic, and other viruses infection in this population. CMV infection is bilateral and interstitial on x-ray films of the chest, cough is nonproductive, chest pain is absent, and the patient is not usually toxic. *Pneumocystis carinii* infection may present in a similar manner. Polymicrobial disease may be present in these patients. It is suspected that bacterial and fungal infections are enhanced by the neutropenia that can accompany CMV infection. Infection of the gastrointestinal tract is diagnosed by endoscopy. This will exclude candidal and herpes simplex infections and allows tissue confirmation of CMV-induced mucosal ulcerations.

Treatment & Prognosis

Blood donors should be screened to exclude those with prior CMV infection, or blood should be filtered. Ideally, seronegative transplant recipients should receive organs from seronegative donors. Severe symptoms, most commonly pneumonitis, often respond to early therapy with intravenous ganciclovir (5 mg/kg every 12 hours for 14–21 days). Neutropenia is a frequent side effect of this therapy. Foscarnet is an alternative antiviral therapy. Prophylactic use of oral acyclovir or intravenous ganciclovir may prevent CMV infections in organ transplant recipients. "Preemptive" therapy can be utilized in some high-risk transplant recipients who are monitored for CMV antigen or DNA in their plasma or mononuclear cells, and who receive antivirals when these tests are positive regardless of clinical signs or symptoms. CMV-seropositive children with AIDS and low CD4 counts ($< 50/\mu L$) should have funduscopic examinations every 3 months.

Boppana SB et al: Symptomatic congenital cytomegalovirus infection: Neonatal morbidity and mortality. Pediatr Infect Dis J 1992;11:93.

Fowler KB et al: Progressive and fluctuating sensorineural hearing loss in children with asymptomatic congenital cytomegalovirus infection. J Pediatr 1997;130:624.

Ivarsson SA, Lernmark B, Svanberg L: Ten-year clinical, developmental, and intellectual followup of children with congenital cytomegalovirus infection without neurologic symptoms at one year of age. Pediatrics 1997;99:800.

Jordan CJ et al: Spontaneous cytomegalovirus mononucleosis. Ann Intern Med 1973;79:153.

Lynch L et al: Prenatal diagnosis of fetal cytomegalovirus infection. Am J Obstet Gynecol 1991;165:714.

Stagno S, Whitley RJ: Herpesvirus infections of pregnancy: Part 1. Cytomegalovirus and Epstein-Barr virus infections. N Engl J Med 1985;313:1270.

INFECTIOUS MONONUCLEOSIS

Mononucleosis is the most characteristic syndrome produced by infection with Epstein-Barr virus (EBV). Its elements are fever, pharyngitis, lymphadenopathy, splenomegaly, atypical lymphocytosis, and the presence of heterophil antibodies. Young children infected with EBV have either no symptoms or a mild nonspecific febrile illness. As the age of the host increases, EBV infection is more likely to produce the mononucleosis syndrome, occurring in 20–25% of infected adolescents. Epstein-Barr virus is readily acquired from asymptomatic carriers (15–20% of whom excrete the virus on any given day) and from recently ill patients, who excrete virus for many months. Young children are infected from the saliva of playmates and family members. Adolescents may be infected through sexual activity. Epstein-Barr virus can also be transmitted by blood transfusion and organ transplantation.

Clinical Findings

A. Symptoms and Signs: After an incubation period of 1–2 months, a 2- to 3-day prodrome of malaise and anorexia yields, abruptly or insidiously, to a febrile illness with temperatures exceeding 39 °C. The major complaint is pharyngitis, which is often (50%) exudative. Lymph nodes are enlarged, firm, and mildly tender. Any area may be affected, but posterior and anterior cervical nodes are almost always enlarged. Splenomegaly is present in 50–75% of patients. Hepatomegaly is common (30%), and the liver is frequently tender. Five percent of patients have a rash, which can be macular, scarlatiniform, or urticarial. Rash is almost universal in patients taking penicillin or ampicillin. Soft palate petechiae and eyelid edema are also observed.

B. Laboratory Findings:

1. Peripheral blood–Leukopenia may occur early, but an atypical lymphocytosis (comprising over 10% of the total leukocytes at some time in the illness) is most notable. Hematologic changes may not be seen until the third week of illness and may be entirely absent in some EBV syndromes, eg, neurologic ones.

2. Heterophil antibodies–These nonspecific antibodies appear in over 90% of older patients with mononucleosis but in fewer than 50% of children under age 5. They may not be detectable until the second week of illness and may persist for up to 12 months after recovery. Rapid screening tests (slide agglutination) are usually positive if the titer is sig-nificant; a positive result strongly suggests but does not prove EBV infection.

3. Anti-EBV antibodies–It may be necessary to measure specific antibody titers when heterophil antibodies fail to appear, as in young children. Epstein-Barr virus infection is established by detecting IgM antibody to the viral capsid antigen (VCA) or by detecting a fall over several weeks of IgG antibody to the antigen (IgG antibody peaks by the time symptoms appear). Seroconversion of antibody to Epstein-Barr nuclear antigen (EBNA) confirms the above indicators.

4. Aminotransferase, γ-glutamyl transferase, and bilirubin levels–Aminotransferase and γ-glutamyl transferase levels are mildly elevated in 80% of patients; bilirubin is mildly elevated in 25%.

Differential Diagnosis

Severe pharyngitis may suggest group A streptococcal infection. Enlargement of only the anterior cervical lymph nodes, a neutrophilic leukocytosis, and the absence of splenomegaly suggest bacterial infection. Although a child with a positive throat culture usually requires therapy, up to 10% of children with mononucleosis are asymptomatic streptococcal carriers. In this group, penicillin therapy is unnecessary and often causes a rash. Severe primary herpes simplex pharyngitis, occurring in adolescence, may also mimic infectious mononucleosis. In this type of pharyngitis, some anterior mouth ulcerations should suggest the correct diagnosis. EBV infection should be considered in the differential diagnosis of any perplexing prolonged febrile illness. Some similar illnesses that produce atypical lymphocytosis include rubella (pharyngitis not prominent, shorter illness, less adenopathy and splenomegaly), adenovirus (upper respiratory symptoms and cough, conjunctivitis, less adenopathy, fewer atypical lymphocytes), hepatitis A or B (more severe liver function abnormalities, no pharyngitis or splenomegaly), and toxoplasmosis (negative heterophil test and less pharyngitis). Serum sickness-like drug reactions and leukemia (smear morphology is important) may be confused with infectious mononucleosis. Cytomegalovirus mononucleosis is a close mimic except for minimal pharyngitis and less adenopathy; it is much less common. Serologic tests for EBV and cytomegalovirus should clarify the correct diagnosis. The acute initial manifestation of HIV infection is a mononucleosis-like syndrome in many patients.

Complications

Splenic rupture is a very rare complication, which usually follows significant trauma. Hematologic complications, including hemolytic anemia, thrombocytopenia, and neutropenia, are more common. Neurologic involvement can include aseptic meningitis, encephalitis, isolated neuropathy such as Bell's palsy, and Guillain-Barré syndrome. Any of these may appear prior to or in the absence of the more typical signs and symptoms of infectious mononucleosis. Rare complications include myocarditis, pericarditis, and atypical pneumonia. Very rarely, EBV infection becomes a progressive lymphoproliferative disorder characterized by persistent fever, multiple organ involvement, neutropenia or pancytopenia, and agammaglobulinemia. Hemocytophagia is often present in the bone marrow. An X-linked genetic defect in immune response has been inferred for some patients (Duncan's syndrome, X-linked lymphoproliferative disorder). Children with other congenital immunodeficiencies or chemotherapy-induced immunosuppression can also develop progressive EBV infection or EBV-induced lymphomas.

Treatment & Prognosis

Bed rest may be necessary in severe cases. Acetaminophen controls high fever. Potential airway obstruction due to swollen pharyngeal lymphoid tissue responds rapidly to systemic corticosteroids. Corticosteroids may also be given for hematologic and neurologic complications, though no controlled trials have proved their efficacy in these conditions. Fever and pharyngitis disappear by 10–14 days. Adenopathy and splenomegaly can persist several weeks longer. Some patients complain of fatigue, malaise, or lack of well-being for several months. Although steroids may shorten the duration of fatigue and malaise, their long-term effects on this potentially oncogenic viral infection are unknown, and indiscriminate use is discouraged. Patients with splenic enlargement should avoid contact sports for 6–8 weeks.

Chetham MM, Roberts KB: Infectious mononucleosis in adolescents. Pediatr Ann 1991;20:206.

Connelly KP, DeWitt LD: Neurologic complications of infectious mononucleosis. Pediatr Neurol 1994;10:181.

Farley DR et al: Spontaneous rupture of the spleen due to infectious mononucleosis. Mayo Clin Proc 1992;67:846.

Khoury M, Kovacs A: Epstein-Barr virus: Specific serology. Rep Pediatr Inf Dis 1994;10:37.

Schaller RJ, Counselman FL: Infectious mononucleosis in young children. Am J Emerg Med 1995;13:438.

Schuster V, Kreth HW: Epstein-Barr virus infection and associated diseases in children: II. Diagnostic and therapeutic strategies. Eur J Pediatr 1992;151:794.

VIRAL INFECTIONS SPREAD BY INSECT VECTORS (Table 34–4)

In the United States, mosquitoes are the most common insect vectors that spread viral infections. As a consequence, these infections—and others which are spread by ticks—tend to occur as summer-fall epidemics that coincide with the seasonal breeding and feeding habits of the vector. Thus, a careful travel and exposure history is critical for correct diagnostic workup. Encephalitis is the common severe manifestation, but for many pathogens the infection is most often subclinical. Mild central nervous system disease, such as meningitis, is also common. There are no specific therapies for these infections. Prevention consists of control of mosquito vectors and precautions with proper clothing and insect repellents to minimize mosquito and tick bites (Table 34–4).

Arboviral disease—United States, 1994. MMWR Morb Mortal Wkly Rep 1995;44:641.

Calisher CH: Medically important arboviruses of the United States and Canada. Clin Microbiol Rev 1994;7:89.

Goodpasture HC et al: Colorado tick fever: Clinical, epidemiologic, and laboratory aspects of 228 cases in Colorado in 1973–74. Ann Intern Med 1978;88:303.

Hayes EB, Gubler DJ: Dengue and dengue hemorrhagic fever. Pediatr Infect Dis J 1992;11:311.

INFECTIONS DUE TO MISCELLANEOUS VIRUSES

ERYTHEMA INFECTIOSUM

This benign exanthematous illness of school-age children is caused by a human parvovirus designated B19. Spread is respiratory, occurring in winter-spring epidemics. A nonspecific mild flu-like illness may occur during the initial viremia at 7–10 days; the characteristic rash occurring at 10–17 days actually represents an immune response. The patient is viremic and contagious prior to—but not after—the onset of rash.

Approximately one-half of infected individuals have a subclinical illness. Most cases (60%) occur in children between the ages of 5 and 15, with an additional 40% occurring later in life. Forty percent of adults are seronegative. The disease is mildly contagious; the secondary attack rate in a school or household setting is 50% among susceptible children and 20–30% among susceptible adults.

Clinical Findings

Owing to the nonspecific nature of the exanthem and the many subclinical cases, a history of contact with an infected individual is often absent or unreliable. Recognition of the illness is easier during outbreaks.

A. Symptoms and Signs: Typically, the first

Table 34–4. Some virus diseases spread by insects in the United States.

Disease	Natural Reservoir (Vector)	Geographic Distribution	Incubation Period	Clinical Presentations	Laboratory Findings	Complications, Sequelae	Diagnosis, Therapy, Comments
FLAVIVIRUSES St. Louis encephalitis (SLE)	Birds (*Culex* mosquitoes)	Southern Canada, Central USA, Caribbean, South America	2–5 days (up to 3 weeks)	Abrupt onset of fever, chills, headache, nausea, vomiting; may develop generalized weakness, seizures, coma, ataxia, cranial nerve palsies. Aseptic meningitis is common in children.	Modest leukocytosis, neutrophilia, elevated liver enzymes. CSF: 100–200 WBC/μL (PMNs predominate early).	Mortality rate 2–5% in children (especially <age 5). Neurologic sequelae in 1–20%.	Most important mosquito-borne encephalitis in USA: 20–500 cases a year, < 2% symptomatic. (Worse in elderly.) Therapy: supportive. Diagnosis: serology. Specific antibody often present within 5 days.
Dengue	Humans (*Aedes* mosquitoes)	Asia, Africa, Central and South America, Caribbean; rarely in southern USA	2–7 days	Fever, headache, myalgia, joint and bone pain, retroocular pain, pharyngitis, cough; maculopapular or petechial rash in 20%, sparing palms and soles; adenopathy. Meningoencephalitis in 5–10% of children.	Leukopenia, thrombocytopenia. CSF: 100–500 mononuclear cells/μL if neurologic signs are present.	Hemorrhagic fever, shock syndrome, prolonged weakness.	High infection rate. Biphasic course may occur. Therapy: supportive. Ribavirin is experimental. Diagnosis: serology.
ALPHA TOGAVIRUSES Western equine encephalitis	Birds (*Culisata* mosquitoes)	Canada, Mexico, and USA west of Mississippi River	2–5 days	Similar to that of St. Louis encephalitis. Most infections are subclinical.	Variable white counts. CSF: 10–300 WBC/μL.	Permanent brain damage, 10% overall; most severe in old adults.	About 50–150 cases a year in USA. Worse in infants. Case/infection is 1:1000 for infants. Equine illness precedes human outbreaks. Therapy: supportive. Diagnosis: serology. Often IgM antibody in first week.
Eastern equine encephalitis	Birds (*Culisata* mosquitoes)	Eastern seaboard USA; Caribbean; South America	2–5 days	Similar to that of St. Louis encephalitis. but more severe. Progresses rapidly in one-third to coma and death.	Leukocytosis with neutrophilia. CSF: 500–2000 WBC/μL; PMNs predominate early.	Mortality rate 20–70%; neurologic sequelae in over 50% of children.	Most severe mosquito-borne encephalitis in USA. Fewer than 20 cases a year. Only 3–10% of cases are symptomatic. Therapy: supportive. Diagnosis: serology. Background seropositivity very low. Titers often positive in first week. Equine deaths may signal an outbreak.
Venezuelan equine encephalitis	Horses (ten species of mosquitoes)	South and Central America; Texas	1–6 days	Similar to that of St. Louis encephalitis.	Lymphopenia, mild thrombocytopenia, abnormal liver function tests. CSF: 50–200 mononuclears/μL.	Severe disease more common in infants; 20% fatality rate for encephalitis.	Most infections do not cause encephalitis. Vaccination of horses will stop epidemic. Therapy: Supportive. Diagnosis: IgM antibody EIA test.

Table 34–4. Some virus diseases spread by insects in the United States.

Disease	Natural Reservoir (Vector)	Geographic Distribution	Incubation Period	Clinical Presentations	Laboratory Findings	Complications, Sequelae	Diagnosis, Therapy, Comments
BUNYAVIRUS							
California encephalitis (La-Crosse, Jamestown Canyon, California)	Chipmunks and other small mammals (*Aedes* mosquitoes)	Northern and mid Central USA, southern Canada	3–7 days	Similar to that of St. Louis encephalitis; sore throat and respiratory symptoms are common; focal neurologic signs in up to 25%. Seizures prominent. Prepubertal children are most likely to have severe disease.	Variable white counts. CSF: 30–200 (up to 600) WBC/µL; variable PMNs; protein often normal.	Mortality rate < 1%. Seizure disorder may begin during acute illness.	About 50–150 cases a year in USA, 5% symptomatic. Therapy: supportive. Diagnosis: serology. Up to 90% have specific IgM antibody in first week; 25% of population has IgG antibody.
COLTIVIRUS							
Colorado tick fever	Small mammals (*Dermacentor andersoni,* or wood tick)	Rocky Mountain region of USA and Canada	3–14 days (range, 1–14 days)	Fever, chills, myalgia, conjunctivitis, headache, retro-orbital pain; rash in < 10%. No respiratory symptoms. Biphasic fever in 50%.	Leukopenia (maximum at 4–6 days), mild thrombocytopenia.	Rare encephalitis, coagulopathy.	Patient may have no known tick bite. Acute illness lasts 7–10 days; prolonged fatigue in adults. Therapy: supportive. Diagnosis: serology, direct FA staining of red cells for viral antigen, PCR.

sign of illness is the rash, which begins as raised, fiery red maculopapular lesions on the cheeks that coalesce to give a "slapped cheek" appearance. The lesions are warm, nontender, and sometimes pruritic. They may be scattered on the forehead, chin, and postauricular areas, but the circumoral region is spared. Within 1–2 days, similar lesions appear on the proximal extensor surfaces of the extremities and spread distally in a symmetric fashion. Palms and soles are usually spared. The trunk, neck, and buttocks are also commonly involved. Central clearing of confluent lesions produces a characteristic lace-like pattern. The rash fades in several days to several weeks but frequently reappears in response to local irritation, heat (bathing), sunlight, and stress. Almost one-half of infected children have some rash remaining (or recurring) for 10 days. Fine desquamation may be present.

Mild systemic symptoms occur in up to 50% of children. These include low-grade fever (38–38.5 °C), mild malaise, sore throat, and coryza. They appear for 2–3 days and are followed by a week-long asymptomatic phase before the rash appears.

B. Laboratory Findings: A mild leukopenia occurs early in some patients, followed by leukocytosis and lymphocytosis. Specific IgM and IgG serum antibody tests are available, but care must be used in choosing a reliable laboratory for this test. Nucleic acid detection tests are often definitive. The disease is not diagnosed by routine viral culture.

Differential Diagnosis

The characteristic rash and the mild nature of the illness distinguish erythema infectiosum from other childhood exanthems. It lacks the prodromal symptoms of measles and the lymphadenopathy of rubella. Systemic symptoms and pharyngitis are more prominent with enteroviral infections and scarlet fever.

Complications & Sequelae

A. Arthritis: This is more common in older patients, beginning with late adolescence. Approximately 10% of children have severe joint symptoms. Girls are affected more commonly than boys. Pain and stiffness occur symmetrically in the peripheral joints. Arthritis usually follows the rash and may persist for 2–6 weeks but resolves without permanent damage.

B. Aplastic Crisis: Parvovirus B19 replicates primarily in erythroid progenitor cells. Consequently, reticulocytopenia occurs for approximately 1 week during the illness. This goes unnoticed in normal individuals but results in severe anemia in patients with chronic hemolytic anemia. The rash of erythema infectiosum follows the hemolysis in these patients.

Pure red cell aplasia, chronic pancytopenia, idiopathic thrombocytopenic purpura, and a hemophagocytic syndrome have also been described. Patients with AIDS and other immunosuppressive illnesses may develop prolonged anemia or pancytopenia. Patients with hemolytic anemia and aplastic crisis or immunosuppressed patients may still be contagious and should be isolated while in the hospital. Parvovirus is under study as a potential cause of a variety of collagen-vascular diseases, neurologic syndromes, and myocarditis.

C. In Utero Infections: Infection of susceptible pregnant women may produce fetal infection with hydrops fetalis; fetal death occurs in about 6%, with most fatalities occurring in the first 20 weeks—compared with a fetal loss of 3.5% in controls. The risk of fetal infection is not known. Congenital anomalies have not been associated with parvovirus B19 infection during pregnancy.

Treatment & Prognosis

Erythema infectiosum is a benign illness for normal individuals. Patients with aplastic crisis may require blood transfusions. It is unlikely that this complication can be prevented by quarantine measures, since acute parvovirus infection in contacts is often unrecognized and is most contagious prior to the rash. Pregnant women who are exposed to erythema infectiosum or who work in a setting where an epidemic occurs should be tested for evidence of prior infection. Susceptible pregnant women should then be followed for evidence of parvovirus infection. Approximately 1.5% of women of childbearing age are infected during pregnancy. If maternal infection occurs, the fetus should be followed by ultrasonography for evidence of hydrops and distress. In utero transfusion or early delivery may salvage some fetuses. Pregnancies should not be terminated because of parvovirus infection. The risk of fetal death among exposed pregnant women of unknown serologic status is less than 2.5% for homemakers and less than 1.5% for schoolteachers.

Intramuscular immune globulin (IGIM) is not protective. High-dose intravenous immune globulin (IGIV) has stopped viremia and led to marrow recovery in some cases of prolonged aplasia. Its role in normal patients and pregnant women is unknown.

Brown KE, Young NS: Parvovirus B19 in human disease. Ann Rev Medicine 1997; 48:59.

Heegaard ED, Hornsleth A: Parvovirus: The expanding spectrum of disease. Acta Paediatr 1995;84:109.

Levy R et al: Infection by parvovirus B19 during pregnancy: A review. Obstet Gynecol Surv 1997;52:254.

HANTAVIRUS INFECTION (Pulmonary Syndrome)

Essentials of Diagnosis & Typical Features

- Influenza-like prodrome (fever, myalgia, headache, cough).

- Rapid onset of unexplained pulmonary edema.
- Residence or travel in epidemic area; exposure to aerosols from deer mouse droppings or secretions.

General Considerations

A new severe viral disease appeared in an epidemic cluster in the Southwestern United States in 1993. This unique viral illness is the first native bunyavirus epidemic in this country. Hantavirus pulmonary syndrome is distinctly different in mode of spread (no arthropod vector) and clinical picture from other bunyavirus diseases.

Clinical Findings

The initial cases of hantavirus pulmonary syndrome involved travel to or residence in an area where New Mexico, Colorado, Utah, and Arizona are contiguous and involved potential exposure to the habitat of the reservoir, ie, the deer mouse. This rodent and other selected rodents that harbor related hantaviruses live in many other locales. Thus, through 1996, 143 cases were confirmed in 20 other states west of the Mississippi River and five additional states in the northeast and southeast. Fewer than 25 were reported in 1997.

A. Symptoms and Signs: Onset is sudden, with a nonspecific virus-like prodrome: fever; back, hip, and leg pain; chills, headache, dry cough, and nausea and vomiting. Abdominal pain may be present. Sore throat, conjunctivitis, rash, and adenopathy are absent. After 1–10 days (usually 4–5), dyspnea, tachypnea, and evidence of a pulmonary capillary leak syndrome appear. This often progresses rapidly over a period of hours. Hypotension is common not only from hypoxemia but also from decreased cardiac output. Decreased cardiac output and elevated systemic vascular resistance distinguish this disease from early bacterial sepsis.

B. Laboratory Findings: The hemogram shows leukocytosis with a prominent left shift, thrombocytopenia, and hemoconcentration. LDH is elevated, as are liver function tests; serum albumin is low. Urinalysis is normal. Lactic acidosis is a poor prognostic sign. A serum IgM ELISA test is positive early in the illness. Otherwise the diagnosis is made by specific staining of tissue or PCR, usually at autopsy.

C. Imaging: Initial chest x-rays are normal. This is followed by bilateral interstitial infiltrates with the typical butterfly pattern of acute pulmonary edema, bibasilar airspace disease, or both. Significant pleural effusions are often present.

Differential Diagnosis

In the same geographic areas, plague and tularemia are possibilities. Infections with viral respiratory pathogens and *Mycoplasma* have a slower tempo, do not elevate the LDH, and do not cause the hematologic changes. Q fever, psittacosis, toxin exposure, legionellosis, and fungal infections are possibilities, but the history and tempo of the illness as well as the exposure history should be distinguishing features. Hantavirus pulmonary syndrome is a consideration in previously healthy persons with a febrile illness that results in unexplained pulmonary edema.

Treatment & Prognosis

When given early for other bunyavirus infections, intravenous ribavirin has been effective, and the agents of the pulmonary syndrome are sensitive in vitro to ribavirin. A trial of this therapy for hantavirus is under way. Management should concentrate on oxygen therapy and mechanical ventilation as required. Because of capillary leakage, Swan-Ganz catheterization to monitor cardiac output and inotropic support—rather than fluid therapy—should be used to maintain perfusion. The role of extracorporeal membrane oxygenation is also under study. The virus is not spread by person-to-person contact. No isolation is required. Thus far, the case fatality rate is approximately 50%. Guidelines are available for reduction of exposure to the infectious agent.

Butler JC, Peters CJ: Hantavirus, and hantavirus pulmonary syndrome. Clin Infect Dis 1994;19:387.

Khan AS et al: Fatal hantavirus pulmonary syndrome in an adolescent. Pediatrics 1995;95:276.

Mertz GJ, Hjelle BL, Bryan RT: Hantavirus infection. Adv Intern Med 1997;42:369.

MUMPS

Essentials of Diagnosis & Typical Features

- No prior mumps immunization; exposure 14–21 days previously.
- Parotid gland swelling.
- Aseptic meningitis with or without parotitis.
- Orchitis, pancreatitis, or oophoritis.

General Considerations

Mumps was one of the classic childhood infections; the virus spread by the respiratory route, attacked almost all unimmunized children (asymptomatically in 30–40% of cases), and produced lifelong immunity. The vaccine is so efficacious that clinical disease is rare in immunized children. As a result of subclinical infections or childhood immunization, 95% of adults are immune. Infected patients can spread the infection from 1–2 days prior to the onset of symptoms and for 5 additional days.

A history of exposure to a child with parotitis is not proof of mumps exposure. In an adequately immunized individual, parotitis is usually due to another cause.

Clinical Findings

A. Symptoms and Signs:

1. Salivary gland disease–Tender swelling of

one or more glands, variable fever, and facial lymphedema are typical. Parotid involvement is most common; signs are bilateral in 70%. The ear is displaced upward and outward; the mandibular angle is obliterated. Systemic toxicity is usually absent. Parotid stimulation with sour foods may be quite painful. The orifice of Stensen's duct may be red and swollen; yellow secretions may be expressed, but pus is absent. Parotid swelling dissipates after 1 week.

2. Meningoencephalitis–Prior to widespread immunization, mumps was the most common cause of aseptic meningitis, which occurs in up to 50% of cases and is usually manifested by mild headache or asymptomatic mononuclear pleocytosis. Fewer than 10% have clinical meningitis or encephalitis. Cerebral symptoms do not correlate with parotid symptoms, which are absent in many patients with meningoencephalitis. Although neck stiffness, nausea, and vomiting can occur, encephalitic symptoms are rare (1:1000 cases of mumps); recovery in 3–10 days is the rule. Vaccine-related meningoencephalitis is very rare with vaccines licensed in the USA.

3. Pancreatitis–Abdominal pain may represent transient pancreatitis. Because salivary gland disease may elevate serum amylase, specific markers of pancreatic function (lipase, amylase isoenzymes) are required for assessing pancreatic involvement.

4. Orchitis, oophoritis–Involvement of the gonads is associated with fever, local tenderness, and swelling. Epididymitis is usually present. Orchitis is unusual in young children but occurs in up to one-third of affected postpubertal males. Usually it is unilateral and resolves in 1–2 weeks. Although one-third of infected testes atrophy, bilateral involvement and sterility are rare.

5. Other–Thyroiditis, mastitis (especially adolescent females), arthritis, and presternal edema (occasionally with dysphagia or hoarseness) may be seen.

B. Laboratory Findings: Peripheral blood leukocyte count is usually normal. Up to 1000 cells/µL (predominantly lymphocytes) may be present in the spinal fluid, with mildly elevated protein and normal to slightly decreased glucose. Viral culture of saliva, throat, urine, or spinal fluid may be positive for at least 1 week after onset. Paired sera assayed by EIA are currently used for diagnosis. Complement-fixing antibody to the soluble antigen disappears in several months; its presence in a single specimen thus indicates recent infection.

Differential Diagnosis

Mumps parotitis may resemble the following: cervical adenitis (the jaw angle may be obliterated, but the ear does not usually protrude; Stensen's duct orifice is normal; leukocytosis and neutrophilia are observed), bacterial parotitis (pus in Stensen's duct, toxicity, exquisite tenderness); recurrent parotitis (idiopathic or associated with calculi), tumors or

leukemia, and tooth infections. Many viruses, including parainfluenza, enteroviruses, Epstein-Barr virus, CMV, and influenza virus, can cause parotitis. Parotid swelling in HIV infection is less painful and tends to be bilateral and chronic.

Unless parotitis is present, mumps meningitis resembles that caused by enteroviruses or early bacterial infection. An elevated amylase is a useful clue in this situation. Isolated pancreatitis is not distinguishable from many other causes of epigastric pain and vomiting. Mumps is a classic cause of orchitis, but torsion, bacterial or chlamydial epididymitis, *Mycoplasma* infection, other viral infections, hematomas, hernias, drugs, and tumors must also be considered.

Complications

The major neurologic complication is nerve deafness (usually unilateral), which may be transient but usually results in inability to hear high tones. It may occur without meningitis. Permanent damage is rare, occurring in less than 0.1% of cases of mumps. Aqueductal stenosis and hydrocephalus (especially following congenital infection), myocarditis, transverse myelitis, and facial paralysis are other rare complications.

Treatment & Prognosis

Treatment is supportive and includes provision of fluids, analgesics, and scrotal support for orchitis. Systemic steroids have been used for orchitis, but their value is anecdotal. Surgery is not recommended.

Harel L et al: Mumps arthritis in children. Pediatr Infect Dis J 1990;9:928.

Hersh BS et al: Mumps outbreak in a highly vaccinated population. J Pediatr 1991;119:187.

Koskiniemi M et al: Clinical appearance and outcome in mumps encephalitis in children. Acta Paediatr Scand 1983;72:603.

Manson AL: Mumps orchitis. Urology 1990;36:355.

McDonald JC, Moore DL, Quennec P: Clinical and epidemiologic features of mumps meningoencephalitis and possible vaccine-related disease. Pediatr Infect Dis J 1989;8:751.

RABIES

Essentials of Diagnosis & Typical Features

- History of animal bite 10 days to 1 year (usually less than 90 days) previously.
- Paresthesias or hyperesthesia in bite area.
- Progressive limb and facial weakness in some patients (dumb rabies; 30%).
- Irritability followed by fever, confusion, combativeness, muscle spasms (especially pharyngeal with swallowing) in all patients (furious rabies).

- Rabies antigen detected in corneal scrapings or tissue obtained by brain or skin biopsy; Negri bodies seen in brain tissue.

General Considerations

Rabies remains a potentially serious public health problem wherever animal immunization is not widely practiced or when humans play or work in areas with sylvan rabies. Although infection does not always follow a bite by a rabid animal (about 40% infection rate following rabid dog bites), infection is almost invariably fatal. Any warm-blooded animal may be infected, but susceptibility and transmissibility vary with different species. Bats may be well yet carry and excrete the virus in saliva or feces for prolonged periods; they are the major cause of rabies in the United States. Dogs and cats are usually clinically ill within 10 days after becoming contagious (the standard quarantine period for suspect animals). Valid quarantine periods or signs of illness are not fully known for many species. Rodents rarely transmit infection. Animal vaccines are very effective when properly administered, but a single inoculation may fail to produce immunity in up to 20% of dogs.

The risk is assessed according to the type of animal (bats always considered rabid; raccoons, skunks, foxes in many areas); wound extent and location (infection more common after head or arm bites, or if wounds have extensive salivary contamination or are not quickly and thoroughly cleaned); geographic area (urban rabies rare to nonexistent in many U.S. cities; rural rabies always possible, especially outside the United States); and animal vaccination history (risk low if documented). Most rabies in this country is with genotypes found in bats, yet a history of bat bite is rarely obtained. Aerosolized virus in caves inhabited by bats has caused infection.

Clinical Findings

A. Symptoms and Signs: Paresthesias at the bite site are usually the first symptom. Nonspecific anxiety, excitability, or depression follows, then muscle spasms, drooling, hydrophobia, delirium, and lethargy. Swallowing or even the sensation of air blown on the face may cause pharyngeal spasms. Seizures, fever, cranial nerve palsies, coma, and death follow within 7–14 days after onset. In a minority of patients, the spastic components are initially absent and the symptoms are primarily flaccid paralysis and cranial nerve defects. Subsequently, the furious components appear.

B. Laboratory Findings: Leukocytosis is common. The spinal fluid is usually normal or may show elevation of protein and mononuclear cell pleocytosis. Cerebral imaging and electroencephalography are not diagnostic.

Infection in an animal may be determined by use of the fluorescent antibody test to examine brain tissue for antigen.

Rabies virus is excreted in the saliva of infected humans, but the diagnosis is usually made by antigen detection in scrapings or tissue samples of richly innervated epithelium, such as the cornea or the hairline of the neck. Classic Negri cytoplasmic inclusion bodies in brain tissue are not always present. Seroconversion occurs after 7–10 days.

Differential Diagnosis

Failure to elicit the bite history in areas where rabies is rare may delay diagnosis. Other disorders to be considered include parainfectious encephalopathy; encephalitis due to herpes simplex, mosquito-borne viruses, other viruses; and Guillain-Barré syndrome.

Prevention

See Chapter 9 for information regarding vaccination and postexposure prophylaxis. Rabies immune globulin and diploid cell vaccine have made prophylaxis more effective and minimally toxic. Since rabies is almost always fatal, presumed exposures must be managed carefully.

Treatment & Prognosis

Survival is rare but has been reported in four patients receiving meticulous intensive care. No antiviral preparations are of proved benefit. Early diagnosis is important for the protection and prophylaxis of individuals exposed to the patient.

Alvaraz L et al: Partial recovery from rabies in a nine-year-old boy. Pediatr Infect Dis J 1994;13:1154.

Fishbein DB, Robinson LE: Rabies. N Engl J Med 1993;329:1632.

Shah U, Jaswal GS: Victims of a rabid wolf in India: Effect of severity and location of bites on development of rabies. J Infect Dis 1976;134:25.

Smith J: New aspects of rabies with emphasis on epidemiology, diagnosis, and prevention of the disease in the United States. Clin Microbiol Rev 1996;9:166.

RUBELLA

Essentials of Diagnosis & Typical Features

- History of rubella vaccination usually absent.
- Prodromal nonspecific respiratory symptoms and adenopathy (postauricular and occipital).
- Maculopapular rash beginning on face, rapidly spreading to entire body, and disappearing by fourth day.
- Few systemic symptoms.

Congenital infection:

- Retarded growth, development.
- Cataracts, retinopathy.
- Purpuric "blueberry muffin" rash at birth, jaundice, thrombocytopenia.
- Deafness.
- Congenital heart defect.

General Considerations

If it were not teratogenic, rubella would be of little clinical importance. Clinical diagnosis is difficult in some cases because of its variable expression. In one study, over 80% of infections were subclinical. Because of inadequate vaccination, outbreaks now occur in adolescents or adults. Rubella is transmitted by aerosolized respiratory secretions. Patients are infectious 5 days before until 5 days after the rash.

Congenital rubella, both in infants of unimmunized women and in some who have apparently been reinfected in pregnancy, is now rare. (Fewer than five cases were reported in 1997.)

Clinical Findings

The incubation period is 14–21 days. The nondistinctive signs may make exposure history unreliable. A history of immunization makes rubella unlikely but still possible.

Congenital rubella usually follows maternal infection in the first trimester.

A. Symptoms and Signs:

1. Infection in children–Young children may only have rash. Older patients often have a nonspecific prodrome of low-grade fever, ocular pain, sore throat, and myalgia. Postauricular and suboccipital adenopathy (sometimes generalized) is characteristic. This often precedes the rash or may occur without rash. The rash consists of erythematous discrete maculopapules beginning on the face. A "slapped cheek" appearance or pruritus may occur. Scarlatiniform or morbilliform rash variants may occur. The rash quickly spreads to the trunk and extremities after it fades from the face; it is gone by the fourth day. Enanthem is usually absent.

2. Congenital infection–More than 80% of women infected in the first 4 months of gestation are delivered of affected infants; congenital disease occurs in less than 5% of those infected later in pregnancy. Later infections can result in isolated defects, such as deafness. The main manifestations are as follows:

a. Growth retardation–Fifty to 85 percent are small at birth and remain so.

b. Cardiac anomalies–Pulmonary artery stenosis, patent ductus arteriosus, ventricular septal defect.

c. Ocular anomalies–Cataracts, microphthalmia, glaucoma, retinitis.

d. Deafness.

e. Cerebral disorders–Chronic encephalitis.

f. Hematologic disorders–Thrombocytopenia, dermal nests of extramedullary hematopoiesis or purpura ("blueberry muffin" rash), lymphopenia.

g. Others–Hepatitis, osteomyelitis, immune disorders, malabsorption, diabetes.

B. Laboratory Findings: Leukopenia is common, and platelet counts may be low. Congenital infection is associated with low platelet counts, abnormal liver function tests, hemolytic anemia, pleocytosis, and very high rubella IgM antibody titers. Total serum IgM is elevated, and IgA and IgG levels may be depressed.

C. Imaging: Pneumonitis and bone metaphysial longitudinal lucencies may be present in films of children with congenital infection.

Diagnosis & Differential Diagnosis

Virus may be isolated from throat or urine from 1 week before to 2 weeks after onset of rash. Children with congenital infection are infectious for months. The virus laboratory must be notified that rubella is suspected. Serologic diagnosis is best made by demonstrating a fourfold rise in antibody titer between specimens drawn 1–2 weeks apart. The first should be drawn promptly, since titers increase rapidly after onset of rash. Both specimens must be tested simultaneously by a single laboratory. Specific IgM antibody can be measured by immunoassay. Because the decision to terminate a pregnancy is usually based on serologic results, testing must be done carefully.

Rubella may resemble infections due to enterovirus, adenovirus, measles, Epstein-Barr virus, roseola, parvovirus, *Toxoplasma gondii,* and *Mycoplasma.* Drug reactions may also mimic rubella. Because public health implications are great, sporadic suspected cases should be serologically or virologically confirmed.

Congenital rubella must be differentiated from congenital CMV infection, toxoplasmosis, and syphilis.

Complications & Sequelae

A. Arthralgia and Arthritis: Both occur more often in adult women. Polyarticular involvement (fingers, knees, wrists), lasting a few days to weeks, is typical. Frank arthritis occurs in a small percentage. It may resemble acute rheumatoid arthritis.

B. Encephalitis: With an incidence of about 1:6000, this is a nonspecific parainfectious encephalitis associated with a low mortality rate. A syndrome resembling subacute sclerosing panencephalitis (see rubeola) has also been described in congenital rubella.

C. Rubella in Pregnancy: Infection in the mother is self-limited and not severe. (See previous text for sequelae.)

Prevention

See Chapter 9 for the indications for and efficacy of rubella vaccine. Standard prenatal care should include rubella antibody testing. Seropositive mothers are at no risk; seronegative mothers are vaccinated after delivery.

A pregnant woman possibly exposed to rubella should be tested immediately; if seropositive, she is immune and need not worry. If she is seronegative, a second specimen should be drawn in 4 weeks, and both specimens should be tested simultaneously. Seroconversion in the first trimester suggests high fetal risk; such women require counseling regarding therapeutic abortion.

When pregnancy termination is not an option, some experts recommend intramuscular administration of 20 mL of immune globulin within 72 hours after exposure in an attempt to prevent infection. (This negates the value of subsequent antibody testing.) The efficacy of this practice is unknown.

Treatment & Prognosis

Symptomatic therapy is sufficient. Arthritis may improve with administration of anti-inflammatory agents. The prognosis is excellent in all children and adults but poor in congenitally infected infants, in whom most defects are irreversible or progressive. The severe cognitive defects seem to correlate closely in these infants with the degree of growth failure.

Chantler JK et al: Persistent rubella virus infection associated with chronic arthritis in children. N Engl J Med 1985;313:1117.

Freij BJ, South MA, Sever JL: Maternal rubella and the congenital rubella syndrome. Clin Perinatol 1988; 15:247.

Kaplan KM et al: A profile of mothers giving birth to infants with congenital rubella syndrome: An assessment of risk factors. Am J Dis Child 1990;144:118.

Weber B et al: Congenital rubella syndrome after maternal reinfection. Infection 1993;21:118.

II. RICKETTSIAL INFECTIONS

Rickettsiae are pleomorphic, gram-negative coccobacilli which are obligate intracellular parasites. Rickettsial diseases are often included in the differential diagnosis of febrile rashes, though some (notably Q fever) are not characterized by rash. Severe headache is a prominent symptom. The endothelium is the primary target tissue, and the ensuing vasculitis is responsible for severe illness.

All rickettsioses except Q fever are transmitted by cutaneous arthropod contact, either by bite or fecal contamination of skin breaks. Evidence of such contact by history or physical examination may be completely lacking, especially in young children. The geographic distribution of the vector is often the primary determinant for suspicion of these infections. Therapy often must be empirical. Most new broad-spectrum antimicrobials are inactive against these cell wall-deficient organisms; chloramphenicol and tetracycline are usually effective.

HUMAN EHRLICHIOSIS

Ehrlichia species are responsible for febrile pancytopenia in animals. In humans, *Ehrlichia sennetsu* is responsible for a mononucleosis-like syndrome seen in Japan and Malaysia. One agent of North American human ehrlichiosis has been identified as a new species, *Ehrlichia chaffeensis.* The reservoir is currently unknown; ticks are the presumed vectors. Most cases caused by this agent are reported in the south central and mid to southern Atlantic states. Almost all cases occur between March and October, when ticks are active. A second ehrlichiosis syndrome, which is seen in the upper Midwest, Connecticut, and northern California, is caused by an organism closely related to *Ehrlichia phagocytophila* or *Ehrlichia equi,* which are known large animal pathogens. *E chaffeensis* has a predilection for mononuclear cells, whereas intracytoplasmic inclusions in granulocytes are common with the *E phagocytophila* and *E equi* infections. Hence, diseases caused by these agents are referred to as human monocytic ehrlichiosis or human granulocytic ehrlichiosis, respectively. Rocky Mountain spotted fever and human monocytic ehrlichiosis share the same vector (Lone Star tick), while Lyme disease and human granulocytic ehrlichiosis are spread by the deer tick. Thus, dual infections are common and should be considered in patients who fail to respond to therapy.

Clinical Findings

In approximately 75% of cases, a history of tick bite can be elicited. The majority of the remaining patients report having been in a tick-infested area. The usual incubation period ranges from 5 to 21 days.

A. Symptoms and Signs: Fever and headache are universally present. Gastrointestinal symptoms (anorexia, nausea and vomiting) are reported in most pediatric cases. Photophobia, conjunctivitis, myalgia, and rash are seen in over 50%. The rash may be erythematous, macular, papular, petechial, scarlatiniform, or vasculitic. Meningitis occurs. Interstitial pneumonitis occurs in severe cases. The physical examination, in addition to rash, reveals mild cervical adenopathy and hepatomegaly.

B. Laboratory Findings: Laboratory abnormalities include leukopenia with left shift, lymphopenia, thrombocytopenia, and elevated aminotransferase levels. Anemia is seen in one-third of cases.

The definitive diagnosis is made serologically. CDC uses appropriate antigens in an immunofluorescent antibody test in order to distinguish between the etiologic agents. Intracytoplasmic inclusions (morulae) may occasionally be observed in mononuclear cells in monocytic ehrlichiosis and are usually observed in polymorphonuclear cells from the peripheral blood or bone marrow in granulocytic ehrlichiosis.

Differential Diagnosis

The differential diagnosis includes septic or toxic shock, other rickettsial infections (especially Rocky Mountain spotted fever), Colorado tick fever, leptospirosis, Epstein-Barr virus, CMV, and other viral infections, Kawasaki disease, systemic lupus erythematosus, and leukemia.

Treatment & Prognosis

Although the disease may last several weeks, it is usually self-limited. Deaths do occur in children. Doxycycline, 2–4 mg/kg/d divided every 12 hours (maximum 100 mg/dose) for 7–10 days, is the treatment of choice.

Barton LL et al: Infection with *Ehrlichia* in childhood. J Pediatr 1992;120:998.

Dawson JE: Human ehrlichiosis in the United States. Curr Clin Top Infect Dis 1996;16:164.

Nadelman RB et al: Simultaneous human granulocytic ehrlichiosis and Lyme borreliosis. N Eng J Med 1997;337:27.

Roland WE et al: Ehrlichiosis: A cause of prolonged fever. Clin Infect Dis 1995;20:212.

Schutze GE: Ehrlichiosis. Rep Ped Infect Dis 1996;6:31.

RICKETTSIALPOX

Rickettsia akari is transmitted by mites from infected house mice. Most cases in the United States have occurred in northeastern cities, particularly New York. The bite site becomes a papule, then a pustule; it ulcerates and then forms a characteristic black eschar at about the time fever develops at 9–14 days. Local adenopathy is the rule. Headache, myalgia, and photophobia are followed in 2–4 days by a generalized maculopapular rash. Palms and soles may be involved. Vesicles develop on the papules and form crusts. The fever lasts about a week.

The differential diagnosis includes varicella, enteroviral infections, other rickettsial spotted fevers, meningococcemia, and gonococcemia. Mild cases require no therapy. Tetracycline or chloramphenicol is effective.

Kass EM et al: Rickettsialpox in a New York City hospital, 1980 to 1989. N Engl J Med 1994;331:1612.

ROCKY MOUNTAIN SPOTTED FEVER

Rickettsia rickettsii causes one of many similar tick-borne illnesses characterized by fever and rash. Most are named for their geographic area. In all except Rocky Mountain spotted fever and murine typhus, there is a characteristic eschar at the bite site, the "tache noire." Dogs and rodents are reservoirs of *R rickettsii*.

Rocky Mountain spotted fever is the most severe of these infections and the most important in the United States. It occurs predominantly in the eastern seaboard, in the southeastern states, and in Arkansas, Texas, Missouri, Kansas, and Oklahoma—rarely in the West. Most cases occur in children exposed in rural areas from April to September. Approximately 350–400 cases are reported yearly. Since tick attachment lasting 6 hours or longer is needed, frequent tick removal is a preventive measure.

Clinical Findings

A. Symptoms and Signs: After the incubation period of 3–12 days (mean, 7 days), there is high fever (over 40 °C, often hectic), usually of abrupt onset, myalgia, severe and persistent headache (less obvious in infants), toxicity, myalgia, photophobia, vomiting, and diarrhea. The characteristic rash occurs in 85–90% of patients and appears 2–6 days after fever onset as macules and papules especially prominent on the palms, soles, and extremities, becoming petechial and spreading centrally. Conjunctivitis, splenomegaly, edema, meningismus, irritability, and confusion may be seen.

B. Laboratory Findings: Laboratory findings are nonspecific and reflect diffuse vasculitis: thrombocytopenia, hyponatremia, early mild leukopenia, proteinuria, abnormal liver function tests, hypoalbuminemia, and hematuria. Cerebrospinal fluid pleocytosis is common. Serologic diagnosis is achieved with indirect fluorescent or latex agglutination antibody methods, but generally only 7–10 days after onset of the illness. Skin biopsy with specific fluorescent staining may give the diagnosis within the first week of the illness.

Differential Diagnosis

The differential diagnosis includes meningococcemia, measles, meningitis, staphylococcal sepsis, enteroviral infection, leptospirosis, Colorado tick fever, scarlet fever, murine typhus, Kawasaki disease, and ehrlichiosis.

Treatment & Prognosis

To be effective, therapy for Rocky Mountain spotted fever must be started early and is often based on a presumptive diagnosis in endemic areas prior to rash onset. It is important to remember that atypical presentations, such as the absence of pathognomonic rash, often lead to delay in appropriate therapy. Chloramphenicol is the agent of choice for children under 8 years of age; a tetracycline is preferable for older children. Treatment should be continued for 2 or 3 days after the temperature has returned to normal for a full day. A minimum of 10 days of therapy is recommended.

Complications and death result from severe vasculitis, especially in the brain, heart, and lung. The mortality rate is 5–7%. Delay in therapy is an important determinant of mortality.

Myers SA, Sexton DJ. Dermatologic manifestations of arthropod-borne diseases. Infect Dis Clin North Am 1994;8:689.

Sexton DJ, Corey CR: Rocky Mountain "spotless" and "almost spotless" fever: A wolf in sheep's clothing. Clin Infect Dis 1992;15:439.

Silber JL. Rocky Mountain spotted fever. Clin Dermatol 1996;14:245.

Walker DH: Rocky Mountain spotted fever: A second alert. Clin Infect Dis 1995;20:1111.

ENDEMIC TYPHUS (Murine Typhus)

Endemic typhus is present in the southern United States, mainly in southern Texas. The disease is transmitted by fleas from infected rodents, either by bite, from their feces in scratches, or by inhalation. Domestic cats and opossums may play a role in the transmission of suburban cases. There is no eschar at the bite, which may go unnoticed. The incubation period is 6–14 days. Headache, myalgia, and chills slowly worsen. Fever may last 10–14 days. After 3–8 days, a rash appears. Truncal macules and papules spread to the extremities; the rash may become petechial.

The centrifugal nature of the rash in typhus, with sparing of the palms and soles, is a distinction from Rocky Mountain spotted fever. Rash may be absent in 20–40% of patients. Hepatomegaly may be present. Intestinal and respiratory symptoms may occur. Mild thrombocytopenia and elevated liver enzymes may be present. The illness is usually self-limited and milder than epidemic typhus. More prolonged neurologic symptoms have been described. Therapy is usually not needed. Doxycycline is the drug of choice. Therapy for 3 days is usually sufficient. Fluorescent antibody and enzyme immunoassay serologic tests are available.

Esperanza L et al: Murine typhus: Forgotten but not gone. South Med J 1992;85:754.

Samra Y, Shaked Y, Maier MK: Delayed neurologic toxicity in murine typhus: Report of two cases. Arch Intern Med 1989;149:949.

Q FEVER

Coxiella burnetii is transmitted by inhalation rather than by an arthropod bite. The birth tissues and excreta of domestic animals and of some rodents are the infectious source. Unpasteurized milk from infected animals may also transmit disease. Q fever is also distinguished from other rickettsial diseases by the absence of cutaneous manifestations and by the prominence of pulmonary disease.

Clinical Findings

A. Symptoms and Signs: Chills, fever, severe headache, and myalgia occur 10–30 days after exposure. Abdominal pain, vomiting, chest pain, and cough are prominent in children. Examination of the lung may produce few findings, as in other atypical pneumonias. Hepatosplenomegaly is common.

B. Laboratory Findings: Leukopenia with left shift is characteristic. Thrombocytopenia is unusual and another distinction from other symptomatic rickettsial diseases. Aminotransferase levels are elevated. Diagnosis is made by finding a complement-fixing antibody response (fourfold rise or single high titer) to the phase II organism. Chronic infection is indicated by antibody against the phase I organism. IgM ELISA is also available.

C. Imaging: Pneumonitis occurs in 50% of patients. Multiple segmental infiltrates are common. Consolidation and pleural effusion are exceptional.

Differential Diagnosis

In the appropriate epidemiologic setting, Q fever should be considered in evaluating causes of atypical pneumonias such as *Mycoplasma pneumoniae,* viruses, and *Chlamydia pneumoniae).* It should also be included among the causes of mild hepatitis without rash or adenopathy.

Treatment & Prognosis

Typically the illness lasts 1–2 weeks without therapy. One complication is chronic disease, which often implies myocarditis or granulomatous hepatitis.

C burnetii is also one of the causes of "culture-negative" endocarditis. Both types of complication are rare. The endocarditis is difficult to treat; mortality approaches 50%. The course of the uncomplicated illness is shortened with tetracycline or chloramphenicol; doxycycline is preferred.

Pinsky RK et al: An outbreak of cat-associated Q fever in the United States. J Infect Dis 1991;164:202.

Ruiz-Contreras J et al: Q fever in children. Am J Dis Child 1993;147:300.

To H et al: Q fever pneumonia in children in Japan. J Clin Microbiol 1996;34:647.

REFERENCES

Drugs for non-HIV viral infections. Med Lett Drugs Ther 1997;39:69.

Feigin RD, Cherry JD (editors): *Textbook of Pediatric Infectious Diseases,* 4th ed. Saunders, 1997.

Myers SA, Sexton DJ: Dermatologic manifestations of arthropod-borne disease. Infect Dis Clin North Am 1994;8:689.

Remington JS, Klein JO: *Infectious Disease of the Fetus and Newborn Infant.* Saunders, 1990.

Human Immunodeficiency Virus (HIV) Infection

35

Elizabeth J. McFarland, MD

Essentials of Diagnosis & Typical Features

Children less than 18 months:
- A child known to be HIV-seropositive or born to an HIV-infected mother.

And
- Has positive results on two separate determinations on blood or tissue (excluding cord blood) for one or more of the following HIV detection tests: HIV culture, HIV polymerase chain reaction, HIV antigen (p24).

Or
- Meets criteria for AIDS diagnosis based on the 1987 CDC AIDS surveillance case (specific opportunistic infections, lymphoid interstitial pneumonitis, Kaposi's sarcoma, primary brain lymphoma, others; see Table 35–1 and CDC case definition, MMWR, 1994).

Or
- Has HIV antibody and evidence of cellular and humoral immunodeficiency (without an obvious cause) and symptoms compatible with HIV infections (multiple serious bacterial infections, encephalopathy, recurrent *Salmonella* septicemia, HIV wasting syndrome, certain non-Hodgkin's lymphomas, disseminated fungal infections, or mycobacterial infections).

Children older than 18 months:
- HIV-seropositive by repeatedly reactive enzyme immunoassay (EIA) and confirmatory test.

Or
- Meets any of the criteria listed for children less than 18 months.

General Considerations

Acquired immunodeficiency syndrome (AIDS) is the result of progression of HIV infection. HIV is a retrovirus that infects mainly helper T lymphocytes (CD4 lymphocytes), monocytes, and macrophages. In general, cells are infected after binding of the virus's glycosylated envelope protein, gp120, to the CD4 protein and a chemokine receptor, both found on the surface of the target cells. Individuals who are homozygous for a rare allele coding for mutation in a chemokine receptor (CCR-5) are highly resistant to HIV infection. The function and the number of helper T lymphocytes are diminished by infection, with profound effects on both humoral and cell-mediated immunity. Without treatment, HIV infection causes generalized immune incompetence and progression to AIDS.

AIDS is a clinical syndrome that was originally defined before HIV was identified as the etiologic agent. The diagnosis is made after an HIV-infected child develops any of the opportunistic infections or malignancies listed in category C (Table 35–1). In adults and adolescents, the criteria for a diagnosis of AIDS also include absolute CD4 lymphocyte counts of 200/μL or less.

AIDS ranks among the top ten causes of death in children aged 1–4 years. In the United States during recent years, 600–900 new cases of perinatally acquired AIDS have occurred each year; this number reflects the larger number of infants newly infected with HIV. Worldwide, an estimated 800,000 children are infected with HIV, most of them in Africa, India, Thailand, and parts of South America.

Perinatal transmission accounts for over 90% of prepubertal AIDS cases and almost all new pediatric HIV infections. Perinatal transmission may occur in utero, at the time of delivery, or via breast feeding. Indirect evidence suggests that about 30% of perinatal infections occur prior to birth. The timing of in utero transmission is currently the subject of active investigation. Formerly, most nonperinatal cases were acquired via transfusion or hemophilia therapy. Of hemophiliacs who received blood products prior to 1985 (when screening began), 65–90% are infected. Sexual activity (both heterosexual and homosexual) and sharing of contaminated needles account for most infections after puberty. During recent years, there has been an increasing incidence of HIV infection in young people aged 13–25 years.

About 84% of HIV-infected women are of childbearing age; 41% are intravenous drug abusers, and most of the remainder are sexual partners of infected

Table 35–1. Clinical categories of children
with HIV infection.[1]

Category N: Not symptomatic
No signs or symptoms or only one of the conditions listed
in category A
Category A: Mildly symptomatic
Having two or more of the following conditions:
Lymphadenopathy
Hepatomegaly
Splenomegaly
Dermatitis
Parotitis
Recurrent or persistent upper respiratory infection,
sinusitis, or otitis media
Category B: Moderately symptomatic
Having symptoms attributed to HIV infections other than
those in category A or C
Examples:
Anemia, neutropenia, thrombocytopenia
Bacterial meningitis, pneumonia, sepsis (single episode)
Candidiasis, oropharyngeal, persisting over 2 months
Cardiomyopathy
Cytomegalovirus infection with onset < 1 month of age
Diarrhea, recurrent or chronic
Hepatitis
Herpes simplex virus recurrent stomatitis, bronchitis,
pneumonitis, esophagitis at < 1 month of age
Herpes zoster, two or more episodes or more than one
dermatome
Leiomyosarcoma
Lymphoid interstitial pneumonia
Nephropathy
Nocardiosis
Persistent fever
Toxoplasmosis with onset < 1 month of age
Varicella, complicated
Category C: Severely symptomatic
Serious bacterial infections, multiple or recurrent
Candidiasis, esophageal or pulmonary
Coccidioidomycosis, disseminated
Cryptosporidiosis or isosporiasis with diarrhea > 1 month
Cytomegalovirus infection with onset > 1 month of age
Encephalopathy
Herpes simplex virus: persistent oral lesions, or bronchitis,
pneumonitis, esophagitis at > 1 month of age
Histoplasmosis
Kaposi's sarcoma
Lymphoma
Mycobacterium tuberculosis, extrapulmonary
Mycobacterium infection, other species, disseminated
Pneumocystis carinii pneumonia
Progressive multifocal leukoencephalopathy
Salmonella septicemia, recurrent
Toxoplasmosis of the brain with onset > 1 month of age
Wasting syndrome

[1]Adapted from MMWR Morb Mortal Wkly Rep 1994;43(RR-
12):6, 8.

men. The incidence of HIV infection in women exposed by heterosexual contact continues to increase.
In the United States, approximately 7000 HIV-infected women deliver live infants each year; without
intervention, 15–30% of these infants would be infected. Risk factors associated with mother-to-infant
transmission include advanced disease stage, high viral burden, low CD4 lymphocyte count, and factors

related to increased exposure to maternal blood or
cervical secretions at the time of delivery (ie, duration of rupture of membranes, presence of blood in
the infant's gastric secretions, first-born twin delivery). The rate of vertical transmission can be reduced
to 5–8% by zidovudine treatment of the mother during pregnancy and delivery and of the infant during
the first 6 weeks after birth.

In the United States, risk factors for HIV infection
among adults include exposure to blood products
from 1978 to the spring of 1985, parenteral illicit
drug use, multiple heterosexual or homosexual contacts, and a partner with one of the above risk factors.
Casual, classroom, or household contact with an
HIV-infected person poses no risk. Many individuals, particularly women, are unaware of their risk
factors. Adolescents are also likely to be unaware of
or unwilling to admit the existence of risk factors. A
high level of suspicion is required for making the diagnosis in such cases.

At the time of initial HIV infection, high levels of
HIV are detected in the bloodstream. In adults, the
level of viremia declines without therapy concurrently with the appearance of an HIV-specific host
immune response. Plasma viremia usually reaches a
steady state level about 6–12 months after primary
infection. The amount of virus present in the plasma
at that point and thereafter is predictive of the rate of
disease progression for the individual. Despite ongoing virus replication, there is usually a period of clinical latency lasting from 1 year to more than 12 years
during which the infected person is generally asymptomatic. The virus and anti-HIV immune responses
are in a steady state, with high levels of virus production and destruction balanced against production and
destruction of CD4 lymphocytes. Eventually, the balance favors the virus, and the viral burden increases
as the CD4 lymphocyte count declines.

Among infants with vertically acquired HIV infection, approximately 30% will have virus detectable in
the blood at birth. The remaining infants will be negative for HIV at birth but will soon have detectable
virus, usually by 2–8 weeks. In either case, the level
of viremia rises steeply, reaching a peak at 1–2
months of age. In contrast with adults, infants will
then have a gradual decline in plasma viremia that
extends beyond 2 years. The peak level of viremia
and the mean plasma virus level over the first year of
life are predictors of the rate of progression. Infants
generally have plasma virus levels ten times higher
than those in adults.

In untreated infections, about 20–30% of HIV-infected infants develop an AIDS-defining illness by 1
year of age and die before age 2–3 years. High levels
of viremia at 1–2 months and high average levels
over the first year of life are observed in these infants. Other predictors of rapid progression are low
absolute counts of CD4 and CD8 T lymphocytes in
the first 6 months. In the remainder, the disease pro-

gresses more slowly, with a mortality rate of 3.5% per year between ages 1 and 7 years, with a median survival greater than 7 years. It is not uncommon for an HIV-infected child to survive into early adolescence. These slow progressors will generally have lower virus levels and a gradual decline in CD4 T lymphocytes. There are rare HIV-infected children and adults who have been infected over 8–10 years with no evidence of immune suppression. It is not yet clear whether these patients will escape disease progression.

Clinical Findings

A. Symptoms and Signs:

1. Primary acute infection–The incubation period for primary infection is 2–4 weeks. Symptoms associated with primary infection are nonspecific ("flu" or mild mononucleosis-like illness) and often subclinical. Infected persons may present with fever, fatigue, malaise, pharyngitis, enlarged lymph nodes, and hepatosplenomegaly. Signs seen more frequently with HIV than with other similar viral syndromes are mild oral ulcerations, a diffuse macular, erythematous rash, and mild encephalopathy. Occasionally, thrush or *Candida* esophagitis is observed. The early symptoms associated with primary infection resolve spontaneously within 1–2 weeks, though some persons have fatigue and depression for weeks or months.

Following perinatal acquisition, a primary infection syndrome is rarely recognized. Newborns with perinatal HIV infection are rarely symptomatic (less than 7%) at birth. Size and physical features are not different from uninfected infants. However, 75–95% will demonstrate some sign (mostly nonspecific signs) by age 1 year.

2. Nonspecific symptoms–The manifestations described below are likely to be observed in children with untreated infection or in those failing to respond to therapy. The CDC has developed disease staging criteria for HIV-infected children (Tables 35–1 and 35–2). The criteria incorporate clinical symptoms ranging from no symptoms to mild, moderate, and severe symptoms (categories N, A, B, C,

respectively) and age-adjusted CD4 lymphocyte counts (immunologic categories 1, 2, 3, corresponding to no evidence of immune suppression, moderate evidence, and severe immune suppression, respectively). Each child is classified both by CD4 count and by clinical category. In general, category C diagnoses are the diseases indicating an AIDS diagnosis, with the exception of lymphoid interstitial pneumonitis, which was included as an AIDS-defining illness but is not a sign of late-stage disease. Initial studies suggest that these criteria are useful in predicting outcome.

Frequent illness (especially recurrent otitis media or sinusitis) is a typical historical feature, in addition to poor weight gain (sometimes progressing to wasting syndrome), chronic cough, chronic diarrhea, recurrent mucocutaneous *Candida* infection, developmental delay, unexplained fevers, night sweats, generalized lymphadenopathy, or hepatosplenomegaly. Delayed growth may be observed as early as 4 months in some infants. These common early findings may be present for years in an otherwise well child.

3. Infections related to immunodeficiency–Progressive immune dysfunction in both humoral and cell-mediated responses results in susceptibility to infections. Children lack prior experience with many bacterial pathogens; hence, recurrent bacterial infections are more common in children than in HIV-infected adults. The most common types of serious bacterial infections are bacteremia, pneumonia, urinary tract infections, cellulitis, abscesses, bone and joint infections, and meningitis. Infections with *Mycobacterium tuberculosis* (usually acquired from adults in the household) may be severe. Persistent candidal mucocutaneous infections (oral, skin, and vaginal) are common. Candidal esophagitis is reported in about 15% of pediatric cases. Cryptococcal infections and histoplasmosis have been described, though much less frequently than among HIV-infected adults.

Abnormal responses to viral infections, particularly herpesviruses, are common. Primary varicella infections may be prolonged or severe, and recur-

Table 35–2. Immunologic categories based on age-specific CD4 T-lymphocyte counts and percentages of total lymphocytes.[1]

Immunologic Category	Age of Child					
	< 12 months		1–5 years		6–12 years	
	/μL	(%)	/μL	(%)	/μL	(%)
1. No evidence of suppression	≥ 1500	(≥ 25)	≥ 1000	(≥ 25)	≥ 500	(≥ 25)
2. Evidence of moderate suppression	750–1499	(15–24)	500–999	(15–24)	200–499	(15–24)
3. Evidence of severe suppression	< 750	(< 15)	< 500	(< 15)	< 200	(< 15)

[1]Adapted from MMWR Morb Mortal Wkly Rep 1994;43(RR-12):4.

rence of infections results with progressive immune dysfunction. Cytomegalovirus (CMV) infections may result in disseminated disease, hepatitis, gastroenteritis, retinitis, and encephalitis. Recurrent herpes simplex lesions may be large, painful, and persistent. Likewise, persistent aphthous ulcers may cause significant morbidity.

Late-stage immunodeficiency is accompanied by susceptibility to a variety of opportunistic pathogens. Pneumonia caused by *Pneumocystis carinii* is the most common, accounting for 30% of AIDS-defining diagnoses among children. The incidence is highest between age 2 months and 6 months, and pneumocystis pneumonia is often fatal during this period. Symptoms are difficult to distinguish from those of viral or atypical pneumonia. Patients typically have fever, tachypnea, intercostal retractions, progressive hypoxemia, and an elevated lactate dehydrogenase (LDH). Disseminated infection with *Mycobacterium avium* complex (MAC) occurs in approximately 11% of HIV-infected children. The rate increases to about 25% in infected children who have CD4 lymphocyte counts under 50–100/μL. Symptoms and signs associated with this opportunistic pathogen include fever, night sweats, weight loss, diarrhea, fatigue, lymphadenopathy, hepatomegaly, anemia, and granulocytopenia. A variety of diarrheal pathogens that cause mild, self-limited symptoms in healthy persons may result in severe, chronic diarrhea in HIV-infected persons. These include rotavirus, *Cryptosporidium, Isospora belli, Giardia,* and bacterial pathogens *(Campylobacter, Salmonella, Shigella, Clostridium difficile).* Chronic parvovirus infection manifested by anemia can occur. Reactivation of toxoplasmosis is uncommon in pediatric HIV but causes encephalitis in up to 28% of HIV-infected adults. It may present as encephalitis, a central nervous system mass lesion, or disseminated disease during early infancy.

4. Organ system disease–HIV infection may cause a variety of organ system symptoms. In most cases, the pathogenesis is not fully understood; however, symptoms occurring in the absence of other pathogens are thought to result from HIV infection itself.

Encephalopathy is a common problem, afflicting 20% or more of HIV-infected children. Following perinatal transmission, affected patients may present with acquired microcephaly, progressive motor deficit, ataxia, pseudobulbar palsy, and failure to attain (or surrender of previously attained) developmental milestones. The affected child may demonstrate a static course associated with steady but below-normal developmental progress; may reach and maintain a developmental plateau; or may lose developmental skills. Children who are older may have symptoms similar to those observed in infected adults, such as gradual mental status changes initially affecting attention span and memory. However, other treatable causes of central nervous system disease should be sought, especially when an acute change in symptoms occurs.

Lymphoid interstitial pneumonitis, which is uncommon among adults, is common in HIV-infected children. Histologically, it is characterized by a diffuse peribronchial and interstitial infiltrate composed of lymphocytes and plasma cells. It may be asymptomatic or associated with dry cough, hypoxemia, dyspnea or wheezing on exertion, and clubbing of the digits. Auscultatory findings may be few. Children with this disorder frequently have enlargement of the parotid glands, generalized lymphadenopathy, and normal LDH.

Hematologic signs are common. Immune thrombocytopenia associated with antiplatelet antibodies occurs but does not correlate with the degree of immune suppression. Many cases are low-grade, with no clinical symptoms and no therapy required. However, some cases result in serious bleeding complications. Anemia is frequently present in late-stage disease. Likewise, granulocytopenia may occur as the disease progresses. Patients are often also taking antiretroviral or prophylactic medication, which may result in bone marrow suppression; distinguishing between the effects of HIV and the drug therapy may be difficult.

Subclinical cardiac abnormalities detectable only by echocardiography are common. Symptomatic cardiomyopathy is also observed in some cases, mainly infants with rapid disease progression. Symptoms are those of congestive heart failure and may respond to diuretics and digitalis.

Mild to moderate elevation of liver enzymes is frequently observed and, more rarely, overt clinical hepatitis due to HIV infection itself. However, patients are often taking medications with potential hepatotoxicity, and superinfection with other pathogens (CMV, EBV, MAC, hepatitis C) that affect the liver is common. Thus, causes other than HIV should be sought in the face of significant liver disease. Chronic diarrhea may occur with HIV infection. However, as with hepatitis, it is commonly associated with other gastrointestinal infections, which may respond to treatment. Severe diarrhea warrants an aggressive evaluation, including cultures, microscopic examinations, and perhaps colonoscopy with biopsy. Lactose intolerance is not infrequent among HIV-infected children. Nephropathy, myopathy, and neuropathy are all recognized in pediatric HIV but are relatively uncommon.

5. Malignancy–Malignancy is AIDS-defining in 2% of HIV-infected children. The tumors most commonly associated with pediatric HIV infection are non-Hodgkin's lymphomas. Unlike non-Hodgkin's lymphomas in immunocompetent persons, in HIV-infected children the disease commonly manifests at extranodal sites (bone, gastrointestinal tract, liver, or lungs) and is usually high-grade and of B cell origin. Central nervous system primary lesions are common, causing symptoms of a mass lesion or increased intracranial pressure. Kaposi's sarcoma, a common malignancy among HIV-infected homosexual males, rarely occurs in children. There is an increased frequency of leiomyosarcomas, a soft tissue tumor not associated with other immunodeficiencies. Cervical neoplasia associated with human papillomavirus is more common in adolescent females with HIV infection.

B. Laboratory Findings: In children older than 18 months (after loss of maternal antibody), HIV antibody is positive by enzyme immunoassay (EIA). A confirmatory test, usually a Western blot, must be performed since individuals occasionally have nonviral cross-reacting antibodies, which result in a false-positive EIA. Rarely (less than 1% of cases) an infected person may fail to make antibody. However, they are usually obviously ill, and tests for virus or viral antigen are positive. During the early weeks after primary infection of adolescents, HIV antibody may be absent; tests for the presence of virus (p24 antigen, HIV culture, or nucleic acid detection) are positive.

Infants born to HIV-infected mothers will have positive tests for HIV antibody—regardless of infection status—owing to transplacental passage of maternal antibody. The median time to loss of maternal HIV antibody is 10 months; all children lose maternal antibody by 18 months. No reliable IgM antibody test is available. A diagnosis of HIV infection can be made in over 95% by age 2–4 months using tests for virus in blood (HIV culture or nucleic acid detection). Detection of viral antigen (p24 antigen) by using an immune complex dissociation step in the assay is an alternative less expensive test requiring only frozen serum and less technical expertise; however, it is 10–20% less sensitive.

Approximately 70% of infected infants will have negative results by these sensitive assays during the first few weeks of life, presumably because of low viral burden, perhaps indicating that the infection was acquired at the time of birth. Hence, negative tests during this early period do not reliably rule out infection. However, an infant who is otherwise well and has had at least two negative HIV cultures or nucleic acid detection tests, both performed at over 1 month of age and at least one performed at over 4 months of age, is unlikely to be infected. These infants can be followed for clinical symptoms and tested at age 15–18 months for reversion to seronegative status to confirm the absence of infection. Some experts recommend a final antibody test at 24 months.

There are rare reports of children who had blood tests that were repeatedly positive for HIV by culture or nucleic acid detection and who demonstrated no symptoms of HIV infection and have subsequently reverted to negative serologic and virologic tests. In most cases, detailed investigation has demonstrated

that the positive tests result from laboratory error. The phenomenon of transient viremia appears to be extremely uncommon and rarely documented.

As the disease progresses, the absolute number and percentage of helper T (CD4) lymphocytes declines; suppressor-killer T (CD8) lymphocytes may be increased. Helper T lymphocyte numbers and percentages in infants are normally much higher than in adults and decline to adult levels by age 6 years. Hence, age-adjusted values must be used in evaluating these tests (Table 35–2).

In the absence of a secondary infection or organ system disease, routine laboratory tests (CBC, blood chemistry profiles) are often normal. Some children will have thrombocytopenia due to autoimmune antibodies at a relatively early stage of disease. As disease progresses, anemia becomes common and granulocytopenia unrelated to drug therapy may occur. Mild elevation of liver enzymes is common. Serum LDH levels are high in children with *P carinii* infection. Hypergammaglobulinemia is characteristic and may be observed as early as 9 months of age. Some children fail to make specific antibody to antigens (eg, *Haemophilus influenzae* type b, *S pneumoniae*), which contributes to subsequent infections. With brain involvement, the cerebrospinal fluid may be normal or the protein elevated and a mononuclear pleocytosis may be present.

C. Imaging: Cerebral images can demonstrate atrophy and calcification in the basal ganglia and frontal lobes in patients with encephalopathy. Chest radiographs of children with lymphoid interstitial pneumonitis show diffuse interstitial reticulonodular infiltrates, occasionally with hilar adenopathy. The chest radiograph in pneumocystis pneumonia typically demonstrates perihilar infiltrates progressing to bilateral diffuse alveolar disease.

Differential Diagnosis

Differential diagnosis of HIV will vary with the presenting sign or symptom. Infants with immunodeficiency may resemble infants with other types of congenital immunodeficiencies such as hypogammaglobulinemia or severe combined immunodeficiency syndrome. When poor growth is a prominent feature of the presentation, HIV may be confused with other causes of growth deficiency. Children or adolescents presenting with generalized lymphadenopathy or hepatosplenomegaly may resemble those infected with viruses such as EBV or CMV. The symptoms of acute primary infection in the adolescent may be similar to those of EBV or CMV infection, toxoplasmosis, rubella, syphilis, or viral hepatitis.

The diagnosis can be made or excluded with HIV antibody testing in a child over 18 months of age. In younger children, a negative result usually excludes HIV infection, but a positive result must be followed by confirmatory testing for the presence of virus. Likewise, an adolescent with symptoms of primary infection should be tested for virus by nucleic acid detection.

Prevention

Awareness of modes of transmission is crucial for prevention of HIV. As a result of careful donor screening and testing of the donated blood, HIV transmission resulting from transfusion of blood products is now an extremely rare event (1:100,000 to 1:40,000 transfusions). An aggressive educational campaign promoted by the gay community resulted in a marked decrease in the annual incidence of HIV infections in that population. However, ongoing and expanded educational efforts are necessary to maintain the decreased rates and to reach other populations at risk. Health care providers should encourage developmentally appropriate AIDS education for children beginning at early ages and continuing into adolescence.

The only 100% effective method of avoiding sexual transmission of HIV infection is abstinence or limiting sexual contact to a mutually monogamous partner who is not HIV-infected. However, condoms—used consistently and correctly—are highly effective in preventing transmission between stable, sexually active couples in which only one partner is HIV-infected. In two studies, seroconversions occurred in 0–2% of discordant couples using condoms consistently compared with 10–15% of couples with inconsistent condom use. A third study reported 1.1 seroconversions per 100 person-years of observation among consistent condom users compared with 9.7 seroconversions among inconsistent users. The CDC provides detailed instructions on correct condom use. Prompt treatment of other STDs also reduces the risk of sexual transmission. Although there are no efficacy data and no official recommendation, some experts have recently begun to offer antiretroviral medications as prophylaxis against HIV infection to people who are exposed to HIV in a circumstance which is not likely to recur (eg, sexual assault, condom rupture).

All medical equipment that can penetrate the skin should be sterile. Infected blood and secretions should be handled according to CDC recommendations. The CDC recommends postexposure prophylaxis following occupational exposure. Recommended therapy is with zidovudine and lamivudine (3TC), with or without a protease inhibitor depending on the degree of risk associated with the exposure.

Vertical transmission can be substantially prevented by antiretroviral therapy of the mother and early prophylaxis of the newborn. A multicenter clinical trial, ACTG 076, compared placebo with zidovudine treatment of the mother and infant during the second or third trimester, at the time of delivery, and during the first 6 weeks of life (Table 35–3). Among HIV-infected asymptomatic women with no prior an-

Table 35–3. Treatment regimen used in ACTG 076 trial of zidovudine for the reduction of mother-to-infant HIV transmission.[1]

Maternal treatment	
During pregnancy, starting at 14–34 weeks' of gestation	Zidovudine, 100 mg orally five times daily
During labor and delivery	Zidovudine, 2 mg/kg IV as loading dose, then continuous infusion of 1 mg/kg/h
Infant treatment	
Begun within 12 hours after delivery and continued for 6 weeks	Zidovudine, 2 mg/kg orally four times daily

[1]Adapted from MMWR Morb Mortal Wkly Rep 1994;43 (RR-11):3.

tiretroviral treatment, a 65% lower transmission rate was observed with zidovudine therapy. Short-term adverse events were minor and reversible. Subsequent trials incorporating the ACTG 076 regimen have reported similar reductions in the expected transmission rates. The CDC and the American College of Obstetrics and Gynecology now recommend offering routine HIV testing with informed consent to all pregnant women. Women found to be infected should be counseled regarding all HIV-related pregnancy care issues, including the risks and benefits of therapy with zidovudine and other antiviral agents. Recommendations regarding the use of combination antiretroviral therapy in pregnant women have recently been published. Trials are ongoing to study the long-term effects on women and infants receiving zidovudine during pregnancy as well as to investigate other dosing regimens and treatment agents.

Since breast milk can carry the virus, breast feeding by HIV-infected mothers is contraindicated when access to safe formula can be ensured, as is the case in the United States.

Treatment

HIV infection calls for specific antiretroviral treatment to prevent progressive deterioration of the immune system as well as prophylactic measures aimed at preventing opportunistic infections. Whenever possible, children should be enrolled in collaborative treatment studies. Current information on clinical trials may be obtained by calling the AIDS Clinical Trials Information Line (1-800-TRIALS-A).

The management of HIV infection has changed markedly in the past few years owing to availability of a greater number of antiretroviral agents and use of the quantitative plasma HIV RNA copy number as a surrogate marker for disease progression and response to therapy. This marker provides information independently of CD4 lymphocyte counts. Both are used in monitoring therapy. Quantitative plasma viremia measurements can be performed by several techniques. The results are positively correlated but are not identical. For that reason, serial tests performed to follow the course of infection should be done by the same technique each time.

Recent studies have validated plasma viral copy number as a surrogate marker in HIV-infected infants and children. One study demonstrated a linear relationship between risk of progression and the baseline RNA copy number (54% risk reduction for each 1 log reduction in baseline RNA). Likewise, response to therapy was predicted both by changes in RNA and by CD4 count after 24 weeks of treatment. High plasma virus loads have been associated with an increased risk of progression in several pediatric studies. Establishing a consensus threshold RNA value above which progression is likely to occur has been difficult owing to considerable overlap in levels of plasma viremia between rapid progressors and slow progressors. However, most experts agree that levels of plasma viremia exceeding 100,000 viral copies per milliliter place the child at high risk of disease progression and fatal outcome.

A working group of pediatric HIV specialists recently convened by the National Pediatric and Family HIV Resource Center generated guidelines for the use of antiretroviral agents in pediatric HIV infection. Antiretroviral therapy is recommended for all children with HIV-related symptoms (clinical categories A, B, C in Table 35–1) or evidence of immune suppression (CD4 lymphocyte counts in category 2 or 3; Table 35–2) and all HIV-infected infants under 12 months of age regardless of clinical stage number of viral RNA copies in plasma. For children over 12 months of age, most experts favored initiating therapy in any child with virus detectable in plasma. An alternative approach for asymptomatic children is close observation, with therapy initiated if rapidly declining CD4 lymphocyte counts or increasing or high HIV plasma RNA copy numbers are observed. Initial therapy should include at least two and preferably three drugs. Effective therapy should result in a greater than 0.5–1 log decline in plasma virus copies after 1–2 months; optimally, plasma virus will decrease to undetectable levels after 4–6 months of treatment. Once therapy has been initiated, the patient should be monitored every 3 months for changes in plasma virus copy number, CD4 lymphocyte count, and symptoms.

HIV has a high spontaneous mutation rate, and emergence of drug resistance during treatment is well documented. Many antiretroviral drugs are likely to induce resistant mutations in the virus within weeks to months when used as monotherapy. For that reason, the use of combinations and strict adherence to dosing regimens is critically important to durable antiretroviral activity. It can be expected that if viral replication is not fully suppressed (ie, plasma virus remains detectable), the potential for emergence of

resistant mutations exists. If increasing plasma viremia is observed after treatment in a compliant patient, viral resistance is likely and selection of a new antiretroviral regimen—most often involving switching at least two drugs—should be considered.

A. Specific Measures: Eleven drugs in three classes have been approved by FDA for the treatment of HIV infection. Additional drugs in each class are under development. Although the testing of these drugs in children has been delayed relative to adults, many are now available in pediatric formulations and with pediatric dosing information.

Combination therapy is recommended for all patients. Selecting a combination of drugs appropriate for an individual patient is a complex process requiring expert understanding of antiretroviral activity, cross-resistance patterns, and drug interactions. Changes in standards of care occur frequently and precede reports in the literature. Decisions regarding antiretroviral therapy should therefore be made in collaboration with the patient and the family by a physician with expertise in HIV treatment.

1. NRTIs–The first FDA-approved antiretroviral drugs were nucleoside reverse transcriptase inhibitors (NRTIs). These drugs are nucleoside analogs that block production of viral DNA, a step preceding productive infection of the cell. The NRTIs vary widely with regard to antiviral activity, rates at which viral resistance is induced, and adverse effects. Zidovudine (AZT) has moderate antiretroviral activity and a relatively long interval prior to development of resistance. Toxicities include anemia, neutropenia, headache, myalgia, and insomnia. Stavudine (d4T) also has moderate antiretroviral activity. It has fewer adverse effects, mainly peripheral neuropathy observed mostly in patients with advanced disease. Time to induction of drug resistance is long. Lamivudine (3TC) is highly active against HIV, but complete resistance develops within weeks when 3TC is used as monotherapy. Didanosine (ddI) has moderate activity and a prolonged time to induction of resistance. However, the drug is poorly absorbed in the presence of gastric acid and must be taken in conjunction with antacid preparations 1–2 hours before and after food. Common side effects include gastrointestinal discomfort, pancreatitis, and peripheral neuropathy. Zalcitabine (ddC) is the least potent of the approved drugs in this class and is frequently associated with peripheral neuropathy in adult patients. This toxicity is less frequent in children.

2. NNRTIs–The second class of drugs to be developed were nonnucleoside reverse transcriptase inhibitors (NNRTIs). These agents also inhibit viral DNA synthesis but act at a different site on the viral reverse transcriptase. The NNRTIs generally have high-level antiretroviral activity, but rapid induction of resistance has limited their use. They are being reconsidered in combination therapy with other highly active drugs with the expectation that development of resistance will be delayed. Their most common toxicity is rash. Stevens-Johnson syndrome has been reported, but rash is usually mild and may resolve without changing therapy. There is pediatric dosing information for nevirapine (age over 2 years: 120 mg/m^2 daily for 14 days, then 120 mg/m^2 twice daily), and a liquid formulation is available by extended access protocol. Pediatric dosing information is not available for delavirdine, the other approved drug in this class.

3. Protease inhibitors–The agents most recently developed are the protease inhibitors. These drugs inhibit viral protease during assembly of viral progeny and result in noninfectious particles. The protease inhibitors are highly active but also induce resistance within months when used as monotherapy. Four drugs in this class have been FDA-approved— nelfinavir, ritonavir, indinavir, and saquinavir—but only the first two are available with pediatric dosing information and in pediatric formulations. Common dose-limiting toxicities include diarrhea (nelfinavir), nausea and perioral paresthesias (ritonavir), nephrolithiasis and nephropathy (indinavir), and elevation of liver enzymes (all). The original formulation of saquinavir had poor bioavailability, and therapeutic levels were best obtained using it in combination with ritonavir, which inhibits saquinavir metabolism. The new soft gel capsule formulation may overcome this problem, but there are no data on its use in children. The protease inhibitors are metabolized by the hepatic P450 cytochrome enzymes, resulting in many interactions with other drugs including other antiretrovirals. Careful attention to drug interactions is necessary when prescribing other medications to a patient taking a protease inhibitor.

B. General Measures:

1. Immunizations–Combined diphtheria-tetanus-pertussis (DPT), conjugated *Haemophilus influenzae* type b (Hib), hepatitis B, pneumococcal, and influenza vaccines should be given at the recommended times (see Chapter 9). Because of the possibility of vaccine-associated poliomyelitis in the patient or in immunodeficient contacts (eg, the mother) after administration of oral poliovirus vaccine, inactivated vaccine is recommended both for the patient and for healthy children in the household. The risk of measles is considered greater than the potential risk of the vaccine in asymptomatic children; thus, measles-mumps-rubella vaccine should be given at 12 months, with a booster dose at more than 1 month later, to children without evidence of severe immunosuppression (category C or category 3). Varicella vaccine, also a live virus, has not been approved for use in immunocompromised patients; studies of its safety and immunogenicity in mildly HIV-infected children are under way. Since antibody titers to vaccines decline with time and progressive immunodeficiency, prophylaxis with immune globulin for measles exposure should be given regardless of immunization status. Varicella-zoster immune globulin should be given to HIV-infected children without prior varicella after each varicella exposure. Infected children with tetanus-prone wounds should receive tetanus immune globulin regardless of immunization status.

2. Prophylaxis for infections–A number of effective prophylactic measures for the prevention of opportunistic infections are available. Since patients taking all potential prophylactic agents require extremely complicated medication regimens—which may result in a reduced quality of life, harmful drug interactions, or synergistic toxicities—caregivers need to prioritize the choice of prophylactic therapies for each child on the basis of specific risk factors or patient desires.

Antibiotic prophylaxis for *P carinii* has been extremely effective. Since this infection has its highest incidence during the first year of life—at a time when the infection status of the infant may still be unknown and during which rapid decline of CD4 lymphocyte count may occur within weeks—current recommendations are to treat all infants born to HIV-infected mothers from 4–6 weeks of age until a reasonably certain determination of HIV infection status can be made, usually by age 4 months. At that time, uninfected infants may discontinue prophylaxis. Infected infants should continue on prophylactic drugs until 12 months, when further treatment is based on assessment of age-adjusted CD4 lymphocyte counts during the first year of life and every 3 months thereafter. Published guidelines from the CDC are summarized in Table 35–4. The first choice for prophylaxis is trimethoprim-sulfamethoxazole. For patients intolerant to trimethoprim-sulfamethoxazole, dapsone, atovaquone (30 mg/kg/d as single daily dose), and pentamidine (aerosolized for older children, intravenous for younger children) are alternative drugs (Table 35–5).

Monthly intravenous immune globulin (IVIG) is effective in reducing the number of bacterial infections and hospitalizations in HIV-infected children who are not receiving *P carinii* prophylaxis with trimethoprim-sulfamethoxazole. Appropriate candidates for IVIG might be children with hypogammaglobulinemia, poor functional antibodies, or a history of serious or multiple bacterial infections.

Clarithromycin, azithromycin, and rifabutin are all effective for MAC prophylaxis in adults. Each drug reduces the frequency of disseminated MAC by approximately 50% in HIV-infected adults with CD4 counts of less than 50/μL, with a slight therapeutic advantage attributed to the macrolides. In one study, a survival benefit of MAC prophylaxis was demonstrated. Prophylaxis for MAC is recommended for HIV-infected children based on age-adjusted CD4 lymphocyte counts: age > 6 years, CD4 count < 50 μL; age 2–6 years, CD4 < 75 count μL; age 1–2 years, CD4 count < 500 μL; age < 1 year, CD4 count < 750 μL.

Table 35–4. *Pneumocystis* pneumonia prophylaxis for HIV-exposed and infected infants by age and HIV infection status.[1]

Birth to 4–6 wk	No prophylaxis
4–6 weeks to 4 months	Prophylaxis
4–12 months	
HIV-infected or indeterminate	Prophylaxis
HIV infection reasonably excluded[2]	No prophylaxis
1–5 years, HIV-infected	Prophylaxis if CD4 count < 500/μL or CD4 < 15%[3,4]
6–12 years, HIV-infected	Prophylaxis if CD4 count < 200/μL or CD4 < 15%[3]

[1]Adapted from MMWR Morb Mortal Wkly Rep 1995; 44(RR-4):6.
[2]Among children who have had two or more negative HIV cultures or PCR tests, both of which are performed at 1 month of age and one of which is performed at 4 months of age or older, or two or more negative HIV IgG antibody tests performed at over 6 months of age among children who have no clinical evidence of HIV disease.
[3]Children 1–2 years of age who were receiving pneumocystis pneumonia prophylaxis and had a CD4 count <750/μL or percentage of < 15% at under 12 months of age should continue prophylaxis.
[4]Prophylaxis should be considered on a case-by-case basis for children who might otherwise be at risk for pneumocystis pneumonia, such as those with rapidly declining CD4 counts or percentages or children with category C conditions; children who have had pneumocystis pneumonia should receive lifelong prophylaxis.

A trial of azithromycin in combination with atovaquone versus trimethoprim-sulfamethoxazole for general prophylaxis is ongoing.

CMV-seropositive children with very low CD4 lymphocyte counts (< 50–100/μL) may benefit from ophthalmologic examinations every 3–6 months for early detection of retinitis, though this practice has

Table 35–5. Drug regimens for *P carinii* prophylaxis for children over 4 weeks of age.[1]

Recommended regimen
  Trimethoprim-sulfamethoxazole, 150 mg TMP/M^2/d plus 750 mg SMX/m^2/d, administered orally, divided into two doses per day 3 days a week on consecutive days
  Alternative (same total daily dosages):
    Single daily dose 3 days a week on consecutive days
    Divided twice-daily doses 7 days a week
    Divided twice-daily doses 3 days a week on alternate days
Alternative if trimethoprim-sulfamethoxazole is not tolerated
  Dapsone, 2 mg/kg/kg (not to exceed 100 mg) orally once daily
  Aerosolized pentamidine (children over 5 years), 300 mg via Respirgard II inhaler monthly
  Intravenous pentamidine 4 mg/kg 2–4 weeks

[1]Adapted from MMWR Morb Mortal Wkly Rep 1995:44(RR-4):6.

not been studied rigorously. After CMV retinitis has been diagnosed, patients require induction treatment with intravenous ganciclovir and subsequent lifelong prophylaxis with ganciclovir.

Recurrent mucocutaneous and esophageal candidiasis can sometimes be prevented with topical treatments such as nystatin or clotrimazole. Some patients require chronic fluconazole treatment for effective control. Unfortunately, chronic treatment with this drug often results in emergence of fluconazole-resistant *Candida* isolates. In that case, high-dose fluconazole, itraconazole, or amphotericin B may be used for symptomatic disease. Some patients suffer recurrent severe herpes simplex or varicella-zoster infections. These may be prevented with oral acyclovir prophylaxis.

HIV-infected children have a higher risk of progression of infections due to *M tuberculosis*. These children should have yearly Mantoux skin tests with several concurrent control skin tests (tetanus, *Candida*, mumps). If the control skin tests are not reactive, the child may be anergic, and results of the tuberculosis skin test are not reliable. Since the child's infection is usually acquired from adult household contacts, other household members should be skin-tested for tuberculosis yearly. Adults and children found to have positive tuberculosis skin tests should be further evaluated for disease and treated according to guidelines for HIV-infected persons.

3. Infections and other conditions–Unusual infections may require invasive diagnostic techniques such as biopsy or bronchoscopy. Bacterial infections should be diagnosed and treated aggressively. Varicella-zoster and herpes simplex virus infections should be treated with acyclovir. Short courses of valacyclovir or famciclovir—drugs with greater bioavailability—may also be effective, but pharmacokinetic data are lacking. Mucocutaneous *Candida* infections that fail to resolve with topical antifungal medications may be treated with fluconazole. Symptomatic CMV infection should be treated with ganciclovir or foscarnet. MAC requires treatment with a multidrug regimen to delay the emergence of resistance. Lymphoid interstitial pneumonitis may respond to corticosteroid therapy. Aphthous ulcers improve with thalidomide treatment. Organ system disease (eg, encephalopathy, cardiomyopathy, and nephropathy) and chronic infections may improve with the initiation of or change in antiretroviral therapy. Zidovudine treatment has been associated with marked improvement in encephalopathic symptoms. Autoimmune thrombocytopenia may improve with IVIG or corticosteroid treatments. Anemia and granulocytopenia, whether drug-induced or HIV-induced, may respond to epoetin alfa (erythropoietin) and filgrastim (granulocyte colony-stimulating factor; G-CSF), respectively. Transfusions may be needed; CMV-seronegative blood should be used. Chronic parvovirus as a cause of anemia should be ruled out and can be treated with IVIG. Most of these conditions are likely to be recurrent or chronic, and most will require either repeated or lifelong treatment.

4. General support–Growth failure (weight and height) is one of the earliest and most sensitive markers of disease progression. The cause is a complex combination of increased metabolic needs related to chronic infection and decreased caloric intake. Although controlled trials of the effects of nutritional intervention have been difficult to conduct, malnutrition is known to contribute to immunodeficiency, and well-nourished HIV-infected children appear to have fewer infections, less fatigue, and a better quality of life. Nutritional evaluation and counseling should be a part of early care before problems arise. When a child's routine diet fails to provide adequate nutrition, supplemental nutrition in the form of oral supplements and nutritious snacks is often required. Supplemental feeding by gastrointestinal tubes may be required for children who are unable to consume sufficient calories by the oral route.

Evaluation and support for psychosocial needs of HIV-affected families is imperative. As with other chronic illnesses, HIV infection affects all family members and carries an additional social stigma. Emotional concerns and financial needs are more prominent than medical needs at many stages of the disease process and influence the family's ability to comply with a medical treatment regimen. Ideally, care should be coordinated by a team of caregivers familiar with this disease, the newest therapies, and community resources.

Prognosis

Prospective natural history studies have demonstrated a median survival of more than 7 years in untreated children. Plasma viremia and CD4 lymphocyte count can be used to assess the risk of progression. Poor prognosis in perinatal infection is associated with encephalopathy, infections with *P carinii,* early development of AIDS, and a rapidly declining helper T lymphocyte count. The presence of lymphoid interstitial pneumonitis or parotitis implies a relatively good prognosis. Some perinatally infected children and many of those infected at older ages by blood products survive into adolescence. Because of the great variability in individual responses to infection and treatment, definite statements regarding the life expectancy or quality of life should not be made.

Public Health Issues

In general, the infant or child who is well enough to attend day care or school should be treated no differently from other children. The exception may be a toddler with uncontrollable biting behavior or bleeding lesions that cannot be adequately covered; in these situations, the child may be withheld from group day care. Routine good hygiene used for the prevention of transmission of other infectious diseases is appropriate for the prevention of common infections, which may be severe in the HIV-infected child. Optimally, the school health care provider and teacher will be aware of the diagnosis, but there is no legal requirement that any individual at the school or day care center be informed. Parents and child may prefer to keep the diagnosis confidential, since the social consequences of HIV infection often overshadow the medical problems.

Horizontal transmission (ie, in the absence of sexual contact or injecting drug use) of HIV is exceedingly rare and is associated with exposure of broken skin or mucous membranes to HIV-infected blood or bloody secretions. Since undiagnosed HIV-infected infants and children might be enrolled, all schools and day care centers should have policies with simple guidelines for blood precautions to prevent transmission of HIV infection in these settings. Saliva, tears, urine, and stool are not contagious if there is no gross blood in these fluids. A barrier protection (eg, latex or rubber gloves, thick pads of fabric, or paper) should be used when possible contact with blood or bloody body fluids may occur. Sharp objects that might be contaminated with blood, such as razors or toothbrushes, should not be shared. No special care is required for dishes, towels, toys, or bedclothes. Blood-soiled clothing may be washed routinely with hot water and detergent. Contaminated surfaces may be easily disinfected with a variety of agents, including household bleach (1:10 dilution), some commercial disinfectants (eg, Lysol), and 70% isopropyl alcohol.

Conclusion

Pediatric HIV infection is a complex and multifaceted disease. Many aspects of care are under intense investigation, and recommendations for clinical care change frequently. Updated information should be sought whenever a child is diagnosed with HIV infection. With recognition of the longer survival time in most infected children, this disease is now approached as a chronic illness. Primary care physicians are encouraged to participate in the care of HIV-infected children in collaboration with centers staffed by personnel with expertise in pediatric HIV issues.

REFERENCES

American Academy of Pediatrics: HIV infection and AIDS. In: *1997 Red Book: Report of the Committee on Infectious Diseases,* 24th ed. Peter G, Hall CB, Orenstein WA (editors). American Academy of Pediatrics, 1997.

Bryson Y et al: Proposed definitions for in utero versus intrapartum transmission of HIV-1. (Letter.) N Engl J Med 1992;327:1246.

Carpenter CCJ et al: Antiretroviral therapy for HIV infection in 1997: Updated recommendations of the International AIDS Society—USA Panel. JAMA 1997;277:1962.

Comans-Bitter WM et al: Immunophenotyping of blood lymphocytes in childhood: Reference values for lymphocyte subpopulations. J Pediatr 1997;130:388.

Connor E et al: Reduction of maternal-infant transmission of human immunodeficiency virus type 1 with zidovudine treatment: Pediatric AIDS Clinical Trials Group Protocol 076 Study Group. N Engl J Med 1994; 331:1173.

Fauci AS et al: Immunopathogenic mechanism of HIV infection. Ann Intern Med 1996;124:654.

Havlir DV et al: Prophylaxis against disseminated *Mycobacterium avium* complex with weekly azithromycin, daily rifabutin or both. California Collaborative Treatment Group. N Engl J Med 1996;335:392.

Havlir DV, Richman DD: Viral dynamics of HIV: Implications for drug development and therapeutic strategies. Ann Intern Med 1996;124:984.

Human immunodeficiency virus transmission in household settings—United States. MMWR Morb Mortal Wkly Rep 1994;43:347, 353.

Kinloch-De Loes S et al: A controlled trial of zidovudine in primary human immunodeficiency virus infection. N Engl J Med 1995;333:408.

McKinney RE Jr, Wilfert C: Growth as a prognostic indicator in children with human immunodeficiency virus infection treated with zidovudine: AIDS Clinical Trials Group Protocol 043 Study Group. J Pediatr 1994; 125:728.

Mofenson LM et al: The relationship between serum human immunodeficiency virus type 1 (HIV-1) RNA level, CD4 lymphocyte count, and long-term mortality risk in HIV-1-infected children. J Infect Dis 1997;175:1029.

1995 Revised guidelines for prophylaxis against *Pneumocystis carinii* pneumonia for children infected with or perinatally exposed to human immunodeficiency virus. MMWR Morb Mortal Wkly Rep 1995;44(RR-4):1.

1994 Revised classification system for human immunodeficiency virus infection in children less than 13 years of age. MMWR Morb Mortal Wkly Rep 1994;43(RR-12):1.

Peckham C, Gibb D: Mother-to-child transmission of the human immunodeficiency virus. N Engl J Med 1995; 333:298.

Recommendations and Reports: 1993 Sexually Transmitted Diseases Treatment Guidelines. MMWR Morb Mortal Wkly Rep 1993;42(RR-14):1.

Recommendations of the U.S. Public Health Service Task Force on the use of zidovudine to reduce perinatal transmission of human immunodeficiency virus. MMWR Morb Mortal Wkly Rep 1994;43:1.

Scarlatti G: Paediatric HIV infection. Lancet 1996;348:863.

Shearer WT et al: Viral load and disease progression in infants infected with human immunodeficiency virus type 1. N Engl J Med 1997;336:1337.

Spector S et al: Pediatric AIDS Clinical Trials Group: A controlled trial of intravenous immune globulin for the prevention of serious bacterial infections in children receiving zidovudine for advanced human immunodeficiency virus infection. N Engl J Med 1994;331:1181.

Task Force on Pediatric AIDS: Pediatric guidelines for infection control of human immunodeficiency virus (acquired immunodeficiency virus) in hospitals, medical offices, schools and other settings. Pediatrics 1988;82:801.

Tovo P et al: Prognostic factors and survival in children with perinatal HIV-1 infection: The Italian Register for HIV infections in children. Lancet 1992;339:1249.

Update: Barrier protection against HIV infection and other sexually transmitted diseases. MMWR Morb Mortal Wkly Rep 1993;43:589.

Update: Provisional public health service recommendations for chemoprophylaxis after occupational exposure to HIV. MMWR Morb Mortal Wkly Rep 1996;45:468.

US Public Health Service recommendations for human immunodeficiency virus counseling and voluntary testing for pregnant women. MMWR Morb Mortal Wkly Rep 1995;44(RR-7):1.

USPHS/IDSA Guidelines for the prevention of opportunistic infections in persons infected with human immunodeficiency virus: A summary. MMWR Morb Mortal Wkly Rep 1995;44(RR-8):1.

36 Infections: Bacterial & Spirochetal

John W. Ogle, MD

I. BACTERIAL INFECTIONS

GROUP A STREPTOCOCCAL INFECTIONS

Essentials of Diagnosis & Typical Features

Streptococcal pharyngitis:
- Clinical diagnosis based entirely on symptoms; signs and physical examination unreliable.
- Throat culture or rapid antigen detection test positive for group A streptococci.

Impetigo:
- Rapidly spreading, highly infectious skin rash.
- Erythematous denuded areas and honey-colored crusts.
- On culture, group A streptococci are grown in most (not all) cases.

General Considerations

Group A streptococci are common gram-positive bacteria capable of producing a wide variety of clinical illnesses. Prominent among these are acute pharyngitis, impetigo, cellulitis, and scarlet fever, the generalized illness caused by strains that elaborate erythrogenic toxin. Group A streptococci can also cause pneumonia, septic arthritis, osteomyelitis, meningitis, and other less common infections. Group A streptococcal infections may also produce nonsuppurative sequelae (rheumatic fever, acute glomerulonephritis).

The cell walls of streptococci contain both carbohydrate and protein antigens. The C-carbohydrate antigen determines the *group* and the M- or T-protein antigens determine the specific *type*. In most strains, the M protein appears to confer virulence, and antibodies developed against the M protein are protective against reinfection with that type.

Group A streptococci are almost all β-hemolytic. These organisms may be carried asymptomatically on the skin and in the pharynx, rectum, and vagina. Ten to 15 percent of school children in some studies are asymptomatic pharyngeal carriers of group A streptococci. Streptococcal carriers are asymptomatic individuals who do not mount an immune response to the organism and are therefore believed to be at low risk for nonsuppurative sequelae. Unfortunately, there are no accepted criteria for identification of streptococcal carriers.

All group A streptococci are sensitive to penicillin. Resistance to erythromycin is common in some countries and has increased in the United States.

Clinical Findings

A. Symptoms and Signs:

1. Respiratory infections—

a. Infancy and early childhood (under 3 years of age)—The onset of infection is insidious, with mild symptoms, eg, low-grade fever, serous nasal discharge, and pallor. Otitis media is common. Pharyngitis with exudate and cervical adenitis are uncommon in this age group.

b. Childhood type—Onset is sudden, with fever and marked malaise and often with repeated vomiting. The pharynx is sore and edematous, and the tonsillar area generally shows exudate. Anterior cervical lymph nodes are tender and enlarged. Small petechiae are frequently seen on the soft palate. Fine discrete petechiae occasionally appear also on the upper abdomen and trunk. In scarlet fever, the skin is diffusely erythematous and appears sunburned and roughened ("sandpaper rash"). The rash is most intense in the axillae and groin and on the abdomen and trunk. It blanches on pressure except in the skin folds, which do not blanch and are pigmented (Pastia's sign). The rash usually appears 24 hours after the onset of fever and rapidly spreads over the next 1–2 days. Desquamation begins on the face at the end of the first week and becomes generalized by the third week. Early, the surface of the tongue is coated white, with the papillae enlarged and bright red ("white strawberry tongue"). Subsequently, desquamation occurs, and the tongue appears beefy red ("red strawberry tongue"). The face generally shows circumoral pallor. Petechiae may be seen on all mucosal surfaces.

c. Adult type–The adult type is characterized by exudative or nonexudative tonsillitis with fewer systemic manifestations, lower fever, and no vomiting. Scarlet fever is uncommon in this age group.

2. Impetigo–Streptococcal impetigo begins as a papule that vesiculates and then breaks, leaving a denuded area covered by a honey-colored crust. Both *Staphylococcus aureus* and group A streptococci are isolated in some cases. The lesions spread readily and diffusely. Local lymph nodes may become swollen and inflamed. Although the affected child often lacks systemic symptoms, occasionally a high fever and toxicity are present. If flaccid bullae are present, the disease is called bullous impetigo and is caused by an epidermolytic toxin-producing strain of *S aureus*.

3. Cellulitis–The portal of entry is often an insect bite or superficial abrasion on an extremity. There is a diffuse and rapidly spreading cellulitis that involves the subcutaneous tissues and extends along the lymphatic pathways with only minimal local suppuration. Local acute lymphadenitis occurs. The child is usually acutely ill, with fever and malaise. In classic erysipelas, the involved area is bright red, swollen, warm, and very tender. The infection may extend rapidly from the lymphatics to the bloodstream.

Streptococcal perianal cellulitis is an entity peculiar to young children. Pain with defecation often leads to constipation, which may be the presenting complaint. The child is afebrile and otherwise well. Perianal erythema and tenderness and painful rectal examination are the only abnormal physical findings. Culture of a perianal swab specimen usually yields a heavy growth of group A streptococcus. A variant of this syndrome is streptococcal vaginitis in prepubertal girls. Symptoms are dysuria and pain; marked erythema and tenderness of the introitus and blood-tinged discharge are seen.

4. Necrotizing fasciitis–This dangerous disease is being more frequently reported, particularly complicating varicella. Only 20–40% of cases are due to group A streptococci. About 30–40% are due to *S aureus* and the rest to mixed bacterial infections. The disease is characterized by extensive necrosis of superficial fasciae, with undermining of surrounding tissue and extreme systemic toxicity. Initially, the skin overlying the infection is tender and pale red without distinct borders, resembling subcutaneous cellulitis. Blisters or bullae may appear. The color deepens to a distinct purple. The involved area may develop mild to massive edema. Early recognition and aggressive debridement of necrotic tissue are essential.

5. Group A streptococcal infections in newborn nurseries–Group A streptococcal epidemics still occasionally occur in nurseries. The organism may be introduced into the nursery from the vaginal tract of a mother or from the throat or nose of a mother or a staff member. The organism then spreads from infant to infant. The umbilical stump is colonized while the infant is in the nursery. As is true also in staphylococcal infections, there may be no or few clinical manifestations while infants are still in the nursery; most often, a colonized infant develops a chronic, oozing omphalitis days later at home. The organism may spread from the infant to other family members. More serious and even fatal infections may develop, including sepsis, meningitis, empyema, septic arthritis, and peritonitis.

6. Streptococcal sepsis–Serious illness from group A streptococcal sepsis is now more common both in children and in adults. Rash and scarlet fever may be present; prostration and shock result in high mortality rates. Pharyngitis is uncommon as an antecedent illness. Underlying disease is a predisposing factor. Some authors hypothesize that a more virulent clone of group A streptococci is responsible for the increase in cases of streptococcal sepsis.

B. Laboratory Findings: Leukocytosis with a marked shift to the left is seen early. Eosinophilia regularly appears during convalescence. Beta-hemolytic streptococci are cultured from the throat. The organism may be cultured from the skin and by needle aspiration from subcutaneous tissues and other involved sites, such as infected nodes. Occasionally, blood cultures are positive. Group A streptococci may be identified most easily by demonstrable sensitivity to bacitracin. Grouping by immunofluorescence or coagglutination studies correlates best with the original precipitin reactions described by Lancefield. M and T typing is not routinely done.

Rapid antigen detection tests are 60–95% sensitive and over 95% specific for detecting group A streptococci in throat swabs. The predictive value of negative tests is about 80%, meaning that one in five patients with a positive throat culture will have a negative rapid antigen test. Rapid tests may be useful when early antibiotic therapy is considered, but because the currently available tests lack sensitivity, a standard culture should be done on specimens testing negative.

Antistreptolysin O (ASO) titers rise about 150 units within 2 weeks after an acute infection. Elevated ASO and anti-DNase B titers are useful in documenting prior throat infections in cases of acute rheumatic fever. However, elevated anti-DNase B and antihyaluronidase titers are most useful in associating pyoderma and acute glomerulonephritis. The streptozyme test is a 2-minute slide test that detects antibodies to streptolysin O, hyaluronidase, streptokinase, DNase B, and NADase. It is somewhat more sensitive than the measurement of ASO titers.

Proteinuria, cylindruria, and minimal hematuria may be seen early in children with streptococcal infection. True poststreptococcal glomerulonephritis is seen 1–4 weeks after the respiratory or skin infection.

Differential Diagnosis

Streptococcal infection in early childhood must be differentiated from adenovirus and other respiratory virus infections.

Adenoviruses, coxsackieviruses (both A and B), echoviruses, Epstein-Barr virus (infectious mononucleosis), and many respiratory viruses can produce pharyngitis. The pharyngitis in herpangina (coxsackie A viruses) is vesicular or ulcerative. Herpes simplex also causes ulcerative lesions, which most commonly involve the anterior pharynx, tongue, and gums. With other viruses (coxsackieviruses and echoviruses), rashes are common. In infectious mononucleosis, the pharyngitis is also exudative, but splenomegaly and generalized adenopathy are typical, and laboratory findings are often diagnostic (atypical lymphocytes, elevated liver enzymes, and a positive heterophil or other serologic test for mononucleosis). Uncomplicated streptococcal pharyngitis improves within 24–48 hours if penicillin is given and by 72–96 hours without antimicrobials.

Group G and group C streptococci are uncommon causes of pharyngitis but have been implicated in epidemics of sore throat in college students. Acute rheumatic fever does not occur following group G or C infection, though acute glomerulonephritis is a complication.

Arcanobacterium hemolyticum is also a cause of pharyngitis. Scarlatinal or maculopapular truncal rashes may be been seen.

In diphtheria, systemic symptoms, vomiting, and fever are less marked; pharyngeal pseudomembrane is confluent and adherent; the throat is less red; and cervical adenopathy is prominent.

Pharyngeal tularemia causes white rather than yellow exudate. There is little erythema, and cultures for β-hemolytic streptococci are negative. A history of exposure to rabbits and a failure to respond to antimicrobials may suggest the diagnosis. Response to specific antibiotic therapy is prompt.

Leukemia and agranulocytosis may present with pharyngitis and are diagnosed by bone marrow examination.

Scarlet fever must be differentiated from other exanthematous diseases (principally rubella), erythema due to sunburn, drug reactions, Kawasaki disease, toxic shock syndrome, and staphylococcal scalded skin syndrome. (See also Table 34–3.)

Complications

Suppurative complications of group A streptococcal infections include sinusitis, otitis, mastoiditis, cervical lymphadenitis, pneumonia, empyema, septic arthritis, and meningitis. Spread of streptococcal infection from the throat to other sites—principally the skin (impetigo) and vagina—is common and should

be considered in every instance of chronic vaginal discharge or chronic skin infection, such as that complicating childhood eczema.

Both acute rheumatic fever and acute glomerulonephritis are nonsuppurative complications of group A streptococcal infections.

A. Acute Rheumatic Fever: See Chapter 18.

B. Acute Glomerulonephritis: Acute nephritis can follow streptococcal infections of either the pharynx or the skin—in contrast to rheumatic fever, which follows pharyngeal infection only. Glomerulonephritis may occur at any age, including infancy. In most reported series of acute glomerulonephritis, males predominate by a ratio of 2:1, whereas acute rheumatic fever occurs with equal frequency in both sexes. Certain M types are strongly associated with poststreptococcal glomerulonephritis ("nephritogenic types"). Moreover, the serotypes resident on or producing disease on the skin often differ from those found in the pharynx.

The incidence of acute glomerulonephritis after streptococcal infection is variable and has ranged from nil to 28%. Several outbreaks of acute glomerulonephritis in families have involved 50–75% of siblings of affected patients in 1- to 7-week periods. Second attacks of glomerulonephritis are rare. The median latent period between infection and the development of glomerulonephritis is 10 days. This contrasts with acute rheumatic fever, which occurs after a median latent period of 18 days.

Treatment

A. Specific Measures: Treatment is directed not only toward eradication of acute infection but also toward the prevention of rheumatic fever. In patients with pharyngitis, antibiotics should be started early to relieve symptoms and should be continued for 10 days to prevent rheumatic fever. Although early therapy has not been shown to prevent glomerulonephritis, it seems advisable to treat impetigo promptly in sibling contacts of patients with poststreptococcal nephritis. Neither sulfonamides nor trimethoprim-sulfamethoxazole is effective in the treatment of streptococcal infections.

Although topical therapy for impetigo with antimicrobial ointments (especially mupirocin) is as effective as systemic therapy, it does not eradicate pharyngeal carriage and is less practical for extensive disease.

1. Penicillin–A single dose of benzathine penicillin G given intramuscularly (0.6 million units for children weighing under 60 lb and 1.2 million units for children weighing over 60 lb) is preferred for treatment of pharyngitis and impetigo. Phenoxymethyl penicillin (penicillin V) (250 mg for children weighing less than 40 lb and 500 mg for children weighing over 40 lb) administered orally three or four times daily between meals for 10 days is successful in about 90% of cases. Giving penicillin

V (250 mg) twice daily is as effective as more frequent oral administration or intramuscular therapy and may achieve better compliance, but a single daily dose results in a higher failure rate. Parenteral therapy is indicated if there is vomiting or sepsis. Mild cellulitis may be similarly treated. Cellulitis requiring hospitalization should be treated with aqueous penicillin G (150,000 units/kg/d intravenously in four to six divided doses) or procaine penicillin (50,000 units/kg intramuscularly once or twice a day) until there is marked improvement. Penicillin V, 125–250 mg every 6 hours, may then be given orally to complete a 10-day course. Acute cervical lymphadenitis may require incision and drainage. Treatment of necrotizing fasciitis requires emergency surgical debridement followed by high-dose parenteral antibiotics appropriate to the organisms cultured.

2. Other antibiotics–For pharyngitis or impetigo, erythromycin estolate (20–40 mg/kg/d in two to four divided doses) should be given for 10 days. Erythromycin ethyl succinate (40–50 mg/kg/d) is best tolerated if given in four divided doses. Both erythromycin preparations are best absorbed and tolerated when taken with food. Clarithromycin (15 mg/kg/d in two divided doses for 10 days) and azithromycin (12 mg/kg/d once daily for 5 days) are alternatives for patients intolerant to erythromycin. Although much more expensive, compliance may be better. Clindamycin, cephalexin, cefuroxime, cefaclor, loracarbef, cefprozil, cefpodoxime, ceftibuten, cefixime, and cefadroxil are also effective oral antimicrobials. Cefixime and cefadroxil may be given once daily, whereas cefuroxime, loracarbef, cefprozil, and cefaclor may be used twice daily. In most studies, bacteriologic failures after cephalosporin therapy are less frequent than failures following penicillin. However, cephalosporins are far more expensive than penicillin, and penicillin currently remains the agent of choice. The dosage of clindamycin is 10–20 mg/kg/d orally in four divided doses. Each of these drugs should be given for 10 days. Many strains are resistant to tetracycline. For serious infections in patients with known penicillin allergy, cefazolin (100–150 mg/kg/d intravenously or intramuscularly in three divided doses), clindamycin (25–40 mg/kg/d intravenously in four divided doses), or vancomycin (40 mg/kg/d intravenously in four divided doses) should be given. Clindamycin is preferred by many and may be superior to penicillin for necrotizing fasciitis.

3. Treatment failure–Even when compliance is perfect, organisms will be found cultures in 5–15% of children after cessation of therapy. Reculture is indicated only in the patient with pharyngitis who has a personal or family history of rheumatic fever. Repeat treatment at least once with an oral cephalosporin or clindamycin is indicated in patients with recurrent culture-positive pharyngitis.

4. Prevention of recurrences in rheumatic individuals–The preferred prophylaxis for rheumatic individuals is benzathine penicillin G, 1.2 million units intramuscularly every 4 weeks. If the risk of streptococcal exposure is high, every 3 week dosing is preferred. One of the following alternative oral prophylactic regimens may be used: sulfadiazine, 0.5–1 g daily; penicillin G, 200,000 units twice daily; or erythromycin, 250 mg twice daily. Prophylaxis is continued for five years or until age 21 if carditis is absent. In the presence of carditis, a minimum of ten years and well into adulthood is the minimum duration. If residual heart disease persists, many recommend lifelong prophylaxis. A similar approach to the prevention of recurrences of glomerulonephritis is debatable but may be indicated during childhood when there is a suspicion that repeated streptococcal infections coincide with flare-ups of acute glomerulonephritis.

B. General Measures: Analgesic lozenges or gargles with 30% glucose or warm saline solution may be used for relief of sore throat. A soft, bland diet that includes noncarbonated high-glucose drinks (such as apple, grape, and pear juice) and iced milk or sherbet is helpful. Acetaminophen is useful for pain or fever.

With impetigo, local treatment may promote earlier healing. Crusts should first be soaked off; areas beneath the crusts should then be washed with soap daily.

C. Treatment of Complications: Acute complications are best treated with penicillin. Rheumatic fever is best prevented by early and adequate penicillin treatment of the streptococcal infection (see above).

D. Treatment of Carriers: Identification and management of group A streptococcal carriers is difficult. There are no established clinical or serologic criteria for differentiating carriers from the truly infected. Some children receive multiple courses of antimicrobials, with persistence of group A streptococci in the throat, leading to a "streptococcal neurosis" on the part of families.

Clindamycin (20 mg/kg/d in four divided doses) given orally or a combination of rifampin (20 mg/kg/d for 4 days) given orally and penicillin in standard dosage given orally has been used to improve bacteriologic cure rates after streptococcal pharyngitis and may be useful in selected streptococcal carriers.

Prognosis

Death is rare except in infants or young children with sepsis or pneumonia. The febrile course is shortened and complications eliminated by early and adequate treatment with penicillin.

Bisno AL, Stevens DL: Streptococcal infections of skin and soft tissues. N Engl J Med 1996;334:240.

Dajani A et al: Treatment of acute streptococcal pharyngitis and prevention of rheumatic fever: A statement for health professionals. Pediatrics 1995;96:758.

Kaplan EL: Clinical guidelines for group A streptococcal throat infections. Lancet 1997;350:899.

Moses AE et al: Increased incidence and severity of *Streptococcus pyogenes* bacteremia in young children. Pediatr Infect Dis J 1995;14:767.

Orrling A et al: Clindamycin in persisting streptococcal pharyngotonsillitis after penicillin treatment. Scand J Infect Dis 1994;26:535.

Shiffman RN: Guideline maintenance and revision: 50 years of the Jones criteria for diagnosis of rheumatic fever. Arch Pediatr Adolesc Med 1995;149:727.

Shulman ST et al: Streptococcal pharyngitis: The case for penicillin. Pediatr Infect Dis J 1994;13:1.

Veasy LG, Hill HR: Immunologic and clinical correlations in rheumatic fever and rheumatic heart disease. Pediatr Infect Dis J 1997;16:400.

GROUP B STREPTOCOCCAL INFECTIONS

Essentials of Diagnosis & Typical Features

Early-onset neonatal infection:

- Newborn, birth to 7 days, with rapidly progressing overwhelming sepsis, with or without meningitis.
- Pneumonia with respiratory failure frequently present; chest x-ray resembles that seen in hyaline membrane disease.
- Leukopenia with a shift to the left.
- Blood or spinal fluid cultures growing group B streptococci.

Late-onset infection:

- Meningitis, sepsis, or other focal infection in a child 1–16 weeks old with spinal fluid or blood cultures growing group B streptococci.

General Considerations

Although most patients with group B streptococcal disease are infants under 3 months of age, cases are seen in infants 4–5 months of age. Serious infection also occurs in women with puerperal sepsis, in immunocompromised patients, in patients with cirrhosis and spontaneous peritonitis, and in diabetics with cellulitis. Group B streptococcal infections occur as frequently as gram-negative infections in the newborn period. Two distinct clinical syndromes distinguished by differing perinatal events, age at onset, and serotype of the infecting strain occur in these infants.

Clinical Findings

Early-onset illness is observed in newborns less than 7 days old. The onset of symptoms in the majority of these infants occurs in the first 48 hours of life, and most are ill within 6 hours. Apnea is often the first sign. There is a high incidence of associated maternal obstetric complications, especially premature labor and prolonged rupture of the membranes. Newborns with early-onset disease are severely ill at the time of diagnosis, and more than 50% die. Although most infants with early-onset infections are full-term, premature infants are at increased risk for the disease. Newborns with early-onset infection acquire group B streptococci in utero as an ascending infection or during passage through the birth canal. When early-onset infection is complicated by meningitis, as occurs in approximately 30% of cases, more than 80% of the bacterial isolates belong to serotype III. Postmortem examination of infants with early-onset disease almost always reveals pulmonary inflammatory infiltrates and hyaline membranes containing large numbers of group B streptococci.

Late-onset infection occurs in infants between 7 days and 4 months of age; the median age at onset is about 4 weeks. Maternal obstetric complications are infrequently associated with late-onset infection. These infants are usually not as severely ill at the time of diagnosis as those with early-onset disease, and the mortality rate is significantly lower. In recent series, about 37% of patients have meningitis and 46% have sepsis. Other clinical manifestations, such as septic arthritis and osteomyelitis, "occult" bacteremia, otitis media, ethmoiditis, conjunctivitis, cellulitis (particularly of the face or submandibular area), lymphadenitis, breast abscess, empyema, and impetigo, have been described. Strains of group B streptococci possessing the capsular type III polysaccharide antigen are isolated from more than 95% of infants with late-onset disease, regardless of clinical manifestations. The exact mode of transmission of the organisms is not well defined.

Type III group B streptococci that cause neonatal disease are genetically closely related. Dissemination of a clone of high virulence in neonates is responsible for the increase in cases reported from many nurseries in the 1970s and 1980s.

Diagnosis

Culture of group B streptococci from a normally sterile site such as blood or cerebrospinal fluid provides proof of diagnosis. Frequent false-positive results limit the usefulness of testing for group B streptococcal antigen.

Prevention

Many women of childbearing age possess circulating antibody to the polysaccharide antigen of type III group B streptococci. This antibody is transferred to the newborn via the placental circulation. Carriers delivering healthy infants have significant serum levels of IgG antibody to this antigen. In contrast, women delivering infants who develop type III group B streptococcal disease of either the early- or late-onset type rarely have detectable antibody in their sera. Similar findings have recently been described for type Ia infections.

A vaccine prepared with type III polysaccharide has been evaluated in pregnant women. Although the vaccine is not optimally immunogenic, 63% of mothers produced IgG antibody.

The American Academy of Pediatrics and the

American College of Obstetrics and Gynecology, in cooperation with Centers for Disease Control, have developed two equally acceptable approaches to prevention of early-onset group B streptococcal disease.

In the approach based on risk factors, women are given intrapartum penicillin if one or more risk factors are present. The risk factors are (1) a previously delivered infant with invasive group B streptococcal disease, (2) group B streptococcal disease, (3) group B streptococcal bacteriuria during pregnancy, (4) delivery at less than 37 weeks of gestation, (5) rupture of the membranes greater than 18 hours, and (6) intrapartum temperature ≥ 38 °C.

In the approach based on screening, women with one or more of the risk factors numbered (1) to (3) above are given penicillin during delivery. All other women are screened at 34–36 weeks for group B streptococcal colonization by obtaining rectal and lower vaginal cultures using a selective broth media. If the culture is positive, intrapartum penicillin is offered. If the culture result is unknown or unavailable and if the intrapartum temperature is ≥ 38 °C or if rupture of membranes greater than 18 hours is present, then intrapartum penicillin is given.

The risk factor approach is preferred by some because it is simpler and cheaper. The screening approach should theoretically prevent more cases of neonatal group B streptococcal disease. Sufficient comparative studies of the cost, practicality and efficacy of these two approaches are not available.

Treatment

Penicillin G is the drug of choice. Group B streptococci are less susceptible than other streptococci to penicillin, and high doses are recommended, especially for meningitis (at least 250,000 units/kg/d, given in three doses per day to infants less than 1 week old and in four doses per day to older infants). Aminoglycosides act synergistically with penicillin in vitro; for this reason, both penicillin and gentamicin should be used for meningitis and other serious infections. Penicillin dosage for nonmeningeal infections is 50,000 units/kg/d (in divided doses every 12 hours) for infants less than 1 week old and 75,000–100,000 units/kg/d (in divided doses every 8 hours) for older infants. Duration of therapy is 3 weeks for meningitis, at least 4 weeks for osteomyelitis or endocarditis, and 10–14 days for other infections. Therapy does not eradicate carriage of the organism. Ceftriaxone is active in vitro against group B streptococci, and because of its long serum half-life it may be given once or twice daily intramuscularly or intravenously. Ceftriaxone is sometimes used to complete a course of therapy when intravenous access has become difficult. Ceftriaxone is usually not used in newborns because of associated cholestasis.

Baker CJ et al: Immunization of pregnant women with a polysaccharide vaccine of group B streptococcus. N Engl J Med 1988;319:1180.

Green PA et al: Recurrent group B streptococcal infections in infants: Clinical and microbiologic aspects. J Pediatr 1994;125:931.

Halsey NA et al: The 1997 AAP guidelines for prevention of early-onset group b streptococcal disease. Pediatrics 1997;100:383.

Hussain SM et al: Invasive group B streptococcal disease in children beyond infancy. Pediatr Infect Dis J 1995; 14:278.

Katz V et al: Group B streptococci: Results of a protocol of antepartum screening and intrapartum treatment. Am J Obstet Gynecol 1994;170:521.

Perkins MD, Mirrett S, Reller LB: Rapid bacterial antigen detection is not clinically useful. J Clin Microbiol 1995;33:1486.

STREPTOCOCCAL INFECTIONS WITH ORGANISMS OTHER THAN GROUP A OR B

Streptococci of groups other than A and B are part of the normal flora of humans and can cause disease. Group C or G organisms occasionally produce pharyngitis (with an ASO rise) but without risk of subsequent rheumatic fever, though acute glomerulonephritis may occasionally occur. Group D streptococci and *Enterococcus* species are normal inhabitants of the gastrointestinal tract and may produce urinary tract infections, meningitis and sepsis in the newborn, and endocarditis. Nosocomial infections caused by *Enterococcus* are frequent in neonatal and oncology units. Nonhemolytic aerobic streptococci and α-hemolytic streptococci are normal flora of the mouth. They are involved in the production of dental plaque and probably dental caries and are the most common cause of subacute infective endocarditis. Finally, there are numerous anaerobic and microaerophilic streptococci, normal flora of the mouth, skin, and gastrointestinal tract, which alone or in combination with other bacteria may cause sinusitis, dental abscesses, brain abscesses, and intra-abdominal or lung abscesses.

Treatment

A. Enterococcal Infections: Urinary tract infections can be treated with oral amoxicillin alone. Sepsis or meningitis in the newborn should be treated intravenously with a combination of ampicillin (100–200 mg/kg/d in three divided doses) and gentamicin (6–7.5 mg/kg/d in three divided doses). Endocarditis requires 4–6 weeks of intravenous treatment. Penicillin G (250,000 units/kg/d in six to eight divided doses) plus streptomycin (30 mg/kg/d) or gentamicin (6–7.5 mg/kg/d in three divided doses) is most often used. Third-generation cephalosporins are not effective. Ampicillin-resistant enterococci are usually susceptible to vancomycin (40–60 mg/kg/d in four divided doses). Careful monitoring of aminoglycoside levels is required, both to avoid toxicity and to ensure therapeutic levels.

Whenever endocarditis is being treated, peak and trough serum killing powers should be obtained. A bactericidal level of 1:8 or greater immediately before the next antibiotic dose should be maintained.

High-level resistance to aminoglycosides (MIC > 1000 μg/mL) is an increasing problem in many hospitals. Vancomycin-resistant enterococci are a serious problem in many hospitals. Patients with serious enterococcal infections require consultation with infectious disease experts and with the clinical microbiology laboratory to determine the optimal combination of antimicrobials.

B. Viridans Streptococcal Infections (Subacute Infective Endocarditis): It is important to determine the penicillin sensitivity of the infecting strain as early as possible in the treatment of viridans streptococcal endocarditis. Resistant organisms are most commonly seen in patients receiving chronic penicillin prophylaxis for rheumatic heart disease. Strains sensitive to penicillin G (MIC < 0.1 μg/μL) may be treated for 4 weeks with penicillin, 150,000–200,000 units/kg/d intravenously, with gentamicin added during the first 2 weeks. There is considerable experience with 2-week therapy in adult patients using penicillin and gentamicin. Similarly, excellent results have been obtained with ceftriaxone once daily for 4 weeks. If the MIC is 0.5 μg/mL or higher, longer therapy and higher doses of penicillin G must be used (200,000–300,000 units/kg/d intravenously in combination with streptomycin or gentamicin for 4–6 weeks). If the MIC is 0.1–0.5 μg/mL, penicillin G at the higher dose for a minimum of 4 weeks is recommended, with gentamicin added for the first 2 weeks. Vancomycin, 40 mg/kg/d, is usually preferred for resistant strains and patients allergic to penicillin.

Murray BE: What can we do about vancomycin-resistant enterococci? (Editorial Response.) Clin Infect Dis 1995;20:1134.

Norris AN et al: Chloramphenicol for vancomycin-resistant enterococcal infections. Clin Infect Dis 1995;20:1137.

Rice LB, Shales DM: Vancomycin resistance in the *Enterococcus*: Relevance in Pediatrics. Pediatr Clin North Am 1995;42:601.

Shay, DK, Goldmann DA, Jarvis WR: Reducing the spread of antimicrobial-resistant microorganisms. Pediatr Clin North Am 1995;42:703.

Wilson WR et al: Antibiotic treatment of adults with infective endocarditis due to streptococci, enterococci, staphylococci, and HACEK microorganisms. JAMA 1995;274:1706.

PNEUMOCOCCAL INFECTIONS

Essentials of Diagnosis
& Typical Features

Bacteremia:
- High fever (≥ 39.4 °C).

- Leukocytosis (≥ 15,000/μL).
- Age 6–24 months.

Pneumonia:
- Fever, leukocytosis, and tachypnea.
- Localized chest pain.
- Localized or diffuse rales. Chest x-ray may show lobar infiltrate (with effusion).

Meningitis:
- Fever, leukocytosis.
- Bulging fontanelle, neck stiffness.
- Irritability and lethargy.

All types:
- Diagnosis confirmed by cultures of blood, spinal fluid, pleural fluid, or other body fluid.

General Considerations

Pneumococcal sepsis, sinusitis, otitis media, pneumonitis, meningitis, osteomyelitis, cellulitis, arthritis, vaginitis, and peritonitis are all part of a spectrum of pneumococcal infection. Clinical findings that correlate with occult bacteremia in ambulatory patients include age (6–24 months), degree of temperature elevation (≥ 39.4 °C), and leukocytosis (≥ 15,000/μL). Although each of these findings is in itself nonspecific, a combination of them should arouse suspicion. This constellation of findings in a child who has no focus of infection may be an indication for blood cultures and antibiotic therapy. The cause of most of such bacteremic episodes is pneumococci.

Streptococcus pneumoniae is the most common cause of acute purulent otitis media.

Pneumococci are the organisms responsible for most cases of acute bacterial pneumonia in children. The disease is indistinguishable on clinical grounds from other bacterial pneumonias. Effusions are common, though frank empyema is less common. Abscesses also occasionally occur.

Pneumococcal meningitis is more common than *H influenzae* type b meningitis because of widespread vaccination. Pneumococcal meningitis, sometimes recurrent, may complicate serious head trauma, particularly if there is persistent leakage of cerebrospinal fluid. This has led some physicians to recommend the prophylactic administration of penicillin or other antimicrobials in such cases.

Children with sickle cell disease, other hemoglobinopathies, congenital or acquired asplenia, and some immunoglobulin and complement deficiencies are unusually susceptible to overwhelming pneumococcal sepsis and meningitis. These children often have a catastrophic illness with shock and disseminated intravascular coagulation. Even with excellent supportive care, the mortality rate is 20–50%. The spleen is important in the control of pneumococcal infection by clearing organisms from the blood and producing an opsonin that enhances phagocytosis. Autosplenectomy may explain why children with sickle cell disease are at increased risk for developing serious pneumococcal infections.

S pneumoniae rarely causes serious disease in the neonate. Although *S pneumoniae* does not normally colonize the vagina, transient colonization does occur. Serious neonatal disease—including pneumonia, sepsis, and meningitis—may occur and clinically is similar to group B streptococcal infection.

For more than 30 years, penicillin has been the agent of choice for pneumococcal infections. Many strains are still highly susceptible to penicillin; however, there have been increasing reports of pneumococci with moderately increased resistance to penicillin and reports of treatment failure, particularly in meningitis. The prevalence of these relatively penicillin-resistant strains in North America varies from 3% to 35%. Pneumococci with high-level resistance to penicillin and multiple other drugs are increasingly encountered throughout the United States. Pneumococci from normally sterile body fluids should be screened routinely for susceptibility to penicillin as well as other drugs.

Pneumococci have been classified into 83 serotypes based on capsular polysaccharide antigens. Serotypes 6, 14, 18, 19, and 23 cause most pneumococcal infections in children. The frequency distribution of serotypes varies at different times, in different geographic areas, and with different sites of infection. The most recently developed polyvalent pneumococcal vaccine contains capsular polysaccharides of 23 serotypes and is discussed in Chapter 9. Specific antibody induced by the vaccine protects only against the serotypes included in the vaccine. Children under age 18–24 months generally do not have a good antibody response to this vaccine, and the protective efficacy of the vaccine in older children is controversial. Despite these limitations, the vaccine is recommended for high-risk children over 2 years of age. The successful development of conjugate vaccines that protect against *H influenzae* type b has spurred the development of protein-polysaccharide conjugates to protect against pneumococci.

Clinical Findings

A. Symptoms and Signs: In pneumococcal sepsis, fever usually appears abruptly, often accompanied by chills. There may be no respiratory symptoms. In pneumococcal sinusitis, mucopurulent nasal discharge may occur. In infants and young children with pneumonia, fever, and tachypnea without auscultatory changes are the usual presenting signs. Respiratory distress is manifested by flaring of the alae nasi, chest retractions, and tachypnea. Abdominal pain is common. In older children, the adult form of pneumococcal pneumonia with signs of lobar consolidation may occur, but sputum is rarely bloody. Thoracic pain resulting from pleural involvement is sometimes present, but less often in children than in adults. With involvement of the right hemidiaphragm, pain may be referred to the right lower quadrant, suggesting appendicitis. Vomiting is common at onset but seldom persists. Convulsions are relatively common at onset in infants.

Meningitis is characterized by fever, irritability, convulsions, and neck stiffness. The most important sign in very young infants is a tense, bulging anterior fontanelle. In older children, fever, chills, headache, and vomiting are common symptoms. Classic signs are nuchal rigidity associated with positive Brudzinski and Kernig signs. With progression of untreated disease, the child may develop opisthotonos, stupor, and coma.

B. Laboratory Findings: Leukocytosis is often pronounced ($20{,}000$–$45{,}000/\mu L$), with 80–90% polymorphonuclear neutrophils. Neutropenia may be seen early in very serious infections. The presence of pneumococci in the nasopharynx is not a helpful finding, because up to 40% of normal children carry pneumococci in the upper respiratory tract. Large numbers of organisms are seen on gram-stained smears of endotracheal aspirates from patients with pneumonia. In meningitis, cerebrospinal fluid usually shows an elevated white cell count of several thousand, chiefly polymorphonuclear neutrophils, with decreased glucose and elevated protein levels. Gram-positive diplococci are seen on stained smears of cerebrospinal fluid sediment in 70–90% of cases in young children but are positive in only 50–65% of adolescents and adults. Antigen detection tests are not useful.

Differential Diagnosis

There are many causes of high fever and leukocytosis in young infants; 90% of children presenting with these signs have a disease other than pneumococcal bacteremia, such as herpesvirus 6, enterovirus, or other viral infection, urinary tract infection, unrecognized focal infection elsewhere in the body, or early acute shigellosis (diarrhea will appear later).

Infants with upper respiratory tract infection who subsequently develop signs of lower respiratory disease are most likely to be infected with a respiratory virus. Hoarseness or wheezing is often present. X-ray of the chest typically shows perihilar infiltrates and increased bronchovascular markings. It must be remembered, however, that viral respiratory infection often precedes pneumococcal pneumonia and that the clinical picture may be mixed.

Staphylococcal pneumonia frequently causes cavities and empyema, but it may be indistinguishable early in its course from pneumococcal pneumonia. It is most common in infants.

In primary pulmonary tuberculosis, children are not toxic, and x-rays show a primary focus associated with hilar adenopathy and often with pleural involvement. Miliary tuberculosis presents a classic x-ray appearance.

Pneumonia caused by *Mycoplasma pneumoniae* is most common in children 5 years of age and older. Onset is insidious, with infrequent chills, low-grade fever, prominent headache and malaise, cough, and, often, striking x-ray changes. Marked leukocytosis (eg, > 18,000/μL) is unusual.

Pneumococcal meningitis is diagnosed by lumbar puncture. Without a gram-stained smear and culture of spinal fluid, it is not distinguishable from other types of acute bacterial meningitis.

Complications

Complications of sepsis include meningitis and osteomyelitis; complications of pneumonia include empyema, parapneumonic effusion, and, rarely, lung abscess. Mastoiditis, subdural empyema, and brain abscess may follow untreated pneumococcal otitis media. Both pneumococcal meningitis and peritonitis are more likely to occur independently without coexisting pneumonia. Shock, disseminated intravascular coagulation, and Waterhouse-Friderichsen syndrome resembling meningococcemia are occasionally seen in pneumococcal sepsis, particularly in asplenic patients. Hemolytic-uremic syndrome may be seen as a complication of pneumococcal pneumonia or sepsis.

Treatment

A. Specific Measures: All *S pneumoniae* isolated from normally sterile sites should be tested for susceptibility to penicillin. Susceptible strains should be treated with penicillin or amoxicillin. Absolute or relatively penicillin-resistant strains should be tested for susceptibility to cephalosporins, vancomycin, and selected other drugs. Therapy with penicillin, amoxicillin, or cephalosporins will usually succeed in cases of bacteremia or pneumonia despite the demonstration of resistance because serum levels in excess of the MIC can be achieved.

Therapy of meningitis, empyema, osteomyelitis, and endocarditis due to resistant *S pneumoniae* is more difficult, because penetration of antimicrobials to these sites is limited. Vancomycin and third-generation cephalosporins are indicated pending susceptibility test results.

1. Sepsis–Presumptive therapy of children under 2 years of age who present with fever and leukocytosis is controversial. Three to 5 percent of blood cultures will yield *S pneumoniae*. Many experts treat with ceftriaxone (50 mg/kg intramuscularly). In comparison to therapy with oral amoxicillin (50–75 mg/kg/d), fever and the need for hospitalization may be reduced. However, meningitis occurs with the same frequency despite the choice of presumptive therapy. The widespread treatment of young children with ceftriaxone has contributed significantly to resistance in *S pneumoniae*. All children with blood cultures that grow pneumococci must be reexamined as soon as possible. The child who has a focal infection such as meningitis or who appears septic should be admitted to the hospital and should receive parenteral antimicrobials. Only if the child is afebrile and appears well should management on an ambula-

tory basis be considered. If the physician is confident that close follow-up can be achieved, lumbar puncture is not mandatory.

2. Pneumonia–For infants, severely ill patients, and immunocompromised hosts, aqueous penicillin G is given (150,000–200,000 units/kg/d intravenously in four to six divided doses). Mild pneumonia may be treated with phenoxymethyl penicillin (50 mg/kg/d orally in four divided doses for 7–10 days). Erythromycin (40–50 mg/kg/d orally in two to four divided doses) is given to patients allergic to penicillin. Oral cephalosporins may be used.

3. Otitis media–Treat with oral ampicillin, amoxicillin, trimethoprim-sulfamethoxazole, or erythromycin-sulfisoxazole for 10 days.

4. Meningitis–Until bacteriologic confirmation and susceptibility testing are completed, vancomycin (60 mg/kg/d intravenously in four divided doses) and cefotaxime (200 mg/kg/d intravenously in four divided doses) or ceftriaxone (100 mg/kg/d intravenously) should be given. Corticosteroids (dexamethasone, 0.6 mg/kg/d in four divided doses for 2 days) are recommended by many as adjunctive therapy for pneumococcal meningitis, but they are controversial because they may reduce the entry of vancomycin into the cerebrospinal fluid. Repeated lumbar puncture at 24–48 hours is indicated to ensure sterility of the cerebrospinal fluid if dexamethasone is given or if resistant pneumococci are isolated. After bacteriologic confirmation of susceptibility, aqueous penicillin G (300,000 units/kg/d intravenously in six divided doses for 10–14 days) should be given. Third-generation cephalosporins are acceptable alternative therapy though more expensive.

B. General Measures: Supportive and symptomatic care is required.

Prognosis

In children, case fatality rates of less than 1% should be achieved except in meningitis, in which rates of 5–20% still prevail. The presence of large numbers of organisms without a prominent cerebrospinal fluid inflammatory response or meningitis due to a penicillin-resistant strain indicates a poor prognosis. Serious neurologic sequelae, particularly hearing loss, are frequent following pneumococcal meningitis.

Adcock PM, Paul RI, Marshall GS: Effect of urine latex agglutination tests on the treatment of children at risk for invasive bacterial infection. Pediatrics 1995;96:951.

American Academy of Pediatrics Committee on Infectious Diseases: Therapy for children with invasive pneumococcal infections. Pediatrics 1997;99:289.

Baraff LJ et al: Practice guideline for management of infants and children 0 to 36 months of age with fever without source. Pediatrics 1993;92:1.

Barnett E, Klein J: The problem of resistant bacteria for the management of acute otitis media. Pediatr Clin North Am 1995;42;509.

Kilpi T et al: Oral glycerol and intravenous dexamethasone in preventing neurologic and audiologic sequelae of childhood bacterial meningitis. Pediatr Infect Dis J 1995;14:270.

Kornelisse RF et al: Pneumococcal meningitis in children: Prognostic indicators and outcome. Clin Infect Dis 1995;21:1390.

Schreiber JR, Jacobs MR: Antibiotic-resistant pneumococci. Pediatr Clin North Am 1995;42:519.

Schuchat A et al: Bacterial meningitis in the United States in 1995. N Engl J Med 1997;337:970.

Tuomanen EI, Austrian R, Masure HR: Pathogenesis of pneumococcal infections. N Engl J Med 1995;332:1280.

Wald EER et al: Dexamethasone therapy for children with bacterial meningitis. Pediatrics 1995;95:21.

STAPHYLOCOCCAL INFECTIONS

Staphylococcal infections are common and important in childhood. Staphylococcal skin infections range from minor furuncles to the varied syndromes now collectively referred to as "scalded skin syndrome." Staphylococci are the major cause of osteomyelitis and of septic arthritis. They are an uncommon but important cause of bacterial pneumonia. A toxin produced by certain strains causes staphylococcal food poisoning. Staphylococci are now responsible for most infections of artificial heart valves. They cause toxic shock syndrome (see below). Finally, they are found in infections at all ages and in multiple sites, particularly when infection is introduced from the skin or upper respiratory tract or when closed compartments become infected (pericarditis, sinusitis, cervical adenitis, surgical wounds, abscesses in the liver or brain, and abscesses elsewhere in the body).

Staphylococci, which do not produce the enzyme coagulase, are termed coagulase-negative but are seldom speciated in the clinical microbiology laboratory. Most *Staphylococcus aureus* strains produce coagulase. *S aureus* and coagulase-negative staphylococci are normal flora of the skin and respiratory tract. The latter rarely causes disease except in compromised hosts, the newborn, or patients with plastic indwelling lines.

Most strains of *S aureus* elaborate β-lactamase that confers penicillin resistance. This can be overcome in clinical practice by the use of a nonpenicillin antibiotic, a cephalosporin, or a penicillinase-resistant penicillin such as methicillin, oxacillin, nafcillin, cloxacillin, or dicloxacillin. Methicillin-resistant strains are found worldwide and are now common in certain hospitals and areas in the United States. Most of these strains retain β-lactamase production, and many are resistant to other antibiotics as well. Methicillin-resistant strains are also resistant in vivo to all of the penicillinase-resistant penicillins and cephalosporins. Strains with reduced susceptibility to vancomycin have been recovered in the United

States and Japan. This is of concern because of the inherent virulence of most strains of *S aureus* and because vancomycin is frequently the only effective antibiotic for methicillin-resistant strains.

S aureus produces a variety of exotoxins, most of which are of uncertain importance. Two toxins are recognized as playing a central role in specific diseases: exfoliatin and staphylococcal enterotoxin. The former is largely responsible for the various clinical presentations of the scalded skin syndrome. Most strains that elaborate exfoliatin are of phage group II. Enterotoxin causes staphylococcal food poisoning. The exoprotein toxin most commonly associated with toxic shock syndrome has been termed TSST-1. However, *S aureus* strains isolated from patients with toxic shock syndrome who have focal infections do not produce detectable TSST-1. Their organisms have been found to produce enterotoxins B or C, suggesting that the syndrome may be caused by more than one *S aureus* exoprotein.

Clinical Findings

A. Symptoms and Signs:

1. Staphylococcal skin diseases–Dermal infection with *S aureus* causes furuncles or cellulitis.

S aureus are often found along with streptococci in impetigo. If the strains produce exfoliatin, localized lesions become bullous (bullous impetigo).

Generalized exfoliative disease (scalded skin syndrome) is thought to result from systemic spread of exfoliatin. The infection may begin at any site but appears to be introduced through the respiratory tract in most cases. There is a prodromal phase of erythema, often beginning around the mouth, accompanied by fever and irritability. The involved skin becomes tender, and a sick infant will cry when picked up or touched. A day or so later, exfoliation begins, usually around the mouth. The inside of the mouth is red, and a peeling rash is present around the lips, often in a radial pattern resembling rhagades. Generalized, painful peeling may follow, involving the limbs and trunk but often sparing the feet. More commonly, peeling is confined to areas around body orifices. If erythematous but unpeeled skin is rubbed sideways, superficial epidermal layers separate from deeper ones and sloughs (Nikolsky's sign). In the newborn, the disease is termed Ritter's disease and may be fulminant. If there is tender erythema but not exfoliation, the disease is termed nonstreptococcal scarlet fever. The scarlatiniform rash is sandpaper-like, but strawberry tongue is not seen, and cultures grow *S aureus* rather than streptococci.

2. Osteomyelitis and septic arthritis–See Chapter 23.

3. Staphylococcal pneumonia–Staphylococcal pneumonia in infancy is characterized by abdominal distention, high fever, respiratory distress, and toxemia. It often occurs without predisposing factors or after minor skin infections. The organism is necrotizing, producing bronchoalveolar destruction. Pneumatoceles, pyopneumothorax, and empyema are frequently encountered. Rapid progression of disease is characteristic. Frequent chest x-rays to monitor the progress of disease are indicated. Presenting symptoms may be typical of paralytic ileus, suggestive of an abdominal catastrophe.

Staphylococcal pneumonia usually is peribronchial and diffuse and begins with a focal infiltrative lesion progressing to patchy consolidation. Most often only one lung is involved (80%), more often the right. Purulent pericarditis occurs by direct extension in about 10% of cases, with or without empyema.

4. Staphylococcal food poisoning–Staphylococcal food poisoning is produced by enterotoxin. The most common source is poorly refrigerated and contaminated food. The disease is characterized by vomiting, prostration, and diarrhea occurring 2–6 hours after ingestion of contaminated foods.

5. Staphylococcal endocarditis–*S aureus* may produce infection of normal heart valves, of valves or endocardium in children with congenital or rheumatic heart disease, or of artificial valves. About 25% of all cases of endocarditis are due to *S aureus*. The great majority of artificial heart valve infections involve either *S aureus* or coagulase-negative staphylococci. Infection usually begins in an extracardiac focus, often the skin. Involvement of the endocardium must be suspected in every case of *S aureus* bacteremia, regardless of initial signs. Suspicion must be highest in the presence of congenital heart disease, particularly ventricular septal defects with aortic insufficiency but also simple ventricular septal defect, patent ductus arteriosus, and tetralogy of Fallot.

The presenting symptoms in staphylococcal endocarditis are fever, weight loss, weakness, muscle pain or diffuse skeletal pain, poor feeding, pallor, and cardiac decompensation. Signs include splenomegaly, cardiomegaly, petechiae, hematuria, and a new or changing murmur. The course of *S aureus* endocarditis is rapid, though subacute disease is occasionally seen. Peripheral septic embolization and uncontrollable cardiac failure are common, even when optimal antibiotic therapy is administered, and may be indications for surgical intervention (see below).

6. Toxic shock syndrome–Toxic shock syndrome is characterized by fever, blanching erythroderma, diarrhea, vomiting, myalgia, prostration, hypotension, and multiple organ dysfunction. It is due to *S aureus* focal infection without bacteremia. Large numbers of cases have been described in menstruating adolescents and young women using vaginal tampons. Toxic shock syndrome has also been seen in both boys and girls with focal staphylococcal infections as well as in individuals with postoperative wound infections due to *S aureus*. Additional clinical features include sudden onset; conjunctival suffusion; mucosal hyperemia; desquamation of skin on the palms, soles, fingers, and toes during convalescence; disseminated intravascular coagulation in severe cases; renal and hepatic functional abnormalities; and evidence of myolysis. The mortality rate with early treatment is now about 2%. Recurrences were seen during subsequent menstrual periods in as many as 60% of untreated women who continued to use tampons. Recurrences were reported in up to 15% of those who were treated with antistaphylococcal antibiotics and stopped using tampons. The disease is caused by strains of *S aureus* that produce TSST-1 or one of the related enterotoxins.

7. Coagulase-negative staphylococcal infections–Localized and systemic coagulase-negative staphylococcal infections occur primarily in immunocompromised patients, high-risk newborns, and patients with plastic prostheses or catheters. In low-birth-weight infants, coagulase-negative staphylococci are the commonest nosocomial pathogen in nurseries in the United States. Intravenous administration of lipid emulsions and indwelling central venous catheters are risk factors contributing to coagulase-negative staphylococcal bacteremia in newborn infants. In patients with an artificial heart valve, Dacron patch, ventriculoperitoneal shunt for hydrocephalus, or a Hickman or Broviac vascular catheter, coagulase-negative staphylococci are a common cause of sepsis or catheter infection, often necessitating removal of the foreign material and protracted antibiotic therapy. Because blood cultures are frequently contaminated by this organism, diagnosis of genuine localized or systemic infection is often difficult or uncertain.

B. Laboratory Findings: Moderate leukocytosis (15,000–20,000/μL) with a shift to the left is occasionally found, though normal counts are common, particularly in infants. The sedimentation rate is elevated. Blood cultures are frequently positive in systemic staphylococcal disease and should always be obtained when it is suspected. Similarly, pus from sites of infection should always be aspirated or obtained surgically, examined with Gram's stain, and cultured both aerobically and anaerobically.

There are no useful serologic tests for staphylococcal disease.

Differential Diagnosis

Staphylococcal skin disease has many morphologic forms and therefore many differential diagnoses. Bullous impetigo must be differentiated from chemical or thermal burns, from drug reactions, and, in the very young, from the various congenital epidermolytic syndromes or even herpes simplex infections. Staphylococcal scalded skin syndrome resembles scarlet fever in some instances and in others appears similar to Kawasaki disease, Stevens-Johnson syndrome, erythema multiforme, and other drug reactions. A skin biopsy may be critical in establish-

ing the correct diagnosis. The skin lesions of varicella may become superinfected with exfoliatin-pro-
ducing staphylococci and produce a combination of
the two diseases (bullous varicella).

Osteomyelitis of the long bones and septic arthritis
must often be differentiated (see Chapter 23).

Severe, rapidly progressing pneumonia is typical
of *S aureus* infection and group A streptococci but
may occasionally be produced by pneumococci. Abscesses and pneumatoceles may be seen in pneumonia due to pneumococci, *Haemophilus influenzae,*
and group A streptococci. Empyema formation occurs with all bacterial pneumonias.

Staphylococcal food poisoning is often epidemic. It
is differentiated from other common-source gastroenteritis syndromes (*Salmonella, Clostridium perfringens, Vibrio parahaemolyticus*) by the short incubation period (2–6 hours), the prominence of vomiting
(as opposed to diarrhea), and the absence of fever.

Endocarditis must be suspected in any instance of
S aureus bacteremia, particularly when there is a significant heart murmur or preexisting cardiac disease
(see Chapter 18).

Newborn infections with *S aureus* can resemble
infections with streptococci and a variety of gram-
negative organisms. Umbilical and respiratory tract
colonization occurs with many pathogenic organisms
(group B streptococci, *Escherichia coli, Klebsiella*),
and both skin and systemic infections occur with virtually all of these.

Toxic shock syndrome must be differentiated from
Rocky Mountain spotted fever, leptospirosis, Kawa-
saki disease, drug reactions, adenovirus, and measles.
(See also Table 34–3.)

Treatment

A. Specific Measures: Since 85% of *S aureus*
strains are penicillin-resistant, it is important to use a
β-lactamase-resistant penicillin as the first drug in
treatment. In serious systemic disease, in osteomyelitis, and in the treatment of large abscesses,
intravenous therapy is indicated initially (oxacillin or
nafcillin, 100–200 mg/kg/d in four divided doses, or
methicillin, 200–300 mg/kg/d in four divided doses).
When high doses over a long period are required, it is
preferable not to use methicillin, because of the frequency with which interstitial nephritis is seen. In
life-threatening illness, an aminoglycoside antibiotic
(gentamicin or tobramycin) or rifampin may be used
in addition for its possible synergistic action. If *S aureus* is penicillin-sensitive, penicillin G may be used
for treatment.

When children with established penicillin sensitivity are treated, cephalosporins may be used (cefazolin, 100–150 mg/kg/d intravenously in three divided doses; or cephalexin, 50–100 mg/kg/d orally
in four divided doses). The third-generation cephalosporins should not generally be used for staphylococcal infections.

For methicillin-resistant infections, vancomycin
(40 mg/kg/d intravenously in three or four divided
doses) should be used. Infections due to methicillin-
resistant staphylococci frequently do not respond to
cephalosporins despite in vitro testing that suggests
susceptibility. For treatment of meningitis, vancomycin must be given in higher doses (60 mg/kg/d
divided into four doses). Combinations including
rifampin may be either synergistic or antagonistic.

1. Skin infections–See Chapter 13.

2. Osteomyelitis and septic arthritis–Treatment should be begun intravenously, with antibiotics
selected to cover the most likely organisms (staphylococci in hematogenous osteomyelitis; meningococci, pneumococci, staphylococci in children with
septic arthritis under the age of 3 years; staphylococci and gonococci in arthritis in older children).
Antibiotic levels should be kept high at all times.

In osteomyelitis, clinical studies support the use of
intravenous treatment until fever and local symptoms
and signs have subsided—usually after at least 1
week—followed by oral therapy (dicloxacillin,
100–150 mg/kg/d in four divided doses; or cephalexin, 100–150 mg/kg/d in four divided doses) for at
least 3 additional weeks. Longer treatment may be
required, particularly when x-rays show extensive involvement. In arthritis, where drug diffusion into
synovial fluid is good, intravenous therapy need be
given only for a few days, followed by adequate oral
therapy for at least 3 weeks. In all instances, oral
therapy should be administered under careful supervision, either in the hospital or at home with frequent
support and reinforcement from physicians or visiting nurses. Monitoring serum bactericidal concentrations is recommended by some experts, but has not
been proved necessary in all cases. The erythrocyte
sedimentation rate is a good indicator of response to
therapy. Surgical drainage of osteomyelitis or septic
arthritis is often required (see Chapter 23).

3. Staphylococcal pneumonia–Antibiotic
therapy should consist of a parenteral penicillinase-
resistant penicillin with or without an aminoglycoside. Empyema or pyopneumothorax require chest
tube drainage. The tube should be removed as soon
as drainage has become clinically insignificant. If
staphylococcal pneumonia is promptly treated and
empyema promptly drained, resolution in children is
almost always complete—despite evidence of widespread parenchymal destruction and the persistence
of bullae, blebs, and even pockets of empyema or abscess fluid well into convalescence. Surgical decortication or segmental resection is usually not required.

4. Staphylococcal food poisoning–Therapy
is supportive and usually not required except in severe cases or for small infants with marked dehydration.

5. Staphylococcal endocarditis–As outlined
above, high-dose, prolonged, parenteral treatment
with oxacillin, nafcillin, or methicillin plus genta-

micin or tobramycin is indicated. In penicillin-allergic patients, vancomycin should be used. With penicillin-sensitive organisms, penicillin G is the drug of choice. Therapy lasts in all instances for at least 6 weeks.

In some patients, medical treatment may fail. Signs of this are (1) recurrent fever without apparent treatable other cause (eg, thrombophlebitis, incidental respiratory or urinary tract infection, drug fever), (2) persistently positive blood cultures, (3) intractable and progressive congestive heart failure, and (4) recurrent (septic) embolization. In such circumstances—particularly (2), (3), and (4)—valve replacement becomes necessary. Antibiotics are continued for at least another 4 weeks. Persistent or recurrent infection may require a second surgical procedure.

6. Toxic shock syndrome–Treatment is first with volume expansion and inotropic agents and later with oxacillin, nafcillin, or cephalosporins. If a tampon is in place, it should be removed. All focal staphylococcal infections should be drained without delay. Some experts feel that corticosteroid therapy may be effective if given to patients with severe illness early in the course of their disease. Antibiotic treatment reduces risk of recurrence.

7. Coagulase-negative staphylococcal infections–Bacteremia and other serious coagulase-negative staphylococcal infections are treated initially with vancomycin. Coagulase-negative staphylococci are uncommonly resistant to vancomycin (see Chapter 34 for dosing). Strains susceptible to penicillin or oxacillin are treated with those agents.

B. General Measures: Localized pus should be drained. Oxygen, intravenous fluids, and other supportive care are indicated in staphylococcal pneumonia and other systemic infections. Blood transfusion may be indicated if the patient is severely anemic.

Prognosis

Septicemia, endocarditis, and widespread pneumonitis in infancy all have a serious prognosis. Infants and children who recover from serious staphylococcal pneumonia have a good long-term prognosis without development of chronic respiratory disease. Osteomyelitis is never fatal if promptly treated.

Baltimore RS: Infective endocarditis in children. Pediatr Infect Dis J 1992;11:907.

Bamberger DM: Outcome of medical treatment of bacterial abscesses without therapeutic drainage: Review of cases reported in the literature. Clin Infect Dis 1996;23:592.

Choux M et al: Shunt implantation: Reducing the incidence of shunt infection. J Neurosurg 1992;77:875.

Dagan R: Management of acute hematogenous osteomyelitis and septic arthritis in the pediatric patient. Pediatr Infect Dis J 1993;12:88.

Edmond MB, Wenzel RP, Pasculle AW: Vancomycin resistant *Staphylococcus aureus:* Perspectives on measures needed for control. Ann Intern Med 1996;124:329.

Freeman J et al: Extra hospital stay and antibiotic usage with nosocomial coagulase-negative staphylococcal bacteremia in two neonatal intensive care unit populations. Am J Dis Child 1990;144:324.

Friedland IR, du Plessis J, Cilliers A: Cardiac complications in children with *Staphylococcus aureus* bacteremia. J Pediatr 1995;127:746.

Lew DP, Waldvogel FA: Osteomyelitis. N Engl J Med 1997;336:999.

Moreira BM, Daum RS: Antimicrobial resistance in *Staphylococcus.* Pediatr Clin North Am 1995;42:619.

Raad II, Sabbagh MF: Optimal duration of therapy for catheter-related *Staphylococcus aureus* bacteremia: A study of 35 cases and review. Clin Infect Dis 1992; 14:75.

Tolan RW Jr et al: Operative intervention in active endocarditis in children: Report of a series of cases and review. Clin Infect Dis 1992;14:852.

Update: *Staphylococcus aureus* with reduced susceptibility to vancomycin—United States 1997. MMWR Morb Mortal Wkly Rep 1997;46:813.

Van Lierde S et al: Toxic shock syndrome without rash in a young child: Link with syndrome of hemorrhagic shock and encephalopathy? J Pediatr 1997;131:130.

MENINGOCOCCAL INFECTIONS

Essentials of Diagnosis & Typical Features

- Fever, headache, vomiting, convulsions, shock (meningitis).
- Fever, shock, petechial or purpuric skin rash (meningococcemia).
- Diagnosis confirmed by culture of normally sterile body fluids.

General Considerations

Meningococci may be carried asymptomatically for many months in the upper respiratory tract. Fewer than 1% of carriers develop disease. Meningitis and sepsis are the two commonest forms of illness, but septic arthritis, pericarditis, pneumonia, chronic meningococcemia, otitis media, conjunctivitis, and vaginitis also occur. The highest attack rate for meningococcal meningitis is in the first year of life. The incidence in the United States is about 1.2 cases per 100,000 people. There were nearly 3300 reported cases in 1995.

Meningococci are classified serologically into groups A, B, C, D, X, Y, Z, 29-E, and W-135. The serologic groups serve as specific markers for studying outbreaks and transmission of disease. Major epidemics of meningococcal disease in the United States prior to 1950 were caused by group A strains. In recent years, however, group A organisms have accounted for only about 2% of meningococcal isolates. Many small outbreaks of serotype C are reported. Serotype C now comprises about 45% of isolates; serotype B accounts for about 45% of isolates. Sulfonamide resistance is common in non-group A strains. *N meningitidis* with increased MICs to penicillin G are reported from South Africa and Spain. A small number of these isolates are reported in the United States; they are serotype B, but unrelated by molecular typing. The resistance in these strains is low-level and not due to β-lactamase. Resistant isolates are susceptible to third-generation cephalosporins. Few isolates are resistant to rifampin.

Children develop immunity from asymptomatic carriage of meningococci (usually nontypable, nonpathogenic strains) or other cross-reacting bacteria. Patients deficient in one of the late components of complement (C6, C7, or C8) are uniquely susceptible to meningococcal infection, particularly group A meningococci. Deficiencies of early and alternate pathway complement components are also associated with increased susceptibility.

Meningococci are gram-negative organisms containing endotoxin in their cell walls. Endotoxins may cause capillary vascular injury and leak and may also cause disseminated intravascular coagulation. The development of irreversible shock with multiple organ failure is a significant factor in the fatal outcome of acute meningococcal infections.

Vaccines prepared from purified meningococcal polysaccharides (A, C, Y, and W-135) are available for controlling outbreaks and preventing spread in special high-risk groups such as household contacts and military recruits. Unfortunately, the vaccines, except for the A component, are ineffective in children under 2 years of age (see Chapter 9).

Clinical Findings

A. Symptoms and Signs: Many children with clinical meningococcemia also have meningitis, and some may have other foci of infection. All children with suspected meningococcemia should have a lumbar puncture.

1. Meningococcemia—A prodrome of upper respiratory infection is followed by high fever, headache, nausea, marked toxicity, and hypotension. Purpura, petechiae, and occasionally bright pink, tender macules or papules over the extremities and trunk are seen. The rash usually progresses rapidly. Occasional cases lack rash.

Fulminant meningococcemia (Waterhouse-Friderichsen syndrome) progresses rapidly and is characterized by disseminated intravascular coagulation, massive skin and mucosal hemorrhages, and shock. This syndrome also may be due to *H influenzae, S pneumoniae,* or other bacteria.

Chronic meningococcemia is characterized by periodic bouts of fever, arthralgia or arthritis, and recurrent petechiae. Splenomegaly is often present. The patient may be free of symptoms between bouts. Chronic meningococcemia occurs primarily in adults and mimics Henoch-Schönlein purpura.

2. Meningitis—In many children, meningococcemia is followed within a few hours to several days by symptoms and signs of acute purulent meningitis, with severe headache, stiff neck, nausea, vomiting, and stupor. Children with meningitis generally fare better than children with meningococcemia alone, probably because they have survived long enough to develop clinical signs of meningitis.

B. Laboratory Findings: The peripheral white blood cell count may be either low or elevated. Thrombocytopenia may be present with or without disseminated intravascular coagulation (see Chapter 25). If petechial or hemorrhagic lesions are present, meningococci can sometimes be demonstrated on smear by puncturing the lesions and expressing a drop of tissue fluid. Organisms may be demonstrated by Gram's stain of buffy coat preparations of blood. The spinal fluid is generally cloudy and contains more than 1000 white cells/μL, with many polymorphonuclear cells and gram-negative intracellular diplococci.

A total hemolytic complement assay may reveal absence of late components as an underlying cause.

Differential Diagnosis

The skin lesions of *H influenzae* or pneumococci, enterovirus infection, endocarditis, leptospirosis, Rocky Mountain spotted fever, other rickettsial diseases, Henoch-Schönlein purpura, and blood dyscrasias, may be very similar to meningococcemia. Other causes of sepsis and meningitis are distinguished by appropriate Gram's stain and cultures. Most children with fever and petechial skin rash do not have meningococcemia, which increases the difficulty of clinical decision making.

Complications

Meningitis may lead to permanent central nervous system damage, with deafness, convulsions, paralysis, or impairment of intellectual function. Hydrocephalus may develop and requires ventriculo-peritoneal shunt. Subdural collections of fluid are common but usually resolve spontaneously. Extensive skin necrosis, loss of digits or extremities, intestinal hemorrhage, and late adrenal insufficiency may complicate fulminant meningococcemia.

Prevention

Household contacts, day care center contacts, and hospital personnel directly exposed to the respiratory secretions of patients are at increased risk of developing meningococcal infection and should be given chemoprophylaxis with rifampin. The secondary attack rate among household members is 1–5% during epidemics and less than 1% in nonepidemic situations. Children 3 months to 2 years of age are at greatest risk, presumably because they lack protective antibodies. Secondary cases are reported in day care centers and in some school classrooms. Hospital personnel are not at increased risk unless they have had contact with a patient's oral secretions, eg, during mouth-to-mouth resuscitation, intubation, or suctioning procedures. Approximately 50% of secondary cases in households have their onset within 24 hours of identification of the index case. Exposed contacts should be examined promptly. If they are febrile, they should be fully evaluated and treated with high doses of penicillin or another effective antimicrobial pending the results of blood cultures.

All intimate contacts should receive chemoprophylaxis with rifampin given orally in the following dosages twice daily for 2 days: 600 mg for adults, 10 mg/kg for children 1 month to 12 years of age, and 5 mg/kg for infants under 1 month of age. An alternative dosing schedule for rifampin is 20 mg/kg/d (maximum adult dose, 600 mg/d) once daily for 4 days. If the organism is sensitive to sulfonamides, sulfadiazine may be used. Penicillin and most other antibiotics (even with parenteral administration) are not effective chemoprophylactic agents, since they do not eradicate upper respiratory tract carriage of meningococci. Cephalosporins such as ceftriaxone intramuscularly and cefixime orally are effective for prophylaxis. Ciprofloxacin effectively eradicates nasopharyngeal carriage in adults and children but is not approved for use in children. Throat cultures to identify carriers are not useful. Meningococcal vaccine has been used increasingly for control of outbreaks. Patients with complement deficiencies should also be vaccinated.

Treatment

Blood cultures should be obtained for all children with fever and purpura or other signs of meningococcemia, and antibiotics should be administered immediately as an emergency procedure. There is a good correlation between survival rates and initiation of prompt antibiotic therapy. Purpura and fever should be considered a medical emergency.

Children with meningococcemia or meningococcal meningitis should be managed as though shock were imminent even if their vital signs are stable when they are first seen. If hypotension already is present, supportive measures should be aggressive, because the prognosis is grave in such situations. It is optimal to initiate treatment in an intensive care setting. Treatment should not be delayed for the sake of transporting the patient. Shock may worsen following antimicrobial therapy due to endotoxin release. To minimize the risk of nosocomial transmission, patients should be treated in respiratory isolation for the first 24 hours of antibiotic treatment.

A. Specific Measures: Antibiotics should be begun promptly. Since other bacteria, such as *S pneumoniae, S aureus,* or other gram-negative organisms, can cause identical syndromes, initial therapy should be broadly effective. Cefotaxime or ceftriaxone are preferred (see Chapter 33 for dosages). When the diagnosis is confirmed, penicillin G (250,000 units/kg/d in six doses) intravenously for 7 days is the drug of choice. Relative penicillin resistance is uncommon.

B. General Measures:

1. Cardiovascular–See Chapter 11 for management of septic shock. Corticosteroids are not beneficial. Sympathetic blockade and topically applied nitroglycerin have been used locally to improve perfusion.

2. Hematologic–Since hypercoagulability is frequently present in patients with meningococcemia, administration of heparin should be considered for patients with disseminated intravascular coagulation. A loading dose of 100 units/kg is followed by 15 units/kg/h as a continuous drip. The patient is monitored by following the partial thromboplastin time. Recombinant tissue plasminogen activator and concentrated antithrombin III have been tried experimentally to reverse coagulopathy. See Chapter 25 for the management of disseminated intravascular coagulation.

Prognosis

Unfavorable prognostic features include shock, disseminated intravascular coagulation, and extensive skin lesions. The case fatality rate in fulminant meningococcemia is over 50%. In uncomplicated meningococcal meningitis, the fatality rate is much lower (10–20%).

American Academy of Pediatrics, Committee on Infectious Diseases: Meningococcal disease prevention and control strategies for practice-based physicians. Pediatrics 1996;97:404.

Boyer D, Gordon RC, Baker T: Lack of clinical usefulness of a positive latex agglutination test for *Neisseria meningitidis/Escherichia coli* antigens in the urine. Pediatr Infect Dis J 1993;12:779.

Control and prevention of meningococcal disease and control and prevention of serogroup C meningococcal disease: Evaluation and management of suspected outbreaks. MMWR Morb Mortal Wkly Rep 1997;46:1.

Cuevas LE et al: Eradication of nasopharyngeal carriage of *Neisseria meningitidis* in children and adults in rural Africa: A comparison of ciprofloxacin and rifampicin. J Infect Dis 1995;171:728.

Jackson LA et al: Prevalence of *Neisseria meningitidis* relatively resistant to penicillin in the United States, 1991. J Infect Dis 1994;169:438.

Kornelisse RF et al: Meningococcal septic shock in children: Clinical and laboratory features, outcome, and development of a prognostic score. Clin Infect Dis 1997;25:640.

Mandt KD, Stack AM, Fleisher GR: Incidence of bacteremia in infants and children with fever and petechiae. J Pediatr 1997;131:398.

Reido FX, Plikaytis BD, Broome CV: Epidemiology and prevention of meningococcal disease. Pediatr Infect Dis J 1995;14:643.

Rivard GE et al: Treatment of purpura fulminans in meningococcemia with protein C concentrate. J Pediatr 1995;126:646.

Schlesinger M et al: Killing of meningococci by neutrophils: Effect of vaccination on patients with complement deficiency. J Infect Dis 1994;170:449.

Shay DK, Goldman DA, Jarvis WR: Reducing the spread of meningococcemia. Pediatrics 1995;96:144.

Zangwill KM et al: School-based clusters of meningococcal disease in the United States. JAMA 1997;277:389.

Zens W et al: Recombinant tissue plasminogen activator treatment in two infants with fulminant meningococcemia. Pediatrics 1995;96:144.

GONOCOCCAL INFECTIONS

Essentials of Diagnosis & Typical Features

- Purulent urethral discharge showing intracellular gram-negative diplococci on smear in male patient (usually adolescent).
- Purulent, edematous, sometimes hemorrhagic conjunctivitis showing intracellular gram-negative diplococci on smear in infant 2–4 days of age.
- Fever, arthritis (often polyarticular) or tenosynovitis, and maculopapular peripheral rash that may be vesiculopustular or hemorrhagic.
- Positive culture of blood or pharyngeal or genital secretions.

General Considerations

Neisseria gonorrhoeae is a gram-negative diplococcus. Although morphologically similar to other neisseriae, it differs in its ability to grow on selective media and to ferment carbohydrates. The cell wall of *N gonorrhoeae* contains endotoxin, which is liberated when the organism dies and is responsible for the production of a cellular exudate. The incubation period is short, usually 2–5 days.

Antimicrobial-resistant gonococci are now a serious problem. *N gonorrhoeae* is resistant to tetracyclines (20%), penicillins (22%), or both (5%). About 1.5% of strains are resistant to ciprofloxacin.

Gonococcal disease in children may be transmitted sexually or nonsexually. Prepubertal gonococcal infection outside the neonatal period should be considered presumptive evidence of sexual contact or child abuse. Prepubertal girls usually manifest gonococcal vulvovaginitis because of the neutral-alkaline pH of the vagina and thin vaginal mucosa.

In the adolescent or adult, the workup of every case of gonorrhea should include a careful and accurate inquiry into sexual practices, since pharyngeal infection must be detected if present and may be difficult to eradicate. In addition, efforts should be made to identify and treat all sexual contacts. When prepubertal children are infected, all family members should be cultured, and epidemiologic investigation should be thorough.

Clinical Findings

A. Symptoms and Signs:

1. Asymptomatic gonorrhea–The ratio of asymptomatic to symptomatic gonorrheal infections in adolescents and adults is probably 3–4:1 in women and 0.5–1:1 in men. Asymptomatic infections are considered as infectious as symptomatic ones.

2. Uncomplicated genital gonorrhea–

a. Male with urethritis–Urethral discharge is sometimes painful and bloody and may be white, yellow, or green. There may be associated dysuria. The patient is usually afebrile.

b. Prepubertal female with vaginitis–The only clinical findings initially may be dysuria and polymorphonuclear neutrophils in the urine. Vulvitis characterized by erythema, edema, and excoriation accompanied by a purulent discharge may follow.

c. Postpubertal female with cervicitis–Symptomatic disease is characterized by a purulent discharge, dysuria, and, occasionally, dyspareunia. Lower abdominal pain is absent. Physical examination reveals an afebrile patient with a yellow, foul-smelling discharge. The cervix is frequently hyperemic and tender when touched by the examining finger. This tenderness is not worsened by moving the cervix, nor are the adnexa tender to palpation.

d. Rectal gonorrhea–Rectal gonorrhea is often asymptomatic. There may be purulent discharge, edema, and pain during evacuation.

3. Pharyngeal gonorrhea–Pharyngeal involvement is usually asymptomatic. There may be some sore throat and, rarely, acute exudative tonsillitis with bilateral cervical lymphadenopathy and fever.

4. Conjunctivitis and iridocyclitis–Copious exudate is characteristic of gonococcal conjunctivitis. Newborns are symptomatic on days 2–4. In the adolescent or adult eye, infection probably is spread from infected genital secretions by the fingers.

5. Pelvic inflammatory disease (salpingitis)–The interval between initiation of genital infection and its ascent to the uterine tubes is variable and may range from days to months; menses frequently are the initiating factor. With the onset of a menstrual period, gonococci invade the endometrium, causing transient endometritis. Subsequently, salpingitis may occur, resulting in pyosalpinx or hydrosalpinx; rarely, it leads to peritonitis or perihepatitis. Gonococcal salpingitis occurs in an acute, subacute, or chronic form. All three forms have in common tenderness on gentle movement of the cervix and bilateral tubal tenderness during pelvic examination.

Gonococci or *Chlamydia trachomatis* are the cause of about 50% of cases of pelvic inflammatory disease. A mixed infection caused by enteric bacilli, *Bacteroides fragilis,* or other anaerobes occurs in the other 50%.

6. Gonococcal perihepatitis (Fitz-Hugh and Curtis syndrome)–In the typical clinical pattern, there is right upper quadrant tenderness in association with signs of acute or subacute salpingitis. Pain may be pleuritic and referred to the shoulder. Hepatic friction rub is a valuable but inconstant sign.

7. Disseminated gonorrhea–Dissemination follows asymptomatic more often than symptomatic genital infection and often results from gonococcal pharyngitis or anorectal gonorrhea. The most common form of disseminated gonorrhea is polyarthritis or polytenosynovitis, with or without dermatitis. Monarticular arthritis is less common, and gonococcal endocarditis and meningitis are fortunately rare.

a. Polyarthritis–Disease usually begins with the simultaneous onset of low-grade fever, polyarthralgia, and general malaise. After a day or so, the joint symptoms become acute, and swelling, redness, and tenderness occur, frequently over the wrists, ankles, and knees but also in the fingers, feet, and other peripheral joints. Skin lesions may be noted at the same time: individual, tender, evolving maculopapular lesions 5–8 mm in diameter that may become vesicular, pustular, and then hemorrhagic. They are few in number and noted on the fingers, palms, feet, and other distal surfaces and may be single or multiple. In patients with this form of the disease, blood cultures are often positive, but joint fluid rarely yields organisms. Skin lesions often are positive by Gram's stain but rarely by culture. Genital, rectal, and pharyngeal cultures must always be performed.

b. Monarticular arthritis–In this somewhat less common form of disseminated gonorrhea, fever is often absent. Arthritis evolves in a single joint. Dermatitis usually does not occur. Systemic symptoms are minimal. Blood cultures are negative, but joint aspirates may yield gonococci on smear and culture. Genital, rectal, and pharyngeal cultures must always be performed.

B. Laboratory Findings: Demonstration of gram-negative, kidney bean-shaped diplococci on smears of urethral exudate in males is presumptive evidence of gonorrhea. Positive culture confirms the diagnosis. Negative smears do not rule out gonorrhea. Gram-stained smears of cervical or vaginal discharge in girls are more difficult to interpret because of normal gram-negative flora, but they may be useful when technical personnel are experienced. In girls with suspected gonorrhea, both the cervical os and the anus should be cultured. Gonococcal pharyngitis requires culture for diagnosis.

Cultures for *N gonorrhoeae* are plated on a selective chocolate agar containing antibiotics (eg, Thayer-Martin agar) to suppress normal flora. If bacteriologic diagnosis is critical, suspected material should be cultured on chocolate agar as well. Since gonococci are labile, agar plates should be inoculated immediately and placed without delay in an atmosphere containing CO_2 (candle jar). When transportation is necessary, material should be directly inoculated into Transgrow medium prior to shipment to an appropriate laboratory. In cases of possible sexual molestation, notify the laboratory that definite speciation is needed, since nongonococcal *Neisseria* species can grow on the selective media.

All children or adolescents with a suspected or established diagnosis of gonorrhea should have serologic tests for syphilis and HIV.

Differential Diagnosis

Urethritis in the male may be gonococcal or "nonspecific." The latter is a syndrome characterized by discharge (rarely painful), mild dysuria, and a subacute course. The discharge is usually scant or moderate in amount but may be profuse. The responsible microorganisms cannot all be identified, but about half of cases are due to *C trachomatis*. The remainder are probably due to *Ureaplasma,* trichomonads, or other as yet unknown agents. Most cases respond to tetracycline therapy (500 mg orally four times a day for 7 days in adolescents). Single-dose azithromycin 1 g orally may achieve better compliance. *C trachomatis* has been shown to cause epididymitis in males and salpingitis in females.

Vulvovaginitis in a prepubertal female may be due to infection caused by miscellaneous bacteria, including *Shigella* and group A streptococci, *Candida,* and herpes simplex; discharges may be caused by trichomonads, *Enterobius vermicularis* (pinworm), or foreign bodies. Symptom-free discharge (leukorrhea) normally accompanies rising estrogen levels.

Cervicitis in a postpubertal female, alone or in association with urethritis and involvement of Skene's and Bartholin's glands, may be due to infection caused by *Candida,* herpes simplex, *Trichomonas,* or discharge resulting from inflammation caused by foreign bodies (usually some form of contraceptive device). Leukorrhea may be associated with birth control pills.

Salpingitis may be due to infection with other organisms. The symptoms must be differentiated from those of appendicitis, urinary tract infection, ectopic pregnancy, endometriosis, or ovarian cysts or torsion.

Disseminated gonorrhea presents a wide differential diagnosis that must include meningococcemia, acute rheumatic fever, Henoch-Schönlein purpura, juvenile rheumatoid arthritis, lupus erythematosus, leptospirosis, secondary syphilis, certain viral infections (particularly rubella, but also enteroviruses and parvovirus), serum sickness, type B hepatitis (in the prodromal phase), infective endocarditis, and even acute leukemia and other types of cancer. The fully evolved skin lesions of disseminated gonorrhea are remarkably specific, and genital, rectal, or pharyngeal cultures, plus cultures of blood and joint fluid, usually yield gonococci from at least one source.

Prevention

Prevention of gonorrhea is principally a problem of sex education, use of condoms, and treatment of contacts.

Treatment

A. Uncomplicated Urethral, Endocervical,

or Rectal Gonococcal Infections in Adolescents: Owing to increasing penicillin resistance, current recommended therapy is ceftriaxone (125 mg or 250 mg intramuscularly once) plus, for potential concurrent *Chlamydia trachomatis* infection, doxycycline (100 mg orally twice daily for 7 days). Erythromycin base (500 mg orally four times daily for 7 days) should be substituted for the doxycycline in pregnant patients. Azithromycin, 1 g orally as a single dose, is efficacious in treatment of both *N gonorrhoeae* and *C trachomatis* and may be preferred because of the cost and convenience. Alternatives to ceftriaxone include cefixime, 400 mg orally; ciprofloxacin, 500 mg orally; or ofloxacin, 400 mg orally—each given in one dose. Spectinomycin (2 g intramuscular once) is used for penicillin- and cephalosporin-allergic patients. Quinolone antibiotics should not be used in pregnant women and are not approved for children. Quinolone resistance has been recognized in several cities. If the contact's infecting strain was proved susceptible to penicillin, the patient may be treated orally with amoxicillin, 50 mg/kg to a maximum of 3 g, and probenecid, 25 mg/kg to a maximum of 1 g, taken together as a single dose. A "test of cure" culture is not necessary in asymptomatic adolescents after the ceftriaxone-doxycycline regimen; repeat screening in 1–2 months is preferable. Infants and children should be recultured.

B. Pharyngeal Gonococcal Infection: Ceftriaxone (125 mg or 250 mg intramuscularly once) should be used; ciprofloxacin (0.5 g orally once) is an alternative for adults and older adolescents. Neither spectinomycin nor amoxicillin is recommended. A repeat culture is recommended 4–7 days after therapy.

C. Disseminated Gonorrhea: Recommended regimens include ceftriaxone (1 g intramuscularly or intravenously once daily) or cefotaxime (1 g intravenously every 8 hours). Proved penicillin-sensitive organisms may be treated with ampicillin (1 g intravenously every 6 hours) or an equivalent penicillin regimen. Oral therapy may follow parenteral therapy after clinical resolution. Recommended regimens include cefixime (400 mg orally twice daily) or ciprofloxacin (0.5 g twice daily; not used for pregnant patients) to complete 7 days of therapy. If concurrent infection with *Chlamydia* is present or has not been excluded, a course of doxycycline, azithromycin, or erythromycin should also be prescribed.

Total duration of therapy is 7 days for disseminated infections.

D. Pelvic Inflammatory Disease: Therapy is given with cefoxitin (2 g intramuscularly or intravenously every 6 hours) and doxycycline (100 mg twice daily orally.) until the patient is clinically improved, then continued with doxycycline to complete 7 days. Clindamycin and gentamicin given intravenously until the patient is clinically improved may be used rather than cefoxitin.

E. Prepubertal Gonococcal Infections:
1. Uncomplicated genitourinary, rectal, or pharyngeal infections–These infections may be treated with ceftriaxone (25–50 mg/kg/d to a maximum of 125 mg intramuscularly once). Children over 8 years of age should also receive doxycycline (100 mg orally twice daily for 7 days). The physician should evaluate all children for evidence of sexual abuse and coinfection with syphilis, *Chlamydia,* and HIV.
2. Disseminated gonorrhea–This should be treated with ceftriaxone (50 mg/kg once daily parenterally for 7 days).

Fluoroquinolone resistance in *Neisseria gonorrhoeae*: Colorado and Washington, 1995. MMWR Morb Mortal Wkly Rep 1995;44:761.

Gonorrhea among men who have sex with men. Sexually Transmitted Disease Clinics, 1993–1996. MMWR Morb Mortal Wkly Rep 1997;46:889.

Handsfield HH et al: A comparison of single-dose cefixime with ceftriaxone as treatment for uncomplicated gonorrhea. N Engl J Med 1991;325:1337.

McCormack W: Pelvic inflammatory disease. N Engl J Med 1994;320:115.

Sexually transmitted diseases: Treatment guidelines MMWR Morb Mortal Wkly Rep 1998;47(RR-1):1.

Siegel RM et al: The prevalence of sexually transmitted diseases in children and adolescents evaluated for sexual abuse in Cincinnati: Rationale for limited STD testing in prepubertal girls. Pediatrics 1995;96:1090.

Steingrimsson O et al: Single dose azithromycin treatment of gonorrhea and infections caused by *C. trachomatis* and *U. urealyticum* in men. Sex Transm Dis 1994;21:43.

BOTULISM

Essentials of Diagnosis & Typical Features

- Dry mucous membranes.
- Nausea and vomiting.
- Diplopia; dilated, unreactive pupils.
- Descending paralysis.
- Difficulty in swallowing and speech occurring within 12–36 hours after ingestion of toxin-contaminated home-canned food.
- Multiple cases in a family or group.
- Hypotonia and constipation in infants.
- Diagnosis by clinical findings and identification of toxin in blood, stool, or implicated food.

General Considerations

Botulism is a paralytic disease caused by *Clostridium botulinum,* an anaerobic, gram-positive, spore-forming bacillus normally found in soil. The organism produces an extremely potent neurotoxin. Of the seven types of toxin (A–G), types A, B, and E cause most human diseases. The toxin, a polypeptide, is so potent that 0.1 mg is lethal for humans.

Food-borne botulism usually results from ingestion of toxin-containing food. Preformed toxin is absorbed from the gut and produces paralysis by preventing acetylcholine release from cholinergic fibers at myoneural junctions.

In the United States, home-canned vegetables are usually the cause. Commercially canned foods rarely are responsible. Virtually any food will support the growth of *C botulinum* spores into vegetative toxin-producing bacilli if an anaerobic, nonacid environment is provided. The food may not appear or taste spoiled. The toxin is heat-labile, but the spores are heat-resistant. Inadequate heating during processing (temperature < 115 °C) allows the spores to survive and later resume toxin production. Boiling of foods for 10 minutes or heating at 80 °C for 30 minutes before eating will destroy the toxin.

Infant botulism is seen in infants less than 6 months of age. About 80 cases were reported in 1994. It usually presents as constipation and severe hypotonia at a median age of 10 weeks. Uncommonly, infants less than 2 weeks of age develop botulism. The toxin appears to be produced by *C botulinum* organisms residing in the gastrointestinal tract. In some instances, honey has been the source of spores. Clinical findings include constipation, weak suck and cry, pooled oral secretions, cranial nerve deficits, generalized weakness, and, on occasion, sudden apnea. A characteristic electromyographic pattern termed "brief, small, abundant motor-unit action potentials" (BSAP) is observed.

Wound botulism was recognized in 11 (21%) of 53 adult botulism cases reported in 1994. All occurred in drug users at the injection site.

Clinical Findings

A. Symptoms and Signs: The incubation period for food-borne botulism is 8–36 hours. Initially, there is lassitude or fatigue, generally with headache. This is followed by double vision, dilated pupils, ptosis, and, within a few hours, difficulty in swallowing and in speech. Pharyngeal paralysis occurs in some cases, and food may be regurgitated. The mucous membranes often are very dry. Descending skeletal muscle paralysis may be seen. The sensorium is clear, and the temperature normal. Death usually results from respiratory failure.

B. Laboratory Findings: Feces, vomitus, serum, and suspect food should be examined for the presence of toxin by injection into mice. The organism also may be cultured from feces or the suspect food. Laboratory findings, including cerebrospinal fluid examination, are usually normal. Electromyography suggests the diagnosis if the characteristic abnormalities—small amplitude, brief polyphasic potentials with an incremental response to repeated stimuli—are seen. A nondiagnostic EMG does not exclude the diagnosis and should be repeated.

Differential Diagnosis

Carbon monoxide poisoning causes unconscious-

ness without cranial nerve paralysis, and carboxyhemoglobin can be detected in blood. Guillain-Barré syndrome is characterized by ascending paralysis, sensory deficits, and elevated cerebrospinal fluid protein without pleocytosis.

Other illnesses that should be considered include poliomyelitis, postdiphtheritic polyneuritis, certain chemical intoxications, tick paralysis, and myasthenia gravis. The history and elevated cerebrospinal fluid protein characterize postdiphtheritic polyneuritis. Poisoning with methyl alcohol, organic phosphorus compounds, methyl chloride, sodium fluoride, or atropine may have to be ruled out. Tick paralysis is characterized by a flaccid ascending motor paralysis that begins in the legs. An attached tick should be sought. Myasthenia gravis usually occurs in adolescent girls. It is characterized by ocular and bulbar symptoms, with normal pupils, fluctuating weakness, absence of other neurologic signs, and clinical response to cholinesterase inhibitors.

Complications

Difficulty in swallowing leads to aspiration pneumonia. Serious respiratory paralysis may be fatal despite assisted ventilation and modern intensive supportive measures.

Treatment

A. Specific Measures: Equine botulism antitoxin is of probable value in the treatment of botulism. Trivalent antitoxin (types A, B, and E) should be given intramuscularly as soon as the diagnosis is made after skin testing for horse serum sensitivity. The antitoxin, 24-hour diagnostic consultation, epidemic assistance, and laboratory testing services are available from the CDC. Botulism immune globulin is available in California under a study protocol from the Infant Botulism Prevention Program (510-540-2646). A clinical trial is under way to evaluate this product. Guanidine hydrochloride, 15–35 mg/kg/d orally in three doses, may reverse the neuromuscular block, but its efficacy is questionable.

B. General Measures: General and supportive therapy consists of bed rest, ventilatory support (if necessary), fluid therapy, and administration of purgatives and high enemas. In cases of infant botulism, some authorities recommend penicillin to eliminate organisms continuing to produce toxin within the gastrointestinal tract. Aminoglycoside antimicrobials may exacerbate neuromuscular blockage and should be avoided.

Prognosis

The mortality rate (about 25%) is lower in children than adults. In nonfatal cases, symptoms subside over 2–3 months and recovery is complete.

Graf WD et al: Electrodiagnosis reliability in the diagnosis of infant botulism. J Pediatr 1992;120:747.

Infant Botulism Prevention Program. Wound botulism—California, 1995. MMWR Morb Mortal Wkly Rep 1995;44:889.

Schreiner MS et al: Infant botulism: A review of 12 years experience at the Children's Hospital of Philadelphia. Pediatrics 1991;87:159.

Schwartz PJ, Arnon SS: Botulism immune globulin for infant botulism arrives: One year and a Gulf war later. West J Med 1992;156:197.

Thilo EH, Townsend SF: Infant botulism at 1 week of age: Report of two cases. Pediatrics 1993;92:151.

Wilcox P et al: Long-term follow-up of symptoms, pulmonary function, respiratory muscle strength, and exercise performance after botulism. Am Rev Respir Dis 1989; 139:157.

TETANUS

Essentials of Diagnosis & Typical Features

- Unimmunized or partially immunized patient.
- History of skin wound.
- Spasms of jaw muscles (trismus).
- Stiffness of neck, back, and abdominal muscles, with hyperirritability and hyperreflexia.
- Episodic, generalized muscle contractions.
- Diagnosis is based on clinical findings and the immunization history.

General Considerations

Tetanus is caused by *Clostridium tetani,* an anaerobic, gram-positive bacillus that produces a potent neurotoxin. In unimmunized or incompletely immunized individuals, infection follows contamination of a wound by soil containing clostridial spores from animal manure. The toxin reaches the central nervous system by retrograde axon transport, is bound to cerebral gangliosides, and is thought to increase reflex excitability in neurons of the spinal cord by blocking function of inhibitory synapses. Intense muscle spasms result. Two-thirds of cases in the United States follow minor puncture wounds of the hands or feet. In many cases, no history of a wound can be obtained. In the newborn, usually in underdeveloped countries, infection generally results from contamination of the umbilical cord. The incubation period typically is 4–14 days but may be longer.

Although 41 cases of tetanus were reported in the United States in 1995, an estimated 1 million cases occur globally.

Clinical Findings

A. Symptoms and Signs: In children and adults, the first symptom is often minimal pain at the site of inoculation, followed by hypertonicity and spasm of the regional muscles. Characteristically, difficulty in opening the mouth (trismus) is evident within 48 hours. In newborns, the first signs are irritability and inability to suck at the breast. The disease may then progress to stiffness of the jaw and neck, increasing dysphagia, and generalized hyperreflexia with extreme rigidity and spasms of all muscles of the abdomen and back (opisthotonos). The facial distortion resembles a grimace (risus sardonicus). Difficulty in swallowing and convulsions triggered by minimal stimuli such as sound, light, or movement may occur. Individual spasms may last seconds or minutes. Recurrent spasms are seen several times each hour, or they may be almost continuous. In most cases, the temperature is normal or only mildly elevated. A high or subnormal temperature is a bad prognostic sign. Patients are fully conscious and lucid. A profound circulatory disturbance associated with sympathetic overactivity may occur on the second to fourth day, which may contribute to the mortality rate. This is characterized by elevated blood pressure, increased cardiac output, tachycardia (> 20 beats/min), and arrhythmia.

B. Laboratory Findings: The diagnosis is made on clinical grounds. There may be a mild polymorphonuclear leukocytosis. The cerebrospinal fluid is normal with the exception of some elevation of pressure. Serum muscle enzymes may be elevated. Transient electrocardiographic and electroencephalographic abnormalities may occur. Anaerobic culture and microscopic examination of pus from the wound can be helpful, but *C tetani* is difficult to grow, and the drumstick-shaped gram-positive bacilli often cannot be found.

Differential Diagnosis

In areas where tetanus is rarely seen, physicians may not recognize the infection until classic findings are present. Poliomyelitis is characterized by asymmetric paralysis in an incompletely immunized child. The history of an animal bite, absence of trismus, and cerebrospinal fluid pleocytosis suggest rabies. Local infections of the throat and jaw should be easily recognized. Bacterial meningitis, phenothiazine reactions, decerebrate posturing, narcotic withdrawal, spondylitis, and hypocalcemic tetany may be confused with tetanus.

Complications

Complications include sepsis, malnutrition, pneumonia, atelectasis, asphyxial spasms, decubitus ulcers, and fractures of the spine due to intense contractions. They can be prevented in part by skilled supportive care.

Prevention

A. Tetanus Toxoid: Active immunization with tetanus toxoid is the cornerstone of prevention of tetanus (see Chapter 9) and almost always is achieved after the third dose of vaccine. A booster at the time of injury is needed if none has been given in the past 10 years—or within 5 years in case of a heavily contaminated wound. Nearly all cases of tetanus (99%) in the United States are in unimmunized or incompletely immunized individuals. Many adolescents and adults lack protective antibody.

B. Tetanus Antitoxin: Human tetanus immune globulin (TIG) should be used in nonimmunized individuals with soil-contaminated wounds. For children who have had no or one tetanus toxoid immunization, 250–500 units should be given intramuscularly. Tetanus toxoid and TIG should be administered concurrently at different sites using different syringes.

C. Treatment of Wounds: Proper surgical cleansing and debridement of contaminated wounds will decrease the risk of tetanus.

D. Prophylactic Antimicrobials: Prophylactic antimicrobials are useful if the child is unimmunized and TIG is not available.

Treatment

A. Specific Measures: Serotherapy lowers the mortality rate from tetanus, but not dramatically. TIG in a single dose of 3000–6000 units is given to children and adults. Doses of 500 units have been used in infants. Surgical debridement of wounds is indicated, but more extensive surgery or amputation to eliminate the site of infection is not necessary. Penicillin G and tetanus toxin are both GABA antagonists; therefore, some experts prefer metronidazole.

B. General Measures: The patient is kept in a quiet room with minimal stimulation. Control of spasms and prevention of hypoxic episodes are crucial. Diazepam is useful (0.6–1.2 mg/kg/d intravenously in six divided doses). In the newborn, two or three divided doses should be given. Large doses (up to 25 mg/kg/d) may be required for older children. Diazepam is given intravenously until muscular spasms become infrequent and the generalized muscular rigidity much less prominent. The drug may then be given orally and the dose reduced as the child improves. Barbiturates, chlorpromazine, and paraldehyde may also be useful. Mechanical ventilation and muscle paralysis are necessary in severe cases.

Prognosis

The fatality rate in newborns and heroin addicts is high (70–90%). The overall mortality rate in the United States is 65%. In a recent series of 44 neonates treated in Mexico City, the mortality rate was 25%. The fatality rate depends primarily on the quality of supportive care. Many deaths are due to pneumonia or respiratory failure. If the patient survives 1 week, recovery is likely.

Abrutyn E and Berlin JA: Intrathecal therapy in tetanus. JAMA 1991;266:2262.

Craig AS et al: Neonatal tetanus in the United States: A sentinel event in the foreign-born. Pediatr Infect Dis J 1997;16:955.

Gergen PJ et al: A population based serologic survey of immunity to tetanus in the United States. N Engl J Med 1995;332:761.

Sanford JP: Tetanus: Forgotten but not gone. N Engl J Med 1995;322:812.

Simental PS et al: Neonatal tetanus experience at the National Institute of Pediatrics in Mexico City. Pediatr Infect Dis J 1993;12:722.

Sutton DN: Management of autonomic dysfunction in severe tetanus: The use of magnesium sulphate and clonidine. Intensive Care Med 1990;16:75.

GAS GANGRENE

Essentials of Diagnosis & Typical Features

- Contamination of a wound with soil or feces.
- Massive edema, skin discoloration, bleb formation, and pain in an area of trauma.
- Serosanguineous exudate from wound.
- Crepitation of subcutaneous tissue.
- Rapid progression of signs and symptoms.
- Clostridia cultured or seen on stained smears.

General Considerations

Gas gangrene (clostridial myonecrosis) is a necrotizing infection that follows trauma or surgery and is caused by several anaerobic, gram-positive, spore-forming bacilli of the genus *Clostridium.* These are soil, genital tract (female), and fecal organisms. In devitalized tissue, the spores germinate into vegetative bacilli that proliferate and produce toxins causing thrombosis, hemolysis, and tissue necrosis. *Clostridium perfringens,* the species causing approximately 80% of cases of gas gangrene, produces at least 8 such toxins. The areas involved most often are the extremities, abdomen, and uterus. *Clostridium septicum* may also cause myonecrosis and causes septicemia in patients with neutropenia. Nonclostridial infections with gas formation can mimic clostridial infections and are more common.

Clinical Findings

A. Symptoms and Signs: The onset of gas gangrene is sudden, usually 1–20 days (mean, 3–4 days) after trauma or surgery. The skin around the wound becomes discolored, with hemorrhagic bullae, serosanguineous exudate, and crepitation in the subcutaneous tissues. Pain and swelling are usually intense. Systemic illness appears early and progresses rapidly to intravascular hemolysis, jaundice, shock, toxic delirium, and renal failure.

B. Laboratory Findings: Isolation of the organism requires anaerobic culture. Gram-stained smears may demonstrate many gram-positive rods and few inflammatory cells.

C. Imaging: X-ray films may demonstrate gas in tissues, but this is a late finding and is also seen in infections with other gas-forming organisms or may be due to air introduced into tissues during trauma or surgery.

D. Operative Findings: Direct visualization of the muscle at surgery may be necessary to diagnose gas gangrene. Early, the muscle is pale and edematous and does not contract normally; later, the muscle may be frankly gangrenous.

Differential Diagnosis

Gangrene and cellulitis caused by other organisms and clostridial cellulitis (not myonecrosis) must be distinguished. Necrotizing fasciitis may resemble gas gangrene.

Prevention

Gas gangrene can be prevented by the adequate cleansing and debridement of all wounds. It is essential that foreign bodies and dead tissue be removed. A clean wound does not provide a suitable anaerobic environment for the growth of clostridial species.

Treatment

A. Specific Measures: Penicillin G (300,000–400,000 units/kg/d intravenously in six divided doses) should be given. Clindamycin, metronidazole, and chloramphenicol are alternatives for penicillin-allergic patients.

B. Surgical Measures: Surgery should be prompt and extensive, with removal of all necrotic tissue.

C. Hyperbaric Oxygen: Hyperbaric oxygen therapy has been shown to be effective, but it is not a substitute for surgery. A patient may be exposed to 2–3 atm in pure oxygen for 1- to 2-hour periods for as many sessions as necessary until there is clinical remission.

Prognosis

Clostridial myonecrosis is fatal if untreated. With early diagnosis, antibiotics, and surgery, the mortality rate is about 20–60%. Involvement of the abdominal wall, leukopenia, intravascular hemolysis, renal failure, and shock are ominous prognostic findings.

Bratton SL et al: *Clostridium septicum* infections in children. Pediatr Infect Dis J 1992;11:569.

Rudge FW: The role of hyperbaric oxygen in the treatment of clostridial myonecrosis. Mil Med 1993;158:80.

Stevens DL et al: Comparison of clindamycin, rifampin, tetracycline, metronidazole, and penicillin for efficacy in prevention of experimental gas gangrene due to *Clostridium perfringens*. J Infect Dis 1987;155:220.

DIPHTHERIA

Essentials of Diagnosis & Typical Features

- A gray, adherent pseudomembrane, most often in the pharynx but also in the nasopharynx or trachea.

- Sore throat, serosanguineous nasal discharge, hoarseness, and fever in a nonimmunized child.
- Peripheral neuritis or myocarditis.
- Positive culture.
- Treatment should *not* be withheld pending culture results.

General Considerations

Diphtheria is an acute infection of the upper respiratory tract or skin caused by toxin-producing *Corynebacterium diphtheriae*. Diphtheria in the United States is rare; only 42 cases were reported from 1980 to 1995. However, significant numbers of elderly adults and unimmunized children are susceptible to infection. Travelers to foreign countries such as the former Soviet Union, where an epidemic of diphtheria occurred involving nearly 40,000 cases in 1994, may also acquire the disease. Corynebacteria are gram-positive club-shaped rods with a beaded appearance on Gram's stain.

The capacity to produce exotoxin is conferred by a lysogenic bacteriophage and is not present in all strains of *C diphtheriae*. In immunized communities, infection probably occurs through spread of the phage among carriers of susceptible bacteria rather than through spread of phage-containing bacteria themselves. Diphtheria toxin kills susceptible cells by irreversible inhibition of protein synthesis.

The toxin is absorbed into the mucous membranes and causes destruction of epithelium and a superficial inflammatory response. The necrotic epithelium becomes embedded in exuding fibrin and red and white cells, forming a grayish "pseudomembrane" commonly present over the tonsils, pharynx, or larynx. Any attempt to remove the membrane exposes and tears the capillaries, resulting in bleeding. The diphtheria bacilli within the membrane continue to produce toxin, which is absorbed and may result in toxic injury to heart muscle, liver, kidneys, and adrenals, and is sometimes accompanied by hemorrhage. The toxin also produces neuritis, resulting in paralysis of the soft palate, eye muscles, or extremities. Death may occur as a result of respiratory obstruction or toxemia and circulatory collapse. The patient may succumb after a somewhat longer time as a result of cardiac damage. The incubation period is 1–6 days.

Clinical Findings

A. Symptoms and Signs:

1. Pharyngeal diphtheria–Early manifestations of diphtheritic pharyngitis are mild sore throat, moderate fever, and malaise, followed fairly rapidly by severe prostration and circulatory collapse. The pulse is more rapid than the fever would seem to justify. A pharyngeal membrane forms and may spread into the nasopharynx or the trachea, producing respiratory obstruction. The membrane is tenacious and gray and is surrounded by a narrow zone of erythema and a broader zone of edema. The cervical lymph nodes become swollen, and swelling is associated with brawny edema of the neck ("bull neck"). Laryngeal diphtheria presents with stridor, which can lead to obstruction of the airway.

2. Other forms–Cutaneous, vaginal, and wound diphtheria account for up to one-third of cases and are characterized by ulcerative lesions with membrane formation.

B. Laboratory Findings: Diagnosis is clinical. Direct smears are unreliable. Material is obtained from the nose, throat, or skin lesions, if present, for culture on Loeffler's and tellurite agar. Sixteen to 48 hours are required before identification of the organism. A toxigenicity test is then performed. Cultures may be negative in individuals who have received antibiotics. The white blood cell count is usually normal, but hemolytic anemia and thrombocytopenia are frequent. The red blood cell count may reflect rapid destruction of erythrocytes. Thrombocytopenia due to peripheral destruction is frequent.

Differential Diagnosis

Pharyngeal diphtheria resembles acute streptococcal pharyngitis, mononucleosis, and occasionally, other viral pharyngitis. Nasal diphtheria may be mimicked by a foreign body or purulent sinusitis. Other causes of laryngeal obstruction are epiglottitis and viral croup. Neuropathy may mimic Guillain-Barré syndrome, poliomyelitis, or acute poisoning.

Complications

A. Myocarditis: Diphtheritic myocarditis is characterized by a rapid, thready pulse; indistinct heart sounds, ST–T wave changes, conduction abnormalities, dysrhythmias, or cardiac failure; hepatomegaly; and fluid retention. Myocardial dysfunction may occur from 2 to 40 days after the onset of pharyngitis.

B. Polyneuritis: Neuritis of the nerves innervating the palate and pharyngeal muscles occurs during the first or second week. Nasal speech and regurgitation of food through the nose are seen. Diplopia and strabismus occur during the third week or later. Neuritis may also involve peripheral motor nerves supplying the intercostal muscles and diaphragm and other muscle groups. Generalized paresis usually occurs after the fourth week.

C. Bronchopneumonia: Secondary pneumonia is common in fatal cases.

Prevention

A. Immunization: Immunization with diphtheria toxoid combined with pertussis and tetanus toxoids (DTP) should be used routinely for infants and children (see Chapter 9).

B. Care of Exposed Susceptibles: Children exposed to diphtheria should be examined, and nose and throat cultures obtained. If signs and symptoms of early diphtheria are found, treatment should be as for diphtheria. Immunized asymptomatic individuals should receive diphtheria toxoid if a booster has not been received within 5 years. Unimmunized close contacts should receive either erythromycin orally (40 mg/kg/d in four divided doses) for 7 days or benzathine penicillin G intramuscularly (25,000 units/kg), active immunization with diphtheria toxoid and be observed daily.

Treatment

A. Specific Measures:\eh6

1. Antitoxin–Diphtheria antitoxin should be administered within 48 hours to be effective (see Chapter 9).

2. Antibiotics–Penicillin G (150,000 units/kg/d intravenously) should be given for 10 days. For the patient allergic to penicillin, erythromycin, 40 mg/kg/d, is given orally for 10 days.

B. General Measures: Bed rest in the hospital for 10–14 days is usually required. All patients must be strictly isolated for 1–7 days until respiratory secretions are noncontagious. Isolation may be discontinued when three successive nose and throat cultures at 24-hour intervals are negative. These cultures should not be taken until at least 24 hours have elapsed since the cessation of antibiotic treatment.

C. Treatment of Carriers: All carriers should be treated. Erythromycin (40 mg/kg/d orally in three or four divided doses), penicillin V potassium (50 mg/kg/d for 10 days), or benzathine penicillin G (600,000–1,200,000 units intramuscularly) should be given. All carriers must be confined at home. Before they can be released, carriers must have three negative cultures of both the nose and the throat taken 24 hours apart and obtained at least 24 hours after the cessation of antibiotic therapy.

Prognosis

Mortality rates vary from 3% to 25% and are particularly high in the presence of early myocarditis. Neuritis is reversible; it is fatal only if an intact airway and adequate respiration cannot be maintained. Permanent damage due to myocarditis occurs rarely.

Bethell DB et al: Prognostic value of electrocardiographic monitoring of patients with severe diphtheria. Clin Infect Dis 1995;20:1259.

Diphtheria acquired by US citizens in the Russian Federation and Ukraine—1994. MMWR Morb Mortal Wkly Rep 1995;44:237.

English PC: Diphtheria and theories of infectious disease: Centennial appreciation of the critical role of diphtheria in the history of medicine. Pediatrics 1985;76:1.

Respiratory diphtheria caused by *Corynebacterium ulcerans*—Terre Haute, Indiana, 1996. MMWR Morb Mortal Wkly Rep 1997;46:330.

Thisyakorn US, Wongvanich J, Kumpeng V: Failure of corticosteroid therapy to prevent diphtheritic myocarditis or neuritis. Pediatr Infect Dis 1984;3:126.

INFECTIONS DUE TO ENTEROBACTERIACEAE

Essentials of Diagnosis & Typical Features

- Diarrhea by several different mechanisms due to *Escherichia coli.*
- Hemorrhagic colitis and hemolytic-uremic syndrome.
- Neonatal sepsis or meningitis.
- Urinary tract infection.
- Opportunistic infections.
- Diagnosis confirmed by culture.

General Considerations

Enterobacteriaceae are a family of gram-negative bacilli that are part of the normal flora of the gastrointestinal tract and are also found in water and soil. They cause gastroenteritis, urinary tract infections, neonatal sepsis and meningitis, opportunistic infections, and, occasionally, other infections. *Escherichia coli* is the organism in this family that most commonly causes infection in children, but *Klebsiella, Morganella, Enterobacter, Serratia, Proteus,* and other genera are also important, particularly in the compromised host. *Shigella* and *Salmonella* are discussed in separate sections.

E coli strains capable of causing diarrhea were originally termed enteropathogenic and were recognized by serotype. It is now known that *E coli* may cause diarrhea by several distinct mechanisms. Classic EPEC strains cause a characteristic histologic injury in the small bowel termed adherence and effacement. Enterotoxigenic *E coli* (ETEC) causes a secretory, watery diarrhea. ETEC adheres to enterocytes and secretes one or more plasmid-encoded enterotoxins. One of these toxins resembles cholera toxin in structure, function, and mechanism of action. Enteroinvasive *E coli* is very similar to *Shigella* in pathogenetic mechanism. Enterohemorrhagic *E coli* (EHEC) is the cause of hemorrhagic colitis and the hemolytic-uremic syndrome. The most common EHEC serotype is O157:H7, though several other serotypes cause the same syndrome. These strains elaborate one of several cytotoxins, closely related to Shiga toxin produced by *S dysenteriae*. Several outbreaks of hemolytic-uremic syndrome associated with EHEC have followed consumption of inadequately cooked ground beef. Thorough heating to 68–71 °C is necessary. Unpasteurized fruit juice, various uncooked vegetables, and contaminated water have also caused infections and epidemics.

Eighty percent of *E coli* strains causing neonatal meningitis possess specific capsular polysaccharide (K1 antigen), which, alone or in association with specific somatic antigens, confers virulence. K1 antigen is also present on approximately 40% of strains causing neonatal septicemia. The *E coli* K1 organisms do not appear to cause gastrointestinal disease.

Approximately 90% of urinary tract infections in children are caused by *E coli. E coli* binds to the uroepithelium by P-fimbria, which are present in greater than 90% of *E coli* that cause pyelonephritis. Other bacterial cell surface structures, such as O and K antigens, and host factors are also important in the pathogenesis of urinary tract infections.

Klebsiella, Enterobacter, Serratia, and *Morganella* are normally found in the gastrointestinal tract and in soil and water. *Klebsiella* may cause a bronchopneumonia with cavity formation. *Klebsiella, Enterobacter,* and *Serratia* are often hospital-acquired opportunists associated with antibiotic usage, debilitating states, and chronic respiratory conditions. They frequently cause urinary tract infection or sepsis. In many newborn nurseries, nosocomial outbreaks caused by aminoglycoside-resistant *Klebsiella pneumoniae* are a major problem.

Many of these infections are difficult to treat because of antibiotic resistance. Antibiotic susceptibility tests are necessary. Parenteral third-generation cephalosporins are usually more active than ampicillin, but resistance due to high-level production of chromosomal cephalosporinase may occur. *Enterobacter* and *Serratia* strains broadly resistant to cephalosporins also cause infections in hospitalized newborns and children. Aminoglycoside antibiotics are usually effective but require monitoring of serum levels to ensure therapeutic and nontoxic levels.

Clinical Findings

A. Symptoms and Signs:

1. *E coli* gastroenteritis–*E coli* may cause diarrhea of varying types and severity. Enterotoxigenic *E coli* usually produce mild, self-limiting illness without significant fever or systemic toxicity, often known as traveler's diarrhea. However, diarrhea may be severe in newborns and infants, and occasionally an older child or adult will have a cholera-like syndrome. Enteroinvasive strains cause a shigellosis-like illness characterized by fever, systemic symptoms, blood and mucus in the stool, and leukocytosis, but currently are uncommon in the United States. Enterohemorrhagic strains cause hemorrhagic colitis. Diarrhea is initially watery, and fever is usually absent. Abdominal pain and cramping occur, and diarrhea progresses to blood streaking or grossly bloody stools. Hemolytic-uremic syndrome occurs within a few days of diarrhea in 2–5% of children and is characterized by microangiopathic hemolytic anemia, thrombocytopenia, and renal failure (see Chapter 22).

E coli are transmitted from person to person and in food and water. Spread of *E coli* in day care centers is probably common. Undercooked ground beef, unpasteurized apple juice, and contaminated vegetables may transmit enterohemorrhagic *E coli*.

2. Neonatal sepsis–Findings include jaundice, hepatosplenomegaly, fever, temperature lability, apneic spells, irritability, and failure to suck vigorously.

Meningitis is associated with sepsis in 25–40% of cases. Other metastatic foci of infection may be present, including pneumonia and pyelonephritis. Sepsis may lead to severe metabolic acidosis, shock, disseminated intravascular coagulation, and death.

3. Neonatal meningitis–Findings include high fever, full fontanelles, vomiting, coma, convulsions, pareses or paralyses, poor or absent Moro reflex, opisthotonos, and, occasionally, hypertonia or hypotonia. Sepsis coexists or precedes meningitis in most cases. Thus, signs of sepsis often accompany those of meningitis. Cerebrospinal fluid usually shows a cell count of over 1000/μL, mostly polymorphonuclear neutrophils, and bacteria on Gram's stain. Cerebrospinal fluid glucose concentration is low (usually less than half that of blood), and the protein is elevated above the levels normally seen in newborns and premature infants (> 150 mg/dL).

4. Acute urinary tract infection–Symptoms include dysuria, increased urinary frequency, and fever in the older child. Nonspecific symptoms such as anorexia, vomiting, irritability, failure to thrive, and unexplained fever are seen in children under 2 years of age. Young infants may present with jaundice. As many as 1% of girls of school age and 0.05% of boys have asymptomatic bacteriuria. Screening for and treatment of asymptomatic bacteriuria is not recommended.

B. Laboratory Findings: Because *E coli* are normal flora in the stool, a positive stool culture alone does not prove that the *E coli* in the stool are causing disease. Serotyping, tests for enterotoxin production or invasiveness, and tests for P-fimbriae are performed in research laboratories. MacConkey's agar with sorbitol substituted for lactose (SMAC agar) is useful to screen stool for enterohemorrhagic *E coli.* Serotyping and testing for enterotoxin are available at many state health departments. Blood cultures are positive in neonatal sepsis. Cultures of cerebrospinal fluid and urine should also be obtained. The diagnosis of urinary tract infections is discussed in Chapter 21.

Differential Diagnosis

The clinical picture of enteropathogenic *E coli* infection may resemble that of salmonellosis, shigellosis, or viral gastroenteritis.

Neonatal sepsis and meningitis caused by *E coli* can be differentiated from other causes of neonatal infection only by blood and cerebrospinal fluid culture.

Treatment

A. Specific Measures:

1. *E coli* gastroenteritis–Gastroenteritis due to enteropathogenic *E coli* seldom requires antimicrobial treatment. Fluid and electrolyte therapy, preferably given orally, may be required to avoid dehydration. Bismuth subsalicylate reduces stool volume by about one-third in infants with watery diarrhea, probably including toxigenic *E coli.* In nursery outbreaks, infants have been treated with neomycin (100 mg/kg/d orally in three divided doses for 5 days) or colistin (10–15 mg/kg/d orally in three divided doses for 5 days). Clinical efficacy is not established. Traveler's diarrhea may be treated with trimethoprim-sulfamethoxazole in children and with fluoroquinolones in adults. It is not clear whether the risk of hemolytic-uremic syndrome increases or decreases following treatment of enterohemorrhagic colitis, but many experts withhold antimicrobials in this setting.

2. *E coli* sepsis, pneumonia, or pyelonephritis–The drugs of choice are ampicillin (150–200 mg/kg/d intravenously or intramuscularly in divided doses every 4–6 hours), cefotaxime (150–200 mg/kg/d intravenously or intramuscularly in divided doses every 6–8 hours), ceftriaxone (50–100 mg/kg/d intramuscularly as single dose or in two divided doses), and gentamicin (5–7.5 mg/kg/d intramuscularly or intravenously in divided doses every 8 hours). Treatment is for 10–14 days. Amikacin or tobramycin may be used instead of gentamicin if the strain is susceptible. Third-generation cephalosporins are often an attractive alternative as single-drug therapy and do not require monitoring for toxicity.

3. *E coli* meningitis–Third-generation cephalosporins such as cefotaxime (200 mg/kg/d intravenously in four divided doses) are given for a minimum of 3 weeks. Ampicillin (200–300 mg/kg/d intravenously in four to six divided doses) and gentamicin (5–7.5 mg/kg/d intramuscularly or intravenously in three divided doses) are also effective. Treatment with intrathecal and intraventricular aminoglycosides does not improve outcome. Serum levels need to be monitored.

4. Acute urinary tract infection–See Chapter 21.

Prognosis

Death due to gastroenteritis leading to dehydration can be prevented by early fluid and electrolyte therapy. Neonatal sepsis with meningitis is still associated with a mortality rate of over 50%. Most children with recurrent urinary tract infections do well if they have no serious underlying anatomic defects. The mortality rate in opportunistic infections usually depends on the severity of infection and the underlying condition.

Boyce TG, Swerdlow DL, Griffin PM: *Escherichia coli* 0157:H7 and the hemolytic-uremic syndrome. N Engl J Med 1995;333:364.

Cohen MB: *Escherichia coli* O157:H7 infections: A frequent cause of bloody diarrhea and the hemolytic-uremic syndrome. Adv Pediatr 1996;43:171

Ericsson CD, DuPont HL: Travelers' diarrhea: Approaches to prevention and treatment. Clin Infect Dis 1993; 16:616.

Figueroa-Quintanilla D et al: A controlled trial of bismuth subsalicylate in infants with acute watery diarrheal disease. N Engl J Med 1993;328:1654.

Gallagher PG: *Enterobacter* bacteremia in pediatric patients. Rev Infect Dis 1990;12:808.

Keene WE et al: A swimming-associated outbreak of hemorrhagic colitis caused by *Escherichia coli* 0157:H7 and *Shigella sonnei*. N Engl J Med 1994;331:579.

Siitonen A et al: Invasive *Escherichia coli* infections in children: bacterial characteristics in different age groups and clinical entities. Pediatr Infect Dis J 1993;12:606.

Stull TL: Epidemiology and natural history of urinary tract infections in children. Med Clin North Am 1991;75:287.

PSEUDOMONAS INFECTIONS

Essentials of Diagnosis & Typical Features

- Opportunistic infection.
- Confirmed by cultures.

General Considerations

Pseudomonas aeruginosa is an important cause of infection in children with cystic fibrosis, neoplastic disease, neutropenia, or extensive burns and in those receiving antibiotic therapy. Infections of the urinary and respiratory tracts, ears, mastoids, paranasal sinuses, eyes, skin, meninges, and bones are seen. *Pseudomonas* pneumonia is a common nosocomial infection in patients receiving assisted ventilation.

P aeruginosa sepsis may be accompanied by characteristic peripheral lesions called ecthyma gangrenosum. Ecthyma gangrenosum also may occur by direct invasion through intact skin in the groin, axilla, or other skinfolds. *P aeruginosa* is an infrequent cause of sepsis in previously healthy infants, and may be the initial sign of underlying medical problems. *P aeruginosa* osteomyelitis often complicates puncture wounds of the feet. *P aeruginosa* is a frequent cause of malignant external otitis media and of chronic suppurative otitis media. Outbreaks of vesiculopustular skin rash have been associated with exposure to contaminated water in whirlpool baths and hot tubs.

P aeruginosa is an aerobic gram-negative rod with versatile metabolic requirements. *P aeruginosa* may grow in distilled water and in commonly used disinfectants, complicating the problem of infection control. *P aeruginosa* is both invasive and destructive to tissue, and toxigenic due to secreted exotoxins, which contribute to virulence. Other *Pseudomonas* species occasionally cause nosocomial infections. *Stenotrophomonas maltophilia* (previously *P maltophilia*) and *Burkholderia cepacia* (previously *P cepacia*) are the most frequent.

P aeruginosa infects the tracheobronchial tree of nearly all patients with cystic fibrosis. Mucoid exopolysaccharide, an exuberant capsule, is characteristically overproduced by isolates from patients with cystic fibrosis. Although bacteremia seldom occurs, patients with cystic fibrosis ultimately succumb to chronic lung infection with *P aeruginosa*. Infection due to *B cepacia* has caused a rapidly progressive pulmonary disease in some colonized patients and may be spread by close contact.

Clinical Findings

The clinical findings depend on the site of infection and the patient's underlying disease. Sepsis with these organisms resembles gram-negative sepsis with other organisms, though the presence of ecthyma gangrenosa suggests the diagnosis. The diagnosis is made by culture. *Pseudomonas* infection should be suspected in neonates and neutropenic patients with clinical sepsis. A severe necrotizing pneumonia occurs in patients on ventilators.

Patients with cystic fibrosis have a persistent bronchitis which progresses to bronchiectasis and ultimately to respiratory failure. During exacerbations of illness, cough and sputum production increase with low grade fever, malaise, and diminished energy.

The purulent aural drainage without fever in patients with chronic suppurative otitis media is not distinguishable from that due to other cause.

Prevention

A. Infections in Debilitated Patients: Colonization of extensive second- and third-degree burns by *P aeruginosa* can lead to fatal septicemia. Aggressive debridement and topical treatment with 0.5% silver nitrate solution, 10% mafenide cream, or gentamicin ointment will greatly inhibit *P aeruginosa* contamination of burns. (See Chapter 11 for a discussion of burn wound infections and prevention.)

B. Nosocomial Infections: Faucet aerators, communal soap dispensers, disinfectants, improperly cleaned inhalation therapy equipment, infant incubators, and back rub lotions have all been associated with *Pseudomonas* epidemics. Infant-to-infant transmission by nursery personnel carrying *Pseudomonas* on the hands is frequent in neonatal units. Careful maintenance of equipment and enforcement of infection control procedures are essential to minimize nosocomial transmission.

C. Patients With Cystic Fibrosis: Chronic infection of the lower respiratory tract occurs in nearly all patients with cystic fibrosis. The infecting organism is seldom cleared from the respiratory tract, even with intensive antimicrobial therapy, and the resultant injury to the lung eventually leads to pulmonary insufficiency. Treatment is aimed at controlling signs and symptoms of the infection.

Treatment

P aeruginosa is inherently resistant to many antimicrobials and may develop resistance during therapy. Mortality rates in hospitalized patients exceed 50%, due both to the severity of underlying illnesses in patients predisposed to *Pseudomonas* infection and to the limitations of therapy. Aminoglycoside antimicrobials; ureidopenicillins such as ticarcillin or piperacillin; the combination of β-lactamase inhibitor with a ureidopenicillin such as ticarcillin-clavulanate or piperacillin-tazobactam; expanded-spectrum cephalosporins such as ceftazidime or cefepime; imipenem; and the fluoroquinolones are active against most *P aeruginosa* strains as well as other enteric gram-negative rods. However, antimicrobial susceptibility patterns vary from area to area, and resistance tends to appear as new drugs become popular. Treatment of infections is best guided by clinical response and susceptibility tests.

Use of gentamicin or tobramycin (5–7.5 mg/kg/d intramuscularly or intravenously in three divided doses) or amikacin (15–22 mg/kg/d in two or three divided doses) in combination with ticarcillin (200–300 mg/kg/d intravenously in six divided doses) or with another anti-*Pseudomonas* β-lactam antibiotic is recommended for treatment of serious *Pseudomonas* infections. Ceftazidime (150–200 mg/kg/d in four divided doses) is a third-generation cephalosporin with excellent activity against *P aeruginosa.* Treatment should be continued for 10–14 days. Treatment with two active drugs is recommended for all serious infections.

Pseudomonas osteomyelitis requires surgical debridement and antimicrobial therapy for 2 weeks. *Pseudomonas* folliculitis does not require antibiotic therapy.

Chronic suppurative otitis media responds to intravenous ceftazidime (150–200 mg/kg/d in three or four divided doses) given until the drainage has ceased for 3 days. Twice-daily ceftazidime with aural debridement and cleaning given on an outpatient basis has also been successful. Oral ciprofloxacin is also effective but is not FDA-approved in children because of concerns about skeletal toxicity.

Swimmer's ear may be caused by *P aeruginosa* and responds well to topical drying agents (alcohol-vinegar mix) and cleansing.

Prognosis

Because debilitated patients are most frequently affected, the mortality rate is high. These infections may have a protracted course, and eradication of the organisms may be difficult.

Agger WA, Mardan A: *Pseudomonas aeruginosa* infections of intact skin. Clin Infect Dis 1995;20:302.

Dagan R et al: Outpatient management of chronic suppurative otitis media without cholesteatoma in children. Pediatr Infect Dis J 1992;11:542.

Fergie JE, Patrick CC, Lott L: *Pseudomonas aeruginosa* cellulitis and ecthyma gangrenosum in immunocompromised children. Pediatr Infect Dis J 1991;10:469.

Fiel SB: Clinical management of pulmonary disease in cystic fibrosis. Lancet 1993;341:1070.

Flores G, Stavola JJ, Noel GJ: Bacteremia due to *Pseudomonas aeruginosa* in children with AIDS. Clin Infect Dis 1993;16:706.

Jacobs RF, McCarthy RE, Elser JM: *Pseudomonas* osteochondritis complicating wound punctures of the foot in children: A ten year evaluation. J Infect Dis 1989; 160:657.

Leigh I et al: *Pseudomonas aeruginosa* infection in very low birth weight infants: A case-control study. Pediatr Infect Dis J 1995;12:367.

Martin-Ancel A, Borque C, del Castillo F: *Pseudomonas* sepsis in children without previous medical problems. Pediatr Infect Dis J 1993;12:258.

SALMONELLA GASTROENTERITIS

Essentials of Diagnosis & Typical Features
- Nausea, vomiting, headache, meningismus.
- Fever, diarrhea, abdominal pain.
- Culture or organism from stool, blood, or other specimens.

General Considerations

Salmonellae are gram-negative rods that frequently cause food-borne gastroenteritis and occasionally bacteremic infection of bone, meninges, and other foci. Three species—*Salmonella typhi, Salmonella choleraesuis,* and *Salmonella enteritidis*—and approximately 2000 serotypes are recognized. *S typhimurium* is the most frequently isolated serotype in most parts of the world. An estimated 4 million cases of salmonellosis occur yearly in the United States, but only 45,000 are reported.

Salmonellae are able to penetrate the mucin layer of the small bowel and attach to epithelial cells. Organisms penetrate the epithelial cells and multiply in the submucosa. Infection results in fever, vomiting, watery diarrhea, and occasionally mucus with some polymorphonuclear leukocytes in the stool. Although the small intestine is generally regarded as the principal site of infection, colitis also occurs. *S typhimurium* frequently involves the large bowel.

Salmonella infections in childhood occur in two major forms: (1) gastroenteritis (including food poisoning), which may be complicated by sepsis and focal suppurative complications; and (2) enteric fever (typhoid fever and paratyphoid fever). (See next section.) Although the incidence of typhoid fever has decreased in the United States, the incidence of *Salmonella* gastroenteritis has greatly increased in the past 15–20 years. The highest attack rates occur in children under 6 years of age, with a peak in the age group from 6 months to 2 years old.

Salmonellae are widespread in nature, infecting domestic and wild animals. Fowl and reptiles have a particularly high carriage rate. Transmission results primarily from ingestion of contaminated food. Transmission from human to human occurs by the fecal-oral route via contaminated food, water, and fomites. Numerous foods are associated with outbreaks including meats, milk, cheese, ice cream, chocolate and other foods. Contaminated egg powder and frozen whole egg preparations used to make ice cream, custards, and mayonnaise are responsible for outbreaks. Eggs with contaminated shells that are consumed raw or undercooked have been incriminated in outbreaks and sporadic cases.

Salmonellae are susceptible to gastric acidity and, therefore, the elderly, infants, and patients treated with antacids or H_2 blocking drugs are at increased risk of infection. Most cases of *Salmonella* meningitis (80%) and bacteremia occur in infancy. Newborns may acquire the infection from their mothers during delivery and may precipitate outbreaks in nurseries. Newborns are at special risk of developing meningitis.

Clinical Findings

A. Symptoms and Signs: Infants usually develop fever, vomiting, and diarrhea. The older child may also complain of headache, nausea, and abdominal pain. Stools are often watery or may contain mucus and, in some instances, blood, suggesting shigellosis. Drowsiness and disorientation may be associated with meningismus. Convulsions occur less frequently than with shigellosis. Splenomegaly is occasionally noted. In the usual case, diarrhea is moderate and subsides after 4–5 days, but it may be protracted.

B. Laboratory Findings: Diagnosis is made by isolation of the organism from stool, blood, or, in some cases, from urine, cerebrospinal fluid, or pus from a suppurative lesion. The white blood cell count usually shows a polymorphonuclear leukocytosis but may show leukopenia. Typing of isolates is done with specific antisera. *Salmonella* isolates should be reported to public health authorities for epidemiologic purposes.

Differential Diagnosis

In staphylococcal food poisoning, the incubation period is shorter (2–4 hours) than in *Salmonella* food poisoning (12–24 hours). Fever is absent, and vomiting rather than diarrhea is the main symptom. In shigellosis, many pus cells are likely to be seen on a stained smear of stool and there is more apt to be a marked shift to the left in the peripheral white count, though some cases of salmonellosis are indistinguishable from shigellosis. *Campylobacter* gastroenteritis commonly resembles salmonellosis clinically. (Organisms previously classified as *Arizona* are considered *Salmonella* and cause a similar illness.) Culture of the stools is necessary to distinguish the causes of bacterial gastroenteritis.

Complications

Unlike most types of infectious diarrhea, salmonellosis is frequently accompanied by bacteremia, especially in newborns and infants. Septicemia with extraintestinal infection is seen, most commonly with *S choleraesuis* but also with *S enteritidis, S typhimurium,* and *S paratyphi* B and C. The organism may localize in any tissue and may cause arthritis, osteomyelitis, cholecystitis, endocarditis, meningitis, pericarditis, pneumonia, or pyelonephritis. In patients with sickle cell anemia or other hemoglobinopathies, there is a predilection for osteomyelitis to develop. Severe dehydration and shock are more likely to occur with shigellosis but may occur with *Salmonella* gastroenteritis.

Prevention

Measures for the prevention of *Salmonella* infections include thorough cooking of foodstuffs derived from potentially infected sources; proper refrigeration during storage; and recognition and control of infection among domestic animals, combined with proper meat and poultry inspections. Raw and undercooked fresh eggs should be avoided. Adults with salmonellosis who are food handlers or who have occupations involving care of young children should have three negative stool cultures before resuming work.

Treatment

A. Specific Measures: In uncomplicated *Salmonella* gastroenteritis, antibiotic treatment does not shorten the course of the clinical illness and may prolong convalescent carriage of the organism. Colitis or secretory diarrhea due to *Salmonella* may improve with antibiotic therapy.

However, to prevent sepsis and focal disease, antibiotic treatment is recommended for newborns and infants less than 3 months of age, for severely ill children, and for children with sickle cell disease, liver disease, recent gastrointestinal surgery, cancer, depressed immunity, and chronic renal or cardiac disease. Infants with positive stool cultures or suspected salmonellosis sepsis at less than 3 months of age should be admitted to hospital, evaluated for focal infection including blood culture and cerebrospinal fluid examination, and treated intravenously. Ampicillin (150–200 mg/kg/d intravenously in four divided doses for 5–10 days) or trimethoprim-sulfamethoxazole is recommended. Older patients developing bacteremia during the course of gastroenteritis should receive parenteral treatment initially, and a careful search should be made for additional foci of infection. After signs and symptoms subside, these patients should receive oral medication. Parenteral and oral treatment should last a total of 7–10 days. Longer treatment is indicated for specific complications. If susceptibility tests indicate resistance to ampicillin, chloramphenicol, third-generation cephalosporins, or trimethoprim-sulfamethoxazole should be given. Fluoroquinolones also are efficacious but are not FDA-approved for administration to children.

Salmonella meningitis is best treated with a combination of chloramphenicol (100 mg/kg/d intravenously in four divided doses) and ampicillin (200–300 mg/kg/d intravenously in four to six divided doses) for 3 weeks or a third-generation cephalosporin (cefotaxime, ceftriaxone) for 3 weeks. If the child improves rapidly and the cerebrospinal fluid is sterile, treatment may be completed with a single drug, the choice guided by results of susceptibility tests.

Outbreaks on pediatric wards are difficult to control. Strict hand washing, cohorting of patients and personnel, and ultimate closure of the unit may be necessary.

B. Treatment of the Carrier States: About half of patients are still infectious after 4 weeks. Infants tend to remain convalescent carriers for up to a year. Antibiotic treatment of carriers is not effective.

C. General Measures: Careful attention must be given to maintaining fluid and electrolyte balance, especially in infants.

Prognosis

In gastroenteritis, the prognosis is good. In sepsis with focal suppurative complications, the prognosis is more guarded.

The case fatality rate of *Salmonella* meningitis is high in infants. There is a strong tendency to relapse if treatment is not continued for at least 14–21 days.

Ackman DM et al: Reptile-associated salmonellosis in New York State. Pediatr Infect Dis J 1995;14:955.

Herikstad H et al: Ceftriaxone-resistant *Salmonella* in the United States. Pediatr Infect Dis J 1997;16:904.

Mermin J, Hoar B, Angulo FJ: Iguanas and *Salmonella marina* infection in children: A reflection of the increasing incidence of reptile-associated salmonellosis in the United States. Pediatrics 1997;99:399.

Sanchez C et al: Ciprofloxacin and trimethoprim-sulfamethoxazole versus placebo in acute uncomplicated *Salmonella* enteritis: A double blind trial. J Infect Dis 1993;168:1304.

St Geme JW III et al: Consensus: management of *Salmonella* infection in the first year of life. Pediatr Infect Dis J 1988;7:615.

Wright J, Thomas P, Serjeant GR: Septicemia caused by *Salmonella* infection: An overlooked complication of sickle cell disease. J Pediatr 1997;130:394.

TYPHOID FEVER & PARATYPHOID FEVER

Essentials of Diagnosis & Typical Features

- Insidious or acute onset of headache, anorexia, vomiting, constipation or diarrhea, ileus, and high fever.
- Meningismus, splenomegaly, and rose spots.
- Leukopenia; positive blood, stool, bone marrow, and urine cultures.

General Considerations

Typhoid fever is caused by the gram-negative bacillus *Salmonella typhi;* paratyphoid fevers, which are usually milder but may be clinically indistinguishable, are caused by *Salmonella paratyphi* A, *Salmonella schottülleri,* or *Salmonella hirschfeldii* (formerly *Salmonella paratyphi* A, B, and C). Children have a shorter incubation period than do adults (usually 5–8 days instead of 8–14 days). The organism enters the body through the walls of the intestinal tract and, following a transient bacteremia, multiplies in the reticuloendothelial cells of the liver and spleen.

Persistent bacteremia and symptoms then follow. Reinfection of the intestine occurs as organisms are excreted in the bile. Bacterial emboli produce the characteristic skin lesions (rose spots). Symptoms in children may be mild or severe, but children younger than age 5 uncommonly have clinically severe typhoid fever.

Typhoid fever is transmitted by the fecal-oral route and by contamination of food or water. Unlike other *Salmonella* species, there are no animal reservoirs of *S typhi;* each case is the result of direct or indirect contact with the organism or with an individual who is actively infected or a chronic carrier.

About 500 cases per year are reported in the United States, 60% of which are acquired during foreign travel.

Clinical Findings

A. Symptoms and Signs: In children, the onset of typhoid fever is apt to be sudden rather than insidious, with malaise, headache, crampy abdominal pains and distention, and sometimes constipation followed within 48 hours by diarrhea, high fever, and toxemia. An encephalopathy may be seen with irritability, confusion, delirium, and stupor. Vomiting and meningismus may be prominent in the young. The classic prolonged three-stage disease seen in adult patients is often shortened in children. The prodrome may be only 2–4 days; the toxic stage may last only 2–3 days; and the defervescence stage may last 1–2 weeks.

During the prodromal stage, physical findings may be absent, or there may merely be some abdominal distention and tenderness, meningismus, mild hepatomegaly, and minimal splenomegaly. The typical typhoidal rash (rose spots) is present in 10–15% of children. It appears during the second week of the disease and may erupt in crops for the succeeding 10–14 days. Rose spots are erythematous maculopapular lesions 2–3 mm in diameter that fade on pressure. They are found principally on the trunk and chest, and they generally disappear within 3–4 days. The lesions usually number less than 20.

B. Laboratory Findings: Typhoid bacilli can be isolated from many sites, including blood, stool, urine, and bone marrow. Blood cultures are positive in 50–80% of cases during the first week and less often later in the illness. Stool cultures are positive in about 50% of cases after the first week. Urine and bone marrow cultures are also valuable. Most patients will have negative cultures (including stool) by the end of a 6-week period. Serologic tests (Widal reaction) are not as useful as cultures because both false-positive and false-negative results occur. A fourfold rise in titer of O (somatic) agglutinins is suggestive but not diagnostic of infection.

Leukopenia is common in the second week of the disease, but in the first week, leukocytosis may be seen. Proteinuria, mild elevation of liver enzymes, thrombocytopenia, and disseminated intravascular coagulation are common.

Differential Diagnosis

Typhoid and paratyphoid fevers must be distinguished from other serious prolonged fevers. These include typhus, brucellosis, tularemia, miliary tuberculosis, psittacosis, vasculitis, lymphoma, mononucleosis, and Kawasaki disease.

The diagnosis of typhoid fever if often made clinically in developing countries. In developed countries, where typhoid fever is uncommon and physicians are unfamiliar with the clinical picture, the diagnosis is often not suspected until late. Positive cultures confirm the diagnosis.

Complications

The most important complications of typhoid fever are gastrointestinal hemorrhage (2–10%) and perforation (1–3%). They occur toward the end of the second week or during the third week of the disease.

Intestinal perforation is one of the principal causes of death. The site of perforation generally is the terminal ileum or cecum. The clinical manifestations are indistinguishable from those of acute appendicitis, with pain, tenderness, and rigidity in the right lower quadrant. The x-ray finding of free air in the peritoneal cavity is diagnostic.

Bacterial pneumonia, meningitis, septic arthritis, abscesses, and osteomyelitis are uncommon complications, particularly if specific treatment is given promptly. Shock and electrolyte disturbances may lead to death.

About 1–3% of patients become chronic carriers of *S typhi*. Chronic carriage is defined as excretion of typhoid bacilli for more than a year, but carriage is often lifelong. Adults with underlying biliary or urinary tract disease are much more likely than children to become chronic carriers.

Prevention

Routine typhoid vaccine is not recommended in the United States but should be considered for foreign travel to endemic areas. An attenuated oral typhoid vaccine produced from strain Ty21a has better efficacy and causes minimal side effects but is not approved for children under 6 years. A newly licensed capsular polysaccharide vaccine (ViCPS) requires one intramuscular injection and may be given to children 2 years and older (see Chapter 9).

Treatment

A. Specific Measures: Equally effective regimens for susceptible strains include the following: trimethoprim-sulfamethoxazole (10 mg/kg trimethoprim and 50 mg/kg sulfamethoxazole per day orally in two or three divided doses), amoxicillin (100 mg/kg/d orally in four divided doses), and ampicillin (100–200 mg/kg/d intravenously in four divided doses). Aminoglycosides and first- and second-generation cephalosporins are clinically ineffective regardless of in vitro susceptibility results. Third-generation cephalosporins are used for resistant strains. Ceftriaxone and cefotaxime may be used parenterally. Cefixime is efficacious orally. Occasionally, the presence of multiple resistant strains requires the use of chloramphenicol (50–100 mg/kg/d orally or intravenously in four doses).

Treatment duration is 14–21 days. Patients remain febrile for 3–5 days even with appropriate therapy.

B. General Measures: General support of the patient is exceedingly important and includes rest, good nutrition, and careful observation, with particular regard to evidence of intestinal bleeding or perforation. Blood transfusions may be needed even in the absence of frank hemorrhage.

Prognosis

A prolonged convalescent carrier stage may occur in children. Three negative cultures off all antibiotics are required before contact precautions are stopped.

With early antibiotic therapy, the prognosis is excellent. With early treatment, the mortality rate is less than 1%. Relapse occurs 1–3 weeks later in 10–20% of cases despite appropriate antibiotic treatment.

Butler T et al: Patterns of morbidity and mortality in typhoid fever dependent on age and gender: Review of 552 hospitalized patients with diarrhea. Rev Infect Dis 1991;13:85.

Girgis NI et al: Comparison of the efficacy, safety, and cost of cefixime, ceftriaxone, and aztreonam in the treatment of multi-drug-resistant *Salmonella typhi* septicemia in children. Pediatr Infect Dis J 1995;14:603.

Hall CB: A single shot of *Salmonella typhi:* A new typhoid vaccine with pediatric advantages. Pediatrics 1995;96:348.

Mahle WT, Levine MM: *Salmonella typhi* infection in children younger than five years of age. Pediatr Infect Dis J 1993;12:627.

Meloni T et al: Ceftriaxone treatment of *Salmonella* enteric fever. Pediatr Infect Dis J 1988;7:734.

Stormon M et al: Typhoid fever in children: Diagnostic and therapeutic difficulties. Pediatr Infect Dis J 1997;16:713.

SHIGELLOSIS
(Bacillary Dysentery)

Essentials of Diagnosis & Typical Features

- Cramps and bloody diarrhea.
- High fever, malaise, convulsions.
- Pus and blood in diarrheal stools examined microscopically.
- Diagnosis confirmed by stool culture.

General Considerations

Shigellae are nonmotile gram-negative rods of the family Enterobacteriaceae and are closely related to *Escherichia coli*. The genus *Shigella* is divided into four major groups, A–D: *Shigella dysenteriae, Shigella flexneri, Shigella boydii,* and *Shigella sonnei.* Approximately 30,000 cases of shigellosis are reported each year in the United States. *S sonnei* followed by *S flexneri* are the most common isolates.

S dysenteriae, which causes the most severe diarrhea of all species and the greatest number of extraintestinal complications, accounts for fewer than 1% of all *Shigella* infections in the United States.

Shigellosis is often a serious disease, particularly in children under 2 years of age, and without supportive treatment there is an appreciable mortality rate. In older children and adults, the disease tends to be self-limited and milder. Shigellosis is unusual in infants under 3 months of age, though in rare cases shigellae may be transmitted from the mother to the newborn during delivery. Diarrhea and refusal to take feedings are the most common symptoms in neonatal shigellosis, and bloody diarrhea and fever occur less frequently. Vomiting, convulsions, or high fever is almost never encountered.

Shigella is usually transmitted by the fecal-oral route. Food- and water-borne outbreaks occur but are less important overall than person-to-person transmission. The disease is very communicable—as few as 200 bacteria can produce illness in an adult. The secondary attack rate in families is high, and shigellosis is a serious problem in day care centers and custodial institutions. *Shigella* organisms produce disease by invading the colonic mucosa, causing mucosal ulcerations and microabscesses. A plasmid-encoded gene is required for enterotoxin production, chromosomal genes are required for invasiveness, and smooth lipopolysaccharide are required for virulence.

Clinical Findings

A. Symptoms and Signs: The incubation period of shigellosis usually is 2–4 days. Onset is abrupt, with abdominal cramps, urgency, tenesmus, chills, fever, malaise, and diarrhea. In severe forms, blood and mucus are seen in small volume in the watery stool (dysentery), and meningismus and convulsions may occur. In older children, the disease may be mild and may be characterized by watery diarrhea without blood. In young children, a fever of 39.4–40 °C is common. Rarely, there is rectal prolapse. Symptoms generally last 3–7 days.

B. Laboratory Findings: The total white blood cell count varies, but often there is a marked shift to the left. The stool may contain gross blood and mucus, and many neutrophils are seen if mucus from the stool is examined microscopically. Stool cultures usually are positive; however, they may be negative because the organism is somewhat fragile and present in small numbers late in the disease, and because laboratory techniques are suboptimal for the recovery of shigellae.

Differential Diagnosis

Diarrhea due to rotavirus infection is a winter rather than a summer disease, usually children are not as febrile or toxic, and stool does not contain gross blood or neutrophils. Intestinal infections caused by *Salmonella* or *Campylobacter* are differentiated by culture. Amebic dysentery is diagnosed by microscopic examination of fresh stools or sigmoidoscopy specimens; intussusception is characterized by an abdominal mass, "currant jelly" stools without leukocytes, and absence of fever. Mild shigellosis is not distinguishable clinically from other forms of infectious diarrhea.

Complications

Dehydration, acidosis, shock, and renal failure are the major complications. In some cases, a chronic form of dysentery occurs, characterized by mucoid stools and poor nutrition. Bacteremia and metastatic infections are rare but serious complications. Febrile seizures are common. Fulminating fatal dysentery and hemolytic-uremic syndrome occur rarely.

Treatment

A. Specific Measures: Trimethoprim-sulfamethoxazole (10 mg/kg/d trimethoprim and 50 mg/kg/d sulfamethoxazole, in two divided doses orally for 5 days) is the treatment of choice. Amoxicillin is not effective. Ampicillin (100 mg/kg/d in four divided doses) is also efficacious if the strain is sensitive. Ceftriaxone parenterally or cefixime orally is effective and should be used for resistant strains. Ciprofloxacin, 500 mg twice daily for 5 days, is efficacious in adults but is not approved in children. Successful treatment results in reduced duration of fever, cramping, and diarrhea and in termination of fecal excretion of *Shigella.* Strains resistant to ampicillin and trimethoprim-sulfamethoxazole are common in Mexico and underdeveloped countries, and are increasingly common in the United States. Most isolates are resistant to ampicillin, and many are resistant to trimethoprim-sulfamethoxazole. Tetracycline and chloramphenicol are also effective, but resistance is common. Presumptive therapy should be based on the susceptibility pattern of recent local isolates.

B. General Measures: In severe cases, immediate rehydration is critical. A mild form of chronic malabsorption syndrome may supervene and require prolonged dietary control.

Prognosis

The prognosis is excellent if vascular collapse is treated promptly by adequate fluid therapy. The mortality rate is high in very young, malnourished infants who do not receive fluid and electrolyte therapy. Convalescent fecal excretion of *Shigella* lasts 1–4 weeks in patients not receiving antimicrobial therapy. Long-term carriers are rare.

Ashkenazi S et al: A randomized, double-blind study comparing cefixime and trimethoprim-sulfamethoxazole in the treatment of childhood shigellosis. J Pediatr 1993;123:817.

Bennish ML: Potentially lethal complications of shigellosis. Rev Infect Dis 1991;13:5319.

Church DL et al: Practice guidelines for ordering stool cultures in a pediatric population. Am J Clin Pathol 1995;103:149

Eidlitz-Marcus T et al: Comparative efficacy of two- and five-day courses of ceftriaxone for treatment of severe shigellosis in children. J Pediatr 1993;123:822.

Huskins WC et al: Shigellosis in neonates and young infants. J Pediatr 1994;125:14.

Tauxe RV et al: Antimicrobial resistance of *Shigella* isolates in the United States: The importance of international travelers. J Infect Dis 1990;162:1107.

CHOLERA

Essentials of Diagnosis & Typical Features

- Sudden onset of severe watery diarrhea.
- Persistent vomiting without nausea or fever.
- Extreme and rapid dehydration and electrolyte loss, with rapid development of vascular collapse.
- Contact with a case of cholera, with shellfish, or the presence of cholera in the community.
- Diagnosis confirmed by stool culture.

General Considerations

Cholera is an acute diarrheal disease caused by the gram-negative organism *Vibrio cholerae*. It is transmitted by contaminated water or food, especially contaminated shellfish. The disease is generally so dramatic that in endemic areas the diagnosis is obvious. Individuals with mild illness and young children may play an important role in transmission of the infection.

Asymptomatic infection is far more common than clinical disease. In endemic areas, rising titers of vibriocidal antibody are seen with increasing age; infection occurs in individuals with low titers. The age-specific attack rate is highest in children under 5 years and declines with age. Cholera is unusual in infancy.

Cholera toxin is a protein enterotoxin that is primarily responsible for symptoms. Cholera toxin binds to a regulatory subunit of adenylyl cyclase in enterocytes, causing increased cAMP and an outpouring of NaCl and water into the lumen of the small bowel.

Nutritional status is an important factor determining the severity of the diarrhea. Duration of diarrhea is prolonged in adults and children suffering from severe malnutrition.

Cholera is endemic in India and southern and Southeast Asia and in parts of Africa. The most recent pandemic, caused by the El Tor biotype of *V cholerae* 01, began in 1961 in Indonesia. In 1982, thirty-seven countries were affected and 54,000 cases were reported. Epidemic cholera spread in Central and South America, with a total of 1 million cases and 9500 deaths reported through 1994. Cases in the United States occurred in the course of foreign travel or as a result of consumption of contaminated imported food. Cholera is increasingly associated with consumption of shellfish. Interstate shipment of oysters has resulted in cholera in several inland states.

Several recent studies provide evidence that *V cholerae* is a natural inhabitant of shellfish and copepods in estuarine environments. Seasonal multiplication of *V cholerae* may provide a source of outbreaks in endemic areas. Chronic cholera carriers are rare. The incubation period is short, usually 1–3 days.

Clinical Findings

A. Symptoms and Signs: Many patients infected with *V cholerae* have mild disease, with 1–2% developing severe diarrhea. During severe cholera, there is a sudden onset of massive, frequent, watery stools, generally light gray in color ("rice-water") and containing some mucus but no pus. Vomiting may be projectile and is not accompanied by nausea. Within 2–3 hours, the tremendous loss of fluids results in life-threatening dehydration, hypochloremia, and hypokalemia, with marked weakness and collapse. Renal failure with uremia and irreversible peripheral vascular collapse will occur if fluid therapy is not administered. The illness lasts 1–7 days and is shortened by appropriate antibiotic therapy.

B. Laboratory Findings: Markedly elevated hemoglobin (20 g/dL) and marked acidosis, hypochloremia, and hyponatremia are seen, and marked acidosis may complicate isotonic dehydration.

Cultural confirmation using thiosulfate-citrate-bile salt-sucrose (TCBS) agar takes 16–18 hours for a presumptive diagnosis and 36–48 hours for a definitive bacteriologic diagnosis.

Prevention

Cholera vaccine is available and provides 50% efficacy. Protection lasts 3–6 months. Cholera vaccine is not generally recommended for travelers. In endemic areas, all water and milk must be boiled, food protected from flies, and sanitary precautions observed. Thorough cooking of shellfish prevents transmission. All patients with cholera should be isolated.

Chemoprophylaxis is indicated for household and other close contacts of cholera patients. It should be initiated as soon as possible after the onset of the disease in the index patient. Tetracycline (500 mg daily for 5 days) is effective in preventing infection. Trimethoprim-sulfamethoxazole may be substituted in children.

Tourists visiting endemic areas are at little risk if they exercise common sense in what they eat and drink and maintain good personal hygiene.

Treatment

Physiologic saline or lactated Ringer's solution should be administered intravenously in large amounts to restore blood volume and urine output and prevent irreversible shock. Potassium supplements are required. Sodium bicarbonate, given intravenously, may also be needed initially to overcome profound acidosis. Moderate dehydration and acidosis can be corrected in 3–6 hours by oral therapy alone, because the active glucose transport system of the small bowel is normally functional. The optimal composition of the oral solution (in mEq/L) is as follows: Na^+ 90, Cl^- 80, and K^+ 20—with glucose, 110 mmol/L.

Treatment of children with tetracycline (50 mg/kg/d orally in four divided doses for 2–5 days) shortens the duration of the disease and prevents clinical relapse but is not as important as fluid and electrolyte therapy. Tetracycline resistance occurs in some regions, and ciprofloxacin may be used. Trimethoprim-sulfamethoxazole should be used in children under 9 years of age.

Prognosis

With early and rapid replacement of fluids and electrolytes, the case fatality rate is 1–2% in children. If significant symptoms appear and no treatment is given, the mortality rate is over 50%.

Birmingham ME et al: Epidemic cholera in Burundi: Patterns of transmission in the Great Rift Valley Lake region. Lancet 1997;349:981.

Carpenter CC: The treatment of cholera: Clinical science at the bedside. J Infect Dis 1992;166:2.

Fukuda JM et al: Clinical characteristics and risk factors for *Vibrio cholerae* infection in children. J Pediatr 1995;126:882.

Gotuzzo E et al: Ciprofloxacin for the treatment of cholera: A randomized, double-blind, controlled clinical trial of a single daily dose in Peruvian adults. Clin Infect Dis 1995;20:1485.

Lacey SW: Cholera: Calamitous past, ominous future. Clin Infect Dis 1995;20:1409.

Update: *Vibrio cholerae* 01—Western Hemisphere, 1991–1994, and *V cholerae* 0139—Asia, 1994. MMWR Morb Mortal Wkly Rep 1995;44:215.

CAMPYLOBACTER INFECTION

Essentials of Diagnosis & Typical Features

- Fever, vomiting, abdominal pain, diarrhea.
- Blood, mucus, pus in stools (dysentery).
- Presumptive diagnosis by darkfield or phase contrast microscopy of stool wet mount or modified Gram's stain.
- Definitive diagnosis by stool culture.

General Considerations

Campylobacter species are small gram-negative, curved or spiral bacilli that are commensals or pathogens in many animals. *Campylobacter jejuni* frequently causes acute enteritis in humans, and *Campylobacter fetus* causes bacteremia and meningitis in immunocompromised patients. *C fetus* may cause maternal fever, abortion, stillbirth, and severe neonatal infection. *Helicobacter pylori* (previously called *Campylobacter pylori*) causes most cases of gastritis and peptic ulcer disease in both adults and children (see Chapter 19).

In the past decade, *C jejuni* has been responsible for 3–11% of cases of acute gastroenteritis in North America and Europe; in many areas, enteritis due to *C jejuni* is more common than that due to *Salmonella* or *Shigella*.

Campylobacter colonizes domestic and wild animals, especially poultry. Numerous cases have been associated with sick puppies or other animal contacts. Contaminated food and water, improperly cooked poultry, and person-to-person spread by the fecal-oral route are important in transmission. Outbreaks associated with day care centers, contaminated water supplies, and raw milk have been reported. Raw milk consumption, often during visits to dairy farms, was responsible for 20 outbreaks involving nearly 500 children from 1981 to 1990. Newborns may acquire the organism from their mothers at delivery.

Clinical Findings

A. Symptoms and Signs: *C jejuni* enteritis can be mild or severe. In tropical countries, asymptomatic stool carriage is common. The incubation period is usually 1–7 days. The disease usually begins with sudden onset of high fever, malaise, headache, abdominal cramps, nausea, and vomiting. Diarrhea follows and may be watery or bile-stained, mucoid, and bloody. Passage of up to 20 stools per day is not uncommon. The illness is self-limiting, lasting 2–7 days, but relapses occur in 15–25% of cases. Without antimicrobial treatment, the organism remains in the stool for 1–6 weeks.

B. Laboratory Findings: The peripheral white blood cell count generally is elevated, with many band forms. Microscopic examination of stool reveals erythrocytes and pus cells, and darkfield or phase contrast microscopic examination of wet mounts may reveal darting bacilli characteristic of *Campylobacter.* Other bacteria, particularly *Vibrio* species, may exhibit similar motility, but in areas where cholera and *Vibrio parahaemolyticus* diarrhea are rare, a positive darkfield examination has a predictive value of about 90%. Isolation of *C jejuni* from stool is not difficult but requires selective agar, incubation at 42 °C rather than 35 °C, and incubation in an atmosphere of about 5% oxygen and 5% CO_2 (candle jar is satisfactory).

Differential Diagnosis

Campylobacter enteritis may resemble viral gastroenteritis, salmonellosis, shigellosis, amebiasis, or other infectious diarrheas. Because it also mimics ulcerative colitis, Crohn's disease, intussusception, and appendicitis, mistaken diagnosis can lead to unnecessary surgery.

Complications

The most important complications are dehydration and inappropriate treatment due to misdiagnosis as inflammatory bowel disease. Other uncommon complications include erythema nodosum, convulsions, reactive arthritis, bacteremia, urinary tract infection, and cholecystitis. Guillain-Barré syndrome may follow *C jejuni* infection by 1–3 weeks.

Prevention

No vaccine is available. Hand washing and adherence to basic food sanitation practices help prevent disease. Hand washing and cleaning of kitchen utensils after contact with raw poultry are important.

Treatment

Treatment of fluid and electrolyte disturbances is most important. Antimicrobial treatment with erythromycin in children (30–50 mg/kg/d orally in four divided doses for 5 days) or with ciprofloxacin in adults terminates fecal excretion and may prevent relapses. Therapy given early in the course of the illness will shorten the duration of symptoms but is unnecessary if given later. Antimicrobials used for shigellosis, such as trimethoprim-sulfamethoxazole and ampicillin, are inactive against *Campylobacter.* Supportive therapy is sufficient in most cases.

Prognosis

The outlook is excellent if dehydration is corrected and misdiagnosis does not lead to inappropriate diagnostic or surgical procedures.

Allos BM, Blaser MJ: *Campylobacter jejuni* and the expanding spectrum of related infections. Clin Infect Dis 1995;20:1092.

Rees JH et al: *Campylobacter jejuni* infection and Guillain-Barré syndrome. N Engl J Med 1995;333:1374.

Wong S-N et al: *Campylobacter* infection in the neonate: Case report and review of the literature. Pediatr Infect Dis J 1990;9:665.

Wood RC et al: *Campylobacter* enteritis outbreaks associated with drinking raw milk during youth activities. JAMA 1992;268:3228.

TULAREMIA

Essentials of Diagnosis & Typical Features

- A cutaneous or mucous membrane lesion at the site of inoculation and regional lymph node enlargement.
- Sudden onset of fever, chills, and prostration.
- History of contact with infected animals, principally wild rabbits, or history of tick exposure.
- Positive culture or immunofluorescence from mucocutaneous ulcer or regional lymph nodes.
- High serum antibody titer.

General Considerations

Tularemia is caused by *Francisella tularensis,* a gram-negative organism usually acquired directly from infected animals, principally wild rabbits; occasionally from infected domestic dogs or cats; by contamination of the skin or mucous membranes with infected blood or tissues; by inhalation of infected material; by bites of ticks, fleas, or deer flies that have been in contact with infected animals; or by ingestion of contaminated meat or water. Strains of high virulence for humans and rabbits (Jellison type A) and strains with lowered virulence (Jellison type B) for humans, which are avirulent in rabbits, are present throughout the United States. The incubation period is short, usually 3–7 days, but may vary from 2 to 25 days.

Ticks are the most important vector. Rabbits are the classic vectors of tularemia. It is important to seek a history of rabbit hunting, skinning, or food preparation in any patient who has a febrile illness with tender lymphadenopathy, often in the region of a draining skin ulcer.

Clinical Findings

A. Symptoms and Signs: Several clinical types of tularemia are seen in children. Sixty percent of infections are of the ulceroglandular form and start as a reddened papule that may be pruritic, quickly ulcerates, and is not very painful. Shortly thereafter, the regional lymph nodes become large and tender. Fluctuance quickly follows. At the same time, there may be marked systemic manifestations, including high fever, chills, weakness, and vomiting. Pneumonitis occasionally accompanies the ulceroglandular form or may be seen as the sole manifestation of infection (pneumonic form). A detectable skin lesion is occasionally absent, and localized lymphoid enlargement exists alone (glandular form). Oculoglandular and oropharyngeal forms also occur in children. The latter is characterized by tonsillitis, often with membrane formation, cervical adenopathy, and high fever. In the absence of any primary ulcer or localized lymphadenitis, a prolonged febrile disease reminiscent of typhoid fever can be seen (typhoidal form). Splenomegaly is common in all forms.

B. Laboratory Findings: *F tularensis* can be recovered from ulcers, regional lymph nodes, and sputum of patients with the pneumonic form. However, the organism grows only on an enriched medium (blood-cystine-glucose agar), and laboratory handling is dangerous owing to the risk of airborne transmission to laboratory personnel. Immunofluorescent staining of biopsy material or aspirates of involved lymph nodes is diagnostic, although it is not widely available.

The white blood cell count is not remarkable. Agglutinins are present after the second week of illness, and in the absence of a positive culture their development confirms the diagnosis. An agglutination titer of 1:160 or higher is considered positive.

Differential Diagnosis

The typhoidal form of tularemia may mimic typhoid, brucellosis, miliary tuberculosis, Rocky Mountain spotted fever, and infectious mononucleosis. Pneumonic tularemia resembles atypical or mycotic pneumonitis. The ulceroglandular type of tularemia resembles pyoderma caused by staphylococci or streptococci, rat-bite fever, plague, anthrax, and cat-scratch fever. The oropharyngeal type must be distinguished from streptococcal or diphtheritic pharyngitis, infectious mononucleosis, herpangina, or other viral pharyngitides.

Prevention

Reasonable attempts should be made to protect children from bites of insects, principally ticks, fleas, and deer flies, by the use of proper clothing and repellents. Since rabbits are the source of most human infections, the dressing and handling of such game should be performed with great care. If contact occurs, thorough washing with soap and water is indicated.

Treatment

A. Specific Measures: Streptomycin (30 mg/kg/d intramuscularly in two divided doses for 8–10 days; maximum dose 1 g) is the drug of choice, though gentamicin is efficacious, more available, and familiar to clinicians. Tetracycline is effective, but relapse rates are higher. Chloramphenicol is less effective. Failures occur with ceftriaxone.

B. General Measures: Antipyretics and analgesics may be given as necessary. Skin lesions are best left open. Glandular lesions occasionally require incision and drainage.

Prognosis

The prognosis is excellent with appropriate therapy in patients recognized early.

Cross JT, Jacobs RF: Tularemia: Treatment failures with outpatient use of ceftriaxone. Clin Infect Dis 1993; 17:976.

Enderlin G et al: Streptomycin and alternative agents for the treatment of tularemia: Review of the literature. Clin Infect Dis 1994;19:42.

Liles WC, Burger RJ: Tularemia from domestic cats. West J Med 1993;158:619.

Spach DH et al: Tick-borne diseases in the United States. N Engl J Med 1993;329:936.

PLAGUE

Essentials of Diagnosis & Typical Features

- Sudden onset of fever, chills, and prostration.
- Regional lymphadenitis with suppuration of nodes (bubonic form).
- Hemorrhage into skin and mucous membranes and shock (septicemia).
- Cough, dyspnea, cyanosis, and hemoptysis (pneumonia).
- History of exposure to infected animals.

General Considerations

Plague is an extremely serious acute infection caused by a gram-negative bacillus, *Yersinia pestis.* It is a disease of rodents that is transmitted to humans by the bites of fleas. Plague bacilli have been isolated from rodents in 15 of the western states in the United States. Direct contact with rodents, rabbits, or domestic cats may transmit fleas infected with plague bacilli. During the 1980s, a mean of 18 cases per year was reported in the United States, primarily from the southwestern region. Most cases occur from June through September.

Human plague in the United States appears to occur in cycles that reflect cycles in wild animal reservoirs.

Clinical Findings

A. Symptoms and Signs: Plague assumes several clinical forms, the two most common being bubonic and septicemic. Pneumonic plague, the form that occurs when organisms enter the body through the respiratory tract, is now very uncommon.

1. Bubonic plague–Bubonic plague begins after an incubation period of 6 days with a sudden onset of high fever, chills, headache, vomiting, and marked delirium or clouding of consciousness. A less severe form also exists, with a less precipitous onset, but with progression over several days to severe symptoms. Although the flea bite is rarely seen, the regional lymph node, usually inguinal and unilateral, is painful and tender, 1–5 cm in diameter. The node usually suppurates and drains spontaneously after 1 week. The plague bacillus produces endotoxin that causes vascular necrosis. Bacilli may overwhelm regional lymph nodes and enter the circulation to produce septicemia. Severe vascular necrosis results in widely disseminated hemorrhage in skin, mucous membranes, liver, and spleen. Myocarditis and circulatory collapse may result from damage by the endotoxin.

Plague meningitis or pneumonia may occur following bacteremic spread from an infected lymph node.

2. Septicemic plague–The septicemic form is defined as any case of plague without evidence of lymphadenopathy. Regional lymphadenopathy and bubo formation occur after 3–5 days. This form is less common than bubonic plague but carries a worse prognosis, largely because it is less likely to be recognized and treated early. Patients may present initially with a nonspecific febrile illness characterized by fever, myalgia, chills, and anorexia. It is frequently complicated by pneumonia.

B. Laboratory Findings: Aspiration of a bubo leads to visualization of bipolar staining gram-negative bacilli on a stained smear. Pus, sputum, and blood all yield the organism, though laboratory infections are common enough to make isolation dangerous. A buffy coat Gram stain may reveal the organism, and blood-agar cultures yield positive results in 48 hours. The white blood cell count is markedly elevated, with a shift to the left. Paired acute and convalescent sera may be tested for a significant antibody rise in those cases with negative cultures.

Differential Diagnosis

The septic phase of the disease may be confused with such illnesses as meningococcemia, sepsis, and rickettsioses. The bubonic form resembles tularemia, anthrax, cat-scratch fever, streptococcal adenitis, and cellulitis. Primary gastroenteritis and appendicitis may have to be distinguished.

Prevention

Proper disposal of household and commercial wastes and chemical control of rats are basic for control of plague. Flea control is instituted and maintained with liberal use of insecticides. Children vacationing in remote camping areas should be warned not to handle dead or dying animals. Domestic cats that roam freely in suburban areas may contact infected wild animals and acquire infected fleas. Travelers to wild areas in the enzootic western states are at low risk of infection, and immunization of visitors to these areas is not recommended. Vaccination is recommended for those traveling to or living in areas of high incidence (see Chapter 9).

Treatment

A. Specific Measures: Streptomycin (20–40 mg/kg/d intramuscularly) or gentamicin (7.5 mg/kg/d) in three divided doses for 5–7 days is effective. For patients not requiring parenteral therapy, tetracycline (20–30 mg/kg/d in four divided doses) or chloramphenicol (75–100 mg/kg/d intravenously or orally in four divided doses) may be given for 10–14 days. Tetracycline is not recommended for children under 9 years of age. Plague bacilli that are multiply resistant to antimicrobials are uncommon but of serious concern.

In septicemic and pneumonic plague, specific antibiotic treatment must be started in the first 24 hours of the disease if survival is to be expected.

Bubonic plague is not highly contagious. Every effort is made to effect resolution of buboes without resorting to surgery. Pus from draining lymph nodes should be handled with gloves.

B. General Measures: Pneumonic plague is highly infectious, and strict isolation is required. All contacts should receive prophylaxis with sulfadiazine (100–200 mg/kg/d orally in four divided doses for 7 days) or tetracycline (30 mg/kg/d in four divided doses for 7 days).

Prognosis

The mortality rate in untreated bubonic plague is about 50%; it is 90% in the septicemic form and nearly 100% in the pneumonic form. Recent mortality rates in New Mexico were 3% for bubonic plague and 71% for the septicemic form.

Craven BB, Barnes AM: Plague and tularemia. Infect Dis Clin North Am 1991;5:165.

Crook LD: Plague: A clinical review of 27 cases. Arch Intern Med 1992;152:1253.

Fatal human plague—Arizona and Colorado, 1996. MMWR Morb Mortal Wkly Rep 1997;46:617.

Galimand M et al: Multidrug resistance in *Yersinia pestis* mediated by a transferable plasmid. N Engl J Med 1997;337:667.

HAEMOPHILUS INFLUENZAE TYPE b INFECTIONS

Essentials of Diagnosis & Typical Features

- Purulent meningitis in children under age 4 years with direct smears of cerebrospinal fluid showing gram-negative pleomorphic rods.
- Acute epiglottitis: High fever, drooling, dysphagia, aphonia, and stridor.
- Septic arthritis: Fever, local redness, swelling, heat, and pain with active or passive motion of the involved joint in a child 4 months to 4 years of age.
- Cellulitis: Sudden onset of fever and distinctive

cellulitis in an infant, often involving the cheek or periorbital area.
- In all cases, a positive culture from the blood, cerebrospinal fluid, or aspirated pus confirm the diagnosis.

General Considerations

H influenzae type b (Hib) has become uncommon because of widespread immunization in early infancy. The 95% reduction in incidence seen in many parts of the United States is due to high rates of vaccine coverage and reduced nasopharyngeal carriage after vaccination. Although the incidence is reduced, Hib remains important because of its potential for serious invasive disease. Three hundred and seventeen cases of Hib were reported in the United States in 1995. It causes meningitis, bacteremia, epiglottitis (supraglottic croup), septic arthritis, periorbital and facial cellulitis, pneumonia, and pericarditis. Hib infections occur most frequently in the age group from 4 months to 4 years (epiglottitis: 2–5 years). Recognition and prompt therapy of the many serious manifestations of Hib infection will become more challenging as physicians encounter fewer infections.

Antibody to the Hib capsular polysaccharide polyribose phosphate (PRP) is protective against invasive disease. PRP is a poor immunogen, particularly in infants less than 2 years old. Vaccines consisting of PRP chemically conjugated to protein are far more immunogenic and raise protective levels of antibody in infants beginning at age 2 months. Four separate interchangeable PRP protein conjugate vaccines are available (see Chapter 9).

Disease due to *H influenzae* types A, C, D, E, F, or unencapsulated strains is uncommonly seen but now comprises a larger proportion of positive cultures. Third-generation cephalosporins are preferred for initial therapy of suspected Hib infections. Ampicillin is adequate for culture-proved Hib where susceptibility to ampicillin has been proved by the microbiology laboratory.

Unencapsulated, nontypable *H influenzae* frequently colonizes the mucous membranes and causes otitis media, sinusitis, bronchitis, and pneumonia in both children and adults. Bacteremia is uncommon but does occur. Neonatal sepsis similar to early-onset group B streptococci is recognized. Obstetric complications of chorioamnionitis and bacteremia are associated with these neonatal cases.

Ampicillin resistance occurs in 25–40% of nontypable *H influenzae.*

Clinical Findings

A. Symptoms and Signs:

1. Meningitis–In the United States, Hib is an uncommon cause of bacterial meningitis except in unimmunized children. Infants usually present with fever, irritability, lethargy, poor feeding with or without vomiting, and a high-pitched cry.

2. Acute epiglottitis–The most useful clinical finding in the early diagnosis of Hib epiglottitis is evidence of dysphagia, characterized by a refusal to eat or swallow saliva and by drooling. This finding, plus the presence of a high fever in a "toxic" child—even in the absence of a cherry-red epiglottis on direct examination—should strongly suggest the diagnosis and lead to prompt intubation. Stridor is a late sign. (See Chapter 16 for details.)

3. Septic arthritis–Hib is a common cause of septic arthritis in unimmunized children under 4 years of age in the United States. The child is febrile and refuses to move the involved joint and limb because of pain. Examination reveals swelling, warmth, redness, tenderness on palpation, and severe pain on attempted movement of the joint.

4. Cellulitis–Cellulitis due to Hib occurs almost exclusively in the age group from 3 months to 4 years but is now uncommon as a result of immunization. Fever is usually noted at the same time as the cellulitis, and many infants appear toxic. The cheek or periorbital (preseptal) area is usually involved.

B. Laboratory Findings: The white blood cell count in Hib infections may be high or normal with a shift to the left. Blood culture is frequently positive. Positive culture of aspirated pus or fluid from the involved site proves the diagnosis.

In meningitis (before treatment), spinal fluid smear may show the characteristic pleomorphic gram-negative rods.

C. Imaging: A lateral view of the neck in suspected acute epiglottitis may suggest the diagnosis, but misinterpretation is common. Intubation should not be delayed to obtain films. Haziness of maxillary and ethmoid sinuses occurs with orbital cellulitis.

Differential Diagnosis

A. Meningitis: Meningitis must be differentiated from head injury, brain abscess, tumor, lead encephalopathy, and other forms of meningoencephalitis, including mycobacterial, viral, fungal, and bacterial agents.

B. Acute Epiglottitis: In croup caused by viral agents (parainfluenza 1, 2, and 3, respiratory syncytial virus, influenza A, adenovirus), the child has more definite upper respiratory symptoms, cough, hoarseness, slower progression of obstructive signs, and fever. Spasmodic croup occurs typically at night in a child with a history of previous attacks; these attacks may be of allergic origin. A history of sudden onset of choking and paroxysmal coughing suggests aspiration of a foreign body. Retropharyngeal abscess occasionally or laryngeal diphtheria rarely may have to be differentiated from epiglottitis.

C. Septic Arthritis: Differential diagnosis includes acute osteomyelitis, prepatellar bursitis, cellulitis, rheumatic fever, and fractures and sprains.

D. Cellulitis: Erysipelas, streptococcal cellulitis, insect bites, and trauma (including Popsicle panniculitis or other types of freezing injury) may occur. Periorbital cellulitis must be differentiated from paranasal sinus disease without cellulitis, allergic inflammatory disease of the lids, conjunctivitis, and herpes zoster infection.

Complications
  A. Meningitis: See Chapter 22.
  B. Acute Epiglottitis: The disease may rapidly progress to complete airway obstruction with complications owing to hypoxia. Mediastinal emphysema and pneumothorax may occur.
  C. Septic Arthritis: Septic arthritis may result in rapid destruction of cartilage and ankylosis if diagnosis and treatment are delayed. Even with early treatment, the incidence of residual damage and disability after septic arthritis in weight-bearing joints may be as high as 25%.
  D. Cellulitis: Bacteremia may lead to meningitis or pyarthrosis.

Prevention
  Epidemiologic studies have demonstrated that families and close contacts of patients with Hib infections are at increased risk of acquiring infection. The index case and all household contacts should be given rifampin, 20 mg/kg/d (maximum adult dose 600 mg/d), orally for 4 successive days. There is controversy regarding a recommendation for chemoprophylaxis for day care center contacts. Some authorities recommend rifampin chemoprophylaxis for young contacts (especially children age 2 or less) of a case who regularly attended a day care center. Other authorities believe that the risk to day care center contacts is low and do not recommend prophylaxis unless two cases of systemic Hib disease have occurred in children in the day care center within a 60-day period. Rifampin, if used, should be given to children in the same classroom as the index case and to adults working in that classroom.

Treatment
  All bacteremic or potentially bacteremic Hib diseases require hospitalization for treatment. The drugs of choice in hospitalized cases are a third-generation cephalosporin (cefotaxime or ceftriaxone) until the sensitivity of the organism is known.
  A. Meningitis: Therapy is begun as soon as bacterial meningitis has been identified and cerebrospinal fluid, blood, and other appropriate cultures have been obtained. Therapy is begun with cefotaxime (50 mg/kg intravenously every 6 hours) or ceftriaxone (50 mg/kg intravenously every 12 hours). If the organism is sensitive to ampicillin, it is the drug of choice. Therapy should preferably be given intravenously for the entire course; ceftriaxone may be given intramuscularly if venous access becomes difficult.
  Duration of therapy is 10 days. Although a 7-day

regimen appears effective in most uncomplicated cases, it has not been studied in children who have also been treated with steroids to prevent hearing loss (see below). Longer treatment is reserved for children who respond slowly or in whom septic complications have occurred.
  Repeated lumbar taps are usually not necessary in Hib meningitis. They should be obtained in the following circumstances: unsatisfactory or questionable clinical response, seizure occurring after several days of therapy, and prolonged (7 days) or recurrent fever if the neurologic examination is abnormal or difficult to evaluate. Routine lumbar tap at the end of therapy is not recommended. (See Chapter 22 for additional information.)
  Dexamethasone given immediately after diagnosis and continued for 2–4 days may reduce the incidence of hearing loss in children with Hib meningitis. The use of dexamethasone is controversial, but when it is used the dose is 0.6 mg/kg/d in four divided doses for 2–4 days. Therapy is not recommended for longer than 4 days, for neonates, or for viral meningitis. In animal models, it is important to give dexamethasone prior to beginning antimicrobials; this maximally blocks formation of inflammatory mediators (interleukin-1β and tumor necrosis factor) thought responsible for eighth nerve damage.
  B. Acute Epiglottitis: See Chapter 16.
  C. Septic Arthritis: Initial therapy should include nafcillin (or another effective antistaphylococcal antibiotic), 150 mg/kg/d in four divided doses, and cefotaxime or ceftriaxone (dosage as for meningitis). If the isolate is sensitive to ampicillin, it is given in a dosage of 200–300 mg/kg/d intravenously in four divided doses. If a child is improved following initial intravenous therapy, oral amoxicillin (75–100 mg/kg/d in four divided doses every 6 hours) may be administered under careful supervision to complete a 2-week course. Alternative oral agents for ampicillin-resistant organisms include chloramphenicol, cefaclor, trimethoprim-sulfamethoxazole, amoxicillin-clavulanic acid, and cefixime. Ideally, susceptibility to these agents should be proved prior to use. Drainage of infected joint fluid is an essential part of treatment. In joints other than the hip, this can often be accomplished by one or more needle aspirations. In hip infections—and in arthritis of other joints where treatment is delayed or clinical response is slow—surgical drainage is advised. Local instillation of antibiotics is not necessary and may be injurious. The joint should be immobilized.
  D. Cellulitis, Including Orbital Cellulitis: Initial therapy should include an agent effective against staphylococci in combination with cefotaxime or ceftriaxone. Ampicillin may be used if the isolate is shown to be susceptible. Therapy is given parenterally for 3–7 days, followed by oral treatment as for septic arthritis, and supportive and symptomatic

treatment as required. There is usually marked improvement after 72 hours of treatment. Antibiotics should be given for 10–14 days.

Prognosis

The case fatality rate for Hib meningitis is less than 5%. Young infants have the highest mortality rate. One of the most common neurologic sequelae, which develops in approximately 5–10% of patients with Hib meningitis, is significant sensorineural hearing loss. All patients with Hib meningitis should have their hearing checked at some time during the course of the illness or shortly after recovery.

Children in whom invasive Hib infection develops despite appropriate immunization should have tests to investigate immune function and to rule out HIV.

The case fatality rate in acute epiglottitis is 2–5%; deaths are associated with bacteremia and the rapid development of airway obstruction. The prognosis for the other diseases requiring hospitalization is good with the institution of early and adequate antibiotic therapy.

Gorelick MH, Baker MD: Epiglottitis in children, 1979 through 1992. Arch Pediatr Adolesc Med 1994;148:47.

Haemophilus influenzae: Its role in pediatric infections. Pediatr Infect Dis J 1997;16(Suppl):83.

Kinney JS et al: Early onset Haemophilus influenzae sepsis in the newborn infant. Pediatr Infect Dis J 1993;12:739.

Korones DN, Marshall GS, Shapiro ED: Outcome of children with occult bacteremia caused by Haemophilus influenzae type b. Pediatr Infect Dis J 1992;11:516.

Kostman JR et al: Invasive Haemophilus influenzae infections in older children and adults in Seattle. Clin Infect Dis 1993;17:389.

Progress toward elimination of Haemophilus influenzae type b disease among infants and children—United States, 1987–1995. MMWR Morb Mortal Wkly Rep 1996;45:901.

Haemophilus influenzae. Diagn Microbiol Infect Dis 1995;21:223.

Valdepena HG et al: Epiglottitis and Haemophilus influenzae immunization: The Pittsburgh experience—a five-year review. Pediatrics 1995;96:424.

PERTUSSIS
(Whooping Cough)

Essentials of Diagnosis
& Typical Features

- Prodromal catarrhal stage (1–3 weeks) characterized by mild cough, coryza, and fever.
- Persistent staccato, paroxysmal cough ending with a high-pitched inspiratory "whoop."
- Leukocytosis with absolute lymphocytosis.
- Diagnosis confirmed by fluorescent stain or culture of nasopharyngeal secretions.

General Considerations

Pertussis is an acute, highly communicable infection of the respiratory tract caused by *Bordetella pertussis* and characterized by severe bronchitis. Children usually acquire the disease from symptomatic family contacts. Adults who have mild respiratory illness, not recognized as pertussis, frequently are the source of infection. Asymptomatic carriage of *B pertussis* is not documented. Infectivity is greatest during the catarrhal and early paroxysmal cough stage (for about 4 weeks after onset).

The disease is most common and most severe in early infancy. In 1995, over 5000 cases were reported in the United States. From 1992 to 1994, 41% of cases occurred in children under 1 year of age. Seventy-four percent of hospitalized patients were infants aged 6 months or less. Fifteen percent had pneumonia, 1.9% had seizures, 0.2% had encephalopathy, and 0.6% died.

Active immunity follows natural pertussis. Reinfections occur years to decades later but are usually milder. Immunity following vaccination wanes in 5–10 years. The majority of young adults in the United States are susceptible to pertussis infection, and disease is probably common but unrecognized.

Bordetella parapertussis causes a similar but milder syndrome and is reported frequently in Central Europe.

B pertussis organisms attach to the ciliated respiratory epithelium and multiply there; deeper invasion does not occur. Disease is due to several bacterial toxins; the most potent is pertussis toxin, which is responsible for lymphocytosis and many of the symptoms of pertussis.

Clinical Findings

A. Symptoms and Signs: The onset of pertussis is insidious, with catarrhal upper respiratory tract symptoms (rhinitis, sneezing, and an irritating cough). Slight fever may be present; temperature greater than 38.3 °C suggests bacterial superinfection or another cause of respiratory tract infection. After about 2 weeks, cough becomes paroxysmal, characterized by 10–30 forceful coughs ending with a loud inspiration (the "whoop"). Infants and adults with otherwise typical severe pertussis often lack characteristic whooping. Vomiting commonly follows a paroxysm. Coughing is accompanied by cyanosis, sweating, prostration, and exhaustion. This stage lasts for 2–4 weeks, with gradual improvement. Cough suggestive of chronic bronchitis lasts for another 2–3 weeks. Paroxysmal coughing may continue for some months and may worsen with intercurrent viral respiratory infection. In adults, older children, and partially immunized individuals, symptoms may consist only of irritating cough lasting 1–2 weeks. In the younger unimmunized child, symptoms of pertussis last about 8 weeks or longer. Clinical pertussis is milder in immunized children.

B. Laboratory Findings: White blood cell

counts of 20,000–30,000/μL with 70–80% lymphocytes typically appear near the end of the catarrhal stage. Many older children and adults with mild infections never demonstrate lymphocytosis. The blood picture may resemble lymphocytic leukemia or leukemoid reactions. Identification of *B pertussis* by culture from nasopharyngeal swabs or nasal wash specimens proves the diagnosis. The organism may be found in the respiratory tract in diminishing numbers beginning in the catarrhal stage and ending about 2 weeks after the beginning of the paroxysmal stage. After 4–5 weeks of symptoms, cultures and fluorescent antibody tests are almost always negative. Charcoal agar containing an antimicrobial should be inoculated as soon as possible; *B pertussis* does not tolerate drying or prolonged transport. Enzyme-linked immunosorbent assays for detection of antibody to pertussis toxin or filamentous hemagglutinin may be useful for diagnosis but are currently not widely available. The chest x-ray reveals thickened bronchi and sometimes shows a "shaggy" heart border, indicating bronchopneumonia and patchy atelectasis.

Differential Diagnosis

The differential diagnosis of pertussis includes bacterial, tuberculous, chlamydial, and viral pneumonia. Cystic fibrosis and foreign body aspiration may be considerations. Adenoviruses and respiratory syncytial virus may cause paroxysmal coughing with an associated elevation of lymphocytes in the peripheral blood, mimicking pertussis.

Complications

Bronchopneumonia due to superinfection is the most common serious complication. It is characterized by abrupt clinical deterioration during the paroxysmal stage, accompanied by high fever and sometimes a striking leukemoid reaction with a shift to predominantly polymorphonuclear leukocytes. Atelectasis is a second common pulmonary complication. Atelectasis may be patchy or extensive and may shift rapidly to involve different areas of lung. Intercurrent viral respiratory infection is also a common complication and may provoke worsening or recurrence of paroxysmal coughing. Otitis media is common. Residual chronic bronchiectasis is infrequent despite the severity of the illness. Apnea and sudden death may occur during a particularly severe paroxysm. A diffuse encephalopathy may complicate severe cases and frequently is fatal. It is unclear whether anoxic brain damage, cerebral hemorrhage, or pertussis neurotoxins are to blame, but anoxia is most likely the cause. Epistaxis and subconjunctival hemorrhages are common.

Prevention

Active immunization (see Chapter 9) with pertussis vaccine in combination with diphtheria and tetanus toxoids (DTP) should be given in early infancy. Acellular pertussis (DTaP) vaccines cause less fever and fewer local and febrile systemic reactions and are preferred for all doses. Pertussis cases have greatly increased recently, probably due in part to the large number of children who are not adequately immunized and in part to an increased incidence of the disease in adults.

Chemoprophylaxis with erythromycin should be given to exposed family and hospital contacts, particularly those under age 2 years. Hospitalized children with pertussis should be isolated because of the great risk of transmission to patients and staff. Several large hospital outbreaks have been reported in the last decade.

Treatment

A. Specific Measures: Antibiotics may ameliorate early infections but have no effect on clinical symptoms in the paroxysmal stage. Erythromycin is the drug of choice since it promptly terminates respiratory tract carriage of *B pertussis.* A single resistant strain has been reported. Patients should be treated with erythromycin estolate (40–50 mg/kg/24 h in four divided doses for 14 days). Erythromycin ethylsuccinate is efficacious, but the higher dose recommended causes considerable gastrointestinal intolerance. A recent study suggests that 7 days and 14 days of treatment are equally effective. Clarithromycin for 7 days and azithromycin for 5 days were equal to erythromycin for 14 days in one small study. Ampicillin (100 mg/kg/d divided in four doses) may also be used for erythromycin-intolerant patients. Household or other close contacts such as in day care centers should be treated with erythromycin to reduce secondary transmission. This prophylaxis should be used regardless of age or immunization status.

Corticosteroids reduce the severity of disease but may mask signs of bacterial superinfection. Albuterol (0.3–0.5 mg/kg/d in four doses) has reduced the severity of illness, but tachycardia is common when the drug is given orally, and aerosol administration may precipitate paroxysms.

B. General Measures: Nutritional support during the paroxysmal phase is very important. Frequent small feedings, tube feeding, or parenteral fluid supplementation may be needed. Minimizing stimuli that trigger paroxysms is probably the best way of controlling cough. In general, cough suppressants are of little benefit.

C. Treatment of Complications: Respiratory insufficiency due to pneumonia or other pulmonary complications should be treated with oxygen and assisted ventilation if necessary. Convulsions are treated with oxygen and anticonvulsants. Bacterial pneumonia or otitis media requires additional antibiotics.

Prognosis

The prognosis for patients with pertussis has improved in recent years because of adequate nursing care, treatment of complications, nutrition, and modern intensive care. However, the disease is still very serious in infants under 1 year of age; most deaths occur in this age group. Children with encephalopathy have a poor prognosis.

Aoyama T et al: Efficacy of short-term treatment of pertussis with clarithromycin and azithromycin. J Pediatr 1996;129:761.

Bortolussi R et al: Clinical course of pertussis in immunized children. Pediatr Infect Dis J 1995;14:870.

Christie CDC et al: The 1993 epidemic of pertussis in Cincinnati. N Engl J Med 1994;331:16.

Halperin SA et al: Seven days of erythromycin estolate is as effective as fourteen days for the treatment of *Bordetella pertussis* infections. Pediatrics 1997;100:65.

He Q et al: Sensitive and specific polymerase chain reaction assays for detection of *Bordetella pertussis* in nasopharyngeal specimens. J Pediatr 1994;126:421.

Lewis K et al: Pertussis caused by an erythromycin-resistant strain of *Bordetella pertussis*. Pediatr Infect Dis J 1995;14:388.

Long SS et al: Widespread silent transmission of pertussis in families: Antibody correlates of infection and symptomatology. J Infect Dis 1990;161:480.

Pertussis—United States, January 1992–June 1995. MMWR Morb Mortal Wkly Rep 1995;44:525.

Roberts I, Gavin R, Lennon D: Randomized controlled trial of steroids in pertussis. Pediatr Infect Dis J 1992;11:982.

LISTERIOSIS

Essentials of Diagnosis & Typical Features

Early-onset neonatal disease:

- Signs of sepsis a few hours after birth in an infant born with fetal distress and hepatosplenomegaly; maternal fever.

Late-onset neonatal disease:

- Meningitis, sometimes with monocytosis in the cerebrospinal fluid and peripheral blood. Onset at 9–30 days of age.

General Considerations

Listeria monocytogenes is a gram-positive, nonspore-forming aerobic rod distributed widely in the animal kingdom and in food, dust, and soil. It causes systemic infections in newborn infants and immunosuppressed older children. In pregnant women, infection is relatively mild, with fever, aches, and chills, but is accompanied by bacteremia and sometimes results in intrauterine or perinatal infection with grave consequences for the fetus or newborn. One-fourth of the cases occurred in pregnant women, and 20% of their pregnancies ended in stillbirth or neonatal death. *Listeria* is present in the stool of approximately 10% of the normal population. Persons in contact with animals are at greater risk. Recent large food-borne outbreaks have been traced to contaminated cabbage in coleslaw, contaminated soft cheese, and milk. The role of contaminated food in sporadic listeriosis is now recognized.

Like group B streptococcal infections, *Listeria* infections in the newborn can be divided into early and late forms. Early infections are more common, leading to a severe congenital form of infection. Later infections are often characterized by meningitis.

Clinical Findings

A. Symptoms and Signs: In the early neonatal form, symptoms of listeriosis usually appear on the first day of life and always by the third day. Fetal distress is common, and infants frequently have signs of severe disease at birth. Respiratory distress, diarrhea, and fever occur. On examination, hepatosplenomegaly and a papular rash are found. A history of maternal fever is common. Meningitis may accompany the septic course.

The late neonatal form usually occurs after 9 days of age and can occur as late as 5 weeks. Meningitis is common, characterized by irritability, fever, and poor feeding.

Listeria infections occur rarely in older children, usually in those with animal contact or those who are immunosuppressed. Signs and symptoms are those of meningitis, usually with insidious onset.

B. Laboratory Findings: In all patients except those receiving white cell depressant drugs, the white blood cell count is elevated, with 10–20% monocytes. When meningitis is found, the characteristic cerebrospinal fluid cell count is high (> 500/μL) with a predominance of polymorphonuclear leukocytes in 70% of cases; monocytes predominate in up to 30%. Gram-stained smears of cerebrospinal fluid are usually negative, but short gram-positive rods may be seen. The chief pathologic feature in severe neonatal sepsis is miliary granulomatosis with microabscesses in liver, spleen, central nervous system, lung, and bowel.

Cultures are frequently positive from multiple sites, including blood in the infant and the mother. The organisms form small, weakly hemolytic colonies on blood agar which may be mistaken for streptococci.

Differential Diagnosis

Early-onset neonatal disease resembles hemolytic disease of the newborn, group B streptococcal sepsis or severe cytomegalovirus infection, rubella, or toxoplasmosis. Late-onset disease must be differentiated from meningitis due to echovirus and coxsackievirus, group B streptococci, and gram-negative enteric bacteria.

Prevention

Immunosuppressed, pregnant, and elderly patients can decrease the risk of *Listeria* infection by avoiding soft cheeses and by thoroughly reheating or avoiding ready-to-eat foods. These recommendations include avoiding raw meat and milk and thorough washing of vegetables.

Treatment

Ampicillin (150–300 mg/kg/d every 6 hours intravenously) is the drug of choice in most cases of listeriosis. Gentamicin (2.5 mg/kg every 8 hours intravenously) should also be given, since it has a synergistic effect with ampicillin in vitro. If ampicillin cannot be used, trimethoprim-sulfamethoxazole is also effective. Cephalosporins are not effective. Treatment of severe disease should continue for at least 2 weeks.

Prognosis

In a recent outbreak of early-onset neonatal disease, the mortality rate was 27% despite aggressive and appropriate management. Meningitis in older infants has a good prognosis. In immunosuppressed children, prognosis depends to a great extent on that of the underlying illness.

Dalton CG et al: An outbreak of gastroenteritis and fever due to *Listeria monocytogenes* in milk. N Engl J Med 1997;336:100.

Foodborne listeriosis, United States 1988–1990: Update. MMWR Morb Mortal Wkly Rep 1992:41:251.

Gellin BG et al: The epidemiology of listeriosis in the United States—1986. Listeriosis Study Group. Am J Epidemiol 1991;133:392.

Schlech WF III: Listeria gastroenteritis: Old syndrome, new pathogen. N Engl J Med 1997;336:130.

Schuchat A et al: Role of foods in sporadic listeriosis. I. Case-control study of dietary risk factors. JAMA 1992;267:2041.

TUBERCULOSIS

Essentials of Diagnosis
& Typical Features

- All types: Positive tuberculin test in patient or members of household, suspicious chest x-ray, history of contact, and demonstration of organism by stain and culture.
- Pulmonary: Fatigue, irritability, and undernutrition, with or without fever and cough.
- Glandular: Chronic cervical adenitis.
- Miliary: Classic "snowstorm" appearance of chest x-ray; choroidal tubercles.
- Meningitis: Fever and manifestations of meningeal irritation and increased intracranial pressure. Characteristic cerebrospinal fluid.

General Considerations

Tuberculosis is a granulomatous disease caused by *Mycobacterium tuberculosis*. It remains a leading cause of death throughout the world. Children under 3 years of age are most susceptible. Lymphohe-matogenous dissemination through the lungs to extrapulmonary sites, including the brain and meninges, eyes, bones and joints, lymph nodes, kidneys, intestines, larynx, and skin, is more likely to occur in infants. Increased susceptibility occurs again in adolescence, particularly in girls within 2 years of menarche. Tuberculosis in the United States has increased substantially since 1986 following three decades of decline. In 1995, over 22,000 cases were reported. Certain high-risk groups are identified, including ethnic minorities, foreign-born persons, prisoners, residents of nursing homes, indigents, migrant workers, and health care providers. HIV infection is an important risk factor both for development and spread of disease. Pediatric tuberculosis is also increasing, with about 1400 cases in children under age 15 reported in 1995. Exposure to an adult at risk for tuberculosis is the most common risk factor in children. The primary complex in infancy and childhood consists of a small parenchymal lesion in any area of the lung with caseation of regional nodes and calcification. Postprimary tuberculosis in adolescents and adults occurs in the apices of the lungs and is likely to cause chronic progressive cavitary pulmonary disease with less tendency for hematogenous dissemination.

Clinical Findings

A. Symptoms and Signs:

1. Pulmonary–See Chapter 17.

2. Miliary–Diagnosis is made on the basis of a classic snowstorm or millet seed appearance of lung fields on x-ray, though early in the course of disseminated tuberculosis the chest x-ray may show no or only subtle abnormalities. The majority also have a fresh primary complex and pleural effusion. Choroidal tubercles are sometimes seen on funduscopic examination. Other lesions may be present and produce osteomyelitis, arthritis, meningitis, tuberculomas of the brain, enteritis, or infection of the kidneys and liver.

3. Meningitis–Symptoms include fever, vomiting, headache, lethargy, and irritability, with signs of meningeal irritation and increased intracranial pressure, including cranial nerve palsies, convulsions, and coma. Choroidal tubercles are pathognomonic when associated with these signs and symptoms. Otorrhea or acute otitis media may be seen.

4. Glandular–The primary complex may be associated with a skin lesion drained by regional nodes or chronic cervical node enlargement and infection of the tonsils. Involved nodes may become fixed to the overlying skin, suppurate, and drain.

B. Laboratory Findings: The Mantoux test (0.1 mL of intermediate strength PPD [5 TU] inoculated intradermally) is read as positive at 48–72 hours if there is significant induration (Table 36–1). False-negative results are seen in malnourished patients, those with overwhelming disease, and in a few

Table 36–1. Interpretation of tuberculin skin test reactions.[1]

Degree of Risk	Risk Factors	Positive Reaction
High	Recent close contact with a case of active tuberculosis; chest radiograph compatible with tuberculosis; immunocompromise; HIV infection	≥ 5 mm induration
Medium	Current or previous residence in high-prevalence area (Asia, Africa, Latin America); skin test converters within past 2 years; intravenous drug use; homelessness, or residence in a correctional institution; recent weight loss or malnutrition; leukemia, Hodgkin's disease, diabetes mellitus; age < 4 years	≥ 10 mm induration
Low	Children ≥ 4 years without any risk factor	≥ 15 mm induration

[1]Standard intradermal Mantoux test, 5 test units.

percent of children with isolated pulmonary disease. Temporary suppression of tuberculin reactivity may be seen with viral infections (eg, measles, influenza, varicella, mumps), after live virus immunization, and when corticosteroids or other immunosuppressive drugs are present. For this reason, every Mantoux test should be accompanied by intradermal injection of control antigens such as *Candida* or diphtheria-tetanus toxoids. Unfortunately, some normal children have no reaction to control antigens. When tuberculosis is suspected and the child is anergic, household members and adult contacts (eg, teachers, caretakers) should also be tested immediately. Multiple puncture tests (tine tests) are associated with false-negative and false-positive reactions. Furthermore, a positive tine test is not sufficient for diagnosis, necessitating a Mantoux test. The subsequent Mantoux test may lead to "boosting" and a false-positive reaction. Because of these problems, tine tests should not be used. The two commercially available reagents for Mantoux testing give discrepant results in some cases.

The erythrocyte sedimentation rate is usually elevated. Cultures of pooled early morning gastric aspirates from three successive days will yield *M tuberculosis* in about 40% of cases. Biopsy may be necessary to establish the diagnosis in some cases. Therapy should not be delayed in suspected cases. The cerebrospinal fluid in tuberculous meningitis shows slight to moderate pleocytosis (50–300 white blood cells, predominantly lymphocytes), decreased glucose, and increased protein.

The direct detection of mycobacteria in body fluids or discharges is best done by staining specimens with auramine-rhodamine and examining them with fluorescence microscopy; this is superior to the Ziehl-Neelsen method.

C. Imaging: Chest x-ray should be obtained in all children with suspicion of tuberculosis at any site or with a positive skin test. Segmental consolidation with some volume loss and hilar adenopathy are common findings in children. Pleural effusion also occurs with primary infection. Cavities and apical disease are unusual.

Differential Diagnosis

Pulmonary tuberculosis must be differentiated from fungal, parasitic, mycoplasmal, and bacterial pneumonias; lung abscess; foreign body aspiration; lipoid pneumonia; sarcoidosis; and mediastinal cancer. Cervical lymphadenitis is most apt to be due to streptococcal or staphylococcal infections. Cat-scratch fever and infection with atypical mycobacteria may need to be distinguished from tuberculous lymphadenitis. Viral meningoencephalitis, head trauma (battered child), lead poisoning, brain abscess, acute bacterial meningitis, brain tumor, and disseminated fungal infections must be excluded in tuberculous meningitis. The skin test in the patient or family contacts is frequently valuable in differentiating these conditions from tuberculosis.

Prevention

A. BCG Vaccine: BCG vaccines are live attenuated strains of *M bovis*. Although this BCG is often routinely given to infants and children in countries with a high prevalence of tuberculosis, protective efficacy varies greatly with vaccine potency and method of delivery. In the United States, BCG vaccination is considered only for tuberculin-negative children and neonates in high-risk situations who are HIV-negative and who are unlikely to receive isoniazid (INH) prophylaxis or close follow-up—or who are at high risk of exposure to persons infected with *M tuberculosis* resistant to isoniazid and rifampin (see Chapter 9).

B. Isoniazid Chemoprophylaxis: Daily administration of isoniazid (10 mg/kg/d orally; maximum 300 mg) is advised for children who cannot avoid intimate household contact with adolescents or adults with active disease. Isoniazid is given until 3 months after last contact. At the end of this time, a Mantoux test should be done, and therapy should be continued for 3–6 months if it is positive. BCG is not recommended during the period of isoniazid chemoprophylaxis.

C. Other Measures: Tuberculosis in infants and young children is evidence of recent exposure to active infection in an adult. The source contact (index case) should be identified, isolated, and treated to prevent other secondary cases. Reporting cases to local health departments is essential for contact tracing. Exposed tuberculin-negative children should be skin-tested every 2 months for 6 months after contact has been terminated. Routine tuberculin skin testing is advised at 12–15 months of age, prior to school entry, and again in adolescence. Yearly testing of school children is recommended in high-risk populations, including children from socioeconomically deprived neighborhoods and those from high-risk foreign countries.

Treatment

A. Specific Measures: Most children in the United States are hospitalized initially. If the infecting organism has not been isolated for susceptibility testing from the presumed contact, reasonable attempts should be made to obtain it from the child using gastric aspirates, sputum induction, bronchoscopy, thoracentesis, and so on. Cooperation with outpatient therapy must be assured. Direct observed therapy given twice weekly by a trained professional is carried out when compliance cannot be ensured.

All children with positive skin tests (see Table 36–1) without overt disease should receive 6–9 months of isoniazid (10 mg/kg/d orally, maximum 300 mg) therapy. In children with overt pulmonary disease, therapy for 6–9 months using isoniazid (10 mg/kg/d), rifampin (15 mg/kg/d), and pyrazinamide (25–30 mg/kg/d) in a single daily oral dose for 2 months, followed by isoniazid plus rifampin (either in a daily or twice-weekly regimen) for 4 months appears effective for isoniazid-susceptible organisms. For more severe disease, such as miliary or central nervous system infection, duration is increased to 12 months or more, and a fourth drug (streptomycin or ethambutol) is added for the first 2 months. Directly observed therapy is recommended for treatment in the United States.

1. Isoniazid–The hepatotoxicity from isoniazid seen in adults and some adolescents is rare in children. Transient elevation of aminotransferases (up to three times normal) may be seen at 6–12 weeks, but therapy is continued unless clinical illness occurs. Routine monitoring of liver function tests is unnecessary. Peripheral neuropathy associated with pyridoxine deficiency is rare in children, and it is not necessary to add pyridoxine unless significant malnutrition coexists.

2. Rifampin–Although it is an excellent bactericidal agent, rifampin is never used alone owing to rapid development of resistance. Hepatotoxicity may be seen, but rarely with recommended doses. The orange discoloration of secretions is benign.

3. Pyrazinamide–This excellent sterilizing agent has most effect during the first 2 months of therapy; with the recommended duration and dosing, it is well tolerated. Although it elevates the uric acid level, it rarely causes symptoms of hyperuricemia in children. Use of this drug is now common for tuberculous disease in children; resistance is almost unknown. Oral acceptance and central nervous system penetration are good.

4. Ethambutol–Since color blindness and optic neuritis are the major side effects, ethambutol is usually given only to children who can be reliably vision tested every 2 months. This complication occurs in a small percentage of patients, usually those receiving more than the recommended dosage of 15 mg/kg/d.

5. Streptomycin–Streptomycin (20–30 mg/kg/d intramuscularly in one or two doses) should be given for 1 or 2 months in severe disease. Hearing should be tested periodically during use.

B. Chemotherapy for Drug-Resistant Tuberculosis: The incidence of drug resistance is increasing and reaches 10–20% in some areas of the United States. Transmission of multiply resistant strains to contacts has occurred in some epidemics. For all cases with resistant strains, at least two effective drugs should be given. In areas with high rates of resistance, it may be necessary to begin therapy with four drugs pending susceptibility testing. Consultation of local laboratories or experts in treating tuberculosis is important. Therapy should continue for 12 months or longer.

C. General Measures:

1. Corticosteroids–These drugs may be used for suppressing inflammatory reactions in meningeal, pleural, and pericardial tuberculosis and for the relief of bronchial obstruction due to hilar adenopathy. Prednisone is given orally, 1 mg/kg/d for 6–8 weeks, with gradual withdrawal at the end of that time. The use of corticosteroids may mask progression of disease. Accordingly, the clinician needs to be sure that an effective regimen is being used.

2. Bed rest–Rest in bed is indicated only while the child feels ill. Isolation is necessary only for children with draining lesions or renal disease and those with chronic pulmonary tuberculosis. Most children with tuberculosis are noninfectious and can attend school while being treated.

Prognosis

If bacteria are sensitive and treatment is completed, most patients make lasting recovery. Repeat treatment is more difficult and less successful. With antituberculosis chemotherapy (especially isoniazid), there should now be nearly 100% recovery in miliary tuberculosis. Without treatment, the mortality rate in both miliary tuberculosis and tuberculous meningitis is almost 100%. In the latter form, about two-thirds of treated patients survive. There may be a high incidence of neurologic abnormalities among survivors if treatment is started late.

Cieslak TJ et al: A pseudoepidemic of tuberculin skin test conversions caused by a particular lot of purified protein derivative of tuberculin test solution. Pediatr Infect Dis J 1995;14:392.

Essential components of a tuberculosis prevention and control program: Screening for tuberculosis and tuberculosis infection in high-risk populations. MMWR Morb Mortal Wkly Rep 1995;44(RR-11):1.

Kent SJ et al: Tuberculous meningitis: A 30-year review. Clin Infect Dis 1993;17:987.

Schaaf HS et al: Respiratory tuberculosis in childhood: The diagnostic value of clinical features and special investigations. Pediatr Infect Dis J 1995;14:189.

Schoeman JF et al: Effect of corticosteroids on intracranial pressure, computed tomographic findings, and clinical outcome in young with tuberculous meningitis. Pediatrics 1997;99:226.

Serwint JR et al: Outcomes of annual tuberculosis screening by Mantoux test in children considered to be at high risk: Results from one urban clinic. Pediatrics 1997;99:529.

Starke JR, Correa AG: Management of mycobacterial infection and disease in children. Pediatr Infect Dis J 1994;14:455.

Swanson DS, Starke JR: Drug-resistant tuberculosis in pediatrics. Pediatr Clin North Am 1995;42:553.

INFECTIONS WITH NONTUBERCULOUS MYCOBACTERIA

Essentials of Diagnosis & Typical Features

- Chronic unilateral cervical lymphadenitis.
- Granulomas of the skin.
- Chronic bone lesion with draining sinus (chronic osteomyelitis).
- Reaction to PPD-S (standard) of 5–8 mm, negative chest x-ray, and negative history of contact with tuberculosis.
- Positive skin reaction to a specific atypical antigen.
- Diagnosis by positive acid-fast stain or culture.
- Disseminated infection in patients with AIDS.

General Considerations

Various species of acid-fast mycobacteria other than *Mycobacterium tuberculosis* may cause subclinical infections and, occasionally, clinical disease closely simulating tuberculosis. Strains of nontuberculous mycobacteria are common in soil, food, and water. Organisms enter the host by small abrasions in skin, oral mucosa, or gastrointestinal mucosa. Strain cross-reactivity with *M tuberculosis* can be demonstrated by simultaneous skin testing (Mantoux) with PPD-S (standard) and PPD prepared from one of the atypical antigens. The larger skin reaction suggests infection with the homologous strain.

The Runyon classification of mycobacteria includes the following:

Group I. Photochromogens (PPD-Y): (*Mycobacterium kansasii* and *Mycobacterium marinum*) Yellow color develops upon exposure to light in previously white colony grown 2–4 weeks in the dark.

Group II. Scotochromogens (PPD-G): (*Mycobacterium scrofulaceum*) Colonies are definitely yellow-orange after incubation in the dark. Organisms may be found in small numbers in the normal flora of some human saliva and gastric contents. Subclinical infection is widespread in the United States, but clinical disease appears rarely.

Group III. Nonphotochromogens (PPD-B): "Battey avian-swine group" grows as small white colonies after incubation in the dark, with no significant development of pigment upon exposure to light. Infection with *Mycobacterium avium* complex is prevalent on the East Coast of the United States, particularly the Southeast, and in patients with AIDS.

Group IV. "Rapid growers": (*Mycobacterium fortuitum, Mycobacterium chelonei*) Within 1 week after inoculation they form colonies closely resembling *M tuberculosis* morphologically.

Clinical Findings

A. Symptoms and Signs:

1. Lymphadenitis–In children, the commonest form of infection due to mycobacteria other than *M tuberculosis* is cervical lymphadenitis. *M scrofulaceum* or *M avium* complex (MAC) is almost always the cause. A submandibular node swells slowly and is firm and initially somewhat tender. Low-grade fever may occur. Over time, the node suppurates and may drain chronically. Nodes in other areas of the head and neck and elsewhere are sometimes involved.

2. Pulmonary disease–In the western United States, this is usually due to *M kansasii;* in the eastern United States, it may be due to MAC. In other countries, disease is usually caused by MAC. In adults, (but not in children), there is usually underlying chronic pulmonary disease. Immunologic deficiency may be present. Presentation is clinically indistinguishable from that of tuberculosis. Patients with cystic fibrosis may be infected with nontuberculous mycobacteria. It may be difficult to differentiate infection from colonization in these patients with chronic symptoms.

3. Swimming pool granuloma–This is due to *M marinum.* A solitary chronic granulomatous lesion, frequently on the elbow, develops after minor trauma in infected swimming pools. Minor trauma in home aquariums or other aquatic environments also may lead to infection.

4. Chronic osteomyelitis–Osteomyelitis is caused by *M kansasii, M scrofulaceum,* or "rapid growers." Findings include swelling and pain over a distal extremity, radiolucent defects in bone, fever, and clinical and x-ray evidence of bronchopneumonia. Such cases are rare.

5. Meningitis–Disease is due to *M kansasii* and may be indistinguishable from tuberculous meningitis.

6. Disseminated infection–Rarely, apparently immunologically normal children develop disseminated infection due to nontuberculous mycobacteria. Children are ill, with fever and hepatosplenomegaly, and organisms are demonstrated in bone lesions, lymph nodes, or liver. Chest x-rays are usually normal. Sixty to 80 percent of patients with AIDS will acquire *M avium* complex infection, characterized by fever, night sweats, weight loss, and diarrhea. Infection usually indicates severe immune dysfunction and is associated with CD4 lymphocyte counts less than 50/µL.

B. Laboratory Findings: In most cases, there is a small reaction (< 10 mm) when Mantoux testing is done. Larger reactions may be seen. The chest x-ray is negative, and there is no history of contact with tuberculosis. Needle aspiration of the node excludes bacterial infection and may yield acid-fast bacilli on stain or culture. Fistulization should not be a problem because total excision follows if the infection is due to atypical mycobacteria. If other organisms are found, formal excision may be avoided. Excision is usually required if aspiration is nondiagnostic and the clinical findings support the diagnosis.

Cultures of any normally sterile body site will yield *M avium* complex in immunocompromised patients with disseminated disease. Blood cultures are positive, with a large density of bacteria.

Differential Diagnosis

See section on differential diagnosis in the previous discussion of tuberculosis and in Chapter 17.

Treatment

A. Specific Measures: The usual treatment of lymphadenitis is complete surgical excision. Chemotherapy is neither necessary nor sufficient for cure. Occasionally, excision is impossible because of proximity to branches of the facial nerve. Chemotherapy may then be necessary. Occasionally, resolution of the adenopathy is under way when the diagnosis is made. In these cases, careful follow-up is adequate.

Response of extensive adenopathy or other forms of infection varies according to the infecting species and susceptibility. Recent data suggest that isoniazid, rifampin, and streptomycin with or without ethambutol (depending on sensitivity to isoniazid) will result in a favorable response in almost all patients with *M kansasii* infection. Chemotherapeutic treatment of *M avium* complex is much less satisfactory as resistance to isoniazid, rifampin, and pyrazinamide is usual. Susceptibility testing is necessary to optimize therapy. Most clinicians favor surgical excision of involved tissue if possible and treatment with at least three drugs to which the organism has been shown to be sensitive. Disseminated disease in patients with AIDS calls for a combination of three or more active drugs. Clarithromycin and ethambutol, in addition to one or more of the following drugs, is started immediately: ethionamide, capreomycin, amikacin, rifabutin, or ciprofloxacin. *M fortuitum* and *M chelonei* are usually susceptible to amikacin plus erythromycin or doxycycline and may be successfully

treated with such combinations. Swimming pool granuloma due to *M marinum* is usually treated with tetracycline (in children over 9 years of age) or rifampin, ethambutol, clarithromycin, or trimethoprim-sulfamethoxazole for a minimum of 3 months. Surgery may also be beneficial.

B. General Measures: Isolation of the patient is usually not necessary. General supportive care is indicated for the child with disseminated disease.

Prognosis

The prognosis is good for localized disease, though fatalities occur in immunocompromised children with disseminated disease.

Askew GL et al: *Mycobacterium tuberculosis* transmission from a pediatrician to patients. Pediatrics 1997;100:19.

Burns JL et al: Unusual presentations of nontuberculous mycobacterial infections in children. Pediatr Infect Dis J 1997;16:802.

Hofer M et al: Disseminated osteomyelitis from *Mycobacterium ulcerans* after a snakebite. N Engl J Med 1993;328:1007.

Horsburgh CR Jr: *Mycobacterium avium* complex infection in the acquired immunodeficiency syndrome. N Engl J Med 1991;324:1332.

Margileth AM: Nontuberculous (atypical) mycobacterial disease. Semin Pediatr Infect Dis 1993;4:307.

Smith S et al: A window on the ontogeny of cellular immunity. J Pediatr 1997;131:16.

Starke JR, Correa AB: Management of mycobacterial infection and disease in children. Pediatr Infect Dis J 1995;14:455.

LEGIONELLA INFECTION

Essentials of Diagnosis
& Typical Features

- Severe progressive pneumonia in a child with compromised immunity.
- Diarrhea and neurologic signs are common.
- Positive culture requires buffered charcoal yeast extract media and proves infection.
- Direct fluorescent antibody staining of respiratory secretions proves infection.

General Considerations

Legionella pneumophila is a ubiquitous gram-negative bacillus that causes two distinct clinical syndromes: Legionnaire's disease and Pontiac fever. Legionnaire's disease is an acute, severe pneumonia that is frequently fatal in immunocompromised patients. Pontiac fever is a mild, nonpneumonic, flu-like illness characterized by fever, headache, myalgia, and arthralgia. The disease is self-limited and is described in outbreaks in otherwise healthy adults.

Forty species of *Legionella* have been discovered, but not all cause disease in humans. *L pneumophila* causes most infections. *Legionella* is present in many natural water sources as well as domestic water supplies (faucets, showers). Contaminated cooling towers and heat exchangers have been implicated in several large institutional outbreaks. Sporadic community-acquired cases also occur, and the source of infection is not usually clear. Person-to-person transmission has not been documented.

Few cases of Legionnaire's disease have been reported in children. Most were in children with compromised cellular immunity. In adults, risk factors include smoking, underlying cardiopulmonary or renal disease, alcoholism, and diabetes.

L pneumophila is thought to be acquired by inhalation of a contaminated aerosol. The bacteria are phagocytosed but proliferate within macrophages. Cell-mediated immunity is necessary to activate macrophages to kill intracellular bacteria.

Clinical Findings

A. Symptoms and Signs: Onset of fever, chills, anorexia, and headache is abrupt. Pulmonary symptoms appear within 2–3 days and progress rapidly. The cough is nonproductive early; purulent sputum occurs late. Hemoptysis, diarrhea, and neurologic signs (including lethargy, irritability, tremors, and delirium) are seen.

B. Laboratory Findings: White blood count is usually elevated. Chest radiographs show rapidly progressive patchy consolidation. Cavitation and large pleural effusions are uncommon. Cultures from sputum, tracheal aspirates, or bronchoscopic specimens, when grown on buffered yeast charcoal extract media, are positive in 70–80% of patients at 3–7 days. Direct fluorescent antibody staining of sputum or other respiratory specimens is only 50–70% sensitive but 95% specific. As such, a negative culture or direct fluorescent antibody staining of sputum or tracheal secretions does not rule out Legionnaire's disease. A urine test for *Legionella* antigen detects 80% of infecting species. Serologic tests are available and aid in diagnosis, but a maximum rise in titer may require 6–8 weeks.

Differential Diagnosis

Legionnaire's disease is usually a rapidly progressive pneumonia in a patient who appears very ill with unremitting fevers. Other bacterial pneumonias, viral pneumonias, *Mycoplasma* pneumonia, and fungal disease are all possibilities and may be difficult to differentiate on clinical grounds in an immunocompromised patient.

Complications

In sporadic untreated cases, mortality rates are 5–25%. In untreated immunocompromised patients, mortality approaches 80%. Hematogenous dissemination may result in extrapulmonary foci of infection, including pericardium, myocardium, and renal involvement. *Legionella* may present as "culture-negative" endocarditis.

Prevention

No vaccine is available. Hyperchlorination and periodic superheating of water supplies in hospitals have been shown to reduce the number of organisms and the frequency of cases.

Treatment

Erythromycin (40–50 mg/kg/d in four divided doses, orally or intravenously) results in clinical improvement in 48–72 hours. Clarithromycin, azithromycin, and ciprofloxacin or ofloxacin (in adult patients) are also effective and may be better tolerated than erythromycin. Rifampin (20 mg/kg/d divided in two doses) is very active in vitro and is also given to gravely ill patients. Therapy is continued for 21 days to reduce the likelihood of relapse.

Prognosis

Mortality rate is high if treatment is delayed. Malaise, problems with memory, and fatigue are common problems in patients after recovery.

Carlson NC et al: Legionellosis in children: An expanding spectrum. Pediatr Infect Dis J 1990;9:133.

Lowry PW et al: A cluster of *Legionella* sternal wound infections due to postoperative topical exposure to contaminated tap water. N Engl J Med 1991;324:109.

Plouffe JF et al: Reevaluation of the definition of Legionnaires' disease: Use of the urinary antigen assay. Clin Infect Dis 1995;20:1286.

Stout JE, Yu VL: Legionellosis. N Engl J Med 1997; 337:682.

PSITTACOSIS (ORNITHOSIS) & *CHLAMYDIA PNEUMONIAE* INFECTION*

Essentials of Diagnosis & Typical Features

- Fever, cough, malaise, chills, headache.
- Diffuse rales; no consolidation.
- Long-lasting x-ray findings of bronchopneumonia.
- Isolation of the organism or rising titer of complement-fixing antibodies.
- Exposure to infected birds (ornithosis).

General Considerations

Psittacosis is caused by *Chlamydia psittaci*. When the agent is transmitted to humans from psittacine birds (parrots, parakeets, cockatoos, and budgerigars), the disease is often called psittacosis or parrot fever. However, other avian genera (pigeons, turkeys) are common sources of infection in the United States, and the general term ornithosis is often used. A total of 1132 cases were reported from 1985 to 1995. The agent is an obligate intracellular para-

---

*Chlamydia trachomatis infections are discussed in Chapter 14 (conjunctivitis) and Chapter 17 (pneumonia).

site. Human-to-human spread occurs rarely. The incubation period is 5–14 days. The bird from which the disease was transmitted may not be clinically ill.

Chlamydia pneumoniae may cause atypical pneumonia similar to that due to *Mycoplasma pneumoniae*. Transmission is by respiratory spread. Infection appears to be most prevalent during the second decade; half of surveyed adults are seropositive. Only a small percentage of infections result in clinical pneumonia. The disease may be more common than atypical pneumonia due to *M pneumoniae*. Lower respiratory tract infection due to *C pneumoniae* is uncommon in infants and young children.

Clinical Findings

A. Symptoms and Signs:

1. *C psittaci*–The disease is extremely variable but tends to be mild in children. The onset is rapid or insidious, with fever, chills, headache, backache, malaise, myalgia, and dry cough. Signs include pneumonitis, alteration of percussion note and breath sounds, and rales. Pulmonary findings may be absent early. Dyspnea and cyanosis may occur later. Splenomegaly, epistaxis, prostration, and meningismus are occasionally seen. Delirium, constipation or diarrhea, and abdominal distress may occur.

2. *C pneumoniae*–Clinically, *C pneumoniae* infection is very similar to *M pneumoniae* infection. Most are mild upper respiratory infections. Lower tract infection is characterized by fever, sore throat (perhaps more severe with *C pneumoniae*), cough, and bilateral pulmonary findings and infiltrates. Prolonged symptoms in some patients suggest that therapy with erythromycin or tetracycline should be continued longer than what is usually ordered for mycoplasmal pneumonia.

B. Laboratory Findings:
In psittacosis, the white blood cell count is normal or decreased, often with a shift to the left. Proteinuria is frequently present. *C psittaci* is present in the blood and sputum during the first 2 weeks of illness and can be isolated by inoculation of clinical specimens into mice or embryonated eggs, but culture is available only in research laboratories. A fourfold rise to 1:32 or higher in the microimmunofluorescence or complement fixation tests in specimens obtained at least 2 weeks apart—or IgM antibody ≥ 1:16 in the microimmunofluorescence test—suggests the diagnosis. The rise in titer may be minimized or delayed by early chemotherapy. Infection with *C pneumoniae* may lead to diagnostic confusion because cross-reactive antibody may cause falsely positive *C psittaci* titers. Serologic tests for *C pneumoniae* are now available in reference laboratories. A fourfold rise in microimmunofluorescence or complement-fixing antibody, IgM titers of 1:16 or more, or a single titer greater than 1:512 supports the diagnosis.

C. Imaging:
The x-ray findings in psittacosis are those of central pneumonia, which later becomes widespread or migratory. Psittacosis is indistinguishable from viral pneumonias by x-ray. Signs of pneumonitis may appear on x-ray in the absence of clinical suspicion of pulmonary involvement.

Differential Diagnosis

Psittacosis can be differentiated from acute viral or mycoplasmal pneumonias only by the history of contact with potentially infected birds. In severe or prolonged cases with extrapulmonary involvement, the differential diagnosis includes a wide spectrum of diseases including typhoid fever, brucellosis, and rheumatic fever.

Complications

Complications of psittacosis include myocarditis, endocarditis, hepatitis, pancreatitis, and secondary bacterial pneumonia. *C pneumoniae* infection may be prolonged or may recur.

Treatment

For psittacosis, tetracyclines in full doses should be given for 14 days. Erythromycin is an alternative for children under 9 years of age. Supportive oxygen may be needed. The patient should be kept in isolation. The role of the expanded-spectrum macrolides is not yet clear. *C pneumoniae* responds to either erythromycin or tetracycline.

Block S et al: *Mycoplasma pneumoniae* and *Chlamydia pneumoniae* in pediatric community acquired pneumonia: Comparative efficacy and safety of clarithromycin vs erythromycin ethylsuccinate. Pediatr Infect Dis J 1995;14:471.

Compendium of psittacosis (chlamydiosis) control, 1997. MMWR Morb Mortal Wkly Rep 1997;46:1.

Crosse BA: Psittacosis: A clinical review. J Infect 1990;21:251.

Falck G, Gnarpe J, Gnarpe H: Prevalence of *Chlamydia pneumoniae* in healthy children and in children with respiratory tract infections. Pediatr Infect Dis J 1997; 16:549.

Grayston JT: *Chlamydia pneumoniae* (TWAR) infections in children. Pediatr Infect Dis J 1994;13:675.

Jantos CA et al: Infection with *Chlamydia pneumoniae* in infants and children with acute lower respiratory tract disease. Pediatr Infect Dis J 1995;14:117.

CAT-SCRATCH DISEASE

Essentials of Diagnosis & Typical Features

- History of a cat scratch or cat contact.
- Primary lesion (papule, pustule, conjunctivitis) at site of inoculation.
- Acute or subacute regional lymphadenopathy.
- Aspiration of sterile pus from a node.
- Laboratory studies excluding other causes.
- Biopsy of node or papule showing histopathologic

findings consistent with cat-scratch disease and occasionally characteristic bacilli on Warthin-Starry stain.

- Positive cat-scratch serology (antibody to *Bartonella henselae*).

General Considerations

Cat-scratch disease is a benign, self-limited form of lymphadenitis. Patients often report a cat scratch (67%) or contact with a cat or kitten (90%). The cat almost invariably is healthy. The clinical picture is that of a regional lymphadenitis associated with an erythematous papular skin lesion without intervening lymphangitis. The disease occurs worldwide and is more common in the fall and winter. It is estimated that more than 20,000 cases per year occur in the United States. The most common systemic complication is encephalitis.

The etiologic agent of cat-scratch disease has now been identified as *Bartonella henselae,* a gram-negative bacillus that also causes bacillary angiomatosis.

Clinical Findings

A. Symptoms and Signs: About 50% of patients with cat-scratch disease develop a primary lesion at the site of inoculation, though some authors report a much higher percentage. The lesion usually is a papule or pustule which appears after 7–10 days and is located most often on the arm or hand (50%), head or leg (30%), or trunk or neck (10%). The lesion may be conjunctival (10%). Regional lymphadenopathy appears 10–50 days later and may be accompanied by mild malaise, lassitude, headache, and fever. Multiple sites are seen in about 10% of cases. Involved nodes may be hard or soft and 1–6 cm in diameter. They are usually tender, and about 25% of them suppurate. The overlying skin may or may not be inflamed. Lymphadenopathy usually resolves in about 2 months, but it may persist for up to 8 months.

Unusual manifestations include nonpruritic maculopapular rash, erythema multiforme or nodosum, purpura, conjunctivitis (Parinaud's oculoglandular fever), parotid swelling, pneumonia, chronic sinus drainage, osteolytic lesions, mesenteric and mediastinal adenitis, peripheral neuritis, hepatosplenomegaly, and encephalitis.

B. Laboratory Findings: A sensitive enzyme immunoassay is specific for *B henselae*. The indirect fluorescent antibody test is available through state health departments. Antigens prepared from pus aspirated from nodes of infected individuals have been used for skin testing. Because they are poorly standardized and are not available commercially, their use is discouraged.

Histopathologic examination of involved nodes shows characteristic changes that are nondiagnostic unless the organism is demonstrated. The lymph node architecture is distorted by multiple areas of central necrosis with acidophilic staining. These areas are surrounded by foci of epithelioid cells and scattered giant cells of the Langhans type. There is usually some elevation in the sedimentation rate. In cases with central nervous system involvement, the cerebrospinal fluid is usually normal but may show a slight pleocytosis and modest elevation of protein.

Differential Diagnosis

Cat-scratch disease must be distinguished from pyogenic adenitis, tuberculosis (typical and atypical), tularemia, plague, brucellosis, Hodgkin's disease, lymphoma, primary toxoplasmosis, infectious mononucleosis, lymphogranuloma venereum, and fungal infections.

Treatment

The best therapy is reassurance that the adenopathy is benign and will subside spontaneously within 4–8 weeks in most cases. In cases of suppuration, node aspiration under local anesthesia with an 18- to 19-gauge needle relieves the pain. Excision of the involved node is indicated in cases of chronic adenitis. Antimicrobial therapy has not been proved to alter the course of illness; gentamicin and ciprofloxacin have been useful anecdotally in a few severe infections, and trimethoprim-sulfamethoxazole and erythromycin have also been useful.

Prognosis

The prognosis is good if complications do not occur.

Adal KA, Cockerell CJ, Petri WAJ: Cat scratch disease, bacillary angiomatosis, and other infections due to *Rochalimaea.* N Engl J Med 1994;330:1509.

Collipp PJ: Cat-scratch disease: Therapy with trimethoprim-sulfamethoxazole. Am J Dis Child 1992;146:397.

Demers DM et al: Cat-scratch disease in Hawaii: Etiology and seroepidemiology. J Pediatr 1995;127:23.

Holley HP Jr: Successful treatment of cat-scratch disease with ciprofloxacin. JAMA 1991;265:1563.

Koehler JE, Glaser CA, Tappero JW: *Rochalimaea henselae* infection. JAMA 1994;271:531.

Malatack JJ, Jaffe R: Granulomatous hepatitis in three children due to cat-scratch disease without peripheral adenopathy: An unrecognized cause of fever of unknown origin. Am J Dis Child 1993;147:949.

Margileth AM, Hayden GF: Cat scratch disease. N Engl J Med 1993;329:53.

II. SPIROCHETAL INFECTIONS

SYPHILIS

Essentials of Diagnosis & Typical Features

Congenital:

- All types: History of untreated maternal syphilis, a positive serologic test, and a positive darkfield examination.
- Newborn: Hepatosplenomegaly, characteristic x-ray bone changes, anemia, increased nucleated red cells, thrombocytopenia, abnormal spinal fluid, jaundice, edema.
- Young infant (3–12 weeks): Snuffles, maculopapular skin rash, mucocutaneous lesions, pseudoparalysis (in addition to x-ray bone changes).
- Children: Stigmas of early congenital syphilis, interstitial keratitis, saber shins, gummas of nose and palate.

Acquired:

- Chancre of genitals, lip, or anus in child or adolescent. History of sexual contact.

General Considerations

Syphilis is a chronic, generalized infectious disease caused by a slender spirochete, *Treponema pallidum.* In the acquired form, the disease is transmitted by sexual contact. Primary syphilis is characterized by the presence of an indurated painless chancre, which heals in 7–10 days. A secondary eruption involving the skin and mucous membranes appears in 4–6 weeks. After a long latency period, late lesions of tertiary syphilis involve the eyes, skin, bones, viscera, central nervous system, and cardiovascular system.

Congenital syphilis results from transplacental infection. Infection may result in stillbirth or manifest as illness in the newborn, in early infancy, or later in childhood. First-trimester fetal infection has been found in the products of conception in therapeutic abortions. Syphilis occurring in the newborn and young infant is comparable to secondary disease in the adult but is more severe and life-threatening. Late congenital syphilis (developing in childhood) is comparable to tertiary disease.

Congenital syphilis is increasing in the United States due to increasing primary and secondary syphilis in women of childbearing age, and perhaps due to inadequate diagnosis and treatment of syphilis in prenatal care programs. Nearly 1500 cases of congenital syphilis and 16,500 cases of primary and secondary syphilis were reported in 1995. Prostitution in women addicted to crack cocaine has been associated with a more than 500% increase in congenital syphilis in New York City.

Clinical Findings

A. Symptoms and Signs:

1. Congenital syphilis–

a. Newborns–Most newborns with congenital syphilis are asymptomatic. If not detected and treated, symptoms develop within several weeks to months. When clinical signs are present, they usually consist of jaundice, anemia with or without thrombocytopenia, increase in nucleated red blood cells, hepatosplenomegaly, and edema. There may be overt signs of meningitis (bulging fontanelle, opisthotonos), but subclinical infection with cerebrospinal fluid abnormalities is more likely.

b. Young infants (3–12 weeks)–The infant may appear normal for the first few weeks of life only to develop mucocutaneous lesions and pseudoparalysis of the arms or legs. Shotty lymphadenopathy may be felt. Hepatomegaly is universal, with splenomegaly in 50%. Other signs of disease similar to those seen in the newborn may be present. Anemia has been reported as the only presenting manifestation of congenital syphilis in this age group. "Snuffles" (rhinitis) is characterized by a profuse mucopurulent discharge that excoriates the upper lip and is present in 25%. A syphilitic rash is common on the palms and soles but may occur anywhere on the body; it consists of bright red, raised maculopapular lesions that gradually fade. Moist lesions occur at the mucocutaneous junctions (nose, mouth, anus, genitals) and lead to fissuring and bleeding.

Syphilis in the young infant may lead to stigmas recognizable in later childhood, such as rhagades (scars) around the mouth or nose, a "saddle" nose, and a high forehead (secondary to mild hydrocephalus associated with low-grade meningitis and frontal periostitis). The permanent upper central incisors may be peg-shaped with a central notch (Hutchinson's teeth), and the cusps of the sixth-year molars may have a lobulated mulberry appearance.

c. Children–Bilateral interstitial keratitis (at 6–12 years) is characterized by photophobia, increased lacrimation, and vascularization of the cornea associated with exudation. Chorioretinitis and optic atrophy may also be seen. Meningovascular syphilis (at 2–10 years) is usually slowly progressive, with mental retardation, spasticity, abnormal pupillary response, speech defects, and abnormal spinal fluid. Deafness sometimes occurs. Thickening of the periosteum of the anterior tibias produces saber shins. A bilateral effusion into the knee joints (Clutton's joints) may occur but is not associated with sequelae. Gummas may develop in the nasal septum, palate, long bones, and subcutaneous tissues.

2. Acquired syphilis–The primary chancre of the genitals, mouth, or anus may occur as a result of intimate sexual contact. If the chancre is missed, signs of secondary syphilis, such as rash, fever, headache, and malaise, may be the first manifestation of the disease.

B. Laboratory Findings:

1. Darkfield microscopy–Treponemes can be seen in scrapings from a chancre and from moist lesions.

2. Serologic tests for syphilis (STS)–There are two general types of serologic tests for syphilis: treponemal and nontreponemal. The latter (Venereal Disease Research Laboratory, or VDRL) is useful for screening and follow-up of known cases. A rapid test (the rapid plasma reagin, or RPR) is useful for screening, but positive sera should be further examined by quantitative nontreponemal and treponemal tests. Positive nontreponemal tests are confirmed with more specific fluorescent treponemal antibody absorbed, or FTA-ABS test. False-positive FTA-ABS tests are uncommon except with other spirochetal disease.

One or 2 weeks after the onset of primary syphilis (chancre), the FTA-ABS test becomes positive. The VDRL or a similar nontreponemal test usually turns positive a few days later. By the time the secondary stage has been reached, virtually all patients show both positive FTA-ABS and positive nontreponemal tests. During latent and tertiary syphilis, the VDRL may become negative, but the FTA-ABS test usually remains positive. The quantitative VDRL or a similar nontreponemal test should be used to follow treated cases (see below).

Positive serologic tests in cord sera may represent passively transferred antibody rather than congenital infection and therefore must be supplemented by a combination of clinical and laboratory data. Elevated total cord IgM is a helpful but nonspecific finding. A specific IgM-FTA-ABS is available, but negative results are not conclusive and should not be relied upon. Demonstration of characteristic treponemes by darkfield examination of material from a moist lesion (skin; nasal or other mucous membranes) is definitive. Serial measurement of quantitative VDRL is also very useful, since passively transferred antibody in the absence of active infection should decay with a normal half-life of about 18 days.

In one study, 15% of infants with congenital syphilis had negative cord blood serology, presumably due to maternal infection late in pregnancy.

C. Imaging: Radiographic abnormalities are present in 90% of infants with symptoms of congenital syphilis and 20% of asymptomatic infants. Metaphysial lucent bands, periostitis, and a widened zone of provisional calcification may be present. Bilateral symmetric osteomyelitis with pathologic fractures of the medial tibial metaphyses (Wimberger's sign) is almost pathognomonic.

Differential Diagnosis

A. Congenital Syphilis:

1. Newborns–Sepsis, congestive heart failure, congenital rubella, toxoplasmosis, disseminated herpes simplex, cytomegalovirus infection, and hemolytic disease of the newborn have to be differentiated. A positive Coombs test and blood group incompatibility distinguish hemolytic disease.

2. Young infants–Injury to the brachial plexus, poliomyelitis, acute osteomyelitis, and septic arthritis must be differentiated from pseudoparalysis. Coryza due to viral infection often responds to symptomatic treatment. Rash (ammoniacal diaper rash) and scabies may be confused with a syphilitic eruption.

3. Children–Interstitial keratitis and bone lesions of tuberculosis are distinguished by positive tuberculin reaction and chest x-ray. Arthritis associated with syphilis is unaccompanied by systemic signs, and joints are not tender. Mental retardation, spasticity, and hyperactivity are shown to be of syphilitic origin by strongly positive serologic tests.

B. Acquired Syphilis: Herpes genitalis, traumatic lesions, and other venereal diseases must be differentiated.

Prevention

A serologic test for syphilis should be performed at the initiation of prenatal care and repeated at delivery. In mothers at high risk of syphilis, repeated tests may be necessary. Serologic tests for syphilis may be negative on both the mother and the baby at the time of birth if the mother acquires syphilis near term. Adequate treatment of mothers with secondary syphilis before the last month of pregnancy reduces the incidence of congenital syphilis from 90% to less than 2%. Examination and serologic testing of sexual partners and siblings should also be done.

Treatment

A. Specific Measures: Penicillin is the drug of choice for *T pallidum* infection. If the patient is allergic to penicillin, erythromycin or one of the tetracyclines may be used.

1. Congenital syphilis–Infants with positive serology should be fully evaluated: history of maternal disease and therapy, CBC, liver function tests, long bone radiographs, cerebrospinal fluid examination, and quantitative serologic tests.

Treatment is indicated for infants with physical signs, abnormal radiographs, elevated cerebrospinal fluid protein or cell counts, or reactive cerebrospinal fluid VDRL. Infants born to inadequately treated mothers, mothers treated less than 1 month before delivery, mothers with undocumented or inadequate serologic response to therapy, or mothers treated with nonpenicillin drugs should be treated as well. If there are no clinical or laboratory signs of syphilis, the infant may be followed at monthly intervals with quantitative serologic tests and physical examinations if follow-up is ensured. Rising titers or clinical signs usually occur within 4 months in infants with infection. Infants with suspected congenital syphilis should have roentgenography of the long bones and a cerebrospinal fluid examination.

Infants with proved or suspected congenital syphilis should receive either of the following: (1) aqueous crystalline penicillin G, 50,000 units/kg/dose intramuscularly or intravenously every 12 hours (if < 1 week old) or every 8 hours (if between 1 and 4 weeks of age) for 10–14 days; or (2) aqueous procaine penicillin G, 50,000 units/kg/d intramuscularly for a minimum of 10 days. All infants diagnosed after 4 weeks of age should receive 50,000 units/kg/dose intramuscularly or intravenously every 6 hours for 10–14 days. Because treatment failures in early congenital syphilis may be due to low levels of benzathine penicillin in the cerebrospinal fluid and the eye—and because cerebrospinal fluid serology may fail to detect central nervous system infection— benzathine penicillin is no longer recommended for proved or strongly suspected congenital syphilis. Asymptomatic seropositive infants with normal cerebrospinal fluid born to adequately treated mothers may be given benzathine penicillin G (50,000 units/kg intramuscularly in a single dose) with follow-up serologic examinations at 1, 2, 3, 6, and 12 months. For larger children, the total dose of penicillin need not exceed the dosage used in adult syphilis of more than 1 year's duration.

Follow-up quantitative VDRL or RPR tests should be performed at 3, 6, and 12 months after the end of therapy or should be repeated until they become nonreactive. Repeat cerebrospinal fluid examination every 6 months for 3 years is indicated for infants with a positive cerebrospinal fluid VDRL reaction. Titers decline with treatment and are usually negative by 12 months. Repeat treatment is indicated for rising titers or stable titers that do not decline.

2. Acquired syphilis–Benzathine penicillin G, 50,000 units/kg up to a maximum of 2.4 million units, is given to adolescents with primary, secondary, or latent disease of less than 1 year's duration. Late latent disease and neurosyphilis require weekly therapy for 3 weeks.

B. General Measures: Care should be given to the maintenance of adequate nutrition. Penicillin treatment of early congenital or secondary syphilis may result in a febrile Jarisch-Herxheimer reaction. Treatment is symptomatic, with careful follow-up and aspirin or acetaminophen, though transfusion may be necessary in infants with severe hemolytic anemia.

Prognosis

Severe disease, if undiagnosed, may be fatal in the newborn. Complete cure can be expected if the young infant is treated with penicillin. Serologic reversal usually occurs within 1 year. Treatment of primary syphilis with penicillin is curative. Permanent neurologic sequelae may be seen with meningovascular syphilis.

Bateman DA et al: The hospital cost of congenital syphilis. J Pediatr 1997;130:752.

Beerman MR et al: Lumbar puncture in the evaluation of possible asymptomatic congenital syphilis in neonates. J Pediatr 1996;128:125.

Dunn RA, Zenker PN: Why radiographs are useful in evaluation of neonates suspected of having congenital syphilis. Radiology 1992;182:639.

Paryani SG et al: Treatment of asymptomatic congenital syphilis: Benzathine versus procaine penicillin G therapy. J Pediatr 1994;125:471.

Rolfs RT et al: A randomized trial of enhanced therapy for early syphilis in patients with and without human immunodeficiency virus infections. N Engl J Med 1997;337:307.

Sanchez PJ: Congenital syphilis. Adv Pediatr Infect Dis 1992;7:161.

Sison CG et al: The resurgence of congenital syphilis: A cocaine-related problem. J Pediatr 1997;130:289.

RELAPSING FEVER

Essentials of Diagnosis & Typical Features

- Episodes of fever, chills, malaise.
- Occasional rash, arthritis, cough, hepatosplenomegaly, conjunctivitis.
- Diagnosis confirmed by direct microscopic identification of spirochetes in smears of peripheral blood.

General Considerations

Relapsing fever is a vector-borne disease caused by spirochetes of the genus *Borrelia.* Epidemic relapsing fever is transmitted to humans by body lice *(Pediculus humanus)* and endemic relapsing fever by soft-bodied ticks (genus *Ornithodoros*).

Tick-borne relapsing fever is endemic in the western United States. Transmission usually takes place during the warm months, when ticks are active and recreation or work brings people into contact with *Ornithodoros* ticks. Mountain camping areas and cabins are sites where infection often is acquired. The ticks are nocturnal feeders and remain attached for only 5–20 minutes. Consequently, the patient seldom remembers a tick bite. Rarely, neonatal relapsing fever results from transplacental transmission of *Borrelia.* Both louse-borne and tick-borne relapsing fever may be acquired during foreign travel.

Clinical Findings

A. Symptoms and Signs: The incubation period is 4–18 days. The attack is sudden, with high fever, chills, tachycardia, nausea and vomiting, headache, myalgia, arthralgia, bronchitis, and a dry, nonproductive cough. Hepatomegaly and splenomegaly appear later. Meningeal irritation may be present. An erythematous rash may be seen over the trunk and extremities, and petechiae may be present.

After 3–10 days, the fever falls by crisis. Jaundice, iritis, conjunctivitis, cranial nerve palsies, and hemorrhage occur, more commonly during relapses.

The disease is characterized by relapses at intervals of 1–2 weeks and lasting 3–5 days. The relapses duplicate the initial attack but become progressively less severe. In louse-borne relapsing fever, there is usually a single relapse; in tick-borne infection, there are two to six relapses.

B. Laboratory Findings: During febrile episodes, the urine contains protein, casts, and, occasionally erythrocytes; there is a marked polymorphonuclear leukocytosis and, in about 25% of cases, a false-positive serologic test for syphilis. Spirochetes can be found in the peripheral blood by direct microscopy in approximately 70% of cases by darkfield examination or by Wright, Giemsa, or acridine orange staining of thick and thin smears. They are not found during afebrile periods. The blood may be injected into young mice and the spirochetes found 1–14 days later in the tail blood. OXK agglutinin titers in serum may be positive.

Differential Diagnosis

Relapsing fever may be confused with malaria, leptospirosis, dengue, typhus, rat-bite fever, Colorado tick fever, Rocky Mountain spotted fever, collagen vascular disease, or any fever of unknown origin.

Complications

Complications include facial paralysis, iridocyclitis, optic atrophy, hypochromic anemia, pneumonia, nephritis, myocarditis, endocarditis, and seizures. Central nervous system involvement is seen in 10–30% of cases.

Treatment

For children under 7 years of age with tick-borne relapsing fever, erythromycin (40–50 mg/kg/d orally in divided doses every 6 hours for 10 days) should be given. Older children may be given tetracycline. Penicillin and chloramphenicol are also efficacious. In louse-borne relapsing fever, a single dose of tetracycline or erythromycin has been effective.

Severely ill patients should be hospitalized. Antibiotic treatment should be started after the fever has dropped; this will lessen the risk of severe Jarisch-Herxheimer reaction. Isolation precautions are not necessary.

Prognosis

The mortality rate in treated cases of relapsing fever is very low, except in debilitated or very young children. With treatment, the initial attack is shortened and relapses prevented. The response to antimicrobial therapy is dramatic.

Le CT: Tick-borne relapsing fever in children. Pediatrics 1980;66:963.

Spach DH et al: Tick-borne diseases in the United States. N Engl J Med 1993;329:936.

LEPTOSPIROSIS

Essentials of Diagnosis & Typical Features

- Biphasic course lasting 2 or 3 weeks.
- Initial phase: high fever, headache, myalgia, and conjunctivitis.
- Apparent recovery for 2–3 days.
- Return of fever associated with meningitis.
- Jaundice, hemorrhages, and renal insufficiency (severe cases).
- Culture of organism from blood and cerebrospinal fluid (early) and from urine (later), or direct microscopy of urine or cerebrospinal fluid.
- Positive leptospiral agglutination test.

General Considerations

Leptospirosis is a zoonosis caused by many antigenically distinct but morphologically similar spirochetes. The organism enters through the skin or respiratory tract. Classically, the severe form (Weil's disease), with jaundice and a high mortality rate, was associated with infection with *Leptospira icterohaemorrhagiae* following immersion in water contaminated with rat urine. It is now known that a variety of animals (dogs, rats, cattle, etc) may serve as reservoirs for pathogenic *Leptospira;* that a given serogroup may have multiple animal species as hosts; and that severe disease may be caused by many different serogroups.

In the United States, leptospirosis occurs in children, students, and housewives due to contact with dogs. Cattle, swine, or rodents may transmit the organism. Sewer workers, farmers, abattoir workers, animal handlers, and soldiers are at risk of occupational exposure. Outbreaks have resulted from swimming in contaminated streams and harvesting field crops. In the United States, about 100 cases are reported yearly, and about one-third are in children.

Clinical Findings

A. Symptoms and Signs:

1. Initial phase–The incubation period is 4–19 days, with a mean of 10 days. Chills, fever, headache, myalgia, conjunctivitis (episcleral injection), photophobia, cervical lymphadenopathy, and pharyngitis occur commonly. This leptospiremic phase lasts for 3–7 days.

2. Phase of apparent recovery–Symptoms typically (but not always) subside for 2–3 days.

3. Systemic phase–Fever reappears and is associated with headache, muscular pain and tenderness in the abdomen and back, and nausea and vomiting. Lung, heart, and joint involvement occasionally occurs. These manifestations are due to extensive vasculitis.

a. Central nervous system involvement– The central nervous system is involved in 50–90% of cases. Severe headache and mild nuchal rigidity are usual, but delirium, coma, and focal neurologic signs may be seen.

b. Renal and hepatic involvement–In about 50% of cases, the kidney or liver is affected. Gross hematuria and oliguria or anuria is sometimes seen. Jaundice may be associated with an enlarged and tender liver.

c. Gallbladder involvement–Leptospirosis may cause acalculous cholecystitis in children, demonstrable by abdominal ultrasound as a dilated, nonfunctioning gallbladder. Pancreatitis is unusual.

d. Hemorrhage–Petechiae, ecchymoses, and gastrointestinal bleeding may be severe.

e. Rash–A rash is seen in 10–30% of cases. It may be maculopapular and generalized or may be petechial or purpuric. Occasionally, erythema nodosum is seen. Peripheral desquamation of the rash may occur. Gangrenous areas are sometimes noted over the distal extremities. In such cases, skin biopsy demonstrates the presence of severe vasculitis involving both the arterial and the venous circulations.

B. Laboratory Findings: Leptospires are present in the blood and cerebrospinal fluid only during the first 10 days of illness. They appear in the urine during the second week, where they may persist for 30 days or longer. The organism can be isolated from blood inoculated into Fletcher's semisolid medium or Ellinghausen-McCullough-Johnson-Harris (EMJH) semisolid medium, but culture techniques are slow (7–10 days), difficult, and not generally available.

The white blood cell count is often elevated, especially when there is liver involvement. Serum bilirubin levels usually remain below 20 mg/dL. Other liver function tests may be abnormal, though the AST usually shows only slight elevation. An elevated serum creatine kinase is frequently found. Cerebrospinal fluid shows moderate pleocytosis (< 500/µL)—predominantly mononuclear cells—increased protein (50–100 mg/dL), and normal glucose. Urine often shows microscopic pyuria, hematuria, and, less often, proteinuria (++ or greater). The erythrocyte sedimentation rate is markedly elevated. Chest x-ray may show pneumonitis.

The serologic test of choice is a microscopic agglutination test using live organisms (performed at the Centers for Disease Control and Prevention, Atlanta, GA 30333). Leptospiral agglutinins generally reach peak levels by the third to fourth weeks. A 1:100 titer is considered suspicious; a fourfold or greater rise is diagnostic.

Differential Diagnosis

Fever and myalgia associated with the characteristic conjunctival (episcleral) injection should suggest leptospirosis. During the prodrome, malaria, typhoid fever, typhus, rheumatoid arthritis, brucellosis, and influenza may be suspected. Later, depending on the organ systems involved, a variety of other diseases need to be distinguished, including encephalitis, viral or tuberculous meningitis, viral hepatitis, glomerulonephritis, viral or bacterial pneumonia, rheumatic fever, subacute infective endocarditis, acute surgical abdomen, and Kawasaki disease (see Table 34–3).

Prevention

Preventive measures include avoidance of contaminated water and soil, rodent control, immunization of dogs and other domestic animals, and good sanitation. Immunization or antimicrobial prophylaxis with doxycycline may be of value to certain high-risk occupational groups.

Treatment

A. Specific Measures: Aqueous penicillin G (150,000 units/kg/d in four to six divided doses intravenously for 7–10 days) should be given when the diagnosis is suspected. Studies in severely ill patients indicate a benefit even if treatment is started 4 days after onset. A Jarisch-Herxheimer reaction may be seen. Tetracycline (40–50 mg/kg/d) may be used for mildly ill patients.

B. General Measures: Symptomatic and supportive care is indicated, particularly for renal and hepatic failure and hemorrhage.

Prognosis

Leptospirosis generally is anicteric and self-limiting. The disease usually lasts 1–3 weeks but may be more prolonged. Relapse may occur.

There are usually no permanent sequelae associated with central nervous system infection, though headache may persist. The mortality rate in reported cases in the United States is 5%, usually from renal failure. The mortality rate may reach 20% or more in elderly patients who have severe kidney and hepatic involvement.

Farr RW: Leptospirosis. Clin Infect Dis 1995;21:1.

Van Crevel R et al: Leptospirosis in travelers. Clin Infect Dis 1994;19:132.

Watt G et al: Limulus lysate positivity and Herxheimer-like reactions in leptospirosis: A placebo controlled study. J Infect Dis 1990;162:564.

Watt G et al: Placebo-controlled trial of intravenous penicillin for severe and late leptospirosis. Lancet 1988; 1:433.

LYME DISEASE

Essentials of Diagnosis & Typical Features

- Characteristic skin lesion (erythema migrans) 3–30 days after tick bite.
- Arthritis, usually pauciarticular, occurring about 4

weeks after appearance of skin lesion. Headache, chills, and fever.

• Residence or travel in an endemic area during the late spring to early fall.

General Considerations

Lyme disease is a subacute or chronic spirochetal infection caused by *Borrelia burgdorferi* and transmitted by the bite of an infected deer tick (*Ixodes* species). The disease was known in Europe for many years as tick-borne encephalomyelitis, often associated with a characteristic rash (erythema migrans). Discovery of the agent and vector followed investigation of an outbreak of pauciarticular arthritis in Lyme, Connecticut, in 1977.

Although cases are reported from many countries and states, endemic areas include the Northeast, upper Midwest, and West Coast in the United States and the northern European countries. Nearly 12,000 cases were reported in 1995. The disease is spreading as a result of increased infection in and distribution of the tick vector. Most cases with rash are recognized in spring and summer, when most tick bites occur. Since the incubation period for joint and neurologic disease may be months, however, cases may present at any time. *Ixodes* ticks are very small, and their bite is often unrecognized.

Clinical Findings

A. Symptoms and Signs: Erythema migrans, the most characteristic feature of Lyme disease, develops in 60–80% of patients. Three to 30 days after the bite, a ring of erythema develops at the site and spreads over days. It may attain a diameter of 20 cm. The center of the lesion may clear (resembling tinea corporis), remain red, or become raised (suggesting a chemical or infectious cellulitis). Many patients are otherwise asymptomatic; some have fever (usually low-grade), headache, and myalgias. Multiple satellite skin lesions, urticaria, or diffuse erythema may occur. Untreated, the rash lasts days to 3 weeks.

In up to 50% of patients, arthritis develops several weeks to months after the bite. Recurrent attacks of migratory, monarticular or pauciarticular arthritis involving the knees and other large joints are seen. Each attack lasts for days to a few weeks. Fever is common and may be high. Complete resolution between attacks is typical. Chronic arthritis develops in less than 10%, more often in those with the DR4 haplotype.

Neurologic manifestations develop in up to 20% of cases and usually consist of Bell's palsy, aseptic meningitis (which may be indistinguishable from viral meningitis), or polyradiculitis. Peripheral neuritis, Guillain-Barré syndrome, encephalitis, ataxia, chorea, and other cranial neuropathies are less common. Seizures suggest another diagnosis. Untreated, the neurologic symptoms are usually self-limited but may be chronic or permanent. Although the fatigue

and nonspecific neurologic symptoms may be prolonged in a few patients, Lyme disease is not proved to be a cause of chronic fatigue syndrome.

Self-limited heart-block or myocardial dysfunction occurs in about 5% of patients.

B. Laboratory Findings: Most patients with only rash have normal laboratory tests. Children with arthritis may have moderately elevated sedimentation rates and white blood cell counts; the ANA and rheumatoid factor are negative or nonspecific; streptococcal antibodies are not elevated. Circulating IgM cryoglobulins may be present. Joint fluid may show up to 100,000 cells with a polymorphonuclear predominance, normal glucose, and elevated protein and immune complexes; Gram's stain and culture are negative. In patients with central nervous system involvement, the spinal fluid may show lymphocytic pleocytosis and elevated protein; the glucose and all cultures and stains are normal or negative. Abnormal nerve conduction may be present with peripheral neuropathy.

Diagnosis

Lyme disease is a clinical diagnosis. History, physical examination, and laboratory features are important to consider. The causative organism is difficult to culture. Serologic testing may support the clinical diagnosis. Antibody testing should be performed in experienced laboratories. The enzyme immunoassay is currently the most accurate test; all positive tests should be confirmed by Western blot, especially in the case of unusual clinical syndromes. Serologic tests are positive in only 30–60% of patients with early disease. Therapy early in disease may blunt antibody titers. Recent studies have shown considerable intralaboratory and interlaboratory variability in titers reported. Overdiagnosis of Lyme disease based on atypical symptoms and "positive" serology appears to be common. Sera from patients with syphilis, HIV, and leptospirosis may give false-positive results for Lyme disease. Diagnosis of central nervous system disease requires both objective abnormalities of the neurologic examination, laboratory or radiographic studies, and consistent positive serology.

Differential Diagnosis

Aside from the disorders already mentioned, the rash may resemble pityriasis, erythema multiforme, a drug eruption, or erythema nodosum. Erythema migrans is nonscaly, minimally tender or nontender, and persists longer in the same place than many of the more common childhood erythematous rashes. The arthritis may resemble juvenile rheumatoid arthritis, reactive arthritis, septic arthritis, reactive effusion from a contiguous osteomyelitis, rheumatic fever, leukemic arthritis, lupus, and Henoch-Schönlein purpura. Spontaneous resolution in a few days to weeks helps differentiate Lyme disease from juvenile rheumatoid arthritis, in which arthritis lasting a minimum of 6 weeks is required for diagnosis. The neurologic signs may suggest idiopathic Bell's palsy, viral or parainfectious meningitis or meningoencephalitis, lead poisoning, psychosomatic illness, and many other conditions.

Prevention

Prevention consists of avoidance of endemic areas, wearing long sleeves and pants, frequent "tick checks," and applications of tick repellents. Ticks usually are attached for 24–48 hours before transmission of Lyme disease occurs. Ticks should be removed by pulling gently without twisting or excessive squeezing, using a tweezer. Permethrin sprayed on clothing decreases tick attachment. Repellents containing high concentrations of DEET may be neurotoxic and should be used cautiously and washed off when tick exposure ends. Prophylactic antibiotics should not be used.

Treatment

Although antimicrobial therapy is beneficial in most cases of Lyme disease, it is most effective if started early; prolonged treatment is important for all forms. Relapses are seen with all regimens in some patients.

A. Rash, Other Early Infections: Amoxicillin (40 mg/kg/d) orally in three divided doses, or penicillin V potassium, 25–50 mg/kg/d in three divided doses—some experts add probenecid, 10 mg/kg/dose—for 2–3 weeks. Use erythromycin (30 mg/kg/d) or cefuroxime in penicillin-allergic children, though erythromycin may be less effective. Doxycycline (100 mg orally twice a day) or tetracycline (250 mg four times daily) may be used in children over age 9.

B. Arthritis: Use the amoxicillin or doxycycline regimen (same dosage as above), but treat for 4 weeks. Parenteral ceftriaxone, 75–100 mg/kg once daily, or penicillin G, 300,000 units/kg/d in four divided doses for 2–3 weeks, is used for persistent arthritis.

C. Bell's Palsy: The same oral drug regimens may be used for 4 weeks.

D. Other Neurologic Disease or Cardiac Disease: Parenteral therapy for 2–3 weeks is recommended with either ceftriaxone, 75–100 kg/d in one daily dose, or penicillin G, 300,000 units/kg/d in four divided doses.

Adams WV et al: Cognitive effects of Lyme disease in children. Pediatrics 1994;94:185.

Bingham PM et al: Neurologic manifestations in children with Lyme disease. Pediatrics 1995;96:1053.

Dattwyler RJ et al: Ceftriaxone compared with doxycycline for the treatment of acute disseminated Lyme disease. N Engl J Med 1997;337:289.

Eckman MH et al: Cost effectiveness of oral as compared with intravenous antibiotic therapy for patients with early Lyme disease or Lyme arthritis. N Engl J Med 1997;337:357.

Nadelman RB et al: Simultaneous human granulocytic ehrlichiosis and Lyme borreliosis. N Engl J Med 1997;337:27.

Shapiro ED et al: A controlled trial of antimicrobial prophylaxis for Lyme disease after deer-tick bites. N Engl J Med 1992;327:1769.

Steere AC et al: The overdiagnosis of Lyme disease. JAMA 1993;269:1812.

Szer IL et al: The long term course of Lyme arthritis in children. N Engl J Med 1991;325:159.

Williams CL et al: Lyme disease in childhood: Clinical and epidemiologic features of 90 cases. Pediatr Infect Dis J 1990;9:10.

REFERENCES

Feigin RD, Cherry JD (editors): *Textbook of Pediatric Infectious Disease,* 3rd ed. Saunders, 1993.

Peter G, Hall CB, Orenstein WA (editors): *1997 Red Book: Report of the Committee on Infectious Diseases,* 24th ed. American Academy of Pediatrics, 1997.

37

Infections: Parasitic & Mycotic

Adriana Weinberg, MD, & Myron J. Levin, MD

I. INFECTIONS: PARASITIC

Parasitic diseases are common and may present clinically in a variety of ways (Table 37–1). Although travel to endemic areas suggests particular infections, many are transmitted through fomites or acquired from contact with human carriers and can occur anywhere. A list of antiparasitic agents is presented in Table 37–2.

Some of the less common parasitic infections and those seen primarily in the developing world are presented in abbreviated form in Table 37–3.

Selection of Patients for Evaluation

The incidence of parasitic infections varies greatly with geographic area. Children who have traveled or lived in endemic areas are at risk of infection with a variety of intestinal and tissue parasites. Children who have resided only in developed countries are usually free of tissue parasites (except *Toxoplasma*). Searching for intestinal parasites is expensive for the patient and time-consuming for the laboratory. More than 90% of ovum and parasite examinations performed in most hospital laboratories in the United States are negative; many have been ordered inappropriately. An approach to determining which children with diarrhea need such examinations is presented in Figure 37–1.

Children with underlying immunodeficiency, in all populations worldwide, are uniquely susceptible to parasites, particularly protozoal intestinal infections. In these patients, normally commensal infestations may become debilitating infections, and multiple pathogens are frequently identified. The yield for diagnostic testing in compromised hosts is higher and the threshold for ordering tests must be lower.

Specimen Processing

For tissue parasites, contact the laboratory for proper collection procedure. Diarrheal stools may contain trophozoites that rapidly die during transport. The specimen should be either examined immediately or placed in a stool fixative such as polyvinyl alcohol. Several types of commercial vials containing fixatives are available and may be sent home with the child for outpatient specimen collection. Since they may contain toxic compounds, the vials should be safely stored. Fixed specimens are stable at room temperature. Formed stools usually contain cysts that are more stable. It is best to fix these also after collection, but they may be reliably examined after room temperature transport.

Eosinophilia & Parasitic Infections

Although parasites commonly cause eosinophilia, in developed countries other causes are much more common and include allergies, drugs, and other infections. Heavy intestinal nematode infections cause eosinophilia; they are easily detected on a single ovum and parasite examination. Light nematode infections and common protozoal infections—giardiasis, cryptosporidiosis, and amebiasis—rarely cause eosinophilia. Eosinophilia is also unusual or minimal in more serious infections such as amebic liver abscess, toxoplasmosis, and malaria.

The most common parasitic infection in the United States that causes significant eosinophilia with negative stool examination is toxocariasis. In a young child with unexplained eosinophilia and a negative stool examination, a serologic test for *Toxocara* may be the next appropriate test. Trichinosis may rarely cause marked eosinophilia; strongyloidiasis may also be difficult to diagnose with stool examinations. Patients with eosinophilia who have lived in or traveled to developing regions of the world have a much broader differential diagnosis.

Table 37–1. Symptoms of parasitic infection.

Sign	Agent	Comments[1]
Abdominal pain	*Anisakis*	Shortly after raw fish ingestion.
	Ascaris	Heavy infection; may obstruct bowel, biliary tract.
	Clonorchis	Heavy, early infection. Hepatomegaly later.
	Entamoeba histolytica	Hematochezia, variable fever, diarrhea.
	Fasciola hepatica	Diarrhea, vomiting.
	Hookworm	Heavy infection. Iron deficiency anemia.
	Strongyloides	Eosinophilia, pruritus. May resemble peptic disease.
	Trichinella	Myalgia, periorbital edema, eosinophilia.
	Trichuris	Diarrhea, dysentery with heavy infection.
Cough	*Ascaris*	Wheezing, eosinophilia during migration phase.
	Paragonimus westermani	Hemoptysis; chronic. May mimic tuberculosis.
	Strongyloides	Wheezing, pruritus, eosinophilia during migration or dissemination.
	Toxocara	Affects ages 1–5; hepatosplenomegaly; eosinophilia.
	Tropical eosinophilia	Pulmonary infiltrates, eosinophilia.
Diarrhea	*Blastocystis*	Possibly with heavy infection in immunosuppressed or normal individuals.
	Cryptosporidium	Watery; prolonged in normals, chronic in immunosuppressed.
	Dientamoeba fragilis	Only with heavy infection.
	Entamoeba histolytica	Hematochezia, variable fever; no eosinophilia.
	Giardia	Afebrile, chronic; anorexia; no hematochezia or eosinophilia.
	Schistosoma	Chronic; hepatosplenomegaly.
	Strongyloides	Abdominal pain; eosinophilia.
	Trichinella	Myalgia, periorbital edema, eosinophilia.
	Trichuris	With heavy infection.
Dysentery	*Balantidium coli*	Swine contact.
	Entamoeba histolytica	Few to no leukocytes in stool; fever; hematochezia.
	Schistosoma	During acute infection.
	Trichuris	With heavy infection.
Dysuria	*Enterobius*	Usually girls with worms in urethra, bladder; nocturnal, perianal pruritus.
	Schistosoma	Hematuria. Exclude bacteriuria, stones.
Headache (and other cerebral symptoms)	*Angiostrongylus*	Eosinophilic meningitis.
	Naegleria	Fresh-water swimming; rapidly progressive meningoencephalitis.
	Plasmodium	Fever, chills, jaundice, splenomegaly. Cerebral ischemia (with *P falciparum*).
	Taenia solium	Cysticercosis. Focal seizures, deficits; hydrocephalus, aseptic meningitis.
	Toxoplasma	Meningoencephalitis (especially in the immunosuppressed); hydrocephalus in infants.
	Trypanosoma	African forms. Chronic lethargy (sleeping sickness).
Pruritus	*Ancylostoma braziliense*	Creeping eruption; dermal serpiginous burrow.
	Enterobius	Perianal, nocturnal.
	Filaria	Variable; seen in many filarial disease.
	Hookworm	Local at penetration site in heavy exposure.
	Strongyloides	Diffuse with migration; may be recurrent.
	Trypanosoma	African forms; one of many nonspecific symptoms.

(continued)

Table 37–1. Symptoms of parasitic infection. (continued)

Sign	Agent	Comments[1]
Fever	*Entamoeba histolytica*	With acute dysentery or liver abscess.
	Leishmania donovani	Hepatosplenomegaly, anemia, leukopenia.
	Plasmodium	Chills, headache, jaundice; periodic.
	Toxocara	Cough, hepatosplenomegaly, eosinophilia.
	Toxoplasma	Generalized adenopathy; splenomegaly.
	Trichinella	Myalgia, periorbital edema, eosinophilia.
	Trypanosoma	Early stage, African forms; lymphadenopathy.
Anemia	*Diphyllobothrium*	Megaloblastic due to B_{12} deficiency; rare.
	Hookworm	Iron deficiency.
	Leishmania donovani	Fever, hepatosplenomegaly, leukopenia (kala-azar).
	Plasmodium	Hemolysis.
	Trichuris	Heavy infection, due to iron loss.
Eosinophilia	*Angiostrongylus*	Eosinophilic meningitis.
	Fasciola	Abdominal pain.
	Filaria	Microfilariae in blood. Lymphadenopathy.
	Onchocerca	Nodules, keratitis.
	Schistosoma	Chronic; intestinal or genitourinary symptoms.
	Strongyloides	Abdominal pain, diarrhea.
	Toxocara	Hepatosplenomegaly, cough; affects ages 1–5.
	Trichinella	Myalgia, periorbital edema.
	Tropical pulmonary eosinophilia	Cough.
Hematuria	*Schistosoma*	*S haematobium.* Bladder, urethral granulomas. Exclude stones, bacteriuria.
Hemoptysis	*Paragonimus westermani*	Lung fluke. Variable chest pain; chronic.
Hepatomegaly	*Clonorchis*	Heavy infection. Tenderness early; cirrhosis late.
	Echinococcus	Chronic; cysts.
	Entamoeba histolytica	Toxic hepatitis or abscess. No eosinophilia.
	Leishmania donovani	Splenomegaly, fever, pancytopenia.
	Schistosoma	Chronic; hepatic fibrosis, splenomegaly.
	Toxocara	Splenomegaly, eosinophilia, cough; no adenopathy.
Splenomegaly	*Leishmania donovani*	Hepatomegaly, fever, anemia.
	Plasmodium	Fever, chills, jaundice, headache.
	Schistosoma	Hepatomegaly.
	Toxocara	Eosinophilia, hepatomegaly.
	Toxoplasma	Lymphadenopathy, other symptoms.
Lymphadenopathy	Filaria	Inguinal typical; chronic.
	Leishmania donovani	Hepatosplenomegaly, pancytopenia, fever.
	Schistosoma	Acute infection; fever, rash, arthralgia, heptosplenomegaly.
	Toxoplasma	Cervical common; may involve single site; splenomegaly.
	Trypanosoma	Localized near bite or generalized hepatosplenomegaly (Chagas' disease); generalized (especially posterior cervical) in African forms.

[1]Symptoms usually related to degree of infestation. Infestation with small numbers of organisms is often asymptomatic.

Table 37–2. Commonly used antiparasitic drugs.

[1]Albendazole—*Albenza* (SmithKline Beecham)
[2]Aminosidine (paromomycin)
[2]Artemether
[2]Artesunate
Atovaquone—*Mepron* (Glaxo-Wellcome)
[2]Benznidazole—*Rochagan* (Roche, Brazil)
[3]Bithionol—*Bitin* (Tanabe, Japan)
Chloroquine—*Aralen* (Sanofi Winthrop), others
[1]Diethylcarbamazine—*Hetrazan* (Wyeth-Ayerst)
[3]Diloxanide furoate—*Furamide* (Boots, England)
[1]Eflornithine (difluoromethylornithine, DFMO)—*Ornidyl* (Merrell Dow)
Furazolidone—*Furoxone* (Roberts)
[2]Halofantrine—*Halfan* (SmithKline Beecham)
Hydroxychloroquine—*Plaquenil* (Sanofi Winthrop)
Iodoquinol (diiodohydroxyquin)—*Yodoxin* (Glenwood), others
[3]Ivermectin—*Mectizan* (Merck)
Mebendazole—*Vermox* (Janssen)
Mefloquine—*Lariam* (Roche)
[2]Meglumine antimonate—*Glucantime* (Rhône-Poulenc Rorer, France)
[3]Melarsoprol—*Arsobal* (Rhône-Poulenc Rorer, France)

Metronidazole—*Flagyl* (Searle), others
[3]Nifurtimox—*Lampit* (Bayer, Germany)
Oxamniquine—*Vansil* (Pfizer)
Paromomycin—*Humatin* (Parke-Davis)
Pentamidine isethionate—*Pentam* 300 (Fujisawa), *NebuPent* (Fujisawa)
Praziquantel—*Biltricide* (Miles)
Primaquine phosphate—(Sanofi Winthrop)
[2]Proguanil—*Paludrine* (Ayerst, Canada, ICI, England)
Prantel pamoate—*Antiminth* (Pfizer)
Pyrimethamine—*Daraprim* (Glaxo-Wellcome)
Pyrimethamine-sulfadoxine—*Fansidar* (Roche)
Quinidine gluconate—(Lilly)
[2]Quinine dihydrochloride
Quinine sulfate—many manufacturers
[3]Sodium stibogluconate (antimony sodium gluconate)—*Pentostam* (Glaxo-Wellcome, England)
[1]Spiramycin—*Rovamycine* (Rhône-Poulenc Rorer)
Sulfadiazine—(Eon Labs, and others)
[3]Suramin—(Bayer, Germany)
Thiabendazole—*Mintezol* (Merck)
[2]Tinidazole—*Fasigyn* (Pfizer)
[2]Tryparsamide

Adapted from The Medical Letter 1995;37(961):107.
[1]Available in the United States only from the manufacturer.
[2]Not available in the United States.
[3]Available from the CDC Drug Service, Centers for Disease Control and Prevention, Atlanta, Georgia 30333; 404-639-3670 (evenings, weekends, or holidays: 404-639-2888).

PROTOZOAL INFECTIONS

MALARIA

Essentials of Diagnosis & Typical Features

- Residence in or travel to an endemic area.
- Cyclic paroxysms of chills, fever, and intense diaphoresis.
- Headache, backache, cough, abdominal pain, nausea, vomiting, diarrhea.
- Coma, seizures.
- Splenomegaly, anemia.
- Malaria parasites in peripheral blood smear.

General Considerations

Malaria kills a million children worldwide each year and is undergoing resurgence in areas where it was previously controlled. Imported cases diagnosed in the United States each year number approximately 1000. The female anopheline mosquito transmits the parasites—*Plasmodium vivax* (most common), *Plasmodium falciparum* (most virulent), *Plasmodium ovale* (similar to *P vivax*), and *Plasmodium malariae*. The gametocytes ingested from an infected human form sporozoites in the mosquito; when inoculated into a susceptible host, these sporozoites infect hepa-

tocytes. Antibody—but not drug therapy—decreases sporozoite infectivity. The preerythrocytic phase (hepatic) is about 1–2 weeks for all but *P malariae* infection (3–5 weeks), but the initial symptoms may be delayed for up to a year in *P falciparum,* 4 years in *P vivax,* and decades in *P malariae* infections. Merozoites released into the circulation from hepatocytes infect red cells (young cells by *P vivax* and *P ovale,* old cells by *P malariae,* and all cells by *P falciparum*) and begin the synchronous erythrocytic cycles—rupturing the infected cells at intervals of 48 hours for all but *P malariae,* which has a 72-hour cycle. Asynchronous cycles causing daily fevers are most common in early stages of infection. Survival is associated with a progressive decrease in intensity of cycles; relapses years later may occur as a result of hepatic infection, which persists in *P vivax* and *P ovale* infections. Infection acquired congenitally or from transfusions or needle sticks does not result in a hepatic phase.

Susceptibility varies genetically; certain red cell phenotypes are partially resistant to *P falciparum* infection (hemoglobin S, hemoglobin F, thalassemia, and possibly G6PD deficiency). The worldwide distribution of the four species is determined, to some extent, by host genetic factors. The absence of *P vivax* from Africa reflects the lack of specific Duffy blood group substances among most native Africans. Recurrent infections result in some natural species-specific immunity; this does not prevent sporozoite infection but does decrease parasitemia and symp-

Table 37–3. Some parasitic infections seen less commonly in developed regions.

Agent (Disease)	Geographic Region	Vector	Symptoms and Signs	Laboratory Findings	Diagnosis	Therapy and Comments
Trypanosoma cruzi (Chagas' disease)	South and Central America, Mexico	Reduviid bug	Acute: Painful red nodule at bite site, conjunctivitis, periorbital edema (Romaña's sign), fever, local ± generalized adenitis. Late: Myocarditis, megaesophagus, megacolon.	Mononuclear leukocytosis	Organisms in peripheral blood. Positive serology.	Nifurtimox or benznidazole may help early. No therapy for late disease. May be transmitted by blood transfusion or congenitally.
Trypanosomal brucei (sleeping sickness)	Africa	Tsetse fly	Hepatosplenomegaly, adenopathy. Nodule at bite site (resolves). Recurrent fever, headache, myalgia, progressive encephalitis.	Elevated ESR, anemia, CSF pleocytosis	Organisms in blood, CSF, marrow, nodes. Positive serology.	Suramin for non-CNS disease. Eflornithine promising.
Leishmania donovani (kala-azar)	Mideast, India, Mediterranean, South and Central America	Sandfly	Fever, generalized adenopathy, hepatosplenomegaly weeks to months after infection.	Pancytopenia, hypergammaglobulinemia	Organisms in marrow, nodes, spleen. Positive serology.	Sodium stibogluconate, meglumine antimonate, pentamidine, amphotericin B.
Leishmania tropica (Oriental sore)	Asia, India, North Africa	Sandfly	Papule at bite site (usually on face, limbs) develops after weeks to months, then ulcerates and scars.	…	Organisms in skin biopsy. Positive skin test, serology.	Same as for *L donovani*.
Leishmania braziliensis, L mexicana (chiclero ulcer)	South America	Sandfly	Painful mucocutaneous ulcers or granulomas. Nasolabial lesions common.	…	Skin biopsy. Positive skin test, serology.	Same as for *L donovani; ketoconazole*.
Wuchereria, Brugia (filariasis)	Tropics, subtropics	Mosquito	Chronic adenopathy, often inguinal. Obstructive lymphedema.	Eosinophilia	Concentrated blood smears for larvae. Positive serology.	Ivermectin, diethylcarbamazine kill larvae. Surgery for lymphatic obstruction.
Angiostrongylus cantonensis (eosinophilic meningitis)	Hawaii, Asia, Pacific Islands	Snails, slugs	Ingestion (usually inadvertent) followed in 1–4 weeks by meningitis of variable severity. Paresthesias.	Eosinophils in CSF and blood	Positive serology. Larvae may be present in CSF.	Fever absent or low. No focal lesions on CNS imaging. No specific therapy. Steroids may be beneficial. Mebendazole may help.
Paragonimus westermani (lung fluke infection)	Asia, South America, Africa	Raw crabs, crustaceans	Cough, hemoptysis. Rarely seizures, other CNS signs if migration to brain occurs.	…	Large ova in concentrated specimens, feces. Cystic nodular lesions on chest x-ray or CNS imaging.	Resembles pulmonary tuberculosis. Praziquantel very effective.
Clonorchis sinensis (liver fluke infection)	Asia	Raw fish	Adult flukes obstruct biliary tree. Acute: Hepatomegaly, fever, jaundice, urticaria. Late: cirrhosis, carcinoma.	Variable liver function test abnormalities	Ova in feces.	Praziquantel. Advanced disease not treatable. Liver transplant.

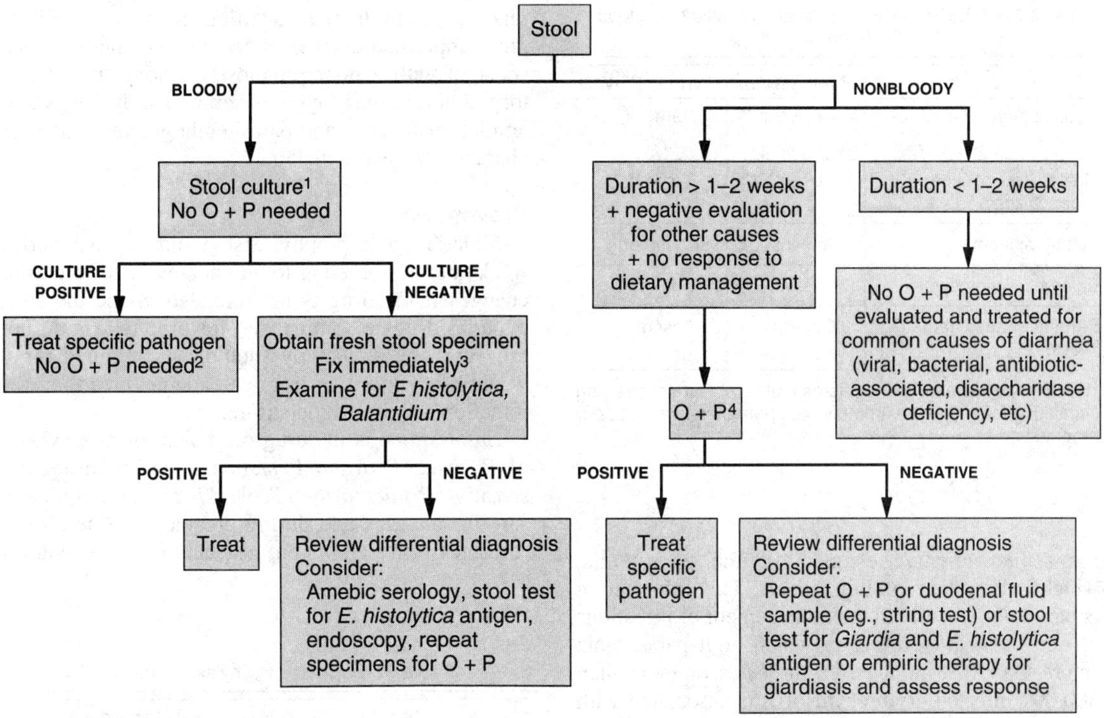

```
                              ┌──────────┐
                              │  Stool   │
                              └─────┬────┘
              BLOODY                │                NONBLOODY
        ┌─────────────────────────────┴────────────────────────────────────┐
        │                                                                    │
┌───────────────────────┐                    ┌─────────────────────┐  ┌──────────────────┐
│ Stool culture¹         │                    │ Duration > 1–2 weeks│  │ Duration < 1–2   │
│ No O + P needed        │                    │ + negative evaluation│  │ weeks            │
└───────────────────────┘                    │ for other causes     │  └────────┬─────────┘
                                              │ + no response to     │           │
 CULTURE                      CULTURE         │ dietary management   │           │
 POSITIVE                     NEGATIVE        └──────────┬──────────┘           │
     │                            │                      │                      │
┌───────────────┐  ┌────────────────────────┐           │            ┌───────────────────────┐
│ Treat specific│  │ Obtain fresh stool      │           │            │ No O + P needed until │
│ pathogen      │  │ specimen                │           │            │ evaluated and treated │
│ No O + P      │  │ Fix immediately³        │      ┌──────────┐      │ for common causes of  │
│ needed²       │  │ Examine for E histolytica,│    │ O + P⁴   │      │ diarrhea (viral,      │
└───────────────┘  │ Balantidium             │      └────┬─────┘      │ bacterial, antibiotic-│
                   └────────────────────────┘           │            │ associated,           │
                                                         │            │ disaccharidase        │
     POSITIVE              NEGATIVE          POSITIVE    │  NEGATIVE  │ deficiency, etc)      │
                                                         │            └───────────────────────┘
```

O + P = Ova and parasite examination.

¹ *Shigella, Salmonella, Campylobacter, E coli (Escherichia coli)* 0157, *Yersinia*; assay for *Clostridium difficile* toxin if recent antimicrobial use.

² Unless critically ill, from endemic area for amebiasis, or unresponsive to standard therapy.

³ In stool fixative, eg, polyvinyl alcohol.

⁴ Include examination for *Cryptosporidium*; immediate stool fixation needed if stool is diarrheal.

Figure 37–1. Parasitologic evaluation of acute diarrhea.

---

toms. Normal splenic function is an important factor because of the immunologic and filter function of the spleen. Asplenic persons develop rapidly progressive malaria with many circulating infected erythrocytes (including mature forms of *P falciparum*). Maternal immunity protects the neonate.

Clinical Findings

A. Symptoms and Signs: Clinical manifestations vary according to species, strain, and host immunity. The infant presents with recurrent bouts of fever, irritability, poor feeding, vomiting, jaundice, and splenomegaly. Exanthem, rash, and significant dehydration are usually absent and help distinguish malaria from viral infections presenting with similar symptoms. Symptoms are similar in older children, with headache, backache, chills, myalgia, and fatigue more easily elicited. Fever may be cyclic (every 48 hours for all but *P malariae* infection, in which it occurs every 72 hours) or irregular (most commonly observed with *P falciparum).* Between attacks, patients may look quite well. If the disease is untreated,

relapses cease within a year in *P falciparum* and within several years in *P vivax* infections, but may recur decades later in *P malariae* infection. Infection during pregnancy often causes intrauterine growth retardation or premature delivery but rarely true fetal infection.

Physical examination in uncomplicated cases may show only mild splenomegaly and anemia.

B. Laboratory Findings: The diagnosis of malaria relies on detecting one or more of the four human plasmodia in blood smears. Most acute infections are caused by either *P vivax, P ovale,* or *P falciparum,* though 5–7% are due to multiple species. Giemsa-stained thick smears offer the highest diagnostic accuracy for malaria parasites. Identification of the *Plasmodium* species relies on morphologic criteria (Table 37–4) and requires an experienced observer.

Alternative techniques of similar or higher diagnostic accuracy for *P falciparum* include ELISA, DNA hybridization, and polymerase chain reactors. A unique feature of the microscopic examination is

Table 37–4. Differentiation of malaria parasites on blood smears.

	P falciparum	P vivax, P ovale
Multiple infected erythro-cytes	Common	Rare
Mature trophozoites or schizonts	Absent[1]	Common
Schüffner's dots	Absent	Common
Enlarged erythrocytes	Absent	Common
Banana-shaped gameto-cytes	Common	Absent

[1]Usually sequestered in the microcirculation. Rare cases with circulating forms have extremely high parasitemia and a poor prognosis.

the semiquantitative estimate of the parasitemia, which is best done on thin smears. This information is particularly useful in the management of infections caused by *P falciparum,* in which high parasitemia (more than 10% infected erythrocytes or more than 500,000 infected erythrocytes/μL) is associated with high morbidity and mortality and requires hospitalization. Treatment response of *P falciparum* and chloroquine-resistant *P vivax* infections is best monitored by daily parasitemia assays: constant or increased number of infected erythrocytes after 48 hours of treatment or after the second hemolytic crisis suggest an inadequate therapeutic response. Other laboratory findings that reflect the severity of hemolysis include decreased hematocrit, hemoglobin, and haptoglobin; increased reticulocyte count; and hyperbilirubinemia and increased lactate dehydrogenase (LDH). Thrombocytopenia is common, but the incidence of leukocytosis is variable.

Differential Diagnosis

Relapsing fever may be seen with borreliosis, brucellosis, sequential common infections, Hodgkin's disease, juvenile rheumatoid arthritis, rat-bite fever, or one of the idiopathic periodic fevers. Other common causes of high fever and headache include influenza, *Mycoplasma pneumoniae* or enteroviral infection, sinusitis, meningitis, enteric fever, tuberculosis, occult pneumonia, or bacteremia. Fever, headache, and jaundice in a patient returning from tropical areas should include leptospirosis and yellow fever in the differential diagnosis. Malaria may also coexist with other diseases.

Complications & Sequelae

Severe complications are limited to *P falciparum* infection and result from microvascular obstruction and tissue ischemia. Impaired consciousness and seizures are the most common complications of

malaria in children. In addition, respiratory failure, renal impairment, severe bleeding, and shock are associated with a poor prognosis. Among the laboratory abnormalities, hypoglycemia, acidosis, elevated aminotransferases, and parasitemia greater than 15% characterize severe malaria.

Prevention

Malaria chemoprophylaxis should be instituted 2 weeks before traveling to an endemic area to permit changes if the drug is not tolerated. Since the antimalarial drugs recommended for prophylaxis do not kill sporozoites, therapy should be continued for 4 weeks after returning from an endemic area to cover infection acquired at departure.

Chloroquine is the drug of choice for prophylaxis of *P vivax, P ovale, P malariae,* and chloroquine-sensitive *P falciparum* (Table 37–5). Chloroquine is safe for all ages and during pregnancy. Side effects (dizziness, blurred vision, headache) can be reduced

Table 37–5. Chemoprophylaxis of malaria.[1]

Drug	Dosage
Chloroquine-sensitive areas[2]	
Chloroquine	5 mg base/kg/wk up to 300 mg (adult dose)
Chloroquine-resistant areas	
Mefloquine	0.25 tablet (62.5 mg) once a week (15–19 kg) 0.5 tablet (125 mg) (20–30 kg) 0.75 tablet (187.5 mg) (31–45 kg) 1 tablet (250 mg) (> 45 kg)
Doxycycline	2 mg/kg/d (age > 8 years) up to 100 mg (adult dose)
Chloroquine	5 mg base/kg/wk up to 300 mg (adult dose)
plus	
Proguanil	50 mg daily (age < 2 years) 100 mg (age 2–6 years) 150 mg (age 7–10 years) 200 mg (age > 10 years)
Relapse of *P vivax* or *P ovale*[3]	
Primaquine	0.3 mg base/kg/d up to 15 mg (adult dose) during the last 2 weeks of prophylaxis

[1]Updated malaria chemoprophylaxis information may be obtained by calling the Centers for Disease Control and Prevention Hot Line at 404-332-4555.
[2]Chloroquine-resistant *Plasmodium falciparum* has not yet been identified in Central America west of the Panama Canal zone, Haiti, Dominican Republic, Mexico, and most of the Middle East.
[3]Optional. Observation and prompt initiation of treatment when relapse occurs are sufficient.

by administering 50% of the weekly dose twice per week. Effects of chloroquine on heart rhythm are infrequent and are typically associated with rapid intravenous infusion or overdosage. Chloroquine has immunosuppressive properties and has been reported to impair immunization against rabies, but not against yellow fever.

For chloroquine-resistant *P falciparum,* the drug of choice is mefloquine. The side effects of mefloquine are headache, dizziness, and blurred vision. Daily doxycycline is recommended for patients older than 8 years of age who are unable to tolerate mefloquine. Women on prolonged doxycycline therapy tend to develop yeast vaginitis, and it is advisable to supply them with nystatin suppositories. For children under 15 kg or during pregnancy, when mefloquine is contraindicated, chloroquine plus proguanil is the alternative even though it is less effective than mefloquine. Daily primaquine also effectively prevents chloroquine-resistant *P falciparum,* and is used to prevent relapse of *P vivax* or *P ovale.*

No drug regimen guarantees protection against malaria. If fever develops within 1 year (particularly within 2 months) after travel to an endemic area, patients should be advised to seek medical attention. Insect repellents, insecticide-impregnated bed nets and proper clothing are important adjuncts for malaria prophylaxis.

Treatment

Treatment for malaria includes a variety of supportive strategies in addition to the antimalarial drugs. It is advisable to hospitalize nonimmune patients with *P falciparum* until a response to treatment, defined as a decrease in daily parasitemias is documented. At this time, severe complications are unlikely to occur.

Partially immune patients with uncomplicated *P falciparum* infection and nonimmune persons infected with *P vivax, P ovale,* or *P malariae* can be treated as outpatients if there is reliable follow-up. For children, hydration and treatment of hypoglycemia are of utmost importance. Anemia, seizures, pulmonary edema, and renal failure require conventional management. Corticosteroids are contraindicated for cerebral malaria. In face of severe malaria, exchange transfusion can be a life-saving procedure, particularly in nonimmune persons with parasitemia greater than 15%.

Chloroquine is the drug of choice for treatment of infection with chloroquine-sensitive plasmodia (Table 37–6). In patients unable to take oral medication, treatment can be initiated with chloroquine or quinidine administered as a carefully controlled intravenous infusion (for potential arrhythmogenic effect) and later converted to oral chloroquine. For chloroquine-resistant *P falciparum,* oral therapy includes quinine in association with pyrimethamine-sulfadoxine, tetracycline, doxycycline, or clinda-

Table 37–6. Treatment of malaria.

Drug	Dosage
Chloroquine-susceptible plasmodia	
Chloroquine	10 mg base/kg up to 600 mg, followed either by 5 mg base/kg after 6, 24, and 48 hours, or 5 mg base/kg after 12, 24, and 36 hours
Chloroquine-resistant *P falciparum*	
A. Oral regimens	
1. Quinine sulfate	25 mg/kg/d up to 2g/d in three doses for 3–7 days
plus	
Pyrimethamine-sulfadoxine	¼ tablet on the last day of quinine (age < 1 year) ½ tablet (age 1–3 years) 1 tablet (age 4–8 years) 2 tablets (age 9–14 years) 3 tablets (age >15 years)
or	
Tetracycline	20 mg/kg/d up to 1 g/d in four doses for 7 days
or	
Doxycycline	3 mg/kg/d up to 100 mg as single daily dose for 7 days
or	
Clindamycin	20–40 mg/kg/d up to 2700 mg in three doses for 3 days
2. Mefloquine	25 mg/kg up to 1250 mg as a single dose
3. Halofantrine	8 mg/kg up to 500 mg every 6 hours for three doses; repeat in 1 week
B. Parenteral regimen	
Quinidine gluconate	10 mg/kg up to 600 mg as loading dose IV in normal saline slowly over 1–2 hours followed by continuous infusion of 0.02 mg/kg/min until oral therapy can be started
Chloroquine-resistant *P vivax*	
Mefloquine	25 mg/kg up to 1250 mg in a single dose
Halofantrine	8 mg/kg up to 500 mg/kg every 6 hours for three doses; repeat in 1 week
Prevention of relapse with *P vivax* or *P ovale*	
Primaquine phosphate[1]	0.3 mg base/kg/d up to 15 mg base/d for 14 days

[1]Screen for G6PD deficiency.

mycin; or mefloquine; or halofantrine. Artemether and artesunate, both derivatives of artemisinin, are very effective against *P falciparum* but are not available in the United States. If the patient failed chemoprophylaxis, the same drug should not be used for treatment. Halofantrine is not recommended for persons who failed mefloquine chemoprophylaxis because of cross-resistance. Patients infected with chloroquine-resistant *P falciparum* who cannot take oral medication should be treated with intravenous quinidine.This is two or three times more active than quinine, and serum levels can be measured in most North American hospitals. Chloroquine-resistant *P vivax,* which has been identified in Papua New Guinea, Irian Jaya, Indonesia, India, Brazil, and Colombia, can be treated with mefloquine or halofantrine. Persons with *P vivax* or *P ovale* infection living in nonendemic areas are usually treated with primaquine to prevent late relapse.

Marsh K et al: Indicators of life-threatening malaria in African children. N Engl J Med 1995;332:1399.
White NJ: The Treatment of malaria. N Engl J Med 1996;335:800.

BABESIOSIS

Babesia microti is a malaria-like protozoan that infects and lyses erythrocytes of wild and domestic animals in North America and Europe. In the United States, human babesiosis has been reported in the coastal areas of Massachusetts, Rhode Island, and New York. Humans accidentally enter the cycle when bitten by *Ixodes scapularis,* one of the intermediate hosts and vectors of *B microti.* After inoculation,the protozoan penetrates the erythrocytes and starts an asynchronous cycle that causes hemolysis.

Clinical Findings

The incubation period is 1–3 weeks but may extend up to 6 weeks. However, many times the tick bite is unnoticed. Symptoms are nonspecific and include sustained or cyclic fever up to 40 °C, shaking chills, malaise, myalgias, headache, and dark urine. Hepatosplenomegaly is an uncommon finding. The disease is usually self-limited, but severe cases have been described in asplenic patients. Since *Babesia* and *Borrelia burgdorferi* share the same vector, *Ixodes dammini,* dual infection may occur.

Diagnosis

Microscopic evaluation of thin or thick blood smears reveals the intraerythrocytic organisms that resemble *P falciparum* ring forms. Specific serology is also available through the CDC and IgG titers ≥ 1:1024 are diagnostic of acute infection.

Treatment

A combination of clindamycin (20 mg/kg/d up to 600 mg every 6 hours) and quinine (25 mg/kg/d up to 650 mg every 6–8 hours) taken for 7–10 days is the treatment of choice. Other antimalarial drugs, including chloroquine, have been unsuccessful.

Benach JL et al: Clinical characteristics of human babesiosis. J Infect Dis 1981;144:481.
Clindamycin and quinine treatment for *Babesia microti* infections. MMWR Morb Mortal Wkly Rep 1993;32:65.

AMEBIASIS

Essentials of Diagnosis & Typical Features

- Acute dysentery: diarrhea with blood and mucus, pain, tenderness.
- Chronic nondysenteric diarrhea.
- Hepatic abscess.
- Lung abscess.
- Amebas or cysts in stools or abscesses; serologic evidence of amebic infection.

General Considerations

Amebiasis, caused by *Entamoeba histolytica,* is a common problem in areas with poor hygiene. An estimated 10% of the world's population is infected with *E histolytica* or *E dispar.* Amebiasis should be suspected in patients with a history of travel to or in contact with individuals from endemic areas who may be asymptomatic carriers. In the United States, amebiasis may be seen in homes for the retarded or handicapped, where poor hygiene fosters the spread of enteric pathogens. *E histolytica* has been found in the stools of as many as 30% of homosexual men. Individuals of any age may be infected. Transmission is usually fecal-oral, often from asymptomatic carriers who pass cysts. Trophozoites are killed by stomach acid and are not infectious. Infection with *E dispar,* which is morphologically identical with *E histolytica* but only results in asymptomatic carriage, is ten times more common than infection with *E histolytica.* Furthermore, only 10% of *E histolytica* infections result in gastrointestinal or other symptoms. However, an estimated 100,000 people die of amebic infection each year.

Clinical Findings

Intestinal amebiasis can present as asymptomatic cyst passage, acute amebic proctocolitis, chronic nondysenteric colitis, or ameboma. Since all *E dispar* infections and up to 90% of *E histolytica* infections are asymptomatic, carriage is the most common presentation of amebiasis. Patients with acute amebic colitis typically have a 1- to 2-week history of watery stools containing blood and mucus, abdominal pain, and tenesmus. A minority of patients are febrile or dehydrated. Abdominal examination may reveal pain over the lower abdominal quadrants. Fulminant colitis is an unusual complication of amebic dysentery and is associated with a grave prognosis (more than 50% mortality). Patients with fulminant colitis present with severe bloody diarrhea, fever and diffuse abdominal pain. Children under the age of 2 years appear to be at increased risk for this condition. Chronic amebic colitis is clinically indistinguishable from idiopathic inflammatory bowel disease; patients present with recurrent episodes of bloody diarrhea over a period of years. Ameboma is a localized amebic infection, usually in the cecum or ascending colon, which presents as a painful abdominal mass.

The most common complication of intestinal amebiasis is intestinal perforation and peritonitis. Perianal ulcers, a less common complication, are painful, punched-out lesions that usually respond to medical therapy. Infrequently, colonic strictures may develop following colitis.

Extraintestinal amebiasis includes liver, lung, and cerebral abscesses and, rarely, genitourinary disease. Patients with amebic liver abscess, the most common form of extraintestinal amebiasis, have fever and right upper quadrant tenderness of less than 10 days' duration. The pain may be dull or pleuritic or referred to the right shoulder. Physical examination reveals liver enlargement in less than 50% of affected patients. A subset of patients has a subacute presentation of 2 weeks' to 6 months' duration. In these patients, hepatomegaly, anemia and weight loss are common findings, and fever is less common. Jaundice and diarrhea are rarely associated with an amebic liver abscess.

The most common complication of amebic liver abscess is pleuropulmonary amebiasis due to rupture of a right liver lobe. Lung abscesses may occur from hematogenous spread. Cough, dyspnea, and pleuritic pain can also be caused by the serous pleural effusions and atelectasis that frequently accompany amebic liver abscesses. Rupture of hepatic abscesses can lead to peritonitis and more rarely to pericarditis. Cerebral amebiasis is an infrequent manifestation. Genitourinary amebiasis is also uncommon and results from rupture of a liver abscess, hematogenous dissemination, or lymphatic spread.

Diagnosis

Intestinal amebiasis is diagnosed by observing the parasite on stool examination or mucosal biopsy. The differential diagnosis of acute amebic colitis includes bacillary diarrhea, *Balantidium coli,* and *Dientamoeba fragilis* infection. Chronic amebic colitis has to be distinguished from inflammatory bowel disease, *Cyclospora,* and *B coli.* Occult blood is present in virtually all cases of amebic colitis and can be used as an inexpensive screening test. Fecal leukocytes are uncommon in amebic dysentery. The presence of hematophagous trophozoites in feces indicates pathogenic *E histolytica* infection.

Ideally, a wet mount of the stool should be examined no longer than 20 minutes after collection to detect motile trophozoites. Otherwise, specimens should be fixed with polyvinyl alcohol or refrigerated to avoid disintegration of the trophozoites. Three separate stool examinations have 90% sensitivity for the diagnosis of amebic dysentery. However, infection of the ascending colon, amebomas, and extraintestinal infections frequently yield negative stool examinations. An antigen detection test, currently under clinical evaluation, may be sensitive and more specific, because it detects *E histolytica*-specific antigens that do not cross-react with *E dispar.*

Colonoscopy and biopsy are most helpful in stool-negative amebic colitis. Barium studies are contraindicated for patients with acute amebic colitis because of the risk of perforation.

The presence of antibodies against *E histolytica* can differentiate *E histolytica* from *E dispar* infections. The antibody response follows both intestinal and extraintestinal invasive amebiasis and can be used for diagnostic purposes. ELISA and indirect hemagglutination assays are positive in 85–95% of invasive *E histolytica* colitis or amebic abscess. However, these antibodies persist for years, and a positive result does not distinguish between acute or past infection. Noninvasive imaging studies have greatly improved the diagnosis of hepatic abscesses. Ultrasonographic examination and computed tomography (CT) are sensitive techniques and can guide fine-needle aspiration to obtain specimens for the definitive diagnosis. Because an amebic abscess may take up to 2 years to completely resolve on CT scans, imaging techniques are not recommended for therapeutic evaluation.

Treatment & Prevention

Treatment of amebic infection is complex because different agents are required for eradicating the parasite from the bowel or from tissue (Table 37–7). Whether treatment of asymptomatic cyst passers is indicated at all is a controversial issue. Currently, the prevalent opinion among experts is that asymptomatic infection with *E histolytica,* as evidenced by the presence of amebic cysts in the stool and a positive serologic test, should be treated in nonendemic

Table 37–7. Treatment of amebiasis.

Type of Infection	Drug of Choice	Dosage
Asymptomatic	Iodoquinol	30–40 mg/kg/d up to 2 g/d in three doses for 20 days
	or	
	Paromomycin	25–35 mg/kg/d in three doses for 7 days
	or	
	Diloxanide furoate[1]	20 mg/kg/d up to 1.5 g/d in three doses for 10 days
Intestinal disease and hepatic abscess[2]	Metronidazole **or** Tinidazole[3]	35–50 mg/kg/d up to 2.25 g/d in three doses for 10 days 50 or 60 mg/kg up to 2 g/d for 3 days

[1]Diloxanide furoate is available from the CDC Drug Service, 404-639-3670.
[2]Treatment should be followed by iodoquinol or other intraluminal cysticidal agent.
[3]Not marketed in the United States; higher dosage is for hepatic abscess.

areas. If serology is negative, the cysts are more likely to represent infection with the nonpathogenic *E dispar,* which does not require treatment. Among the drugs active against intraluminal cysts, iodoquinol is the most readily available, but also the most toxic (causes prominent gastrointestinal side effects, interferes with thyroid function, causes dose-dependent optic neuritis). Paromomycin, a nonabsorbable aminoglycoside, can be safely used during pregnancy and has only mild intestinal side effects including flatulence and increased number of stools. Diloxanide furoate is relatively nontoxic and widely used outside of the United States. The treatment of invasive amebiasis requires metronidazole. Metronidazole has a disulfiram-like effect and should be avoided in patients receiving ethanol-containing medications. Tinidazole, a more potent nitro-imidazole against amebic infection can be used for shorter treatment courses and is well tolerated in children.

In patients who cannot tolerate metronidazole or tinidazole, erythromycin and tetracycline are active against intestinal trophozoites, but are inactive against trophozoites in liver abscesses. Conversely, chloroquine is active only against hepatic amebiasis. Treatment of invasive amebiasis should always be followed with an intraluminal cysticidal agent, even if the stool examination is negative. Patients with large, thin-walled hepatic abscesses may need therapeutic aspiration to avoid abscess rupture. Patients with amebiasis should be placed under enteric precautions. Travelers to endemic areas need to follow the same precautions that apply to prevention of enteric infections—drink bottled or boiled water and eat cooked or peeled vegetables and fruits.

Merritt RJ et al: Spectrum of amebiasis in children. Am J Dis Child 1982;136:785.
Ravdin JI: Amebiasis. Clin Infect Dis 1995;20:1453.

FREE-LIVING AMEBAS

Essentials of Diagnosis & Typical Features

- Acute meningoencephalitis: fever, headache, meningismus, acute mental deterioration.
- Swimming in warm, fresh water in endemic areas.
- Chronic granulomatous encephalitis: insidious onset of focal neurologic deficits.
- Keratitis: pain, photophobia, conjunctivitis, blurred vision.

General Considerations

Infection with free-living amebas is uncommon. *Naegleria* species, *Acanthamoeba* species, and *Balamuthia* (leptomyxid) amebas have been associated with human disease.

Acute meningoencephalitis, caused by *N fowleri,* has been observed, especially in children and young adults. Patients present with abrupt fever, headache, nausea and vomiting, meningismus, and decreased mental status usually 3–5 days after swimming in warm freshwater lakes. Swimming history may be absent. Central nervous system invasion occurs after nasal inoculation of *N fowleri.* The disease is rapidly progressive, and death ensues within 1 week of onset of symptoms.

Chronic granulomatous encephalitis, caused by *Acanthamoeba* or leptomyxid amebas, occurs most commonly in patients who are immunocompromised from corticosteroids, chemotherapy, or AIDS. There is no association with fresh water swimming. This disease has an insidious onset of focal neurologic deficits, and approximately 50% of patients present with headache. Skin, sinus, or lung infections with *Acanthamoeba* precede many of the central nervous system infections and may still be present at the onset of neurologic disease. The granulomatous encephalitis progresses to fatal outcome over a period of weeks to months (average 6 weeks).

Acanthamoeba keratitis is a corneal infection associated with minor trauma or use of soft contact lenses in otherwise healthy persons. Frequently misdiagnosed as herpes simplex or bacterial keratitis, *Acanthamoeba* keratitis has a characteristic dendriform epithelial pattern that suggests the diagnosis.

Diagnosis

Amebic encephalitis should be included in the differential diagnosis of acute meningoencephalitis in children with a history of recent fresh water swimming. The cerebrospinal fluid is usually hemorrhagic, with leukocyte counts that may be normal early in the disease but later range from 400 to 2600/μL with neutrophil predominance, low to normal glucose, and elevated protein. The etiologic diagnosis relies on finding trophozoites on a wet mount of the cerebrospinal fluid.

Granulomatous encephalitis is diagnosed by brain biopsy of CT-identified nonenhancing lucent areas. The cerebrospinal fluid of these patients is usually nondiagnostic with intermediate blood cell counts, elevated protein, and decreased glucose. *Acanthamoeba* or leptomyxid amebas have not been found in the cerebrospinal fluid; however, they can be visualized in biopsies or grown from brain or other infected tissues.

Acanthamoeba keratitis is diagnosed by finding the trophozoites in corneal scrapings or by isolating the parasite from corneal specimens or contact lens cultures.

Treatment & Prevention

The few patients who have survived acute amebic meningoencephalitis received high-dose intravenous and intrathecal amphotericin B, accompanied by miconazole, rifampin, and sulfisoxazole in some cases.

Little is known about the therapeutic response of

granulomatous encephalitis because most cases have been diagnosed at autopsy. In vitro, *Acanthamoeba* is most sensitive to diamidine derivatives (pentamidine) followed by the azoles (miconazole, ketoconazole), paromomycin, neomycin, flucytosine, and amphotericin B. Leptomyxid amebas are particularly sensitive to ketoconazole. Whenever an isolate is obtained, it is advisable to test for antimicrobial susceptibility.

Acanthamoeba keratitis responds well to surgical debridement followed by 3–4 weeks of topical 1% miconazole, 0.1% propamidine isethionate, and Neosporin.

Because primary amebic meningitis occurs infrequently, active surveillance of lakes for *N fowleri* is not warranted. However, in the presence of a documented case, it is advisable to close the implicated lake to swimming. *Acanthamoeba* keratitis can be prevented by heat disinfection of contact lenses, by storage of lenses in sterile solutions, and by not wearing lenses when swimming in fresh water.

Sotelo-Avila C: *Naegleria* and *Acanthamoeba*. Free living amebas pathogenic for man. Perspect Pediatr Pathol 1987;10:51.

Visvesvara GS et al: Leptomyxid ameba, a new agent of amebic meningoencephalitis in humans and animals. J Clin Microbiol 1990;28:2750.

BALANTIDIASIS

Balantidium coli rarely produces human disease. Patients with achlorhydria, poor nutritional status, or poor hygiene are at increased risk of developing invasion of the colonic mucosa with this organism. Patients typically present with chronic intermittent watery diarrhea or with acute colitis with blood and mucus. Complications include intestinal perforation and more rarely extraintestinal spread of *B coli* to mesenteric lymph nodes, liver, or pleura. The diagnosis is made by the finding of large, motile trophozoites in fresh stool or in scrapings taken from the periphery of ulcers on endoscopic examination. Cysts in stool is a less common finding. Tetracycline is the treatment of choice: 40 mg/kg/d up to 2 g/d in four divided doses for 10 days. For children less than 8 years of age, iodoquinol for 20 days or metronidazole for 10 days are acceptable alternatives.

Ladas SD et al: Invasive balantidiasis presented as chronic colitis and lung involvement. Dig Dis Sci 1989;34:1621.

DIENTAMOEBA FRAGILIS INFECTION

The pathogenicity of *Dientamoeba fragilis* is controversial. Purported symptoms include abdominal pain, diarrhea, nausea, anorexia, vomiting, and fatigue. Iodoquinol for 20 days has been used with suc-

cess. Paromomycin and tetracycline (10 days) are alternative drugs.

Spencer MJ, Garcia LS, Chapin MR: *Dientamoeba fragilis:* An intestinal pathogen in children? Am J Dis Child 1979;133:390.

Turner JA: Giardiasis and infections with *Dientamoeba fragilis*. Pediatr Clin North Am 1985;32:865.

GIARDIASIS

Essentials of Diagnosis & Typical Features

- Chronic relapsing diarrhea, flatulence, bloating, anorexia, poor weight gain.
- Absence of fever and hematochezia.
- Detection of trophozoites, cysts, or *Giardia* antigens in stool.

General Considerations

Giardiasis is the most common intestinal protozoal infection in children in the United States and in most areas around the world. It is caused by *Giardia lamblia*. Endemic worldwide, it is classically associated with drinking contaminated water, either in rural areas or in areas with faulty purification systems. Acquisition in swimming pools has occurred. Because even ostensibly clean urban water supplies can be intermittently contaminated, giardiasis can be acquired by almost any traveler. Fecal-oral contamination allows person-to-person spread. Recently, day care centers have been recognized as major sources, with an incidence of up to 50% reported in some centers. Asymptomatic infections occur in 25% of infected persons and facilitate spread to household contacts. Food-borne outbreaks have also occurred. Although infection is rare in neonates, it may occur at any age.

Clinical Findings

A. Symptoms and Signs: *Giardia* infection is followed by asymptomatic cyst passage, acute self-limited diarrhea, and a chronic syndrome of diarrhea, malabsorption, and weight loss. Acute diarrhea occurs 1–2 weeks after infection and is characterized by abrupt onset of diarrhea with greasy, malodorous stools; malaise; flatulence; bloating; and nausea. Fever and vomiting occur in a minority of patients. Urticaria, reactive arthritis, biliary tract disease, gastric infection, and constipation have occasionally been reported. The disease has a protracted course (more than 1 week) and frequently leads to weight loss. Patients who develop chronic diarrhea complain of profound malaise, lassitude, headache, and diffuse abdominal pain in association with bouts of diarrhea—most typically foul-smelling, greasy stools—intercalated with periods of constipation or normal bowel habits. This syndrome can persist for months until specific therapy is administered or until it spontaneously subsides. Chronic diarrhea frequently leads to malabsorption, steatorrhea, vitamin A and vitamin B_{12} deficiencies, and disaccharidase depletion. Lactose intolerance, which develops in 20–40% of patients, can persist for several weeks after treatment and needs to be differentiated from relapsing giardiasis or reinfection.

B. Laboratory Findings: The diagnosis of giardiasis relies on finding the parasite in stool or duodenal aspirates or detecting *Giardia* antigen in feces. For ova and parasite examination, a fresh stool provides the best examination results. Liquid stools have the highest yield of trophozoites. These are more readily found on wet mounts of fresh specimens. With semiformed stools, the examiner should look for cysts in fresh or fixed specimens, preferably using a concentration technique. When these techniques are carefully applied, one ova and parasite examination has a 50–70% sensitivity; three examinations increase the sensitivity to 90%. Antigen assays detect *Giardia* by means of immunofluorescence or enzyme-linked immunoassay. They are comparable in cost to a stool ova and parasite examination and are 85–90% sensitive and 95–100% specific. The antigen detection assays are limited to ruling in or ruling out giardiasis and are best applied for mass screening or testing patients after completion of therapy. With a careful stool ova and parasite examination or with the use of a new antigen test, direct sampling of the duodenal contents should be restricted to particularly difficult cases. Three methods are currently available: the string test (Entero-Test), duodenal aspiration, and duodenal biopsy.

Treatment & Prevention

The drug of choice for giardiasis is metronidazole. When given at 5 mg/kg (up to 250 mg) three times daily for 5 days, metronidazole has an efficacy of 80–95%. The drug is well tolerated in children. It has a disulfiram-like effect and should be avoided in patients receiving ethanol-containing medication. Furazolidone is frequently used in children as an alternative drug because it is available in suspension. Administered at 1.5 mg/kg (up to 100 mg) four times daily for 7–10 days, it has only 80% efficacy. Furazolidone may cause gastrointestinal side effects, turn urine red, and cause mild hemolysis in patients with G6PD deficiency. For pregnant women with giardiasis, paromomycin, a nonabsorbable aminoglycoside, constitutes a safe but only marginally effective alternative (efficacy 60–70%). For patients who fail one drug or suffer relapse, a second course with the same drug or switching to another drug is equally effective.

The prevention of giardiasis requires proper treatment of the water supply and interruption of person-to-person transmission. For travelers to developing countries or in wilderness areas, it is recommended to halogenate or boil (for over 10 minutes) the drink-ing water and avoid uncooked foods that might have been washed with contaminated water. Sexual transmission is prevented by avoiding oral-anal and oral-genital sex. Interrupting fecal-oral transmission requires strict hand washing. However, outbreaks of diarrhea in day care centers might be particularly difficult to eradicate, and reinforcing hand washing and treating both symptomatic and asymptomatic carriers may be necessary.

Addiss DG, Juranek DD, Spencer HC: Treatment of children with asymptomatic and non-diarrheal *Giardia* infection. Pediatr Infect Dis J 1991;10:843.
Babb RR: Giardiasis: Taming this pervasive parasitic infection. Postgrad Med 1995;98:155.
Thompson SC: *Giardia lamblia* in children and the child care setting: A review of the literature. J Paediatr Child Health 1994;30:202.
Wolf MS: Giardiasis. Clin Microbiol Rev 1992;5:93.

CRYPTOSPORIDIOSIS

Cryptosporidium parvum is an intracellular protozoan that has gained importance because it causes severe diarrhea in patients with AIDS and in other immunodeficient persons. The parasite is ubiquitous and infects and reproduces itself in the epithelial cell lining of the digestive and respiratory tracts of humans and most other vertebrate animals. Humans acquire the infection from contaminated water supplies or from close contact with infected humans or animals.

Clinical Findings

A. Symptoms and Signs: Immunocompetent persons infected with *Cryptosporidium* usually develop self-limited diarrhea (2–26 days' duration) with or without abdominal cramps. Diarrhea is intermittent and scant, or continuous, watery, and voluminous. Low-grade fever, nausea, vomiting, loss of appetite, and malaise may accompany the diarrhea. Other clinical manifestations associated with cryptosporidiosis include cholecystitis, pancreatitis, hepatitis, and respiratory symptoms. Young children (younger than 2 years of age) appear more susceptible to infection. Immunocompromised patients (either cellular or humoral deficiency) tend to develop prolonged disease, which usually subsides only after correcting the immunodeficiency.

B. Laboratory Findings: There are no characteristic laboratory features of cryptosporidiosis other than identification of the microorganism in feces or on biopsy. Examination of multiple stool specimens by at least two techniques (concentration and staining) may be necessary.

Treatment & Prevention

There is currently no reliable treatment for cryptosporidiosis. Immunocompetent patients and those with temporary immunodeficiencies do not require specific therapy but may benefit from antidiarrheal agents and hydration. Immunocompromised patients usually require more intense supportive care with parenteral nutrition in addition to hydration and nonspecific antidiarrheal agents. Octreotide acetate, a synthetic analogue of somatostatin that inhibits secretory diarrhea has been associated with symptomatic improvement, but not with parasitologic cure. Among the antiparasitic agents, paromomycin, azithromycin, nitazoxanide (an antiparasitic drug available from Unimed on a compassionate use basis), and hyperimmune bovine colostrum have been successfully used in some patients. In patients with AIDS, institution of effective antiretroviral therapy seems to have a positive impact on the outcome of cryptosporidiosis. Prevention of *Cryptosporidium* infection is limited by oocyst resistance to some of the standard water purification procedures and to common disinfectants. Enteric precautions are recommended for infected persons. Boiled or bottled drinking water may be considered for those at high risk for developing chronic infection (eg, patients with AIDS whose CD4 cells are less than 200/μL).

Current WL, Garcia LS: Cryptosporidiosis. Clin Microbiol Rev 1991;4:325.
Fraser D: Epidemiology of *Giardia lamblia* and *Cryptosporidium* infection in childhood. Isr J Med Sci 1994;30:356.
Goldstein ST et al: Cryptosporidiosis: An outbreak associated with drinking water despite state-of-the-art water treatment. Ann Intern Med 1996;124: 459.

CYCLOSPORIASIS

Cyclospora is a coccidian with worldwide distribution that infects both human and animals. It has recently caused several food-associated outbreaks, characterized by an incubation period of 2–11 days followed by watery diarrhea in relapsing patterns, sometimes alternating with constipation. Other symptoms include profound fatigue, vomiting, and myalgias. Although the illness is self-limited, it may last for several weeks. Diagnosis is based on finding oocysts 8–10 μm in diameter on examination of stool specimens stained with acid-fast stain. The drug of choice for treatment is trimethoprim-sulfamethoxazole for 7 days.

Outbreaks of cyclosporiasis—United States and Canada, 1997. MMWR Morb Mortal Wkly Rep 1997;46:521.
Soave R: *Cyclospora:* An overview. Clin Infect Dis 1996;23:429.

TRICHOMONIASIS

Trichomonas vaginalis resides in the genitourinary tract as an extracellular protozoan. It can damage the underlying epithelial cells through direct contact, leading to ulcerations. Because it is sexually transmitted, *Trichomonas* is commonly associated with other venereal diseases. Thus, patients found to harbor *Trichomonas* should be screened for syphilis (in areas of high endemicity), *N gonorrhoeae, C trachomatis,* hepatitis B virus, and HIV, which may be clinically silent. Newborn females can acquire trichomoniasis at birth. Thereafter, trichomoniasis is rare until menarche. Although finding *Trichomonas* in a prepubertal child suggests sexual abuse, it cannot be used as definite proof because nonsexual transmission of the protozoan has been documented. The clinical features of vaginal trichomoniasis and its management are discussed in Chapter 38.

Graves A, Gardner WA Jr: Pathogenicity of *Trichomonas vaginalis.* Clin Obstet Gynecol 1993;36:145.
Lossick JG: Treatment of sexually transmitted vaginosis/vaginitis. Rev Infect Dis 1990;12:S665.

TOXOPLASMOSIS

Essentials of Diagnosis & Typical Features

- Congenital toxoplasmosis: chorioretinitis, icterus, hepatosplenomegaly, abnormal blood count, microcephaly, hydrocephaly, convulsions, psychomotor retardation, abnormal cerebrospinal fluid, intracranial calcifications, microphthalmia, strabismus.
- Acquired toxoplasmosis in an immunocompetent host: lymphadenopathy sometimes accompanied by fever, hepatosplenomegaly, rash, and myalgias.
- Acquired or reactivated toxoplasmosis in an immunocompromised host: encephalitis, chorioretinitis, myocarditis, and pneumonitis.
- Ocular toxoplasmosis: chorioretinitis.
- Serologic evidence of infection with *Toxoplasma gondii* or demonstration of the agent in tissue or body fluids.

General Considerations

Toxoplasma gondii is a worldwide parasite of animals and birds. Felines, the definitive hosts, excrete oocysts in their feces. Ingested mature oocysts or tissue cysts lead to tachyzoite invasion of the intestinal cells. Intracellular replication of the tachyzoites determine cell lysis and spread of the infection to adjacent cells or to other tissues via the bloodstream. Extracellular tachyzoites are lysed by complement fixing antibodies and interferon-g-activated macrophages. In chronic infection, *T gondii* appears as bradyzoite-containing tissue cysts that do not trigger an inflammatory reaction. Under special circumstances such as immunodepression, tachyzoites are released from the cysts and begin a new cycle of infection. Interferon-g and other cytokines seem to be important in keeping the chronic infection quiescent.

The two major routes of *Toxoplasma* transmission to humans are oral (including pica) and congenital. Oocysts survive for up to 18 months in moist soil. Oral infection occurs after ingestion of cyst-containing undercooked meat or other food products. Oocyst survival is limited in dry, very cold, or very hot conditions, and at high altitude, which probably accounts for the lower incidence of toxoplasmosis in these climatic regions. In the United States, less than 1% of cattle and 25% of sheep and pigs are infected with toxoplasmosis. In humans in different geographic areas, seropositivity increases with age from nil–10% in children under 10 years of age to 3–70% in adults. Congenital transmission occurs during acute infection of the pregnant woman; this occurs in 0.2–1% of all pregnancies in the United States. Rarely, fetal infection has been documented in immunocompromised mothers with chronic toxoplasmosis. The rate of vertical transmission in untreated patients increases from 10% in the first trimester to 60% in the third. Symptomatic disease, however, is more likely to follow infection in early gestation (20–25%) compared with late gestation (less than 11%). Treatment during pregnancy decreases transmission by about 60%.

Clinical Findings

A. Congenital Toxoplasmosis: Congenital toxoplasmosis has a wide variety of manifestations, including miscarriage, prematurity, and stillbirth. Most frequently, symptomatic infants present with a combination of fever, microcephaly or hydrocephaly, hepatosplenomegaly, jaundice, chorioretinitis, convulsions, abnormal cerebrospinal fluid (xanthochromia and mononuclear pleocytosis), and cerebral calcifications. Other findings include strabismus, palsy, maculopapular rash, pneumonitis, myocarditis thrombocytopenia, lymphocytosis, monocytosis, and a erythroblastosis-like syndrome. The overall mortality rate for congenital toxoplasmosis is approximately 10% and is higher in neonates who are asymptomatic at birth. Congenital toxoplasmosis must be differentiated from cytomegalovirus infection, rubella, herpes simplex, syphilis, Lyme disease, listeriosis, erythroblastosis, and the encephalopathies that accompany degenerative diseases.

B. Acquired *Toxoplasma* Infection in the Immunocompetent Host: Only 10–20% of acute *Toxoplasma* infections produce symptoms, and patients usually present with lymphadenopathy without fever. The nodes are discrete, may or may not be tender, and do no suppurate. Cervical lymph nodes are most frequently involved, but any nodes may be enlarged. Less common findings include fever, malaise, myalgias, fatigue, hepatosplenomegaly, atypical lymphocytes (usually less than 10%), and liver enzyme elevations. Unilateral chorioretinitis may occur. The disease is self-limited, although lymph node enlargement may persist or may wax and wane for a few months to 1 year or even longer. Rarely, an apparently healthy child may develop severe disseminated disease with myocarditis, pneumonitis, or encephalitis.

Toxoplasmic lymphadenitis must be distinguished from other causes of infectious mononucleosis-like syndromes (less than 1% are caused by *Toxoplasma*), particularly Epstein-Barr virus and cytomegalovirus, cat-scratch disease, tuberculosis, tularemia, and lymphoma.

C. Acute Toxoplasmosis in the Immunodeficient Host: Immunocompromised hosts tend to develop severe disease following acute infection or reactivation. Children born to HIV- and *Toxoplasma*-infected mothers may acquire both pathogens in utero. Most of these patients who acquire toxoplasmosis after birth develop encephalitis, chorioretinitis, and pneumonia. Patients with lymphoma, leukemia, or transplantation are at high risk for acquiring *Toxoplasma* encephalitis, myocarditis, and pneumonitis.

D. Ocular Toxoplasmosis: In active congenital toxoplasmosis, chorioretinitis is usually bilateral and shows acute inflammatory foci on funduscopic examination. This generally resolves, leaving depigmented scars of the retina surrounded by areas of hyperpigmentation. Chorioretinitis may reactivate in a single eye later in life. The appearance of the ocular lesion is not specific and mimics other granulomatous ocular diseases.

Diagnosis

Active infection is diagnosed by isolation of *T gondii* from blood or body fluids; demonstration of tachyzoites in histologic sections or cytology preparations; demonstration of cysts in placenta or fetal tissues; characteristic lymph node histology; and demonstration of specific serologic test results. Serology is most commonly used. IgG antibodies are reliably measured by the Sabin-Feldman dye test, immunofluorescence, ELISA, and particle agglutination. Using these tests, IgG anti-*Toxoplasma* is first detected 1–2 weeks after infection, peaks at 1–2 months, and, after decreasing at variable speed, persists for life. IgM antibodies are reliably measured by ELISA or particle agglutination. These antibodies appear earlier and decline faster than IgG antibodies. Absence of both serum IgG and IgM virtually rules out the diagnosis of toxoplasmosis. Acute toxoplasmosis in an immunocompetent host is best documented by analyzing IgG and IgM in paired blood samples drawn 3 weeks apart. Since high antibody titers (IgM or IgG) can persist for several months after acute infection, a single high-titer determination is nonspecific. However, seroconversion or a fourfold increase in titer confirms the diagnosis.

In the immunocompromised host, serology is not sensitive, and active infection should be documented by polymerase chain reaction (PCR) or local anti-body production in body fluids or by demonstration of tachyzoites.

Patients with *Toxoplasma* chorioretinitis typically have low levels of specific IgG and absent IgM. The diagnosis can be confirmed by demonstrating high antibody titers in aqueous fluid.

Congenital neonatal infection is documented by detecting anti-*Toxoplasma* IgM or IgA in the blood. Prenatal diagnosis of congenital infection requires a combination of ultrasonography (to detect ventricle enlargement), PCR in amniotic fluid, and serology in cord blood. Recent studies indicate that sampling the cord blood might be unnecessary by virtue of the high PCR sensitivity.

Differential Diagnosis

Congenital infection may resemble that due to cytomegalovirus, syphilis, rubella, or other agents. Acquired infection mimics a number of viral or lymphoproliferative diseases.

Prevention

Pregnant women and immunocompromised patients should wash hands thoroughly after handling raw meat. Cook meat to 66 °C or greater, wash fruits and vegetables before consumption, and avoid contact with cat feces. Serologic screening of pregnant women is warranted in areas of high prevalence. A first test should be performed by 10–12 weeks of pregnancy. Seronegative patients should be retested at 20–22 weeks and near term. Seroconverters require specific therapy.

Treatment

Although therapy does not alter established central nervous system damage, it does markedly decrease late sequelae. A year of treatment is recommended for all congenitally infected infants; symptomatic patients receive 6 months of pyrimethamine and sulfadiazine, followed by alternating spiramycin and pyrimethamine-sulfadiazine monthly for the next 6 months. Subclinical infection is treated with pyrimethamine and sulfadiazine for 6 weeks, followed by alternating spiramycin for 6 weeks with pyrimethamine-sulfadiazine for 4 weeks.

Pyrimethamine is given orally at a dosage of 1 mg/kg/d (maximum 25 mg); gastrointestinal upset, leukopenia, thrombocytopenia, and, rarely, agranulocytosis are side effects. Frequent blood counts should be performed and the drug stopped if the counts fall very low. Leucovorin calcium (folinic acid), 5 mg intramuscularly every 3 days, decreases the myelotoxicity. The dosage of sulfadiazine or trisulfapyrimidines is 40–45 mg/kg twice a day orally (maximum 8 g/d). Clindamycin can be substituted for sulfadiazine in patients who cannot tolerate sulfonamides. Spiramycin and trimethoprim-sulfamethoxazole are less active.

In acquired infection, usually self-limited, the po-tentially toxic therapy should be prescribed with discretion, only if the illness is complicated.

In chorioretinitis, antimicrobial therapy is used for 4 weeks. A course of corticosteroids (prednisone, 1.5 mg/kg up to 75 mg) is recommended when lesions involve the macula or the optic nerve. Lesions tend to improve after 10 days of therapy.

In pregnancy, spiramycin should be started immediately. Pyrimethamine plus sulfadiazine, alternating every 3 weeks with spiramycin, are used when fetal infection has been documented, because, although they are toxic, only the first two drugs ameliorate severity of the disease in the infected fetus.

Freij BG, Sever HL: Toxoplasmosis. Pediatr Rev 1991; 12:227.

McAuley J et al: Early and longitudinal evaluations of treated infants and children and untreated historical patients with congenital toxoplasmosis: The Chicago collaborative treatment trial. Clin Infect Dis 1994;18:38.

McCabe RE et al: Clinical spectrum in 107 cases of toxoplasmic lymphadenopathy. Rev Infect Dis 1987;9:754.

Wong SY, Remington JS: Toxoplasmosis in pregnancy. Clin Infect Dis 1994;18:853.

METAZOAL INFECTIONS

NEMATODE INFECTIONS

1. ENTEROBIASIS (Pinworms)

Essentials of Diagnosis & Typical Features
- Nocturnal anal pruritus.
- Worms in the stool or eggs on perianal skin.

General Considerations

This worldwide infection is caused by *Enterobius vermicularis*. The adult worms are about 5–10 mm long and live in the colon; females deposit eggs on the perianal area, primarily at night, causing intense pruritus. Scratching contaminates the fingers and allows transmission back to the host (autoinfection) or to contacts.

Clinical Findings

A. Symptoms and Signs: Although blamed for a myriad of symptoms, pinworms are definitely associated only with localized pruritus. Adult worms may migrate within the colon or up the urethra or vagina in girls. They can be found within the bowel wall, in the lumen of the appendix (usually an incidental finding by the pathologist), in the bladder, and even the peritoneal cavity of girls. The granulomatous reaction that may be present around these ectopic worms is usually asymptomatic. Worm eradication may correspond with the cure of recurrent urinary tract infections in some young girls.

B. Laboratory Findings: The usual diagnostic test consists of pressing a piece of transparent tape on the child's anus in the morning prior to bathing, then placing it on a drop of xylene on a slide. Microscopic examination under low power usually demonstrates the ova. Occasionally, eggs or adult worms are seen in fecal specimens. Parents may also notice adult worms.

Differential Diagnosis

Nonspecific irritation or vaginitis, streptococcal perianal cellulitis (usually painful), and vaginal or urinary bacterial infections may at times resemble pinworm infection, although the symptoms of pinworms are often so suggestive that a therapeutic trial is justified without a confirmed diagnosis.

Treatment

A. Specific Measures: Treat all household members at the same time to prevent reinfections. Since the drugs are not active against the eggs, therapy should be repeated after 2 weeks to kill the recently hatched adults.

1. Pyrantel pamoate–This drug is given as a single dose (11 mg/kg, maximum 1 g); it is safe and very effective.

2. Mebendazole, albendazole–These drugs are also highly effective for this infection as well as for other helminthiases. A single oral dose of 100 mg mebendazole or 400 mg albendazole is used for all ages.

B. General Measures: Personal hygiene must be emphasized. Nails should be kept short and clean. Children should wear undergarments to bed to diminish contamination of fingers; bedclothes should be laundered frequently. Although eggs may be widely dispersed in the house and multiple family members infected, the disease is mild and treatable. Avoid creating "pinworm psychosis" in the parents.

Tornieporth NG et al: Ectopic enterobiasis: A case report and review. J Infect 1992;24:87.

2. ASCARIASIS

Essentials of Diagnosis & Typical Features

- Abdominal cramps and discomfort.
- Large, white or reddish, round worms or ova in the feces.

General Considerations

Ascaris lumbricoides is a worldwide human parasite. Ova passed by carriers may remain viable for months under the proper soil conditions. The ova contaminate food or fingers and are subsequently ingested by a new host. The larvae hatch, penetrate the intestinal wall, enter the venous system, reach the alveoli, are coughed up, and return to the small intestine, where they mature. The female lays thousands of eggs daily.

Clinical Findings

A. Symptoms and Signs: Infections usually remain asymptomatic; severe cases, however, can be associated with pain, weight loss, anorexia, diarrhea, or vomiting. Adult worms may be seen in feces or vomitus. Rarely, they perforate or obstruct the small bowel, biliary system, or appendix.

Large numbers of larvae migrating through the lungs may cause an acute, transient eosinophilic pneumonia (Löffler's syndrome). Otitis media has been occasionally reported.

B. Laboratory Findings: The diagnosis is made by observing the large round worms in the stool or by microscopic detection of the ova.

Treatment

Because the adult worms live less than a year, asymptomatic infection need not be treated. Mebendazole (100 mg twice daily for 3 days), pyrantel pamoate (a single dose of 11 mg/kg, maximum 1 g), and albendazole (400 mg in a single dose) are highly and equally effective. In cases of intestinal or biliary obstruction, piperazine (150 mg/kg initially, followed by six doses of 65 mg/kg every 12 hours by nasogastric tube) is recommended because it narcotizes the worms and helps relieve obstruction. However, surgical removal is occasionally required.

Bratton RL, Nesse RE: Ascariasis: An infection to watch in immigrants. Postgrad Med 1993;1:171.

3. TRICHURIASIS (Whipworm)

Trichuris trichiura is a widespread human and animal parasite common in poor children living in warm, humid areas conducive to survival of the ova. The adult worms live in the cecum and colon; the ova are passed and become infectious after several weeks in the soil. Ingested infective eggs hatch in the upper small intestine. Unlike *Ascaris, Trichuris* does not have a migratory tissue phase. No symptoms are usually present unless the infection is severe, in which case it can cause pain, diarrhea, and mild abdominal distention. Massive infections may also cause rectal prolapse and dysentery. Detecting the characteristic barrel-shaped ova in the feces makes the diagnosis. Adult worms may be seen in the prolapsed rectum or at proctoscopy; their thin heads are buried in the mucosa, and the thicker posterior portions extrude. Mild to moderate eosinophilia may be present.

Mebendazole (100 mg orally twice daily for 3 days) or albendazole (400 mg in a single dose) improve gastrointestinal symptoms as well as constitutional effects.

Nokes C et al: Parasitic helminth infection and cognitive function in school children. Proc R Soc Lond B Biol Sci 1992;247:77.

Robertson LJ et al: Trichuris trichiura and the growth of primary school children in Panama. Trans R Soc Trop Med Hyg 1992;86:656.

4. HOOKWORM

Essentials of Diagnosis & Typical Features
- Iron deficiency anemia.
- Hematochezia.
- Abdominal discomfort, weight loss.
- Ova in the feces.

General Considerations

The common human hookworms are *Ancylostoma duodenale* and *Necator americanus*. Both are widespread in the tropics and subtropics. The larger *Ancylostoma* is more pathogenic because it consumes more blood, up to 0.5 mL per worm per day.

The adults live in the jejunum. Eggs are passed in the feces and develop and hatch into infective larvae in warm, damp soil within 2 weeks. The larvae penetrate human skin on contact, enter the blood, reach the alveoli, are coughed up and swallowed, and develop into adults in the intestine. The adult worms attach with their mouth parts to the mucosa from which they suck blood. Blood loss is the major sequel of infection. Infection rates reach 90% in areas without sanitation.

A separate species, *Ancylostoma braziliense* (the dog or cat hookworm), causes creeping eruption (cutaneous larva migrans). This disease is seen mainly on the warm-water American coasts.

Clinical Findings

A. Symptoms and Signs: The larvae usually penetrate the skin of the feet and cause intense local itching ("ground itch"). This subsides as the larvae continue their migration. In creeping eruption, the nonhuman larvae migrate blindly in the skin before dying, creating serpiginous burrows. Löffler's syndrome may supervene during lung migration.

Mild intestinal infections produce no symptoms. Severe infections cause pain, iron deficiency anemia, and malnutrition. Occasionally, abdominal pain and diarrhea may be observed.

B. Laboratory Findings: The large ova of both species of hookworm are found in feces and are indis-

tinguishable. Microcytic anemia, hypoalbuminemia, eosinophilia, and hematochezia are seen in severe cases.

Prevention

Fecal contamination of soil should be prevented; skin contact with potentially contaminated soil should also be avoided.

Treatment

A. Specific Measures: Mebendazole (100 mg orally twice daily for 3 days) or pyrantel pamoate (11 mg/kg, maximum 1 g, daily for 3 days) are the drugs of choice. Topical thiabendazole and albendazole and oral thiabendazole are useful for creeping eruption.

B. General Measures: Iron therapy may be more important than worm eradication. Parenteral iron or transfusions may be needed in severe cases.

Prognosis

The outcome is usually excellent.

Hotez PJ: Hookworm disease in children. Pediatr Infect Dis J 1989;8:516.

5. STRONGYLOIDIASIS

Essentials of Diagnosis & Typical Features
- Abdominal pain, diarrhea.
- Eosinophilia.
- Larvae in stools and duodenal aspirates.
- Serum antibodies.

General Considerations

The responsible parasite, *Strongyloides stercoralis,* is unique in having both parasitic and free-living forms; the latter can survive in the soil for several generations. The parasite is found in most tropical and subtropical regions of the world. The adults live in the submucosal tissue of the duodenum and occasionally in the whole intestine. Eggs deposited in the mucosa hatch rapidly; the first-stage (rhabditiform) larvae, therefore, are the predominant form found in duodenal aspirates and feces. The larvae rapidly mature to the tissue-penetrating filariform stage and initiate internal autoinfection. The filariform larvae also inhabit the soil and can penetrate the skin of another host, subsequently migrating into veins and pulmonary alveoli and reaching the intestine when coughed up and swallowed.

Older children and adults are more often infected than young children. Even low worm burden can result in significant clinical symptoms. Infestations due to poor sanitation and hygiene in homes for the retarded are noteworthy. Immunosuppressed patients may develop fatal disseminated strongyloidiasis, known as the **hyperinfection syndrome.**

Clinical Findings

A. Symptoms and Signs: At the site of the skin penetration, there may be a pruritic rash. Large numbers of migrating larvae can cause wheezing, cough, and hemoptysis. Although one third of intestinal infections are asymptomatic, the most prominent features of strongyloidiasis include abdominal pain, distention, diarrhea, vomiting, and occasionally malabsorption.

Patients with cellular immunodeficiencies may develop disseminated infection involving the intestine, the lungs, and the meninges. Gram-negative sepsis may complicate disseminated strongyloidiasis.

B. Laboratory Findings: Finding larvae in the feces, in duodenal aspirates, or on a string test (Entero-Test) is diagnostic. IgG antibodies measured by ELISA or immunoblot are sensitive and specific for *Strongyloides* infection, but persist after successful therapy. Marked eosinophilia is common.

Differential Diagnosis

Strongyloidiasis should be differentiated from peptic disease, celiac disease, regional or tuberculous enteritis, hookworm infection, and other causes of intestinal symptoms or malabsorption. The pulmonary phase may mimic asthma or bronchopneumonia. Severe infection can present as an acute abdomen.

Treatment & Prevention

Thiabendazole (25 mg/kg orally twice daily for 2 days; maximum 3 g/d) and ivermectin (200 mg/kg/d for 1 or 2 days) are the drugs of choice. Relapses are common. In the hyperinfection syndrome, 2–3 weeks of therapy may be necessary. Patients from endemic areas should be tested for specific antibodies and treated before undergoing immunosuppression.

Mahmoud AAF: Strongyloidiasis. Clin Infect Dis 1996;23:949.

6. VISCERAL LARVA MIGRANS (Toxocariasis)

Essentials of Diagnosis & Typical Features

- Visceral involvement including hepatomegaly, marked eosinophilia, and anemia.
- Posterior or peripheral ocular inflammatory mass.
- Elevated antibody titers in serum or aqueous fluid; demonstration of *Toxocara* larvae on biopsy.

General Considerations

Visceral larva migrans is a worldwide disease. The agent is the cosmopolitan intestinal ascarid of dogs and cats, *Toxocara canis* or *Toxocara cati*. The eggs passed by infected animals contaminate parks and other areas that young children frequent. Children with pica are more at risk. In the United States,

seropositivity ranges from 2.8% in unselected populations to 23% in southern United States to 54% in rural areas. Ingested eggs hatch and penetrate the intestinal wall, then migrate to the liver, lungs, eyes, and other organs, where they die and incite a granulomatous inflammatory reaction.

Clinical Findings & Diagnosis

A. Visceral Larva Migrans: Toxocariasis is usually asymptomatic, but young children (1–5 years of age) sometimes present with anorexia, fever, fatigue, pallor, abdominal distention, abdominal pain, nausea, vomiting, and cough. Hepatomegaly is common, splenomegaly is unusual, and adenopathy is absent. Lung involvement, usually asymptomatic, can be readily demonstrated by radiologic examination. Seizures are common, but more severe neurologic abnormalities are infrequent. Eosinophilia with leukocytosis and anemia are typical laboratory findings. Most patients recover spontaneously, but disease may last up to 6 months.

B. Ocular Larva Migrans: This condition occurs in older children and adults who present with a unilateral posterior or peripheral inflammatory mass. Present or past history of viscera larva migrans and eosinophilia are typically absent. Anti-*Toxocara* antibody titers are low in the serum and high in vitreous and aqueous fluids.

Hypergammaglobulinemia and elevated isohemagglutinins sometimes occur in consequence to cross-reactivity between *Toxocara* antigens and human group A and B blood antigens. The diagnosis is confirmed by finding larvae in granulomatous lesions. Positive serology in high titers (optical density > 0.5) and the exclusion of other causes of hypereosinophilia allow a presumptive diagnosis to be made in typical cases.

Differential Diagnosis

Diseases with hypereosinophilia must be considered. These include trichinosis (large liver and spleen not usually seen, muscle tenderness common), eosinophilic leukemia (rare in children; eosinophils are abnormal in appearance), collagen-vascular disease (those associated with eosinophilia are rare in young children), strongyloidiasis (no organomegaly; enteric symptoms are common), early ascariasis, and tropical eosinophilia (seen mainly in India), allergies, and hypersensitivity syndromes.

Treatment & Prevention

A. Specific Measures: The clinical benefit of specific anthelmintic therapy is not defined. Treatment with thiabendazole (25 mg/kg—maximum 3 g/d—orally twice a day for 5–7 days), diethylcarbamazine (2 mg/kg three times a day orally for 7–10 days), albendazole (400 mg twice a day for 3–5 days), or mebendazole (100–200 mg twice a day for 5 days) is indicated for severe complications of brain, lung, or heart viscera larva migrans.

B. General Measures: Treating any cause of pica, such as iron deficiency, is important. Corticosteroids are used for marked inflammation of lung, eye, or other organs. Pets should be dewormed routinely. Other children in the household may be infected. Mild eosinophilia and positive serologic tests may be the only clue to their infection. Therapy is not necessary for these patients.

Blatia V, Sarin SK: Hepatic visceral larva migrans: Evolution of the lesion, diagnosis and role of high-dose albendazole. Am J Gastroenterol 1994;89:624.

Magnaval YF: Comparative efficacy of diethylcarbamazine and mebendazole for the treatment of human toxocariasis. Parasitology 1995;110:529.

Taylor MR et al: The expanded spectrum of toxocaral disease. Lancet 1988;1:692.

7. TRICHINOSIS

Essentials of Diagnosis & Typical Features

- Vomiting, diarrhea, and pain within 1 week of eating infected meat.
- Fever, periorbital edema, myalgia, and marked eosinophilia.

General Considerations

Trichinella spiralis is a small roundworm. The adults inhabit the intestines of hogs and several other meat-eating animals. The cycle begins when the larvae in the muscle of hogs, bear, walrus, and other animals are ingested; they then enter the bowel mucosa, develop into adults, reemerge into the intestine, mate, and reenter the mucosa. The hundreds of larvae produced by each female over the next weeks enter the bloodstream and encyst in the striated muscle. Their migration causes marked inflammation. Humans are usually infected by eating undercooked pork. Smoking, salting, or drying the meat does not kill the larvae. Machines used to grind infected pork may contaminate other meat, such as beef.

Clinical Findings

A. Symptoms and Signs: Most infections are asymptomatic. The initial bowel penetration may cause nausea, vomiting, diarrhea, and cramps within 1 week after ingestion of contaminated meat. This may progress to the classic myopathic form, which consists of fever, periorbital edema, myalgia, and weakness. Many organs may be infected by the migrating larvae—diaphragm, heart, lungs, kidneys, spleen, skin, and brain. Severe cerebral involvement may be fatal. Myocarditis may also be severe or fatal. Symptoms usually peak after 2–3 weeks, but may last months. Another syndrome of chronic diarrhea has been described in the Inuit population in Canada.

B. Laboratory Findings: Marked eosinophilia

is the rule. Serology confirms the diagnosis. Muscle biopsy is rarely necessary.

Differential Diagnosis

The classic symptoms are pathognomonic if one is aware of this disease. It has to be distinguished from influenza, dermatomyositis, typhoid fever, sinusitis, and angioneurotic edema.

Prevention

Because a microscopic examination must be performed, meat in the United States is not inspected for trichinosis. Although all states require the cooking of hog swill, hog-to-hog or hog-to-rat cycles may continue. All pork and sylvatic meat (such as bear or walrus) should be heated to at least 65 °C. Freezing meat to at least –15 °C for 3 weeks may also prevent transmission. Animals used for food should not be fed or allowed access to raw meat.

Treatment

Mebendazole has activity against the intestinal, circulating, and tissue stages of infection. The adult dose is 200–400 mg three times daily for 3 days followed by 400–500 mg three times daily for 10 days. Pediatric dosing has not been standardized. Concurrent corticosteroids are used in attempt to prevent the Herxheimer reaction associated with treatment.

Prognosis

Death may occur within the first weeks, but most infections are self-limited.

MacLean JD et al: Trichinosis in the Canadian Arctic: Report of five outbreaks and a new clinical syndrome. J Infect Dis 1989;160:513.

Santos Duran-Ortiz J et al: Trichinosis with severe myopathic involvement mimicking polymyositis. Report of a family outbreak. J Rheumatol 1992;19:310.

CESTODE INFECTIONS (Flukes)

1. TAENIASIS & CYSTICERCOSIS

Essentials of Diagnosis & Typical Features

- Mild abdominal pain; passage of worm segments (taeniasis).
- Focal seizures, headaches (neurocysticercosis).
- Cysticerci present in biopsy specimens, on plain films (as calcified masses), or on CT or MRI.
- Proglottids and eggs in feces; specific antibodies in serum or CSF.

General Considerations

Both the beef tapeworm (*Taenia saginata*) and the pork (*Taenia solium*) tapeworm cause taeniasis. The adults live in the intestines of humans; the egg-laden distal segments, or proglottids, break off and are passed in feces, disintegrating and releasing the ova in the soil. After ingestion in food or water by cattle or pigs, the eggs hatch and the larvae migrate to and encyst in skeletal muscle. When ingested by humans, these larvae mature into adults.

Humans can be an intermediate host for *T solium* (but not *T saginata*), and the larvae released from ingested eggs encyst in a variety of tissues, especially muscle and brain. Full larval maturation occurs in 2 months, but the cysts cause little inflammation until they die months to years later. Inflammatory edema ensues with calcification or disappearance of the cyst. A slowly expanding mass of sterile cysts at the base of the brain may cause obstructive hydrocephalus (racemose cysticercosis).

Both parasites are distributed worldwide. Contamination of foods by eggs in human feces allows infection without exposure to meat or travel to endemic areas. Asymptomatic cases are common, but neurocysticercosis is a leading cause of seizures in endemic areas.

Person-to-person spread may occur, resulting in infection of individuals with no exposure to infected meat.

Clinical Findings

A. Symptoms and Signs:

1. Taeniasis–In most tapeworm infections, the only clinical manifestation is the passage of fecal proglottids—white, motile bodies 1×2 cm in size. They occasionally crawl out onto the skin and down the leg, especially the larger *T saginata*.

Children may harbor the adult worm for years and complain of abdominal pain, anorexia, and diarrhea.

2. Cysticercosis–Most cases are asymptomatic. Subcutaneous nodules of 1–2 cm may be the only sign. After several years, the cysticerci calcify and appear as radiographic opacities. Brain cysts may remain silent or cause seizures, headache, hydrocephalus, and basilar meningitis. Rarely, the spinal cord is involved. Neurocysticercosis becomes manifest an average of 5 years after exposure but may cause symptoms in the first year of life. In the eye, cysts cause bleeding, retinal detachment, and uveitis. Definitive diagnosis requires histologic demonstration of larvae or cyst membrane. Presumptive diagnosis is often made by the characteristics of the cysts seen on CT or MRI studies; the differential diagnosis may include tuberculoma, brain abscess, arachnoid cyst, and tumor. The presence of *T solium* eggs in feces is uncommon but supports the diagnosis.

B. Laboratory Findings:

Eggs or proglottids may be found in feces or on the perianal skin (using the tape method employed for pinworms). Eggs of both *Taenia* species are identical. The species are identified by examination of proglottids; more than 18 lateral uterine branches are present in *T saginata,* less than 12 branches in *T solium.*

Peripheral eosinophilia is minimal or absent. Spinal fluid eosinophilia is seen in 10–75% of cases of neurocysticercosis; its presence supports an otherwise presumptive diagnosis.

Enzyme immunoassay (EIA) antibody titers are eventually positive in up to 98% of serum specimens and over 75% of cerebrospinal fluid specimens from patients with neurocysticercosis. Solitary cysts are less often associated with seropositivity than are multiple cysts. High titers tend to correlate with more severe disease. Cerebrospinal fluid titers are higher if cysts are near the meninges.

Treatment

A. Taeniasis: Praziquantel (5–10 mg/kg once) is the drug of choice. Feces free of segments or ova for 3 months suggest cure.

B. Cysticercosis: Specific treatment is reserved for patients with meningitis or parenchymal cysts. In contrast, those with inactive disease require only symptomatic treatment (anticonvulsants). Praziquantel and albendazole cause disappearance of noninflamed cysts and possibly more rapid resolution of inflamed ring-enhancing cysts. The recommended dose of praziquantel is 50 mg/kg/d in three divided doses for 2 weeks; that for albendazole is 15 mg/kg divided into three doses daily for 8 days. Albendazole is more effective than praziquantel (and is the drug of choice). Larval death may result in clinical worsening due to inflammatory edema. A short course of dexamethasone may decrease these symptoms. The racemose cysts contain no viable larvae and do not respond to medical therapy. Follow-up scans every several months help assess the response to therapy.

Prevention

The incidence in the United States is low, because beef and pork are inspected for taeniasis. Prevention requires proper cooking of meat, careful washing of raw vegetables and fruits, treatment of intestinal carriers, avoiding the use of human excrement for fertilizer, and providing proper sanitary facilities.

Prognosis

The prognosis is good in intestinal taeniasis. Symptoms associated with a few cerebral cysts may disappear in a few months; heavy infections may cause death or chronic neurologic impairment.

Del Brutto OH et al: Therapy for neurocysticercosis: A reappraisal. Clin Infect Dis 1993;17:730.

Sorvillo FJ et al: Cysticercosis surveillance: Locally acquired and travel-related infections and detection of intestinal tapeworm carriers in Los Angeles County. Am J Trop Med Hyg 1992;47:365.

St. Geme III JW et al: Consensus: Diagnosis and management of neurocysticercosis in children. Pediatr Infect Dis J 1993;12:455,

White, AC: Neurocysticercosis: A major cause of neurological disease worldwide. Clin Infect Dies 1997; 24: 101.

2. HYMENOLEPIASIS

Hymenolepis nana, the cosmopolitan human tapeworm, is a common parasite of children; *Hymenolepis diminuta,* the rat tapeworm, is rare. The former is capable of causing autoinfection, because the entire life cycle may take place in the human intestine. The larvae hatched from the ingested eggs penetrate the intestinal wall and then reenter the lumen to mature into adults. Their eggs are immediately infectious for the same or a new host. The adult is only a few centimeters long. Finding the characteristic eggs in feces is diagnostic.

H diminuta has an intermediate stage in rat fleas and other insects; children are infected when they ingest these insects.

Light infections with either tapeworm are usually asymptomatic; heavy infection can cause diarrhea and abdominal pain. Therapy is with praziquantel (25 mg/kg once).

Drugs for parasitic infections. Med Lett Drugs Ther 1995;37:117.

Tanowitz HB et al: Diagnosis and treatment of intestinal helminths. I. Common intestinal cestodes. Gastroenterologist 1993;1:265.

3. ECHINOCOCCOSIS

Essentials of Diagnosis & Typical Features
- Cystic tumors of liver, lung, kidney, bone, brain, and other organs.
- Eosinophilia.
- Urticaria and pruritus if cysts rupture.
- Protoscoleces or daughter cysts in the primary cyst.
- Positive serology.

General Considerations
Dogs, cats, and other carnivores are the hosts for *Echinococcus granulosus.* Endemic areas include Australia, New Zealand, and southwestern United States, including Native American reservations where shepherding is practiced. The adult tapeworm lives in sheep intestines, and eggs are passed in the feces. When ingested by humans, the eggs hatch, and the larvae penetrate the intestinal mucosa and disseminate in the bloodstream. The larvae produce cysts; the primary sites of involvement are the liver (60–70%) and the lungs (20–25%). A unilocular cyst is most common. Over years, it may reach 25 cm in

diameter, although most are much smaller. The cysts of *Echinococcus multilocularis* are multilocular and demonstrate more rapid growth.

Clinical Findings
A. Symptoms and Signs: Clinical disease is due to pressure from the enlarging cysts, vessel erosion, and sensitization to cyst or worm antigens. Liver cysts present as slowly expanding tumors that may cause biliary obstruction. Most are in the right lobe and extend inferiorly; 25% are on the upper surface and may be asymptomatic for years. Omental torsion or hemorrhage from vessel erosion may occur.

Rupture of a pulmonary cyst causes coughing, dyspnea, wheezing, urticaria, chest pain, and hemoptysis; cyst and worm remnants are found in sputum. Brain cysts may cause focal neurologic signs and convulsions; renal cysts cause pain and hematuria; bone cysts cause pain.

B. Laboratory Findings: Presumptive diagnosis is made by a combination of radiographic, cytologic, and serologic findings. The appropriate body fluid (tracheal aspirate, ascitic or pleural fluid, spinal fluid, or urine, depending on the site of the cyst) should be examined for protoscoleces. Passing a large amount of fluid through a 5 μm filter and then looking for protoscoleces with an acid-fast stain or other stain has been found to be a sensitive method.

Eosinophilia is variable and may be absent. Serologic tests are useful for diagnosis and follow-up of therapy.

Diagnostic titers vary among laboratories. The bentonite flocculation test is positive at a titer of 1:5, and the indirect hemagglutination test is positive at 1:128. Titers are much higher in secondary echinococcosis (due to cyst rupture). Titers remain high at least a year after surgery. They are usually negative by 10 years. Persistently elevated titers suggest persistent infection.

The skin test for echinococcosis (Casoni test) should not be used. It has never been standardized, and many false-positive results are seen.

C. Imaging: Pulmonary or bone cysts may be visible on plain films. Other imaging techniques are preferred for cysts in other organs. Visualization of daughter cysts is highly suggestive of echinococcosis.

Differential Diagnosis
Tumors, bacterial or amebic abscess, and tuberculosis (pulmonary) must be considered.

Complications
Sudden cyst rupture with anaphylaxis and death is the worst complication. If the patient survives, secondary infections from seeding of daughter cysts may occur. Segmental lung collapse, secondary bacterial infections, effects of increased intracranial

pressure, and severe renal damage due to renal cysts are other potential complications.

Treatment

Definitive therapy of *E multilocularis* requires meticulous surgical removal of the cysts, preceded by careful injection of the cyst with formalin, iodine, or 95% alcohol solution to sterilize infectious protoscoleces. Freezing the cyst wall and injecting silver nitrate prior to removal is another technique. A surgeon familiar with this disease should be consulted. Medical therapy (see below) may be of some benefit. If the cyst leaks or ruptures, the allergic symptoms must be managed immediately.

Albendazole (15 mg/kg/d for 28 days with repeat courses as necessary following a 14-day "rest period") is effective in many, but not all, cases of *E granulosus* infection (hydatid disease).

Prognosis

Large liver cysts may be asymptomatic for years. Surgery is often curative for lung and liver cysts but not always for cysts in other locations. Secondary disease has a much worse prognosis; about 15% of patients with this disease die.

Ersahin Y, Mutluer S, Guzelbag E: Intracranial hydatid cysts in children. Neurosurgery 1993;33:219.

Force L et al: Evaluation of eight serological tests in the diagnosis of human echinococcosis and follow-up. Clin Infect Dis 1992;15:473.

Morris DL et al: Albendazole: Objective evidence of response in human hydatid disease. JAMA 1985;253:2053.

TREMATODE INFECTIONS

1. SCHISTOSOMIASIS

Essentials of Diagnosis & Typical Features

- Transient pruritic rash after exposure to fresh water.
- Fever, urticaria, arthralgias, cough, lymphadenitis, and eosinophilia.
- Weight loss, anorexia, hepatosplenomegaly.
- Hematuria, dysuria.
- Eggs in stool, urine, or rectal biopsy specimens.

General Considerations

One of the most common serious parasitic diseases, schistosomiasis, is caused by several species of *Schistosoma* flukes. *Schistosoma japonicum, Schistosoma mekongi,* and *Schistosoma mansoni* involve the intestines and *Schistosoma haematobium* the urinary tract. The first two are found in eastern and southeastern Asia; *S mansoni* in tropical Africa, the Caribbean, and parts of South America; and *S haematobium* in northern Africa.

Infection is caused by free-swimming larvae (cercariae), which emerge from the intermediate hosts, certain species of fresh-water snails. The cercariae penetrate human skin, migrate to the liver, and mature into adults, which then migrate through the portal vein to lodge in the bladder veins (*S haematobium*), superior mesenteric veins (*S mekongi, S japonicum*), or inferior mesenteric veins (*S mansoni*). Clinical disease results primarily from the inflammation caused by the many eggs that are laid in the perivascular tissues or embolize to the liver. Escape of ova into bowel or bladder lumen allows microscopic visualization and diagnosis from stool or urine specimens, as well as contamination of fresh water and infection of the snail hosts that ingest them.

Clinical Findings

Much of the population in endemic areas is infected but asymptomatic. Only heavy infections produce symptoms.

A. Symptoms and Signs: The cercarial penetration may cause a pruritic rash; larval migration may cause fever, urticaria, and cough; the maturation phase may cause tender hepatosplenomegaly followed by days to weeks of fever and malaise as the worms migrate to their final destination. Bladder infection results in dysuria, hematuria, reflux, stones, and incontinence. Secondary pyelonephritis and ureteral obstruction may occur. Intestinal infection is usually asymptomatic. The final stages of disease are characterized by hepatic fibrosis, portal hypertension, splenomegaly, ascites, and bleeding from esophageal varices. The chronic inflammation in the urinary tract associated with *S haematobium* infections may result in obstructive uropathy, stones, infection, bladder cancer, fistulas, and anemia due to chronic hematuria. Spinal cord granulomas and paraplegia due to egg embolization into Batson's plexus have been reported.

B. Laboratory Findings: The diagnosis is made by finding the species-specific eggs in feces (*S japonicum, S mekongi, S mansoni,* and occasionally *S haematobium*) or urine (*S haematobium,* occasionally *S mansoni*). A rectal biopsy may reveal *S mansoni* and should be done if other specimens are negative. Peripheral eosinophilia is common, and eosinophils may be seen in urine.

Prevention

The best prevention is to avoid contact with contaminated fresh water in endemic areas. Efforts to destroy the snail hosts have been successful in areas of accelerated economic development.

Treatment

A. Specific Measures: Praziquantel is the drug of choice for schistosomiasis. A dose of 40 mg/kg/d in two divided doses (*S mansoni* or *S haematobium*) or 20 mg/kg three times in 1 day (*S japonicum* or *S* *mekongi)* is very effective and nontoxic. Oxamniquine (20 mg/kg/d in two doses once per day) is an alternative regimen for *S mansoni.*

B. General Measures: Medical therapy of nutritional deficiency or secondary bacterial infections may be needed. The urinary tract should be carefully evaluated in *S haematobium* infections; reconstructive surgery may be needed. Hepatic fibrosis requires careful evaluation of the portal venous system and surgical management of the portal hypertension when appropriate.

Prognosis

Medical therapy decreases the worm infection and liver size, despite continued exposure in endemic areas. Early disease responds well to therapy, but once significant scarring or severe inflammation has occurred, eradication of the parasites is of little benefit.

Dunn DW et al: Prospects for immunological control of schistosomiasis. Lancet 1995;345:1488.
Mahmoud AAF: Schistosomiasis: An overview. Immunol Invest 1992;21:383.
McGarvey ST et al: Child growth and schistosomiasis japonica in northeastern Leyte, the Philippines: Cross-sectional results. Am J Trop Med Hyg 1992;46:571.

II. INFECTIONS: MYCOTIC

Fungi can be classified as yeasts, which are unicellular and reproduce by budding; as molds, which are multicellular and consist of tubular structures (hyphae) and grow by elongation and branching; or as dimorphic fungi, which can exist either as yeasts or molds depending on environmental conditions. Fungal infections can be categorized as shown in Table 37–8. In the United States, systemic disease in normal hosts is commonly caused by three organisms—*Coccidioides, Histoplasma,* and *Blastomyces*—which are restricted to certain geographic areas. Prior residence in or travel to these areas, even for a brief time, is a prerequisite for inclusion in a differential diagnosis. Of these three, *Histoplasma* most often relapses years later in patients who are immunosuppressed.

Immunosuppression, foreign bodies (eg, central catheters), ulceration of gastrointestinal and respiratory mucosae, broad-spectrum antimicrobial therapy, malnutrition, HIV infection, and neutrophil defects are major risk factors for opportunistic fungal disease.

Laboratory diagnosis may be difficult because of the small number of fungi present in some lesions, slow growth of some of the organisms, and difficulty in distinguishing colonization of mucosal surfaces

Table 37–8. Pediatric fungal infections.

Type	Agents	Incidence	Diagnosis	Diagnostic Tests	Therapy	Prognosis
Superficial	*Candida* Dermatophytes *Sporothrix* *Malassezia*	Very common	Simple[1]	KOH prep	Topical[2]	Good
Systemic: Normal host	*Coccidioides* *Histoplasma* *Blastomyces*	Common: regional	Often presumptive	Chest x-ray Serology, antigen detection (histoplasmosis) Histology Culture examination of body fluids or tissue	None[3] or systemic	Good
Systemic: Opportunistic infection	*Candida* *Pneumocystis*[4] *Aspergillus* *Malassezia* *Pseudallescheria* *Cryptococcus*	Uncommon	Difficult[5]	Tissue biopsy, culture, antigen detection (cryptococcosis)	Systemic, prolonged	Poor if therapy delayed and in severely immunocompromised patients

[1]Sporotrichosis may require biopsy for diagnosis and is treated with systemic therapy.
[2]*Candida* and *Sporothrix* in immunocompromised patients may cause severe, rapidly progressive disease and require systemic therapy.
[3]Often self-limited in normal host.
[4]Now reclassified as a fungus. May infect many normal hosts.
[5]Except *Cryptococcus,* which is often diagnosed by antigen detection.

from infection. A tissue biopsy with fungal stains and culture is the best method for diagnosing systemic disease. Repeat blood cultures may be negative even in the presence of intravascular infections. Tests for antibody and antigen are currently too insensitive to diagnose most systemic infections, but serology is useful for coccidioidomycosis and histoplasmosis and antigen detection is useful in histoplasmosis and cryptococcosis.

The risk of empiric treatment is greater for fungal than for bacterial infections because of the toxicity of some antifungals (especially amphotericin B), the frequent need for prolonged parenteral administration, and the limited data available for choosing the best dose or regimen. Delay in treating systemic disease, however, may prove fatal.

Susceptibility testing of fungi, especially of molds, is not well standardized, and the correlation of in vitro susceptibility to clinical response is not well defined.

Several less common fungal infections, most of which occur only in severely immunocompromised children, are presented in Table 37–9. The common superficial fungal infections of the hair and skin are discussed in Chapter 13.

BLASTOMYCOSIS

The causative fungus, *Blastomyces dermatitidis*, is found in soil primarily in the Mississippi and Ohio River Valleys and the states bordering the Great Lakes.

Table 37–9. Unusual fungal infections in children.

Organism	Predisposing Factors	Route of Infection	Clinical Disease	Diagnostic Tests	Therapy and Comments
Aspergillus species	None	Inhalation of spores	Allergic bronchopulmonary aspergillosis; wheezing, cough, migratory infiltrates, eosinophilia.	Organisms in sputum; positive skin test; specific IgE antibody; elevated IgE levels.	Hypersensitivity to fungal antigens. Use steroids. No antifungals needed.
	Immuno-suppression	Inhalation of spores	Progressive pulmonary disease: consolidation, nodules, abscesses. Sinusitis Disseminated disease: usually lung, brain; occasionally intestine, kidney, heart, bone. Invades blood vessels.	Demonstrate fungus in tissues by stain or culture; septate hyphae branching at 45-degree angle.	Amphotericin B for 4–6 weeks. Concomitant itraconazole may improve outcome.
Malassezia furfur, M pachydermatis	Central venous catheter, usually lipid infusion (can occur in the absence of lipid)	Line infection from skin colonization	Sepsis; pneumonitis, thrombocytopenia	Culture of catheter or blood on lipid-enriched media (for *M furfur; M pachydermatis* does not need lipid). Fungus may be seen in buffy coat.	Discontinuation of lipid may be sufficient. Remove catheter. Short-term amphotericin B may be added. Organism ubiquitous on normal skin; requires long-chain fatty acids for growth.
Mucorales (*Mucor, Rhizopus, Absidia*)	Immunosuppression, diabetic acidosis	Inhalation, mucosal colonization, invasion of vessels or tissue	Rhinocerebral: sinus, nose, nose, necrotizing vasculitis; central nervous system spread. Pulmonary Disseminated: Any organ.	Broad aseptate hyphae branching at 90-degree angles seen on tissue stains. Culture: rapidly growing, fluffy fungus.	Amphotericin B, surgical debridement; itraconazole may be a second agent for combined therapy. Poor prognosis.
Pseudallescheria boydii	Immuno-suppression	Inhalation	Disseminated abscesses (lung, brain, liver, spleen, other)	Culture of pus or tissue.	Surgical drainage; itraconazole.
	Minor trauma	Cutaneous	Mycetoma (most common)	Yellow-white granules in pus. Culture.	Aggressive surgery. Amputation may be needed.
Sporothrix schenkii	Minor trauma (thorns, splinters)	Cutaneous	Chronic skin ulcers, subcutaneous nodules along lymphatics. Rarely pneumonia, osteomyelitis, arthritis.	Gram or fungal stain of pus or tissue may show "hockey stick" organisms. Culture of pus, tissue.	Itraconazole, drainage, debridement. Disseminated disease in immunocompromised host.

Transmission is by inhalation of spores. Outbreaks associated with construction have occurred. Severe disease is much more common in adults and males. In children, infection rates are similar in both sexes.

Primary infection is unrecognized or produces pneumonia. Acute symptoms include cough, chest pain, headache, weight loss, and fever occurring several weeks to months after inoculation. Infection is usually self-limited in normal patients. Progressive pulmonary disease may occur. Radiographic consolidation is typical; effusions, nodules, hilar nodes, and cavities are less common. Lower lobe disease is more common with acute infection. Chronic disease can develop in the upper lobes, with cavities and fibronodular infiltrations similar to that seen in tuberculosis, but, unlike tuberculosis or histoplasmosis, these lesions rarely caseate or calcify.

Cutaneous lesions usually represent disseminated disease; local primary inoculation is rare. Slowly progressive ulcerating nodules are typical. Verrucous lesions may be seen. Bone disease resembles other forms of chronic osteomyelitis. Lytic skull lesions in children are typical, but long bones, vertebrae, and the pelvis may be involved. A total body radiographic examination is advisable when blastomycosis is diagnosed. The genitourinary tract involvement characteristic of dissemination in adults is rare in prepubertal children. Lymph nodes, brain, and kidneys may be involved.

Diagnosis requires isolation or visualization of the fungus. Pulmonary specimens (sputum, tracheal aspirates, lung biopsy) may be positive with conventional stains or fungal cell wall stains. Microscopically, the budding yeasts are thick-walled, have refractile walls, and are large and very distinctive. Sputum specimens are positive in 50–80% of cases; skin lesions are positive in 80–100%. The fungus can be grown readily in most laboratories, but 2 weeks or more are required. Antibody measured by several immunoassays is sensitive for detecting infection. Blastomycosis should be considered when a significant pulmonary infection in an endemic area fails to respond to antibiotic therapy.

Recommended therapy for life-threatening or central nervous system infections is amphotericin B. Itraconazole is preferred for other forms of blastomycosis. Surgical debridement of devitalized bone or drainage of large abscesses is also important.

Alkrinawi S, Reed MH, Pastarkamp H: Pulmonary blastomycosis in children: Findings on chest radiographs. Am J Roentgenol 1995;165:651.
Bradshaw RW: Histoplasmosis and blastomycosis, 1996. Clin Infect Dis 1996;22(Suppl):S102.
Brown LR et al: Roentgenographic features of pulmonary blastomycosis. Mayo Clin Proc 1991;66:29.
Dismukes ED et al: Itraconazole therapy for blastomycosis and histoplasmosis. Am J Med 1992;93:489.
Maxson S, Jacobs RF: Community-acquired fungal pneumonia in children. Semin Respir Infect 1996;11:196.
Schutze GE et al: Blastomycosis in children. Clin Infect Dis 1996;22:496.

CANDIDIASIS

Essentials of Diagnosis & Typical Features

- Superficial infections in normal or immunosuppressed individuals: Oral thrush or ulcerations; vulvovaginitis; erythematous intertriginous rash with satellite lesions.
- Systemic infection in the immunosuppressed: Renal, hepatic, splenic, pulmonary, or cerebral abscesses; "cotton-wool" retinal lesions; cutaneous nodules.
- Budding yeast and pseudohyphae seen in biopsy specimens, fluid, or scrapings of lesions; positive culture.

General Considerations

Disease due to *Candida* is caused by *Candida albicans* in 60–80% of cases; similar systemic infection may be due to *C tropicalis, C parapsilosis, C glabrata,* and a few other *Candida* species. Speciation is important because of differences in pathogenicity and sensitivity for azole therapy. In tissue, pseudohyphae are seen as well as the budding yeast phase. *Candida* grows on routine media more slowly than bacteria; growth is usually evident on agar after 2–3 days and in blood culture media in 2–7 days.

C albicans is ubiquitous and often present in small numbers on skin, mucous membranes, or in the intestinal tract. Normal bacterial flora, intact epithelial barriers, neutrophils and macrophages in conjunction with antibody and complement, and normal lymphocyte function (manifested by skin test reactivity) are all factors in preventing invasion. Disseminated infection is almost always preceded by prolonged broad-spectrum antibiotic therapy, instrumentation, or immunosuppression. Patients with diabetes mellitus are especially prone to superficial *Candida* infection; thrush and vaginitis are most common. *Candida* is the third most common blood isolate in hospitals in the United States.

Clinical Findings

A. Symptoms and Signs:

1. Oral candidiasis (thrush)–Adherent creamy white plaques on the buccal, gingival, or lingual mucosa are seen. Lesions may be few and asymptomatic, or they may be extensive, extending into the esophagus. Thrush is very common in otherwise normal infants in the first weeks of life; it may last weeks despite topical therapy. Spontaneous thrush in older children is unusual unless they have recently received antimicrobials. Steroid inhalation for asthma predisposes patients to thrush. Infection with HIV should be considered if there is no other reason for oral thrush, or if it is persistent or recurrent.

2. Skin infection–

a. Diaper dermatitis is often due entirely or partly to *Candida.* Pronounced erythema with a sharply defined margin, and satellite lesions is typical. Pustules, vesicles, papules, or scales may be seen. Weeping, eroded lesions with a scalloped border are common. Any moist area, such as axillae or neck folds, may be involved.

b. Congenital skin lesions may be seen in infants born to women with *Candida* amnionitis. A red maculopapular or pustular rash is seen. Dissemination may occur.

c. Vulvovaginitis is seen in sexually active girls or diabetics, and occurs at any age in girls receiving antibiotics. Thick, cheesy discharge with intense pruritus is typical. The vagina and labia are usually erythematous.

d. Scattered red papules or nodules may represent cutaneous dissemination.

e. Chronic mucocutaneous candidiasis may be associated with a specific lack of T-cell response to *Candida.*

f. Paronychia and onychomycosis occur in normal children, but are often associated with immunosuppression, hypoparathyroidism, and adrenal insufficiency.

g. Chronic draining otitis media in patients who have received multiple courses of antibiotics may be superinfected with *C albicans.*

3. Enteric infection–Esophageal involvement in immunosuppressed patients is the most common enteric manifestation. It is manifested by substernal pain, dysphagia, painful swallowing, and anorexia. Nausea and vomiting are common in young children. Only 50% of the patients have thrush. Stomach or intestinal ulcers also occur. A syndrome of mild diarrhea in normal individuals who have predominant *Candida* on stool culture has also been described, though *Candida* is not considered a true enteric pathogen. Its presence more often reflects recent antimicrobial therapy.

4. Pulmonary infection–Since the organism frequently colonizes the respiratory tract, it is commonly isolated from respiratory secretions. Thus, demonstration of tissue invasion is needed to diagnose *Candida* pneumonia or tracheitis. It is rare, being seen in immunosuppressed patients and patients intubated for long periods. The infection may cause fever, cough, abscesses, nodular infiltrates, and effusion.

5. Renal infection–Candiduria may be the only manifestation of disseminated disease. More often, candiduria is associated with instrumentation, an indwelling catheter, or anatomic abnormality of the urinary tract. Symptoms of cystitis may be present. Masses of *Candida* may obstruct ureters and cause obstructive nephropathy. *Candida* casts in the urine suggest renal tissue infection.

6. Other infections–Endocarditis, myocarditis, meningitis, and osteomyelitis are usually only seen in compromised patients or neonates.

7. Disseminated candidiasis–Mucosal colonization precedes but does not predict dissemination. Too often, dissemination mimics bacterial sepsis. It is common in neonates—especially premature infants—in an ICU setting, and is recognized when the infant fails to respond to antibiotics. A careful search should be carried out for lesions highly suggestive of disseminated *Candida* (retinal "cotton-wool" spots or nodular dermal abscesses). If these findings are absent, diagnosis is often presumptively based on the presence of a compatible disease in a compromised patient, a burn patient, or a patient with prolonged postsurgical or ICU course, who has no other cause for the symptoms; who fails to respond to antimicrobials; and who usually has *Candida* colonization of mucosal surfaces. This approach is necessary because candidemia is not appreciated antemortem in many such patients.

Hepatosplenic candidiasis is increasingly recognized in immunosuppressed patients. The typical case consists of a severely neutropenic patient who develops chronic fever, variable abdominal pain, and abnormal liver function tests. No bacteria are isolated, and there is no response to antimicrobials. Symptoms persist even when neutrophils return. Ultrasound or CT scan of the liver and spleen demonstrates multiple round lesions. Biopsy is needed to confirm the diagnosis.

B. Laboratory Findings: Budding yeast cells are easily seen in scrapings or other samples. The presence of pseudohyphae is suggestive of tissue invasion. Culture is definitive. Blood cultures may take 3 or more days to yield positive results or they may remain negative (10–40%), even with disseminated disease or endocarditis. *Candida* should never be considered a contaminant in cultures from normally sterile sites. *Candida* in any number in the urine may represent true infection. Antigen tests are not sensitive or specific enough for clinical use. Antibody tests are not useful. The ability of a yeast to form germ tubes when incubated in human serum gives a presumptive speciation for *C albicans.*

Differential Diagnosis

Thrush may resemble formula (which can be easily wiped away with a tongue blade or swab, revealing normal mucosa without underlying erosion), other types of ulcers (including herpes), or burns. Skin lesions may resemble contact, allergic, chemical, or bacterial dermatitis, miliaria, folliculitis, or eczema. Candidemia and systemic infection should be considered in any seriously ill patient with the risk factors previously mentioned.

Complications

Failure to recognize disseminated disease early is

the greatest complication. Osteoarthritis and meningitis occur more often in neonates than older children. Blindness from retinitis, massive emboli from large vegetations of endocarditis, intestinal perforation, and abscesses in any organ are other complications; the greater the length or degree of immunosuppression, and the longer the delay before therapy, the more complications are seen.

Treatment

A. Oral Candidiasis: In infants, oral nystatin suspension (100,000 units four to six times a day in the buccal fold after feeding until resolution) usually suffices. It must come in contact with the lesions because it is not systemically absorbed. Older children may use it as a mouthwash (200,000–500,000 units four times a day), though it is poorly tolerated because of its taste. Clotrimazole troches (10 mg) four times a day are an alternative in older children. Prolonged therapy with either agent and more frequent dosing may be needed. Painting the lesions with a cotton swab dipped in gentian violet (0.5–1%) is visually dramatic and messy but may help refractory cases. Eradication of *Candida* from pacifiers, bottle nipples, toys, or the mother's breasts (if the infant is breast feeding and there is candidal infection of the nipples) may be helpful.

Oral azoles—ketoconazole (200 mg/m^2 in divided doses every 12 hours for 5–7 days) or fluconazole (6 mg/kg/d)—are effective in older children with candidal infection refractory to nystatin. Discontinuation of antibiotics or corticosteroids is advised when possible.

B. Skin Infection: Cutaneous infection usually responds to a cream or lotion containing nystatin, amphotericin B, or an imidazole. Associated inflammation, such as severe diaper dermatitis, is also helped by concurrent use of a topical mild corticosteroid cream, such as 1% hydrocortisone. One approach is to keep the involved area dry; a heat lamp and nystatin powder may be used. Cornstarch is a yeast nutrient and should not be used as a drying agent.

Suppression of intestinal *Candida* with nystatin and eradicating thrush may speed recovery and prevent recurrence of the diaper dermatitis.

C. Vaginal Infections: Vaginal infection is treated with clotrimazole, miconazole, or nystatin (cheapest if generic is used) suppositories or creams, usually applied once nightly for 7–14 days. One high-dose clotrimazole formulation need be given for only a single night. *Candida* balanitis in sexual partners should be treated. Oral azole therapy is equally effective. A single oral dose of fluconazole is effective for vaginitis. It is more expensive, but very convenient. No controlled study has shown that treating colonization of male sexual partners prevents recurrence in females.

D. Renal Infection: Candiduria limited to the bladder may be treated with amphotericin B bladder irrigation (if a catheter is already in place), or a short course of oral flucytosine or fluconazole. Removal of an indwelling catheter is imperative. Renal abscesses or ureteral fungus balls require amphotericin B therapy and surgical debridement in many cases. Amphotericin B may improve poor renal function due to renal candidiasis, even though the drug is nephrotoxic. Fluconazole, which is excreted in urine, is an acceptable alternative.

E. Systemic Infection: Systemic infection is dangerous and resistant to therapy. Surgical drainage of abscesses and removal of all infected tissue (such as a heart valve) are required for cure. Hepatosplenic candidiasis should be treated until all lesions have disappeared or are calcified on imaging studies. Systemic infection is optimally treated with amphotericin B at a dosage of 0.75–1 mg/kg/d infused over 2–4 hours. It is continued for at least 4 weeks, depending on disease response. Correcting predisposing factors is important (eg, discontinuing antibiotics and immunosuppressives, and improving control of diabetes). Addition of flucytosine (50–75 mg/kg/d orally in four doses; keep serum levels below 75 mg/mL) may help. This is frequently done for neonatal infections, but clinical outcome seems to be similar when amphotericin is used alone. Unlike amphotericin B, flucytosine penetrates tissues well; it is also synergistic with amphotericin B against many organisms. It should not be used as a single agent in serious infections because resistance develops rapidly. Fluconazole is an acceptable alternative for serious *C albicans* infections in nonneutropenic patients and is used more frequently in immunocompromised patients. However, the decision to use fluconazole must include consideration of the significant incidence of fluconazole-resistant *Candida* in some hospitals. Infected central venous lines must be removed immediately; this alone often is curative. Persistent fever and candidemia suggest infected thrombus, endocarditis, or tissue infection. If the infection is considered limited to the line and environs, 10–14 days of an antifungal such as amphotericin B or fluconazole following line removal is recommended in compromised patients. Fluconazole should also be considered for immunocompetent patients because of the late occurrence of focal *Candida* infection in some cases.

Fluconazole is well absorbed (oral and intravenous therapy are equivalent), reasonably nontoxic, and effective for a variety of *Candida* infections. It is the drug of choice if amphotericin B is not tolerated. The dosage is 8–12 mg/kg/d in a single daily dose for initial therapy of severely ill children.

Prognosis

Superficial disease in normal hosts has a good prognosis; in abnormal hosts, it may be quite refractory to therapy. Early therapy of systemic disease is often curative if the underlying immune response is adequate. The outcome is poor when therapy is delayed or when host response is inadequate.

Faix RG: Invasive neonatal candidiasis: comparison of albicans and parapsilosis infection. Pediatr Infect Dis J 1992;11:88.

Gigliotti F: Candida: A significant emerging nosocomial neonatal pathogen. Rep Pediatr Infect Dis 1995;5:40.

Nguyen MM et al: The changing face of candidemia: Emergence of non-*Candida albicans* species and antifungal resistance. Am J Med 1996;100:617.

Rex JH et al: A randomized trial comparing fluconazole with amphotericin B for the treatment of candidemia in patients without neutropenia. N Engl J Med 1994; 331:1325.

Stamos JK: Candidemia in a pediatric population. Clin Infect Dis 1995;20:571.

Swerdloff JN, Filler SG, Edwards JE Jr: Severe candidal infections in neutropenic patients. Clin Infect Dis 1993;17:S457.

COCCIDIOIDOMYCOSIS

Essentials of Diagnosis & Typical Features

- Residence in or travel to an endemic area.
- Primary pulmonary form: fever, chest pain, cough, anorexia, weight loss, and often a macular rash or erythema nodosum or multiforme.
- Primary cutaneous form: trauma followed in 1–3 weeks by an ulcer and regional adenopathy.
- Spherules seen in pus, sputum, cerebrospinal fluid, joint fluid; positive culture.
- Positive coccidioidin skin test.
- Appearance of precipitating and complement-fixing antibodies.

General Considerations

This disease is caused by the dimorphic fungus *Coccidioides immitis,* which is endemic in the Sonoran Desert areas of western and southern Texas, New Mexico, Arizona, southern California, northern Mexico, and South America. Infection results from inhalation or inoculation of arthrospores (highly contagious and readily airborne in the dry climate). Even brief travel in or through an endemic area, especially during windy seasons, may allow infection. Human-to-human transmission does not occur. More than half of all infections are asymptomatic, and fewer than 5% have significant pulmonary disease. Dissemination occurs in less than 1% of cases; the risk is much higher in Filipinos, Hispanics, and blacks, especially in older males.

Clinical Findings

A. Symptoms and Signs:

1. Primary disease–The incubation period is 10–16 days (range, 7–28 days). Symptoms vary from those of a mild fever and arthralgia to severe influenza-like illness with high fever, nonproductive cough, pleurisy, myalgias, arthralgias, headache, and anorexia. Upper respiratory tract signs are not common. Severe pleuritic chest pain suggests this diagnosis. Signs vary from none to rash, rales, pleural rubs, hilar adenopathy and signs of pulmonary consolidation. Weight loss may occur.

2. Skin disease–Up to 10% of children develop erythema nodosum or multiforme. These imply a favorable host response to the organism. Less specific maculopapular eruptions occur in a larger number of children. Skin lesions can occur following fungemia. Primary skin inoculation sites develop indurated ulcers with local adenopathy. Contiguous involvement of skin from deep infection in nodes or bone also occurs.

3. Chronic pulmonary disease–This is uncommon in children. Chronic disease is manifested by chronic cough (occasionally with hemoptysis), weight loss, pulmonary consolidation, effusion, cavitation, or pneumothorax.

4. Disseminated disease–This is less common in children than adults. It is more common in infants, neonates, pregnant women (especially during the third trimester), blacks, and Filipinos—or with HIV or any other type of immunosuppression. One or more organs may be involved. The most common sites involved are bone or joint (subacute or chronic swelling, pain, redness), nodes, meninges (slowly progressive meningeal signs, ataxia, vomiting, headache, cranial neuropathies), and kidney (dysuria, urinary frequency). As with most fungal diseases, the evolution of the illness is usually slow.

B. Laboratory Findings: Direct examination of respiratory secretions, pus, spinal fluid, or tissue may reveal large spherules (30–60 μm) containing endospores. These are the product of coccidioidal spores germinated in the lung. Phase-contrast microscopy is useful for demonstrating these refractile bodies; Gram or methylene blue stains are not helpful, but PAS, methenamine silver, and calcofluor stains are.

The fluffy, gray-white colonies grow within 2–5 days on routine fungal or other media. They are highly infectious. Spinal fluid cultures are often negative.

Routine laboratory tests are nonspecific. The sedimentation rate is usually elevated. Eosinophilia may occur, particularly prior to dissemination and is more common in coccidioidomycosis than in many other conditions with similar symptoms. Meningitis causes a mononuclear pleocytosis with elevated protein and mild hypoglycorrhachia.

Within 2–21 days, most patients develop a delayed hypersensitivity reaction to coccidioidin skin test antigen (Spherulin 0.1 mL, intradermally, should produce 5 mm induration at 48 hours). Erythema nodosum predicts strong reactivity; when this is present the antigen should be diluted 10–100 times before use. The skin test may be negative in compromised patients or those with disseminated disease. Positive reactions may remain for years and do not prove active infection.

Antibodies consist of precipitins (usually measurable by 2–3 weeks in 90% of cases and gone by 12 weeks) and complement-fixing antibodies (elevated by several weeks and gone by 8 months, unless dissemination occurs). The extent of the complement-fixing antibody response reflects the severity of infection. Persistent high levels suggest dissemination. Serum precipitins usually indicate acute infection. Excellent ELISA assays are now available to detect IgM and IgG antibodies against the precipitin and complement-fixing antigens. The presence of antibody in spinal fluid indicates central nervous system infection.

C. Imaging: Pulmonary consolidation, hilar adenopathy, effusion, thin-walled cavities, or solitary granulomas (coin lesions) may be seen. About 5% of infected people have asymptomatic nodules or cysts after recovery. Unlike reactivation tuberculosis, apical disease is not prominent. Bone infection causes osteolysis that enhances with technetium. Cerebral imaging may show hydrocephalus and meningitis; intracranial abscesses and calcifications are unusual. Radiographic evolution of all lesions is slow.

Differential Diagnosis

Primary pulmonary infection resembles acute viral, bacterial, or mycoplasmal infections; subacute presentation mimics tuberculosis, histoplasmosis, and blastomycosis. Chronic pulmonary or disseminated disease must be differentiated from cancer, tuberculosis, or other fungal infections.

Complications

Dissemination of primary pulmonary disease is associated with ethnic background, prolonged fever (> 1 month), a negative skin test, high complement fixation antibody titer, and marked hilar adenopathy. Local pulmonary complications include effusion, empyema, and pneumothorax. Cerebral infection can cause noncommunicating hydrocephalus due to basilar meningitis.

Treatment

A. Specific Measures: Mild pulmonary infections require no therapy. Antifungal therapy is used for prolonged fever, severe pneumonitis lasting 4–6 weeks, and mediastinal adenopathy, or any form of disseminated disease. Neonates, those with genetic risk factors, and those with high antibody titer are also treated.

Amphotericin B is used for severe disease (1 mg/kg/d until better; then reduce dose; total duration, 2–3 months). For less severe disease and for meningeal disease, fluconazole is preferred (duration of therapy is more than 6 months). Long-term suppressive therapy is likely to be required after treating coccidioidal meningitis. Refractory meningitis may require prolonged intrathecal or intraventricular amphotericin B therapy.

B. General Measures: Most pulmonary infections require only symptomatic therapy, self-limited activity, and good nutrition. They are not contagious. Secondary bacterial infection is unusual.

C. Surgical Measures: Excision of pulmonary cavities or abscesses may be needed. Infected nodes, sinus tracts, and bone are other operable lesions. Azole therapy should be given prior to surgery to prevent dissemination; it is continued for 4 weeks arbitrarily or until other criteria for cure are met.

Prognosis

Most patients recover. Even with amphotericin B, however, disseminated disease may be fatal, especially in those racially predisposed to severe disease. Reversion of the skin test to negative or a rising complement-fixing antibody titer is an ominous sign. Meningitis may require lifetime therapy to prevent progression or relapse.

Catanzaro A et al: Fluconazole in the treatment of chronic pulmonary and nonmeningeal disseminated coccidioidomycosis. Am J Med 1995;98:249.
Child DC et al: Radiologic findings of pulmonary coccidioidomycosis in neonates and infants. Am J Radiol 1989;145:261.
Galgiani JN et al: Fluconazole therapy for coccidioidal meningitis. Ann Int Med 1993;119:28.
Kafka JA, Catanzaro A: Disseminated coccidioidomycosis in children. J Pediatr 1981;98:355.
Maxson S, Jacobs RF: Community-acquired fungal pneumonia in children. Semin Respir Infect 1996;11:196.
Stevens DA: Coccidioidomycosis. N Engl J Med 1995; 332:1077.

CRYPTOCOCCOSIS

Essentials of Diagnosis & Typical Features

- Mainly a problem for immunosuppressed individuals.
- Meningitis: headache, vomiting, cranial nerve palsies, meningeal signs; mononuclear cell pleocytosis.
- Cryptococcal antigen detected in cerebrospinal fluid; also in serum and urine in some patients.
- Readily isolated on routine media.

General Considerations

Cryptococcus neoformans is a ubiquitous soil yeast. It appears to survive better in soil contaminated with bird excrement, especially that of pigeons. However, most human cases are not associated with a history of significant contact with birds. Inhalation is the presumed route of inoculation. Infections in children are quite rare, even in heavily immunocompromised patients such as those with HIV infection. Normal individuals can also be infected. Asymptomatic carriage is not seen.

Clinical Findings

A. Symptoms and Signs:

1. Meningitis–The most common clinical disease is meningitis, following hematogenous spread from a pulmonary focus. Symptoms of headache, vomiting, and fever occur over days to months. Meningeal signs and papilledema are common. Cranial nerve dysfunction and seizures may occur.

2. Pulmonary disease–Pulmonary infection precedes dissemination to other organs. It is frequently asymptomatic and less often clinically apparent than cryptococcal meningitis. Cryptococcal pneumonia may coexist with cerebral involvement. Symptoms are nonspecific and subacute—cough, weight loss, and fatigue. Radiographic findings are usually lower lobe infiltrates or nodular densities, less often effusions, and rarely cavitation, hilar adenopathy, or calcification.

3. Other forms–Cutaneous forms are usually secondary to dissemination. Papules, pustules, and ulcerating nodules are typical. Bones (rarely joints) may be infected; osteolytic areas are seen, and the process may resemble osteosarcoma. Many other organs can be involved with dissemination.

B. Laboratory Findings:
The spinal fluid usually has a lymphocytic pleocytosis; it may be completely normal in immunosuppressed patients with cryptococcal meningitis. Direct microscopy may reveal organisms in sputum, spinal fluid, or other specimens. The India ink stain demonstrates the capsules nicely, but it is insensitive; artifacts may give false-positive results. The capsular antigen can be detected by latex agglutination or enzyme immunoassay tests, which are both sensitive (> 90%) and specific. Serum, spinal fluid, and urine may be tested. False-negative cerebrospinal fluid tests have occurred. The organism grows well after several days on many routine media; for optimal culture, collecting and concentrating a large amount of spinal fluid (up to 10 mL) is recommended, because the number of organisms may be low.

Differential Diagnosis

Cryptococcal meningitis may mimic tuberculosis, viral meningoencephalitis, meningitis due to other fungi, or a space-occupying central nervous system lesion.

Complications

Hydrocephalus may occur from chronic basilar meningitis. Significant pulmonary or osseous disease may accompany the primary infection or dissemination.

Treatment

Amphotericin B (0.7 mg/kg) and flucytosine (100 mg/kg/d) are used for most systemic infections, including meningitis. The combination is synergistic and allows lower doses of amphotericin B to be used. Therapy is usually 6 weeks for cerebral infections (or for 1 month after sterilization) and 8 weeks for osteomyelitis. Fluconazole (400 mg/d) is an alternative therapy, which may be as efficacious in patients with AIDS. Combinations of fluconazole with flucytosine or amphotericin B are under investigation. Fluconazole (200 mg/d) is the preferred maintenance therapy to prevent relapses in high-risk patients. Relapses occur in up to 25–50% of meningitis cases, especially with continued immunosuppression. Antigen levels should be followed every few weeks to assess the response.

Prognosis

Treatment failure, including death, is common in immunosuppressed patients, especially those with AIDS. Lifelong maintenance therapy is required in these patients. Poor prognostic signs are the presence of extrameningeal disease; fewer than 20 cells/μL of initial cerebrospinal fluid; initial cerebrospinal fluid antigen titer greater than 1:32.

Dismukes WE: Management of cryptococcoses. Clin Infect Dis 1993;17(Suppl 2):S507.

Leggiadro RJ, Barrett FF, Hughes WT: Extrapulmonary cryptococcosis in immunocompromised infants and children. Pediatr Infect Dis J 1992;11:43.

Nelson MR, Fisher M: The role of azoles in the treatment and prophylaxis of cryptococcal disease in HIV infection. AIDS 1994;8:651.

Nightingale SD: Initial therapy for acquired immunodeficiency syndrome-associated cryptococcosis with fluconazole. Ann Intern Med 1995;155:538.

HISTOPLASMOSIS

Essentials of Diagnosis & Typical Features

- Residence in or travel to endemic areas.
- Pneumonia with flu-like illness.
- Hepatosplenomegaly, anemia, leukopenia.
- Positive skin test.
- Detection of the organism in smears or tissue or by culture.

General Considerations

The dimorphic fungus, *Histoplasma capsulatum*, is found in the central and eastern United States (Ohio and Mississippi River Valleys). The small yeast form (2–4 mm) is seen in tissue, especially within macrophages; the mycelial form is a slowly growing, fluffy, gray-white fungus. Endemic infections are very common at all ages and are usually asymptomatic. Over two-thirds of children are infected in endemic areas. Reactivation is very rare in children; it may occur years later, usually due to significant immunosuppression. Reinfection also occurs. Infection is acquired by inhaling spores that transform into the pathogenic yeast phase. Soil contamination is enhanced by the presence of bat or bird feces.

Clinical Findings

Because human-to-human transmission does not occur, infection requires exposure to the endemic area—usually within prior weeks or months. Congenital infection is not seen.

A. Symptoms and Signs:

1. Asymptomatic infection (50% of infections)–This is usually diagnosed by the presence of scattered calcifications in lungs or spleen and a positive skin test. The calcification may resemble that due to tuberculosis but may be more extensive than the usual Ghon complex.

2. Pneumonia–Approximately 45% of patients have mild to moderate disease. Most of these are not recognized as a histoplasmal infection. Acute pulmonary disease may resemble influenza, with fever, myalgia, arthralgia, and cough occurring 1–3 weeks after exposure; the subacute form resembles infections such as tuberculosis, with weight loss, night sweats, and pleurisy. Chronic disease is unusual in children. Physical examination may be normal, or rales may be heard. Mediastinal nodes may be greatly enlarged. Effusion is uncommon. A small number of patients may have immune-mediated signs such as arthritis, pericarditis, and erythema nodosum. The usual duration of the disease is less than 2 weeks, followed by complete resolution. Symptoms may last several months and still resolve without antifungal therapy.

3. Disseminated infection (5% of infections)–Fungemia during primary infection is probably common; transient hepatosplenomegaly may occur, but resolution is the rule in normal individuals. Heavy infection, severe pulmonary disease, and immunosuppression may be followed by progressive reticuloendothelial cell infection, with anemia, fever, weight loss, organomegaly, bone marrow involvement, and death. Dissemination may occur in otherwise normal children; usually they are less than 2 years of age.

4. Other–Ocular involvement consists of multifocal choroiditis. This is usually seen in normal adults with other evidence of disseminated disease. Brain, heart valve, pericardium, intestine, and skin (oral ulcers, nodules) are other involved sites. Adrenal gland involvement is common with systemic disease.

B. Laboratory Findings: Routine tests are normal or nonspecific in the benign forms. Pancytopenia is present in many cases of dissemination. The diagnosis can be made by demonstrating the organism by histology or culture. Tissue yeast forms are small and may be mistaken for artifact. They are usually found in macrophages, occasionally in peripheral blood leukocytes in severe disease, but rarely in sputum,

urine, or spinal fluid. Cultures of infected fluids or tissues may yield the organism after 1–6 weeks of incubation on fungal media, but even cultures of bronchoalveolar lavage or transbronchial biopsy specimens in immunocompromised patients are often negative. Thus, bone marrow and tissue specimens are needed. Detection of histoplasmal antigen in blood, urine, cerebrospinal fluid, and bronchoalveolar lavage is probably the most sensitive diagnostic test. The level of antigen correlates with the extent of the infection, and antigen levels can be used to follow the response to therapy and to indicate low-grade infection, which becomes apparent after completion of therapy (eg, in a child with HIV infection).

Antibodies may be detected by immunodiffusion, complement fixation, and precipitation; the latter two rise in the first few weeks of illness and fall unless dissemination occurs. A single high titer or rising titer indicates a high likelihood of disease. Antigen detection has replaced serology as a rapid diagnostic test. Skin test reactivity to the yeast phase is a sensitive test of infection, but it is not useful in endemic disease, and patients with disseminated disease often have a negative test. Some antigens may induce a serologic response that may invalidate the use of serology for diagnosis. Thus, skin tests play no role in the management of individual cases.

C. Imaging: Scattered pulmonary calcifications in a well child is typical of past infection. Bronchopneumonia (focal mid lung infiltrates) occurs with acute disease, often with hilar adenopathy, occasionally with nodules, but seldom with effusion or cavity formation.

Differential Diagnosis

Pulmonary disease resembles viral infection, tuberculosis, coccidioidomycosis, and blastomycosis. Systemic disease resembles disseminated fungal or mycobacterial infection or leukemia, histiocytosis, or cancer.

Treatment

Mild infections do not require therapy. Disseminated disease in infants may respond to as little as 10 days of amphotericin B, although 4–6 weeks (or 30 mg/kg total dose) is usually recommended. Amphotericin B is the preferred therapy for moderately severe forms of the disease. Surgical excision of chronic pulmonary lesions is rarely required. Itraconazole appears to be equivalent to amphotericin B therapy for mild disease and can be substituted for amphotericin B in severe disease after a favorable initial response has occurred. With chronic pulmonary or disseminated disease therapy may be required for prolonged periods.

Quantification of fungal antigen is useful for directing therapy. Chronically immunosuppressed patients (eg, those with HIV) may require lifelong maintenance therapy with an azole.

Prognosis

Mild infections have a good prognosis. With early diagnosis and treatment, infants with disseminated disease usually recover; the prognosis worsens if the immune response is poor.

Bradsher RW: Histoplasmosis and blastomycosis. Clin Infect Dis 1996;22(Suppl 2):S102.

Fojtasek MF et al: The *Histoplasma* capsulation antigen assay in disseminated histoplasmosis in children. Pediatr Infect Dis J 1994;13:801.

Leggiadro RJ, Barrett FF, Hughes WT: Disseminated histoplasmosis of infancy. Pediatr Infect Dis J 1988;7:799.

Wheat J: Histoplasmosis: Recognition and treatment. Clin Infect Dis 1994;19(Suppl 1):519.

Wheat J: Itraconazole: Treatment for disseminated histoplasmosis in patients with the acquired immuno-deficiency syndrome. Am J Med 1995;98:336.

PNEUMOCYSTIS CARINII INFECTION

Essentials of Diagnosis & Typical Features

- Significant immunosuppression.
- Fever, tachypnea, cough, dyspnea.
- Hypoxemia; diffuse interstitial infiltrates.

General Considerations

Although classified as a fungus on the basis of structural and nucleic acid characteristics, *Pneumocystis* responds readily to antiprotozoal drugs and antifols. It is a ubiquitous pathogen. Infection is presumed to occur via inhalation, usually in early childhood. With normal immune function, there is rarely any clinical disease. A syndrome of afebrile pneumonia similar to that caused by *Chlamydia trachomatis* in normal infants has been described but is rarely diagnosed. Organisms dormant in the lung may be reactivated in heavily immunosuppressed children, chiefly those with abnormal T cell function such as occurs with HIV infection and hematologic malignancies. Environmental exposure is also presumed to occur in immunocompromised children. Prolonged, high-dose corticosteroid therapy is a risk factor; onset of illness as steroids are tapered is a typical presentation. Severely malnourished infants with no underlying illness may also develop this infection, as can those with congenital humoral or cellular immune deficiency. The incubation period is usually at least a month after onset of immunosuppression.

Pneumocystis pneumonia is a common complication of advanced HIV infection and is one of the diseases that defines AIDS. Careful prophylaxis may prevent this infection (see Chapter 35).

Infection is generally limited to the lower respiratory tract. In advanced disease, spread to other organs occurs.

Clinical Findings:

A. Symptoms and Signs: In most patients with HIV infection there is a gradual onset of fever, tachypnea, dyspnea, and mild cough over 1–4 weeks. Initially, the chest is clear, although retractions and nasal flaring are present. At this stage, the illness is nonspecific. Hypoxemia out of proportion to the clinical and radiographic signs is an early finding, however, and even minimally decreased arterial PO_2 values should suggest this diagnosis in immunosuppressed children. Tachypnea, nonproductive cough, and dyspnea progress. Respiratory failure and death occur without treatment. In some children with AIDS or severe immunosuppression from chemotherapy or organ transplantation, the onset may be abrupt and progression more rapid.

The general examination is unremarkable. There are no upper respiratory signs, conjunctivitis, organomegaly, enanthem, or rash.

B. Laboratory Findings: These reflect the individual child's underlying illness and are not specific. Serum lactate dehydrogenase may be markedly elevated from pulmonary damage. In moderately severe cases, the PaO_2 is less than 70 mm Hg.

C. Imaging: Early chest radiographs are normal. The classic pattern in later films is that of bilateral, interstitial, lower lobe alveolar disease starting in the perihilar regions, without effusion, consolidation, or hilar adenopathy. Older HIV-infected patients may present with other patterns, including nodular infiltrates, lobar pneumonia, cavities, and upper lobe infiltrates—especially those receiving aerosolized pentamidine for prophylaxis.

Diagnosis

Diagnosis requires finding the round (6–8 μm) cysts in a lung biopsy specimen, bronchial brushings or alveolar washings, induced sputum, or tracheal aspirates. The latter specimens are less sensitive but are more rapidly and easily obtained. They are more often negative in children with leukemia compared to those with HIV infection; presumably, greater immunosuppression results in larger numbers of organisms. Since immunosuppressed patients may have many causes of pneumonia, negative results from tracheal secretions should prompt more aggressive diagnostic attempts. Bronchial washing using fiberoptic bronchoscopy is usually well tolerated and rapidly performed.

Several rapid stains—as well as the standard methenamine silver stain—are useful. The indirect fluorescent antibody method is most sensitive. All require competent laboratory evaluation, because few organisms may be present and there are many artifacts.

Differential Diagnosis

In normal infants, *Chlamydia trachomatis* and cytomegalovirus pneumonia are the most common causes of the afebrile pneumonia syndrome described for *Pneumocystis*. In older immunocompromised children, the differential diagnosis includes influenza, respiratory syncytial virus, adenovirus, and other viral infections; bacterial and fungal pneumonia; pulmonary emboli or hemorrhage; congestive heart failure; and *Chlamydia pneumoniae* and *Mycoplasma* pneumonia. Lymphoid interstitial pneumonitis, which is seen in older infants with HIV infection, is more indolent and the lactate dehydrogenase is normal (see Chapter 36). *Pneumocystis* pneumonia is uncommon in children who are complying with prophylactic regimens.

Prevention

Children at high risk of developing *Pneumocystis* infection should receive prophylactic therapy. This includes all with hematologic malignancies or other reasons for receiving intensive chemotherapy or high-dose corticosteroids and many children with organ transplants or advanced HIV infection. All children born to HIV-infected mothers should receive prophylaxis against *Pneumocystis* starting at 6 weeks of age. This should be maintained until the HIV infection status and immunologic status are clarified (see Chapter 35). The drug of choice is trimethoprim-sulfamethoxazole (5 mg/kg/d of trimethoprim and 25 mg/kg/d of sulfamethoxazole) for 3 consecutive days of each week.

Many patients with HIV infection have rashes and other adverse reactions that preclude use of sulfonamides. Intravenous pentamidine every 2–4 weeks is a substitute. Aerosolized pentamidine (300 mg per dose via a jet nebulizer) every 4 weeks is a less toxic alternative in older children. It is a lung irritant in some children. Breakthrough infections, particularly in the upper lobes, are seen much more commonly than with trimethoprim-sulfamethoxazole prophylaxis. Dapsone and atovaquone are alternative agents for prophylaxis.

Treatment

A. General Measures: Supplemental oxygen and nutritional support may be needed. Bronchodila-

tors may be tried but are usually not helpful. The patient should be in respiratory isolation.

B. Specific Measures: Trimethoprim-sulfamethoxazole (20 mg/kg/d of trimethoprim and 100 mg/kg of sulfamethoxazole in four divided doses intravenously or orally if well tolerated) is the drug of choice. Improvement may not be seen for 3–5 days. Duration of treatment is 3 weeks in HIV-infected children. Methylprednisolone (2–4 mg/kg/d in four divided doses intravenously) should also be given to HIV-infected patients with moderate to severe infection. If trimethoprim-sulfamethoxazole is not tolerated or there is no clinical response in 5 days, pentamidine isethionate (4 mg/kg once daily by slow intravenous infusion) should be given. Clinical efficacy is similar with pentamidine, but adverse reactions are more common. These include dysglycemias, pancreatitis, nephrotoxicity, and leukopenia. Other effective alternatives in adults include atovaquone, trimethoprim-dapsone, and primaquine plus clindamycin.

Prognosis

The mortality rate is high in immunosuppressed patients who are treated late in the illness.

Hughes WT: *Pneumocystis carinii* pneumonia. Rep Pediatr Infect Dis 1995;5:19.

Masur H: Prevention and treatment of pneumocystis pneumonia. N Engl J Med 1992;327:1853.

Sattler FR et al: Trimethoprim-sulfamethoxazole compared with pentamidine for treatment of *Pneumocystis carinii* pneumonia in the acquired immunodeficiency syndrome: A prospective, noncrossover study. Ann Intern Med 1988;109:280.

Simonds RJ: *Pneumocystis carinii* pneumonia among US children with perinatally acquired HIV infection. JAMA 1993;270:470.

Simonds RJ et al: Prophylaxis against *Pneumocystis carinii* pneumonia among children with perinatally acquired human immunodeficiency virus infection in the United States. N Engl J Med 1995;332:786.

Sleasman JW et al: Corticosteroids improve survival of children with AIDS and *Pneumocystis carinii* pneumonia. Am J Dis Child 1993;147(1):30–34.

REFERENCES

PARASITIC INFECTIONS

Drugs for parasitic infections. Med Lett Drugs Ther 1995;37:99.

Liu LY, Weller PF: Antiparasitic drugs. N Engl J Med 1996;334:1178.

MYCOTIC INFECTIONS

Barber GR et al: Catheter-related *Malassezia furfur* fungemia in immunocompromised patients. Am J Med 1993;95:365.

Cross JT Jr: Antifungal drugs. Pediatr Rev 1995;16:123.

Gallis HA et al: Amphotericin B: 30 years of clinical experience. Rev Infect Dis 1990;12:329.

Gupta AK et al: Antifungal agents: An overview. J Am Acad Dermatol 1994;30(Part I):677,30(Part II):911.

Kauffman CA: Newer developments in therapy for endemic mycoses. Clin Infect Dis 1994;19(Suppl): 528.

Marcon MJ, Powell DA: Human infections due to Malassezia spp. Clin Microbiol Rev 1992;5:101.

Systemic antifungal drugs. Med Lett Drugs Ther 1994; 36:11.

38

Sexually Transmitted Diseases

Eric J. Sigel, MD

The rate of sexually transmitted diseases (STDs) during adolescence continues to rise despite recent public health initiatives that encourage safer sex practices. By age 18 years, 56% of females and 76% of males have initiated sexual activity, and 25% will develop an STD—an estimated 3 million teenagers per year. Adolescents contract STDs at a higher rate than adults because of both sexual risk taking and biologic factors. Practitioners need to carefully screen sexually active adolescents for STDs and use this opportunity to discuss risk reduction.

ADOLESCENT SEXUALITY

Adolescents continue to engage in sexual activity despite the threat of the human immunodeficiency virus (HIV) infection. The average age of sexual debut has steadily declined, with about one-third of all teenagers having initiated sex by age 15. Sixty-six percent of 12th graders and 37% of 9th graders have initiated sexual activity. Racial differences exist, with 73% of African-Americans, 57% of Hispanics and 49% of Caucasians having had sex by the 12th grade. A small but significant number (9%) of preteens have also begun having intercourse, often imitating older siblings and modeling behavior suggested by the media. Condom use is sporadic, though increasing. Fifty-four percent of teens overall used a condom during their last intercourse in 1995 compared with 43% in 1993. Ninth graders are more likely to use a condom (63%) compared with 12th graders (50%). A significant number of teenagers engage in risk-taking sexual activity; 23% of seniors have had four or more sexual partners. One million teenagers become pregnant annually. Anal intercourse occurs in both heterosexual and homosexual populations. Up to 20% of Hispanic girls practice anal intercourse, often with the intent to preserve virginity.

Anywhere from 10% to 30% of males experiment with same-sex partners in some fashion, with 4–10% practicing anal sex. Teenage males often have their first homosexual experience with partners who are significantly older, which puts them at higher risk for STDs. Homosexual women often experiment with male partners during their teen years, placing them at risk for STDs.

Unsafe sexual experimentation sometimes is related to alcohol and drug inebriation; 82% of high school students have experimented with alcohol, whereas 50% of high school senior boys have been drunk in the last 30 days. Twenty-five percent of adolescents used alcohol or marijuana during their last sexual encounter, resulting in decreased condom use as well as an increased incidence of date rape.

RISK FACTORS

Certain behaviors and experiences put the adolescent at higher risk for developing STDs. Early age at sexual debut, lack of condom use, multiple partners, prior STD, history of STD in a partner, and having sex with a partner who is 3 or more years older are risk factors that predispose a teenager to an STD. Other risk-taking behaviors associated with STDs in adolescents are smoking, alcohol use, drug use, dropping out of school, and pregnancy. A thorough history will help elicit these risk factors.

The cervix of the adolescent female is predisposed to certain STDs, such as chlamydial infection, gonorrhea, and human papillomavirus infection. The columnar cells, which divide rapidly at the exposed squamocolumnar junction, are susceptible to infection. During early to mid puberty, this junction slowly invaginates as the uterus and cervix mature, and by the late teens to early 20s the columnar cells are inside the cervix, making it more difficult for organisms to attach.

PREVENTION

Primary prevention focuses largely on education and risk reduction techniques. Primary care providers need to discuss these as part of well adolescent check-ups. Although adolescents are aware of HIV, they may not have much information about other more common STDs. Discussing the prevalence, symptoms, and sequelae of STDs can raise awareness and help teenagers make informed decisions about whether to initiate sexual activity and about what kind of safer sex techniques they should use. Making condoms available reiterates the message that safe sex is vital to health, and this also facilitates safer sex practices.

Secondary prevention requires identifying patients with an STD (see Screening, below) and treating them before they infect others. Risk reduction and safer sex practices need to be discussed. Identifying partners is also essential in order to limit the continued spread of STDs. Working with the state or county health department proves valuable, since these agencies assume the responsibility for locating the contacts of infected persons and ensure appropriate treatment. Gonorrhea, syphilis, HIV, hepatitis B, and chancroid are reportable to government agencies.

Tertiary prevention is prevention of complications of a specific illness, such as treating pelvic inflammatory disease before infertility develops; following the serologic response to syphilis to ensure that secondary or neurosyphilis does not develop; treating cervicitis to prevent pelvic inflammatory disease; or treating a chlamydial infection before orchitis ensues.

SCREENING

Many STDs are asymptomatic; thus, a comprehensive approach to screening adolescents is essential. This begins during the interview; asking open-ended questions about sexual experience is essential. One must be explicit and make sure that the teen understands what is being asked. If the adolescent has ever engaged in sexual activity, the practitioner needs to determine what kind of sexual activity (mutual masturbation; oral, anal, or vaginal sex); whether it has been heterosexual, homosexual, or both; whether birth control devices or condoms were used; and whether sexual activity has been consensual or forced.

During the interview, while trying to assess the degree of risk, an opportunity should be taken to discuss risk reduction techniques. After the practitioner has determined that a patient has engaged in sex—or if the patient denies having had sex but is presenting with STD symptoms, or if a patient reports that a partner has an STD—a thorough clinical screening process is warranted.

For males, the first 10 mL of voided urine should be collected after not voiding for 2 hours. If results are positive for leukocyte esterase, urethritis is likely. Testing for gonorrhea (culture or nucleic acid amplification) and chlamydiae (nucleic acid amplification, culture, or ELISA) is necessary and can be done from spun urine or from a urethral swab. A patient

with urethritis needs evaluation for *Trichomonas*—a wet preparation for *Trichomonas* can be made from the spun urine or from urethral discharge. If high-risk behavior is present (three or more partners in the last 6 months, or more than two partners per year for several years), screening for hepatitis B surface antigen is warranted.

In communities with a high prevalence of hepatitis B, practitioners need to suspect hepatitis B even in patients who have received the hepatitis B vaccine since they may have contracted the infection before receiving the vaccine. A hepatitis B surface antigen test will detect either the carrier state or active infection.

In areas with a relatively high prevalence of syphilis (certain urban areas), an RPR or VDRL test (rapid plasma reagin/Venereal Disease Research Laboratory) should be drawn yearly. Screening for syphilis should be done in all cases in which any STD is present. HIV antibody should be evaluated in all high-risk patients and those requesting an HIV test.

For females, screening criteria for syphilis, hepatitis B, and HIV are the same as for males. Cervical culture for gonorrhea and nucleic acid amplification, culture, or ELISA for chlamydiae should be performed. A wet mount of the vaginal secretions should be performed to check for the presence of bacterial vaginosis and trichomoniasis. The Papanicolaou smear serves to evaluate the cervix for the presence of human papillomavirus. This should be done yearly for teenagers who are asymptomatic and in a monogamous relationship and for all females who are 18 years old. If a patient demonstrates high-risk sexual behavior or has frequent STDs, cervical cytology should be done every 6 months.

Orr DP: Urine based diagnosis of sexually transmitted infections using amplified DNA techniques: A shift in paradigms? J Adolesc Health 1997;20:3.

SYMPTOMS & SIGNS

For males, the most common symptom of an STD is urethritis, with dysuria and penile discharge. Less common symptoms are scrotal pain, hematuria, proctitis, and pruritus in the pubic region. Signs include epididymitis, orchitis, and urethral discharge. Rarely do males develop systemic symptoms.

For females, the most common symptoms are vaginal discharge and dysuria. Vaginal itching and irregular menses or spotting are also common. Abdominal pain, fever, and vomiting, though less common, are signs of pelvic inflammatory disease. Pain in the genital region and dyspareunia may also be present.

Manifestations that can be found in both males and females with an STD include ulcerations, adenopathy, pruritus, and genital warts.

THE SPECTRUM OF STDS

Treatment is summarized in Table 38–1.

CHLAMYDIA TRACHOMATIS INFECTION

Chlamydia trachomatis is the most common bacterial cause of STD, with 4 million cases annually. The highest prevalence and incidence (10–20%) occurs in the sexually active teenager; a recent study found chlamydiae to be present in a first-void urine specimen in 13% of asymptomatic adolescent females. *Chlamydia* is an obligate intracellular organism that is present without causing symptoms in 50% of cases. It presents most commonly as cervicitis but also causes proctitis, or pelvic inflammatory disease. The presence of mucopus at the cervical os (mucopurulent cervicitis) is a sign of chlamydial infection or gonorrhea. Nucleic acid amplification (polymerase or ligase chain reaction) is now recognized as the most sensitive (93–97%) way to detect chlamydial infection, though culture is still mandated for suspected sexual abuse cases. ELISA or direct fluorescence antibody tests are less sensitive but may be the only testing option in some centers.

A cervical sample should be obtained after the gonorrhea culture and the Papanicolaou test, using the manufacturer's swab provided with the specific test. If symptoms are present, a rectal specimen should be obtained. To optimize detection, columnar cells need to be collected by inserting the swab in the os and rotating it 360 degrees. Alternatively, nucleic acid testing of a first-voided urine sample has been approved and recognized as equivalent to endocervical testing, though this testing technique is just beginning to gain acceptance. Since mucopurulent cervicitis indicates either gonorrhea or chlamydial infection or both—and since 30% of patients have both infections—treatment for both is necessary.

In males, chlamydial infection may be asymptomatic or may be manifested as dysuria, urethritis, or epididymitis. Fifty percent may complain of urethral discharge, though an additional 30% have evidence of a discharge after milking the penis. The discharge is usually cloudy white. When urinary tract infection has been ruled out, all males with a discharge, pyuria or urethritis, or complaints of dysuria should be evaluated and treated for both gonorrhea and chlamydial infection. A thorough genital examination will disclose any evidence of epididymitis or orchitis. Reiter's syndrome is a complication of chlamydial urethritis, which should be suspected in males who are sexually active and present with low back pain (sacroiliitis), arthritis (polyarticular), and conjunctivitis.

The first-voided urine for leukocyte esterase is appropriate screening for asymptomatic sexually active males. This test has a high false-positive rate but is the easiest way of screening large numbers of patients. Examination of the urine sediment for white blood cells is similar in sensitivity but more labor-intensive. If either test is positive, a test for chlamydiae should be performed. Because of the false-positive rate of the screening test, patients should be told that there is a chance they have an STD and will need further evaluation.

Patients who are symptomatic and their asymptomatic contacts, regardless of physical signs, need to be treated. Evaluation of the symptomatic patient or the asymptomatic contact includes either a urethral swab inserted 2–4 cm and rotated 360 degrees or a swab of a spun sample of the first-voided urine sent for culture or PCR.

Biro FM et al: A comparison of diagnostic methods in adolescent girls with and without symptoms of *Chlamydia* urogenital infection. Pediatrics 1994;93:476.

Recommendations for prevention and management of *Chlamydia trachomatis* infections. MMWR Morb Mortal Wkly Rep 1998;47(RR-1):1.

Shafer MA et al: Evaluation of urine-based screening strategies to detect *Chlamydia trachomatis* among sexually active asymptomatic young males. JAMA 1993; 270:2065.

NEISSERIA GONORRHOEAE INFECTION

Gonorrhea is the second most prevalent bacterial STD—117 of 100,000 adolescent females and 954 of 100,000 adolescent males report having had gonorrhea. Rates of gonorrhea have steadily declined, from nearly 1 million infections in 1985 to 350,000 in 1995. Sites of infection include the cervix, urethra, rectum, and pharynx. Gonorrhea is also a cause of pelvic inflammatory disease. In uncomplicated gonococcal cervicitis, females are symptomatic 57% of the time, presenting with vaginal discharge and dysuria. Urethritis and pyuria may be present. Mucopurulent cervicitis with a yellowish discharge may be found on examination. The cervical swab should be cultured on Thayer-Martin agar. Gram's stain of the cervical discharge is not used as a diagnostic tool because nongonococcal *Neisseria* species reside in the vagina, confounding the interpretation of the stain. DNA probes to test for gonorrhea have recently been developed and can be performed on endocervical samples as well as on urine samples but are not readily available in all laboratories. If mucopurulent cervicitis is present, the patient should be treated presumptively for gonorrhea and chlamydial infection.

Ninety-five percent of males with gonorrhea are symptomatic, with a yellowish-green urethral discharge and burning on urination. Culture confirmation

Table 38–1. Treatment regimens for sexually transmitted diseases.[1,2]
(**Note:** Alternative regimens are not as effective but are clinically useful if the recommended regimens cannot be used owing
to allergy or pregnancy.)

Disease	Recommended Regimens	Pregnancy
Gonorrhea, uncomplicated		
Cervicitis, urethritis proctitis	Cefixime, 400 mg PO as single dose	Safe
	or	
	Ofloxacin, 400 mg PO as single dose	Contraindicated
	or	
	Ciprofloxacin, 500 mg PO as single dose	Safe
	or	
	Ceftriaxone, 125 mg IM as single dose	Safe
	plus	
	Azithromycin, 1 g PO bid for 7 days	Safe
	or	
	Azithromycin, 2 g PO as single dose	Safe
	or	
	Doxycycline, 100 mg PO bid for 7 days	Contraindicated
Pharyngitis	As above, except that cefixime is not effective	
Epididymitis	Ceftriaxone, 250 mg IM	
Gonorrhea, disseminated	Ceftriaxone, 1 g IV every 24 hours	Safe
	or	
	Cefotaxime, 1 g IV every 8 hours or ceftizoxime, 1 g IV every 8 hours, or ciprofloxacin, 500 mg IV every 8 hours until clinically improved (usually about 48 hours, then switch to oral dosing followed by completion of 10-day course with–	Safe
	Cefixime, 400 mg PO BID	Safe
	or	
	Ciprofloxacin, 500 mg PO bid	Contraindicated
***Chlamydia trachomatis* infection**		
Cervicitis/urethritis	Azithromycin, 1 g PO in a single dose	Safe
	or	
	Doxycycline, 100 mg PO bid for 7 days	Contraindicated
Alternative regimen	Erythromycin, 500 mg PO qid for 7 days	Safe
	or	
	Ofloxacin, 300 mg PO bid for 7 days	Contraindicated
Epididymitis	Doxycycline, 100 mg PO bid for 7 days	
	or	
	Azithromycin, 1 g PO as single dose	
Nongonococcal, nonchlamydial urethritis (male)		
	Doxycycline, 100 mg PO bid for 7 days	
	or	
	Azithromycin, 1 g PO once if no response to doxycycline	
	or	
	Erythromycin, 500 mg PO qid for 7 days	
***Trichomonas vaginalis* infection**		
Vaginitis, urethritis	Metronidazole, 2 g PO as single dose	Contraindicated in first trimester
	or	
	Metronidazole, 500 mg PO bid for 7 days	Contraindicated
Bacterial vaginosis	Metronidazole, 2 g PO in a single dose	Contraindicated in the first trimester
	or	
	Metronidazole, 500 mg PO bid for 7 days	Contraindicated
	or	
	Clindamycin cream, 2%, one full applicator intravaginally at night for 7 days	Safe
	or	
	Metronidazole, 0.75% gel, 5 g intravaginally bid for 5 days	Contraindicated
Syphilis		

Early (primary, secondary, or latent less than 1 year)	Benzathine penicillin G
	  Patients < 40 kg: 50,000 units/kg IM
	  Patients > 40 kg: 2.4 million units IM
		Safe

Alternative Regimen	Doxycycline, 100 mg PO bid for 14 days	Contraindicated

(continued)

Table 38–1. Treatment regimens for sexually transmitted diseases.[1,2]
(**Note:** Alternative regimens are not as effective but are clinically useful if the recommended regimens cannot be used owing to allergy or pregnancy.) (continued)

Disease	Recommended Regimens	Pregnancy
Late (more than 1 year)	Benzathine penicillin G Patients < 40 kg: 50,000 units/kg IM once weekly for 3 consecutive weeks Patients > 40 kg: 2.4 million units IM once weekly for 3 consecutive weeks	Safe
Chancroid	Azithromycin, 1 g PO once	Safe
	or	
	Ceftriaxone 250 mg IM once	Safe
	or	
	Erythromycin 500 mg PO qid for 7 days	Safe
	or	
	Ciprofloxacin, 500 mg PO bid daily for 3 days	Contraindicated
Herpes Simplex First episode genital	Acyclovir, 400 mg PO tid for 7 days	Safe
	or	
	Famciclovir, 250 mg PO tid for 7–10 days	No experience in pregnancy
	or	
	Valacyclovir, 1 g PO bid for 7–10 days.	
First episode proctitis	Acyclovir, 400 mg PO 5 times daily for 7–10 days	Safe
Recurrent	Acyclovir, 400 mg PO tid for 5 days	Safe
	or	
	Famciclovir, 125 mg PO bid for 5 days	No experience in pregnancy
	or	
	Valacyclovir, 500 mg PO bid for 5 days	Safe
Suppression	Acyclovir, 400 mg PO bid	Safe
	or	
	Famciclovir, 250 mg PO bid	No experience in pregnancy
	or	
	Valacyclovir, 500 mg PO daily (if ≤ nine recurrence per year; if ≥ 9 recurrences per year, use 1 g daily)	Safe
Human papillomavirus infection External lesions (penile, vulvar) and intravaginal lesions, uncomplicated	Podophyllum resin, 25% in benzoin tincture, applied directly to warts and washed off in 1–4 hours	Contraindicated
	or	
	Trichloroacetic acid (85%) applied directly to warts and washed off in 6–8 hours	Safe
	or	
	Podofilox, 0.5% solution, applied twice daily for 3 days. Used by the patient at home. Practitioner needs to demonstrate how compound is applied. (To be used only on external lesions.)	Contraindicated
	or	
	Imiquimod, 5% cream, applied by patient 3 times a week at night for up to 16 weeks	Contraindicated
	or	
	Cryotherapy: liquid nitrogen, cryoprobe	Safe
	Note: Topical therapies usually require weekly treatments for 4 consecutive weeks. If patients fail to respond, alternative therapies by experienced clinicians include electrocautery (safe), electrodesiccation (safe), and intralesional interferon alfa (contraindicated).	
Cervical lesions	Laser therapy, cryotherapy, or trichloroacetic acid (85%)	Safe
	or	
	Podophyllum resin, 25% in benzoin tincture; applied only by experienced practitioners	Contraindicated
Arthropod infections Pediculosis pubis	Lindane 1% shampoo applied for 4 minutes, then washed off	Contraindicated
	or	
	Permethrin 1% cream rinse, washed off after 10 minutes	Safe
	Note: Bedding and clothing need to be decontaminated by washing in hot water or by dry-cleaning. Regimen may be repeated in 1 week if complete response is not achieved.	

(continued)

Table 38–1. Treatment regimens for sexually transmitted diseases.[1,2]
(***Note:*** Alternative regimens are not as effective but are clinically useful if the recommended regimens cannot be used owing to allergy or pregnancy.) (continued)

Disease	Recommended Regimens	Pregnancy
Scabies	Permethrin cream 5% applied to entire body from the neck down and washed off in 8–12 hours or Lindane 1%, 1 oz lotion or 30 g cream, applied thinly to all areas of the body from the neck down and washed off in 8 hours.	Safe Contraindicated
	Note: Bedding and clothing need to be decontaminated as outlined above. Re-treatment may be necessary in 1 week.	
Pelvic inflammatory disease Inpatient therapy	**Regimen A** Cefoxitin, 2 g IV every 6 hours or Cefotetan, 2 g IV every 12 hours plus Doxycycline, 100 mg PO or IV every 12 hours	 Safe Safe Contraindicated[3]
	Note: Once clinically improved for 48 hours, patients can be discharged and continue doxycycline, 100 mg bid for 14 days total.[3]	
	Regimen B Clindamycin, 900 mg IV every 8 hours plus Gentamicin, 2 mg/kg IV as loading dose, then 1.5 mg/kg IV every 8 hours	 Safe Safe
	Note: Once clinically improved for 48 hours, patients can be discharged and continue doxycycline, 100 mg PO bid for 14 days total.[3]	
Outpatient therapy	***Note:*** Pregnant patients with PID should be hospitalized and treated with parenteral antibiotics. **Regimen A** Ceftriaxone, 250 mg IM once or Cefoxitin, 2 g IM once plus Probenecid, 1 g PO plus Doxycycline, 100 mg PO bid for 14 days **Regimen B** Ofloxacin, 400 mg PO bid for 14 days plus Metronidazole, 500 mg PO bid for 14 days	 Safe Safe Contraindicated[3] Contraindicated

[1]Adapted from 1998 sexually transmitted treatment guidelines. MMWR Morb Mortal Wkly Rep 1998;42(RR-1):1.
[2]Intravenous or intramuscular therapy should be continued for 24–48 hours after the patient has improved and can then be switched to either oral regimen to complete a 7-day course.
[3]During pregnancy, treat for chlamydial infection with azithromycin, 1 g PO, or erythromycin, 500 mg PO, qid for 7 days.

of gonorrhea can be achieved with a swab of the urethra or urine sediment plated on Thayer-Martin agar. Gram's stain of the discharge showing gram-negative intracellular diplococci indicates gonorrhea. Rarely does gonorrhea cause systemic symptoms in males.

Both males and females can develop proctitis and pharyngitis. If proctitis is present, appropriate cultures should be obtained and treatment administered for both gonorrhea and chlamydial infection. In the case of pharyngitis, streptococcal infection and infectious mononucleosis should be ruled out. If the history is strongly suggestive of oral sex exposure, the patient should be cultured and empirically treated for

gonorrhea. Otherwise, it is appropriate to await culture results (24–48 hours).

Disseminated gonococcal infection occurs in a minority (0.5–3%) of patients with untreated gonorrhea. Hematogenous spread can lead directly to systemic symptoms, most commonly arthritis and dermatitis. Joints most frequently involved are the wrists, the metacarpophalangeal joints, the knees, and the ankles. Skin lesions are typically tender necrotic pustules on an erythematous base occurring on the distal extremities. Disseminated disease occurs more frequently in women, and risk factors include pregnancy and gonococcal pharyngitis. Treatment requires hospitalization.

Test of cure is considered only for patients who remain symptomatic.

NONGONOCOCCAL NONCHLAMYDIAL URETHRITIS

About 15% of males with urethritis have cultures negative for *Neisseria gonorrhoeae* and *Chlamydia trachomatis* but continue to have symptoms despite empiric treatment for infection with these organisms. *Ureaplasma urealyticum* has been identified as a causative organism in urethritis. Routine culture is not done, but studies have shown an increased detection of *U urealyticum* in a first-voided urine specimen. Other organisms that have been implicated but not definitively proved to cause urethritis are *Mycoplasma* species and *Bacteroides ureolyticus*. Coliforms may cause urethritis in males practicing anal intercourse.

A patient with urethritis needs to be evaluated for gonorrhea, chlamydial infection, and trichomoniasis infection. If negative for *Trichomonas,* empiric therapy is given for gonorrhea and chlamydial infection. If symptoms persist after adequate therapy and cultures are negative, then nongonococcal, nonchlamydial urethritis (NGU) should be assumed and treated presumptively.

Stamm WE et al: Azithromycin for empirical treatment of the nongonococcal urethritis syndrome in men: A randomized double blind study. JAMA 1995;274:545.

TRICHOMONAS VAGINALIS INFECTION

Trichomonas vaginalis is a flagellated protozoan that infects 2.5–3 million people annually. Fifty percent of females with *Trichomonas* infection develop a symptomatic vaginitis with vaginal itching, a green-gray, malodorous frothy discharge, and dysuria. Occasionally, postcoital bleeding and dyspareunia may be present. The vulva may be erythematous, with evidence of a discharge. The cervix may be friable. Vaginitis is the most common manifestation of trichomoniasis; rarely does pelvic inflammatory disease result from *Trichomonas* infection. Wet preparation—mixing the discharge with normal saline—permits the flagellated protozoan to be seen on microscopic examination. Seventy-five percent of symptomatic and 64% of asymptomatic patients who have documented trichomoniasis by culture will have a positive wet preparation. This infection also may be detected by the pathologist when reviewing the Papanicolaou smear. Culture and antigen detection are more sensitive (more than 95% and 80–90%, respectively), but these procedures are expensive and not readily available.

Males with urethral discharge should be evaluated for trichomoniasis since 11% have the infection. Almost 50% of males with *Trichomonas* infection have a discharge, typically cloudy white, without being coinfected with other organisms. *Trichomonas* urethritis is frequently associated with a positive urine leukocyte esterase test or the presence of white blood cells on urethral smear. A wet preparation permits detection of the trichomonad. Male partners of females diagnosed with trichomoniasis have a 22% chance of having the infection. Treatment is necessary for the symptomatic person as well as an asymptomatic contact.

Krieger JN: Trichomoniasis in men: Old issues and new data. Sex Transm Dis 1995;22:83.
Wolner-Hanssen P et al: Clinical manifestations of vaginal trichomoniasis. JAMA 1989;261:571.

BACTERIAL VAGINOSIS

Women typically develop bacterial vaginosis after an alteration in normal vaginal flora. A decrease in the number of lactobacilli, the predominant bacteria that reside normally in the vagina, is associated with an overgrowth of *Gardnerella vaginalis, Bacteroides* species, *Mobiluncus* species, or genital mycoplasmas. It is unclear whether bacterial vaginosis is sexually transmitted. The presenting symptom is a malodorous vaginal discharge, though 50% of patients are asymptomatic. Patients may report vaginal itching or dysuria. Risk factors for developing bacterial vaginosis include frequent sexual activity, multiple partners, uncircumcised partners, prior STDs, low socioeconomic status, use of an intrauterine device, and smoking. Diagnosis can be made by finding three of the four following features: presence of a malodorous ("fishy") vaginal discharge, vaginal pH higher than 4.5, a positive "whiff" test (mixing the discharge with potassium hydroxide releases an amine or fishy odor), and 20% of squamous cells positive for clue cells on wet preparation. Clue cells are squamous epithelial cells that have multiple bacteria adhering to them, making their borders irregular and giving them a speckled appearance.

Whether to treat patients who do not complain of vaginal discharge or itching but demonstrate bacterial vaginosis on routine pelvic examination is a matter of debate. Some studies associate bacterial vaginosis and pelvic inflammatory disease. Because of this relationship, the recommendation is to have a low threshold for treating bacterial vaginosis in the asymptomatic patient.

Joesoef MR, Schmid GP: Bacterial vaginosis: Review of treatment options and potential clinical indications for therapy. Clin Infect Dis 1995;20(Suppl 1):S72.
Thomason JL: Bacterial vaginosis: Current review with in-

dications for asymptomatic therapy. Am J Obstet Gynecol 1991;165:1210.

GENITAL ULCERATIONS

A variety of microorganisms—bacterial and viral—cause sexually transmitted genital ulcers. A careful history, physical examination, and appropriate laboratory tests contribute to making the correct diagnosis. Associated pain, adenopathy (nature and duration), a history of recurrence, the number of lesions, and the presence of systemic symptoms are differential points, as is the exposure history.

HERPES SIMPLEX

Herpes simplex virus (HSV) is the most common cause of visible genital lesions. An estimated 30 million people are infected in the United States. As with oral HSV infections, many primary genital infections are asymptomatic or not recognizable as herpetic in origin. Symptomatic initial HSV infection causes vesicles of the external genitalia, quickly followed by painful shallow ulcerations. These may occur in the vulva, vagina, penis, rectum, and urethra. Atypical presentation of herpes infection includes vulvar erythema and fissures. Urethritis may occur. Initial infection can be severe, lasting up to 3 weeks and may be associated with fever and malaise as well as localized tender adenopathy. The pain and dysuria can be extremely uncomfortable, requiring sitz baths, topical anesthetics, and occasionally catheterization for urinary retention.

HSV type 2 is the most common cause of genital herpes (80–90%). Symptoms tend to be more severe in females. Viral meningitis occurs in 10–20% of females with primary genital herpes. Recurrence in the genital area with HSV-2 is likely (65–80%). Recurrent genital herpes is of shorter duration (7–10 days), with a smaller number of lesions and usually no systemic symptoms. Prodromal pain in the genital, buttock, or pelvic region is common prior to recurrences.

Diagnosis of genital herpes is often made presumptively. Culture of the vesicles confirms the diagnosis; recurrent attacks are suggestive. Acyclovir, valacyclovir, or famciclovir administered within the first 5 days of primary infection decreases the duration and severity of HSV infection. The effect of antivirals on the severity or duration of recurrent disease is limited. For best results, therapy should be started with the prodrome or during the first day of the attack (patient has medicine at home). If recur-

rences are frequent and cause significant physical or emotional discomfort, patients can take antiviral prophylaxis on a daily basis for suppression to reduce the number and duration of recurrences.

HSV type 1, which accounts for 10–20% of genital herpes infections, is usually the consequence of oral-genital sex. Primary infection is as severe as with HSV type 2, and treatment is the same. However, this virus is much less often associated with recurrent disease. Thus, determining the type of virus can be useful for prognosis.

Any genital ulcer should be cultured for HSV and differentiated from syphilis and chancroid ulcers. HSV is distinguished from syphilis by the pain associated with the ulcerations. All patients with active lesions should be counseled to abstain from sexual contact. Because most patients have periodic asymptomatic shedding of HSV—an important source of the current epidemic—herpes-infected individuals should be encouraged to use condoms to protect susceptible partners.

Barton SE et al: Asymptomatic shedding of herpes simplex virus from the genital tract: Uncertainty and its consequences for patient management. The Herpes Simplex Advisory Panel. Int J STD AIDS 1996;7:229.

Koutsky LA et al: Underdiagnosis of genital herpes by current clinical and viral isolation procedures. N Engl J Med 1992;326:1533.

Lavoie SR, Kaplowitz L: Management of genital herpes infection. Semin Dermatol 1994;13:248.

Mertz G: Epidemiology of genital herpes infections. Infect Dis Clin North Am 1993;7:825.

SYPHILIS

The incidence of syphilis had risen steadily from the 1940s to 1991, when approximately 50,000 people were infected with either primary or secondary syphilis. The rate of syphilis has steadily declined since its peak, infecting only 15,000 in 1995—a rate about the same as in 1960. Although the absolute number of patients with syphilis has declined, incidence in the teen population is third highest of all age groups, with 10–12% of all syphilis occurring in adolescence and poor urban teenagers being the most susceptible.

Primary syphilis presents as a chancre—a painless ulcer with an indurated base—usually solitary, with associated nontender, firm adenopathy. The chancre appears 10–90 days after exposure and spontaneously resolves 4–8 weeks later. Since it is painless it may go undetected, especially if the lesion is within the vagina. Chancres may occur on the genitalia, lips, or anus. Secondary syphilis occurs 4–10 weeks after the chancre appears, presenting with generalized malaise, adenopathy, and a nonpruritic maculopapular rash that may include the palms and soles. Secondary syphilis resolves in 1–3 months but can recur. Verrucous lesions known as condylomata lata may develop on the genitalia. These must be distinguished from genital warts.

If the patient has a lesion, is at high risk, or is a contact—or if secondary syphilis is suspected—a nontreponemal serum screen, either RPR or VDRL, should be drawn. If the nontreponemal test is positive, then a specific treponemal test, FTA-ABS or MHA-TP, is done to confirm the diagnosis. Titers from the RPR or VDRL are used to evaluate the severity of infection and are repeated at 3, 6, and 12 months to ensure that they fall at least fourfold as a measure of therapeutic response. If the response is not adequate, re-treatment is necessary. An additional diagnostic tool is darkfield microscopy, which can be used to detect spirochetes in scrapings from the base of the chancre.

If a patient is engaging in high-risk sexual behavior or is living in an urban area in which syphilis is endemic, yearly RPRs should be drawn to screen for asymptomatic infections.

Syphilis is reportable to all state health departments, and all contacts need to be evaluated. Patients also need to be evaluated for other STDs, including HIV.

Untreated syphilis can lead to serious complications such as tertiary syphilis, which can in turn lead to serious multiorgan involvement including aortitis and neurosyphilis. Transmission to the fetus can occur from an untreated pregnant woman with syphilis. (See also Chapter 36.)

Martin DH, DiCarlo RP: Recent changes in the epidemiology of genital ulcer disease in the United States: The crack cocaine connection. Sex Transm Dis 1994;21(2 Suppl):S76.

CHANCROID

Chancroid is a relatively rare ulceration caused by *Haemophilus ducreyi.* It is endemic in many urban areas and has been associated with HIV infection, drug use, and prostitution. Ten percent of patients with *H ducreyi* are coinfected with HSV or syphilis. Typically, the lesion begins as a papule and after 24–48 hours erodes into an ulcer, which has ragged, sharply demarcated edges and a purulent base. The ulcer is painful, solitary, and somewhat deeper than HSV infection. Tender fluctuant inguinal adenopathy is usually present. Chancroid is distinguished from syphilis by the painful nature of the ulcer and the associated tender adenopathy. Diagnosis of chancroid is made by ruling out the aforementioned infections and by Gram's stain showing gram-positive cocci arranged in a boxcar formation. Culture can be performed, but the test is not usually available.

After treatment, symptoms improve within 3 days.

Most ulcers resolve in 7 days, though large ulcers may take 2 weeks to heal. All sexual contacts need to be examined and treated even if asymptomatic.

Joseph AK, Rosen T: Laboratory techniques used in the diagnosis of chancroid, granuloma inguinale, and lymphogranuloma venereum. Dermatol Clin 1994;12:1.
Morse SA: Chancroid and *Haemophilus ducreyi.* Clin Microbiol Rev 1989;2:137.

OTHER ULCERATIONS

Lymphogranuloma venereum (LGV), caused by *Chlamydia trachomatis* serovars L1, L2, or L3, is rare in the United States. It presents as a painless vesicle or ulcer that heals spontaneously, followed by development of tender adenopathy, either unilateral or bilateral. A classic finding is the "groove sign"—a crease that forms due to concomitant involvement of inguinal and femoral nodes, which become matted and fluctuant and may rupture. LGV can cause proctocolitis, fistulas, and strictures in those patients with anal involvement. Diagnosis can be made by culturing a node aspirate for *Chlamydia.* Differential diagnosis during the adenopathy phase includes bacterial adenitis, lymphoma, and cat-scratch disease. The differential during the ulcerative phase encompasses all the genital ulcers. Treatment is with doxycycline, 100 mg twice daily for 21 days.

Granuloma inguinale is caused by *Calymmatobacterium granulomatis,* a gram-negative bacillus that is also rare in the United States. An indurated subcutaneous nodule erodes to form a painless, friable ulcer with granulation tissue. Diagnosis is made by clinical suspicion and supported by a Wright- or Giemsa-stained smear of the granulation tissue that reveals intracytoplasmic rods (Donovan bodies) in mononuclear cells. Treatment is with tetracycline, 500 mg four times daily for 2–3 weeks.

Goens JL et al: Mucocutaneous manifestations of chancroid, lymphogranuloma venereum and granuloma inguinale. Am Fam Physician 1994;49:415.
Mroczkowski TF, Martin DH: Genital ulcer disease. Dermatol Clin 1994;12:753.

GENITAL WARTS

Condylomata acuminata, or genital warts, is caused by the human papillomavirus (HPV). Genital warts are the most common STD: 12–40 million people are estimated to be infected. There are multiple serotypes of HPV. Types 6 and 11 are detected most frequently, whereas 16 and 18 are most commonly implicated in the etiology of cervical dysplasia. The infection is more common in persons with multiple sex partners and in women who have previously had an abnormal Papanicolaou smear. HPV is relatively more common in the adolescent population—the exposed and actively dividing cells of the cervical transition zone make teenagers more susceptible. The infection is usually asymptomatic in women and is often detected by cytology or by physical examination. Females may develop verrucous lesions on any genital mucosal surface. Lesions typically are fleshy, soft, and vascular. They can be flat or papular and solitary or clustered, and may range in size from microscopic to several centimeters in diameter. Visible, external lesions and internal vaginal lesions can be treated topically. Internal and cervical lesions should be treated by an experienced practitioner.

If a Papanicolaou smear shows signs of inflammation only and there is concomitant infection such as vaginitis or cervicitis, the smear should be repeated after the infection has cleared. Abnormal findings range from atypical squamous cells of undetermined significance to high-grade squamous interepithelial lesions. Follow-up for atypical cells is controversial, as 25% progress to dysplasia, while the remainder either regress or demonstrate no progression; general recommendations are to repeat Papanicolaou smears in 3–6 months. If the presence of atypical cells persists or if low-grade or high-grade squamous interepithelial lesions are detected, referral for colposcopy is necessary to determine the presence of dysplasia and for treatment if indicated.

HPV is transmitted sexually; 30–60% of males whose partners have HPV have some evidence of genital warts on examination. Verrucous lesions may be found on the shaft or corona of the penis. Lesions may develop also in the urethra or rectum. Condylomata acuminata can be distinguished from condylomas lata (syphilis), skin tags, and molluscum contagiosum by application of 5% acetic acid solution. HPV lesions turn white. Microscopic lesions can be detected by wrapping the penis in gauze soaked with acetic acid. After 5 minutes, one may be able to detect small white papules, which represent HPV. All penile lesions need to be treated topically, and both males and females need weekly treatment for 4 consecutive weeks to clear the infection. If the lesions do not resolve, referral to a dermatologist or gynecologist is necessary. Insistence on condom use is essential to prevent the continued spread of HPV.

Baken L et al: Genital human papillomavirus infection among male and female sex partners: Prevalence and type-specific concordance. J Infect Dis 1995;171:429.

Eltabakh GH: Value of wet mount and cervical cultures at the time of cervical cytology in asymptomatic women. Obstet Gynecol 1995;85:499.

Gutman LT: Human papillomavirus infections of the genital tract in adolescents. Adolescent Medicine: State of the Art Reviews 1995;6:115.

OTHER VIRAL INFECTIONS

HEPATITIS B & C

Hepatitis B and hepatitis C are often sexually transmitted infections. Hepatitis B is at least ten times more common than HIV in the adolescent population. It was the first STD to be prevented by immunization—and, since the sequelae of HBV include hepatocellular carcinoma—the first instance of a malignant neoplasm that can be prevented by immunization. Symptoms, diagnosis, and treatment are described in Chapter 20. Since HBV is an important STD in adolescents, high-risk teenagers need to be screened for HBV (see Screening, above). If HBsAg-positive, follow up to determine persistence of infection and hepatitis needs to be done.

Hepatitis C generally is transmitted through blood products and by the sharing of intravenous needles, though about 10% of infections has been linked to sexual transmission. Hepatitis C needs to be considered in teenagers who are symptomatic and have demonstrated high-risk sexual behavior or intravenous drug use.

Nowicki MJ, Baliestreri WF: Viral hepatitis. Principles Pract Pediatr Updates 1993;1(4):1.

Thomas D et al: Hepatitis C, hepatitis B and human immunodeficiency virus infections among non-intravenous drug using patients attending clinics for sexually transmitted diseases. J Infect Dis 1994;169:990.

HUMAN IMMUNODEFICIENCY VIRUS INFECTION

AIDS is the sixth leading cause of death among persons 15–24 years of age in the USA. Although the incidence in the teen population is relatively small—2754 cases in 1996, representing less than 1% of the overall AIDS rate—the numbers of people in their 20s with AIDS infection is substantial, with approximately 100,000 documented cases. Because of the long latency period between infection with HIV and progression to AIDS, it is believed that many HIV-positive young adults contracted HIV during adolescence. Blinded seroprevalence studies in certain urban areas show that 1% of teens and 2.7% of young adults are HIV-positive.

Risk factors for HIV infection include a prior STD, infrequent condom use, practicing both active and receptive anal sex (both males and females), practicing survival sex (trading sex for money or drugs), intravenous drug use or using crack cocaine, homelessness, and being the victim of sexual abuse (males). The number of females who are becoming HIV-positive has increased dramatically, representing 37% of teenagers with HIV. HIV infection should be considered in all young people who practice unsafe sex, whether it be heterosexual or homosexual.

Screening for HIV is indicated for risk-taking young people and those with any STD. Adolescents may also come requesting an HIV test. In either case, a careful history of sexual behavior should be obtained to assess risk and offer risk reduction counseling. It is necessary also to determine how teens may respond to being told they are HIV-positive and what support systems they have in place. If the adolescent is homeless; does not have emotional support from family, friends, or a counselor; or threatens suicide or homicide in response to the idea of being HIV-positive, testing should be deferred until the practitioner is confident that the youth will be safe if the test is positive.

If a patient has experienced a recent high-risk exposure, one should consider initiating prophylactic therapy. Antiretroviral therapy with a two-drug or three-drug regimen should be started—ideally within 2 hours after exposure, but might be started up to 2 weeks after exposure. Antivirals used in prophylaxis include AZT, 3TC, and indinavir. Guidelines can be found in the 1997 *Redbook.* An HIV PCR should be done 3 weeks postexposure—if negative, prophylactic therapy can be stopped. A repeat PCR should then be done 1 month after stopping therapy—and if negative, blood for HIV antibody testing should be drawn at 6 and 12 months postexposure. If any test becomes positive, referral to an infectious disease specialist is indicated.

One should also consider the possibility of an acute HIV infection presenting in the high-risk population. Symptoms which may mimic mononucleosis, include fever, malaise, lymphadenopathy, rash, and upper respiratory symptoms (see Chapter 35). If symptomatic, a p24 antigen or HIV PCR test should be performed and appropriate referrals made if positive.

Hein K et al: Comparison of HIV+ and HIV− adolescents: Risk factors and psychosocial determinants. Pediatrics 1995;95:96.
Neil J et al: Trends in heterosexually acquired AIDS in the United States, 1988–1995. J Acquir Immune Defic Syndr Hum Retrovirol 1997;14:465.

ARTHROPOD INFESTATIONS

See Chapter 14 for discussion of skin diseases.

Pediculosis pubis, or pubic lice, live in the pubic hair. Either the louse itself or the nits can be transmitted by close contact from person to person. Patients complain of itching and may report having seen the insects. Examination of the pubic hair may reveal the louse crawling around or attached to the hair. Closer inspection may reveal the nit or sack of eggs, which is a gelatinous material (1–2 mm) stuck to the hair shaft.

Sarcoptes scabiei is an organism smaller than the louse. It can be identified by the classic burrow created by the organism laying eggs and traveling just below the skin surface. Scabies can be sexually transmitted by close contact and can be found in the pubic region, groin, lower abdomen, or upper thighs. The rash is intensely pruritic, erythematous, and scaly.

Both infestations can be treated with either permethrin or lindane. The entire area needs to be covered with the lotion or shampoo for the time specified by the manufacturer. One treatment usually clears the infestation, though a second treatment may be necessary. Partners should be treated also. In the case of pubic lice, bedding and clothing should be decontaminated (ie, either machine-washed or machine-dried using the heat cycle or dry-cleaned) or separated from body contact for at least 72 hours.

PELVIC INFLAMMATORY DISEASE

Pelvic inflammatory disease (PID) is a potential complication of STDs caused by infection ascending from the vagina or cervix to the uterus, uterine tubes, or ovaries. Causative agents include gonorrhea, *Chlamydia trachomatis,* and anaerobic bacteria that reside in the vagina. Over 1 million women develop PID annually, and 275,000 are hospitalized. The incidence is highest in the teen population. Teenage girls have a 1:8 chance of developing PID, whereas women in their 20s have a 1:80 chance. Predisposing risk factors include number of sexual partners, younger age of initiating sexual intercourse, and lack of condom use. Low levels of protective antibody from lack of previous exposure to sexually transmitted organisms and cervical ectopy contribute to the risk of developing PID.

Vaginal douching may increase the risk of PID by promoting the access of lower genital tract organisms to internal pelvic organs. There is also an association between recent menses and development of PID.

Clinical Findings

A. Symptoms and Signs: Diagnosis of PID is usually made clinically. Typical patients have lower abdominal pain, nausea, vomiting, and fever. Vaginal discharge may or may not be present. Recent genital infection and menses may be associated. On physical

Table 38–2. Diagnostic criteria for PID.[1]

Minimum criteria: Empiric treatment of PID should be instituted on the basis of the presence of all of the following three minimum clinical criteria for pelvic inflammation and in the absence of an established cause other than PID:
    Lower abdominal tenderness
    Adnexal tenderness
    Cervical motion tenderness
Additional criteria: For women with severe clinical signs, more elaborate diagnostic evaluation is warranted because incorrect diagnosis and management may cause unnecessary morbidity. These additional criteria may be used to increase the specificity of the diagnosis.
  1. The following are the routine criteria for diagnosing PID:
      Oral temperature > 38.3 °C
      Abnormal cervical or vaginal discharge
      Elevated erythrocyte sedimentation rate
      Elevated C-reactive protein
      Laboratory documentation of cervical infection with
        Neisseria gonorrhoeae or *Chlamydia trachomatis*
  2. The following are the elaborate criteria for diagnosing PID:
      Histopathologic evidence of endometritis on endome
        trial biopsy
      Tubo-ovarian abscess on sonography or other
        radiologic tests
      Laparoscopic abnormalities consistent with PID
Although initial treatment decisions can be made before bacteriologic diagnosis of *C trachomatis* or *N gonorrhoeae* infection, such a diagnosis emphasizes the need to treat sex partners.

[1]Adapted from 1998 sexually transmitted diseases treatment guidelines. MMWR Morb Mortal Wkly Rep 1998;47(RR-1):1.

examination, affected patients have lower abdominal, cervical motion, and adnexal tenderness. A pelvic or ovarian mass may be palpated. Signs of peritonitis may be present. Mucopurulent cervicitis is present in 50% of patients. Laparoscopy is the standard method for detecting salpingitis; it can be used if the diagnosis is in question or to help differentiate between an ectopic pregnancy and ovarian cysts or torsion. Pelvic ultrasonography also is helpful in detecting tubo-ovarian abscesses. These are found in almost 20% of teens with PID (Table 38–2).

B. Laboratory Findings: Laboratory findings include leukocytosis with a left shift and an elevated erythrocyte sedimentation rate. A positive cervical culture for *N gonorrhoeae* or *C trachomatis* is supportive of the diagnosis, though in one-fourth of cases neither is detected. Aerobic and anaerobic organisms that normally reside in the vagina are found to be causative or contributory agents in many cases of PID. Pregnancy needs to be ruled out, since ectopic pregnancy can present with abdominal pain.

Treatment

PID is being managed at the outpatient level with increasing frequency. Some argue that all adolescents should be hospitalized because of the significant rate of complications. Severe systemic symptoms and

toxicity, signs of peritonitis, inability to take fluids, pregnancy, and elevated white counts and sedimentation rates support the decision to recommend hospitalization. If the practitioner believes the patient will not comply with medication, hospitalization is further advised. Treatment regimens for hospitalized patients are set forth in Table 38–1. Outpatient management should be reserved for compliant patients who have classic signs of PID without systemic symptoms. Close follow-up is mandatory to detect persistent disease or treatment failure.

Sequelae

Scarring of the uterine tubes is one of the major sequelae of PID. With one episode of PID, 17% of patients become infertile, 17% develop chronic pelvic pain, and 10% will have an ectopic pregnancy. Infertility rates increase with each episode of PID—three episodes result in a 73% infertility rate. Fitz-Hugh and Curtis syndrome is inflammation of the liver capsule (perihepatitis) from either hematogenous or lymphatic spread of the precipitating organism from the uterine tubes. This causes right upper quadrant pain; liver function tests may be elevated. Symptoms resolve with therapy, but subsequent adhesions from the liver capsule to surrounding tissue can develop.

Tubo-ovarian abscesses, another sequela of PID, can be detected by careful physical examination (palpation of a mass or fullness in the adnexa) and confirmed by pelvic ultrasonography. Surgical drainage may be required to ensure adequate treatment.

McCormack WM: Pelvic inflammatory disease. N Engl J Med 1994;330:115.
Rome E: Pelvic inflammatory disease in the adolescent. Curr Opin Pediatr 1994;6:383.

EVALUATION OF STD IN SEXUAL ABUSE

Unfortunately, sexual abuse is more common than we recognize. Twenty-five percent of females and 12% of males will have suffered some form of sexual violence by age 18. Fifty percent of rape victims are under 18. Rape is both a medical and psychologic emergency—evaluation and management vary with the age of the patient, the individual's ability to communicate what occurred, and the timing of the abuse.

Teenagers usually can describe the kind of abuse (oral, anal, vaginal; receptive or insertive), and evaluation directed accordingly. If the abuse has occurred in the preceding 72 hours, most states require a rape kit to be utilized for forensic reasons. All practitioners should have access to such a kit. The kit guides the practitioner through a stepwise collection of evidence and cultures. A thorough physical examination is indicated to evaluate for other signs of trauma.

Beyond 72 hours, evaluation is tailored according to the history provided. In addition to culturing the involved orifices for *N gonorrhoeae* and *C trachomatis* and evaluating vaginal secretions for *T vaginalis,* samples for RPR, hepatitis B, and HIV testing should be drawn at baseline and repeated in 2–3 months. It should be noted that nucleic acid amplification is not admissible in court, so that cultures need to be done instead. Pregnancy testing should be done or not depending on the clinical situation.

Prophylactic therapy should be offered when patients present within the incubation time of any of the disease processes—cefixime or ceftriaxone for gonorrhea and azithromycin or doxycycline for chlamydial infection. HIV prophylaxis should be considered as well (above). Evaluating the perpetrator for STD, if possible, can help determine risk exposure and guide prophylaxis. Emergency contraception should be given if the abuse occurred within the past 72 hours. Psychologic assessment at the time of presentation as well as over the next several months is a top priority. Any abuse that is suspected needs to be reported to the appropriate authority.

For younger children, especially those unable to communicate, the rape kit is required if the patient presents within 72 hours. All younger children should be referred to child abuse specialists who have multidisciplinary teams that help tremendously with the psychologic aspect of the abuse and are competent in helping children communicate what may have occurred. Colposcopic examination is critical to help determine the extent of damage as well as to provide documentation for the legal system.

Neinstein LS et al: Rape and sexual abuse. In: *Adolescent Health Care.* Neinstein LS (editor). Williams & Wilkins, 1997.

Sirotnak AP: Testing sexually abused children for sexually transmitted diseases: Who to test, when to test, and why. Pediatr Ann 1994;23:370.

REFERENCES

Drugs for sexually transmitted diseases. Med Lett Drugs Ther 1995;37:117.

1998 Sexually transmitted diseases treatment guidelines. MMWR Morb Mortal Wkly Rep 1998;47(RR-1):1

Peter G, Hall CB, Orenstein WA (editors): *1997 Red Book: Report of the Committee on Infectious Diseases,* 24th ed. American Academy of Pediatrics, 1997.

Sexually transmitted diseases in the united states. *Facts in Brief.* Alan Guttmacher Institute, 1993.

Youth risk behavior surveillance—United States, 1995. MMWR Surveillance Summaries 1996;45(4):1.

Fluid, Electrolyte, & Acid-Base Disorders & Therapy

39

Douglas M. Ford, MD

REGULATION OF BODY FLUIDS, ELECTROLYTES, & TONICITY

Total body water (TBW) comprises 50–75% of the total body mass depending on age, sex, and fat content. After an initial postnatal diuresis, the TBW slowly decreases to the adult range near puberty (Figure 39–1). Total body water is divided into the intracellular and extracellular spaces. **Intracellular fluid (ICF)** accounts for two-thirds of the TBW, or roughly 50% of total body mass. **Extracellular fluid (ECF)** comprises one-third of the TBW and 25% of total body mass. The ECF is further compartmentalized into plasma (intravascular) volume and **interstitial fluid (ISF).**

The principal constituents of plasma are sodium, chloride, bicarbonate, and protein (primarily albumin). The ISF is similar to plasma but lacks significant amounts of protein (Figure 39–2). Conversely, the ICF is rich in potassium, magnesium, phosphates, sulfates, and protein.

An understanding of osmotic shifts between the ECF and ICF is fundamental to understanding disorders of fluid balance. Isosmolality is generally maintained between fluid compartments. Because the cell membrane is water-permeable, abnormal fluid shifts occur if there is inequality between the ECF and ICF in the concentration of solutes that cannot permeate the cell membrane. Thus, NaCl, mannitol, and glucose (in the setting of hyperglycemia) remain restricted to the ECF space and contribute "effective osmoles" by obligating water to remain in the ECF compartment. In contrast, a freely permeable solute, such as urea, does not contribute "effective osmoles" since it is not restricted to the ECF and readily crosses cell membranes. **Tonicity, or effective osmolality,** differs from measured osmolality in that it accounts only for osmotically active impermeable solutes rather than all osmotically active solutes, including those that are permeable to cell membranes. Osmolality may be estimated by the following formula:

$$mOsm/kg = 2(Na^+, mEq/L) + \frac{Glucose, mg/dL}{18} + \frac{BUN, mg/dL}{2.8}$$

Although osmolality and osmolarity differ, the former being an expression of osmotic activity per weight (kg) and the latter per volume (L) of solution, for clinical purposes they are similar and occasionally used interchangeably. **Oncotic pressure** represents the osmotic activity of macromolecular constituents such as albumin in the plasma and body fluids.

The principal mechanisms that regulate ECF volume and tonicity are **antidiuretic hormone (ADH), thirst, aldosterone,** and **atrial natriuretic factor (ANF).**

In the kidney, **ADH** increases water reabsorption in the cortical and medullary collecting ducts, leading to formation of a concentrated urine. In the absence of ADH, a dilute urine is produced. Under normal conditions, ADH secretion is regulated by the tonicity of body fluids rather than the fluid volume and becomes detectable at a plasma osmolality of 280 mOsm/kg or greater. However, tonicity may be sacrificed to preserve ECF volume, as in the case of hyponatremic dehydration, wherein ADH secretion and renal water retention are maximal.

Water intake is commonly determined by cultural factors rather than by thirst. **Thirst** is not physiologically stimulated until plasma osmolality reaches 290 mOsm/kg, a level at which ADH levels are sufficient to induce maximal antidiuresis. Thirst provides control over a wide range of fluid volumes and can even be a response to absence of ADH with attendant production of copious and dilute urine. One who cannot perceive thirst develops profound problems with fluid balance.

Aldosterone—released from the adrenal cortex in response to decreased effective circulating volume and stimulation of the renin-angiotensin-aldosterone axis or in response to increasing plasma K^+—en-

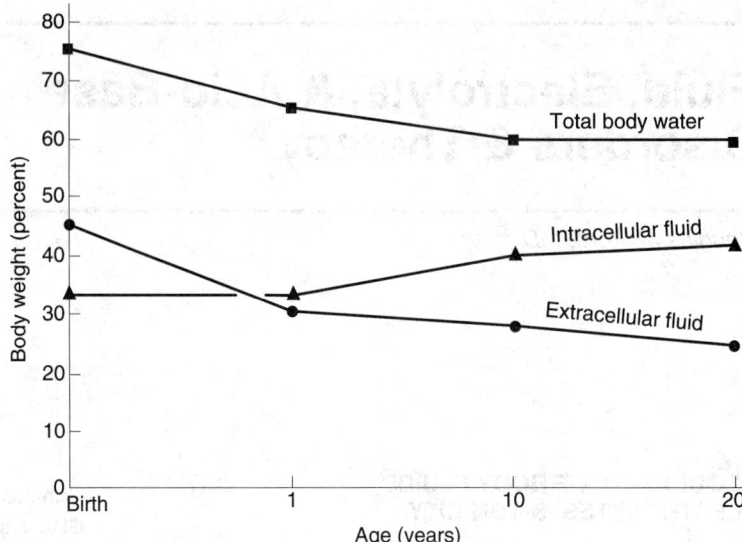

Figure 39–1. Body water compartments related to age. (Modified from Friis-Hansen B: Pediatrics 1961;28:169.)

hances renal tubular reabsorption of Na$^+$ in exchange for K$^+$ and, to a lesser degree, H$^+$. At a constant osmolality, retention of Na$^+$ leads to expansion of ECF volume and suppression of aldosterone release.

Atrial natriuretic factor (ANF), a polypeptide hormone secreted principally by the cardiac atria in response to atrial stretch, plays an important role in regulation of blood volume and blood pressure. ANF inhibits renin secretion and aldosterone synthesis and causes an increase in glomerular filtration rate and renal sodium excretion. ANF also guards against excessive plasma volume expansion in the face of increased ECF volume by shifting fluid from the vascular to the interstitial compartment. ANF inhibits

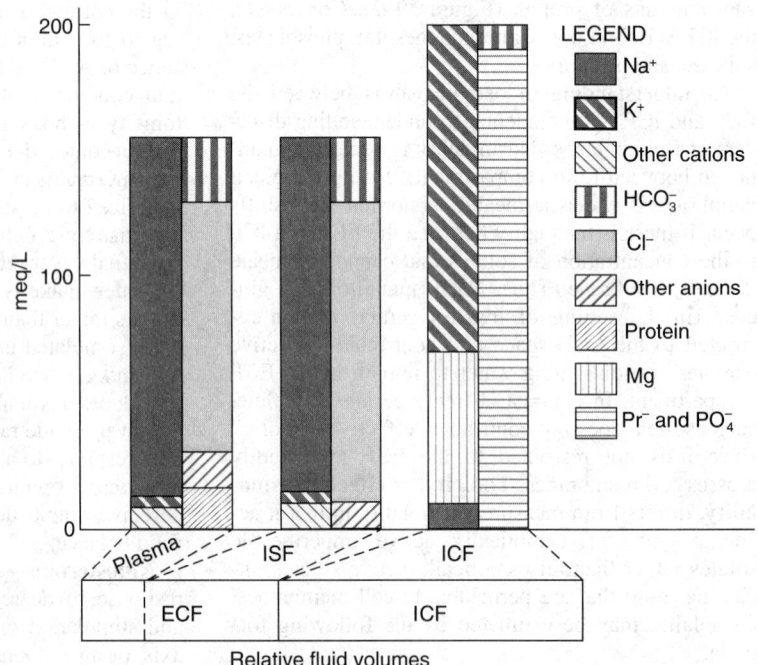

Figure 39–2. Composition of body fluids. (ICF = intracellular fluid, ISF = interstitial fluid.)

angiotensin II- and norepinephrine-induced vasoconstriction and acts in the brain to decrease the desire for salt and inhibit the release of ADH. Thus, the net effect of ANF is a decrease in blood volume and blood pressure associated with natriuresis and diuresis.

ACID-BASE BALANCE

The pH of arterial blood is maintained between 7.38 and 7.42 to ensure that pH-sensitive enzyme systems function normally. Acid-base balance is maintained by interaction of the lungs, kidneys, and systemic buffering systems. Over 50% of the blood's buffering capacity is provided by the carbonic acid-bicarbonate system, roughly 30% by hemoglobin and the remainder by phosphates and ammonium. The carbonic acid-bicarbonate system, depicted chemically as

$$CO_2 + H_2O \leftrightarrow H_2CO_3 \leftrightarrow H^+ + HCO_3^-$$

interacts with the lungs, kidneys, and nonbicarbonate systems to stabilize systemic pH. The concentration of dissolved CO_2 in blood is established by the respiratory system and that of HCO_3^- by the kidneys. Disturbances in acid-base balance are initially stabilized by chemical buffering, compensated for by pulmonary or renal regulation of CO_2 or HCO_3^-, and ultimately corrected when the primary cause of the acid-base disturbance is eliminated.

Renal regulation of acid-base balance is accomplished by the reabsorption of filtered HCO_3^-, and the excretion of H^+ or HCO_3^- to match the net input of acid or base. When urine is alkalinized, HCO_3^- enters the kidney and is ultimately lost in the urine. Alkalinization of the urine may occur when there is an absolute or relative excess of bicarbonate. However, urinary alkalinization will not occur if there is a deficiency of Na^+ or K^+, as HCO_3^- must also be retained to maintain electroneutrality. In contrast, the urine may be acidified if there is an absolute or relative decrease in systemic HCO_3^-. In this setting, proximal tubular HCO_3^- reabsorption and distal tubular H^+ excretion are maximal. Some of the processes involved in acid-base regulation are shown in Figure 39–3.

FLUID & ELECTROLYTE MANAGEMENT

Therapy of fluid and electrolyte disorders is directed toward providing maintenance fluid and elec-

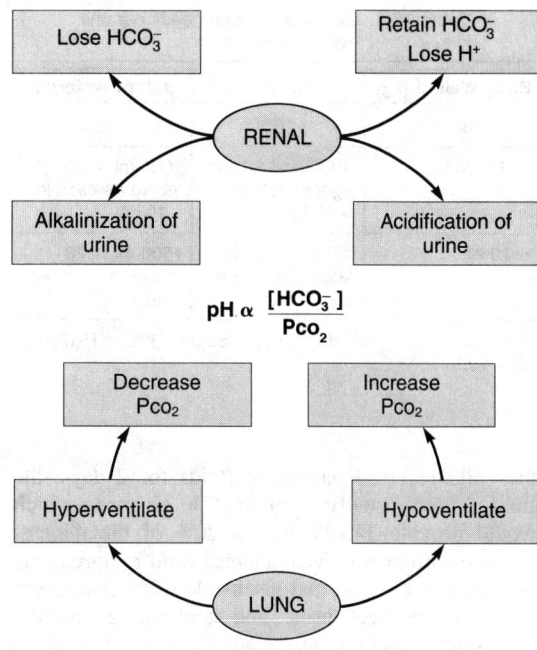

Figure 39–3. Maintaining metabolic stability via compensatory mechanisms.

trolyte requirements, replenishing prior losses, and replacing persistent abnormal losses. Therapy should be phased to (1) rapidly expand the ECF volume and restore tissue perfusion, (2) replenish fluid and electrolyte deficits while correcting attendant acid-base abnormalities, (3) meet the patient's nutritional needs, and (4) replace ongoing losses.

The cornerstone of therapy involves an understanding of "maintenance" fluid and electrolyte requirements. **Maintenance requirements** call for provision of enough water, glucose, and electrolytes to prevent deterioration of body stores. During short-term parenteral therapy, sufficient glucose is provided to prevent ketosis and limit protein catabolism, though this is usually little more than 20% of the patient's true caloric needs. Prior to the administration of maintenance fluids, it is important to consider the patient's volume status and to determine whether intravenous fluids are needed at all.

Various models have been devised to facilitate calculation of maintenance requirements based on body surface area, weight, and caloric expenditure. A system based on caloric expenditure is most helpful, since 1 mL of water is needed for each kilocalorie expended. The system presented in Table 39–1 is based on caloric needs and is applicable to children weighing more than 3 kg.

As depicted in Table 39–1, a child weighing 30 kg would need 1700 kcal and 1700 mL of water daily. If

Table 39–1. Caloric and water needs per unit of body weight.[1]

Body Weight (kg)	kcal/kg	mL of Water/kg
3–10 kg	100	100
11–20 kg	1000 kcal + kcal/kg for each kg > 10 kg	1000 mL + 50 mL/kg for each kg > 10 kg
>20 kg	1500 kcal + 20 kcal/kg for each kg > 20 kg	1500 mL + 20 mL/kg for each kg > 20 kg

[1]Adapted from Holliday MA, Segar WE: Pediatrics 1957;19:823.

the child received parenteral fluids for 2 days, the fluid would usually contain 5% glucose, which would provide 340 kcal/d, or 20% of the maintenance caloric needs. Maintenance fluid requirements take into account normal insensible water losses and water lost in sweat, urine, and stool and assume the patient to be afebrile and relatively inactive. Maintenance requirements are greater for low birth weight and preterm infants. Table 39–2 lists other factors that commonly alter fluid and caloric needs.

Electrolyte losses occur primarily through the urinary tract and to a lesser degree via the skin and stool. Although maintenance electrolyte estimates vary, reasonable approximations for maintenance needs are 3 mEq Na^+/100 kcal and 2 mEq K^+/100 kcal, or 30 mEq Na^+/L and 20 mEq K^+/L, respectively, of intravenous fluid.

It is helpful to monitor the patient's daily weight, urinary output, fluid input, and urine specific gravity. If there is an abnormality in fluid or electrolyte balance, serial determination of electrolyte concentrations, blood urea nitrogen (BUN), and creatinine may be necessary. In patients with significant burns, anuria, oliguria, or persistent abnormal losses (eg, from a stoma, or polyuria secondary to a renal concentrating defect, etc), it is important to measure out-

Table 39–2. Alterations of maintenance fluid requirements.

Factor	Altered Requirement
Fever	12% per °C[1]
Hyperventilation	10–60 mL/100 kcal
Sweating	10–25 mL/100 kcal
Hyperthyroidism	Variable: 25–50%
Gastrointestinal loss and renal disease	Monitor and analyze output. Adjust therapy accordingly.

[1]Do not correct for 38 °C; correct 24% for 39 °C.

put and, if needed, its components so that appropriate replacement can be provided.

DEHYDRATION

Depletion of body fluids is one of the most commonly encountered problems in clinical pediatrics. Children have a high incidence of gastrointestinal diseases, including gastroenteritis, and may demonstrate gastrointestinal symptoms in nongastrointestinal conditions. Infants and young children often decrease their oral intake when ill, and their high ratio of surface area to weight promotes significant evaporative losses. Renal concentrating mechanisms do not maximally conserve water in early life, and fever may significantly increase fluid needs. Dehydration decreases ECF volume, leading to decreased tissue perfusion, impaired renal function, compensatory tachycardia, and lactic acidosis. The clinical effects of dehydration relate to the degree of dehydration and to the relative amounts of salt and water lost. Caregivers must be particularly aware of dehydration occurring in breast-fed newborn infants who go home soon after birth and whose mothers fail to produce enough milk. This problem is more common in the hot summer months and has been associated with severe dehydration, brain damage, and death.

The clinical evaluation of a child with dehydration should focus on the composition and volume of fluid intake; the frequency and amount of vomiting, diarrhea, and urine output; the degree and duration of fever; the nature of any administered medications; and the existence of underlying medical conditions. A recently recorded weight, if known, can be very helpful in calculating the magnitude of dehydration. Important clinical features in estimating the degree of dehydration include the capillary refill time, postural blood pressure, and heart rate changes; dryness of the lips and mucous membranes; lack of tears; lack of external jugular venous filling when supine; a sunken fontanelle in an infant; oliguria; and altered mental status (see Table 39–3). Children generally respond to a decrease in circulating volume with a compensatory increase in pulse rate and may maintain their blood pressure in the face of severe dehydration. A low or falling blood pressure is, therefore, a late sign of shock in children, and when present should prompt emergent treatment. Salient laboratory parameters include a high urine specific gravity (in the absence of an underlying renal concentrating defect), a relatively greater elevation in BUN than creatinine, a low urinary Na^+ excretion (< 15 mEq/L), and an elevated hematocrit or serum albumin level secondary to hemoconcentration.

Emergent intravenous therapy is indicated when there is evidence of compromised perfusion (inadequate capillary refill, tachycardia, poor color, oliguria, or hypotension). The initial goal is to rapidly expand

Table 39–3. Clinical manifestations of dehydration.

Clinical Signs	Degree of Dehydration		
	Mild	Moderate	Severe
Decrease in body weight	3–5%	6–10%	11–15%
Skin Turgor	Normal (+/–)	Decreased	Markedly decreased
Color	Normal	Pale	Markedly decreased
Mucous membranes	Dry ⟶		Mottled or gray; parched
Hemodynamic signs Pulse	Normal	Slight increse	Tachycardia
Capillary refill	2–3 seconds	3–4 seconds	> 4 seconds
Blood pressure	Normal ⟶		Low
Perfusion	Normal ⟶		Circulatory collapse
Fluid loss Urinary output	Mild oliguria	Oliguria	Anuria
Tears	Decreased ⟶		Absent
Urinary indices Specific gravity	> 1.020 ⟶		Anuria
Urine [Na^+]	< 20 mEq/L ⟶		Anuria

the plasma volume and to prevent circulatory collapse. A 20-mL/kg bolus of isotonic fluid should be given intravenously as rapidly as possible. Either colloid (5% albumin) or crystalloid (normal saline or Ringer's lactate) may be used. Colloid is particularly useful in hypernatremic patients in shock, in malnourished infants, and in neonates. If no intravenous site is available, fluid may be administered intraosseously through the marrow space of the tibia. If there is no response to the first fluid bolus, a second bolus may be given. When adequate tissue perfusion is demonstrated by improved capillary refill, decreased pulse rate and urine output, and improved mental status, deficit replacement may be instituted. If adequate perfusion is not restored after 40 mL/kg of isotonic fluids, other processes must be considered such as sepsis, occult hemorrhage, or cardiogenic shock. **Isotonic dehydration** may be treated by providing half of the remaining fluid deficit over 8 hours and the second half over the ensuing 16 hours in the form of 5% dextrose with 0.2–0.45% saline containing 20 mEq/L KCl. In the presence of metabolic acidosis, K^+ acetate may be considered. Maintenance fluids and replacement of ongoing losses should also be provided. Typical electrolyte compositions of various body fluids are depicted in Table 39–4, though it may be necessary to measure the specific constituents of a patient's fluid losses to guide therapy. If the patient is unable to eat for a prolonged period, nutritional needs must be met through hyperalimentation or enteral tube feedings.

Oral rehydration may be provided to children with mild to moderate dehydration. Clear liquid beverages found in the home, such as broths, sodas, juices, and tea, are inappropriate for the treatment of dehydration. Commercially available solutions provide 45–75 mEq/L of Na^+, 20–25 mEq/L of K^+, 30–34 mEq/L of citrate or bicarbonate, and 2–2.5% glucose. Frequent small aliquots (5–15 mL) should be given to provide approximately 50 mL/kg over 4 hours for mild dehydration and up to 100 mL/kg over 6 hours for moderate dehydration. Oral rehydration is contraindicated in children with altered levels of consciousness or respiratory distress who cannot drink freely, in children with the suspicion of an acute sur-

Table 39–4. Typical electrolyte compositions of various body fluids.[1]

	Na^+ (mEq/kg)	K^+ (mEq/kg)	HCO_3^- (mEq/kg)
Diarrhea	10–90	10–80	40
Gastric	20–80	5–20	0
Small intestine	100–140	5–15	40
Ileostomy	45–135	3–15	40

[1]Adapted, with permission, from winters RW: *Principles of Pediatric Fluid Therapy.* Little, Brown, 1973.

gical abdomen; in infants with > 10% volume depletion; in children with hemodynamic instability; and in the setting of severe hyponatremia ($[Na^+]$ < 120 mEq/L) or hypernatremia ($[Na^+]$ > 160 mEq/L). Failure of oral rehydration due to persistent vomiting or inability to keep up with losses mandates intravenous therapy. Successful oral rehydration requires explicit instructions to caregivers.

The type of dehydration is characterized by the serum Na^+ concentration. If relatively more solute is lost than water, the Na^+ concentration falls, and **hyponatremic dehydration** ($[Na^+]$ < 130 mEq/L) ensues. This is important clinically because hypotonicity of the plasma contributes to further volume loss from the ECF into the intracellular space. Thus, tissue perfusion is more significantly impaired for a given degree of hyponatremic dehydration than for a comparable degree of isotonic or hypertonic dehydration. It is important to note, however, that significant solute losses also occur in hypernatremic dehydration. Furthermore, because plasma volume is somewhat protected in hypernatremic dehydration, it poses the risk of underestimating the severity of dehydration. Typical fluid and electrolyte losses associated with each form of dehydration are shown in Table 39–5.

HYPONATREMIA

Hyponatremia may be factitious in the presence of high plasma lipids or proteins, which decrease the percentage of plasma volume that is water. Hyponatremia in the absence of hypotonicity also occurs when an osmotically active solute, such as glucose or mannitol, is added to the ECF. Water drawn from the ICF dilutes the serum $[Na^+]$ despite iso- or hypertonicity.

Patients with **hyponatremic dehydration** generally demonstrate typical signs and symptoms of dehydration (shown in Table 39–3), since the vascular space is compromised as water leaves the ECF to maintain osmotic neutrality. The treatment of hyponatremic dehydration is fairly straightforward. The

magnitude of the sodium deficit may be calculated by the following formula:

$$Na^+ \text{ deficit} = (Na^+ \text{ desired} - Na^+ \text{ observed}) \times \text{Body weight (kg)} \times -0.6$$

One-half the deficits are administered in the first 8 hours of therapy, and the remainder is given over the following 16 hours. Maintenance and replacement fluids should also be provided. The deficit plus maintenance calculations generally approximate 5% dextrose with 0.45% saline. The rise in serum $[Na^+]$ should not exceed 2 meq/L/h. The dangers of too rapid correction of hyponatremia include cerebral dehydration and injury due to fluid shifts from the ICF compartment.

Hypovolemic hyponatremia is also seen in cerebral salt wasting associated with CNS insults, a condition characterized by high urine output and elevated urinary $[Na^+]$ (> 80 mEq/L) due to an increase in atrial natriuretic factor. This must be distinguished from the **syndrome of inappropriate ADH (SIADH),** which may also become manifest in CNS conditions and certain pulmonary disorders. In contrast to cerebral salt wasting, SIADH is characterized by euvolemia or mild volume expansion and relatively low urine output due to ADH-induced water retention. Urinary $[Na^+]$ is high in both conditions, though generally not as high in SIADH. It is important to distinguish between these two conditions, as the treatment of the former involves replacement of urinary salt and water losses while the treatment of SIADH involves water restriction.

In cases of severe hyponatremia (serum $[Na^+]$ < 120 meq/L) with CNS symptoms, intravenous 3% NaCl may be given over 1 hour to raise the $[Na^+]$ to 120 mEq/L, to alleviate CNS manifestations and sequelae. In general, 6 mL/kg of 3% NaCl will raise the serum $[Na^+]$ by 5 meq/L. If 3% NaCl is administered, estimated Na^+ and fluid deficits should be adjusted accordingly. Further correction should proceed slowly, as outlined above.

Hypervolemic hyponatremia may occur in edematous disorders such as nephrotic syndrome, congestive heart failure, or cirrhosis, wherein water is retained in excess of salt. Treatment involves restriction of Na^+ and water and correction of the underlying disorder. Hypervolemic hyponatremia due to water intoxication is characterized by a maximally dilute urine (specific gravity < 1.003) and is also treated with water restriction.

Table 39–5. Estimated water and electrolyte deficits in dehydration (moderate to severe).[1]

Type of Dehydration	H_2O (mL/kg)	Na^+ (mEq/kg)	K^+ (mEq/kg)	Cl^- and HCO_3^- (mEq/kg)
Isotonic	100–150	8–10	8–10	16–20
Hypotonic	50–100	10–14	10–14	20–28
Hypertonic	120–180	2–5	2–5	4–10

[1]Adapted, with permission, from Winters RW: *Principles of Pediatric Fluid Therapy.* Little, Brown, 1982.

HYPERNATREMIA

Although diarrhea is commonly associated with hypo- or isonatremic dehydration, hypernatremia may develop in the presence of persistent fever or decreased fluid intake or in response to improperly mixed rehydration solutions. Extreme care is required to treat hypernatremic dehydration appropriately. If the serum [Na^+] falls precipitously, the osmolality of the ECF drops more rapidly than that of the CNS. Water shifts from the ECF compartment into the CNS to maintain osmotic neutrality. If hypertonicity is corrected too rapidly (a drop in [Na^+] of > 0.5–1 mEq/L/h), cerebral edema, seizures, and CNS injury may occur. Thus, following the initial restoration of adequate tissue perfusion using isotonic fluids, a gradual decrease in serum [Na^+] is desired (10–15 mEq/L/d). This is commonly achieved using 5% dextrose with 0.2% saline to replace the calculated fluid deficit over 48 hours. Maintenance and replacement fluids should also be provided. If the serum [Na^+] is not correcting appropriately, the free water deficit may be estimated as 4 mL/kg of free water for each milliequivalent of serum [Na^+] above 145 and provided as 5% dextrose over 48 hours. If metabolic acidosis is also present, it must be corrected slowly to avoid CNS irritability. Potassium is provided as indicated—as the acetate salt if necessary. Electrolyte concentrations should be assessed every 2 hours in order to control the decline in serum [Na^+]. Elevations of blood glucose and BUN may worsen the hyperosmolar state in hypernatremic dehydration and should also be monitored closely. Hyperglycemia is often seen in hypernatremic dehydration and may necessitate lower intravenous glucose concentrations (eg, 2.5%).

Patients with **diabetes insipidus,** whether nephrogenic or central in origin, are prone to develop profound hypernatremic dehydration as a result of unremitting urinary free water losses (urine specific gravity < 1.010), particularly during superimposed gastrointestinal illnesses associated with vomiting or diarrhea. Treatment involves restoration of fluid and electrolyte deficits as described above as well as replacement of excessive water losses, with subsequent water deprivation testing during daylight hours to distinguish responsiveness to ADH. The evaluation and treatment of nephrogenic and central diabetes insipidus are discussed in detail in Chapters 21 and 28, respectively.

Hypervolemic hypernatremia ("salt poisoning"), associated with excess total body salt and water, may be seen as a consequence of providing improperly mixed formula, of NaCl or $NaHCO_3$ administration, or as a feature of primary hyperaldosteronism. Treatment includes the use of diuretics and, potentially, concomitant water replacement or even dialysis.

POTASSIUM DISORDERS

The predominantly intracellular distribution of potassium is maintained by the actions of Na^+/K^+ ATPase in the cell membranes. Potassium is shifted into the ECF and plasma by acidemia and into the ICF in the setting of alkalosis, hypochloremia, or insulin-induced tissue glucose uptake. The ratio of intracellular to extracellular K^+ is the major determinant of the cellular resting membrane potential and contributes to the action potential in neural and muscular tissue. Abnormalities of K^+ balance are potentially life-threatening. In the kidney, K^+ is filtered at the glomerulus, reabsorbed in the proximal tubule, and excreted in the distal tubule. Distal tubular K^+ excretion is regulated primarily by aldosterone. Renal K^+ excretion continues for significant periods even after the intake of K^+ is decreased. Thus, by the time urinary K^+ decreases, the systemic K^+ pool has been significantly depleted.

The causes of net K^+ loss are primarily renal in origin. Gastrointestinal losses through nasogastric suction or vomiting reduce total body K^+ to some degree. However, the attendant volume depletion results in an increase in plasma aldosterone, promoting renal excretion of K^+ in exchange for Na^+. Diuretics (especially thiazides), mineralocorticoids, and intrinsic renal tubular diseases (such as Bartter's syndrome) enhance the renal excretion of K^+. Clinically, **hypokalemia** is associated with neuromuscular excitability, decreased peristalsis or ileus, hyporeflexia, paralysis, rhabdomyolysis, and arrhythmias. Electrocardiographic changes include flattened T waves, a shortened PR interval, and the appearance of U waves. Arrhythmias associated with hypokalemia include premature ventricular contractions; atrial, nodal, or ventricular tachycardia; and ventricular fibrillation. Hypokalemia increases responsiveness to digitalis and may precipitate overt digitalis toxicity. In the presence of arrhythmias, extreme muscle weakness, or respiratory compromise, intravenous K^+ should be given. If the patient is hypophosphatemic ([PO_4^{2-}] < 2 mg/dL), a phosphate salt may be used. The first priority in the treatment of hypokalemia is the restoration of an adequate serum [K^+]. Providing maintenance amounts of K^+ is usually sufficient; however, when the serum [K^+] is dangerously low and K^+ must be administered intravenously, it is imperative that the patient have a cardiac monitor. Intravenous K^+ should generally not be given faster than at a rate of 0.5 mEq/kg/h. Oral K^+ supplements may be needed for weeks to replenish depleted body stores.

Hyperkalemia, due to decreased renal K^+ excretion, mineralocorticoid deficiency or unresponsiveness, or due to K^+ release from the ICF compartment, is characterized by muscle weakness, paresthesias, and tetany, ascending paralysis, and arrhythmias. Electrocardiographic changes associated with hyperkalemia include peaked T waves, widening of the QRS complex, and arrhythmias such as sinus bradycardia or sinus arrest, atrioventricular block, nodal or idioventricular rhythms, and ventricular tachycardia or fibrillation. The severity of hyperkalemia depends on the electrocardiographic changes, the status of the other electrolytes, and the stability of the underlying disorder. A rhythm strip should be obtained whenever significant hyperkalemia is suspected. If the serum $[K^+]$ is less than 6.5 meq/L, discontinuing K^+ supplementation is usually sufficient. If the serum $[K^+]$ is greater than 7 meq/L or if potentiating factors such as hyponatremia, digitalis toxicity, or renal failure are present, more aggressive therapy is needed. If electrocardiographic changes or arrhythmias are present, treatment must be initiated promptly. Intravenous 10% calcium gluconate (0.2–0.5 mL/kg over 2–10 minutes) will rapidly ameliorate depolarization and may be repeated after 5 minutes if electrocardiographic changes persist. Calcium should only be given with a cardiac monitor in place and should be discontinued if bradycardia develops. The intravenous administration of a diuretic that acts in the loop of Henle, such as furosemide (1–2 mg/kg), will augment renal K^+ excretion and can be very helpful in lowering serum and total body $[K^+]$. Administering Na^+ and increasing systemic pH with bicarbonate therapy (1–2 meq/kg) will shift K^+ from the ECF to the ICF compartment, as will therapy with a β-agonist such as albuterol. In nondiabetics, 0.5 g/kg of glucose over 1–2 hours will enhance endogenous insulin secretion, lowering serum $[K^+]$ 1–2 meq/L. Administration of intravenous glucose and insulin may be needed as a simultaneous drip (0.5–1 g/kg glucose and 0.3 units of regular insulin per gram of glucose) given over 2 hours with monitoring of the serum glucose level every 15 minutes.

The therapies outlined provide transient benefits. Ultimately, K^+ must be reduced to normal by reestablishing adequate renal excretion using diuretics or optimizing urinary flow, using ion exchange resins such as sodium polystyrene sulfonate orally or as a retention enema (0.2–0.5 g/kg orally or 1 g/kg as an enema), or by dialysis.

ACID-BASE DISTURBANCES

When evaluating a disturbance in acid-base balance, the systemic pH, PCO_2, serum $[HCO_3^-]$, and anion gap must be considered. The anion gap—Na^+ – $(Cl^- + HCO_3^-)$—is an expression of the unmeasured anions in the plasma and is normally 12 ± 4 mEq/L. An increase above normal suggests the presence of an unmeasured anion, such as seen in diabetic ketoacidosis, lactic acidosis, salicylate intoxication, etc. Although the base excess (or deficit) is also used clinically, it is important to recall that this expression of acid-base balance is influenced by the renal response to respiratory disorders and cannot be interpreted independently (as in a compensated respiratory acidosis, wherein the base excess may be quite large).

METABOLIC ACIDOSIS

Metabolic acidosis is characterized by a primary decrease in serum $[HCO_3^-]$ and systemic pH due to the loss of HCO_3^- from the kidneys or gastrointestinal tract, the addition of an acid (from external sources or via altered metabolic processes), or the rapid dilution of the ECF with nonbicarbonate containing solution (usually normal saline). When HCO_3^- is lost through the kidneys or gastrointestinal tract, Cl^- must be reabsorbed with Na^+ disproportionately, resulting in a hyperchloremic acidosis with a normal anion gap. Thus, a normal anion gap acidosis in the absence of diarrhea or other bicarbonate-rich gastrointestinal losses suggests the possibility of renal tubular acidosis and should be evaluated appropriately (see Chapter 21). In contrast, acidosis that results from addition of an unmeasured acid is associated with a widened anion gap—examples are diabetic ketoacidosis, lactic acidosis, starvation, uremia, toxin ingestion (salicylates, ethylene glycol, methanol), and certain inborn errors of organic or amino acid metabolism. Dehydration may also result in a widened anion gap acidosis as a result of inadequate tissue perfusion, decreased O_2 delivery, and subsequent lactic and keto acid production. Respiratory compensation is accomplished through an increase in minute ventilation and decrease in PCO_2. The patient's history, physical findings, and laboratory features should lead to the appropriate diagnosis.

The ingestion of unknown toxins or the possibility of an inborn error of metabolism (see Chapter 30) must be considered in children without an obvious cause for a widened anion gap acidosis. Unfortunately, some hospital laboratories fail to include ethylene glycol or methanol in their standard toxicology screens, so that these toxins must be specifically requested. This is of grave importance when therapy with ethanol must be considered for either ingestion—and instituted quickly to head off profound toxicity. Ethylene glycol (eg, antifreeze) is particularly worrisome because of its sweet taste and accounts for a significant number of toxin ingestions. Screening by fluorescence of urine under Wood's lamp is relatively simple but does not replace specific laboratory assessment. Salicylate intoxication has a stimulatory effect on the respiratory center of the CNS and thus may initially present with respiratory alkalosis or mixed respiratory alkalosis and widened anion gap acidosis.

Most types of metabolic acidosis will resolve with correction of the underlying disorder, improved renal perfusion, and acid excretion. Intravenous $NaHCO_3$ administration may be considered in the setting of metabolic acidosis when the pH is less than 7.0 or the $[HCO_3^-]$ is less than 5 mEq/L, but *only if adequate ventilation is ensured.* The dose (in meq) of $NaHCO_3$ may be calculated as

Weight (kg) $\times$ **Base deficit** $\times$ **0.3**

and given as a continuous infusion over 1 hour. The effect of $NaHCO_3$ in lowering serum potassium and ionized calcium concentrations must also be considered and monitored.

METABOLIC ALKALOSIS

Metabolic alkalosis is characterized by a primary increase in $[HCO_3^-]$ and pH resulting from a loss of strong acid or gain of buffer base. The most common cause for a metabolic alkalosis is the loss of gastric juice via nasogastric suction or vomiting. This results in a Cl^- responsive alkalosis, characterized by a low urinary Cl^- (< 20 mEq/L) indicative of a volume contracted state that will be responsive to the provision of adequate Cl^- salt (usually in the form of normal saline). Cystic fibrosis is also commonly associated with a Cl^- responsive alkalosis due to the high losses of NaCl through the sweat, while congenital Cl^- losing diarrhea is a rare cause of Cl^--responsive alkalosis. Chloride-resistant alkalosis is characterized by a urinary $Cl^- > 20$ mEq/L and include Bartter's syndrome, Cushing's syndrome, and primary hyperaldosteronism, conditions associated with primary increases in urinary Cl^- or volume-expanded states lacking stimuli for Cl^- reabsorption. Thus, the urinary Cl^- is helpful in distinguishing the nature of a metabolic alkalosis, but must be specifically requested in many laboratories as it is not routinely included in urine electrolyte screens. The serum $[K^+]$ is also low in these settings (hypokalemic metabolic alkalosis) due to a combination of increased mineralocorticoid activity associated with volume contraction, the shift of K^+ to the ICF compartment, preferential reabsorption of Na^+ rather than K^+ to preserve intravascular volume, or primary mineralocorticoid excess.

RESPIRATORY ACIDOSIS

Respiratory acidosis develops when alveolar ventilation is decreased, increasing PCO_2 and lowering systemic pH. The kidneys compensate for a respiratory acidosis by increasing HCO_3^- reabsorption, a process that takes several days to manifest. Patients with acute respiratory acidoses frequently demonstrate air-hunger with retractions and the use of accessory respiratory muscles. Respiratory acidoses occur in upper or lower airway obstruction, ventilation/perfusion disturbances, CNS depression and neuromuscular defects. Hypercapnia is not as detrimental as the hypoxia that usually accompanies these disorders. The goal of therapy is to correct or compensate for the underlying pathologic process, to improve alveolar ventilation. Bicarbonate therapy is not indicated in a pure respiratory acidosis, as it will worsen the acidosis by shifting the equilibrium of the carbonic acid-bicarbonate buffer system to increase PCO_2.

RESPIRATORY ALKALOSIS

Respiratory alkalosis occurs when hyperventilation results in a decrease in PCO_2 and an increase in pH. Patients may experience tingling, paresthesias, dizziness, palpitations, syncope, or even tetany and seizures due to the associated decrease in ionized calcium. Causes of respiratory alkalosis include psychobehavioral disturbances, CNS irritation from meningitis or encephalitis, and salicylate intoxication. Therapy is directed toward the causal process. Rebreathing into a paper bag will decrease the severity of symptoms in acute hyperventilation.

REFERENCES

Avner ED: Clinical disorders of water metabolism: Hyponatremia and hypernatremia. Pediatr Ann 1995;24:23.

Finberg L et al: *Water and Electrolytes in Pediatrics: Physiology, Pathophysiology and Treatment,* 2nd ed. Saunders, 1993.

Hellerstein S: Fluids and electrolytes: Physiology. Pediatr Rev 1993;14:70.

Jospe N, Forbes G: Fluids and electrolytes: Clinical aspects. Pediatr Rev 1996;17:395.

Kappy MS, Ganong CA: Cerebral salt wasting in children: The role of atrial natriuretic hormone. Adv Pediatr 1996;43:271.

McDonald RA: Disorders of potassium balance. Pediatr Ann 1995;24:31.

Watkins SL: The basics of fluid and electrolyte therapy. Pediatric Ann 1995;24:16.

40

Drug Therapy

Susan Miller, PharmD, & Christopher M. Paap, PharmD, BCPS

Drug therapy in pediatric patients can be a rational and safe process when the concepts of developmental physiology, physical assessment, and pharmacology are understood and taken into consideration. Treatment must be based on the acuteness of the patient's age and clinical condition, the physical examination, the pharmacology of the drugs being considered, and the desired outcome.

DEVELOPING A PEDIATRIC DRUG REGIMEN

Drug Selection

A. Patient-Specific Factors: The age of the patient is one of the most important parameters to consider when developing a drug therapy regimen. Both physiologic and psychologic age should influence the choice of drug, the route of administration, the dosing regimen, and the monitoring parameters. Physiologic factors such as the inability of newborns and infants to reliably absorb oral medications limit this route of administration. Psychologic issues are more important when considering treatment in older children and adolescents or when the parents of a young child have limited cognitive functioning. The ability of the patient or parent to accurately use a drug therapy can affect its efficacy and safety. Factors to keep in mind when selecting drug therapy are given in Table 40–1.

Since nearly all drugs are eliminated from the body by the liver and kidneys, organ function should be assessed both before selecting drug therapy and during the treatment course. Renal function can be easily assessed by monitoring serum creatinine concentrations to estimate glomerular filtration rate (GFR), also known as creatinine clearance (CLcr).

$$\text{Clcr} = \frac{0.48 \times \text{Ht(cm)}}{\text{Serum creatinine}} = \text{mL/min/1.73m}^2$$

Since there are few data regarding drug dosage adjustment in children with renal dysfunction, generalization from the adult literature is commonly done.

Since the GFR calculated from the equation is based on body surface area (BSA), extrapolation from the adult literature can be more reliably assumed. Many of the metabolites of drugs that are primarily degraded by liver enzyme systems are ultimately excreted by the kidneys and can accumulate in patients with renal dysfunction.

Assessment of liver function is difficult clinically. Decreased drug metabolism via the liver has not been correlated with elevated aminotransferases (AST, ALT) or decreased albumin. In late stages of liver dysfunction, changes in bleeding times (prothrombin time, partial thromboplastin time) are strong indicators that hepatic drug metabolism may be impaired. However, this cannot be reliably quantified. Therefore, close monitoring for drug toxicity is necessary when decreased hepatic metabolism is suspected in patients being treated with hepatically metabolized drugs. Table 40–2 lists some commonly used drugs and their primary route of elimination.

The acuteness of the patient's condition should always be taken into consideration. Children who appear toxic warrant more aggressive therapy, which may include administration of several drugs, invasive (eg, intravenous) administration, and close monitoring (hospitalization). Likewise, children with conditions characterized by limited physiologic reserve can deteriorate more rapidly. Alternatively, drug therapy may not be appropriate when the child has mild symptoms since drug side effects may be worse than the disease (eg, decongestant use in infants with a cold).

As the child's condition improves, drug therapy should be changed appropriately. Table 40–3 provides examples of changes in clinical acuteness that may call for a change in drug therapy.

B. Drug-Specific Factors: Individualization of drug therapy requires specific knowledge about the patient and the potential drug treatment alternatives. The **therapeutic index** (Figure 40–1) is the ratio of the maximum tolerated dose to the minimum curative dose. It is a measure of the relative benefits and risks of a selected drug regimen. A drug with a wide therapeutic index has a greater margin of safety than one with a narrow index. (See Table 40–4.)

Table 40–1. Physiologic and psychologic factors that can affect drug therapy.

Factors	Drug and Interactions
Physiologic	
Hyperbilirubinemia	Drugs such as ceftriaxone or sulfisoxazole can displace bilirubin and induce kernicterus in newborns.
Newborn immaturity	
GI malabsorption	Oral antibiotics are unreliably absorbed during the first month of life but may otherwise be useful in older infants and children.
Renal insufficiency	Renally eliminated drugs such as the penicillins and aminoglycosides in newborns require extended dosing intervals.
Hepatic insufficiency	Hepatically eliminated drugs such as phenobarbital, morphine, and diazepam require lower doses and extended intervals.
Malnutrition (decreased albumin)	Drugs such a phenytoin, warfarin, and ibuprofen can have enhanced pharmacologic action due to decreased protein binding and increased "free" drug concentrations.
Short bowel syndrome	Oral medications of all types can have erratic absorption when the amount of bowel available to absorb the drug is reduced.
Cerebral palsy or mental retardation	Drugs such as narcotics, anticonvulsants, and anticholinergics can produce central nervous system side effects that are difficult to recognize.
Psychologic	
Addictive personality	Older children or parents given narcotics, stimulants, or tranquilizers such as codeine, methylphenidate, or diazepam may abuse or misuse these drugs at home.
Limited cognitive functioning	Decreased understanding of directions, indications, or monitoring of drug therapy can lead to noncompliance or delayed recognition of side effects.

Compliance

Drug therapy can be successful only if the patient is amenable to it. In pediatric dosing, the palatability and frequency of administration affect primarily compliance. Cost of medications, undesirable side effects, and comprehension of drug regimen (ie, the importance of drug schedule) also influence patient compliance. Although efficacy of drug therapy is of major importance, the drug regimen is effective only if the patient takes it as prescribed.

Drug Dosing

A. Methods Based on Weight: Nearly every drug that has been safely used in pediatric patients

Table 40–2. Primary route of elimination for drugs commonly used in pediatrics.

Renal Elimination	Hepatic Elimination
Penicillins	Anticonvulsants (phenytoin, carbamazepine)
Cephalosporins	
Aminoglycosides	Acetaminophen
Digoxin	Theophylline
Ranitidine and cimetidine	Antidepressants (imipramine, fluoxetine)
Furosemide	Steroids (anti-inflammatory and hormonal)
Fluconazole	Opiates (morphine, codeine)
Acyclovir	Benzodiazepines (diazepam, lorazepam)
	Erythromycin
	Clindamycin

has an established milligram per kilogram dosing range. Drug dosing based on a child's weight in kilograms is simple, convenient, and widely accepted. Depending on the therapeutic index of the drug, dosing may fall within a range or require a specific initial dose (Figure 40–1; Table 40–5). In general, drugs with a wide therapeutic index have wider dosing ranges, and rounding of doses to a standard dose (eg, amoxicillin 250 mg rather than 236 mg) is recommended.

Drugs with a narrow therapeutic index should be dosed based on the specific mg/kg dosing guidelines and adjusted during therapy with serum drug level monitoring. Frequent recalculation of dosages should be incorporated into the care of children receiving long-term drug therapy since their growth will eventually necessitate increased dosages.

In older children over 40–50 kg, in whom pediatric doses based on body weight might exceed the normal adult dose, it is recommended that the normal adult dosage be used as the upper limit to prevent toxicity and achieve desired efficacy.

B. Methods Based on BSA: Drug dosing based on body surface area may be more accurate. Many drugs with a narrow therapeutic index have dosing guidelines based on patient BSA. Pediatric anticancer chemotherapeutic agents, antiretroviral drugs, and some other antiviral agents are a few of the commonly prescribed pediatric drugs that are dosed according to BSA measurements. There are several different methods for estimating BSA. The

Table 40–3. Effect of changing clinical acuity on drug selection.

Initial Acuity Level	Subsequent Acuity Level	Impact on Drug Selection
Serious bacterial infection with lethargy, decreased oral intake, and fever	Resolving fever, increased oral intake, normal play activities	Initial therapy with intravenous medications may be switched to oral.
Mild bacterial infection with low-grade fever, cough, and sore throat	Persistent fever, decreased activity, focal signs of infection, worsened cough and tachypnea	Initial oral therapy may be switched to intravenous therapy and hospitalization.
Wheezing patient with asthma, with tachypnea, dyspnea, and retractions requiring supplemental oxygen	Asthma, wheezing with normal respiratory rate, breathing room air	Initial aggressive nebulization and intravenous corticosteroids may be switched to metered-dose inhaler and oral or inhaled corticosteroids.
Active generalized seizure	No seizure activity for 24–48 hours	Change from intravenous to oral therapy with same or different anticonvulsant.

nomogram in Figure 40–2 is simple to use. An equation can be easily programmed into a calculator or a computerized database spreadsheet to produce a rapid estimate of BSA for a medical record.

$$BSA\ (m^2) = wt\ (kg)^{0.51436} \times ht\ (cm)^{0.42246} \times 0.0235$$

With some drugs (eg, acyclovir), dosing recommendations are based both on mg/kg and BSA, and the calculated dosages by the two methods can be discrepant. There are limited data evaluating the differences in efficacy and safety of drugs dosed by each method; however, many clinicians believe that dosing based on the BSA is a more accurate method.

Although extrapolation of adult doses to pediatric patients is not recommended, this is best done by dosage adjustment on the basis of BSA.

$$\text{Approximate dose for child} = \frac{\text{BSA of child } (m^2)}{1.73\ m^2\ (\text{normal BSA for adult})} \times \text{Average adult dose } (mg/\text{dose or } mg/d)$$

C. Dosing Intervals: The frequency with which a drug must be given is dictated by pharmacokinetic parameters. The time it takes for the body to eliminate the drug or the time the drug is concentrated intracellularly or in the plasma defines its half-life. The longer the half-life of a drug, the less frequently must it be given. For example, azithromycin has an exceptionally long intracellular half-life and thus is given once a day—compared with eryth-

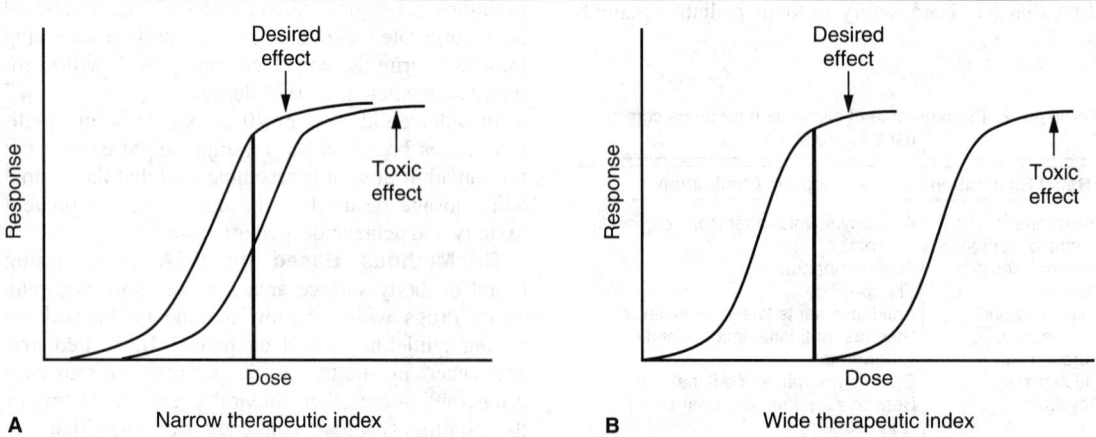

Figure 40–1. Graphs of therapeutic index defined as the difference between desired (therapeutic) effect and toxic effect of a drug at a given dose. **A:** Narrow therapeutic index. **B:** Wide therapeutic index.

Table 40–4. Therapeutic indices of selected drugs.

Wide[1]	Narrow[2]
Penicillins	Aminoglycosides
Cephalosporins	Anticonvulsants
Acetaminophen	Cancer chemotherapy agents
Ibuprofen	Catecholamines (dopamine, epi-
Decongestants and	nephrine)
antihistamines	Amphotericin B
Sucralfate	Opiate narcotics (morphine, codeine)
Benzodiazepines	Heparin and warfarin
Ranitidine and	Lidocaine
cimetidine	Digoxin
	Theophylline
	Vancomycin and immunosuppressants
	(cyclosporine)

[1]Relatively safe; can round doses.
[2]Increased toxicity; requires specific dosing.

romycin, which does not attain similar intracellular concentrations and is given four times a day.

Another variable that determines the frequency of dosing is pharmacodynamics, ie, how the drug and the target organ or organism interact to maximize drug effect. The killing effect of aminoglycosides is maximized when large plasma concentrations of the drug are achieved rapidly, such that the plasma concentration is 15–20 times the minimum inhibitory concentration of the microbe (concentration-dependent killing). Once this is attained, more effective killing and a very long drug effect occurs. This permits dosing once-daily instead of every 8 hours. The opposite occurs with cephalosporins, which kill effectively when constant blood levels—not maximal blood levels—are achieved (time-dependent killing), so that more frequent dosing (every 8 hours or every 6 hours) provides an optimal pharmacodynamic setting.

D. Individualization: Many factors can affect a patient's response to a medication, and individualized dosage adjustments may be necessary to achieve the desired response or outcome. Drugs that require routine blood concentration monitoring should have doses adjusted to achieve therapeutic and nontoxic concentrations (Table 40–5). Three important pharmacokinetic principles govern appropriate individualization of drug doses based on blood concentration determinations.

Steady state is the time it takes for the drug concentration to reach equilibrium in the body and is directly related to the elimination half-life of the drug. In general, a drug is considered to be at steady state after it has been continuously administered at the same dosage and interval (eg, gentamicin, 25 mg every 8 hours) for at least five half-lives. For some drugs, the half-life may be short (eg, gentamicin's half-life is 2–4 hours), and steady state is achieved in 1 day. Some drugs have a long half-life (eg, phenobarbital's half-life is 24–36 hours) and require days

or weeks to achieve steady state. Interpreting drug levels and making dosage adjustments on the basis of blood concentrations that are not at steady state can lead to overdosing and toxicity. Likewise, after a dosage adjustment has been made, a new steady state must be achieved and an additional five half-lives are needed before rechecking the blood concentration.

A second principle is the "linear" relation between blood concentration of the drug and dosing rate and body clearance.

$$\begin{array}{c} \text{Drug} \\ \text{Concentration} \\ \text{(mg/L, } \mu\text{g/mL)} \end{array} = \frac{\begin{array}{c}\text{Dosing rate} \\ \text{(mg/d, mg/kg/d, etc)}\end{array}}{\begin{array}{c}\text{Total body clearance} \\ \text{(renal and hepatic)} \\ \text{(mL/d, mL/kg/d, etc)}\end{array}}$$

The blood concentration of a given drug is directly related to the dosing rate at steady state. Therefore, if a steady state blood concentration is 50% of that desired, doubling the dosage will achieve the desired concentration after it achieves its new steady state.

A third concept is the "nonlinear" relation between clearance, dosing rate, and blood concentration, which exists for a select group of drugs (salicylates, ethanol, phenytoin, and theophylline). These drugs do not have predictable correlation between dosing rate and steady state blood concentration and require close drug monitoring by clinicians experienced with their pharmacokinetics (Figure 40–3).

Dosage individualization and close monitoring of drug concentrations can also be useful in evaluating suspected malabsorption of oral medications or noncompliance. This is encountered during long-term therapy in which oral drugs are preferred, such as in the treatment of HIV infection, osteomyelitis, and seizure disorders. Assessment of oral drug absorption by means of blood concentration monitoring allows for safe dose escalation to overcome decreased absorption.

E. Routes of Administration:

1. Oral route–Oral administration is the easiest, least expensive, and most convenient route of drug administration in children. Oral therapy is not appropriate in very young infants (under 1–2 months of age) or in children with short bowel syndrome because of unpredictable bioavailability (absorption). Oral therapy is also inappropriate in a severely ill child. When oral therapy is indicated and desired, the appropriate dosage form for the age of the child should be selected. Oral suspensions and liquids are available for many medications and are preferred for infants and young children, though most adolescents prefer tablets and capsules. A number of drugs are not available in liquid formulations but can be compounded by pharmacies (Table 40–6). There are several "sprinkle" formulations, that can be added to

Table 40–5. Therapeutic blood levels.[1]

Drug	Expressed as Fraction of g/mL	Expressed as Fraction of mol/L (SI Units)
Acetaminophen	10–20 µg/mL[2]	65–130 µmol/L
Amikacin	15–30 µg/mL (peak) < 5 µg/mL (trough)	
Aspirin	150–300 µg/mL	1–2.2 mmol/L
Carbamazepine	4–12 µg/mL	16–48 µmol/L
Chloramphenicol	15–25 µg/mL	40–75 µmol/L
Cyclosporine	50–250 mg/mL[2]	(trough)
Digoxin	0.9–2.4 ng/mL	1–2 nmol/L
Ethanol	1000 µg/mL	20 mmol/L
Ethosuximide	40–100 µg/mL	280–700 µmol/L
Flucytosine	< 100 µg/mL < 80 µg/mL in newborns and infants	
Gentamicin	6–10 µg/mL (peak) < 2 µg/mL (trough)	
Lidocaine	< 100 ng/mL (newborn) 1.5–2.5 µg/mL (adult)	< 0.4 µmol/L (newborn) 6–9 µmol/L (adult)
Methsuximide as the metabolite of N-des-methsuximide	10–40 µg/mL	50–200 µmol/L
Phenobarbital	15–40 µg/mL	60–160 µmol/L
Phenytoin	10–20 µg/mL	40–80 µmol/L
Primidone	4–12 µg/mL	20–55 µmol/L
Procainamide	4–6 µg/mL	15–20 nmol/L
Quinidine	3–5 µg/mL	10–15 µmol/L
Theophylline	5–20 µg/mL	25–110 µmol/L
Tobramycin	6–10 µg/mL (peak) < 2 µg/mL (trough)	17–21 µmol/L (peak)
Valproic acid	50–120 µg/mL	350–800 µmol/L
Vancomycin	20–40 µg/mL (peak) 4–12 µg/mL (trough)	

[1]Therapeutic level or range for drugs that can be routinely analyzed.
[2]Therapeutic ranges will differ depending on type of cyclosporine assay used (eg, monoclonal versus polyclonal whole boood TDx assays).

foods. Chewable tablets can be used beginning at about 12–18 months of age.

Absorption of orally administered medications can be affected by dietary factors. Recommendations for administration with or without food are specific for each drug and should be followed. Drugs that require administration on an empty stomach generally have significantly decreased absorption when given with food. Giving a drug with food is generally for the purpose of decreasing gastrointestinal upset and not to improve absorption. Thus, most drugs can be taken on an empty stomach to achieve therapeutic response, but some are best administered with food to decrease gastrointestinal complaints.

2. Rectal route–Rectal administration of medications should be reserved for children who cannot take oral medications. It is important to stress to the parent or child the need to remove the wrapping from suppositories prior to insertion. Incomplete dose administration can occur if the suppository does not re-

NOMOGRAM

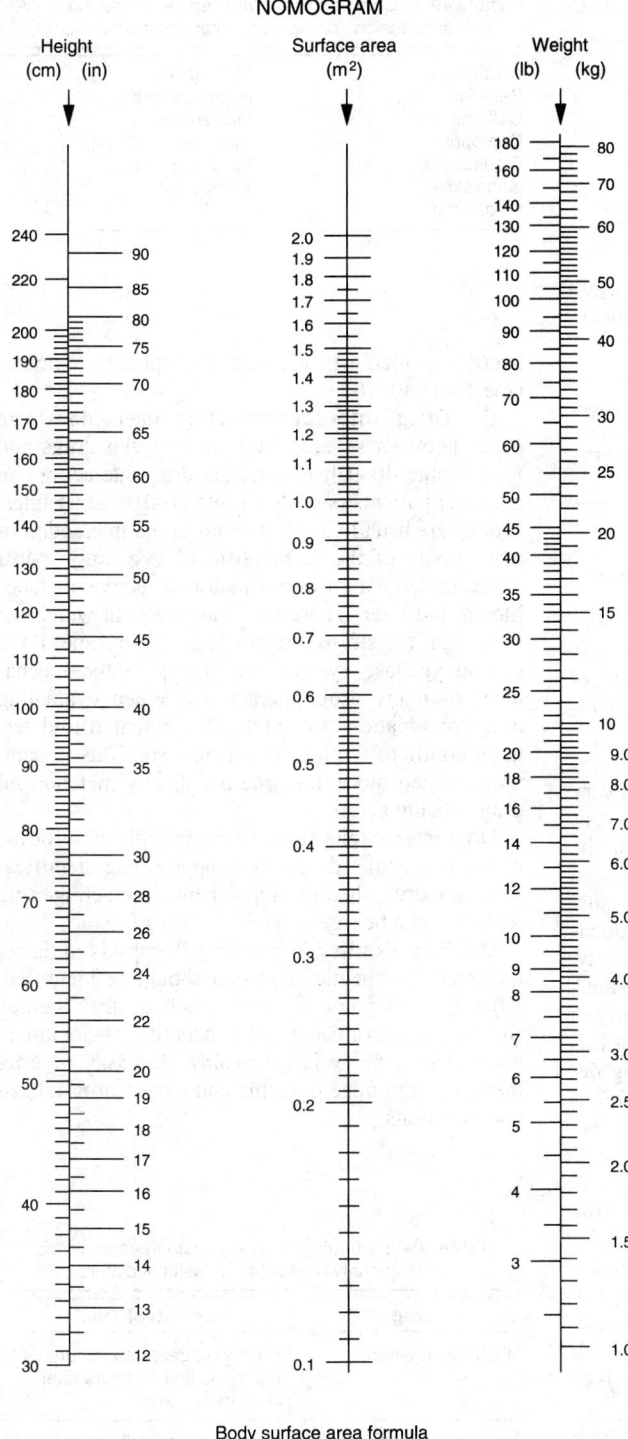

Height
(cm)   (in)

Surface area
(m²)

Weight
(lb)   (kg)

Body surface area formula
(Adult and Pediatric)

$$BSA\ (m^2) = \sqrt{\frac{Ht\ (in)\ x\ Wt\ (lb)}{3131}} \quad \text{or, in metric:}\quad BSA\ (m^2) = \sqrt{\frac{Ht\ (cm)\ x\ Wt\ (kg)}{3600}}$$

Figure 40–2. Body surface area: Children. To determine the body surface area in a child, use a straightedge to connect the height and mass. The point of intersection on the body surface line gives the area in meters squared. (Reproduced, with permission, from *Geigy Scientific Tables,* 8th ed, vol 1. Lentner C [editor]. Ciba-Geigy, 1981.)

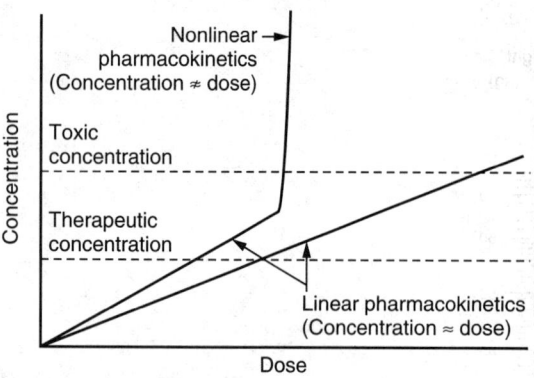

Figure 40–3. Differences between linear and nonlinear concentration-dose profiles. Drugs with nonlinear pharmacokinetics can produce unexpected toxic concentrations with only small incremental changes in dose.

main in the rectum for sufficient time. Drug distribution within a suppository may not be uniform and therefore administering half of a suppository may not provide half the dose, leading to either a subtherapeutic or a toxic response in the child.

3. Parenteral route–Intravenous administration of drugs is the most reliable method of delivery and is preferred in severely ill children. Many physical incompatibilities have been identified with the coadministration of intravenous medications and maintenance fluids. If an incompatibility is suspected, a pharmacist should be contacted for documentation and management of the incompatibility. The site of drug administration into an intravenous line should be as proximal as possible, particularly in infants who have maintenance fluid flow rates of less than 40 mL/h, because significant delay in drug delivery can occur from more distal sites in the intravenous system.

Monitoring Drug Therapy

A. Efficacy: The efficacy of a particular drug regimen should be continuously evaluated. Resolution of signs and symptoms is an excellent indicator of therapeutic effectiveness. Therapy must be given an adequate trial before it is considered ineffective. The time course of response to therapy defines an adequate therapeutic trial. Several examples are given in Table 40–7.

B. Safety: Monitoring the safety of a drug regimen requires knowledge of the specific toxicities of the medication and continuous evaluation of the patient for toxic signs and symptoms. Toxicities are generally categorized by organ system effects. Monitoring parameters for specific organ system dysfunction is summarized in Table 40–8. It is important for clinicians to have appropriate drug information re-

Table 40–6. Common drugs that can be compounded into suspensions or liquids for oral administration.

Azathioprine	Metolazone
Baclofen	Metronidazole
Caffeine	Midazolam
Captopril	Rifampin
Clonazepam	Spironolactone
Ganciclovir	Verapamil
Lorazepam	

sources available to identify drug-specific toxicities (see Table 40–10).

C. Drug Interactions: Drug interactions can occur between several drugs or between drugs and food. Table 40–9 lists common drug interactions in pediatric patients (see also Table 40–10). Drug interactions are usually a direct result of the interaction or overlapping of the metabolism of two drugs. Most drugs undergo biotransformation to active metabolites in the liver. There are many ways in which the liver can transform drugs. The cytochrome P450 monooxygenase system contributes to the mechanism of many drug interactions. When evaluating drug combinations for safety, it is essential to determine conflicting routes of metabolism. This is paramount when more than one hepatically metabolized drug is being given.

Drug interactions are not a contraindication for the use of interacting drugs. With appropriate identification and drug therapy adjustment, interacting drug regimens can be safely used.

D. End Points: When drug therapy is initiated, a desired therapeutic end point should be identified. After the end point has been reached, drug therapy should be reevaluated. The benefits of treatment must always be weighed against the risks of drug therapy to optimize outcome and reduce drug-related complications.

Table 40–7. Duration of an adequate therapeutic trial for commonly prescribed drugs in pediatrics.

Drug	Length of Trial
Albuterol (inhaled)	Response generally occurs within the first 12 hours after starting therapy.
Antibacterial antibiotics	Response generally occurs within 48–72 hours after starting therapy.
Corticosteroids (inhaled)	Maximal response takes 1–2 weeks of continuous therapy.
Antidepressants	Maximal response takes 3–6 weeks of continuous therapy.

Table 40–8. Monitoring parameters for organ toxicities from drug therapy.

Organ-Specific Toxicity	Parameters
Gastrointestinal	Frequency of nausea, vomiting, diarrhea, cramping, abdominal pain, and decrease in oral intake
Renal	Blood urea nitrogen (BUN), creatinine, urinalysis (casts, enzymes, electrolytes), urine output
Hepatic	Liver function tests (AST, ALT, bilirubin/alkaline phosphatase); scleral coloring, bleeding times (PT, PTT), nausea, vomiting, pruritus, mental status, jaundice, liver size
Neurologic	Lethargy, anxiety, irritability, orientation, hallucinations, confusion, mental status
Dermatologic	Type of rash (eg, macular, papular, vesicular), location and extent, itching, temporal onset
Hematologic	Complete blood count with differential, bleeding time (PT/PTT), platelet count, bruising, infection

Table 40–10. Important drug information resources for pediatric practitioners.

Resource	Information Content
Harriet Lane Handbook (Johns Hopkins Hospital and Year Book Medical Publishers)	Drug dosing for standard indications; some side effects information. Available dosage forms; plenty of other useful clinical information not related to drug therapy. Pocket size.
Pediatric Dosing Handbook (American Pharmaceutical Association and Lexicomp Publishing)	Comprehensive dosing and side effect information. Available dosage forms, drug interactions, and pharmacokinetics; useful appendices. Pocket size.
American Hospital Formulary Service (American Society of Health-System Pharmacists)	Most pediatric dosing, comprehensive side effects, dosage forms, drug interactions, and pharmacokinetics. Large book.
Physicians' Desk Reference (Medical Economics)	Incomplete or no pediatric dosing for many drugs. Little or no pediatric pharmacokinetics or side effects. Contains available dosage forms. Large book.
Drugs During Pregnancy and Lactation (Williams & Wilkins)	"The book" on drug use during pregnancy and lactation. No dosing, but well referenced with primary literature. Large book.

Table 40–9. Common pediatric drugs associated with drug interactions.

Drug	Potential Interaction	Comments
Carbamazepine	Increases hepatic metabolism of other drugs, causing decreased levels	Can increase its own metabolism. Has an active epoxide metabolite.
Phenobarbital	Increases hepatic metabolism of other drugs, causing decreased levels	No effect on phenytoin. Primidone is metabolized to phenobarbital and can cause similar interactions.
Phenytoin	Increases hepatic metabolism of other drugs, causing decreased levels	Has nonlinear pharmacokinetics.
Rifampin	Increases hepatic metabolism of other drugs, causing decreased levels	Rapid onset. Can occur with 4-day prophylaxis regimens. Decreases efficacy of oral contraceptives.
Erythromycin Clarithromycin	Decreases hepatic metabolism of other drugs, causing increased levels	Erythromycin is a component of Pediazole suspension. Azithromycin can be used as an alternative to erythromycin without interactions.
Cimetidine	Decreases hepatic metabolism of other drugs, causing increased levels	Can use ranitidine or famotidine as alternatives without interactions
Valproate	Decreases hepatic metabolism of other drugs, causing increased levels	
Antacids	Increases gastric pH and decreases oral absorption of some drugs	All H_2 blockers can cause the same interaction. Decreases ketoconazole and itraconazole absorption.
Mg^{2+}, Ca^{2+}, and Fe^{2+} salts	Bind to some drugs and inactivates or decreases oral absorption	Tetracyclines and fluoroquinolones should not be given within 2 hours of these salts.

SOURCES OF PEDIATRIC DRUG INFORMATION

The Pharmacist

Pharmacists—particularly those who practice in a pediatric care environment—are extremely useful sources of drug information. They often know drug doses and side effects as well as practical issues regarding the appropriate therapeutic uses of pharmaceuticals. Their services are usually available at any hour, 7 days a week, at no cost to the patient.

Reference Works

Table 40–10 summarizes several useful drug references. Clinicians who care for pediatric patients should be familiar with these resources.

Computerized Sources

There is a trend toward use of computerized drug information databases in institutional and managed care settings. Several of these databases also provide specific citations from the primary literature from which the information is derived. Access to these drug information sources will facilitate rapid development of drug therapy decisions. Examples are Drugdex from Micromedex, Inc, and Clinical Pharmacology from Gold Standard.

REFERENCES

Bates RD, Nahata M: Once-daily administration of aminoglycosides. Ann Pharmacother 1994;28:757.

Gelman CR, Rumack BH (editors): *DRUGDEX Information Systems.* Micromedex, 1995.

Gilman AG et al: Goodman & Gilman's The Pharmacological Basis of Therapeutics, 8th ed. Pergamon, 1990.

Radde IC, MacLeod SM: *Pediatric Pharmacology & Therapeutics,* 2nd ed. Mosby, 1993.

Yaffe SJ, Aranda JV: *Pediatric Pharmacology.* Saunders, 1992.

Normal Biochemical & Hematologic Values

41

Keith B. Hammond, MS, FIMLS

Pediatricians and other health professionals caring for children have the responsibility to insist on accurate, rapid, and comprehensive laboratory testing. Collecting large blood samples for biochemical assay is not suitable for the proper care of children—especially for premature infants or older children in intensive care units, where repetitive sampling may be essential. Technology for performing biochemical assays on blood samples of 100 mL or less has been available for 40 years or more. Most of the earlier automated systems for assay were better adapted to larger samples. However, the newest automated systems have the capacity to work with small volumes.

In infants and young children, blood samples taken by heel-prick are better collected by laboratory personnel than by physicians or nurses.

INTERPRETATION OF LABORATORY VALUES

Accreditation by the College of American Pathologists and by state or federal agencies has done much to ensure standardized laboratory performance. Methods used in various laboratories differ, as do normal values for the methods. Normal range is, of course, a combination of biologic variation and intrinsic laboratory variation; thus, an acceptable range of normal values should ideally be composed of data developed within the laboratory for the population it serves. Any laboratory should be able to provide information on the coefficient of variation and standard deviation applicable to each test performed in that laboratory. Each laboratory should maintain a rigorous procedure of checks with daily standards and control specimens. Errors may still occur but can usually be detected by retesting before a questionable result is reported. Fortunately, errors occur much less commonly today than in the past.

The clinical value of a test is related to its sensitivity and specificity. **Sensitivity** is an expression of the incidence of positive test results in those who have the disease. **Specificity** is an expression of the incidence of negative test results in those free of the disease. Sensitivity and specificity are calculated as follows:

$$\textbf{Sensitivity (\%)} = \frac{\textbf{TP}}{\textbf{TP + FN}} \times \textbf{100}$$

(ie, how many TP are missed)

$$\textbf{Specificity (\%)} = \frac{\textbf{TN}}{\textbf{TN + FP}} \times \textbf{100}$$

(ie, how many TN are missed)

where TP = a true-positive result, FP = a false-positive result, TN = a true-negative result, and FN = a false-negative result.

Screening tests must be interpreted with appreciation of sensitivity and specificity. These expressions are illustrated in Figure 41–1 in terms of a screening test for phenylketonuria in newborns. The values are not strictly correct but serve the purpose of illustration. According to Figure 41–1, a blood phenylalanine level of 4 mg/dL is the discriminating point above which all infants are presumed to have the disease and below which they are presumed to be normal. However, no test is ever quite that exact. Some normal infants will have levels above 4 mg/dL; the test results in these will be false-positive. Some abnormal infants will have levels below 4 mg/dL; the test results in these will be false-negative. The discriminating point is a compromise between sensitivity and specificity. Moving the point to 2 mg/dL would effect 100% sensitivity, but there would be a large increase in the number of false-positive results. Moving it to 6 mg/dL would make it very specific, but this would increase the number of false-negative responses, which would result in failure to detect phenylketonuria in a much larger proportion of affected children.

These concepts can be viewed in yet another way. Suppose that this test were set at a specificity of 99.9%. This would mean that in a sample of 10,000 tests, there would be ten false-positive results. In a

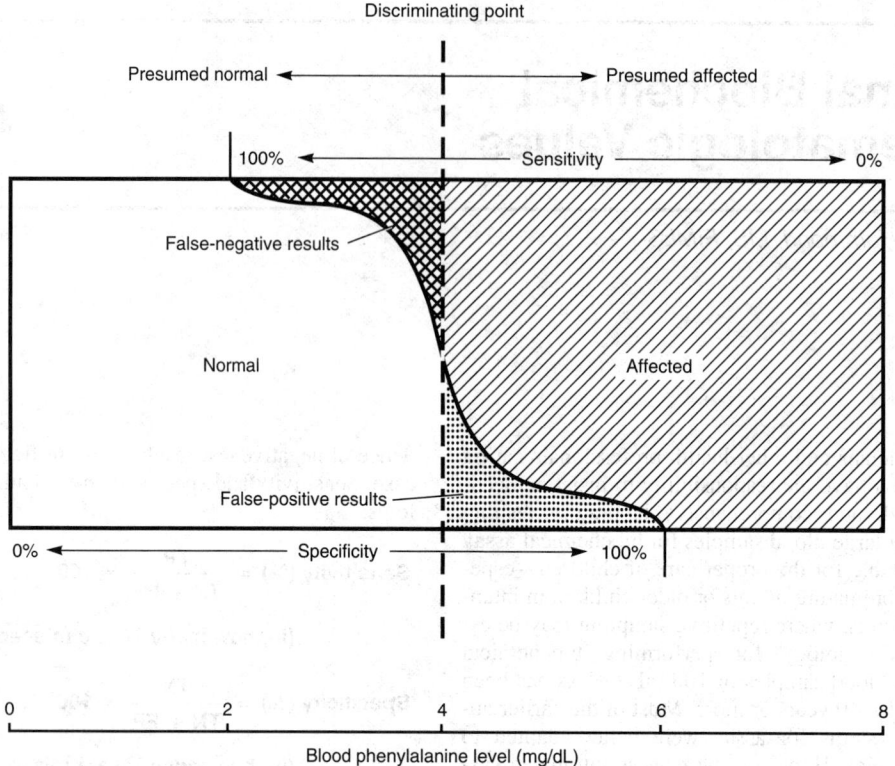

Figure 41–1. Screening test for phenylketonuria in newborns. Data have been simplified to illustrate the concepts of sensitivity and specificity (see text).

rare condition such as phenylketonuria, however, the true incidence of the disease may be only 1:12,000. The ratio of true-positive to false-positive results is thus 1:12; this is a reflection of the low incidence of the disease and the relatively high incidence of false-positive results because of the nature of the assay. These considerations, of course, apply to the interpretation of all laboratory tests.

LABORATORY VALUES

Normal blood chemistry values and miscellaneous other laboratory values are shown in Tables 41–1 to 41–3.

Table 41–1. Normal blood chemistry values and miscellaneous other hematologic values.[1]
(Values may vary with the procedure used.)

Determinations for		
(S) = Serum	(P)	= Plasma
(B) = Whole blood	(RBC)	= Red blood cells

Acid-Base Measurements (B)
pH: 7.38–7.42 from 14 min of age and older
PaO_2: 65–76 mm Hg (8.66–10.13 kPa)
$PaCO_2$: 36–38 mm Hg (4.8–5.07 kPa)
Base excess: –2 to +2 mEq/L, except in newborns (range,
   –4 to –0)

Acid Phosphatase (S, P)
Values using *p*-nitrophenyl phosphate buffered with citrate
   (end-point determination)
Newborns: 7.4–19.4 IU/L at 37 °C
2–13 y: 6.4–15.2 IU/L at 37 °C
Adult males: 0.5–11 IU/L at 37 °C
Adult females: 0.2–9.5 IU/L at 37 °C

Alanine Aminotransferase (ALT, SGPT) (S)
Newborns (1–3 d): 1–25 IU/L at 37 °C
Adult males: 7–46 IU/L at 37 °C
Adult females: 4–35 IU/L at 37 °C

Alkaline Phosphatase (S)
Values in IU/L at 37 °C using *p*-nitrophenyl phosphate
   buffered with AMP (kinetic)

Group	Males	Females
Newborns (1–3 d)	95–368	95–368
2–24 mo	115–460	115–460
2–5 y	115–391	115–391
6–7 y	115–460	115–460
8–9 y	115–345	115–345
10–11 y	115–336	115–437
12–13 y	127–403	92–336
14–15 y	79–446	78–212
16–18 y	58–331	35–124
Adults	41–137	39–118

Ammonia (P)
Newborns: 90–150 µg/dL (53–88 µmol/L); higher in
   premature and jaundiced infants
Thereafter: 0–60 µg/dL (0–35 µmol/L) when blood is
   drawn with proper precautions

Amylase (S)
Values using maltotetrose substrate (kinetic)
Neonates: Undetectable
2–12 mo: Levels increase slowly to adult levels
Adults: 28–108 IU/L at 37 °C

Anticoagulation Factors (P)
Values in U/mL. Shown are mean values and –2 SD or
   lower range (in parentheses)

Factor	Preterm (25–32 wk)	Term Infant	Infant (6 mo)	Adult
AT III	0.35 (0.20)	0.56 (0.32)	1.04 (0.84)	1.0 (0.8)
PC	0.29 (0.20)	0.50 (0.30)	0.59 (0.37)	1.0 (0.6)
PS, total	. . .	0.24 (0.10)	0.87 (0.55)	1.0 (0.6)
PS, free	0.48	0.42	. . .	1.0 (0.5)
HcF II	0.25 (0.10)	0.49 (0.36)	0.97 (0.59)	1.0 (0.7)

AT III = antithrombin III, PC = protein C, PS = protein S,
Hcf II = heparin cofactor II.

α₁-Antitrypsin (antiprotease) (S)
1–3 mo: 127–404 mg/dL
3–12 mo: 145–362 mg/dL
1–2 y: 160–382 mg/dL
2–15 y: 148–394 mg/dL

Ascorbic Acid: See Vitamin C.

Aspartate Aminotransferase (AST, SGOT) (S)
Newborns (1–3 d): 16–74 IU/L at 37 °C
Adult males: 8–46 IU/L at 37 °C
Adult females: 7–34 IU/L at 37 °C

Base Excess: See Acid-Base Measurements.

Bicarbonate, Actual (P)
Calculated from pH and $PaCO_2$
Newborns: 17.2–23.6 mmol/L
2 mo–2 y: 19–24 mmol/L
Children: 18–25 mmol/L
Adult males: 20.1–28.9 mmol/L
Adult females: 18.4–28.8 mmol/L

Bilirubin (S)
Values in mg/dL (µmol/L)
Levels after 1 mo are as follows:
Conjugated: 0–0.3 mg/dL (0–5 µmol/L)
Unconjugated: 0.1–0.7 mg/dL (2–12 µmol/L)

Peak Newborn Level	Percentage of Newborns (Birth Weight) Exceeding Peak Level		
	< 2001 g	2001–2500 g	> 2500 g
20 (342)	8.2%	2.6%	0.8%
18 (308)	13.5%	4.6%	1.5%
16 (274)	20.3%	7.6%	2.6%
14 (239)	33.0%	12.0%	4.4%
11 (188)	53.8%	23.0%	9.3%
8 (137)	77.0%	45.4%	26.1%

Bleeding Time (Simplate)
2–9 min

Blood Volume
Premature infants: 98 mL/kg
At 1 y: 86 mL/kg (range, 69–112 mL/kg)
Older children: 70 mL/kg (range, 51–86 mL/kg)

BUN: See Urea Nitrogen.

C Peptide (S)
5–15 y (8:00 AM fasting): 1–4 ng/mL
Adults (8:00 AM fasting): < 4 ng/mL
Adults (nonfasting): < 8 ng/mL

C-Reactive Protein (S)
3–16 y: 0.1–1.5 mg/dL

Calcium, Ionized (P)
0–2 d: 1.1–1.4 mmol/L
3–4 d: 1.1–1.5 mmol/L
5–8 d: 1.2–1.5 mmol/L
9–14 d: 1.3–1.6 mmol/L
2 mo–18 y: 1.2–1.4 mmol/L

(continued)

Table 41–1. Normal blood chemistry values and miscellaneous other hematologic values.[1]
(Values may vary with the procedure used.) (continued)

Calcium, Total (S)
Premature infants (first week): 3.5–4.5 meq/L (1.7–2.3 mmol/L)
Full-term infants (first week): 4–5 meq/L (2–2.5 mmol/L)
Thereafter: 4.4–5.3 meq/L (2.2–2.7 mmol/L)

Carbon Dioxide, Total (S, P)
Cord blood: 15–20.2 mmol/L
Children: 18–27 mmol/L
Adults: 24–35 mmol/L

Carnitine (P)
Values in mmol/L, measured by an enzymatic radioisotopic method

Age	Total Carnitine	Free Carnitine	Acyl-carnitine	AC/FC Ratio
1 day	23.3–67.9	11.5–36.0	7.0–36.6	0.37–1.68
2–7 days	17.4–40.6	10.1–21.0	2.9–23.8	0.15–1.44
8–28 days	18.5–58.7	12.3–46.2	4.1–14.5	0.11–0.65
1 month to 1 year	38.1–68.0	26.9–49.0	7.4–19.0	0.23–0.50
1–6 years	34.6–83.6	24.3–62.5	4.0–28.3	0.11–0.83
6–10 years	27.8–82.9	21.7–66.4	3.1–32.1	0.08–0.87
10–17 years	33.7–77.0	21.6–64.5	3.7–29.2	0.09–0.88
22–60 years	33.8–77.5	25.4–54.1	5.4–30.1	0.11–0.78

Cation-Anion Gap (S, P)
5–15 mmol/L

Ceruloplasmin (Copper Oxidase) (S, P)
21–43 mg/dL (1.3–2.7 μmol/L)

Chloride (S, P)
Premature infants: 95–110 mmol/L
Full-term infants: 96–116 mmol/L
Children: 98–105 mmol/L
Adults: 98–108 mmol/L

Cholesterol, Total (S, P)
Values in mg/dL (mmol/L)

Group	Males	Females
6–7 y	115–197 (2.97–5.09)	126–199 (3.25–5.14)
8–9 y	112–199 (2.89–5.14)	124–208 (3.20–5.37)
10–11 y	108–220 (2.79–5.68)	115–208 (2.97–5.37)
12–13 y	117–202 (3.02–5.21)	114–207 (2.94–5.34)
14–15 y	103–207 (2.66–5.34)	102–208 (2.63–5.37)
16–17 y	107–198 (2.76–5.11)	106–213 (2.73–5.50)

Coagulation Factors (P)
Values in U/mL. Shown are mean values and –2 SD or lower range (in parentheses).

Factor	Preterm (25–32 wk)	Term Infant	Infant (6 mo)	Adult
II	0.32 (0.18)	0.52 (0.25)	0.88 (0.60)	1.0 (0.7)
V	0.80 (0.43)	1.00 (0.54)	0.91 (0.55)	1.0 (0.6)
VII	0.37 (0.24)	0.57 (0.35)	0.87 (0.50)	1.0 (0.6)
VIII	0.75 (0.40)	1.50 (0.55)	0.90 (0.50)	1.0 (0.6)
vWF	1.50 (0.90)	1.60 (0.84)	1.07 (0.60)	1.0 (0.6)
IX	0.22 (0.17)	0.35 (0.15)	0.86 (0.36)	1.0 (0.5)
X	0.38 (0.20)	0.45 (0.30)	0.78 (0.38)	1.0 (0.6)
XI	0.20 (0.12)	0.42 (0.20)	0.86 (0.38)	1.0 (0.6)
XII	0.22 (0.09)	0.44 (0.16)	0.77 (0.39)	1.0 (0.6)
XIII	. . .	0.61 (0.36)	1.04 (0.50)	1.0 (0.6)
PreK	0.26 (0.14)	0.35 (0.16)	0.86 (0.56)	1.1 (0.6)

vWF = von Willebrand factor, PreK = prekallikrein.

Complement (S)
C3: 96–195 mg/dL
C4: 15–20 mg/dL

Copper (S)
Cord blood: 26–32 μg/dL (4.1–5.2 μmol/L)
Newborns: 26–32 μg/dL (4.1–5.2 μmol/L)
1 mo: 73–93 μg/dL (11.5–14.6 μmol/L)
2 mo: 59–69 μg/dL (9.3–10.9 μmol/L)
6 mo–5 y: 27–153 μg/dL (4.2–24.1 μmol/L)
5–17 y: 94–234 μg/dL (14.8–36.8 μmol/L)
Adults: 70–118 μg/dL (11–18.6 μmol/L)

Copper Oxidase: See Ceruloplasmin.

Cortisol (S, P)
Morning (8:00 AM): 5–25 μg/dL (0.14–0.68 μmol/L)
Evening: 5–15 μg/dL (0.14–0.41 μmol/L)

Creatine (S, P)
0.2–0.8 mg/dL (15.2–61 mmol/L)

Creatine Kinase (S, P)
Newborns (1–3 d): 40–474 IU/L at 37 °C
Adult males: 30–210 IU/L at 37 °C
Adult females: 20–128 IU/L at 37 °C

Creatinine (S,P)
Values in mg/dL (μmol/L)

Group	Males	Females
Newborns (1–3 d)[1]	0.2–1.0 (17.7–88.4)	0.2–1.0 (17.7–88.4)
1 y	0.2–0.6 (17.7–53.0)	0.2–0.5 (17.7–44.2)
2–3 y	0.2–0.7 (17.7–61.9)	0.3–0.6 (26.5–53.0)
4–7 y	0.2–0.8 (17.7–70.7)	0.2–0.7 (17.7–61.9)
8–10 y	0.3–0.9 (26.5–79.6)	0.3–0.8 (26.5–70.7)
11–12 y	0.3–1.0 (26.5–88.4)	0.3–0.9 (26.5–79.6)
13–17 y	0.3–1.2 (26.5–106.1)	0.3–1.1 (26.5–97.2)
18–20 y	0.5–1.3 (44.2–115.0)	0.3–1.1 (26.5–97.2)

[1]Values may be higher in premature newborns.

Creatinine Clearance
Values show great variability and depend on the specificity of the analytical methods used.
Newborns (1 d): 5–50 mL/min/1.73 m (mean, 18 mL/min/1.73 m)
Newborns (6 d): 15–90 mL/min/1.73 m^2 (mean, 36 mL/min/1.73 m^2)
Adult males: 85–125 mL/min/1.73 m^2
Adult females: 75–115 mL/min/1.73 m^2

2,3-Diphosphoglycerate (B)
Values vary with the method used and with altitude.
4.5–6 mmol/L

Factor: See Anticoagulation Factors and Coagulation Factors.

Fatty Acids, "Free" (P)
Newborns: 435–1375 μEq/L
4 mo–10 y (14-h fast): 500–900 μEq/L
4 mo–10 y (19-h fast): 730–1200 μEq/L
Adults (14-h fast): 310–590 μEq/L
Adults (19-h fast): 405–720 μEq/L

(continued)

Table 41–1. Normal blood chemistry values and miscellaneous other hematologic values.[1]
(Values may vary with the procedure used.) (continued)

Ferritin (S)
Newborns: 20–200 ng/mL (mean, 117 ng/mL)
1 mo: 60–550 ng/mL (mean, 350 ng/mL)
1–15 y: 7–140 ng/mL (mean, 31 ng/mL)
Adult males: 50–225 ng/mL (mean, 140 ng/mL)
Adult females: 10–150 ng/mL (mean, 40 ng/mL)

Fibrinogen (P)
200–500 mg/dL (5.9–14.7 μmol/L)

Galactose (S, P)
1.1–2.1 mg/dL (0.06–0.12 mmol/L)

Galactose 1-Phosphate (RBC)
Normal: 1 mg/dL of packed erythrocyte lysate; slightly
    higher in cord blood
Infants with congenital galactosemia on a milk-free diet:
    < 2 mg/dL
Infants with congenital galactosemia taking milk:
    9–20 mg/dL

Galactose-1-Phosphate Uridyl Transferase (RBC)
Normal: 308–475 mIU/g of hemoglobin
Heterozygous for Duarte variant: 225–308 mIU/g of
    hemoglobin
Homozygous for Duarte variant: 142–225 mIU/g of
    hemoglobin
Heterozygous for congenital galactosemia: 142–225 mIU/g
    of hemoglobin
Homozygous for congenital galactosemia: <8 mIU/g of
    hemoglobin

Glomerular Filtration Rate
Newborns: About 50% of values for older children and
    adults
Older children and adults: 75–165 mL/min/1.73 m² (levels
    reached by about 6 mo)

Glucose (S, P)
Premature infants: 20–80 mg/dL (1.11–4.44 mmol/L)
Full-term infants: 30–100 mg/dL (1.67–5.56 mmol/L)
Children and adults (fasting): 60–105 mg/dL
    (3.33–5.88 mmol/L)

Glucose-6-Phosphate Dehydrogenase (RBC)
150–215 U/dL

Glucose Tolerance Test (S): SeeTable below.

γ-Glutamyl Transpeptidase (S)
0–1 mo: 12–271 IU/L at 37 °C (kinetic)
1–2 mo: 9–159 IU/L at 37 °C (kinetic)
2–4 mo: 7–98 IU/L at 37 °C (kinetic)
4–7 mo: 5–45 IU/L at 37 °C (kinetic)
7–12 mo: 4–27 IU/L at 37 °C (kinetic)
1–15 y: 3–30 IU/L at 37 °C (kinetic)
Adult males: 9–69 IU/L at 37 °C (kinetic)
Adult females: 3–33 IU/L at 37 °C (kinetic)

Glycohemoglobin (Hemoglobin A$_{1c}$) (B)
Normal: 6.3–8.2% of total hemoglobin
Diabetic patients in good control of their condition
    ordinarily have levels < 10%
Values tend to be lower during pregnancy; they also vary
    with technique

Growth Hormone (GH) (S)
After infancy (fasting specimen): 0–5 ng/mL
In response to natural and artificial provocation (eg, sleep,
    arginine, insulin, hypoglycemia): > 8 ng/mL
During the newborn period (fasting specimen), GH levels
    are high (15–40 ng/mL) and responses to provocation
    are variable

Haptoglobin (S)
50–150 mg/dL has hemoglobin-binding capacity.

Hematocrit (B)
At birth: 44–64%
14–90 d: 35–49%
6 mo–1 y: 30–40%
4–10 y: 31–43%

Hemoglobin A$_{1c}$: See Glycohemoglobin

Hemoglobin Electrophoresis (B)
A$_1$ hemoglobin: 96–98.5% of total hemoglobin
A$_2$ hemoglobin: 1.5–4% of total hemoglobin

Hemoglobin, Fetal (B)
At birth: 50–85% of total hemoglobin
At 1 y: < 15% of total hemoglobin
Up to 2 y: Up to 5% of total hemoglobin
Thereafter: < 2% of total hemoglobin

Glucose tolerance test results in serum.

Normal levels based on results in 13 normal children given glucose.
1.75 g/kg orally in one dose, after 2 wk on a high-carbohydrate diet.

Time	Glucose		Insulin		Phosphorus	
	mg/dL	mmol/L	μU/mL	pmol/L	mg/dL	mmol/L
Fasting	59–96	3.11–5.33	5–40	36–287	3.2–4.9	1.03–1.58
30 min	91–185	5.05–10.27	36–110	258–789	2.0–4.4	0.64–1.42
60 min	66–164	3.66–9.10	22–124	158–890	1.8–3.6	0.58–1.16
90 min	68–148	3.77–8.22	17–105	122–753	1.8–3.6	0.58–1.16
2 h	66–122	3.66–6.77	6–84	43–603	1.8–4.2	0.58–1.36
3 h	47–99	2.61–5.49	2–46	14–330	2.0–4.6	0.64–1.48
4 h	61–93	3.39–5.16	3–32	21–230	2.7–4.3	0.87–1.39
5 h	63–86	3.50–4.77	5–37	36–265	2.9–4.4	0.94–1.42

(continued)

Table 41–1. Normal blood chemistry values and miscellaneous other hematologic values.[1]
(Values may vary with the procedure used.) (continued)

Immunoglobulins (S)
Values in mg/dL

Group	IgG	IgA	IgM
Cord blood	766–1693	0.04–9	4–26
2 wk–3 mo	299–852	3–66	15–149
3–6 mo	142–988	4–90	18–118
6–12 mo	418–1142	14–95	43–223
1–2 y	356–1204	13–118	37–239
2–3 y	492–1269	23–137	49–204
3–6 y	564–1381	35–209	51–214
6–9 y	658–1535	29–384	50–228
9–12 y	625–1598	60–294	64–278
12–16 y	660–1548	81–252	45–256

Insulin: See table at bottom of preceding page.

Inulin Clearance
< 1 mo: 29–88 mL/min/1.73 m^2
1–6 mo: 40–112 mL/min/1.73 m^2
6–12 mo: 62–121 mL/min/1.73 m^2
< 1 y: 78–164 mL/min/1.73 m^2

Iron (S, P)
Newborns: 20–157 μg/dL (3.6–28.1 μmol/L)
6 wk–3 y: 20–115 μg/dL (3.6–20.6 μmol/L)
3–9 y: 20–141 μg/dL (3.6–25.2 μmol/L)
9–14 y: 21–151 μg/dL (3.8–27 μmol/L)
14–16 y: 20–181 μg/dL (3.6–32.4 μmol/L)
Adults: 44–196 μg/dL (7.2–31.3 μmol/L)

Iron-Binding Capacity (S, P)
Newborns: 59–175 μg/dL (10.6–31.3 μmol/L)
Children and adults: 275–458 μg/dL (45–72 μmol/L)

Lactate (B)
Venous blood: 5–18 mg/dL (0.5–2 mmol/L)
Arterial blood: 3–7 mg/dL (0.3–0.8 mmol/L)

Lactate Dehydrogenase (LDH) (S, P)
Values using lactate substrate (kinetic)
Newborns (1–3 d): 40–348 IU/L at 37 °C
1 mo–5 y: 150–360 IU/L at 37 °C
5–8 y: 150–300 IU/L at 37 °C
8–12 y: 130–300 IU/L at 37 °C
12–14 y: 130–280 IU/L at 37 °C
14–16 y: 130–230 IU/L at 37 °C
Adult males: 70–178 IU/L at 37 °C
Adult females: 42–166 IU/L at 37 °C

LDH: See Lactate Dehydrogenase.

Lead (B)
< 10 μg/dL (< 0.48 μmol/L)
When a large proportion of a population of children have
blood lead levels in the range of 10–19 μg/dL
(0.48–0.92 μmol/L), communitywide childhood lead poisoning activities are warranted.
Levels > 20 μg/dL (> 0.97 μmol/L) indicate the need for
medical and environmental evaluation and possible
pharmalogic intervention.
Levels > 70 μg/dL (> 3.38 μmol/L) indicate the immediate
need for medical and environmental management.

Lipase (S, P)
20–136 IU/L based on 4-h incubation

Lipoprotein Cholesterol, High-Density (HDL) (S)
Values in mg/dL (mmol/L)

Group	Males	Females
6–7 y	35–77 (0.90–1.98)	24–76 (0.62–1.96)
8–9 y	31–80 (0.80–2.06)	34–77 (0.87–1.98)
10–11 y	34–81 (0.87–1.09)	30–74 (0.77–1.91)
12–13 y	30–82 (0.77–2.11)	33–73 (0.85–1.88)
14–15 y	26–72 (0.67–1.86)	29–73 (0.74–1.88)
16–17 y	25–66 (0.72–1.70)	27–78 (0.69–2.01)

Lipoprotein Cholesterol, Low-Density (LDL) (S)
Values in mg/dL (mmol/L)

Group	Males	Females
6–7 y	56–134 (1.44–3.46)	52–149 (1.34–3.85)
8–9 y	52–129 (1.34–3.33)	57–143 (1.47–3.69)
10–11 y	45–149 (1.16–3.85)	56–140 (1.44–3.61)
12–13 y	55–135 (1.42–3.48)	58–138 (1.49–3.56)
14–15 y	48–143 (1.24–3.69)	47–140 (1.21–3.61)
16–17 y	53–134 (1.36–3.36)	44–147 (1.13–3.79)

Magnesium (S, P)
Newborns: 1.5–2.3 mEq/L (0.75–1.15 mmol/L)
Adults: 1.4–2 mEq/L (0.7–1 mmol/L)

Methemoglobin (B)
0–0.3 g/dL (0–186 μmol/L)

Osmolality (S, P)
270–290 mosm/kg

Oxygen Capacity (B)
1.34 mL/g of hemoglobin

Oxygen Saturation (B)
Newborns: 30–80% (0.3–0.8 mol/mol of venous blood)
Thereafter: 65–85% (0.65–0.85 mol/mol of venous blood)

Paco$_2$: See Acid-Base Measurements.

Pao$_2$: See Acid-Base Measurements.

Partial Thromboplastin Time (P)
Children: 42–54 s

pH: See Acid-Base Measurements.

Phenylalanine (S, P)
0.7–3.5 mg/dL (0.04–0.21 mmol/L)

Phosphatase: See Acid Phosphatase and Alkaline
Phosphatase.

Phosphorus, Inorganic (S, P)
Premature infants:
At birth: 5.6–8 mg/dL (1.81–2.58 mmol/L)
6–10 d: 6.1–11.7 mg/dL (1.97–3.78 mmol/L)
20–25 d: 6.6–9.4 mg/dL (2.13–3.04 mmol/L)
Full-term infants:
At birth: 5–7.8 mg/dL (1.61–2.52 mmol/L)
3 d: 5.8–9 mg/dL (1.87–2.91 mmol/L)
6–12 d: 4.9–8.9 mg/dL (1.58–2.87 mmol/L)
Children:
1 y: 3.8–6.2 mg/dL (1.23–2 mmol/L)
10 y: 3.6–5.6 mg/dL (1.16–1.81 mmol/L)
Adults: 3.1–5.1 mg/dL (1–1.65 mmol/L)
(See also Glucose Tolerance Test.)

(continued)

Table 41–1. Normal blood chemistry values and miscellaneous other hematologic values.[1]
(Values may vary with the procedure used.) (continued)

Proteins in serum.

Values are for cellulose acetate electrophoresis and are
in g/dL. SI conversion factor: g/dL × 10 = g/L.

Group	Total Protein	Albumin	α_1-Globulin	α_2-Globulin	β-Globulin	λ-Globulin
At birth	4.6–7.0	3.2–4.8	0.1–0.3	0.2–0.3	0.3–0.6	0.6–1.2
3 mo	4.5–6.5	3.2–4.8	0.1–0.3	0.3–0.7	0.3–0.7	0.2–0.7
1 y	5.4–7.5	3.7–5.7	0.1–0.3	0.5–1.1	0.4–1.0	0.2–0.9
> 4 y	5.9–8.0	3.8–5.4	0.1–0.3	0.4–0.8	0.5–1.0	0.4–1.3

Potassium (S, P)
Premature infants: 4.5–7.2 mmol/L
Full-term infants: 3.7–5.2 mmol/L
Children: 3.5–5.8 mmol/L
Adults: 3.5–5.5 mmol/L

Prealbumin: See Transthyretin.

Proteins (S): See table (top of page).

Prothrombin Time (P)
Children: 11–15 s

Protoporphyrin, "Free" (FEP, ZPP) (B)
Values for free erythrocyte protoporphyrin (FEP) and zinc
protoporphyrin (ZPP) are 1.2–2.7 µg/g of hemoglobin.

Pyruvate (B)
Resting adult males (arterial blood): 50.5–60.1 µmol/L
Adults (venous blood): 34–102 µmol/L

Retinol-Binding Protein (S)

3–5 y	1.0–5.0 mg/dL
6–8 y	1.5–5.9 mg/dL
9–11 y	1.5–6.5 mg/dL
12–16 y	1.5–7.0 mg/dL

Sedimentation Rate (Micro) (B)
< 2 y: 1–5 mm/h
> 2 y: 1–8 mm/h

SGOT: See Aspartate Aminotransferase.

SGPT: See Alanine Aminotransferase.

Sodium (S, P)
Children and adults: 135–148 mmol/L

Sugar: See Glucose.

T_3: See Triiodothyronine.

T_4: See Thyroxine.

TBG: See Thyroxine-Binding Globulin.

Thrombin Time (P)
Children: 12–16 s

Thyroid-Stimulating Hormone (TSH) (S)
Values in µIU/mL

	Males	Females
1–30 d	0.52–16.0	0.72–13.1
1 mo–5 y	0.55–7.1	0.46–8.1
6–18 y	0.37–6.0	0.36–5.8

Thyroxine (T_4) (S)
1–2 d: 11.4–25.5 µg/dL (147–328 nmol/L)
3–4 d: 9.8–25.2 µg/dL (126–324 nmol/L)
1–6 y: 5–15.2 µg/dL (64–196 nmol/L)
11–13 y: 4–13 µg/dL (51–167 nmol/L)
> 18 y: 4.7–11 µg/dL (60–142 nmol/L)

Thyroxine, "Free" (Free T_4) (S)
1–2.3 ng/dL

Thyroxine-Binding Globulin (TBG) (S)
1–7 mo: 2.9–6 mg/dL
7–12 mo: 2.1–5.9 mg/dL
Prepubertal children: 2–5.3 mg/dL
Pubertal children and adults: 1.8–4.2 mg/dL

α-Tocopherol: See Vitamin E.

Transaminase: See Alanine Aminotransferase and
Aspartate Aminotransferase.

Transthyretin (S, P)
2–5 mo: 14–33 mg/dL
6–11 mo: 12–27 mg/dL
12–17 mo: 11–26 mg/dL
18–23 mo: 14–24 mg/dL
24–36 mo: 11–26 mg/dL
3–5 y: 9.1–33.0 mg/dL
6–8 y: 15.3–45.5 mg/dL
9–11 y: 16.0–47.6 mg/dL
12–16 y: 19.0–50.0 mg/dL

Triglyceride (S, P)
Fasting (> 12 h) values in mg/mL (mmol/L)

Group	Males	Females
6–7 y	32–79 (0.36–0.89)	24–128 (0.27–1.44)
8–9 y	28–105 (0.31–1.18)	34–115 (0.38–1.29)
10–11 y	30–115 (0.33–1.29)	39–131 (0.44–1.48)
12–13 y	33–112 (0.37–1.26)	36–125 (0.40–1.41)
14–15 y	35–136 (0.39–1.53)	36–122 (0.40–1.37)
16–17 y	38–167 (0.42–1.88)	34–136 (0.38–1.53)

Note: Lower values represent the 5th percentile, whereas
upper values are calculated from the mean + 2 SD.

Triiodothyronine (T_3) (S)
1–3 d: 89–405 ng/dL
1 wk: 91–300 ng/dL
1–12 mo: 85–250 ng/dL
Prepubertal children: 119–218 ng/dL
Pubertal children and adults: 55–170 ng/dL

(continued)

Table 41–1. Normal blood chemistry values and miscellaneous other hematologic values.[1]
(Values may vary with the procedure used.) (continued)

Tyrosine (S, P)
Premature infants: 3–30.2 mg/dL (0.17–1.67 mmol/L)
Full-term infants: 1.7–4.7 mg/dL (0.09–0.26 mmol/L)
1–12 y: 1.4–3.4 mg/dL (0.08–0.19 mmol/L)
Adults: 0.6–1.6 mg/dL (0.03–0.09 mmol/L)

Urea Clearance
Premature infants: 3.5–17.3 mL/min/1.73 m^2
Newborns: 8.7–33 mL/min/1.73 m^2
2–12 mo: 40–95 mL/min/1.73 m^2
$\geq$ 2 y: > 52 mL/min/1.73 m^2

Urea Nitrogen (S, P)
1–2 y: 5–15 mg/dL (1.8–5.4 mmol/L)
Thereafter: 10–20 mg/dL (3.5–7.1 mmol/L)

Uric Acid (S, P)
Males:
0–14 y: 2–7 mg/dL (119–416 μmol/L)
> 14 y: 3–8 mg/dL (178–476 μmol/L)
Females:
0–14 y: 2–7 mg/dL (119–416 μmol/L)
> 14 y: 2–7 mg/dL (119–416 μmol/L)

Vitamin A (S, P)
Total vitamin A: 19–81 μg/dL (0.66–2.82 μmol/L)
Retinol: 19–77 μg/dL (0.66–2.68 μmol/L)
Retinyl esters: 0.1–4.7 μg/dL (0.01–0.16 μmol/L)

Vitamin C (Ascorbic Acid) (S, P)
0.2–2 mg/dL (11–114 μmol/L)

Vitamin D (S)
1,25-Dihydroxycholecalciferol:
Normal: 37 ± 12 pg/mL
X-linked vitamin D–resistant disease: 16 ± 8 pg/mL
Vitamin D dependency: 9.5 ± 3 pg/mL in type I. Normal in type II.
Hypophosphatemic bone disease: 30 ± 6 pg/mL
Lead poisoning: 20 ± 1 pg/mL
25-Hydroxycholecalciferol:
Normal: 26–31 ng/mL

Vitamin E (Tocopherol) (S, P)
α-Tocopherol:
<12 y: 3.8–15.5 μg/mL (9.1–37.2 μmol/L)
>12 y: 4.7–203 μg/mL (11.3–48.7 μmol/L)
γ-Tocopherol:

The γ isomer contributes 10–20% of the total tocopherols in plasma but is only 10% as active as the α form in vivo.
Vitamin E status is best assessed by performing chromatographic separation of the isomers and determining both α- and γ-tocopherol levels. Levels should be expressed in terms of vitamin E/total lipid ratio:
< 12 y: > 0.6 mg/g (> 1.4 μmol/g)
> 12 y: > 0.8 mg/g (> 1.9 μmol/g)

Volume (B)
Premature infants: 98 mL/kg (mean)
Full-term infants: 75–100 mL/kg
1 y: 69–112 mL/kg (mean, 86 mL/kg)
Older children: 51–86 mL/kg (mean, 70 mL/kg)

Volume (P)
Full-term neonates: 39–77 mL/kg
Infants: 40–50 mL/kg
Older children: 30–54 mL/kg

Water (B, S, RBC)
Whole blood: 79–81 g/dL
Serum: 91–92 g/dL
Red blood cells: 64–65 g/dL

Xylose Absorption Test (B)
Following a 5-g loading dose, the laboratory will report the D-xylose concentration of the baseline and 60-min samples in mg/dL. The difference between these two values should be corrected to a constant surface area of 1.73 m^2 according to the formula shown below.
The actual surface area can be derived from a number of available nomograms using the patient's weight and height.
Normal corrected blood values[2]: 9.8–20 mg/dL
Effect of age and sex: No significant differences between males and females. No significant differences in ages 14–92 y.

Zinc (S)
Males: 83–88 μg/dL (12.7–13.5 μmol/L)
Females: 85–91 μg/dL (13–13.9 μmol/L)
Females taking oral contraceptives: 86–93 μg/dL (13.2–14.2 μmol/L)
At 16 wk of gestation: 66–70 μg/dL (10.1–10.7 μmol/L)
At 38 wk of gestation: 54–58 μg/dL (8.3–8.9 μmol/L)

---

[1]Adapted from Meites S (editor): *Pediatric Clinical Chemistry,* 2nd ed. American Association for Clinical Chemistry, 1982, and many other sources.

[2]
$$\text{Corrected blood value} = \frac{(\text{Value}_{60\ \min} - \text{Value}_{\text{baseline}}) \times \text{Actual surface area}}{1.73}$$

Table 41–2. Normal values: urine, duodenal fluid, feces, sweat, and miscellaneous.[1]

URINE

Acidity, Titratable
20–50 mEq/d

Addis Count
Red blood cells (12-h specimen): < 1 million
White blood cells (12-h specimen): < 2 million
Casts (12-h specimen): < 10,000
Protein (12-h specimen): < 55 mg

Albumin
First mo: 1–100 mg/L
Second month: 0.2–34 mg/L
2–12 mo: 0.5–19 mg/L

δ-**Aminolevulinic Acid:** See Porphyrins.

Ammonia
2–12 mo: 4–20 µEq/min/m^2
1–16 y: 6–16 µEq/min/m^2

Calcium
4–12 y: 4–8 meq/L (2–4 mmol/L)

Catecholamines (Norepinephrine, Epinephrine)
Values in µg/24 h (nmol/24 h)
(See Table, bottom of page.)

Chloride
Infants: 1.7–8.5 mmol/24 h
Children: 17–34 mmol/24 h
Adults: 140–240 mmol/24 h

Copper
0–30 µg/24 h

Coproporphyrin: See Porphyrins.

Creatine
18–58 mg/L (1.37–4.42 mmol/L)

Creatinine
Newborns: 7–10 mg/kg/24 h
Children: 20–30 mg/kg/24 h
Adult males: 21–26 mg/kg/24 h
Adult females: 16–22 mg/kg/24 h

Epinephrine: See Catecholamines.

Homovanillic Acid
Children: 3–16 µg/mg of creatinine
Adults: 2–4 µg/mg of creatinine

5-Hydroxyindoleacetic Acid
0.11–0.61 µmol/kg/7 h, based on results in 15 well-nourished, apparently healthy, mentally defective children on a tryptophan load

Hydroxyproline, Total
5–14 y: 38–126 mg/24 h (290–961 µmol/24 h)

Mercury
<50 µg/24 h (249 nmol/24 h)

Metanephrine and Normetanephrine
<2 y: <4.6 µg/mg of creatinine (23.3 nmol)
2–10 y: <3 µg/mg of creatinine (15.2 nmol)
10–15 y: <2 µg/mg of creatinine (10.3 nmol)
>15 y: <1 µg/mg of creatinine (5.1 nmol)

Mucopolysaccharides
Acid mucopolysaccharide screen should yield negative results. Positive results after dialysis of the urine should be followed up with a thin-layer chromatogram for evaluation of the acid mucopolysaccharide excretion pattern.

Norepinephrine: See Catecholamines.

Normetanephrine: See Metanephrine and Normetanephrine.

Osmolality
Infants: 50–600 mosm/L
Older children: 50–1400 mosm/L

Phosphorus, Tubular Reabsorption
78–97%

Porphobilinogen: See Porphyrins.

Porphyrins
δ-Aminolevulinic acid: 0–7 mg/24 h (0–53.4 µmol/24 h)
Porphobilinogen: 0–2 mg/24 h (0–8.8 µmol/24 h)
Coproporphyrin: 0–160 µg/24 h (0–244 nmol/24 h)
Uroporphyrin: 0–26 µg/24 h (0–31 nmol/24 h)

Potassium
26–123 mmol/L

Sodium
Infants: 0.3–3.5 mmol/24 h (6–10 mmol/m^2)
Children and adults: 5.6–17 mmol/24 h

Urobilinogen
< 3 mg/24 h (< 5.1 µmol/24 h)

Uroporphyrin: See Porphyrins.

Vanilmandelic Acid (VMA)
Because of the difficulty in obtaining an accurately timed 24-h collection, values based on micrograms per milligram of creatinine are the most reliable indications of VMA excretion in young children.
1–12 mo: 1–35 µg/mg of creatinine (31–135 µg/kg/24 h)

Catecholamines in urine.

Group	Total Catecholamines	Norepinephrine	Epinephrine
< 1 y	20	5.4–15.9 (32–94)	0.1–4.3 (0.5–23.5)
1–5 y	40	8.1–30.8 (48–182)	0.8–9.1 (4.4–49.7)
6–15 y	80	19.0–71.1 (112–421)	1.3–10.5 (7.1–57.3)
> 15 y	100	34.4–87.0 (203–514)	3.5–13.2 (19.1–72.1)

(continued)

Table 41–2. Normal values: urine, duodenal fluid, feces, sweat, and miscellaneous.[1] (continued)

1–2 y: 1–30 µg/mg of creatinine
2–5 y: 1–15 µg/mg of creatinine
5–10 y: 1–14 µg/mg of creatinine
10–15 y: 1–10 µg/mg of creatinine (1–7 mg/24 h;
   5–35 µmol/24 h)
Adults: 1–7 µg/mg of creatinine (1–7 mg/24 h;
   5–35 µmol/24 h)

VMA: See Vanilmandelic Acid.

Xylose Absorption Test
Mean 5-h excretion expressed as a percentage
   of the ingested load
< 6 mo: 11–30%
6–12 mo: 20–32%
1–3 y: 20–42%
3–10 y: 25–45%
> 10 y: 25–50%
Or: % excretion > (0.2 × age [mo]) + 12

DUODENAL FLUID VALUE

Enzymes
Amylase: (Anderson)
   0–2 mo: 0–10 U/mL
   2–6 mo: 10–20 U/mL
   6–12 mo: 40–150 U/mL
   1–2 y: 100–225 U/mL
   2–5 y: 125–275 U/mL
Carboxypeptidase:
   0.4–1 U (Ravin)
Chymotrypsin:
   11–65 U (Ravin)
Protease:
   18–70 U (Free-Meyers)
Trypsin: (Anderson or as noted)
   0–2 mo: 110–160 U/mL
   2–6 mo: 115–160 U/mL
   6–12 mo: 120–290 U/mL; 3–10 U
     (Nothman et al)
   1–2 y: 200–300 U/mL
   2–5 y: 200–275 U/mL

pH
6–8.4

FECES

Chymotrypsin
3–14 mg/kg 72 h

Fat, Total
2–6 mo: 0.3–1.3 g/d
6 mo–1 y: < 4 g/d
Children: < 3 g/d
Adolescents: < 5 g/d
Adults: < 7 g/d

Lipids, Split Fat
Adults: > 40% of total lipids

Lipids, Total
Adults: Up to 7 g/d on normal diet, 10–27% of dry weight

Nitrogen
Infants: < 1 g/d
Children: < 1.2 g/d
Adults: < 3 g/d

SWEAT

Electrolytes
Values for chloride. Elevated values in the presence of a
   family history or clinical findings of cystic fibrosis are
   diagnostic of cystic fibrosis.
Normal: < 40 mmol/L
Borderline: 40–60 mmol/L
Elevated: > 60 mmol/L

MISCELLANEOUS

Amylo-1,6-Glucosidase Debrancher (Liver)
>1 µmol/min/g of wet tissue

Chloride
Breast milk: 2.5–30 mmol/L
Cow's milk: 20–80 mmol/L
Muscle: 20–26 mmol/kg of wet fat-free tissue
Spinal fluid: 120–128 mmol/L

Copper (Liver)
< 20 µg/g of wet tissue

Glucose-6-Phosphatase (Liver)
> 5 µmol/min/g of wet tissue

Lactate Dehydrogenase (LDH) (Cerebrospinal Fluid)
17–59 IU/L at 37 °C

Potassium
Breast milk: 12–17 mmol/L
Cow's milk: 20–45 mmol/L
Muscle: 160–180 mmol/kg of wet fat-free tissue

Proteins (Cerebrospinal Fluid)
Total proteins:
   Newborn: 40–120 mg/dL (0.4–1.2 g/L)
   1 mo: 20–70 mg/dL (0.2–0.7 g/L)
   Thereafter: 15–40 mg/dL (0.15–0.4 g/L)
Gamma globulin:
   Children: Up to 9% of total
   Adults: Up to 14% of total

Sodium
Breast milk: 4.7–8.3 mmol/L
Cow's milk: 22–26 mmol/L
Muscle: 33–43 mmol/kg of wet fat-free tissue

[1]Adapted from Meites S (editor): *Pediatric Clinical Chemistry,* 2nd ed. American Association for Clinical Chemistry, 1982, and many other sources.

Table 41–3. Normal values: common hematologic measurements and indices.

RED BLOOD CELL VALUES AT VARIOUS AGES: MEAN AND LOWER LIMIT OF NORMAL (–2 SD)[1]

Age	Hemoglobin (g/dL)		Hematocrit (%)		Red Cell Count (10^{12}/L)		MCV (fl)		MCH (pg)		MCHC (g/dL)	
	Mean	*–2 SD*	*Mean*	*–2 SD*	*Mean*	*–2 SD*	*Mean*	*–2 SD*	*Mean*	*–2 SD*	*Mean*	*–2 SD*
Birth (cord blood)	16.5	13.5	51	42	4.7	3.9	108	98	34	31	33	30
1 to 3 d (capillary)	18.5	14.5	56	45	5.3	4.0	108	95	34	31	33	29
1 wk	17.5	13.5	54	42	5.1	3.9	107	88	34	28	33	28
2 wk	16.5	12.5	51	39	4.9	3.6	105	86	34	28	33	28
1 mo	14.0	10.0	43	31	4.2	3.0	104	85	34	28	33	29
2 mo	11.5	9.0	35	28	3.8	2.7	96	77	30	26	33	29
3–6 mo	11.5	9.5	35	29	3.8	3.1	91	74	30	25	33	30
0.5–2 y	12.0	10.5	36	33	4.5	3.7	78	70	27	23	33	30
2–6 y	12.5	11.5	37	34	4.6	3.9	81	75	27	24	34	31
6–12 y	13.5	11.5	40	35	4.6	4.0	86	77	29	25	34	31
12–18 y												
Female	14.0	12.0	41	36	4.6	4.1	90	78	30	25	34	31
Male	14.5	13.0	43	37	4.9	4.5	88	78	30	25	34	31
18–49 y												
Female	14.0	12.0	41	36	4.6	4.0	90	80	30	26	34	31
Male	15.5	13.5	47	41	5.2	4.5	90	80	30	26	34	31

NORMAL LEUKOCYTE COUNTS[2]

Age	Total Leukocytes		Neutrophils			Lymphocytes			Monocytes		Eosinophils	
	Mean	*(Range)*	*Mean*	*(Range)*	*%*	*Mean*	*(Range)*	*%*	*Mean*	*%*	*Mean*	*%*
Birth	18.1	(9.0–30.0)	11.0	(6.0–26.0)	61	5.5	(2.0–11.0)	31	1.1	6	0.4	2
12 h	22.8	(13.0–38.0)	15.5	(6.0–28.0)	68	5.5	(2.0–11.0)	24	1.2	5	0.5	2
24 h	18.9	(9.4–34.0)	11.5	(5.0–21.0)	61	5.8	(2.0–11.5)	31	1.1	6	0.5	2
1 wk	12.2	(5.0–21.0)	5.5	(1.5–10.0)	45	5.0	(2.0–17.0)	41	1.1	9	0.5	4
2 wk	11.4	(5.0–20.0)	4.5	(1.0–9.5)	40	5.5	(2.0–17.0)	48	1.0	9	0.4	3
1 mo	10.8	(5.0–19.5)	3.8	(1.0–9.0)	35	6.0	(2.5–16.5)	56	0.7	7	0.3	3
6 mo	11.9	(6.0–17.5)	3.8	(1.0–8.5)	32	7.3	(4.0–13.5)	61	0.6	5	0.3	3
1 y	11.4	(6.0–17.5)	3.5	(1.5–8.5)	31	7.0	(4.0–10.5)	61	0.6	5	0.3	3
2 y	10.6	(6.0–17.0)	3.5	(1.5–8.5)	33	6.3	(3.0–9.5)	59	0.5	5	0.3	3
4 y	9.1	(5.5–15.5)	3.8	(1.5–8.5)	42	4.5	(2.0–8.0)	50	0.5	5	0.3	3
6 y	8.5	(5.0–14.5)	4.3	(1.5–8.0)	51	3.5	(1.5–7.0)	42	0.4	5	0.2	3
8 y	8.3	(4.5–13.5)	4.4	(1.5–8.0)	53	3.3	(1.5–6.8)	39	0.4	4	0.2	2
10 y	8.1	(4.5–13.5)	4.4	(1.8–8.0)	54	3.1	(1.5–6.5)	38	0.4	4	0.2	2
16 y	7.8	(4.5–13.0)	4.4	(1.8–8.0)	57	2.8	(1.2–5.2)	35	0.4	5	0.2	3
21 y	7.4	(4.5–11.0)	4.4	(1.8–7.7)	59	2.5	(1.0–4.8)	34	0.3	4	0.2	3

[1]These data have been compiled from several sources. Emphasis is given to recent studies using electronic counters and to the selection of populations that are likely to exclude individuals with iron deficiency. The mean ± 2 SD can be expected to include 95% of the observations in a normal population. MCV = mean corpuscular volume, MCH = mean corpuscular hemoglobin, MCHC = mean corpuscular hemoglobin concentration. (Based on Cairo MS: In: *Pediatrics,* 20th ed. Rudolph AM [editor]. Appleton & Lange, 1996:1222. As modified in Lubin BH: Reference values in infancy and childhood. In: *Hematology of Infancy and Childhood,* 4th ed. Nathan DG, Oski FA [editors]. Saunders, 1993:Appendix iii.)

[2]Numbers of leukocytes are in thousands per cubic millimeter, ranges are estimates of 95% confidence limits, and percentages refer to differential counts. Neutrophils include band cells at all ages and a small number of metamyelocytes and myelocytes in the first few days of life. (From Cairo MS: In: *Pediatrics,* 20th ed. Rudolph AM [editor]. Appleton & Lange, 1996. As modified in Lubin BH: Reference values in infancy and childhood. In: *Hematology of Infancy and Childhood,* 4th ed. Nathan DG, Oski FA [editors]. Saunders, 1993:Appendix xi.)

Index

Page numbers in **boldface** indicate major discussions. Page numbers followed by *t* and *f* indicate tables and figures, respectively.

Cholestyramine
  for cholestasis, 560
  for chronic nonspecific
      diarrhea, 544
  for Crigler-Najjar syndrome, 569
  for intrahepatic cholestasis, 561t
  for pruritus, 565
  for "toxic" cholestasis, 563
Choline, in breast milk, 263t
Cholinergic crisis, in myasthenia
    gravis, 687
Chondroblastoma, 712
Chondrodystrophy, classic. See
    Achondroplasia
Chorea
  and rheumatic fever, 507
  Sydenham's postrheumatic, **672**
Choreoathetosis, 692t, 693–694
Chorioamnionitis, maternal, and
    periventricular
    leukomalacia, 52
Choriocarcinoma, ovarian, 838
Chorionic villus sampling, 915
  indications for, 915–916
Chorioretinitis, in newborns, 24
Choroiditis, 372
Choroid plexus tumors, 781
Christmas disease, **759**
"Christmas tree" deformity, 533
Chromatids, 881
Chromium, nutritional requirements for,
    in intravenous nutrition, 268
Chromosome(s), **881.** See also
    Autosomes; Sex
    chromosomes
  abnormalities of, **884–886**
    in cancer, 890–891
    in children, **909–910**
    clinical significance of, 886
    and mental retardation, 97
    numerical, 884
    recurrence risk, **889**
    structural, 884, 884f
  analysis
    high-resolution, 882
    indications for, 889
    preparation for, 882–883
    procedure for, 882–883
  breaks, assessment of, 883
  deletion, 884, 884f
    interstitial, 884
    terminal, 884
  fragile X study, 889–890
  fragility, syndromes associated
      with, 890
  homologous, 881
  inversion, 884–885
    paracentric, 884f, 885
    pericentric, 884f, 885
  nomenclature for, 883
  nondisjunction, 884
  number of, 881, 882f
  translocation, 884
    balanced, 884
    reciprocal, 884, 884f

  robertsonian, 884, 884f
  unbalanced, 884
Chromosome painting, 883
Chronic autoimmune thyroiditis, **824**
Chronic fatigue syndrome, **721**
Chronic granulomatous disease, 751t,
    799
Chronic illness, **183–184**
  anemia of, **732–733**
  floppy infant syndrome with, 692t
  follow up visit for, **212–213,** 213f
  immunization and, 222
  patterns of coping with, 184t
Chronic mucocutaneous candidiasis,
    807, 1088–1090
Chronic myelogenous leukemia,
    778–779
  juvenile and adult, comparison of,
      778t, 778–779
Chronic renal failure. See Renal failure,
    chronic
Chronotropic incompetence, 516
Chvostek sign, in hypoparathyroidism,
    829
Chyle, in pleural space, 458–459
Chylothorax, **458–459,** 536
  pleural, 457
Chylous ascites, **536**
Chymotrypsin, normal laboratory
    values for
  duodenal fluid, 1136t
  feces, 1136t
Cigarettes, abuse, prevalence
    of, 150t
Cigarette smoking. See Smoking
Cimetidine
  drug interactions with, 1125t
  for peptic ulcer disease, 532
Cineangiocardiography, 474
  in aortic stenosis, 492
  in endocardial fibroelastosis, 496
  in Fallot's tetralogy, 498
  in pulmonary atresia, 499
  for pulmonary stenosis, 488
  in total anomalous pulmonary venous
      return, 505
Cinefluoroscopy, for esophageal achala-
    sia, 529
Ciprofloxacin
  adverse effects and side effects
      of, 947t
  for Crohn's disease, 558
  for mycoplasmal pneumonia, 445
  organisms resistant to, 947t
  organisms susceptible to, 947t
Circulation
  assessment of
    in resuscitation, 274–275
    in trauma patient, 282
  fetal, **475**
  neonatal, **475–476**
  prenatal, **475–476**
  pulmonary, diseases of, **453–456**
Circumcision, **28**
  benefits of, 28

  contraindications for, 28
  risks of, 28
Cirrhosis, **578–579**
  ascites in, 536
  biliary, in cystic fibrosis, 596t
  postnecrotic, 577
Cisapride, for esophageal motor
    function, 529
Citrullinemia, 866–867
Clarithromycin
  adverse effects and side effects
      of, 947t
  drug interactions with, 1125t
  for group A streptococcal
      infection, 1009
  oral, for children ≥ 1 month of age,
      950t
  organisms resistant to, 947t
  organisms susceptible to, 947t, 956
Clatworthy's sign, in portal
    hypertension, 586
Clavicle, fractures of, **706**
Cleft lip, 417, **900–901**
  nonsyndrome, 900–901
  risk for, 900t
  syndromic, 901, 901t
Cleft palate, 386, 387f, 417, **900–901**
  nonsyndrome, 900–901
  risk for, 900t
  submucous, 417
  syndromic, 901, 901t
Clemastine, 927
Clindamycin, 947t, **956**
  adverse effects and side effects
      of, 947t
  for aspiration pneumonia, 447
  for bacterial vaginosis, 144
  diarrhea with, 544
  for group A streptococcal
      infection, 1009
  for impetigo, 349
  for malaria treatment, 1069, 1069t
  for odontogenic infection, 391
  oral, for children ≥ 1 month of age,
      950t
  organisms resistant to, 947t
  organisms susceptible to, 947t
  parenteral, for children ≥ 1 month of
      age, 949t
  for pneumonia, 442
  use in newborns, 951t
Clindamycin phosphate, for acne, 348
Clinical Interview to Assess Suicide
    Risk, in adolescence, 118
Clinitest Tablet poisoning, 300
Clobetasol propionate, for skin
    disorders, 343t
Clomiphene citrate, and incidence of
    twinning, 39
Clomipramine, 188–189
Clonazepam (Klonopin), 644t
Clonidine, 192–193
  for posttraumatic stress
      disorder, 178
Clonorchis, 1063t–1064t

Methemoglobin, normal laboratory
values for (blood), 1132*t*
Methemoglobinemia, **746–747**
acquired, **746–747**
congenital, due to enzyme
deficiencies, **747**
in nitrite poisoning, 308
Methicillin, **954**
adverse effects and side effects
of, 947*t*
apparent volume of distribution
for, 291*t*
organisms resistant to, 947*t*
organisms susceptible to, 947*t*
parenteral, for children ≥ 1 month of
age, 949*t*
pK$_a$ for, 291*t*
use in newborns, 951*t*
Methimazole, for hyperthyroidism, 825
Methotrexate
for iritis, 372
for juvenile rheumatoid arthritis, 717
pulmonary complications of,
795–796
Methsuximide, 645*t*
therapeutic blood levels, 1122*t*
3-Methylcrotonyl-CoA carboxylase deficiency, 872*t*
Methyldopa, for sustained hypertension,
614, 616*t*
Methylene blue
for acquired methemoglobinemia, 747
for anesthetic poisoning, 298
Methylenetetrahydrofolate reductase, deficiency, 870
Methylmalonic acidemia, **871,** 872*t*
Methylmalonyl-CoA mutase, 871, 873*f*
Methylphenidate, for attention-deficit
hyperactivity disorder,
101, 187
Methylprednisolone
for anaphylaxis, 935
for asthma, 326
for inflammatory bowel disease, 557
for laryngeal edema, 530
potency equivalents for
adrenocorticosteroids, 747*t*
systemic, for asthma, 922
Methylxanthines, for apnea, in preterm
infants, 48
Metoclopramide, for esophageal motor
function, 529
Metronidazole, **958**
for amebiasis, 1071*t*, 1072
for amebic liver abscess, 584
for bacterial vaginosis, 144
for Crohn's disease, 558
in fulminant hepatitis, 576
for giardiasis, 1074
oral, for children ≥ 1 month of age,
950*t*
parenteral, for children ≥ 1 month of
age, 949*t*
Metyrapone test, 842
Mezlocillin, **954**

MIC. *See* Minimal inhibitory concentration
Micatin. *See* Miconazole
Miconazole
for candidal vaginitis, 144
for dermatophyte infection, 351
Microcephaly, 662*t*, **662–663,** 693
differential diagnosis of, 663
prognosis for, 663
treatment of, 663
Microcornea, 374
Microgallbladder, in cystic fibrosis, 596*t*
Microhematuria, 600
Microsporum canis, 350, 350*t*
Midazolam (Versed)
for pain control in critically ill child,
338, 338*t*
for status epilepticus, 646*t*
Middle ear
aspiration of secretions into, in otitis
media, 396
effusion, 394
inflammation of, **394–402.** *See also*
Otitis media
trauma to, **403**
Midgut volvulus, 534
Midrin, for migraine, 650
Migraine, 642*t*, 649*t*, 649–650
Milia, 23, 343
Miliaria, 23, 344
crystallina, 344
rubra, 344
Milk
cow's, pulmonary hemosiderosis
induced by, 453
human. *See* Breast milk
requirements in prudent diet, 211
Milk intolerance/allergy, **555**
Miller-Dieker syndrome, 891*t*, 907
Mineralocorticoid(s)
actions of, 841
for adrenocortical insufficiency, 843
for congenital adrenal
hyperplasia, 846
excess, 846
potency equivalents for, 848, 848*t*
Minerals
absorption of, 250
in intravenous nutrition, 267
major, nutritional requirements for,
251*t*, **251–253**
suggested dietary intakes of, 251*t*
Minimal brain dysfunction, 95
and attention-deficit hyperactivity disorder, 100
Minimal change disease. *See* Nephrotic
syndrome, idiopathic
Minimal inhibitory concentration, 944
Minipill, 139
Minnesota Child Development
Inventory, 90*t*
Minocycline
for acne, 349
adverse effects and side effects
of, 948*t*

organisms resistant to, 948*t*
organisms susceptible to, 948*t*, 957
Minoxidil, for sustained hypertension,
614, 616*t*
Mist therapy, for viral croup, 425
Mitochondrial DNA, mutations, 899
Mitochondrial dysfunction, Reye's
syndrome associated
with, 590
Mitochondrial inheritance, **899**
Mitochondrial respiratory chain, defects
of, 865–866
Mitosis, 881–882, 882*f*
Mitral dysfunction syndrome, 510
Mitral insufficiency, 510
Mitral regurgitation, congenital, 494
Mitral stenosis, 510
congenital, 494
Mitral valve prolapse, **493**
Mittelschmerz, **135–137**
Mixed connective tissue disease, 718
Mixed hearing loss, 404
MMFR. *See* Maximum midexpiratory
flow rate
MMR vaccine, 230
administration schedule for,
225*t*–226*t*, 230–231
adverse effects of, 232
contraindications to/precautions with,
220–221*t*
MM vaccine, 230
Mobitz type I (Wenckebach) heart
block, **523**
Mobitz type II, **523,** 524*f*
Möbius' syndrome, 380, 688
Moisturizers, for atopic dermatitis, 930
Molds, 1085
Molecular genetics, 891–892
Molecular genetic testing, 912*t*, 913
Molluscum contagiosum, 348, 352
Molybdenum, nutritional requirements
for, in intravenous
nutrition, 268
Mometasone furoate, for skin
disorders, 343*t*
Mongolian spot, 23, 344
Monkshood, poisoning due to, 310*t*
Monocytes, normal laboratory values
for, age-related, 1137*t*
Mononucleosis spot test, 410
Monoplegia, cerebral palsy and, 693
Monosaccharide intolerance, diarrhea
in, 545*t*
Monosomy, 884
Montelukast, for asthma, 922
Mood disorders, **172–174**
Mood stabilizers, **191–192**
Mood swings, normal, in
adolescence, 118
Moraxella catarrhalis
antimicrobial susceptibility of, 945*t*
dacryocystitis, 368
Morbidity, in adolescence, **102–103**
Morbilliform eruption, drug-
induced, 358*t*

Morganella, 1029
Moro reflex, 9, 25
Morphine
    abuse, physiologic effects of, 148–149
    for acute pulmonary edema, 478
    for cyanotic spells in Fallot's
        tetralogy, 497
    overdose, 309
    for pain control in critically ill child,
        338*t,* 339–340
    poisoning, 309
Morquio's disease. *See* Osteochondrody-
        strophy
Morquio syndrome, 877*t*
Mortality, in adolescence, **102**
Mosaicism, **885**
    in Down syndrome, 886
    germ cell, 894
Mosquitoes
    bites, skin reactions to, 941
    viral infections spread by, 984,
        985*t*–986*t*
Mothballs, poisoning with, 303
Motivation, assessment of, 92
Motor coordination, during
        adolescence, 113
Motor dexterity, in first three years, 10
Motor functions, evaluation of, 623
Motor handicaps, **99**
    in development, **99**
Motor vehicle injuries, prevention
        of, 211
Mottling, in newborn, 344
Mouth
    congenital anomalies/malformations
        of, **416–417**
    in newborn, 385*f*
        examination of, 24
        soft tissue variations in, 386–387
Mouth breathing, **414**
    and recurrent pharyngitis, 412
MRI. *See* Magnetic resonance imaging
MRSA. *See* Staphylococcus aureus, me-
        thicillin-resistant
MR vaccine, 230
MTHR. *See* Methylenetetrahydrofolate
        reductase
Mucocele, 415
Mucocutaneous candidiasis, in
        autoimmune polyglandular
        syndrome, 820
Mucocutaneous diseases. *See also*
        specific type
    conjunctivitis in, 370
Mucocutaneous lymph node syndrome
        (Kawasaki disease), **515**
Mucolipidoses, 877*t*
Mucopolysaccharides, urine
    measurement of, specimen collection
        and handling for, 862*f*
    normal laboratory values for, 1135*t*
Mucopolysaccharidoses, 877*t*
Mucor, 1086*t*
    pneumonia in immunocompromised
        host, 448

Mucorales, 1086*t*
Multifactorial inheritance, **899–903**
Multiple births, **39–40**
    complications of, 39–40
    increased birth defects in, 39
    obstetric complications of, 39–40
Multiple endocrine neoplasia
    and pheochromocytoma, 850
    type 1, 831
    type 2, 826, 831
    type 2b, 826
Multiple sclerosis, 670*t*
Mumps, **988–989**
    arthritis, 989
    diagnosis of, 962*t,* 988–989
    immunization against, **231–232**
    mastitis, 989
    meningoencephalitis, 989
    myocarditis, 510
    oophoritis, 989
    orchitis, 989
    pancreatitis, 989
    parotitis, 988–989
    presternal edema in, 989
    thyroiditis, 989
    vaccine. *See also* MMR vaccine
        administration schedule for,
            231–232
        adverse effects of, 232
Munchausen syndrome by proxy,
        196, 198
    life-threatening, differential diagnosis
        of, 460*t*
Mupirocin, for impetigo, 349
Murphy's sign, in cholelithiasis, 580
Muscle(s)
    biopsy, 681
    childhood disorders affecting,
        681–689
    imaging, in muscle disease, 681
Muscle relaxants, for controlled
        intubation, 320*t*
Muscular dystrophy, 682*t*–685*t*
    congenital
        Fukuyama, 684*t*–685*t,* 691, 691*t*
        occidental, 684*t*–685*t,* 691, 691*t*
Musculature, during adolescence, 113
Musculoskeletal system
    degenerative problems of, **703–704**
    growth disturbances of, **700–703**
    neoplasia of, **712–713**
    neurologic disorders involving,
        711–712
    in shock, 328
    vascular lesions and avascular
        necrosis, 710–711
Mushrooms
    abuse, physiologic effects of,
        148–149
    poisoning with, 308
Mustard procedure, for transposition of
        great arteries, 503
Mutagens, 905
Myalgia, pneumonia and, 443
Myalgia cruris epidemica, 686

Myasthenia gravis, **686–687,** 691
    congenital (persistent), 684*t*–685*t,*
        686–687, 691*t*
    juvenile, 686–687
    neonatal (transient), 682*t*–683*t,*
        686–687, 691*t*
Myasthenic crisis, 687
Mycobacteria
    "Battey avian-swine group," 1050
    central nervous system infection, 677
    nonphotochromogens, 1050
    photochromogens, 1050
    "rapid growers," 1050
    Runyon classification of, 1050
    scotochromogens, 1050
Mycobacterial infection(s). *See also* Tu-
        berculosis
    disseminated, 1050–1051
    nontuberculous, **1050–1051**
    pulmonary, 1050
Mycobacterium avium complex,
        1050–1051
    cervical lymphadenitis, 413
    in HIV-infected (AIDS) patients
        disseminated, 998
        prophylaxis for, 1002
Mycobacterium bovis, immunization
        against, 243
Mycobacterium chelonei, 1050–1051
Mycobacterium fortuitum, 1050–1051
Mycobacterium kansasii, 1050–1051
Mycobacterium marinum, 1050–1051
Mycobacterium scrofulaceum, 1050
Mycobacterium tuberculosis,
        1047–1048. *See also* Tuber-
        culosis
    antimicrobial prophylaxis for, 952*t*
Mycoplasma
    antimicrobial susceptibility of, 945*t*
    central nervous system infection,
        677–678
Mycoplasma pneumoniae, 1053
    empyema, 457
    pneumonia, 442, 444–445
Mycotic infections, 1085*t,* **1085–1095**
Myelinization, 4
Myelodysplasia, orthopedic aspects of,
        711–712
Myelography, 629
Myelomeningocele, 901
    orthopedic aspects of, **711–712**
Myeloperoxidase deficiency, 751*t*
Myocarditis, **510–511**
    bacterial, 510
    diphtheritic, 1028
    fungal, 510
    treatment of, 511
    viral, 510, 972
Myocardium
    abnormalities of, ventricular tachycar-
        dia caused by, 523
    depolarization of, 469*f*
    diseases of, **495–496.** *See also specific*
        type
Myoclonus, benign nocturnal, 642*t*

Otoscopy
in otitis media, 394–395
pneumatic, in otitis media,
396–397, 397f
Ovarian cysts, **138**
Ovarian follicle(s), 130t, 834
Ovarian hormones, in menstruation, 130t
Ovaries
cancer therapy and, 795
cysts of, 838
disorders of, and amenorrhea, 131t
function, abnormalities of, **834–838**
hormone production by, 834, 835f
polycystic ovary syndrome
and, 838
streak, in Turner's syndrome, 833
tumors of, **838**
Overflow incontinence. *See* Encopresis
Overgrowth syndromes, **910**
Overhydration, in topical therapy of skin
disorders, 341
Oxacillin, **954**
adverse effects and side effects
of, 947t
oral, for children ≥ 1 month of age,
950t
organisms resistant to, 947t
organisms susceptible to, 947t
use in newborns, 951t
Oxalic acid, in dumb cane, poisoning
due to, 310t
Oximetry, 420
in oxygen therapy, 422
Oxygen, partial pressure of. *See* PaO$_2$
Oxygen administration, in
resuscitation, 273
Oxygen capacity, normal laboratory values for, 1132t
Oxygen consumption, effect of
environmental temperature
on, 46f
Oxygen saturation
assessment of, noninvasive, **419–420**
in atrial septal defect, 481
cardiac catheterization data on,
473–474, 474f
monitoring, 422
in adult respiratory distress
syndrome, 324
noninvasive, 472
preterm/high-risk infant, 45
normal laboratory values for, 1132t
respiratory failure and, 316
Oxygen tension
assessment of, noninvasive, **419–420**
in cardiovascular disorders, 473
oxygen therapy monitored with, 422
Oxygen therapy, **422.** *See also* Mechanical ventilation
for acute respiratory failure,
318–319, 319t
for asthma, 326
for bronchiolitis, 434
for bronchopulmonary dysplasia, 435
for carbon monoxide poisoning, 299

for cyanotic spells in Fallot's
tetralogy, 497
for heart failure, 478
monitoring, 422
for neuromuscular disorders, of respiratory muscles, 457
for pancreatitis, 593
for pneumonia, 442
for pulmonary edema, 455
for pulmonary embolism, 455
for viral croup, 425
Oxyhood, for oxygen therapy, 319t

P
P$_2$, 466
Pachygyria, 660–661
Pacing, transesophageal atrial, for
supraventricular
tachycardia, 520
Packed red cells
characteristics of, 768t
transfusion, 771
PaCO$_2$
in acute respiratory failure, 316, 317t
normal, 420t
Pain
abdominal. *See* Abdominal pain
in cholelithiasis, 580
in eye, 360
of fibromyalgia, 721
and food refusal, in infants and young
children, 80
of hypermobility syndrome, 721
management of, **337–340**
nonrheumatic, **720–721**
odontogenic, 391
in pericarditis, 512
in peritonitis, 538
of reflex sympathetic dystrophy,
720–721
Pain control
after cardiac surgery, 327
in critical care, **337–340**, 338t
Palate
cleft. *See* Cleft palate
high-arched, 417
in newborn, 385f, 385–386, 387f
short, tonsillectomy/adenoidectomy
contraindicated in children
with, 414
Pallor
at birth, 22
in infants, 459
Palmar grasp, 25
Pancreas, **592–598**
annular, 533
in cystic fibrosis, 595–596t
disorders of, **592–598.** *See also*
specific type
secretion of enzymes, in
malabsorption, 547
tumors of, **597**, 597t
Pancreatic amylase, deficiency of,
diarrhea and, 544

Pancreatic cholera, diarrhea
and, 545t
Pancreatic enzymes
for pancreatic exocrine
insufficiency, 594
supplementation, 593
in cystic fibrosis, 437
Pancreatic exocrine insufficiency, **594**
Pancreatic lipase deficiency,
congenital, 597
Pancreaticojejunostomy, for
pancreatitis, 594
Pancreatitis
acute, **592–593**
chronic, **593–594**
diarrhea in, 545t
in cystic fibrosis, 596t
hemorrhagic, 592
Pancreatogram, for chronic
pancreatitis, 593
Pancuronium, for controlled
intubation, 320t
Panendoscopy, in gastrointestinal bleeding, 550
Panic disorder
in children and adolescents, 177t
psychopharmacologic interventions
in, indications for, 186t
Panner's disease, 710t
Pantothenic acid
biologic role of, 259t
in breast milk, 263t
causes of deficiencies of, 260t
dietary sources of, 259t
suggested intake of, 256t
toxicity of, 256t
PaO$_2$
in acute respiratory failure, 316, 317t
in cardiovascular disorders, 472
normal, 420t
Papanicolaou (Pap) smear, 129, 209
Papilledema, 377, 377f, 674
in hypoparathyroidism, 829
in intracranial hypertension, 285
Papillitis, 377–378
Papilloma/papillomatosis
of larynx, **428**
in lung, 452
Papular urticaria, 353
Papule, 342t
Papulosquamous eruptions, 356t,
356–357
pityriasis rosea, **356**
psoriasis, **357**
Paracetamol. *See* Acetaminophen
Paradoxic pulse, in cardiac
tamponade, 513
Paraesophageal hernia, 530
Paragonimus westermani,
1063t–1064t, 1066t
Parainfectious encephalopathies,
677–678
cerebrospinal fluid analysis in, 625t
Parainfluenza virus/infection, **967**
croup, 967

LANGE medical books...

LANGE medical books are available at your local health science bookstore or by calling

1-800-423-1359

in CT (203)406-4500.

...a smart investment in your medical career.

Basic Science Textbooks

Color Atlas of Basic Histology, 2/e
Berman
1998, ISBN 0-8385-0445-0, A0445-5

Jawetz, Melnick, & Adelberg's Medical Microbiology, 21/e
Brooks, Butel, & Ornston
1998, ISBN 0-8385-6316-3, A6316-2

Concise Pathology, 3/e
Chandrasoma & Taylor
1997, ISBN 0-8385-1499-5, A1499-1

Basic Methods in Molecular Biology, 2/e
Davis, Kuehl, & Battey
1994, ISBN 0-8385-0642-9, A0642-7

Basic & Clinical Biostatistics
Dawson & Trapp
1994, ISBN 0-8385-0542-2, A0542-9

Medical Biostatistics & Epidemiology
Essex-Sorlie
1995, ISBN 0-8385-6219-1, A6219-8

Molecular Basis of Medical Cell Biology
Fuller & Shields
1998, ISBN 0-8385-1384-0, A1384-5

Review of Medical Physiology, 18/e
Ganong
1997, ISBN 0-8385-8443-8, A8443-2

Basic Histology, 9/e
Junqueira, Carniero, & Kelley
1998, ISBN 0-8385-0590-2, A0590-8

Basic & Clinical Pharmacology, 7/e
Katzung
1998, ISBN 0-8385-0565-1, A0565-0

Pharmacology
Examination & Board Review, 5/e
Katzung & Trevor
1998, ISBN 0-8385-7708-3, A7708-9

Medical Microbiology & Immunology
Examination & Board Review, 5/e
Levinson & Jawetz
1998, ISBN 0-8385-6287-6, A6287-5

Clinical Anatomy
Lindner
1989, ISBN 0-8385-1259-3, A1259-9

Pathophysiology of Disease, 2/e
An Introduction to Clinical Medicine
McPhee, Lingappa, Lange, & Ganong
1997, ISBN 0-8385-7678-8, A7678-4

Color Atlas of Basic Histopathology
Milikowski & Berman
1997, ISBN 0-8385-1382-4, A1382-9

Harper's Biochemistry, 24/e
Murray, Granner, Mayes, & Rodwell
1996, ISBN 0-8385-3611-5, A3611-9

Basic Clinical Parasitology, 6/e
Neva & Brown
1994, ISBN 0-8385-0624-9, A0624-5

Pathology
Examination & Board Review
Newland
1995, ISBN 0-8385-7719-9, A7719-6

Basic Histology
Examination & Board Review, 3/e
Paulsen
1996, ISBN 0-8385-2282-3, A2282-0

Laboratory Medicine Case Book
An Introduction to Clinical Reasoning
Raskova, Mikhail, Shea, & Skvara
1997, ISBN 0-8385-5574-8, A5574-7

Medical Immunology, 9/e
Stites, Terr, & Parslow
1997, ISBN 0-8385-0586-4, A0586-6

Correlative Neuroanatomy, 23/e
Waxman
1997, ISBN 0-8385-1477-4, A1477-7

Clinical Science Textbooks

Clinical Neurology, 3/e
Aminoff, Greenberg, & Simon
1996, ISBN 0-8385-1383-2, A1383-2

Clinical Cardiology, 6/e
Cheitlin, Sokolow, & McIlroy
1993, ISBN 0-8385-1093-0, A1093-2

Fluid & Electrolytes
Physiology & Pathophysiology
Cogan
1991, ISBN 0-8385-2546-6, A2546-8

Basic and Clinical Biostatistics, 2/e
Dawson-Saunders & Trapp
1994, ISBN 0-8385-0542-2, A0542-9

Introduction to Clinical Psychiatry
Elkin
1998, ISBN 0-8385-4333-2, A4333-9

Behavioral Medicine in Primary Care
Feldman & Christensen
1997, ISBN 0-8385-0636-4, A0636-9

Evidence-Based Medicine
Friedland et al.
1998, ISBN 0-8385-2476-1, A2476-8

Basic Gynecology and Obstetrics
Gant & Cunningham
1993, ISBN 0-8385-9633-9, A9633-7

Review of General Psychiatry, 4/e
Goldman
1995, ISBN 0-8385-8421-7, A8421-8

(more on reverse)

Medical Epidemiology, 2/e
Greenberg et al.
1995, ISBN 0-8385-6206-X, A6206-5

Basic & Clinical Endocrinology, 5/e
Greenspan & Strewler
1997, ISBN 0-8385-0588-0, A0588-2

Occupational & Environmental Medicine, 2/e
LaDou
1997, ISBN 0-8385-7216-2, A7216-3

Primary Care of Women
Lemcke et al.
1995, ISBN 0-8385-9813-7, A9813-5

Clinical Anesthesiology, 2/e
Morgan & Mikhail
1996, ISBN 0-8385-1381-6, A1381-1

Fundamentals of Surgery
Niederhuber
1998, ISBN 0-8385-0509-0, A0509-8

Dermatology
Orkin, Maibach, & Dahl
1991, ISBN 0-8385-1288-7, A1288-8

Rudolph's Fundamentals of Pediatrics, 2/e
Rudolph & Kamei
1998, ISBN 0-8385-8236-2, A8236-0

Genetics in Primary Care & Clinical Medicine
Seashore
1995, ISBN 0-8385-3128-8, A3128-4

The Principles and Practice of Medicine, 23/e
Stobo et al.
1996, ISBN 0-8385-7963-9, A7963-0

Smith's General Urology, 14/e
Tanagho & McAninch
1995, ISBN 0-8385-8612-0, A8612-2

General Ophthalmology, 15/e
Vaughan, Asbury, & Riordan-Eva
1998, ISBN 0-8385-3137-7, A3137-5

Clinical Oncology
Weiss
1993, ISBN 0-8385-1325-5, A1325-8

CURRENT Clinical References

CURRENT Critical Care Diagnosis & Treatment
Bongard & Sue
1994, ISBN 0-8385-1443-X, A1443-9

CURRENT Diagnosis & Treatment in Cardiology
Crawford
1995, ISBN 0-8385-1444-8, A1444-7

CURRENT Diagnosis & Treatment in Vascular Surgery
Dean, Yao, & Brewster
1995, ISBN 0-8385-1351-4, A1351-4

CURRENT Obstetric & Gynecologic Diagnosis & Treatment, 8/e
DeCherney
1994, ISBN 0-8385-1447-2, A1447-0

CURRENT Diagnosis & Treatment in Gastroenterology
Grendell, McQuaid, & Friedman
1996, ISBN 0-8385-1448-0, A1448-8

CURRENT Pediatric Diagnosis & Treatment, 14/e
Hay, Groothius, Hayward, & Levin
1998, ISBN 0-8385-1254-2, A1254-0

CURRENT Emergency Diagnosis & Treatment, 4/e
Saunders & Ho
1992, ISBN 0-8385-1347-6, A1347-2

CURRENT Diagnosis & Treatment in Orthopedics
Skinner
1995, ISBN 0-8385-1009-4, A1009-8

CURRENT Medical Diagnosis & Treatment 1999, 38/e
Tierney, McPhee, & Papadakis
1999, ISBN 0-8385-1550-9, A1550-1

CURRENT Surgical Diagnosis & Treatment, 10/e
Way
1994, ISBN 0-8385-1439-1, A1439-7

LANGE Clinical Manuals

Dermatology
Diagnosis and Therapy
Bondi, Jegasothy, & Lazarus
1991, ISBN 0-8385-1274-7, A1274-8

Manual for Human Dissection
Callas
1994, ISBN 0-8385-6133-0, A6133-1

Practical Oncology
Cameron
1994, ISBN 0-8385-1326-3, A1326-6

Office & Bedside Procedures
Chesnutt, Dewar, & Locksley
1993, ISBN 0-8385-1095-7, A1095-7

Psychiatry
Diagnosis & Treatment, 2/e
Flaherty, Davis, & Janicak
1993, ISBN 0-8385-1267-4, A126 7-2

Practical Gynecology
Jacobs & Gast
1994, ISBN 0-8385-1336-0, A1336-5

Geriatrics
Lonergan
1996, ISBN 0-8385-1094-9, A1094-0

Ambulatory Medicine
The Primary Care of Families, 2/e
Mengel & Schwiebert
1996, ISBN 0-8385-1466-9, A1466-0

Poisoning & Drug Overdose, 3/e
Olson
1999, ISBN 0-8385-0260-1, A0260-8

Internal Medicine
Diagnosis and Therapy, 3/e
Stein
1993, ISBN 0-8385-1112-0, A1112-0

Surgery
Diagnosis and Therapy
Stillman
1989, ISBN 0-8385-1283-6, A1283-9

Medical Perioperative Management
Wolfsthal
1989, ISBN 0-8385-1298-4, A1298-7

LANGE Handbooks

Handbook of Gynecology & Obstetrics
Brown & Crombleholme
1993, ISBN 0-8385-3608-5, A3608-5

HIV/AIDS Primary Care Handbook
Carmichael, Carmichael, & Fischl
1995, ISBN 0-8385-3557-7, A3557-4

Clinician's Pocket Reference, 8/e
Gomella
1997, ISBN 0-8385-1476-6, A1476-9

Neonatology
Management, Procedures, On-Call Problems, Diseases, and Drugs, 3/e
Gomella
1995, ISBN 0-8385-1331-X, A1331-6

Surgery on Call, 2/e
Gomella & Lefor
1996, ISBN 0-8385-8746-1, A8746-8

Internal Medicine On Call, 2/e
Haist, Robbins, & Gomella
1997, ISBN 0-8385-4056-2, A4056-6

Obstetrics & Gynecology On Call
Horowitz & Gomella
1993, ISBN 0-8385-7174-3, A7174-4

Pocket Guide to Commonly Prescribed Drugs, 2/e
Levine
1996, ISBN 0-8385-8099-8, A8099-2

Handbook of Pediatrics, 18/e
Merenstein, Kaplan, & Rosenberg
1997, ISBN 0-8385-3625-5, A3625-9

Pocket Guide to Diagnostic Tests, 2/e
Nicoll, McPhee, Chou, & Detmer
1997, ISBN 0-8385-8100-5, A8100-8

Quick Medical Spanish, 2/e
Rogers
1997, ISBN 0-8385-8258-3, A8258-4

How to Examine the Nervous System
Ross
1998, ISBN 0-8385-3852-5, A3852-9

Pocket Guide to the Essentials of Diagnosis & Treatment
Tierney
1997, ISBN 0-8385-3605-0, A3605-1

Appleton & Lange • P.O. Box 120041 • Stamford, CT • 06912-0041 • 1-800-423-1359